FUNDAMENTALS OF NURSING

Concepts, Process, and Practice

SEVENTH EDITION

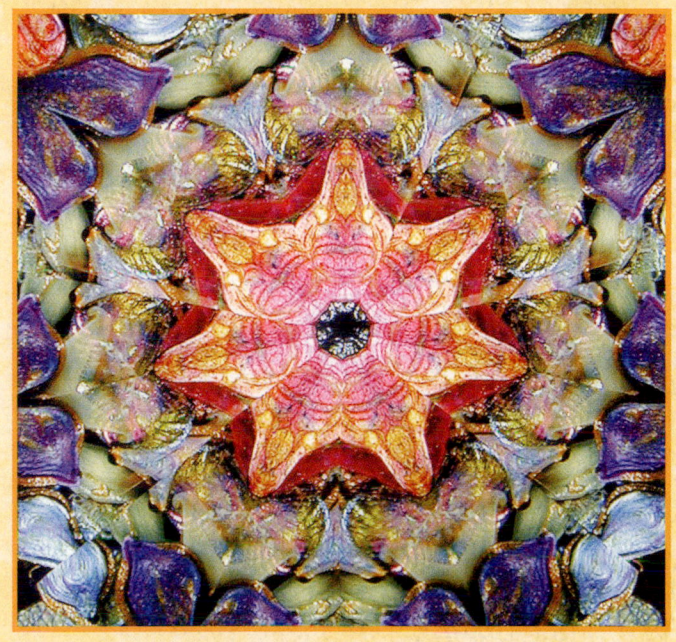

BARBARA KOZIER MN, RN

GLENORA ERB, BSN, RN

AUDREY BERMAN, PhD, RN, AOCN

SHIRLEE J. SNYDER, EdD, RN

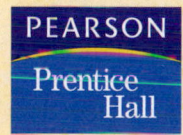

PEARSON

Prentice Hall

Upper Saddle River,
New Jersey 07458

Library of Congress Cataloging-in-Publication Data
Fundamentals of nursing: concepts, process, and practice/Barbara Kozier . . . [et al.]—
7th ed.
p. cm.
Includes bibliographical references and index.
ISBN 0-13-045529-6
1. Nursing. I. Kozier, Barbara.
[DNLM: 1. Nursing Process. 2. Nursing Care.]
RT41.F8813 2004
610.73—dc21
2003043868

Publisher: Julie Levin Alexander
Executive Assistant & Supervisor: Regina Bruno
Editor-in-Chief: Maura Connor
Senior Acquisitions Editor: Nancy Anselment
Development Editor: Teri Zak
Managing Development Editor: Marilyn Meserve
Managing Editor: Patrick Walsh
Production Liaison: Cathy O'Connell
Director of Manufacturing and Production: Bruce Johnson
Manufacturing Buyer: Pat Brown
Production Editor: Amy Gehl, Carlisle Publishers Services
Design Director: Cheryl Asherman
Cover Designer: Cheryl Asherman
Interior Designer: Janice Bielawa
Senior Design Coordinator: Maria Guglielmo Walsh
Senior Marketing Manager: Nicole Benson
Channel Marketing Manager: Rachele Strober
Marketing Coordinator: Janet Ryerson
Supplements Editor: Sladjana Repic
Media Editor: John Jordan
Media Production Manager: Amy Peltier
Media Project Manager: Stephen Hartner
Composition: Carlisle Communications
Printer/Binder: RR Donnelley, Willard
Cover Printer: Lehigh

Cover and interior illustrations: Dreamdrops by Sherry Moser, as seen in *Kaleidoscope Artistry* by Cozy Baker.

Pearson Education LTD.
Pearson Education Australia PTY, Limited
Pearson Education Singapore, Pte. Ltd
Pearson Education North Asia Ltd
Pearson Education Canada, Ltd.

Pearson Educación de Mexico, S.A. de C.V.
Pearson Education—Japan
Pearson Education Malaysia, Pte. Ltd
Pearson Education, Upper Saddle River, NJ

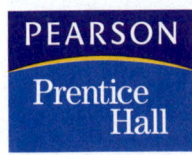

10 9 8 7 6 5 4 3
ISBN 0-13-045529-6

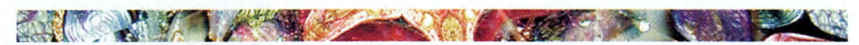

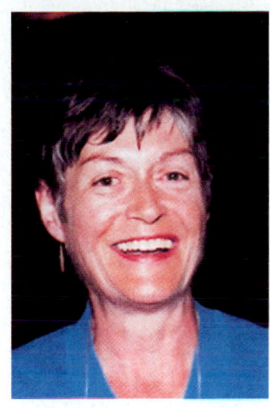

*In loving memory of Glenora Erb,
1937–2001, one of the founding authors of
this textbook*

Contents

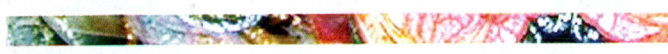

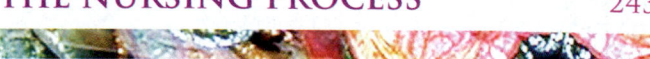

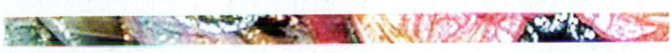

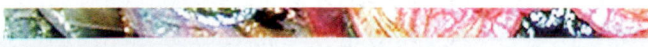

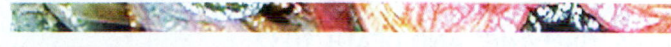

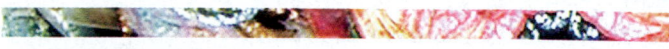

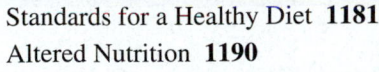

Preface for the Seventh Edition

The practice of nursing continues to evolve . . . the practice of caring is timeless.

Nurses today must be able to grow and evolve in order to meet the demands of a dramatically changing health care system. They need skills in technology, communication, and interpersonal relations to be effective members of the collaborative health care team. They need to think critically and be creative in implementing nursing strategies with clients of diverse cultural backgrounds in increasingly varied settings. They need skills in teaching, leading, managing, and the process of change. They need to be prepared to provide home- and community-based nursing care to clients across the life span—especially to the increasing numbers of elders. They need to understand holistic healing modalities and complementary therapies. And, they need to continue their unique role that demands a blend of nurturance, sensitivity, caring, empathy, commitment, and skill founded on a broad base of knowledge.

Fundamentals of Nursing: Concepts, Process, and Practice, Seventh Edition, addresses the concepts of contemporary professional nursing. These concepts include but are not limited to caring, wellness, health promotion, disease prevention, holistic care, multiculturalism, nursing theories, nursing informatics, nursing research, ethics, and advocacy. With this edition, every chapter has been extensively revised. The content has been updated to reflect the latest nursing research and the increasing emphasis on aging, wellness, and home- and community-based care. Many of the changes are in response to suggestions and comments from reviewers and nursing students using the text. We developed this text so that it can be used with a variety of nursing theories and conceptual frameworks.

ORGANIZATION

The detailed table of contents at the beginning of the book makes its clear organization easy to follow. Continuing with a strong focus on nursing care, the new edition of this book is divided into ten units. Unit 1, The Nature of Nursing, clusters five chapters that provide comprehensive coverage of introductory concepts of nursing. In Unit 2, Contemporary Health Care, five chapters cover contemporary health care topics such as health care delivery systems, community-based care, health promotion, home care, and informatics. This textbook has always been known for its emphasis on wellness and the nurse's role in health promotion. In the new Seventh edition, we include two chapters on these topics: Chapter 8, Health Promotion, and Chapter 11, Health, Wellness, and Illness. These are important concepts for students to learn and to be able to teach their clients. In Unit 3, Health Beliefs and Practices, four chapters cover health-related beliefs and practices for individuals and families from a variety of different cultural backgrounds. Unit 4, The Nursing Process, introduces students to this important framework with each chapter dedicated to a specific step of the nursing process. Chapter 15 applies critical thinking and the nursing process. A *Nursing in Action* case study is used as the frame of reference for applying content in all phases of the nursing process

in Chapter 16, Assessing; Chapter 17, Diagnosing; Chapter 18, Planning; and Chapter 19, Implementing and Evaluating. Starting in this unit and incorporated throughout the book, we refer to the new NANDA 2003–2004 diagnoses. Unit 5, Life Span and Development, consists of three chapters that discuss life span and development from conception to older adults. For the Seventh Edition of this textbook, we involved a gerontology consultant who reviewed every chapter to ensure that the textbook adequately addresses gerontology and the needs of elders. Unit 6, Integral Aspects of Nursing, discusses topics such as caring, comfort, communication, teaching, delegating, managing, and leading. These topics are all crucial elements for providing competent nursing care. Unit 7, Assessing Health, covers vital signs and health assessment in two separate chapters, so beginning students can understand normal assessment findings before they learn what is abnormal. Chapter 27, Vital Signs, begins to introduce students to the clinical procedures that they need to learn to perform. In Unit 8, Integral Components of Client Care, the focus shifts to those components of client care that are universal to all clients including asepsis, safety, hygiene, diagnostic testing, medication, wound care, and preoperative care. Chapter 32, Diagnostic Testing, is a new chapter that was added in this edition to familiarize students with the role of nursing care for clients undergoing tests and procedures. Unit 9, Promoting Psychosocial Health, includes six chapters that cover a wide range of areas that affect one's health. Sensory perception, self-concept, sexuality, spirituality, stress, and loss are all things that a nurse needs to consider in order to properly care for a client. Unit 10, Promoting Physiologic Health, discusses a variety of physiologic concepts that provide the foundations for nursing care. These include activity, rest, pain, nutrition, elimination, oxygenation, fluid and electrolyte balance, and a new chapter on circulation, Chapter 49.

HALLMARK FEATURES

For years, Kozier and Erb's *Fundamentals of Nursing: Concepts, Process, and Practice* has been the leading textbook that helps students embark on their careers in nursing. This new edition retains many of the features that have made this textbook the number one choice of nursing students and faculty for years.

- **Focus on Critical Thinking.** Critical thinking questions throughout the text encourage the introductory nursing student to apply critical thinking skills, that is, analyzing, comparing, contemplating, interpreting, evaluating, and so forth. *Focus on Critical Thinking* boxes contain questions derived from brief case studies. A set of questions follows most nursing care plan. Because there are no discrete right or wrong answers to the critical thinking questions, *Critical Thinking Possibilities* for each question are provided in Appendix A for each question.
- **Identifying Nursing Diagnoses, Outcomes, and Interventions.** Nursing Interventions Classification (NIC) and Nursing Outcomes Classification (NOC) are included in the care plans and in *Identifying Nursing Diagnoses, Outcomes,*

and Interventions features throughout the text. In Chapter 18, Planning, we explain these classification systems and provide tables that outline the domains and classes of the NIC taxonomy with examples to familiarize beginning students with the most current nursing language.

- **Home Care Assessment.** The expansion in home health care delivery has emphasized the need for early discharge planning and continuity of care in the home. *Home Care Assessments* in the clinical chapters direct the nurse to assess (a) the client: self-care abilities, level of knowledge, needs for assistive devices, and so on; (b) the family/caregiver: abilities and responses to assist the client; and (c) community resources available, such as home health agencies, support groups, and equipment and supply companies.

- **Teaching Boxes.** There are three types of *Teaching* boxes: *Wellness Care, Client Care,* and *Home Care.* These guides give students the tools and concepts they need to help clients facilitate self-care, monitor problems, understand medication effects, perform prescribed therapies, and modify lifestyle patterns.

- **Procedures.** This edition incorporates nursing procedures throughout, all established within the framework of the nursing process. Each procedure provides the student with a purpose statement, an assessment focus, planning—including consideration of whether the procedure can be delegated to unlicensed assistive personnel, a list of equipment, step-by-step interventions describing how to perform the procedure, and evaluation.

- **Lifespan Considerations.** These boxes highlight how nursing care is adapted for infants, children, adolescents, and elders.

- **Home Care Considerations.** In this feature, the nurse is guided in modifying care needed when the client is in a home care setting.

- **Practice Guidelines.** These features provide instant-access summaries of clinical do's and don'ts. These offer introductory nursing students clinical pearls of wisdom and reminders as they set forth in their first clinical experiences.

- **Research Notes.** These notes highlight nursing research and evidence-based practices as they apply to clinical nursing practice.

NEW FEATURES

To further enhance this popular fundamentals textbook, we invited nursing faculty and students to provide suggestions. Based on their recommendations, we added several new features to make this new edition of Kozier and Erb's *Fundamentals of Nursing* the most current and engaging textbook that helps all students succeed in their first nursing courses.

- **Nursing Care Plans.** These care plans appear in selected clinical chapters and provide assessment data, NANDA nursing diagnoses, and evaluation, desired outcomes, nursing interventions, relevant to a specific clinical scenario. New to this edition, we include a set of critical thinking questions at the end of most nursing care plans.

- **Concept Maps.** A *Concept Map* follows each *Nursing Care Plan.* These decision-making graphics provide a unique method for viewing a client's plan of care, and the visual presentation reinforces the care plan priorities for beginning students.

- **MediaLinks.** At the beginning of each chapter, the *MediaLink* box identifies chapter-specific topics, animations, videos, NCLEX review questions, tools, and other interactive exercises that appear on the accompanying Student CD-ROM and the Companion Website. Special *MediaLink* icons appear in the margins throughout the chapter to refer students to those topics and activities available on the media supplements. At the end of each chapter, *EXPLORE MediaLink* sections encourage students to use the CD-ROM and the Companion Website to apply what they have learned from the text in additional case studies, to practice NCLEX questions, and to use additional resources. The purpose of the *MediaLink* feature is to further enhance the student experience, build on knowledge gained from the textbook, prepare students for the NCLEX, and foster critical thinking.

- **Clinical Alerts.** These alerts highlight information that requires special attention from the nurse, such as safety.

- **Providing Culturally Competent Care.** These boxes are care related and focus on suggested answers to the question "What may the nurse do differently in a situation in consideration of a client's cultural background?"

- **Functional Health Patterns Concept Maps.** Concept maps are graphic illustrations that show relationships between information. The technique can be used to explore, organize, examine, or explain information related to a concept or idea. The Functional Health Patterns Concept Maps included in the insert of this text are selected patterns from Gordon's Typology of 11 Functional Health Patterns. The boxes around the perimeter highlight each of the 11 patterns and key areas to be assessed within the pattern. Arrows between the patterns show the interconnectedness of each pattern to the whole, representing how the patterns can yield a holistic view of an individual, family, or community.

  The first map illustrates the connection between the patterns and some of the nursing diagnoses that can derive from data collected using the Functional Health Patterns Framework. The other maps highlight a specific pattern and a grouping of relevant diagnoses. These can assist the student or nurse by organizing the relationship between specific data and diagnosis.

- **Chapter Review.** A new section at the end of each chapter focuses students after they complete the chapter reading assignment. *EXPLORE MediaLink* encourages students to use the CD-ROM and the Companion Website to apply what they have learned from the text in additional case studies, practice NCLEX questions, and additional resources. *Chapter Highlights* offer students a bulleted summary of chapter concepts for review. Students who read these concepts before reading the chapter will find them helpful in focusing their attention. *Chapter Highlights* are also an appropriate tool to quickly review the content after reading each chapter. Finally, *Review Questions* provide students with a quick review consisting of multiple-choice questions. These test the students' knowledge of the material and reinforce what they have learned from reading the chapter. Answers are found in Appendix C.

SUPPLEMENTS THAT INSPIRE SUCCESS FOR THE STUDENT AND THE INSTRUCTOR

To supplement the textbook and facilitate active student learning, we include a variety of student learning aids in our comprehensive supplements package.

Student CD-ROM. This CD-ROM is packaged *free* with the textbook. It provides an interactive study program that allows students to practice answering NCLEX-style questions with rationales for right and wrong answers. It also contains an audio glossary, animations and anatomy and physiology reviews, and a link to the Companion Website.

Study Guide. This workbook includes case studies, NCLEX review, and other review exercises. *MediaLinks* refer students to activities on the CD-ROM and Companion Website.

Clinical Companion. This clinical companion serves as a portable, quick-reference to fundamentals of nursing. Topics include lab values, diagnostic tests, Standard Precautions documentation, NANDA diagnoses, and much more. This handbook will allow students to bring the information they learn from class into any clinical setting.

Companion Website. This *free* online study guide, at http://www.prenhall.com/kozier, is designed to help students apply the concepts presented in the book. Each chapter-specific module features objectives, audio glossary, chapter summary for lecture notes, NCLEX review questions, case studies, care plan activities, *MediaLink* applications, web links, and nursing tools, such as *Functional Health Patterns Concept Maps, Assessment Guides,* and more.

Instructor's Resource Manual. This manual contains a wealth of material to help faculty plan and manage the *Fundamentals of Nursing* course. It includes chapter overviews, detailed lecture suggestions and outlines, learning objectives, a complete test bank, answers to the textbook critical thinking exercises, teaching tips, and more for each chapter. It also guides faculty how to incorporate and assign the various media supplements accompanying this textbook, including

- Text-specific Companion Website, http://www.prenhall.com/kozier
- Student CD-ROM animations and activities
- Prentice Hall's *Research Navigator,* featuring online access to nursing journals and nursing research
- Prentice Hall's online *Syllabus Manager* at http://www.prenhall.com, facilitating the students' use of the Companion Website, and allowing faculty to post syllabi and course information online for their students.

Instructor's Resource CD-ROM. This cross-platform CD-ROM provides *Discussion Points* and illustrations in PowerPoint from the new Seventh Edition of this textbook for use in classroom lectures. It also contains an electronic test bank, answers to the textbook critical thinking exercises, and animations from the Student CD-ROM. This supplement is available to faculty free on adoption of the textbook.

Online Course Management Systems. Also available are online companions for schools using *WebCT, Blackboard,* or *CourseCompass* course management systems. The online course management solutions feature interactive modules, electronic test banks, PowerPoint images and text slides, animations, assessment activities, and more. For more information about adopting an online course management system to accompany Kozier and Erb's *Fundamentals of Nursing,* please contact your Prentice Hall Health Sales Representative. Or go online to the appropriate website below and select Courses and Nursing to access a free preview of our online course companions:

WebCT: http://cms.prenhall.com/webct/index.html

Blackboard: http://cms.prenhall.com/blackboard/index.html

CourseCompass: http://cms.prenhall.com/coursecompass/

ACKNOWLEDGMENTS

We wish to extend a sincere thank you to the talented team involved in the Seventh Edition of this book: the contributors and reviewers who provide content and very helpful feedback; the nursing students, for their questioning minds and motivation; and the nursing instructors, who provided many valuable suggestions for this edition.

We would like to thank the editorial team at Prentice Hall including Nancy Anselment, Senior Acquisitions Editor, for keeping our noses to the grindstone; Marilyn Meserve, Managing Editor, who can multitask with the best of them; Teri Zak, Development Editor, for her attention to detail that promoted an excellent outcome; and Sladjana Repic for managing all of the reviews and media supplements with enthusiasm. Many thanks to the production team of Patrick Walsh, Production Manager; Cathy O'Connell, Production Liason, and Amy Gehl, Production Editor, for producing this book with precision, and to the design team led by Cheryl Asherman, Creative Director, for providing a truly beautiful design for this textbook. Many of the new photos in the Seventh Edition were photographed by Al Dodge in the clinical setting courtesy of Beth Israel Deaconess Medical Center, Boston, Massachusetts.

Finally, the kaleidoscope image used on the cover and throughout this textbook was designed by Sherry Moser, a former pediatric oncology nurse. A kaleidoscope is an ever changing piece of art with its colors, light, and form. As a kaleidoscope turns, it represents new opportunities for beautiful new designs. Seeking light and reflections to form new shapes allows you to open your mind to all of the possibilities a kaleidoscope has to offer. It is more expansive than you first imagined. As a nursing student begins on the path of a career in nursing, he or she also finds new opportunities unfolding as a light from within that brightens the path ahead. As students learn more about the field of nursing, they will explore and pursue areas of the field that they may have never imagined at the beginning of their journey. Now is your beginning—open your eyes and your mind to all of the wonderful opportunities in the field of nursing that are waiting to be pursued.

Barbara Kozier

Glenora Erb

Audrey Berman

Shirlee Snyder

Contributors

Sylvia Bertram, DNSc, RN
Kaiser Permanente
Professional Nursing Education Consultant
Oakland, California

Roseann Colosimo, PhD, RN
Assistant Professor
University of Nevada Las Vegas
Las Vegas, Nevada

Cecily Cosby, PhD, FNP
Associate Professor and/FNP Program Director
Samuel Merritt College
Oakland, California
Nurse Practitioner II
Emergency Department
University of California San Francisco
San Francisco, California

Karen Lee Fontaine, MSN, RN, ASSECT
Professor
Purdue University Calumet
Hammond, Indiana

Judith Johnstone, AB
Johnstone Associates
Austin, Texas

Richard MacIntyre, PhD, RN
Professor and Chairman of Health Sciences
Mercy College
Dobbs Ferry, New York

Grace Miller, MSN, RN
Assistant Professor
College of Saint Mary
Omaha, Nebraska

Judy A. Scott, MSN, RN
Pediatric Instructor
Community College Southern Nevada
Las Vegas, Nevada

Rachel Spector, PhD, RN, FAAN
Associate Professor
Boston College School of Nursing
Chestnut Hill, Massachusetts

Barbara T. Steuble, MSN, RN, CPHQ
Assistant Professor
Samuel Merritt College School of Nursing
Sacramento, California

Elizabeth Johnston Taylor, PhD, RN
Associate Professor
School of Nursing
Loma Linda University
Loma Linda, California

Reviewers

JoAnn Abegglen, MS, APRN, PNP
Brigham Young University
Provo, Utah

Marianne Adam, MSN, CRNP
Assistant Professor
Moravian College
Blandon, Pennsylvania

Ruth R. Alteneder, PhD, CNM
Interim Director
Lourdes College
Sylvania, Ohio

Gina M. Ankner, MSN, RN, ANP
Instructor
University of Massachusetts, Dartmouth
College of Nursing
N. Dartmouth, Massachusetts

Joan H. Baldwin, DNSc, MSN, MA, RN
Professor
Brigham Young University College of
Nursing
Provo, Utah

Kathleen Barta, EdD, RN
University of Arkansas Eleanor Mann
School of Nursing
Fayatteville, Arkansas

Debra Bass-Chambless, MSN, RN, CS,
ANP, GNP
Clinical Instructor
Texas Woman's University
Dallas, Texas

Margaret Bellek, MN, RN
Associate Professor
Indiana University of Pennsylvania
Indiana, Pennsylvania

Diane Benefiel, MSN, RN
Instructor
California State University at Fresno
Fresno, California

Beverly Bowers, PhD, RNC
Assistant Professor of Nursing
The University of Oklahoma Health
Sciences Center, College of Nursing
Oklahoma City, Oklahoma

L. Adrienne Bowlus, MSN, RN
New York Medical College—Graduate
School of Nursing
New York, New York

Josie M. Bowman, DSN, RN
Associate Professor
East Carolina University
Greenville, North Carolina

Sabita Busch, DNSc, RN
Associate Professor
Chicago State University
Chicago, Illinois

Mary D. Calabro, MSN, RNC, PNP
Lecturer, Lead Faculty
Kent State University
Kent, Ohio

Susan Carlson, MS, RN, CS NPP
Instructor of Nursing
Monroe Community College
Rochester, New York

Barbara M. Craig, MS, RN
Associate Professor ADN Program
Pasco-Hernando Community College
Dade City, Florida

Barbara P. Daniel, MEd, MS, RNCS,
CRNP
Professor of Nursing
Cecil Community College
North East, Maryland

Sharon Decker, MSN, RN, CS, CCRN
Professor of Clinical Nursing, Director of
Clinical Simulations
Texas Tech University Health Sciences
Center School of Nursing
Lubbock, Texas

Linda Elsik, MS, RN
Instructor
Lewis University College of Nursing and
Health Professions
Romeoville, Illinois

Tara N. Fedric, MS, RN, CNS, OCR
Adjunct Clinical Professor
Texas Woman's University
Dallas, Texas

Carol E. Feingold, MS, RN
Clinical Associate Professor
University of Arizona College of Nursing
Tucson, Arizona

Lisa Fiorentino, PhD, RN, CRNP
Assistant Professor of Nursing and Chair,
Department of Nursing
University of Pittsburgh at Bradford
Bradford, Pennsylvania

Jane H. Freeman, EdD, RN
Professor in Nursing
Jacksonville State University, College of
Nursing and Health Sciences
Jacksonville, Alabama

Diana Girdley, MS, RN
Assistant Clinical Professor
University of Wisconsin School of Nursing
Madison, Wisconsin

Rebecca Crews Gruener, MSN
Associate Professor of Nursing
Louisiana State University at Alexandria
Alexandria, Louisiana

Kathy L. Ham, EdD, RN
Assistant Professor of Nursing
Southeast Missouri State University
Cape Girardeau, Missouri

Janice D. Hausauer, MS, RN, FNP
Adjunct Assistant Professor
Montana State University College of
Nursing
Bozeman, Montana

Peggy L. Hawkins, PhD, RN
Associate Professor
College of Saint Mary
Omaha, Nebraska

Laura J. Higgs, MSN, MEd, RNC
Associate Professor in Nursing
Chesapeake College
Wye Mills, Maryland

Beverly Hogan, RN, APRN, BC
University of Alabama School of Nursing
Birmingham, Alabama

Mary Jane Hopkins, MSN, ARNP
Assistant Professor
Indian River Community College
Fort Pierce, Florida

June A. Ige, BSN, RN, MA
Nursing Instructor
North Hennepin Community College
Brooklyn Park, Minnesota

Cherry Ann Karl, MSN, MA, RN
Associate Professor
Anne Arondel Community College
Arnold, Maryland

M. Frances Keen, DNSc, RNC
Associate Professor
Villanova University College of Nursing
Villanova, Pennsylvania

Pamela D. Korte, MS, RN
Associate Professor of Nursing
Monroe Community College
Rochester, New York

Sylvia Kubsch, PhD, RN
Associate Professor Nursing
University of Wisconsin–Green Bay
Green Bay, Wisconsin

Marjorie J. Kurt, BSN, RN
Clinical Professor
Indiana University School of Nursing
Indianapolis, Indiana

Patricia K. Leary, MA Ed
Mecosta–Osceola Career Center
Big Rapids, Michigan

Kenyann Lucas, MS, RN, CNS, P/MH
Associate Professor Associate Degree
Program
Texarkana College
Texarkana, Texas

Rosemary Macy, MS, RN
Assistant Professor
Boise State University
Boise, Idaho

Kim Meyer, MSN, RN
Associate Professor of Nursing
Bethel College
St. Paul, Minnesota

Carma K. Miller, MSN, RN
Nursing Instructor
Brigham Young University
Provo, Utah

Judith P. Moore, MS, RN
Lecturer, Course Coordinator
University of North Carolina at Wilmington
School of Nursing
Wilmington, North Carolina

Ruth E. Novitt-Schumacher, RN, MSN
Instructor
University of Illinois at Chicago
Chicago, Illinois

Rebecca Otten, MSN
Director, ADN Program
Mt. St. Mary's College, Doheny Campus
Los Angeles, California

Penelope Overby, MSN, RN
Faculty
Florence-Darlington Technical College
Florence, South Carolina

Mimi Padgett, MSN
Director RN Studies
Husson College
Bangor, Maine

Laurie J. Palmer, MS, RN
Associate Professor
Monroe Community College
Rochester, New York

Annette M. Peacock-Johnson, MSN, RNC
Assistant Professor of Nursing
Saint Mary's College Department of
Nursing
Notre Dame, Indiana

Sandra M. Peacock, MS, RN
Assistant Professor
McNeese State University, College of
Nursing
Lake Charles, Louisiana

Cathy J. Pimple, MS, RN
Assistant Professor
Emporia Sate University
Emporia, Kansas

Deborah A. Roberts, EdD, RN
Nursing Faculty
Humboldt State University
Arcata, California

Brenda Routh, MS, RN, BSN
Nursing Faculty
Dallas County Community
College–Brookhaven College
Dallas, Texas

Arlene Saliba, MS, RN, CS-FNP
Assistant Professor
Andrews University Nursing Department
Berrien Springs, Michigan

Donna J. Sauls, PhD, RN
Assistant Professor
Texas Woman's University
Denton, Texas

Grace E. Saylor, MSN, RN
Nursing Instructor
York Technical College/USCL
Rock Hill, South Carolina

Maria Seidel, MS, ARNP
Assistant Professor
Indian River Community College
Ft. Pierce, Florida

Nancy D. Severance, MS, RN
Instructor
Boise State University
Boise, Idaho

Martha Tafoya, MSN, RNC
Professional Specialist
Angelo State University
San Angelo, Texas

Ann B. Tritak, RN, EdD
Associate Professor
Fairleigh Dickinson University
Teaneck, New Jersey

Jean Urick, MSN
Assistant Professor of Nursing
Southeastern Louisiana University
Hammond, Louisiana

Stephanie Valdes, MS, RN
Associate Professor of Nursing
Black Hawk College
Moline, Illinois

Vicky C. Walley, MN
Instructor
The University of Southern Mississippi
College of Nursing
Hattiesburg, Mississippi

Iris Walliser, MSN, RN
ADN Program Coordinator
University of South Carolina Aiken
Aiken, South Carolina

Mary Ann Ware, EdD, RN
Dean, School of Nursing
William Carey College
Hattiesburg, Mississippi

Robin Y. Wood, EdD, RN
Assistant Professor, Coordinator Learning
Resource Center
Boston College, School of Nursing
Chestnut Hill, Massachusetts

Lucia Yiu, MScN, BA
Associate Professor
University of Windsor
Windsor, Ontario, Canada

Supplement and Media Contributors

Susan Barnes, MSN, RN
Instructor, Durham Technical Community College
Durham, North Carolina
Student Study Guide

Mary T. Boylston, MSN, RN, CCRN
Associate Professor, Nursing Informatics Coordinator, Eastern University
St Davids, Pennsylvania
Companion Website

Janet Witucki Brown, PhD, RN
Assistant Professor, University of Tennessee
Knoxville, Tennessee
Companion Website

Vera Dauffenbach, EdD, MSN, RN
Associate Professor of Nursing, Bellin College of Nursing
Green Bay, Wisconsin
Companion Website

Lourdes A. D. de la Cruz, MHSc, MScCHN
Professor of Nursing, Sheridan College
Brampton, Ontario, Canada
Student CD-ROM

Joseann Helmes DeWitt, MSN, RN, BC, CLNC
Assistant Professor, Alcorn State University School of Nursing
Natchez, Mississippi
Student Study Guide

Laurie Gasperi Kaudewitz, MSN, RNC
Assistant Professor of Nursing, East Tennessee State University
Johnson City, Tennessee
Companion Website

Dawna Martich, MSN, RN
Education, American Healthways
Pittsburgh, Pennsylvania
Instructor's Resource Manual
Instructor's Resource CD-ROM

Duane F. Napier, MSN, RN, C
Assistant Professor of Nursing, St. Mary's School of Nursing
Huntington, West Virginia
Companion Website

Phyllis G. Peterson, MN, RN, AOCN
Assistant Professor, Division of Nursing, Our Lady of Holy Cross College
New Orleans, Louisiana
Companion Website

Pamela Pranke, MSN, RNC, SANE
Clinical Coordinator–Nursing
S.A.F.E. Shelter/ Jamestown College, Campus Violence Intervention Advocate
Jamestown, North Dakota
Companion Website

Georgianna M. Thomas, EdD, RN
Associate Professor, West Suburban College of Nursing
Oak Park, Illinois
Per Diem Staff Nurse, Stat Resources
Chicago, Illinois
Companion Website

Golden M. Tradewell, PhD, RN
Associate Professor, College of Nursing, McNeese State University
Lake Charles, Louisiana
Student Study Guide

Kim Webb, MN, RN
Nursing Chair, Northern Oklahoma College
Tonkawa, Oklahoma
Companion Website

About the Authors

Glenora Erb

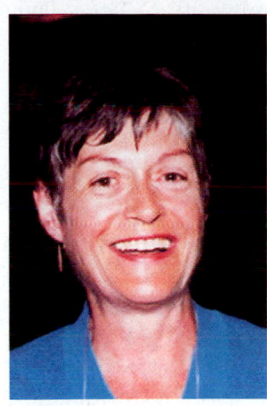

Glenora Lea Erb was born in Calgary, Alberta, Canada. All of her schooling took place in Calgary and, with her identical twin sister, she attended the Nursing School of Calgary General Hospital. She was awarded a gold medal when she graduated and was recognized as an outstanding bedside nurse.

Following two years traveling in Asia, Europe, India, Australia, and New Zealand, Ms. Erb returned to Vancouver and taught nursing at St. Paul's Hospital School of Nursing, and later at a two-year program at the B.C. Institute of Technology. At this time she also wrote textbooks on *Fundamentals of Nursing, Techniques of Clinical Nursing, Concepts and Issues in Nursing Practice,* and *Essentials of Nursing Practice.*

Glen was diagnosed with cancer of the breast 15 years ago. She died at home December 24, 2001. Her death has meant that nursing has lost a highly skilled clinical nurse and her friends and family have lost a sensitive and giving person.

Barbara Kozier

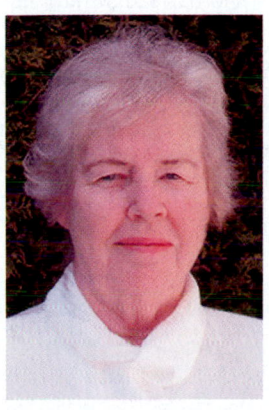

Barbara Kozier was educated in Vancouver, British Columbia, Canada. After obtaining a bachelor of arts degree from the University of British Columbia, she entered the nursing program at that institution. After four years of study she graduated with a bachelor's degree in nursing. She obtained a position at Bella Bella, an aboriginal settlement on the northern coast of British Columbia. She then nursed with the Victorian Order of Nurses providing home care. Following a position with a large general hospital as an acute care nurse in a medical surgical unit, she taught medical and surgical nursing, pediatric nursing, psychiatric, and community nursing courses at the Vancouver General Hospital School of Nursing. Ms. Kozier then enrolled at the University of Washington where she studied for two years, taught part time, and obtained her master of nursing title.

Barbara is a member of three honor societies: Sigma Theta Tau (nursing), Pi Lambda Theta (education), and Delta Sigma Pi (Canadian Honor Society for University Women). Barbara was a member and a chair of many nursing and government committees. She wrote a number of texts and collaborated with Glenora Erb on four books: *Techniques of Clinical Nursing, Fundamentals of Nursing, Concepts and Issues in Nursing Practice,* and *Essentials of Nursing Practice.*

Audrey Berman

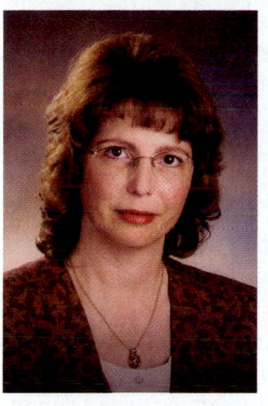

Audrey Berman received her BSN from the University of California–San Francisco and later returned to that campus to obtain her MS in physiologic nursing and her PhD in nursing. Her dissertation was entitled *Sailing a Course through Chemotherapy: The Experience of Women with Breast Cancer.* She worked in oncology at Samuel Merritt Hospital prior to beginning her teaching career in the diploma program at Samuel Merritt Hospital School of Nursing in 1976. As a faculty member, she participated in the transition of that program into a baccalaureate degree and in the development of the master of science in nursing program. Over the years, she has taught a variety of medical-surgical nursing courses in the prelicensure programs. She currently serves as the associate dean of nursing, at the Sacramento Regional Center campus of Samuel Merritt College (an affiliate of Sutter Health) where students are enrolled in an entry-level MSN curriculum. She also serves as coordinator of academic computing for the college.

Dr. Berman has traveled extensively, visiting nursing and health care institutions in Germany, Israel, Spain, Korea, Botswana, Australia, and Brazil. She serves on the board of directors for the Bay Area Tumor Institute and has been active with the American Cancer Society. She is a member of the American Nurses Association, Case Management Society of America, Oncology Nursing Society, and Sigma Theta Tau and is a site visitor for the Commission on Collegiate Nursing Education. She has twice participated as an NCLEX-RN item writer for the National Council of State Boards of Nursing. She is certified as an advanced oncology nurse and as an AIDS educator and has presented locally, nationally, and internationally on topics related to nursing education, breast cancer, and technology in health care.

Dr. Berman authored the scripts for more than 35 nursing skills videotapes in the 1990s. She is currently a manuscript reviewer for the *Journal of Nursing Scholarship.* She was a coauthor of the sixth edition of *Fundamentals of Nursing* and, with Shirlee Snyder, coauthor of the fifth edition of Kozier and Erb's *Techniques in Clinical Nursing.*

Audrey dedicates this textbook in gratitude to the strong women who have mentored and encouraged her all along the way; her mother, sister Lynn, Andrea, Carol, Darlene, Elizabeth, Helen, and Susie.

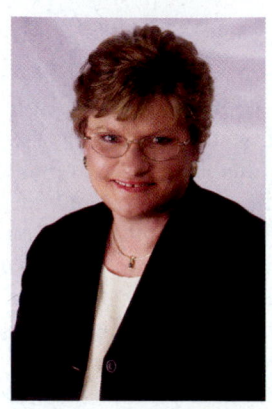

Shirlee J. Snyder

Shirlee Snyder graduated from Columbia Hospital School of Nursing in Milwaukee, Wisconsin, and subsequently received a bachelor of science in nursing from University of Wisconsin–Milwaukee. She was an RN in a medical-surgical nursing unit and transitioned to the first critical care/coronary care unit at Columbia Hospital. Because of her interest in cardiac nursing and teaching, she earned a master of science in nursing with a minor in cardiovascular clinical specialist and teaching from the University of Alabama in Birmingham. A move to California resulted in becoming a faculty member at Samuel Merritt Hospital School of Nursing in Oakland, California. Shirlee was fortunate to be involved in the phasing out of the diploma and ADN programs and development of a baccalaureate intercollegiate nursing program. She held numerous positions during her 15-year tenure at Samuel Merritt College including curriculum coordinator, assistant director–instruction, dean of instruction, and associate dean of the Intercollegiate Nursing Program. She is associate professor alumnus at Samuel Merritt College and periodically returns to teach graduate courses in Curriculum Development and Foundations in Education. Her interest and experiences in nursing education resulted in Shirlee obtaining a doctorate of education focused in curriculum and instruction from the University of San Francisco. Her dissertation was entitled *Comparing Training Effects of Field Independence–Dependence to Adaptive Flexibility on Nurse Problem Solving.*

Dr. Snyder moved to Portland, Oregon, in 1990 and taught in the ADN program at Portland Community College. During this teaching experience she became interested in computer-assisted instruction (CAI) and developed CAI modules in cardiac and respiratory assessment and initiated web-based assessment testing for student learning. She presented locally and nationally on topics related to using multimedia in the classroom and promoting ethnic and minority student success.

Another career opportunity in 1998 led her to Community College of Southern Nevada in Las Vegas, Nevada, where Dr. Snyder presently is the nursing program director with responsibilities for the associate degree and practical nursing programs. During this time she became involved in coauthoring the fifth edition of Kozier and Erb's *Techniques in Clinical Nursing* with Audrey Berman. Dr. Snyder is an advisory board member for the Nevada Geriatric Education Center and a member of the National League for Nursing, American Nurses Association, Sigma Theta Tau, and a variety of task groups addressing the Southern Nevada nursing shortage. She is a site visitor for the National League for Nursing Accrediting Commission and the Northwest Association of Schools and Colleges.

Dr. Snyder's experiences in nursing education and teaching keep her current in nursing and nursing education. She appreciates all she learns from the students she has taught and her past and present faculty colleagues.

Shirlee dedicates this textbook to her mother, Jean Snyder of Madison, Wisconsin, and in loving memory of her late father, Everett Snyder, and finally to her husband, Terry J. Schnitter, for his unconditional love and support.

GUIDE TO
FUNDAMENTALS OF NURSING

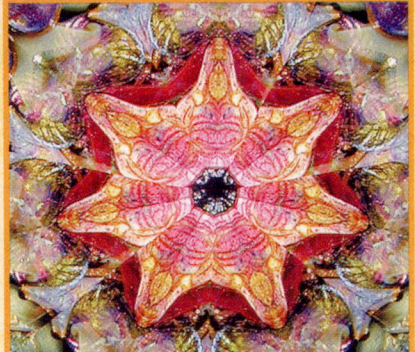

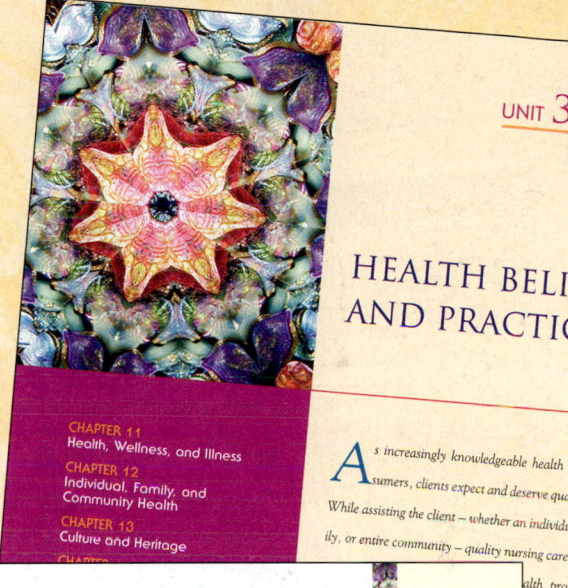

UNIT **3**

HEALTH BELIEFS AND PRACTICES

CHAPTER 11
Health, Wellness, and Illness

CHAPTER 12
Individual, Family, and Community Health

CHAPTER 13
Culture and Heritage

*A*s increasingly knowledgeable health care consumers, clients expect and deserve quality care. While assisting the client – whether an individual, family, or entire community – quality nursing care seeks to

---

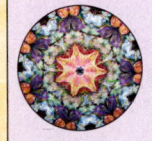

CHAPTER 29

ASEPSIS

LEARNING OUTCOMES

After completing this chapter, you will be able to:

- Explain the concepts of medical and surgical asepsis.
- Identify risks for nosocomial infections.
- Identify signs of localized and systemic infections.
- Identify factors influencing a microorganism's capability to produce an infectious process.
- Identify anatomic and physiologic barriers that defend the body against microorganisms.
- Differentiate active from passive immunity.
- Identify relevant nursing diagnoses and contributing factors for clients at risk for infection and who have an infection.
- Identify interventions to reduce risks for infections.
- Identify measures that break each link in the chain of infection.
- Compare and contrast category-specific, disease-specific, universal, body substance, standard, and transmission-based isolation precaution systems.
- Describe the steps to take in the event of a bloodborne pathogen exposure.
- Correctly implement aseptic practices, including hand washing, donning and removing a facemask, gowning, donning and removing disposable gloves, bagging articles, and managing equipment used for isolation clients.

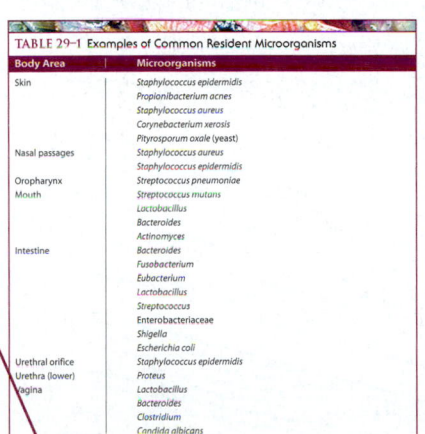

MediaLink

www.prenhall.com/kozier

Additional resources for this chapter can be found on the Student CD-ROM accompanying this textbook, and on the Companion Website at www.prenhall.com/kozier. Click on Chapter 29 to select the activities for this chapter.

CD-ROM
- Audio Glossary
- NCLEX Review

Companion Website
- Additional NCLEX Review
- Case Study: Client with Mycoplasma Pneumonia
- Care Plan Activity: Client on Radiation Therapy and Medication
- MediaLink Application: Go to "Infection Control Today"
- Links to Resources

Nurses are directly involved in providing a biologically safe environment. Microorganisms exist everywhere: in water, in soil, and on body surfaces such as the skin, intestinal tract, and other areas open to the outside (e.g., mouth, upper respiratory tract, vagina, and lower urinary tract). Most microorganisms are harmless, and some are even beneficial in that they perform essential functions in the body. Some microorganisms found in the intestines (e.g., enterobacteria) produce substances called **bacteriocins**, which are lethal to related strains of bacteria. Others produce antibiotic-like substances and toxic metabolites that repress the growth of other microorganisms. Some microorganisms are normal **resident flora** (the collective vegetation in a given area) in one part of the body, yet produce infection in another. For example, *Escherichia coli* is a normal inhabitant of the large intestine but a common cause of infection of the urinary tract. Table 29–1 provides a list of common resident microorganisms.

An **infection** is an invasion of body tissue by microorganisms and their proliferation there. Such a microorganism is called an *infectious agent*. If the microorganism produces no clinical evidence of disease, the infection is called *asymptomatic* or *subclinical*. Some subclinical infections can cause significant damage, for example, cytomegalovirus (CMV) infection in a pregnant woman can lead to significant disease in the unborn child. A detectable alteration in normal tissue function, however, is called **disease.**

Microorganisms vary in their **virulence** (i.e., their ability to produce disease). Microorganisms also vary in the severity of the diseases they produce and their degree of communicability. For example, the common cold virus is more readily transmitted than the bacillus that causes leprosy (*Mycobacterium leprae*). If the infectious agent can be transmitted to an individual by direct or

TABLE 29–1 Examples of Common Resident Microorganisms

Body Area	Microorganisms
Skin	Staphylococcus epidermidis
	Propionibacterium acnes
	Staphylococcus aureus
	Corynebacterium xerosis
	Pityrosporum oxale (yeast)
Nasal passages	Staphylococcus aureus
	Staphylococcus epidermidis
Oropharynx	Streptococcus pneumoniae
Mouth	Streptococcus mutans
	Lactobacillus
	Bacteroides
	Actinomyces
Intestine	Bacteroides
	Fusobacterium
	Eubacterium
	Lactobacillus
	Streptococcus
	Enterobacteriaceae
	Shigella
	Escherichia coli
Urethral orifice	Staphylococcus epidermidis
Urethra (lower)	Proteus
Vagina	Lactobacillus
	Bacteroides
	Clostridium
	Candida albicans

acquired immunity, 635
active immunity, 635
acute infections, 630
Airborne Precautions, 648
airborne transmission, 633
antibodies, 635
antigen, 635
antiseptics, 646
asepsis, 630
autoantigen, 635
bacteremia, 630
bacteria, 630
bacteriocins, 629
bloodborne pathogens, 648
body substance isolation (BSI), 648
carrier, 632
cell-mediated defenses, 635
cellular immunity, 635
chemotaxis, 634
chronic infections, 630
cicatrix, 635
circulating immunity, 635
clean, 630
colonization, 630
communicable disease, 630
compromised host, 633
Contact Precautions, 650
cultures, 639
diapedesis, 634
dirty, 630
disease, 629
disinfectants, 646
droplet nuclei, 633
Droplet Precautions, 650
emigration, 634
endogenous, 631
exogenous, 631
exudate, 634
fibrinogen, 634
fibrous (scar) tissue, 654
fungi, 630
granulation tissue, 634
humoral immunity, 635
hyperemia, 634
iatrogenic infections, 631
immune defenses, 633
immunity, 635
immunoglobulins, 635
infection, 629
inflammation, 634
isolation, 648
leukocytes, 634

629

Learning Outcomes
Learning Outcomes identify the most critical points in the chapter that students should understand at the chapter's conclusion.

MediaLink
MediaLink introduces each chapter of the text and lists additional specific content, animations, NCLEX Review, tools, and other interactive exercises, which appear on the accompanying Student CD-ROM and the Companion Website.

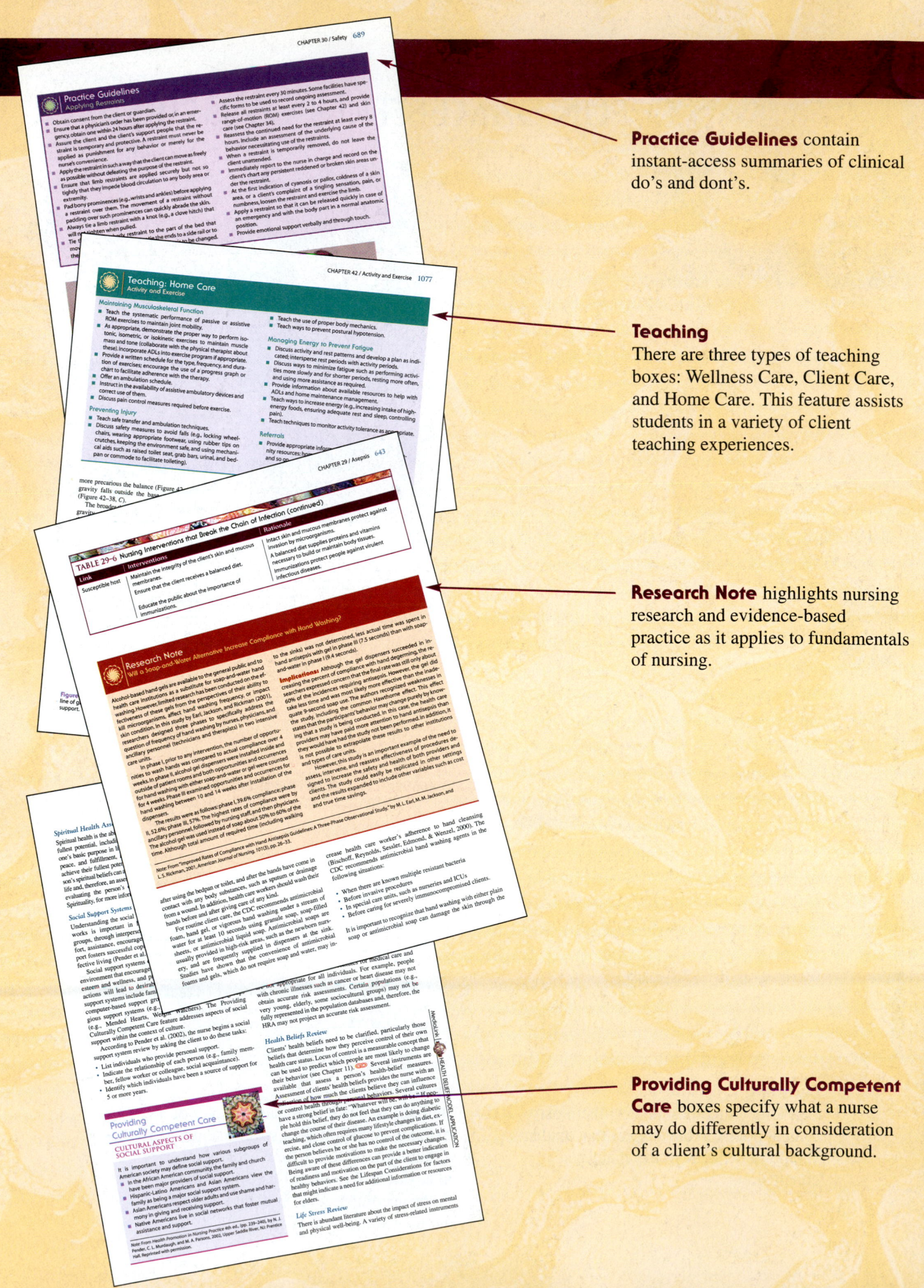

Practice Guidelines contain instant-access summaries of clinical do's and dont's.

Teaching

There are three types of teaching boxes: Wellness Care, Client Care, and Home Care. This feature assists students in a variety of client teaching experiences.

Research Note highlights nursing research and evidence-based practice as it applies to fundamentals of nursing.

Providing Culturally Competent Care boxes specify what a nurse may do differently in consideration of a client's cultural background.

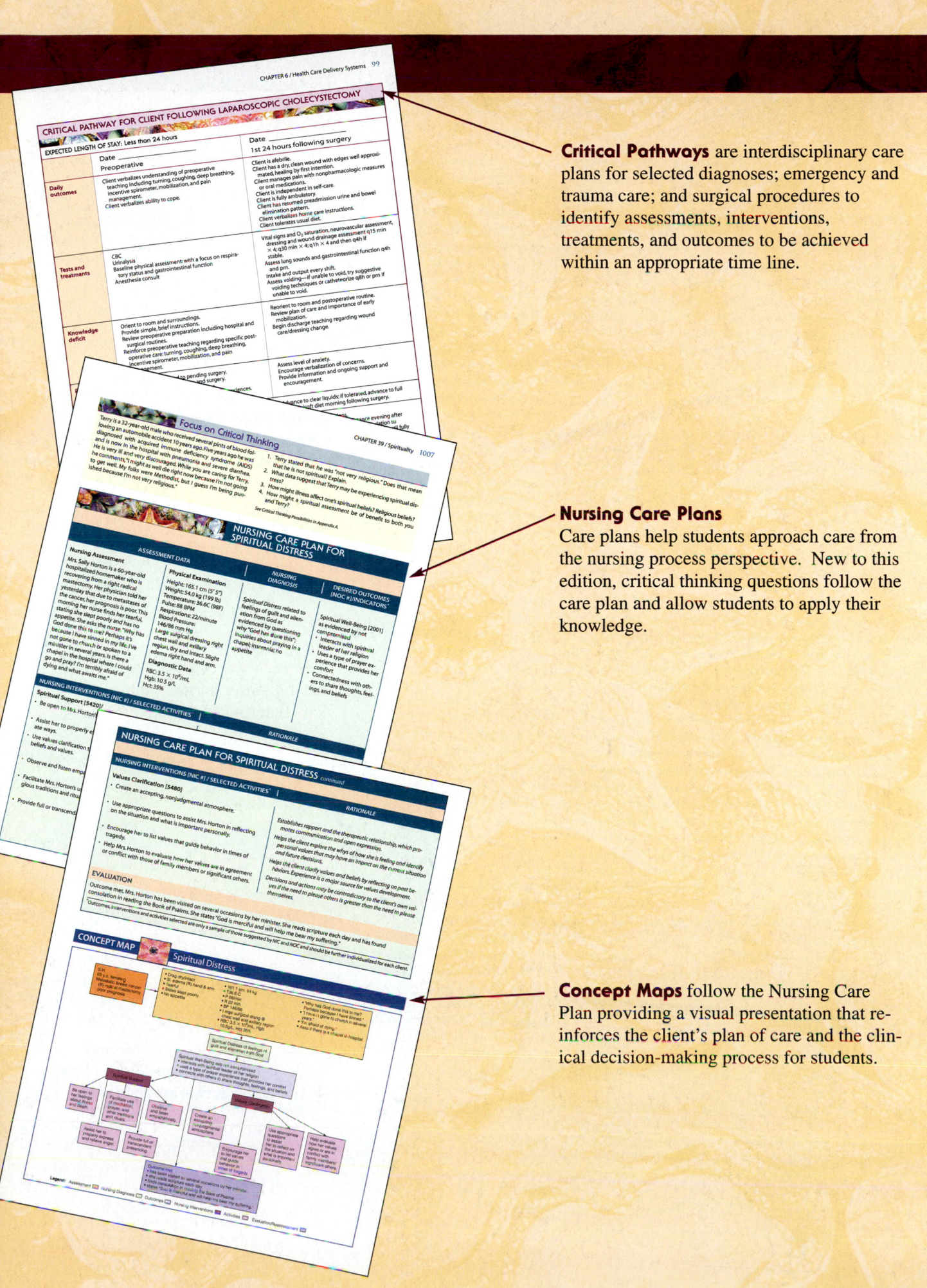

CRITICAL PATHWAY FOR CLIENT FOLLOWING LAPAROSCOPIC CHOLECYSTECTOMY

EXPECTED LENGTH OF STAY: Less than 24 hours

	Date _____ Preoperative	Date _____ 1st 24 hours following surgery
Daily outcomes	Client verbalizes understanding of preoperative teaching including turning, coughing, deep breathing, incentive spirometer, mobilization, and pain management. Client verbalizes ability to cope.	Client is afebrile. Client has a dry, clean wound with edges well approximated, healing by first intention. Client manages pain with nonpharmacologic measures or oral medications. Client is independent in self-care. Client is fully ambulatory. Client has resumed preadmission urine and bowel elimination pattern. Client verbalizes home care instructions. Client tolerates usual diet.
Tests and treatments	CBC Urinalysis Baseline physical assessment with a focus on respiratory status and gastrointestinal function Anesthesia consult	Vital signs and O₂ saturation, neurovascular assessment, dressing and wound drainage assessment q15 min × 4, q30 min × 4; q1h × 4 and then q4h if stable. Assess lung sounds and gastrointestinal function q4h and prn. Intake and output every shift. Assess voiding—if unable to void, try suggestive voiding techniques or catheterize q8h or prn if unable to void.
Knowledge deficit	Orient to room and surroundings. Provide simple, brief instructions. Review preoperative preparation including hospital and surgical routines. Reinforce preoperative teaching regarding specific postoperative care: turning, coughing, deep breathing, incentive spirometer, mobilization, and pain management.	Reorient to room and postoperative routine. Review plan of care and importance of early mobilization. Begin discharge teaching regarding wound care/dressing change. Assess level of anxiety. Encourage verbalization of concerns. Provide information and ongoing support and encouragement. Advance to clear liquids; if tolerated, advance to full ... soft diet morning following surgery.

Focus on Critical Thinking

Terry is a 32-year-old male who received several pints of blood following an automobile accident 10 years ago. Five years ago he was diagnosed with acquired immune deficiency syndrome (AIDS) and is now in the hospital with pneumonia and severe diarrhea. He is very ill and very discouraged. While you are caring for Terry, he comments, "I might as well die right now because I'm not going to get well. My folks were Methodist, but I guess I'm being punished because I'm not very religious."

1. Terry stated that he was "not very religious." Does that mean that he is not spiritual? Explain.
2. What data suggest that Terry may be experiencing spiritual distress?
3. How might illness affect one's spiritual beliefs? Religious beliefs?
4. How might a spiritual assessment be of benefit to both you and Terry?

See Critical Thinking Possibilities in Appendix A.

NURSING CARE PLAN FOR SPIRITUAL DISTRESS

ASSESSMENT DATA

Nursing Assessment
Mrs. Sally Horton is a 60-year-old hospitalized homemaker who is recovering from a right radical mastectomy. Her physician told her yesterday that due to metastases of the cancer, her prognosis is poor. This morning her nurse finds her tearful, stating she slept poorly and has no appetite. She asks the nurse, "Why has God done this to me? Perhaps it's because I have sinned in my life. I've not gone to church or spoken to a minister in several years. Is there a chapel in the hospital where I could go and pray? I'm terribly afraid of dying and what awaits me."

Physical Examination
Height: 165.1 cm (5' 5")
Weight: 54.0 kg (199 lb)
Temperature: 36.6C (98F)
Pulse: 88 BPM
Respirations: 22/minute
Blood Pressure: 146/86 mm Hg
Large surgical dressing right chest wall and axillary region, dry and intact. Slight edema right hand and arm.

Diagnostic Data
RBC: 3.5 × 10⁶/mL
Hgb: 10.5 g/L
Hct: 35%

NURSING DIAGNOSIS
Spiritual Distress related to feelings of guilt and alienation from God as evidenced by questioning why "God has done this": inquiries about praying in a chapel; insomnia; no appetite

DESIRED OUTCOMES [NOC #]/INDICATORS*
Spiritual Well-Being [2001] as evidenced by not compromised
• Interacts with spiritual leader of her religion
• Uses a type of prayer experience that provides her comfort
• Connectedness with others to share thoughts, feelings, and beliefs

NURSING INTERVENTIONS [NIC #] / SELECTED ACTIVITIES*

Spiritual Support [5420]/
• Be open to Mrs. Horton's ...
• Assist her to properly e... ate ways.
• Use values clarification t... beliefs and values.
• Observe and listen emp...
• Facilitate Mrs. Horton's u... gious traditions and ritu...
• Provide full or transcend...

RATIONALE

NURSING CARE PLAN FOR SPIRITUAL DISTRESS continued

NURSING INTERVENTIONS [NIC #] / SELECTED ACTIVITIES* continued

Values Clarification [5480]
• Create an accepting, nonjudgmental atmosphere.
• Use appropriate questions to assist Mrs. Horton in reflecting on the situation and what is important personally.
• Encourage her to list values that guide behavior in times of tragedy.
• Help Mrs. Horton to evaluate how her values are in agreement or conflict with those of family members or significant others.

RATIONALE
Establishes rapport and the therapeutic relationship, which promotes communication and open expression.
Helps the client explore the whys of how she is feeling and identify personal values that may have an impact on the current situation and future decisions.
Helps the client clarify values and beliefs by reflecting on past behaviors. Experience is a major source for values development.
Decisions and actions may be contradictory to the client's own values if the need to please others is greater than the need to please themselves.

EVALUATION
Outcome met. Mrs. Horton has been visited on several occasions by her minister. She reads scripture each day and has found consolation in reading the Book of Psalms. She states "God is merciful and will help me bear my suffering."

*Outcomes, interventions and activities selected are only a sample of those suggested by NIC and NOC and should be further individualized for each client.

CONCEPT MAP

Spiritual Distress

Legend: Assessment ☐ Nursing Diagnosis ☐ Outcomes ☐ Nursing Interventions ☐ Activities ☐ Evaluation/Reassessment ☐

Critical Pathways are interdisciplinary care plans for selected diagnoses; emergency and trauma care; and surgical procedures to identify assessments, interventions, treatments, and outcomes to be achieved within an appropriate time line.

Nursing Care Plans
Care plans help students approach care from the nursing process perspective. New to this edition, critical thinking questions follow the care plan and allow students to apply their knowledge.

Concept Maps follow the Nursing Care Plan providing a visual presentation that reinforces the client's plan of care and the clinical decision-making process for students.

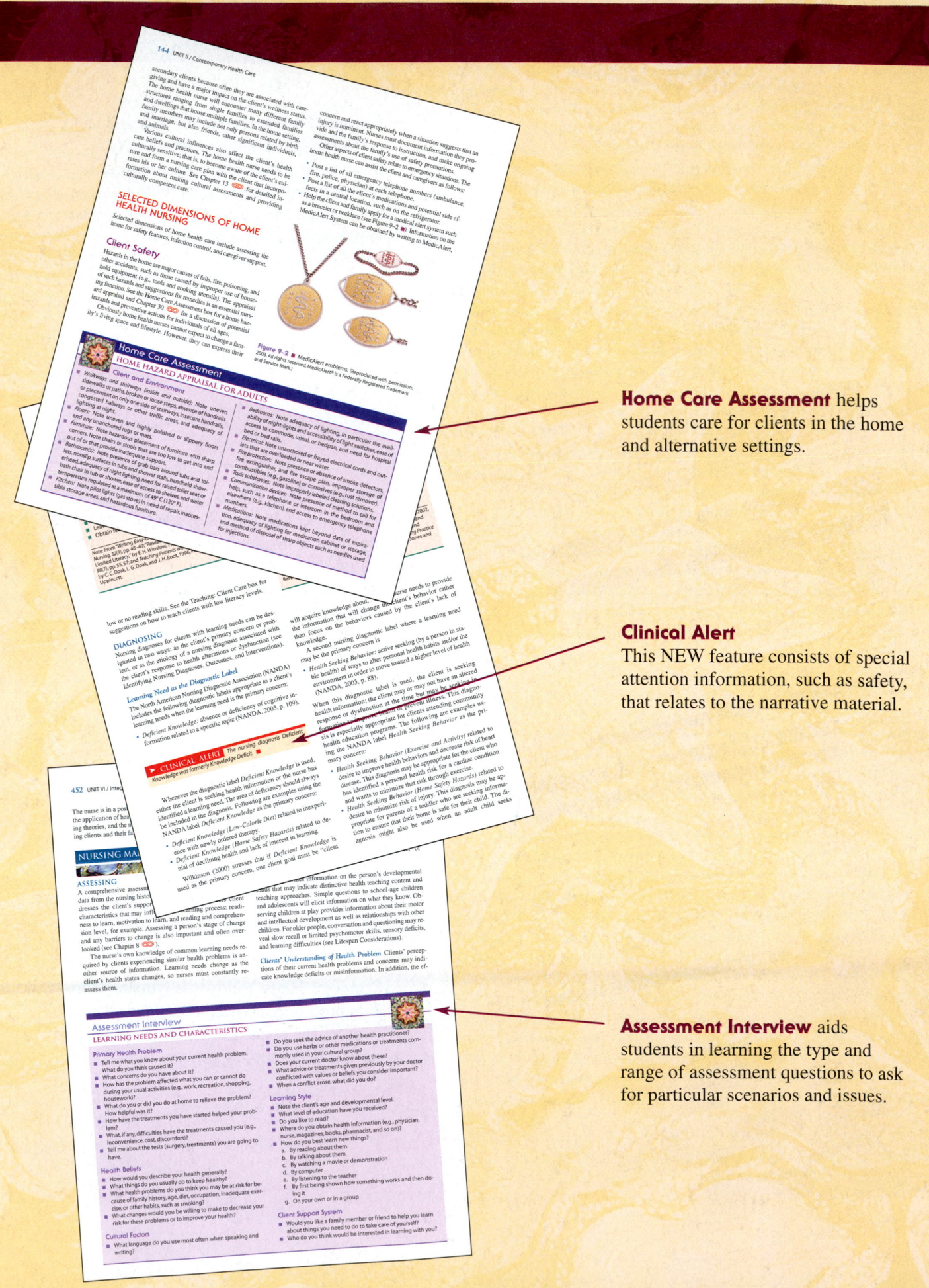

Home Care Assessment helps students care for clients in the home and alternative settings.

Clinical Alert
This NEW feature consists of special attention information, such as safety, that relates to the narrative material.

Assessment Interview aids students in learning the type and range of assessment questions to ask for particular scenarios and issues.

---

144 UNIT II / Contemporary Health Care

secondary clients because often they are associated with caregiving and have a major impact on the client's wellness care.

The home health nurse will encounter many different family structures ranging from single families to extended families and dwellings that house multiple families. In the home setting, family members may include not only persons related by birth and marriage, but also friends, other significant individuals, and animals.

Various cultural influences also affect the client's health care beliefs and practices. The home health nurse needs to be culturally sensitive; that is, to become aware of the client's culture and form a nursing care plan with the client that incorporates his or her culture. See Chapter 13 [CD] for detailed information about making cultural assessments and providing culturally competent care.

SELECTED DIMENSIONS OF HOME HEALTH NURSING

Selected dimensions of home health care include assessing the home for safety features, infection control, and caregiver support.

Client Safety

Hazards in the home are major causes of falls, fire, poisoning, and other accidents, such as those caused by improper use of household equipment (e.g., tools and cooking utensils). The appraisal of such hazards and suggestions for remedies is an essential nursing function. See the Home Care Assessment box for a review of hazards and preventive actions for individuals of all ages. Obviously home health nurses cannot expect to change a family's living space and lifestyle. However, they can express their

concern and react appropriately when a situation suggests that an injury is imminent. Nurses must document information they provide and the family's response to instruction, and make ongoing assessments about the family's use of safety precautions. The home health nurse can assist the client and caregivers as follows:

- Post a list of all emergency telephone numbers (ambulance, fire, police, physician) at each telephone.
- Post a list of all the client's medications and potential side effects in a central location, such as on the refrigerator.
- Help the client and family apply for a medical alert system such as a bracelet or necklace (see Figure 9–2 ■). Information on the MedicAlert System can be obtained by writing to MedicAlert,

Figure 9–2 ■ MedicAlert emblems. (Reproduced with permission, 2003. All rights reserved. MedicAlert® is a Federally Registered Trademark and Service Mark.)

Home Care Assessment
HOME HAZARD APPRAISAL FOR ADULTS

Client and Environment
- *Walkways and stairways (inside and outside):* Note uneven sidewalks or paths, broken or loose steps, absence of handrails or placement on only one side of stairways, insecure handrails, congested hallways or other traffic areas, and adequacy of lighting at night.
- *Floors:* Note uneven and highly polished or slippery floors and any unanchored rugs or mats.
- *Furniture:* Note hazardous placement of furniture with sharp corners. Note chairs or stools that are too low to get into and out of or that provide inadequate support.
- *Bathroom(s):* Note presence of grab bars around tubs and toilets, nonslip surfaces in tubs and shower stalls, handheld showerhead, adequacy of night lighting, need for raised toilet seat or bath chair in tub or shower, ease of access to shelves, and water temperature regulated at a maximum of 49° C (120° F).
- *Kitchen:* Note pilot lights (gas stove) in need of repair, inaccessible storage areas, and hazardous furniture.

- *Bedrooms:* Note adequacy of lighting, in particular the availability of night-lights and accessibility of light switches, ease of access to commode, urinal, or bedpan, and need for hospital bed or bed rails.
- *Electrical:* Note unanchored or frayed electrical cords and outlets that are overloaded or near water.
- *Fire protection:* Note presence or absence of smoke detectors, fire extinguisher, and fire escape plan, improper storage of combustibles (e.g., gasoline) or corrosives (e.g., rust removers).
- *Toxic substances:* Note improperly labeled cleaning solutions.
- *Communication devices:* Note presence of method to call for help, such as a telephone or intercom in the bedroom and elsewhere (e.g., kitchen), and access to emergency telephone numbers.
- *Medications:* Note medications kept beyond date of expiration, adequacy of lighting for medication cabinet or storage, and method of disposal of sharp objects such as needles used for injections.

---

low or no reading skills. See the Teaching: Client Care box for suggestions on how to teach clients with low literacy levels.

DIAGNOSING

Nursing diagnoses for clients with learning needs can be designated in two ways: as the client's primary concern or problem, or as the etiology of a nursing diagnosis associated with the client's response to health alterations or dysfunction (see Identifying Nursing Diagnoses, Outcomes, and Interventions).

Learning Need as the Diagnostic Label

The North American Nursing Diagnosis Association (NANDA) includes the following diagnostic labels appropriate to a client's learning needs when the learning need is the primary concern:

- *Deficient Knowledge:* absence or deficiency of cognitive information related to a specific topic (NANDA, 2003, p. 109).

▶ CLINICAL ALERT The nursing diagnosis Deficient Knowledge was formerly Knowledge Deficit. ■

Whenever the diagnostic label *Deficient Knowledge* is used, either the client is seeking health information or the nurse has identified a learning need. The area of deficiency should always be included in the diagnosis. Following are examples using the NANDA label *Deficient Knowledge* as the primary concern:

- *Deficient Knowledge (Low-Calorie Diet)* related to inexperience with newly ordered therapy.
- *Deficient Knowledge (Home Safety Hazards)* related to declining health and lack of interest in learning.

Wilkinson (2000) stresses that if *Deficient Knowledge* is used as the primary concern, one client goal must be "client

nurse needs to provide than focus on the behaviors caused by the client's lack of knowledge.

A second nursing diagnostic label where a learning need may be the primary concern is

- *Health Seeking Behavior:* active seeking (by a person in stable health) of ways to alter personal health habits and/or the environment in order to move toward a higher level of health (NANDA, 2003, p. 88).

When this diagnostic label is used, the client is seeking health information; the client may or may not have an altered response or dysfunction at the time but may be seeking information to promote health or prevent illness. This diagnosis is especially appropriate for clients attending community health education programs. The following are examples using the NANDA label *Health Seeking Behavior* as the primary concern:

- *Health Seeking Behavior (Exercise and Activity)* related to desire to improve health behaviors and decrease risk of heart disease. This diagnosis may be appropriate for the client who has identified a personal health risk for a cardiac condition and wants to minimize that risk through exercise.
- *Health Seeking Behavior (Home Safety Hazards)* related to desire to minimize risk of injury. This diagnosis may be appropriate for parents of a toddler who are seeking information to ensure that their home is safe for their child. The diagnosis might also be used when an adult child seeks

---

452 UNIT VI / Integ

The nurse is in a po the application of he ing theories, and the ing clients and their fa

ASSESSING

A comprehensive assessm data from the nursing histo dresses the client's suppor characteristics that may infl ness to learn, motivation to learn, and reading and comprehension level, for example. Assessing a person's stage of change and any barriers to change is also important and often overlooked (see Chapter 8 [CD]).

The nurse's own knowledge of common learning needs required by clients experiencing similar health problems is another source of information. Learning needs change as the client's health status changes, so nurses must constantly reassess them.

mation on the person's developmental that may indicate distinctive health teaching content and teaching approaches. Simple questions to school-age children and adolescents will elicit information on what they know. Observing children at play provides information about their motor and intellectual development as well as relationships with other children. For older people, conversation and questioning may reveal slow recall or limited psychomotor skills, sensory deficits, and learning difficulties (see Lifespan Considerations).

Clients' Understanding of Health Problem Clients' perceptions of their current health problems and concerns may indicate knowledge deficits or misinformation. In addition, the ef-

Assessment Interview
LEARNING NEEDS AND CHARACTERISTICS

Primary Health Problem
- Tell me what you know about your current health problem.
  What do you think caused it?
- What concerns do you have about it?
- How has the problem affected what you can or cannot do during your usual activities (e.g., work, recreation, shopping, housework)?
- What do you or did you do at home to relieve the problem?
  How helpful was it?
- How have the treatments you have started helped your problem?
- What, if any, difficulties have the treatments caused you (e.g., inconvenience, cost, discomfort)?
- Tell me about the tests (surgery, treatments) you are going to have.

Health Beliefs
- How would you describe your health generally?
- What things do you usually do to keep healthy?
- What health problems do you think you may be at risk for because of family history, age, diet, occupation, inadequate exercise, or other habits, such as smoking?
- What changes would you be willing to make to decrease your risk for these problems or to improve your health?

Cultural Factors
- What language do you use most often when speaking and writing?

- Do you seek the advice of another health practitioner?
- Do you use herbs or other medications or treatments commonly used in your cultural group?
- Does your current doctor know about these?
- What advice or treatments given previously by your doctor conflicted with values or beliefs you consider important?
- When a conflict arose, what did you do?

Learning Style
- Note the client's age and developmental level.
- What level of education have you received?
- Do you like to read?
- Where do you obtain health information (e.g., physician, nurse, magazines, books, pharmacist, and so on)?
- How do you best learn new things?
  a. By reading about them
  b. By talking about them
  c. By watching a movie or demonstration
  d. By computer
  e. By listening to the teacher
  f. By first being shown how something works and then doing it
  g. On your own or in a group

Client Support System
- Would you like a family member or friend to help you learn about things you need to do to take care of yourself?
- Who do you think would be interested in learning with you?

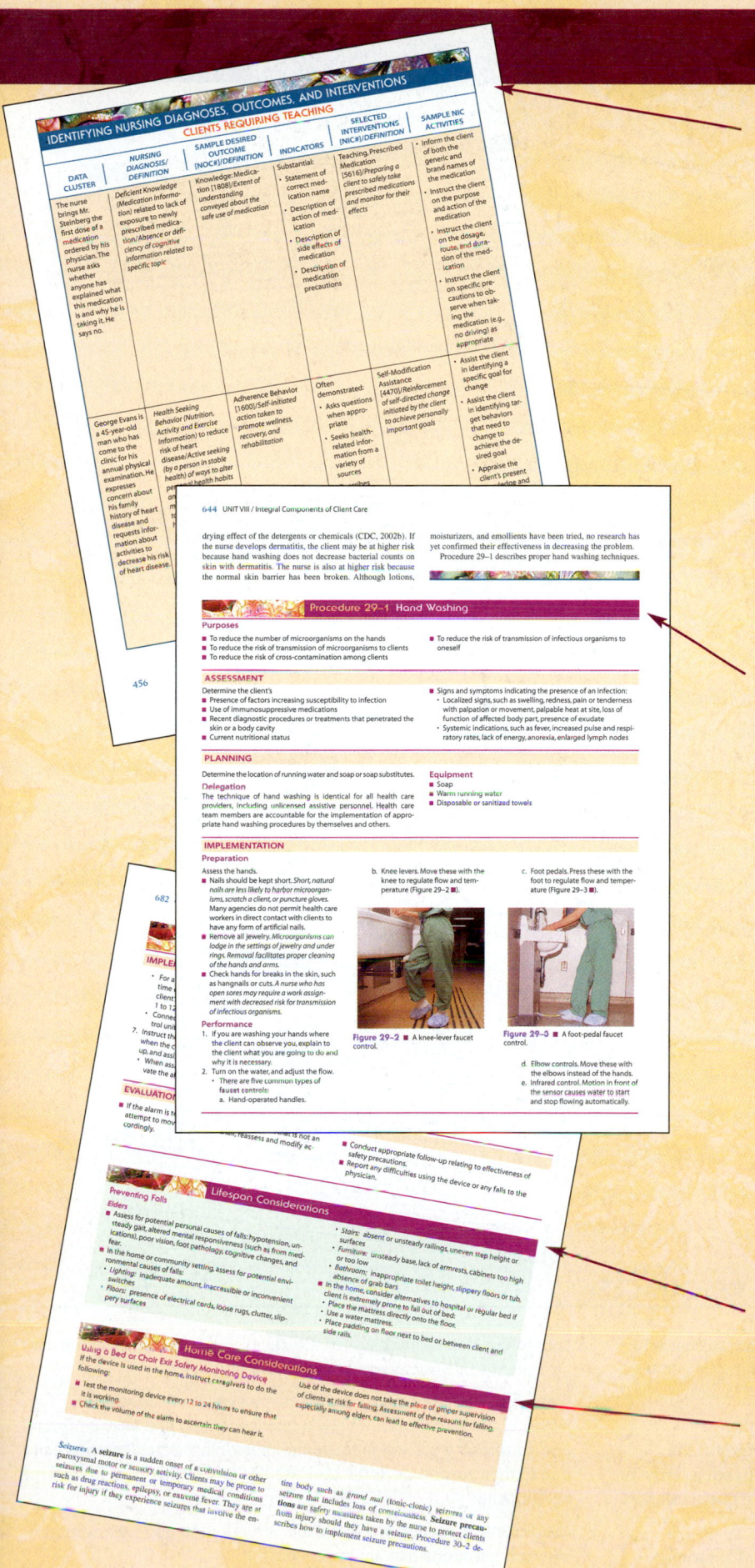

Identifying Nursing Diagnoses, Outcomes, and Interventions

These boxes provide guidelines for establishing nursing diagnoses, outcomes, and interventions and will include data clusters and the most current NOC and NIC language for the specific nursing diagnoses being discussed in the chapter.

Procedures

Presented in a step-by-step format, these are clinical nursing skills that students will have to perform on patients. Framed in the context of the nursing process, the steps of the skills also provide rationales for the nurse's actions in italic type.

Lifespan Considerations focus on applying a particular skill or procedure for clients of different ages.

Home Care Considerations show variations for different skills performed in the home setting.

CHAPTER REVIEW

Focus on Critical Thinking

provides a brief case study followed by approximately five questions that stimulate critical thinking. The Focus on Critical Thinking box is always located at the end of the chapter. Suggested answers are found in Appendix A.

EXPLORE MediaLink

Found at the end of every chapter, EXPLORE MediaLink encourages students to use the CD-ROM and the Companion Website to apply what they have learned from the text in case studies, practice NCLEX questions, and additional resources.

Chapter Highlights is a summary of chapter content. Students who read these concepts before reading the chapter will find them helpful in focusing their attention. Chapter Highlights is also an appropriate tool to quickly review the content after reading the chapter.

Review Questions

These review questions, written in multiple-choice format test the students' knowledge of the material and reinforce what they have learned from the chapter readings.

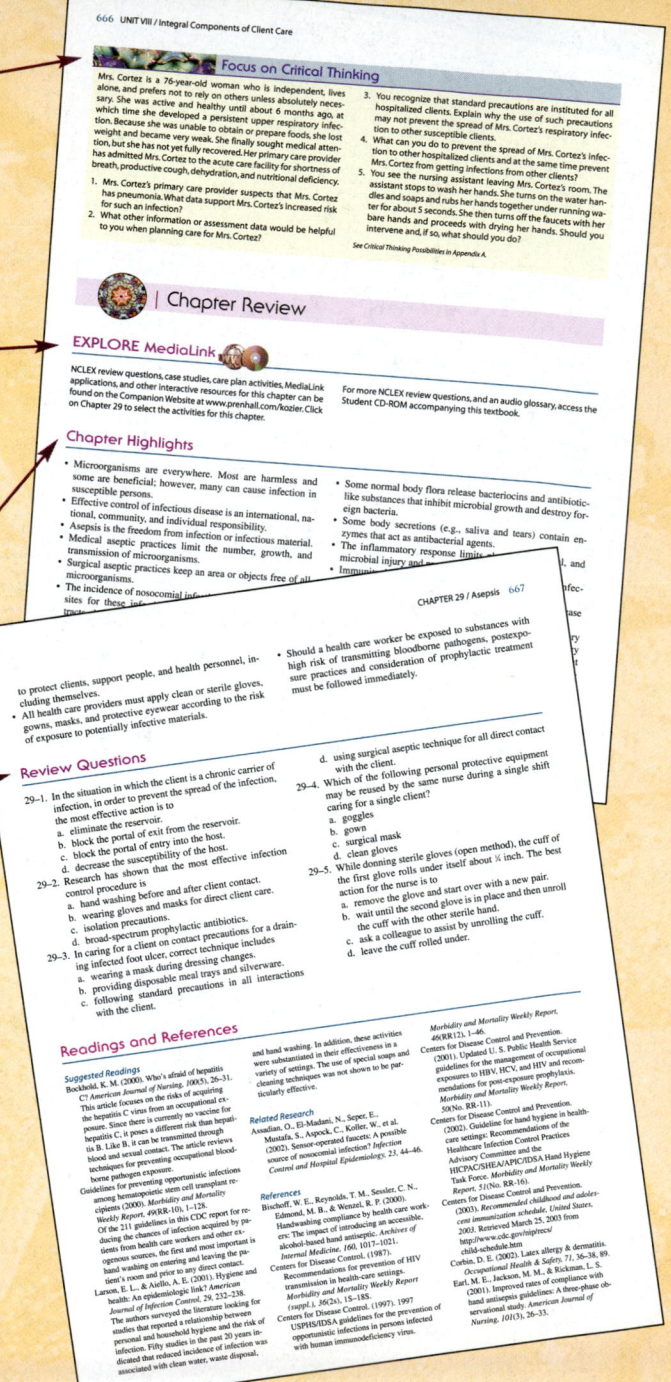

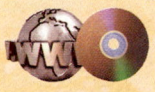 **ADDITIONAL MEDIA RESOURCES:**

Animation Tutorials—On the Student CD-ROM, the student will find animations illustrating difficult concepts or reinforcing content from the text.

NCLEX Reviews—Both the Student CD-ROM and the free Companion Website offer the student an abundance of NCLEX review questions for each chapter of the book. The questions provide comprehensive rationales, as well as identify how the questions correlate to the NCLEX test plan.

Care Plan Activities—Each clinical chapter on the Companion Website provides the student with a case scenario and asks the stu-

dent to develop a care plan for the client. Students can e-mail these care plans to instructors as homework assignments.

Case Studies—For each clinical chapter on the Companion Website, the student can review a client scenario and answer several critical thinking questions related to that client's care. Students can e-mail their responses to the case studies to instructors as homework assignments.

MediaLink Application—Students are asked to go to the web to research questions that are presented.

SPECIAL FEATURES

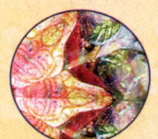

PROVIDING CULTURALLY COMPETENT CARE

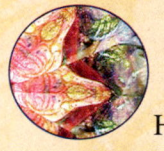

IDENTIFYING NURSING DIAGNOSES, OUTCOMES, AND INTERVENTIONS

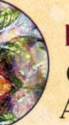

LIFESPAN CONSIDERATIONS

TEACHING: WELLNESS CARE

TEACHING: CLIENT CARE

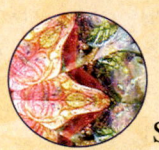
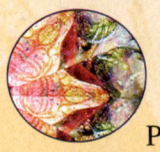

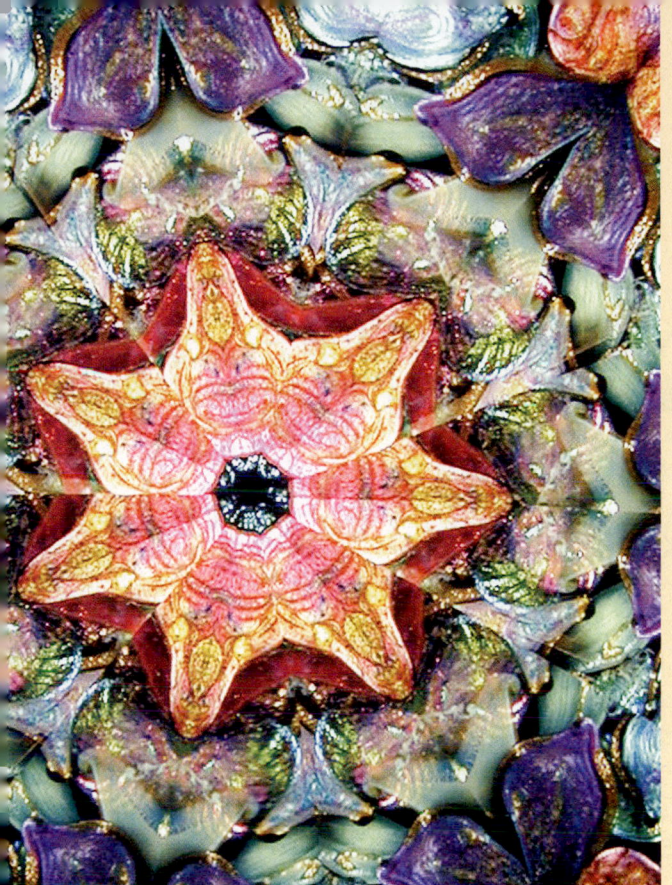

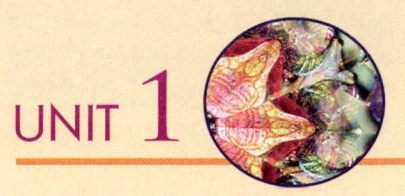

THE NATURE OF NURSING

Throughout its distinguished history, nursing has had a significant effect on people's lives. As rapid change continues to transform the profession of nursing and the health care system with which it is intricately linked, nurses embrace broader opportunities to influence human well-being. Today, nurses bring knowledge, leadership, spirit, and vital expertise to expanding roles that afford increased participation, responsibility, and rewards. However nursing continues to evolve, underlying all is a time-honored, fervent, and profound commitment to caring.

CHAPTER | 1

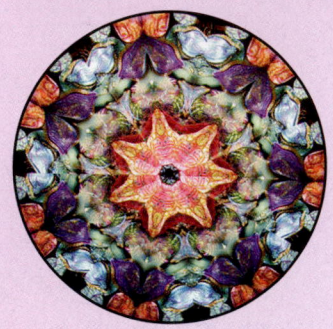

HISTORICAL AND CONTEMPORARY NURSING PRACTICE

LEARNING OUTCOMES

After completing this chapter, you will be able to:

- Discuss historical and contemporary factors influencing the development of nursing.

- Identify the essential aspects of nursing.

- Identify four major areas within the scope of nursing practice.

- Identify the purposes of nurse practice acts and standards for nursing practice.

- Describe the roles of nurses.

- Describe the expanded career roles and their functions.

- Discuss the criteria of a profession and the professionalization of nursing.

- Discuss Benner's levels of nursing proficiency.

- Relate essential nursing values to attitudes, personal qualities, and professional behaviors.

- Explain the functions of national and international nurses' associations.

MediaLink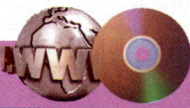

www.prenhall.com/kozier

Additional resources for this chapter can be found on the Student CD-ROM accompanying this textbook, and on the Companion Website at www.prenhall.com/kozier. Click on Chapter 1 to select the activities for this chapter.

CD-ROM
- Audio Glossary
- NCLEX Review

Companion Website
- Additional NCLEX Review
- Case Study: Evolution of Nursing
- MediaLink Applications:
    Florence Nightingale
    American Association of Colleges of Nursing
    Sigma Theta Tau
- Links to Resources

Nursing today is far different from nursing as it was practiced years ago, and it is expected to continue changing during the 21st century. To comprehend present-day nursing and at the same time prepare for the future, one must understand not only past events but also contemporary nursing practice and the sociological and historical factors that affect it.

HISTORICAL PERSPECTIVES

Nursing has undergone dramatic change in response to societal needs and influences. A look at nursing's beginnings reveals its continuing struggle for autonomy and professionalization. In recent decades, a renewed interest in nursing history has produced a growing amount of related literature. This section highlights only selected aspects of events that have influenced nursing practice. Recurring themes of women's roles and status, religious (Christian) values, war, societal attitudes, and visionary nursing leadership have influenced nursing practice in the past. Many of these factors still exert their influence today.

Women's Roles

Traditional female roles of wife, mother, daughter, and sister have always included the care and nurturing of other family members. From the beginning of time, women have cared for infants and children; thus, nursing could be said to have its roots in "the home." Additionally, women, who in general occupied a subservient and dependent role, were called on to care for others in the community who were ill. Generally, the care provided was related to physical maintenance and comfort. Thus, the traditional nursing role has always entailed humanistic caring, nurturing, comforting, and supporting.

Religion

Religion has also played a significant role in the development of nursing. Although many of the world's religions encourage benevolence, it was the Christian value of "love thy neighbor as thyself" and Christ's parable of the Good Samaritan that had a significant impact on the development of Western nursing. During the third and fourth centuries, several wealthy matrons of the Roman Empire, such as **Fabiola** converted to Christianity and used their wealth to provide houses of care and healing (the forerunner of hospitals) for the poor, the sick, and the homeless. Women were not, however, the sole providers of nursing services.

The Crusades saw the formation of several orders of knights, including the Knights of Saint John of Jerusalem (also known as the Knights Hospitalers), the Teutonic Knights, and the Knights of Saint Lazarus (Figure 1–1 ■). These brothers in arms provided nursing care to their sick and injured comrades. These orders also built hospitals, the organization and management of which set a standard for the administration of hospitals throughout Europe at that time. The **Knights of Saint Lazarus** dedicated themselves to the care of people with leprosy, syphilis, and chronic skin conditions.

The deaconess groups, which had their origins in the Roman Empire of the third and fourth centuries, were suppressed during the Middle Ages by the Western churches. However, these groups of nursing providers resurfaced occasionally throughout the centuries, most notably in 1836, when Theodore Fliedner reinstituted the Order of Deaconesses and opened a small hospital and training school in Kaiserswerth, Germany. Florence Nightingale received her "training" in nursing at the Kaiserswerth School.

Early religious values, such as self-denial, spiritual calling, and devotion to duty and hard work, have dominated nursing throughout its history. Nurses' commitment to these values often resulted in exploitation and few monetary rewards. For some time, nurses themselves believed it was inappropriate to expect economic gain from their "calling."

War

Throughout history, wars have accentuated the need for nurses. During the Crimean War (1854–1856), the inadequacy of care given to soldiers led to a public outcry in Great Britain. The role Florence Nightingale played in addressing this problem is well known. She was asked by Sir Sidney Herbert of the British War Department to recruit a contingent of female nurses to provide care to the sick and injured in the Crimea. Nightingale and her nurses transformed the military

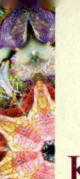

KEY TERMS

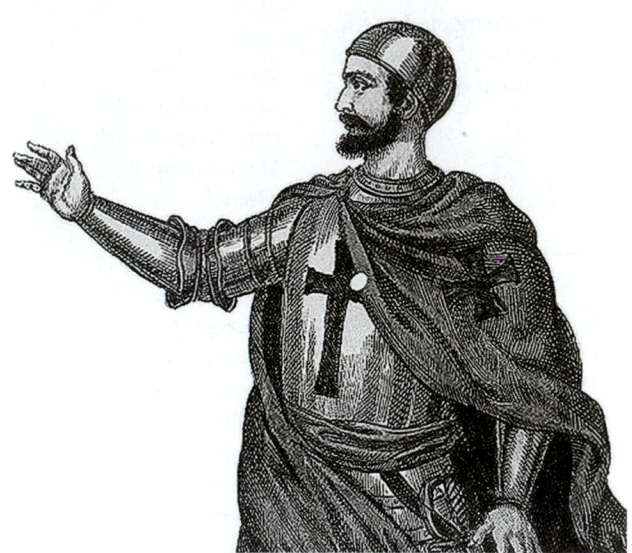

Figure 1–1 ■ The Knights of Saint Lazarus (established circa 1200) dedicated themselves to the care of people with leprosy, syphilis, and chronic skin conditions. From the time of Christ to the mid-13th century, leprosy was viewed as an incurable and terminal disease. (CORBIS Images.)

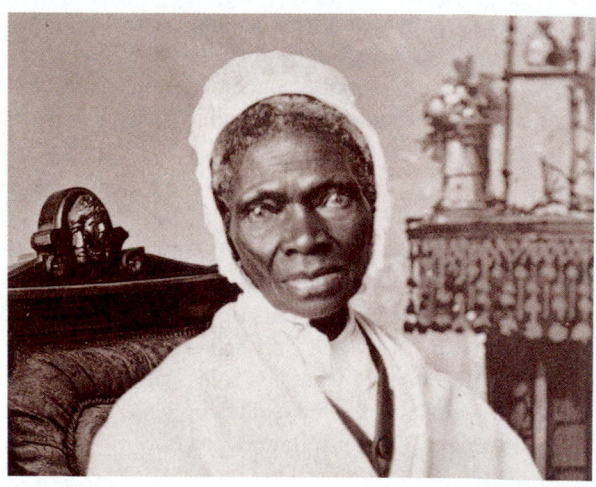

Figure 1–3 ■ Sojourner Truth (1797–1883), abolitionist, Underground Railroad agent, preacher, and women's rights advocate, was a nurse for over 4 years during the Civil War and worked as a nurse and counselor for the Freedmen's Relief Association after the war. (Randall Studio (1805–1875) Sojourner Truth (c. 1797–18--), abolitionist. © 1870. Photograph, Albumen Silver Print. Copyright National Portrait Gallery, Smithsonian Institution/Art Resources, NY.)

hospitals by setting up sanitation practices, such as hand washing and washing clothing regularly. Nightingale is credited with performing miracles; the mortality rate in the Barrack Hospital in Turkey, for example, was reduced from 42 to 2 percent (Donahue, 1996, p. 197).

During the American Civil War (1861–1865), several nurses emerged who were notable for their contributions to a country torn by internal strife. **Harriet Tubman** and **Sojourner Truth** (Figures 1–2 ■ and 1–3 ■) provided care and safety to slaves fleeing to the North on the Underground Railroad. Mother Biekerdyke and Clara Barton searched the battlefields and gave care to injured and dying soldiers. Noted authors Walt Whitman and Louisa May Alcott volunteered as nurses to give care to injured soldiers in military hospitals.

World War II casualties created an acute shortage of care and the Cadet Nurse Corps was established in response to a marked shortage of nurses (Figure 1–4 ■). Also at that time, auxiliary health care workers became prominent. "Practical" nurses, aides, and technicians provided much of the actual nursing care under the instruction and supervision of better prepared nurses. Medical specialties also arose at that time to meet the needs of hospitalized clients.

Societal Attitudes

Society's attitudes about nurses and nursing have significantly influenced professional nursing.

Before the mid-1800s, nursing was without organization, education, or social status; the prevailing attitude was that a woman's place was in the home and that no respectable woman should have a career. The role for the Victorian middle-class woman was that of wife and mother, and any education she obtained was for the purpose of making her a pleasant companion to her husband and a responsible mother to her children. Nurses in hospitals during this period were poorly educated; some were even incarcerated criminals. Society's attitudes about nursing during this period are reflected in the writings of Charles Dickens. In his book *Martin Chuzzlewit* (1896), Dickens reflected his attitude toward nurses through his character **Sairy Gamp** (Figure 1–5 ■). She "cared" for the sick by neglecting them, stealing from them, and physically abusing them (Donahue, 1996, p. 192). This literary portrayal of nurses greatly influenced the negative image and attitude toward nurses up to contemporary times.

In contrast, the *Guardian Angel* or *Angel of Mercy* image arose in the latter part of the 19th century, largely because of the work of Florence Nightingale during the Crimean War. After Nightingale brought respectability to the nursing profes-

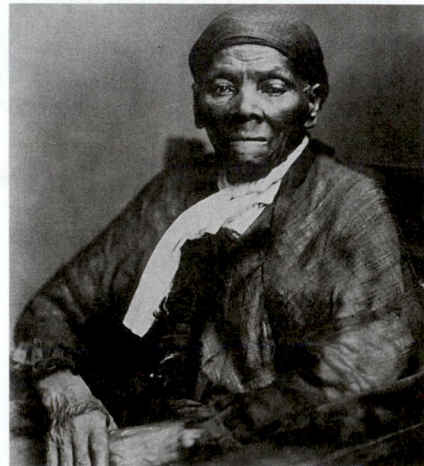

Figure 1–2 ■ Harriet Tubman (1820–1913) was known as "The Moses of Her People" for her work with the Underground Railroad. During the Civil War (1861–1865), she nursed the sick and suffering of her own race. (© CORBIS.)

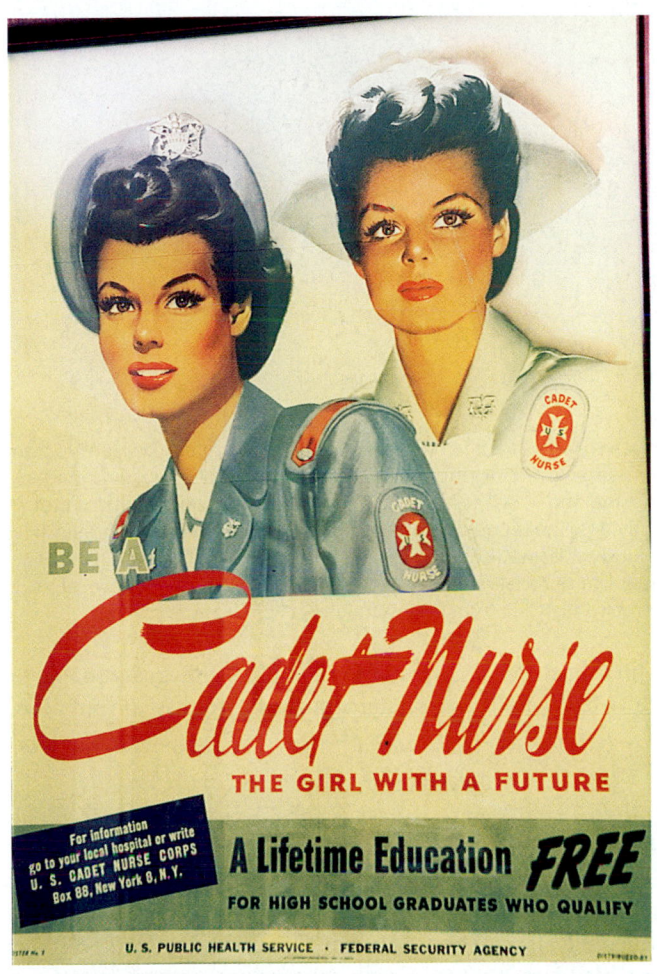

Figure 1–4 ■ Recruiting poster for the Cadet Nurse Corps during WWII. (Courtesy of Illinois State Library digital archives.)

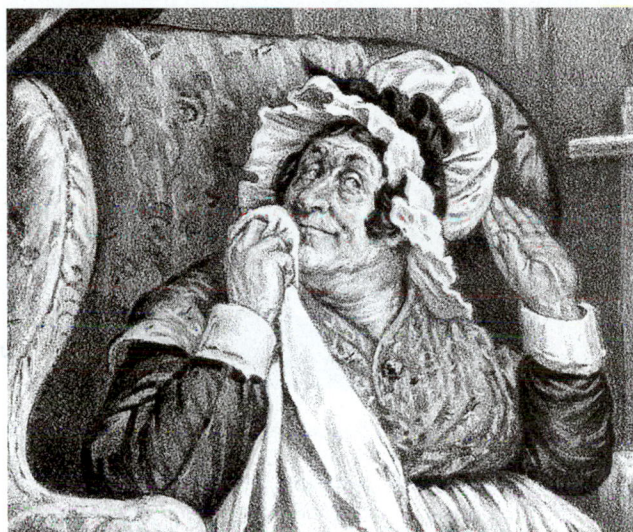

Figure 1–5 ■ Sairy Gamp, a character in Dickens' book *Martin Chuzzlewit*, represented the negative image of nurses in the early 1800s. (CORBIS Images.)

Nursing Leaders

Florence Nightingale, Clara Barton, Lillian Wald, Lavinia Dock, Margaret Sanger, and Mary Breckinridge are among the leaders who have made notable contributions both to nursing's history and to women's history. These women were all politically astute pioneers. Their skills at influencing others and bringing about change remain models for political nurse activists today. Contemporary nursing leaders, such as Virginia Henderson, who created a modern worldwide definition of nursing, and Martha Rogers, a catalyst for theory development, are discussed in Chapter 3.

Nightingale (1820–1910)

Florence Nightingale's contributions to nursing are well documented. Her achievements in improving the standards for the care of war casualties in the Crimea earned her the title "Lady with the Lamp." Her efforts in reforming hospitals and in producing and implementing public health policies also made her an accomplished political nurse: She was the first nurse to exert political pressure on government. Through her contributions to nursing education—perhaps her greatest achievement—she is also recognized as nursing's first scientist-theorist for her work *Notes on Nursing: What It Is, and What It Is Not* (1860/1969).

Nightingale (Figure 1–6 ■) was born to a wealthy and intellectual family. She believed she was "called by God to help others . . . [and] to improve the well-being of mankind" (Schuyler, 1992, p. 4). She was determined to become a nurse in spite of opposition from her family and the restrictive societal code for affluent young English women. As a well-traveled young woman of the day, she visited Kaiserswerth in 1847, where she received three months' training in nursing. In 1853 she studied in Paris with the Sisters of Charity, after which she returned to England to assume the position of superintendent of a charity hospital for ill governesses.

sion, nurses were viewed as noble, compassionate, moral, religious, dedicated, and self-sacrificing.

Another image arising in the early 19th century that has affected subsequent generations of nurses and the public and other professionals working with nurses is the image of *doctor's handmaiden*. This image evolved when women had yet to obtain the right to vote, when family structures were largely paternalistic, and when the medical profession portrayed increasing use of scientific knowledge that, at that time, was viewed as a male domain. Since that time, several images of nursing have been portrayed. The *heroine* portrayal evolved from nurses' acts of bravery in World War II and their contributions in fighting poliomyelitis—in particular, the work of the Australian nurse Elizabeth Kenney. Other images in the late 1900s include the nurse as sex object, surrogate mother, tyrannical mother, and body expert or body minder.

During the past few decades, the nursing profession has taken steps to improve the image of the nurse. In the early 1990s, the Tri-Council for Nursing (the American Association of Colleges of Nursing, the American Nurses Association, the American Organization of Nurse Executives, and the National League for Nursing) initiated a national effort (titled "Nurses of America") to improve the image of nursing.

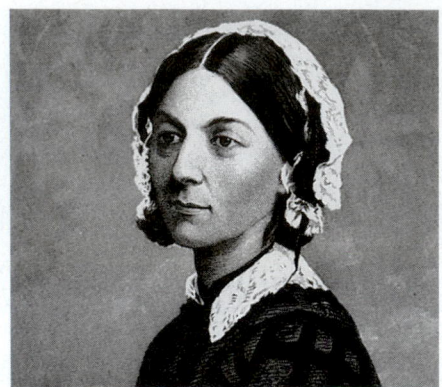

Figure 1–6 ■ Considered the founder of modern nursing, Florence Nightingale (1820–1910) was influential in developing nursing education, practice, and administration. Her publication, *Notes on Nursing: What It Is, and What It Is Not,* first published in England in 1859 and in the U.S. in 1860, was intended for all women. (© Bettman/CORBIS.)

When she returned to England from the Crimea, a grateful English public gave Nightingale an honorarium of £ 4500. She later used this money to develop the Nightingale Training School for Nurses, which opened in 1860. The school served as a model for other training schools. Its graduates traveled to other countries to manage hospitals and institute nurse-training programs.

Nightingale's vision of nursing, which included public health and health promotion roles for nurses, was only partially addressed in the early days of nursing. The focus tended to be on developing the profession within hospitals.

Barton (1812–1912)

Clara Barton (Figure 1–7 ■) was a schoolteacher who volunteered as a nurse during the American Civil War. Her responsibility was to organize the nursing services. Barton is noted for her role in establishing the American Red Cross, which linked with the International Red Cross when the U.S. Congress ratified the Treaty of Geneva (Geneva Convention). It was Barton

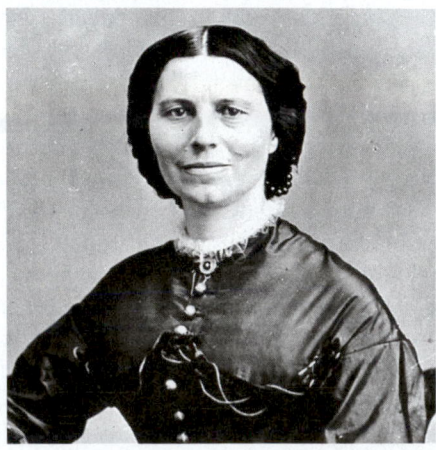

Figure 1–7 ■ Clara Barton (1812–1912) organized the American Red Cross, which linked with the International Red Cross when the U.S. Congress ratified the Geneva Convention in 1882. (© Bettman/CORBIS.)

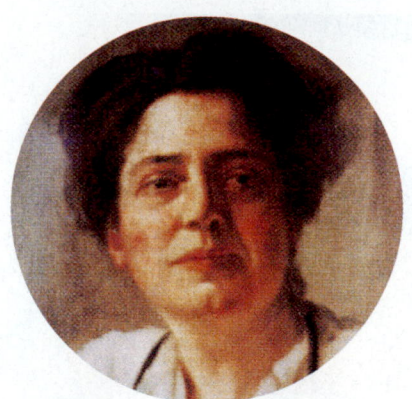

Figure 1–8 ■ Lillian Wald (1867–1940) founded the Henry Street Settlement and Visiting Nurse Service (circa 1893), which provided nursing and social services and organized educational and cultural activities. She is considered the founder of public health nursing. (Schevill, William Valentine (1864–1951). Lillian D. Wald (1867–1940). Public health nurse, social worker. 1919. *Oil on Cardboard.* Copyright National Portrait Gallery, Smithsonian Institution/Art Resources, NY.)

who persuaded Congress in 1882 to ratify this treaty so that the Red Cross could perform humanitarian efforts in time of peace.

Wald (1867–1940)

Lillian Wald (Figure 1–8 ■) is considered the founder of public health nursing. Wald and Mary Brewster were the first to offer trained nursing services to the poor in the New York slums. Their home among the poor on the upper floor of a tenement, called the Henry Street Settlement and Visiting Nurse Service, provided nursing services, social services, and organized educational and cultural activities. Soon after the founding of the Henry Street Settlement, school nursing was established as an adjunct to visiting nursing.

Dock (1858–1956)

Lavinia L. Dock (Figure 1–9 ■) was a feminist, prolific writer, political activist, suffragette, and friend of Wald. She partici-

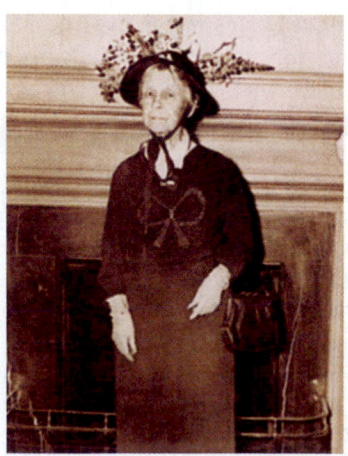

Figure 1–9 ■ Nursing leader and suffragist Lavinia L. Dock (1858–1956) was active in the protest movement for women's rights that resulted in the U.S. Constitution amendment allowing women to vote in 1920. (Courtesy of Teachers College, Columbia University.)

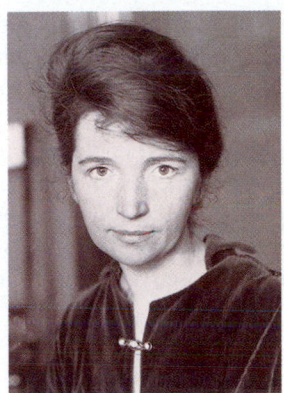

Figure 1–10 ■ Nurse activist Margaret Sanger, considered the founder of Planned Parenthood, was imprisoned for opening the first birth control information clinic in Baltimore in 1916. (© Bettman/CORBIS.)

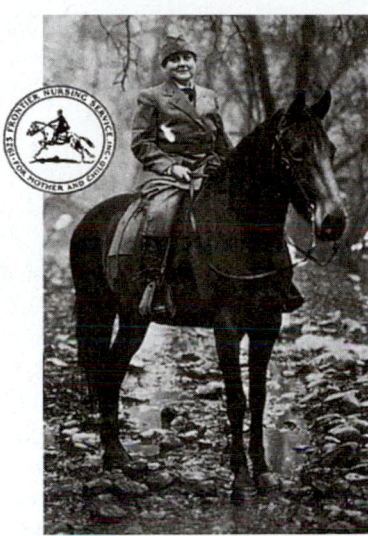

Figure 1–11 ■ Mary Breckinridge, a nurse who practiced midwifery in England, Australia, and New Zealand, founded the Frontier Nursing Service in Kentucky in 1925 to provide family-centered primary health care to rural populations. (Courtesy of Frontier Nursing Service, Inc., Wandover, KY.)

pated in protest movements for women's rights that resulted in the 1920 passage of the 19th Amendment to the U.S. Constitution, which granted women the right to vote. In addition, Dock campaigned for legislation to allow nurses rather than physicians to control their profession. In 1893, Dock, with the assistance of Mary Adelaide Nutting and Isabel Hampton Robb, founded the American Society of Superintendents of Training Schools for Nurses of the United States and Canada, a precursor to the current National League for Nursing.

Sanger (1879–1966)

Margaret Higgins Sanger (Figure 1–10 ■), a public health nurse in New York, has had a lasting impact on women's health care. Imprisoned for opening the first birth control information clinic in America, she is considered the founder of Planned Parenthood. Her experience with the large number of unwanted pregnancies among the working poor was instrumental in addressing this problem.

Breckinridge (1881–1965)

After World War I, **Mary Breckinridge** (Figure 1–11 ■), a notable pioneer nurse, established the Frontier Nursing Service (FNS). In 1918, she worked with the American Committee for Devastated France, distributing food, clothing, and supplies to rural villages and taking care of sick children. In 1921, Breckinridge returned to the United States with plans to provide health care to the people of rural America. In 1925, Breckinridge and two other nurses began the FNS in Leslie County, Kentucky. Within this organization, Breckinridge started one of the first midwifery training schools in the United States.

CONTEMPORARY NURSING PRACTICE

An understanding of contemporary nursing practice includes a look at definitions of nursing, recipients of nursing, scope of nursing, settings for nursing practice, nurse practice acts, and current standards of clinical nursing practice.

Definitions of Nursing

Florence Nightingale defined nursing over 100 years ago as "the act of utilizing the environment of the patient to assist him in his recovery" (Nightingale, 1860). Nightingale considered a clean, well-ventilated, and quiet environment essential for recovery. Often considered the first nurse theorist, Nightingale raised the status of nursing through education. Nurses were no longer untrained housekeepers but people educated in the care of the sick.

Virginia Henderson was one of the first modern nurses to define nursing. She wrote, "The unique function of the nurse is to assist the individual, sick or well, in the performance of those activities contributing to health or its recovery (or to peaceful death) that he would perform unaided if he had the necessary strength, will, or knowledge, and to do this in such a way as to help him gain independence as rapidly as possible" (Henderson, 1966, p. 3). Like Nightingale, Henderson described nursing in relation to the client and the client's environment. Unlike Nightingale, Henderson saw the nurse as concerned with both healthy and ill individuals, acknowledged that nurses interact with clients even when recovery may not be feasible, and mentioned the teaching and advocacy roles of the nurse.

In 1987, the Canadian Nurses Association (CNA) described nursing practice as a dynamic, caring, helping relationship in which the nurse assists the client to achieve and obtain optimal health (CNA, 1987). In the latter half of the 20th century, a number of nurse theorists developed their own theoretical definitions of nursing. Theoretical definitions are important because they go beyond simplistic common definitions. They describe what nursing is and the interrelationship among nurses, nursing, the client, the environment, and the intended client outcome: health (see Chapter 3). ∞

Certain themes are common to many of these definitions:

- Nursing is caring.
- Nursing is an art.

- Nursing is a science.
- Nursing is client centered.
- Nursing is holistic.
- Nursing is adaptive.
- Nursing is concerned with health promotion, health mainte-
  nance, and health restoration.
- Nursing is a helping profession.

Professional nursing associations have also examined nursing and developed their definitions of it. In 1973, the American
Nurses Association (ANA) described nursing practice as "direct, goal oriented, and adaptable to the needs of the individual,
the family, and community during health and illness" (ANA,
1973, p. 2). In 1980, the ANA changed this definition of nursing to this: "Nursing is the diagnosis and treatment of human
responses to actual or potential health problems" (ANA, 1980,
p. 9). In 1995, the ANA recognized the influence and contribution of the science of caring to nursing philosophy and practice.
Their most recent definition of nursing acknowledges four essential features of contemporary nursing practice:

- Attention to the full range of human experiences and responses to health and illness without restriction to a problem-
  focused orientation
- Integration of objective data with knowledge gained from an
  understanding of the client or group's subjective experience
- Application of scientific knowledge to the processes of diagnosis and treatment
- Provision of a caring relationship that facilitates health and
  healing (ANA, 1995)

Research to explore the meaning of caring in nursing has been
increasing. For example, Sherwood (1997) conducted a meta-
synthesis of qualitative studies describing caring from the perspective of clients. Likewise, Beck (2001) analyzed qualitative
studies that researched caring within schools of nursing. Details
about caring are discussed in Chapter 24. ∞ See also Watson's
"Assumptions of Caring" (Box 3–1) in Chapter 3. ∞

Recipients of Nursing

The recipients of nursing are sometimes called consumers,
sometimes patients, and sometimes clients. A **consumer** is an
individual, a group of people, or a community that uses a service or commodity. People who use health care products or services are consumers of health care.

A **patient** is a person who is waiting for or undergoing medical treatment and care. The word *patient* comes from a Latin
word meaning "to suffer" or "to bear." Traditionally, the person
receiving health care has been called a patient. Usually, people
become patients when they seek assistance because of illness
or for surgery. Some nurses believe that the word *patient* implies passive acceptance of the decisions and care of health professionals. Additionally, with the emphasis on health promotion and prevention of illness, many recipients of nursing care
are not ill. Moreover, nurses interact with family members and
significant others to provide support, information, and comfort
in addition to caring for the patient.

For these reasons, nurses increasingly refer to recipients of
health care as *clients*. A **client** is a person who engages the advice or services of another who is qualified to provide this service. The term *client* presents the receivers of health care as collaborators in the care, that is, as people who are also responsible
for their own health. Thus, the health status of a client is the responsibility of the individual in collaboration with health professionals. In this book, *client* is the preferred term, although
consumer and *patient* are used in some instances.

Scope of Nursing

Nurses provide care for three types of clients: individuals, families, and communities. Theoretical frameworks applicable to
these client types, as well as assessments of individual, family,
and community health are discussed in detail in Chapter 12. ∞
Nursing practice involves four areas: promoting health
and wellness, preventing illness, restoring health, and care of
the dying.

Promoting Health and Wellness

Wellness is a state of well-being. It means engaging in attitudes
and behavior that enhance the quality of life and maximize personal potential (Anspaugh, Hamrick, & Rosata, 2001). Nurses
promote wellness in clients who are both healthy and ill. This
may involve individual and community activities to enhance
healthy lifestyles, such as improving nutrition and physical fitness, preventing drug and alcohol misuse, restricting smoking,
and preventing accidents and injury in the home and workplace. See Chapter 8 ∞ for details.

Preventing Illness

The goal of illness prevention programs is to maintain optimal
health by preventing disease. Nursing activities that prevent illness include immunizations, prenatal and infant care, and prevention of sexually transmitted disease.

Restoring Health

Restoring health focuses on the ill client and it extends from
early detection of disease through helping the client during the
recovery period. Nursing activities include the following:

- Providing direct care to the ill person, such as administering
  medications, baths, and specific procedures and treatments
- Performing diagnostic and assessment procedures, such as
  measuring blood pressure and examining feces for occult
  blood
- Consulting with other health care professionals about client
  problems
- Teaching clients about recovery activities, such as exercises
  that will accelerate recovery after a stroke
- Rehabilitating clients to their optimal functional level following physical or mental illness, injury, or chemical addiction

Care of the Dying

This area of nursing practice involves comforting and caring for
people of all ages who are dying. It includes helping clients live

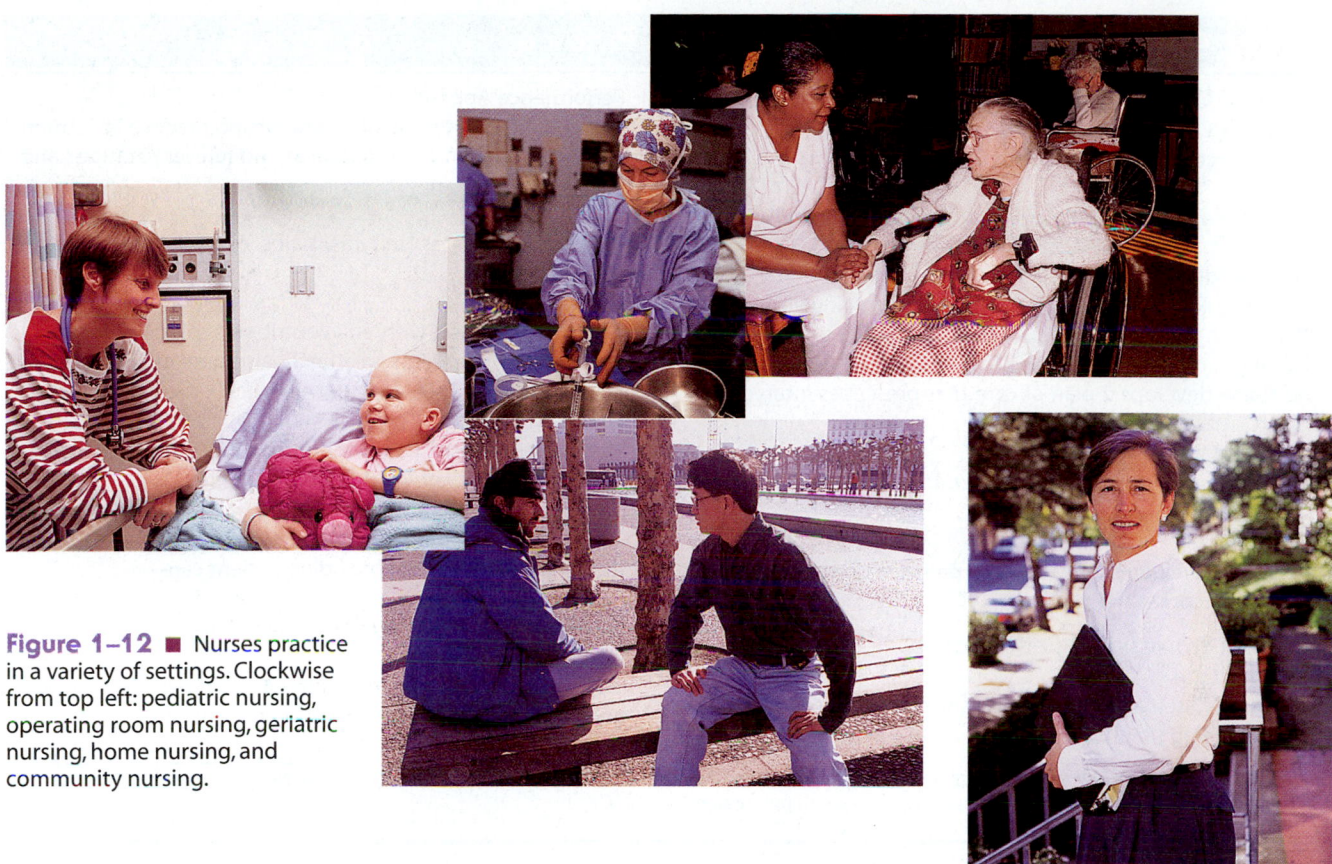

Figure 1–12 ■ Nurses practice in a variety of settings. Clockwise from top left: pediatric nursing, operating room nursing, geriatric nursing, home nursing, and community nursing.

as comfortably as possible until death and helping support persons cope with death. Nurses carrying out these activities work in homes, hospitals, and extended care facilities. Some agencies, called *hospices*, are specifically designed for this purpose.

Settings for Nursing

In the past, the acute care hospital was the main practice setting open to most nurses. Today many nurses work in hospitals, but increasingly they work in clients' homes, community agencies, ambulatory clinics, long-term care, health maintenance organizations (HMOs), and nursing practice centers (see Figure 1–12 ■).

Nurses have different degrees of nursing autonomy and nursing responsibility in the various settings. They may provide direct care, teach clients and support persons, serve as nursing advocates and agents of change, and help determine health policies affecting consumers in the community and in hospitals. For information about the models for delivery of nursing, see Chapter 6. ⊖⊘

Nurse Practice Acts

Nurse practice acts, or legal acts for professional nursing practice, regulate the practice of nursing in the United States and Canada. Each state in the United States and each province in Canada has its own act. Although nurse practice acts differ in various jurisdictions, they all have a common purpose: to protect the public. Nurses are responsible for knowing their state's nurse practice act as it governs their practice. For additional information, see Chapter 4. ⊖⊘

Standards of Clinical Nursing Practice

Establishing and implementing standards of practice are major functions of a professional organization. The purpose of **standards of clinical nursing practice** is to describe the responsibilities for which nurses are accountable (see Box 1–1). The standards (a) reflect the values and priorities of the nursing profession, (b) provide direction for professional nursing practice, (c) provide a framework for the evaluation of nursing practice, and (d) define the profession's accountability to the public and the client outcomes for which nurses are responsible (ANA, 1998). The American Nurses Association developed standards of clinical nursing practice that are generic in nature and provide for the practice of nursing regardless of area of specialization. Various specialty nursing organizations have further developed specific standards of nursing practice for their area. For nurses in Canada, each province or territory establishes its own standards of practice.

ROLES AND FUNCTIONS OF THE NURSE

Nurses assume a number of roles when they provide care to clients. Nurses often carry out these roles concurrently, not exclusively of one another. For example, the nurse may act as a counselor while providing physical care and teaching aspects of that care. The roles required at a specific time depend on the needs of the client and aspects of the particular environment.

BOX 1–1   ■ ANA Standards of Clinical Nursing Practice

Standards of Care

I. Assessment
The Nurse collects patient health data.
II. Diagnosis
The Nurse analyzes the assessment data in determining diagnoses.
III. Outcome Identification
The Nurse identifies expected outcomes individualized to the patient.
IV. Planning
The Nurse develops a plan of care that prescribes interventions to attain expected outcomes.
V. Implementation
The Nurse implements the interventions identified in the plan of care.
VI. Evaluation
The Nurse evaluates the patient's progress toward attainment of outcomes.

Standards of Professional Performance

I. Quality of Care
The Nurse systematically evaluates the quality and effectiveness of nursing practice.

II. Performance Appraisal
The Nurse evaluates his/her own nursing practice in relation to professional practice standards and relevant statutes and regulations.
III. Education
The Nurse acquires and maintains current knowledge in nursing practice.
IV. Collegiality
The Nurse interacts with, and contributes to the professional development of, peers and other health care providers as colleagues.
V. Ethics
The Nurse's decisions and actions on behalf of patients are determined in an ethical manner.
VI. Collaboration
The Nurse collaborates with the patient, family, and other health care providers in providing patient care.
VII. Research
The Nurse uses research findings in practice.
VIII. Resource Utilization
The Nurse considers factors related to safety, effectiveness, and cost in planning and delivering patient care.

Note: From *Standards of Clinical Nursing Practice,* 2nd ed., by American Nurses Association, 1998, Washington, DC: American Nurses Publishing, American Nurses Foundation/American Nurses Association. Reprinted with permission.

Caregiver

The **caregiver** role has traditionally included those activities that assist the client physically and psychologically while preserving the client's dignity. The required nursing actions may involve full care for the completely dependent client, partial care for the partially dependent client, and supportive-educative care to assist clients in attaining their highest possible level of health and wellness. Caregiving encompasses the physical, psychosocial, developmental, cultural, and spiritual levels. The nursing process provides nurses with a framework for providing care (see Chapters 15–19). 🔗 A nurse may provide care directly or delegate it to other caregivers.

Communicator

Communication is integral to all nursing roles. Nurses communicate with the client, support persons, other health professionals, and people in the community.

In the role of **communicator,** nurses identify client problems and then communicate these verbally or in writing to other members of the health team. The quality of a nurse's communication is an important factor in nursing care. The nurse must be able to communicate clearly and accurately in order for a client's health care needs to be met (see Chapters 20 and 24). 🔗

Teacher

As a **teacher,** the nurse helps clients learn about their health and the health care procedures they need to perform to restore or maintain their health. The nurse assesses the client's learning

needs and readiness to learn, sets specific learning goals in conjunction with the client, enacts teaching strategies, and measures learning. Nurses also teach unlicensed assistive personnel (UAP) to whom they delegate care, and they share their expertise with other nurses and health professionals. See Chapter 25 🔗 for additional details about the teaching/learning process.

Client Advocate

A **client advocate** acts to protect the client. In this role the nurse may represent the client's needs and wishes to other health professionals, such as relaying the client's wishes for information to the physician. They also assist clients in exercising their rights and help them speak up for themselves (see Chapter 5). 🔗

Counselor

Counseling is the process of helping a client to recognize and cope with stressful psychologic or social problems, to develop improved interpersonal relationships, and to promote personal growth. It involves providing emotional, intellectual, and psychologic support. The nurse counsels primarily healthy individuals with normal adjustment difficulties and focuses on helping the person develop new attitudes, feelings, and behaviors by encouraging the client to look at alternative behaviors, recognize the choices, and develop a sense of control.

Change Agent

The nurse acts as a **change agent** when assisting others, that is, clients, to make modifications in their own behavior. Nurses also often act to make changes in a system, such as clinical care, if it is not helping a client return to health. Nurses are continually dealing with change in the health care system. Technological change, change in the age of the client population, and changes in medications are just a few of the changes nurses deal with daily. See Chapter 26 for additional information about change.

Leader

A **leader** influences others to work together to accomplish a specific goal. The leader role can be employed at different levels: individual client, family, groups of clients, colleagues, or the community. Effective leadership is a learned process requiring an understanding of the needs and goals that motivate people, the knowledge to apply the leadership skills, and the interpersonal skills to influence others. The leadership role of the nurse is discussed in Chapter 26.

Manager

The nurse manages the nursing care of individuals, families, and communities. The nurse-**manager** also delegates nursing activities to ancillary workers and other nurses, and supervises and evaluates their performance. Managing requires knowledge about organizational structure and dynamics, authority and accountability, leadership, change theory, advocacy, delegation, and supervision and evaluation. See Chapter 26 for additional details.

Case Manager

Nurse case managers work with the multidisciplinary health care team to measure the effectiveness of the case management plan and to monitor outcomes. Each agency or unit specifies the role of the nurse **case manager.** In some institutions, the case manager works with primary or staff nurses to oversee the care of a specific caseload. In other agencies, the case manager is the primary nurse or provides some level of direct care to the client and family. Insurance companies have also developed a number of roles for nurse case managers, and responsibilities may vary from managing acute hospitalizations to managing high-cost clients or case types. Regardless of the setting, case managers help ensure that care is oriented to the client, while controlling costs.

Research Consumer

Nurses often use research to improve client care. In a clinical area, nurses need to (a) have some awareness of the process and language of research, (b) be sensitive to issues related to protecting the rights of human subjects, (c) participate in the identification of significant researchable problems, and (d) be a discriminating consumer of research findings.

Expanded Career Roles

Nurses are fulfilling expanded career roles, such as those of nurse practitioner, clinical nurse specialist, nurse midwife, nurse educator, nurse researcher, and nurse anesthetist, all of which allow greater independence and autonomy (see Box 1–2).

CRITERIA OF A PROFESSION

Nursing is gaining recognition as a profession. **Profession** has been defined as an occupation that requires extensive education or a calling that requires special knowledge, skill, and preparation. A profession is generally distinguished from other kinds of occupations by (a) its requirement of prolonged, specialized training to acquire a body of knowledge pertinent to the role to be performed; (b) an orientation of the individual toward service, either to a community or to an organization; (c) ongoing research; (d) code of ethics; (e) autonomy; and (f) professional organization.

Two terms related to profession need to be differentiated: professionalism and professionalization. **Professionalism** refers to professional character, spirit, or methods. It is a set of attributes, a way of life that implies responsibility and commitment. Nursing professionalism owes much to the influence of Florence Nightingale. **Professionalization** is the process of becoming professional, that is, of acquiring characteristics considered to be professional.

Specialized Education

Specialized education is an important aspect of professional status. In modern times, the trend in education for the professions has shifted toward programs in colleges and universities. Many nursing educators believe that the undergraduate nursing curriculum should include liberal arts education in addition to the biologic and social sciences and the nursing discipline.

In the United States today, there are five means of entry into registered nursing: hospital diploma, associate degree, baccalaureate degree, master's degree, and doctoral degree. These programs are discussed in Chapter 2. The ANA recommends the baccalaureate degree as the entry level for professional practice. Conversely, the National Organization for Associate Degree Nursing (N-OADN) supports ADN preparation as the entry level into registered nursing (NOADN, 2002).

Body of Knowledge

As a profession, nursing is establishing a well-defined body of knowledge and expertise. A number of nursing conceptual frameworks (discussed in Chapter 3) contribute to the knowledge base of nursing and give direction to nursing practice, education, and ongoing research.

Service Orientation

A service orientation differentiates nursing from an occupation pursued primarily for profit. Many consider altruism (selfless concern for others) the hallmark of a profession. Nursing has a tradition of service to others. This service, however, must be guided by certain rules, policies, or codes of ethics. Today, nursing is also an important component of the health care delivery system.

Ongoing Research

Increasing research in nursing is contributing to nursing practice. In the 1940s nursing research was at a very early stage of development. In the 1950s increased federal funding and professional

BOX 1–2 ■ Selected Expanded Career Roles for Nurses

Nurse Practitioner

A nurse who has an advanced education and is a graduate of a nurse practitioner program. These nurses are certified by the American Nurses Credentialing Center in areas such as adult nurse practitioner, family nurse practitioner, school nurse practitioner, pediatric nurse practitioner, or gerontology nurse practitioner. They are employed in health care agencies or community-based settings. They usually deal with nonemergency acute or chronic illness and provide primary ambulatory care.

Clinical Nurse Specialist

A nurse who has an advanced degree or expertise and is considered to be an expert in a specialized area of practice (e.g., gerontology, oncology). The nurse provides direct client care, educates others, consults, conducts research, and manages care. The American Nurses Credentialing Center provides national certification of clinical specialists.

Nurse Anesthetist

A nurse who has completed advanced education in an accredited program in anesthesiology. The nurse anesthetist carries out preoperative visits and assessments, and administers general anesthetics for surgery under the supervision of a physician prepared in anesthesiology. The nurse anesthetist also assesses the postoperative status of clients.

Nurse Midwife

An RN who has completed a program in midwifery and is certified by the American College of Nurse Midwives. The nurse gives prenatal and postnatal care and manages deliveries in normal pregnancies. The midwife practices in association with a health care agency and can obtain medical services if complications occur.

The nurse midwife may also conduct routine Papanicolaou smears, family planning, and routine breast examinations.

Nurse Researcher

Nurse researchers investigate nursing problems to improve nursing care and to refine and expand nursing knowledge. They are employed in academic institutions, teaching hospitals, and research centers such as the National Institute for Nursing Research in Bethesda, Maryland. Nurse-researchers usually have advanced education at the doctoral level.

Nurse Administrator

The nurse administrator manages client care, including the delivery of nursing services. The administrator may have a middle management position, such as head nurse or supervisor, or a more senior management position, such as director of nursing services. The functions of nurse-administrators include budgeting, staffing, and planning programs. The educational preparation for nurse-administrator positions is at least a baccalaureate degree in nursing and frequently a master's or doctoral degree.

Nurse Educator

Nurse educators are employed in nursing programs, at educational institutions, and in hospital staff education. The nurse educator usually has a baccalaureate degree or more advanced preparation and frequently has expertise in a particular area of practice. The nurse educator is responsible for classroom and often clinical teaching.

Nurse Entrepreneur

A nurse who usually has an advanced degree and manages a health-related business. The nurse may be involved in education, consultation, or research, for example.

---

support helped establish centers for nursing research. Most early research was directed to the study of nursing education. In the 1960s, studies were often related to the nature of the knowledge base underlying nursing practice. Since the 1970s, nursing research has focused on practice-related issues. Nursing research as a dimension of the nurse's role is discussed further in Chapter 2. 🔗

Code of Ethics

Nurses have traditionally placed a high value on the worth and dignity of others. The nursing profession requires integrity of its members; that is, a member is expected to do what is considered right regardless of the personal cost.

Ethical codes change as the needs and values of society change. Nursing has developed its own codes of ethics and in most instances has set up means to monitor the professional behavior of its members. See Chapter 5 🔗 for additional information on ethics.

Autonomy

A profession is autonomous if it regulates itself and sets standards for its members. Providing autonomy is one of the purposes of a professional association. If nursing is to have professional status,

it must function autonomously in the formation of policy and in the control of its activity. To be autonomous, a professional group must be granted legal authority to define the scope of its practice, describe its particular functions and roles, and determine its goals and responsibilities in delivery of its services.

To practitioners of nursing, autonomy means independence at work, responsibility, and accountability for one's actions. Autonomy is more easily achieved and maintained from a position of authority. Therefore, some nurses seek administrative positions rather than expanded clinical competence as a means to ensure their autonomy in the workplace.

Professional Organization

Operation under the umbrella of a professional organization differentiates a profession from an occupation. **Governance** is the establishment and maintenance of social, political, and economic arrangements by which practitioners control their practice, their self-discipline, their working conditions, and their professional affairs. Nurses, therefore, need to work within their professional organizations.

The American Nurses Association is a professional organization that "advances the nursing profession by fostering high standards of nursing practice, promoting the economic and general welfare of nurses in the workplace, projecting a positive and realistic view of nursing, and by lobbying the Congress and regulatory agencies on health care issues affecting nurses and the public" (ANA, 2002).

SOCIALIZATION TO NURSING

The standards of education and practice for the profession are determined by the members of the profession, rather than by outsiders. The education of the professional involves a complete socialization process, more far reaching in its social and attitudinal aspects and its technical features than is usually required in other kinds of occupations.

Socialization can be defined simply as the process by which people (a) learn to become members of groups and society and (b) learn the social rules defining relationships into which they will enter. Socialization involves learning to behave, feel, and see the world in a manner similar to other persons occupying the same role as oneself (Hardy & Conway, 1988, p. 261). The goal of professional socialization is to instill in individuals the norms, values, attitudes, and behaviors deemed essential for the survival of the profession.

Various models of the socialization process have been developed. Benner's model (2001) describes five levels of proficiency in nursing based on the Dreyfus general model of skill acquisition. The five stages, which have implications for teaching and learning, are novice, advanced beginner, competent, proficient, and expert. Benner writes that experience is essential for the development of professional expertise (see Box 1–3).

One of the most powerful mechanisms of professional socialization is interaction with fellow students. Within this student culture, students collectively set the level and direction of their scholastic efforts. They develop perspectives about the situation in which they are involved, the goals they are trying to achieve, and the kinds of activities that are expedient and proper, and they establish a set of practices congruent with all of these. Students become bound together by feelings of mutual cooperation, support, and solidarity.

Critical Values of Nursing

It is within the nursing educational program that the nurse develops, clarifies, and internalizes professional values. Specific professional nursing values are stated in nursing codes of ethics (see Chapter 5) 🔗, in standards of nursing practice (discussed earlier in this chapter), and in the legal system itself (see Chapter 4). 🔗 Additionally, in 2001, the National Student Nurses' Association (NSNA) adopted a code of academic and clinical conduct (see Box 1–4).

FACTORS INFLUENCING CONTEMPORARY NURSING PRACTICE

To understand nursing as it is practiced today and as it will be practiced tomorrow requires an understanding of some of the social forces currently influencing this profession. These forces usually affect the entire health care system, and nursing, as a major component of that system, cannot avoid the effects.

Economics

Greater financial support provided through public and private health insurance programs has increased the demand for nursing care. As a result, people who could not afford health care in the past are increasingly using such health services as emergency room care, mental health counseling, and preventive physical examinations.

Costs of health care have also increased during the past two decades. In 1982, the Medicare payment system to hospitals and physicians was revised to establish reimbursement fees according to the client's medical diagnosis. This classification system is known as **diagnostic-related groups (DRGs)**. The system has categories that establish pretreatment diagnosis billing categories. With the implementation of this legislation, clients in hospitals are more acutely ill than before and clients once considered sufficiently ill to be hospitalized are now treated at home; however, health care costs continue to rise.

BOX 1–3	■ Benner's Stages of Nursing Expertise

Stage I, Novice
No experience (e.g., nursing student). Performance is limited, inflexible, and governed by context-free rules and regulations rather than experience.

Stage II, Advanced Beginner
Demonstrates marginally acceptable performance. Recognizes the meaningful "aspects" of a real situation. Has experienced enough real situations to make judgments about them.

Stage III, Competent
Has 2 or 3 years of experience. Demonstrates organizational and planning abilities. Differentiates important factors from less important aspects of care. Coordinates multiple complex care demands.

Stage IV, Proficient
Has 3 to 5 years of experience. Perceives situations as wholes rather than in terms of parts, as in Stage II. Uses maxims as guides for what to consider in a situation. Has holistic understanding of the client, which improves decision making. Focuses on long-term goals.

Stage V, Expert
Performance is fluid, flexible, and highly proficient; no longer requires rules, guidelines, or maxims to connect an understanding of the situation to appropriate action. Demonstrates highly skilled intuitive and analytic ability in new situations. Is inclined to take a certain action because "it felt right."

Note: From *Novice to Expert: Excellence and Power in Clinical Nursing Practice,* Commemorative Edition (pp. 20–34), by P. Benner, 2001, Upper Saddle River, NJ: Prentice Hall Health. Adapted with permission.

Research Note
Why Women and Men Choose Nursing

Using grounded theory methodology, a study by Boughn (2001) revisited data from two previous studies to compare and contrast why women and men selected nursing. The analysis of the data focused on three main constructs: caring, power, and practical motivations.

The subjects included 12 males and 16 females who were enrolled in the same baccalaureate nursing program. Each of the four class levels was represented. Except for two men and two women, all subjects were under 23 years of age and single.

Both female and male subjects expressed that the desire to care for others motivated their decision to become a nurse. Likewise, both sexes indicated a strong interest in power and empowerment for themselves by expressing such statements as desiring to be the best or advancing to a management position. A difference did exist between the two groups, however, in the desire to empower others. The female subjects were more interested in empowering others while the male subjects were more interested in empowering the profession and themselves as professionals. Another difference between

the two groups concerned the third construct: practical motivation or expectations regarding salary and working conditions. The men clearly chose nursing based on financial expectations while only one of the female subjects mentioned finances as a motivating factor in choosing nursing as a profession.

Implications: Both male and female nursing students were motivated by the desire to care for others. The differences in the focus of power and empowerment could complement each other. The author discusses that caring theory points out that caring for self is needed in order to care for others. Male and female nurses need to incorporate both values into their thinking. Salary and working conditions have been and continue to be chronic complaints among nurses. The author suggests that female nursing students be socialized to become assertive and proactive and to subsequently expect financial rewards and favorable working conditions.

Note: From "Why Women and Men Choose Nursing," by S. Boughn, 2001, *Nursing and Health Care Perspectives, 22* (1), pp. 14–19. Reprinted with permission from the National League for Nursing.

BOX 1–4   ■ National Student Nurses' Association, Inc., Code of Academic and Clinical Conduct

Preamble
Students of nursing have a responsibility to society in learning the academic theory and clinical skills needed to provide nursing care. The clinical setting presents unique challenges and responsibilities while caring for human beings in a variety of health care environments.

The Code of Academic and Clinical Conduct is based on an understanding that to practice nursing as a student is an agreement to uphold the trust with which society has placed in us. The statements of the Code provide guidance for the nursing student in the personal development of an ethical foundation and need not be limited strictly to the academic or clinical environment but can assist in the holistic development of the person.

A Code for Nursing Students
As students are involved in the clinical and academic environments we believe that ethical principles are a necessary guide to professional development. Therefore within these environments we:

1. Advocate for the rights of all clients.
2. Maintain client confidentiality.
3. Take appropriate action to ensure the safety of clients, self, and others.
4. Provide care for the client in a timely, compassionate and professional manner.
5. Communicate client care in a truthful, timely and accurate manner.
6. Actively promote the highest level of moral and ethical principles and accept responsibility for our actions.
7. Promote excellence in nursing by encouraging lifelong learning and professional development.
8. Treat others with respect and promote an environment that respects human rights, values and choice of cultural and spiritual beliefs.
9. Collaborate in every reasonable manner with the academic faculty and clinical staff to ensure the highest quality of client care.
10. Use every opportunity to improve faculty and clinical staff understanding of the learning needs of nursing students.
11. Encourage faculty, clinical staff, and peers to mentor nursing students.
12. Refrain from performing any technique or procedure for which the student has not been adequately trained.
13. Refrain from any deliberate action or omission of care in the academic or clinical setting that creates unnecessary risk of injury to the client, self, or others.
14. Assist the staff nurse or preceptor in ensuring that there is full disclosure and that proper authorizations are obtained from clients regarding any form of treatment or research.
15. Abstain from the use of alcoholic beverages or any substances in the academic and clinical setting that impair judgment.
16. Strive to achieve and maintain an optimal level of personal health.
17. Support access to treatment and rehabilitation for students who are experiencing impairments related to substance abuse and mental or physical health issues.
18. Uphold school policies and regulations related to academic and clinical performance, reserving the right to challenge and critique rules and regulations as per school grievance policy.

Note: Adopted by the NSNA House of Delegates, Nashville, TN, on April 6, 2001. Reprinted with permission.

These changes present challenges to nurses. Currently, the health care industry is shifting its emphasis from inpatient to outpatient care with preadmission testing, increased outpatient same-day surgery, post-hospitalization rehabilitation, home health care, health maintenance, physical fitness programs, and community health education programs. As a result, more nurses are being employed in community-based health settings, such as home health agencies, hospices, and community clinics. These changes in employment for nurses have implications for nursing education, nursing research, and nursing practice.

Consumer Demands

Consumers of nursing services (the public) have become an increasingly effective force in changing nursing practice. On the whole, people are better educated and have more knowledge about health and illness than in the past. Consumers also have become more aware of others' needs for care. The ethical and moral issues raised by poverty and neglect have made people more vocal about the needs of minority groups and the poor.

The public's concepts of health and nursing have also changed. Most now believe that health is a right of all people, not just a privilege of the rich. The media emphasize the message that individuals must assume responsibility for their own health by obtaining a physical examination regularly, checking for the seven danger signals of cancer, and maintaining their mental well-being by balancing work and recreation. Interest in health and nursing services is therefore greater than ever. Furthermore, many people now want more than freedom from disease—they want energy, vitality, and a feeling of wellness.

Increasingly, the consumer has become an active participant in making decisions about health and nursing care. Planning committees concerned with providing nursing services to a community usually have active consumer membership. Recognizing the legitimacy of public input, many state nursing associations and regulatory agencies have consumer representatives on their governing boards.

Family Structure

New family structures are influencing the need for and provision of nursing services. More people are living away from the extended family and the nuclear family, and the family breadwinner is no longer necessarily the husband. Today, many single men and women rear children, and in many two-parent families both parents work. It is also common for young parents to live at great distances from their own parents. These young families need support services, such as day-care centers. For additional information about the family, see Chapter 12. ∞

Adolescent mothers also need specialized nursing services, both while they are pregnant and after their babies are born. These young mothers usually have the normal needs of teenagers as well as those of new mothers. Many teenage mothers are raising their children alone with little, if any, assistance from the child's father. This type of single-parent family is especially vulnerable because motherhood compounds the difficulties of adolescence. And because many of these families live in poverty, the children often do not receive preventive immunizations and are at increased risk for nutritional and other health problems.

Science and Technology

Advances in science and technology affect nursing practice. For example, people with acquired immune deficiency syndrome (AIDS) are receiving new drug therapies to prolong life and delay the onset of AIDS-associated diseases. Nurses must be knowledgeable about the action of such drugs and the needs of clients receiving them. Biotechnology is affecting health care. For example, DNA-based vaccines are replacing conventional ones (Kim, 2000). Nurses will need to expand their knowledge base and technical skills as they adapt to meet the new needs of clients.

In some settings, technologic advances have required that nurses be highly specialized. Nurses frequently have to use sophisticated computerized equipment to monitor or treat clients. As technologies change, nursing education changes, and nurses require increasing education to provide effective, safe nursing practice.

The space program has developed advanced technologies for space travel based on the need for long-distance monitoring of astronauts and spacecraft, lighter materials, and miniaturization of equipment. Health care has benefited as this new technology has been adapted in such health care aids as Viewstar (an aid for the visually impaired), the insulin infusion pump, the voice-controlled wheelchair, magnetic resonance imaging, laser surgery, filtering devices for intravenous fluid control devices, and monitoring systems for intensive care.

Information and Telecommunications

The Information Superhighway or Internet has already impacted health care, with more and more clients becoming well informed about their health concerns. No longer the sole provider of health information, physicians and nurses may need to interpret Internet sources of information to clients and their families. Because not all of the Internet-based information is accurate, nurses need to become information brokers so they can help people to access high-quality, valid websites; interpret the information; and then help clients evaluate the information and determine if it is useful to them. Clark (2000) predicts that the difference between the future novice and expert nurse will be in knowing where to look for information and how to use it.

Telecommunications is the transmission of information from one site to another, using equipment to transmit information in the form of signs, signals, words, or pictures by cable, radio, or other systems (Chaffee, 1999, p. 27). Telehealth uses telecommunication technology to provide long-distance health care. It can include using videoconferencing, computers, or telephones. Telenursing occurs when the nurse delivers care through a telecommunication system. Examples of telenursing include the nurse who telephones clients at home to assess their progress or to answer questions and the nurse who participates in a video teleconference where consultants or experts at various sites discuss a client's health care plan.

Telehealth recognizes no state boundaries and, subsequently, licensure issues have been raised. For example, if a nurse licensed in one state provides health information to a client in another state, does the nurse need to maintain licensure in both states? The National Council of State Boards of Nursing endorses a change from single-state licensure to a mutual recognition model. Many state legislatures have adopted mutual recognition language into statute and are currently implementing it (see Chapter 4). ✇

Legislation

Legislation about nursing practice and health matters affects both the public and nursing. Legislation related to nursing is discussed in Chapter 4. ✇ Changes in legislation relating to health also affect nursing. For example, the **Patient Self-Determination Act (PSDA)** requires that every competent adult be informed in writing on admission to a health care institution about his or her rights to accept or refuse medical care and to use advance directives. See Chapter 41 ✇ for more information about the PSDA and advance directives. This law, which in many institutions is implemented by nurses, affects the nurse's role in supporting clients and their families.

Demography

Demography is the study of population, including statistics about distribution by age and place of residence, mortality (death), and morbidity (incidence of disease). From demographic data, needs of the population for nursing services can be assessed. For example:

- The total population in North America is increasing. The proportion of elderly people has also increased, creating an increased need for nursing services for this group.
- The population is shifting from rural to urban settings. This shift signals an increased need for nursing related to prob-

lems caused by pollution and by the effects on the environment of concentrations of people. Thus, most nursing services are now provided in urban settings.
- Mortality and morbidity studies reveal the presence of risk factors. Many of these risk factors (e.g., smoking) are major causes of death and disease that can be prevented through changes in lifestyle. The nurse's role in assessing risk factors and helping clients make healthy lifestyle changes is discussed in Chapter 8. ✇

The New Nursing Shortage

Multiple factors influence the new nursing shortage (see Box 1–5) and these factors contribute to the current nursing shortage being different from previous shortages. Registered nurses make up the largest group of health care providers. Fewer nurses, however, are entering the workforce and certain geographic areas are experiencing acute nursing shortages. The supply is inadequate to meet the demand, especially for specialized nurses (e.g., critical care) and it is anticipated to worsen during the next 20 years (Tri-Council for Nursing Policy Statement, 2001).

Addressing the nursing shortage requires collaborative activities among health care systems, policy makers, nursing education, and professional organizations. Recommendations include, but are not limited to these:

- Develop mechanisms for nursing student's to progress to and through educational programs more efficiently and quickly.
- Recruit young people to nursing early (e.g., grade school).
- Improve the nurse's work environment: Provide greater flexibility in work hours, reward experienced nurses who serve as mentors, ensure adequate staffing, and increase salaries.
- Increase nursing education funding.

BOX 1–5	■ Factors Affecting the Nursing Shortage

- Aging Nurse Workforce
  - Number of nurses under 30 decreasing
  - Number of nurses age 40–49 increasing with 40% older than 50 by 2010
  - New graduates entering workforce at an older age and will have fewer years to work

- Aging of Nursing Faculty
  - As nursing faculty retire, nursing programs may have fewer faculty to educate future nurses

- Reduced Entry of Younger People into Nursing
  - Reduction in nursing program enrollments

- Aging Population
  - Individuals 65 and older to double between 2000 and 2030

- Increasing health care needs of aging population

- Increased Demand for Nurses
  - Increased acuity of hospital clients requiring skilled and specialized nurses
  - Shorter hospital stays resulting in transfer of clients to long-term care and community settings, creating increased demand for nurses in the community

- Workplace Issues
  - Inadequate staffing
  - Heavy workloads
  - Increased use of overtime
  - Lack of sufficient support staff
  - Inadequate wages
  - Difficulty recruiting and retaining nurses

Note: From *"Tri-Council for Nursing Policy Statement: Strategies to Reverse the New Nursing Shortage."* Retrieved March 5, 2003, from http://www.nln.org/aboutnln/news_tricouncil2.htm; *"Nursing Workforce: Emerging Nurse Shortages Due to Multiple Factors"* (Publication No. GAO-01-944). U.S. General Accounting Office, 2001. Retrieved March 5, 2003, from http://www.aacn.nche.edu/Government/GAO%20Report.pdf(2001); *"Nurses for a Healthier Tomorrow. Facts about the Nursing Shortage,"* by Honor Society of Nursing, Sigma Theta Tau International. Retrieved March 5, 2003, from http://www.nursesource.org/facts_shortage.html.

Collective Bargaining

More nurses are using collective bargaining to deal with their concerns. The ANA participates in collective bargaining on behalf of nurses through its economic and general welfare programs. Today, some nurses are joining other labor organizations that represent them at the bargaining table. Nurses have gone on strike over economic concerns and over issues about safe care for clients and safety for themselves.

Nursing Associations

Professional nursing associations have provided leadership that affects many areas of nursing. Voluntary accreditation of nursing education programs by the National League for Nursing Accrediting Commission (NLNAC) and Commission on Collegiate Nursing Education (CCNE) has also influenced nursing. Many nursing programs have steadily improved to meet the standards for accreditation over the years. As a result, nurse graduates are better prepared to meet the demands of society.

To influence policy making for health care, a group of professional nurses organized formally to promote political action in the nursing and health care arenas. Nurses for Political Action (NPA) formed in 1971 and became an arm of the ANA in 1974, when its name changed to Nurses Coalition for Action in Politics (N-CAP). In 1986, the name was changed to American Nurses Association—Political Action Committee (ANA-PAC). Through this group, nurses have lobbied actively for legislation affecting health care. A number of nursing leaders hold positions of authority in government. Attaining such positions is essential if nurses hope to exert ongoing political influence.

NURSING ORGANIZATIONS

As nursing has developed, an increasing number of nursing organizations have formed. These organizations are at the local, state, national, and international levels. The organizations that involve most North American nurses are the American Nurses Association, the Canadian Nurses Association, the National League for Nursing, the International Council of Nurses, and the National Student Nurses' Association. The number of nursing specialty organizations is also increasing, for example, the Academy of Medical Surgical Nursing, the American Association of Nurse Anesthetists, and the National Black Nurses Association. Participation in the activities of nursing associations enhances the growth of involved individuals and helps nurses collectively influence policies affecting nursing practice.

American Nurses Association

The American Nurses Association (ANA) is the national professional organization for nursing in the United States. It was founded in 1896 as the Nurses Associated Alumnae of the United States and Canada. In 1911 the name was changed to the American Nurses Association. It was a charter member of the International Council of Nurses, along with organizations in Great Britain and Germany, in 1899. The purposes of the ANA are to foster high standards of nursing practice and to promote the educational and professional advancement of nurses so that all people may have better nursing care.

In 1982, the organization became a federation of state nurses' associations. Individuals participate in the ANA by joining their state nurses' associations. The official journal of the ANA is the *American Journal of Nursing,* and *American Nurse* is the official newspaper.

Canadian Nurses Association

The Canadian Nurses Association (CNA) is the national nursing association in Canada. Nurses do not join the CNA independently but obtain membership by paying a fee to the provincial chapters. The CNA has developed standards and a code of ethics, and it offers support to all provincial associations. The CNA prepares licensure examinations and offers research grants, fellowships, and scholarships to Canadian nurses. The official journal of the CNA, *The Canadian Nurse,* is published monthly.

National League for Nursing

The National League for Nursing (NLN), formed in 1952, is an organization of both individuals and agencies. Its objective is to foster the development and improvement of all nursing services and nursing education. People who are not nurses but have an interest in nursing services, for example, hospital administrators, can be members of the league. This feature of the NLN—involving non-nurse members, consumers, and nurses from all levels of practice—is unique.

The NLN presents continuing education workshops and seminars for its members. For schools of nursing, the NLN offers testing services including preadmission testing for potential students, and achievement testing throughout the program. The NLN also conducts yearly surveys of nursing schools, newly registered nurses, and post-basic graduates. These surveys serve as a primary source of research data about nursing education in the United States. The National League for Nursing Accrediting Commission, an independent body within the NLN, provides voluntary accreditation for educational programs in nursing. The official journal of the NLN is *Nursing and Health Care Perspectives.*

International Council of Nurses

The International Council of Nurses (ICN) was established in 1899. Nurses from Great Britain, the United States, and Canada were among the founding members. The council is a federation of national nurses' associations, such as the ANA and CNA.

The ICN provides an organization through which member national associations can work together for the mission of representing nursing worldwide, advancing the profession and influencing health policy. The five core values of ICN are visionary leadership, inclusiveness, flexibility, partnership, and achievement (ICN, n.d.). The official journal of the ICN is *International Nursing Review.*

National Student Nurses' Association

The National Student Nurses' Association (NSNA) is the official preprofessional organization for nursing students. Formed in 1953 and incorporated in 1959, the NSNA originally functioned under the aegis of the ANA and NLN; however, in 1968 the NSNA became an autonomous body, although it communicates with the NLN and the ANA. To qualify for membership in the NSNA, a student must be enrolled in a state-approved nursing education program. The official organ of the NSNA is *Imprint* magazine.

In Canada, nursing students have a similar organization, the Canadian University Student Nurses Association. The provincial student nurses' associations also have programs related to the needs of nursing students and to concerns within the health field in general.

International Honor Society: Sigma Theta Tau

Sigma Theta Tau, the international honor society in nursing, was founded in 1922 and is headquartered in Indianapolis,

Indiana. The Greek letters stand for the Greek words *storga, tharos,* and *tima,* meaning "love," "courage," and "honor." The society is a member of the Association of College Honor Societies. The society's purpose is professional rather than social. Membership is attained through academic achievement. Students in baccalaureate programs in nursing and nurses in master's, doctoral, and postdoctoral programs are eligible to be selected for membership. Potential members, who hold a minimum of a bachelor's degree, and have demonstrated achievement in nursing can apply for membership as a nurse leader in the community.

The official journal of Sigma Theta Tau, *Journal of Nursing Scholarship,* is published quarterly. The journal publishes scholarly articles of interest to nurses. The society also publishes *Reflections,* a quarterly newsletter that provides information about the organization and its various chapters.

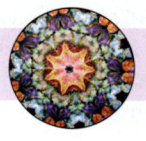 | Chapter Review

EXPLORE MediaLink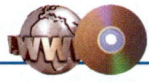

NCLEX review questions, case studies, MediaLink applications, and other interactive resources for this chapter can be found on the Companion Website at www.prenhall.com/kozier. Click on Chapter 1 to select the activities for this chapter.

For more NCLEX review questions, and an audio glossary, access the Student CD-ROM accompanying this textbook.

Chapter Highlights

- Historical perspectives of nursing practice reveal recurring themes or influencing factors. For example, women have traditionally cared for others, but often in subservient roles. Religious orders left an imprint on nursing by instilling such values as compassion, devotion to duty, and hard work. Wars created an increased need for nurses and medical specialties. Societal attitudes have influenced nursing's image. Visionary leaders have made notable contributions to improve the status of nursing.
- The scope of nursing practice includes promoting wellness, preventing illness, restoring health, and care of the dying.
- Although traditionally the majority of nurses were employed in hospital settings, today the numbers of nurses working in home health care, ambulatory care, and community health settings are increasing.

- Nurse practice acts vary among states and nurses are responsible for knowing the act that governs their practice.
- Standards of clinical nursing practice provide criteria against which the effectiveness of nursing care and professional performance behaviors can be evaluated.
- Every nurse may function in a variety of roles that are not exclusive of one another; in reality, they often occur together and serve to clarify the nurse's activities. These roles include caregiver, communicator, teacher, client advocate, counselor, change agent, leader, manager, case manager, and research consumer.
- With advanced education and experience, nurses can fulfill advanced practice roles such as clinical nurse specialist, nurse practitioner, nurse midwife, nurse anesthetist, educator, administrator, and researcher.

- A desired goal of nursing is professionalism, which necessitates specialized education; a unique body of knowledge, including specific skills and abilities; ongoing research; a code of ethics; autonomy; a service orientation; and a professional organization.
- Socialization is a lifelong process by which people become functioning participants of a society or a group. It is a reciprocal learning process that is brought about by interaction with other people and established boundaries of behavior. Socialization to professional nursing practice is the process whereby the values and norms of the nursing profession are internalized into the nurse's own behavior and self-concept. The nurse acquires the knowledge, skill, and attitudes characteristic of the profession.
- Although several models of the socialization process have been developed, Benner's five stages of novice, advanced beginner, competent, proficient, and expert may serve as guidelines to establish the phase and extent of an individual's socialization.
- Contemporary nursing practice is influenced by economics, changing demands for nurses, consumer demand, family structure, science and technology, information and telecommunications, legislation, demographic and social changes, the new nursing shortage, collective bargaining, and the work of nursing associations.
- Participation in the activities of nursing associations enhances the growth of involved individuals and helps nurses collectively influence policies that affect nursing practice.

Review Questions

1–1. Which recipient of nursing is perceived as a person who accepts responsibility for their health?
 a. individual
 b. patient
 c. consumer
 d. client

1–2. Which activity is an example of health promotion by the nurse?
 a. administering immunizations
 b. giving a bath
 c. preventing accidents in the home
 d. performing diagnostic procedures

1–3. Which of the following nurses usually provides primary ambulatory care?
 a. clinical nurse specialist
 b. nurse practitioner
 c. nurse midwife
 d. nurse entrepreneur

1–4. According to Benner's states of nursing expertise, a nurse with 2 to 3 years of experience who can coordinate multiple complex nursing care demands is at which stage?
 a. advanced beginner
 b. competent
 c. proficient
 d. expert

1–5. Which professional organization developed a code for nursing students?
 a. ANA
 b. NLN
 c. AACN
 d. NSNA

1–6. Which of the following social forces will impact the future supply and demand for nurses?
 a. aging
 b. economics
 c. science/technology
 d. telecommunications

Readings and References

Suggested Readings

McDonald, L. (2001). Florence Nightingale and the early origins of evidence-based nursing [Electronic version]. *Evidence-Based Nursing, 4*, 68–69.
 The author outlines how Florence Nightingale's work reflected an evidence-based framework. Examples include her knowledge-based leadership style, passion for statistics, development of survey instruments, pioneering presentations of data by using color-coded graphics, and landmark study of maternal mortality from puerperal fever.

Related Research

Judkins, S. K., Barr, W. J., Clark, D., & Okimi, P. (2000). Consumer perception of the professional nursing role: Development and testing of a scale. *Nurse Researcher, 7*(3), 32–39.

References

American Nurses Association. (1973). *Standards of nursing practice.* Kansas City, MO: Author.
American Nurses Association. (1980). *Nursing: A social policy statement.* Kansas City, MO: Author.
American Nurses Association. (1995). *Nursing vs social policy statement.* Washington, DC: American Nurses Publishing.
American Nurses Association. (1998). *Standards of clinical nursing practice* (2nd ed.). Washington, DC: Author.
American Nurses Association. (2002). About us. Retrieved March 5, 2003, from http://nursingworld.org/about/index.htm
Anspaugh, D. J., Hamrick, M. H., & Rosata, F. D. (2001). *Wellness: Fundamental concepts and applications.* New York: McGraw-Hill.

Beck, C. T. (2001). Caring within nursing education: A metasynthesis. *Journal of Nursing Education, 40*(3), 101–109.
Benner, P. (2001). *From novice to expert: Excellence and power in clinical nursing practice* (commemorative ed.). Upper Saddle River, NJ: Prentice Hall Health.
Boughn, S. (2001). Why women and men choose nursing. *Nursing and Health Care Perspectives, 22*(1), 14–19.
Chaffee, M. (1999). A telehealth odyssey. *American Journal of Nursing, 99*(7), 27–32.
Clark, D. J. (2000). Old wine in new bottles: Delivering nursing in the 21st century. *Journal of Nursing Scholarship, 32*(1), 11–15.
Donahue, M. P. (1996). *Nursing: The finest art. An illustrated history* (2nd ed.). St. Louis, MO: Mosby.

Hardy, M. E., & Conway, M. E. (1988). *Role theory: Perspectives for healthy professionals* (2nd ed.). Norwalk, CT: Appleton & Lange.

Henderson, V. (1966). *The nature of nursing: A definition and its implications for practice, research, and education.* New York: Macmillan.

Honor Society of Nursing, Sigma Theta Tau International. (2001). *Nurses for a Healthier Tomorrow. Facts about the Nursing Shortage.* Retrieved March 5, 2003 from http://www. nursesource.org/facts_shortage.html.

Humphreys, K. (2002). Guide to 2002 nursing organizations. *Nursing, 32*(5), 46–48.

International Council of Nurses. (n.d.). About the International Council of Nurses. Retrieved March 5, 2003, from http://www.icn.ch/abouticn.htm

Kim, M. (2000). Meeting the challenges of the 21st century. *Journal of Nursing Scholarship, 32*(1), 7–9.

National Organization for Associate Degree Nursing. (2002). Position statement in support of associate degree as preparation for the entry-level registered nurse. Retrieved March 5, 2003, from http://www.noadn.org/positionstatement. htm

National Student Nurses' Association House of Delegates. (2001). *The Code of Academic and Clinical Conduct.* Nashville, TN: Author.

Nightingale, F. (1969). *Notes on nursing: What it is, and what it is not.* New York: Dover. (original work published 1860).

Schuyler, C. B. (1992). Florence Nightingale. In F. Nightingale, *Notes on nursing: What it is, and what it is not* (commemorative ed., pp. 3–17). Philadelphia: Lippincott.

Sherwood, G. (1997). Meta-synthesis of qualitative analyses of caring: Defining a therapeutic model of nursing. *Advances in Practice of Nursing Quarterly, 3,* 32–42.

Tri-council for Nursing policy statement: Strategies to reverse the new nursing shortage. Retrieved March 5, 2003, from http://www.nln.org/aboutnln/news_tricouncil2.htm

U. S. General Accounting Office. (2001). *Nursing workforce: Emerging nurse shortages due to multiple factors* (Publication No. GAO-01-944). Report to the Chairman, Subcommittee on Health, Committee on Ways and Means, House of Representatives. Retrieved March 5, 2003, from http://www. aacn.nche.edu/Government/GAO%20Report.pdf

Selected Bibliography

Ballou, K. A. (2000). A historical-philosophical analysis of the professional nurse obligation to participate in sociopolitical activities. *Policy Politics and Nursing Practice, 1*(3), 172–184.

Burggraf, V., & Barry, R. (1998). Tomorrow: Gerontological nursing in the 21st century. *Journal of Gerontological Nursing, 24*(4), 29–35.

Dossey, B. M. (2000). *Florence Nightingale: Mystic, visionary, healer.* Springhouse, PA: Springhouse Corp.

Fondiller, S. H. (2000). From the archives. The legacy of the great triumvirate: Annie Goodrich, Adelaide Nutting, and Lillian Wald. *Nursing and Health Care Perspectives, 21*(4), 164–167.

Fondiller, S. H. (2001). From the archives. Pioneers in the forefront of integration. *Nursing and Health Care Perspectives, 22*(2), 64–66.

Frantz, A. K. (1998). Nursing pride: Clara Barton in the Spanish-American war. *American Journal of Nursing, 98*(10), 39–41.

Gennaro, S. (2000). International nursing: The past 25 years and beyond. *American Journal of Maternal/Child Nursing, 25*(6), 296–299.

Hinshaw, A. A. (2001, January 31). A continuing challenge: The shortage of educationally prepared nursing faculty. *Online Journal of Issues in Nursing, 6*(1), Article 3. Retrieved March 5, 2003, from http://www.nursingworld.org/ojin/topic14/tpc14_3.html

Overbay, J. D., & Aaltonen, P. M. (2001). A comparison of NLNAC and CCNE accreditation. *Nurse Educator, 26*(1), 17–22.

Peterson, C. A. (2001, January 31). Nursing shortage: Not a simple problem—no easy answers. *Online Journal of Issues in Nursing, 6*(1), Article 1. Retrieved March 5, 2003 from http://www.nursingworld.org/ojin/topic14/tpc14_1.htm.

Sarnecky, M. T. (2001). Nurses at Pearl Harbor. The real story. . . . *Reflections on Nursing Leadership, 27*(4), 18–20.

Should you join a professional association? (2002). *American Nursing Student, 3*(4), 6–7.

Staggers, N., Thompson, C. B., & Snyder-Halpern, R. (2001). History and trends in clinical information systems in the United States. *Journal of Nursing Scholarship, 33*(1), 75–81.

Tanner, C. A., & Bellack, J. P. (2001). Resolving the nursing shortage: Replacement plus one! *Journal of Nursing Education, 40*(3), 99–100.

Tracing Nightingale's steps: A pictorial tribute. (2001). *Nursing, 31*(1), 44–47.

CHAPTER 2

NURSING EDUCATION AND RESEARCH

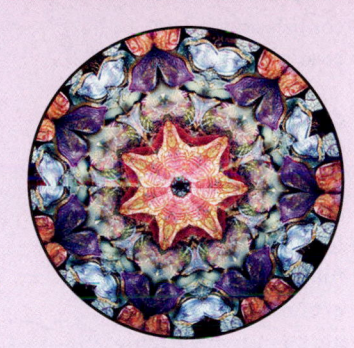

LEARNING OUTCOMES

After completing this chapter, you will be able to:

- Describe the different types of educational nursing programs.

- Discuss aspects of entry to professional nursing practice.

- Explain the importance of continuing nursing education.

- Identify ways the nurse can participate in research activities in practice.

- Differentiate the quantitative approach from the qualitative approach in nursing research.

- Describe the nurse's role in protecting the rights of human subjects in research.

- Identify the steps of the research process.

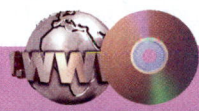

MediaLink

www.prenhall.com/kozier

Additional resources for this chapter can be found on the Student CD-ROM accompanying this textbook, and on the Companion Website at www.prenhall.com/kozier. Click on Chapter 2 to select the activities for this chapter.

CD-ROM
- Audio Glossary
- NCLEX Review

Companion Website
- Additional NCLEX Review
- Case Study: Nursing Profession
- MediaLink Application:
  Entry into Practice
- Links to Resources

Nursing education is controlled from within the profession through state boards of nursing and national accrediting bodies. The traditional focus of nursing education was to teach the knowledge and skills that would enable a nurse to practice in the hospital setting. However, as nursing responds to new scientific knowledge and technological, cultural, political, and socioeconomic changes in society, nursing education curricula are continually revised to meet the needs of nurses working in a changing environment. Programs of nursing study are increasingly based on a broad knowledge of biologic, social, and physical sciences as well as the liberal arts and humanities. Nursing curricula now have a greater focus on critical thinking and the application of nursing and supporting knowledge to health promotion, health maintenance, and health restoration as provided in both community and hospital settings (see Figure 2–1 ■).

Nursing research entails developing and expanding knowledge about human responses to actual or potential health problems and investigating the effects of nursing actions on those responses. The major goal of nursing research is to improve client care.

NURSING EDUCATION

At the present time, state laws recognize two types of nurses: the registered nurse (RN), and the licensed practical or vocational nurse (LPN, LVN). These designations have been used since licensure laws for each level were first enacted. Responsibilities differ for these two levels.

There are also generic master's and doctoral programs leading to RN licensure. For example, students entering a generic master's program already have a baccalaureate degree from a discipline other than nursing. On completion of the program, generally 2 years in length, the graduates obtain their initial professional degree in nursing. Graduates of these master's programs demonstrate the same entry-level competencies as do graduates from baccalaureate programs and are eligible to take the licensure examinations to become an RN.

Although these programs vary considerably, graduates of all programs take the same licensing examinations and, if successful, are licensed as registered nurses. Graduates take the National Council Licensure Examination (NCLEX), which is administered by each state. The successful candidate becomes licensed in that particular state even though the examinations are of national origin. To practice nursing in another state, the nurse must receive reciprocal licensure by applying to that state's board of nursing. Some state legislatures are creating a regulatory model called *mutual recognition* that allows for multistate licensure under one license (see Chapter 4). Nurses from other countries are granted registration by endorsement after successfully completing the NCLEX. Both licensure and registration must be renewed on an annual basis (in some states, every 2 years) to remain valid. For additional information about licensure and registration, see Chapter 4.

The legal right to practice nursing requires not only passing the licensing examination but also verification that the graduate has completed a prescribed course of study from an approved program in nursing. Individual states may have additional requirements. All nursing programs require state approval by the State Board of Nursing.

In addition to state approval, the National League for Nursing Accrediting Commission (NLNAC) provides accreditation standards for all types of nursing programs. Accreditation by the NLNAC signifies excellence in nursing education. A second accrediting body was established in 1996. The Commission on Collegiate Nursing Education (CCNE) accredits baccalaureate and graduate degree nursing programs, thereby, allowing these programs a choice between two professional accrediting agencies.

TYPES OF EDUCATIONAL PROGRAMS

Several educational programs are available for nurses including practical or vocational, registered nursing, graduate nursing, continuing education, and in-service.

Licensed Practical (Vocational) Nursing Programs

Approved practical or vocational nursing programs are provided by community colleges, vocational schools, hospitals, or other independent health agencies. These programs usually last 9 or

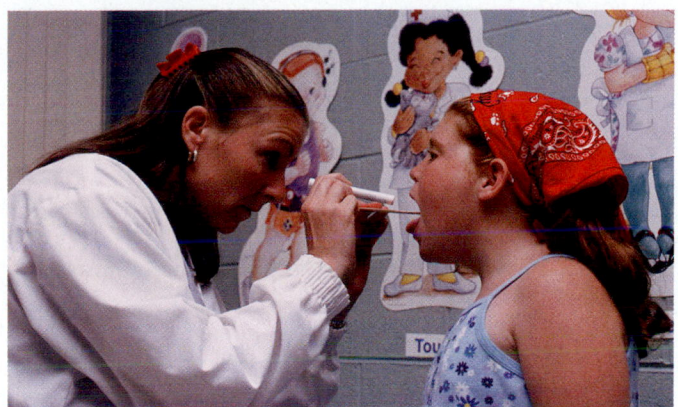

Figure 2–1 ■ Nursing students learn to care for clients in community settings.

12 months and provide both classroom and clinical experiences. In some areas of the United States, LPN programs are being expanded to the associate degree level. At the end of the program, the graduate takes the NCLEX-PN to obtain a license as a practical or vocational nurse.

Licensed practical nurses practice under the supervision of a registered nurse in a hospital, nursing home, rehabilitation center, or home health agency. LPNs (LVNs) usually provide basic direct technical care to clients. The registered nurse, who has the knowledge and skill to make more sophisticated nursing judgments, is responsible for assessing the client's condition, planning care, and evaluating the effect of the care provided.

Registered Nursing Programs

Currently, three major educational routes lead to RN licensure: diploma, associate degree, and baccalaureate programs.

Diploma Programs

After Florence Nightingale established the Nightingale Training School for Nurses at St. Thomas's Hospital in England in 1860, the concept traveled quickly to North America. Hospital administrators welcomed the idea of training schools as a source of free or inexpensive staffing for the hospital. Nursing education in the early years largely took the form of apprenticeships. With little formal classroom instruction, students learned by doing, that is, by providing care to clients in hospitals. There was no standardization of curriculum and no accreditation. Programs were designed to meet the service needs of the hospital, not the educational needs of the students.

The first training programs for nurses at US hospital schools were opened in the 1860s at the New England Hospital for Women and Children in Boston, at Women's Hospital in Philadelphia, at Bellevue Hospital in New York, and at Johns Hopkins in Baltimore. The number of diploma programs rose quickly after these initial programs.

The three-year diploma programs were the dominant nursing programs from the late 1800s and were the major source of graduates until the mid-1960s. Today's diploma nursing pro-

grams have changed markedly from the original Nightingale model. In the United States, diploma programs are hospital-based educational programs that provide a rich clinical experience for nursing students. These programs are often associated with colleges or universities. Almost 70 NLNAC accredited diploma programs provide this avenue for students desiring an education in nursing (NLNAC, 2002).

The number of diploma nursing programs has declined since the ANA resolution in 1965 which recommended that "education for those who work in nursing should be placed in institutions of learning within the general system of education," that "minimal preparation for beginning professional nursing practice at the present time should be the baccalaureate degree education in nursing," and that "associate degree education in nursing should be the minimum preparation for beginning technical nursing practice" (ANA, 1965, p. 107).

Community College/Associate Degree Programs

Community college/associate degree nursing programs, which arose in the early 1950s, were the first and only educational programs for nursing that were systematically developed from planned research and controlled experimentation. Several trends and events influenced the development of these programs: (a) the Cadet Nurse Corps, (b) the community college movement, (c) earlier nursing studies, and (d) Dr. Montag's proposal for an associate degree.

The Cadet Nurse Corps of the United States was legislated and financed during World War II to provide additional nurses to meet both military and civilian nursing needs. The corps proved that qualified nurses could be educated in less time than the traditional 3 years.

After World War II, the number of community colleges in the United States grew rapidly. The low tuition and open-door policy of these colleges made higher education more accessible to all by offering the first 2 years of a 4-year college program.

Studies of nursing education, such as the Goldmark report in 1923, the Committee on the Grading of Schools of Nursing in 1934, and the Brown report in 1948, also had a significant influence on the development of 2-year programs. The recommendations in all of these reports supported independent schools of nursing in institutions of higher learning separate from hospitals.

In the United States, associate degree programs were started after Mildred Montag published her doctoral dissertation in 1951, "The Education of Nursing Technicians," which proposed a 2-year education program for RNs in the community colleges. Dr. Montag made the suggestion as a solution to the acute shortage of nurses that came about because of World War II. She conceptualized a "nursing technician" or "bedside nurse" able to perform nursing functions broader than those of the practical nurse and smaller in scope than those of the professional nurse. The emphasis was to be on education. At the end of 2 years, the student was to be awarded an associate degree in nursing and be eligible to take the state board examination for registered nurse licensure. The first associate degree in nursing (ADN) program started at Columbia University Teachers' College in 1952 under the direction of Mildred Montag. The number of ADN programs has grown from seven in 1958 to more than 880 in 2001 (National Organization for Associate Degree Nursing [NOADN], 2001).

Dr. Montag's original idea that these graduates be nursing technicians and that the degree become a terminal one did not last, however. In 1978, the ANA proposed a resolution that associate degree programs were no longer to be considered terminal but part of a career upward-mobility plan. Today many students enter an associate degree program with the intention of continuing their education in nursing to the baccalaureate or higher level.

Associate degree programs are offered in the United States primarily in community colleges although some 4-year colleges also have ADN programs. The graduating student receives an ADN or an associate of arts (AA), associate of science (AS), or associate in applied science (AAS) degree with a major in nursing.

Because ADN-prepared and bachelor of science in nursing-prepared nurses currently function under the same practice acts, the need for differentiated competencies has been debated for years. Brady et al. (2001) point out that clear and specific information about the type of knowledge, skills, and abilities of each type of nursing education program would "assure that the right nurse with the right competencies is in the right job at the right cost" (p. 34).

The Pew Health Professions Commission (O'Neill, 1998) developed a set of competencies needed by all health professional groups for successful practice in the 21st century (see Box 2–1). In addition, The Pew commission challenges nursing to address a number of issues, among them, to define the various competencies for each educational level. On another front, the Robert Wood Foundation funded 20 nationwide Colleagues in Caring (CIC) projects to "facilitate a statewide collaborative approach to nursing workforce development" (Brady et al., 2001, p. 30). The various CIC projects focus on providing seamless articulation, in which graduates of one nursing program type can easily transition to the next educational level (Lusk & Decker, 2001) or on differentiating competencies between the nursing educational levels (Brady et al., 2001).

Baccalaureate Degree Programs

The first school of nursing in a university setting was established at the University of Minnesota in 1909. This program's curriculum, however, differed little from a 3-year hospital program. It was not until 1919 that the University of Minnesota established its undergraduate baccalaureate degree in nursing.

Most of the early baccalaureate programs were 5 years in length. They consisted of the basic 3-year diploma program in addition to 2 years of liberal arts.

It was not until the 1960s that the number of students enrolled in these baccalaureate programs increased markedly. Almost 700 baccalaureate programs of nursing are in existence in the United States.

Today baccalaureate nursing programs are located in 4-year colleges and universities and are 4 to 5 years in length. The cur-

---

BOX 2–1	■ Twenty-One Competencies for the 21st Century

- ■ Embrace a personal ethic of social responsibility and service.
- ■ Exhibit ethical behavior in all professional activities.
- ■ Provide evidence-based, clinically competent care.
- ■ Incorporate the multiple determinants of health in clinical care.
- ■ Apply knowledge of the new sciences.
- ■ Demonstrate critical thinking, reflection, and problem-solving skills.
- ■ Understand the role of primary care.
- ■ Rigorously practice preventive health care.
- ■ Integrate population-based care and services into practice.
- ■ Improve access to health care for those with unmet health needs.
- ■ Practice relationship-centered care with individuals and families.
- ■ Provide culturally sensitive care to a diverse society.
- ■ Partner with communities in health care decisions.
- ■ Use communication and information technology effectively and appropriately.
- ■ Work in interdisciplinary teams.
- ■ Ensure care that balances individual, professional, system, and societal needs.
- ■ Practice leadership.
- ■ Take responsibility for quality of care and health outcomes at all levels.
- ■ Contribute to continuous improvement of the health care system.
- ■ Advocate for public policy that promotes and protects the health of the public.
- ■ Continue to learn and help others learn.

Note: From *Recreating Health Professional Practice for a New Century,* by E. H. O'Neil and the Pew Health Professions Commission, 1998, San Francisco: Pew Health Professionals. Reprinted with permission.

---

ricula offer courses in the liberal arts, sciences, humanities, and nursing. Graduates must fulfill both the degree requirements of the college or university and the nursing program before being awarded a baccalaureate degree. The usual degree awarded is a bachelor of science in nursing (BSN).

Most baccalaureate programs also admit registered nurses who have diplomas or associate degrees. Some programs have a special curriculum to meet the needs of these students. Some universities also offer nursing students the opportunity to pursue a self-paced, independent study, or online program. Many accept transfer credits from other accredited colleges and universities and offer students the opportunity to take challenge examinations when the students believe they have the knowledge or skills taught in a course. These programs are referred to as BSN completion, BSN transition, 2 + 2, or RN-BSN programs.

Because of changes in the practice environment, the nurse who holds a baccalaureate degree is beginning to reap the rewards of greater autonomy, responsibility, participation in institutional decision making, and career advancement. These changes provide an incentive for nurses with diplomas and associate degrees to continue their formal preparation in baccalaureate completion (transition) programs.

Graduate Nursing Education

Most graduate programs are conducted by departments within the graduate school of a university, and the applicant must first meet requirements established by the graduate school. Although graduate schools differ, common requirements for admission to graduate programs in nursing include the following:

- The applicant must be a registered nurse licensed or eligible for licensure within the program's state.
- The applicant generally must hold a baccalaureate degree in nursing from an approved college or university and have had an acceptable upper division major in nursing at the baccalaureate level. In some regions, however, master's degree programs accept applicants with an ADN.
- The applicant must give evidence of scholastic ability (usually a minimum grade point average of 2.7 to 3.0 on a 4.0 scale).
- The applicant must demonstrate satisfactory achievement on a qualifying examination, such as the Graduate Record Examination (GRE) or the Miller Analogy Test (MAT).
- The applicant must have letters of recommendation from supervisors, nursing faculty, or nursing colleagues indicating the applicant's ability to do graduate study.

Master's Programs

The growth of university nursing programs encouraged the development of graduate study in nursing. In 1953, the newly established National League for Nursing encouraged educators to develop programs for master's degrees in nursing. The major emphasis of the programs was to be research and specialization for teaching and administration. The first "clinical" master's degree (in psychiatric nursing) was offered at Rutgers University in New Jersey in 1954.

Today master's programs generally take from 1.5 to 2 years to complete. Degrees granted are the master of arts (MA), master in nursing (MN), master of science in nursing (MSN), and master of science (MS).

Master's degree programs provide specialized knowledge and skills that enable nurses to assume advanced roles in practice, education, administration, and research (see Figure 2–2 ■).

Doctoral Programs

Doctoral programs in nursing, which award the degrees of doctor of philosophy (PhD), doctor of nursing science (DNS or DNSc), or nursing doctorate (ND), began in the 1960s in the United States. These programs further prepare the nurse for advanced clinical practice, administration, education, and research. Before 1960, nurses acquired doctoral degrees in such related fields as psychology, sociology, physiology, and education.

Content and approach vary among doctoral programs. Some focus on the usual clinical areas, such as medical-surgical nursing, and others emphasize such nontraditional areas as transcultural nursing. Some programs emphasize theory development, but all emphasize research.

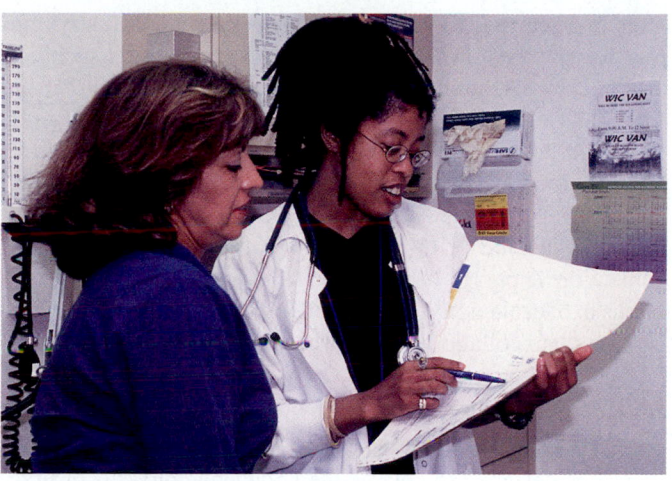

Figure 2–2 ■ A nurse practitioner usually holds a master's degree and assumes an advanced practice role.

Entry to Practice

In 1985, the ANA endorsed the BSN in nursing as the entry level for professional practice. According to the ANA's proposal, only the baccalaureate graduate would be licensed under the legal title registered nurse. The graduate with an associate degree in nursing would be considered a technical nurse and be licensed under the legal title associate nurse (AN).

The ANA proposal sparked sharp debates among graduates, students, and educators, some of whom perceive that it undervalues associate degree (AD) graduates. As a result, the National League for Nursing (NLN) has suggested that the title of associate nurse be replaced by registered associate nurse. However, this suggestion has not eliminated the controversy; many argue that AD graduates have held the title registered nurse since the inception of these ADN programs and should retain that title.

As a professional organization, the ANA cannot legislate these changes. It is the responsibility of each state to define the legal boundaries of nursing practice and to designate the title to be used by those practitioners who meet the individual state's criteria for licensure. If the ANA's proposal is to be accepted nationally, each state will need to adopt the proposal and implement its own changes in its licensure law.

If the ANA proposal is implemented, a grandfather clause would need to be considered for registered nurses who were educated in associate degree or diploma programs before the date of change. Under a grandfather clause, these nurses would continue to be licensed and practice as registered nurses provided that their performance meets established standards. Note, however, that a grandfather clause would protect only the nurse's license: If, for example, an institution required a minimum of a baccalaureate degree for the position of head nurse, an RN who is currently employed as a head nurse but who does not hold the baccalaureate degree would have no guarantee of retaining that position.

Licensure law changes also have major implications for diploma nurses and LPNs because their status is not discussed in the proposal. In addition, this proposal entails that new standardized examinations must be developed to test the two levels of competence.

It is important to note that perspectives about entry into practice are changing. For example, the American Association of Colleges of Nursing (AACN), a national organization that represents colleges and universities with baccalaureate, master's, and doctoral programs in nursing, provides a fact sheet that informs of AACN's support for articulation (AACN, 2002). This fact sheet states that AACN does not advocate for removing the title of RN from ADN program graduates. The organization supports articulation from associate degree programs to baccalaureate and higher degree programs and desires to strengthen collaboration between ADN and BSN programs.

Continuing Education

The term **continuing education (CE)** refers to formalized experiences designed to enlarge the knowledge or skills of practitioners. Compared to advanced education programs, which result in an academic degree, CE courses tend to be more specific and shorter. Participants may receive certificates of completion or specialization.

Continuing education is the responsibility of each practicing nurse. Constant updating and growth are essential to keep abreast of scientific and technological change and changes within the nursing profession. A variety of educational and health care institutions conduct continuing education programs. They are usually designed to meet one or more of the following needs: (a) to keep nurses abreast of new techniques and knowledge; (b) to help nurses attain expertise in a specialized area of practice, such as intensive care nursing; and (c) to provide nurses with information essential to nursing practice, for example, knowledge about the legal aspects of nursing.

Some state laws require nurses to obtain a certain number of CE credits to renew their licenses. In these states, required CE contact hours vary from 15 to 30 hours for every 2-year relicensure period. All, some, or none of these hours may be acquired through home study. Some home study courses are offered through professional journals. The ANA offers online CE programs to nurses. A few states also require a certain number of hours of practice, either independently or in lieu of study hours, before license renewal.

In-Service Education

An **in-service education** program is administered by an employer; it is designed to upgrade the knowledge or skills of employees. For example, an employer might offer an in-service program to inform nurses about a new piece of equipment, specific isolation practices, or methods of implementing a nurse theorist's conceptual framework for nursing. Some in-service programs are mandatory, such as cardiopulmonary resuscitation and fire safety programs.

NURSING RESEARCH

Today, nurses are actively generating, publishing, and applying research in practice to improve client care and enhance nursing's scientific knowledge base. The *Standards of Clinical Nursing Practice* published by the ANA (1998) include research as one of the standards of professional performance (see Box 2–2).

BOX 2–2 ■ **American Nurses Association's Standards of Professional Performance Pertaining to Research**

Standard VII: Research
The nurse uses research findings in practice.

Measurement Criteria
1. The nurse utilizes best available evidence, preferably research data, to develop the plan of care and interventions.
2. The nurse participates in research activities as appropriate to the nurse's education and position. Such activities may include:
   - identifying clinical problems suitable for nursing research.
   - participating in data collection.
   - participating in a unit, organization, or community research committee or program.
   - sharing research activities with others.
   - conducting research.
   - critiquing research for application to practice.
   - using research findings in the development of policies, procedures, and practice guidelines for patient care.

Note: From *Standards of Clinical Nursing Practice,* 2nd ed. by the American Nurses Association, 1998, Washington, D. C: Author. Reprinted with permission.

Although the focus for all nurses is use of research findings in practice, the degree of participation in research depends on the nurse's educational level, position, experience, and practical environment.

As early as 1854, Florence Nightingale demonstrated the importance of research in the delivery of nursing care. When Nightingale arrived in the Crimea in November 1854, she found the military hospital barracks overcrowded, filthy, rat and flea infested, and lacking in food, drugs, and essential medical supplies. As a result of these conditions, men died from starvation and such diseases as dysentery, cholera, and typhus (Woodham-Smith, 1950, pp. 151–167). By systematically collecting, organizing, and reporting data, Nightingale was able to institute sanitary reforms and significantly reduce mortality rates from contagious disease.

Although the Nightingale tradition influenced the establishment of American nursing schools, the research approach did not take hold until the beginning of the 20th century. Since that time, the concept of research was introduced into nursing education programs, research journals in nursing were developed, and an Institute for Nursing Research was established.

The journal *Nursing Research* was established in 1952 to serve as a vehicle to communicate nurses' research and scholarly productivity. The publication of many other nursing research journals followed, some dedicated to research and others combining clinical and research manuscripts (see Box 2–3). The breadth and diversity of nursing research is reflected in the examples of nursing studies shown in Box 2–4.

In 1985, the U.S. Congress passed a bill creating a National Center for Nursing Research in the National Institutes of Health (NIH) to house the research activities conducted by the Division of Nursing at the Department of Health and Human

BOX 2–3 ■ Nursing Research Journals

Examples of Research Journals in Nursing
Advances in Nursing Science
Applied Nursing Research
International Journal of Nursing Studies
Nursing Research
Research in Nursing and Health
Scholarly Inquiry for Nursing Practice
The Journal of Nursing Scholarship
Western Journal of Nursing Research

Examples of Clinical and Specialty Nursing Journals That Publish Research
American Journal of Critical Care
American Journal of Nursing
Heart and Lung
Journal of Gerontologic Nursing
Journal of Neuroscience Nursing
Journal of Nursing Administration
Journal of Nursing Education
Journal of Pediatric Nursing
Journal of Professional Nursing
MedSurg Nursing
Nursing Administration Quarterly
Nursing Outlook

BOX 2–4 ■ Examples of Nursing Studies

- Ugarriza (2002) conducted a qualitative study of elderly women's explanation of depression and found that their major symptoms of depression differed from the criteria for major depression outlined in the DSM-IV.
- Tilden, Tolle, Nelson, and Fields (2001) assessed factors that affect levels of family stress associated with making decisions to withdraw life-sustaining treatments from a dying hospitalized client.
- Metheny, Smith, and Stewart (2000) tested the effectiveness of using a combination of pH and bilirubin test strips for predicting feeding tube placement. Reliable and valid tools are needed to assist nurses to accurately assess feeding tube placement at the bedside.
- Bliss et al. (2001) compared the effects of using fiber supplements containing psyllium or gum Arabic, or a placebo in three groups of adults who were incontinent of loose or liquid stools to determine if a fiber supplement decreases the percentage of incontinent stools.
- Bauer, Geront, and Huynh (2001) compared instructional strategies for teaching blood pressure measurement. The instructional strategies consisted of CD-ROM versus classroom instruction versus a combination of both.
- Hupcey (2000) conducted qualitative research to investigate and describe the psychosocial needs of critically ill clients.

BOX 2–5 ■ Research Opportunities of the National Institute of Nursing Research for 2000–2004

Support research opportunities and provide leadership in:

- *End of life/palliative care research.* NINR is currently the lead institute at NIH for this area of research and is focusing on clinical management of physical and psychological symptom management, communication, ethics and clinical decision making, caregiver support, and care delivery issues.
- *Chronic illness experiences,* such as managing symptoms, avoiding complications of disease and disability, supporting family caregivers, promoting adherence and self-management activities, and promoting healthy behaviors within the context of the chronic condition.
- *Cultural and ethnic considerations* in health and illness, including culturally sensitive interventions to decrease *health disparities* among groups by focusing upon health promotion activities and chronic illness management strategies.
- *Health promotion and disease prevention research,* particularly as it relates to lifestyle changes and healthy behavior maintenance across the life span.
- *Implications of genetic advances,* including reducing factors that increase risk of disease, issues related to genetic screening, and subsequent gene therapy techniques.
- *Quality of life and quality of care,* to include cost savings for the patient, health care system, and society.
- *Symptom management* of illness and treatment, such as pain, cognitive impairment, fatigue, nausea and vomiting, and sleep problems.
- *Telehealth interventions and monitoring* or other emerging technologies to promote patient education and treatment.

Note: From "Mission of the National Institute of Nursing Research. Scientific Goals and Objectives (Objective 1.1)," by National Institute of Nursing Research, 2000. Retrieved May 26, 2002, at http://www.nih.gov/ninr/research/diversity/mission.html Reprinted with permission.

Approaches to Nursing Research

There are two major approaches to investigating diverse phenomena in nursing research. These approaches originate from different philosophical perspectives and use different methods for collection and analysis of data.

Quantitative Research

Quantitative research progresses through systematic, logical steps according to a specific plan to collect numerical information, often under conditions of considerable control, that is analyzed using statistical procedures. The quantitative approach is most frequently associated with positivism or logical positivism, a philosophical doctrine that emphasizes the rational and the scientific (Polit & Hungler, 1999, p. 10). Quantitative research is often viewed as "hard" science and uses deductive reasoning and the measurable attributes of human experience.

Services (DHHS). In 1993, the Center for Nursing Research was promoted to the National Institute for Nursing Research (NINR), gaining equal status with other institutes within the NIH. Research opportunities identified by NINR for the years 2000 to 2004 are listed in Box 2–5.

The following are examples of research questions that lend themselves to a quantitative approach:

- What are the differential effects of continuous versus intermittent application of negative pressure on tracheal tissue during endotracheal suctioning?
- Is the auscultatory method effective in validating the location of a feeding tube?

Qualitative Research

The qualitative approach is often associated with naturalistic inquiry, which explores the subjective and complex experiences of human beings. Qualitative research investigates "the human experience as it is lived through careful collection and analysis of narrative, subjective materials" (Polit & Hungler, 1999, p. 13). Data collection and its analysis occur concurrently. Using the inductive method, data are analyzed by identifying themes and patterns to develop a theory or framework that helps explain the processes under observation (Polit & Hungler, 1999, p. 14). The qualitative approach would be appropriate for the following types of research questions:

- What is the nature of the bereavement process in spouses of clients with terminal cancer?
- What is the nature of coping and adjustment after a radical prostatectomy?
- What is the process of family caregiving for elderly family relatives with Alzheimer's dementia as experienced by the caregiver?

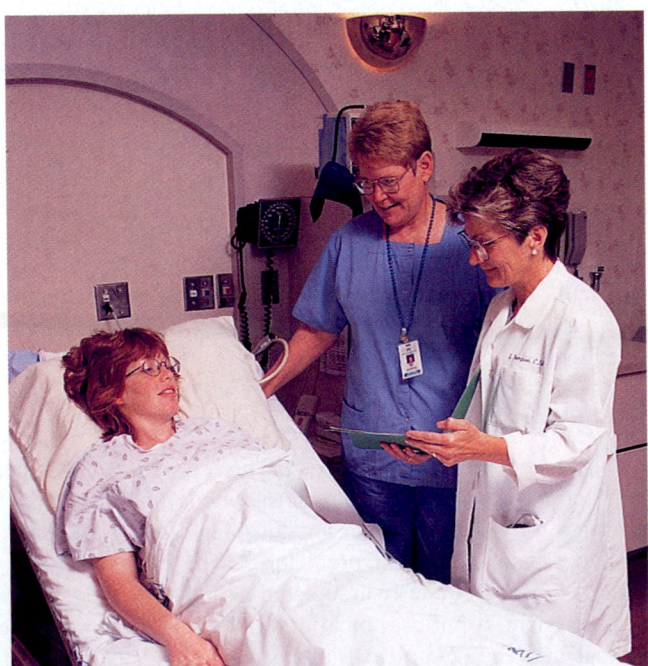

Figure 2–3 ■ Clients must be fully informed before they participate in a research study.

Protecting the Rights of Human Subjects

Because nursing research usually focuses on humans, a major nursing responsibility is to be aware of and to advocate on behalf of clients' rights. All clients must be informed and understand the consequences of consenting to serve as research subjects. The client needs to be able to assess whether an appropriate balance exists between the risks of participating in a study and the potential benefits, either to the client or to the development of knowledge (Figure 2–3 ■).

All nurses who practice in settings where research is being conducted with human subjects or who participate in such research as data collectors or collaborators play an important role in safeguarding the following rights.

Right Not to Be Harmed

The Department of Health and Human Services defines **risk of harm** to a research subject as exposure to the possibility of injury going beyond everyday situations. The risk can be physical, emotional, legal, financial, or social. For instance, withholding standard care from a client in labor for the purpose of studying the course of natural childbirth clearly poses a potential physical danger. Risks can be less overt and involve psychologic factors, such as exposure to stress or anxiety, or social factors, such as loss of confidentiality or loss of privacy.

Right to Full Disclosure

Even though it may be possible to collect data about a client as part of everyday care without the client's particular knowledge or consent, to do so is considered unethical. **Full disclosure** is a basic right. It means that deception, either by withholding information about a client's participation in a study or by giving the client false or misleading information about what participating in the study will involve, must not occur.

Right of Self-Determination

Many clients in dependent positions, such as people in nursing homes, feel pressured to participate in studies. They feel that they must please the doctors and nurses who are responsible for their treatment and care. The **right of self-determination** means that subjects should feel free from constraints, coercion, or any undue influence to participate in a study. Masked inducements, for instance, suggesting to potential participants that by taking part in the study they might become famous, make an important contribution to science, or receive special attention, must be strictly avoided. Nurses must be assertive in advocating for this essential right.

Right of Privacy and Confidentiality

Privacy enables a client to participate without worrying about later embarrassment. The anonymity of a study participant is ensured if even the investigator cannot link a specific subject to the information reported. **Confidentiality** means that any information a subject relates will not be made public or available to others without the subject's consent. Investigators must inform research subjects about the measures that provide for these rights. Such measures may include the use of pseudonyms or code numbers or reporting only aggregate or group data in published research.

The Quantitative Research Process

Polit, Beck, and Hungler (2001) define research as "systematic inquiry that uses disciplined methods to answer questions or solve problems" (p. 4). Research is the application of the scientific approach to generate empirical knowledge. The steps in the research process are discussed next.

State a Research Question or Problem

The investigator's initial task is to narrow a broad area of interest to a circumscribed problem that specifies exactly the intent of the study. The ideas for research may arise from recurrent problems encountered in practice, questions that are difficult to resolve because of contradictions in the literature, or areas in which minimal or no research has been done.

In formulating a research problem, Polit and Hungler (1999, pp. 55–58) suggest that four criteria be used: significance, researchability, feasibility, and interest to the researcher. A research problem has **significance** if it has the potential to contribute to nursing science by enhancing client care, testing or generating a theory, or resolving a day-to-day clinical problem. The question "So what?" must be answered adequately to determine if a research problem is significant.

Researchability means that the problem can be subjected to scientific investigation. Many significant problems that produce ambiguity and uncertainty in clinical situations may not be amenable to research. For instance, "Should nurses support voluntary euthanasia?" is a relevant, timely, and difficult question, but it cannot be answered through research.

Feasibility pertains to the availability of time as well as the material and human resources needed to investigate a research problem or question. Conducting a study involves the use of space, money, equipment, supplies, computers, subjects, research assistants, and consultants.

A researcher spends much time and energy while conducting a research project. It is important, therefore, that the researcher be genuinely interested in and curious about the research problem because the researcher's enthusiasm can be a factor for successful completion of the research.

Research problems contain dependent and independent variables, except for descriptive research, which has no dependent variables. The **dependent variable** is the behavior, characteristic, or outcome that the researcher wishes to explain or predict. The **independent variable** is the presumed cause of or influence on the dependent variable.

Define the Study's Purpose or Rationale

The statement of the study's purpose indicates what the researcher intends to do with the research problem identified. The study purpose includes what the researcher will do, who the subjects will be, and where the data will be collected.

Review the Related Literature

Before progressing with the development of the research design, the investigator determines what is known and what is not known about the problem. A thorough review of the literature provides the foundation on which to build new knowledge. Through a literature review, a researcher may also acquire information about available techniques, instruments, and methods of data analysis that have been used in prior research, as well as potential flaws or problems and how to avoid them.

Formulate Hypotheses and Define Variables

Some studies are intended to develop hypotheses, whereas others are intended to test hypotheses using statistical procedures. Hypothesis formulation requires not only sufficient knowledge about a topic to predict the outcome of the study but also **operational definitions,** definitions that specify the instruments or procedures by which concepts will be measured.

Select a Research Design to Test the Hypothesis

A research design is "the overall plan for answering the research questions or testing the research hypotheses" (Polit et al., 2001, p. 167). The research design includes the study setting, the sample, and the type of data to be collected, as well as strategies to control extraneous variables and reduce bias. There are three major types of research design:

- *Experimental design.* The investigator manipulates the independent variable by administering an experimental treatment to some subjects while withholding it from others.
- *Quasi-experimental design.* The investigator manipulates the independent variable but without either the randomization or control that characterizes true experiments.
- *Nonexperimental design.* The investigator does no manipulation of the independent variable.

Select the Population, Sample, and Setting

At this stage, the researcher chooses the study population, selects a sample, and decides on the setting where the sample can be found. The **population** includes all possible members of the group who meet the criteria for the study. The **sample** is the segment of the population from whom the data will actually be collected.

Conduct a Pilot Study

A pilot study is a "dress rehearsal" before the actual study begins. A trial run of the research procedure is conducted on a few subjects to assess the adequacy of the data collection plan (Polit & Hungler, 1999, p. 38). By identifying any problems or flaws during the pilot study, the investigators can refine the proposed plan and strengthen the research methodology.

Collect the Data

The research process relies on **empirical data,** or information collected from the observable world. Conclusions and generalizations are derived from collected data. The most commonly used methods of collecting data in nursing are questionnaires, rating scales, interviews, observation, and biophysical measures.

The validity and reliability of measurement tools need to be established prior to the start of data collection. **Validity** is the degree to which an instrument measures what it is supposed to measure. If a nurse measures anxiety, how would the nurse be sure that what is being measured is not fear or stress, which are related concepts? **Reliability** is the degree of consistency with which an instrument measures a concept or variable. If an instrument is reliable, repeated measurement of the same variable should yield similar or nearly similar results.

Analyze the Data

In this step, the collected data are organized, coded, and analyzed for the purpose of answering the research question or testing the hypotheses. Even before data collection is initiated, a systematic plan must be in place for analyzing the results. Data analysis may involve descriptive or inferential statistics. **Descriptive statistics,** procedures that summarize large volumes of data, are used to describe and synthesize data, showing patterns and trends. Descriptive statistics include measures of central tendency and measures of variability.

Measures of central tendency describe the center of a distribution of data, denoting where most of the subjects lie. These include the **mean, median,** and **mode. Measures of variability** indicate the degree of dispersion or spread of the data. These include the **range, variance,** and **standard deviation.** See Box 2–6 for definitions of these measures. Typically in a research report, the mean (a measure of central tendency) and standard deviation (a measure of variability) are reported together to give the reader an idea of the nature of the data distribution. The following is an example:

Systolic blood pressure

$$130 \pm 30 \text{ mm Hg}$$

BOX 2–6	■ Definitions of Measures of Central Tendency and Variability

Central Tendency
mean   A measure of central tendency, computed by summing all scores and dividing by the number of subjects; commonly symbolized as $\bar{X}$ or *M*.
median   A measure of central tendency, representing the exact middle score or value in a distribution of scores; the median is the value above and below which 50 percent of the scores lie.
mode   The score or value that occurs most frequently in a distribution of scores.

Variability
range   A measure of variability, consisting of the difference between the highest and lowest values in a distribution of scores.
variance   A measure of variance or dispersion, equal to the square of the standard deviation.
standard deviation   The most frequently used measure of variability, indicating the average to which scores deviate from the mean; commonly symbolized as *SD* or *S*.

The two statistics reported are the mean and the standard deviation. The number 130 indicates the mean systolic blood pressure, whereas 30 represents 1 standard deviation (SD) from the mean. Hence, 1 SD from the mean would include blood pressure from 100 mm Hg to 160 mm Hg (1 SD below to 1 SD above the mean).

After data have been analyzed, nurse researchers attempt to determine whether the results were **statistically significant.** Underlying this statement is the notion of probability. By convention, *p* (probability) less than 0.05 is considered the acceptable level of significance. A *p* value greater than 0.05 is considered statistically insignificant. In research, the desire is to generalize beyond the sample, so there is a need to determine the probability that the results were due to chance or a "fluke" rather than a true occurrence in the population. Hence, a *p* value of 0.05 means that the probability of the findings being caused by chance alone is 5 in 100 (Polit et al., 2001, p. 350).

Communicate Conclusions and Implications

Implicit in conducting research is the requirement to share the knowledge generated with others, either through publication in professional journals or by reporting the results at professional conferences. Interpreting the results, communicating the findings, and suggesting directions for further study conclude the research process.

The Qualitative Research Process

In contrast, qualitative research is not linear like quantitative research. Qualitative researchers do not use independent and dependent variables or manipulate some aspect of the study to test a hypothesis.

The intent of qualitative research is to thoroughly describe and explain a phenomenon (Polit et al., 2001, p. 209). The researchers collect their data through interviews, which are often in the same setting (e.g., home of the participants in the study). These interviews are transcribed and often result in hundreds to thousands of pages of narrative that need to be organized and interpreted. These narrative data are organized around some type of categorization scheme such as concepts, actions, or themes. Finally, the themes of the data are integrated to present a description or theory.

Polit et al. (2001, pp. 211–217) describe three common qualitative research traditions:

- **Ethnography:** Research that provides a framework to focus on the culture of a group of people
- **Phenomenology:** Research that investigates people's life experiences and how they interpret those experiences
- **Grounded theory:** Research to understand social structures and social processes. This method focuses on generation of categories or hypotheses that explain patterns of behavior of the people in the study.

Critiquing Research Reports

If nurses are to use research, they must first learn to conduct a critical appraisal of research reports published in the literature. A research critique enables the nurse as a research consumer to evaluate the scientific merit of the study and decide how the results may be useful in practice. Critiquing involves intensive scrutiny of a study, including its strengths and weaknesses, statistical and clinical significance, and the generalizability of the results.

Polit et al. (2001, pp. 416–421) proposed that the following elements be considered in conducting a research critique: substantive and theoretical dimensions, methodologic dimensions, ethical dimensions, interpretive dimensions, and presentation and stylistic dimensions.

- *Substantive and theoretical dimensions.* For these dimensions, the nurse needs to evaluate the significance of the research problem, the appropriateness of the conceptualizations and the theoretical framework of the study, and the congruence between the research question and the methods used to address it.
- *Methodologic dimensions.* The methodologic dimensions pertain to the appropriateness of the research design, the size and representativeness of the study sample as well as the sampling design, validity and reliability of the instruments, adequacy of the research procedures, and the appropriateness of data analytic techniques used in the study.
- *Ethical dimensions.* The nurse must determine whether the rights of human subjects were protected during the course of the study and whether any ethical problems compromised the scientific merit of the study or the well-being of the subjects.
- *Interpretive dimensions.* For these dimensions, the nurse needs to ascertain the accuracy of the discussion, conclusions, and implications of the study results. The findings must be related back to the original hypotheses and the conceptual framework of the study. The implications and limitations of the study should be reviewed, together with the potential for replication or generalizability of the findings to similar populations.
- *Presentation and stylistic dimensions.* The manner in which the research plan and results are communicated refers to the presentation and stylistic dimensions. The research report must be detailed, logically organized, concise, and well written.

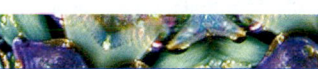 ## Focus on Critical Thinking

A friend, knowing that you are a nursing student, tells you that s/he is considering nursing school and wants your advice.

1. What questions would you ask before responding?

2. What went into your decision making to choose your nursing educational program?

See Critical Thinking Possibilities in Appendix A.

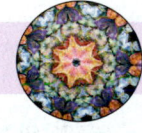 # | Chapter Review

EXPLORE MediaLink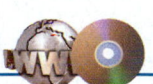

NCLEX review questions, case studies, MediaLink applications, and other interactive resources for this chapter can be found on the Companion Website at www.prenhall.com/kozier. Click on Chapter 2 to select the activities for this chapter.

For more NCLEX review questions, and an audio glossary, access the Student CD-ROM accompanying this textbook.

Chapter Highlights

- Nursing education curricula are continually undergoing revisions in response to new scientific knowledge and technological, cultural, political, and socioeconomic changes in society.
- Nursing education has changed dramatically since the mid-1800s. Early apprenticeship programs established in the 1800s were designed to meet the service needs of the hospital, not the educational needs of the students. Today, nursing education is provided primarily in college and university settings independent of hospitals' needs—a concept proposed by Florence Nightingale.
- Growth of ADN programs in community colleges began in the 1950s after Mildred Montag's proposal supported a 2-year education program for RNs.

- Continuing education is the responsibility of each practicing nurse to keep abreast of scientific and technological change and changes within the nursing profession.
- Nursing research began in North America in the early 1900s. Since that time, the concept of research has been introduced into nursing education programs, research journals in nursing have been developed, and the National Institute for Nursing Research has been established.
- All nurses practicing in settings where research is conducted have a role in safeguarding their clients' rights.

Review Questions

2–1. Which of the following is an example of continuing education for nurses?
   a. attending the hospital's fire safety program
   b. talking with a company representative about a new piece of equipment
   c. receiving a certificate of completion for a workshop on legal aspects of nursing
   d. obtaining information about the facility's new computer charting system

2–2. Which type of research inquiry investigates the issues of human complexity (e.g., understanding the human experience)?
   a. positivism
   b. naturalistic inquiry
   c. logical positivism
   d. quantitative research

2–3. Which of the following studies is based on quantitative research?
   a. a study measuring the effects of sleep deprivation on wound healing
   b. a study examining the bereavement process in spouses of clients with terminal cancer
   c. a study exploring factors influencing weight control behavior
   d. a study examining a client's feelings before and after a bone marrow aspiration

2–4. Which of the following studies is based on qualitative research?
   a. a study measuring nutrition and weight loss or gain in clients with cancer
   b. a study examining oxygen levels after endotracheal suctioning
   c. a study examining client reactions to stress after open heart surgery
   d. a study measuring differences in blood pressure before, during, and after a procedure

2–5. An 85-year-old client in a nursing home tells a nurse, "I signed the papers for that research study because the doctor was so insistent and I want him to continue taking care of me." Which client right is being violated?
   a. right not to be harmed
   b. right to full disclosure
   c. right of privacy and confidentiality
   d. right of self-determination

Readings and References

Suggested Readings

Brady, M., Leuner, J. D., Bellack, J. P., Loquist, R. S., Cipriano, P. F., & O'Neil, E. H. (2001). A proposed framework for differentiating the 21 Pew competencies by level of nursing education. *Nursing and Health Care Perspectives, 22*(1), 30–35.
Based on the Pew commission's list of competencies (abilities and attitudes) required by health professionals to meet the nation's health care needs, the authors describe the South Carolina Colleagues in Caring project. This project differentiated the Pew competencies by level of nursing education and recommended teaching–learning strategies for nurse educators to use as guidelines to assist students in achieving the competencies. The document of differentiated competencies is available at the following website: http://www.sc.edu/nursing/cic

Heller, B. R., Oros, M. T., & Durney-Crowley, J. (2000). The future of nursing education: Ten trends to watch. *Nursing and Health Care Perspectives, 21*(1), 9–13.
The authors describe 10 trends that will impact nursing education: changing demographics, increasing diversity, globalization, the educated consumer, population-based care, health care costs, health policy and regulation, interdisciplinary education, current nursing shortage, and advances in nursing science and research.

References

American Association of Colleges of Nursing. (2002). *Fact sheet: Associate degree in nursing programs and AACN's support for articulation.* Retrieved March 5, 2003, from http://www.aacn.nche.edu/Media/Backgrounders/medback.htm

American Nurses Association. (1965). ANA's first position on education for nursing. *American Journal of Nursing, 65*(12), 106–111.

American Nurses Association. (1998). *Standards of clinical nursing practice* (2nd ed.). Washington, DC: Author.

Bauer, M., Geront, M., & Huynh, M. (2001). Teaching blood pressure measurement: CD-ROM versus conventional classroom instruction. *Journal of Nursing Education, 40*(3), 138–141.

Bliss, D. Z., Jung, H. J., Savik, K., Lowry, A., LeMoine, M. Jensen, L., et al. (2001). Supplementation with dietary fiber improves fecal incontinence. *Nursing Research, 50*(4), 203–213.

Brady, M., Leuner, J. D., Bellack, J. P., Loquist, R. S., Cipriano, P. F., & O'Neil, E. H. (2001). A proposed framework for differentiating the 21 Pew competencies by level of nursing education. *Nursing and Health Care Perspectives, 22*(1), 30–35.

Brown, E. L. (1948). *Nursing for the future: A report prepared for the National Nursing Council.* New York: Russell Sage Foundation.

Committee on the Grading of Nursing Schools. (1934). *Nursing Schools today and tomorrow.* New York: National League of Nursing Education.

Goldmark, J. (1923). *Nursing and nursing education in the United States.* New York: Macmillan.

Hupcey, J. E. (2000). Feeling safe: The psychosocial needs of ICU patients. *Journal of Nursing Scholarship, 32*(4), 361–367.

Lusk, M., & Decker, I. (2001). Moving toward a model for nursing education and practice. *Nursing and Health Care Perspectives, 22*(2), 81–84.

Metheny, N. A., Smith, L., & Stewart, B. J. (2000). Development of a reliable and valid bedside test for bilirubin and its utility for improving prediction of feeding tube location. *Nursing Research, 49*(6), 302–309.

Montag, M. L. (1951). *The education of nursing technicians.* New York: Putnam.

National Institute of Nursing Research. (2000). *About NINR. Mission of the National Institute of Nursing Research. Scientific goals and objectives.* (Objective 1.1). Retrieved March 5, 2003, from http://www.nih.gov/ninr/research/diversity/mission.html

National League for Nursing Accreditating Commission, Inc. (2002). *Directory of accredited nursing programs.* New York: Author.

National Organization for Associate Degree Nursing. (2001). Associate degree nursing

(ADN) facts. Retrieved May 26, 2002, from http://www.noadn.org/about.html

O'Neil, E. H., & the Pew Health Professions Commission. (1998). *Recreating health professional practice for a new century.* San Francisco: Pew Health Professions Commission.

Polit, D. F., Beck, C. T., & Hungler, B. P. (2001). *Essentials of nursing research: Methods, appraisal, and utilization* (5th ed.). Philadelphia: Lippincott.

Polit, D. F., & Hungler, B. P. (1999). *Nursing research: Principles and methods* (5th ed.). Philadelphia: Lippincott.

Tilden, V. P., Tolle, S. W., Nelson, C. A., & Fields, J. (2001). Family decision making to withdraw life-sustaining treatments from hospitalized patients. *Nursing Research, 50*(2), 105–115.

Ugarriza, D. N. (2002). Elderly women's explanation of depression. *Journal of Gerontological Nursing, 28*(5), 22–29.

Woodham-Smith, C. (1950). *Florence Nightingale.* London: Constable & Co.

Selected Bibliography

American Association of Colleges of Nursing. (1998). *The essentials of baccalaureate education for professional nursing practice.* Washington, DC: Author.

American Nurses Association, Cabinet on Nursing Research. (1985). *Directions for nursing research: Toward the twenty-first century.* Kansas City, MO: Author.

ANA delegates vote to limit RN title to BSN grads: "Associate nurse": wins vote for technical level. (1985). *American Journal of Nursing, 85*(9), 1016, 1017, 1020, 1022, 1024, 1025.

Donahue, M. P. (1996). *Nursing: The finest art.* St. Louis, MO: Mosby.

Fondiller, S. H. (2001). From the archives: Nursing's pioneers in the associate degree movement. *Nursing and Health Care Perspectives, 22*(4), 172–174.

Loquist, R. S., & Bellack, J. P. (1999). A model for differentiated entry-level nursing practice by educational program type. *Journal of Nursing Education, 38*(6), 301–303.

Mills, N. M., Haun, L. L., & Daldrup, D. (2000). Kansas City colleagues in caring: Giving new meaning to networking. *Journal of Nursing Education, 39*(2), 54–56.

National Commission on Nursing Implementation Project. (NCNIP). (1987). *Timeline for transition into the future: Nursing education system for two categories of nurse.* Milwaukee: Author.

National League for Nursing. (1996). *Entry-level competencies of graduates of educational programs in practical nursing.* New York: Author.

National League for Nursing. (2000). *Educational competencies for graduates of associate degree nursing programs.* Sudbury, MA: Jones and Bartlett Publishers.

Overbay, J. D., & Aaltonen, P. M. (2001). A comparison of NLNAC and CCNE accreditation. *Nurse Educator, 26*(1), 17–22.

Rapson, M. F. (2000). Colleagues in caring: Statewide nursing articulation model design: Politics or academics? *Journal of Nursing Education, 39*(7), 294–301.

Rolince, P., Giesser, N., Greig, J., Knittel, K., Mahowald, J. F., McAloney-Madden, L., et al. (2001). A regional collaboration for educational and career mobility: The nursing education mobility action group. *Nursing and Health Care Perspectives, 22*(2), 75–80.

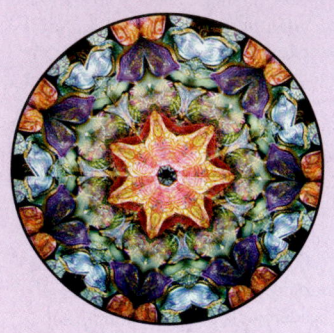

CHAPTER 3

NURSING THEORIES AND CONCEPTUAL FRAMEWORKS

LEARNING OUTCOMES

After completing this chapter, you will be able to:

- Differentiate the terms *concept, conceptual framework, theory, paradigm*, and *metaparadigm for nursing*.

- Identify the purposes of nursing theory in nursing education, research, and clinical practice.

- Identify the components of the metaparadigm for nursing.

- Describe the major purpose of theory in the natural sciences.

- Describe the major purpose of theory in the social sciences and practice disciplines.

- Identify one positive and one negative effect of using theory to understand clinical practice.

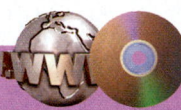

MediaLink

www.prenhall.com/kozier

Additional resources for this chapter can be found on the Student CD-ROM accompanying this textbook, and on the Companion Website at www.prenhall. com/kozier. Click on Chapter 3 to select the activities for this chapter.

CD-ROM
- Audio Glossary
- NCLEX Review

Companion Website
- Additional NCLEX Review
- Case Study: Theories
- MediaLink Applications:
    Nursing Theory Growth
    Shaping Watson's Theory
- Links to Resources

Nursing is involved in identifying its own unique knowledge base—that is, the body of knowledge essential to nursing practice, or a so-called nursing science. To identify this knowledge base, nurses must develop and recognize concepts and theories that are specific to nursing.

INTRODUCTION TO THEORIES IN OTHER DISCIPLINES

Theory has been defined as a supposition or system of ideas that is proposed to explain a given phenomenon. For now, think of theory as a major, very well articulated idea about something important. The four most influential theories from the 20th century were Marx's theory of alienation, Freud's theory of the unconscious, Darwin's theory of evolution, and Einstein's theory of relativity. Most undergraduate students are introduced to the major theories in their disciplines. Psychology majors study Freud and Jung's theories of the unconscious, Sullivan and Piaget's theories of development, and Skinner's theory of behaviorism. Psychology majors are also introduced to critiques of those theories. Sociology majors study Marx's theory of alienation and Weber's theories of modern work, as well as the critiques of their theories. Both sociology and psychology majors spend the majority of their time studying theories and approaches to research.

Biology majors are introduced to Darwin's theory of evolution, but also to Stephen Jay Gould's critique and modification of evolutionary theory. Gould's interpretation of the fossil record proposes that instead of being a slow, gradual process, evolution proceeds in uneven leaps. Physics majors are introduced to a historical progression of theorists including Copernicus, Newton, Einstein, and a new group of theorists in quantum mechanics. Students majoring in the natural sciences also spend the majority of their time studying theories and approaches to research.

The extent to which theories build on or modify previous theories varies with the discipline, as does the importance of theory in the discipline. Undergraduate music and art majors often take some courses in theory, but these students generally focus on creating art or performing music. This is also true of students in nursing, teaching, and management. Management students study management theories, but the relationship between the theory of management and the practice of management is not nearly as strong as the relationship between the theory of physics and the practice of physics. This is because the practice of physics *is* theory and research, whereas the practice of management, teaching, nursing, art, music, law, clinical psychology, and pastoral care is something else entirely. The term **practice discipline** is used for fields of study in which the central focus is performance of a professional role (nursing, teaching, management, music). Practice disciplines are differentiated from the disciplines that have research and theory development as their central focus, for example, the natural sciences. In the practice disciplines, the main function of theory (and research) is to provide new possibilities for understanding the discipline's focus (music, art, management, nursing).

Context for Theory Development in American Universities

In the 19th century, Florence Nightingale thought that the people of Great Britain needed to know more about how to maintain healthy homes and to care for sick family members. Nightingale's *Notes on Nursing: What It Is, and What It Is Not* (1860/1969) was our first textbook on home care and community health. However, the audience for that text was the public at large, not a separate discipline or profession. To Nightingale, the knowledge to provide good nursing was neither unique nor specialized. Rather, Nightingale viewed nursing as a central human activity grounded in observation, reason, and commonsense health practices.

In the 20th century, nursing education in the United States took a different path from nursing education in Great Britain and Europe. The drive to establish nursing departments in colleges and universities exposed American nursing to the dominant ideas and pressures in American higher education at the time. During the latter half of the 20th century, disciplines seeking to establish themselves in universities had to demonstrate something that Nightingale had not envisioned for nursing—a unique body of theoretical knowledge.

The natural and technological sciences were often seen as role models in this regard. Theories in the natural sciences provided a foundation and direction for research. Research in these disciplines often produced tangible results: knowledge that could be used in our efforts to control nature, disease, and foreign threats. Scientifically produced knowledge resulted in a stronger national security and economy.

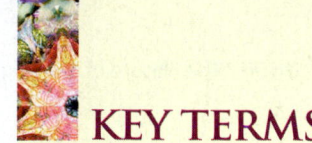

The term *practice discipline* was not in common use until the very end of the 20th century. Disciplines without a strong theory and research base were referred to as "soft," a negative comparison with the "hard" natural sciences. Many of the soft disciplines attempted to emulate the sciences, so theory and scientific research became a more important part of academic life, both in the practice disciplines and in the humanities.

Whereas theories in the natural sciences provide a suitable framework for productive research, theories serve a different purpose in the social sciences and practice disciplines such as nursing. In these disciplines, theories work like lenses through which we are invited to interpret things like market forces, industrial efficiency, the human mind, pain, and suffering. Their usefulness comes from helping us interpret phenomena from unique perspectives, building new understandings, relationships, and possibilities.

Defining Terms

Concepts are often called the building blocks of theories. Concepts are hard to define because the definition has to include everything from the speed of light to the unconscious. Concepts are easier to understand by example. Einstein's theory of relativity consists of a beautiful mathematical relationship between three concepts in physics: mass, energy, and the speed of light. However, theories are not always built like houses out of block-like concepts. Freud's theory of the unconscious not only required some new concepts, it required a completely new model. Freud needed a model for the mind that could bring a host of human experiences (or concepts or phenomena) together under one mental roof: dreams, wishes, decisions, behaviors, feelings, anxieties, sexuality. Freud's theory of the mind included three new concepts: the ego, the id, and the superego. It would not be right to say that Freud's theory of the unconscious evolved out of these concepts. Rather, these new concepts helped him create a model in which his larger idea, the unconscious, might be understood.

A **conceptual framework** is a group of related ideas, statements, or concepts. Freud's structure of the mind (id, ego, superego) could be considered a conceptual framework or model. The term **conceptual model** is often used interchangeably with conceptual framework, and sometimes with **grand theories,** those that articulate a broad range of the significant relationships among the concepts of a discipline.

No scientific theory is purely objective, because each is developed in cultures and expressed in language. Theories offer ways of looking at or conceptualizing the central interests of a discipline. In the natural sciences, theories are often expressed in mathematical terms, but Darwin's *Origin of Species* is a short book. In the social and behavioral sciences, theories attempt to explain relationships between concepts. Although it is helpful when these theories are presented in clear, specific, nonambiguous language, they are most often presented in books that in turn generate other books of critique and explanation.

Broadly speaking, a **paradigm** refers to a pattern of shared understandings and assumptions about reality and the world.

Paradigms include our notions of reality that are largely unconscious or taken for granted. However, the term *paradigm* is used in a variety of ways by different authors and its everyday usage varies considerably.

We become aware of paradigms when realities clash. The paradigm of 16th century Europe, informed largely by established religious doctrines and practices, clashed with the emerging discoveries in astronomy. The Industrial Revolution clashed with the long-standing feudal order, disrupting social and class relationships. In the 20th century, the ideals of socialism clashed with ideals of capitalism, and religious fundamentalism clashed with evolution. The next paradigm clash is likely to be between commonsense notions of space and time and the emerging field of quantum mechanics.

THE METAPARADIGM FOR NURSING

In the late 20th century, much of the theoretical work in nursing focused on articulating relationships among four major concepts: person, environment, health, and nursing. Because these four concepts can be superimposed on almost any work in nursing, they are sometimes collectively referred to as a **metaparadigm** for nursing. The term originates from two Greek words: *meta,* meaning "with," and *paradigm,* meaning "pattern."

Many consider the following four concepts to be central to nursing.

1. Person or **client,** the recipient of nursing care (includes individuals, families, groups, and communities).
2. **Environment,** the internal and external surroundings that affect the client. This includes people in the physical environment, such as families, friends, and significant others.
3. **Health,** the degree of wellness or well-being that the client experiences.
4. **Nursing,** the attributes, characteristics, and actions of the nurse providing care on behalf of, or in conjunction with, the client.

The work of American nurse theorists reflects a wide range of ideas about people, health, values, and the world. Each nurse theorist's definitions of these four major concepts vary in accordance with scientific and philosophical orientation, experience in nursing, and the effects of that experience on the theorist's view of nursing. A single metaparadigm may be impossible given the divergence in world views expressed in nursing models.

Nursing theories fall into one of two paradigms. One view reflects prevailing understandings in medicine and the health care system. The other view reflects emerging understandings in transpersonal psychology. Leddy and Pepper (1998) refer to the dominant view as the "stability model" and the emerging view as the "growth model" (p. 167). Leddy and Pepper place the theories of Imogene King, Betty Neuman, and Callista Roy in the stability model and the theories of Dorothea Orem, Jean Watson, Hildegard Peplau, Martha Rogers, and Rosemarie Parse in the emerging growth model.

It is important to remember that any organized approach to understanding the world—including theories, social practices, and people—can both illuminate and obscure what is of central importance to nurses.

PURPOSES OF NURSING THEORY

Direct links exist among theory, education, research, and clinical practice.

In Education

Because nursing theory was used primarily to establish the profession's place in the university, it is not surprising that nursing theory became more firmly established in academia than in clinical practice. In the 1970s and 1980s, many nursing programs identified the major concepts in one or two nursing models, organized these concepts into a conceptual framework, and attempted to organize the entire curriculum around that framework. The unique language in these models was typically introduced into program objectives, course objectives, course descriptions, and clinical performance criteria. The purpose was to elucidate the central meanings of the profession and to gain status vis-à-vis other professions. Occasionally, the language of nursing syllabi became so torturous that neither the faculty nor the students had a clear understanding of what was meant. Many nursing programs have abandoned theory-driven conceptual frameworks.

In Research

Nurse scholars have repeatedly insisted that nursing research identifies the philosophical assumptions or theoretical frameworks from which it proceeds. That is because all thinking, writing, and speaking is based on previous assumptions about people and the world. New theoretical perspectives provide an essential service by identifying gaps in the way we approach specific fields of study such as symptom management or quality of life. Different theoretical perspectives can also help generate new ideas, research questions, and interpretations.

Grand theories only occasionally direct nursing research. Nursing research is more often informed by **midlevel theories** that focus on the exploration of concepts such as pain, self-esteem, learning, and hardiness. Qualitative research in nursing and the social sciences can also be grounded in theories from philosophy or the social sciences. The term **critical theory** is used in academia to describe theories that help elucidate how social structures affect a wide variety of human experiences from art to social practices. In nursing, critical theory helps explain how these structures such as race, gender, sexual orientation, and economic class affect patient experiences and health outcomes.

In Clinical Practice

Where nursing theory has been employed in a clinical setting, its primary contribution has been the facilitation of reflection, questioning, and thinking about what nurses do. Because nurses and nursing practice are often subordinated to powerful

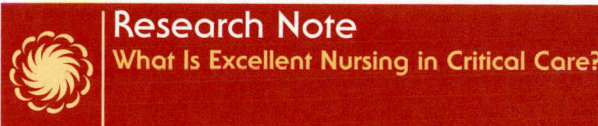

Research Note
What Is Excellent Nursing in Critical Care?

Researchers Benner, Hooper-Kyriakidis, and Stannard (1999) used theories from philosophy and the social sciences to ground a study into the nature of expert nursing in critical care settings. The work of several theorists provided a foundation for the qualitative study. This allowed the researchers to develop a "thick" ethnography of excellent nursing in critical care units through observational interviews and storytelling. The authors knew that the kinds of clinical judgments required in critical care could "not be as certain or predicted and controlled to the degree that scientific experiments can" (p. 5) and so required another theoretical framework for a scholarly investigation of their question.

From a careful analysis of the nurses' stories about their patients, the researchers reported that experienced, expert critical care nurses recognized subtle pattern changes and cues that were indicative of untoward events such as pulmonary emboli and bleeding aneurysms. These were not the routine signs and symptoms that nursing students learn in their educational programs or that can be printed in standard care plans, but rather nuanced interpretations that in part depended on rich and varied experiences with similar patients. The stories also showed a multitude of impressive interventions nurses made to preserve the dignity and humanity of this vulnerable population of patients.

Note: From Clinical Wisdom and Interventions in Critical Care, by P. Benner, P. Hooper-Kyriakidis, and D. Stannard, 1999, Philadelphia: W. B. Saunders.

institutional forces and traditions, the introduction of any framework that encourages nurses to reflect on, think about, and question what they do provides an invaluable service.

An increasing body of theoretical scholarship in nursing has been outside the framework of the formal theories presented in the next section. Benner (2000) and MacIntyre (2001) argue that formalistic theories are too often superimposed on the life-worlds of patients, overshadowing core values of the profession and our patients' humanity. Philosophy is used to explore both clinical and theoretical issues in the journal *Nursing Philosophy*. Family theorists and critical theorists have encouraged the profession to move the focus from individuals to families and social structures. Debates about the role of theory in nursing practice provide evidence that nursing is maturing, both as an academic discipline and as a clinical profession.

OVERVIEW OF SELECTED NURSING THEORIES

The nursing theories discussed in this chapter vary considerably (a) in their level of abstraction; (b) in their conceptualization of the client, health/illness, environment, and nursing; and (c) in their ability to describe, explain, or predict. Some theories are broad in scope; others are limited. The works presented in this chapter may be categorized as philosophies, conceptual frameworks or grand theories, or midlevel theories (Tomey & Alligood, 1998). A **philosophy** is often an early effort to define nursing phenomena and serves as the basis for later theoretical formulations. Examples of philosophies are those of Nightingale, Henderson, and Watson. Conceptual models/grand theories include those of Orem, Rogers, Roy, and King, whereas midlevel theorists are Peplau, Leininger, Parse, and Neuman. Only brief summaries of the author's central theme and basic assumptions are included here.

Nightingale's Environmental Theory

Florence Nightingale, often considered the first nurse theorist, defined nursing more than 100 years ago as "the act of utilizing the environment of the patient to assist him in his recovery" (Nightingale, 1860/1969). She linked health with five environmental factors: (1) pure or fresh air, (2) pure water, (3) efficient drainage, (4) cleanliness, and (5) light, especially direct sunlight. Deficiencies in these five factors produced lack of health or illness.

These environmental factors attain significance when one considers that sanitation conditions in the hospitals of the mid-1800s were extremely poor and that women working in the hospitals were often unreliable, uneducated, and incompetent to care for the ill. In addition to those factors, Nightingale also stressed the importance of keeping the client warm, maintaining a noise-free environment, and attending to the client's diet in terms of assessing intake, timeliness of the food, and its effect on the person.

Nightingale set the stage for further work in the development of nursing theories. Her general concepts about ventilation, cleanliness, quiet, warmth, and diet remain integral parts of nursing and health care today.

Peplau's Interpersonal Relations Model

Hildegard Peplau, a psychiatric nurse, introduced her interpersonal concepts in 1952. Central to Peplau's theory is the use of a therapeutic relationship between the nurse and the client.

Nurses enter into a personal relationship with an individual when a need is present. The nurse–client relationship evolves in four phases:

1. *Orientation.* During this phase, the client seeks help, and the nurse assists the client to understand the problem and the extent of the need for help.
2. *Identification.* During this phase, the client assumes a posture of dependence, interdependence, or independence in relation to the nurse (relatedness). The nurse's focus is to assure the person that the nurse understands the interpersonal meaning of the client's situation.
3. *Exploitation.* In this phase, the client derives full value from what the nurse offers through the relationship. The client uses available services based on self-interest and needs. Power shifts from the nurse to the client.
4. *Resolution.* In this final phase, old needs and goals are put aside and new ones adopted. Once older needs are resolved, newer and more mature ones emerge.

To help clients fulfill their needs, nurses assume many roles: stranger, teacher, resource person, surrogate, leader, and coun-

selor. Peplau's model continues to be used by clinicians when working with individuals who have psychologic problems.

Henderson's Definition of Nursing

In 1966, Virginia Henderson's definition of the unique function of nursing was a major stepping stone in the emergence of nursing as a discipline separate from medicine. Like Nightingale, Henderson described nursing in relation to the client and the client's environment. Unlike Nightingale, Henderson saw the nurse as concerned with both healthy and ill individuals, acknowledged that nurses interact with clients even when recovery may not be feasible, and mentioned the teaching and advocacy roles of the nurse.

Henderson (1966) conceptualized the nurse's role as assisting sick or healthy individuals to gain independence in meeting 14 fundamental needs:

1. Breathing normally
2. Eating and drinking adequately
3. Eliminating body wastes
4. Moving and maintaining a desirable position
5. Sleeping and resting
6. Selecting suitable clothes
7. Maintaining body temperature within normal range by adjusting clothing and modifying the environment
8. Keeping the body clean and well groomed to protect the integument
9. Avoiding dangers in the environment and avoiding injuring others
10. Communicating with others in expressing emotions, needs, fears, or opinions
11. Worshipping according to one's faith
12. Working in such a way that one feels a sense of accomplishment
13. Playing or participating in various forms of recreation
14. Learning, discovering, or satisfying the curiosity that leads to normal development and health, and using available health facilities

Henderson has published many works and continues to be cited in current nursing literature. Her emphasis on the importance of nursing's independence from, and interdependence with, other health care disciplines is well recognized.

Rogers's Science of Unitary Human Beings

Martha Rogers first presented her theory of unitary human beings in 1970. It contains complex conceptualizations related to multiple scientific disciplines (e.g., Einstein's theory of relativity, Burr and Northrop's electrodynamic theory of life; von Bertalanffy's general systems theory; and many other disciplines, such as anthropology, psychology, sociology, astronomy, religion, philosophy, history, biology, and literature).

Rogers views the person as an irreducible whole, the whole being greater than the sum of its parts. *Whole* is differentiated from *holistic,* the latter often being used to mean only the sum of all parts. She states that humans are dynamic energy fields in continuous exchange with environmental fields, both of which are infinite. The "human field image" perspective surpasses that of the physical body. Both human and environmental fields are characterized by pattern, a universe of open systems, and four dimensionality. According to Rogers, unitary man

- Is an irreducible, four-dimensional energy field identified by pattern
- Manifests characteristics different from the sum of the parts
- Interacts continuously and creatively with the environment
- Behaves as a totality
- As a sentient being, participates creatively in change.

Nurses applying Rogers's theory in practice (a) focus on the person's wholeness, (b) seek to promote symphonic interaction between the two energy fields (human and environment) to strengthen the coherence and integrity of the person, (c) coordinate the human field with the rhythmicities of the environmental field, and (d) direct and redirect patterns of interaction between the two energy fields to promote maximum health potential.

Nurses' use of noncontact therapeutic touch is based on the concept of human energy fields. The qualities of the field vary from person to person and are affected by pain and illness. Although the field is infinite, realistically it is most clearly "felt" within several feet of the body. Nurses trained in noncontact therapeutic touch claim they can assess and feel the energy field and manipulate it to enhance the healing process of people who are ill or injured.

Orem's General Theory of Nursing

Dorothea Orem's theory, first published in 1971, includes three related concepts: self-care, self-care deficit, and nursing systems. Self-care theory is based on four concepts: self-care, self-care agency, self-care requisites, and therapeutic self-care demand. Self-care refers to those activities an individual performs independently throughout life to promote and maintain personal well-being. Self-care agency is the individual's ability to perform self-care activities. It consists of two agents: a self-care agent (an individual who performs self-care independently) and a dependent care agent (a person other than the individual who provides the care). Most adults care for themselves, whereas infants and people weakened by illness or disability require assistance with self-care activities.

Self-care requisites, also called self-care needs, are measures or actions taken to provide self-care. There are three categories of self-care requisites:

1. Universal requisites are common to all people. They include maintaining intake and elimination of air, water, and food; balancing rest, solitude, and social interaction; preventing hazards to life and well-being; and promoting normal human functioning.
2. Developmental requisites result from maturation or are associated with conditions or events, such as adjusting to a change in body image or to the loss of a spouse.
3. Health deviation requisites result from illness, injury, or disease or its treatment. They include actions such as

seeking health care assistance, carrying out prescribed therapies, and learning to live with the effects of illness or treatment.

Therapeutic self-care demand refers to all self-care activities required to meet existing self-care requisites, or in other words, actions to maintain health and well-being (see Figure 3–1 ■).

Self-care deficit results when self-care agency is not adequate to meet the known self-care demand. Orem's self-care deficit theory explains not only when nursing is needed but also how people can be assisted through five methods of helping: acting or doing for, guiding, teaching, supporting, and providing an environment that promotes the individual's abilities to meet current and future demands.

Orem identifies three types of nursing systems:

1. Wholly compensatory systems are required for individuals who are unable to control and monitor their environment and process information.
2. Partly compensatory systems are designed for individuals who are unable to perform some, but not all, self-care activities.
3. Supportive-educative (developmental) systems are designed for persons who need to learn to perform self-care measures and need assistance to do so.

The five methods of helping discussed for self-care deficit can be used in each nursing system.

King's Goal Attainment Theory

Imogene King's theory of goal attainment (1981) was derived from her conceptual framework (Figure 3–2 ■). King's framework shows the relationship of operational systems (individuals), interpersonal systems (groups such as nurse-patient), and social systems (such as educational system, health care system). She selected 15 concepts from the nursing literature (self, role, perception, communication, interaction, transaction, growth and development, stress, time, personal space, organization, status, power, authority, and decision making) as essential knowledge for use by nurses.

Ten of the concepts in the framework were selected (self, role, perception, communication, interaction, transaction, growth and development, stress, time, and personal space) as essential knowledge for use by nurses in concrete nursing situations. Within this theory, a transaction process model was designed (Figure 3–3 ■). This process describes the nature of and standard for nurse–patient interactions that leads to goal attainment—that nurses purposefully interact and mutually set, explore, and agree to means to achieve goals. Goal attainment represents outcomes. When this information is recorded in the patient record, nurses have data that represent evidence-based nursing practice.

King's theory offers insight into nurses' interactions with individuals and groups within the environment. It highlights the importance of a client's participation in decisions that influence care and focuses on both the process of nurse–client interaction and the outcomes of care.

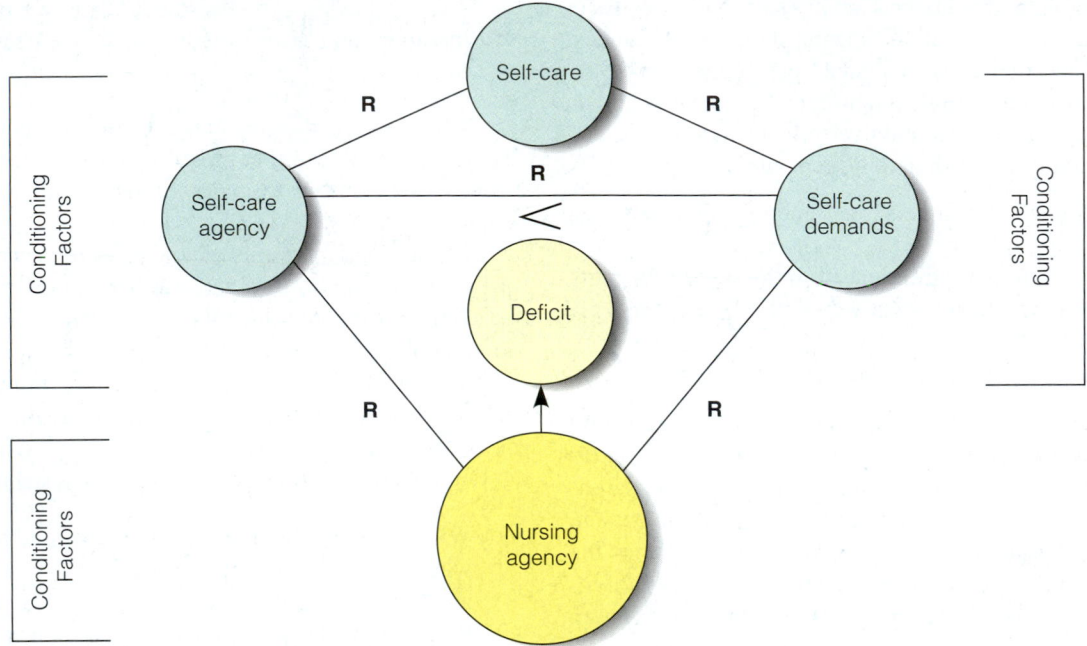

Figure 3–1 ■ The major components of Orem's self-care deficit theory. R indicates a relationship between components; < indicates a current or potential deficit where nursing would be required. (*Note:* From *Nursing Concepts of Practice,* 6th ed. (p. 491), by D.E. Orem, 2001, St. Louis, MO: Mosby. Reprinted with permission from Elsevier Science.)

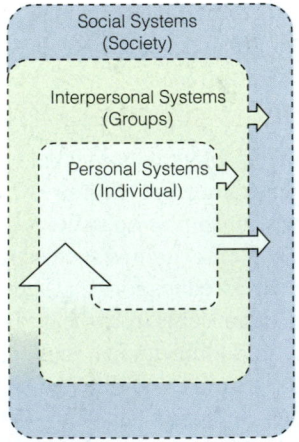

Figure 3–2 ■ King's conceptual framework for nursing: dynamic interacting systems. (*Note:* From *A Theory for Nursing: Systems, Concepts, Process* (p. 11), by I. M. King, 1981, Albany, NY: Delmar. Copyright Imogene M. King. Used with permission.)

Neuman's Systems Model

Betty Neuman (Neuman & Fawcett, 2002), a community health nurse and clinical psychologist, developed a model based on the individual's relationship to stress, the reaction to it, and reconstitution factors that are dynamic in nature. Reconstitution is the state of adaptation to stressors.

Neuman views the client as an open system consisting of a basic structure or central core of energy resources (physiologic, psychologic, sociocultural, developmental, and spiritual) surrounded by two concentric boundaries or rings referred to as lines of resistance (see Figure 3–4 ■). The lines of resistance

represent internal factors that help the client defend against a stressor; one example is an increase in the body's leukocyte count to combat an infection. Outside the lines of resistance are two lines of defense. The inner or normal line of defense, depicted as a solid line, represents the person's state of equilibrium or the state of adaptation developed and maintained over time and considered normal for that person. The flexible line of defense, depicted as a broken line, is dynamic and can be rapidly altered over a short period of time. It is a protective buffer that prevents stressors from penetrating the normal line of defense. Certain variables (e.g., sleep deprivation) can create rapid changes in the flexible line of defense.

Neuman categorizes stressors as intra-personal stressors, those that occur within the individual (e.g., an infection); inter-personal stressors, those that occur between individuals (e.g., unrealistic role expectations); and extrapersonal stressors, those that occur outside the person (e.g., financial concerns). The individual's reaction to stressors depends on the strength of the lines of defense. When the lines of defense fail, the resulting reaction depends on the strength of the lines of resistance. As part of the reaction, a person's system can adapt to a stressor, an effect known as reconstitution.

Nursing interventions focus on retaining or maintaining system stability. These interventions are carried out on three preventive levels: primary, secondary, and tertiary.

1. Primary prevention focuses on protecting the normal line of defense and strengthening the flexible line of defense.
2. Secondary prevention focuses on strengthening internal lines of resistance, reducing the reaction, and increasing resistance factors.

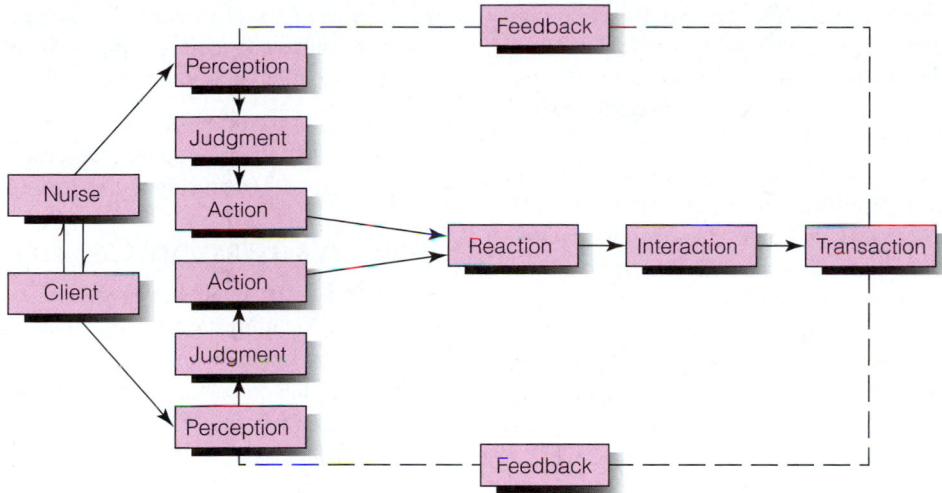

Figure 3–3 ■ King's model of transactions. (*Note:* From *A Theory for Nursing: Systems, Concepts, Process* (p. 145), by I. M. King, 1981, Albany, NY: Delmar. Copyright Imogene M. King. Reprinted with permission.)

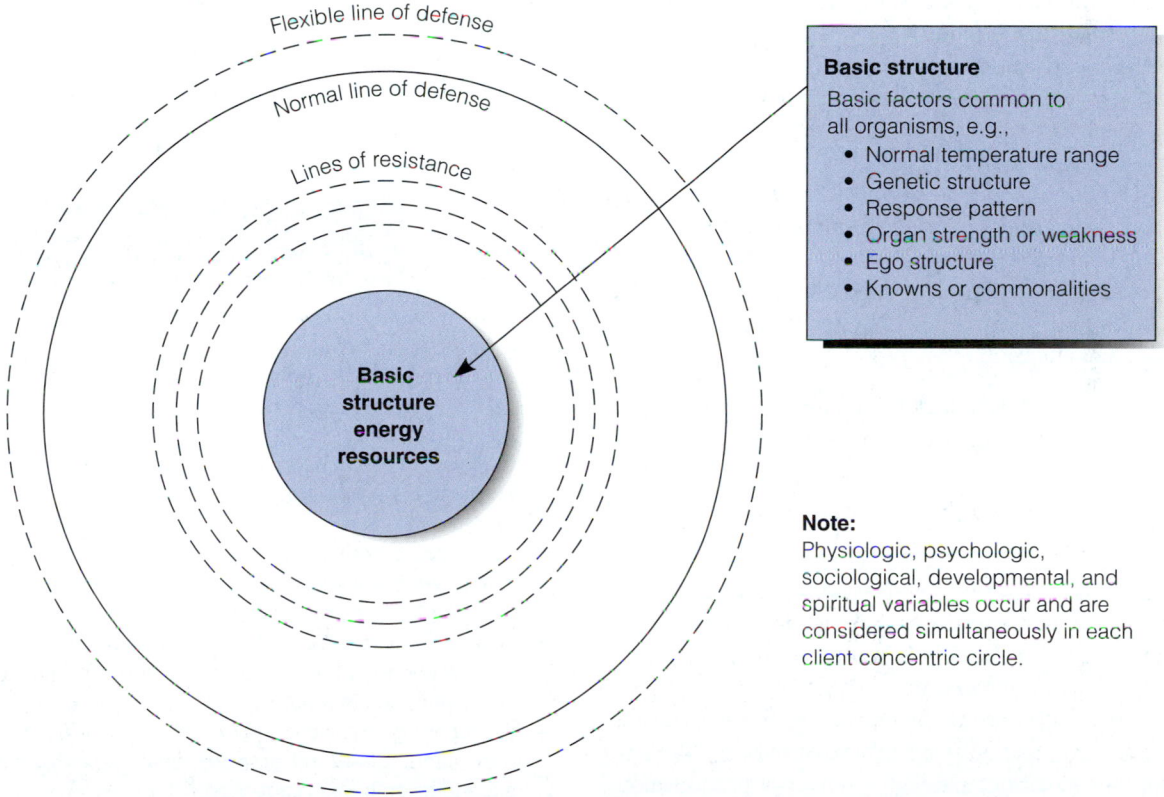

Figure 3–4 ■ Neuman's client system. (*Note:* From *The Neuman Systems Model,* 4th ed. (p. 15), by B. Neuman and J. Fawcett, 2002, Upper Saddle River, NJ: Prentice Hall. Reprinted with permission.)

3. Tertiary prevention focuses on readaptation and stability and protects reconstitution or return to wellness following treatment.

Betty Neuman's model of nursing is applicable to a variety of nursing practice settings involving individuals, families, groups, and communities.

Roy's Adaptation Model

Sister Callista Roy (1997) defines adaptation as "the process and outcome whereby the thinking and feeling person uses conscious awareness and choice to create human and environmental integration" (p. 44).

Roy's work focuses on the increasing complexity of person and environment self-organization, and on the relationship between and among persons, universe, and what can be considered a supreme being or God. Her philosophical assumptions have been refined using major characteristics of "creation spirituality"—a view that "persons and the earth are one, and that they are in God and of God" (Roy, 1997, p. 46).

Roy focuses on the individual as a biopsychosocial adaptive system that employs a feedback cycle of input (stimuli), throughput (control processes), and output (behaviors or adaptive responses). Both the individual and the environment are sources of stimuli that require modification to promote adaptation, an ongoing purposive response. Adaptive responses contribute to health, which she defines as the process of being and becoming integrated; ineffective or maladaptive responses do not contribute to health. Each person's adaptation level is unique and constantly changing.

Individuals respond to needs (stimuli) in one of four modes:

1. The physiologic mode involves the body's basic physiologic needs and ways of adapting with regard to fluid and electrolytes, activity and rest, circulation and oxygen, nutrition and elimination, protection, the senses, and neurologic and endocrine function.
2. The self-concept mode includes two components: the physical self, which involves sensation and body image, and the personal self, which involves self-ideal, self-consistency, and the moral-ethical self.
3. The role function mode is determined by the need for social integrity and refers to the performance of duties based on given positions within society.
4. The interdependence mode involves one's relations with significant others and support systems that provide help, affection, and attention.

The goal of Callista Roy's model is to enhance life processes through adaptation in the four adaptive modes.

Leininger's Cultural Care Diversity and Universality Theory

Madeleine Leininger, a well-known nurse anthropologist, put her views on transcultural nursing in print in the 1970s and then in 1991 published her book *Culture Care Diversity and Universality: A Theory of Nursing.*

Leininger states that care is the essence of nursing and the dominant, distinctive, and unifying feature of nursing. She emphasizes that human caring, although a universal phenomenon, varies among cultures in its expressions, processes, and patterns; it is largely culturally derived. Leininger produced the Sunrise model to depict her theory of cultural care diversity and universality. This model emphasizes that health and care are influenced by elements of the social structure, such as technology, religious and philosophical factors, kinship and social systems, cultural values, political and legal factors, economic factors, and educational factors. These social factors are addressed within environmental contexts, language expressions, and ethnohistory. Each of these systems is part of the social structure of any society; health care expressions, patterns, and practices are also integral parts of

these aspects of social structure (Leininger & McFarland, 2002). In order for nurses to assist people of diverse cultures, Leininger presents three intervention modes:

- Culture care preservation and maintenance
- Culture care accommodation, negotiation, or both
- Culture care restructuring and repatterning.

Watson's Human Caring Theory

Jean Watson (1979) believes the practice of caring is central to nursing; it is the unifying focus for practice. Her major assumptions about caring are shown in Box 3–1. Nursing interventions related to human care are referred to as *carative factors,* a guide Watson refers to as the "Core of Nursing." Watson outlines the following 10 factors:

- Forming a humanistic-altruistic system of values
- Instilling faith and hope
- Cultivating sensitivity to one's self and others
- Developing a helping-trust (human care) relationship
- Promoting and accepting the expression of positive and negative feelings
- Systematically using the scientific problem-solving method for decision making

---

BOX 3–1   ■   Watson's Assumptions of Caring

- Human caring in nursing is not just an emotion, concern, attitude, or benevolent desire. Caring connotes a personal response.
- Caring is an intersubjective human process and is the moral ideal of nursing.
- Caring can be effectively demonstrated only interpersonally.
- Effective caring promotes health and individual or family growth.
- Caring promotes health more than does curing.
- Caring responses accept a person not only as they are now, but also for what the person may become.
- A caring environment offers the development of potential while allowing the person to choose the best action for the self at a given point in time.
- Caring occasions involve action and choice by nurse and client. If the caring occasion is transpersonal, the limits of openness expand, as do human capacities.
- The most abstract characteristic of a caring person is that the person is somehow responsive to another person as a unique individual, perceives the other's feelings, and sets one person apart from another.
- Human caring involves values, a will and a commitment to care, knowledge, caring actions, and consequences.
- The ideal and value of caring is a starting point, a stance, and an attitude that has to become a will, an intention, a commitment, and a conscious judgment that manifests itself in concrete acts.

Note: From J. Watson, personal communication, September 22, 2002.

MediaLink · SHAPING WATSON'S THEORY APPLICATION

- Promoting interpersonal teaching–learning
- Providing a supportive, protective, or corrective mental, physical, sociocultural, and spiritual environment
- Assisting with the gratification of human needs
- Allowing for existential-phenomenologic forces.

Watson's theory of human caring has received worldwide recognition and is a major force in redefining nursing as a caring-healing health model.

Parse's Human Becoming Theory

Parse (1995) proposes three assumptions about *human becoming*:

1. Human becoming is freely choosing personal meaning in situations in the intersubjective process of relating value priorities.
2. Human becoming is cocreating rhythmic patterns or relating in mutual process with the universe.
3. Human becoming is cotranscending multidimensionally with the emerging possibles (p. 6).

These three assumptions focus on meaning, rhythmicity, and cotranscendence.

- Meaning arises from a person's interrelationship with the world and refers to happenings to which the person attaches varying degrees of significance.
- Rhythmicity is the movement toward greater diversity.
- Cotranscendence is the process of reaching out beyond the self.

Parse's model of human becoming emphasizes how individuals choose and bear responsibility for patterns of personal health. Parse contends that the client, not the nurse, is the authority figure and decision maker. The nurse's role involves helping individuals and families in choosing the possibilities for changing the health process. Specifically, the nurse's role consists of illuminating meaning (uncovering what was and what will be), synchronizing rhythms (leading through discussion to recognize harmony), and mobilizing transcendence (dreaming of possibilities and planning to reach them).

The Parse nurse uses "true presence" in the nurse–client process. "In true presence the nurse's whole being is immersed with the client as the other illuminates the meanings of his or her situation and moves beyond the moment" (Parse, 1994, p. 18).

CRITIQUE OF NURSING THEORY

Several nurse scholars have developed strong critiques of 20th-century nursing theories, choosing to ground their work in philosophy or the social sciences (Benner, 2000; Munhall, 2001). The best theories in philosophy and the social sciences are often used in the humanities for the insights and perspectives that can be brought to literature and art. So far, other disciplines have not discovered a sufficiently unique or interesting perspective on the human condition in nursing theories.

Nursing scholars continue to debate whether grounding our research in the best theories from other disciplines is good or bad. Some think this detracts from the development of nursing as a separate discipline; others argue that nursing research becomes more relevant when informed by scholarship that addresses larger social concerns.

Most things in the world have both positive and negative implications. Technology can be used for good or for evil. Theory can be used to broaden our perspectives in nursing and facilitate the altruistic and humanistic values of the profession. At the same time, rational and predictive theory can produce language and social practices that are superimposed onto the lives of vulnerable patients and do violence to the fragility of human dignity. As a lens, theory can either illuminate or obscure. As a tool, theory can either liberate or enslave.

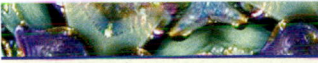 **Focus on Critical Thinking**

Tony is a 32-year-old man with HIV. His first AIDS-defining illness caused his weight to drop from 175 to 116 pounds due to intractable diarrhea. The physician thought caloric intake was of primary importance and urged Tony to eat whatever he wanted. He also prescribed tincture of opium for the diarrhea, but Tony hated the tincture of opium because it made him feel out of control. Because Tony was getting worse, his nurse argued that he needed intravenous nutrition and should eat only bananas, rice, applesauce, and weak tea until the diarrhea stopped. The nurse suggested adding other foods one at a time and only as tolerated. Tony's family and friends offered to take control of Tony's food preparation.

The physician compared AIDS to advanced cancer and argued he would not prescribe intravenous nutrition for advanced cancer. The nurse argued that this was Tony's first AIDS infection and that his prognosis was better than someone with advanced cancer. The nurse's primary focus was on stopping the diarrhea, and used the analogy of pouring gas into a leaking tank. Tony's friends preferred the nurse's approach, but Tony was not as easily convinced.

1. What concepts are present in this case?
2. What appear to be the perspectives or views represented by the MD and the nurse (how might you say they are defining the metaparadigm)?
3. How might Florence Nightingale analyze this situation?
4. Which of the nursing models in this chapter best supports the physician's plan of care? The nurse's plan of care?

See Critical Thinking Possibilities in Appendix A.

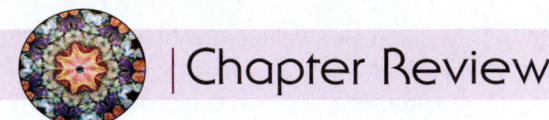 | Chapter Review

EXPLORE MediaLink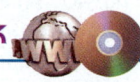

NCLEX review questions, case studies, care plan activities, MediaLink applications, and other interactive resources for this chapter can be found on the Companion Website at www.prenhall.com/kozier. Click on Chapter 3 to select the activities for this chapter.

For animations, video clips, more NCLEX review questions, and an audio glossary, access the Student CD-ROM accompanying this textbook.

Chapter Highlights

- In the natural sciences, the main function of theory is to guide research. In the practice disciplines, the main function of theory (and research) is to provide new possibilities for understanding the discipline's focus (music, art, management, nursing).
- To Nightingale, the knowledge required to provide good nursing was neither unique nor specialized. Rather, Nightingale viewed nursing as a central human activity grounded in observation, reason, and commonsense health practices.
- During the latter half of the 20th century, disciplines seeking to establish themselves in universities had to demonstrate something that Nightingale had not envisioned for nursing—a unique body of theoretical knowledge.
- Theories articulate significant relationships between concepts in order to point to something larger, such as gravity, the unconscious, or the experience of pain.

- Paradigms include our notions of reality that are largely unconscious or taken for granted. Most theories reflect the dominant paradigm of a culture, although some may grow out of a developing rival paradigm.
- In the late 20th century, much of the theoretical work in nursing focused on articulating relationships between four major concepts: person, environment, health, and nursing. Because these four concepts can be superimposed on almost any work in nursing, they are sometimes collectively referred to as a "metaparadigm" for nursing.
- It is important to remember that any organized approach to understanding the world—including theories, social practices, and people—can both illuminate and obscure what is of central importance to nurses.
- Debates about the role of theory in nursing practice provide evidence that nursing is maturing, as both an academic discipline and a clinical profession.

Review Questions

3–1. "A supposition or system of ideas that is proposed to explain a given phenomenon" best defines
   a. a concept.
   b. a conceptual framework.
   c. a theory.
   d. a paradigm.
3–2. "A group of related ideas or statements" is a definition for
   a. a philosophy.
   b. a conceptual framework.
   c. a theory.
   d. a paradigm.
3–3. "A set of shared understandings and assumptions about reality and the world" is a definition for
   a. a concept.

   b. a conceptual framework.
   c. a practice discipline.
   d. a paradigm.
3–4. Which of the following is NOT considered a practice discipline?
   a. physics
   b. psychology
   c. nursing
   d. management
3–5. Which of the following constitute the metaparadigm for nursing?
   a. nursing process, nursing diagnosis, nursing theory, nursing research
   b. person, environment, health, nursing
   c. assessment, diagnosis, planning, evaluation
   d. individual, family, group, community

Readings and References

Suggested Readings

Fawcett, J., Watson, J., Neuman, B., Walker, P. H., & Fitzpatrick, J. (2001). On nursing theories and evidence. *Journal of Nursing Scholarship, 33,* 115–119.

This article, written by five of the most prominent nurses in the field of nursing theory, challenges the reader to engage in considering what is required to state that practice is guided by theory and based on research. They propose that there are four patterns of nursing knowledge and each can be considered a type of theory: empirics, ethics, personal, and aesthetics. Further, each requires unique approaches to gathering, interpreting, and naming evidence. Their perspective is significantly broader than that which generally limits evidence to the results of empirical study.

Related Research

Forbes, M. (1999). Hope in the older adult with chronic illness: A comparison of two research methods in theory building. *Advances in Nursing Science, 22,* 74–87.

Madrid, M., Windstead-Fry, P., & Malinski, V. M. (2001). Nursing research on the health patterning modalities of therapeutic touch and imagery. *Nursing Science Quarterly, 14,* 187–193.

Schafer, P. (1999). Working with Dave: Application of Peplau's interpersonal nursing theory in the correctional environment. *Journal of Psychosocial Nursing & Mental Health Services, 37*(9), 19–24.

References

Benner, P. (2000). The roles of embodiment, emotion and lifeworld for rationality and agency in nursing practice. *Nursing Philosophy, 1*(1), 5–19.

Benner, P., Hooper-Kyriakidis, P., & Stannard, D. (1999). *Clinical wisdom and interventions in critical care.* Philadelphia: W. B. Saunders.

Henderson, V. A. (1966). *The nature of nursing: A definition and its implications for practice, research, and education.* Riverside, NJ: Macmillan.

King, I. M. (1981). *A theory for nursing: Systems, concepts, process.* Albany, NY: Delmar.

Leddy, S., & Pepper, J. M. (1998). *Conceptual bases of professional nursing* (4th ed.). Philadelphia: Lippincott.

Leininger, M. M. (Ed.). (1991). *Culture care diversity and universality: A theory of nursing.* New York: National League for Nursing Press.

Leininger, M., & McFarland, M. R. (2002). *Culture care diversity and universality: A theory of nursing* (3rd ed.). New York: McGraw-Hill.

MacIntyre, R. C. (2001). Interpretive analysis. In P. Munhall (Ed.). *Nursing research: A qualitative perspective* (3rd ed., pp. 439–466). Boston: Jones and Bartlett.

Munhall, P. L. (Ed.). (2001). *Nursing research: A qualitative perspective* (3rd ed.). Boston: Jones and Bartlett.

Neuman, B., & Fawcett, J. (2002). *The Neuman systems model* (4th ed.). Upper Saddle River, NJ: Prentice Hall.

Nightingale, F. (1969). *Notes on nursing: What it is, and what it is not.* New York: Dover. (Original work published in 1860.)

Orem, D. E. (1971). *Nursing: Concepts of practice.* Hightstown, NJ: McGraw-Hill.

Orem, D. E., Taylor, S. G., & Renpenning, K. M. (2001). *Nursing: Concepts of practice* (6th ed.). St. Louis, MO: Mosby.

Parse, R. R. (1994). Quality of life: Sciencing and living the art of human becoming. *Nursing Science Quarterly, 7*(1), 16–21.

Parse, R. R. (Ed.). (1995). *Illumination: The human becoming theory in practice and research.* New York: National League for Nursing Press.

Peplau, H. E. (1952). *Interpersonal relations in nursing.* New York: Putnam.

Rogers, M. E. (1970). *An introduction to the theoretical basis of nursing.* Philadelphia: F. A. Davis.

Roy, C. (1997). Future of the Roy model: Challenge to redefine adaptation. *Nursing Science Quarterly, 10*(1), 42–48.

Tomey, A. M., & Alligood, M. R. (1998). *Nursing theorists and their work* (4th ed.). St. Louis, MO: Mosby.

Watson, J. (1979). *Nursing: The philosophy and science of caring.* Boston: Little, Brown.

Selected Bibliography

Benner, P., Tanner, C. A., & Chesla, C. A. (1996). *Expertise in nursing practice: Caring, clinical judgment and ethics.* New York: Springer.

Bettelheim, B. (1983). *Freud and man's soul.* New York: Alfred A. Knopf.

Fawcett, J. (2001). The nurse theorists: 21st-century updates—Betty Neuman. *Nursing Science Quarterly, 14,* 211–214.

Freud, S. (1949). *An outline of psycho-analysis* (J. Strachey, Trans.). New York: W.W. Norton. (Original work published 1940.)

Henderson, V. A. (1991). *The nature of nursing: Reflections after 25 years.* New York: National League for Nursing Press.

Im, E., & Meleis, A. I. (2001). An international imperative for gender-sensitive theories in women's health. *Journal of Nursing Scholarship, 33,* 309–314.

Parse, R. R. (1981). *Man–living–health: A theory of nursing.* New York: Wiley.

Parse, R. R. (1997). The human becoming theory: The was, is, and will be. *Nursing Science Quarterly, 10*(1), 32–37.

Riehl, J. P., & Roy, C. (Eds.). (1989). *Conceptual models for nursing practice* (2nd ed.). New York: Appleton-Century-Crofts.

Rogers, M. E. (1994). The science of unitary human beings: Current perspectives. *Nursing Science Quarterly, 7*(1), 33–35.

Roy, C. (1976). *Introduction to nursing: An adaptation model.* Englewood Cliffs, NJ: Prentice Hall.

Roy, C. (1999). *The Roy adaptation model* (2nd ed.). Upper Saddle River, NJ: Prentice Hall.

Watson, J. (1997). The theory of human caring: Retrospective and prospective. *Nursing Science Quarterly, 10,* 49–52.

Watson, J. (2002). Intentionality and caring-healing consciousness: A practice of transpersonal nursing. *Holistic Nursing Practice, 16*(4), 12–19.

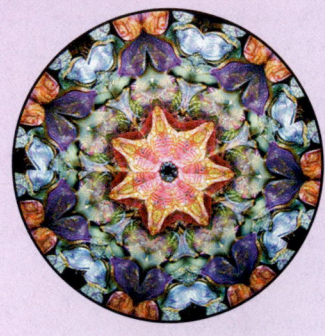

CHAPTER 4

LEGAL ASPECTS OF NURSING

LEARNING OUTCOMES

After completing this chapter, you will be able to:

- List sources of law and types of laws.

- Describe ways nurse practice acts, standards of care, and agency policies and procedures affect the scope of nursing practice.

- Compare and contrast the state-based licensure model and the mutual recognition model for multistate licensure.

- Describe the purpose and essential elements of informed consent.

- Describe the purpose of the following legislated acts: Good Samaritan acts and Americans with Disabilities Act.

- Discuss the impaired nurse and available diversion or peer assistance programs.

- Recognize the nurse's legal responsibilities with selected aspects of nursing practice.

- Differentiate crimes from torts and give examples in nursing.

- Discriminate between negligence and malpractice.

- Delineate the elements of malpractice.

- Compare and contrast intentional torts (assault/battery, false imprisonment, invasion of privacy, defamation) and unintentional torts (negligence, malpractice).

- Describe the purpose of professional liability insurance.

- List information that needs to be included in an incident report.

- Identify ways nurses and nursing students can minimize their chances of liability.

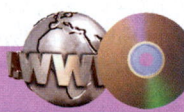

MediaLink

www.prenhall.com/kozier

Additional resources for this chapter can be found on the Student CD-ROM accompanying this textbook, and on the Companion Website at www.prenhall.com/kozier. Click on Chapter 4 to select the activities for this chapter.

CD-ROM
- Audio Glossary
- NCLEX Review

Companion Website
- Additional NCLEX Review
- Case Study: Obstetrics
- MediaLink Applications:
  Nurse Practice Act
  Collective Bargaining
  Liability

Nursing practice is governed by many legal concepts. It is important for nurses to know the basics of legal concepts, because nurses are accountable for their professional judgments and actions. Accountability is an essential concept of professional nursing practice and the law. Knowledge of laws that regulate and affect nursing practice is needed for two reasons:

1. To ensure that the nurse's decisions and actions are consistent with current legal principles.
2. To protect the nurse from liability.

GENERAL LEGAL CONCEPTS

Law can be defined as "the sum total of rules and regulations by which a society is governed. As such, law is created by people and exists to regulate all persons" (Guido, 2001, p. 2).

Functions of the Law in Nursing

The law serves a number of functions in nursing:

- It provides a framework for establishing which nursing actions in the care of clients are legal.
- It differentiates the nurse's responsibilities from those of other health professionals.
- It helps establish the boundaries of independent nursing action.
- It assists in maintaining a standard of nursing practice by making nurses accountable under the law.

Sources of Law

The legal system in the United States has its origin in the English common law system. Figure 4–1 ■ provides an overview of the primary sources of law: constitutions, statutes, administrative agencies, and decisions of courts (common law).

Constitutional Law

The Constitution of the United States is the supreme law of the country. It establishes the general organization of the federal government, grants certain powers to the government, and places limits on what federal and state governments may do. The constitution creates legal rights and responsibilities and is the foundation for a system of justice. For example, the constitution ensures each U.S. citizen the right to due process of law.

Legislation (Statutory Law)

Laws enacted by any legislative body are called **statutory laws.** When federal and state laws conflict, federal law supersedes. Likewise, state laws supersede local laws.

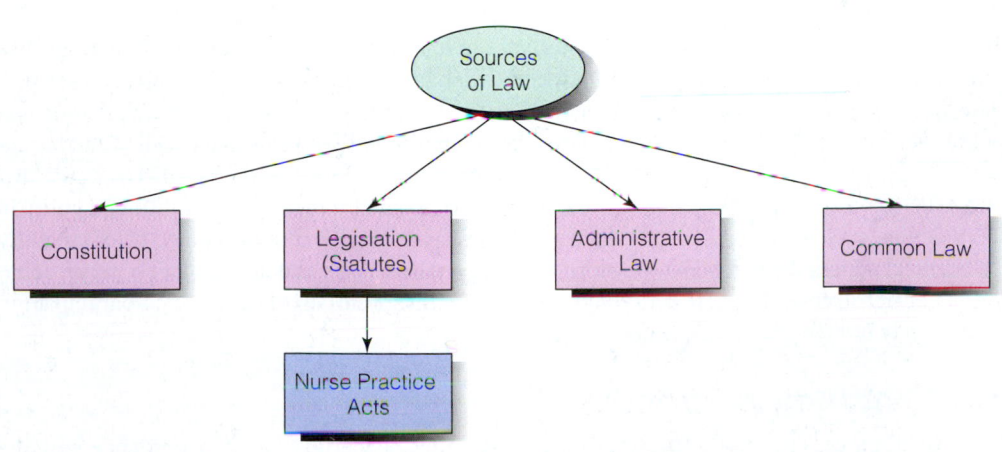

Figure 4–1 ■ Overview of sources of law.

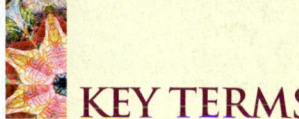

The regulation of nursing is a function of state law. State legislatures pass statutes that define and regulate nursing, that is, nurse practice acts. These acts, however, must be consistent with constitutional and federal provisions.

> ► **CLINICAL ALERT**   *It is important for nurses to keep their legislators informed about nursing because it is the legislature that passes laws that impact nursing practice.* ■

Administrative Law

When a state legislature passes a statute, an administrative agency is given the authority to create rules and regulations to enforce the statutory laws. For example, state boards of nursing write rules and regulations to implement and enforce a nurse practice act, which was created through statutory law (Guido, 2001).

Common Law

Laws evolving from court decisions are referred to as **common law.** In addition to interpreting and applying constitutional or statutory law, courts also are asked to resolve disputes between two parties. Common law is continually being adapted and expanded. In deciding specific controversies, courts generally adhere to the doctrine of *stare decisis*—"to stand by things decided"—usually referred to as "following precedent." In other words, to arrive at a ruling in a particular case, the court applies the same rules and principles applied in previous, similar cases.

Types of Laws

Laws govern the relationship of private individuals with government and with each other.

Public law refers to the body of law that deals with relationships between individuals and the government and governmental agencies. An important segment of public law is **criminal law,** which deals with actions against the safety and welfare of the public. Examples are homicide, manslaughter, and theft. Crimes can be classified as either felonies or misdemeanors, which are described in more detail later in this chapter.

Private law, or **civil law,** is the body of law that deals with relationships among private individuals. It can be categorized into a variety of legal specialties such as contract law and tort law. **Contract law** involves the enforcement of agreements among private individuals or the payment of compensation for failure to fulfill the agreements. **Tort law** defines and enforces duties and rights among private individuals that are not based on contractual agreements. Some examples of tort laws applicable to nurses are negligence and malpractice, invasion of privacy, and assault and battery, which are discussed in more detail later in this chapter. See Table 4–1 for selected categories of law affecting nurses.

Kinds of Legal Actions

There are two kinds of legal actions: civil or private actions and criminal actions. **Civil actions** deal with the relationships among individuals in society; for example, a man may file a suit against a person who he believes cheated him. Civil actions that are of concern to nurses include the torts and contracts listed in Table 4–1. **Criminal actions** deal with disputes between an individual and the society as a whole; for example, if a man shoots a person, society brings him to trial. The major difference between civil and criminal law is the potential outcome for the defendant. If found guilty in a civil action, such as malpractice, the defendant will have to pay a sum of money. If found guilty in a criminal action, the defendant may lose money, be jailed, or be executed and, if a nurse, could lose his or her license. The action of a lawsuit is called **litigation** and lawyers who participate in lawsuits may be referred to as litigators.

The Civil Judicial Process

The judicial process primarily functions to settle disputes peacefully and in accordance with the law. A lawsuit has strict procedural rules. There are generally five steps:

TABLE 4–1 Selected Categories of Laws Affecting Nurses

Category	Examples
Constitutional	Due process
	Equal protection
Statutory (legislative)	Nurse practice acts
	Good Samaritan acts
	Child and adult abuse laws
	Living wills
	Sexual harassment laws
	Americans with Disabilities Act
Criminal (public)	Homicide, manslaughter
	Theft
	Arson
	Active euthanasia
	Sexual assault
	Illegal possession of controlled drugs
Contracts (private/civil)	Nurse and client
	Nurse and employer
	Nurse and insurance
	Client and agency
Torts (private/civil)	Negligence/malpractice
	Libel and slander
	Invasion of privacy
	Assault and battery
	False imprisonment
	Abandonment

MediaLink   NURSE PRACTICE ACT APPLICATION

1. A document, called a **complaint,** is filed by a person referred to as the **plaintiff,** who claims that his or her legal rights have been infringed on by one or more other persons or entities, referred to as **defendants.**
2. A written response, called an **answer,** is made by the defendants.
3. Both parties engage in pretrial activities, referred to as **discovery,** in an effort to obtain all the facts of the situation.
4. In the **trial** of the case, all the relevant facts are presented to a jury or only a judge.
5. The judge renders a **decision,** or the jury renders a **verdict.** If the outcome is not acceptable to one of the parties, an appeal can be made for another trial.

During a trial, a plaintiff must offer evidence of the defendant's wrongdoing. This duty of proving an assertion or wrongdoing is called the **burden of proof.**

Nurses as Witnesses

A nurse may be called to testify in a legal action. It is advisable that any nurse who is asked to testify in such a situation seek the advice of an attorney before providing testimony. In most cases, the attorney for the employer will provide support and counsel during the legal case. If the nurse is the defendant, however, it is advisable for the nurse to retain an attorney to protect the nurse's own interests.

A nurse may also be asked to provide testimony as an expert witness. An **expert witness** has special training, experience, or skill in a relevant area and is allowed by the court to offer an opinion on some issue within their area of expertise. Such a witness is usually called to help a judge or jury understand evidence pertaining to the extent of damage or the standard of care.

REGULATION OF NURSING PRACTICE

The purpose of legal controls for the scope of nursing practice, licensing requirements for nurses, and standards of care is to protect the public. Nurses who know and follow their nurse practice act and standards of care provide safe, competent nursing care.

Nurse Practice Acts

Each state has a nurse practice act, which protects the public by legally defining and describing the scope of nursing practice. State nurse practice acts also legally control nursing practice through licensing requirements. For advanced nursing practice, many states require a different license or have an additional clause that pertains to actions that may be performed only by nurses with advanced education. For example, an additional license may be required to practice as a nurse midwife, nurse anesthetist, or nurse practitioner. The advanced practice nurse also requires a license to be able to prescribe medication or order treatments from physical therapists or other health professionals.

Credentialing

Credentialing is the process of determining and maintaining competence in nursing practice. The credentialing process is one way in which the nursing profession maintains standards of practice and accountability for the educational preparation of its members. Credentialing includes licensure, certification, and accreditation.

Licensure

A **license** is a legal permit that a government agency grants to individuals to engage in the practice of a profession and to use a particular title. Nursing licensure is mandatory in all states. For a profession or occupation to obtain the right to license its members, it generally must meet three criteria:

1. There is a need to protect the public's safety or welfare.
2. The occupation is clearly delineated as a separate, distinct area of work.
3. There is a proper authority to assume the obligations of the licensing process, for example, in nursing, state boards of nursing.

Each state has a mechanism by which licenses can be revoked for just cause (e.g., incompetent nursing practice, professional misconduct, conviction of a crime such as using illegal drugs or selling drugs illegally). In each situation, a committee at a hearing reviews all the facts. Nurses are entitled to be represented by legal counsel at such a hearing. If the nurse's license is revoked as a result of the hearing, either the nurse can appeal the decision to a court of law or, in some states, an agency is designated to review the decision before any court action is initiated.

Mutual Recognition Model

Historically, licensure for nurses has been state based; that is, the state's board of nursing licensed all nurses practicing in the state. Changes, however, in health care delivery and telecommunication technology advances (e.g., telehealth) have raised questions about the state-based model. The American Nurses Association (1998) describes telehealth as the removal of time and distance barriers for the delivery of health care services and related health care activities. Thus, according to the state-based model, a nurse who electronically interacts with a client in another state to provide health information or intervention is practicing across state lines without a license in the other state.

In response to these recent changes, the National Council of State Boards of Nursing (NCSBN) developed a new regulatory model named the **mutual recognition model,** which allows for multistate licensure. With mutual recognition, a nurse who is not under discipline or a monitoring agreement can practice in person or electronically across state lines under one license.

An **interstate compact** (an agreement between two or more states) is the mechanism used to create mutual recognition among states. The state legislature initiates and decides on the establishment of an interstate compact. As of 2002, 18 states had passed the compact but 3 of the 18 have not yet implemented it (Harrington, 2002). The NCSBN website (http://www.ncsbn. org) provides current information about the number of states that have passed compact legislation. See Box 4–1 for additional information about the mutual recognition model.

BOX 4–1   ■ Mutual Recognition Model

- Each state has to enter into an interstate compact that allows nurses to practice in more than one state.
- Multistate licensure privilege means the authority to practice nursing in another state that has signed an interstate compact. It is not an additional license.
- A nurse must have a license in his or her primary state of residency.
- The states continue to have authority in determining licensure requirements and disciplinary actions.
- The nurse is held accountable for the nursing practice laws and regulations in the state where the client is located at the time of care.
- Enactment does not change a state's nurse practice act.
- Complaints and/or violations would be addressed by the home state (place of residence) and the remote (practice) state.
- RNs and LPNs/LVNs are included in the interstate compact; advanced practice nurses are not.

Note: From "Interstate Compact Opens New Opportunities" by C. Lindsay, 2001, *Nursing Spectrum West Region Metro Edition, 2*(8), Reprinted with permission.

Certification

Certification is the voluntary practice of validating that an individual nurse has met minimum standards of nursing competence in specialty areas such as maternal–child health, pediatrics, mental health, gerontology, and school nursing. National certification may be required in order to become licensed as an advanced practice nurse. Certification programs are conducted by the ANA and by specialty nursing organizations.

Accreditation/Approval of Basic Nursing Education Programs

One of the functions of a state board of nursing is to ensure that schools preparing nurses maintain minimum standards of education. Depending on the state, a state board of nursing must either approve or accredit a nursing program. This is a legal requirement.

Nursing programs can also choose to seek voluntary accreditation from a private organization such as the National League for Nursing Accrediting Commission (NLNAC) and the Commission on Collegiate Nursing Education (CCNE). Maintaining voluntary accreditation is a means of informing the public and prospective students that the nursing program has met certain criteria.

All states require approval/accreditation by the state board of nursing. Some states require that nursing programs be both state approved/accredited and accredited by a national accrediting agency such as NLNAC or CCNE.

Standards of Care

Standards of care are the skills and learning commonly possessed by members of a profession (Guido, 2001, p. 63). The purpose of standards of care is to protect the consumer. These standards are used to evaluate the quality of care nurses provide and, therefore, become legal guidelines for nursing practice.

Nursing standards of care can be classified into two categories: internal and external standards. Internal standards of care include "the nurse's job description, education, and expertise as well as individual institutional policies and procedures" (Guido, 2001, p. 64).

External standards consist of:

- Nurse practice acts
- Professional organizations (e.g., American Nurses Association)
- Nursing speciality-practice organizations (e.g., Emergency Nurses Association, Oncology Nursing Society)
- Federal organizations and federal guidelines (e.g., Joint Commission on Accreditation of Healthcare Organizations and Medicare).

In a lawsuit, the nursing expert witness testifies to those standards that nurses are accountable for on a national level and in the local community. It is important, therefore, for nurses to remain competent through reading professional journals and attending continuing education and in-service programs.

CONTRACTUAL ARRANGEMENTS IN NURSING

A contract is the basis of the relationship between a nurse and an employer—for example, a nurse and a hospital or a nurse and a physician. A **contract** is an agreement between two or more competent persons, on sufficient consideration (remuneration), to do or not to do some lawful act. A contract may be written or oral. An oral contract is as equally binding as a written contract. The terms of the oral contract, however, may be more difficult to prove in a court of law. A written contract cannot be changed legally by an oral agreement. If two people wish to change some aspect of a written contract, the change must be written into the contract, because one party cannot hold the other to an oral agreement that differs from the written one.

A contract is considered to be *expressed* when the two parties discuss and agree, orally or in writing, to terms and conditions during the creation of the contract. For example, a nurse will work at a hospital for a stated length of time and under stated conditions. An **implied contract** is one that has not been explicitly agreed to by the parties but that the law nevertheless considers to exist. For example, the nurse is expected to be competent and to follow hospital policies and procedures even though these expectations were not written or discussed. Likewise, the hospital is expected to provide the necessary supplies and equipment needed to provide competent nursing care.

A lawful contract requires the following four features (Guido, 2001):

1. Promise or agreement between two or more persons for the performance of an action or restraint from certain actions
2. Mutual understanding of the terms and meaning of the contract by all
3. A lawful purpose (the activity must be legal)
4. Compensation in the form of something of value—in most cases, compensation is monetary.

Legal Roles of Nurses

Nurses have three separate, interdependent legal roles, each with rights and associated responsibilities: provider of service, employee or contractor for service, and citizen.

Provider of Service

The nurse is expected to provide safe and competent care. Implicit in this role are several legal concepts: liability, standards of care, and contractual obligations.

Liability is the quality or state of being legally responsible for one's obligations and actions and to make financial restitution for wrongful acts. A nurse, for example, has an obligation to practice and direct the practice of others under the nurse's supervision so that harm or injury to the client is prevented and standards of care are maintained. Even when a nurse carries out treatments ordered by the physician, the responsibility for the nursing activity belongs to the nurse. When a nurse is asked to carry out an activity that the nurse believes will be injurious to the client, the nurse's responsibility is to refuse to carry out the order and report this to the nurse's supervisor.

The standards of care by which a nurse acts or fails to act are legally defined by nurse practice acts and by the rule of reasonable and prudent action—what a reasonable and prudent professional with similar preparation and experience would do in similar circumstances. **Contractual obligations** refer to the nurse's duty of care, that is, duty to render care, established by the presence of an expressed or implied contract.

Employee or Contractor for Service

A nurse who is employed by an agency works as a representative of the agency, and the nurse's contract with clients is an implied one. However, a nurse who is employed directly by a client, for example, a private nurse, may have a written contract with that client in which the nurse agrees to provide professional services for a certain fee. A nurse might be prevented from carrying out the terms of the contract because of illness or death. However, personal inconvenience and personal problems, such as the nurse's car failure, are not legitimate reasons for failing to fulfill a contract.

Contractual relationships vary among practice settings. An independent nurse practitioner is a contractor for service whose contractual relationship with the client is an independent one. The nurse employed by a hospital functions within an employer–employee relationship in which the nurse represents and acts for the hospital and therefore must function within the policies of the employing agency. This type of legal relationship creates the ancient legal doctrine known as ***respondeat superior*** ("let the master answer"). In other words, the master (employer) assumes responsibility for the conduct of the servant (employee) and can also be held responsible for malpractice by the employee. By virtue of the employee role, therefore, the nurse's conduct is the hospital's responsibility.

This doctrine does not imply that the nurse cannot be held liable as an individual. Nor does it imply that the doctrine will prevail if the employee's actions are extraordinarily inappropriate, that is, beyond those expected or foreseen by the employer. For example, if the nurse hits a client in the face, the employer could disclaim responsibility because this behavior is beyond the bounds of expected behavior. Criminal acts, such as assisting with criminal abortions or taking tranquilizers from a client's supply for personal use, would also be considered extraordinarily inappropriate behavior. Nurses can be held liable for failure to act as well. For example, a nurse who sees another nurse hitting a client and fails to do anything to protect the client may be considered negligent.

The nurse in the role of employee or contractor for service has obligations to the employer, the client, and other personnel. The nursing care provided must be within the limitations and terms specified. The nurse has an obligation to contract only for those responsibilities that the nurse is competent to discharge. For example, the nurse must practice according to the state's nurse practice act and the policies and procedures of the facility or organization.

The nurse is expected to respect the rights and responsibilities of other health care participants. For example, although the nurse has a responsibility to explain nursing activities to a

TABLE 4–2 Legal Roles, Rights, and Responsibilities

Role	Responsibilities	Rights
Provider of service	To provide safe and competent care commensurate with the nurse's preparation, experience, and circumstances	Right to adequate and qualified assistance as necessary
	To inform clients of the consequences of various alternatives and outcomes of care	Right to reasonable and prudent conduct from clients (e.g., provision of accurate information as required)
	To provide adequate supervision and evaluation of others for whom the nurse is responsible	
	To remain competent	
Employee or contractor for service	To fulfill the obligations of contracted service with the employer	Right to adequate working conditions (e.g., safe equipment and facilities)
	To respect the employer	Right to compensation for services rendered
	To respect the rights and responsibilities of other health care providers	Right to reasonable and prudent conduct by other health care providers
Citizen	To protect the rights of the recipients of care	Right to respect by others of the nurse's own rights and responsibilities
		Right to physical safety

client, the nurse does not have the right to comment on medical practice in a way that disturbs the client or denounces the physician. At the same time, the nurse has the right to expect reasonable and prudent conduct from other health professionals.

Citizen

The rights and responsibilities of the nurse in the role of citizen are the same as those of any individual under the legal system. Rights of citizenship protect clients from harm and ensure consideration for their personal property rights, rights to privacy, confidentiality, and other rights discussed later in this chapter. These same rights apply to nurses.

Nurses move in and out of these roles when carrying out professional and personal responsibilities. An understanding of these roles and the rights and responsibilities associated with them promotes legally responsible conduct and practice by nurses. A **right** is a privilege or fundamental power to which an individual is entitled unless it is revoked by law or given up voluntarily; a **responsibility** is the obligation associated with a right. See Table 4–2 for examples of the responsibilities and rights associated with each role.

Collective Bargaining

Collective bargaining is the formalized decision-making process between representatives of management (employer) and representatives of labor (employee) to negotiate wages and conditions of employment, including work hours, working environment, and fringe benefits of employment (e.g., vacation time, sick leave, and personal leave). Through a written agreement, both management and employees legally commit themselves to observe the terms and conditions of employment.

The collective bargaining process involves the recognition of a certified bargaining agent for the employees. This agent can be a union, a trade association, or a professional organiza-

tion. The agent represents the employees in negotiating a contract with management. The ANA, through its state constituent associations, has represented the interests of nurses within individual states.

When collective bargaining breaks down because an agreement cannot be reached, the employees usually call a strike. A **strike** is an organized work stoppage by a group of employees to express a grievance, enforce a demand for changes in conditions of employment, or solve a dispute with management.

Because nursing practice is a service to people who are often ill or vulnerable, striking presents a moral dilemma to many nurses. Actions taken by nurses can affect the safety of people. When faced with a strike, each nurse must make an individual decision to cross or not to cross a picket line. Nursing students may also be faced with decisions about crossing picket lines in the event of a strike at a clinical agency used for learning experiences. The ANA supports striking as a means of achieving economic and general welfare.

SELECTED LEGAL ASPECTS OF NURSING PRACTICE

Nurses need to know and apply legal aspects in their many different roles. For example, as client advocates, nurses ensure the client's right to informed consent or refusal, and they identify and report violent behavior and neglect of vulnerable clients. Legal aspects also include the duty to report the nurse suspected of chemical impairment.

Informed Consent

Informed consent is an agreement by a client to accept a course of treatment or a procedure after being provided complete information, including the benefits and risks of treatment, alternatives to the treatment, and prognosis if not treated by a

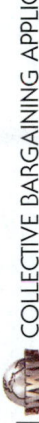

MediaLink   COLLECTIVE BARGAINING APPLICATION

health care provider. Usually the client signs a form provided by the agency. The form is a record of the informed consent, not the informed consent itself.

There are two types of consent: express and implied. **Express consent** may be either an oral or written agreement. Usually, the more invasive a procedure and/or the greater the potential for risk to the client, the greater the need for written permission. **Implied consent** exists when the individual's non-verbal behavior indicates agreement. For example, clients who position their bodies for an injection or cooperate with the taking of vital signs infer implied consent. Consent is also implied in a medical emergency when an individual cannot provide express consent because of physical condition.

Obtaining informed consent for specific medical and surgical treatments is the responsibility of the person who is going to perform the procedure. Generally it is the physician; however, it could also be a nurse practitioner, nurse-anesthetist, or nurse-midwife who is performing procedures in their advanced practices.

Informed consent also applies to nurses who are not independent practitioners and are performing direct nursing care for such procedures as nasogastric tube insertion or medication administration. The nurse relies on orally expressed consent or implied consent for most nursing interventions. It is imperative to remember the importance of communicating with the client by explaining nursing procedures, ensuring the client understands, and obtaining permission.

The law says that a "reasonable amount" of information required for the client to make an informed decision is what any other reasonable physician or practitioner would disclose under similar circumstances (Dunn, 1999, p.42). General guidelines include the following:

- The purposes of the treatment
- What the client can expect to feel or experience
- The intended benefits of the treatment
- Possible risks or negative outcomes of the treatment
- Advantages and disadvantages of possible alternatives to the treatment (including no treatment).

There are three major elements of informed consent:

1. The consent must be given voluntarily.
2. The consent must be given by a client or individual with the capacity and competence to understand.
3. The client or individual must be given enough information to be the ultimate decision maker.

To give informed consent voluntarily, the client must not feel coerced. Sometimes fear of disapproval by a health professional can be the motivation for giving consent; such consent is not voluntarily given. Coercion invalidates the consent. It is important, therefore, for the person obtaining the consent to invite and answer client questions. Cultural perspective also needs to be considered when clients are asked to make decisions about a procedure or treatment (see Providing Culturally Competent Care).

It is also important that the client understand. Technical words and language barriers can inhibit understanding. If a

Providing Culturally Competent Care

INFORMED CONSENT

An individual's rights are emphasized in the United States. Clients have the autonomy to make their own decisions about their health care. The family is not included in informed consent unless the person is legally unable to make the decision. Individuals from certain cultures (e.g., Korean, Southeast Asian, American Indian) may have a group perspective rather than the individual orientation in the United States. Cultures with a group orientation may believe that another member of the family, group, or tribe should make the decision or be involved in hearing the information or making the decision.

The nurse needs to assess whether the client wishes others to be involved. It is suggested that the nurse ask, "Do you wish to have someone present when information or discussion of your health care occurs?" or "Is there anyone we can contact to be with you while you are deciding which course of treatments you prefer?"

Note: From "Informed Consent and Truth-Telling: Cultural Directions for Healthcare Providers," by K. Crow, L. Matheson, and A. Steel, 2000, *Journal of Nursing Administration, 30*(3), pp. 148–152. Reprinted with permission.

client cannot read, the consent form must be read to the client and the client must state understanding before the form is signed. If the client does not speak the same language as the health professional who is providing the information, an interpreter must be present.

If given sufficient information, a competent adult can make decisions regarding health. A competent adult is a person over 18 years of age who is conscious and oriented. A client who is confused, disoriented, or sedated is not considered functionally competent. A legal guardian or representative can provide or refuse consent for the incompetent adult.

Informed consent regulations were originally written with acute care settings in mind. Nonetheless, ensuring informed consent is equally important in providing nursing care in the home. Because the provision of home care often occurs over an extended period of time, the nurse has multiple opportunities to ensure that the client agrees to the plan of treatment. A challenge to informed consent in the home, however, is that the plan may affect other members of the family and, if so, they need to be consulted.

Exceptions

Three groups of people cannot provide consent. The first is minors. In most areas, a parent or guardian must give consent before minors can obtain treatment. The same is true of an adult who has the mental capacity of a child and who has an appointed guardian. In some states, however, minors are allowed to give consent for such procedures as blood donations, treatment for substance abuse, mental health problems, and reproductive health concerns such as sexually transmitted diseases or pregnancy (Brent, 2001; Sullivan, 1998). In addition, certain groups of minors are often legally permitted to provide their own consent. These include those who are married, pregnant, parents, members of the military, or emancipated (living on their own). These statutes may vary by state.

The second group is persons who are unconscious or injured in such a way that they are unable to give consent. In these situations, consent is usually obtained from the closest adult relative if existing statutes permit. In a life-threatening emergency, if consent cannot be obtained from the client or a relative, then the law generally agrees that consent is implied to provide necessary care for the client's emergency condition.

The third group is mentally ill persons who have been judged by professionals to be incompetent. State and provincial mental health acts or similar statutes generally provide definitions of mental illness and specify the rights of the mentally ill under the law as well as the rights of the staff caring for such clients.

Nurse's Role

Often the nurse is asked to obtain a signed consent form. The nurse is not responsible for explaining the procedure but for witnessing the client's signature on the form (see Figure 4–2 ■). Sullivan (1998) states that the nurse's signature confirms three things:

- Client gave consent voluntarily.
- Signature is authentic.
- Client appears competent to give consent.

The nurse advocates for the client by verifying that the client received enough information to give consent. If the client has questions or if the nurse has doubts about the client's understanding, the nurse must notify the health provider. Again, the nurse is not responsible for explaining the medical or surgical procedure. In fact, the nurse could be liable for giving incorrect or incomplete information or interfering with the client–provider relationship (Dunn, 1999).

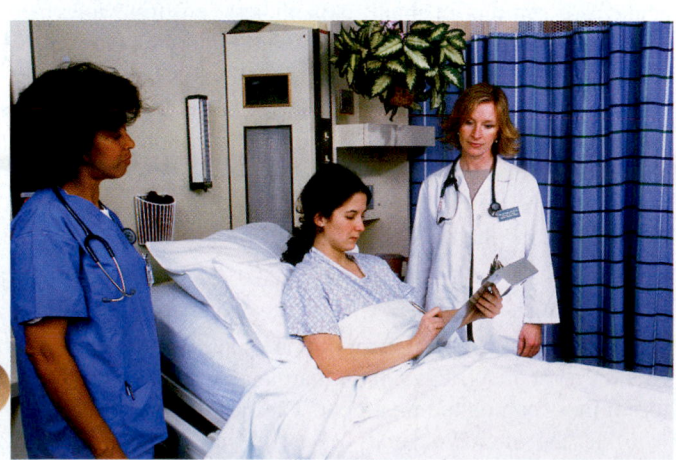

Figure 4–2 ■ Obtaining informed consent is the responsibility of the person performing the procedure. The nurse may be asked to witness the client's signature on the consent form.

According to Guido (2001), the right of consent also involves the right of refusal. Remind clients that they can change their minds and cancel the procedure at any time because the right to refuse continues even after signing the consent. Similar to informed consent, it is important to verify that the client is aware of the pros and cons of refusal and is making an informed decision. The nurse needs to notify the health provider of the client's refusal and document the refusal in the chart.

Documentation is an important aspect to informed consent. A client's concerns or questions must be documented along with the notification of the health care provider. Sullivan (1998) suggests also documenting when the client states understanding. Record any teaching as a result of nursing-related questions by the client. Any special circumstances, such as use of an interpreter, should be documented.

Delegation

The National Council of State Boards of Nursing (1995) defines **delegation** as "transferring to a competent individual the authority to perform a selected nursing task in a selected situation". Competent unlicensed assistive personnel (UAP) can be of assistance to the nurse, which allows the nurse to perform those functions appropriate to the nurse's scope of practice. From a legal perspective, however, the nurse's authority to delegate is based on laws and regulations. Therefore, nurses must be familiar with their nurse practice act (NPA). Sheehan (2001) states that the nurse needs to determine the answers to these questions:

- Does the NPA permit delegation?
- Does the NPA include a list of what the nurse can delegate?
- Has the state board of nursing issued any guidelines explaining the nurse's responsibilities when delegating?

Nurses must know not only their own scope of practice but also the scope of practice of the UAP, which may vary depending on the facilities' policies and procedures. Thus, the nurse must know the employer's policies and procedures for delegation, the UAP's job description, and the UAP's skill level. Is the UAP competent to perform the delegated task? The NCSBN has provided "five rights of delegation" to help nurses make delegation decisions (see Chapter 26). ◐ It is important to remember that the nurse may delegate a task to a UAP; however, the responsibility for action or inaction of the nurse and UAP remains with the nurse (Fisher, 2000).

Violence, Abuse, and Neglect

Violent behavior can include domestic violence, child abuse, elder abuse, and sexual abuse. Neglect is the absence of care necessary to maintain the health and safety of a vulnerable individual such as a child or elder. Nurses, in their many roles (e.g., home health nurse, pediatric nurse, emergency department nurse), can often identify and assess cases of violence against others. As a result, they are often included as **mandated reporters.** Brent (2001) states that "when an identified instance of injury appears to be present and the result of abuse, neglect or exploitation, the mandated reporter must report the situation to the proper authorities" (p. 281). See Chapter 22 for additional information about child abuse and Chapter 23 for elder abuse.

The Americans with Disabilities Act

The Americans with Disabilities Act (ADA), passed by the U.S. Congress in 1990 and fully implemented in 1994, prohibits discrimination on the basis of disability in employment, public services, and public accommodations. The purposes of the act are as follows:

- To provide a clear and comprehensive national mandate for eliminating discrimination against individuals with disabilities
- To provide clear, strong, consistent, enforceable standards addressing discrimination against individuals with disabilities
- To ensure that the federal government plays a central role in enforcing standards established under the act.

The ADA is about productivity, economic independence, and the ability to move about freely in society. The nurse plays a key part in helping individuals with disabilities comprehend the opportunities provided by the law (Watson, 2000, p. 199). For example, nurses working in a variety of settings may be involved in educating clients with disabilities about accessing and using public transportation, communicating through telecommunications devices for individuals with speech and hearing impairments, and patronizing public accommodations such as grocery stores, restaurants, and theaters. Furthermore, an employer may not refuse to hire a nurse with disabilities if the nurse is qualified and able to fulfill the essential functions of the work role. Box 4–2 lists the criteria for ADA eligibility. The ADA also enables individuals of normal intelligence who have a physical or learning disability to pursue a nursing curriculum through alternative learning methods.

Court cases have challenged the definition of a qualified individual with a disability. For example, early challenges to the ADA concerned HIV-infected individuals. A landmark 1998 Supreme Court decision, *Bragdon v. Abbott,* ruled that an asymptomatic HIV-positive individual is considered to have a disability and is protected by the ADA (Guido, 2001). In contrast, courts have also held that a variety of conditions do not constitute a disability under ADA. Examples include a nurse with a lifting disability, depression and anxiety, inability to handle the stress of a specific job, migraine headaches and nonlatex allergies, a short-term condition, and pregnancy (Guido, 2001).

It is the employer's responsibility to provide reasonable accommodations that would allow the person with a disability to perform the job satisfactorily. The employer, however, can claim undue hardship if the accommodation is extremely expensive or difficult to implement.

Controlled Substances

U.S. laws regulate the distribution and use of controlled substances such as narcotics, depressants, stimulants, and hallucinogens. Misuse of controlled substances leads to criminal penalties (see Chapter 33).

The Impaired Nurse

The term **impaired nurse** refers to a nurse whose practice has been affected because of chemical abuse, specifically the use of alcohol and drugs. Chemical dependence in health care workers has become a problem because of the high levels of stress involved in many health care settings and the easy access to addictive drugs.

Data from state boards of nursing support the premise that chemical dependency is a serious problem in the nursing profession. For example, a national survey of state boards of nursing reported that 67% of *disciplinary actions* related to chemical dependency. Some states report higher percentages (e.g., 80% to 93%) of disciplinary cases that were alcohol and drug related (Grover & Floyd, 1998). Recently, schools of nursing have begun to develop policies and procedures related to drug testing of students.

Between 10% and 15% of nurses are estimated to be chemically impaired—about the same percentage as in the general population (Grover & Floyd, 1998). Employers must have sound policies and procedures for identifying and intervening in situations involving a possibly impaired nurse. The primary concern is for the protection of clients, but it is also critically important that the nurse's problem be identified quickly so that appropriate treatment may be instituted. Box 4–3 lists behaviors that may be seen in the impaired nurse. The accompanying Practice Guidelines box can be used to report the nurse suspected of chemical impairment.

BOX 4–2   ■ Meeting ADA Eligibility

The employee or applicant for employment must show:
- A disability
  - A physical or mental impairment that substantially limits one or more major life activities
  - A record of the impairment *or* be regarded as having the impairment
- Ability to perform the essential functions of the position

Note: From *Legal and Ethical Issues in Nursing*, 3rd ed. (pp. 441–442), by G. W. Guido, 2001, Upper Saddle River, NJ: Prentice Hall. Reprinted with permission.

► CLINICAL ALERT   *It is important that student nurses and nurses become knowledgeable about the risk factors of chemical abuse and its early identification and interventions.* ■

A variety of programs have been developed to assist impaired nurses to recover. In many states, impaired nurses who voluntarily enter a diversion program (sometimes called a peer assistance

BOX 4–3   ■ Warning Signs of Impairment

The following patterns or changes in behavior are warning signs that a nurse may be impaired by chemical dependence or a mental health disorder.

Alcoholism
■ Irritability, mood swings
■ Elaborate excuses for behavior; unkempt appearance
■ Blackouts (periods of temporary amnesia)
■ Impaired motor coordination, slurred speech, flushed face, bloodshot eyes
■ Numerous injuries, burns, bruises, etc., with vague explanations
■ Smell of alcohol on breath, or excessive use of mouthwash, mints, etc.
■ Increased isolation from others

Drug Addiction
■ Rapid changes in mood and/or performance
■ Frequent absence from unit; frequent use of restroom
■ May work a lot of overtime, usually arriving early and staying late
■ Increased somatic complaints necessitating prescriptions of pain medications

■ Consistently signs out more or larger amounts of controlled drugs than anyone else; excessive wasting of drugs
■ Often volunteers to medicate other nurses' clients may wear long sleeves all of the time
■ Increased isolation from others
■ Clients complain that pain medication is not effective or they deny receiving medication
■ Excessive discrepancies in signing and documentation procedures of controlled substances

Mental Health Disorder
■ Depressed, lethargic, unable to focus or concentrate, apathetic
■ Makes many mistakes at work
■ Erratic behavior or mood swings
■ Inappropriate or bizarre behavior or speech
■ May also exhibit some of the same or similar characteristics as chemically dependent nurses

Note: From "Texas Peer Assistance Program for Nurses," by Texas Nurses Association. Retrieved February 5, 2003, from *www.texasnurses.org/foundation/tpapn/warningsigns.html* Reprinted with permission.

Practice Guidelines
Reporting a Crime, Tort, or Unsafe Practice

■ Write a clear description of the situation you believe you should report.
■ Make sure that your statements are factual and complete.
■ Make sure you are credible.
■ Obtain support from at least one trustworthy person before filing the report.
■ Report the matter starting at the lowest possible level in the agency hierarchy.
■ Assume responsibility for reporting the individual by being open about it. Sign your name to the letter.
■ See the problem through once you have reported it.

program) do not have their nursing license revoked if they follow treatment requirements. Their practice, however, is closely supervised within specific guidelines (e.g., working on a general nursing unit versus critical care area, no overtime, work only day shift, not allowed to administer or have access to narcotics). The programs require counseling and ongoing participation in support groups with periodic progress reports that may include random drug screening. The nurse may petition the state board of nursing for reinstatement of full licensure after a specified amount of time and evidence of recovery as determined by the state board. Diversion programs allow for rehabilitation of the nurse while still being able to work in the profession. They also allow the state board to protect the public while complying with the ADA. According to Brent (2001), "the nurse who is in a treatment program or has successfully completed one is protected under the ADA as an individual with a disability" (p. 352).

Sexual Harassment

Sexual harassment is a violation of the individual's rights and a form of discrimination. In 1987, the law prohibiting sexual discrimination was clarified to apply to all educational and employing institutions receiving federal funding. The Equal Employment Opportunity Commission (EEOC) defines sexual harassment as "unwelcome sexual advances, requests for sexual favors, and other verbal or physical conduct of a sexual nature" occurring in the following circumstances (EEOC, 2000, section 1604.11):

• When submission to such conduct is considered, either explicitly or implicitly, a condition of an individual's employment
• When submission to or rejection of such conduct is used as the basis for employment decisions affecting the individual
• When such conduct interferes with an individual's work performance or creates an "intimidating, hostile, or offensive working environment."

The victim or the harasser may be male or female. The victim does not have to be of the opposite sex. Nurses must develop skills of assertiveness to deter sexual harassment in the workplace. In addition, nurses must be familiar with the sexual harassment policy and procedures that must be in place in every institution. These will include information regarding the reporting procedure, to whom incidents should be reported, the investigative process, and how confidentiality will be protected to the extent possible (Monarch, 2000).

Abortions

Abortion laws provide specific guidelines for nurses about what is legally permissible. In 1973, when the *Roe v. Wade* and *Doe v. Bolton* cases were decided, the Supreme Court of the United States held that the constitutional rights of privacy give a woman the right to control her own body to the extent that she can abort her fetus in the early stages of pregnancy.

In 1989, the Supreme Court's decision in *Webster v. Reproductive Health Services* upheld a Missouri law banning the use of public funds or facilities for performing or assisting with abortions. In 1992, President Clinton rescinded the *Rust v. Sullivan* 1991 decision, dubbed the "gag rule," that prevented health care providers from discussing abortion services with clients in nonprofit agencies. The Supreme Court and state legislatures continue to struggle with the issue of abortion.

Many statutes also include conscience clauses, upheld by the Supreme Court, designed to protect nurses and hospitals. These clauses give hospitals the right to deny admission to abortion clients and give health care personnel, including nurses, the right to refuse to participate in abortions. When these rights are exercised, the statutes also protect the agency and employee from discrimination or retaliation.

Death and Related Issues

Legal issues associated with death include advance directives, euthanasia, do not resuscitate (DNR) orders, certification of death, autopsy, inquest, and organ donation (see Chapter 41). 🔗

AREAS OF POTENTIAL LIABILITY IN NURSING

Nursing liability is usually involved with tort law. It is important for the nurse to know the differences between malpractice (an unintentional tort) and intentional torts. Nurses must also recognize those nursing situations in which negligent actions are most likely to occur and to take measures to prevent them.

Crimes and Torts

A **crime** is an act committed in violation of public (criminal) law and punishable by a fine or imprisonment. A crime does *not* have to be intended in order to be a crime. For example, a nurse may accidentally give a client an additional and lethal dose of a narcotic to relieve discomfort.

Crimes are classified as either felonies or misdemeanors. A **felony** is a crime of a serious nature, such as murder, punishable by a term in prison. In some areas, second-degree murder is called **manslaughter.** A nurse who accidentally gives an additional and lethal dose of a narcotic can be accused of manslaughter.

Crimes are punished through criminal action by the state against an individual. A **misdemeanor** is an offense of a less serious nature and is usually punishable by a fine or short-term jail sentence, or both. A nurse who slaps a client's face could be charged with a misdemeanor.

A **tort** is a civil wrong committed against a person or a person's property. Torts are usually litigated in court by civil action between individuals. In other words, the person or persons claimed to be responsible for the tort are sued for damages. Tort liability almost always is based on fault, which is something that was done incorrectly (an unreasonable act of commission) or something that should have been done but was not (act of omission).

Torts may be classified as unintentional or intentional.

Unintentional Torts

Negligence and malpractice are examples of unintentional torts that may occur in the health care setting. **Negligence** is misconduct or practice that is below the standard expected of an ordinary, reasonable, and prudent person. Such conduct places another person at risk for harm. Both nonmedical and professional persons can be liable for negligent acts. **Gross negligence** involves extreme lack of knowledge, skill, or decision making that the person clearly should have known would put others at risk for harm. **Malpractice** is "professional negligence," that is, negligence that occurred while the person was performing as a professional. Malpractice applies to physicians, dentists, lawyers, and generally includes nurses. Six elements must be present for a case of nursing malpractice to be proven.

- **Duty.** The nurse must have (or should have had) a relationship with the client that involves providing care and following an acceptable standard of care. Such duty, for example, is evident when the nurse has been assigned to care for a client in the home or hospital. A nurse also has a general duty of care, even if not specifically assigned to a client, and if the client needs help.

> **► CLINICAL ALERT**   *It is a nurse's duty to respond to all clients' call lights, not just those of assigned client(s).* ■

- **Breach of duty.** There must be a standard of care that is expected in the specific situation but that the nurse did not observe. For example, something was done that should not have been done or nothing was done when it should have been done. This is the failure to act as a reasonable, prudent nurse under the circumstances. The standard can come from documents published by national or professional organizations, boards of nursing, institutional policies and procedures, or textbooks or journals, or it may be stated by expert witnesses.
- **Foreseeability.** A link must exist between the nurse's act and the injury suffered.
- **Causation.** It must be proved that the harm occurred as a direct result of the nurse's failure to follow the standard of care and the nurse could have (or should have) known that failure to follow the standard of care could result in such harm.

- **Harm or injury.** The client or plaintiff must demonstrate some type of harm or injury (physical, financial, or emotional) as a result of the breach of duty owed the client. The plaintiff will be asked to document physical injury, medical costs, loss of wages, "pain and suffering," and any other damages.
- **Damages.** If malpractice caused the injury, the nurse is held liable for damages that may be compensated. The goal of awarding damages is to assist the injured party to his or her original position so far as financially possible (Guido, 2001).

> ➤ **CLINICAL ALERT** *The best defense against a malpractice claim is to know your nursing responsibilities and the scope of practice of members of your health team (e.g., LPN/LVN, UAP).* ■

Several legal doctrines are related to negligence. One such doctrine is *respondeat superior.* A lawsuit for a negligent act performed by a nurse will also name the nurse's employer. In addition, employers may be held liable for negligence if they fail to provide adequate human and material resources for nursing care, fail to properly educate nurses on the use of new equipment or procedures, or fail to orient nurses to the facility. Another doctrine is *res ipsa loquitur* ("the thing speaks for itself"). In some cases, the harm cannot be traced to a specific health care provider or standard but does not normally occur unless there has been a negligent act. An example is harm that results when surgical instruments or bandages are accidentally left in a client during surgery.

To defend against a malpractice lawsuit, the nurse must prove that one or more of the required elements is not met. There is also a limit to the amount of time that can pass between recognition of harm and the bringing of a suit. This is referred to as the statute of limitations. The exact time limitation varies by type of suit and state but typically plaintiffs have 1 to 2 years from the time that they knew of the injury or had reason to believe that an injury was sustained to file a malpractice lawsuit. In some cases, an additional defense is "contributory or comparative negligence" on the part of the injured client. In these situations, the client was at least partly responsible for his or her own injury. When clients choose not to follow health care advice, such as remaining in bed while recovering from a treatment, the court may reduce any verdict against the nurse by an amount considered to be the plaintiff's own contribution.

To avoid charges of malpractice, nurses must recognize those nursing situations in which negligent actions are most likely to occur and to take measures to prevent them (see Box 4–4). The most common situation is the *medication error.* Because of the large number of medications on the market today and the variety of methods of administration, these errors may be on the increase. Nursing errors include failing to read the medication label, misreading or incorrectly calculating the dosage, failing to correctly identify the client, preparing the wrong concentration, or administering a medication by the wrong route (e.g., intravenously instead of intramuscularly). Some medication errors are very serious and can result in death. For example, administering dicumarol, an anticoagu-

---

BOX 4–4 ■ Basic Nursing Care Errors Resulting in Malpractice

Assessment Errors
Failing to

- Assess whether a client is unsteady on his feet
- Recognize the significance of certain information (e.g., laboratory values, vital signs)
- Monitor clients who are using equipment

Planning Errors
Failing to

- Be aware of the client's medications and knowing whether drowsiness or impaired judgment are potential adverse effects
- Bring questionable orders or protocols to the attention of the physician and the supervisor
- Give discharge instructions that the client understands

Intervention Errors
Failing to

- Document all nursing interventions
- Understand the medications being administered
- Always monitor the client as the condition warrants and as ordered
- Document the frequency of client monitoring and client status
- Promptly bring distressing symptoms and changes in client status to the attention of the physician
- Document the time and content of all telephone conversations with the physician

Note: From "Seven Common Legal Pitfalls in Nursing," by T. R. Eskreis, 1998, *American Journal of Nursing, 98*(4), pp. 34–40. Adapted with permission.

---

lant, to a client recently returned from surgery could cause the client to have a hemorrhage. Nurses always must check medications very carefully. Even after checking, the nurse is wise to recheck the medication order and the medication before administering it if the client states, for example, "I did not have a green pill before."

> ➤ **CLINICAL ALERT** *To be a client advocate, you must know about the medications being administered. Know why the client is receiving the medication, the dosage range, possible adverse effects, toxicity levels, and contraindications.* ■

A relatively frequent malpractice action attributed to nurses is *burning a client.* Hot water bottles, heating pads, and solutions that are too hot for application may cause burns. Elderly, comatose, or diabetic people are particularly vulnerable to burns because of their decreased sensitivity to pain and temperature. Hot objects can burn these people before they notice it. A nurse may also be held negligent for leaving a client without taking precautions (giving warnings or providing protections), for example, when using a steam vaporizer.

Clients often fall accidentally, sometimes with resultant injury. Some falls can be prevented by elevating the side rails on the cribs, beds, and stretchers of babies and small children and, when necessary, of adults. If a nurse leaves the rails down or leaves a baby unattended on a bath table, that nurse is guilty of malpractice if the client falls and is injured as a direct result. Most hospitals and nursing homes have policies regarding the use of safety devices such as side rails and restraints. The nurse needs to be familiar with these policies and to take indicated precautions to prevent accidents (see Chapter 30). 🔗

> ► **CLINICAL ALERT**   *Assess clients for fall potential. Document all nursing measures taken to protect the client (e.g., instructed client on how to use the call light).* ■

In some instances, ignoring a client's complaints can constitute malpractice. This type of malpractice is termed *failure to observe and take appropriate action.* The nurse who does not report a client's complaint of acute abdominal pain is negligent and may be found guilty of malpractice if ensuing appendix rupture and death occur. By failing to take the blood pressure and pulse and to check the dressing of a client who has just had abdominal surgery, a nurse omits important assessments. If the client hemorrhages and dies, the nurse may be held responsible for the death as a result of this malpractice.

> ► **CLINICAL ALERT**   *Monitor both physical and psychosocial status of the client. Document observations and interventions.* ■

Incorrectly identifying clients is a problem, particularly in busy hospital units. Unfortunate occurrences, such as removal of a healthy gallbladder from the wrong person, have resulted from nurses' preparing the wrong client for surgery. Cases of *mistaken identity* are costly to the client and render the nurse liable for malpractice.

Intentional Torts

Several differences distinguish unintentional torts from intentional torts. Unintentional torts (e.g., negligence, malpractice) do not require intent but do require the element of harm. In contrast, with intentional torts, the defendant executed the act on purpose or with intent. No harm need be caused by intentional torts for liability to exist. Also, since no standard is involved, no expert witnesses are needed. Four intentional torts related to nursing will be discussed: assault/battery, false imprisonment, invasion of privacy, and defamation (libel/slander). Figure 4–3 ■ provides an overview of the types of law in nursing.

The terms *assault* and *battery* are often heard together, but each has its own meaning. **Assault** can be described as an attempt or threat to touch another person unjustifiably. Assault precedes battery; it is the act that causes the person to believe a battery is about to occur. For example, the person who threatens someone by making a menacing gesture with a club or a closed fist is guilty of assault. In nursing, a nurse who threatens a client with an injection after the client refuses to take the medication orally would be committing assault.

Battery is the willful touching of a person (or the person's clothes or even something the person is carrying) that may or may not cause harm. To be actionable at law, however, the touching must be wrong in some way; for example, touching done without permission, that is embarrassing, or that causes injury. In the previous example, if the nurse followed through on the threat and gave the injection without the client's consent, the nurse would be committing battery. Liability applies even though the physician ordered the medication or the activity and even if the client benefits from the nurse's action.

Consent is required before procedures are performed. Battery exists when there is no consent, even if the plaintiff was not asked for consent. Unless there is implied consent, such as in life-threatening emergencies, a procedure performed on an unconscious client without informed consent is battery. Another requirement for consent is that the client be competent to give consent. It can be very difficult to determine if clients who are elderly, who have specific mental disorders, or who take particular medications are competent to agree to treatments. If the nurse is uncertain whether a client refusing a treatment is competent, the supervisor and physician should be consulted so that ethical treatment that does not constitute battery can be provided. Determination of competency is not a medical decision; it is one made through court hearings.

False imprisonment is the "unjustifiable detention of a person without legal warrant to confine the person" (Guido, 2001, p. 98). False imprisonment accompanied by forceful restraint or threat of restraint is battery.

Although nurses may suggest under certain circumstances that a client remain in the hospital room or in bed, the client must not be detained against the client's will. The client has a right to insist on leaving even though it may be detrimental to health. In this instance, the client can leave by signing an AWA (absence without authority) or AMA (against medical advice) form. As with assault or battery, client competency is a factor in determining whether there is a case of false imprisonment or a situation of protecting a client from injury. To guide nurses in such dilemmas, agencies usually have clear policies regarding the application of restraints (see Chapter 30). 🔗

Invasion of privacy is a direct wrong of a personal nature. It injures the feelings of the person and does not take into account the effect of revealed information on the standing of the person in the community. The right to privacy is the right of individuals to withhold themselves and their lives from public scrutiny. It can also be described as the right to be left alone. Liability can result if the nurse breaches confidentiality by passing along confidential client information to others or intrudes into the client's private domain.

In this context, there is a delicate balance between the need of a number of people to contribute to the diagnosis and treatment of a client and the client's right to confidentiality. In most situations, necessary discussion about a client's medical condition is considered appropriate, but unnecessary discussions and gossip are considered a breach of confidentiality. Necessary discussion involves only those engaged in the client's care.

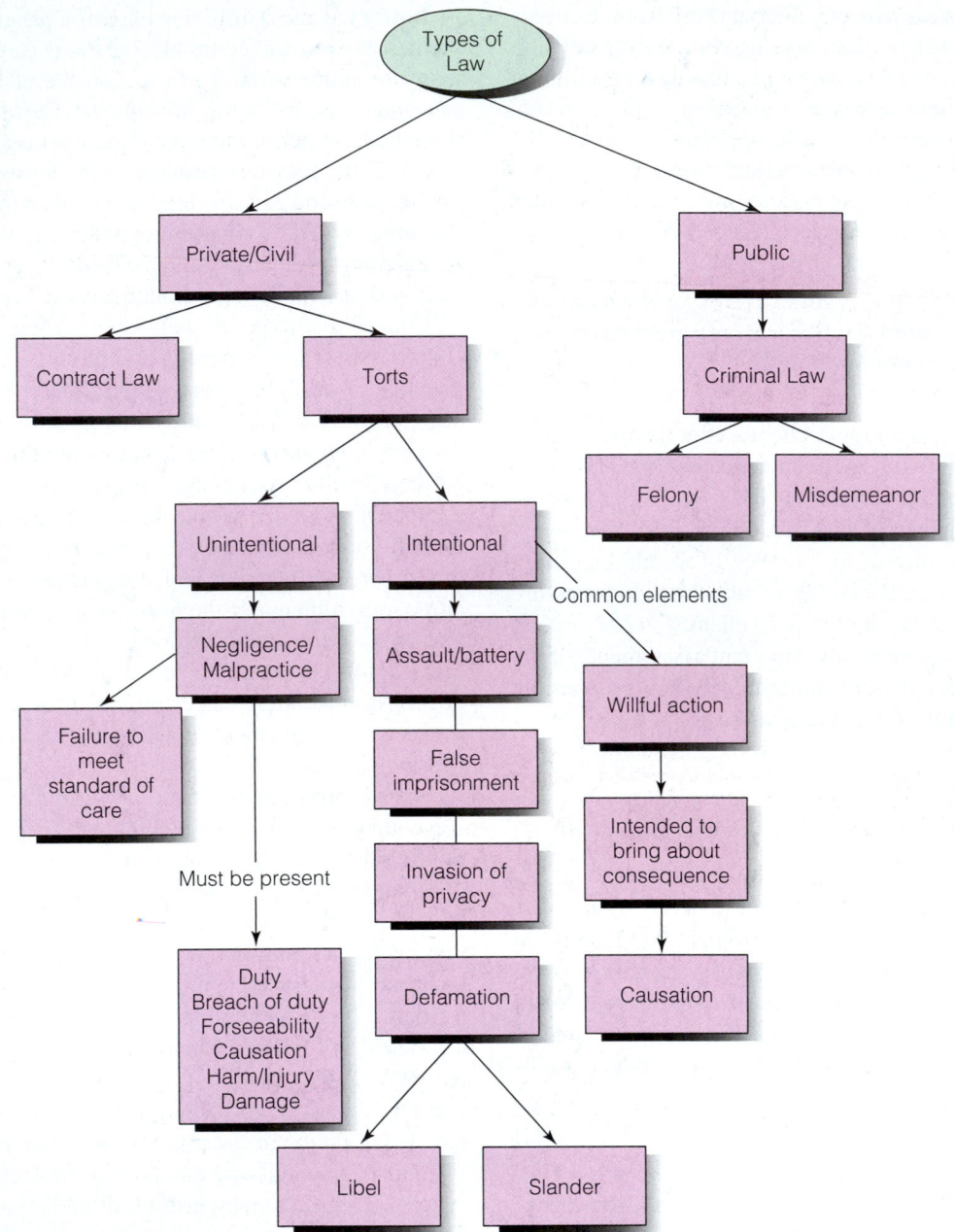

Figure 4–3 ■ An overview of the types of law in nursing practice.

> ➤ **CLINICAL ALERT**   *Never discuss client situations in the elevator, cafeteria, or other public areas.* ■

Most jurisdictions of the country have a variety of statutes that impose a duty to report certain confidential client information. Four major categories are (a) vital statistics, such as births and deaths; (b) infections and communicable diseases, such as diphtheria, syphilis, and typhoid fever; (c) child or elder abuse; and (d) violent incidents, such as gunshot wounds and knife wounds.

The client must be protected from four types of invasion:

- *Use of the client's name or likeness for profit, without consent.* This refers to use of identifiable photographs or names

such as advertising for the health care agency or provider without the client's permission.

- *Unreasonable intrusion.* Observation of client care (such as by nursing students) or taking of photographs for any purpose without the client's consent.
- *Public disclosure of private facts.* Private information is given to others who have no legitimate need for that information.
- *Putting a person in a false light.* This type of invasion involves publishing information that is normally considered offensive but which is not true.

Defamation is communication that is false, or made with a careless disregard for the truth, and results in injury to the reputation of a person. Both libel and slander are wrongful actions that come under the heading of defamation. **Libel** is defamation by means of print, writing, or pictures. Writing in the nurse's notes that a physician is incompetent because he didn't respond immediately to a call is an example of libel. **Slander** is defamation by the spoken word, stating unprivileged (not legally protected) or false words by which a reputation is damaged. An example of slander would be for the nurse to tell a client that another nurse is incompetent.

Only the person defamed may bring the lawsuit. The defamatory material must be communicated to a third party such that the person's reputation may be harmed. For example, a comment made in private criticizing that person's competence is not defamation since a third party did not hear it.

Nurses have a qualified privilege to make statements that could be considered defamatory, but only as a part of nursing practice and only to a physician or another health team member caring directly for the client. The communication must be made in good faith with the intent to protect the quality of client care.

Loss of Client Property

Loss of client property, such as jewelry, money, eyeglasses, and dentures, is a constant concern to hospital personnel. Today, agencies are taking less responsibility for property and are generally requesting clients to sign a waiver on admission relieving the hospital and its employees of any responsibility for property. Situations arise, however, in which the client cannot sign a waiver and the nursing staff must follow prescribed policies for safeguarding the client's property. Nurses are expected to take reasonable precautions to safeguard a client's property, and they can be held liable for its loss or damage if they do not exercise reasonable care.

Unprofessional Conduct

According to most nurse practice acts, unprofessional conduct is considered one of the grounds for action against the nurse's license. **Unprofessional conduct** includes incompetence or gross negligence, conviction for practicing without a license, falsification of client records, and illegally obtaining, using, or possessing controlled substances. Having a personal relationship with a client, especially a vulnerable client, may be considered unprofessional conduct because the *Code of Ethics for Nurses* states that nurses are responsible for retaining their professional boundaries (ANA, 2001, p.11). Certain acts may constitute a tort or crime in addition to being unprofessional conduct.

Unethical conduct may also be addressed in nurse practice acts. Unethical conduct includes violation of professional ethical codes, breach of confidentiality, fraud, or refusing to care for clients of specific socioeconomic or cultural origins (see Chapter 5). ∞

Nurses, at all levels of nursing practice, can be reported to national data banks. The Healthcare Integrity and Protection Data Bank (HIPDB) was created for the reporting of civil judgments or criminal convictions related to health care and licensure or certification actions (Sloan, 2001). Another data bank, the National Practitioner Data Bank (NPDB), was established to identify incompetent and unprofessional health care practitioners. The information in these two data banks is not accessible by the public. It can be accessed, however, by state licensing boards, HMOs, hospitals, and professional organizations. The data banks are examples of a nationwide effort to protect the public and to identify and track professionals found liable of malpractice or actions taken against their license.

LEGAL PROTECTIONS IN NURSING PRACTICE

Laws and strategies are in place to protect the nurse against litigation. Good Samaritan acts are an example of laws designed to help protect nurses when assisting at the scene of an accident. Providing safe, competent practice by following the nurse practice act and standards of practice is a major legal safeguard for nurses. Accurate and complete documentation is also a critical component of legal protection for the nurse.

Good Samaritan Acts

Good Samaritan acts are laws designed to protect health care providers who provide assistance at the scene of an emergency against claims of malpractice unless it can be shown that there was a gross departure from the normal standard of care or willful wrongdoing on their part. Gross negligence usually involves further injury or harm to the person. For example, an automobile may strike an injured child left on the side of the road when the nurse leaves to obtain help.

Most state statutes do not require citizens to render aid to people in distress. Such assistance is considered more of an ethical than a legal duty. To encourage citizens to be Good Samaritans, most states have now enacted legislation releasing a Good Samaritan from legal liability for injuries caused under such circumstances, even if the injuries resulted from negligence of the person offering emergency aid. It is important, however, to check your state's statute since some states (e.g., Vermont) require people to stop and aid persons in danger.

It is generally believed that a person who renders help in an emergency, at a level that would be provided by any reasonably prudent person under similar circumstances, cannot be held liable. The same reasoning applies to nurses, who are among the people best prepared to help at the scene of an accident. If the level of care a nurse provides is of the caliber that would have been provided by any other nurse, then the nurse will not be held liable.

Guidelines for nurses who choose to render emergency care are as follows:

- Limit actions to those normally considered first aid, if possible.
- Do not perform actions that you do not know how to do.
- Offer assistance, but do not insist.
- Have someone call or go for additional help.
- Do not leave the scene until the injured person leaves or another qualified person takes over.
- Do not accept any compensation.

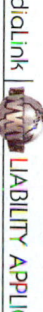

MediaLink | LIABILITY APPLICATION

Professional Liability Insurance

Because of the increase in the number of malpractice lawsuits against health professionals, nurses are advised to carry their own liability insurance. Most hospitals have liability insurance that covers all employees, including all nurses. However, some smaller facilities, such as walk-in clinics, may not. Thus, the nurse should always check with the employer at the time of hiring to see what coverage the facility provides. A physician or a hospital can be sued because of the negligent conduct of a nurse, and the nurse can also be sued and held liable for negligence or malpractice. Because hospitals have been known to countersue nurses when they have been found negligent and the hospital was required to pay, nurses are advised to provide their own insurance coverage and not rely on hospital-provided insurance.

Additionally, nurses often provide nursing services outside of employment-related activities, such as being available for first aid at childrens' sport or social activities or providing health screening and education at health fairs. Neighbors or friends may seek advice about illnesses or treatment for themselves or family members. In the latter situation, the nurse may be tempted to give advice; however, it is always advisable for the nurse to refer the friend or neighbor to their family physician. The nurse may be protected from liability under Good Samaritan acts when nursing service is volunteered; however, if the nurse receives any compensation or if there is a written or verbal agreement outlining the nurse's responsibility to the group, the nurse needs liability coverage for legal expenses in the event that the nurse is sued.

Liability insurance coverage usually defrays all costs of defending a nurse, including the costs of retaining an attorney. The insurance also covers all costs incurred by the nurse up to the face value of the policy, including a settlement made out of court. In return, the insurance company may have the right to make the decisions about the claim and the settlement.

Nursing faculty and nursing students are also vulnerable to lawsuits. Students and teachers of nursing employed by community colleges and universities are not likely to be covered by the insurance carried by hospitals and health agencies. It is advisable for nursing students to check with their school about the coverage that applies to them. Increasingly, faculty carry their own malpractice insurance. Liability insurance can be obtained through the ANA or private insurance companies. Nursing students can also obtain insurance through the National Student Nurses' Association. In some states, hospitals do not allow nursing students to provide nursing care without liability insurance.

Carrying Out a Physician's Orders

Nurses are expected to analyze procedures and medications ordered by the physician. It is the nurse's responsibility to seek clarification of ambiguous or seemingly erroneous orders from the prescribing physician. Clarification from any other source is unacceptable and regarded as a departure from competent nursing practice.

If the order is neither ambiguous nor apparently erroneous, the nurse is responsible for carrying it out. For example, if the physician orders oxygen to be administered at 4 liters per minute, the nurse must administer oxygen at that rate, and not at 2 or 6 liters per minute. If the orders state that the client is not to have solid food after a bowel resection, the nurse must ensure that no solid food is given to the client.

There are several categories of orders that nurses must question to protect themselves legally:

- *Question any order a client questions.* For example, if a client who has been receiving an intramuscular injection tells the nurse that the doctor changed the order from an injectable to an oral medication, the nurse must recheck the order before giving the medication.
- *Question any order if the client's condition has changed.* The nurse is considered responsible for notifying the physician of any significant changes in the client's condition, whether the physician requests notification or not. For example, if a client who is receiving an intravenous infusion suddenly develops a rapid pulse, chest pain, and a cough, the nurse must notify the physician immediately and question continuance of the ordered rate of infusion. If a client who is receiving morphine for pain develops severely depressed respirations, the nurse must withhold the medication and notify the physician.
- *Question and record verbal orders to avoid miscommunications.* In addition to recording the time, the date, the physician's name, and the orders, the nurse documents the circumstances that occasioned the call to the physician, reads the orders back to the physician, and documents that the physician confirmed the orders as the nurse read them back.
- *Question any order that is illegible, unclear, or incomplete.* Misinterpretations in the name of a drug or in dose, for example, can easily occur with handwritten orders. The nurse is responsible for ensuring that the order is interpreted the way it was intended and that it is a safe and appropriate order.

Providing Competent Nursing Care

Competent practice is a major legal safeguard for nurses. Nurses need to provide care that is within the legal boundaries of their practice and within the boundaries of agency policies and procedures. Nurses therefore must be familiar with their various job descriptions, which may be different from agency to agency. Every nurse is responsible for ensuring that his or her education and experience are adequate to meet the responsibilities delineated in the job description.

Competency also involves care that protects clients from harm. Nurses need to anticipate sources of client injury, educate clients about hazards, and implement measures to prevent injury.

Application of the nursing process is another essential aspect of providing safe and effective client care. Clients need to be assessed and monitored appropriately and involved in care decisions. All assessments and care must be documented accurately. Effective communication can also protect the nurse from negligence claims. Nurses need to approach every client with sincere concern and include the client in conversations. In addition, nurses should always acknowledge when they do not

Practice Guidelines
Legal Protection for Nurses

- Function within the scope of your education, job description, and nurse practice act.
- Follow the procedures and policies of the employing agency.
- Build and maintain good rapport with clients.
- Always check the identity of a client to make sure it is the right client.
- Observe and monitor the client accurately. Communicate and record significant changes in the client's condition to the physician.
- Promptly and accurately document all assessments and care given.
- Be alert when implementing nursing interventions and give each task your full attention and skill.
- Perform procedures correctly and appropriately.
- Make sure the correct medications are given in the correct dose, by the right route, at the scheduled time, and to the right client.
- When delegating nursing responsibilities, make sure that the person who is delegated a task understands what to do and that the person has the required knowledge and skill.
- Protect clients from injury.
- Report all incidents involving clients.
- Always check any order that a client questions.
- Know your own strengths and weaknesses. Ask for assistance and supervision in situations for which you feel inadequately prepared.
- Maintain your clinical competence. For students, this demands study and practice before caring for clients. For graduate nurses, it means continued study to maintain and update clinical knowledge and skills.

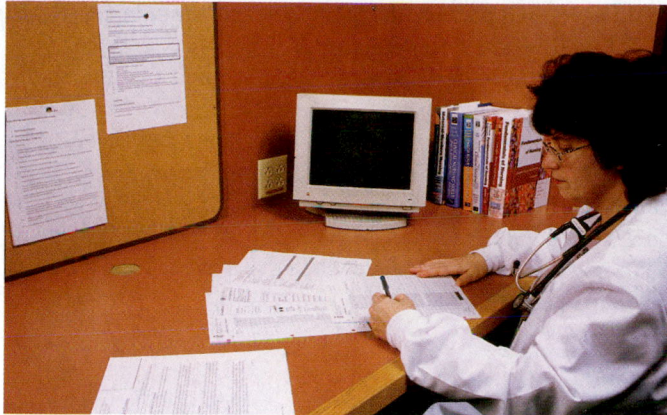

Figure 4–4 ■ Clear and accurate documentation is the nurse's best defense against potential liability.

know the answer to a client's questions, telling the client they will find out the answer and then follow through.

Methods of legal protection are summarized in the accompanying Practice Guidelines.

Record Keeping

The client's medical record is a legal document and can be produced in court as evidence. Often, the record is used to remind a witness of events surrounding a lawsuit, because several months or years usually elapse before the suit goes to trial. The effectiveness of a witness's testimony can depend on the accuracy of such records. Nurses, therefore, need to keep accurate and complete records of nursing care provided to clients. Failure to keep proper records can constitute negligence and be the basis for tort liability. Insufficient or inaccurate assessments and documentation can hinder proper diagnosis and treatment and result in injury to the client (see Figure 4–4 ■). See Chapter 20 🔗 for types of records and facts about recording.

The Incident Report

An incident report (also called an unusual occurrence report) is an agency record of an accident or unusual occurrence. Incident reports are used to make all the facts available to agency personnel, to contribute to statistical data about accidents or incidents, and to help health personnel prevent future incidents or accidents. All accidents are usually reported on incident forms. Some agencies also report other incidents, such as the occurrence of client infection or the loss of personal effects.

The nurse includes the following information in an incident report:

- Identify the client by name, initials, and hospital or identification number.
- Give the date, time, and place of the incident.
- Describe the facts of the incident. Avoid any conclusions or blame. Describe the incident as you saw it even if your impressions differ from those of others.
- Incorporate the client's account of the incident. State the client's comments by using direct quotes.
- Identify all witnesses to the incident.
- Identify any equipment by number and any medication by name and dosage.

The report should be completed as soon as possible and filed according to agency policy. Because incident reports are not part of the client's medical record, the facts of the incident should also be noted in the medical record. Do not record in the client record that an incident report has been completed because the facts are already documented in the chart. The purpose of the report form is to alert the risk manager to the event.

The person who identifies that the incident occurred should complete the incident report. This may not be the same person actually involved with the incident. For example, the nurse who discovers that an incorrect medication has been administered completes the form even if it was another nurse who administered the medication. In addition, all witnesses to an incident, such as a client fall, are listed on the incident form even if they were not directly involved.

Incident reports are often reviewed by an agency risk management committee, which decides whether to investigate the incident further. Nurses may be required to answer such questions as what they believe precipitated the accident, how it could have been prevented, and whether any equipment should be adjusted.

When an accident occurs, the nurse should first assess the client and intervene to prevent injury. If a client is injured, nurses must take steps to protect the client, themselves, and their employer. Most agencies have policies regarding accidents. It is important to follow these policies and not to assume one is negligent. Although negligence may be involved, accidents can and do happen even when every precaution has been taken to prevent them.

REPORTING CRIMES, TORTS, AND UNSAFE PRACTICES

Nurses may need to report nursing colleagues or other health professionals for practices that endanger the health and safety of clients. For instance, alcohol and drug use, theft from a client or agency, and unsafe nursing practice should be reported. Reporting a colleague is not easy. The person reporting may feel disloyal, incur the disapproval of others, or perceive chances for promotion are endangered. When reporting an incident or series of incidents, the nurse must be careful to describe observed behavior only and not make inferences as to what might be happening.

Guidelines for reporting a crime, tort, or unsafe practice include these:

- Write a clear description of the situation you believe you should report.
- Make sure that your statements are factual and complete.
- Make sure you are credible.
- Obtain support from at least one trustworthy person before filing the report.
- Report the matter starting at the lowest possible level in the agency hierarchy.
- Assume responsibility for reporting the individual by being open about it. Sign your name to the letter.
- See the problem through once you have reported it.

Reporting these events is referred to as "whistle-blowing." Many states have laws that prevent wrongful termination of whistle-blowers by employers. In some states, it is mandatory for a nurse with knowledge of unprofessional conduct to report that behavior to the state board of nursing. In addition, reporting illegal, unethical, or incompetent performance is an expectation found in the ANA code of ethics.

LEGAL RESPONSIBILITIES OF STUDENTS

Nursing students are responsible for their own actions and liable for their own acts of negligence committed during the course of clinical experiences. When they perform duties that are within the scope of professional nursing, such as administering an injection, they are legally held to the same standard of skill and competence as a registered professional nurse. Lower standards are not applied to the actions of nursing students.

► **CLINICAL ALERT**   *Students do not practice on their instructor's or another nurse's license. Each nurse and nursing student is responsible and accountable for providing safe client care.* ■

In cases arising from negligent acts by nursing students, the student has traditionally been treated as an employee of the hospital, which was held liable under the doctrine of *respondeat superior*. Today, associate degree and baccalaureate nursing students are not usually considered employees of the agencies in which they receive clinical experience because these nursing programs contract with agencies to provide clinical experiences for students. In cases of negligence involving such students, the hospital or agency (e.g., public health agency) and the educational institution will be held potentially liable for negligent actions by students. Some nursing schools require students to carry individual professional liability insurance.

Nursing students need to be aware that most state boards of nursing require a reporting of prior criminal history when applying for licensure. A person with past felony and some misdemeanor offenses may be denied licensure even though that individual graduated from an approved nursing program. Nursing students who are unsure of their personal situation are advised to contact their state board of nursing for more information.

Students in clinical situations must be assigned learning experiences within their capabilities and be given reasonable guidance and supervision. Nursing instructors are responsible for assigning students to the care of clients and for providing reasonable supervision. Failure to provide reasonable supervision or the assignment of a client to a student who is not prepared and competent can be a basis for liability.

To fulfill responsibilities to clients and to minimize chances for liability, nursing students need to:

- Make sure they are prepared to carry out the necessary care for assigned clients.
- Ask for additional help or supervision in situations for which they feel inadequately prepared.
- Comply with the policies of the agency in which they obtain their clinical experience.
- Comply with the policies and definitions of responsibility supplied by the school of nursing.

Students who work as part-time or temporary nursing assistants or aides must also remember that legally they can perform only those tasks that appear in the job description of a nurse's aide or assistant. Even though a student may have received instruction and acquired competence in administering injections or suctioning a tracheostomy tube, the student cannot legally perform these tasks while employed as an aide or assistant. While acting as a paid employee, the student is covered for negligent acts by the employer, not the school of nursing.

Lifespan Considerations

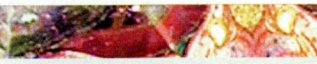

Legal issues such as self-determination and advance directives are discussed in Chapter 41. These issues relate to persons making health care decisions for themselves, or appointing someone to make decisions for them, if they become unable to do so.

The Omnibus Budget Reconciliation Act (OBRA) was passed in 1990 and lists requirements for ensuring quality of care in skilled nursing facilities. These requirements mainly affect elders, but also pertain to any resident in a long-term or skilled nursing facility. These standards were developed to enhance the quality of life of each resident and to focus on achieving the highest practical physical, mental, and psychosocial well-being for residents of these facilities. Some of the important requirements from OBRA are summarized below:

- A quality assessment and assurance committee must meet at least quarterly to discuss the resident's condition and make appropriate revisions.

- A physician is to visit every 30 days for 3 months, and then every 90 days.
- The facility must employ a registered nurse who works there 40 hours a week.
- Rehabilitation services and activities must be available for each resident.
- Nurse aides must have special training and also be given information concerning abuse and neglect.
- Social work requirements were increased.
- The use of psychotropic drugs is strictly monitored and reevaluated at regular intervals. Documentation of behaviors is required to support the need for prescribing these drugs.
- Residents' rights must be recognized and honored.

Focus on Critical Thinking

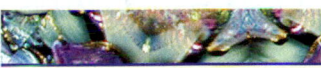

A female adult client, who has been blind since birth, is admitted to the surgical unit. She is to have surgery the next morning. The physician has written an order for the client to sign the surgical consent form. The husband is in the client's room when the nurse approaches the client to sign the consent form. The husband says that he will sign for his wife.

1. What question(s) should the nurse be asking before addressing the signing of the form?

2. Can someone who is blind give consent?
3. How can the nurse ensure that the client is aware of what she is signing?
4. What else should the nurse consider when obtaining a signature?
5. What would the nurse include in the documentation?

See Critical Thinking Possibilities in Appendix A.

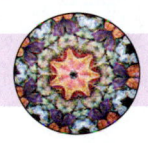 | Chapter Review

EXPLORE MediaLink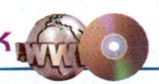

NCLEX review questions, case studies, MediaLink applications, and other interactive resources for this chapter can be found on the Companion Website at www.prenhall.com/kozier. Click on Chapter 4 to select the activities for this chapter.

For more NCLEX review questions, and an audio glossary, access the Student CD-ROM accompanying this textbook.

Chapter Highlights

- Accountability is an essential concept of professional nursing practice under the law.
- Nurses need to understand laws that regulate and affect nursing practice to ensure that the nurses' actions are consistent with current legal principles and to protect the nurse from liability.

- Nurse practice acts legally define and describe the scope of nursing practice that the law seeks to regulate.
- Competence in nursing practice is determined and maintained by various credentialing methods, such as licensure, certification, and accreditation, that protect the public's welfare and safety.

- Standards of practice published by national and state nursing associations, agency policies and procedures, and job descriptions further delineate the scope of a nurse's practice.
- The nurse has specific legal obligations and responsibilities to clients and employers. As a citizen, the nurse has the rights and responsibilities shared by all individuals in the society.
- Collective bargaining is one way nurses can improve their working conditions and economic welfare.
- Informed consent implies that (a) the consent was given voluntarily, (b) the client was of age and had the capacity and competency to understand, and (c) the client was given enough information on which to make an informed decision.
- The Americans with Disabilities Act of 1990 prohibits discrimination on the basis of disability in employment, public services, and public accommodations. Nurses need to know how the ADA affects nursing practice.
- Chemical dependence in health care workers is a problem, in part, because of the high levels of stress involved in many health care settings and the easy access to addictive drugs. Chemical impairment includes abuse of alcohol and addictive drugs. The nurse needs to know the proper reporting of nursing colleagues whose practice is chemically impaired.
- Nurse malpractice, an unintentional tort, can be established when the following criteria are met: (a) the nurse (defendant) owed a duty to the client, (b) the nurse failed to carry out that duty according to standards, (c) foreseeability of harm, (d) causation, where the client's injury was caused by the nurse's failure to follow the standard, and (e) the client (plaintiff) was injured. The nurse is liable for damages that may be compensated.
- Nurses can be held liable for intentional torts, such as assault and battery, false imprisonment, invasion of privacy, and defamation.
- Good Samaritan acts protect health professionals from claims of malpractice when they offer assistance at the scene of an emergency, provided that there is no willful wrongdoing or gross departure from normal standards of care.
- Nursing students and practicing nurses can obtain professional liability insurance through professional nursing associations.
- When a client is accidentally injured or involved in an unusual situation, the nurse's first responsibility is to take steps to protect the client and then to notify appropriate agency personnel.
- Nursing students are held to the same standard as licensed nurses and, therefore, need to make certain that they are prepared to provide the necessary care to assigned clients. It is important that students ask for help or supervision in situations for which they feel inadequately prepared.

Review Questions

4–1. You were not present when the physician discussed a surgical procedure with the client. The doctor's orders indicate that the consent form needs to be signed. Which statement *best* reflects the nurse being an advocate for the client?
   a. "The doctor has asked that you sign this consent form."
   b. "Do you have any questions about the procedure?"
   c. "What were you told about the procedure you are going to have?"
   d. "Remember that you can change your mind and cancel the procedure."

4–2. A nurse inserts a nasogastric tube even though the client refused the procedure. The nurse told the client "this tube is necessary in order for you to feel better." In spite of the nurse's good intention, the nurse is liable for:
   a. an unintentional tort
   b. assault
   c. invasion of privacy
   d. battery

4–3. The nurse is to give a medication she has not given before. When checking the drug handbook, she reads that the ordered amount is an unusually large dose. A nurse who is aware of nursing liability would do which of the following actions?

   a. Give the medication.
   b. Call the physician.
   c. Call the pharmacist.
   d. Not give the medication.

4–4. The nurse gives two pills instead of the ordered one pill. The physician is notified. The client is carefully monitored and no untoward effects happen. Can the client sue the nurse for malpractice?
   a. No, the client was not harmed.
   b. No, the nurse notified the physician.
   c. Yes, a breach of duty exists.
   d. Yes, foreseeability is present.

4–5. A nursing student is employed and working as a UAP on a busy surgical unit. The nurses know that the UAP is enrolled in a nursing program and will be graduating soon. A nurse asks the UAP if he has performed a urinary catheterization on clients while in the nursing program. When the UAP says "Yes," the nurse asks him to help her out by doing a urinary catheterization on a postsurgical client. What is the best response by the UAP?
   a. "Let me get permission from the client first."
   b. "Sure. Which client is it?"
   c. "I can't do it unless you supervise me."
   d. "I can't do it. Is there something else I can help you with?"

Readings and References

Suggested Readings

Crow, K., Matheson, L., & Steed, A. (2000). Informed consent and truth-telling. Cultural directions for healthcare providers. *Journal of Nursing Administration, 30*(3), 148–152. Providing culturally sensitive nursing care includes understanding that there are different approaches to truth telling. The U.S. health care model emphasizes the individual's right to know and to make their own health care decisions, and health care providers have a duty to give all information—to "tell the truth." Conflicts occur, however, when the client is from a cultural group that holds a group-oriented worldview. The authors present three case studies involving group-oriented persons or families and how they responded to informed consent provided by health care providers with individual-oriented perspectives.

Sloan, A., & Vernarec, E. (2001). Impaired nurses: Reclaiming careers. *RN, 64*(2), 58–63. Instead of a punitive disciplinary approach that may jeopardize a nurse's license, many state boards of nursing are adopting diversion programs focused on rehabilitation of impaired nurses. The authors describe the general pattern of the programs, the benefit to nurses and the public, and how nurses can get help or help a colleague.

Wilkinson, A. P. (1998). Nursing malpractice. *Nursing, 28*(6), 34–39. This author differentiates malpractice from professional negligence, uses case examples to emphasize essential ways to prevent lawsuits, provides seven reasons nurses can become involved in a malpractice claim, and discusses the two types of liability insurance.

Related Research

Trinkoff, A. M., & Storr, C. L. (1998). Substance use among nurses: Differences between specialties. *Journal of Addictions Nursing, 10*(2), 77–84.

References

American Nurses Association. (1998). *Competencies for telehealth technologies in nursing.* Washington, DC: Author.

American Nurses Association. (2001). *Code of ethics for nurses with interpretive statements.* Washington, DC: Author.

Brent, N. J. (2001). *Nurses and the law* (2nd ed.). Philadelphia: W. B. Saunders.

Crow, K., Matheson, L., & Steed, A. (2000). Informed consent and truth-telling. Cultural directions for healthcare providers. *Journal of Nursing Administration, 30*(3), 148–152.

Dunn, D. (1999). Exploring the gray areas of consent. *Nursing, 29*(7), 41–44.

Equal Employment Opportunity Commission. (2000). Guidelines on discrimination because of sex. (Section 1604.11, Sexual harassment. Code of Federal Regulations, Title 29, Vol. 4). Retrieved February 5, 2003 from http://www.access.gpo.gov/nara/cfr/waisidx_99/29cfr1604_99.html

Eskreis, T. R. (1998). Seven common legal pitfalls in nursing. *American Journal of Nursing, 98*(4), 34–40.

Fisher, M. (2000). Do you have delegation savvy? *Nursing, 30*(12), 58–59.

Grover, S. M., & Floyd, M. R. (1998). Nurses' attitudes toward impaired practice and knowledge of peer assistance programs. *Journal of Addictions Nursing, 10*(2), 70–76.

Guido, G. W. (2001). *Legal and ethical issues in nursing* (3rd ed.). Upper Saddle River, NJ: Prentice Hall.

Harrington, S. (2002). Advanced practitioners build strong foundation. *Nursing Spectrum.* Retrieved January 29, 2003, from http://community.nursingspectrum.com/magazinearticles/article.cfm?aid-7959

Lindsay, C. (2001). Interstate compact opens new opportunities. *Spectrum, West Region, Metro Edition, 2*(8), 10.

Monarch, K. (2000). Workplace rights: Protect yourself from sexual harassment. *American Journal of Nursing, 100*(5), 75.

National Council of State Boards of Nursing. (1995). Delegation concepts and decision-making process. Retrieved February 3, 2003, from http://www.ncsbn.org/public/regulation/delegation_documents_delegati.htm#definiti

Sheehan, J. P. (2001). Legally speaking: Delegating to UAPs—a practical guide. *RN, 64*(11), 65–66.

Sloan, A. (2001). Legally speaking: The national data bank nurses need to know about. *RN, 64*(7), 65–69.

Sullivan, G. H. (1998). Legally speaking: Getting informed consent. *RN, 61*(4), 59–62.

Texas Nurses Foundation/Texas Nurses Association. (n.d.). Texas peer assistance program for nurses. Retrieved February 5, 2003, from http://www.texasnurses.org/tpapn/warningsigns.html

Omnibus Budget Reconciliation Act, 42 U.S.C.S. Sec. 1395(i)(3) (2002).

Watson, P. G. (2000). The Americans with Disabilities Act: More rights for people with disabilities. *Rehabilitation Nursing, 25*(4), 145–147.

Wilkinson, A. P. (1998). Nursing malpractice. *Nursing, 28*(6), 34–39.

Selected Bibliography

American Nurses Association. (1997). Position statement: Sexual harassment. Retrieved March 9, 2003, from http://www.nursingworld.org/readroom/position/workplac/wkharass.htm

Boucher, M. A. (1998). Delegation alert. How to delegate effectively while maintaining your nursing presence with patients. *American Journal of Nursing, 98*(2), 26–32.

Bronder, E. (2001). Issues update: Collective bargaining agreements. *American Journal of Nursing, 101*(8), 59–60.

Carson, W. Y. (2001). Nursing malpractice: Protect yourself. *American Journal of Nursing, 101*(12), 81.

Crawford, L. (2001). Regulation of registered nursing: The American perspective. *Reflections on Nursing Leadership, 27*(4), 28–29, 34.

Dempski, K. (2000). Legally speaking: Serving as an expert witness. *RN, 63*(2), 65–68.

Fiesta, J. (1999). Nursing malpractice: Cause for consideration. *Nursing Management, 30*(2), 12–13.

Gaffney, T. (1999, May 31). The regulatory dilemma surrounding interstate practice. *Online Journal of Issues in Nursing, 4*(1), Article 1. Retrieved March 9, 2003, from http://www.nursingworld.org/ojin/topic9/topic9_1.htm

Gassert, C. A. (2000). Telehealth: A challenge to the regulation of multistate practice. *Policy, Politics, & Nursing Practice, 1*(2), 85–92.

Helm, A. (1998). Liability, UAPs, and you. *Nursing, 29*(11), 52–53.

Helm, A., & Kihm, N. C. (2001). Is professional liability insurance for you? Before you say no, weigh these considerations. *Nursing, 31*(1), 48–49.

Hutcherson, C., Sheets, V. R., & Williamson, S. H. (1998). What five regulatory trends mean to you. *Nursing, 28*(5), 54–57.

Hutcherson, C., & Williamson, S. (1999, May 31). Nursing regulation for the new millennium: The mutual recognition model. *Online Journal of Issues in Nursing, 4*(1), Article 2. Retrieved March 9, 2003, from http://www.nursingworld.org/ojin/topic9/topic9_2.htm

Kuther, T. L. (1999). Competency to provide informed consent in older adulthood. *Gerontology & Geriatrics Education, 20*(1), 15–30.

LaDuke, S. (1999). What you should expect from your attorney . . . *Nursing, 29*(6), 62–64.

Laskowski-Jones, L. (1998). Reaching beyond the rules: Understanding—and influencing—your scope of practice. *Nursing, 28*(9), 42–47.

Martin, K., & Cepero, K. (1999). You're being deposed? Remain calm. *Nursing, 29*(3), 60–61.

Nguyen, B. (1999). Workplace protections: When are you protected under the Americans with Disabilities Act? *American Journal of Nursing, 99*(6), 70.

Olsen-Chavarriaga, D. (2000). Informed consent: Do you know your role? *Nursing, 30*(5), 60–61.

Polston, M. D. (1999). Whistleblowing: Does the law protect you? *American Journal of Nursing, 99*(1), 26–31.

Sheehan, J. P. (1998). Legally speaking: Directing UAPs—safely. *RN, 61*(6), 53–55.

Showers, J. L. (2000). What you need to know about negligence lawsuits. *Nursing, 30*(2), 45–48.

Sloan, A. J. (2002). Legally speaking: Whistleblowing: Proceed with caution. *RN, 65*(1), 67–70.

Sosin, J. (2002). Legally speaking: Careful with that equipment. *RN, 65*(2), 59–62.

Spital, J. K. (1999). . . . And what your attorney expects from you. *Nursing, 29*(6), 62–64.

White, G. (2000). Workplace rights: Informed consent. *American Journal of Nursing, 100*(9), 83.

Wilkinson, A. P. (1998). Nursing malpractice. *Nursing, 28*(8), 34–39.

Wysoker, A. (2000). Informed consent: The ultimate right. *Journal of the American Psychiatric Nurses Association, 6*(3), 100–102.

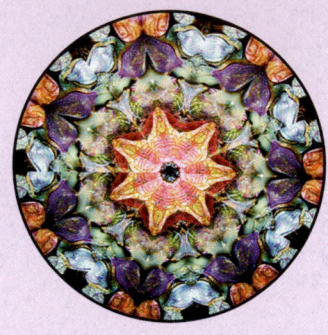

CHAPTER 5

VALUES, ETHICS, AND ADVOCACY

LEARNING OUTCOMES

After completing this chapter, you will be able to:

- Explain how cognitive development, values, moral frameworks, and codes of ethics affect moral decisions.

- Explain how nurses use knowledge of values transmission and values clarification to make ethical decisions and facilitate ethical decision making by clients.

- When presented with an ethical situation, identify the moral issues and principles involved.

- Explain the uses and limitations of professional codes of ethics.

- Discuss common ethical issues currently facing health care professionals.

- Describe ways in which nurses can enhance their ethical decision making and practice.

- Discuss the advocacy role of the nurse.

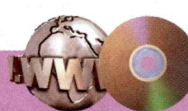

MediaLink

www.prenhall.com/kozier

Additional resources for this chapter can be found on the Student CD-ROM accompanying this textbook, and on the Companion Website at www.prenhall.com/kozier. Click on Chapter 5 to select the activities for this chapter.

CD-ROM
• Audio Glossary
• NCLEX Review

Companion Website
• Additional NCLEX Review
• Case Study: Ethics Committee
• MediaLink Applications:
  AIDS Resources
  Privacy
• Links to Resources

In their daily work, nurses deal with intimate and fundamental human events such as birth, death, and suffering. They must decide the morality of their own actions when they face the many ethical issues that surround such sensitive areas. Because of the special nurse–client relationship, nurses are the ones who are there to support and advocate for clients and families who are facing hard difficult choices, and for those who are living out the results of choices that others make for and about them.

The present cost-driven environment of managed care tends to give highest priority to business values. This creates new moral problems and intensifies old ones, making it more critical than ever for nurses to make sound moral decisions. Therefore, nurses need to (a) develop sensitivity to the ethical dimensions of nursing practice, (b) examine their own and clients' values, (c) understand how values influence their decisions, and (d) think ahead about the kinds of moral problems they are likely to face. This chapter explores the influences of values and moral frameworks on the ethical dimensions of nursing practice and on the nurse's role as a client advocate.

VALUES

Values are freely chosen, enduring beliefs or attitudes about the worth of a person, object, idea, or action. Values are important because they influence decisions and actions, including nurses' ethical decision making. Even though they may be unspoken and perhaps even unconsciously held, questions of value underlie all moral dilemmas. Of course, not all values are moral values. For example, people hold values about work, family, religion, politics, money, and relationships, to name just a few. Values are often taken for granted. In the same way that people are not aware of their breathing, they usually do not think about their values; they simply accept them and act on them.

A **value set** is the small group of values held by an individual. People organize their set of values internally along a continuum from most important to least important, forming a **value system.** Value systems are basic to a way of life, give direction to life, and form the basis of behavior— especially behavior that is based on decisions or choices.

Values consist of beliefs and attitudes, which are related, but not identical, to values. People have many different beliefs and attitudes, but only a small number of values. **Beliefs** (or opinions) are interpretations or conclusions that people accept as true. They are based more on faith than fact and may or may not be true. Beliefs do not necessarily involve values. For example, the statement "I believe if I study hard I will get a good grade" expresses a belief that does not involve a value. By contrast, the statement "Good grades are really important to me. I believe I must study hard to obtain good grades" involves both a belief and a value.

Attitudes are mental positions or feelings toward a person, object, or idea (e.g., acceptance, compassion, openness). Typically an attitude continues over time, whereas a belief may last only briefly. Attitudes are often judged as bad or good, positive or negative, whereas beliefs are judged as correct or incorrect. Attitudes have thinking and behavioral aspects, but feelings are an especially important component because they vary so greatly among individuals. For example, some clients may feel strongly about their need for privacy, whereas others may dismiss it as unimportant.

Values Transmission

Values are learned through observation and experience. As a result, they are heavily influenced by a person's sociocultural environment—that is, by societal traditions; by cultural, ethnic, and religious groups; and by family and peer groups. For example, if a parent consistently demonstrates honesty in dealing with others, the child will probably begin to value honesty. Nurses should keep in mind the influence of values on health. For example, some cultures value treatment by a folk healer over that by a physician. For additional information about cultural values related to health and illness, see Chapter 13. ⌘

Personal Values

Although people derive values from society and their individual subgroups, they internalize some or all of these values and perceive them as **personal values.** People need societal values to feel accepted, and they need personal values to have a sense of individuality.

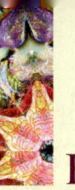

TABLE 5–1 Essential Nursing Values and Behaviors

Values	Professional Behaviors
Altruism is a concern for the welfare and well-being of others. In professional practice, altruism is reflected by the nurse's concern for the welfare of patients, other nurses, and other health care providers. *Autonomy* is the right to self-determination. Professional practice reflects autonomy when the nurse respects patients' rights to make decisions about their health care. *Human dignity* is respect for the inherent worth and uniqueness of individuals and populations. In professional practice, human dignity is reflected when the nurse values and respects all patients and colleagues. *Integrity* is acting in accordance with an appropriate code of ethics and accepted standards of practice. Integrity is reflected in professional practice when the nurse is honest and provides care based on an ethical framework that is accepted within the profession. *Social justice* is upholding moral, legal, and humanistic principles. This value is reflected in professional practice when the nurse works to ensure equal treatment under the law and equal access to quality health care.	• Demonstrates understanding of cultures, beliefs, and perspectives of others. • Advocates for patients, particularly the most vulnerable. • Takes risks on behalf of patients and colleagues. • Mentors other professionals. • Plans care in partnership with patients. • Honors the right of patients and families to make decisions about health care. • Provides information so patients can make informed choices. • Provides culturally competent and sensitive care. • Protects the patient's privacy. • Preserves the confidentiality of patients and health care providers. • Designs care with sensitivity to individual patient needs. • Provides honest information to patients and the public. • Documents care accurately and honestly. • Seeks to remedy errors made by self or others. • Demonstrates accountability for own actions. • Supports fairness and nondiscrimination in the delivery of care. • Promotes universal access to health care. • Encourages legislation and policy consistent with the advancement of nursing care and health care.

Note: From *The Essentials of Baccalaureate Education for Professional Nursing Practice* (pp.8–9), American Association of Colleges of Nursing, 1998, Washington, DC: Author. Reprinted with permission.

Professional Values

Nurses' **professional values** are acquired during socialization into nursing from codes of ethics, nursing experiences, teachers, and peers. Watson (1981, pp. 20–21) outlined four important values of nursing.

1. Strong commitment to service
2. Belief in the dignity and worth of each person
3. Commitment to education
4. Professional autonomy.

In comparison, the American Association of Colleges of Nursing (AACN, 1998) identified five values essential for the professional nurse: altruism, autonomy, human dignity, integrity, and social justice. Table 5–1 lists the values and professional behaviors associated with these values.

Values Clarification

Values clarification is a process by which people identify, examine, and develop their own individual values. A principle of values clarification is that no one set of values is right for everyone. When people can identify their values, they can retain or change them and thus act on the basis of freely chosen, rather than unconscious, values. Values clarification promotes

personal growth by fostering awareness, empathy, and insight. Therefore, it is an important step for nurses to take in dealing with ethical problems.

One widely used theory of values clarification was developed by Raths, Harmin, and Simon (1978). They described a "valuing process" of thinking, feeling, and behavior that they termed "choosing," "prizing," and "acting " (see Box 5–1).

BOX 5–1	■ Values Clarification
Choosing (cognitive)	Beliefs are chosen ■ Freely, without outside pressure ■ From among alternatives ■ After reflecting and considering consequences
Prizing (affective)	Chosen beliefs are prized and cherished
Acting (behavioral)	Chosen beliefs are ■ Affirmed to others ■ Incorporated into one's behavior ■ Repeated consistently in one's life

Note: From *Values and Teaching,* 2nd ed. (p. 47), by L. Raths, M. Harmin, and S. Simon, copyright 1978. Adapted and reprinted with permission of the authors.

Clarifying the Nurse's Values

Nurses and nursing students need to examine the values they hold about life, death, health, and illness. One strategy for gaining awareness of personal values is to consider one's attitudes about specific issues such as abortion or euthanasia, asking: "Can I accept this, or live with this?" "Why does this bother me?" "What would I do or want done in this situation?"

Clarifying Client Values

To plan effective care, nurses need to identify clients' values as they influence and relate to a particular health problem. For example, a client with failing eyesight will probably place a high value on the ability to see, and a client with chronic pain will value comfort. Normally, people take such things for granted. For information about health beliefs and values, see Chapter 11. When clients hold unclear or conflicting values that are detrimental to their health, the nurse should use values clarification as an intervention. Examples of behaviors that may indicate the need for values clarification are listed in Table 5–2.

The following process may help clients clarify their values.

1. *List alternatives.* Make sure that the client is aware of all alternative actions. Ask "Are you considering other courses of action?" "Tell me about them."

2. *Examine possible consequences of choices.* Make sure the client has thought about possible results of each action. Ask "What do you think you will gain from doing that?" "What benefits do you foresee from doing that?"

3. *Choose freely.* To determine whether the client chose freely, ask "Did you have any say in that decision?" "Do you have a choice?"

4. *Feel good about the choice.* To determine how the client feels, ask "How do you feel about that decision (or action)?" Because some clients may not feel satisfied with their decision, a more sensitive question may be "Some people feel good after a decision is made; others feel bad. How do you feel?"

5. *Affirm the choice.* Ask "What will you say to others (family, friends) about this?"

6. *Act on the choice.* To determine whether the client is prepared to act on the decisions, ask, for example, "Will it be difficult to tell your wife about this?"

7. *Act with a pattern.* To determine whether the client consistently behaves in a certain way, ask "How many times have you done that before?" or "Would you act that way again?"

When implementing these seven steps to clarify values, the nurse assists the client to think each question through, but does not impose personal values. The nurse offers an opinion only when the client asks for it—and then only with care.

MORALITY AND ETHICS

The term **ethics** has several meanings in common use. It refers to (a) a method of inquiry that helps people to understand the morality of human behavior (i.e., it is the study of morality), (b) the practices or beliefs of a certain group (e.g., medical ethics, nursing ethics), and (c) the expected standards of moral behavior of a particular group as described in the group's formal code of professional ethics. **Bioethics** is ethics as applied to life (e.g., to decisions about abortion or euthanasia). **Nursing ethics** refers to ethical issues that occur in nursing practice. The American Nurses Association (ANA) revised *Standards of Clinical Nursing Practice* (1998) holds nurses accountable for their ethical conduct. Professional Performance Standard V relates to ethics (see Box 5–2).

Morality (or morals) is similar to ethics and many use the terms interchangeably. **Morality** usually refers to private, personal standards of what is right and wrong in conduct, character, and attitude. Sometimes the first clue to the moral nature of

TABLE 5–2	Behaviors that May Indicate Unclear Values
Behavior	**Example**
Ignoring a health professional's advice	A client with heart disease who values hard work ignores advice to exercise regularly.
Inconsistent communication or behavior	A pregnant woman says she wants a healthy baby, but continues to drink alcohol and smoke tobacco.
Numerous admissions to a health agency for the same problem	A middle-aged, obese woman repeatedly seeks help for back pain but does not lose weight.
Confusion or uncertainty about which course of action to take	A woman wants to obtain a job to meet financial obligations, but also wants to stay at home to care for an ailing husband.

BOX 5–2   ■ ANA Standards of Professional Performance

Standard V: Ethics
The nurse's decisions and actions on behalf of patients are determined in an ethical manner.

Measurement Criteria

1. The nurse's practice is guided by the Code for Nurses.
2. The nurse maintains patient confidentiality within legal and regulatory parameters.
3. The nurse acts as a patient advocate and assists patients in developing skills so they can advocate for themselves.
4. The nurse delivers care in a nonjudgmental and nondiscriminatory manner that is sensitive to patient diversity.
5. The nurse delivers care in a manner that preserves patient autonomy, dignity, and rights.
6. The nurse seeks available resources in formulating ethical decisions.

Note: From *Standards of Clinical Nursing Practice*, 2nd ed. (pp. 13–14), by American Nurses Association, 1998, Washington, DC: Author. Reprinted by permission.

a situation is an aroused conscience or an awareness of feelings such as guilt, hope, or shame. Another indicator is the tendency to respond to the situation with words such as *ought, should, right, wrong, good,* and *bad.* Moral issues are concerned with important social values and norms; they are not about trivial things.

Nurses should distinguish between morality and law. Laws do reflect the moral values of a society, and they offer guidance in determining what is moral. However, an action can be legal but not moral. For example, an order for full resuscitation of a dying client is legal, but one could still question whether the act is moral. On the other hand, an action can be moral but illegal. For example, if a child at home stops breathing, it is moral but not legal to exceed the speed limit when driving to the hospital. Legal aspects of nursing practice are covered in Chapter 4.

Nurses should also distinguish between morality and religion, although the two concepts are related. For example, according to some religious beliefs, women should undergo procedures such as female circumcision that may cause physical mutilation. Other religions or groups may consider this practice to be a violation of human rights (Sala & Manara, 2001).

> **► CLINICAL ALERT** *Confucian religious beliefs do not consider a fetus a human being. However, Buddhists believe the fetus is a form of life. Thus, Chinese people vary in their views on abortion depending on religious affiliation.* ■

Moral Development

Ethical decisions require nurses to think and reason. Reasoning is a cognitive function and is, therefore, developmental. **Moral development** is the process of learning to tell the difference between right and wrong and of learning what ought and ought not to be done. It is a complex process that begins in childhood and continues throughout life.

Theories of moral development attempt to answer questions such as these: How does a person become moral? What factors influence the way a person behaves in a moral situation? Two well-known theorists of moral development are Lawrence Kohlberg (1969) and Carol Gilligan (1982). Kohlberg's theory emphasizes rights and formal reasoning; Gilligan's theory emphasizes care and responsibility, although it points out that people use the concepts of both theorists in their moral reasoning. For a full discussion of these two theories, see Chapter 22.

Moral Frameworks

Moral theories provide different frameworks through which nurses can view and clarify disturbing client care situations. Nurses can use moral theories in developing explanations for their ethical decisions and actions and in discussing problem situations with others. Three types of moral theories are widely used, and they can be differentiated by their emphasis on either (a) consequences, (b) principles and duties, or (c) relationships.

Consequence-based (teleological) theories look to the consequences of an action in judging whether that action is right or wrong. **Utilitarianism,** one form of consequentialist theory, views a good act as one that brings the most good and the least harm for the greatest number of people. This is called the principle of **utility.** This approach is often used in making decisions about the funding and delivery of health care.

Principles-based (deontological) theories emphasize individual rights, duties, and obligations. The morality of an action is determined not by its consequences but by whether it is done according to an impartial, objective principle. For example, following the rule "Do not lie," a nurse might believe she should tell the truth to a dying client, even though the physician has given instruction not to do so. There are many deontological theories; each justifies the rules of acceptable behavior differently.

Relationships-based (caring) theories stress courage, generosity, commitment, and the need to nurture and maintain relationships. Unlike the two preceding theories, which frame problems in terms of justice (fairness) and formal reasoning, caring theories (Watson, 1997) judge actions according to a perspective of caring and responsibility. Principles-based theories stress individual rights, but caring theories promote the common good or the welfare of the group.

Caring is a central force in the client–nurse relationship, and a force for protecting and enhancing client dignity. For example, guided by this framework, nurses use touch and truth telling to affirm clients as persons, not objects, and to help them make choices and find meaning in their illness experiences. Watson (1988) and Benner and Wrubel (1989) proposed caring as the central goal for nursing as well as a basis for nursing ethics. However, caring is not unique to nursing, and some have criticized the caring perspective for reinforcing the stereotype of women as caretakers, while overlooking other important moral principles such as fairness and autonomy (Bowden, 1995).

A moral framework guides moral decisions, but it does not determine the outcome. This can be illustrated by imagining a situation in which a frail, elderly client has insisted that he does not want further surgery, but the family and surgeon insist. Three nurses have each decided that they will not help with preparations for surgery and that they will work through proper channels to try to prevent it. Using consequence-based reasoning, Nurse A thinks, "Surgery will cause him more suffering; he probably will not survive it anyway; and the family may even feel guilty later." Using principles-based reasoning, Nurse B thinks, "This violates the principle of autonomy. This man has a right to decide what happens to his body." Using caring-based reasoning, Nurse C thinks, "My relationship to this client commits me to protecting him and meeting his needs; and I feel such compassion for him. I must try to help the family understand that he needs their support."

Moral Principles

Moral principles are statements about broad, general, philosophic concepts such as autonomy and justice. They provide the foundation for **moral rules,** which are specific prescriptions for actions. For example, the rule "People should not lie" is based on the moral principle of respect for persons (autonomy). Principles are useful in ethical discussions because even if people disagree about which action is right in a situation, they may be able to agree on the principles that apply. Such an agreement can serve as the basis for a solution that is acceptable to all parties. For example, most people would agree to the principle that nurses are obligated to respect their clients, even if they disagree as to whether the nurse should deceive a particular client about his or her prognosis.

Autonomy refers to the right to make one's own decisions. Nurses who follow this principle recognize that each client is unique, has the right to be what that person is, and has the right to choose personal goals. People have "inward autonomy" if they have the ability to make choices; they have "outward autonomy" if their choices are not limited or imposed by others.

Honoring the principle of autonomy means that the nurse respects a client's right to make decisions even when those choices seem to the nurse not to be in the client's best interest. It also means treating others with consideration. In a health care setting this principle is violated, for example, when a nurse disregards clients' subjective accounts of their symptoms (e.g., pain). Finally, respect for autonomy means that people should not be treated as an impersonal source of knowledge or training. This principle comes into play, for example, in the requirement that clients provide informed consent before tests, procedures, research, or being a teaching subject can be carried out. See "Informed Consent" in Chapter 4. 🔗

Nonmaleficence is duty to "do no harm." Although this would seem to be a simple principle to follow, in reality it is complex. Harm can mean intentionally causing harm, placing someone at risk of harm, and unintentionally causing harm. In nursing, intentional harm is never acceptable. However, placing a person at risk of harm has many facets. A client may be at risk of harm as a known consequence of a nursing intervention that is intended to be helpful. For example, a client may react adversely to a medication. Caregivers do not always agree on the degree of risk that is morally permissible in order to attempt the beneficial result. Unintentional harm occurs when the risk could not have been anticipated. For example, while catching a client who is falling, the nurse grips the client tightly enough to cause bruises to the client's arm.

Beneficence means "doing good." Nurses are obligated to do good, that is, to implement actions that benefit clients and their support persons. However, doing good can also pose a risk of doing harm. For example, a nurse may advise a client about a strenuous exercise program to improve general health, but should not do so if the client is at risk of a heart attack.

Justice is often referred to as fairness. Nurses often face decisions in which a sense of justice should prevail. For example, a nurse making home visits finds one client tearful and depressed, and knows she could help by staying for 30 more minutes to talk. However, that would take time from her next client, who is a diabetic who needs a great deal of teaching and observation. The nurse will need to weigh the facts carefully in order to divide her time justly among her clients.

Fidelity means to be faithful to agreements and promises. By virtue of their standing as professional caregivers, nurses have responsibilities to clients, employers, government, and society, as well as to themselves. Nurses often make promises such as "I'll be right back with your pain medication" or "I'll

find out for you." Clients take such promises seriously, and so should nurses.

Veracity refers to telling the truth. Although this seems straightforward, in practice choices are not always clear. Should a nurse tell the truth when it is known that it will cause harm? Does a nurse tell a lie when it is known that the lie will relieve anxiety and fear? Lying to sick or dying people is rarely justified. The loss of trust in the nurse and the anxiety caused by not knowing the truth, for example, usually outweigh any benefits derived from lying.

Nurses must also have professional accountability and responsibility. According to the *Code of Ethics for Nurses* (ANA, 2001), **accountability** means "answerable to oneself and others for one's own actions," while **responsibility** refers to "the specific accountability or liability associated with the performance of duties of a particular role." Thus, the ethical nurse is able to explain the rationale behind every action and recognizes the standards to which he or she will be held.

NURSING ETHICS

In the past, nurses looked on ethical decision making as the physician's responsibility. However, no one profession is responsible for ethical decisions, nor does expertise in one discipline such as medicine or nursing necessarily make a person an expert in ethics. As situations become more complex, input from all caregivers becomes increasingly important.

Ethical standards of the Joint Commission on Accreditation of Healthcare Organizations (JCAHO) mandate that health care institutions provide ethics committees or a similar structure to write guidelines and policies and to provide education, counseling, and support on ethical issues (JCAHO, 1996). These multidisciplinary committees include nurses and can be asked to review a case and provide guidance to a competent client, an incompetent client's family, or health care providers. They ensure that relevant facts of a case are brought out, provide a forum in which diverse views can be expressed, provide support for caregivers, and can reduce the institution's legal risks. In some settings, ethics rounds are held. In these meetings, ethical dilemmas from real or simulated cases are presented from a more theoretical perspective, introducing those present to the issues and processes used in analyzing such dilemmas (see Figure 5–1 ■).

Nursing Codes of Ethics

A **code of ethics** is a formal statement of a group's ideals and values. It is a set of ethical principles that (a) is shared by members of the group, (b) reflects their moral judgments over time, and (c) serves as a standard for their professional actions. Codes of ethics usually have higher requirements than legal standards, and they are never lower than the legal standards of the profession. Nurses are responsible for being familiar with the code that governs their practice.

International, national, and state nursing associations have established codes of ethics. The International Council of Nurses (ICN) first adopted a code of ethics in 1953 and the most recent revisions are shown in Box 5–3. The ANA first adopted a *Code for*

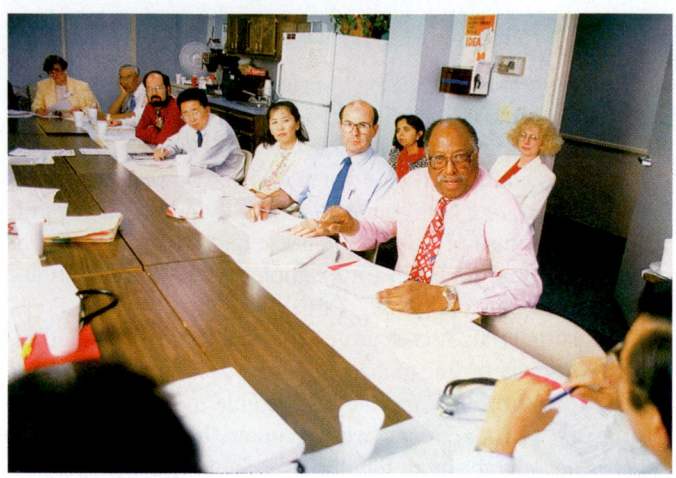

Figure 5–1 ■ An ethics committee considers all aspects of the case being considered. (Mark Richards/PhotoEdit.)

Nurses in 1950. The current version (Box 5–4) reflects several major changes in the code (now called the *Code of Ethics for Nurses*). A statement on compassion has been added and the duty to protect patients has been broadened to include all patient rights. Several previous provisions have been collapsed and the provision on delegation has been significantly enhanced to reflect the increased use of unlicensed assistive personnel. The Canadian Nurses Association (CNA) adopted a code of ethics in 1980 (see Box 5–5).

Nursing codes of ethics have the following purposes:

1. Inform the public about the minimum standards of the profession and help them understand professional nursing conduct.
2. Provide a sign of the profession's commitment to the public it serves.
3. Outline the major ethical considerations of the profession.
4. Provide ethical standards for professional behavior.
5. Guide the profession in self-regulation.
6. Remind nurses of the special responsibility they assume when caring for the sick.

BOX 5–3 ■ International Council of Nurses Code of Ethics

Preamble

Nurses have four fundamental responsibilities: to promote health, to prevent illness, to restore health and to alleviate suffering. The need for nursing is universal.

Inherent in nursing is respect for human rights, including the right to life, to dignity and to be treated with respect. Nursing care is unrestricted by considerations of age, colour, creed, culture, disability or illness, gender, nationality, politics, race or social status.

Nurses render health services to the individual, the family and the community and coordinate their services with those of related groups.

The Code

The *ICN Code of Ethics for Nurses* has four principal elements that outline the standards of ethical conduct.

Elements of the Code

1. Nurses and people
   The nurse's primary professional responsibility is to people requiring nursing care.
   In providing care, the nurse promotes an environment in which the human rights, values, customs and spiritual beliefs of the individual, family and community are respected.
   The nurse ensures that the individual receives sufficient information on which to base consent for care and related treatment.
   The nurse holds in confidence personal information and uses judgement in sharing this information.
   The nurse shares with society the responsibility for initiating and supporting action to meet the health and social needs of the public, in particular those of vulnerable populations.

The nurse also shares responsibility to sustain and protect the natural environment from depletion, pollution, degradation and destruction.

2. Nurses and practice
   The nurse carries personal responsibility and accountability for nursing practice, and for maintaining competence by continual learning.
   The nurse maintains a standard of personal health such that the ability to provide care is not compromised.
   The nurse uses judgement regarding individual competence when accepting and delegating responsibility.
   The nurse at all times maintains standards of personal conduct that reflect well on the profession and enhance public confidence.
   The nurse, in providing care, ensures that use of technology and scientific advances are compatible with the safety, dignity and rights of people.

3. Nurses and the profession
   The nurse assumes the major role in determining and implementing acceptable standards of clinical nursing practice, management, research and education.
   The nurse is active in developing a core of research-based professional knowledge.
   The nurse, acting through the professional organisation, participates in creating and maintaining equitable social and economic working conditions in nursing.

4. Nurses and co-workers
   The nurse sustains a cooperative relationship with co-workers in nursing and other fields.
   The nurse takes appropriate action to safeguard individuals when their care is endangered by a co-worker or any other person.

Note: From *ICN Code of Ethics for Nurses,* International Council of Nurses, 2000, Geneva: Imprimeries Populaires. Reprinted with permission.

Origins of Ethical Problems in Nursing

Nurses' growing awareness of ethical problems has occurred largely because of (a) social and technological changes and (b) nurses' conflicting loyalties and obligations.

Social and Technological Changes

Social changes, such as the women's movement and a growing consumerism, also expose problems. The large number of people without health insurance, the high cost of health care, and workplace redesign under managed care all raise issues of fairness and allocation of resources.

Technology creates new issues that did not exist in earlier times. Before monitors, respirators, and parenteral feedings, there was no question about whether to "allow" an 800-gram premature infant to die. Before organ transplantation, death did not require a legal definition that might still permit viable tissues to be removed and given to other living persons. Advances in the ability to decode and control the growth of tissues through gene manipulation present new potential ethical dilemmas related to cloning organisms and altering the course of hereditary diseases and biological characteristics. Today, with treatments that can prolong and enhance biologic life, these questions arise: Should we do what we know we can? Who

---

BOX 5–4   ■ American Nurses Association Code of Ethics for Nurses (Approved July 2001)

MediaLink | PRIVACY APPLICATION

1. The nurse, in all professional relationships, practices with compassion and respect for the inherent dignity, worth and uniqueness of every individual, unrestricted by considerations of social or economic status, personal attributes, or the nature of health problems.
   1.1. Respect for human dignity
   1.2. Relationships to patients
   1.3. The nature of health problems
   1.4. The right to self-determination
   1.5. Relationships with colleagues and others
2. The nurse's primary commitment is to the patient, whether an individual, family, group, or community.
   2.1. Primacy of patient's interests
   2.2. Conflict of interest for nurses
   2.3. Collaboration
   2.4. Professional boundaries
3. The nurse promotes, advocates for and strives to protect the health, safety and rights of the patient.
   3.1. Privacy
   3.2. Confidentiality
   3.3. Protection of participants in research
   3.4. Standards and review mechanisms
   3.5. Acting on questionable practice
   3.6. Addressing impaired practice
4. The nurse is responsible and accountable for individual nursing practice and determines the appropriate delegation of tasks consistent with the nurse's obligation to provide optimum patient care.
   4.1. Acceptance of accountability and responsibility
   4.2. Accountability for nursing judgment and action
   4.3. Responsibility for nursing judgment and action
   4.4. Delegation of nursing activities
5. The nurse owes the same duties to self as to others, including the responsibility to preserve integrity and safety, to maintain competence and to continue personal and professional growth.
   5.1. Moral self-respect
   5.2. Professional growth and maintenance of competence
   5.3. Wholeness of character
   5.4. Preservation of integrity
6. The nurse participates in establishing, maintaining and improving healthcare environments and conditions of employment conducive to the provision of quality healthcare and consistent with the values of the profession through individual and collective action.
   6.1. Influence of the environment on moral virtues and values
   6.2. Influence of the environment on ethical obligations
   6.3. Responsibility for the healthcare environment
7. The nurse participates in the advancement of the profession through contributions to practice, education, administration and knowledge development.
   7.1. Advancing the profession through active involvement in nursing and healthcare policy
   7.2. Advancing the profession by developing, maintaining, and implementing professional standards in clinical, administrative, and educational practice
   7.3. Advancing the profession through knowledge development, dissemination, and application to practice
8. The nurse collaborates with other health professionals and the public in promoting community, national, and international efforts to meet health needs.
   8.1. Health needs and concerns
   8.2. Responsibilities to the public
9. The profession of nursing, as represented by associations and their members, is responsible for articulating nursing values, for maintaining the integrity of the profession and its practice and for shaping social policy.
   9.1. Assertion of values
   9.2. The profession carries out its collective responsibility through professional associations
   9.3. Intraprofessional integrity
   9.4. Social reform

Note: From *Code of Ethics for Nurses,* American Nurses Association, 2001, Washington, DC: American Nurses Publishing. Retrieved March 11, 2003, from http://nursingworld.org/ethics/code/ethicscode150.htm Reprinted with permission.

BOX 5–5	■ Canadian Nurses Association Code of Ethics for Nursing
Health and well-being	Nurses value health and well-being and assist persons to achieve their optimum level of health in situations of normal health, illness, injury, or in the process of dying.
Choice	Nurses respect and promote the autonomy of clients and help them to express their health needs and values, and to obtain appropriate information and services.
Dignity	Nurses value and advocate the dignity and self-respect of human beings.
Confidentiality	Nurses safeguard the trust of clients that information learned in the context of a professional relationship is shared outside the health care team only with the client's permission or as legally required.
Fairness	Nurses apply and promote principles of equity and fairness to assist clients in receiving unbiased treatment and a share of health services and resources proportionate to their needs.
Accountability	Nurses act in a manner consistent with their professional responsibilities and standards of practice.
Practice environments conducive to safe, competent, and ethical care	Nurses advocate practice environments that have the organizational and human support systems, and the resource allocations necessary for safe, competent, and ethical nursing care.

The code is organized around the seven values listed above. Each value is articulated by responsibility statements that clarify its application and provide more direct guidance.

Note: From *Code of Ethics for Nursing*, Canadian Nurses' Association, 1997, Ottawa: Author. Reprinted with permission.

BOX 5–6	■ Ethical Decision-Making Models

Thompson and Thompson (1985)
- Review the situation to determine health problems, decision needs, ethical components, and key individuals.
- Gather additional information to clarify the situation.
- Identify the ethical issues in the situation.
- Define personal and professional moral positions.
- Identify moral positions of key individuals involved.
- Identify value conflicts, if any.
- Determine who should make the decision.
- Identify range of actions with anticipated outcomes.
- Decide on a course of action and carry it out.
- Evaluate/review results of decision/action.

Cassells and Redman (1989)
- Identify the moral aspects of nursing care.
- Gather relevant facts related to a moral issue.
- Clarify and apply personal values.
- Understand ethical theories and principles (e.g., autonomy and justice).
- Utilize competent interdisciplinary resources (e.g., clergy, literature, family, other caregivers, and consultants).
- Propose alternative actions.
- Apply nursing codes of ethics to help guide actions.
- Choose and implement resolutive action.
- Participate actively in resolving the issue.
- Apply state and federal laws governing nursing practice.
- Evaluate the action taken.

Note: From *Bioethical Decision-Making for Nurses*, (p. 99), by J. B. Thompson and H. O. Thompson, 1985, Norwalk, CT: Appleton-Century-Crofts, and "Preparing Students to be Moral Agents in Clinical Nursing Practice," by J. Cassells and B. Redman, 1989, *Nursing Clinics of North America, 24*(2), pp. 463–473. Reprinted with permission.

should be treated—everyone, only those who can pay, only those who have a chance to improve?

Conflicting Loyalties and Obligations

Because of their unique position in the health care system, nurses experience conflicts among their loyalties and obligations to clients, families, physicians, employing institutions, and licensing bodies. Client needs may conflict with institutional policies, physician preferences, needs of the client's family, or even laws of the state. According to the nursing code of ethics, the nurse's first loyalty is to the client. However, it is not always easy to determine which action best serves the client's needs. For instance, the nurse may be aware that marijuana has been shown to be effective for a condition a client has that has not responded to mainstream therapies. Although legal issues are involved, the nurse must determine if, ethically, the client should be made aware of a potentially effective alternative.

Making Ethical Decisions

Responsible ethical reasoning is rational and systematic. It should be based on ethical principles and codes rather than on emotions, intuition, fixed policies, or precedent (that is, an earlier similar occurrence). Two decision-making models are shown in Box 5–6.

BOX 5–7	■ Examples of Nurses' Obligations in Ethical Decisions

- Maximize the client's well-being.
- Balance the client's need for autonomy with family members' responsibilities for the client's well-being.
- Support each family member and enhance the family support system.
- Carry out hospital policies.
- Protect other clients' well-being.
- Protect the nurse's own standards of care.

A good decision is one that is in the client's best interest and at the same time preserves the integrity of all involved. Nurses have ethical obligations to their clients, to the agency that employs them, and to physicians. Therefore, nurses must weigh competing factors when making ethical decisions. See Box 5–7 for examples. Although ethical reasoning is principle based and has the client's well-being at center, being involved in ethical problems and dilemmas is stressful for the nurse. The nurse may feel torn between obligations to the client, the family, and the employer. What is in the client's best interest may be contrary to the nurse's personal belief system. In settings in which ethical issues arise frequently, nurses should establish support systems such as team conferences and use of counseling professionals to allow expression of their feelings.

Many nursing problems are not moral problems at all, but simply questions of good nursing practice. An important first step in ethical decision making is to determine whether a moral situation exists. The following criteria may be used:

- A difficult choice exists between actions that conflict with the needs of one or more persons.
- Moral principles or frameworks exist that can be used to provide some justification for the action.
- The choice is guided by a process of weighing reasons.
- The decision must be freely and consciously chosen.
- The choice is affected by personal feelings and by the particular context of the situation.

Box 5–8 presents an example of ethical decision making using the model proposed by Cassells and Redman (1989).

Although the nurse's input is important, in reality several people are usually involved in making an ethical decision. Therefore, collaboration, communication, and compromise are important skills for health professionals. When nurses do not have the autonomy to act on their moral or ethical choices, compromise becomes essential.

> **CLINICAL ALERT** *Ethical behavior is contextual— what is an ethical action or decision in one situation may not be ethical in a different situation.* ■

Strategies to Enhance Ethical Decisions and Practice

Several strategies help nurses overcome possible organizational and social constraints that may hinder the ethical practice of nursing and create moral distress for nurses. You as a nurse should do the following:

- Become aware of your own values and the ethical aspects of nursing.
- Be familiar with nursing codes of ethics.
- Respect the values, opinions, and responsibilities of other health care professionals that may be different from your own.
- Participate in or establish ethics rounds. Ethics rounds use hypothetical or real cases that focus on the ethical dimensions of client care rather than the client's clinical diagnosis and treatment.
- Serve on institutional ethics committees.
- Strive for collaborative practice in which nurses function effectively in cooperation with other health care professionals.

SPECIFIC ETHICAL ISSUES

Some of the ethical problems nurses encounter most frequently are issues in the care of HIV/AIDS clients, abortion, organ transplantation, end-of-life decisions, cost-containment issues that jeopardize client welfare and access to health care (resource allocation), and breaches of client confidentiality (e.g., computerized information management).

Acquired Immune Deficiency Syndrome (AIDS)

Because of its association with sexual behavior, illicit drug use, and physical decline and death, AIDS bears a social stigma. According to an ANA position statement, the moral obligation to care for an HIV-infected client cannot be set aside unless the risk exceeds the responsibility. "Not only must nursing care be readily available, . . . but nurses must be advised of the risks and responsibilities they face in providing care. . . . Accepting personal risk which exceeds the limits of duty is not morally obligatory; it is a moral option" (ANA, 1988, p. 310).

Other ethical issues center on testing for HIV status and for the presence of AIDS in health professionals and clients. Questions arise as to whether testing of all providers and patients should be mandatory or voluntary and whether test results should be released to insurance companies, sexual partners, or caregivers. As with all ethical dilemmas, there are both positive and negative implications of each possibility for specific individuals (see Figure 5–2 ■).

Abortion

Abortion is a highly publicized issue about which many people feel very strongly. Debate continues, pitting the principle of sanctity of life against the principle of autonomy and the woman's right to control her own body. This is an especially volatile issue because no public consensus has yet been reached.

MediaLink | AIDS RESOURCES APPLICATION

BOX 5–8   ■ Application of a Bioethical Decision-Making Model

Situation

Mrs. L, a 67-year-old woman, is hospitalized with multiple fractures and lacerations caused by an automobile accident. Her husband, who was killed in the accident, was taken to the same hospital. Mrs. L, who had been driving the automobile, constantly questions her primary nurse about her husband. The surgeon has told the nurse not to tell Mrs. L about the death of her husband; however, he does not give the nurse any reason for these instructions. The nurse expresses concern to the charge nurse, who says the surgeon's orders must be followed. However, the nurse is not comfortable with this and wonders what should be done.

Nursing Actions	Considerations
1. Identify the moral aspects. See the criteria provided on page 76 to determine whether a moral situation exists.	The alternative actions are to tell the truth or withhold it. The moral principles involved are honesty and loyalty. These principles conflict because the primary nurse wants to be honest with Mrs. L without being disloyal to the surgeon and the charge nurse. The nurse will weigh reasons in making a freely and consciously chosen choice. The choice will probably be affected by feelings of concern for Mrs. L and a context that includes the surgeon's incomplete communication with the client and the nurse.
2. Gather relevant facts that relate to the issue.	Data should include information about the client's health problems. Determine who is involved, the nature of their involvement, and their motives for acting. In this case, the people involved are the client (who is concerned about her husband), the husband (who is deceased), the surgeon, the charge nurse, and the primary nurse. Motives are not known. Perhaps the nurse wishes to protect her therapeutic relationship with Mrs. L; possibly the physician believes this action protects Mrs. L from psychologic trauma and consequent physical deterioration.
3. Determine ownership of the decision. For example, for whom is the decision being made? Who should decide and why?	In this case, the decision is being made for Mrs. L. The surgeon obviously believes that a physician should be the one to decide, and the charge nurse agrees. It would be helpful if caregivers agreed on criteria for deciding who the decision maker should be.
4. Clarify and apply personal values.	We can infer from this situation that Mrs. L values her husband's welfare, that the charge nurse values policy and procedure, and that the nurse seems to value a client's right to have information. The nurse needs to clarify his or her own and the surgeon's values, as well as confirm the values of Mrs. L and the charge nurse.
5. Identify ethical theories and principles.	For example, failing to tell Mrs. L the truth can negate her autonomy. The nurse would uphold the principle of honesty by telling Mrs. L. The principles of beneficence and nonmaleficence are also involved because of the possible effects of the alternative actions on Mrs. L's physical and psychologic well-being.
6. Identify applicable laws or agency policies.	Because the surgeon simply "gave instructions" rather than an actual order, agency policies might not require the nurse to follow the instructions. The nurse should clarify this with the charge nurse and be familiar with the nurse practice act in that state.
7. Use competent interdisciplinary resources.	In this case, the nurse might consult literature to find out whether clients are harmed by receiving bad news when they are injured and might also consult with the chaplain.
8. Develop alternative actions and project their outcomes on the client and family. Possibly because of the limited time available for ethical deliberations in the clinical setting, nurses tend to identify two opposing, either-or alternatives (e.g., to tell or not to tell) instead of generating multiple options. This creates a dilemma even when none exists.	Two alternative actions, with possible outcomes, follow (others may also be appropriate): 1. Follow the charge nurse's advice and do as the surgeon says. Possible outcomes: (a) Mrs. L might become anxious and angry when she finds out that information has been withheld from her; or (b) by waiting until Mrs. L is stronger to give her the bad news, the health care team may avoid harming Mrs. L's health. 2. Discuss the situation further with the charge nurse and surgeon, pointing out Mrs. L's right to autonomy and information. Possible outcomes: (a) The surgeon acknowledges Mrs. L's right to be informed, or (b) the surgeon states that Mrs. L's health is at risk and insists that she not be informed until a later time. Regardless of whether the action is congruent with the nurse's personal value system, Mrs. L's best interests take precedence.
9. Apply nursing codes of ethics to help guide actions. (Codes of nursing usually support autonomy and nursing advocacy.)	If the nurse believes strongly that Mrs. L should hear the truth, then as a client advocate, the nurse should choose to confer again with the charge nurse and surgeon.

BOX 5–8   ■   Application of a Bioethical Decision-Making Model continued

Nursing Actions	Considerations
10. For each alternative action, identify the risk and seriousness of consequences for the nurse. (Some employers may not support nursing autonomy and advocacy in ethical situations.)	If the nurse tells Mrs. L the truth without the agreement of the charge nurse and surgeon, the nurse risks the surgeon's anger and a reprimand from the charge nurse. If the nurse follows the charge nurse's advice, the nurse will receive approval from the charge nurse and surgeon; however, the nurse risks being seen as unassertive, and the nurse violates a personal value of truthfulness. If the nurse requests a conference, the nurse may gain respect for assertiveness and professionalism, but the nurse risks the surgeon's annoyance at having the instructions questioned.
11. Participate actively in resolving the issue. Recommend actions that can be ethically supported, recognizing that all actions have positive and negative aspects.	The appropriate degree of nursing input varies with the situation. Sometimes nurses participate in choosing what will be done; sometimes they merely support a client who is making the decision. In this situation, if an action cannot be agreed on, the nurse must decide whether this issue is important enough to merit the personal risks involved.
12. Implement the action.	The nurse will carry out one of the actions developed in step 8.
13. Evaluate the action taken. Involve the client, family, and other health members in the evaluation, if possible.	The nurse can begin by asking, "Did I do the right thing?" Would the nurse make the same decisions again if the situation were repeated? If the nurse is not satisfied, the nurse can review other alternatives and work through the process again.

Note: From "Preparing Students to be Moral Agents in Clinical Nursing Practice," by J. Cassells and B. Redman, 1989, *Nursing Clinics of North America, 24*(2), pp. 463–473. Reprinted with permission.

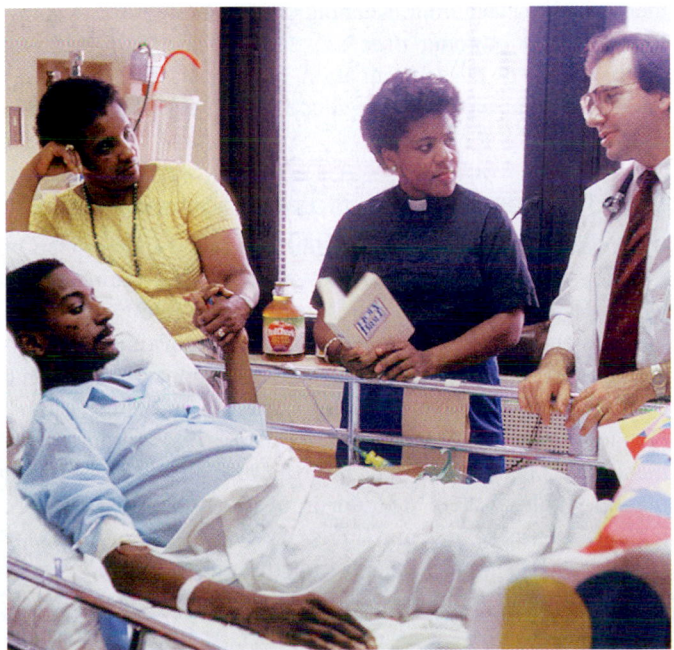

Figure 5–2 ■ Spiritual issues often arise when there is a need for ethical decisions or client advocacy. (A. Ramsey/PhotoEdit.)

Most state and provincial laws have provisions known as conscience clauses that permit individual physicians and nurses, as well as institutions, to refuse to assist with an abortion if doing so violates their religious or moral principles. However, nurses have no right to impose their values on a client. Nursing codes of ethics support clients' rights to information and counseling in making decisions.

Organ Transplantation

Organs for transplantation may come from living donors or from donors who have just died. Many living people choose to become donors by giving consent under the Uniform Anatomical Gift Act (see Chapter 41). Ethical issues related to organ transplantation include allocation of organs, selling of body parts, involvement of children as potential donors, consent, clear definition of death, and conflicts of interest between potential donors and recipients. In some situations, a person's religious belief may also present conflict. For example, certain religions forbid the mutilation of the body, even for the benefit of another person.

End-of-Life Issues

The increase in technological advances and the growing number of elderly people have expanded the ethical dilemmas faced by elders and the health care professions. Providing them with information and professional assistance, as well as the highest quality of care and caring, is of the utmost importance during these times. Some of the most frequent disturbing ethical problems for nurses involve issues that arise around death and dying. These include euthanasia, assisted suicide, termination of life-sustaining treatment, and withdrawing or withholding of food and fluids.

Advance Directives

Many moral problems surrounding the end of life can be resolved if clients complete advance directives. Presently, all 50

Research Note

How Do Nurses, Patients, and Families Feel about Making Bioethical Decisions?

Using the phenomenological research methodology, 15 nurses, 5 patients, and 11 family members were interviewed about their experiences and feelings of being involved in a bioethical decision. Significant statements were reviewed and collapsed into themes. The 10 themes that resulted for the nurses were frustration, guilt, anger, sadness, confidence, support from colleagues, advocacy, knowledge, contentedness with outcomes, and power. The themes for patients/families were frustration, guilt, anger, hope, ability to make decisions, support from staff, control, knowledge, agreement with decisions, and power. The author developed a visual analog scale that allows the nurse/client to indicate their feelings along the line between the polar opposites, for example, anger/no anger, power/powerlessness. Most participants reported that their experiences were negative.

Implications: The author concluded that the negative feelings of nurses and clients in making bioethical decisions could not exist if the environment in which they functioned was more caring and concerned. Clearly, if clients rate their support from staff, control, knowledge, agreement with decisions, and power on the negative end of the spectrum, nurses have a great deal of work to do in better sustaining, communicating with, and educating clients and families. In addition, the health care setting has a responsibility to investigate the specific source of the nurses' feelings of lack of support from colleagues, confidence, and knowledge.

Note: From "The Feelings Nurses/Families Experience When Faced with the Need to Make Bioethical Decisions," by G. L. Husted, 2001, *Nursing Administration Quarterly, 25*(3), pp. 46–54.

of the United States have enacted advance directive legislation. Advance directives direct caregivers as to the client's wishes about treatments, providing an ongoing voice for clients when they have lost the capacity to make or communicate their decisions. See Chapter 41 ∞ for a full discussion of advance directives.

Euthanasia and Assisted Suicide

Euthanasia, a Greek word meaning "good death," is popularly known as "mercy killing." **Active euthanasia** involves actions to directly bring about the client's death, with or without client consent. An example of this would be the administration of a lethal medication to end the client's suffering. Regardless of the caregiver's intent, active euthanasia is forbidden by law and can result in criminal charges of murder.

Active euthanasia includes **assisted suicide,** or giving clients the means to kill themselves if they request it (e.g., providing pills or a weapon). Some countries or states have laws permitting assisted suicide for clients who are severely ill, near death, and who wish to commit suicide. In any case, the nurse should recall that legality and morality are not one and the same. Determining whether an action is legal is only one aspect

of deciding whether it is ethical. The questions of suicide and assisted suicide are still controversial in our society. The American Nurses Association's position statement on assisted suicide (ANA, 1995) states that active euthanasia and assisted suicide are in violation of the *Code for Nurses.*

Passive euthanasia involves the withdrawal of extraordinary means of life support, such as removing a ventilator or withholding special attempts to revive a client (e.g., giving the client "no code" status).

Termination of Life-Sustaining Treatment

Antibiotics, organ transplants, and technological advances (e.g., ventilators) help to prolong life, but not necessarily to restore health. Clients may specify that they wish to have life-sustaining measures withdrawn, they may have advance directives on this matter, or they may appoint a surrogate decision maker. However, it is usually more troubling for health care professionals to withdraw a treatment than to decide initially not to begin it. Nurses must understand that a decision to withdraw treatment is not a decision to withdraw care. As the primary caregivers, nurses must ensure that sensitive care and comfort measures are given as the client's illness progresses.

It is difficult for families to withdraw treatment, which makes it very important that they fully understand the treatment. They often have misunderstandings about which treatments are life sustaining. Keeping clients and families well informed is an ongoing process, allowing them time to ask questions and discuss the situation. It is also essential that they understand that they can reevaluate and change their decision if they wish

Withdrawing or Withholding Food and Fluids

It is generally accepted that providing food and fluids is part of ordinary nursing practice and, therefore, a moral duty. However, when food and fluids are administered by tube to a dying client, or are given over a long period of time to an unconscious client who is not expected to improve, then some consider it to be an extraordinary, or heroic, measure. A nurse is morally obligated to withhold food and fluids (or any treatment) if it is determined to be more harmful to administer them than to withhold them. The nurse must also honor competent patients' refusal of food and fluids. The ANA *Code of Ethics for Nurses* (2001) supports this position through the nurse's role as a client advocate and through the moral principle of autonomy.

Allocation of Scarce Health Resources

Allocation of limited supplies of health care goods and services, including organ transplants, artificial joints, and the services of specialists, has become an especially urgent issue as medical costs continue to rise and more stringent cost-containment measures are implemented.

Nursing care is also a health resource. Most institutions have been implementing "workplace redesign" in order to cut costs. As a result, nursing units are staffed with fewer RNs and more unlicensed caregivers. Some nurses are concerned that staffing in their institutions is not adequate to give the level of care they value. Nurses must continue to look for ways to balance economics and caring in the allocation of health resources.

Management of Computerized Information

In keeping with the principle of autonomy, nurses are obligated to respect clients' privacy and confidentiality. Clients must be able to trust that nurses will reveal details of their situations only as appropriate and will communicate only the information necessary to provide for their health care. Computerized client records make sensitive data accessible to more people and accent issues of confidentiality. Nurses should help develop and follow security measures and policies to ensure appropriate use of client data. For example, nurses should not give their system security codes to unauthorized persons to allow access to computer files.

ADVOCACY

When people are ill, they are frequently unable to assert their rights as they would if they were healthy. An **advocate** is one who expresses and defends the cause of another. A **client advocate** is an advocate for clients' rights. The health care system is complex and many clients are too ill to deal with it. If they are to keep from "falling through the cracks," clients need an advocate to cut through the layers of bureaucracy and help them get what they require. Values basic to client advocacy are shown in Box 5–9. Clients may also advocate for themselves. Today, clients are seeking more self-determination and control over their own bodies when they are ill.

Several versions of a patient's bill of rights have been published by consumer organizations. The most commonly used was originally adopted by the American Hospital Association in 1973 and last revised in 1992 (see Box 5–10). A national patients' bill of rights, the McCain-Edwards-Kennedy/Ganske-Dingell bill (S. 1052/H.R. 526), passed the United States Senate in July 2001. It contains a number of different issues including shared decision making, the right to be informed of all medical options, and the right to refuse treatment. One controversial aspect of the proposed bill is the right to file suit against insurance companies.

If a client lacks decision-making capacity, is legally incompetent, or is a minor, these rights can be exercised on the client's behalf by a designated surrogate or proxy decision maker. It is important, however, for the nurse to remember that client control over health decisions is a Western view. In other countries and societies, such decisions may normally be made by the head of the family or another member of the community. The nurse must ascertain the client and family's views and honor their traditions regarding the locus of decision making.

The Advocate's Role

The overall goal of the client advocate is to protect clients' rights. An advocate informs clients about their rights and provides them with the information they need to make informed decisions.

An advocate supports clients in their decisions, giving them full or at least mutual responsibility in decision making when they are capable of it. The advocate must be careful to remain objective and not convey approval or disapproval of the client's choices. Advocacy requires accepting and respecting the client's right to decide, even if the nurse believes the decision to be wrong.

In mediating, the advocate directly intervenes on the client's behalf, often by influencing others. An example of acting on behalf of a client is asking a physician to review with the client the reasons for and the expected duration of therapy because the client says he always forgets to ask the physician.

Advocacy in Home Care

Although the goals of advocacy remain the same, home care poses unique concerns for the nurse advocate. For example, while in the hospital, people may operate from the values of the nurses and physicians. When they are at home they tend to operate from their own personal values, and may revert to old habits and ways of doing things that may not be beneficial to their health. The nurse may see this as noncompliance; nevertheless, client autonomy must be respected.

In home care, limited resources and a lack of client care services may shift the focus from client welfare to concerns about resource allocation. Financial considerations can limit the availability of services and materials, making it difficult to ensure that client needs are met.

Professional and Public Advocacy

Advocacy is needed for the nursing profession as well as for the public. Gains that nursing makes in developing and improving health policy at the institutional and government levels help to achieve better health care for the public.

Nurses who function responsibly as professional and public advocates are in a position to effect change. To act as an advocate in this arena, the nurse needs an understanding of the ethical issues in nursing and health care, as well as knowledge of the laws and regulations that affect nursing practice and the health of society (see Chapter 4).

BOX 5–9	■ Values Basic to Client Advocacy

- The client is a holistic, autonomous being who has the right to make choices and decisions.
- Clients have the right to expect a nurse–client relationship that is based on shared respect, trust, collaboration in solving problems related to health and health care needs, and consideration of their thoughts and feelings.
- It is the nurse's responsibility to ensure the client has access to health care services that meet health needs.

BOX 5–10   ■ A Patient's Bill of Rights

A Patient's Bill of Rights was first adopted by the American Hospital Association in 1973.
This revision was approved by the AHA Board of Trustees on October 21, 1992.

Introduction

Effective health care requires collaboration between patients and physicians and other health care professionals. Open and honest communication, respect for personal and professional values, and sensitivity to differences are integral to optimal patient care. As the setting for the provision of health services, hospitals must provide a foundation for understanding and respecting the rights and responsibilities of patients, their families, physicians, and other caregivers. Hospitals must ensure a health care ethic that respects the role of patients in decision making about treatment choices and other aspects of their care. Hospitals must be sensitive to cultural, racial, linguistic, religious, age, gender, and other differences as well as the needs of persons with disabilities.

The American Hospital Association presents *A Patient's Bill of Rights* with the expectation that it will contribute to more effective patient care and be supported by the hospital on behalf of the institution, its medical staff, employees, and patients. The American Hospital Association encourages health care institutions to tailor this bill of rights to their patient community by translating and/or simplifying the language of this bill of rights as may be necessary to ensure that patients and their families understand their rights and responsibilities.

Bill of Rights

These rights can be exercised on the patient's behalf by a designated surrogate or proxy decision maker if the patient lacks decision-making capacity, is legally incompetent, or is a minor.

1. The patient has the right to considerate and respectful care.
2. The patient has the right to and is encouraged to obtain from physicians and other direct caregivers relevant, current, and understandable information concerning diagnosis, treatment, and prognosis.

    Except in emergencies when the patient lacks decision-making capacity and the need for treatment is urgent, the patient is entitled to the opportunity to discuss and request information related to the specific procedures and/or treatments, the risks involved, the possible length of recuperation, and the medically reasonable alternatives and their accompanying risks and benefits.

    Patients have the right to know the identity of physicians, nurses, and others involved in their care, as well as when those involved are students, residents, or other trainees. The patient also has the right to know the immediate and long-term financial implications of treatment choices, insofar as they are known.
3. The patient has the right to make decisions about the plan of care prior to and during the course of treatment and to refuse a recommended treatment or plan of care to the extent permitted by law and hospital policy and to be informed of the medical consequences of this action. In case of such refusal, the patient is entitled to other appropriate care and services that the hospital provides or transfer to another hospital. The hospital should notify patients of any policy that might affect patient choice within the institution.
4. The patient has the right to have an advance directive (such as a living will, health care proxy, or durable power of attorney for health care) concerning treatment or designating a surrogate decision maker with the expectation that the hospital will honor the intent of that directive to the extent permitted by law and hospital policy.

    Health care institutions must advise patients of their rights under state law and hospital policy to make informed medical choices, ask if the patient has an advance directive, and include that information in patient records. The patient has the right to timely information about hospital policy that may limit its ability to implement fully a legally valid advance directive.
5. The patient has the right to every consideration of privacy. Case discussion, consultation, examination, and treatment should be conducted so as to protect each patient's privacy.
6. The patient has the right to expect that all communications and records pertaining to his/her care will be treated as confidential by the hospital, except in cases such as suspected abuse and public health hazards when reporting is permitted or required by law. The patient has the right to expect that the hospital will emphasize the confidentiality of this information when it releases it to any other parties entitled to review information in these records.
7. The patient has the right to review the records pertaining to his/her medical care and to have the information explained or interpreted as necessary, except when restricted by law.
8. The patient has the right to expect that, within its capacity and policies, a hospital will make reasonable response to the request of a patient for appropriate and medically indicated care and services. The hospital must provide evaluation, service, and/or referral as indicated by the urgency of the case. When medically appropriate and legally permissible, or when a patient has so requested, a patient may be transferred to another facility. The institution to which the patient is to be transferred must first have accepted the patient for transfer. The patient must also have the benefit of complete information and explanation concerning the need for, risks, benefits, and alternatives to such a transfer.
9. The patient has the right to ask and be informed of the existence of business relationships among the hospital, educational institutions, other health care providers, or payers that may influence the patient's treatment and care.
10. The patient has the right to consent to or decline to participate in proposed research studies or human experimentation affecting care and treatment or requiring direct patient involvement, and to have those studies fully explained prior

BOX 5–10   ■ A Patient's Bill of Rights continued

to consent. A patient who declines to participate in research or experimentation is entitled to the most effective care that the hospital can otherwise provide.

11. The patient has the right to expect reasonable continuity of care when appropriate and to be informed by physicians and other caregivers of available and realistic patient care options when hospital care is no longer appropriate.

12. The patient has the right to be informed of hospital policies and practices that relate to patient care, treatment, and responsibilities. The patient has the right to be informed of available resources for resolving disputes, grievances, and conflicts, such as ethics committees, patient representatives, or other mechanisms available in the institution. The patient has the right to be informed of the hospital's charges for services and available payment methods.

The collaborative nature of health care requires that patients, or their families/surrogates, participate in their care. The effectiveness of care and patient satisfaction with the course of treatment depend, in part, on the patient fulfilling certain responsibilities. Patients are responsible for providing information about past illnesses, hospitalizations, medications, and other matters related to health status. To participate effectively in decision making, patients must be encouraged to take responsibility for requesting additional information or clarification about their health status or treatment when they do not fully understand information and in-

structions. Patients are also responsible for ensuring that the health care institution has a copy of their written advance directive if they have one. Patients are responsible for informing their physicians and other caregivers if they anticipate problems in following prescribed treatment.

Patients should also be aware of the hospital's obligation to be reasonably efficient and equitable in providing care to other patients and the community. The hospital's rules and regulations are designed to help the hospital meet this obligation. Patients and their families are responsible for making reasonable accommodations to the needs of the hospital, other patients, medical staff, and hospital employees. Patients are responsible for providing necessary information for insurance claims and for working with the hospital to make payment arrangements, when necessary.

A person's health depends on much more than health care services. Patients are responsible for recognizing the impact of their life-style on their personal health.

Conclusion

Hospitals have many functions to perform, including the enhancement of health status, health promotion, and the prevention and treatment of injury and disease; the immediate and ongoing care and rehabilitation of patients; the education of health professionals, patients, and the community; and research. All these activities must be conducted with an overriding concern for the values and dignity of patients.

Being an effective client advocate involves the following:

- Being assertive
- Recognizing that the rights and values of clients and families must take precedence when they conflict with those of health care providers
- Being aware that conflicts may arise over issues that require consultation, confrontation, or negotiation between the nurse

and administrative personnel or between the nurse and physician
- Working with community agencies and lay practitioners
- Knowing that advocacy may require political action—communicating a client's health care needs to government and other officials who have the authority to do something about these needs.

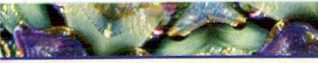 **Focus on Critical Thinking**

A 79-year-old man with severe peripheral vascular disease has been told that a nonhealing lesion on his foot must be treated either with vascular bypass surgery or amputation of the foot. Although the surgeon believes the foot can be saved with bypass, the man elects to have the amputation. His main reason is that the site will heal more quickly and allow him to resume normal activities sooner. He asks for the nurse's opinion.

1. What values and beliefs does the client seem to embrace?
2. What additional information might the nurse need to gather from the client or the surgeon?

3. Does the nurse have an ethical/moral responsibility in this instance?
4. Does the nurse face any conflicting loyalties and obligations?
6. Of what value is the *Code of Ethics for Nurses* to the nurse in solving this dilemma?

See Critical Thinking Possibilities in Appendix A.

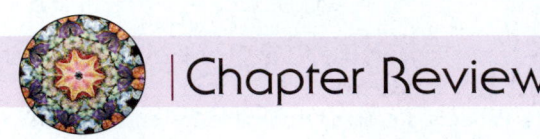

Chapter Review

EXPLORE MediaLink

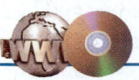

NCLEX review questions, case studies, MediaLink applications, and other interactive resources for this chapter can be found on the Companion Website at www.prenhall.com/kozier. Click on Chapter 5 to select the activities for this chapter.

For more NCLEX review questions, and an audio glossary, access the Student CD-ROM accompanying this textbook.

Chapter Highlights

- Values give direction and meaning to life and guide a person's behavior.
- Values are freely chosen, prized, and cherished, affirmed to others, and consistently incorporated into one's behavior.
- Values clarification is a process in which people identify, examine, and develop their own values.
- Nursing ethics refers to the moral problems that arise in nursing practice and to ethical decisions that nurses make.
- Morality refers to what is right and wrong in conduct, character, or attitude.
- Moral issues are those that arouse conscience, are concerned with important values and norms, and evoke words such as *good, bad, right, wrong, should,* and *ought.*
- Three common moral frameworks (approaches) are consequence-based (teleologic), principles-based (deontologic), and relationships-based (caring-based) theories.
- Moral principles (e.g., autonomy, beneficence, nonmaleficence, justice, fidelity, and veracity) are broad, general philosophical concepts that can be used to make and explain moral choices.
- A professional code of ethics is a formal statement of a group's ideals and values that serves as a standard and guideline for the group's professional actions and informs the public of its commitment.

- Ethical problems are created as a result of changes in society, advances in technology, conflicts within nursing itself, and nurses' conflicting loyalties and obligations (e.g., to clients, families, employers, physicians, and other nurses).
- Nurses' ethical decisions are influenced by their moral theories and principles, levels of cognitive development, personal and professional values, and nursing codes of ethics.
- The goal of ethical reasoning, in the context of nursing, is to reach a mutual, peaceful agreement that is in the best interests of the client; reaching the agreement may require compromise.
- Nurses are responsible for determining their own actions and for supporting clients who are making moral decisions or for whom decisions are being made by others.
- Nurses can enhance their ethical practice and client advocacy by clarifying their own values, understanding the values of other health care professionals, becoming familiar with nursing codes of ethics, and participating in ethics committees and rounds.
- Client advocacy involves concern for and actions on behalf of another person or organization in order to bring about change.
- The functions of the advocacy role are to inform, support, and mediate.

Review Questions

5–1. The most important nursing responsibility in patient care ethical situations is to
   a. be able to defend the morality of one's own actions.
   b. remain neutral and detached in ethical decisions.
   c. ensure that a team is responsible for deciding ethical questions.
   d. follow exactly the client and family wishes.

5–2. Which of the following is most clearly a question of nursing ethics?
   a. The hospital policy permits use of internal fetal monitoring during labor. However, there is literature both to support and refute the value of this practice.
   b. When asked about the purpose of a medication, a nurse colleague responds, "Oh, I never look them up. I just give what the doctor orders."
   c. The nurses on the unit agree to sponsor a fund-raising event to support striking fellow nurses at another facility.
   d. A client reports that he didn't quite tell the doctor the truth when asked if he was following his therapeutic diet at home.

5–3. A child who has been in a car accident has been shown to have no brain function. The parents refuse to allow life support to be withdrawn. Although the nurse believes the child should be allowed to die and organ donation considered, once the parents have decided, the nurse supports their decision. Which moral principle provides the best basis for the nurse's actions?
   a. respect for autonomy
   b. nonmaleficence
   c. beneficence
   d. justice

5–4. Which of the following statements by the nurse would be *most* helpful to assist clients in clarifying their values?
   a. "That was not a good decision. Why did you think it would work?"
   b. "The most important thing is to follow the plan of care. Did you follow all your doctor's orders?"
   c. "Some people might have made a different decision. What led you to make your decision?"
   d. "If you had asked me, I would have given you my opinion about what to do. Now, how do you feel about your choice?"

5–5. An elderly client wants to go home after recovering from her hip replacement. The family wants her to go to a nursing home. Acting as a client advocate, the nurse
   a. informs the family that the client has a right to decide on her own.
   b. asks the physician to discharge the client to home.
   c. suggests the client hire a lawyer to protect her rights.
   d. helps the client and family communicate their views to each other.

Readings and References

Suggested Readings

Haddad, A. (2001). Ethics in action. *RN, 64*(1), 29–30, 32.
   An ethics committee was asked to consider a hypothetical scenario in which a dying woman declines to take pain medication due to her belief in suffering as a religious experience. The nurses' discussion regarding the interfaces between ethics, religion/spirituality, and decision making is presented and the implications for practice are explored.

Meaney, M. E. (2001). More on confidentiality and disclosure: A case study in ethical conflict. *The Case Manager, 12,* 40–42.
   Issues of confidentiality, disclosure, and privacy arise in the attempt to balance individual rights and the legal need for information to be shared among insurance companies, employers, and other entities. The nurse case manager may be caught directly in the middle of this—called upon to assist with the allocation of scarce health resources and yet protect the client's privacy. What is the case manager's obligation to disclose to employers confidential information shared by the client? This and similar dilemmas are discussed as they relate to medical information privacy regulations and ethical principles.

Related Research

Hedel, T., & Wagner, N. (1998). Nursing ethics from a bi-cultural perspective: A comparative survey. *Journal of Multicultural Nursing & Health, 4*(1), 16–21.
McDaniel, C. (1998). Enhancing nurses' ethical practice: Development of a clinical ethics program. *Nursing Clinics of North America, 33,* 299–311.

References

American Association of Colleges of Nursing. (1998). *The essentials of baccalaureat education for professional nursing practice.* Washington, DC: Author.
American Hospital Association. (1992). *A patient's bill of rights.* Chicago: Author.
American Nurses Association. (1988). *Nursing and the human immunodeficiency virus: A guide for nursing's response to AIDS.* Kansas City, MO: Author.
American Nurses Association. (1995). American Nurses Association: Position statement on assisted suicide. *Health Care Law Ethics, 10*(1–2), 125–127.
American Nurses Association. (1998). *Standards of clinical nursing practice* (2nd ed.). Washington, DC: Author.
American Nurses Association. (2001). *Code of ethics for nurses.* Kansas City, MO: Author. Retrieved March 11, 2003, from http://www. nursingworld. org/ethics/code/ ethicscode150.htm
Benner, P., & Wrubel, J. (1989). *The primacy of caring.* Redwood City, CA: Addison-Wesley Nursing.
Bowden, P. L. (1995). The ethics of nursing care and "the ethic of care." *Nursing Inquiry, 2*(1), 10–21.
Canadian Nurses Association. (1997). *Code of ethics for nursing.* Ottawa. Author.
Cassells, J., & Redman, B. (1989). Preparing students to be moral agents in clinical nursing practice. *Nursing Clinics of North America, 24*(2), 463–473.
Gilligan, C. (1982). *In a different voice.* Cambridge, MA: Harvard University Press.
Husted, G. L. (2001). The feelings nurses and patients/families experience when faced with the need to make bioethical decisions. *Nursing Administration Quarterly, 25*(3), 46–54.
International Council of Nurses. (2000). *ICN code for nurses: Ethical concepts applied to nursing.* Geneva: Imprimeries Populaires.
Joint Commission on Accreditation of Healthcare Organizations. (1996). *1997 Accreditation manual for hospitals.* Oakbrook Terrace, IL: Author.
Kohlberg, L. (1969). Stage and sequence: The cognitive-developmental approach to socialization. In D. A. Goslin, (Ed.), *Handbook of socialization theory and research* (pp. 347–480). Chicago: Rand McNally.
Raths, L., Harmin, M., & Simon, S. (1978). *Values and teaching: Working with values in the classroom* (2nd ed.). Columbus, OH: Merrill
Sala, R., & Manara, D. (2001). Nurses and requests for female genital mutilation: Cultural rights versus human rights. *Nursing Ethics, 8,* 247–258.
Thompson, J. B., & Thompson, H. O. (1985). *Bioethical decision-making for nurses.* Norwalk, CT: Appleton-Century-Crofts.
Watson, J. (1981, Summer). Socialization of the nursing student in a professional nursing education programme. *Nursing Papers, 13,* 19–24.
Watson, J. (1988). *Nursing: Human science and human care. A theory of nursing.* New York: National League for Nursing.
Watson, J. (1997). The theory of human caring: Retrospective and prospective. *Nursing Science Quarterly, 10,* 49–52.
O'Connor, A. M., Wells, G. A., Tugwell, P., Laupacis, A., Elmslie, T., & Drake, E. (1999). The effects of an "explicit" values clarification exercise in a woman's decision aid regarding postmenopausal hormone therapy. *Health Expectations, 2*(1), 21–32.

Selected Bibliography

Annas, G. J. (1998). A national patients' bill of rights. *New England Journal of Medicine, 338,* 695–699.

Burkhardt, M. A., & Nathaniel, A. K. (1998). *Ethics and issues in contemporary nursing.* Albany, NY: Delmar.

Catalano, J. T., & Aiken, T. D. (2001). *Legal, ethical, and political issues in nursing* (2nd ed.). Philadelphia: F. A. Davis.

Corey, G., Corey, M., & Callahan, P. (1997). *Issues and ethics in the helping professions* (5th ed.). Stamford, CT: Wadsworth.

Fry, A. T., & Veatch, R. M. (2000). *Case studies in nursing ethics* (2nd ed.). Boston: Jones & Bartlett.

Guido, G. W. (2001). *Legal and ethical issues in nursing* (3rd ed.). Upper Saddle River, NJ: Prentice Hall.

Jecker, N. S., Jonson, A. R., & Pearlman, R. A. (1997). *Bioethics: An introduction to the history, methods, and practice.* Boston: Jones & Bartlett.

Kinsella, L. (2001). Truthtelling in patient care. *Nursing, 31*(12), 52–55.

Purtillo, R. (1999). *Ethical dimensions in the health professions* (3rd ed). Philadelphia: W. B. Saunders.

Saewyc, E. M. (2000). Nursing theories of caring: A paradigm for adolescent nursing practice. *Journal of Holistic Nursing, 18,* 114–128.

Veatch, R. M. (2000). *Cross-cultural perspectives in medical ethics* (2nd ed.). Boston: Jones & Bartlett.

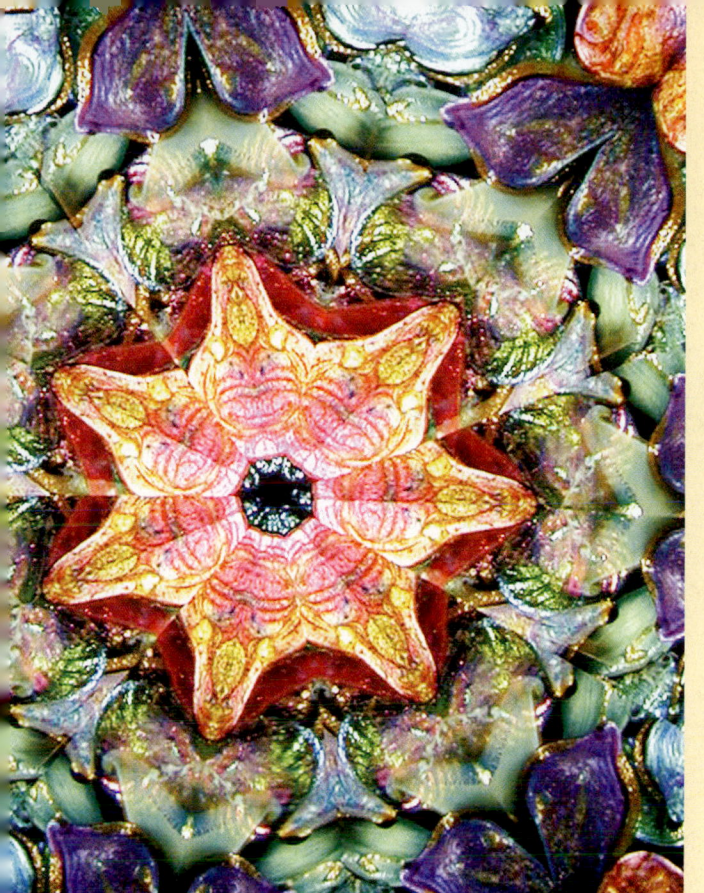

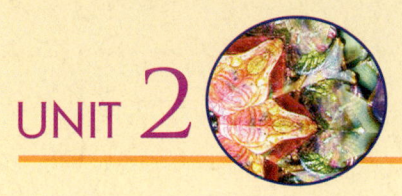

CONTEMPORARY HEALTH CARE

To be effective within a dynamic, complex health care system and to help clients achieve outcomes, nurses need to be knowledgeable, resourceful, and able to work well with other health care practitioners. The nurse is a key participant within interdisciplinary teams whose members share expertise, establish collaborative strategies, and use information technology to support quality care. Nursing care requires even greater flexibility and creativity as it continues to move beyond the hospital into outpatient centers, client homes, and community-based settings.

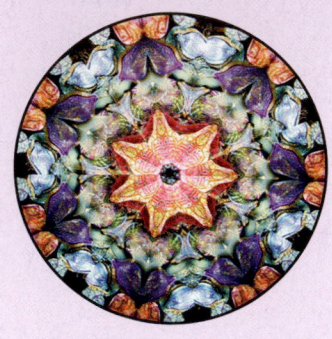

CHAPTER 6

HEALTH CARE DELIVERY SYSTEMS

LEARNING OUTCOMES

After completing this chapter, you will be able to:

- Differentiate primary, secondary, and tertiary health care services.

- Describe the functions and purposes of the health care agencies outlined in this chapter.

- Identify the roles of various health care professionals.

- Describe the factors that affect health care delivery.

- Compare various systems of payment for health care services.

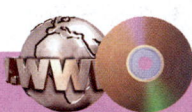

MediaLink

www.prenhall.com/kozier

Additional resources for this chapter can be found on the Student CD-ROM accompanying this textbook, and on the Companion Website at www.prenhall.com/kozier. Click on Chapter 6 to select the activities for this chapter.

CD-ROM
- Audio Glossary
- NCLEX Review

Companion Website
- Additional NCLEX Review
- Case Study: Delivery Systems
- MediaLink Applications:
    Where Do Elders Live?
    Issues Plaguing Women and Children
    Health Care and the Homeless and Poor
    The Competent Case Manager
- Links to Resources

A **health care system** is the totality of services offered by all health disciplines. It is one of the largest industries in the United States. Previously, the primary purpose of a health care system was to provide care to the ill and injured. However, with increasing awareness of health promotion, illness prevention, and levels of wellness, health care systems are changing, as are the roles of nurses in these areas. The services provided by a health care system are commonly categorized according to type and level.

TYPES OF HEALTH CARE SERVICES

Three types of health care services are often described in a way correlated with levels of disease prevention: (a) health promotion and illness prevention (primary prevention), (b) diagnosis and treatment (secondary prevention), and (c) rehabilitation and health restoration (tertiary prevention).

Health Promotion and Illness Prevention

Based on the notion of maintaining an optimum level of wellness, the World Health Organization (WHO) developed a project called Healthy People. The U.S. Department of Health and Human Services (2000) project that evolved from the original work is called *Healthy People 2010* and has two primary goals: (a) increase quality and years of health life and (b) eliminate health disparities.

Health promotion was slow to develop until the 1980s. Since that time more and more people are recognizing the advantages of staying healthy and avoiding illness. Health-promotion programs address areas such as adequate and proper nutrition, weight control and exercise, and stress reduction. Health-promotion activities emphasize the important role clients play in maintaining their own health and encourage them to maintain the highest level of wellness they can achieve.

> ► **CLINICAL ALERT** *As insurance companies have realized that keeping people healthy is less expensive than treating illnesses, their insurance plans have begun to pay for preventive health care activities.* ■

Illness prevention programs may be directed at the client or the community and involve such practices as providing immunizations, identifying risk factors for illnesses, and helping people take measures to prevent these illnesses from occurring. Illness prevention also includes environmental programs that can reduce the incidence of illness or disability. For example, steps to decrease air pollution include requiring inspection of automobile exhaust systems to ensure acceptable levels of fumes. Environmental protective measures are frequently legislated by governments and lobbied for by citizens groups.

Also included as a health-promotion service is early detection of disease. This is accomplished through routine screening of the population and focused screening of those at increased risk of developing certain conditions. Examples of early detection services include regular dental exams from childhood throughout life and bone density studies for women at menopause to evaluate for early osteoporosis. Community-based agencies have become instrumental in providing these services. For example, clinics in some communities provide mammograms and education regarding the early detection of cancer of the breast. Voluntary HIV testing and counseling is another example of the shift in services to community-based agencies. Some shopping malls and shopping centers have walk-in clinics that provide diagnostic screening tests, such as screening for cholesterol and high blood pressure.

Diagnosis and Treatment

In the past, the largest segment of the health care services has been dedicated to the diagnosis and treatment of illness. Hospitals and physicians' offices have been the major agencies offering these complex services. Hospitals continue to focus significant resources on patients requiring emergency, intensive, and round-the-clock acute care.

Freestanding diagnostic and treatment facilities have also evolved and serve ever-growing numbers of clients. For example, magnetic resonance imaging (MRI) and related radiological diagnostic procedures are commonly performed at physician- or corporate-owned centers. Similar structures exist in outpatient surgical units (surgi-centers).

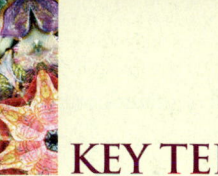

Rehabilitation, Health Restoration, and Palliative Care

Rehabilitation is a process of restoring ill or injured people to optimum and functional levels of wellness. Rehabilitative care emphasizes the importance of assisting clients to function adequately in the physical, mental, social, economic, and vocational areas of their lives. The goal of rehabilitation is to help people move to their previous level of health (i.e., to their previous capabilities) or to the highest level they are capable of given their current health status. Rehabilitation may begin in the hospital, but will eventually lead clients back into the community for further treatment and follow-up once health has been restored.

Sometimes, people cannot be returned to health. A growing field of nursing and health care services is that of palliative care—providing comfort and treatment for symptoms. End-of-life care may be conducted in many settings including the home.

TYPES OF HEALTH CARE AGENCIES AND SERVICES

Health care agencies and services in the United States and Canada are both varied and numerous. Some health care agencies or systems provide services in different settings; for example, a hospital may provide acute inpatient services, outpatient clinic or ambulatory care services, and emergency room services. Hospice services may be provided in the hospital, in the home, or in another agency within the community (see Figure 6–1 ■). Because the array of health care agencies and services is so great, nurses often need to help clients choose that which best suits their needs. Clients may be seen by any number and type of providers depending on their care and ability to pay for the services.

Public Health

Government (official) agencies are established at the local, state or provincial, and federal levels to provide public health services. Health agencies at the state, county, or city level vary according to the need of the area. Their funds, generally from taxes, are administered by elected or appointed officials. Local health departments have responsibility for developing programs to meet the health needs of the people, providing the necessary staff and facilities to carry out these programs, continually evaluating the effectiveness of the programs, and monitoring changing needs. State health organizations are responsible for assisting the local health departments. In some remote areas, state departments also provide direct services to people.

The Public Health Service (PHS) of the U.S. Department of Health and Human Services is an official agency at the federal level. Its functions include conducting research and providing training in the health field, providing assistance to communities in planning and developing health facilities, and assisting states and local communities through financing and provision of trained personnel. Also at the national level in the United States are research institutions such as the National Institutes of Health (NIH). The National Institute on Drug Abuse, the National Institute on Alcohol Abuse and Alcoholism, and the National Institute of Mental Health work with federal, regional, and state agencies. The Centers for Disease Control and Prevention

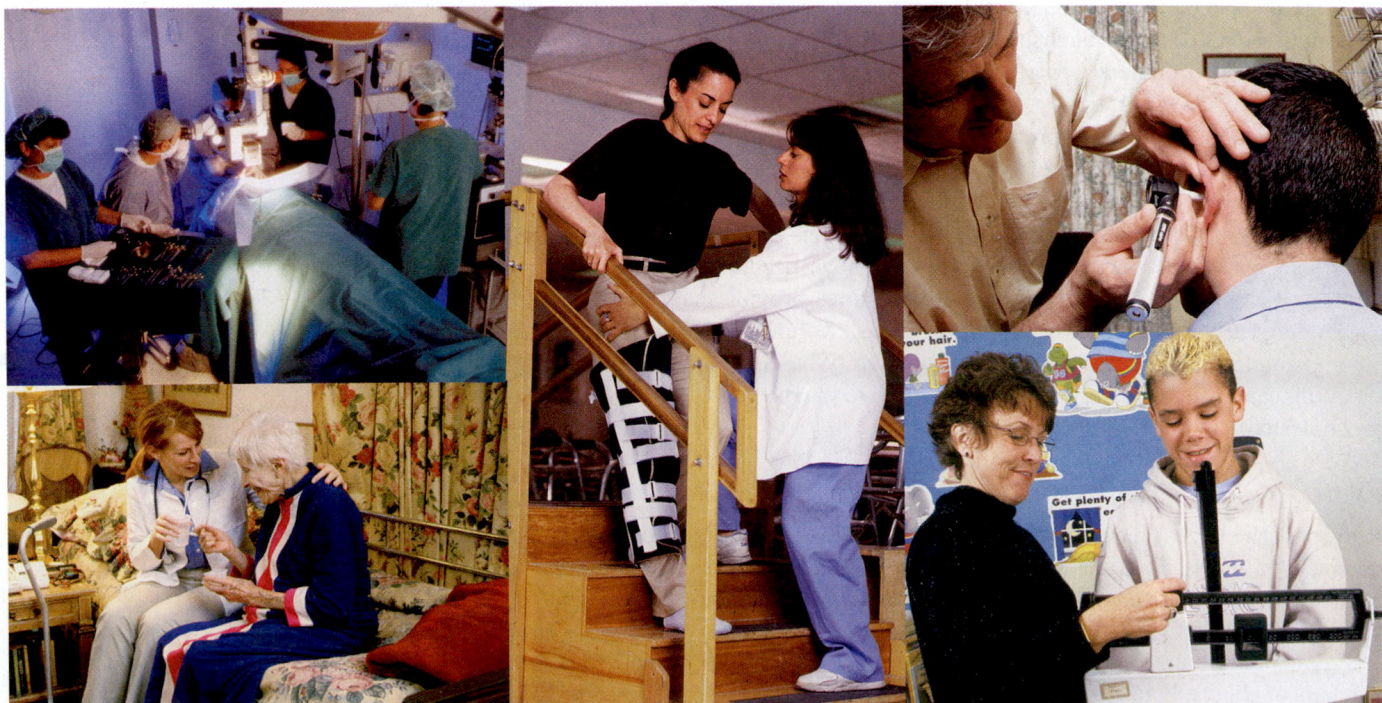

Figure 6–1 ■ Various health care settings. (a-Collection/CNRI/Phototake; b-Mednet/Phototake; c-Mark Thomas/Science Photo Library/Photo Researchers, Inc.; d-David M. Grossman/Phototake; e-Michelle Bridwell/PhotoEdit.)

(CDC) in Atlanta, Georgia, administer a broad program related to surveillance of diseases and behaviors that lead to disease and disability. By means of laboratory and epidemiological investigations, data are made available to the appropriate authorities. The CDC also publishes recommendations about the prevention and control of infections and administers a national health program. The federal government also administers a number of Veterans Administration (VA) services in the United States.

The Canadian Department of Health and Welfare administers such federal programs as native health in the north and health care in the territories. However, provincial governments generally have responsibility for administering health services to the people of each province.

Physicians' Offices

In North America, the physician's office is a primary care setting. The majority of physicians either have their own offices or work with several other physicians in a group practice. Clients usually go to a physician's office for routine health screening, illness diagnosis, and treatment. People often seek consultation from physicians when they are experiencing symptoms of illness or when a significant other considers the person to be ill.

Often, physician's offices do not require the expertise of registered nurses. Where there are RNs, they have a variety of roles and responsibilities including client registration, preparing the client for an examination, obtaining health information, and providing information. Other functions may include obtaining specimens, assisting with procedures, and providing some treatments. In offices without RNs, these tasks may be performed by medical assistants.

Ambulatory Care Centers

Ambulatory care centers are used frequently in many communities. Most ambulatory care centers have diagnostic and treatment facilities providing medical, nursing, laboratory, and radiological services, and they may or may not be attached to or associated with an acute care hospital. Some ambulatory care centers provide services to people who require minor surgical procedures that can be performed outside the hospital. After surgery, the client returns home, often the same day. These centers offer two advantages: They permit the client to live at home while obtaining necessary health care, and they free costly hospital beds for seriously ill clients. The term *ambulatory care center* has replaced the term *clinic* in many places.

Occupational Health Clinics

The industrial (occupational) clinic is gaining importance as a setting for employee health care. Employee health has long been recognized as important to productivity. Today, more companies recognize the value of healthy employees and encourage healthy lifestyles by providing exercise facilities and coordinating health-promotion activities.

Community health nurses in the occupational setting have a variety of roles. Worker safety has always been a concern of occupational nurses. Today, nursing functions in industrial health care include work safety and health education, annual employee health screening for tuberculosis, and maintaining immunization information. Other functions may include screening for such health problems as hypertension and obesity, caring for employees following injury, and counseling.

Hospitals

Hospitals vary in size from the 12-bed rural hospital to the 1,500-bed metropolitan hospital. Hospitals can be classified according to their ownership or control as governmental (public) or nongovernmental (private). In the United States, governmental hospitals are either federal, state, city, or county hospitals; in Canada, they are federal or provincial hospitals. The federal government provides hospital facilities for veterans and merchant mariners (VA hospitals). Military hospitals provide care to military personnel and their families. Private hospitals are often operated by churches, companies, communities, and charitable organizations. Private hospitals may be for-profit or not-for-profit. Although hospitals are chiefly viewed as institutions that provide care, they have other functions, such as providing sources for health-related research and teaching.

Hospitals are also classified by the services they provide. General hospitals admit clients requiring a variety of services, such as medical, surgical, obstetric, pediatric, and psychiatric services. Other hospitals offer only specialty services, such as psychiatric or pediatric care. Hospitals can be further described as acute care or chronic (long-term) care. An acute care hospital provides assistance to clients who are acutely ill or whose illness and need for hospitalization are relatively short term, for example, 2 days. Long-term care hospitals provide services for longer periods, sometimes for years or the remainder of the client's life.

The variety of health care services hospitals provide usually depends on their size and location. The large urban hospitals usually have inpatient beds, emergency services, diagnostic facilities, ambulatory surgery centers, pharmacy services, intensive and coronary care services, and multiple outpatient services provided by clinics. Some large hospitals have other specialized services such as spinal cord injury and burn units, oncology services, and infusion and dialysis units. In addition, some hospitals have substance abuse treatment units and health-promotion units. Small rural hospitals often are limited to inpatient beds, radiology and laboratory services, and basic emergency services. The number of services a rural hospital provides is usually directly related to its size and its distance from an urban center.

Hospitals in the United States have undergone organizational changes in order to contain costs or to attract clients. Some hospitals have merged with other hospitals or have been sold to large multihospital for-profit corporations (e.g., Columbia/HCA Healthcare Corporation, Humana, and Tenet, Inc.). Other hospitals are providing innovative outpatient services, such as fitness classes, day care for elderly people, nutrition classes, and alternative birth centers.

Extended Care (Long-Term Care) Facilities

Extended care facilities, formerly nursing homes, are now often multilevel campuses that include independent living quarters for seniors and assisted living facilities, skilled nursing facilities (intermediate care), and extended care facilities (long-term care) that provide levels of personal care for those who are chronically ill or are unable to care for themselves without assistance. Traditionally, extended care facilities only provided care for elderly clients, but they now provide care to clients of all ages who require rehabilitation or custodial care. Because clients are being discharged earlier from acute care hospitals, some clients may still require supplemental care in a skilled nursing or extended care facility before they return home.

Because long-term illness occurs most often in the elderly, long-term care facilities have programs that are oriented to the needs of this age group. These facilities are intended for people who require not only personal services (bathing, hygiene, assistance with daily activities, and so on) but also some regular nursing care and occasional medical attention. However, the type of care provided varies considerably. Some facilities admit and retain only residents who are able to dress themselves and are ambulatory. Other extended care facilities provide bed care for clients who are more incapacitated. These facilities can, in effect, become the client's home, and consequently the people who live there are frequently referred to as residents rather than patients or clients.

Specific guidelines govern the admission procedures for clients admitted to an extended care facility. Insurance criteria, treatment needs, and nursing care requirements must all be assessed beforehand. Extended care and skilled nursing facilities are becoming increasingly popular means for managing the health care needs of clients who require additional care but do not meet the criteria for remaining in the hospital. Nurses in extended-care facilities assist clients with their daily activities, provide care when necessary, and coordinate rehabilitation activities.

> ▶ CLINICAL ALERT *Elder adults may move among levels of care several times—from independent living, to a hospital, to a rehabilitation center, to long-term care, and hopefully back to independent or assisted living. The sequence varies as will the length of time in each setting.* ◼

Retirement and Assisted-Living Centers

Retirement or assisted-living centers consist of separate houses, condominiums, or apartments for residents. Residents live relatively independently; however, many of these facilities offer meals, laundry services, nursing care, transportation, and social activities. Some centers have a separate hospital to care for residents with short-term or long-term illnesses. Often these centers also work collaboratively with other community services including case managers, social services, and a hospice to meet the needs of the residents who live there. The retirement or assisted-living center is intended to meet the needs of people who are unable to remain at home but do not require hospital or nursing home care. Nurses in retirement and assisted-living centers provide limited care to residents, usually related to the administration of medications and minor treatments and health promotion.

Rehabilitation Centers

Rehabilitation centers usually are independent community centers or special units. However, because rehabilitation ideally starts the moment the client enters the health care system, nurses who are employed on pediatric, psychiatric, or surgical units of hospitals also help to rehabilitate clients. Rehabilitation centers play an important role in assisting clients to restore their health and recuperate. Drug and alcohol rehabilitation centers, for example, help free clients of drug and alcohol dependence and assist them to reenter the community and function to the best of their ability. Today, the concept of rehabilitation is applied to all illness and injury (physical and mental). Nurses in the rehabilitation setting coordinate client activities and ensure that clients are complying with their treatments. This type of nursing often requires specialized skills and knowledge.

Home Health Care Agencies

The implementation of prospective payment (discussed later in this chapter) and the resulting earlier discharge of clients from hospitals have made home care an essential aspect of the health care delivery system. As concerns about the cost of health care have escalated, the use of the home as a care delivery site has increased. In addition, the scope of services offered in the home has broadened. Home health care agencies offer education to clients and families and also provide comprehensive care to acute, chronic, and terminally ill clients.

Day-Care Centers

Day-care centers serve many functions and many age groups. Some day-care centers provide care for infants and children while parents work. Other centers provide care and nutrition for adults who cannot be left at home alone but do not need to be in an institution. Elder care centers often provide care involving socializing, exercise programs, and stimulation. Some centers provide counseling and physical therapy. Nurses who are employed in day-care centers may provide medications, treatments, and counseling, thereby facilitating continuity between day care and home care.

Rural Care

Rural primary care hospitals were created as a result of the 1987 Omnibus Budget Reconciliation Act to provide emergency care to clients in rural areas. In 1997, the Balanced Budget Act authorized the Medicare Rural Hospital Flexibility Program in order to continue to make available primary care access and improve emergency care for rural residents. This program established a new classification called critical access hospitals, which receive federal funding to remain open and provide the breadth of services needed for rural residents, including interfaces with regional tertiary care centers. Each state has an Office of Rural Health Programs that assesses and identifies interventions for the health care needs of the local population. Nurses in rural settings must be generalists who are able to manage a wide variety of clients and health care problems. Nurse practitioners are particularly suited to these roles.

Hospice Services

Originally, a hospice was a place for travelers to rest. Recently the term has come to mean interdisciplinary health care service for the dying provided in the home or another health care setting. The hospice movement subsumes a variety of services given to the terminally ill, their families, and support persons. The central concept of the hospice movement, as distinct from the acute care model, is not saving life but improving or maintaining the quality of life until death. Hospice nurses serve primarily as case managers and supervise the delivery of direct care by other members of the team. Clients in hospice programs are cared for at home, in the hospital, or in skilled nursing facilities. The place of health care delivery may vary as the client's condition declines or the ability of the family to care for the client changes. The hospice nurse does ongoing assessments of needs of the client and family and helps to find the appropriate resources and additional services for them as needed.

Crisis Centers

Crisis centers provide emergency services to clients experiencing life crises. These centers may operate out of a hospital or in the community, and most provide 24-hour telephone service. Some also provide direct counseling to people at the center or in their homes. The primary purpose of a crisis center is to help people cope with an immediate crisis and then provide guidance and support for long-term therapy.

Nurses working in crisis centers need well-developed communication and counseling skills. The nurse must immediately identify the person's problem, offer assistance to help the person cope, and perhaps later direct the person to resources for long-term support.

Mutual Support and Self-Help Groups

In North America today, there are more than 500 mutual support or self-help groups that focus on nearly every major health problem or life crisis people experience. Such groups arose largely because people felt their needs were not being met by the existing health care system. Alcoholics Anonymous, which formed in 1935, served as the model for many of these groups. The National Self-Help Clearinghouse provides information on current support groups and guidelines about how to start a self-help group. The nurse's role in self-help groups is discussed in Chapter 25.

PROVIDERS OF HEALTH CARE

The providers of health care, also referred to as the health care team or health professionals, are health personnel from different disciplines who coordinate their skills to assist clients and their support persons. Their mutual goal is to restore a client's health and promote wellness. The choice of personnel for a particular client depends on the needs of the client. Health teams commonly include the nurse and some or all of the personnel that follow (in alphabetical order).

Nurse

The role of the nurse varies with the needs of the client, the nurse's credentials, and the type of employment setting. A registered nurse (RN) assesses a client's health status, identifies health problems, and develops and coordinates care. A **licensed vocational nurse (LVN),** in some states known as a **licensed practical nurse (LPN),** provides direct client care under the direction of a registered nurse, physician, or other licensed practitioner. As nursing roles have expanded, new dimensions for nursing practice have been established. Nurses can pursue a variety of practice specialties (e.g., critical care, mental health, oncology). Advance practice nurses (APNs) provide direct client care as nurse practitioners, nurse-midwives, certified registered nurse-anesthetists, and clinical nurse specialists. These nurses have education and certifications that—depending on state regulations—may allow them to provide primary care, prescribe medications, and receive third-party (insurance) reimbursement directly for their services.

Alternative Care Provider

Chiropractors, herbalists, acupuncturists, massage therapists, reflexologists, holistic health healers, and other nontraditional health care providers are playing increasing roles in the contemporary health care system. These providers may practice alongside Western health care providers, or clients may use their services in conjunction with, or in lieu of, Western therapies.

Case Manager

The case manager's role is to ensure that clients receive fiscally sound, appropriate care in the best setting. This role is often filled by the member of the health care team who is most involved in the client's care. Depending on the nature of the client's concerns, the case manager may be a nurse, a social worker, an occupational therapist, a physical therapist, or any other member of the health care team.

Dentist

Dentists diagnose and treat dental problems. Dentists are also actively involved in preventive measures to maintain healthy oral structures (e.g., teeth and gums). Many hospitals, especially long-term care facilities, have dentists on staff.

Dietitian or Nutritionist

When dietary and nutritional services are required, the dietitian or nutritionist may be a member of a health team. A dietitian, often a registered dietitian, has special knowledge about the diets required to maintain health and to treat disease. Dietitians in hospitals generally are concerned with therapeutic diets, may design special diets to meet the nutritional needs of individual clients, and supervise the preparation of meals to ensure that clients receive the proper diet.

A nutritionist is a person who has special knowledge about nutrition and food. The nutritionist in a community setting recommends healthy diets and gives broad advisory services about the purchase and preparation of foods. Community nutritionists often function at the preventive level. They promote health and prevent disease, for example, by advising families about balanced diets for growing children and pregnant women.

Occupational Therapist

An occupational therapist (OT) assists clients with an impaired function to gain the skills to perform activities of daily living. For example, an occupational therapist might teach a man with severe arthritis in his arms and hands how to adjust his kitchen utensils so that he can continue to cook. The occupational therapist teaches skills that are therapeutic and at the same time provide some fulfillment. For example, weaving is a recreational activity but also exercises the arthritic man's arms and hands.

OT practitioners can be credentialed at either the professional (occupational therapist) or technical (occupational therapy assistant) level after completing a baccalaureate or entry-level master's degree (OT) or 2-year associate degree (OT assistant) program. In some states, California for example, recent legislation requires that OTs become licensed (they are currently registered). OT assistants are certified.

Paramedical Technologist

Laboratory technologists, radiological technologists, and nuclear medicine technologists are just three kinds of paramedical technologists in the expanding field of medical technology. *Paramedical* means having some connection with medicine. Laboratory technologists examine specimens such as urine, feces, blood, and discharges from wounds to provide exact information that facilitates the medical diagnosis and the prescription of a therapeutic regimen. The radiologic technologist assists with a wide variety of x-ray film procedures, from simple chest radiography to more complex fluoroscopy. The nuclear medicine technologist uses radioactive substances to provide diagnostic information and can administer therapeutic doses of radioactive materials as part of a therapeutic regimen. These technologists have highly specialized skills and knowledge important to client care.

Pharmacist

A pharmacist prepares and dispenses pharmaceuticals in hospital and community settings. The role of the pharmacist in monitoring and evaluating the actions and effects of medica-

tions on clients is becoming increasingly prominent. A clinical pharmacist is a specialist who guides physicians in prescribing medications. A pharmacy assistant is also recognized in some states. This person administers medications to clients or works in the pharmacy under the direction of the pharmacist.

> ► **CLINICAL ALERT** *Significant overlap may occur among those providers who can perform certain health care activities. For example, an anesthesiologist (MD), a neonatal care nurse, or a respiratory therapist may be responsible for assisting a newborn baby with breathing problems. All providers perform client teaching.* ■

Physical Therapist

The licensed physical therapist (PT) assists clients with musculoskeletal problems. Physical therapists treat movement dysfunctions by means of heat, water, exercise, massage, and electric current. The physical therapist's functions include assessing client mobility and strength, providing therapeutic measures (e.g., exercises and heat applications to improve mobility and strength), and teaching new skills (e.g., how to walk with an artificial leg). Some physical therapists provide their services in hospitals; however, independent practitioners establish offices in communities and serve clients either at the office or in the home. Physical therapy aides also work with PTs and clients.

Physician

The physician is responsible for medical diagnosis and for determining the therapy required by a person who has a disease or injury. The physician's role has traditionally been the treatment of disease and trauma (injury); however, many physicians are now including health promotion and disease prevention in their practice. Some physicians are surgeons, oncologists, orthopedists, pediatricians, or psychiatrists.

Physician Assistant

Physician assistants (PAs) perform certain tasks under the direction of a physician. They diagnose and treat certain diseases, conditions, and injuries. In many states, nurses are not legally permitted to follow a PA's orders unless they are cosigned by a physician. In some settings, PAs and nurse practitioners have similar job descriptions.

Podiatrist

Doctors of podiatric medicine (DPM) diagnose and treat foot conditions. They are licensed to perform surgery and prescribe medications.

Respiratory Therapist

A respiratory therapist is skilled in therapeutic measures used in the care of clients with respiratory problems. These therapists are knowledgeable about oxygen therapy devices, intermittent positive pressure breathing respirators, artificial mechanical ventilators, and accessory devices used in inhalation therapy. Respiratory therapists administer many of the pulmonary function tests.

Respiratory therapists are required to complete either a 2-year associate's degree or a 4-year baccalaureate degree. Upon graduation they are eligible to take a national voluntary examination that, upon passing, leads to the credential Certified Respiratory Therapist. Subsequently they may take two more examinations that lead to the Registered Respiratory Therapist credential. Some settings also use respiratory therapy aides.

Social Worker

A social worker counsels clients and support persons regarding social problems, such as finances, marital difficulties, and adoption of children. It is not unusual for health problems to produce problems in living and vice versa. For example, an elderly woman who lives alone and has a stroke resulting in impaired walking may find it impossible to continue to live in her third-floor apartment. Finding a more suitable living arrangement can be the responsibility of the social worker if the client has no support network in place.

Spiritual Support Person

Chaplains, pastors, rabbis, priests, and other religious or spiritual advisors serve as part of the health care team by attending to the spiritual needs of clients. In most facilities, local clergy volunteer their services on a regular or on-call basis. Hospitals affiliated with specific religions, as well as many large medical centers, have full-time chaplains on staff. They usually offer regularly scheduled religious services. The nurse is often instrumental in identifying the client's desire for spiritual support and notifying the appropriate person.

Unlicensed Assistive Personnel

Unlicensed assistive personnel (UAPs) are health care staff who assume delegated aspects of client care. These tasks include bathing, assisting with feeding, and collecting specimens. Their titles include certified nurse assistants, hospital attendants, nurse technicians, patient care technicians, and orderlies. Some of these persons may have standardized education and job duties (e.g., certified nurse assistants), while others do not. The parameters regarding nurse delegation to UAPs are delineated by the state boards of nursing.

FACTORS AFFECTING HEALTH CARE DELIVERY

Today's health care consumers have greater knowledge about their health than in previous years and they are increasingly influencing health care delivery. Formerly, people expected a physician to make decisions about their care; today, however, consumers expect to be involved in making any decisions. Consumers have also become aware of how lifestyle affects health. As a result, they desire more information and services related to health promotion and illness prevention. A number of other factors affect the health care delivery system.

Increasing Number of Elderly

By the year 2020 it is estimated that the number of U.S. adults over the age of 65 years will be more than 53 million (U.S. Census Bureau, 2000). Long-term illnesses are prevalent among this group and frequently require special housing, treatment services, financial support, and social networks. The frail elderly, considered to be people over age 85, are projected to be the fastest growing population in the United States and will number over 76.5 million by 2020 and almost 90 million by 2030 (U.S. Census Bureau). Because only 5% of older people are institutionalized with health problems, substantial home management and nursing support services are required to assist those living in their homes and communities.

Older people also need to feel they are part of a community even though they are approaching the end of their lives. The feeling of being a useful, wanted, and productive citizen is essential to every person's health. Special programs are being designed in communities so that the talents and skills of this group will be used and not lost to society.

Advances in Technology

Scientific knowledge and technology related to health care are rapidly increasing. Improved diagnostic procedures and sophisticated equipment permit early recognition of diseases that might otherwise have remained undetected. New antibiotics and medications are continually being manufactured to treat infections and multiple drug-resistant organisms. Surgical procedures involving the heart, lungs, and liver that were nonexistent 20 years ago are common today. Laser and microscopic procedures streamline the treatment of diseases that required surgery in the past.

Computers, bedside charting, and the ability to store and retrieve large volumes of information in databases are commonplace in health care organizations. In addition, as a result of the Internet and World Wide Web access from numerous public and private locations, clients now have access to medical information similar to that of health care providers (although not all websites provide accurate information).

These discoveries have changed the profile of the client. Clients are now more likely to be treated in the community, utilizing resources, technology, and treatments outside the hospital. For example, years ago a person having cataract surgery had to remain in bed in the hospital for 10 days; today, most cataract removals are performed on an outpatient basis in outpatient surgery centers. These technological advances and specialized treatments and procedures may come, unfortunately, with a high price tag.

Economics

Paying for health care services is becoming a greater problem. The health care delivery system is very much affected by a country's total economic status. According to the National Center for Health Statistics (2000), by 1998 the United States was spending more than $3 billion a day on health care, which is equal to over $4,000 per year for every man, woman, and child. Approximately 55% of these costs were paid through private funds and 45% through public programs. Medical care costs more than doubled from 1985 to 1995 and continue to increase at a rate of approximately 5% each year.

The major reasons for cost increases are as follows:

- Existing equipment and facilities are continually becoming obsolete as research uncovers new and better methods in health care. Health care providers and patients want the newest and the best, and these cost more each year.
- Inflation increases all costs.
- The total population is growing, especially the segment of older adults who tend to have greater health care needs than younger persons.
- As more people recognize that health is everyone's right, large numbers of people are seeking assistance in health matters. The average American sees a doctor five times per year and over 16% of the population is admitted to a hospital annually (Kovner & Jonas, 1999).
- The relative number of people who provide health care services has increased.
- The numbers of uninsured persons are rising: 44 million in 2000 (Agency for Healthcare Research and Quality [AHRQ], 2001a).
- The cost of prescription drugs is increasing. In 2000, these costs increased 14.5% and represented 27% of the total increase in healthcare costs in the United States (Gundling, 2002).

Women's Health

The women's movement has been instrumental in changing health care practices. Examples are the provision of childbirth services in more relaxed settings such as birthing centers, and the provision of overnight facilities for parents in children's hospitals. Until recently, women's health issues focused on the reproductive aspects of health, disregarding many health care concerns that are unique to women. Investigators are beginning to recognize the need for research that examines women equally to men in health issues such as osteoporosis, heart disease, and responses to various treatment modalities. Current provision of health care shows an increased emphasis on the psychosocial aspects of women's health including the impact of career, delayed childbearing, role of caregiver to older family members, and extended life span.

Uneven Distribution of Services

Serious problems in the distribution of health services exist in the United States. Two facets of this problem are (a) uneven distribution and (b) increased specialization. In some areas, particularly remote and rural locations, there are insufficient health care professionals and services available to meet the health care needs of individuals. Rural clients may need to drive large distances to obtain the services they require. Uneven distribution is evidenced by the relatively higher number of nurses per capita in the New England states and the lowest number in California and Nevada (see Figure 6–2 ■). Physicians are also unevenly distributed: In 1998, Mississippi, Alaska, Idaho, Iowa, Wyoming, and Nevada had the fewest

physicians per 100,000 people, whereas the District of Columbia, Massachusetts, and New York had the most (National Center for Health Statistics, 2000).

An increasing number of health care personnel provide specialized services. Specialization can lead to fragmentation of care and, often, increased cost of care. To clients, it may mean receiving care from 5 to 30 people during their hospital experience. This seemingly endless stream of personnel is often confusing and frightening.

Access to Health Care

Another problem plaguing individuals is access to health care. It has been estimated that 44 million Americans have no health insurance (AHRQ, 2001a). Lack of health insurance is related to income. Where only 3.9% of persons who earned more than $50,000 per year in 2000 were without insurance, 17.6% of those earning less than $15,000 per year were uninsured (CDC, 2001). Low income has been associated with relatively higher rates of infectious diseases (e.g., tuberculosis, AIDS), problems with substance abuse, rape, violence, and chronic diseases. The use of health care services is also affected by unemployment and poverty. Even though some government assistance is available, eligibility for government insurance programs and benefits varies considerably from state to state and is continually being reevaluated.

The Homeless and the Poor

It has been estimated that in the 5-year period from 1995 to 2000, 5.7 million Americans had been homeless for at least some period of time (National Health Care for the Homeless Council, 2000). Because of the conditions in which homeless people live (in shelters, on the streets, in parks, in tents, under temporary covers and dwellings, in transportation terminals, or in cars), their health problems are often exacerbated and sometimes become chronic.

Physical, mental, social, and emotional factors create health care challenges for the homeless and the poor (see Box 6–1). Limited access to health care services significantly contributes

BOX 6–1 ■ Factors Contributing to Health Problems of the Homeless and the Poor

- Poor physical environment resulting in increased susceptibility to infections
- Inadequate rest and privacy
- Improper nutrition
- Poor access to facilities for personal hygiene
- Exposure to the elements
- Lack of social support
- Few personal resources
- Questionable personal safety (physical assault is a constant threat for the homeless)
- Inconsistent health care
- Difficulty with adherence to treatment plans

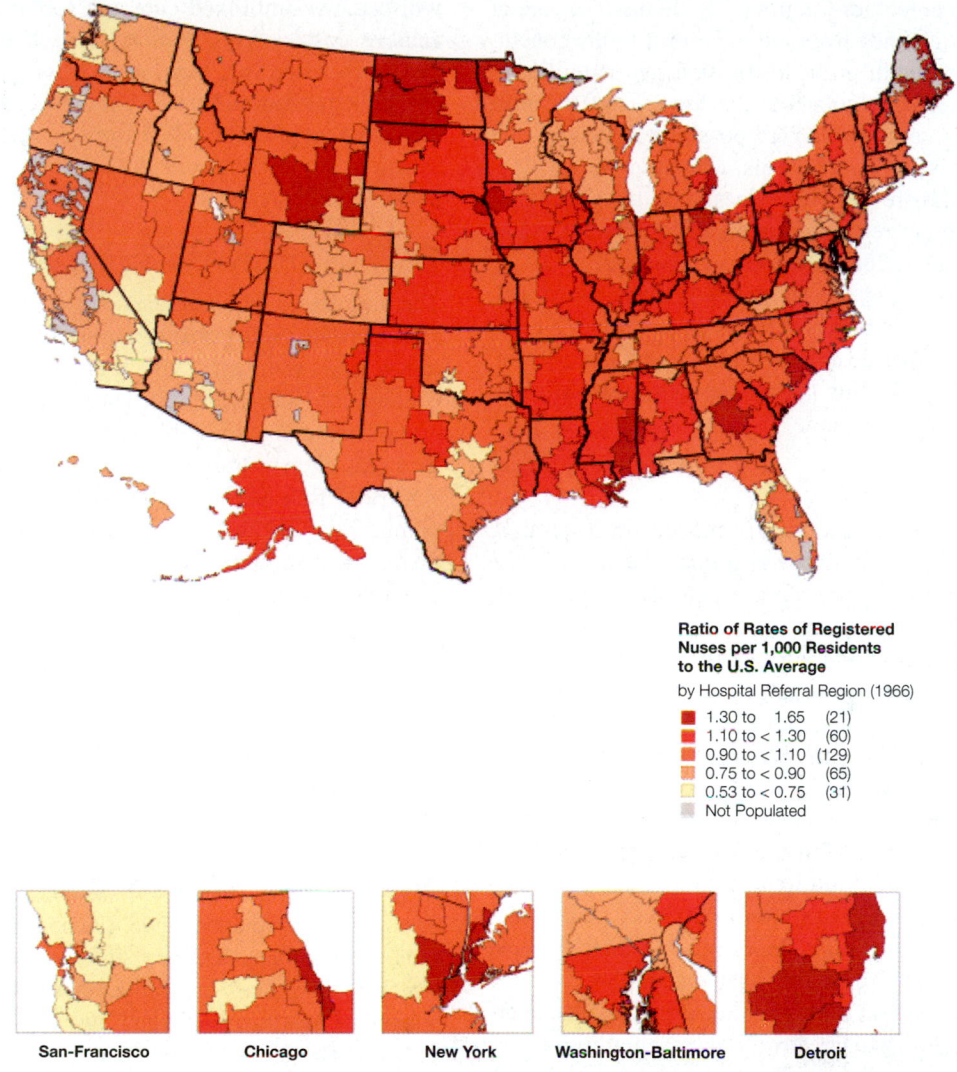

Ratio of Rates of Registered Nuses per 1,000 Residents to the U.S. Average

by Hospital Referral Region (1966)

- 1.30 to   1.65   (21)
- 1.10 to < 1.30   (60)
- 0.90 to < 1.10   (129)
- 0.75 to < 0.90   (65)
- 0.53 to < 0.75   (31)
- Not Populated

San-Francisco   Chicago   New York   Washington-Baltimore   Detroit

Figure 6–2 ■ Nurses per population map. (*Note:* From Center for the Evaluative Clinical Sciences at Dartmouth Medical School, Hanover, NH, http://www.dartmouthatlas.org/99us/chap_2_sec_4.php#. Copyright 2002.)

to the general poor health of the homeless and poor in the United States.

Demographic Changes

The characteristics of the North American family have changed considerably in the last few decades. The numbers of single-parent families and alternative family structures have increased markedly. Most of the single-parent families are headed by women, many of whom work and require assistance with child care or when a child is sick at home.

Recognition of the cultural and ethnic diversity of the United States and Canada is also increasing. Health care professionals and agencies are aware of this diversity and are employing means to meet the challenges it presents. For example, more agencies are employing nurses who are bilingual and who can communicate with clients whose primary language is not English.

FRAMEWORKS FOR CARE

A number of configurations for the delivery of nursing care support continuity of care and cost effectiveness. These include managed care, case management, patient-focused care, differentiated practice, shared governance, the case method, the functional method, team nursing, and primary nursing. These have evolved, some from each other, for reasons such as the need to decrease health care costs and to improve the utilization of limited human and physical resources. A particular agency may use more than one configuration, for example, team nursing on the medical-surgical units and primary nursing on the cardiac surgery unit.

Managed Care

Managed care describes a health care system whose goals are to provide cost-effective, quality care that focuses on decreased costs and improved outcomes for groups of clients. The care of a client is carefully planned from initial contact to the conclusion of the specific health problem. In managed care, health care providers and agencies collaborate so as to render the most appropriate, fiscally responsible care possible. Managed care denotes an emphasis on cost controls, customer satisfaction, health promotion, and preventive services. Health maintenance organizations and preferred provider organizations are examples of provider systems committed to managed care.

Managed care can be used with primary, team, functional, and alternative nursing care delivery systems. Although managed care has been embraced as a model for health care reform, many question the application of this business approach to a commodity as precious as health.

Case Management

Case management describes a range of models for integrating health care services for individuals or groups. Generally, case management involves multidisciplinary teams that assume collaborative responsibility for planning, assessing needs, and coordinating, implementing, and evaluating care for groups of clients from preadmission to discharge or transfer and recuperation. A case manager, however, may be a nurse, social worker, or other appropriate professional. Key responsibilities for case managers are shown in Box 6–2.

Case management may be used as a cost-containment strategy in managed care. Both case management and managed care systems often use **critical pathways** to track the client's progress. A critical pathway is an interdisciplinary plan or tool that specifies interdisciplinary assessments, interventions, treatments, and outcomes for health-related conditions across a time line. Critical pathways are also called critical paths, interdisciplinary plans, anticipated recovery plans, interdisciplinary action plans, and action plans (see the accompanying Critical Pathways box).

Patient-Focused Care

Patient-focused care is a delivery model that brings all services and care providers to the clients. It has been proposed as one of the 10 primary challenges for nursing care in the 21st century (Vandenberg, 1999). The supposition is that if activities normally provided by auxiliary personnel (e.g., physical therapy, respiratory therapy, ECG testing, and phlebotomy) are moved closer to the client, the number of personnel involved and the number of steps involved to get the work done are decreased. Proponents of this type of system believe that clients

will perceive improved care and service and the agency will achieve cost savings. Patient-focused care units often have their own admitting, pharmacy, laboratory, and radiology areas, although variations exist among agencies. Cross-training, development of multiskilled workers who can perform tasks or functions in more than one discipline, is an essential element of patient-focused care.

Differentiated Practice

The purpose of differentiated practice is to make the best possible use of nursing personnel based on their educational preparation and resultant skill sets (American Association of Colleges of Nursing, 1995). Thus, differentiated practice models consist of specific job descriptions for nurses according to their education or training, for example, LVN, associate degree RN, BSN RN, MSN RN, or APN. The model is customized within each health care institution by the nurses employed there. The institution must first identify the nursing competencies required by the clients within the specific practice environment. This model further requires the delineation of roles between both licensed nursing personnel and UAPs. This enables nurses to progress and assume roles and responsibilities appropriate to their level of experience, capability, and education. As with managed care and case management, differentiated nursing practice seeks to provide quality care at an affordable cost.

Shared Governance

The shared governance model can be used in concert with other models of nursing delivery. It is an organizational model in which nursing staff are cooperative with administrative personnel in making, implementing, and evaluating client care policies. The focus of this model is to encourage participation of nurses in decision making at all levels of the organization. Individuals may participate either at their own request or as part of their job role criteria. More commonly, nurses participate through serving in decision-making groups, such as committees and task forces. The decisions made may also address employment conditions, cost effectiveness, long-range planning, productivity, and wages and benefits. The underlying principle of shared governance is that employees will be more committed to the organizational goals if they have had input into planning and decision making.

Case Method

The case method, also referred to as total care, is one of the earliest nursing models developed. In this client-centered method, one nurse is assigned to and is responsible for the comprehensive care of a group of clients during an 8- or 12-hour shift. For each client, the nurse assesses needs, makes nursing plans, formulates diagnoses, implements care, and evaluates the effectiveness of care. In this method, a client has consistent contact with one nurse during a shift but may have different nurses on other shifts. The case method, considered the precursor of primary nursing, continues to be used in a variety of practice settings such as intensive care nursing.

BOX 6–2	■ Responsibilities of Case Managers

- Assessing clients and their homes and communities
- Coordinating and planning client care
- Collaborating with other health professionals
- Monitoring clients' progress
- Evaluating client outcomes

CRITICAL PATHWAY FOR CLIENT FOLLOWING LAPAROSCOPIC CHOLECYSTECTOMY

EXPECTED LENGTH OF STAY: Less than 24 hours

	Date _____ Preoperative	Date _____ 1st 24 hours following surgery
Daily outcomes	Client verbalizes understanding of preoperative teaching including turning, coughing, deep breathing, incentive spirometer, mobilization, and pain management. Client verbalizes ability to cope.	Client is afebrile. Client has a dry, clean wound with edges well approximated, healing by first intention. Client manages pain with nonpharmacologic measures or oral medications. Client is independent in self-care. Client is fully ambulatory. Client has resumed preadmission urine and bowel elimination pattern. Client verbalizes home care instructions. Client tolerates usual diet.
Tests and treatments	CBC Urinalysis Baseline physical assessment: with a focus on respiratory status and gastrointestinal function Anesthesia consult	Vital signs and O_2 saturation, neurovascular assessment, dressing and wound drainage assessment q15 min × 4; q30 min × 4; q1h × 4 and then q4h if stable. Assess lung sounds and gastrointestinal function q4h and prn. Intake and output every shift. Assess voiding—if unable to void, try suggestive voiding techniques or catheterize q8h or prn if unable to void.
Knowledge deficit	Orient to room and surroundings. Provide simple, brief instructions. Review preoperative preparation including hospital and surgical routines. Reinforce preoperative teaching regarding specific postoperative care: turning, coughing, deep breathing, incentive spirometer, mobilization, and pain management.	Reorient to room and postoperative routine. Review plan of care and importance of early mobilization. Begin discharge teaching regarding wound care/dressing change.
Psychosocial	Assess anxiety related to pending surgery. Assess fears of the unknown and surgery. Encourage verbalization of concerns. Provide information regarding surgical experiences. Minimize external stimuli (e.g., noise, movement).	Assess level of anxiety. Encourage verbalization of concerns. Provide information and ongoing support and encouragement.
Diet	NPO Baseline nutritional assessment	Advance to clear liquids; if tolerated, advance to full liquids/soft diet morning following surgery.
Activity	OOB ad lib until premedicated for surgery.	Provide safety precautions. Bathroom privileges with assistance evening after surgery and begin progressive ambulation to tolerance the morning following surgery until fully ambulatory.
Medications	NPO except ordered medications.	IM or PO analgesics Antibiotics if ordered IV fluids until adequate PO intake, then intermittent IV device Discontinue prior to discharge
Transfer/ Discharge plans	Assess discharge plans and support system.	Probable discharge within 24 hours of surgery. Complete discharge home care teaching when fully awake and oriented and before discharge. Provide a written copy of discharge instructions.

Note: From *Critical Pathways for Collaborative Care*, (pp. 111–112) by S.C. Beyea, 1996, Menlo Park, CA: Addison-Wesley Nursing. Adapted with permission.

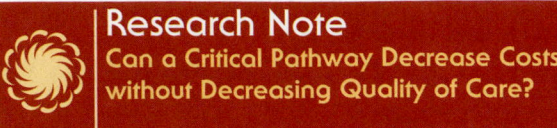

Research Note
Can a Critical Pathway Decrease Costs without Decreasing Quality of Care?

A total of 1,743 clients who presented at the study hospitals' emergency rooms with specific symptoms of pneumonia were treated by conventional plan (10 hospitals) or using the critical pathway (9 hospitals). Outcomes were measured using a quality-of-life instrument 6 weeks following treatment, occurrence of complications, mortality, admission of low-risk clients, and number of days of hospitalization per client.

The only statistically significant differences between the control and treatment groups were a 10% reduction in the number of hospital admissions for low-risk clients and a shorter length of stay for clients with more severe disease in the treatment hospitals. The authors estimated a cost savings of $1,700 per client.

Implications: Although this study had a large sample, it is not known if the same results would be seen if the study were conducted in different areas of the country. Use and acceptability of critical pathways vary geographically. Also, penetration of managed care could lead to similar outcome results without use of a critical path. That is, institutions that have been encouraged to avoid admissions and reduce length of stay due to economic disadvantages associated with increased care may show similar cost savings. Emphasis on future research must be on client and caregiver satisfaction, long-term reductions in complications, and prevention of (re)admission in situations where effective therapy can be provided on an outpatient basis.

Note: From "A Controlled Trial of a Critical Pathway for Treatment of Community-Acquired Pneumonia," by T. J. Marrie, C. Y. Lau, S. L. Wheeler, C. J. Wong, M. K. Vandervort, and B. J. Feagen, 2000, *Journal of the American Medical Association, 283,* pp. 749–755.

Functional Method

The functional nursing method focuses on the jobs to be completed (e.g., bed making, temperature measurement). In this task-oriented approach, personnel with less preparation than the professional nurse perform less complex care requirements. It is based on a production and efficiency model that gives authority and responsibility to the person assigning the work, for example, the head nurse. Clearly defined job descriptions, procedures, policies, and lines of communication are required. The functional approach to nursing is economical and efficient and permits centralized direction and control. Its disadvantages are fragmentation of care and the possibility that nonquantifiable aspects of care, such as meeting the client's emotional needs, may be overlooked.

Team Nursing

Team nursing is the delivery of individualized nursing care to clients by a team led by a professional nurse. A nursing team consists of registered nurses, licensed practical nurses, and unlicensed assistive personnel. This team is responsible for providing coordinated nursing care to a group of clients.

The registered nurse retains responsibility and authority for client care but delegates appropriate tasks to the other team members. Proponents of this model believe the team approach increases the efficiency of the registered nurse. Opponents state that inpatients' high acuity of illness leaves little to be delegated.

Primary Nursing

Primary nursing is a system in which one nurse is responsible for total care of a number of clients 24 hours a day, 7 days a week. It is a method of providing comprehensive, individualized, and consistent care.

Primary nursing uses the nurse's technical knowledge and management skills. The primary nurse assesses and prioritizes each client's needs, identifies nursing diagnoses, develops a plan of care with the client, and evaluates the effectiveness of care. Associates provide some care, but the primary nurse coordinates it and communicates information about the client's health to other nurses and other health professionals. Primary nursing encompasses all aspects of the professional role, including teaching, advocacy, decision making, and continuity of care. The primary nurse is the first-line manager of the client's care with all its inherent accountabilities and responsibilities.

FINANCING HEALTH CARE

Although efforts have been made to control the costs of health care, these costs continue to increase. Employers, legislators, insurers, and health care providers continue to collaborate in efforts to resolve the issues surrounding how to best finance health care costs. Among these efforts, the United States has implemented some cost-containment strategies including health-promotion and illness prevention activities, managed care systems, and alternative insurance delivery systems. Based on reports from the Institute for Medicine, the AHRQ (2001b) identified two research priorities: "Impact of Payment and Organization on Cost, Quality, and Equity" will focus on studies able to demonstrate if payment and reimbursement methods provide efficient and coordinated care. "Patient-Centered Care: Customizing Care to Meet Patients' Needs" emphasizes research into client empowerment, access to health care, and communication with providers.

Payment Sources in the United States

In most situations, a health care agency receives funding from several of the available payment sources. For example, an elderly client may have Medicare coverage and supplement Medicare with private insurance plus the need to pay some out-of-pocket expenses (see Figure 6–3 ■). Almost all insurance plans include a per-visit or per-prescription copayment.

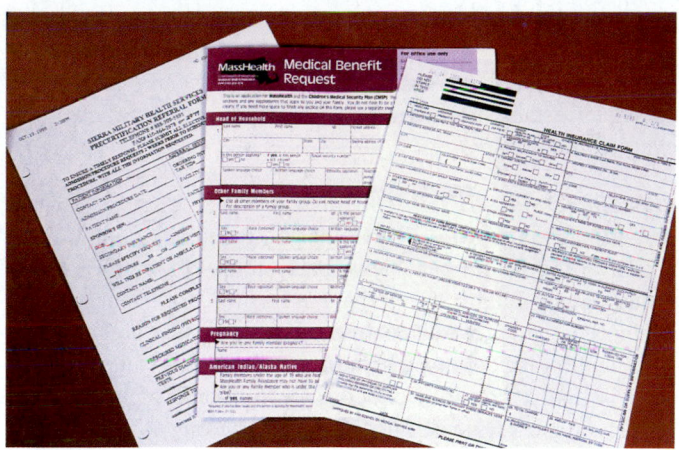

Figure 6–3 ■ Medicare helps defray the costs of health care for elders.

Medicare and Medicaid

In the United States, the 1965 **Medicare** amendments (Title 18) to the Social Security Act provided a national and state health insurance program for older adults. By the mid-1970s, virtually everyone over 65 years old was protected by hospital insurance under Part A, which also includes post-hospital extended care and home health benefits. In 1972, its coverage was broadened to include workers with permanent disabilities and their dependents who are eligible for disability insurance under Social Security. In 1988, Congress expanded Medicare to include extremely expensive hospital care, "catastrophic care," and expensive drugs.

The Medicare plan is divided into two parts: Part A is available to people with disabilities and people 65 years and over. It provides insurance toward hospitalization, home care, and hospice care. Part B is voluntary and provides partial coverage of physician services to people eligible for Part A. Clients pay a monthly premium for this coverage.

All Medicare clients pay a deductible and coinsurance. **Coinsurance** is the 20% share of a government-approved charge that is paid by the client; the other 80% is paid by the plan.

Medicare does not cover dental care, dentures, eyeglasses, hearing aids, or examinations to prescribe and fit hearing aids. Most preventive care, including routine physical examinations and associated diagnostic tests, is also not included.

Medicaid was also established in 1965 under Title 19 of the Social Security Act. Medicaid is a federal public assistance program paid out of general taxes to people who require financial assistance, such as people with low incomes. Medicaid is paid by federal and state governments. Each state program is distinct. Some states provide very limited coverage, whereas others pay for dental care, eyeglasses, and prescription drugs.

In 1972, Congress directed the Department of Health, Education, and Welfare to create professional standards review organizations to monitor the appropriateness of hospital use under the Medicare and Medicaid programs. In 1974, the National Health Planning and Resources Development Act established health systems agencies throughout the United States for comprehensive health planning. In 1978, the Rural Health Clinics Act provided for the development of health care in medically underserved rural areas. This act opened the door for nurse practitioners to provide primary care.

Supplemental Security Income

Persons with disabilities or those who are blind may be eligible for special payments called **Supplemental Security Income (SSI)** benefits. These benefits are also available to people not eligible for Social Security, and payments are not restricted to health care costs. Clients often use this money to purchase medicines or to cover costs of extended health care.

Prospective Payment System

To curtail health care costs in the United States, Congress in 1983 passed legislation putting the prospective payment system into effect. This legislation limits the amount paid to hospitals that are reimbursed by Medicare. Reimbursement is made according to a classification system known as **diagnosis-related groups (DRGs).** The system has categories that establish pretreatment diagnosis billing categories.

Under this system, the hospital is paid a predetermined amount for clients with a specific diagnosis. For example, a hospital that admits a client with a diagnosis of uncomplicated asthma is reimbursed a specified amount, such as $1,300, regardless of the cost of services, the length of the stay, or the acuity or complexity of the client's illness. Prospective payment or billing is formulated before the client is even admitted to the hospital; thus, the record of admission, rather than the record of treatment, now governs payment. DRG rates are set in advance of the prospective year during which they apply and are considered fixed except for major, uncontrollable occurrences.

Payment Sources in Canada

The Canadian National Hospital Insurance program was started in 1958, and the National Medical Care Insurance program (Medicare) began in 1968. Through these programs, every Canadian can obtain health insurance. Not all hospital and medical services are covered by provincial hospital insurance or Medicare plans; there are slight differences between provinces. The Canada Health Act was passed in 1984 by Parliament to provide federal government reimbursements to provincial governments for health services they provide. Through this act, Canadians can be hospitalized without client cost; the hospitals are financed through taxation.

Insurance Plans

A variety of plans have come into existence to finance health care in the United States. These include private insurance and group insurance. Each individual and group plan offers different options for consumers to consider when choosing a prepaid health care program.

Private Insurance

In the United States, numerous commercial health insurance carriers offer a wide range of coverage plans. There are two types of private insurance: not-for-profit (e.g., Blue Shield) and for-profit (e.g., commercial companies such as Metropolitan Life, Travelers, and Aetna). Private health insurance is known as third-party reimbursement because the insurance company pays either the entire bill or, more often, 80% of the costs of health care services. With private insurance health plans, the insurance company reimburses the health care provider a fee for each service provided (fee-for-service).

These insurance plans may be purchased either as an individual plan or as part of a group plan through a person's employer, union, student association, or similar organization. For private insurance not covered by an employer, the individual usually pays a monthly premium for health care insurance. Group plans offer lower premiums that may be paid for completely by the employer, completely by group members, or some combination of the two.

Group Plans

Health care group plans provide blanket medical service in exchange for a predetermined monthly payment. A variety of group plans have come into existence to finance health care in the United States. These include health maintenance organizations, preferred provider organizations, preferred provider arrangements, independent practice associations, and physician/hospital organizations. Each group plan offers different options for consumers to consider when choosing a prepaid health care program.

HEALTH MAINTENANCE ORGANIZATIONS. A **health maintenance organization (HMO)** is a group health care agency that provides basic and supplemental health maintenance and treatment services to voluntary enrollees. A fee is set without regard to the amount or kind of services provided.

The HMO plan emphasizes client wellness; the better the health of the person, the fewer HMO services are needed and the greater the agency's profit. Members of HMOs choose a primary care provider (PCP), an internal medicine physician, general practitioner, or nurse practitioner who evaluates their health status and coordinates their care. If the primary care physician cannot treat a particular problem because of its special nature, he or she may decide to make a referral to a specialist physician. For example, a client with a skin problem sees a PCP. After evaluating the client, the PCP has two options: treat the condition or refer the client to a dermatologist. To reduce costs, HMOs will pay for a specialty physician's services only if the PCP has made a referral to the specialist. It is an expectation between the HMO and physicians being reimbursed under their plans that PCPs will treat clients and reduce costs whenever possible.

Thus, under HMO plans, clients are limited in their ability to select health care providers and services. Because health promotion and illness prevention are highly emphasized in HMOs, nurses in HMOs focus on these aspects of care. Companies that provide HMO plans such as Kaiser Permanente Medical Group, United Healthcare, and Aetna have been established across the United States, although not in every community.

PREFERRED PROVIDER ORGANIZATIONS. The **preferred provider organization (PPO)** has emerged as another alternative in the health care delivery system. PPOs consist of a group of physicians and perhaps a health care agency (often hospitals) that provide an insurance company or employer with health services at a discounted rate. One advantage of the PPO is that it provides clients with a choice of health care providers and services. Physicians can belong to one or several PPOs, and the client can choose among the physicians belonging to the PPO. A disadvantage of PPOs is that they tend to be slightly more expensive than HMO plans and if individuals wish to join a PPO, they might have to pay more for the additional choices.

PREFERRED PROVIDER ARRANGEMENTS. **Preferred provider arrangements (PPAs)** are similar to PPOs. The main difference is that the PPAs can be contracted with individual health care providers, whereas PPOs involve an organization of health care providers. A PPA plan can be limited or unlimited. A limited PPA restricts the client to using only preferred providers of health care; an unlimited PPA permits the client to use any health care provider in the area who accepts the contractual agreement of the plan. Again, with PPAs, more choices in health care providers may mean more cost to the enrollee.

INDEPENDENT PRACTICE ASSOCIATIONS. **Independent practice associations (IPAs)** are somewhat like HMOs and PPOs. The IPA provides care in offices, just as the providers belonging to a PPO do. The difference is that clients pay a fixed prospective payment to the IPA, and the IPA pays the provider. In some instances, the health care provider bills the IPA for services; in others, the provider receives a fixed fee for services given. At the end of the fiscal year, any surplus money is divided among the providers; any loss is assumed by the IPA.

PHYSICIAN/HOSPITAL ORGANIZATIONS. Physician/hospital organizations (PHOs) are joint ventures between a group of private practice physicians and a hospital. PHOs combine both resources and personnel to provide managed care alternatives and medical services. PHOs work with a variety of insurers to provide services. A typical PHO will include primary care providers and specialists.

A PHO may be part of an **integrated delivery system (IDS).** Such a system incorporates acute care services, home health care, extended and skilled care facilities, and outpatient services. Most integrated delivery systems provide care throughout the life span. Insurers can contract with IDSs to provide all required services, rather than the insurer contracting with multiple agencies for the same services. Ideally, an IDS enhances continuity of care and communication between professionals and various agencies providing managed care.

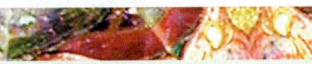

Lifespan Considerations

Elders

Assessing the functional levels of elders on an ongoing basis will provide guidelines for detecting needs for special care, resources, and services. It helps to determine their level of independence and changes as they occur. The two most common assessments are to evaluate activities of daily living and instrumental activities of daily living as follow:

Activities of Daily Living

- Bathing
- Dressing
- Toileting
- Transferring
- Continence
- Feeding

Instrumental Activities of Daily Living

- Ability to use the telephone
- Shopping
- Food preparation
- Housekeeping
- Laundry
- Mode of transportation
- Responsibility for own medication
- Ability to handle finances

The case study in this chapter in the Focus on Critical Thinking feature is an example of how these assessments and needs might change for elders. Mobilizing appropriate resources to help maintain elders' functioning ability is important in providing nursing care.

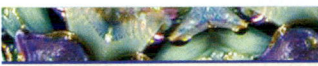

Focus on Critical Thinking

Mr. Mendel is an 83-year-old married man. He has a history of severe osteoarthritis leading to bilateral hip replacements and one knee replacement. He has mild hypertension controlled by oral medication. His last orthopedic surgery was done to replace a hip component that failed due to repeated dislocations experienced when getting out of his car. At that time, he developed a severe urinary tract infection resulting in weight loss, fatigue, and weakness. After stabilizing, he was sent to the skilled nursing unit of the hospital for 2 weeks until ready to go back home. Occupational therapists consulted with him and his wife during his hospitalization.

He lives in a three-story house with the bedrooms on the top floor, kitchen and living room on the middle/main floor, and family room on the bottom floor. He has not driven since the last operation, but would like to. He has smoked cigars for years and sits on the front porch to smoke. Physical therapists have come to the house three times a week for several months. A home health nurse has also been consulted periodically to assist with nutrition and elimination difficulties.

1. In what ways has Mr. Mendel used (a) health promotion and illness prevention (primary prevention), (b) diagnosis and treatment (secondary prevention), and (c) rehabilitation and health restoration (tertiary prevention) health care services?
2. Name three types of health care agencies he has used. What are the strengths of each of these?
3. Mr. Mendel's insurance company has assigned him a case manager. What would this person's responsibilities be in his particular case?
4. What other members of the health care profession would most likely be on the case manager's team and why?

See Critical Thinking Possibilities in Appendix A.

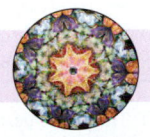 ## |Chapter Review

EXPLORE MediaLink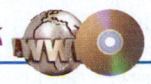

NCLEX review questions, case studies, MediaLink applications, and other interactive resources for this chapter can be found on the Companion Website at www.prenhall.com/kozier. Click on Chapter 6 to select the activities for this chapter.

For more NCLEX review questions, and an audio glossary, access the Student CD-ROM accompanying this textbook.

Chapter Highlights

- Health care delivery services can be categorized as primary, secondary, or tertiary and, generally, they can also be grouped by the type of service: (1) health promotion and illness prevention, (2) diagnosis and treatment, and (3) rehabilitation.

- Hospitals provide a wide variety of services on an inpatient and outpatient basis. Hospitals can be categorized as for-profit or not-for-profit, public or private, acute care or long-term care. Many other settings, such as clinics, offices, and day-care centers, also provide care.
- Various providers of health care coordinate their skills to assist a client. Their mutual goal is to restore a client's health and promote wellness.
- The many factors affecting health care delivery include the increasing number of elderly people, advances in knowledge and technology, economics, increased emphasis on women's health, uneven distribution of health services, access to health care, health care of the homeless and poor, and demographic changes.
- There are a number of frameworks for client health care, including managed care, case management, and patient-focused care.
- In the United States, health care is financed largely through government agencies and private organizations that provide health care insurance, prepaid plans, and federally funded programs. Government-financed plans include Medicare and Medicaid. Private plans include Blue Cross and Blue Shield. Prepaid group plans include HMOs, PPOs, PPAs, IPAs, and PHOs.

Review Questions

6–1. Cost-effective health care emphasizes the primary prevention of illness. Which of the following is an example of a primary prevention activity?
   a. antibiotic treatment of a suspected urinary tract infection
   b. occupational therapy to assist a client in adapting his or her home environment following a stroke
   c. nutrition counseling for young adults with a strong family history of high cholesterol
   d. removal of tonsils for client with recurrent tonsilitis

6–2. Which of the following statements is true regarding types of health care agencies and services?
   a. Hospitals provide only acute, inpatient services.
   b. Public health agencies are funded by governments to research and provide health programs.
   c. Surgery can only be performed inside a hospital setting.
   d. Skilled nursing, extended care, and long-term care facilities provide care for the elderly whose insurance no longer covers hospital stays.

6–3. In many cases, clients must have a primary care provider in order to receive health insurance benefits. Which of the following might the nurse suggest for a client as a primary care provider?

   a. family practice physician
   b. hospital
   c. case manager
   d. pharmacist

6–4. Health care costs in the United States continue to increase. At least one way to influence cost would be to stop the increasing
   a. number of older adults.
   b. numbers of uninsured and underinsured persons.
   c. number of physicians and nurses nationwide.
   d. competition among drug and medical equipment manufacturers.

6–5. A client is seeking to control his or her health care costs for both preventive and illness care. Although no system guarantees exact out-of-pocket expenditures, the most prepaid and predictable client contribution would be seen with
   a. Medicare.
   b. an individual fee-for-service insurance.
   c. a preferred provider organization (PPO).
   d. a health maintenance organization (HMO).

Readings and References

Suggested Readings

Elder, K. N., O'Hara, N., Crutcher, T., Wells, N., Graham, C., & Heflin, W. (1998). Managed care: The value you bring. American Journal of Nursing, 98(6), 34–39.
   This continuing education article discusses how nurses can preserve the quality of care within a managed care environment. They include changing mind-sets, learning to refocus, collaborating with colleagues, acquiring systems savvy, solving problems through teaching, and working together.

Mitchell, G. J., Closson, T., Coulis, N., Flint, F., & Gray, B. (2000). Patient-focused care and human becoming thought: Connecting the right stuff. Nursing Science Quarterly, 13, 216–224.

The history of patient-focused care is reviewed and related to the theoretical precepts of Rosemarie Parse (see Chapter 3). A hospital in Canada implemented this model in efforts to improve client satisfaction. A client, staff nurse, professional practice leader, and president/CEO share their point of view about this process through stories.

Plociak, B. J., Lato, A., & Palumbo, M. (1999). Case study: A fractured ankle. Orthopedic Nursing, 18, 21–26.

The Clinical Quality Improvement Team from a hospital emergency room developed a critical path for clients who presented with a fractured ankle but who could not undergo surgery at that time. The team included physicians, case man-

agers, and home care staff. The article describes the application of the path to a sample client.

Related Research

Shi, L. (2000). Vulnerable populations and health insurance. Medical Care Research and Review, 57, 110–134.

References

Agency for Healthcare Research and Quality. (2001a). 2000 statistics for U.S. health insurance coverage. Retrieved February 5, 2003 from http://www.meps.ahrq.gov/Pubdoc/H022/HIC2000stats.htm

Agency for Healthcare Research and Quality. (2001b). AHRQ announces new research *priorities: Patient-centered care and payment and organization.* Press release. Retrieved February 5, 2003, from http://www.ahrq.gov/news/press/ pr2001/2newpapr.htm

American Association of Colleges of Nursing. (1995). *A model for differentiated nursing practice.* Washington, DC: Author.

Beyea, S. C. (1996). *Critical pathways for collaborative care.* Menlo Park, CA: Addison-Wesley Nursing.

Center for the Evaluative Clinical Sciences at Dartmouth Medical School. (1999). Ratio of rates of registered nurses per 1,000 residents to the U.S. average: By hospital region (1996). *Dartmouth atlas of healthcare.* Retrieved February 5, 2003, from http://www.dartmouthatlas.org/99US/chap_2_sec_4.php#

Centers for Disease Control and Prevention (2001). Behavioral risk factor surveillance system: Prevalence data. Retrieved January 3, 2003, from http://apps.nccd.cdc.gov/brfss/income.asp?cat_hc.&yr_2000&qkey_7335&state_US

Gundling, R. L. (2002). Rising healthcare spending gives pause to Congress and the public. *Healthcare Financial Management, 56*(3), 76–78.

Kovner, A. R., & Jonas, S. (1999). *Health care delivery in the United States* (6th ed.). New York: Springer.

Marrie, T. J., Lau, C. Y., Wheeler, S. L., Wong, C. J., Vandervort, M. K., & Feagen, B. G. (2000). A controlled trial of a critical pathway for treatment of community-acquired pneumonia. *Journal of the American Medical Association, 283*, 749–755.

National Center for Health Statistics. (2000). *Health: United States, 2000.* Hyattsville, MD: Author.

National Health Care for the Homeless Council. (2000). *Homelessness in America today.* Retrieved March 15, 2003, from http://www.nhchc.org/Publications/basics_of_homelessness.htm.

U.S. Census Bureau, Population Division. (2000). *National population projections.* Retrieved February 5, 2003 from http://www.census.gov/population/www/projections/natsum-T3.html

U.S. Department of Health and Human Services (2000). *Healthy people 2010: Understanding and improving health* (2nd ed.) Washington, DC: U.S. Government Printing Office.

Vandenberg, B. (1999). Nursing's future: Past the year 2000. *ANNA Journal, 26,* 362–363.

Selected Bibliography

Hansten, R., & Washburn, M. J. (1998). Professional practice: Facts and impact. *American Journal of Nursing, 98*(3) 42–45.

Harrington, C., & Estes, C. L. (Eds.). (1999). *Health policy and nursing: Crisis and reform in the U.S. health care delivery system.* Boston: Jones and Bartlett.

Reschovsky, J. D., Kemper, P., & Tu, H. (2000). Does type of health insurance affect health care use and assessments of care among the privately insured? *Health Services Research, 35*(1, Part 2), 219–237.

Ruflin, P., Matlock, R., Holy, C., Sorbello, S., Nadzan, L., & Selden, T. (1999). Closed-unit staffing speaks volumes. *Nursing Management, 30*(6), 37–39.

Thompson, E. J., & Roda, P. I. (1999). Ensuring competencies of multidisciplinary staff in patient-focused care. *Dimensions of Critical Care Nursing, 18*(4), 36–44.

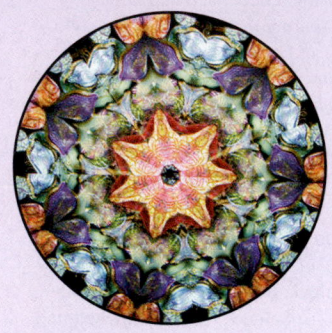

CHAPTER 7

COMMUNITY-BASED NURSING AND CARE CONTINUITY

LEARNING OUTCOMES

After completing this chapter, you will be able to:

- Discuss factors influencing health care reform.

- Describe community-based health care including the Pew Health Professions Commission recommendations for health care systems.

- Describe various community-based frameworks including integrated health care systems, community initiatives and conditions, and case management.

- Differentiate community-based health care settings from traditional settings.

- Differentiate community-based nursing from traditional institutional-based nursing.

- Discuss competencies community-based nurses need for practice.

- Explain essential aspects of collaborative health care: definitions, objectives, benefits, and the nurse's role.

- Describe the role of the nurse in providing continuity of care.

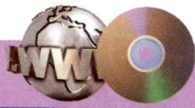

MediaLink

www.prenhall.com/kozier

Additional resources for this chapter can be found on the Student CD-ROM accompanying this textbook, and on the Companion Website at www.prenhall.com/kozier. Click on Chapter 7 to select the activities for this chapter.

CD-ROM
- Audio Glossary
- NCLEX Review

Companion Website
- Additional NCLEX Review
- Case Study: Community Health Nursing
- MediaLink Applications:
    Community Nursing Standards
    Government Services
- Link to Resources

The health care system is undergoing change. Escalating health care costs, expanding technology, changing patterns of demographics, shorter hospital stays, increased patient acuity, and diminishing access to health care are some of the factors motivating change. Client care is moving out of traditional settings into community/neighborhood locations. For example, health care once considered safe only in hospital settings is now provided in homes (see Chapter 9 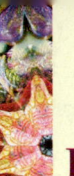) and in ambulatory surgical, rehabilitation, and dialysis centers. Although hospitals and other health care institutions will remain components of the health care system of the future, they will likely have less prominence. The trend is toward an integrated health care system—one that is community based. The shift from institutional to community-based care also brings changes in the roles and responsibilities of health care professionals.

HEALTH CARE REFORM

Both consumers and health care professionals have major areas of concern about the current health care system. Although plans to reform the health care system have been proposed nationally and internationally, no single plan has been adopted. Drafts of legislative reform in the United States include initiatives directed at cost control through managed care competition, providing health insurance for the poor, and transforming the insurance industry.

In addition to legislative influences, nurses, professional organizations, and consumers are affecting health care reform. Nurses provide a unique perspective on the health care system because of their constant presence in a variety of settings and their contact both with consumers who receive the benefits of the system's most complex services and with those who have problems with the system's inefficiencies. The greater numbers of advanced practice nurses in recent years has resulted in the provision of primary care to many consumers who have previously been neglected—those living in rural areas, the poor, older adults, and women and infants.

Through nurses' major organizations, nursing has presented a strong voice in describing what a new system should include and what nursing's contributions should be. In 1991, the American Nurses Association (ANA) published *Nursing's Agenda for Health Care Reform,* which set forth the ANA's recommendations for health care reform. These recommendations are summarized in Box 7–1. Although the agenda called for "immediate" changes, the majority of the recommendations have still not been implemented over a dozen years later.

Another major influence promoting health care reform has been the work on *Healthy People 2000* and *Healthy People 2010* (U.S. Department of Health and Human Services [USDHHS], 1990, 2000). These projects present health-related objectives that provide a framework for national health promotion, health protection, and disease prevention. Details of *Healthy People 2000* are discussed in Chapter 8.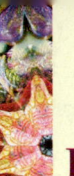

The forerunner of *Healthy People 2000* and *Nursing's Agenda for Health Care Reform* was the 1978 World Health Organization (WHO) report *Primary Health Care.* The term *primary health care* (PHC) was coined in the World Health Assembly by WHO and the United Nations International Children's Emergency Fund (UNICEF).

Primary health care (PHC) is defined as

> essential health care based on practical, scientifically sound and socially acceptable methods and technology made universally accessible to individuals and families in the community through their full participation and at a cost that the community and country can afford to maintain at every stage of their development in the spirit of self-reliance and self-determination. (WHO, 1978, p. 35)

Primary health care incorporates five principles:

- Equitable distribution
- Appropriate technology
- A focus on health promotion and disease prevention
- Community participation
- A multisectoral approach.

Deep concern about health care for the majority of the world's population, specifically low life expectancies and high mortality rates among children, led to the global health strategy of primary health care. The WHO declaration emphasized health or well-being as a fundamental right and a

---

BOX 7–1   ■ Nursing's Agenda for Health Care Reform

- A restructured health care system that (a) enhances consumer access to services by delivering primary health care in community-based settings, (b) fosters consumer responsibility for personal health, self-care, and informed decision making in selecting health care services, and (c) facilitates using the most cost-effective providers and therapeutic options in the most appropriate settings
- A federally defined standard package of essential health care services available to all citizens and residents of the United

States, provided and financed through an integration of public and private plans and sources
- A phase-in of essential services
- Planned change to anticipate health service needs that correlate with changing national demographics
- Steps to reduce health care costs
- Case management for those with continuing health care needs
- Provisions for long-term care
- Insurance reforms to improve access to coverage

Note: From *Nursing's Agenda for Health Care Reform,* by American Nurse Publishing of the American Nurses Foundation, 1991, Kansas City, MO: American Nurses Association. Adapted with permission.

---

worldwide social goal. It attempted to address inequality in health status of persons in all countries and to target government responsibility for policies that would promote economic, social, and health development. Both economic and social development were considered basic to the achievement of health for all. Thus, PHC extends beyond the boundaries of traditional health care services. It involves issues of the environment, agriculture, housing, and other social, economic, and political issues such as poverty, transportation, unemployment, economic development to sustain the population, and so on. A major feature of PHC is that consumers, governments, and public institutions such as public health departments and city councils should be involved in the planning and delivery of health care.

PHC differs from primary care (PC). Primary care addresses personal health services and not population-based public health services. **Primary care (PC),** according to the Institute of Medicine (IOM), is "the provision of integrated, accessible health care services by clinicians who are accountable for addressing a large majority of personal health services, developing a sustained partnership with patients, and practicing in the context of family and community" (IOM, 1994, p. 15).

PHC is community driven and involves an approach that requires active community involvement in making decisions to improve health. It is community based. PC, on the other hand, is expert driven and involves an approach by health professionals who advise individuals and communities about what is best for their health. Other differences are shown in Table 7–1.

There are also similarities between PHC and PC. Both systems acknowledge the prevention and promotion components of health and well-being. Both systems strive for universal access to and affordability of health care, support empowerment of the client, and target those at risk for preventable health problems.

Consumers are also effecting major changes in health care delivery systems. Consumers are adopting health-related values that include the following:

- Health means more than the absence of disease; it encompasses well-being and quality of life.
- Quality of life is related to a healthy community that includes healthy families and a healthy environment.
- Individuals can actively participate in promoting and maintaining their health through behavior and lifestyle changes.
- Disease prevention is important.

These values indicate that consumers support an increased emphasis on health care services and programs that promote wellness and restoration and prevent disease.

COMMUNITY-BASED HEALTH CARE

Community-based health care (CBHC) is a PHC system that provides health-related services within the context of people's daily lives—that is, in places where people spend their time, for example, in the home, in shelters, in long-term care residences,

---

TABLE 7–1   Differences between Primary Care and Primary Health Care

Primary Care	Primary Health Care
• Community participation is provider directed.	• Community participation is client directed.
• The professional's role is expert, provider, authority, team leader.	• The professional's role is facilitator, consultant, resource.
• Collaboration occurs among members of the health care team.	• Collaboration goes beyond the health care sector.
• The individual or family is the focus.	• The community or some aggregate is the focus.
• Access is limited.	• Access is universal.
• Health care is available within given health care institutions.	• Health care is available where people live and work.
• Empowerment is a provider-assisted process.	• Empowerment is a collaborative, enabling process.

Note: From "Primary Health Care and Primary Care: A Confusion of Philosophies," by D. Barnes, et al., 1995, *Nursing Outlook, 43*(1), pp. 7–16. Adapted with permission.

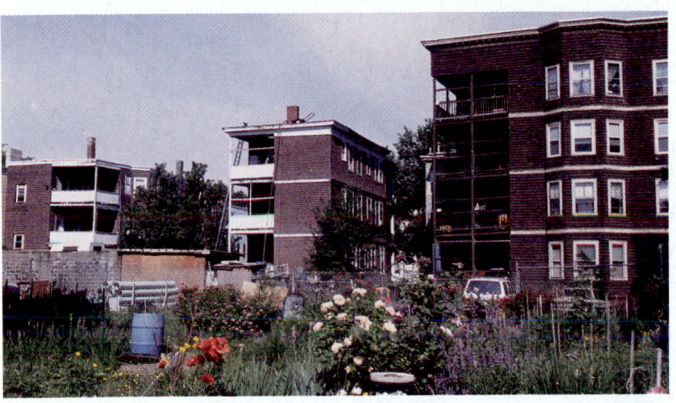

Figure 7–1 ■ Communities may consist of several types of neighborhoods.

at work, in schools, in senior citizens centers, in ambulatory settings, and in hospitals. Care is provided to individuals who have common needs and live within a defined region. The care is directed toward a specific group within the geographical neighborhood (see Figure 7–1 ■). The group may be established by a physical boundary, an employer, a school district, a managed care insurance provider, or a specific medical need or category. In contrast to the traditional health care system that focused primarily on the ill and the injured, community-based care is holistic. It involves a broad range of services designed not only to restore health but also to promote health, prevent illness, and protect the public.

To be truly effective, a community-based health care system needs to (a) provide easy access to the system, (b) be flexible in responding to the care needs that individuals and families identify, (c) promote care between and among health care agencies through improved communication mechanisms, (d) provide appropriate support for family caregivers, and (e) be affordable.

The ideal CBHC system is consistent with the nine characteristics identified by the Pew Health Professions Commission needed to build any new health care system. According to deTornyay (1992), that ideal health care system would accomplish these goals:

- Be more oriented to health and emphasize health promotion and disease prevention.
- Focus on individual responsibility for health practices and behavior.
- Be population based and focus more attention on risk factors in the physical and social environment.
- Use electronic information systems for client histories and research findings to support diagnostic decisions and treatment recommendations.
- Have a stronger focus on consumers who would have increased information and be informed participants in decisions about their health care.
- Base decisions on outcomes.
- Provide care more efficiently by means of integrated or coordinated teams of providers.
- Balance technology with nontechnical interventions and weigh the benefits against its effects on human values and interpersonal processes.

- Have health care providers who will be increasingly accountable to consumers and society for a wider range of outcomes of care.

A decade later, only some of these characteristics can be found in health care systems.

Community-Based Frameworks

Various approaches are emerging to address this concept. Some of these are an integrated health care system, community initiatives, community coalitions, managed care, case management, and outreach programs using lay health workers.

An **integrated health care system** is one that makes all levels of care available in an integrated form—primary care, secondary care, and tertiary care (see Figure 7–2 ■). Its goals are to facilitate care across settings, recovery, positive health outcomes, and the long-term benefits of modifying harmful lifestyles through health promotion and disease prevention. In many parts of the country, hospitals are reflecting this concept by changing their names to *health care organization* or *integrated health care system.* This type of system is sometimes referred to as *seamless care.*

Community initiatives are being sponsored by some hospitals or local community agencies. These initiatives, called *healthy cities* and *healthier communities,* involve members of the community to establish health priorities, set measurable goals, and determine actions to reach these goals. If a community agency is initiating this project, the associated hospital generally contributes human resources to assist in this endeavor.

Community coalitions bring together individuals and groups for the shared purpose of improving the community's health. Nurses are major participants and contributors in these coalitions and often assume leadership positions. Community coalitions may focus on a single or multifaceted problem. Examples include establishment of an abuse program, a gang prevention program, an older adults assessment program, or an immunization program for a high-risk group.

In managed care, a common model in health care restructuring, health care providers (hospitals, physicians, nurse practitioners, insurance carriers, and so on) join to meet health needs across the care continuum.

Case management is an integrative health care model that tracks client needs and services through a variety of care settings to ensure continuity.

Outreach programs using lay health workers are a method of linking underserved or high-risk populations with the formal health care system. They can minimize or reduce barriers to health care, increase access to services, and thus improve the health status of the community. They involve partnerships between nurses and members of the community. Interested and committed lay health workers are identified who will assist their neighbors through outreach networks. Nurses provide training, consultation, and support to these individuals.

Community-Based Settings

Traditionally, community nursing services have been provided in county and state health departments (public health nursing), in

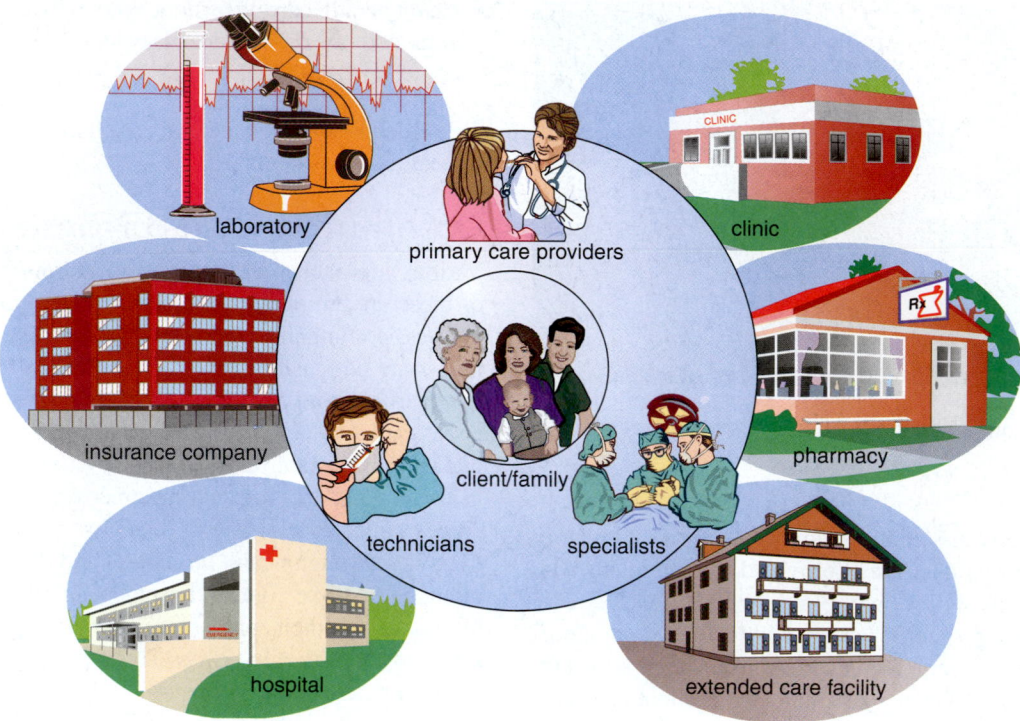

Figure 7–2 ■ Model of an integrated health care delivery system.

schools (school nursing), in workplaces (occupational nursing), and in homes (home health care and hospice nursing). Over the years numerous other settings have been established including day-care centers, senior centers, storefront clinics, homeless shelters, mental health centers, crisis centers, drug rehabilitation programs, and ambulatory care centers. More recent settings for community-based nursing practice include nurse-managed community nursing centers, parish nursing, and telehealth projects.

Community Nursing Centers

Community nursing centers provide primary care to specific populations and are staffed by nurse practitioners and community health nurses. Although the nurses are the primary providers of care to clients visiting the center, a physician's consultation is available as needed. Nursing centers may be located in schools, workplaces, other community agencies, or be free standing. Nursing centers must interface with nurse-managed services in other settings across the health care continuum, that is, services being provided to clients in their home, hospital, or long-term care facility. There are various categories of community nursing centers:

- *Community outreach centers.* Relatively small freestanding clinics providing services similar to those traditionally provided by large public health clinics but focused on a narrower population
- *Institution-based centers.* Associated with a large parent organization such as a hospital, corporation, or university or college
- *Wellness centers.* Provide services such as health promotion, health maintenance, education, counseling, and screen-

ing. In some settings, wellness centers are staffed by members of the health care team other than nurses (e.g., physical therapists or occupational therapists).

Parish Nursing

Parish nursing was founded in the United States in Illinois in the mid-1980s by Reverend Granger Westberg (Metzger, 2000) and became a specialty recognized by the ANA in 1998. The International Parish Nurse Resource Center describes the roles of the parish nurse as follows:

- Personal health counselor who discusses health issues and problems with individuals and makes home, hospital, and nursing home visits as needed
- Health educator who educates and supports individuals through health education activities that promote an understanding of the relationship between values, attitudes, lifestyle, faith, and well-being
- Referral source who acts as a liaison to other congregational and community resources
- Facilitator who recruits and coordinates volunteers within the congregation and develops support groups
- Integrator of faith and health.

An estimated 3,000 parish nurses serve churches, synagogues, and temples in the United States (see Figure 7–3 ■). Most parish nurses are volunteers, but some are employees paid by the congregation or an affiliated institution such as a health system or community agency. Parish nursing is nondenominational and includes nurses of all religious faiths. Parish

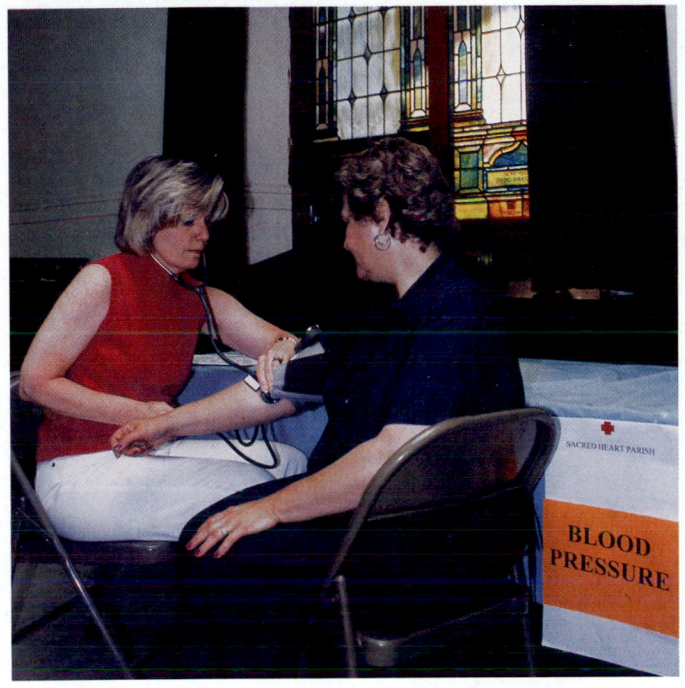

Figure 7–3 ■ Some parish-based health services provide care to community residents in addition to members of the congregation.

nursing is one of the few community-based nursing roles found with a similar structure and focus in nations around the world.

Telehealth

Telehealth projects use communication and information technology to provide health information and health care services to people in rural, remote, or underserviced areas. Video conferences or "video clinics" enable health care workers to provide distant consultation to assess and treat ambulatory clients who have a variety of health care needs. These video conferences are similar to any outpatient clinic visit except that the client and health care specialist are miles apart. A related development to telehealth is telenursing, in which nurses provide client teaching and health promotion to distant clients.

COMMUNITY-BASED NURSING

Community-based nursing (CBN) is nursing care directed toward specific individuals. However, community-based nursing involves nursing care that is not confined to one practice setting. It extends beyond institutional boundaries and involves a network of nursing services: nursing wellness centers, ambulatory care, acute care, long-term care nursing services, telephone advice, home health, and hospice services. For example, a nurse case manager may be involved in (a) visiting a newly admitted client in the hospital to take a detailed nursing history, confer with the primary nurse, and begin discharge planning; (b) making several home visits to monitor a client recently transferred from a hospital to a long-term care agency to discuss the client's progress with the nursing staff; or (c) making

consultative telephone calls to other health professionals (physicians, social workers, respiratory therapists, and so on) and to clients who are managing self-care independently but who may need support.

> ► **CLINICAL ALERT**   *Community-based nursing and community health nursing are not the same concept. Community-based nursing focuses on care of individuals in geographically local settings, whereas community health nursing (Chapter 12 ∞) emphasizes the promotion and preservation of the health of groups (populations or aggregates).* ■

Other nurses who work in community-based settings, such as case managers, occupational health nurses, school nurses, and public health department nurses, need to be prepared to make home visits. Home visits can provide information that is not obtainable in other ways.

Competencies Required for Community-Based Care

Nurses practicing in community-based integrated health care systems need to have specific knowledge and skills. In 1991, the Pew Health Professions Commission, in a report entitled *Healthy America: Practitioners for 2005* (as cited in de Tornyay, 1992), identified 17 competencies (skills) that future health professionals would require (see Box 7–2). These competencies have given direction to schools preparing future health professionals for practice. To achieve these competencies, nurses need the following knowledge: (a) determinants of a healthy community; (b) primary and secondary preventive strategies for people of all ages; (c) health-promotion strategies for individuals, families, and communities; (d) how to participate in collaborative and interdisciplinary teamwork; (e) determinants of an accessible, cost-effective, integrated health care system; (f) decision-making processes that involve active participation by consumers and balance cost and quality care; and (g) concepts of information management. Community-based nurses also require up-to-date clinical skills and knowledge of complex technology, public health policy, and strategies to influence and effect change.

Collaborative Health Care

Collaboration among health care professionals becomes increasingly important as more practitioners specialize in progressively more narrow areas of expertise while others take on the generalist role. Over time, the boundaries and legal scope of practice of each health care profession may change. To deliver optimal health care for the client, nurses must work as a member of the team providing comprehensive health care.

In 1992, the ANA Congress on Nursing Practice adopted the following operational definition of the concept of collaboration:

> **Collaboration** means a collegial working relationship with another health care provider in the provision of (to supply) patient care. Collaborative practice requires (may

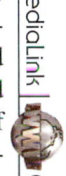

MediaLink | COMMUNITY NURSING STANDARDS APPLICATION

BOX 7–2	■ Pew Commission Competencies for Future Practitioners

1. Care for the community's health.
2. Expand access to effective care.
3. Provide contemporary clinical care.
4. Emphasize primary care.
5. Participate in coordinated care.
6. Ensure cost-effective and appropriate care.
7. Practice prevention.
8. Involve patients and families in decision-making processes.
9. Promote healthy lifestyles.
10. Access and use technology appropriately.
11. Improve the health care system.
12. Manage information.
13. Understand the role of the physical environment.
14. Practice counseling on ethical issues.
15. Accommodate expanded accountability.
16. Participate in a racially and culturally diverse society.
17. Continue to learn.

Note: From "Reconsidering Nursing Education: The Report of the Pew Health Professional Commission," by R. De Tornyay, 1992, *Journal of Nursing Education, 31,* pp. 296–301. Adapted with permission.

include) the discussion of patient diagnosis and cooperation in the management and delivery of care. Each collaborator is available to the other for consultation either in person or by communication device, but need not be physically present on the premises at the time the actions are performed. The patient-designated health care provider is responsible for the overall direction and management of patient care. (ANA, 1992)

The Nurse as a Collaborator

Nurses collaborate with nurse colleagues and other health care professionals. They frequently collaborate about client care but may also be involved, for example, in collaborating on bioethical issues, on legislation, on health-related research, and with professional organizations. Box 7–3 outlines selected aspects of the nurse's role as a collaborator.

To fulfill a collaborative role, nurses need to assume accountability and increased authority in practice areas. Education is integral to ensuring that the members of each professional group understand the collaborative nature of their roles, specific contributions, and the importance of working to-

gether. Each professional needs to understand how an integrated delivery system centers on the client's health care needs rather than on the particular care given by one group.

Competencies Basic to Collaboration

Key elements necessary for collaboration include effective communication skills, mutual respect, trust, and a decision-making process.

COMMUNICATION. Collaborating to solve complex problems requires effective communication skills. Effective communication can occur only if the involved parties are committed to understanding each other's professional roles and appreciating each other as individuals. Additionally, they must be sensitive to differences among communication styles. Instead of focusing on distinctions, a group of professionals needs to center on their common ground: the client's needs.

MUTUAL RESPECT AND TRUST. Mutual respect occurs when two or more people show or feel honor or esteem toward one another. Trust occurs when a person is confident in the actions

BOX 7–3	■ The Nurse as a Collaborator

With Nurse Colleagues
- Shares personal expertise with other nurses and elicits the expertise of others to ensure quality client care.
- Develops a sense of trust and mutual respect with peers that recognizes their unique contributions.

With Other Health Care Professionals
- Recognizes the contribution that each member of the interdisciplinary team can make by virtue of his or her expertise and view of the situation.
- Listens to each individual's views.
- Shares health care responsibilities in exploring options, setting goals, and making decisions with clients and families.
- Participates in collaborative interdisciplinary research to increase knowledge of a clinical problem or situation.

With Professional Nursing Organizations
- Seeks opportunities to collaborate with and within professional organizations.
- Serves on committees in state (or provincial) and national nursing organizations or specialty groups.
- Supports professional organizations in political action to create solutions for professional and health care concerns.

With Legislators
- Offers expert opinions on legislative initiatives related to health care.
- Collaborates with other health care providers and consumers on health care legislation to best serve the needs of the public.

Research Note
Does Primary Care Result in Better Care for Children with Diabetes?

In the state of Washington, 250 children with Type 1 diabetes who were cared for under the Medicaid public system were studied retrospectively to determine if there was a relationship between their degree of primary care/care continuity and (a) their use of appropriate health services and (b) the incidence of certain diabetic complications. Those children considered to have had high or medium continuity of care were found to have statistically significant reduced incidence of diabetic ketoacidosis (DKA), fewer hospitalizations for DKA, and an increased likelihood of having been seen by an ophthalmologist.

Implications: It is intuitively apparent that children with chronic conditions who are followed consistently by health care providers would have more preventive care and earlier detection and minimization of complications than children with fragmented care. However, it may not be as intuitive that this would apply to clients receiving their care from welfare systems serving the working poor and uninsured. This research indicates that increased quality of care can be demonstrated as an outcome of continuity of care—even within the Medicaid system.

Note: From "Continuity and Quality of Care for Children with Diabetes Who Are Covered by Medicaid," by D. A. Christakis, C. Feudtner, C. Pihoker, and F. A. Connell, 2001, *Ambulatory Pediatrics, 1,* pp. 99–103.

of another person. Both mutual respect and trust imply a mutual process and outcome. They must be expressed both verbally and nonverbally.

DECISION MAKING. The decision-making process at the team level involves shared responsibility for the outcome. Obviously, to create a solution the team must follow each step of the decision-making process, beginning with a clear definition of the problem. Team decision making must be directed at the objectives of the specific effort. It requires full consideration and respect of diverse viewpoints. Members must be able to verbalize their perspectives in a nonthreatening environment.

An important aspect of decision making is satisfied when the interdisciplinary team focuses on the client's priority needs and organizing interventions accordingly. The discipline best able to address the client's needs is given priority in planning and is responsible for providing its interventions in a timely manner. For example, a social worker may first direct attention to a client's social needs when these needs interfere with the client's ability to respond to therapy. Nurses, by the nature of their holistic practice, are often able to help the team identify priorities and areas requiring further attention.

CONTINUITY OF CARE

A major responsibility of the nurse is to ensure continuity of care. **Continuity of care** is the coordination of health care services by health care providers for clients moving from one health care setting to another and between and among health care professionals. Continuity ensures uninterrupted and consistent services for the client from one level of care to another, and when coordinated appropriately, it maintains client-focused individualized care and helps optimize the client's health status. To provide continuity of care, nurses need to accomplish the following:

- Initiate discharge planning for all clients when they are admitted to any health care setting.
- Involve the client and the client's family or support persons in the planning process.
- Collaborate with other health care professionals as needed to ensure that biopsychosocial, cultural, and spiritual needs are met.

However, achieving continuity assumes that needed client data are shared with other providers while implementing strategies to protect client privacy. The American Health Insurance Portability and Accountability Act (HIPAA), passed in 1996, requires that health information about clients be secured in such a way that only those with the right and need to acquire the information are able to do so. In the computer age, this has become a complex requirement since standards for coding and transmitting data are not universal and authentication of authority to access may be breached. Health plan and provider compliance with the privacy aspect of HIPAA was required as of April 2003. It will result in a balance between protecting disclosure of confidential client information and the need for certain data to be released to specific agencies. Ultimately, clients will have increased control over their own information and those who violate the rule face significant penalties.

Discharge Planning

Discharge planning is the process of preparing a client to leave one level of care for another within or outside the current health care agency. Usually, discharge planning refers to the client leaving the hospital for home. However, discharges occur among many other settings. Within a facility it can occur from one unit to another. For example, a client with a cerebral vascular accident may move from a medical unit to a rehabilitation unit, or a client with multiple traumas may move from emergency to an intensive care unit. Clients may also move from a hospital to a long-term care agency, from a rehabilitation center to home, or from a home health care setting to a hospital, and so on.

Each agency generally has its own policies and procedures related to discharge. Many agencies have discharge planners, a health or social services professional who coordinates the transition and acts as a link between the discharging agency and the receiving facility. Often, a nurse assumes this responsibility of providing continuity of care.

Discharge planning needs to begin when a client is admitted to an agency, especially in hospitals where length of stays are considerably shortened. Effective discharge planning involves (a) ongoing assessment to obtain comprehensive information about the client's ongoing needs, (b) statements of nursing diagnoses, and (c) plans to ensure the client's and caregivers'

MediaLink   COMMUNITY NURSING CASE STUDY

BOX 7–4 ■ Discharge Planning: Home Assessment Parameters

Personal and Health Data
Age; sex; height and weight; cultural beliefs and practices; medical history; current health status; prognosis; surgery.

Abilities to Perform Activities of Daily Living (ADLs)
Abilities for dressing; eating; toileting; bathing (tub, shower, sponge); ambulating (with or without aids such as a cane, crutches, walker, wheelchair); transferring (from bed to chair, in and out of bath, in and out of car); meal preparation; transportation; and shopping

Disabilities/Limitations
Sensory losses (auditory, visual); motor losses (paralysis, amputation); communication disorder; mental confusion or depression; incontinence

Caregivers' Responses/Abilities
Principle caregiver's relationship to client; thoughts and feelings about client's discharge; expectations for recovery; health and coping abilities; comfort with performing needed care

Financial Resources
Financial resources and needs (note equipment, supplies, medications, special foods required)

Community Supports
Family members, friends, neighbors, volunteers; resources such as Medicaid; food stamps; nutrition services; health centers; community health nurses; day programs; legal assistance; home care; respite care

Home Hazard Appraisal
Safety precautions (stairs with or without handrails; lighting in rooms, hallways, stairways; nightlights in hallways or bathroom; grab bars near toilet and tub; firmly attached carpets and rugs); self-care barriers (lack of running water, lack of wheelchair access to bathroom or home, lack of space for required equipment, lack of elevator) (A detailed home hazard appraisal is provided in Chapter 9.)

Need for Health Care Assistance
Home-delivered meals; special dietary needs; volunteers for telephone reassurance, friendly visiting, transportation, shopping; assistance with bathing; assistance with housekeeping; assistance with wound care, ostomies, tubes, intravenous medications

---

needs are met. In some situations discharge planning necessitates health team conferences and family conferences. At a health team conference, health team professionals focus on ways to individualize care for the client. At a family conference, both health professionals and the family discuss family issues related to the client. Both types of conferences give the client, family, and health care professionals the opportunity to mutually plan care and set goals.

Preparing Clients to Go Home

Nurses preparing to send clients home need to assess the following parameters in their clients: personal and health data, abilities to perform the activities of daily living (ADLs), any physical, cognitive, or other functional limitations, caregiver's responses and abilities, adequacy of financial resources, community supports, hazards or barriers that the home environment presents, and need for health care assistance in the home. Box 7–4 outlines details about each of these parameters.

Assessment data may lead to the development of both actual and potential nursing diagnostic labels, including these examples:

- *Activity Intolerance*
- *Impaired Health Maintenance*
- *Anxiety*
- *Impaired Home Maintenance*
- *Deficient Knowledge (Specify)*
- *Risk for Caregiver Role Strain*
- *Risk for Injury*
- *Self-Care Deficits: Bathing/Hygiene, Dressing/Grooming, Feeding, Toileting*
- *Social Isolation.*

The diagnoses and database establish nursing activities that are needed before the client is discharged. These activities most often include (a) teaching the client to cope with continuing self-care at home and (b) a home care referral.

Home Health Care Teaching

Clients need help to understand their situation, to make health care decisions, and to learn new health behaviors. Because of today's shortened hospital stays, it is often unrealistic to teach clients everything they need to know. Referral to a home health agency for follow-up teaching may be necessary. Essential information before discharge includes information about medications, dietary and activity restrictions, signs of complications that need to be reported to the physician, follow-up appointments and telephone numbers, and where supplies can be obtained. Clients or caregivers also need to demonstrate safe performance of any necessary treatments. Information needs to be provided verbally and in writing. Details about effective teaching strategies are provided in Chapter 25.

Referrals

The referral process is a systematic problem-solving approach that helps clients to use resources that meet their health care needs. The process involves knowledge of community resources and an ability to solve problems, set priorities, coordinate, and collaborate. Home care referrals are often made before discharge for the following clients:

- Elders
- Children with complex conditions
- Frail persons who live alone
- Those who lack or have a limited support system

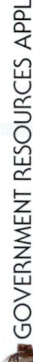

- Those who have a caregiver whose health is failing
- Those whose home presents barriers to their safety (e.g., stairs).

Referrals need to present as much information as possible about the client and the hospitalization. Most agencies have well-established protocols and detailed referral forms. The assessment parameters in Box 7–4 can also be used as a guide.

To ensure appropriate reimbursement to the home health agency, the physician must provide a written order for a home care referral and subsequent home visits. Clients must meet specific criteria to have Medicare or other third-party payers reimburse them for home care services. Chapter 9 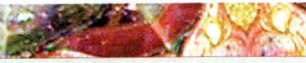 provides details about home health nursing.

Lifespan Considerations

Elders

Due to the changes caused by aging and the increase of chronic illnesses in elders, various levels of health care delivery are often required. Clients may go back and forth between these levels as their needs fluctuate. At various times and situations, they might need care from hospitals, home care, extended care facilities, ambulatory care, and assisted living. Maintaining communications and providing continuity of care during these changes are essential.

Caregivers of elders are often older themselves and may have health problems of their own. Attention should be given to signs of emotional and physical fatigue and other problems that might arise for them. Community health nurses have the opportunity to do ongoing assessments of this as they see clients and caregivers in their home environment. They can then provide support and resources as needed.

Focus on Critical Thinking

Nurses are, and should be, taking an active role in influencing the direction of health care. Recognizing that there are finite limits to the amount of money and health care providers available, desirable outcomes often compete for resources. Consider a clinical situation such as the so-called "drive-through (or 24-hour) mastectomies" in which clients are moved through the acute care (hospital) system extremely quickly compared to previously. *Nursing's Agenda for Health Care Reform* (ANA, 1991) stated that there should be (a) increased access to care via primary health care provided in community-based settings, (b) an emphasis on consumer self-care and decision making, and (c) cost-effective care provided in the most appropriate setting.

1. How does this clinical example reflect or not reflect the agenda?
2. Which of the three agenda items listed above do you consider the most important and why?
3. How might different community-based frameworks manage the clinical example?
4. How would the nurse use collaboration with insurance payers, women, or surgeons to resolve any concerns with the clinical example?

See Critical Thinking Possibilities in Appendix A.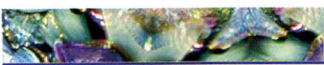

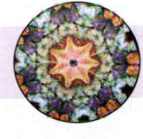 # Chapter Review

Explore MediaLink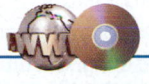

NCLEX review questions, case studies, MediaLink applications, and other interactive resources for this chapter can be found on the Companion Website at www.prenhall.com/kozier. Click on Chapter 7 to select the activities for this chapter.

For more NCLEX review questions, and an audio glossary, access the Student CD-ROM accompanying this textbook.

Chapter Highlights

- Health care costs, access to health care, and the quality of health care are major areas of concern about the current health care system.
- *Nursing's Agenda for Health Care Reform* by the ANA (1991) and *Healthy People 2000* and *Healthy People 2010*

by the USDHHS (1990, 2000) have set forth recommendations for health care reform. These focus on accessibility of health care services, health promotion and disease prevention, and steps to consider how health care costs can be reduced.

- Consumers support an increased emphasis on health care measures that promote wellness.
- Community-based health care, akin to primary health care, provides health-related services in places where people spend their time—in homes, in shelters, in long-term care residences, at work, in schools, in senior citizen centers, and so on.
- Approaches are emerging to address community-based care. These include an integrated health care system, community initiatives, community coalitions, managed care, case management, and outreach programs using lay health workers.
- Numerous community-based settings have been established. More recent ones include nurse-managed community nursing centers, parish nursing, and telehealth projects.
- Community-based nursing directs nursing care toward specific individuals. It is not confined to one practice setting; it extends beyond institutional boundaries involving a network of nursing services: nursing wellness centers, ambulatory care, long-term care, home health, and hospice care.
- To practice in community-based health care systems, nurses need knowledge and competencies such as determinants of a

healthy community, primary and secondary preventive strategies, health-promotion strategies, collaborative and interdisciplinary teamwork, determinants of an accessible, cost-effective health care system, a decision-making process that involves consumers, and information management. Education in public health policy and strategies to influence and effect change are essential.
- Collaboration among health care providers is key to maintaining continuity of care as clients move through the health care system.
- A major responsibility of the nurse is to ensure continuity of care as clients move from one level of care to another.
- Continuity of care involves (a) discharge planning that begins when clients are admitted to an agency, (b) cooperation with the client and support persons, and (c) interdisciplinary collaboration.
- Nurses need to ensure that clients have essential information and skills to manage self-care before being discharged to their homes. In some situations referral to a home health agency is necessary.

Review Questions

7–1. *Nursing's Agenda for Health Care Reform* (ANA, 1991) recommended that
   a. primary health care should be based in acute care hospitals.
   b. a minimum standard of health care for all persons should be paid for with public funds.
   c. case management be focused on clients with enduring healthcare needs.
   d. indicated that essential services should be initiated simultaneously to avoid gaps.

7–2. A category of the Pew Commission *Competencies for Future Practitioners* emphasized the need for providers to become skilled in
   a. use of technology.
   b. budgetary and financial management strategies.
   c. traditional clinical approaches.
   d. making decisions for incompetent clients.

7–3. A characteristic of community-based health care is that the nurse provides client care
   a. primarily to clients with identified illnesses.
   b. to individuals in groups according to their geographical commonalities.

   c. that is paid for by the community as a whole rather than by individuals.
   d. in which all clients are case managed.

7–4. Collaborative health care necessitates that the nurse
   a. assume a leadership role in directing the health care team.
   b. demonstrate respect for the opinions of the client, peers, and other health care providers.
   c. be physically present for the implementation of all aspects of the care plan.
   d. pass decision-making authority to each health care provider in turn.

7–5. The nurse can conclude that effective discharge planning (hospital to home) has been conducted when the client states
   a. "As soon as I get home, the nurse will come out, look at where I live, and see what kind of care I will need."
   b. "All I need are my medications and a ride home. Then I'm all ready for discharge."
   c. "When I visit my doctor in 10 days, they will show me how to change my bandages."
   d. "I have the phone numbers of the home care nurse and the therapist who will visit me at home tomorrow."

Readings and References

Suggested Readings
Trofino, J. (2000). Primary care parish nursing: Academic, service, and parish partnership. *Nursing Administration Quarterly, 25*(1), 59–74. The authors represent a university, major medical center, and the community who collaborated to create a health care program within their faith community. The goals were to provide care for the underserved with a focus on prevention and

early detection of illness. Nurse practitioners and nurse case managers were the primary care providers. The article describes the history and models of parish nursing as well as an approach to performing health outcomes research.

Related Research
Anderson, M. A., & Helms, L. B. (1998). Comparison of continuing care communica-

tion. *Image: Journal of Nursing Scholarship, 30,* 255–260.

References
American Nurses Association. (1991). *Nursing's agenda for health care reform.* Kansas City, MO: Author.
American Nurses Association. (1992). *House of delegates report: 1992 convention, Las Vegas,*

Nevada (pp. 104–120). Kansas City, MO: Author.

Barnes, D., Eribes, C. Juarbe, T., Nelson, M., Proctor, S., Sawyer, L., et al. (1995). Primary health care and primary care: A confusion of philosophies. *Nursing Outlook, 43*(1), 7–16.

Christakis, D. A., Feudtner, C., Pihoker, C., & Connell, F. A. (2001). Continuity and quality of care for children with diabetes who are covered by Medicaid. *Ambulatory Pediatrics, 1,* 99–103.

deTornyay, R. (1992). Reconsidering nursing education: The report of the Pew Health Professions Commission. *Journal of Nursing Education, 31,* 296–301.

Institute of Medicine. (1994). *Defining primary care: An interim report.* Washington, DC: National Academy Press.

Metzger, S. M. (2000). Parish nursing: Integrating body, mind, and spirit. *Nursing, 30*(12), 64HH6–64HH7.

U.S. Department of Health and Human Services. (1990). *Healthy people 2000: National health promotion and disease prevention objectives* (DHHS Pub. No. PHS 91-50212). Washington, DC: U.S. Government Printing Office.

U.S. Department of Health and Human Services. (2000). *Healthy people 2010: Understanding and improving health* (2nd ed.). Washington, DC: U.S. Government Printing Office.

World Health Organization. (1978). *Primary health care: Report of the international conference on primary health care.* Geneva: Author.

Selected Bibliography

Armentrout, G. (1998). *Community based nursing: Foundation for practice.* Upper Saddle River, NJ: Prentice Hall.

Ayers, M., Bruno, A. A., & Langford, R. W. (1998). *Community-based nursing care: Making the transition.* St. Louis, MO: Mosby.

Bellack, J. P. (1998). Community-based nursing practice: Necessary but not sufficient. *Journal of Nursing Education, 37,* 99–100.

Hunt, R. (2001). *Introduction to community based nursing.* Philadelphia: Lippincott Williams & Wilkins.

Kiehl, E. M., & Wink, D. M. (2000). Nursing students as change agents and problem solvers in the community: Community-based nursing education in practice. *Nursing and Health Care Perspectives, 21,* 293–297.

McEwen, M., & Eoyang, T. (Eds.) (1998). *Community-based nursing: An introduction.* Philadelphia: W. B. Saunders.

Payne, J. (1999). *Researching health needs: A community-based approach.* Thousand Oaks, CA: Sage.

Pew Health Professions Commission. (1991). *Healthy America: Practitioners for 2005. An agenda for action for U.S. health professional schools.* San Francisco: Author.

Van Ort, S., & Townsend, J. (2000). Community-based nursing education and nursing accreditation by the Commission on Collegiate Nursing Education. *Journal of Professional Nursing, 16,* 330–335.

Whisnant, S. (1999). The parish nurse: Tending to the spiritual side of health. *Holistic Nursing Practice, 14*(1), 84–86.

CHAPTER | 8

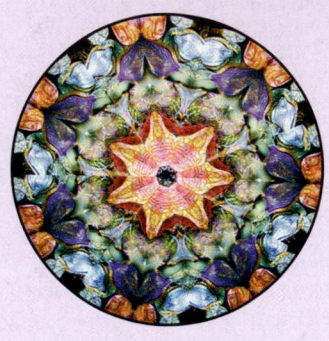

HEALTH PROMOTION

LEARNING OUTCOMES

After completing this chapter, you will be able to:

- Describe how the *Healthy People 2010* leading health indicators can help improve the health of a community.

- Differentiate health promotion from health protection or illness prevention.

- Discuss essential components of health promotion.

- Identify various types and sites of health-promotion programs.

- Discuss the Health Promotion model.

- Explain the stages of health behavior change.

- Discuss the nurse's role in health promotion.

- Assess the health of individuals.

- Develop, implement, and evaluate plans for health promotion.

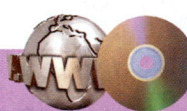

MediaLink

www.prenhall.com/kozier

Additional resources for this chapter can be found on the Student CD-ROM accompanying this textbook, and on the Companion Website at www.prenhall.com/kozier. Click on Chapter 8 to select the activities for this chapter.

CD-ROM
- Audio Glossary
- NCLEX Review

Companion Website
- Additional NCLEX Review
- Case Study: Health Promotion Program
- MediaLink Applications:
    Health Belief Model
    Community Services
- Links to Resources

Health promotion is an important component of nursing practice. It is a way of thinking that revolves around a philosophy of wholeness, wellness, and well-being. In the past two decades, the public has become increasingly aware of and interested in health promotion. Many people are aware of the relationship between lifestyle and illness and are developing health-promoting habits, such as getting adequate exercise, rest, and relaxation; maintaining good nutrition; and controlling the use of tobacco, alcohol, and other drugs.

HEALTHY PEOPLE 2010

The vision of health promotion was expressed in 1979 with the surgeon general's report *Healthy People*, which emphasized health promotion and disease prevention. *Healthy People 2000* followed in 1990 and provided a framework for national health promotion, health protection, and preventive service strategy (U.S. Department of Health and Human Services [USDHHS], 1990). *Healthy People 2010: Understanding and Improving Health* (USDHHS, 2000) presents a comprehensive 10-year strategy for promoting health and preventing illness, disability, and premature death. The two major goals of *Healthy People 2010* reflect the nation's changing demographics:

- "Increase quality and years of healthy life" indicates the aging or "graying" of the population.
- "Eliminate health disparities" reflects the diversity of the population.

To support these goals, *Healthy People 2010* contains 467 objectives to improve health. These objectives are organized into 28 focus areas (see Box 8–1). *Healthy People 2010* also establishes a set of leading health indicators that reflect the major public health concerns in the United States at the beginning of the 21st century (see Box 8–2). Each indicator relates to a number of the health objectives. It is expected that these indicators will help develop action plans to improve the health of both individuals and communities.

The foundation for *Healthy People 2010* is the belief that individual health is closely linked to community health and the reverse. For example, community health is affected by the beliefs, attitudes, and behaviors of the individuals who live in the community. Thus, the vision for *Healthy People 2010* is "Healthy People in Healthy Communities" (USDHHS, 2000, p. 3). As a result, partnerships are important to improve individual and community health. Businesses, local government, and civic, professional, and religious organizations can all participate. Examples include sponsoring a health fair, establishing fitness programs, beginning community recycling, and printing immunization schedules.

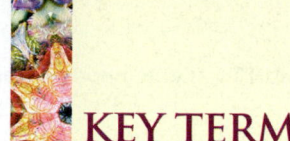

KEY TERMS

action stage, 125
contemplation stage, 125
health promotion, 120
health protection, 120
health risk assessment
    (HRA), 131
maintenance stage, 125
precontemplation stage, 125
preparation stage, 125
primary prevention, 120
secondary prevention, 120
termination stage, 125
tertiary prevention, 120
wellness diagnosis, 133

BOX 8–1	■ The 28 Focus Areas in Healthy People 2010

- Access to quality health services
- Arthritis, osteoporosis, and chronic back conditions
- Cancer
- Chronic kidney disease
- Diabetes
- Disability and secondary conditions
- Educational and community-based programs
- Environmental health
- Family planning
- Food safety
- Health communication
- Heart disease and stroke
- HIV
- Immunization and infectious diseases
- Injury and violence prevention
- Maternal, infant, and child health
- Medical product safety
- Mental health and mental disorders
- Nutrition and overweight
- Occupational safety and health
- Oral health
- Physical activity and fitness
- Public health infrastructure
- Respiratory diseases
- Sexually transmitted diseases
- Substance abuse
- Tobacco use
- Vision and hearing

Note: From *Healthy People 2010: Understanding and Improving Health*, 2nd ed., by U. S. Department of Health and Human Services, 2000, Washington, DC: U.S. Government Printing Office.

BOX 8–2   ■ The Leading Health Indicators in Healthy People 2010

■ **Physical Activity**
  • Regular physical activity throughout life is important for maintaining a healthy body, enhancing psychological well-being, and preventing premature death (p. 26).

■ **Overweight and Obesity**
  • Overweight and obesity are major contributors to many preventable causes of death. On average, higher body weights are associated with higher death rates. The number of overweight children, adolescents, and adults has risen over the past four decades (p. 28).

■ **Tobacco Use**
  • Cigarette smoking is the single most preventable cause of disease and death in the United States (p. 30).

■ **Substance Abuse**
  • Alcohol and illicit drug use are associated with many of this country's most serious problems, including violence, injury, and HIV infection (p. 32).

■ **Responsible Sexual Behavior**
  • Unintended pregnancies and sexually transmitted diseases (STDs), including infection with the human immunodeficiency virus that causes AIDS, can result from unprotected sexual behaviors (p. 34).

■ **Mental Health**
  • Approximately 20 percent of the U.S. population is affected by mental illness during a given year; no one is immune. Of all mental illnesses, depression is the most common disorder. Major depression is the leading cause of disability and is the cause of more than two-thirds of suicides each year (p. 36).

■ **Injury and Violence**
  • More than 400 Americans die each day from injuries due primarily to motor vehicle crashes, firearms, poisonings, suffocation, falls, fires, and drowning (p. 38).

■ **Environmental Quality**
  • An estimated 25 percent of preventable illnesses worldwide can be attributed to poor environmental quality. Two indicators of air quality are ozone (outdoor) and environmental tobacco smoke (indoor) (p. 40).

■ **Immunization**
  • Vaccines are among the greatest public health achievements of the 20th century. Immunizations can prevent disability and death from infectious diseases for individuals and can help control the spread of infections within communities (p. 42).

■ **Access to Health Care**
  • Strong predictors of access to quality health care include having health insurance, a higher income level, and a regular primary care provider or other source of ongoing health care. Use of clinical preventive services, such as early prenatal care, can serve as indicators of access to quality health care services (p. 44).

Note: From *Healthy People 2010: Understanding and Improving Health,* 2nd ed., by U.S. Department of Health and Human Services, 2000, Washington, DC: U.S. Government Printing Office.

Health promotion, then, includes programs that modify both the environment and the behavior of individuals. It involves education in lifestyle and behavioral change, community development, organizational change, and—at the political level—legislation.

DEFINING HEALTH PROMOTION

Considerable differences appear in the literature regarding the use of the terms *health promotion, primary prevention, health protection,* and *illness prevention.* Edelman and Mandle (2002) state that "prevention, in a narrow sense, means avoiding the development of disease in the future, and, in the broader sense, consists of all interventions to limit progression of a disease" (p. 14). The levels of prevention occur at various points of a course of disease progression. Leavell and Clark (1965) define three levels of prevention: primary, secondary, and tertiary. Five steps describe these levels: **Primary prevention** focuses on (a) health promotion and (b) protection against specific health problems (e.g., immunization against hepatitis B). The purpose of primary prevention is to decrease the risk or exposure of the individual or community to disease. **Secondary prevention** focuses on (a) early identification of health problems and (b) prompt intervention to alleviate health problems. Its goal is to identify individuals in an early stage of a disease process and to limit future disability. **Tertiary prevention** focuses on restoration and rehabilitation with the goal of returning the individual to an optimal level of functioning. Table 8–1 provides examples of activities for each level of prevention. The three levels of prevention may overlap in practice. For example, a client may have experienced a heart attack and a goal of secondary prevention is to limit disability. The teaching (e.g., lifestyle changes) for the client's rehabilitation will be similar to health education activities in primary prevention.

Pender, Murdaugh, and Parsons (2002) consider health promotion to be different from health protection or illness prevention. They define **health promotion** as "behavior motivated by the desire to increase well-being and actualize human health potential," and **health protection** or illness prevention as "behavior motivated by a desire to actively avoid illness, detect it early, or maintain functioning within the constraints of illness" (p. 7). The individual's underlying motivation for the behavior is the major difference. Box 8–3 provides an overview of the differences between health promotion and health protection.

The difficulty in separating the terms *health promotion* and *health protection* lies in the fact that an activity may be carried out for numerous reasons. For example, a 40-year-old male may begin a program of walking 3 miles each day. If the goal of his program were to "decrease the risk of cardiovascular disease," then the activity would be considered health protection. By contrast, if the motivation for his walking regimen were to "increase his overall health and feeling of well-being," then the

TABLE 8–1 Levels of Prevention

Level and Description	Examples
Primary prevention Generalized health promotion and specific protection against disease. It precedes disease or dysfunction and is applied to generally healthy individuals or groups.	• Health education about accident and poisoning prevention, standards of nutrition and of growth and development for each stage of life, exercise requirements, stress management, protection against occupational hazards, and so on • Immunizations • Risk assessments for specific disease • Family planning services and marriage counseling • Environmental sanitation and provision of adequate housing, recreation, and work conditions
Secondary prevention Emphasizes early detection of disease, prompt intervention, and health maintenance for individuals experiencing health problems. Includes prevention of complications and disabilities.	• Screening surveys and procedures of any type (e.g., Denver Developmental Screening Test, hypertension screening) • Encouraging regular medical and dental checkups • Teaching self-examination for breast and testicular cancer • Assessing the growth and development of children • Nursing assessments and care provided in home, hospital, or other agency to prevent complications (e.g., maintaining skin integrity; turning, positioning, and exercising clients; ensuring adequate rest, food, and fluid intake; promoting fecal and urinary elimination; administering medical therapies such as medications; and so on)
Tertiary prevention Begins after an illness, when a defect or disability is fixed, stabilized, or determined to be irreversible. Its focus is to help rehabilitate individuals and restore them to an optimum level of functioning within the constraints of the disability.	• Referring a client who has had a colostomy to a support group • Teaching a client who has diabetes to identify and prevent complications • Referring a client with a spinal cord injury to a rehabilitation center to receive training that will maximize use of remaining abilities

---

BOX 8–3   ■ Differences between Health Promotion and Health Protection

Health Promotion	Health Protection
Not disease oriented	Illness or injury specific
Motivated by personal, positive "approach" to wellness	Motivated by "avoidance" of illness
Seeks to expand positive potential for health	Seeks to thwart the occurrence of insults to health and well-being

Note: From *Health Promotion in Nursing Practice,* 4th ed. (pp. 120–122), by N. J. Pender, C. L. Murdaugh, and M. A. Parsons, 2002. Upper Saddle River, NJ: Prentice Hall. Reprinted with permission.

activity would be considered a health-promotion behavior. It is most helpful to think of health promotion and health protection as being complementary processes because both impact quality of health.

Health promotion can be offered to all clients regardless of their health and illness status or age. For example, weight-control measures can benefit both overweight clients without disease and clients with cardiac or joint disease. Age-specific health-promotion activities are discussed in Chapters 22 and 23. 🔗 See Lifespan Considerations for examples of health-promotion topics.

SITES FOR HEALTH-PROMOTION ACTIVITIES

Health-promotion programs are found in many settings. Programs and activities may be offered to individuals and families in the home or in the community setting and at schools, hospitals, or worksites. Some individuals may feel more comfortable having a nurse, diet counselor, or fitness expert come to their home for teaching and follow-up on individual needs. This type of program, however, is not cost effective for most individuals. Many people prefer the group approach, find it more motivating, and enjoy the socializing and support. Most programs offered in the community are group oriented.

Community programs are frequently offered by cities and towns. The type of program depends on the current concerns and the expertise of the sponsoring department or group. Program offerings may include health promotion, specific protection, and screening for early detection of disease. The local

Lifespan Considerations

Health-Promotion Topics

Infants
- Infant–parent attachment/bonding
- Breastfeeding
- Sleep patterns
- Playful activity to stimulate development
- Immunizations
- Safety promotion and injury control

Children
- Nutrition
- Dental checkups
- Rest and exercise
- Immunizations
- Safety promotion and injury control

Adolescents
- Communicating with the teen
- Hormonal changes
- Nutrition
- Exercise and rest
- Peer group influences
- Self-concept and body image
- Sexuality
- Safety promotion and accident prevention

Elders
- Adequate sleep
- Appropriate use of alcohol
- Dental/oral health
- Drug management
- Exercise
- Foot health
- Health screening recommendations
- Hearing aid use
- Immunizations
- Medication instruction
- Mental health
- Nutrition
- Physical fitness
- Preventive health services
- Safety precautions
- Smoking cessation
- Weight control

---

health department may offer a townwide immunization program or blood pressure screening. The fire department may disseminate fire prevention information; the police may offer a bicycle safety program for children or a safe-driving campaign for young adults.

Hospitals began the emphasis on health promotion and prevention by focusing on the health of their employees. Because of the stress involved in caring for the sick and the various shifts that nurses and other health care workers must work, the lifestyles and health habits of health care employees were given priority.

Programs offered by health care organizations initially began with a specific focus on prevention. Examples include infection control, fire prevention and fire drills, limiting exposure to x-rays, and the prevention of back injuries. Gradually, issues related to the health and lifestyle of the employee were addressed with programs on topics such as smoking cessation, exercise and fitness, stress reduction, and time management. Increasingly, hospitals have offered a variety of these programs and others (e.g., women's health) to the community as well as to their employees. Such community activities enhance the public image of the hospital, increase the health of the surrounding population, and generate some additional income.

School health-promotion programs may serve as a foundation for children of all ages to gain basic knowledge about personal hygiene and issues in the health sciences. Because school is the focus of a child's life for so many years, the school provides a cost-effective and convenient setting for health-focused programs. The school nurse may teach programs about basic nutrition, dental care, activity and play, drug and alcohol abuse, domestic violence, child abuse, and issues related to sexuality and pregnancy. Classroom teachers may include health-related top-

ics in their lesson plans, for example, the way the normal heart functions or the need for clean air and water in the environment.

Worksite programs for health promotion have developed out of the need for businesses to control the rising cost of health care and employee absenteeism. Many industries feel that both employers and employees benefit from healthy lifestyles and behaviors. The convenience of the worksite setting makes these programs particularly attractive to many adults who would otherwise not be aware of them or motivated to attend them. Health-promotion programs may be held in the company cafeteria so that employees can watch a film or attend a discussion group during their lunch break. Worksite programs may include programs that address air quality standards for the office, classroom, or plant; programs aimed at specific populations, such as accident prevention for the machine worker or back-saver programs for the individual involved in heavy lifting; programs to screen for high blood pressure; or health enhancement programs, such as fitness information and relaxation techniques. Benefits to the worker may include an increased feeling of well-being, fitness, weight control, and decreased stress. Benefits to the employer may include an increase in employee motivation and productivity, an increase in employee morale, a decrease in absenteeism, and a lower rate of employee turnover, all of which may decrease business and health care costs.

Older adults who have retired often have more time for health-promotion activities than they did before retirement. The nurse can inform elders of available community resources such as walking groups. Nurses can address the need for health protection and health promotion through teaching classes at retirement communities and other community resource centers for elders.

HEALTH PROMOTION MODEL

The initial version of the Health Promotion Model (HPM) appeared in the nursing literature in the early 1980s and focused on health-promoting behaviors rather than health protection or illness prevention behaviors. The initial model has recently been replaced by the Health Promotion Model (Revised) as shown in Figure 8–1 ■. The HPM is a competence- or approach-oriented model that depicts the multidimensional nature of persons interacting with their interpersonal and physical environments as they pursue health (Pender et al., 2002, p. 61). The assumptions of the HPM are stated in Box 8–4. The variables in the revised HPM and their interrelationships are described next.

Individual Characteristics and Experiences

The importance of an individual's unique personal factors or characteristics and experiences will depend on the target behavior for health promotion. There is flexibility in the HPM to select those characteristics that are relevant to the particular health behavior. Personal factors are categorized as biological (e.g., age, strength, balance), psychological (e.g., self-esteem, self-motivation), and sociocultural (e.g., race, ethnicity, education, socioeconomic status). Some personal factors can influence health behaviors while others, such as age, cannot be changed. Prior related behavior includes previous experience, knowledge, and skill in health-promoting actions. Individuals who made a habit of a previous health-promoting behavior and received a positive benefit as a result will engage in future health-promoting behaviors. In contrast, a person with a history of barriers to achieving the behavior remembers the "hurdles," which creates a negative effect. The nurse can assist by focusing on the positive benefits of the behavior, teaching how to overcome the hurdles and providing positive feedback for the client's successes.

Nursing interventions usually focus on factors that can be modified. It is just as important, however, to also focus on factors that cannot be changed, such as family history. For instance, if a woman has a strong family history of breast cancer, she may neglect self-care practices such as performing breast self-exams and having regular mammograms. She may do this

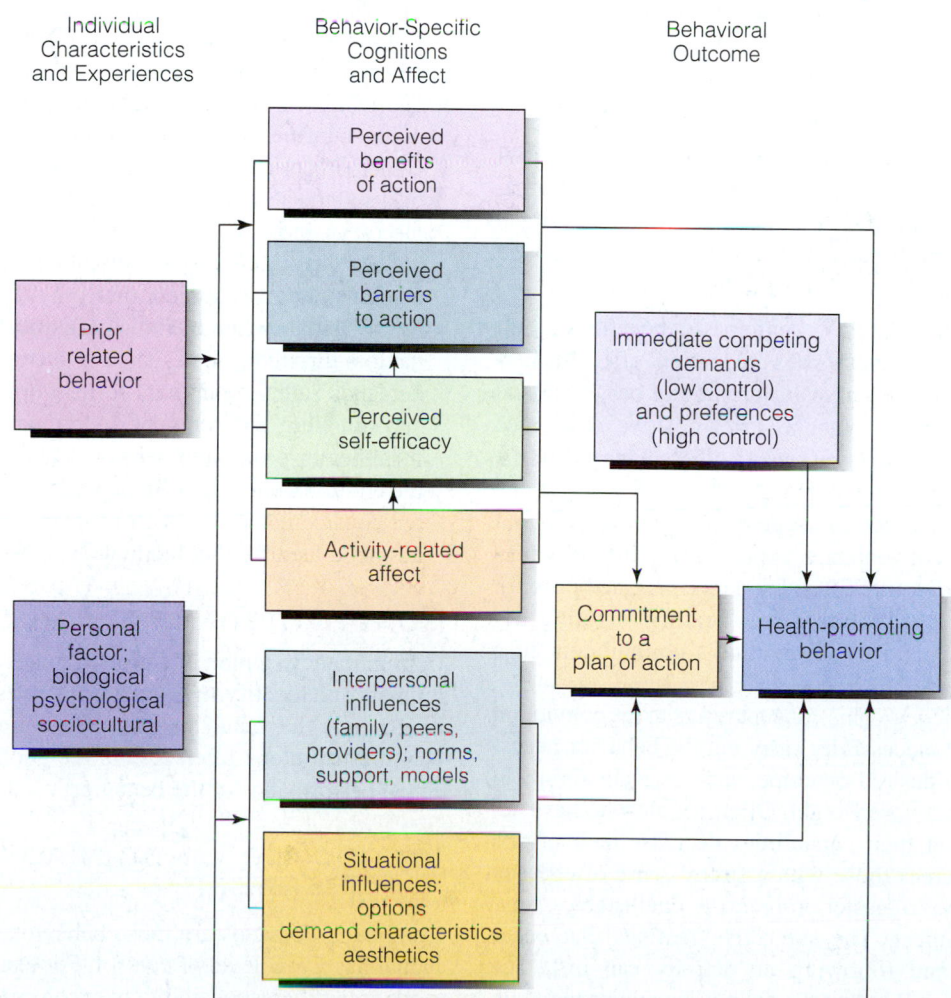

Figure 8–1 ■ The Health Promotion Model (Revised). (*Note:* From *Health Promotion in Nursing Practice*, 4th ed. (p. 60), by N. J. Pender, C. L. Murdaugh, and M. A. Parsons, 2002, Upper Saddle River, NJ: Prentice Hall. Reprinted with permission.)

BOX 8–4   ■ Assumptions of the Health Promotion Model

- Persons seek to create conditions of living through which they can express their unique human health potential.
- Persons have the capacity for reflective self-awareness, including assessment of their own competencies.
- Persons value growth in directions viewed as positive and attempt to achieve a personally acceptable balance between change and stability.
- Individuals seek to actively regulate their own behavior.

- Individuals in all their biopsychosocial complexity interact with the environment, progressively transforming the environment and being transformed over time.
- Health professionals constitute a part of the interpersonal environment, which exerts influence on persons throughout their life span.
- Self-initiated reconfiguration of person–environment interactive patterns is essential to behavior change.

Note: From *Health Promotion in Nursing Practice,* 4th ed. (pp. 120–122), by N. J. Pender, C. L. Murdaugh, and M. A. Parsons, 2002, Upper Saddle River, NJ: Prentice Hall. Reprinted with permission.

---

out of fear of finding a lump, or just feeling that with her family history, it is inevitable that she will have breast cancer. Nurses should recognize this and direct more support and information to this group of women, reinforcing the idea that even with a strong family history, early detection and treatment are especially important and offer more hope for a cure. Helping to transform that fear into hope for early detection can make a difference in health attitudes and behaviors.

Behavior-Specific Cognitions and Affect

This set of variables is considered to be of major motivational significance for acquiring and maintaining health-promoting behaviors. Behavior-specific cognitions constitute a critical "core" for intervention because they can be modified through nursing interventions. They include the following:

- *Perceived benefits of action.* Anticipated benefits or outcomes (e.g., physical fitness, stress reduction) affect the person's plan to participate in health-promoting behaviors and may facilitate continued practice. Prior positive experience with the behavior or observations of others engaged in the behavior is a motivational factor.
- *Perceived barriers to action.* A person's perceptions about available time, inconvenience, expense, and difficulty performing the activity may act as barriers (imagined or real). Perceived barriers to action affect health-promoting behaviors by decreasing the individual's commitment to a plan of action.
- *Perceived self-efficacy.* This concept refers to the conviction that a person can successfully carry out the behavior necessary to achieve a desired outcome, such as maintaining an exercise program to lose weight. Often people who have serious doubts about their capabilities decrease their efforts and give up, whereas those with a strong sense of efficacy exert greater effort to master problems or challenges.
- *Activity-related affect.* The subjective feelings that occur before, during, and following an activity can influence whether a person will repeat the behavior again or maintain the behavior. What is the individual's reaction to the thought of the behavior? Is it perceived as fun, enjoyable, or unpleasant? A positive affect or emotional response to a behav-

ior is likely to be repeated and behaviors associated with a negative affect are usually avoided.
- *Interpersonal influences.* Interpersonal influences are a person's perceptions concerning the behaviors, beliefs, or attitudes of others. Family, peers, and health professionals are sources of interpersonal influences that can influence a person's health-promoting behaviors. Interpersonal influences include expectation of significant others, social support (e.g., emotional encouragement), and learning through observing others or modeling.
- *Situational influences.* Situational influences are direct and indirect influences on health-promoting behaviors and include perceptions of available options, demand characteristics, and the aesthetic features of the environment. An example of an individual's perception of available options can include easy access to healthy alternatives such as vending machines and restaurants that provide healthful menu options. Demand characteristics can directly affect healthy behaviors through policies such as a company regulation that demands safety equipment to be worn or that establishes a "no smoking" environment. Individuals are more apt to perform health-promotion behaviors if they are comfortable in the environment versus feeling alienated. Environments that are considered safe as well as interesting are also desirable aesthetic features that facilitate health-promotion behaviors.

Commitment to a Plan of Action

Commitment to a plan of action involves two processes: commitment and identifying specific strategies for carrying out and reinforcing the behavior. Strategies are important because commitment alone often results in "good intentions" and not actual performance of the behavior.

Immediate Competing Demands and Preferences

Competing demands are those behaviors over which an individual has a low level of control. For example, an unexpected work or family responsibility may compete with a planned visit to the health club and not responding to this responsibility may cause a more negative outcome than missing the exercise routine. Competing preferences are behaviors over which an individual has a high level of control, however, this control depends on the individual's ability to be self-regulating or to not "give in." For example, a person who chooses a high-fat food over a low-fat food because it tastes better has "given in" to an urge based on a competing preference.

Behavioral Outcome

Health-promoting behavior, the outcome of the Health Promotion Model, is directed toward attaining positive health outcomes for the client. Health-promoting behaviors should result in improved health, enhanced functional ability, and better quality of life at all stages of development (Pender et al., 2002, p. 74).

STAGES OF HEALTH BEHAVIOR CHANGE

Health behavior change is a cyclic phenomenon in which people progress through several stages. In the first stage, the person does not think seriously about changing a behavior; by the time the person reaches the final stage, he or she is successfully maintaining the change in behavior. Several behavior change models have been proposed. The stage model proposed by Prochaska, Norcross, and DiClemente (1994) is discussed here. As shown in Figure 8–2 ■, the stages are (a) precontemplation, (b) contemplation, (c) preparation, (d) action, (e) maintenance, and (f) termination. If the person does not succeed in changing behavior, relapse occurs.

Precontemplation Stage

In the **precontemplation stage,** the person typically denies having a problem, views others as having a problem, and, therefore, wants others to change *their* behavior. They do not think about changing behavior, nor are they interested in information about the behavior. Some people believe the behavior is not under their control and may become defensive when confronted with information because they believe the situation is hopeless. The person may have tried changing previously and was unsuccessful and now sees the behavior as their "fate" or that change is hopeless.

Contemplation Stage

During the **contemplation stage,** the person acknowledges having a problem, seriously considers changing a specific behavior, actively gathers information, and verbalizes plans to change the behavior in the near future. The person, however, may not be ready to commit to action. Some people may stay in the contemplative stage for months or years before taking action. When comtemplators begin the transition to the preparation stage, their thinking is clearly marked by two changes: focusing on the solution rather than the problem and thinking more about the future than the past (Prochaska et al., 1994, p. 43).

Preparation Stage

The **preparation stage** occurs when the person undertakes cognitive and behavioral activities that prepare the person for change. At this stage, the person makes the final specific plans to accomplish the change. Some people in this stage may have already started making small behavioral changes, such as eliminating sugar in their coffee.

Action Stage

The **action stage** occurs when the person actively implements behavioral and cognitive strategies to interrupt previous behavior patterns and adopt new ones. This stage requires the greatest commitment of time and energy.

Maintenance Stage

During the **maintenance stage,** the person integrates newly adopted behavior patterns into his or her lifestyle. This stage lasts until the person no longer experiences temptation to return to previous unhealthy behaviors. Without a strong commitment to maintenance, there will be a relapse, usually to the precontemplation or contemplation stage (Prochaska et al., 1994, p. 45).

Termination Stage

The **termination stage** is the ultimate goal where the individual has complete confidence that the problem is no longer a temptation or threat. Experts debate whether some behaviors can be terminated versus requiring continual maintenance.

These six stages are cyclical; people generally move through one stage before progressing to the next. However, at any point a person may relapse or recycle to any previous stage. In fact, the average successful self-changer recycles through the stages several times before they make it to the top and exit the cycle (Prochaska et al., 1994, pp. 47–48). The majority of individuals who relapse return to the contemplation stage. During this time they can think about what they learned and plan for the next action attempt. Box 8–5 on page 127 suggests a method to assess your stage of change for a health behavior.

THE NURSE'S ROLE IN HEALTH PROMOTION

Individuals and communities who seek to increase their responsibility for personal health and self-care require health education. The trend toward health promotion has created the opportunity for nurses to strengthen the profession's influence on health promotion, disseminate information that promotes an educated public, and assist individuals and communities to change long-standing health behaviors.

A variety of programs can be used for the promotion of health, including (a) information dissemination, (b) health risk appraisal and wellness assessment, (c) lifestyle and behavior change, and (d) environmental control programs.

Information dissemination is the most basic type of health-promotion program. This method makes use of a variety of media to offer information to the public about the risk of particular lifestyle choices and personal behavior, as well as the benefits of changing that behavior and improving the quality of life. Billboards, posters, brochures, newspaper features, books, and health fairs all offer opportunities for the dissemination of

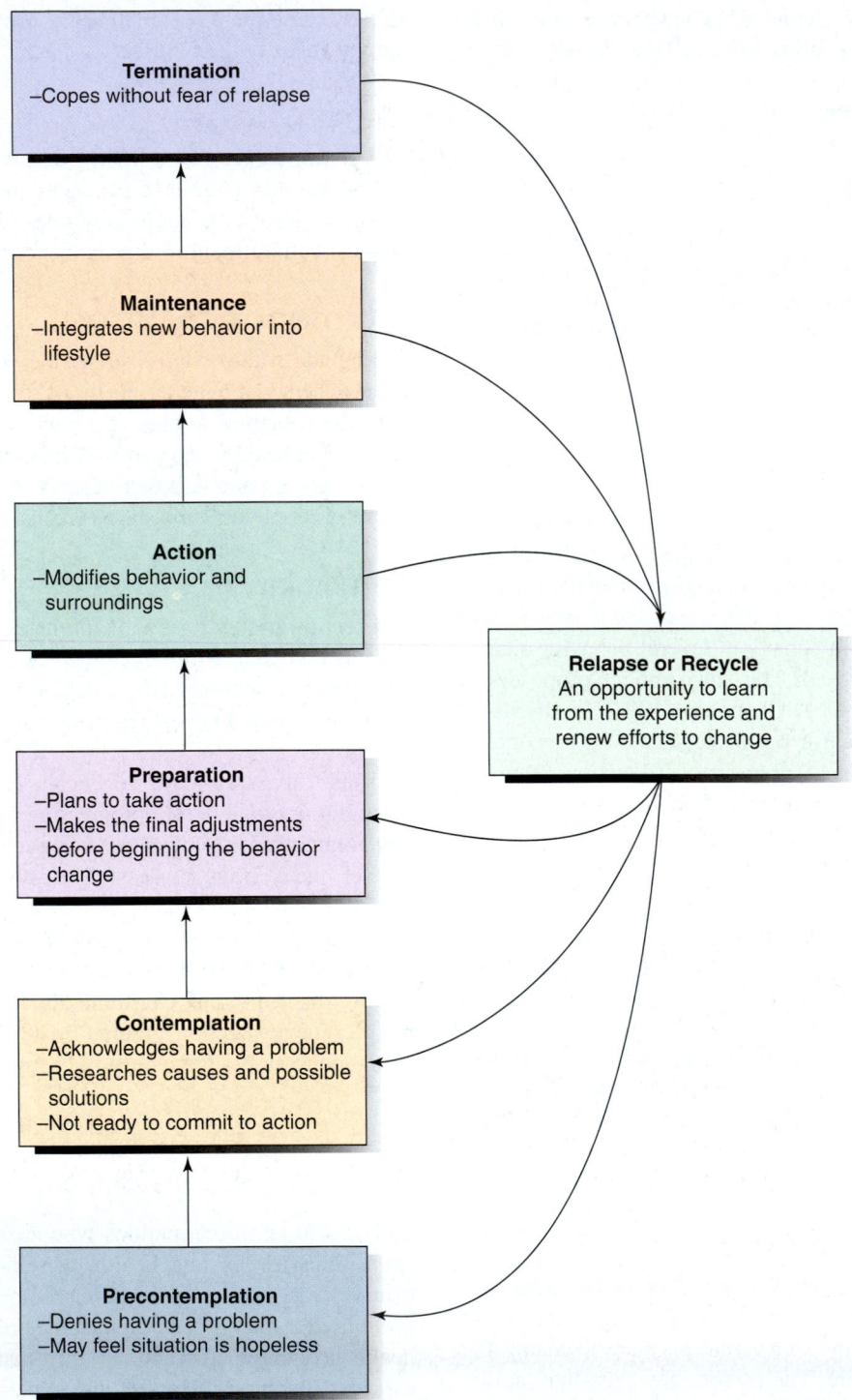

Figure 8–2 ■ The stages of change are rarely linear. It is more common for people to recycle several times through the stages. The person who takes action and has a relapse (recycles through some or all of the stages again) is more apt to be successful the next time than the individual who never takes action. (Diagram based on content from *Changing for Good* by James O. Prochaska, John C. Norcross, and Carlo C. DiClemente. Copyright 1994 by James O. Prochaska, John C. Norcross, and Carlo C. Dilemente. Reprinted by permission of HarperCollins Publishers, Inc.)

health-promotion information. Alcohol and drug abuse, driving under the influence of alcohol, hypertension, and the need for immunizations are some of the topics frequently discussed. Information dissemination is a useful strategy for raising the level of knowledge and awareness of individuals and groups about health habits.

When planning information dissemination, it is important to consider factors such as cultural factors and different age groups. Knowing the best place and method to distribute information will increase the effectiveness. For example, older African Americans usually have strong ties to their churches for social support as well as religious practices. Knowing this, the church

---

BOX 8–5	■ Assessing Your Stage of Change

Respond to the following statements to assess the stage you are in for a particular problem behavior.

1. I solved my problem more than six months ago.
2. I have taken action on my problem within the past six months.
3. I am intending to take action in the next month.
4. I am intending to take action in the next six months.

If you answered . . .

No to all the statements → precontemplation stage
Yes to statement 4 and no to all others → contemplation stage
Yes to statements 3 and 4 and no to the others → preparation stage
No to statement 1 and yes to statement 2 → action stage
Yes to statement 1 → maintenance stage

Note: From *Changing for Good* (p. 68) by James O. Prochaska, John C. Norcross, and Carlo C. DiClemente, copyright 1994, by James O. Prochaska, John C. Norcross, and Carlo C. DiClemente. Reprinted by permission of HarperCollins Publishers, Inc.

---

can often be the appropriate place to hold health fairs or even small group discussions on various health topics. It provides a stepping stone for providing information and suggesting resources for special needs—all done in a comfortable, nonthreatening environment for persons in that age group and culture.

It is just as critical to know where people get "misinformation." Sending multiple mailings has become a marketing ploy for advertising "miracle" vitamins, herbs, and food supplements. These are heavily directed toward elders who may choose this route of purchasing items due to transportation problems that they may have.

Health risk appraisal and wellness assessment programs are used to apprise individuals of the risk factors that are inherent in their lives in order to motivate them to reduce specific risks and develop positive health habits. Wellness assessment programs are focused on more positive methods of enhancement, in contrast to the risk factor approach used in the health appraisal. A variety of tools are available to facilitate these assessments. Some of these tools are computer based and can therefore be offered to educational institutions and industries at a reasonable cost.

Lifestyle and behavior change programs require the participation of the individual and are geared toward enhancing the quality of life and extending the life span. Individuals generally consider lifestyle changes after they have been informed of the need to change their health behavior and have become aware of the potential benefits of the process. Many programs are available to the public, both on a group and individual basis, some of which address stress management, nutrition awareness, weight control, smoking cessation, and exercise.

Environmental control programs have been developed in response to the continuing increase of contaminants of human origin that have been introduced into our environment. The amounts of contaminants that are already present in the air, food, and water will affect the health of our descendants for several generations. The most common concerns of community groups are toxic and nuclear wastes, nuclear power plants, air and water pollution, and herbicide and pesticide use.

Health-promotion activities, such as the variety of programs previously discussed, involve collaborative relationships with both clients and physicians. The role of the nurse is to work *with* people, not *for* them—that is, to act as a facilitator of the process of assessing, evaluating, and understanding health. The nurse may act as advocate, consultant, teacher, or coordinator of services. For examples of the nurse's role in health promotion, see Box 8–6.

In these roles, the nurse may work with individuals of all age groups and diverse family units or concentrate on a specific population, such as new parents, school-age children, or older adults. In any case, the nursing process is a basic tool for the nurse in a health-promotion role. Although the process is the same, the nurse emphasizes teaching the client (who can be either an individual or a family unit) self-care responsibility. Adult clients decide the goals, determine the health-promotion plans, and take the responsibility for the success of the plans.

THE NURSING PROCESS AND HEALTH PROMOTION

A thorough assessment of the individual's health status is basic to health promotion. As nurses move toward greater autonomy in providing client care, expanded assessment skills are essential to provide the meaningful data needed for health planning.

BOX 8–6	■ The Nurse's Role in Health Promotion

- Model healthy lifestyle behaviors and attitudes.
- Facilitate client involvement in the assessment, implementation, and evaluation of health goals.
- Teach clients self-care strategies to enhance fitness, improve nutrition, manage stress, and enhance relationships.
- Assist individuals, families, and communities to increase their levels of health.
- Educate clients to be effective health care consumers.

- Assist clients, families, and communities to develop and choose health-promoting options.
- Guide clients' development in effective problem solving and decision making.
- Reinforce clients' personal and family health-promoting behaviors.
- Advocate in the community for changes that promote a healthy environment.

NURSING MANAGEMENT

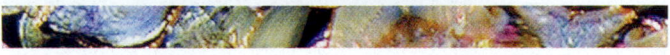

ASSESSING

Components of this assessment are the health history and physical examination, physical fitness assessment, lifestyle assessment, spiritual assessment, social support systems review, health risk assessment, health beliefs review, and life-stress review.

Health History and Physical Examination

The health history and physical examination discussed in Chapter 28 ⊙⊙ provide a means for detecting any existing problems. The age of the individual must be considered when collecting data. For example, an environmental safety assessment and immunization history must be appropriate to the person's age. A nutritional assessment is an important part of the health history. The nurse must consider both age and body build of the client when gathering information on dietary patterns. See Chapter 45 ⊙⊙ for more information about nutritional assessment.

Physical Fitness Assessment

During an evaluation of physical fitness, the nurse assesses several components of the body's physical functioning: muscle endurance, flexibility, body composition, and cardiorespiratory endurance. Specific guidelines for obtaining measurements and the optimal values for men, women, and children can be found in physical fitness texts (see Table 8–2). Elders need to be monitored carefully for fatigue during strength and endurance tests.

A common test for muscular endurance is performing sit-ups with knees bent (bent-knee situps) for 1 minute. The number of sit-ups performed during that time is compared to standardized charts.

Flexibility of the joints and muscles greatly increases an individual's ability to move about with ease and comfort. Trunk flexion is one test used to measure the client's ability to stretch the back and thigh muscles. In this test the client sits on an examining table or the floor with the legs fully extended, the feet placed flat against a box, and the arms and hands stretched forward as far as possible and holds for a count of three. The distance the client can reach beyond the near edge of the box is measured in inches or, if the client is unable to reach the box, the distance between the fingertips and the box is measured and recorded as a negative number.

Body composition indicates the ratio of body fat to muscle and is estimated through skinfold measurements. Skinfold measurements are obtained by grasping the skinfold (skin layers and subcutaneous fat) between the thumb and forefinger and measuring the skinfold at subcutaneous sites (chest, midaxillary, triceps, subscapula, abdomen, suprailiac, and thigh) with special calipers. Generally three measurements are taken at each site and the average values summed. The technique for measuring skin folds is described in Chapter 45. ⊙⊙

One test for cardiorespiratory endurance is the step test. Individuals step up and down on a 16- to 17-inch step for 3 minutes at a prescribed rate (e.g., 22 to 24 steps per minute). After the test, the client sits in a chair while the nurse assesses the apical or carotid pulse rate from 5 to 20 seconds into recovery.

Lifestyle Assessment

Lifestyle assessment focuses on the personal lifestyle and habits of the client as they affect health. Categories of lifestyle generally assessed are physical activity, nutritional practices, stress management, and such habits as smoking, alcohol consumption, and drug use. Other categories may be included. The goals of lifestyle assessment tools are to provide the following:

1. An opportunity for clients to assess the impact of their present lifestyle on their health
2. A basis for decisions related to desired behavior and lifestyle change

Several tools are available to assess lifestyle. A form for self-assessment of lifestyle is shown in Figure 8–3 ■.

TABLE 8–2 Physical Fitness Values

Test	Age	Desired Outcomes	Undesired Outcomes
Sit-ups	36 to 45 years	Men: 42 or more	21 or less
		Women: 39 or more	12 or less
	Over 46 years	Men: 38 or more	18 or less
		Women: 24 or more	11 or less
Trunk flexion		Men: 11 to 15 inches	Below –6 inches
		Women: 12 to 16 inches	Below –4 inches
Skin folds		Men: 21 mm	Marked deviations
		Women: 30 mm	above or below desired ratings
Step test		Men: recovery pulse rate 124	Men: recovery pulse rate 178
		Women: recovery pulse rate 140	Women: recovery pulse rate 184
		(95th percentile rankings)	(10th percentile rankings)

Note: From Health Promotion in Nursing Practice 4th ed. (pp. 120–122) by N. J. Pender, C. L. Murdaugh, and M. A. Parsons, 2002, Upper Saddle River, NJ: Prentice Hall. Reprinted with permission.

Healthstyle: A Self-Test

Everyone wants good health. But many of us don't know how to be as healthy as possible. Health experts describe *lifestyle* as one of the most important factors affecting our health. In fact, it is estimated that 7 of the 10 leading causes of death could be reduced through common-sense changes in lifestyle. The first step in a healthier lifestyle is thinking about what we are doing now.

This brief self-test, developed by the Public Health Service, will let you know how well you are doing to stay healthy. The behaviors included in the test are recommended for most adult Americans. Some behaviors may not apply to persons with certain chronic diseases or handicaps, or to pregnant women. Such persons may need special advice from their doctor or other health care provider.

Cigarette Smoking

If you never smoke, enter a score of 10 for this section and go to the next section on *Alcohol and Drugs*.

	Almost Always	Sometimes	Almost Never
1. I avoid smoking cigarettes.	2	1	0
2. I smoke only low tar and nicotine cigarettes *OR* I smoke a pipe or cigars.	2	1	0

Smoking Score: _____

Alcohol and Drugs

	Almost Always	Sometimes	Almost Never
1. I avoid drinking alcoholic beverages or I drink no more than 1 or 2 drinks a day.	4	1	0
2. I avoid using alcohol or other drugs (especially illegal drugs) as a way of handling stressful situations or the problems.	2	1	0
3. I am careful not to drink alcohol when taking certain medicines (for example, medicine for sleeping, pain, colds, and allergies) or when pregnant.	2	1	0
4. I read and follow the label directions when using prescribed and over-the-counter drugs.	2	1	0

Alcohol and Drugs Score: _____

Eating Habits

	Almost Always	Sometimes	Almost Never
1. I eat a variety of foods each day, such as fruits and vegetables; whole grain breads and cereals; lean meats; dairy products; dry peas; beans; nuts and seeds.	4	1	0
2. I limit the amount of fat, saturated fat, and cholesterol I eat (including fat on meats, eggs, butter, cream, shortenings, and organ meats such as liver).	2	1	0
3. I limit the amount of salt I eat by cooking with only small amounts, not adding salt at the table, and avoiding salty snacks.	2	1	0
4. I avoid eating too much sugar (especially frequent snacks of sticky candy or soft drinks).	2	1	0

Eating Habits Score: _____

Exercise/Fitness

	Almost Always	Sometimes	Almost Never
1. I do vigorous exercises for 20–30 minutes a day at least 3 times a week (examples include jogging, swimming, brisk walking, bicycling).	4	2	0
2. I do exercises that enhance my muscle tone for 15–30 minutes at least 3 times a week (examples include using weight machines or free weights, yoga and calisthenics).	3	1	0
3. I use part of my leisure time participating in individual, family, or team activities that increase my level of fitness (such as gardening, dancing, bowling, golf, baseball).	3	1	0

Exercise/Fitness Score: _____

Stress Control

	Almost Always	Sometimes	Almost Never
1. I have a job or do other work that I enjoy.	2	1	0
2. I find it easy to relax and express my feelings freely.	2	1	0
3. I recognize early, and prepare for, events or situations likely to be stressful for me.	2	1	0
4. I have close friends, relatives, or others whom I can talk to about personal matters and call on for help when needed.	2	1	0
5. I participate in group activities (such as religious worship and community organizations) and/or have hobbies that I enjoy.	2	1	0

Stress Control Score: _____

Safety

	Almost Always	Sometimes	Almost Never
1. I wear a seat belt while riding in a car.	2	1	0
2. I avoid driving while under the influence of alcohol and other drugs.	2	1	0
3. I obey traffic rules and the speed limit when driving.	2	1	0
4. I am careful when using potentially harmful products or substances (such as household cleaners, poisons, and electrical devices).	2	1	0
5. I avoid smoking in bed.	2	1	0

Safety Score: _____

(continued)

Figure 8–3 ■ Healthstyle: A Self-Test

Note: From "Healthstyle: A Self-Test," by L. B. Bobroff, 1999, University of Florida, Institute of Food and Agricultural Sciences (UF/IFAS). Retrieved March 23, 2003, from http://edis.ifas.ufl.edu/BODY_HE778. Copyright 1999 by UF/IFAS. Reprinted with permission.

Your Lifestyle Scores

After you have figured your scores for each of the six sections, circle the number in each column that matches your score for that section of the test. Remember: There is no total score for this self-test. Think about each section separately. You are identifying aspects of your lifestyle that you an improve in order to be healthier. So let's see what your scores reveal.

What Your Score Means to You (By Section)

Scores of 9 and 10

Excellent! Your answers show that you are aware of the importance of this area to your health. More important, you are putting your knowledge to work for you by practicing good health habits. As long as you continue to do so, this area should not pose a serious health risk. It's likely that you are setting an example for the rest of your family and friends to follow. Since you got a very high test score on this part of the test, you may want to consider other areas where your scores indicate room for improvement.

Scores of 6 to 8

Your health practices in this area are good, but there is room for improvement. Look again at the items you answered with a "Sometimes" or "Almost Never." What changes can you make to improve your score? Even a small change can help you achieve better health.

Scores of 3 to 5

Your health risks are showing. Would you like more information about the risks you are facing? Do you want to know why it is important for you to change these behaviors? Perhaps you need help in deciding how to make the changes you desire. In either case, help is available.

Scores of 0 to 2

Obviously, you were concerned enough about your health to take this test. But your answers show that you may be taking serious risks with your health. Perhaps you were not aware of the risks and what to do about them. You can easily get the information and help you need to reduce your health risks and have a healthier lifestyle if you wish. The next step is up to you.

YOU CAN START RIGHT NOW

The test you just completed included many suggestions to help you reduce your risk of disease and premature death. Here are some of the most significant:

Avoid cigarettes.

Cigarette smoking is the single most important preventable cause of illness and early death. It is especially risky for pregnant women and their unborn babies. Persons who stop smoking reduce their risk of getting heart disease and cancer. So if you're a cigarette smoker, think twice before lighting that next cigarette. If you choose to continue smoking, try decreasing the number of cigarettes you smoke and switching to a low tar and nicotine brand.

Follow sensible drinking habits.

Alcohol produces changes in mood and behavior. Most people who drink are able to control their intake of alcohol and to avoid undesired, and often harmful, effects. Heavy, regular use of alcohol can lead to cirrhosis of the liver, a leading cause of death. Also, statistics clearly show that mixing drinking and driving is often the cause of fatal or crippling accidents. So, if you drink, do it wisely and in moderation.

Use care in taking drugs.

Today's greater use of drugs—both legal and illegal—is one of our most serious health risks. Even some drugs prescribed by your doctor can be dangerous if taken when drinking alcohol or before driving. Use prescription drugs as directed and discard out-dated medications. Excessive or continued use of tranquilizers (or "pep pills") can cause physical and mental problems. Using or experimenting with illicit drugs such as marijuana, heroin, cocaine, and other street drugs may lead to a number of damaging effects or even death.

Eat sensibly.

Your eating habits are related to risk for high blood pressure, heart disease, and many forms of cancer. Good eating habits mean holding down the amount of fat (especially saturated fat), cholesterol, sugar, and salt in your diet. Include a wide variety of plant foods like whole grain foods, beans, nuts, fresh fruits, and vegetables in your daily diet. They contain nutrients as well as protective factors that may reduce your risk of chronic diseases. You'll feel better.

Exercise regularly.

Almost everyone can benefit from exercise—and there's some form of exercise almost everyone can do. (If you have any doubt, check first with your doctor). Usually as little as 20–30 minutes of vigorous exercise a day three times a week will help you have a healthier heart, tone up sagging muscles, and sleep better. Think about how these changes can improve the way you feel.

Learn how to handle stress.

Stress is a normal part of living. The causes of stress can be good (like a promotion on the job) or bad (loss of a spouse). Properly handled, stress does not need to be a problem. But unhealthy responses to stress—such as driving too fast, drinking too much, or prolonged anger or grief—can cause a variety of physical and mental problems. Even on a very busy day, find a few minutes to slow down and relax. Talking over a problem with someone you trust can often help you find a satisfactory solution. Learn to distinguish between things that are "worth fighting about" and things that are less important.

Be safety conscious.

Think "safety first" at home, at work, at school, at play, and on the highway. Buckle seat belts and place young children in child restraint seats. Children under 12 should sit in the back seat. Obey traffic rules. Keep posions and weapons out of the reach of children, and follow label directions for care and use. Keep emergency numbers by your telephone—when the unexpected happens, you'll be prepared.

Figure 8–3 ■ Healthstyle: A Self-Test (continued)

Spiritual Health Assessment

Spiritual health is the ability to develop one's spiritual nature to its fullest potential, including the ability to discover and articulate one's basic purpose in life, to learn how to experience love, joy, peace, and fulfillment, and how to help ourselves and others achieve their fullest potential (Pender et al., 2002, p. 132). A person's spiritual beliefs can affect their interpretation of events in their life and, therefore, an assessment of spiritual well-being is a part of evaluating the person's overall health. See Chapter 39 🔗, Spirituality, for more information.

Social Support Systems Review

Understanding the social context in which a person lives and works is important in health promotion. Individuals and groups, through interpersonal relationships, can provide comfort, assistance, encouragement, and information. Social support fosters successful coping and promotes satisfying and effective living (Pender et al., 2002, p. 238).

Social support systems contribute to health by creating an environment that encourages healthy behaviors, promotes self-esteem and wellness, and provides feedback that the person's actions will lead to desirable outcomes. Examples of social support systems include family, peer support groups (including computer-based support groups), community-organized religious support systems (e.g., churches), and self-help groups (e.g., Mended Hearts, Weight Watchers). The Providing Culturally Competent Care feature addresses aspects of social support within the context of culture.

According to Pender et al. (2002), the nurse begins a social support system review by asking the client to do these tasks:

- List individuals who provide personal support.
- Indicate the relationship of each person (e.g., family member, fellow worker or colleague, social acquaintance).
- Identify which individuals have been a source of support for 5 or more years.

Providing Culturally Competent Care

CULTURAL ASPECTS OF SOCIAL SUPPORT

It is important to understand how various subgroups of American society may define social support.

- In the African American community, the family and church have been major providers of social support.
- Hispanic-Latino Americans and Asian Americans view the family as being a major social support system.
- Asian Americans respect older adults and use shame and harmony in giving and receiving support.
- Native Americans live in social networks that foster mutual assistance and support.

Note: From *Health Promotion in Nursing Practice* 4th ed., (pp. 239–240), by N. J. Pender, C. L. Murdaugh, and M. A. Parsons, 2002, Upper Saddle River, NJ: Prentice Hall. Reprinted with permission.

This assessment allows the nurse and client to discuss and evaluate the adequacy of the client's support system together and, if necessary, plan options for enhancing the support system.

Health Risk Assessment

A **health risk assessment (HRA)** is an assessment and educational tool that indicates a client's risk for disease or injury during the next 10 years by comparing the client's risk with the mortality risk of the corresponding age, sex, and racial group. The client's general health, lifestyle behaviors, and demographic data are compared to data from a large national sample. Individual risk reports are based on statistics for the population group that matches the individual's surveyed characteristics. The HRA includes a summary of the person's health risks and lifestyle behaviors with educational suggestions on how to reduce the risk.

Many HRA instruments are available today in paper-and-pencil as well as computerized forms. Recently, HRAs have begun to reflect a broader approach to health as companies use the HRA as a means to begin a health-promotion and risk reduction program. Occupational health nurses can identify risk factors and subsequently plan interventions aimed to decrease illness, absenteeism, and disability.

HRAs are helpful for assessing individual and group health risks. They are not, however, substitutes for medical care and are not appropriate for all individuals. For example, people with chronic illnesses such as cancer or heart disease may not obtain accurate risk assessments. Certain populations (e.g., very young, elderly, some sociocultural groups) may not be fully represented in the population databases and, therefore, the HRA may not project an accurate risk assessment.

Health Beliefs Review

Clients' health beliefs need to be clarified, particularly those beliefs that determine how they perceive control of their own health care status. Locus of control is a measurable concept that can be used to predict which people are most likely to change their behavior (see Chapter 11). 🔗 Several instruments are available that assess a person's health-belief measures. Assessment of clients' health beliefs provides the nurse with an indication of how much the clients believe they can influence or control health through personal behaviors. Several cultures have a strong belief in fate: "Whatever will be, will be." If people hold this belief, they do not feel that they can do anything to change the course of their disease. An example is doing diabetic teaching, which often requires many lifestyle changes in diet, exercise, and close control of glucose to prevent complications. If the person believes he or she has no control of the outcome, it is difficult to provide motivations to make the necessary changes. Being aware of these differences can provide a better indication of readiness and motivation on the part of the client to engage in healthy behaviors. See the Lifespan Considerations for factors that might indicate a need for additional information or resources for elders.

Life Stress Review

There is abundant literature about the impact of stress on mental and physical well-being. A variety of stress-related instruments

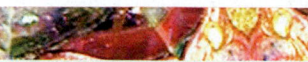

Lifespan Considerations

Factors Impacting Health Promotion and Illness Prevention

Elders

In elders, health promotion and illness prevention are important, but often the focus is on learning to adapt to and live with increasing changes and limitations. Maximizing strengths continues to be of prime importance in maintaining optimal function and quality of life. Factors to be aware of that might indicate a need for additional information or resources include these:

- An increase in physical limitations
- Presence of one or more chronic illnesses
- Change in cognitive status
- Difficulty in accessing health care services due to transportation problems
- Poor support system
- Need for environmental modifications for safety and to maintain independence
- Attitude of hopelessness and depression, which decreases the motivation to use resources or learn new information.

---

have been found in the literature. For example, Holmes and Rahe (1967, p. 213) developed a Life-Change Index, a tool that assigns numerical values to life events (see Box 8–7). Studies have shown that a high score is associated with the increased possibility of illness in an individual.

Validating Assessment Data

Following the collection of assessment data, the nurse and client need to review, validate, and summarize the informa-

tion. This step is carried out jointly by the nurse and the client. During this process, the nurse verbally reviews the current practices and attitudes of the client. This allows validation of the information by the client and may increase awareness of the need to change behavior. The nurse and client need to consider:

- Any existing health problems
- The client's perceived degree of control over health status
- Key health beliefs

BOX 8–7   ■ Life-Change Index

Life Event	Impact Score	Life Event	Impact Score
Death of spouse	100	Begin or end school	26
Divorce	73	Change in living conditions	25
Marital separation	65	Revisions of personal habits	24
Jail term	63	Trouble with boss	23
Death of close family member	63	Change in work hours or conditions	20
Personal injury or illness	53	Change in residence	20
Marriage	50	Change in schools	20
Fired at work	47	Change in recreations	19
Marital reconciliation	45	Change in church activities	19
Retirement	45	Change in social activities	19
Change in health of family member	44	Mortgage or loan less than $20,000	17
Pregnancy	40	Change in sleeping habits	16
Sex difficulties	39	Change in number of family get-togethers	15
Gain of a new family member	39	Change in eating habits	15
Business readjustment	39	Vacation	13
Change in financial state	38	Christmas approaching	11
Death of a close friend	37	Minor violation of the law	11
Change to a different line of work	36		
Change in number of arguments with spouse	35		
Mortgage over $20,000	31		

Life Change Units	Likelihood of Illness in Near Future
300+	About 80%
150–299	About 50%
Less than 150	About 30%

Life Event	Impact Score
Foreclosure of mortgage or loan	30
Change in responsibilities at work	29
Son or daughter leaving home	29
Trouble with in-laws	29
Outstanding personal achievement	28
Spouse begins or stops work	26

The higher your life change score, the harder you have to work to get yourself back into a state of good health.

- Level of physical fitness and nutritional status
- Illnesses for which the client is at risk
- Current positive health practices
- Spirituality
- Sources of life stress and ability to handle stress
- Social support systems
- Information needed to enhance health care practices.

DIAGNOSING

Nursing diagnoses accepted by the North American Nursing Diagnosis Association (NANDA) have generally focused on impaired or imbalanced health patterns or problems. The definition, however, of the NANDA **wellness diagnoses** states: "Describes human responses to levels of wellness in an individual, family, or community that have a readiness for enhancement" (2003, p. 263).

Wellness diagnoses can be applied at all levels of prevention but are particularly useful for healthy clients who require teaching for health promotion, disease prevention, and personal growth. When the nurse and client conclude that the client has positive function in a certain pattern area, such as adequate nutrition or effective coping, the nurse can use this information to help the client reach a higher level of functioning.

A wellness diagnosis is preceded by the modifier "readiness for enhanced" (NANDA, 2003, p. 227). The following examples are included in the NANDA taxonomy:

- *Readiness for Enhanced Spiritual Well-being*
- *Readiness for Enhanced Coping*
- *Readiness for Enhanced Nutrition*
- *Readiness for Enhanced Knowledge (Specify)*
- *Readiness for Enhanced Parenting*
- *Readiness for Enhanced Self-concept.*

Wellness diagnoses provide a clear focus for planning interventions without indicating that a problem exists (Wilkinson, 2001, p. 222).

PLANNING

Health-promotion plans need to be developed according to the needs, desires, and priorities of the client. The client decides on health-promotion goals, the activities or interventions to achieve those goals, the frequency and duration of the activities, and the method of evaluation. During the planning process the nurse acts as a resource person rather than as an advisor or counselor. The nurse provides information when asked, emphasizes the importance of small steps to behavioral change, and reviews the client's goals and plans to make sure they are realistic, measurable, and acceptable to the client.

Steps in Planning

Pender et al. (2002, pp. 147–166) outline several steps in the process of developing a joint health protection promotion plan

(see Box 8–8). These steps are carried out jointly by the nurse and the client:

1. *Identify health goals and related behavior-change options.* The client selects two or three top priority health goals, prioritizes them, and reviews behavior-change options. Common goals follow:
   a. To reduce the risk of cardiovascular disease.
   b. To achieve or maintain a desired weight.
   c. To increase knowledge of safety practices in the home.
2. *Identify behavioral or health outcomes.* For each of the selected goals or areas in step 1, determine what specific behavioral changes are needed to bring about the desired outcome. For example, to reduce the risk of cardiovascular disease, the client may need to change behaviors such as stop smoking, lose weight, and increase activity level.
3. *Develop a behavior-change plan.* A constructive program of change is based on client "ownership" of those behavior changes selected for implementation within everyday life (Pender et al., 2002, p. 156). Clients may need to be assisted in examining value-behavior inconsistencies and in selecting behavioral options that are most appealing and that they are most willing to try. The client's priorities will reflect personal values, activity preferences, and expectations for success.
4. *Reiterate benefits of change.* The benefits will probably need to be reiterated by both the nurse and the client even though the client is committed to the change. The health-related and non–health-related benefits should be kept before the client as central motivating factors.
5. *Address environmental and interpersonal facilitators and barriers to change.* Environmental and interpersonal factors that support positive change should be used to reinforce the client's efforts to change lifestyle. All people experience barriers, some of which can be anticipated and planned for, thereby making the change more likely to occur.
6. *Determine a time frame for implementation.* By developing a time frame, the appropriate knowledge and skills can be developed before a new behavior is implemented. The time frame may be several weeks or months. Scheduling short-term goals and rewards can offer encouragement to achieve long-term objectives. Clients may need help to be realistic and to deal with one behavior at a time.
7. *Commit to behavior-change goals.* In the past, commitments to changing behaviors have usually been verbal. Increasingly, a formal, written behavioral contract is being used to motivate the client to follow through with selected actions (see Chapter 25). Motivation to follow through is provided by a positive reinforcement or reward stated in the contract. Contracting is based on the belief that all people have the potential for growth and the right of self-determination, even though their choices may be different from the norm.

| BOX 8–8 | ■ Example of an Individual Health Protection Promotion Plan |

Designed for: James Moore
Home Address: 714 George
Home Telephone Number: 222-3333
Occupation (if employed): Building services supervisor
Work Telephone Number: 445-6666
Cultural Identification: African American
Birth Date: 3/14/57   Date of Initial Plan: 1/15/2003

Client strengths	Satisfactory peer relationships, spiritual strength, adequate sleep pattern
Major risk factors	Elevated cholesterol, mild obesity, sedentary lifestyle, moderate life change, multiple daily hassles, few reported uplifts
Nursing diagnoses	Deficient Diversional Activity
(derived from assessment	Imbalanced Nutrition: More than Body Requirements
of functional health patterns)	Caregiver Role Strain (elderly mother)
Medical diagnoses (if any)	Mild hypertension
Age-specific screening recommendations	Blood pressure, cholesterol, fecal occult blood, malignant skin lesions, depression
Desired behavioral and health outcomes	Become a regular exerciser (3X/week), lower my blood pressure, weigh 165 lb

Personal Health Goals (1 = highest priority)	Selected Behaviors to Accomplish Goals	Stage of Change	Strategies/Interventions for Change
1. Achieve desired body weight	Begin a progressive walking program	Planning	Counterconditioning Reinforcement management Client contracting
	Decrease caloric intake while maintaining good nutrition	Action (eating 2 fruits and 2 vegetables daily; using low-fat dairy products for last 2 months)	Stimulus control Cognitive restructuring
2. Decrease risk for hypertension-related disorders	Change from high- to low-sodium snacks	Contemplation	Consciousness raising Learning facilitation
3. Learn to manage stress effectively	Attend relaxation classes and use home relaxation tapes	Contemplation	Consciousness raising Self-reevaluation Simple relaxation therapy
4. Increase leisure-time activities	Join a local bowling league	Contemplation	Support system enhancement

Note: From Health Promotion in Nursing Practice, 4th ed. (pp. 151–152), by N. J. Pender, C. L. Murdaugh, and M. A. Parsons, 2002, Upper Saddle River, NJ: Prentice Hall. Reprinted with permission.

Exploring Available Resources

Another essential aspect of planning is identifying support resources available to the client. These may be community resources, such as a fitness program at a local gymnasium or educational programs, such as stress management, breast self-examination, nutrition, smoking cessation, and health lectures.

IMPLEMENTING

Implementing is the "doing" part of behavior change. Self-responsibility is emphasized for implementing the plan. Depending on the client's needs, the nursing interventions may include supporting, counseling, facilitating, teaching, consulting, enhancing the behavior change, and modeling.

Providing and Facilitating Support

A major nursing role is to support the client. A vital component of lifestyle change is ongoing support that focuses on the desired behavior change and is provided in a nonjudgmental manner. Support can be offered by the nurse on an individual basis or in a group setting. The nurse can also facilitate the development of support networks for the client, such as family members and friends.

Individual Counseling Sessions.
Counseling sessions may be routinely scheduled as part of the plan or may be provided if the client encounters difficulty in carrying out interventions or meets insurmountable barriers to change. In a counseling relationship, the nurse and client share ideas. In this sharing relationship, the nurse acts as a facilitator, promoting the client's decision making in regard to the health-promotion plan.

Telephone Counseling.
Regular telephone sessions may be provided to the client to help in answering questions, reviewing goals and strategies, and reinforcing progress. The

Research Note

Do Nursing Students Practice Healthy Lifestyles that Would Help Them Prepare to Be Effective Advocates for Health Promotion and Disease Prevention?

The problem addressed in this research study was "Does exposure to nursing theory content and client interactions make any difference in the regular practice of positive health behaviors in nursing students when compared to non-nursing students?"

The literature review conducted by the researchers indicated inconclusive results. Some studies found nursing students to have greater stress and burnout than other college students and other findings disagreed. A longitudinal study was done to determine if nursing students improved their personal health behaviors to a greater degree than non-nursing students between their sophomore and senior years. Health habits were measured using the Health Habits Inventory (HHI). Data were collected at the beginning of their sophomore year and senior year.

Study findings revealed that many of the student nurses improved their health habits during their 2 years in nursing school (e.g., increased number performing monthly self-breast exam for female students and monthly testicular exam for male students). The behaviors that became more negative in nursing students were smoking, practicing safe sex, and knowing their current cholesterol level. Nursing students, even though they started out at a higher level in health habits than non-nursing students, improved in their health habits to a greater degree.

Implications: The findings support the idea that nursing students learn the importance of healthy lifestyles from nursing theory classes and clinical experiences. The authors stress the importance of faculty encouraging nursing students to make health priorities for themselves and a commitment to practice positive health behaviors. They also point out that healthy behaviors help decrease burnout in the professional workforce.

Note: From "Health Habits of Nursing Versus Non-Nursing Students: A Longitudinal Study," by C. B. Shriver and A. Scott-Stiles, 2000, *Journal of Nursing Education, 39*(7), pp. 308–314.

Facilitating Social Support. Social networks, such as family and friends, can facilitate or impede the efforts directed toward health promotion and prevention. The nurse's role is to assist the client to assess, modify, and develop the social support necessary to achieve the desired change. To provide the necessary support, families must communicate effectively, be aware of and support each other's needs and goals, and provide help and assistance to one another to achieve those goals. The client may wish the nurse to meet with the family or significant others and help enlist their understanding and support.

Providing Health Education

Health education programs on a variety of topics discussed earlier can be provided to groups, individuals, or communities. Group programs need to be planned carefully before they are implemented. The decision to establish a health-promotion program must be based on the health needs of the people; also, specific health-promotion goals must be set. After the program is implemented, outcomes must be evaluated.

Enhancing Behavior Change

Whether people will make and maintain changes to improve health or prevent disease depends on many interrelated factors. To help clients succeed in implementing behavior changes, the nurse needs to understand the stages of change and effective interventions that focus on progressing the individual through the stages of change. Guidelines for assisting the client toward behavior change are offered in the Practice Guidelines. Figure 8–4 ■ provides suggested strategies to assist clients depending on their stage of change. As Saarmann, Daugherty, and Riegel (2000) point out, the nursing goal is not necessarily to change behavior but to advance the client to the next stage of change (p. 285).

Modeling

Through observing a model, the client acquires ideas for behavior and coping strategies that can be used with specific problems. The client is not expected to mimic the sequence of actions or behavior patterns of the model. The nurse and client should mutually select models with whom the client can identify, since the cultural and ethnic backgrounds and age of the nurse and client often differ. Models should be people the client respects. Nurses should also serve as models of wellness. To model effectively, nurses need to have a philosophy and lifestyle that demonstrate good health habits.

EVALUATING

Evaluation takes place on an ongoing basis, both during the attainment of short-term goals and after the completion of long-term goals. Goals are written during the planning phase and a date determined for attaining the specific results or behaviors that are desired to promote health or prevent illness. During evaluation, the client may decide to continue with the plan, reorder priorities, change strategies, or revise the health protection promotion contract. Evaluation of the plan is a collaborative effort between the nurse and the client.

client may find that scheduling a weekly telephone session is helpful or may wish to initiate a call if a problem occurs. The client is asked, "Is your plan working?" If the plan is not working, the nurse asks, "What would you like to do?" The client may wish to continue or may wish to change the plan to a more realistic one. Telephone support is efficient for the busy client who may not have the time for regular, in-person sessions.

Group Support. Group sessions provide an opportunity for participants to learn the experiences of others in changing behavior. Group contact gives individuals a renewed commitment to their goals. Groups can be scheduled at monthly or less frequent intervals for over a year.

Establish Rapport

- Provide privacy and a perception of a collaborative, equal-power relationship.
- If time allows, ask the client to describe a "typical" day. Usually the problematic behavior is described; however, even if it is not, the listening will strengthen rapport and the personal information may be helpful in understanding the client's current situation

Set Agenda

- Allow the client to identify concerns. If there are multiple concerns (e.g., smoking, exercise, diet, stress), it is best to focus on one specific behavior at a time. Ask the client which behavior he or she feels most ready to *think* about changing.

Assess Importance, Confidence, and Readiness

- A client's readiness to change is often influenced by his or her perception of importance and confidence.
- Importance refers to the personal value of change. Questions that obtain this information can include: "How do you feel at the moment about [state the change]?" "How important is it to you to [state the change]?" "On a scale of 1 to 10 with 1 being 'not important' and 10 'very important,' what number would you give yourself?"
- Confidence relates to the mastering of the skills needed to achieve the behavior and the situations in which behavior change will be challenging to the client. A potential question to

use to assess confidence is "If you decided right now to change, how confident would you feel about succeeding with this?"

Exchange Information and Reduce Resistance

- These two tasks are performed throughout the various stages of behavior change.
- Ask clients if they would like information and about what.
- When presenting information, present it in a neutral tone of voice, and avoid using the word "you" too much. Referring to other people (versus "you") and what happens to them makes the information less threatening to the client.
- After presenting the information, ask for the client's interpretation of the information.
- Three *traps* that increase resistance and *strategies to avoid the traps* include:
  - Take control away. *Instead,* emphasize personal choice and control.
  - Misjudge importance, confidence, or readiness. Often this results in talking about action before the client is ready. It is important to *reexamine* the client's feelings about importance and confidence as they influence readiness to make a specific change.
  - Meet force with force. Instead of attacking or defending through argument, sit back and use reflective listening. By understanding how the client is feeling, the resistance usually subsides and the discussion can move in a different direction.

Note: From *Health Behavior Change: A Guide for Practitioners,* by S. Rollnick, P. Mason, and C. Butler, 1999, Edinburgh: Churchill Livingstone. Adapted with permission from Elsevier.

Strategies to Promote Behavioral Change for Each Stage of Change

Precontemplation	Contemplation	Preparation	Action	Maintenance	Termination
Assess confidence, importance & readiness for change. Discuss positive & negative aspects of behavior to assist the person to *consider* changing. Provide information in a caring, non-threatening manner.	Ask client if they would like information and about what. Assist client to increase awareness of behavior by: -Determining specific behavior(s) client wishes to change. -Performing self-evaluation of present view of self versus future view of self without the behavior. -Reflecting on the behavior (e.g., "Why do I want to smoke?") -Examining the pros and cons of change.	Continue to discuss pros and cons of behavior change. Provide support and guidance for the client to: -Set a date to begin action. -Tell family and friends of the intended change and advise them how they can be helpful. -Create a plan of action. -Make change a priority. Remind client of past successes.	Continue to discuss benefits with client. Continue positive reinforcement. Encourage client to: -Substitute healthy responses for problem behaviors (e.g., exercise, and relaxation). -Modify environment to reduce stimulus to a problem behavior (e.g., remove ashtrays from home). -Monitor behavior (e.g., food journal). -Plan rewards.	Continue positive reinforcement of desired behavior. Continue to remind client of previous successes. Encourage client to know the danger signs, which are usually the result of overwhelming stress or insufficient coping skills.	Inform client of criteria for terminators (versus lifetime maintainers): -A new self-image. -No temptation in any situation. -Solid confidence. -A healthier lifestyle.

Figure 8–4 ■ Strategies to promote behavioral change for each stage of change.

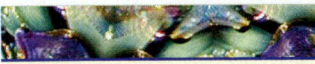

Focus on Critical Thinking

Mr. W., a 50-year-old professional man has pneumonia and is currently being treated with antibiotics. He smokes two packs of cigarettes a day. Since this bout of pneumonia he voices concern about his smoking and wonders if he should try to quit again. He states, "I've tried everything and nothing works. The longest I last is about one month." He admits to being 30 pounds overweight and states that his wife and he have started walking for 30 minutes every evening. His wife has also started making low-fat meals. He is concerned that if he quits smoking he will gain more weight.

1. What information/knowledge is important for the nurse to remember when assisting a client to advance to the next stage of change?
2. Each contact between a nurse and a client is an opportunity for health promotion. Based on the knowledge or key concepts listed above, what question(s) would you ask Mr. W.?
3. Mr. W. is in which stage of change relating to his cigarette smoking and what strategies could you, the nurse, consider?

See Critical Thinking Possibilities in Appendix A.

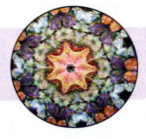 # Chapter Review

Explore MediaLink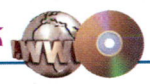

NCLEX review questions, case studies, MediaLink applications, and other interactive resources for this chapter can be found on the Companion Website at www.prenhall.com/kozier. Click on Chapter 8 to select the activities for this chapter.

For more NCLEX review questions, and an audio glossary, access the Student CD-ROM accompanying this textbook.

Chapter Highlights

- *Healthy People 2010* (USDHHS, 2000) presents a comprehensive 10-year strategy for promoting health and preventing illness of both individuals and communities.
- Health promotion is defined as client behavior directed toward developing well-being and actualizing human health potential. Health protection is client behavior geared toward preventing illness, detecting it early, or maintaining function.
- The Health Promotion Model (Pender et al., 2002) is a competence- or approach-oriented model that depicts the multidimensional nature of persons interacting with their interpersonal and physical environments as they pursue health. The major motivational variables that can be modified through nursing interventions include perceived benefits of action, perceived barriers to action, perceived self-efficacy, activity-related affect, interpersonal influences, and situational influences.
- Prochaska, Norcross, and DiClemente (1994) propose a six-stage model for health behavior change. The stages are (a) precontemplation, (b) contemplation, (c) preparation, (d) action, (e) maintenance, and (f) termination. If the person is not successful in changing behavior, relapse occurs. However, at any point in these stages, people may move to any previous stage. An understanding of these stages enables the nurse to provide appropriate nursing interventions.
- The nurse's role in health promotion is to act as a facilitator of the process of assessing, evaluating, and understanding health. It is the opportunity for nurses to strengthen the profession's influence on health promotion, disseminate information that promotes an educated public, and assist individuals and communities to change long-standing adverse health behaviors.
- A complete and accurate assessment of the individual's health status is basic to health promotion. Lifestyle assessment tools give clients the opportunity to assess the impact of their present lifestyle behaviors on their health and to make decisions about specific lifestyle changes. Health risk appraisals provide the data that may influence the individual to adopt healthier life behaviors. Assessments or reviews of a client's spiritual health, social support, health beliefs, and life stress are also important because they impact a person's health.
- Organizing assessment data from individual and family assessments enables the nurse to make wellness diagnoses that identify client strengths, recognize self-care abilities, and enhance health-promotion goals to help the client reach a higher level of functioning.
- Health-promotion plans need to be developed according to the needs, desires, and priorities of the client.
- The nurse acts as a resource person, provides ongoing support, and supplies additional information and education in a nonjudgmental manner in order to help individuals change their lifestyles or health behaviors.
- As role models for their clients, nurses should have a philosophy and lifestyle that demonstrate good health habits.
- During the evaluation phase of the health-promotion process, the nurse assists clients in determining whether they will continue with the plan, reorder priorities, or revise the plan.

Review Questions

8–1. Which of the following statements reflect the contemplation stage of behavior change?
   a. "I currently do not exercise 30 minutes three times a week and do not intend to start in the next six months."
   b. "I have tried several times to exercise 30 minutes three times a week but am seriously thinking of trying again in the next month."
   c. "I currently do not exercise 30 minutes three times a week, but I am thinking about starting to do so in the next six months."
   d. "I have exercised 30 minutes three times a week regularly for more than six months."

8–2. A female client is 46 pounds overweight. She previously attended two programs that "guaranteed" weight loss. Although the weight was lost, more returned after each program. She tells you, "I was just born to be fat. I don't have the willpower." According to the Health Promotion Model, the nurse recognizes which of the behavior-specific cognitions and affect variable in this client?
   a. perceived barriers to action
   b. perceived self-efficacy
   c. interpersonal influences
   d. situational influences

8–3. Which of the following individuals would have an increased possibility of illness in the near future?
   a. a 25-year-old man who recently married his high school sweetheart
   b. a 35-year-old man who was fired from his job
   c. a 40-year-old woman who started a nursing program
   d. a 50-year-old woman whose husband died a month ago

8–4. The nurse who is assisting a client in the action stage of change would use which of the following strategies?
   a. Reinforce the importance of providing rewards for positive behavior.
   b. Ask the client if they would like information.
   c. Guide the client to create a plan of action.
   d. Remind the client of previous successes.

8–5. If a client fails to follow the information or teaching provided, how should the nurse respond?
   a. Give up, as the client doesn't want to change.
   b. Develop a tough approach.
   c. Reteach the information, as the nurse is the expert.
   d. Reassess the client's importance given to the behavior and readiness to change it.

Readings and References

Suggested Readings

Saarmann, L., Daugherty, J., & Riegel, B. (2000). Patient teaching to promote behavioral change. *Nursing Outlook, 48*(6), 281–287.
   The authors review that nursing education programs stress how teaching is an important role of nurses. However, they emphasize the invalidity of the assumption that knowledge gained through teaching will motivate a client to change a behavior. Imparting knowledge rarely motivates behavioral change. Saarmann et al. describe ineffective behavioral change strategies of fear, confrontation and coercion, and paternalism. Effective behavioral change strategies, on the other hand, include acknowledging the person's stage of change, motivational interviewing, and cognitive-behavioral therapy. They conclude by giving examples of how the effective strategies can be used at each stage of change.

Whitehead, D. (2001). Health education, behavioural change and social psychology: Nursing's contribution to health promotion? *Journal of Advanced Nursing, 34*(6), 822–832.
   The author asserts that nurses may believe they promote health when in fact they are more likely performing traditional health teaching. The article challenges the assumption that providing the necessary health information is often viewed as the most effective and, often, the only needed intervention. Then, the client is blamed if noncompliance results. Whitehead argues that client noncompliance or failure of the client to change behavior lies with the nurse. The author's review of the literature reflects the complexities involved in health promotion and modifying health behaviors.

Related Research

Acton, G. J., & Malathum, P. (2000). Basic need status and health-promoting self-care behavior in adults. *Western Journal of Nursing Research, 22*(7), 796–811.
Bock, B., Niaura, R., Fontes, A., & Bock, F. (1999). Acceptability of computer assessments among ethnically diverse, low-income smokers. *American Journal of Health Promotion, 13*(5), 299–304.
Boland, C. S. (2000). Social support and spiritual well-being: Empowering older adults to commit to health-promoting behaviors. *The Journal of Multicultural Nursing & Health, 6*(3), 12–23.
Hagerty, B. M., & Williams, R. A. (1999). The effects of sense of belonging, social support, conflict, and loneliness on depression. *Nursing Research, 48*(4), 215–219.
Heidrich, S. M. (1998). Health promotion in old age. *Annual Review of Nursing Research, 16,* 173–195.
McMahon, S. D., & Jason, L. A. (2000). Social support in a worksite smoking intervention. A test of theoretical models. *Behavior Modification, 24*(2), 184–201.
Shriver, C. B., & Scott-Stiles, A. (2000). Health habits of nursing versus non-nursing students: A longitudinal study. *Journal of Nursing Education, 39*(7), 308–314.

References

Bobroff, L. B. (1999). *Healthstyle: A self-test.* Retrieved March 23, 2003, from University of Florida, Cooperative Extension Service Institute of Food and Agricultural Sciences website: http://edis.ifas.ufl.edu/BODY_HE778
Edelman, C. L., & Mandle, C. L. (2002). *Health promotion throughout the lifespan* (5th ed.). St. Louis, MO: Mosby.
Holmes, T. H., & Rahe, T. H. (1967) The social readjustment rating scale. *Journal of Psychosomatic Research, 11*(8), 213–218.
Leavell, H. R., & Clark, E. G. (1965). *Preventive medicine for the doctor in the community* (3rd ed.). New York: McGraw-Hill.
North American Nursing Diagnosis Association. (2003). *Nursing diagnoses: Definitions & classification 2003–2004.* Philadelphia: Author.
Pender, N. J., Murdaugh, C. L., & Parsons, M. A. (2002). *Health promotion in nursing practice* (4th ed.). Upper Saddle River, NJ: Prentice Hall.
Prochaska, J. O., Norcross, J. C., & DiClemente, C. C. (1994). *Changing for good: A revolutionary six-stage program for overcoming bad habits and moving your life positively forward.* New York: Avon Books/Harper Collins.
Rollnick, S., Mason, P., & Butler, C. (1999). *Health behavior change. A guide for practitioners.* Edinburgh: Churchill Livingstone.

Saarmann, L., Daugherty, J., & Riegel, B. (2000). Patient teaching to promote behavioral change. *Nursing Outlook, 48*(6), 281–287.

Shriver, C. B., & Scott-Stiles, A. (2000). Health habits of nursing versus non-nursing students: A longitudinal study. *Journal of Nursing Education, 39*(7), 308–314.

U.S. Department of Health and Human Services. (1990). *Healthy people 2000: National health promotion and disease prevention objectives* (DHHS Pub. No. PHS 91-50212). Washington, DC: U.S. Government Printing Office.

U.S. Department of Health and Human Services. (2000). *Healthy people 2010: Understanding and improving health* (2nd ed.). Washington, DC: U.S. Government Printing Office.

U.S. Surgeon General. (1979). *Healthy people: The surgeon general's report on health promotion and disease prevention* (DHHS Pub. No. 79-55071). Washington, DC: U.S. Government Printing Office.

Wilkinson, J. M. (2001). *Nursing process & critical thinking* (3rd ed.). Upper Saddle River, NJ: Prentice Hall.

Selected Bibliography

Artinian, N. T. (2001). Best practice: Perceived benefits and barriers of eating heart healthy. *MEDSURG Nursing, 10*(3), 129–138.

Belza, B., & Baker, M. W. (2000). Maintaining health in well older adults: Initiatives for schools of nursing and The John A. Hartford Foundation for the 21st century. *Journal of Gerontological Nursing, 26*(7), 8–17.

Boyd, L. (2001). Healthcare & the net: Monitoring patients. *RN, 64*(2), 53–54.

Buijs, R., & Olson, J. (2001). Parish nurses influencing determinants of health. *Journal of Community Health Nursing, 18*(1), 13–23.

Carpenter, B. D., Van Haitsma, K., Ruckdeschel, K., & Lawton, M. P. (2000). The psychosocial preferences of older adults: A pilot examination of content and structure. *The Gerontologist, 40*(3), 335–348.

Clark, C. (1999). Low self-esteem: A barrier to health promoting behaviour. *Journal of Community Nursing, 13*(1), 7–10.

Cohen, C. (2001). Healthcare & the net: Guiding seniors. *RN, 64*(2), 50–52.

Greenstreet, W. M. (1999). Teaching spirituality in nursing: A literature review. *Nurse Education Today, 19,* 649–658.

Murray, R. B., & Zentner, J. P. (2001). *Health promotion strategies through the life span.* (7th ed.) Upper Saddle River, NJ: Prentice Hall.

Puterbaugh, D. (1999). Lifestyle assessment and changes: Using the health lifestyle worksheet in practice. *Psychiatric Rehabilitation Journal, 23*(1), 70–74.

Waite, P. J., Hawks, S. R., & Gast, J. A. (1999). The correlation between spiritual well-being and health behaviors. *American Journal of Health Promotion, 13,* 159–162.

Walker, L. O., & Wilging, S. (2000). Rediscovering the "M" in "MCH": Maternal health promotion after childbirth. *Journal of Obstetric, Gynecologic, and Neonatal Nursing, 29,* 229–235.

Whitehead, D. (2000). Using mass media within health-promoting practice: A nursing perspective. *Journal of Advanced Nursing, 32,* 807–816.

Wilkinson, J. M. (2000). *Nursing diagnosis handbook with NIC interventions and NOC outcomes* (7th ed.). Upper Saddle River, NJ: Prentice Hall Health.

CHAPTER | 9

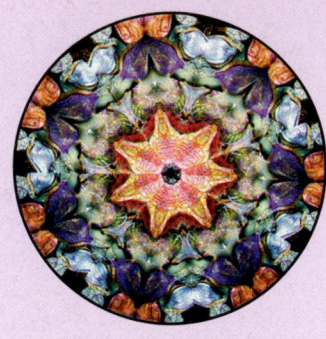

HOME CARE

LEARNING OUTCOMES

After completing this chapter, you will be able to:

- Define home health care.

- Compare the characteristics of home health nursing to those of institutional nursing care.

- Describe the types of home health agencies, including reimbursement and referral sources.

- Describe the roles of the home health nurse.

- Identify the essential aspects of the home visit.

- Discuss the safety and infection control dimensions applicable to the home care setting.

- Identify ways the nurse can recognize and minimize caregiver role strain.

- Apply the nursing process to care of the client in the home.

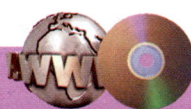

MediaLink

www.prenhall.com/kozier

Additional resources for this chapter can be found on the Student CD-ROM accompanying this textbook, and on the Companion Website at www.prenhall.com/kozier. Click on Chapter 9 to select the activities for this chapter.

CD-ROM
- Audio Glossary
- NCLEX Review

Companion Website
- Additional NCLEX Review
- Case Study: Home Care Nurse
- MediaLink Applications:
    Hospice Nursing
    Nurse Assistant
- Links to Resources

Historically, **home care** consisted primarily of nurses providing private duty care in clients' homes and care of the ill by their own family members. However, the delivery of professional nursing services in home settings has increased in frequency, scope, and complexity in the past two decades. A number of factors have contributed to this trend, among them rising health care costs, an aging population, and a growing emphasis on managing chronic illness and stress, preventing illness, and enhancing the quality of life. In the not-too-distant past, home health care occurred at the end of the client care continuum—that is, after discharge from an acute care facility. Today the trend is changing to use of home health care services to avoid hospitalization.

Because home health nurses must function independently in a variety of home settings and situations, employers generally prefer that the nurse be prepared at the baccalaureate level or above. The American Nurses Credentialing Center (ANCC) provides certification for home health nursing at both the generalist and advanced practice levels. Advanced practice certification requires a master's degree in nursing and recognizes the need for **home health clinical specialists** who can provide direct care, manage client care, and engage in consulting, education, administrative, and research activities.

HOME HEALTH NURSING

Home nursing care is one of the fastest growing sectors of the health care system. Factors that have contributed to the growth of home health care include (1) the increase in the older population, who are frequent recipients of home care; (2) third-party payers who favor home care to control costs; (3) the ability of agencies and institutions to successfully deliver high-technology services in the home; and (4) consumers who prefer to receive care in the home rather than in an institution.

Hospice nursing is often considered a subspecialty of home health nursing because hospice services are frequently delivered to terminally ill clients in their residence. See Chapter 41 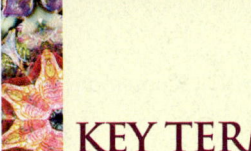 for further information about hospice care.

Definitions of Home Nursing

The delivery of nursing services in the home has been called a variety of terms, including **home health nursing, home care nursing,** and **visiting nursing.** Home health care includes the services and products provided to clients in their homes that are needed to maintain, restore, or promote their physical, psychological, and social well-being. The focus of home health nursing is individuals and their families. This differs somewhat from the focus of community health nursing, which focuses on individuals, families, and groups.

Unique Aspects of Home Health Nursing

Home care nurses must function independently in a variety of unfamiliar home settings and situations. Because the home is the family's territory, power and control issues in delivering nursing care differ from those in the institution. For example, entry into a home is granted, not assumed; the nurse must therefore establish trust and rapport with the client and family. Health care that is provided is often given with other family members present. Families also may feel more free to question advice, to ignore directions, to do things differently, and to set their own priorities and schedules.

Home health nurses have identified significant advantages in caring for individuals and families in the home. The home setting is intimate; this intimacy fosters familiarity, sharing, connections, and caring between clients, families, and their nurse. Behaviors are more natural, cultural beliefs and practices are more visible, and multigenerational interactions tend to be displayed.

Home health nurses have also identified issues that negatively affect care in the home. More than any other care providers, these nurses have firsthand knowledge and experience about the burden of caregiving. In the interest of cutting health care costs, policy makers, third-party payers, and medical providers are placing increasingly complex responsibilities on clients' families and significant other(s). Caregiving demands may go on for months or years, placing the caregivers themselves (many of whom are elders) at risk for physiologic and psychosocial problems. Additionally, nurses enter homes where the living conditions and support systems may be inadequate.

MediaLink HOSPICE NURSING APPLICATION

THE HOME HEALTH CARE SYSTEM

The need for home health care may be identified by any person involved with the client. Clients are referred to a home health agency or private duty nursing agency. Individuals with extremely complex needs beyond those that direct nursing care alone can provide may benefit from the services of an agency with direct connections to a medical equipment company. Payment for home health is accomplished through private pay, third-party reimbursement, or a combination of sources.

Referral Process

Clients may be referred to home health care providers by a physician, nurse, social worker, therapist (e.g., physical therapist), discharge planner, or family member. Families often initiate the process by approaching one of these referral sources or by directly contacting the home health agency to make inquiries. Home care cannot begin, however, without a physician's order and a physician-approved treatment plan. This is a legal and reimbursement requirement.

After an initial set of physician's orders is obtained, a nursing assessment visit is scheduled to identify the client's needs. At this assessment visit the nurse develops a plan of care, which must be reviewed, approved, authorized, and signed by the attending physician before home health agency providers can continue with services.

Home Health Agencies

Home health agencies offer coordinated professional, skilled, and paraprofessional services. Because clients often require the services of several professionals, case coordination (case management) is essential. This responsibility generally rests with the registered nurse. Depending on the agency, additional providers may include nurse practitioners, practical nurses, nursing assistants, home health care aides, physical therapists, occupational therapists, respiratory therapists, speech therapists, social workers, dietitians, and a pastoral care minister or chaplain. In addition, it is not unusual for home health agencies to offer the services of specialized nurses such as wound-ostomy-continence nurses or diabetes educators. The care plan implemented by the home health agency may require services once or twice a day, up to 7 days a week. The minimum time of each episode of care, or visit, is usually 1 hour.

There are several different types of home health agencies. These include the following:

- Official or public agencies are operated by state or local governments and financed primarily by tax funds.
- Voluntary or private not-for-profit agencies are supported by donations, endowments, charities such as the United Way, and third-party reimbursement.
- Private, proprietary agencies are for-profit organizations and are governed by either individual owners or national corporations. Some of these agencies participate in third-party reimbursement; others rely on "private-pay" sources.

- Institution-based agencies operate under a parent organization, such as a hospital, funded by the same sources as the parent.

Regardless of the type of agency, all home health agencies must meet specific standards for licensing, certification, and accreditation.

Private Duty Agencies

This type of agency may be referred to as a *registry*. The agency contracts with individual practitioners (e.g., nurses, home health aides) to care for the client in the home. The client may require care coverage from the agency for 4 to 24 hours a day. However, the agency is not focused uniquely on providing personnel for home care assignments but also supplies staff to hospitals, clinics, and other care settings. Thus, it does not afford the coordinated focus of a home care agency. Private duty care is expensive. Commercial insurance generally provides limited reimbursement. Otherwise, the client must pay privately.

Durable Medical Equipment Companies

A **durable medical equipment (DME) company** provides health care equipment for the client at home. The types of equipment can range from hospital beds and bedside commodes to ventilators and apnea monitors. Because of the cost associated with medical equipment, the nurse needs to ensure that clients have either Medicare/Medicaid or a DME benefit within their commercial insurance or are able to pay privately. Before billing Medicare for any DME, it is wise to consult the list of equipment for which Medicare will reimburse the client. Most DME companies today seek accreditation from the Joint Commission on Accreditation of Healthcare Organizations (JCAHO) to ensure compliance with quality standards for equipment and services.

Reimbursement

Health care agencies in the United States receive reimbursement for services they provide from various sources: Medicare and Medicaid, private insurance companies, and private pay. The Medicare and Medicaid programs have strict guidelines governing reimbursement for home health care. For example, the client must (a) need reasonable and necessary home care including skilled care; (b) be homebound, that is, confined to the home except for occasional outings for medical treatment, for a trip to the barber, or for a drive; and require the use of supportive devices, special transportation, or the escort of another person; (c) have a plan of care that includes all of Medicare's criteria; and (d) need nursing care on an intermittent basis. The agency too must meet specific conditions.

Payers other than Medicare or Medicaid, such as Blue Cross, Blue Shield, and HealthNet, typically negotiate reimbursement rates for home health care services. Voluntary agencies, like the Visiting Nurses of America (VNA) are reimbursed by charitable disbursements to the agency.

All health care agencies need to adhere to established guidelines and provide care within the predetermined reimbursement levels. Treatment plans (developed by the home health agency providers and authorized by the physician) are used by the reimbursement source. Only interventions identified on the treatment plan are paid for. Periodically the reimbursement source may request the home health provider's notes to substantiate what is being done in the home. This is a major reason why accurate documentation is critical.

ROLES OF THE HOME HEALTH NURSE

Historically, nurses who provided direct services in the home were strong generalists who focused on long-term preventive, educational, remedial, and rehabilitative outcomes. Today many home health nurses are generalists or specialists possessing high-technology skills that were formerly used only in acute care settings. For example, nurses provide a variety of intravenous therapies in the home setting and monitor clients who are dependent on technologically complex medical equipment, such as ventilators and central lines. These nurses collaborate with physicians and other health care professionals in providing care.

Major roles of the home health nurse are those of advocate, caregiver (provider of direct care), educator, and case manager or coordinator.

Advocate

Advocacy begins on the first visit. The nurse explores and supports the client's choices in health care; all viable options are considered. Advocacy includes having discussions about the client's rights, advance medical directives, living wills, and durable power of attorney for health care. It also usually involves assistance to access community resources, to make informed decisions, to recognize and cope with necessary changes in lifestyle, to negotiate medical insurance, and to understand ways to effectively use the complex medical system. Advocacy can be a particular challenge when family members' or other caregivers' views differ from those of the client. In the event of conflict, the nurse, being the client's primary advocate, ensures that the client's rights and desires are upheld.

Caregiver

The home health nurse's major role as caregiver is to assess and diagnose the client's actual and potential health problems, plan care, and evaluate the client's outcomes. Direct personal care activities such as bathing, changing linens, feeding, and light housekeeping activities to maintain a clean and safe home environment are usually provided by a family member or a home health aide arranged by the nurse. The home health nurse, however, will provide direct care for specific procedures and treatments such as ostomy care, wound care, intravenous therapy, and so on according to agency policies and practices (see Figure 9–1 ■). Much of the home health nurse's time is spent teaching others to provide required care.

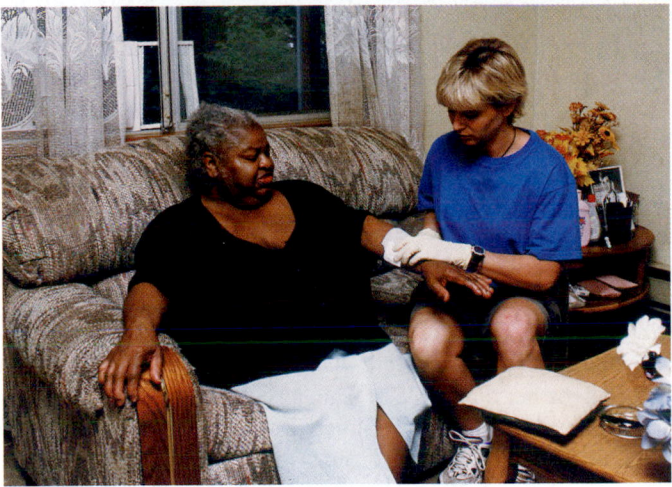

Figure 9–1 ■ Home care nurses perform skilled direct care such as changing dressings.

Educator

The educative role of the home health nurse focuses on illness care, the prevention of problems, and the promotion of optional wellness or well-being. Education is ongoing and can be considered the crux of home care practice; its goal is to help clients learn to manage as independently as possible. All home health nurses need to be skilled in teaching and learning principles and strategies that facilitate learning. (See Chapter 25 ∞ for detailed information.)

Case Manager or Coordinator

The home health nurse coordinates the activities of all other home health team members involved in the client's treatment plan. Coordination can occur individually, in person or by telephone, with a specific team member such as the dietitian or respiratory therapist, or during a team conference where each team member provides information about the client's health status. The nurse is the main contact with the physician or nurse practitioner to report any changes in the client's condition and to bring about a revision in the plan of care as needed. Documentation of care coordination is a legal and reimbursement requirement and must be recorded on the client's medical record.

PERSPECTIVES OF HOME CARE CLIENTS

Home care clients include a diverse population that encompasses all ages, a variety of health problems, and families of different structures and cultural backgrounds. Home care clients have a wide range of health problems that include disabilities, perinatal problems, mental illness, and acute and chronic illnesses. The majority of clients have medical-surgical problems that are similar to those seen in acute or extended care facilities.

Although the person receiving care is considered the primary client in home care, the client's family can be considered

MediaLink | NURSE ASSISTANT APPLICATION

secondary clients because often they are associated with care-giving and have a major impact on the client's wellness status. The home health nurse will encounter many different family structures ranging from single families to extended families and dwellings that house multiple families. In the home setting, family members may include not only persons related by birth and marriage, but also friends, other significant individuals, and animals.

Various cultural influences also affect the client's health care beliefs and practices. The home health nurse needs to be culturally sensitive; that is, to become aware of the client's culture and form a nursing care plan with the client that incorporates his or her culture. See Chapter 13 ∞ for detailed information about making cultural assessments and providing culturally competent care.

SELECTED DIMENSIONS OF HOME HEALTH NURSING

Selected dimensions of home health care include assessing the home for safety features, infection control, and caregiver support.

Client Safety

Hazards in the home are major causes of falls, fire, poisoning, and other accidents, such as those caused by improper use of household equipment (e.g., tools and cooking utensils). The appraisal of such hazards and suggestions for remedies is an essential nursing function. See the Home Care Assessment box for a home hazard appraisal and Chapter 30 ∞ for a discussion of potential hazards and preventive actions for individuals of all ages.

Obviously home health nurses cannot expect to change a family's living space and lifestyle. However, they can express their concern and react appropriately when a situation suggests that an injury is imminent. Nurses must document information they provide and the family's response to instruction, and make ongoing assessments about the family's use of safety precautions.

Other aspects of client safety relate to emergency situations. The home health nurse can assist the client and caregivers as follows:

- Post a list of all emergency telephone numbers (ambulance, fire, police, physician) at each telephone.
- Post a list of all the client's medications and potential side effects in a central location, such as on the refrigerator.
- Help the client and family apply for a medical alert system such as a bracelet or necklace (see Figure 9–2 ■). Information on the MedicAlert System can be obtained by writing to MedicAlert,

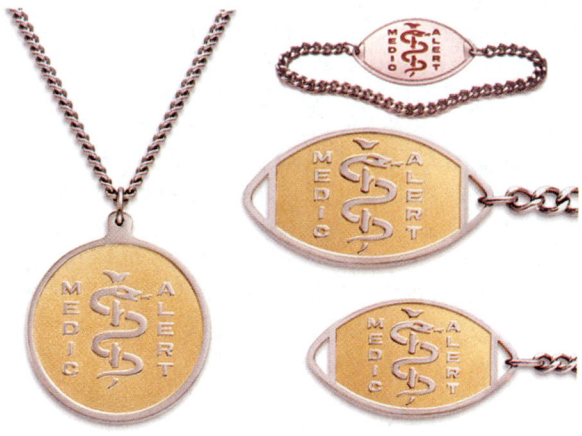

Figure 9–2 ■ MedicAlert emblems. (Reproduced with permission: 2003. All rights reserved. MedicAlert® is a Federally Registered Trademark and Service Mark.)

Home Care Assessment

HOME HAZARD APPRAISAL FOR ADULTS

Client and Environment

- *Walkways and stairways (inside and outside):* Note uneven sidewalks or paths, broken or loose steps, absence of handrails or placement on only one side of stairways, insecure handrails, congested hallways or other traffic areas, and adequacy of lighting at night.
- *Floors:* Note uneven and highly polished or slippery floors and any unanchored rugs or mats.
- *Furniture:* Note hazardous placement of furniture with sharp corners. Note chairs or stools that are too low to get into and out of or that provide inadequate support.
- *Bathroom(s):* Note presence of grab bars around tubs and toilets, nonslip surfaces in tubs and shower stalls, handheld showerhead, adequacy of night lighting, need for raised toilet seat or bath chair in tub or shower, ease of access to shelves, and water temperature regulated at a maximum of 49° C (120° F).
- *Kitchen:* Note pilot lights (gas stove) in need of repair, inaccessible storage areas, and hazardous furniture.

- *Bedrooms:* Note adequacy of lighting, in particular the availability of night-lights and accessibility of light switches, ease of access to commode, urinal, or bedpan, and need for hospital bed or bed rails.
- *Electrical:* Note unanchored or frayed electrical cords and outlets that are overloaded or near water.
- *Fire protection:* Note presence or absence of smoke detectors, fire extinguisher, and fire escape plan, improper storage of combustibles (e.g., gasoline) or corrosives (e.g., rust remover).
- *Toxic substances:* Note improperly labeled cleaning solutions.
- *Communication devices:* Note presence of method to call for help, such as a telephone or intercom in the bedroom and elsewhere (e.g., kitchen), and access to emergency telephone numbers.
- *Medications:* Note medications kept beyond date of expiration, adequacy of lighting for medication cabinet or storage, and method of disposal of sharp objects such as needles used for injections.

Turlock, California 95381-1009, by calling 1-888-633-4298, or by accessing http://www.medicalert. org.

- Enroll the client in a program that places all the client's vital medical information in one place for emergency personnel to have in the event of a life-threatening situation. The program can be obtained through a pharmacy, physician's office, the VNA, or other community support groups. The kit contains a plastic vial, a medical information form, a decal, and an instruction sheet. The information form is filled out, rolled, and placed in the vial. The vial is placed in the refrigerator and emergency personnel are trained to routinely check there. The decal is placed on the refrigerator as a signal that the vial is inside.
- Recommend the client enroll in an emergency response system. These systems provide a small device with a help button that attaches to a wrist or neck chain. The home base station requires the client to send a signal daily that indicates that he or she is OK. If the signal is not sent or if the portable device is activated, the system automatically calls the client and then dials a previously established list of emergency contacts. This system is particularly useful for clients who are alone because if they should fall, for instance, and be unable to reach a telephone, they might be left helpless for extended periods of time.

Nurse Safety

Some less desirable living locations pose additional safety concerns for the nurse. Many home health agencies have contracts with security firms to escort nurses needing to see clients in potentially unsafe neighborhoods. The nurse should avoid taking any personal belongings during these visits and have a preestablished mechanism to signal for help. Home health agencies provide training for nurses in ways to decrease personal risk.

Infection Control

The goal of infection control in the home is to protect clients, caregivers, and the general community from the transmission of disease. This is particularly important for clients who are immunocompromised, who have infectious or communicable diseases, or who have draining wounds, drainage tubes, or other invasive access devices. The nurse's major role in infection control is health teaching. Clients and caregivers need to learn about effective hand washing, use of gloves, handling of linens, disposal of wastes and soiled dressings, and the practice of infection control (Standard Precautions). Infection control can present a challenge to the home health nurse, especially if the home care facilities are not conducive to basic aseptic requirements such as running water for hand washing.

An important aspect of infection control involves handling the home health nurse's equipment and supplies. Supplies may include materials for hand washing; assessment equipment such as stethoscope, blood pressure cuff and monitor, thermometer, and tape measure; infection control items such as gowns, goggles, masks, gloves, and blood spill kit; and antimicrobial cleaning agents. Nurses need to follow agency protocol in regard to aseptic practice with these.

Caregiver Support

Caregiving may be directed to individuals of any age and varies from short term to long term according to the physical or mental disabilities of the care receivers. For example, some children who have permanent disabilities and adults who experience progressive deterioration such as those with Alzheimer's disease or multiple sclerosis require care on a permanent basis. Others who are recovering from a surgical procedure require care only on a temporary basis. Most caregivers have close relationships with the care receiver, that is, a spouse/partner, parent, child, friend, or other significant relationship. Many caregiving relationships, therefore, represent changes from the caring and caregiving intrinsic to all close relationships to an extraordinary and unequal burden for the caregiver. Caregivers, many of whom are older adults, may experience **caregiver role strain** when they have physical, emotional, social, and financial burdens that can seriously jeopardize their own health and well-being.

The home health nurse needs to recognize signs of caregiver role strain and suggest ways to minimize or alleviate this problem. Signs of caregiver overload include the following:

- Difficulty performing routine tasks for the client
- Reports of declining physical energy and insufficient time for caregiving
- Concern that caregiving responsibilities interfere with other roles such as those of parent, spouse, work, friend
- Anxiety about ability to meet future care needs of client
- Feelings of anger and depression
- Dramatic change in the home environment's appearance.

When caregiver role strain is identified, the nurse needs to encourage caregivers to express their feelings and at the same time convey understanding about the difficulties associated with caregiving and acknowledge the caregivers' competence. The nurse can obtain a realistic appraisal of the situation by asking a caregiver to describe a typical day and daily or weekly leisure and social activities. It is also helpful to identify activities for which assistance is desired. These activities may include client care needs such as hygiene, mobility, feeding, or treatments; house cleaning; laundry; shopping; house repairs; yard work; transportation; doctor's or hairdresser's appointments; or respite.

Activities that are commonly done by nurses and aides, such as changing an occupied bed and transferring a client from bed to chair, may be overwhelming to a caregiver who has not performed them before. Demonstrating them in the home and allowing caregivers to perform them with the nurse's supervision increases their confidence and increases the likelihood of them asking for assistance in other situations.

When activities for which assistance is required are identified, the nurse and caregiver need to identify possible sources of help. Both volunteer and agency sources need to be explored. Volunteer sources of help may include family members (cousins, siblings), neighbors, friends, church associates, or caregiver support groups in the community. Other sources include, for example, a home health aide for light housekeeping and grocery shopping, Meals on Wheels, day care, transportation, and counseling and social services. Families with a chronically ill member may benefit from a weekend respite—a program some hospitals provide in which the client is admitted to a skilled unit for observation and care, enabling the caregiver a break from ongoing health care needs.

Caregivers need to be reminded of the importance of caring for themselves by getting adequate rest, eating nutritious meals, asking for help, delegating household chores, and making time for leisure activities or simply some time alone. Family members other than the caregiver also may need help to learn ways to support the caregiver. The nurse may discuss the importance to the caregiver of regular phone calls, cards, letters, and visits; offer encouragement to take day trips or a vacation; listen without giving advice; acknowledge the burden of caregiving and the need to feel appreciated; and so on.

A particular challenge exists when the nurse is in a position to be a caregiver to a family member. Although the nurse's clinical expertise and familiarity with the client and setting can be especially useful, negotiating the professional distancing that is sometimes needed when providing care to clients can be difficult with family. The nurse may feel obligated to provide care, even when this is over and above regular employment responsibilities. The nurse must have the opportunity to be able to step back and experience the role and emotions of being a family member—not always only those of being a nurse.

APPLYING THE NURSING PROCESS IN THE HOME

The application of the nursing process is focused on the needs of individual clients and their caregivers. You will learn more about the nursing process in other chapters.

ASSESSING

The home health nurse assesses not only the health care demands of the client and family but also the home and community environment. Assessment actually begins when the nurse contacts the client for the initial home visit and reviews documents received from the referral agency. The goal of the initial visit is to obtain a comprehensive clinical picture of the client's needs.

Most agencies have an admissions or intake packet that includes forms for consent to treatment; physical, psychosocial, and spiritual assessment; medications; pain assessment; family data; financial assessment including insurance verification; client's bill of rights; care plan; and daily visit notes. During the initial home visit, the home health nurse obtains a health history from the client (see Figure 9–3 ■), examines the client, observes the relationship of the client and caregiver, and assesses the home and community environment. Parameters of assessment of the home environment include client and caregiver mobility, client ability to perform self-care, the cleanliness of the environment, the availability of caregiver support, safety, food preparation, financial supports, and the emotional status of the client and caregiver.

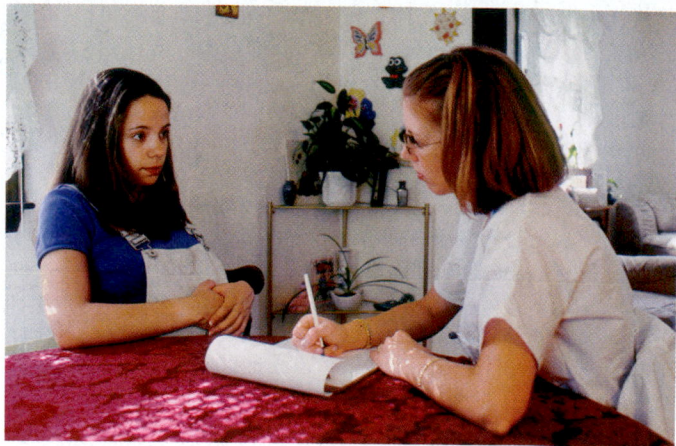

Figure 9–3 ■ Interviewing the home care client.

Following assessment, the nurse determines whether further consults and support personnel are needed. For example, would the client benefit from a dietary consult or Meals on Wheels? Is a home health aide needed to assist with activities of daily living and homemaker tasks? Is a social worker needed to help with financial resources or future care needs such as placement in a nursing home? What additional supplies does the client need?

Before completing this initial assessment interview, the nurse also discusses what the client and family can expect from home care, what other health care providers may be needed to help the client achieve independence, and the frequency of home visits.

DIAGNOSING

As in other care environments, the nurse identifies both actual and potential client problems. Examples of common nursing diagnoses for home care include *Deficient Knowledge (Specify), Impaired Home Maintenance,* and *Risk for Caregiver Role Strain.* See the Identifying Nursing Diagnoses, Outcomes, and Interventions box for an example of applying the nursing process to a home care client. Because client education is considered a skill reimbursed by Medicare and other commercial insurance carriers, it is important for the nurse to include *Deficient Knowledge* in the plan of care. The deficit in knowledge may relate to clients' lack of information about their disease process, medications, self-care skills, and so on.

PLANNING AND IMPLEMENTING

During the planning phase the nurse needs to encourage and permit clients to make their own health management decisions. Alternatives may need to be suggested for some decisions if the nurse identifies potential harm from a chosen course of action.

Strategies to meet goals generally include teaching the client and family techniques of care and identifying appropriate resources to assist the client and family in maintaining self-sufficiency. Box 9–1 lists Medicare's required data for the nursing plan of care.

To implement the plan, the home health nurse performs nursing interventions, including teaching; coordinates and uses referrals and resources; provides and monitors all levels

NURSING MANAGEMENT

IDENTIFYING NURSING DIAGNOSES, OUTCOMES, AND INTERVENTIONS

FOR HOME CARE CLIENTS

DATA CLUSTER	NURSING DIAGNOSIS/ DEFINITION	SAMPLE DESIRED OUTCOMES [NOC#]/DEFINITION	INDICATORS	SELECTED INTERVENTIONS [NIC#]/DEFINITION	SAMPLE NIC ACTIVITIES
Mr. J is a 60-year-old retired engineer who has recently experienced a severe episode of irritable bowel syndrome. He is very weak, needs to remain near the bathroom, and has become unable to perform many of his usual duties in the home. His wife works long hours and now must take on his responsibilities plus some physical care for her husband.	Impaired Home Maintenance/Inability to independently maintain a safe growth-promoting immediate environment	Role Performance [1501]/Congruence of an individual's role behavior with role expectations	Substantially adequate • Ability to meet role expectations • Performance of family role behaviors	Home Maintenance Assistance [7180]/Helping the patient/family to maintain the home as a clean, safe, and pleasant place to live Family Support [7140]/Promotion of family values, interests, and goals	• Involve patient/family in deciding home maintenance requirements • Discuss cost of needed maintenance and available resources • Suggest necessary structural alterations to make home accessible • Teach the nurse's care plans to the family
		Self-Care: Instrumental Activities of Daily Living (IADL) [0306]/Ability to perform activities needed to function in the home or community	Independent with assistive device • Shops for household needs • Performs housework • Prepares meals • Uses telephone	Sustenance Support [7500]/Helping a needy individual to locate food, clothing, or shelter	• Discuss with the individual/family financial aid support available • Inform individual/family of eligibility requirements for food stamps • Arrange transportation as necessary

continued on page 148

IDENTIFYING NURSING DIAGNOSES, OUTCOMES, AND INTERVENTIONS *continued*

FOR HOME CARE CLIENTS

DATA CLUSTER	NURSING DIAGNOSIS/ DEFINITION	SAMPLE DESIRED OUTCOMES [NOC#]/DEFINITION	INDICATORS	SELECTED INTERVENTIONS [NIC#]/DEFINITION	SAMPLE NIC ACTIVITIES
	Risk of Caregiver Role Strain/A caregiver is vulnerable for felt difficulty in performing the family caregiver role	Caregiver Stressors [2208]/*The extent of biopsychosocial pressure on a family care provider caring for a family member or significant other over an extended period of time*	Limited • Psychological limitations for caregiving • Impairment of usual work performance • Severity of care recipient illness	Caregiver Support [7040]/*Provision of the necessary information, advocacy, and support to facilitate patient care by someone other than a health care professional*	• Determine caregiver's level of knowledge • Monitor family interaction problems related to care of patient • Provide information about the patient's condition in accordance with patient preference • Teach caregiver stress management techniques • Teach caregiver strategies to access and maximize health care and community resources
		Caregiver Emotional Health [2506]/*Feelings, attitudes, and emotions of a family care provider while caring for a family member or significant other over an extended period of time*	Mildly compromised • Free of resentment • Perceived social connectedness • Perceived adequacy of resources		• Explore with the caregiver strengths and weaknesses

of technical care; collaborates with other disciplines and providers; identifies clinical problems and solutions from research and other health literature; supervises ancillary personnel; and advocates for the client's right to self-determination. Technical skills commonly performed by home health nurses include blood pressure measurement; body fluid collection (blood, urine, stool, sputum); wound care; respiratory care; all types of intravenous therapy, enteral nutrition, urinary catheterization, enterostomal care, and renal dialysis (see Figure 9–4 ■).

A large part of the nurse's implementing role involves teaching the client and caregiver the necessary skills for self-care—for example, administering insulin injections, measuring blood glucose, and administering medications. Medication instruction about dosage, frequency of administration, and possible side effects is of particular concern for many clients. (See Chapter 33 ⊙⊙ for more information.) Clients who are receiving high-technology interventions are often anxious about their ability to manage such sophisticated equipment. The home health nurse is challenged to alleviate the client's fears and to provide thorough instruction, demonstration, and periodic evaluation of the client and family's performance of such skills. Members of the home care team specially trained in the skill, such as intravenous nurses and respiratory therapists, generally make periodic visits to service the equipment and to monitor the client's skills.

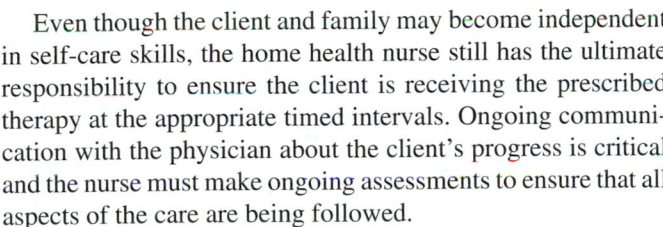

BOX 9–1 ■ Medicare's Required Data for the Nursing Plan of Care

1. All pertinent diagnoses
2. A notation of the beneficiary's mental status
3. Types of services, supplies, and equipment ordered
4. Frequency of visits to be made
5. Client's prognosis
6. Client's rehabilitation potential
7. Client's functional limitations
8. Activities permitted
9. Client's nutritional requirements
10. Client's medications and treatments
11. Safety measures to protect against injuries
12. Discharge plans
13. Any other items the home health agency or physician wishes to include.

Note: From *Medicare Home Health Agency Manual* (HCFA Pub. 11, PB 98-955200), by Centers for Medicare & Medicaid Services. Retrieved March 25, 2003, from http://cms.hhs.gov/manuals/11_hha/hh200.asp.#sect_204_2

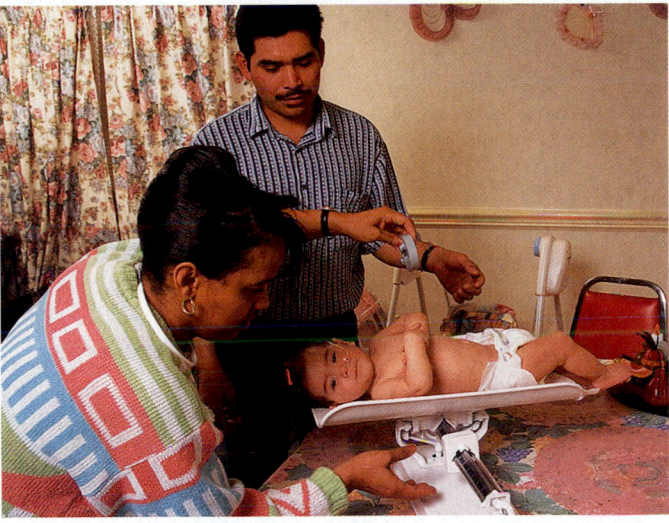

Figure 9–5 ■ Determining the success of the care plan includes comparing assessment findings to previous values. Weighing this tube-fed baby provides critical data about her progress.

Even though the client and family may become independent in self-care skills, the home health nurse still has the ultimate responsibility to ensure the client is receiving the prescribed therapy at the appropriate timed intervals. Ongoing communication with the physician about the client's progress is critical and the nurse must make ongoing assessments to ensure that all aspects of the care are being followed.

EVALUATING AND DOCUMENTING

Evaluation is carried out by the nurse on subsequent home visits, observing the same parameters assessed on the initial home visit and relating findings to the expected outcomes or goals

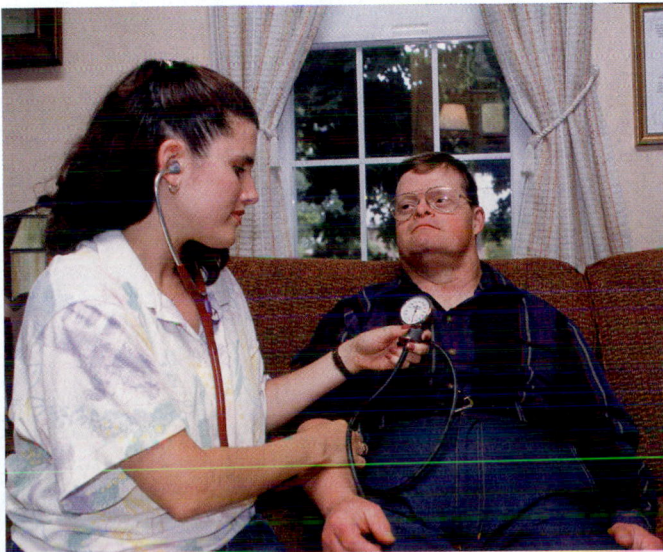

Figure 9–4 ■ The nurse monitors the client's response to treatments and therapy.

(see Figure 9–5 ■). The nurse can also teach caregivers parameters of evaluation so that they can obtain professional intervention if needed. Documentation of care given and the client's progress toward goal achievement at each visit is essential. Notes must also reflect plans for subsequent visits and when the client may be sufficiently prepared for self-care and discharge from the agency.

THE FUTURE OF HOME HEALTH CARE

What is the future for home health care? Experts in the home health care industry have identified some trends:

1. Establishing ethics committees to handle ethical issues that arise in the home. These committees may be necessary for agencies to receive accreditation.
2. Providing third-party reimbursement for community clinical nurse specialists and psychiatric nurse specialists. These advanced practice nurses can provide education, support, counseling, and therapy for clients and their families.
3. Providing third-party reimbursement for social workers. Social workers can assist clients and their families in the home with financial and household problems, freeing the nurse to focus on nursing care.
4. Utilizing nurse pain specialists to assess and manage pain in the home, thus avoiding costly hospitalizations and procedures.
5. Providing pet care for clients who may become too ill to care for them. Clients can make arrangements for the care of a pet if they are hospitalized or die.
6. Utilizing electronic home visits. A computerized system can obtain information, such as blood pressure readings, allowing case managers to review a client's progress from offsite.

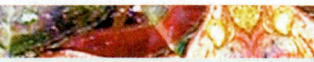

Lifespan Considerations

Elders

Clients who have been hospitalized are often discharged after short stays and are often acutely ill. This becomes a challenge for home health nurses in planning and implementing care. Special areas of concern for elder in this situation include the following:

- Healing time is slower due to changes that normally occur in aging, such as impaired circulation and alteration in immune response.
- Changes in medications or lingering traces of anesthesia may alter cognitive status, even though it is usually temporary.

- Weakness and fatigue create safety issues, such as risk for falling.
- Chronic diseases already present may have been complicated by other conditions acquired while hospitalized.
- Assessment should be initiated while the client is in the hospital to determine the need for assistive devices or environmental changes when the client returns home. Some examples of these devices are walkers, raised toilet seats, safety bars in the bathroom, and better lighting. Good planning eases the transition to home care for the client and caregiver.

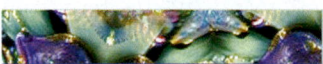

Focus on Critical Thinking

Mr. Madden is a 67-year-old African American male with a 20-year history of hypertension and diabetes mellitus. He has recently undergone amputation of three toes due to poor circulation.

Because he is progressing well and his diabetes is under control, he is being discharged from the acute care setting to go home. He has been referred to the hospital-based home health agency, which will assign a nurse to change his foot dressings, administer IV antibiotics, and monitor his blood glucose levels.

1. When delivering care in the home environment, how will the nurse's role be similar to and different from that of the nurse's role in the acute care environment?

2. What rights does the client have when being cared for at home that may not be afforded him while institutionalized?
3. What factors could negatively impact the care of Mr. Madden in his own home?
4. Speculate about personal and financial savings derived by patients being cared for at home rather than in a hospital or other institution.

See Critical Thinking Possibilities in Appendix A.

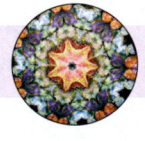

| Chapter Review

Explore MediaLink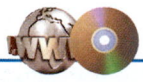

NCLEX review questions, case studies, MediaLink applications, and other interactive resources for this chapter can be found on the Companion Website at www.prenhall.com/kozier. Click on Chapter 9 to select the activities for this chapter.

For more NCLEX review questions, and an audio glossary, access the Student CD-ROM accompanying this textbook.

Chapter Highlights

- Home health care is an alternative to acute and subacute health care facilities. The trend has changed from using home health care after hospitalization to using it to avoid hospitalization.
- Hospice nursing, often considered a subspecialty of home nursing, supports terminally ill clients and their families during the last stages of life and bereavement.
- Home health agencies offer skilled professional and paraprofessional services. Because clients often require the serv-

ices of several professionals simultaneously, case coordination is essential.
- There are several types of home health agencies: official or public agencies, voluntary or private not-for-profit agencies, private proprietary agencies, and institution-based agencies. All home health agencies must meet specific standards for licensing, certification, and accreditation.
- Private duty agencies provide professional nursing and home health aide care for 4 to 24 hours per day.

- Health care agencies in the United States receive reimbursement for services they provide from various sources: Medicare and Medicaid, private insurance companies, and private pay. The Medicare and Medicaid programs have strict guidelines.
- Referrals for home health services may be made by the client's physician, a nurse, social worker, therapist, discharge planner, or family member. Home care requires, however, a physician's order and an approved treatment plan.
- Major roles of the home health nurse are those of advocate, caregiver, educator, and case manager.
- The home health nurse assesses the care needs of clients in their home; plans, implements, and supervises that care; teaches clients and their families self-care; and mobilizes the resources of hospitals, physicians, and community agencies in meeting the needs of the clients and their families.
- Home care clients include a diverse population that encompasses all ages, a variety of health problems, and families of different structures and cultural backgrounds. The home health nurse needs to be culturally sensitive, that is, become aware of the client's culture, and form a nursing care plan with the client that incorporates the client's culture.
- Important dimensions of home health nursing include the home visit in which the nurse assesses the client and they make plans for care; client and nurse safety; infection control; and caregiver support.

Review Questions

9–1. Care in the home is an alternative to hospital placement. A major difference is that in-home care
   a. does not focus on curative and lifesaving approaches.
   b. is less able to manage complex symptoms.
   c. facilitates extensive involvement of significant others/family.
   d. permits use of pain medication regimens not allowed in the hospital.

9–2. If there is a physician's order for all of the following, which can be delegated to the home health aide?
   a. feeding and bathing the client
   b. teaching the client about medications
   c. assessing wound healing progress
   d. adjusting oxygen flow

9–3. The client needs to sit with feet elevated to enhance venous return. However, even after being taught the reasons, the client refuses. Which statement by the nurse would be most useful?
   a. "If you won't cooperate, I can't help you."
   b. "Tell me the reasons you won't put your feet up."
   c. "It is essential that you do this."
   d. " I'll notify your doctor that you are unable to keep your feet up."

9–4. Which of the following may be a sign of caregiver role strain?
   a. caregiver weight and sleep loss
   b. the caregiver asks other family and friends for help
   c. the caregiver asks the nurse what other ways he or she can help the client
   d. the caregiver seems sad whenever the client's prognosis is discussed.

9–5. Which of the following is needed before home nursing care can be started?
   a. insurance coverage
   b. an in-home caregiver
   c. a curable health problem
   d. a physician's authorization

Readings and References

Suggested Readings

Blevins, C. (2001). There really is a difference: Home care competencies. *The Journal of Continuing Education in Nursing, 32,* 114–117. In this article, the author discusses the need for awareness that the knowledge, values, and skills (competencies) required of home care nurses are not the same as those needed by nurses in other settings. She reviews the small amount of research available examining home care nurse competencies and recommends directions for further development.

Wrubel, J., Richards, T. A., Folkman, S., & Acree, M. C. (2001). Tacit definitions of informal caregiving. *Journal of Advanced Nursing, 33,* 175–181. This study focused on the male caregivers of men with AIDS who were interviewed several times over a 2-year period. Three groups of men emerged who varied in their level of understanding about caregiving, their involvement in client decision making, and their sources of stress. Understanding how people differ in their caregiving roles can help nurses provide individualized care and support.

Related Research

Aucoin-Gallant, G. (2001). The utilization and efficiency of the informal caregivers' coping strategies. *Canadian Oncology Nursing Journal, 11*(1), 21–23, 27.

Katz, S. J., Kabeto, M., & Langa, K. M. (2000). Gender disparities in the receipt of home care for elderly people with disability in the United States. *Journal of the American Medical Association, 284,* 3022–3027.

Lee, H. S., Brennan, P. F., & Daly, B. J. (2001). Relationship of empathy to appraisal, depression, life satisfaction, and physical health in informal caregivers of older adults. *Research in Nursing and Health, 24,* 44–56.

Pierce, L. L. (2001). Caring and expressions of stability by urban family caregivers of persons with stroke within African American family systems. *Rehabilitation Nursing, 26,* 100–107, 116, 121.

References

Centers for Medicare & Medicaid Services. (2001). *Medicare home health agency manual* (HCFA Publication No. 11, PB 98-955200). Retrieved March 25, 2003, from http://cms.hhs.gov/ manuals/11_hha/hh200. asp#sect_204_2

Johnson, M., Maas, M., & Moorhead, S. (Eds.) (2000). *Nursing outcomes classification (NOC)* (2nd ed.). St. Louis, MO: Mosby.

McCloskey, J. C., & Bulechek, G. M. (Eds.). (2000). *Nursing interventions classification (NIC)* (3rd ed.). St. Louis, MO: Mosby.

NANDA International. (2003). NANDA *nursing diagnoses: Definitions and classification 2003–2004.* Philadelphia: Author.

Selected Bibliography

American Nurses Association. (1999). *Scope and standards of home health nursing practice.* Washington, DC: American Nurses Publishing.

Beckert, J. (1998). Hospital nurses in home care. *Case Manager, 9*(4), 43–45.

Brown, S. (2000). The legal pitfalls of home care. *RN, 63*(11), 75–80.

Caro, F. G. (2001). Asking the right questions: The key to discovering what works in home care. *The Gerontologist, 41,* 307–308.

Cochran, M., & Brennan, S. J. (1998). Home healthcare nursing in the managed care environment: Part 1—managed care: An overview. *Home Healthcare Nurse, 16,* 214–221.

Davidson, F. G., & Haddock, D. B. (2001). *The caregiver's sourcebook.* New York: McGraw-Hill.

Ebersole, P. (1998). Home care and the elderly. *Home Care Provider, 3*(1), 7–8.

Joint Commission on Accreditation of Healthcare Organizations. (2001). *2001–2002 Comprehensive accreditation manual for home care.* Oakbrook Terrace, IL: Joint Commission Resources.

Marrelli, T. M. (2001). *Handbook of home health standards and documentation—Guidelines for reimbursement.* St. Louis, MO: Mosby.

Murray, T. A. (1998). Using role theory concepts to understand transitions from hospital based nursing practice to home care nursing. *Journal of Continuing Nursing Education, 2,* 105–111.

Rice, R. (1999). *Handbook of home health nursing procedures* (2nd ed.). St. Louis, MO: Mosby.

Stackhouse, J. C. (1998). *Into the community: Nursing in ambulatory and home care.* Philadelphia: Lippincott-Raven.

Young, M. G. (2001). Providing care for the caregiver. *Patient Care for the Nurse Practitioner, 4*(2), 36–40, 43–48.

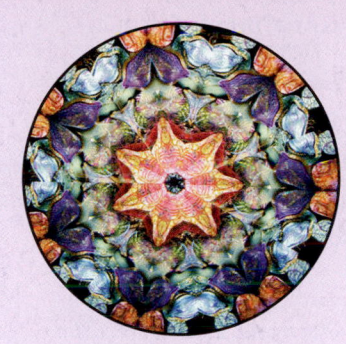

CHAPTER 10

NURSING INFORMATICS

LEARNING OUTCOMES

After completing this chapter, you will be able to:

- Define the terms used to describe the common components of desktop computers.

- Recognize the uses of word processing, database, spreadsheet, and communications software in nursing.

- Describe the uses of computers in nursing education.

- Discuss the advantages of and concerns about computerized patient documentation systems.

- Identify computer applications used in direct client monitoring and diagnosis.

- List ways computers may be used by nurse administrators in the areas of personnel, facilities management, finance, quality assurance, and accreditation.

- Identify the role of computers in each step of the research process.

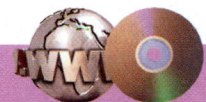

MediaLink

www.prenhall.com/kozier

Additional resources for this chapter can be found on the Student CD-ROM accompanying this textbook, and on the Companion Website at www.prenhall.com/kozier. Click on Chapter 10 to select the activities for this chapter.

CD-ROM
- Audio Glossary
- NCLEX Review

Companion Website
- Additional NCLEX Review
- Case Study:
  Computerizing Clinical Documentation
- MediaLink Applications:
  Confidentiality Laws
  Informatics Certification Exam
- Links to Resources

Computers have become a part of everyday life for many people, including nurses. Computers are used for educating nursing students and clients, assessing and documenting clients' health conditions, managing medical records, communicating among health care providers, and conducting nursing research. All nurses must have a basic level of computer literacy in order to perform their jobs. Advanced practice in nursing informatics is a growing specialty. The first American Nurses Association certification examination in nursing informatics was given in October 1995.

GENERAL CONCEPTS

Informatics refers to the science of computer information systems. **Nursing informatics** is the science of using computer information systems in the practice of nursing. This is a relatively young science—the first Nursing Information Systems conference was held in the United States in 1977. Nurses have taken significant strides since then to design and adapt computer processes to enhance client care, education, administration and management, and nursing research.

The terminology used to describe the parts and functions of computer systems can be confusing. Many of the terms are acronyms, words made up from the first letter of several words or syllables. New terms emerge daily and it is a challenge to keep up with them. This section describes the most common computer hardware and software nurses may come across in the work setting.

Computer Hardware

The term **hardware** refers to the physical parts of the computer. The hardware allows the user to enter data into the computer, performs the actions of the computer's processing, and produces the computer output. Hardware size, shape, and type vary depending on the computer's purpose. Large supercomputers are generally limited to military, industrial, and complex research uses. Mainframe computers are systems used in businesses and many health care agencies to store and process large amounts of information. Users are connected to the mainframe through peripheral terminals. A smaller version of the mainframe is called a minicomputer, or sometimes a server because it "serves" the connected terminals or computers. Microcomputers are typically individual systems referred to as desktop or **personal computers (PCs).** These include portable laptop, notebook, or handheld computers. The basic components of computer hardware include the central processing unit and one or more types of data input and output devices.

Central Processing Unit

The **central processing unit (CPU)** is in the box that contains the computer hardware necessary to process and store data. Also located with the CPU are the power supply, disk drives, chips, and connections for all the other computer hardware, referred to as **peripherals.** The speed of the computer is determined by three components: the CPU processor (measured in megahertz), the amount of RAM (explained shortly), and the speed of data location or transfer rate of the disk drives. For example, at the time of this writing, a reasonably fast desktop computer would have a processing speed of more than 800 mHz, at least 32 MB of RAM, and a hard drive average seek time of less than 10 milliseconds. By the time you read this, standards will have changed.

Computer Memory and Storage

In order for data to be kept for later retrieval, the computer must store the information in an electronic form. Computer information is measured in bytes (usually 1 byte is one letter, digit, or character), kilobytes (1,000 bytes = 1 KB), megabytes (1 million bytes = 1 MB), or gigabytes (1 billion bytes = 1 GB).

While the computer is turned on, data and instructions for the computer are loaded into **random-access memory (RAM).** Storage in RAM is temporary and is lost when the computer is turned off. To save their work, computer users employ other forms of data storage, most commonly magnetic hard disks or drives and "floppy" diskettes. These forms allow both reading and writing of data and can be reused. Inside the computer box are one or more hard disks. Users often transport data from one computer to another or keep extra copies of data using 3.5-inch-diameter diskettes housed in hard plastic. The smaller diskettes can store 1 to 2 MB and hard disks store up to several gigabytes of data. Data can also be stored and retrieved from high-capacity disks (e.g., Zip disks) and magnetic tape cassettes.

For data not created by the user, storage can be in the form of **read-only memory (ROM),** like that found on silicon chips inside the CPU. ROM chips contain programs needed to ensure that the computer functions correctly; ROM cannot be altered by the computer user. A **CD**-ROM is a **compact disc** with read-only memory; it is a thin optical disc that can be read by the laser in a computer's CD-ROM drive. An advantage of CD-ROMs is that they can store hundreds of megabytes of data, including audio and video that have been converted to digital format. Several CD-ROM drives can be linked to allow the user to access huge amounts of data. Computers frequently have drives that can read and write (burn) data on CDs. **Digital video discs (DVDs)** store and play digital information, such as a movie, and are similar in size to the common CD-ROM disc.

Input Devices

There are several ways to get information into a computer. The most common method is to use a keyboard, much like the keyboard of a typewriter but with additional function keys. A *mouse* is a pointing device with buttons used to choose items or initiate an action. Some computer screens respond to touching with a finger or a lightpen or wand. Many computers also have a microphone attached and can respond to voice commands. Other electronic devices used for entering data into a computer are scanners and analog-to-digital converters. Scanners allow data to be copied into the computer from a paper version or other "hardcopy" text or graphics. Analog signals such as those from testing devices can also be converted to digital signals in order to go directly into the computer.

Output Devices

The results of computer data entry or processing are usually displayed first on the computer screen or monitor and then through a printer or plotter as a hardcopy. Both monitors and printers can display text and graphics, and color monitors and printers also show color images. There is a wide spectrum of quality in monitors and printers, primarily depending on the size of the small dots (called *pixels* for monitors and *dots per inch* [dpi] for printers) used to form the shapes. The greater the number of pixels or dots per square inch, the better the resolution.

Communications Devices

Sometimes computer data need to be sent long distances or directly to one or more other computers. The term **online** refers to a computer being connected to other computers in a **network.** The network is often coordinated by one computer, the network server. PCs linked directly to other nearby PCs and servers by wires or wireless communications devices constitute a **local-area network (LAN).** Direct connections between computers are only possible over limited distances. Agencies that need to have distant locations linked do so through a **wide-area network (WAN),** virtual networks, or private networks. These larger distances can be covered by sending the data through a modem that uses standard telephone wires or a high-speed data connection (e.g., cable, digital subscriber line [DSL], or integrated services digital network [ISDN] line). These linked computers can access another computer, printer, or a facsimile (fax) machine. The technology for network connections and devices changes rapidly.

> ► **CLINICAL ALERT**   *Personal digital assistants (PDAs) are handheld computers that can interface with networks. Nurses increasingly use them as data entry and retrieval devices.* ■

Computer Software

Computers are useful because people can instruct the hardware to perform certain tasks. These instructions are called *programs, applications,* or *software.* The most commonly used software programs are word processors, databases, spreadsheets, and utilities such as communications. Other PC software of interest to nurses includes computer-assisted instruction and presentation graphics programs.

Word Processing

The ability to save and manipulate words is probably the most used computer application. Once the material has been typed into the computer (or scanned from an existing document), it is saved onto a hard or floppy disk as a file that can be repeatedly retrieved, changed, and sent to a variety of output devices. The word processing program has numerous options to permit the user to specify the typeface, spacing, and page layout. Words, sentences, and entire documents can be automatically checked for spelling and grammar with the program suggesting modifications. Documents can also be individualized by merging them with name and address lists in a chosen template. Word processing programs are becoming increasingly sophisticated and can include pictures, tables and charts, and many graphical designs.

Databases

Database programs are used to manage a file or group of files of detailed information about people or things. Within a database file are individual records that represent the person, product, or area. The record contains *fields* that are characteristics of the record. For example, a hospital patient database has a record for each client that contains separate fields for age, gender, physician's name, diagnosis, and so on. The pharmacy also has a database that lists each medication it has in stock (a record) and the strength, quantity, location, price, and manufacturer for each (the fields). The power of database programs is their ability to quickly search extremely large numbers of records and fields for commonalities, and then help the user generate detailed and complex reports.

Spreadsheets

Electronic **spreadsheets** are programs that manipulate primarily numbers. The data are arranged in columns and rows and the program can perform many complicated calculations on the data using formulas that are entered or built into the software.

Spreadsheets are used extensively for managing budgets but are also useful for working with staffing, scheduling, invoicing, research, and other analyses.

Communications

Communications devices require software to guide the computer in connecting to a remote device and knowing what data to send or receive. The various communications programs that are available must use one or more standard protocols depending on the form of communication, such as fax or file transfer, in order to communicate effectively with the distant site.

An important type of communications software is electronic mail (e-mail). E-mail has become a standard method of communication worldwide for the technologically endowed user. The e-mail package, combined with some type of network, allows the user to send messages and files to another computer using an e-mail address. The address consists of the person's identifier (name, alias, or number) and the network.

Presentation Graphics Programs

Due in part to advances in color printing and computer display hardware, software programs to create charts, graphs, tables, pictures, and other nontext files have become increasingly popular. Many integrated software packages include graphics programs that can easily exchange materials with word processing and spreadsheet programs. Users can create so-called "slide shows" for use in teaching or research presentations.

Computer Systems

The concept of a computer system—not in the sense of one machine but of a network of computers, users, and procedures in an organization—implies that there is identifiable input, processing, output, and feedback. The two most common types of computer systems used by nurses are management information systems and hospital information systems.

Management Information Systems

A **management information system (MIS)** is designed to facilitate the organization and application of data used to manage an organization or department. The system provides analyses used for planning, decision making, and evaluation of management activities. All levels of management benefit from the ability to access the data.

Hospital Information Systems

A **hospital information system (HIS)** is like an MIS except that it focuses on the types of data needed to manage client care activities and health care organizations. As with any system, the goal is to provide people with the data they need to determine appropriate actions and have control over them. Typically an HIS will have subsystems in the areas of admissions, medical records (Figure 10–1 ■), clinical laboratory, pharmacy, and finance. The personnel in these areas enter the data needed to allow management of billing, quality assurance, scheduling, and inventory both within their own areas and across the insti-

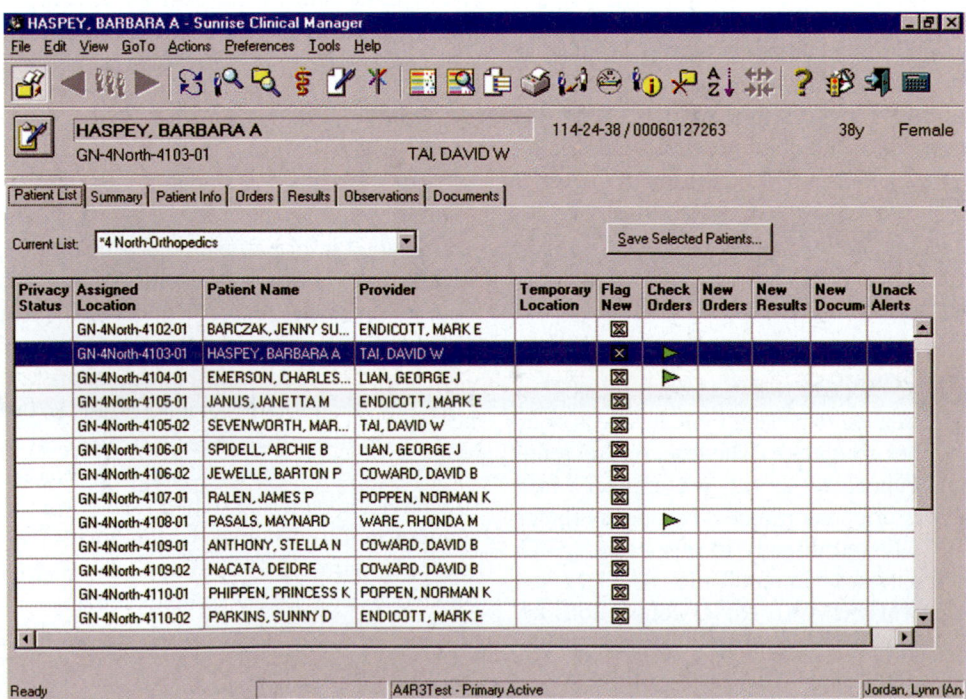

Figure 10–1 ■ Patient list screen. This is the screen that the user sees when logging into an HIS application. It is the "home base" and displays alerts and notifications regarding new orders and new results. It also gives access to other areas of the chart such as documents or results. (Courtesy of Sutter Health.)

tution as a whole. Increasingly, accrediting organizations mandate the use of an HIS and require that reports be submitted using computerized formats. Eventually, integrated HISs will form the center of all record keeping and analysis for interdisciplinary health care.

World Wide Web and the Internet

The **Internet** is a worldwide network that connects other networks. Connections among networks and PCs via the Internet allow for almost instantaneous transmission among distant sites and can include text, audio, and video data. Uses of the Internet for nurses in education, practice, and research are described later in this chapter. The **World Wide Web (WWW)** refers to the complex links among webpages or websites, accessed through "addresses" called universal resource locators (URLs). All URLs begin with the designation *http://,* which is often followed by *www.* URLs end with a designation that denotes the type of site. For example, *.com* is for commercial sites, *.org* for organizations, *.edu* for educational institutions, and *.gov* for government sites.

Tens of thousands of health-related websites exist, many new ones appearing and others becoming "dead links" daily. Consumers can access these from computers in their homes, public libraries, schools, and even cyber cafés. A risk with this extensive availability of sites is that no controls exist to ensure that the information provided is current or accurate. Nurses should evaluate health websites as they access them and assist clients in doing the same. Tools for doing this include (as of this publication) Evaluating Internet Resources from the State University of New York at Albany (http://library.albany.edu/internet/evaluate.html) and Criteria for Assessing the Quality of Health Information on the Internet—Policy Paper from the Health Information Technology Institute of Mitretek Systems Health Summit Working Group (http://hitiweb.mitretek.org/docs/policy.html).

The complexity and breadth of computer applications are expanding exponentially. Computer access is rapidly increasing while the cost tends to decrease over time. Technology is evolving in the areas of virtual reality, remote access, task automation, robotics, and bioengineering. Simultaneously, however, concerns regarding privacy, access by persons with disabilities and in underdeveloped countries, piracy, destructive programs (computer viruses), and ergonomic injuries continue to arise.

COMPUTERS IN NURSING EDUCATION

Just as computers have become standard instructional tools in the primary and secondary school systems, they are used extensively in all aspects of nursing education. Nursing programs require computerized libraries, faculty members use technological teaching strategies in the classroom and for outside assignments, and academic record keeping is facilitated by database programs.

Teaching and Learning

Computers enhance academics for both students and faculty in at least four ways. These include access to literature, CAI, classroom technologies, and strategies for learning at a distance.

Literature Access and Retrieval

In our information age, it is a challenge to keep abreast of the information on any subject. Computers have significantly improved our abilities in this area by presenting catalogs and text of materials in a way that can be searched systematically. Previously, users needed to leaf through multiple collections of printed indexes, one keyword or topic at a time. Now continuously updated cumulative indexes of related materials can be searched electronically in a fraction of the time. These bibliographic retrieval systems may be stored on CD-ROM or on a mainframe computer that can be accessed online. The searcher can specify the recency, language, document type, and other characteristics of the citation for desired materials. Once a list of search matches is displayed on the computer screen, users can select all or certain citations and either print them or store them on their own local computers. Search results can include journals and other magazines, books, videotapes, computer programs, dissertations, or other documents. Box 10–1 lists commonly used bibliographic systems and databases.

In addition to searching lists of documents, actual complete publications and materials are available in computerized formats. These include medical textbooks, the full text of journals, drug references, digitized x-rays or scans, and graphics including clip art. Through the Internet and the World Wide Web, both classic and the most current information can be found on any topic. Users can access statistics from the Centers for Disease Control and Prevention, census data, and the National Library of Medicine.

Computer-Assisted Instruction

Nursing has enjoyed the computer revolution in the form of computer-assisted instruction (CAI). Dozens of software programs help nursing students and nurses learn and demonstrate learning. These have been created by individuals, educational institutions,

---

BOX 10–1 ■ Common Health-Related Bibliographic Systems and Databases

Acquired Immune Deficiency Syndrome information onLINE (AIDSLINE)
CANCER LITerature (CANCER LIT)
Cumulative Index to Nursing and Allied Health Literature (CINAHL)
Educational Resources Information Center (ERIC)
Medical Literature Analysis and Retrieval System (MEDLARS)
Mental Measurements Yearbook
Psychological Abstracts (PsychINFO)

technology companies, or print publishers. Programs cover topics from drug dosage calculations to ethical decision making and are classified according to format: tutorial, drill-and-practice, simulation, or testing. CAI can contain diagrams, graphics, animation, video, and audio. A variation of CAI is interactive videodisc, which combines full motion and sound video with text on a laser videodisc, controlled by the user through the computer. CAI programs on CD-ROMs incorporate digitized video. All forms of CAI allow almost instant access to any section of the program and can be designed to branch to different sections depending on the user's responses.

Tutorials on electrocardiogram (ECG, EKG) interpretation, drug interactions, and legal aspects of nursing are examples of these programs. At some schools, faculties author their own programs to meet the unique needs of their students. Course syllabi that contain worksheets or activities students can complete on the computer may be distributed on disk, through the college network, or via the Internet. Students who become familiar with CAI will also find that they have an easier time adjusting to the software programs many employers require them to complete for annual competency testing mandated by accrediting bodies in certain areas (e.g., bloodborne pathogens and fire safety). Completion of CAI programs may also be an acceptable means of demonstrating continuing education activities required for license renewal.

Classroom Technology

Most new educational buildings are wired to accommodate technology. This includes adequate electric outlets for students to plug in laptop computers and wiring (or wireless technology) for network or Internet access. For the faculty, projectors and liquid crystal display (LCD) panels that allow computer screens to be displayed to the entire classroom are becoming standard. These enhancements allow faculty to use the full text, motion, and audio capabilities of computers instead of overhead transparencies, slides, or writing on the board.

Distance Learning

Computers allow people to communicate effectively across large distances. This technology is extended to nursing education where students at satellite sites participate in educational experiences. There are several different models of **distance learning.** In one model, the student receives course materials, communicates with the faculty and other students, and submits assignments completely through the mail, phone or fax, e-mail, website, and electronic "dropbox" (a server folder accessible from the Internet). This may be referred to as an asynchronous mode because the persons involved are not interacting at the same "real" time. Another model of distance education involves groups of students in classrooms at different sites participating in a class session through two-way audio and video transmission. Computers are used to code and decode the sounds and visuals for transmission. Students who are not at the site where the faculty member is located can also communicate via voice-activated microphones or response pads.

These pads have buttons that permit the students to indicate that they wish to ask a question or even to respond to multiple-choice test questions. As computer technology becomes more cost effective and increases its transmission quality, it is anticipated that more schools will use distance learning strategies to reach students around the globe.

> **CLINICAL ALERT** *Distance education courses held entirely on computer are called* online courses *whereas part computer and part classroom-based courses are often referred to as* web-enhanced courses. ■

Testing

The computer is ideal for conducting certain types of learning evaluations. Surveys can be completed online, including anonymous questionnaires. For testing, large banks of potential items can be written and the computer can generate different exams for each student depending on the selection criteria designated by the faculty. In addition, the students' answers can be scored electronically and the overall exam results analyzed quickly. In 1994, the National Council Licensure Examination for RNs in the United States (NCLEX-RN) moved from paper-and-pencil tests to computer tests. Applicants can complete the computerized exam in less than 5 hours compared to 2 days for the written exam, test results are available in about half the time, and exams can be taken at the applicant's convenience as opposed to two scheduled sessions each year. The computer determines if the applicant passed the examination by using a scoring algorithm that ensures all required competencies have been evaluated fairly.

Student and Course Record Management

Computers are also very useful for maintaining results of students' grades or attendance using spreadsheets. Often faculty are able to scan student exam answer sheets directly into a gradebook on the computer. The program can then calculate percentages, sort student scores in order, and print results for both students and faculty. Grades from multiple exams plus scores on essays or other projects are calculated into final grades.

Students are frequently asked to evaluate faculty and courses using machine-readable forms. These data are also scanned into the computer so that cumulative results can be calculated and stored. Such data can be compared later across different courses, faculty, and terms. That is an example of what is called **data warehousing**—the accumulation of large amounts of data that are stored over time and can be examined for output in different types of reports (charts and tables).

Most schools now have all student records on computer. From the student's initial application to the nursing program through graduation, the registrar's office keeps track of names, addresses, courses taken, grades, and all other pertinent student data. Students may also be able to sign up for classes, check their tuition bills, and see their transcripts on computer terminals on campus or at home. These capabilities are making it much easier for programs to collect and report data for accreditation and internal evaluation purposes.

COMPUTERS IN NURSING PRACTICE

Many activities of the registered nurse involve collecting, recording, and using data. Computers are well suited to assist the nurse in these functions. Specifically, the nurse records client information in computer records that replace or supplement the written medical record, access other departments' information on the client from centralized computers, use computers to manage client scheduling, and use programs for unique applications such as home health nursing and case management.

Documentation of Client Status and Medical Record Keeping

How might a computer assist individual nurses with their daily activities? In the typical 8-hour day of a nurse providing direct client care, as much as one-third of the time may be spent recording in the client's record. Additional time is spent trying to access data about the client that may be somewhere in the medical record or elsewhere in the health care agency. Nurses need access to standardized forms, policies, and procedures. Also, nurses need to be able to gather broader client information such as length of stay for specific diagnoses. Computers can assist with each of these.

Bedside Data Entry

Several different types of computers and systems are designated as bedside data entry or bedside terminals. These allow recording of client assessments, medication administration (Figure 10–2 ■), progress notes, care plan updating, patient acuity, and accrued charges. The terminal can be fixed or hand-held, and hardwired to the central system or cordless with the ability to transmit the data to distant sites, such as from the client's home to the agency office. A slightly different type of bedside terminal is the point-of-care or point-of-service computer. In this case the terminal is located near, but not necessarily at, the client.

Computer-Based Patient Records

Computer-based patient records (CPRs) or **electronic medical records (EMRs)** permit electronic client data retrieval by caregivers, administrators, accreditors, and other persons who require the data. The Computer-Based Patient Record Institute, established in 1992, identified four ways the CPR could improve health care: (a) constant availability of client health information across the life span, (b) ability to monitor quality, (c) access to warehoused (stored) data, and (d) ability for clients to share in knowledge and activities influencing their own health.

Because of the way computers provide access to the CPR, providers can easily retrieve specific data such as trends in vital signs (Figure 10–3 ■), immunization records, and current problems. The system can be designed to warn providers about conflicting medications or client parameters that indicate dangerous conditions (Figure 10–4 ■). Sophisticated systems can also allow replay of audio, graphic, or video data for comparison with current status. All text is legible and can be searched for keywords.

There are several areas of concern with CPRs. Maintaining privacy and security of data is a significant issue. One way that

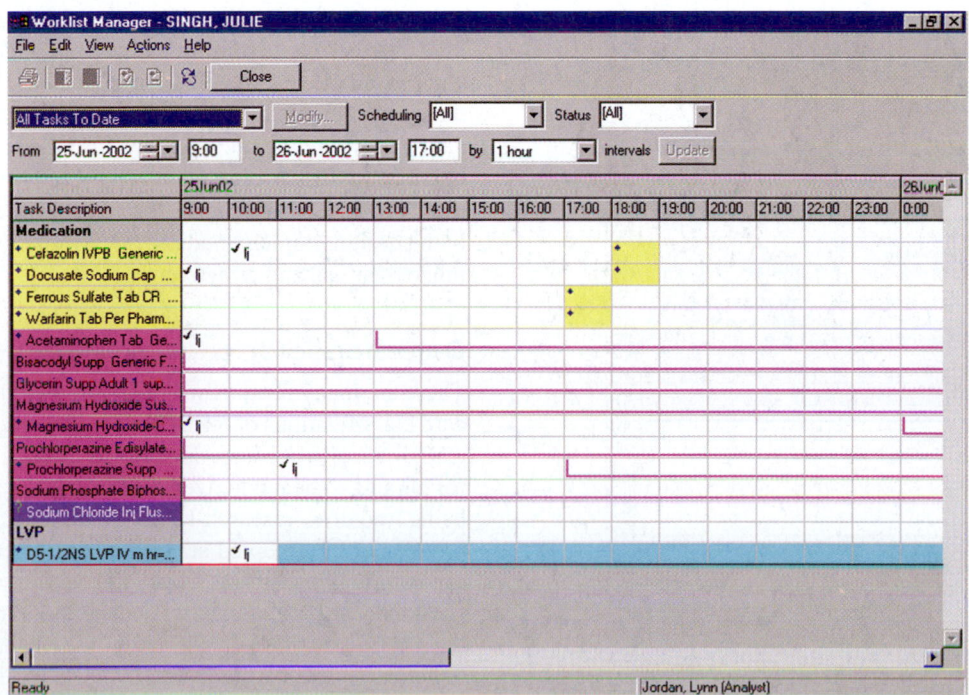

Figure 10–2 ■ This screen shows a MAR (medication administration record) for several regularly scheduled medications. The worksheet displays the next time the medications may be administered. (Courtesy of Sutter Health.)

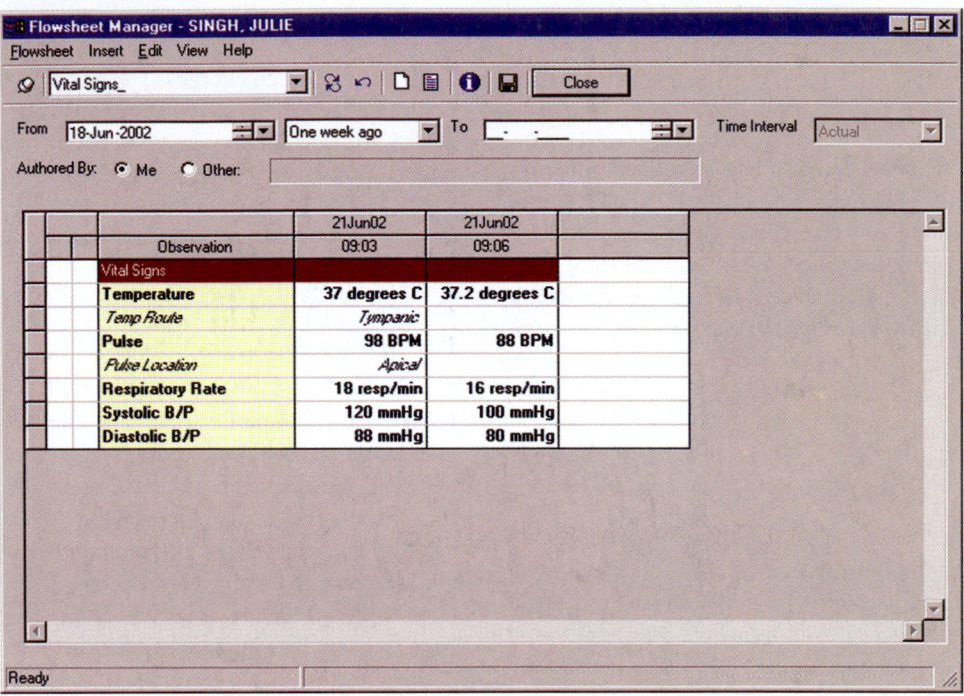

Figure 10–3 ■ This screen displays the client's vital signs. They can be entered by the nurse (or anyone with the security rights to do so) at the bedside, and they can then be displayed wherever needed. (Courtesy of Sutter Health.)

computers can protect data is by the use of passwords—only those persons who have a legitimate need to access the data receive the password. Additional policies and procedures for protecting the confidentiality of CPRs are evolving as the use of computer systems becomes more widespread. Following several previous reports, the American Nurses Association (ANA) developed a position statement on privacy, confidentiality of

medical records, and the nurse's role (see Box 10–2). One role of the **nurse informaticist,** an expert who combines computer, information, and nursing science, is to develop policies and procedures that promote effective use of computerized records by nurses and other health care professionals.

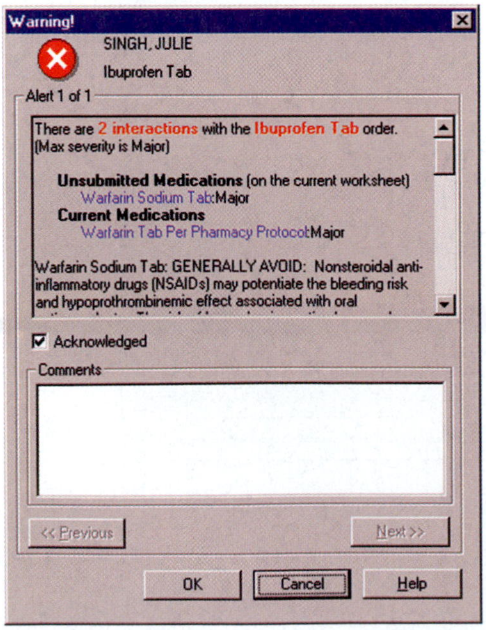

Another concern is the diverse system setups offered by manufacturers and used by health care agencies. To get the greatest benefits from the computer's ability to manage and report data between institutions requires using one set of terms and a standardized organization of database records. Currently, there are no national standards for CPRs: not for the specific data that should be included nor for how the record should be organized. HIPAA regulations (see Chapter 7 🔗) will play a key role in establishing these. Nurses will need to be involved in the design, implementation, and evaluation of CPRs to maximize their use and effectiveness.

Data Standardization and Classifications

There are many reasons why nursing would benefit from standard classifications of terms used to describe and measure clinical, disease, procedure, and outcomes data. One reason is that for nursing to be recognized for the value it adds to client well-being requires research-based findings showing client improvement by accepted standards. This requires agreement to use common, consistent, clear, and rule-based standards.

Standards for clinical data such as laboratory test results and their documentation in the CPR have been proposed by the American National Standards Institute Healthcare Informatics Standards Planning Panel, the American Society for Testing and Materials, the European Technical Committee for Standardization, the International Standards Organization, and

Figure 10–4 ■ One of the strengths of an electronic patient record is its ability to alert the clinician to potential drug interactions using warnings like the one displayed. (Courtesy of Sutter Health.)

BOX 10–2 ■ ANA Position Statement on Privacy

The Role of Nursing in Privacy and Confidentiality Related to Access to Electronic Data
1999 American Nurses Association House of Delegates

Privacy and Confidentiality
EXECUTIVE SUMMARY: Advances in technology have led to the development of computerized medical databases and telehealth systems and have raised serious concerns about patient privacy and the confidentiality of health care information. Threats to confidentiality of medical records and health care information affect the kinds of care that patients seek and potentially undermine the relationship of trust between health professionals and patients that is essential to quality health care. Nurses play a critical role in preserving patient privacy and confidentiality and should participate in the ongoing debate about and development of Federal laws designed to ensure patient privacy/confidentiality.

In keeping with the nursing profession's commitment to patient advocacy and the trust that is essential to the preservation of the high quality of care patients have come to expect from registered nurses, the American Nurses Association supports the following principles with respect to patient privacy and confidentiality:

■ A patient's right to privacy with respect to individually identifiable health information, including genetic information, should be established statutorily. Individuals should retain the right to decide to whom, and under what circumstances, their individually identifiable health information will be disclosed. Confidentiality protections should extend not only to health records, but also to all other individually identifiable health information, including genetic information, clinical research records, and mental health therapy notes.

■ Use and disclosure of individually identifiable health information should be limited.

■ A patient should have the right to access his or her own health information and the right to supplement such information so that they are able to make informed health care decisions, to correct erroneous information, and to address discrepancies that they perceive.

■ Patients should receive written, easily understood notification of how their health records are used and when their individually identifiable health information is disclosed to third parties.

■ The use or disclosure of individually identifiable health information absent an individual's informed consent should be prohibited. Exceptions should be permitted only if a person's life is endangered, if there is a threat to the public, or if there is a compelling law enforcement need. In the case of such exceptions, information should be limited to the minimum amount necessary.

■ Appropriate safeguards should be developed and required for the use, disclosure and storage of personal health information.

■ Legislative or regulatory protections on individually identifiable health information should not unnecessarily impede public health efforts or clinical, medical, nursing, or quality of care research.

■ Strong and enforceable remedies for violations of privacy protections should be established, and health care professionals who report violations should be protected from retaliation.

■ Federal legislation should provide a floor for the protection of individual privacy and confidentiality rights, not a ceiling. Federal legislation should not preempt any other federal or state law or regulation that offers greater protection.

Note: From Position Statement: Privacy and Confidentiality, by American Nurses Association, 1999. Retrieved June 5, 2003, from http://www.nursingworld.org/readroom/position/ethics/etprivcy.htm. Reprinted with permission.

---

the Workgroup for Electronic Data Interchange. Disease classification standards are in use in a variety of forms. The most common are the World Health Organization's *International Classification of Diseases* (ICD-9 and ICD-10); the World Organization of National Colleges *International Classification of Primary Care* (ICPC); and the American Psychiatric Association's *Diagnostic and Statistical Manual of Mental Disorders* (DSM).

In nursing also, classifications or taxonomies have been developed. The Nursing Minimum Data Set (NMDS) contains 16 elements of nursing data, along with their definitions, in three categories: nursing care, client demographics, and service. The NMDS can be used for data collection and documentation and allows sharing of information regarding the quality, cost, and effectiveness of nursing. In the United States, five classification systems are used: the North American Nursing Diagnosis Association (NANDA) taxonomy, the Omaha System, the Home Health Care Classification (HHCC), the Nursing Intervention Classification (NIC), and the Nursing Outcomes Classification (NOC). In addition, the International Council of Nurses has proposed an International Classification for

Nursing Practice, a common language for describing nursing problems (or diagnoses), interventions, and outcomes. It may take years to determine which standards will allow optimal access to and manipulation of computerized records.

Tracking Client Status

Once a CPR has been established, the nurse can retrieve and display a client's physiologic parameters across time (see Figure 10–5 ■). In addition to the rather straightforward viewing of trends in vital signs, for example, the nurse can also track more global client progress. Standardized nursing care plans, care maps, critical pathways, or other prewritten treatment protocols can be stored in the computer and easily placed in the CPR electronically. Then the nurse and other health care personnel can examine progression and variance from the expected plan directly on the computer.

Electronic Access to Client Data

Besides computers designed for record keeping, other computers are used extensively in health care to assess and monitor

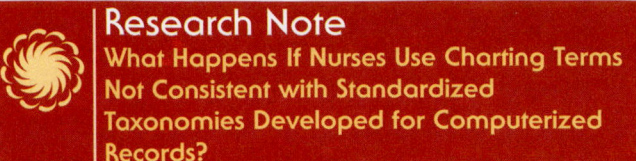

Research Note

What Happens If Nurses Use Charting Terms Not Consistent with Standardized Taxonomies Developed for Computerized Records?

In a Norwegian study, terms from the International Classification for Nursing Practice (ICNP) that relate to elimination and circulation were compared to those found in chart records of hospital critical care and home care clients. About half of the concept terms but only one-third of intervention terms matched. In particular, there were few matches for terms that related to the client's subjective experience. The researchers also did not find the use of the ICNP "user friendly."

Implications: Standardized taxonomies of terms are needed to enhance the ability to benefit from computerization of client records. Nurses can no longer use any terms desired—they must be able to locate and invoke terms that have standardized meaning and, thus, can be tracked, evaluated, researched, and so on. The researchers recommend that the ICNP be reevaluated for ease of navigation and that additional terms be created to match those missing from the taxonomy but found in client records. Further extensive research will be needed in various settings, nationally and internationally, before a substantially complete classification system can exist.

Note: From "Evaluating the Beta Version of the International Classification For Nursing Practice for Domain Completeness, Applicability of Its Axial Structure and Utility in Clinical Practice: A Norwegian Project," by C. M. Ruland, 2001, *International Nursing Review, 48*(1), pp. 9–16.

clients' conditions. The data accumulated from various electronic devices can be part of the CPR and also stored for research purposes. Electronic records take up much less space than paper records and may be stored more securely. Copies can be made easily onto different electronic media (e.g., magnetic tape, microfiche) that tend to be more compact and durable than paper. Data can also be transmitted to a consulting specialist in another location.

Client Monitoring and Computerized Diagnostics

Nursing has benefited greatly from the myriad of client monitors. Examples in everyday practice are the digital or tympanic thermometers, digital scales, pulse oximetry, ECG/telemetry/hemodynamic monitoring, apnea monitors, fetal heart monitors, blood glucose analyzers, ventilators, and intravenous (IV) pumps. These instruments can be used in any care setting, from intensive care to the home. Most keep a record of the most recent values. Some can transmit their data to a more sophisticated computer or print out a paper record. Some have digital displays that "talk" to the user, giving instructions or results. Most also have error detection or alarms that indicate either that the instrument is malfunctioning or that the assessed value is outside predetermined parameters. These devices, with their minute but powerful computer chips, make it possible to extend the nurse's observations and provide valid and reliable data.

In various specialty areas of health care, clients undergo diagnostic procedures in which computers play a major role. Computerized axial tomography (CAT) scans and magnetic resonance imaging (MRI) use computers extensively to perform tests and analyze the findings. Blood gas analyzers, pulmonary

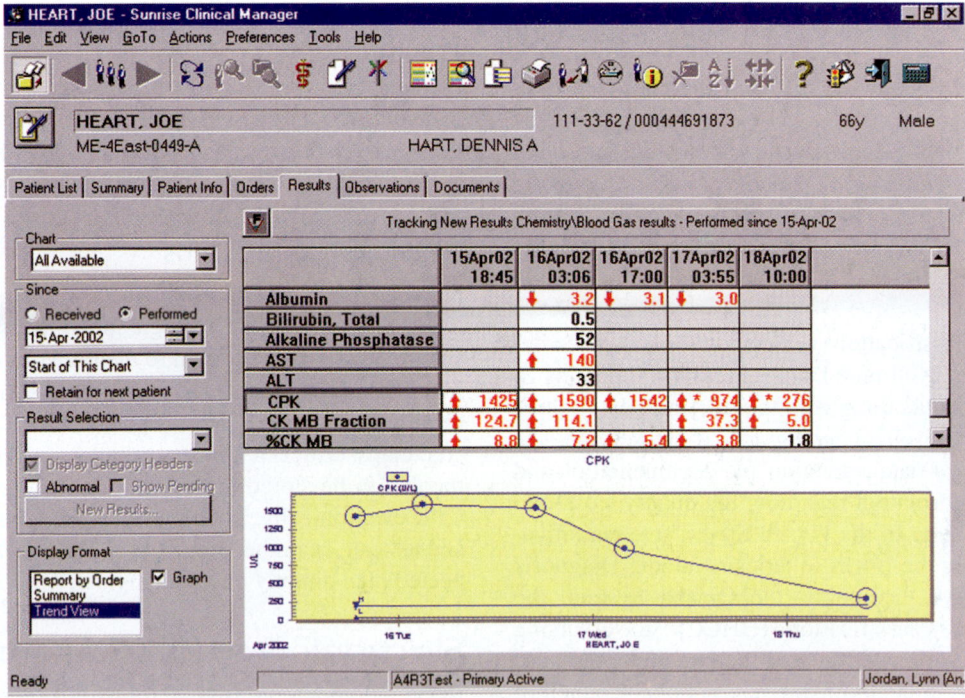

Figure 10–5 ■ Lab results are displayed in a Trend View with a graph. (Courtesy of Sutter Health.)

function test machines, and intracranial pressure monitors all use computer processing. All of these can be linked directly to store data in the CPR (see Figure 10–6 ■). There are many more examples of ways that computers assist us in monitoring and diagnosing client conditions.

Telemedicine/Telehealth

One of the most exciting areas being developed in computer-assisted health care is **telemedicine**. Telemedicine uses technology to transmit electronic data about clients to persons at distant locations. In one example, two-way audiovisual communication allows an international expert to examine and consult on a client's case from thousands of miles away. X-rays, scans, stored computer data, and almost anything imaginable can be "sent" using computers. Another example is the ability for a few providers to provide primary health care to people living in remote areas using the kinds of monitors described previously plus telephone, fax, and other relatively simple equipment in the client's home.

Concerns regarding telehealth relate to legal and ethical issues. Who has responsibility for the client when a teleconsult is used? Does the care provider need to be licensed in the state or province where the client's primary care is given? The National Council of State Boards of Nursing has declared that the applicable regulations are those for where the patient resides and not where the provider is located. This is also one of the reasons for the initiation of the Mutual Recognition Compact that boards of nursing are promulgating to facilitate nurses licensure in several states. How is the client's privacy protected? HIPAA and several other projects are under way to answer these questions and to determine the most effective designs for telehealth programs.

Practice Management

Beyond direct client care, computers also assist nurses in many ways in the management of their work. In hospitals, data terminals are commonly used to order supplies, tests, meals, and services from other departments. Tracking of these orders allows the nursing service to determine the most frequent or most costly items used by a particular nursing unit. This information may lead to decisions to modify a budget, provide different staffing, move supplies to a different location, or make other changes for more efficient and higher quality care.

Computers are used extensively for scheduling. Client appointments can be easily entered or changed. Special notes or tags can be applied to the appointment as a reminder to the provider to perform particular services. The schedule for a single day can be printed so that all personnel have a copy. Staffing patterns must also be coordinated. Special requests for days off or continuing education classes can be entered and the schedule can be viewed for a day, week, month, or year.

Each practice needs to keep track of procedures health care workers perform, client diagnoses, and time spent with clients so that billing can be accurate. With managed care, information tracking is also aimed at determining trends in health problems and the need for providers with specific skills. The use of computerized databases filled with unique codes for each medication, medical and nursing diagnoses, treatment, and supply allows for accurate and timely management of these data.

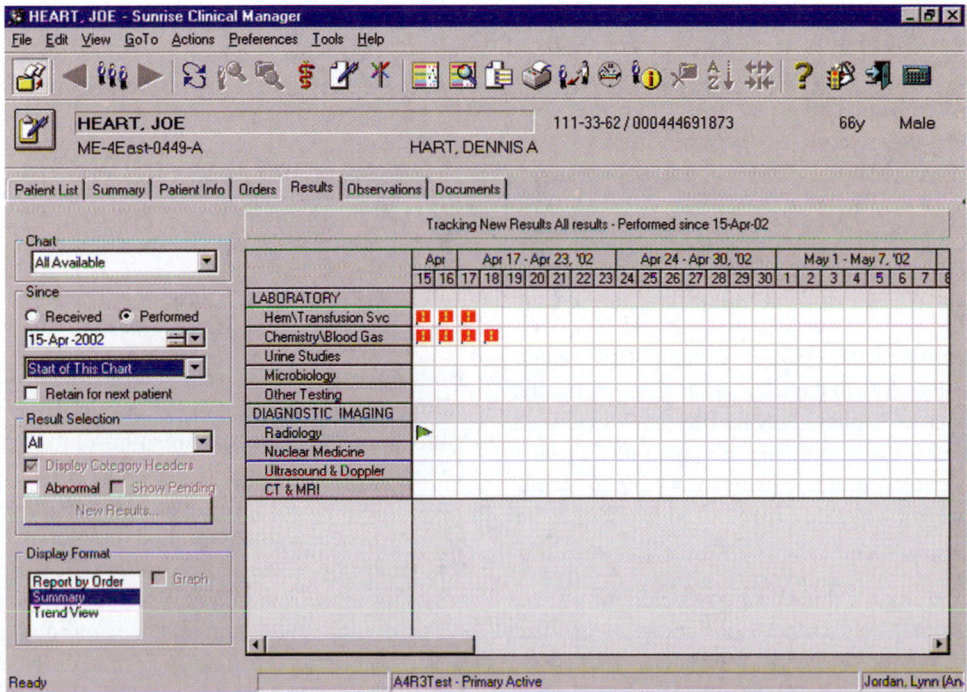

Figure 10–6 ■ This screen displays a summary view of all available results for a particular client. In this case, the red rectangular flag indicates that at least one of the results is normal. The information is always reported from most summarized to most detailed so that the user gets an overview first and can then "drill down" to see the details. (Courtesy of Sutter Health.)

Specific Applications of Computers in Nursing Practice

As previously described, numerous systems are in use for collecting and classifying the various types of data used in nursing practice. Some of these systems have been found particularly useful in specific settings.

Community and Home Health

Computer networks are being used in innovative ways in home settings. A computer terminal placed in a high-risk client's or family's home allows them to access information on a variety of topics, search the Internet, or e-mail a health care provider with questions or concerns. Clients can also record data about their health status that can be transmitted to the health care provider at the central network computer. Examples that have been successful using this approach include monitoring women at risk for preterm labor, persons with AIDS, and Alzheimer's patients. Home alert systems that allow the client to signal the base station in an emergency are also widely used.

Nurses who visit clients in their homes are using notebook computer systems to record assessments and transmit data to the main office. Similar systems have been developed for nursing students in community health courses to communicate with their faculty.

Case Management

Case managers must be able to track a group of clients—the caseload. Software programs allow the case manager to enter client data and integrate this with predesigned care tracking templates. In addition, the case manager must keep abreast of the latest regulations affecting eligibility for health care benefits, the reporting requirements of the payer agencies, and detailed facts about the variety of service providers the client may need to access. All of these data can be placed in integrated computer software programs. Finally, the case manager must document quality; that is, demonstrate client outcomes related to dollars spent.

COMPUTERS IN NURSING ADMINISTRATION

As indicated in the section of this chapter on computers in nursing practice, the volume of data that nurses need to have available and the additional volume of data generated by nurses can and must be managed electronically. Nursing administrators require these data in order to develop strategic plans for the organization.

Human Resources

All employers must maintain a database, computerized or not, on each employee. In addition to the usual demographic and salary data, the database for licensed or certified health care personnel has unique fields for areas such as life support certification, health requirements (e.g., tuberculosis testing, hepatitis immunization, rubella titers), and performance appraisals. Administrators can use this human resources database to communicate with employees, examine staffing patterns, and create budget projections.

Medical Records Management

Costs are inherent in and reflected by medical records. It is expensive to keep records but it is even more expensive not to be able to access what is in them. Therefore, nurses require computer programs that allow client records to be searched for trends such as the most common presenting diagnoses, number of cases by diagnosis-related groups, most expensive cases, length of stay or total number of days the case was open, and client outcomes. Nurse informaticists can assist administrators with the design and implementation of systems that allow for such searches to be generated, analyzed, printed, and distributed.

Facilities Management

Many aspects of managing buildings and non-nursing services can be facilitated by computer. Heating, air conditioning, and ventilation systems are computer controlled. Security devices such as readers that scan identification cards, bar codes, or magnetic strips permit only authorized personnel to enter client or private areas. Computers also manage and report inventory, tracking everything from pillowcases to syringes.

Budget and Finance

Advantages of computerized billing are that claims are transmitted much more quickly and have a greater likelihood of being complete and accurate. If this is the case, claims will be paid sooner and the agency will have control over its financial status. Computers can also effect cost savings by reducing the clerical services time needed for accounts payable and receivable. In cases where nursing can directly bill and be reimbursed by payers, the same benefits of computerized accounting apply.

The budget itself is generally a spreadsheet program. This software allows tracking as well as forecasting and planning. In uncertain times, the ability to perform "what if" calculations is especially valuable.

Quality Assurance and Utilization Reviews

Both internal and external stakeholders in health care organizations need to know that the services and activities of the organization have positive results. Once standards, pathways, key indicators, and other vital data have been identified and described, computers can facilitate the analysis of the data. Quality is considered a process and not an end point. Applying this perspective, computerized systems are ideal for taking a snapshot view of the institution's quality indices at any time.

Utilization review consists of examining trends and proposing advantageous disposition of resources (specifically, length of stay). For example, might clients who have had a fractured hip repaired have equivalent outcomes at lesser cost if transferred from the hospital to a skilled nursing facility sooner? Studies can be conducted with computer analyses to answer such questions.

Accreditation

The Joint Commission on Accreditation of Healthcare Organizations (JCAHO) has mandated that hospitals have online mechanisms to monitor quality indicators, so as to reduce the difficulty and time involved in the accreditation process. JCAHO has also required a move to computer systems that assess outcomes rather than processes.

Another aspect of accreditation review is demonstrating adequate staffing for the number and acuity of clients. Each agency, whether hospital, outpatient, or home care, must use a method of determining the number of hours of nursing care required for their current clients. This method can consider the severity of the clients' illnesses, length of time needed to perform certain procedures, training and expertise of the nursing staff, and any other parameters desired.

COMPUTERS IN NURSING RESEARCH

Computers are invaluable assistants in the conduct of both quantitative and qualitative nursing research. In each step of the research process, computers facilitate generation, refinement, analysis, and output of data. Computer resources are an important component of the planning phase of any research project: The size of the computer and its storage capacity must be adequate for the amount of data that will be collected, and the proper software programs must be in place to manage and analyze the data. Computerized word processing is also an integral component in the publication and dissemination of research.

Problem Identification

The first step of the research process is to identify and describe the problem of interest. The computer can be useful in locating current literature about the problem and related concepts. Perhaps, unknown to the researcher, a solution to the problem has already been found and reported. A search of existing documents, and e-mail to colleagues, may help define the problem.

Literature Review

An exhaustive review of the print literature can be time consuming. Without computer access to online or CD-ROM bibliographic databases, the researcher must wade through huge volumes of publications. The software programs that facilitate searches contain thesauruses so that the most appropriate terms can be selected. If the researcher determines that little has been published on the topic of interest, closely related terms and topics must also be searched. It is not unusual for a researcher to collect more than 100 pertinent research or theoretical references during the literature review. The increase in availability of full-text journal articles online has made the electronic literature search process even more productive.

Research Design

The design of a research study, including the choice of specific research method, is always driven by the research question. At the design stage the investigator determines whether the study will use a qualitative or quantitative approach, what instruments will be used to collect data, and the types of analyses that will be carried out on the data to answer the research questions. Computers may be used during this step to search the literature for instruments that have already been established or to design and test instruments that need to be developed for the particular study. In addition, the investigator would not likely select an instrument or design that requires extensive computer or mathematical analysis if such resources are not available.

Data Collection and Analysis

Once the types of data to be collected have been determined, the investigator will create forms on the computer for collecting the data. These may include the informed consent document, a tool to collect demographic data, and recording forms for research variables. If possible, computer-readable forms are created so that the data can be scanned directly into the computer or the participant can enter responses directly into the computer (e.g., an online survey). This eliminates the errors that may occur if the researcher must enter the data into the computer manually.

It is particularly important that all variables that will be computer analyzed are identified in a way that the computer can recognize and manipulate. This may mean determining how to code the data for optimal manipulation. For example, will age be recorded in specific years or by categories such as 1–10, 11–15, 16–20, and so on? Software programs can assist with the analysis and coding of qualitative data. Such programs as N6 (formerly Nud*ist, an acronym for Non-numerical Unstructured Data with powerful processes of Indexing Searching and Theorizing) and Ethnograph assist the researcher in finding and coding sections of text and organizing coded material.

When the variables have been coded, other programs can be used to calculate descriptive and analytic statistics. Calculations that formerly were extremely time consuming and complex can now be done by computer programs quickly and accurately. Commonly used software programs for quantitative data analysis include SPSS (Statistical Package for the Social Sciences), SAS (Statistical Analysis System), SysSTAT, and MYSTAT. These programs perform analyses and display output in tables, charts, lists, and other easily read formats.

Research Dissemination

Research is of limited value if the findings are not widely dispersed to the practitioners who can use the findings to improve their practice. Computer word processing programs are used to author the final reports of research and to send the reports to various readerships. Many journals now require that manuscripts submitted for publication include both hardcopy and diskette versions. As noted earlier in this chapter, the number of electronic journals is increasing. With the rapid growth of e-mail, authors can also send an article or data to interested persons instantaneously. Computers speed completion of a research project and the availability of the findings to the public.

Computers are frequently used to present research at meetings. Using computer projectors to display screens of data and findings also allows the researcher to highlight, modify, and manipulate content in an instant. In the future, we will see computer conferencing where researchers collaborate on a study from distant locations and can examine and analyze the data simultaneously on screen.

Research Grants

Funds are available from a variety of resources to support the conduct of nursing research. The budget in a grant application may include a request to purchase computers or software needed to carry out the proposed study. Funds may also be requested to pay people to enter data into the computer and to run the statistical analyses.

Information about available grant funding is most easily found online. The U.S. federal government makes all of the grant applications for nursing projects available only by downloading them from Internet sites. Forms to be completed are computer generated and often must be submitted to the funding agency in electronic format.

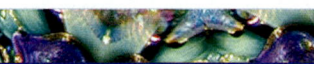

Lifespan Considerations

Elders

Computer classes are being taught to increasing numbers of elders. Use of the computer provides them with an avenue of communication and exposure to a vast amount of health care information. Although nurses have little control over what Internet sites will be accessed, it is important to teach clients and the general public to evaluate information from the site and to be aware that misinformation can also be presented. Important guidelines that increase the validity of a site are as follows:

■ The article or information lists the author and credentials and/or the institution from which the information came.

■ A date is listed that states when information was updated.
■ If health care information is presented, a disclaimer should be included. The disclaimer presents limitations of the information and should say that it is not medical advice.

Computer-assisted programs can be very effective teaching aids for elders. They may provide audio and visual instruction and may even be interactive. They are useful for teaching about medical conditions and medications and for providing information about procedures and surgeries to be performed.

Focus on Critical Thinking

As a nurse working for a home care agency in a small, rural town, you would like your clients to receive up-to-date and accurate health information and care. High-speed computer access is available in your office and many of the residents have computers in their homes since it provides a low-cost way of communicating with friends and relatives who are far away (for example, using e-mail and sending digitized photos).

1. You have a difficult clinical case and want to investigate possible interventions. What are some of the ways computers could assist in this endeavor?

2. You decide that sending photos of the client would be useful to your colleagues in providing input. Since time is an issue, you determine that sending them electronically would be most expeditious. The client agrees to the photos but is worried about privacy in sending them through the computer. How would you handle this?

3. A client shares with you a website that states it can guarantee a cure to the client's illness. How would you respond?

4. You are considering enrolling in an advanced degree program that is offered online. What would be some of the advantages and disadvantages of such a program?

See Critical Thinking Possibilities in Appendix A.

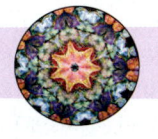 ## | Chapter Review

EXPLORE MediaLink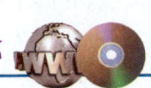

NCLEX review questions, case studies, MediaLink applications, and other interactive resources for this chapter can be found on the Companion Website at www.prenhall.com/kozier. Click on Chapter 10 to select the activities for this chapter.

For more NCLEX review questions, and an audio glossary, access the Student CD-ROM accompanying this textbook.

Chapter Highlights

- Computer hardware consists of the central processing unit, memory, the keyboard and other input devices, and the monitor and other output devices.
- Common computer software programs used in nursing are word processors, databases, spreadsheets, communications, computer-assisted instruction, and presentation graphics.
- A hospital information system (HIS) organizes data from various areas in the hospital such as admissions, medical records, clinical laboratory, pharmacy, and finance.
- Concerns regarding privacy and confidentiality of health records have arisen as electronic databases and communications have proliferated.
- Computers are used extensively to locate and access data through online databases and Internet searching. Many nursing journals are electronic.
- Computer-assisted instruction programs include tutorial, drill-and-practice, and simulations. Programs are also available that simulate the national licensure examination in the United States.
- In distance learning, the faculty and student may be located far apart and communicate via computer, phone, fax, and video technologies.
- Bedside entry of nursing data is becoming more prevalent. Studies on whether these systems save nursing time have conflicting results.
- Computerized patient records (CPRs) enable longitudinal data to be collected on a client and made available to all health care providers who require it. Such data warehousing also enables research to be conducted on quality of care, client outcomes, and a variety of other parameters. However, no national standards exist for the structure or contents of these records.
- Nurses need to participate in the creation of taxonomies and classifications of electronic data. Existing models include the World Health Organization's International Classification of Diseases (ICD-9 and ICD-10), the World Organization of National Colleges' International Classification of Primary Care (ICPC), the American Psychiatric Association's *Diagnostic and Statistical Manual of Mental Disorders* (DSM), the North American Nursing Diagnosis Association (NANDA) taxonomy, the Omaha System, the Home Health Care Classification (HHCC), the Nursing Intervention Classification (NIC), the Nursing Outcomes Classification (NOC), International Council of Nurses' International Classification of Nursing Practice, and the Nursing Minimum Data Set (NMDS).
- Computer monitoring and diagnosing of client conditions is widespread. Examples include digital or tympanic thermometers, digital scales, pulse oximetry, ECG/telemetry/hemodynamic monitoring, apnea monitors, fetal heart monitors, blood glucose analyzers, ventilators, IV pumps, CAT scans, and MRI.
- Telehealth, the conduct of the health care profession using electronic means of communication, is a growing area that generates both excitement and concerns.
- Data terminals in health care settings allow placing of order requests and retrieval of client data and accounts. Appointments can be scheduled on computer.
- Computers are used by home health nurses to record client data and to communicate with the central office. Clients can also have computers in the home that allow them to monitor their own health status and send information about their condition to the nurse.
- Specialized computer software programs enable case managers to track clients' needs, resources, and health care outcomes.
- Computers are used in nursing administration to manage personnel, human resources, facilities, budgets, quality assurance, utilization review, staffing and scheduling, and accreditation.
- Each step of the nursing research process makes use of computer technology. In particular, computers are used to access literature, analyze data, and report findings.

Review Questions

10–1. A textbook publisher wishes to store large amounts of data in a computer format that cannot be changed by other people. Which of the following would best serve this purpose?
   a. CD-ROM
   b. RAM
   c. floppy diskette
   d. network

10–2. The greatest concern about electronic patient records is that of
   a. cost.
   b. accuracy.
   c. privacy.
   d. durability.

10–3. A drawback to using electronic (e.g., Internet-based) courses over face-to-face is
   a. they take longer.
   b. interpersonal communication is not possible.
   c. everyone has to "log on" at the same time.
   d. it is harder to establish a sense of community.

10–4. In research, the major way that computers enhance the speed and accuracy of the process is by assisting the researcher to
   a. locate potential participants.
   b. design the steps of the research plan.
   c. analyze the quantitative data.
   d. disseminate the research findings.

10–5. A client insists that the practitioner use a treatment method the client found on a website. The nurse appropriately responds that
   a. the treatment must be examined to see if it is appropriate.
   b. website treatments have not been studied or researched.
   c. only the person who put the treatment on the website can use it on clients.
   d. websites are like advertising, they are biased and may not be legitimate.

Readings and References

Suggested Readings

Nagelkerk, J., Ritola, P. M., & Vandort, P. J. (1998). Nursing informatics: The trend of the future. *Journal of Continuing Education in Nursing, 29*(1), 17–21.
Nursing informatics is a combination of computer information and nursing sciences. The authors state it is essential to prepare nurses for computerized technology to use the most cost-effective methods. Six essential factors for preparing nurses for computerization are strong leadership, effective communication, organized training sessions, established time frames, planned change, and tailored software.

Sibbald, B. (1998). Nursing informatics for beginners. *Canadian Nurse, 94*(4), 22–30.
Sibbald discusses the significance of nursing informatics for nurses. She emphasizes that through informatics, nurses can make decisions based on the latest research, up-to-the-minute patient data, and on-site consultations with experts worldwide. Informatics can not only help nurses improve quality care, it allows them to document their worth for the first time.

Related Research

Currell, R., Wainwright, P., & Urquhart, C. (2001). Nursing record systems: Effects on nursing practice and health care outcomes. *The Cochrane Library, 2* [Computer software]. Abstract retrieved September 3, 2002 from CINAHL database.

Hardiker, N. R., & Rector, A. L. (2001). Structural validation of nursing terminologies. *Journal of the American Medical Informatics Association, 8*, 212–221.

Larrabee, J. H., Boldreghini, S., Elder-Sorrells, K., Turner, Z. M., Wender, R. G., Hart, J. M., et al. (2001). Evaluation of documentation before and after implementation of a nursing information system in an acute care hospital. *Computers in Nursing, 19*(2), 56–68.

Rosen, E. L., & Routon, C. M. (1998). American Nursing Informatics role survey. *Computers in Nursing, 16*, 171–175.

References

American Nurses Association, (1997). *Position statement: Privacy and confidentiality.* Retrieved October 27, 2002, from http://www.nursingworld.org/readroom/position/ethics/etprivacy.htm.

Computer-Based Patient Record Institute. (1992). Newsletters and membership brochures. Chicago: Author.

Ruland, C. M. (2001) Evaluating the beta version of the International Classification for Nursing Practice for domain completeness, applicability, of its axial structure and utility in clinical practice: A Norwegian project. *International Nursing Review, 48*(1), 9–16.

Selected Bibliography

Anthony, D. (2000).Current issues in nursing informatics, *Nurse Researcher, 8*(2), 18–28.

Ball, M. J., Hannah, K. J., Newbold, S. K., & Douglas, J. V. (Eds.). (2000). *Nursing informatics: Where caring and technology meet.* New York: Springer-Verlag.

Boyd, L. (2001). Healthcare and the net: Monitoring patients. *RN, 64*(2), 53–54.

Burke, L., & Weill, B. (1999). *Information technology for the health professions.* Upper Saddle River, NJ: Prentice Hall.

Carty, B. (2000). *Nursing informatics: Education for practice.* New York: Springer.

Christman, L. P. (2001). Nursing informatics: Education for practice. *Nursing Administration Quarterly, 25*(3), 92.

Clark, P. M., & Gomez, E. G. (2001). Details on demand: Consumers, cancer information, and the Internet. *Clinical Journal of Oncology Nursing, 5*(1), 19–24.

Cohen, C. (2001). Healthcare and the net: Guiding seniors. *RN, 64*(2), 50–52.

Curtin, L., & Simpson, R. L. (2001). Automated billing systems and compliance. *Health Management Technology, 22*(8), 40–41.

Curtin, L., & Simpson, R. L. (2001). Standards of practice for nursing informatics. *Health Management Technology, 22*(4), 52.

Czar, P., Mascara, C. M., & Hebda, T. (2000). *Handbook of informatics for nurses and health care professionals.* Upper Saddle River, NJ: Prentice-Hall.

Detwiler, S. M., Basch, R., & Barrett, S. (2000). *Super searchers on health & medicine: The online secrets of top health & medical researchers.* Medford, NJ: Cyberage Books.

Gilder, R. E. (1999). Enhancing perioperative nursing effectiveness through informatics. *AORN Journal, 69*, 978–987.

Goossen, W. (2000). Nursing informatics research. *Nurse Researcher, 8*(2), 42–54.

Hannah, K. J., Ball, M. J., & Edwards, M. J. A. (1999). *Introduction to nursing informatics* (2nd ed.). New York: Springer-Verlag.

Hebda, T. L., Czar, P., & Mascara, C. (2001). *Handbook of informatics for nursing and health professionals* (2nd ed.). Upper Saddle River, NJ: Prentice Hall Health.

Joos, I. M., Whitman, N., Smith, M., & Nelson, R. (Eds.). (2000). *Computers in small bytes: A workbook for healthcare professionals.* New York: National League for Nursing.

Lehoux, P., Battista, R.N., & Lance, J. (2000). Telehealth: Passing fad or lasting benefits. *Canadian Journal of Public Health, 91*, 277–280.

Lundberg, C. B. (2000). Nursing informatics: Using uniform language in patient care documentation. *Nursing Economics, 18*(1), 38–39.

Mantas, J. (Ed.). (2001). *Textbook in health informatics: A nursing perspective.* Amsterdam: IOS Press.

Mascara, C. M., Czar, P., & Hebda, T. (2000). *Internet resource guide for nurses & health care professionals.* Upper Saddle River, NJ: Prentice-Hall.

Mildon, J., & Cohen, T. (2001). Drivers in the medical records market. *Health Management Technology, 22*(5), 14, 16, 18.

Rewick, D., & Gaffey, E. (2001). Nursing system makes a difference. *Health Management Technology, 22*(8), 24–26.

Saba, V. K., & McCormick, K. A. (Eds.). (2001). *Essentials of computers for nurses: Informatics for the new millennium* (3rd ed.). New York: McGraw-Hill.

Schilp, J. L., & Gilbreath, R. E. (Eds.). (2000). *Health data quest: How to find and use data for performance improvement.* San Francisco: Jossey-Bass.

Shortliffe, E. H., Wiederhold, G., Perreault, L. E., & Fagan, L. M. (Eds.). (2000). *Medical informatics: Computer applications in health care and biomedicine (health informatics).* New York: Springer-Verlag.

Simpson, R. L. (1999). The state of nursing informatics. *Nursing Administration Quarterly, 23*, 90–92.

Simpson, R. L. (2001). Size up the big three. *Nursing Management, 32*(3), 12–14.

Slack, W., Nader, R., & Slack, C. (2001). *Cybermedicine: How computing empowers doctors and patients for better care.* San Francisco: Jossey-Bass.

Staggers, N., Thompson, C. B., & Snyder-Halpern, R. (2001). History and trends in clinical information systems in the United States. *Journal of Nursing Scholarship, 33*, 75–81.

Young, K. M. (Ed.). (2000). *Informatics for health-care professionals.* Philadelphia: F. A. Davis.

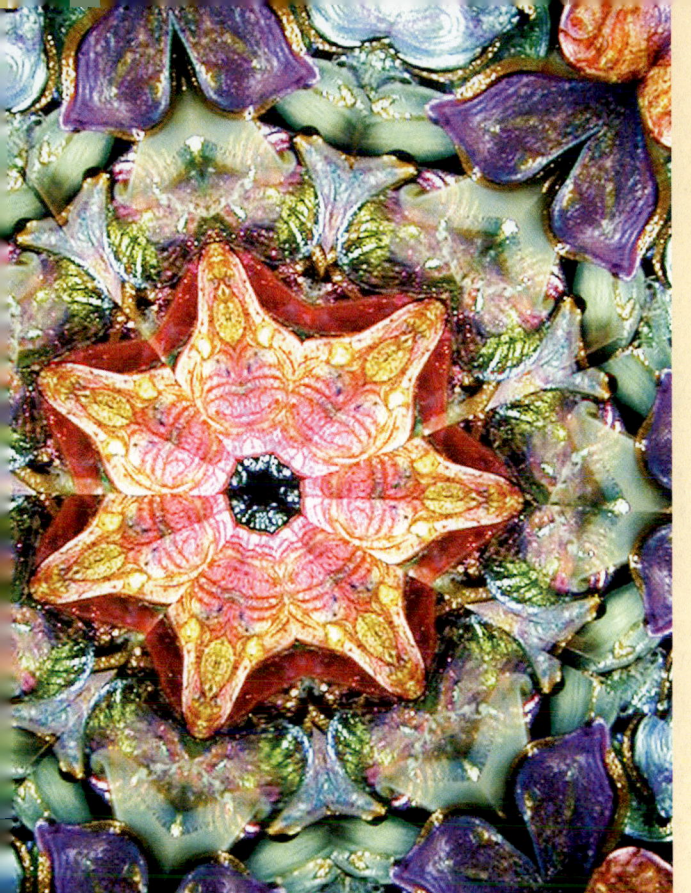

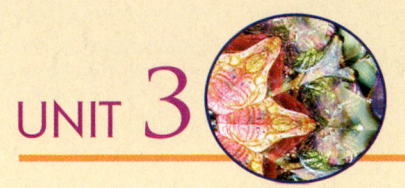

HEALTH BELIEFS AND PRACTICES

As increasingly knowledgeable health care consumers, clients expect and deserve quality care. While assisting the client – whether an individual, family, or entire community – quality nursing care seeks to emphasize illness prevention and health promotion. Nurses recognize that a client's state of health and wellness encompasses many dimensions, including social, spiritual, cultural, sexual, and environmental, as well as physical and psychological. Each client encounter affords the nurse an opportunity to influence and encourage both traditional and innovative health-seeking behaviors.

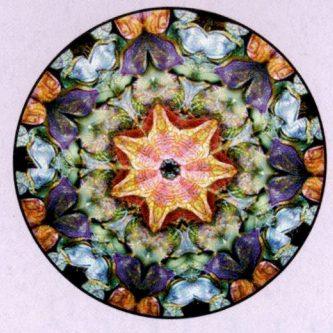

CHAPTER | 11

HEALTH, WELLNESS, AND ILLNESS

LEARNING OUTCOMES

After completing this chapter, you will be able to:

- Differentiate health, wellness, and well-being.
- Describe five dimensions of wellness.
- Compare various models of health outlined in this chapter.
- Identify factors affecting health status, beliefs, and practices.
- Describe factors affecting health care adherence.
- Differentiate illness from disease and acute illness from chronic illness.
- Identify Parsons' four aspects of the sick role.
- Explain Suchman's stages of illness.
- Describe effects of illness on individuals' and family members' roles and functions.

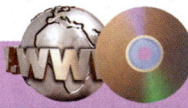

MediaLink

www.prenhall.com/kozier

Additional resources for this chapter can be found on the Student CD-ROM accompanying this textbook, and on the Companion Website at www.prenhall.com/kozier. Click on Chapter 11 to select the activities for this chapter.

CD-ROM
• Audio Glossary
• NCLEX Review

Companion Website
• Additional NCLEX Review
• Case Study: Nonadherent Diabetic Client
• MediaLink Application: Health Beliefs
• Links to Resources

Nurses need to clarify their understanding of health and wellness because their definitions largely determine the scope and nature of nursing practice. Clients' health beliefs also influence their health practices. Some people think of health and wellness (or well-being) as the same thing or, at the very least, as accompanying one another. However, health may not always accompany well-being: A person who has a terminal illness may have a sense of well-being; conversely, another person may lack a sense of well-being yet be in a state of good health. For many years the concept of disease was the yardstick by which health was measured. In the late 19th century the "how" of disease (pathogenesis) was the major concern of health professionals. Currently the emphasis on health and wellness is increasing.

CONCEPTS OF HEALTH, WELLNESS, AND WELL-BEING

Health, wellness, and well-being have many definitions and interpretations. The nurse should be familiar with the most common aspects of the concepts and consider how they may be individualized with specific clients.

Health

There is no consensus about any definition of health. There is knowledge of how to attain a certain level of health, but health itself cannot be measured.

Traditionally **health** has been defined in terms of the presence or absence of disease. Nightingale defined health as a state of being well and using every power the individual possesses to the fullest extent (Nightingale, 1969). The World Health Organization (WHO) takes a more holistic view of health. Its constitution defines health as "a state of complete physical, mental, and social well-being, and not merely the absence of disease or infirmity" (WHO, 1948). This definition

- Reflects concern for the individual as a total person functioning physically, psychologically, and socially. Mental processes determine people's relationship with their physical and social surroundings, their attitudes about life, and their interaction with others.
- Places health in the context of environment. People's lives, and therefore their health, are affected by everything they interact with—not only environmental influences such as climate and the availability of nutritious food, comfortable shelter, clean air to breathe, and pure water to drink, but also other people, including family, lovers, employers, coworkers, friends, and associates of various kinds.
- Equates health with productive and creative living. It focuses on the living state rather than on categories of disease that may cause illness or death.

Health has also been defined in terms of role and performance. Talcott Parsons (1951), an eminent American sociologist and creator of the concept "sick role," conceptualized health as the ability to maintain normal roles.

In 1953, the (United States) President's Commission on Health Needs of the Nation made the following statement about health: "Health is not a condition; it is an adjustment. It is not a state but a process. The process adapts the individual not only to our physical but also our social environments" (President's Commission, 1953, p. 4). This definition emphasizes health as an adaptive process rather than a state.

In 1980, the American Nurses Association (ANA) defined health in its social policy statement as "a dynamic state of being in which the developmental and behavioral potential of an individual is realized to the fullest extent possible" (ANA, 1980, p. 5). In this definition, health is more than a state or the absence of disease; it includes striving toward optimal functioning.

In the past few decades a number of health professionals, including nurse theorists, have provided definitions of health and wellness (see Chapter 3). ᴳᴼ

Personal Definitions of Health

Health is a highly individual perception. Consider the following examples of individuals who would probably say they are healthy even though they have physical impairments that some would consider an illness:

- Devon Dobrowski, a 15-year-old with diabetes, takes injectable insulin each morning. He plays on the school soccer team and is editor of the high school newspaper.
- John Talbot, age 32, is paralyzed from the waist down and needs a wheelchair for mobility. He is taking accounting at a nearby college and uses a specially designed automobile for transportation.
- Susan Helmer, age 72, takes antihypertensive medications to treat high blood pressure. She bowls once a week, is a member of the neighborhood golf club, makes handicrafts for a local charity, and travels 2 months each year.

Most people define and describe health as the following:

- Being free from symptoms of disease and pain as much as possible
- Being able to be active and to do what they want or must
- Being in good spirits most of the time.

These characteristics indicate that health is not something that a person achieves suddenly at a specific time. It is an ongoing process—a way of life—through which a person develops and encourages every aspect of the body, mind, and feelings to interrelate harmoniously as much as possible (see Figure 11–1 ■).

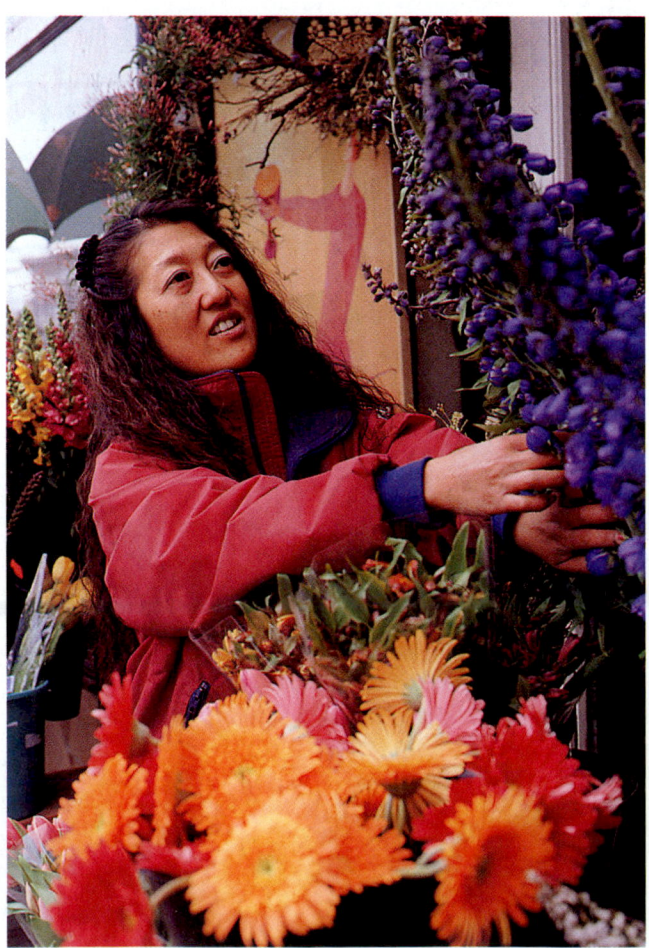

Figure 11–1 ■ Satisfaction with work enhances a sense of well-being and contributes to wellness.

BOX 11-1	■ Developing a Personal Definition of Health

The following questions can help nurses develop a personal definition of health.

- Is a person more than a biophysiologic system?
- Is health more than the absence of disease symptoms?
- Is health the ability of an individual to perform work?
- Is health the ability of an individual to adapt to the environment?
- Is health a condition of a person's actualization?
- Is health a state or a process?
- Is health the effective functioning of self-care activities?
- Is health static or changing?
- Are health and wellness the same?
- Are disease and illness different?
- Are there levels of health?
- Are wellness, health, and illness separate entities or points along a continuum?
- Is health socially determined?
- How do you rate your health and why?

Many factors affect individual definitions of health. Definitions vary according to an individual's previous experiences, expectations of self, age, and sociocultural influences.

Nurses should be aware of their own personal definitions of health and should appreciate that other people have their own individual definitions as well. A person's definition of health influences behavior related to health and illness. By understanding clients' perceptions of health and illness, nurses can provide more meaningful assistance to help them regain or attain a state of health. For aid in developing a personal definition of health, see Box 11–1.

Wellness and Well-Being

Wellness is a state of well-being. Basic concepts of wellness include self-responsibility; an ultimate goal; a dynamic, growing process; daily decision making in the areas of nutrition, stress management, physical fitness, preventive health care, emotional health, and other aspects of health; and, most importantly, the whole being of the individual.

Anspaugh, Hamrick, and Rosato (2003, pp. 3–7) propose seven components of wellness (see Figure 11–2 ■). To realize optimal health and wellness, people must deal with the factors within each component:

- *Physical.* The ability to carry out daily tasks, achieve fitness (e.g., pulmonary, cardiovascular, gastrointestinal), maintain adequate nutrition and proper body fat, avoid abusing drugs and alcohol or using tobacco products, and generally to practice positive lifestyle habits.
- *Social.* The ability to interact successfully with people and within the environment of which each person is a part, to develop and maintain intimacy with significant others, and to develop respect and tolerance for those with different opinions and beliefs.

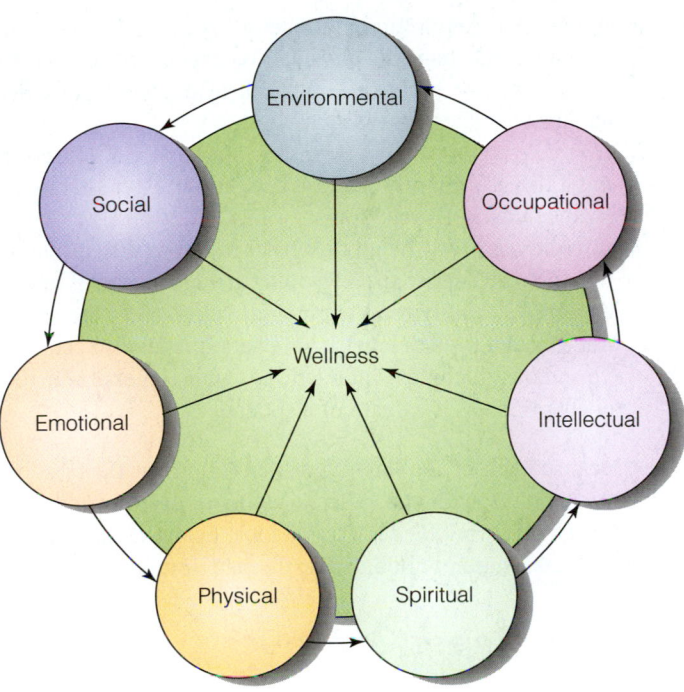

Figure 11–2 ■ The seven components of wellness. (From *Wellness: Concepts and Applications,* 6th ed. (p. 4), by D. J. Anspaugh, M. H. Hamrick, and F. D. Rosato, copyright 2003, New York: McGraw-Hill. Reprinted by permission.)

- *Emotional.* The ability to manage stress and to express emotions appropriately. Emotional wellness involves the ability to recognize, accept, and express feelings and to accept one's limitations.
- *Intellectual.* The ability to learn and use information effectively for personal, family, and career development. Intellectual wellness involves striving for continued growth and learning to deal with new challenges effectively.
- *Spiritual.* The belief in some force (nature, science, religion, or a higher power) that serves to unite human beings and provide meaning and purpose to life. It includes a person's own morals, values, and ethics.
- *Occupational.* The ability to achieve a balance between work and leisure time. A person's beliefs about education, employment, and home influence personal satisfaction and relationships with others.
- *Environmental.* The ability to promote health measures that improve the standard of living and quality of life in the community. This includes influences such as food, water, and air.

The seven components overlap to some extent, and factors in one component often directly affect factors in another. For example, a person who learns to control daily stress levels from a physiologic perspective is also helping to maintain the emotional stamina needed to cope with a crisis. Wellness involves working on all aspects of the model.

"**Well-being** is a subjective perception of vitality and feeling well . . . can be described objectively, experienced, and measured . . . and can be plotted on a continuum" (Hood & Leddy, 2002, p. 264). It is a component of health.

MODELS OF HEALTH AND WELLNESS

Because health is such a complex concept, various researchers have developed models or paradigms to explain health and in some instances its relationship to illness or injury. Models can be helpful in assisting health professionals to meet the health and wellness needs of individuals. Nurses need to clarify their understanding of health, wellness, and illness for the following reasons:

- Nurses' definitions of health largely determine the scope and nature of nursing practice. For example, when health is defined narrowly as a physiologic phenomenon, nurses confine themselves to assisting clients to regain normal physiologic functioning. When health is defined more broadly, the scope of nursing practice increases correspondingly.
- People's health beliefs influence their health practices. Thus a nurse's health values and practices may differ from those of a client. Nurses need to ensure that a plan of care developed for an individual relates to the client's conception of health. Otherwise the client may fail to respond to a health care regimen.

Models of health include the clinical model, the role performance model, the adaptive model, the eudemonistic model, the agent–host–environment model, and health–illness continua.

Clinical Model

The narrowest interpretation of health occurs in the clinical model. People are viewed as physiologic systems with related functions, and health is identified by the absence of signs and symptoms of disease or injury. To laypeople it is considered the state of not being "sick." In this model the opposite of health is disease or injury.

Many medical practitioners use the clinical model in their focus on the relief of signs and symptoms of disease and elimination of malfunction and pain. When these signs and symptoms are no longer present, the medical practitioner considers the individual's health restored.

Role Performance Model

Health is defined in terms of the individual's ability to fulfill societal roles, that is, to perform work. According to this model, people who can fulfill their roles are healthy even if they appear clinically ill. For example, a man who works all day at his job as expected is healthy even though an x-ray film of his lung indicates a tumor.

It is assumed in this model that sickness is the inability to perform one's work. A problem with this model is the assumption that a person's most important role is the work role. People usually fulfill several roles (e.g., mother, daughter, friend), and certain individuals may consider nonwork roles paramount in their lives.

Adaptive Model

The focus of the adaptive model is adaptation. In the adaptive model, health is a creative process; disease is a failure in adaptation, or maladaption. The aim of treatment is to restore the ability of the person to adapt, that is, to cope. According to this model, extreme good health is flexible adaptation to the environment and interaction with the environment to maximum advantage. Sister Callista Roy's adaptation model of nursing (Roy, 1999) views the person as an adaptive system (see Chapter 3). ∞ The focus of this model is stability, although there is also an element of growth and change.

Murray and Zentner (2001) indicate this growth and change in their definition of health: "a state of well-being in which the person is able to use purposeful, adaptive responses and processes, physically, mentally, emotionally, spiritually, and socially, in response to internal and external stimuli (stressors) in order to maintain relative stability and comfort and to strive for personal objectives and cultural goals" (p. 53).

Eudemonistic Model

The eudemonistic model incorporates a comprehensive view of health. Health is seen as a condition of actualization or realization of a person's potential. Actualization is the apex of the fully developed personality, described by Abraham Maslow (see Chapter 12). ∞ In this model the highest aspiration of people is fulfillment and complete development, which is actualization. Illness, in this model, is a condition that prevents self-actualization.

Pender includes stabilizing and actualizing tendencies in her definition of health: "Health is the actualization of inherent and acquired human potential through goal-directed behavior, competent self-care, and satisfying relationships with others while adjustments are made as needed to maintain structural integrity and harmony with relevant environments" (Pender, Murdaugh, & Parsons, 2002, p. 22).

Agent–Host–Environment Model

The agent–host–environment model of health and illness, also called the ecologic model, originated in the community health work of Leavell and Clark (1965) and has been expanded into a general theory of the multiple causes of disease. The model is used primarily in predicting illness rather than in promoting wellness, although identification of risk factors that result from the interactions of agent, host, and environment are helpful in promoting and maintaining health. The model has three dynamic interactive elements (see Figure 11–3 ■):

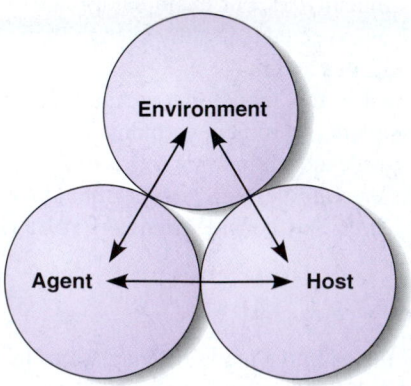

Figure 11–3 ■ The agent–host–environment triangle.

1. *Agent.* Any environmental factor or stressor (biologic, chemical, mechanical, physical, or psychosocial) that by its presence or absence (e.g., lack of essential nutrients) can lead to illness or disease.
2. *Host.* Person(s) who may or may not be at risk of acquiring a disease. Family history, age, and lifestyle habits influence the host's reaction.
3. *Environment.* All factors external to the host that may or may not predispose the person to the development of disease. Physical environment includes climate, living conditions, sound (noise) levels, and economic level. Social environment includes interactions with others and life events, such as the death of a spouse.

Because each of the agent–host–environment factors constantly interacts with the others, health is an ever-changing state. When the variables are in balance, health is maintained; when variables are not in balance, disease occurs.

Health–Illness Continua

Health–illness continua (grids or graduated scales) can be used to measure a person's perceived level of wellness. Health and illness or disease can be viewed as the opposite ends of a health continuum. From a high level of health a person's condition can move through good health, normal health, poor health, and extremely poor health, eventually to death. People move back and forth within this continuum day by day. There is no distinct boundary across which people move from health to illness or from illness back to health. How people perceive themselves and how others see them in terms of health and illness will also affect their placement on the continuum. The ranges in which people can be thought of as healthy or ill are considerable.

Dunn's High-Level Wellness Grid

Dunn (1959) describes a health grid in which a health axis and an environmental axis intersect. The grid demonstrates the interaction of the environment with the illness–wellness continuum (see Figure 11–4 ■). The health axis extends from peak wellness to death, and the environmental axis extends from very favorable to very unfavorable. The intersection of the two axes forms four quadrants of health and wellness:

1. *High-level wellness in a favorable environment.* An example is a person who implements healthy lifestyle behaviors and has the biopsychosocial, spiritual, and economic resources to support this lifestyle.
2. *Emergent high-level wellness in an unfavorable environment.* An example is a woman who has the knowledge to implement healthy lifestyle practices but does not implement adequate self-care practices because of family responsibilities, job demands, or other factors.
3. *Protected poor health in a favorable environment.* An example is an ill person (e.g., one with multiple fractures or severe hypertension) whose needs are met by the health care system and who has access to appropriate medications, diet, and health care instruction.

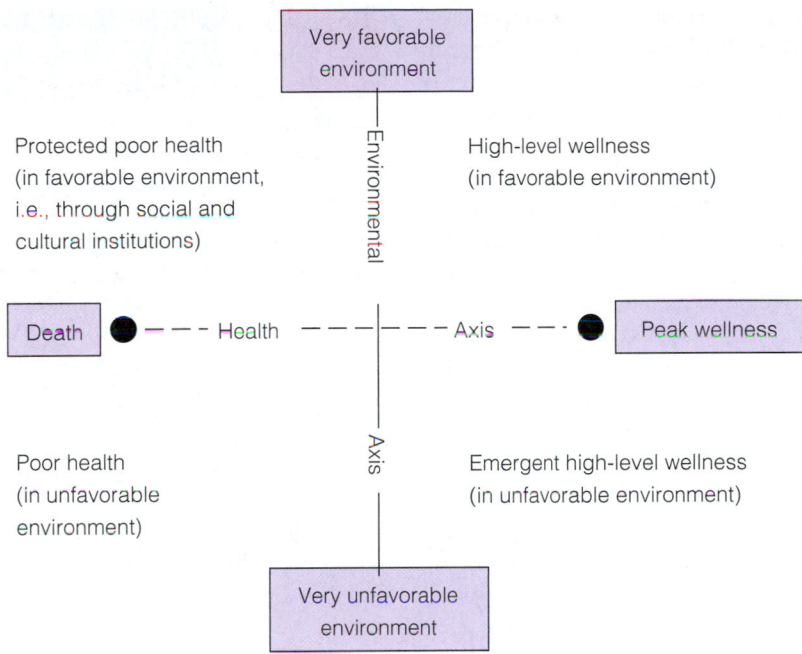

Figure 11–4 ■ Dunn's health grid: its axes and quadrants. (From "High-Level Wellness for Man and Society," by H. L. Dunn, 1959, *American Journal of Public Health, 49,* p. 788. Reprinted with permission of American Public Health Association.)

4. *Poor health in an unfavorable environment.* An example is a young child who is starving in a drought-stricken country.

In his book about high-level wellness in the individual, Dunn (1973) explores the concept of wellness as it relates to family, community, environment, and society. He believes that family wellness enhances wellness in individuals. In a well family that offers trust, love, and support, the individual does not have to expend energy to meet basic needs and can move forward on the wellness continuum. By providing effective sanitation and safe water, disposing of sewage safely, and preserving beauty and wildlife, the community enhances both family and individual wellness. Environmental wellness is related to the premise that humans must be at peace with and guard the environment. Societal wellness is significant because the status of the larger, social group affects the status of smaller groups. Dunn believes that social wellness must be considered on a worldwide basis.

Travis's Illness–Wellness Continuum

The illness–wellness continuum (Figure 11–5 ■) developed by Travis ranges from high-level wellness to premature death (Travis & Ryan, 2001). The model illustrates two arrows pointing in opposite directions and joined at a neutral point. Movement to the right of the neutral point indicates increasing levels of health and well-being for an individual. This is achieved in three steps: (a) awareness, (b) education, and (c) growth. In

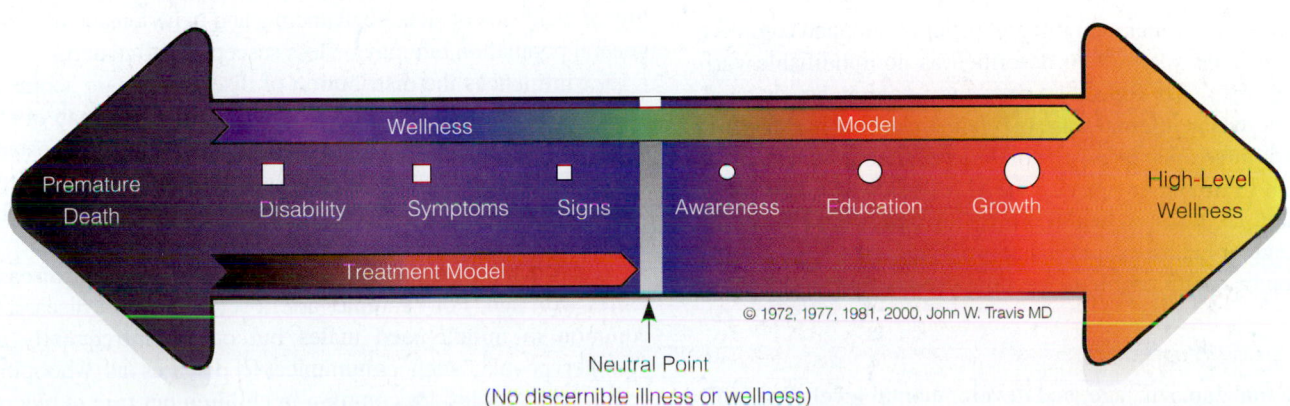

Figure 11–5 ■ Illness–wellness continuum. (Reprinted with permission, *Wellness Workbook,* Travis & Ryan, Ten Speed Press, Berkeley, CA. © 1981, 1988 by John W. Travis, MD. *www.thewellspring.com.*)

contrast, movement to the left of the neutral point indicates progressively decreasing levels of health. Travis and Ryan believe it is possible to be physically ill and at the same time oriented toward wellness, or be physically healthy and at the same time function from an illness mentality.

The model also compares the traditional treatment model with the wellness model. The former can help an individual move from the left only to the neutral point, where symptoms of the illness are alleviated. For example, a man with hypertension who takes an antihypertensive medication to reduce blood pressure and relieve any associated symptoms moves to the neutral point. However, wellness-oriented measures such as reducing weight or ceasing to smoke are needed to move the person beyond the neutral point to a higher level of wellness. Note that wellness interventions can be initiated at any point on the continuum. Thus, both the wellness model and treatment model can work together.

A newer model, the 4+ model of wellness (Baldwin & Conger, 2001), consists of the four domains of the inner self—physical, spiritual, emotional, and intellectual—plus the elements of the outer systems (environment, culture, nutrition, safety, and many other elements). The nurse assesses the inner self for strengths and excesses, sources of nurturing and of depletion, and the interactions between the inner self and the outer systems. This model is useful when working with individuals, families, or communities.

VARIABLES INFLUENCING HEALTH STATUS, BELIEFS, AND PRACTICES

Many variables influence a person's health status, beliefs, and behaviors or practices. Box 11–2 differentiates health status, beliefs, and behaviors or practices. These factors may or may not be under conscious control. People can usually control their health behaviors and can choose healthy or unhealthy activities. In contrast, people have little or no choice over their genetic makeup, age, sex, culture, and sometimes their geographical environments.

Internal Variables

Internal variables include biologic, psychologic, and cognitive dimensions. They are often described as nonmodifiable variables because, for the most part, they cannot be changed. However, when internal variables are linked to health problems, the nurse must be even more diligent about working with the client to influence external variables (such as exercise and diet) that may assist in health promotion and prevention of illness. Regular health exams and appropriate screening for early detection of health problems become even more important.

Biologic Dimension

Genetic makeup, sex, age, and developmental level all significantly influence a person's health.

Genetic makeup influences biologic characteristics, innate temperament, activity level, and intellectual potential. It has

---

BOX 11–2 ■ Differentiating Health Status, Beliefs, and Behaviors

- **Health status.** State of health of an individual at a given time. A report of health status may include anxiety, depression, or acute illness and thus describe the individual's problem in general. Health status can also describe such specifics as pulse rate and body temperature.

- **Health beliefs.** Concepts about health that an individual believes true. Such beliefs may or may not be founded on fact. Some of these are influenced by culture, such as the "hot–cold" system of some Hispanic Americans. In this system, health is viewed as a balance of hot and cold qualities within a person. Citrus fruits and some fowl are considered cold foods, and meats and bread are hot foods. In this context hot and cold do not denote temperature or spiciness but innate qualities of the food. For example, a fever is said to be caused by an excess of hot foods. Another example of a culturally related health belief is the belief that health and illness are closely associated with the amount and quality of blood in the body. For example, some Southerners say that "high blood," meaning too much blood in the body, causes headaches and dizziness. For additional information about cultural views of health and illness, see Chapter 13. ⌖

- **Health behaviors.** The actions people take to understand their health state, maintain an optimal state of health, prevent illness and injury, and reach their maximum physical and mental potential. Behaviors such as eating wisely, exercising, paying attention to signs of illness, following treatment advice, avoiding known health hazards such as smoking, taking time for rest and relaxation, and managing one's time effectively are all examples.

Health behavior is intended to prevent illness or disease or to provide for early detection of disease. Nurses preparing a plan of care with an individual need to consider the person's health beliefs before they suggest a change in health behaviors.

---

been related to susceptibility to specific disease, such as diabetes and breast cancer. In some cases, genetic predisposition for health or illness is enhanced when parents are from the same ethnic genetic pool. For example, people of African heritage have a higher incidence of sickle-cell anemia and hypertension than the general population but may be less susceptible to malaria.

Sex influences the distribution of disease. Certain acquired and genetic diseases are more common in one sex than in the other. Disorders more common among females include osteoporosis and autoimmune disease such as rheumatoid arthritis. Those more common among males are stomach ulcers, abdominal hernias, and respiratory diseases.

Age is also a significant factor. The distribution of disease varies with age. For example, arteriosclerotic heart disease is common in middle-aged males but occurs infrequently in younger people; such communicable diseases as whooping cough and measles are common in children but rare in elders, who have acquired immunity to them.

Developmental level has a major impact on health status. Consider these examples:

- Infants lack physiologic and psychologic maturity so their defenses against disease are lower during the first years of life.
- Toddlers who are learning to walk are more prone to falls and injury.
- Adolescents who need to conform to peers are more prone to risk-taking behavior and subsequent injury.
- Declining physical and sensory-perceptual abilities limit the ability of elders to respond to environmental hazards and stressors.

Psychologic Dimension

Psychologic (emotional) factors influencing health include mind–body interactions and self-concept.

Mind–body interactions can affect health status positively or negatively. Emotional responses to stress affect body function. For example, a student who is extremely anxious before a test may experience urinary frequency and diarrhea. A person worried about the outcome of surgery or about the behavior of a teenager may chain-smoke. Prolonged emotional distress may increase susceptibility to organic disease or precipitate it. Emotional distress may influence the immune system through central nervous system and endocrine alterations. Alterations in the immune system are related to the incidence of infections, cancer, and autoimmune diseases.

Increasing attention is being given to the mind's ability to direct the body's functioning. Relaxation, meditation, and biofeedback techniques are gaining wider recognition by individuals and health care professionals. For example, women often use relaxation techniques to decrease pain during childbirth. Other people may learn biofeedback skills to reduce hypertension.

Emotional reactions also occur in response to body conditions. For example, a person diagnosed with a terminal illness may experience fear and depression. *Self-concept* is how a person feels about self (self-esteem) and perceives the physical self (body image), needs, roles, and abilities. Self-concept affects how people view and handle situations. Such attitudes can affect health practices, responses to stress and illness, and the times when treatment is sought. An example is the anorexic woman who deprives herself of needed nutrients because she believes she is too fat even though she is well below an acceptable weight level. Self-concept is discussed in detail in Chapter 37. Self-perceptions are also associated with a person's definition of health. For example, a 75-year-old man who can no longer move large objects as he was accustomed to do may need to examine and redefine his concept of health in view of his age and abilities.

Cognitive Dimension

Cognitive or intellectual factors influencing health include lifestyle choices and spiritual and religious beliefs.

Lifestyle refers to a person's general way of living, including living conditions and individual patterns of behavior that are influenced by sociocultural factors and personal characteristics. In brief, lifestyle is often considered as behavior and activities over which people have control. Lifestyle choices may

---

BOX 11–3 ■ Examples of Healthy Lifestyle Choices

- Regular exercise
- Weight control
- Avoidance of saturated fats
- Alcohol and smoking avoidance
- Seat belt use
- Bike helmet use
- Immunization updates
- Regular dental checkups
- Regular health maintenance visits for screening examinations or tests

---

have positive or negative effects on health. Practices that have potentially negative effects on health are often referred to as **risk factors.** For example, overeating, getting insufficient exercise, and being overweight are closely related to the incidence of heart disease, arteriosclerosis, diabetes, and hypertension. Excessive use of tobacco is clearly implicated in lung cancer, emphysema, and cardiovascular diseases. See Box 11–3 for examples of healthy lifestyle choices.

Spiritual and religious beliefs can significantly affect health behavior. For example, Jehovah's Witnesses oppose blood transfusions; some fundamentalists believe that a serious illness is a punishment from God; some religious groups are strict vegetarians; and Orthodox Jews perform circumcision on the eighth day of a male baby's life. The influence of spirituality and religion is discussed further in Chapter 39.

External Variables

External variables affecting health include the physical environment, standards of living, family and cultural beliefs, and social support networks.

Environment

People are becoming increasingly aware of their environment and how it affects their health and level of wellness. Geographical location determines climate, and climate affects health. For instance, malaria and malaria-related conditions occur more frequently in tropical rather than temperate climates. Pollution of the water, air, and soil affects the health of cells. Pollution can occur naturally (e.g., lightning-caused fires produce smoke, which pollutes the air). Other substances in the environment, such as asbestos, are considered carcinogenic (i.e., they cause cancer). Cigarette smoke is "hazardous to one's health," with rates of cancer higher among smokers and those who live or work near smokers.

Another environmental hazard is radiation. Two sources of radiation that can be hazardous to health are machines and drugs that emit radiation. The improper use of x-rays, for example, can harm many of the body's organs. Another common source of radiation is the sun's ultraviolet rays. Light-skinned people are more susceptible to the harmful effects of the sun than are dark-skinned people.

The main component of acid rain is sulfur dioxide, produced by ore smelters and related industries. The other components are nitrogen oxides. These emissions are thought by scientists to damage forests, lakes, and rivers.

Another environmental hazard that is receiving more attention is an increase in the "greenhouse effect." The glass roof of a greenhouse permits the sun's radiation to penetrate, but the resulting heat does not escape back through the glass. Carbon dioxide in the earth's atmosphere acts like the glass roof of a greenhouse, and as carbon dioxide levels increase due to industrial and automobile emissions, the surface temperature of the earth may also be increasing.

Other sources of environmental contamination are pesticides and chemicals used to control weeds and plant diseases. These contaminants can be found in some animals and plants that are subsequently ingested by people. In excessive levels, they are harmful to health.

Standards of Living

An individual's standard of living (reflecting occupation, income, and education) is related to health, morbidity, and mortality. Hygiene, food habits, and the propensity to seek health care advice and follow health regimens vary among high-income and low-income groups.

Low-income families often define health in terms of work; if people can work they are healthy. They tend to be fatalistic and believe that illness is not preventable. Because their present problems are so great and all efforts are exerted toward survival, an orientation to the future may be lacking.

The environmental conditions of poverty-stricken areas also have a bearing on overall health. Slum neighborhoods are overcrowded and in a state of deterioration. Sanitation services tend to be inadequate. Many streets are strewn with garbage, and rats overrun alleys. Fires and crime are constant threats. Recreational facilities are almost nonexistent, forcing children to play in streets and alleys.

Occupational roles also predispose people to certain illnesses. For instance, some industrial workers may be exposed to carcinogenic agents. More affluent people may fulfill stressful social or occupational roles that predispose them to stress-related diseases. Such roles may also encourage overeating or social use of drugs or alcohol.

Family and Cultural Beliefs

The family passes on patterns of daily living and lifestyles to offspring. For example, a man who was abused as a child may physically abuse his small son. Physical or emotional abuse may cause long-term health problems. Emotional health depends on a social environment that is free of excessive tension and does not isolate the person from others. A climate of open communication, sharing, and love fosters the fulfillment of the person's optimum potential.

Culture and social interactions also influence how a person perceives, experiences, and copes with health and illness. Each culture has ideas about health, and these are often transmitted from parents to children. Heritage and cultural influences on health are discussed in detail in Chapter 13. 🔗

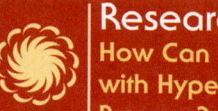

Research Note

How Can Nurses Help African Americans with Hypertension Control Their Blood Pressure?

African Americans have a greater severity and higher prevalence of hypertension than other minorities and Whites. In addition, the rate of control and treatment of hypertension in the United States is actually worsening. Strategies are needed to improve blood pressure control. Artinian, Washington, and Templin (2001) performed a pilot study to compare a nurse-managed home tele-monitoring (HT) plus usual care model and a nurse-managed community-based monitoring (CMB) plus usual care model with a usual care model. The usual care model included strategies typically used to control blood pressure. Twenty-six African Americans with a mean age of 59 years were randomly assigned to one of the three groups and monitored for 3 months. Both the HT and the CMB group had clinically and statistically significant drops in systolic and diastolic blood pressure over the 3-month period, while the usual care group showed little change.

Implications: More than simply the "usual care" is often required to improve outcomes for many clients with chronic disease, especially those taking daily medications. Nurses can contribute in many creative ways to support client adherence and therefore improve both quality of life and health outcomes.

Note: From "Effects of Home Telemonitoring and Community-Based Monitoring on Blood Pressure Control in Urban African Americans: A Pilot Study," by N. T. Artinian, O. G. M. Washington, and T. N. Templin, 2001, *Heart and Lung: The Journal of Acute and Critical Care, 30,* pp. 191–199.

People of certain cultures may perceive home remedies or tribal health customs as superior and more dependable than the health care practices of North American society. For example, a person of Asian origin may prefer to use herbal remedies and acupuncture to treat pain rather than analgesic medications. Cultural rules, values, and beliefs give people a sense of being stable and able to predict outcomes. The challenging of old beliefs and values by second-generation cultural groups may give rise to conflict, instability, and insecurity, in turn contributing to illness.

Social Support Networks

Having a support network (family, friends, or a confidant) and job satisfaction helps people avoid illness. Support people also help the person confirm that illness exists. People with inadequate support networks sometimes allow themselves to become increasingly ill before confirming the illness and seeking therapy. Support people also provide the stimulus for an ill person to become well again (Hurdle, 2001).

HEALTH BELIEF MODELS

Several theories or models of health beliefs and behaviors have been developed to help determine whether an individual is likely to participate in disease prevention and health-promotion activities. These models can be useful tools in developing programs for helping people change to healthier lifestyles and develop a more positive attitude toward preventive health measures (see also Chapter 8). ⌘

Health Locus of Control Model

Locus of control (LOC) is a concept from social learning theory that nurses can use to determine whether clients are likely to take action regarding health, that is, whether clients believe that their health status is under their own or others' control. People who believe that they have a major influence on their own health status—that health is largely self-determined—are called *internals*. People who exercise internal control are more likely than others to take the initiative on their own health care, be more knowledgeable about their health, and adhere to prescribed health care regimens such as taking medication, making and keeping appointments with physicians, maintaining diets, and giving up smoking. By contrast, people who believe their health is largely controlled by outside forces (e.g., chance or powerful others) are referred to as *externals*.

Research has shown that locus of control plays a role in clients' choices about health behaviors. In some cases, externals demonstrate better adherence to medical regimes (e.g., Wong & White, 2002) while in others, internals with appropriate support systems have better adherence (Murphy, Prewitt, Bote, West, & Iber, 2001).

Locus of control is a measurable concept that can be used to predict which people are most likely to change their behavior.

Many measurement instruments are available to assess LOC. One widely used example is the Multidimensional Health Locus of Control (MHLC) Scale (Wallston, Wallston, & DeVellis, 1978), most recently expanded to Form C (Wallston, Stein, & Smith, 1994). Nurses can use LOC results to plan internal reinforcement training if necessary in order to improve client efforts toward better health.

Rosenstock's and Becker's Health Belief Models

In the 1950s Rosenstock (1974) proposed a health belief model intended to predict which individuals would or would not use such preventive measures as screening for early detection of cancer. Becker (1974) modified the health belief model to include these components: individual perceptions, modifying factors, and variables likely to affect initiating action. The health belief model (see Figure 11–6 ■) is based on motivational theory. Rosenstock (1974) assumed that good health is an objective common to all people. Becker added "positive health motivation" as a consideration.

Individual Perceptions

Individual perceptions include the following:

- *Perceived susceptibility.* A family history of a certain disorder, such as diabetes or heart disease, may make the individual feel at high risk.

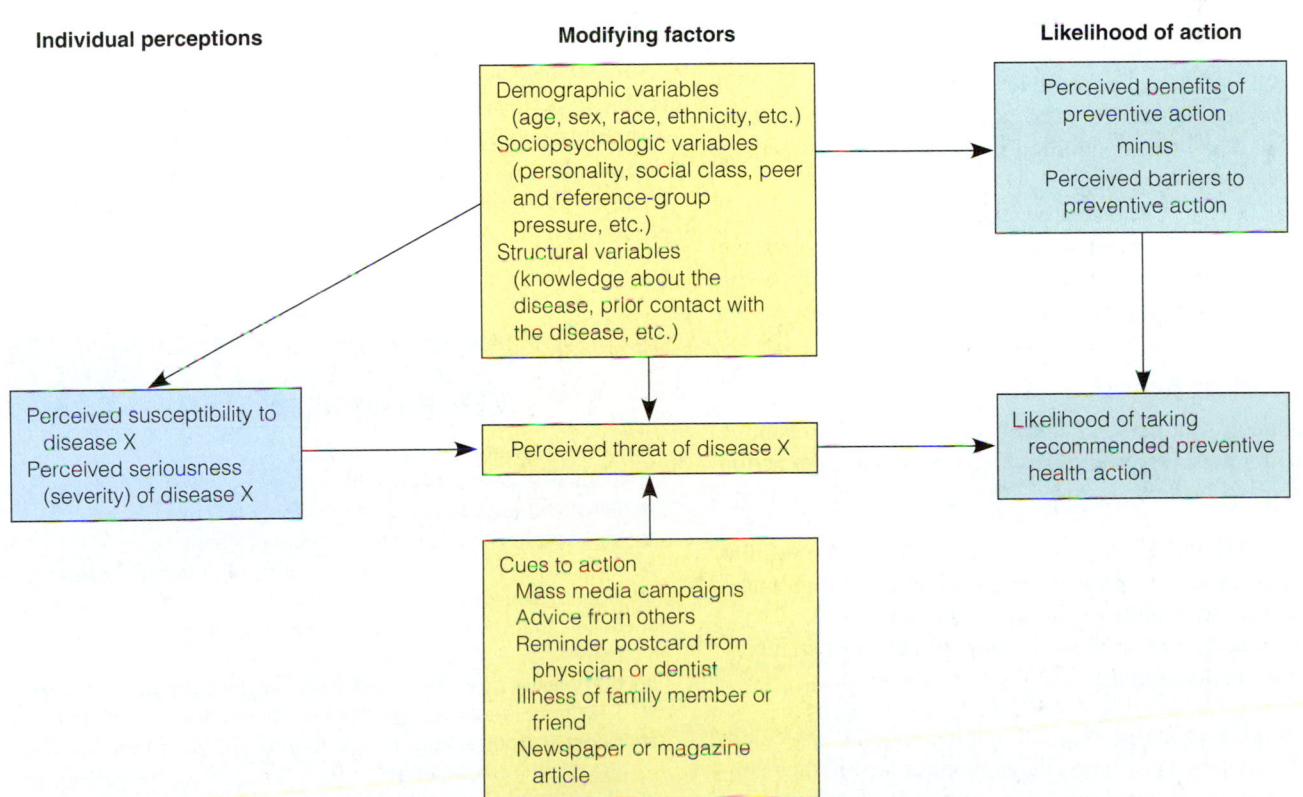

Figure 11–6 ■ The health belief model. (From "Selected Psychosocial Models and Correlates of Individual Health-Related Behaviors," by M. H. Becker, et al.,1977, *Medical Care, 15*(5 Suppl), pp. 27–46. Reprinted with permission.)

- *Perceived seriousness.* The question here is this: In the perception of the individual, does the illness cause death or have serious consequences? Concern about the spread of acquired immune deficiency syndrome (AIDS) reflects the general public's perception of the seriousness of this illness.
- *Perceived threat.* According to Becker (1974), perceived susceptibility and perceived seriousness combine to determine the total perceived threat of an illness to a specific individual. For example, a person who perceives that many individuals in the community have AIDS may not necessarily perceive a threat of the disease; if the person is a drug addict or a homosexual, however, the perceived threat of illness is likely to increase because the susceptibility is combined with seriousness.

Modifying Factors

Factors that modify a person's perceptions include the following:

- *Demographic variables.* Demographic variables include age, sex, race, and ethnicity. An infant, for example, does not perceive the importance of a healthy diet; an adolescent may perceive peer approval as more important than family approval and as a consequence may participate in hazardous activities or adopt unhealthy eating and sleeping patterns.
- *Sociopsychologic variables.* Social pressure or influence from peers or other reference groups (e.g., self-help or vocational groups) may encourage preventive health behaviors even when individual motivation is low. Expectations of others may motivate people, for example, not to drive an automobile after drinking alcohol.
- *Structural variables.* Knowledge about the target disease and prior contact with it are structural variables that are presumed to influence preventive behavior. Becker (1974) found higher adherence rates with prescribed treatments among mothers whose children had frequent ear infections and occurrences of asthma.
- *Cues to action.* Cues can be either internal or external. Internal cues include feelings of fatigue, uncomfortable symptoms, or thoughts about the condition of an ill person who is close. External cues are listed in Figure 11–6.

Likelihood of Action

The likelihood of a person's taking recommended preventive health action depends on the perceived benefits of the action minus the perceived barriers to the action.

- *Perceived benefits of the action.* Examples include refraining from smoking to prevent lung cancer, and eating nutritious foods and avoiding snacks to maintain weight.
- *Perceived barriers to action.* Examples include cost, inconvenience, unpleasantness, and lifestyle changes.

Nurses play a major role in helping clients implement healthy behaviors. They help clients monitor health, they supply anticipatory guidance, and they impart knowledge about health. Nurses can also reduce barriers to action (e.g., by minimizing inconvenience or discomfort) and can support positive actions.

Pender et al. (2002) have modified this health belief model to develop a health-promotion model. According to Pender, HBM explains health-protecting or preventive behaviors but does not emphasize health-promoting behaviors. See Pender's health-promotion model in Chapter 8.

In addition to applying these models, the nurse uses other resources to evaluate options in planning interventions to maximize wellness. Two very useful documents developed by federal agencies are the *Guide to Community Preventive Services* (Truman et al., 2000) from the Centers for Disease Control and Prevention and the 2000–2002 third edition of the *Guide to Clinical Preventive Services* from the U.S. Public Health Service (Berg & Allan, 2001). A major emphasis in both sets of documents is providing evidence-based recommendations for practices and policies aimed at improving health. Both documents are updated as the data become available and can be retrieved from their respective websites: for the *Community Guide,* go to http://www.thecommunityguide.org, and for the *Clinical Guide,* go to http://www.ahrq.gov/clinic/cps3dix.htm.

HEALTH CARE ADHERENCE

Adherence is the extent to which an individual's behavior (for example, taking medications, following diets, or making lifestyle changes) coincides with medical or health advice. Degree of adherence may range from disregarding every aspect of the recommendations to following the total therapeutic plan. There are many reasons why some people adhere and others do not (see Box 11–4).

To enhance adherence, nurses need to ensure that the client is able to perform the prescribed therapy, understands the necessary instructions, is a willing participant in establishing goals of therapy, and values the planned outcomes of behavior changes. Examples of questions to be included in assessment are found in the Assessment Interview box.

BOX 11–4 ■ Factors Influencing Adherence

- Client motivation to become well
- Degree of lifestyle change necessary
- Perceived severity of the health care problem
- Value placed on reducing the threat of illness
- Difficulty in understanding and performing specific behaviors
- Degree of inconvenience of the illness itself or of the regimens
- Beliefs that the prescribed therapy or regimen will or will not help
- Complexity, side effects, and duration of the proposed therapy
- Specific cultural heritage that may make adherence difficult
- Degree of satisfaction and quality and type of relationship with the health care providers
- Overall cost of prescribed therapy

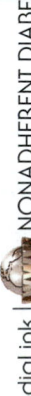

MediaLink NONADHERENT DIABETIC CLIENT CASE STUDY

Assessment Interview

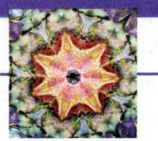

DETERMINING THE RISK FOR MEDICATION NONADHERENCE

- Are you having side effects from any of your medication?
- Do you think your medications are helping?
- Do you have "tools" to remind you to take your medication? Examples could be an alarm, medi-set, or environmental cues (6:00 news).
- Is there someone at home who helps you with your medications?
- How many times per day are your medications prescribed?
- How many pills do you take every day?
- Are there any special storage requirements for your medications?
- How much do your medication requirements interfere with your lifestyle?
- How well are you able to follow special dosing requirements?
- How many doses of your medications have you missed over the last 3 days?

When a nurse identifies nonadherence, it is important to take the following steps:

- *Establish why the client is not following the regimen.* Depending on the reason, the nurse can provide information, correct misconceptions, attempt to decrease expense, or suggest counseling if psychologic problems are interfering with adherence. It is also essential that the nurse reevaluate the suitability of the health advice provided. In situations where the client's cultural beliefs or age conflict with planned therapies, the nurse needs to consider ways to repattern and restructure care that will preserve and accommodate the client's practices. See "Providing Cultural Care" in Chapter 13.

- *Demonstrate caring.* Show sincere concern about the client's problems and decisions and at the same time accept the client's right to a course of action. For example, a nurse might tell a client who is not taking his heart medication, "I can appreciate how you feel about this, but I am very concerned about your heart."

- *Encourage healthy behaviors through positive reinforcement.* If the man who is not taking his heart medication is walking every day, the nurse might say, "You are really doing well with your walking."

- *Use aids to reinforce teaching.* For instance, the nurse can leave pamphlets for the client to read later or make a "pill calendar," a paper with the date and number of pills to be taken.

- *Establish a therapeutic relationship of freedom, mutual understanding, and mutual responsibility with the client and support persons.* By providing knowledge, skills, and information, the nurse gives clients control over their health and establishes a cooperative relationship, which results in greater adherence.

Aspects influencing clients of varying ages are found in the Lifespan Considerations box.

> ➤ **CLINICAL ALERT** *Chronic illness often requires complicated treatment regimens for lengthy periods that may include significant adverse reactions and be very costly. Thus, clients with chronic illnesses may be at increased risk for treatment nonadherence.* ■

Lifespan Considerations

Children

Several causes of nonadherence are specific to teenagers. It is important for the nurse to consider these when working with adolescents, because they

- Don't consider the consequences of their actions
- Are in the early stages of problem solving
- Assert independence by rejecting adult values
- Conform to their peers and don't like being "different"
- Focus on self-concept and body image
- Live in the "here and now"
- May regress developmentally at times of stress or illness
- May be unable to distinguish benefits from disadvantages.

Note: From "Rebels with a Cause: When Adolescents Won't Follow Medical Advice," by M. E. Muscari, 1998, *American Journal of Nursing, 98*(12), pp. 26–31. Adapted with permission.

Elders

Issues that influence the health and well-being of elders include:
- Lifestyle choices and individual responsibility for health maintenance

- Availability of home and community-based services to maximize independence
- Alternative/complimentary therapies
- Housing and home modifications to accommodate the physical aspects of aging
- Affordable and accessible transportation
- Preventive nursing and medical care
- Available mental health services
- The caregiving crisis that overburdens some family and informal caregivers.

Note: From *Gerontological Nursing Care,* by S. R. Tyson, "Elders: Issues That Influence the Health and Well-Being of Elders," p. 9, copyright 1999, with permission from Elsevier.

Other factors affecting elders' adherence include:
- Forgetfulness
- Dementia
- Feeling that they have lived their life and it is time for life to end.

ILLNESS AND DISEASE

Illness is a highly personal state in which the person's physical, emotional, intellectual, social, developmental, or spiritual functioning is thought to be diminished. It is not synonymous with disease and may or may not be related to disease. An individual could have a disease, for example, a growth in the stomach, and not feel ill. Similarly a person can feel ill, that is, feel uncomfortable, yet have no discernible disease. Illness is highly subjective; only the individual person can say he or she is ill.

Disease can be described as an alteration in body functions resulting in a reduction of capacities or a shortening of the normal life span. Traditionally intervention by physicians has the goal of eliminating or ameliorating disease processes. Primitive people thought "forces" or spirits caused disease. Later this belief was replaced by the single-causation theory. Today multiple factors are considered to interact in causing disease and determining an individual's response to treatment.

The causation of a disease is called its **etiology.** A description of the etiology of a disease includes the identification of all causal factors that act together to bring about the particular disease. For example, the tubercle bacillus is designated as the biologic agent of tuberculosis. However, other etiologic factors, such as age, nutritional status, and even occupation, are involved in the development of tuberculosis and influence the course of infection. There are many diseases for which the cause is unknown (e.g., multiple sclerosis).

Nurses have traditionally taken a holistic view of people and base their practice on the multiple-causation theory of health problems.

There are many ways to classify illness and disease; one of the most common is as acute or chronic. **Acute illness** is typically characterized by severe symptoms of relatively short duration. The symptoms often appear abruptly and subside quickly and, depending on the cause, may or may not require intervention by health care professionals. Some acute illnesses are serious (for example, appendicitis may require surgical intervention), but many acute illnesses, such as colds, subside without medical intervention or with the help of over-the-counter medications. Following an acute illness, most people return to their normal level of wellness.

A **chronic illness** is one that lasts for an extended period, usually 6 months or longer, and often for the person's life. Chronic illnesses usually have a slow onset and often have periods of **remission,** when the symptoms disappear, and **exacerbation,** when the symptoms reappear.

Examples of chronic illnesses are arthritis, heart and lung diseases, and diabetes mellitus. Nurses are involved in caring for chronically ill individuals of all ages in all types of settings—homes, nursing homes, hospitals, clinics, and other institutions. Care needs to be focused on promoting the highest level possible of independence, sense of control, and wellness. Clients often need to modify their activities of daily living, social relationships, and perception of self and body image. In addition, many must learn how to live with increasing physical limitations and discomfort.

Illness Behaviors

When people become ill, they behave in certain ways that sociologists refer to as illness behavior. **Illness behavior,** a coping mechanism, involves ways individuals describe, monitor, and interpret their symptoms, take remedial actions, and use the health care system. How people behave when they are ill is highly individualized and affected by many variables, such as age, sex, occupation, socioeconomic status, religion, ethnic origin, psychologic stability, personality, education, and modes of coping.

Parsons (1979) described four aspects of the sick role:

1. Clients are not held responsible for their condition.
2. Clients are excused from certain social roles and tasks.
3. Clients are obliged to try to get well as quickly as possible.
4. Clients or their families are obliged to seek competent help.

Suchman (1979) describes five stages of illness: symptoms, sick role, medical care contact, dependent client role, and recovery or rehabilitation. Not all clients progress through each stage. For example, the client who experiences a sudden heart attack is taken to the emergency room and immediately enters stages 3 and 4, medical care contact and dependent client role. Other clients may progress through only the first two stages and then recover. Details of Suchman's five stages follow.

Stage 1 Symptom Experiences

At this stage the person comes to believe something is wrong. Either someone significant mentions that the person looks unwell, or they experience some symptoms such as pain, rash, cough, fever, or bleeding. Stage 1 has three aspects:

- The physical experience of symptoms
- The cognitive aspect (the interpretation of the symptoms in terms that have some meaning to the person)
- The emotional response (e.g., fear or anxiety).

During this stage, the unwell person usually consults others about the symptoms or feelings, validating with a spouse or support people that the symptoms are real. At this stage the sick person may try home remedies. If self-management is ineffective, the individual enters the next stage.

Stage 2 Assumption of the Sick Role

The individual now accepts the sick role and seeks confirmation from family and friends. Often people continue with self-treatment and delay contact with health care professionals as long as possible. During this stage people may be excused from normal duties and role expectations. Emotional responses such as withdrawal, anxiety, fear, and depression are not uncommon depending on the severity of the illness, perceived degree of disability, and anticipated duration of the illness. When symptoms of illness persist or increase, the person is motivated to seek professional help.

Stage 3 Medical Care Contact

Sick people seek the advice of a health professional either on their own initiative or at the urging of significant others. When people seek professional advice they are really asking for three types of information:

- Validation of real illness
- Explanation of the symptoms in understandable terms
- Reassurance that they will be all right or prediction of what the outcome will be.

The health professional may determine that the client does not have an illness or that an illness is present, and may even be life threatening. The client may accept or deny the diagnosis. If the diagnosis is accepted, the client usually follows the prescribed treatment plan. If the diagnosis is not accepted, the client may seek the advice of other health care professionals or quasi-practitioners who will provide a diagnosis that fits the client's perceptions.

Stage 4 Dependent Client Role

After accepting the illness and seeking treatment, the client becomes dependent on the professional for help. People vary greatly in the degree of ease with which they can give up their independence, particularly in relation to life and death. Role obligations—such as those of wage earner, father, mother, student, baseball team member, or choir member—complicate the decision to give up independence.

Most people accept their dependence on the physician, although they retain varying degrees of control over their own lives. For example, some people request precise information about their disease, their treatment, and the cost of treatment, and they delay the decision to accept treatment until they have all this information. Others prefer that the physician proceed with treatment and do not request additional information.

For some clients illness may meet dependence needs that have never been met and thus provide satisfaction. Other people have minimal dependence needs and do everything possible to return to independent functioning. A few may even try to maintain independence to the detriment of their recovery.

Stage 5 Recovery or Rehabilitation

During this stage the client is expected to relinquish the dependent role and resume former roles and responsibilities. For people with acute illness, the time as an ill person is generally short and recovery is usually rapid. Thus most find it relatively easy to return to their former lifestyles. People who have long-term illnesses and must adjust their lifestyles may find recovery more difficult. For clients with a permanent disability, this final stage may require therapy to learn how to make major adjustments in functioning.

Effects of Illness

Illness brings about changes in both the involved individual and in the family. The changes vary depending on the nature, severity, and duration of the illness, attitudes associated with the illness by the client and others, the financial demands, the lifestyle changes incurred, adjustments to usual roles, and so on.

Impact on the Client

Ill clients may experience behavioral and emotional changes, changes in self-concept and body image, and lifestyle changes. Behavioral and emotional changes associated with short-term illness are generally mild and short lived. The individual, for example, may become irritable and lack the energy or desire to interact in the usual fashion with family members or friends. More acute responses are likely with severe, life-threatening, chronic, or disabling illness. Anxiety, fear, anger, withdrawal, denial, a sense of hopelessness, and feelings of powerlessness are all common responses to severe or disabling illness. For example, a client experiencing a heart attack fears for his life and the financial burden it may place on his family. Another client informed about a diagnosis of cancer or AIDS or crippling neurologic disease may, over time, experience episodes of denial, anger, fear, and hopelessness.

Certain illnesses can also change the client's body image or physical appearance, especially if there is severe scarring or loss of a limb or special sense organ. The client's self-esteem and self-concept may also be affected. Many factors can play a part in low self-esteem and a disturbance in self-concept: loss of body parts and function, pain, disfigurement, dependence on others, unemployment, financial problems, inability to participate in social functions, strained relationships with others, and spiritual distress. Nurses need to help clients express their thoughts and feelings, and to provide care that helps the client effectively cope with change.

Ill individuals are also vulnerable to loss of **autonomy,** the state of being independent and self-directed without outside control. Family interactions may change so that the client may no longer be involved in making family decisions or even decisions about their own health care. Nurses need to support clients' right to self-determination and autonomy as much as possible by providing them with sufficient information to participate in decision-making processes and to maintain a feeling of being in control.

Illness also often necessitates a change in lifestyle. In addition to participating in treatments and taking medications, the ill person may need to change diet, activity and exercise, and rest and sleep patterns.

Nurses can help clients adjust their lifestyles by these means:

- Providing explanations about necessary adjustments
- Making arrangements wherever possible to accommodate the client's lifestyle
- Encouraging other health professionals to become aware of the person's lifestyle practices and to support healthy aspects of that lifestyle
- Reinforcing desirable changes in practices with a view to making them a permanent part of the client's lifestyle.

Impact on the Family

A person's illness affects not only the person who is ill but also the family or significant others. The kind of effect and its extent depend chiefly on three factors: (a) the member of the family who is ill, (b) the seriousness and length of the illness, and (c) the cultural and social customs the family follows.

The changes that can occur in the family include the following:

- Role changes
- Task reassignments and increased demands on time
- Increased stress due to anxiety about the outcome of the illness for the client and conflict about unaccustomed responsibilities

- Financial problems
- Loneliness as a result of separation and pending loss
- Change in social customs.

See Chapter 12 for further information about the effects of illness on the family.

Focus on Critical Thinking

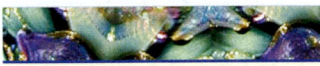

Jerry and Joe have both suffered heart attacks. Jerry, upon advice from his physician, started exercising, changed his dietary intake, entered stress reduction classes, and returned to work 6 weeks after his heart attack. He has a positive outlook, is doing well, and talks about being "well." Joe also changed his dietary habits and started exercising. However, Joe has been unable to quit smoking even though he wants to and has been advised to do so. Joe is frequently despondent, very fearful of having another heart attack, has not yet returned to work, and frequently talks about being "ill."

1. How does Jerry's psychologic dimension of health status differ from Joe's?

2. Both Jerry and Joe have heart disease. Jerry considers himself "well" whereas Joe considers himself "ill." Explain this phenomenon based on the health locus of control model.
3. What external factors may have influenced Jerry's decision to implement positive health behaviors?
4. What factors may have prevented Joe from developing the same positive outlook and actions that Jerry was able to take in regard to his illness?
5. What nursing interventions would be most beneficial to Joe concerning his smoking problem?

See Critical Thinking Possibilities in Appendix A.

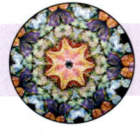 | # Chapter Review

Explore MediaLink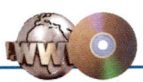

NCLEX review questions, case studies, MediaLink applications, and other interactive resources for this chapter can be found on the Companion Website at www.prenhall.com/kozier. Click on Chapter 11 to select the activities for this chapter.

For more NCLEX review questions, and an audio glossary, access the Student CD-ROM accompanying this textbook.

Chapter Highlights

- Nurses need to clarify their understanding of health because their definitions of health largely determine the scope and nature of nursing practice. Likewise, people's health beliefs influence their health practices.
- The perspective from which health is viewed has changed; instead of absence of disease, health has come to mean a high level of wellness or the fulfillment of one's maximum potential for physical, psychosocial, and spiritual functioning.
- Wellness is an active, seven-dimensional process of becoming aware of and making choices toward a higher level of well-being. The seven dimensions of wellness are the physical, social, emotional, intellectual, spiritual, occupational, and environmental dimensions.
- Well-being is considered a subjective perception of balance, harmony, and vitality. It is a state rather than a process.
- Most people describe health as freedom from symptoms of disease, the ability to be active, and a state of being in good spirits.

- Because notions of health are highly individual, the nurse must determine a client's perception of health in order to provide meaningful assistance. This involves well-developed communication skills. Nurses need to be aware of their own personal definitions of health.
- Various models have been developed to explain health: clinical, role performance, adaptive, and eudemonistic models and Leavell and Clark's agent–host–environment model, Dunn's high-level wellness grid, and Travis's illness–wellness continuum.
- The health status of a person is affected by many internal and external variables over which the person has varying degrees of control.
- Internal variables include biologic, psychologic, and cognitive dimensions. The biologic dimension includes genetic makeup, sex, age, and developmental level. The psychologic dimension includes mind–body interactions and self-concept.

The cognitive dimension includes lifestyle choices and spiritual and religious beliefs.

- External variables influencing health are physical environment, standards of living, family and cultural beliefs, and social support networks.
- Health belief and behavior models have been developed to help determine whether an individual is likely to participate in disease prevention and health-promotion activities. Two of these are the locus of control model and Rosenstock's and Becker's health belief models.
- A person's decision to implement health behaviors or to take action to improve health depends on such factors as the importance of health to the person, perceived threat of a particular disease or severity of the health care problems, perceived benefits of preventive or therapeutic actions, inconvenience and unpleasantness involved, degree of lifestyle change necessary, cultural ramifications, and cost.
- Nurses can enhance health care adherence by identifying the reasons for nonadherence if it occurs, demonstrating caring,

using positive reinforcement to encourage healthy behaviors, using aids to reinforce teaching, and establishing a therapeutic relationship of freedom, mutual understanding, and mutual responsibility with the client and support persons.

- Illness is usually associated with disease but may occur independently of it. Illness is a highly personal state in which the person feels unhealthy or ill. Disease alters body functions and results in a reduction of capacities or a shortened life span.
- Various theorists have described stages and aspects of illness. Parsons describes four aspects of the sick role. Suchman outlines five stages of illness: symptom experience, assumption of the sick role, medical care contact, dependent client role, and recovery or rehabilitation.
- An individual's usual pattern of behavior changes with illness and hospitalization, which disrupt a person's privacy, autonomy, lifestyle, roles, and finances.
- Nurses need to be aware that the illness of one member of a family affects all other members.

Review Questions

11–1. Which of the following examples is an example of the emotional component of wellness?
   a. The client chooses health foods.
   b. A new father decides to take parenting classes.
   c. A client expresses frustration with her partner's substance abuse.
   d. A widow with no family decides to join a bowling league.

11–2. Which of the following individuals appears to have taken on the sick role?
   a. An obese client states "I deserve to have a heart attack."
   b. A mother is ill and says "I won't be able to make your lunch today."
   c. A man with low back pain misses several physical therapy appointments.
   d. An elder states, "My horoscope says I will be well again."

11–3. Mrs. Parajh, a newly diagnosed diabetic, has been taking her medications and testing her blood sugar as instructed. She is confident that she can also improve her blood sugar control with diet and exercise, and recently went to the HMO education center to check out a video

on the management of diabetes. Her actions are most representative of which of the following models:
   a. health belief model
   b. clinical model
   c. role performance model
   d. agent–host–environment model

11–4. A client with HIV infection will be starting on combination medications to manage her disease. As you discuss the medication schedule you know that all of the following predict improved adherence EXCEPT
   a. her educational level
   b. a trusting relationship with her provider
   c. an expectation that the medications will be helpful
   d. being able to take the medications twice daily instead of four times daily

11–5. Which of the following might be the BEST way to measure medication adherence for a patient with diabetes?
   a. direct observation of dosing with insulin
   b. evidence of illness complications or exacerbations
   c. objective measurement of blood sugar and HgbAIC
   d. questioning the client about his or her medication routine

Readings and References

Suggested Readings

Tittle, M., Chiarelli, M., McGough, K., McGee, S. J., & McMillan, S. (2002). Women's health beliefs about breast cancer and health locus of control. *Journal of Gerontological Nursing, 28*(5), 37–45.

This is a research article that examined the relationships among health locus of control, health beliefs, and beliefs about breast cancer in women of different ages. Additional variables examined included the women's educational level and whether or not they had family members or friends who had cancer. They found that women over age 55 believed more in chance and powerful others than younger women and that women with friends/family with cancer felt more susceptible to cancer and were more externally motivated. The article provides particularly useful guidance for nurses working with older women.

Related Research

Muscari, M. E. (1998). Rebels with a cause: When adolescents won't follow medical advice. *American Journal of Nursing, 98*(12), 26–31.

References

American Nurses Association. (1980). *Nursing: A social policy statement.* Kansas City, MO: Author.

Anspaugh, D. J., Hamrick, M., & Rosato, F. D., (2003). *Wellness: Concepts and applications* (5th ed.). New York: McGraw-Hill.

Artinian, N. T., Washington, O. G. M., & Templin, T. N. (2001). Effects of home telemonitoring and community-based monitoring on blood pressure control in urban African Americans: A pilot study. *Heart and Lung: The Journal of Acute and Critical Care, 30,* 191–199.

Baldwin, J. H., & Conger, C. O. (2001). Health promotion and wellness. In K. S. Lundy & S. Janes (Eds.), *Community health nursing: Caring for the public's health* (pp. 286–307). Boston: Jones & Bartlett.

Becker, M. H. (Ed.). (1974). *The health belief model and personal health behavior.* Thorofare, NJ: Charles B. Slack.

Becker, M. H., Haefner, D. P., Kasl, S. V., Kirscht, J. P., Maiman, L. A., & Rosenstock, I. M. (1977). Selected psychosocial models and correlates of individual health-related behaviors. *Medical Care, 15*(5 Suppl), 27–46.

Berg, A. O., & Allan, J. D. (2001). Introducing the Third U.S. Preventive Services Task Force. *American Journal of Preventive Medicine, 20*(3S), 3–4.

Dunn, H. L. (1959). High-level wellness in man and society. *American Journal of Public Health, 48,* 786.

Dunn, H. L. (1973). *High-level wellness* (7th ed.). Arlington, VA: Beatty.

Hood, L., & Leddy, S. K. (2002). *Leddy & Pepper's conceptual basis of professional nursing* (5th ed.). Philadelphia: Lippincott Williams & Wilkins.

Hurdle, D. E. (2001). Social support: A critical factor in women's health and health promotion. *Health & Social Work, 26*(2), 72–79.

Leavell, H. R., & Clark, E. G. (1965). *Preventive medicine for the doctor in his community* (3rd ed.). New York: McGraw-Hill.

Murphy, P. A., Prewitt, T. E., Bote, E., West, B., & Iber, F. L. (2001). Internal locus of control and social support associated with some dietary changes by elderly participants in a diet intervention trial. *Journal of the American Dietetic Association, 101,* 203–208.

Murray, R. B., & Zentner, J. P. (2001). *Health assessment promotion strategies through the life span* (7th ed.). Upper Saddle River, NJ: Prentice Hall.

Muscari, M. E. (1998). Rebels with a cause: When adolescents won't follow medical advice. *American Journal of Nursing, 98*(12), 26–31.

Nightingale, F. (1969). *Notes on nursing: What it is, and what it is not.* New York: Dover Books. (Original work published in 1860.)

Parsons, T. (1951). *The social system.* Glencoe, IL: Free Press.

Parsons, T. (1979). Definitions of health and illness in the light of American values and social structure. In E. G. Jaco (Ed.), *Patients, physicians, and illness* (3rd ed.). New York: Free Press.

Pender, N. J., Murdaugh, C. L., & Parsons, M. J. (2002). *Health promotion in nursing practice* (4th ed.). Upper Saddle River, NJ: Prentice Hall.

President's Commission on Health Needs of the Nation. (1953). *Building Americans' health* (Vol. 2). Washington, DC: U.S. Government Printing Office.

Rosenstock, I. M. (1974). Historical origins of the health belief model. In M. H. Becker (Ed.), *The health belief model and personal health behavior.* Thorofare, NJ: Charles B. Slack.

Roy, C. (1999). *The Roy adaptation model* (2nd ed.). Upper Saddle River, NJ: Prentice Hall.

Suchman, E. A. (1979). Stages of illness and medical care. In E. G. Jaco (Ed.), *Patients, physicians, and illness* (3rd ed.). New York: Free Press.

Travis, J. W., & Ryan, R. S. (2001). *Simply well.* Berkeley, CA: Ten Speed Press.

Truman, B. I., Smith-Akin, C. K., Hinman, A. R., Gebbie, K. M., Brownson, R., Novick, L. F., et al. (2000). Developing the *Guide to Community Preventive Services*—Overview and rationale. *American Journal of Preventive Medicine, 18*(1S), 18–26.

Tyson, S. R. (1999). *Gerontological nursing care.* "Elders: Issues that influence the health and well-being of elders." Philadelphia: W. B. Saunders.

Wallston, K. A., Stein, M. J., & Smith, C. A. (1994). Form C of the MHLC scales: A condition-specific measure of locus of control. *Journal of Personality Assessment, 63,* 534–553.

Wallston, K. A., Wallston, B. S., & DeVellis, R. (1978, Spring). Development of the Multidimensional Locus of Control (MHLC) scales. *Health Education Monographs, 6,* 160–170.

Wong, V. K., & White, M. A. (2002). Family dynamics and health locus of control in adults with ostomies. *Journal of WOCN, 29*(1), 37–44.

World Health Organization. (1948). *Preamble to the constitution of the World Health Organization as adopted by the International Health Conference.* New York, 19–22 June, 1946; signed on 22 July 1946 by the representatives of 61 States (Official Records of the World Health Organization, no. 2, p. 100) and entered into force on 7 April 1948.

Selected Bibliography

Mackey, S. (2000). Towards a definition of wellness. *Australian Journal of Holistic Nursing, 7*(2), 34–38.

Mordacci, R., & Sobel, R. (1998). Health: A comprehensive concept. *Hastings Center Report, 28*(1), 34–37.

Myers, L. B., & Myers, F. (1999). The relationship between control beliefs and self-reported adherence in adults with cystic fibrosis. *Psychology Health and Medicine, 4,* 387–391.

Puschel, K., Thompson, B., Coronado, G. D., Lopez, L. C., & Kimball, A. M. (2001, October). Factors related to cancer screening in Hispanics: A comparison of the perceptions of Hispanic community members, health care providers, and representatives of organizations that serve Hispanics. *Health Education and Behavior, 28,* 573–590.

Stewart, A., & Eales, C. J. (2002, February). Hypertension: Patient adherence, health beliefs, health behavior and modification. *South African Journal of Physiotherapy, 58*(1), 12–17.

Stewart, K. S., & Dearmun, A. K. (2001, Winter). Adherence to health advice amongst young people with chronic illness. *Journal of Child Health Care, 5,* 155–162.

INDIVIDUAL, FAMILY, AND COMMUNITY HEALTH

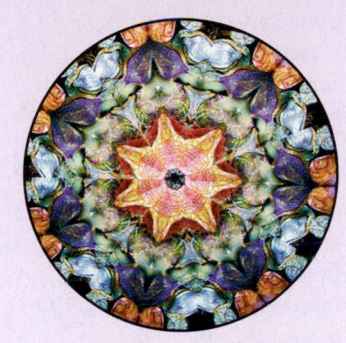

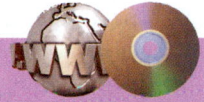
LEARNING OUTCOMES

After completing this chapter, you will be able to:

- Explain the relationship of individuality and holism to nursing practice.

- Give four main characteristics of homeostatic mechanisms.

- Describe the roles and functions of the family.

- Describe different types of families.

- Identify the components of a family health assessment.

- Identify common risk factors regarding family health.

- Develop nursing diagnoses, outcomes, and interventions pertaining to family functioning.

- Develop outcome criteria for specific nursing diagnoses related to family functioning.

- Identify theoretical frameworks used in individual and family health promotion.

- Identify Maslow's characteristics of the self-actualized person.

- Identify various types of communities.

- Describe the use of the nursing process in the community setting.

Nurses assess and plan health care for three types of clients: the individual, the family, and the community. Care of the individual is enhanced when the nurse understands the concepts of individuality, holism, homeostasis, human needs, and systems theory. The beliefs and values of each person and the support he or she receives come in large part from the family and are reinforced by the community. Thus an understanding of family dynamics and the context of the community assists the nurse in planning care. When a family is the client, the nurse determines the health status of the family and its individual members, the level of family functioning, family interaction patterns, and family strengths and weaknesses. When a community is the client, the nurse determines what environmental problems are present, for example, pollution, poor sanitation, waste disposal, incidence of crime, housing conditions, and so on, and intervenes to promote healthful living and prevent health problems.

INDIVIDUAL HEALTH

Dimensions of individuality include the person's total character, self-identity, and perceptions. The person's total character encompasses behaviors, emotional state, attitudes, values, motives, abilities, habits, and appearances. The person's self-identity encompasses perception of self as a separate and distinct entity alone and in interactions with others. The person's perceptions encompass the way the person interprets the environment or situation, directly affecting how the person thinks, feels, and acts in any given situation.

Concept of Individuality

To help clients attain, maintain, or regain an optimal level of health, nurses need to understand clients as individuals. Each individual is a unique being who is different from every other human being, with a different combination of genetics, life experiences, and environmental interactions.

When providing care, nurses need to focus on the client within both a total care and an individualized care context. In the total care context, the nurse considers all the principles and areas that apply when taking care of any client of that age and condition. In the individualized care context, the nurse becomes acquainted with the client as an individual, referring to the total care principles and using those principles that apply to this person at this time. For example, a nurse who is advising the mother of a preschooler understands that the child's desire to explore his world is a developmental stage that all preschoolers experience. However, the preschooler diagnosed with attention deficit hyperactivity disorder may have an increased risk of accidents and injuries when interacting with his environment, due to his impulsivity and poor self-control.

Concept of Holism

Nurses are concerned with the individual as a whole, complete, or holistic person, not as an assembly of parts and processes. When applied in nursing, the concept of **holism** emphasizes that nurses must keep the whole person in mind and strive to understand how one area of concern relates to the whole person. The nurse must also consider the relationship of the individual to the external environment and to others. For example, in helping a man who is grieving over the death of his spouse, the nurse explores the impact of the loss on the whole person (i.e., on the man's appetite, rest and sleep pattern, energy level, sense of well-being, mood, usual activities, family relationships, and relationships with others). Nursing interventions are directed toward restoring overall harmony, so they depend on the man's sense of purpose and meaning of his life. For additional information about holistic practices, see Chapter 14.

Concept of Homeostasis

The concept of **homeostasis** was first introduced by Cannon (1939) to describe the relative constancy of the internal processes of the body, such as blood oxygen and carbon dioxide levels, blood pressure, body temperature, blood glucose, and fluid and electrolyte balance. To Cannon, the word *homeostasis* did not imply something stagnant, set, or immobile; it meant a condition that might vary but remained relatively constant. Cannon viewed the human being as separate from the external environment and constantly endeavoring to maintain physiologic **equilibrium,** or balance, through adaptation to that environment. Homeostasis, then, is the tendency of the body to maintain a state of balance or equilibrium while continually changing.

Physiologic Homeostasis

Physiologic homeostasis means that the internal environment of the body is relatively stable and constant. All cells of the body require a relatively constant environment to function; thus the body's internal environment must be maintained within narrow limits. Homeostatic mechanisms have four main characteristics:

1. They are self-regulating.
2. They are compensatory.
3. They tend to be regulated by negative feedback systems.
4. They may require several feedback mechanisms to correct only one physiologic imbalance.

Self-regulation means that homeostatic mechanisms come into play automatically in the healthy person. However, if a person is ill, or if a respiratory organ such as a lung is injured, the homeostatic mechanisms may not be able to respond to the stimulus as they would normally. Homeostatic mechanisms are **compensatory** (counterbalancing) because they tend to counteract conditions that are abnormal for the person. An example is a sudden drop in air temperature. The compensatory mechanisms are that the peripheral blood vessels constrict, thereby diverting most of the blood internally; and increased muscular activity and shivering occur to create heat. Through these mechanisms the body temperature remains stable despite the cold.

Homeostasis occurs within the physiologic **system,** a set of interacting identifiable parts or components. The fundamental components of a system are matter, energy, and communication. Without any one of these, a system does not exist. The individual is a human system with matter (the body), energy (chemical or thermal), and communication (e.g., the nervous system). The **boundary** of a system, such as the skin in the human system, is a real or imaginary line that differentiates one system from another system or a system from its environment.

There are two general types of systems: closed and open. A **closed system** does not exchange energy, matter, or information with its environment; it receives no input from the environment and gives no output to the environment. An example of a closed system is a chemical reaction that takes place in a test tube. In reality, outside the laboratory, no closed systems exist. In an **open system,** energy, matter, and information move into and out of the system through the system boundary. All living systems, such as plants, animals, people, families, and communities, are open systems, since their survival depends on a continuous exchange of energy. They are, therefore, in a constant state of change.

An open system depends on the quality and quantity of its input, output, and feedback. **Input** consists of information, material, or energy that enters the system. After the input is absorbed by the system, it is processed in a way useful to the system. This transformation is called **throughput.** For example, food is input to the digestive system; it is digested (throughput) so that it can be used by the body. **Output** from a system is en-

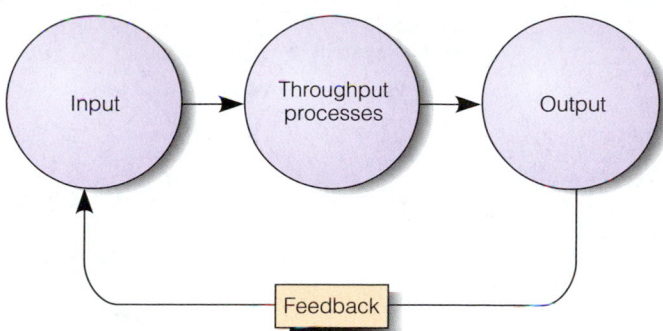

Figure 12–1 ■ An open system with a feedback mechanism.

ergy, matter, or information given out by the system as a result of its processes. Output from the digestive system includes caloric energy, nutrients, urine, and feces.

Feedback is the mechanism by which some of the output of a system is returned to the system as input. Feedback enables a system to regulate itself by redirecting the output of a system back into the system as input, thus forming a feedback loop (see Figure 12–1 ■). This input influences the behavior of the system and its future output. **Negative feedback** inhibits change; **positive feedback** stimulates change. Most biologic systems are controlled by negative feedback to bring the system back to stability. This type of feedback system senses and counteracts any deviations from normal. The deviations may be greater or less than the normal level or range. For example, an increase in the production of parathyroid hormone is stimulated by a drop in blood calcium, but when additional parathyroid hormone raises the level of blood calcium, the hormone's production is then inhibited (see Figure 12–2 ■). With hypoxia (shortage of oxygen), the concentration of red blood cells increases and the heart rate becomes faster to transport the blood and available oxygen around the body adequately. People interact with the environment by adjusting themselves to it or adjusting it to themselves. This premise directs the nurse to look at environmental factors influencing the system and to plan nursing interventions to help the client maintain homeostasis. For example, the individual who is experiencing severe anxiety may be taught a variety of stress management techniques.

Feedback mechanisms are also found within family and community systems. In the family system, parents provide feedback to children to regulate behavior. In the community, laws, rules, and regulations control the behavior of citizens.

Psychologic Homeostasis

The term **psychologic homeostasis** refers to emotional or psychologic balance or a state of mental well-being. It is maintained by a variety of mechanisms. Each person has certain psychologic needs, such as the need for love, security, and self-esteem, which must be met to maintain psychologic homeostasis. When one or more of these needs is not met or is threatened, certain coping mechanisms are activated to protect the person and provide psychologic homeostasis.

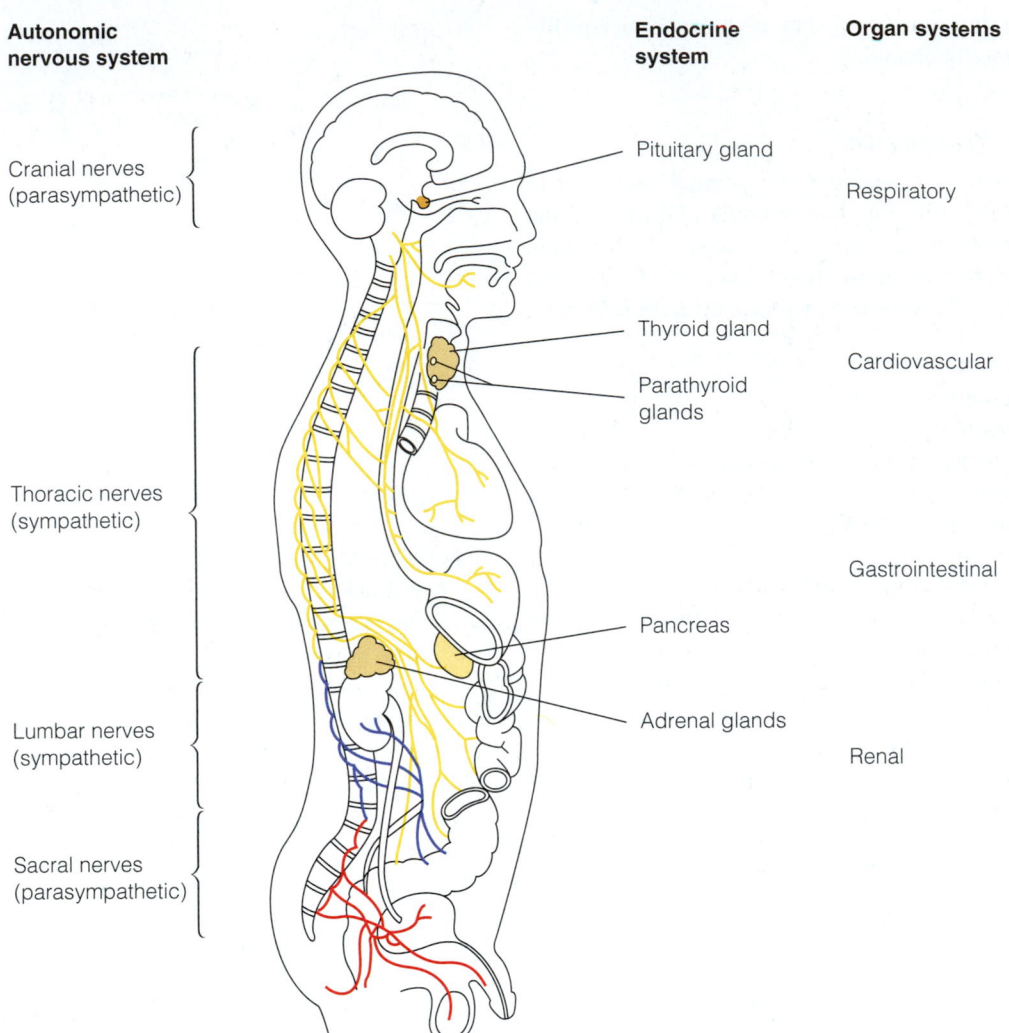

Autonomic nervous system

Cranial nerves (parasympathetic)

Thoracic nerves (sympathetic)

Lumbar nerves (sympathetic)

Sacral nerves (parasympathetic)

Endocrine system

Pituitary gland

Thyroid gland

Parathyroid glands

Pancreas

Adrenal glands

Organ systems

Respiratory

Cardiovascular

Gastrointestinal

Renal

Figure 12–2 ■ The homeostatic regulators of the body: autonomic nervous system, endocrine system, and specific organ systems.

Psychologic homeostasis is acquired or learned through the experience of living and interacting with others. In addition, societal norms and culture influence behavior. Some prerequisites for a person to develop psychologic homeostasis can be summarized as follows:

- A stable physical environment in which the person feels safe and secure. For example, the basic needs for food, shelter, and clothing must be met consistently from birth onward.
- A stable psychologic environment from infancy onward, so that feelings of trust and love develop. Growing children and adolescents also need kind but firm and consistent discipline, encouragement, and support to be their own unique selves.
- A social environment that includes adults who are healthy role models. Children learn the customs and values of society from these individuals.
- A life experience that provides satisfactions. Throughout life, people encounter many frustrations. People deal with these better if enough satisfying experiences have occurred to counterbalance the frustrating ones.

Assessing the Health of Individuals

A thorough assessment of the individual's health status is basic to health promotion. Components of this assessment are the health history and physical examination, physical fitness assessment, lifestyle assessment, health risk appraisal, health beliefs review, and life-stress review. Details about these assessments are discussed in Chapters 8, 16, and 28. ⌘

FAMILY HEALTH

The **family** is a basic unit of society. It consists of those individuals, male or female, youth or adult, legally or not legally related, genetically or not genetically related, who are considered by the others to represent their significant persons. In the nursing profession, interest in the family unit and its impact on the health, values, and productivity of individual family members is expressed by **family-centered nursing:** nursing that considers the health of the family as a unit in addition to the health of individual family members.

Functions of the Family

The economic resources needed by the family are secured by adult members. The family protects the physical health of its members by providing adequate nutrition and health care services. Nutritional and lifestyle practices of the family also directly affect the developing health attitudes and lifestyle practices of the children.

In addition to providing an environment conducive to physical growth and health, the family creates an atmosphere that influences the cognitive and the psychosocial growth of its members. Children and adults in healthy, functional families receive support, understanding, and encouragement as they progress through predictable developmental stages, as they move in or out of the family unit, and as they establish new family units. In families where members are physically and emotionally nurtured, individuals are challenged to achieve their potential in the family unit. As individual needs are met, family members are able to reach out to others in the family and the community, and to society.

Families from different cultures are an integral part of North America's rich heritage. Each family has values and beliefs that are unique to their culture of origin and that shape the family's structure, methods of interaction, health care practices, and coping mechanisms. These factors interact to influence the health of families. Families of a particular culture may cluster to form mutual support systems and to preserve their heritage; however, this practice may isolate them from the larger society (see Figure 12–3 ■).

Becoming acculturated is a slow, stressful process of learning the language and customs of a new country. Children in cultural clusters often have greater contact with the world around them than do adults; through school, children become more proficient in language and more comfortable with new customs and behaviors. Sometimes children create conflict in the family when they bring home new ideas and values. For more information about cultural aspects of health of individuals and families, see Chapter 13. 🔗

Types of Families in Today's Society

Families consist of persons (structure) and their responsibilities within the family (roles). A family structure of parents and their offspring is known as the **nuclear family.** The relatives of nuclear families, such as grandparents or aunts and uncles, compose the **extended family.** In some families, members of the extended family live with the nuclear family. Although members of the extended family may live in different areas, they may be a source of emotional or financial support for the family.

Traditional Family

The traditional family is viewed as an autonomous unit in which both parents reside in the home with their children, the mother often assuming the nurturing role and the father providing the necessary economic resources. In today's society both males and females are less bound to traditional role patterns. For example, fathers are more likely to be involved with the household chores, their children, and family life (see Figure 12–4 ■).

Two-Career Family

In two-career (or dual-career) families, both partners are employed. They may or may not have children. Two-career families have steadily increased since the 1960s because of increased career opportunities for women, a desire to increase their standard

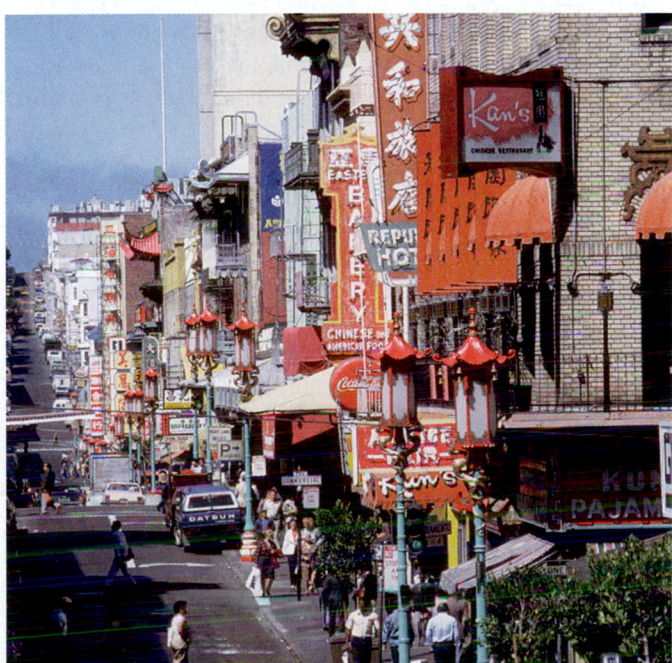

Figure 12–3 ■ Cultural separation. (Morton Beebe/CORBIS.)

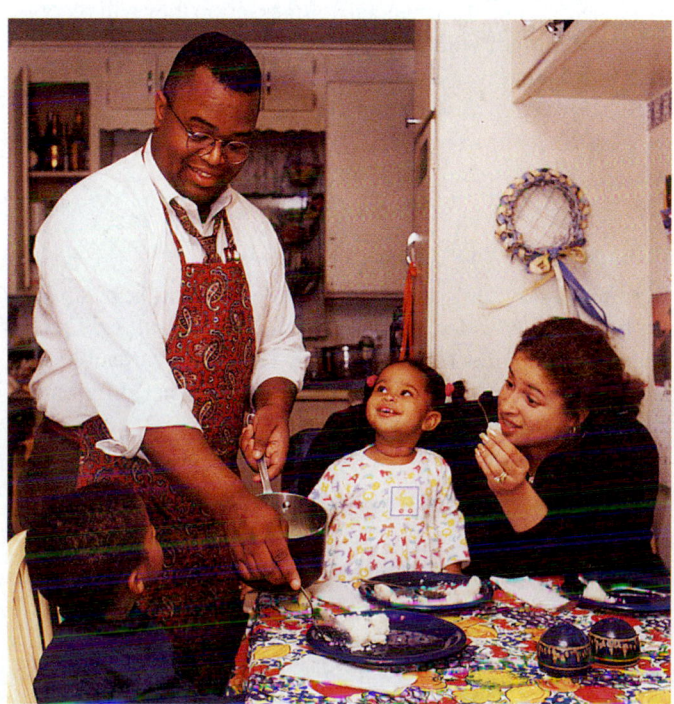

Figure 12–4 ■ Role patterns within traditional families are changing.

of living, and economic necessity. Finding good-quality, affordable child care is one of the greatest stresses faced by working parents.

Single-Parent Family

Approximately 50% of American children live in a single-parent home. There are many reasons for single parenthood, including death of a spouse, separation, divorce, birth of a child to an unmarried woman, or adoption of a child by a single man or woman. About 78% of single-parent families are headed by a female (Simmons & O'Neill, 2001). The stresses of single parenthood are many: child care concerns, financial concerns, role overload and fatigue in managing daily tasks, and social isolation.

Adolescent Family

A growing proportion of infants are born each year to adolescent parents, especially those of minority cultural groups. These young parents are often developmentally, physically, emotionally, and financially ill prepared to undertake the responsibility of parenthood. Adolescent pregnancies frequently interrupt or stop formal education. Children born to an adolescent are often at greater risk for health and social problems, and they have few role models to assist in breaking out of the cycle of poverty.

Foster Family

Children who can no longer live with their birth parents may require placement with a family that has agreed to include them temporarily. The legal agreement between the foster family and the court to care for the child includes the expectations of the foster parents and the financial compensation they will receive. A family (with or without their own children) may house more than one foster child at a time or different children over many years. Hopefully, at some time the fostered child can return to the birth parent(s) or be legally and permanently adopted by other parents.

Blended Family

Existing family units who join together to form new families are known as *blended, step,* or *reconstituted families.* Family integration requires time and effort. Stresses occur as blended families get acquainted with each other, respect differences, and establish new patterns of behavior.

Intragenerational Family

In some cultures, and as people live longer, more than two generations may live together. Children may continue to live with their parents even after having their own children or the grandparents may move in with their grown children's families after some years of living apart. In other situations, a generation is skipped or missing; that is, grandparents live with and care for their grandchildren but the children's parents are not a part of this family. Many life events and choices can lead to this type of family.

Cohabiting Family

Cohabiting (or communal) families consist of unrelated individuals or families who live under one roof. Reasons for cohabiting may be a need for companionship, a desire to achieve a sense of family, testing a relationship or commitment, or sharing expenses and household management. Cohabiting families illustrate the flexibility and creativity of the family unit in adapting to individual challenges and changing societal needs.

Gay and Lesbian Family

Homosexual adults may form gay and lesbian families based on the same goals of caring and commitment seen in heterosexual relationships. Children raised in these family units develop sex role orientations and behaviors similar to children in the general population. The greater danger to children in these families is the prejudice and ridicule expressed by others in society.

Single Adults Living Alone

Individuals who live by themselves represent a significant portion of today's society. Singles include young self-supporting adults who have recently left the nuclear family as well as older adults living alone. Older adults may find themselves single through divorce, separation, or the death of a spouse.

NURSING MANAGEMENT

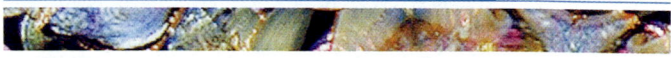

ASSESSING

The purpose of family assessment is to determine the level of family functioning, clarify family interaction patterns, identify family strengths and weaknesses, and describe the health status of the family and its individual members. Also important are family living patterns, including communication, child rearing, coping strategies, and health practices. Family assessment gives an overview of the family process and helps the nurse identify areas that need further investigation. Nurses carry out a detailed assessment in specific target areas as they become more acquainted with the family and begin to understand family needs and strengths more fully. In planning interventions, nurses need to focus not only on problems but also on family strengths and resources as part of the nursing care plan (see Box 12–1).

The assessment begins with a complete health history. The nurse focuses first on the family unit and then on the individuals in that family. The health history is one of the most effective ways of identifying existing or potential health problems. The history is followed by physical assessment of family members. If further evaluation is indicated, a referral is made to the appropriate health care professional. When the focus is on health, the appraisal includes information on lifestyle behaviors and health beliefs. The nurse uses data from the health appraisal to formulate a health profile. The health profile provides the data necessary to determine wellness or to establish a nursing diagnosis and to plan appropriate nursing interventions to promote optimal health through lifestyle modification.

BOX 12–1   ■   Family Assessment Guide

Family Structure
- Size and type: nuclear, extended, or other type of family
- Age and sex of family members

Family Roles and Functions
- Family members working outside the home; type of work and satisfaction with it
- Household roles and responsibilities and how tasks are distributed
- Ways child-rearing responsibilities are shared
- Major decision maker and methods of decision making
- Family members' satisfaction with roles, the way tasks are divided, and the way decisions are made

Physical Health Status
- Current physical health status of each member
- Perceptions of own and other family members' health
- Preventive health practices (e.g., status of immunizations, oral hygiene practices, regularity of visual examinations)
- Routine health care, when and why physician last seen

Interaction Patterns
- Ways of expressing affection, love, sorrow, anger, and so on
- Most significant family member in person's life
- Openness of communication with all family members

Family Values
- Cultural and religious orientations; degree to which cultural practices are followed
- Use of leisure time and whether leisure time is shared with total family unit
- Family's view of education, teachers, and the school system
- Health values: how much emphasis is put on exercise, diet, preventive health care

Coping Resources
- Degree of emotional support offered to one another
- Availability of support persons and affiliations outside the family (e.g., friends, church memberships)
- Sources of stress
- Methods of handling stressful situations and conflicting goals of family members
- Financial ability to meet current and future needs

Health Beliefs

To promote health, the nurse must understand the health beliefs of individuals and families. Health beliefs may reflect a lack of information or misinformation about health or disease. They may also include folklore and practices from different cultures. Because of the many advances in medicine and health care during the last few decades, clients may have outdated information about health, illness, treatment, and prevention. The nurse is frequently in a position to give information or correct misconceptions. This function is an important component of the nursing care plan. For additional information on health beliefs, see Chapter 11. 🔗

Family Communication Patterns

The effectiveness of family communication determines the family's ability to function as a cooperative, growth-producing unit. Messages are constantly being communicated among family members, both verbally and nonverbally. The information transmitted influences how members work together, fulfill their assigned roles in the family, incorporate family values, and develop skills to function in society. Intrafamily communication plays a significant role in the development of self-esteem, which is necessary for the growth of personality.

Families that communicate effectively transmit messages clearly. Members are free to express their feelings without fear of jeopardizing their standing in the family. Family members support one another and have the ability to listen, empathize, and reach out to one another in times of crisis. When the needs of family members are met, they are more able to reach out to meet the needs of others in society.

When patterns of communication among family members are dysfunctional, messages are often communicated unclearly. Verbal communication may be incongruent with nonverbal messages. Power struggles may be evidenced by hostility, anger, or silence. Members may be cautious in expressing their feelings because they cannot predict how others in the family will respond. When family communication is impaired, the growth of individual members is stunted. Members often turn to other systems to seek personal validation and gratification.

The nurse needs to observe intrafamily communication patterns closely. Nurses should pay special attention to who does the talking for the family, which members are silent, how disagreements are handled, and how well the members listen to one another and encourage the participation of others. Nonverbal communication is important because it gives valuable clues about what people are feeling.

Family Coping Mechanisms

Family coping mechanisms are the behaviors families use to deal with stress or changes imposed from either within or without. Coping mechanisms can be viewed as an active method of problem solving developed to meet life's challenges. The coping mechanisms families and individuals develop reflect their individual resourcefulness. Families may use coping patterns rather consistently over time or may change their coping strategies when new demands are made on the family. The success of a family largely depends on how well it copes with the stresses it experiences.

Nurses working with families realize the importance of assessing coping mechanisms as a way of determining how families relate to stress. Also important are the resources available to the family. Internal resources, such as knowledge, skills, effective communication patterns, and a sense of mutuality and purpose within the family, assist in the problem-solving process. In addition, external support systems promote coping and adaptation. These external systems may be extended family, friends, religious affiliations, health care professionals, or social services. The development of social support systems is particularly valuable today because many families, due to stress, mobility, or poverty, are isolated from the resources that would traditionally have helped them cope.

The incidence of family violence has increased in recent years. Statistics are not accurate, because many cases remain unreported. Family violence includes abuse between intimate partners, child abuse, and elder abuse, and may include physical, mental, and verbal abuse, as well as neglect. Early symptoms are evident in burns, cuts, fractures, and even death. Later manifestations often seen are depression, alcohol and substance abuse, and suicide attempts. Nurses should be alert to the symptoms of family violence and take appropriate measures to report it and obtain resources for the family.

Risk for Health Problems

Risk assessment helps the nurse identify individuals and groups at higher risk than the general population of developing specific health problems, such as stroke, diabetes, and lung cancer. The vulnerability of family units to health problems may be based on the maturity level of individual family members, heredity or genetic factors, sex or race, sociologic factors, and lifestyle practices.

Maturity Factors. Families with members at both ends of the age continuum are at risk of developing health problems. Families entering childbearing and child-rearing phases experience many changes in roles, responsibilities, and expectations. The many, often conflicting, demands on the family cause stress and fatigue, which may impede growth of individual family members and the functioning of the group as a unit. Adolescent mothers, because of their developmental level and lack of knowledge about parenthood, and single-parent families, because of role overload experienced by the head of the household, are more likely to develop health problems. Many elderly persons feel a lack of purpose and decreased self-esteem. These feelings in turn reduce their motivation to engage in health-promoting behaviors, such as exercise or community and family involvement.

Hereditary Factors. Persons born into families with a history of certain diseases, such as diabetes or cardiovascular disease, are at greater risk of developing these conditions. A detailed family health history, including genetically transmitted disorders, is crucial to the identification of persons and families at risk. These data are used not only to monitor the health of individual family members but also to recommend modifications in health practices that potentially reduce the risk, minimize the consequences, or postpone the development of genetically related conditions.

Sex or Race. Some family units or family members may be at risk of developing a disease by reason of sex or race. Males, for example, are at greater risk of having cardiovascular disease at an earlier age than females, and females are at greater risk of developing osteoporosis, particularly after menopause. Although it is sometimes difficult to separate genetic factors from cultural factors, certain risk factors seem to be related to race.

Sickle-cell anemia, for example, is a hereditary disease limited to people of African descent and Tay-Sachs is a neurodegenerative disease that occurs primarily in descendents of Eastern European Jews.

Sociologic Factors. Poverty is a major problem that affects not only the family but also the community and society. Poverty is a real concern among the rising number of single-parent families, and as the number of these families increases, poverty will affect a large number of growing children.

When ill, the poor are likely to put off seeking services until the illness reaches an advanced state and requires longer or more complex treatment. Although the health of the people of industrialized nations has improved significantly during the past century, this progress has not benefited all segments of society, particularly the poor.

Lifestyle Factors. Many diseases are preventable, the effects of some diseases can be minimized, or the onset of disease can be delayed through lifestyle modifications. Certain cancers, cardiovascular disease, adult-onset diabetes, and tooth decay are among the lifestyle diseases. The incidence of lung cancer, for example, would be greatly reduced if people stopped smoking. Good nutrition, dental hygiene, and use of fluoride—in the water supply, in toothpaste, as a topical application, or as supplements—have been shown to reduce dental decay or caries, one of America's most prevalent health problems.

Other important lifestyle considerations are exercise, stress management, and rest. Today health professionals have the knowledge to prevent or minimize the effects of some of the main causes of disease, disability, and death. The challenge is to disseminate information about prevention and to motivate families to make lifestyle changes prior to the onset of illness.

DIAGNOSING AND PLANNING

Data gathered during a family assessment may lead to the following nursing diagnoses: *Interrupted Family Processes,* a change in family relationships; *Readiness for Enhanced Family Coping,* effective management of adaptive tasks by family member involved with the client's health challenge, who now exhibits desire and readiness for enhanced health and growth in regard to self and in relation to the client; *Disabled Family Coping,* behavior of significant person (family member or other primary person) that disables his/her capacities to effectively address tasks essential to either person's adaptation to the health challenge; *Impaired Parenting,* inability of the primary caretaker to create, maintain, or regain an environment that promotes the optimum growth and development of the child; *Impaired Home Maintenance,* inability to independently maintain a safe growth-promoting immediate environment; *Caregiver Role Strain,* difficulty in performing family caregiver role. Examples of contributing factors for one selected diagnosis, desired outcomes to evaluate the achievement of client goals, and the effectiveness of nursing interventions are listed in Identifying Nursing Diagnoses, Outcomes, and Interventions.

Being sensitive to cultural differences is important in assessment and planning care. Knowing who makes most of the decisions in the family, especially in health care, helps the nurse know to whom to direct questions in order to obtain in-

IDENTIFYING NURSING DIAGNOSES, OUTCOMES, AND INTERVENTIONS
CLIENTS WITH DISRUPTION IN FAMILY HEALTH

DATA CLUSTER	NURSING DIAGNOSIS/ DEFINITION	SAMPLE DESIRED OUTCOMES [NOC#]/DEFINITION	INDICATORS	SELECTED INTERVENTIONS [NIC#]/DEFINITION	SAMPLE NIC ACTIVITIES
Mr. & Mrs. G's 6-year-old son has just been diagnosed with acute leukemia. They also have a 9-year-old daughter and a 4-year-old son.	Interrupted Family Processes/Change in family relationships	Family Coping [2600]/ Family actions to manage stressors that tax family resources.	Often demonstrated • Involves family members in decision making • Uses stress reduction strategies • Arranges for respite care	Family Integrity Promotion [7100]/ Promotion of family cohesion and unity Normalization Promotion [7200]/ Assisting parents and other family members of children with chronic illness or disabilities in providing normal life experiences for their children and families	• Determine family understanding of illness • Tell family members it is safe and acceptable to use typical expressions of affection • Refer for family therapy, as indicated • De-emphasize uniqueness of child's condition • Involve siblings in care and activities of child as appropriate
		Psychosocial Adjustment: Life Change [1305]/ Psychosocial adaptation of an individual to a life change.	Moderate • Realistic goal setting • Expressions of feeling empowered	Family Process Maintenance [7130]/ Minimization of family process disruption effects	• Determine typical family processes • Discuss strategies for normalizing family life with family members

formation and also to whom to give instructions. The extended family unit is found in many cultures and there may be a difference in health beliefs and health practices within the family. Older members of the family may use their traditional practices, while younger members may have had more exposure to modern practices. Building a trusting relationship with these families is the first step toward planning more effective care by being able to talk to them about their beliefs and practices.

Nursing needs to focus on assisting the family to plan realistic goals/outcomes and strategies that enhance family functioning, such as improving communication skills, identifying and utilizing support systems, and developing and rehearsing parenting skills. For families who are functioning well, anticipatory guidance may assist families in preparing for predictable developmental transitions that occur in the life of families.

The Family Experiencing a Health Crisis

Illness of a family member is a crisis that affects the entire family system. The family is disrupted as members abandon their usual activities and focus their energy on restoring family equilibrium. Roles and responsibilities previously assumed by the ill person are delegated to other family members, or those functions may remain undone for the duration of the illness. The family experiences anxiety because members are concerned about the sick person and the resolution of the illness. This anxiety is compounded by additional responsibilities when there is less time or motivation to complete the normal tasks of daily living. See Box 12–2 for some factors that determine the impact of illness on the family unit.

The family's ability to deal with the stress of illness depends on the members' coping skills. Families with good communication skills are better able to discuss how they feel about the illness and how it affects family functioning. They can plan for the future and are flexible in adapting these plans as the situation changes. An established social support network provides strength, encouragement, and services to the family during the illness. During health crises, families need to realize that it is a strength, not a sign of weakness, to turn to others for support.

BOX 12–2 ■ **Factors Determining the Impact of Illness on the Family**

- The nature of the illness, which can range from minor to life threatening
- The duration of the illness, which ranges from short term to long term
- The residual effects of the illness, including none to permanent disability
- The meaning of the illness to the family and its significance to family systems
- The financial impact of the illness, which is influenced by factors such as insurance and ability of the ill member to return to work
- The effect of the illness on future family functioning (for instance, previous patterns may be restored or new patterns may be established)

Nurses can be part of the support system for families, or they can identify other sources of support in the community.

During a crisis, families are often drawn together by a common purpose. In this time of closeness, family members have the opportunity to reaffirm personal and family values and their commitment to one another. Indeed, illness may provide a unique opportunity for family growth.

The Nurse's Role with Families Experiencing Illness

Nurses committed to family-centered care involve both the ailing individual and the family in the nursing process. Through their interaction with families, nurses can give support and information. Nurses make sure that not only the individual but also each family member understands the disease, its management, and the effect of these two factors on family functioning. The nurse also assesses the family's readiness and ability to provide continued care and supervision at home when warranted. After carefully planned instruction and practice, families are given an opportunity to demonstrate their ability to provide care under the supportive guidance of the nurse. When the care indicated is beyond the capability of the family, nurses work with families to identify available resources that are socially and financially acceptable.

In helping families reintegrate the ill person into the home, nurses use data gathered during family assessment to identify family resources and deficits. By formulating mutually acceptable goals for reintegration, nurses help families cope with the realities of the illness and the changes it may have brought about, which may include new roles and functions of family members or the need to provide continued medical care to the ill or recovering person. Working together, nurses and families can create environments that restore or reorganize family functioning during illness and throughout the recovery process.

Death of a Family Member

The death of a family member often has a profound effect on the family. The structure of the family is altered, and this change may in turn affect how it functions as a unit. Individual members experience a sense of loss. They grieve for the lost person, and they grieve for the family that once was. Family disorganization may occur. However, as the family begins to recover, a new sense of normalcy develops, the family reintegrates its roles and functions, and it comes to grips with the reality of the situation. This painful blow takes time to heal.

After the death of a member, families may need counseling to deal with their feelings and to talk about the person who died. They may also want to talk about their fears and hopes for the future. At this time, families often derive comfort from their religious beliefs and their spiritual advisers. Support groups are also available for families experiencing the pain of death. It is often difficult for nurses to deal with grieving families because the nurses also feel the loss and feel inadequate in knowing what to say or do. By understanding the effect death has on families, nurses can help families resolve their grief and move ahead with life. (See Chapter 41 ∞ for a discussion of loss and grieving.)

IMPLEMENTING AND EVALUATING

Nursing interventions are based on the medical diagnoses, nursing diagnoses, and selected goals or outcomes (see Identifying Nursing Diagnoses, Outcomes, and Interventions). In evaluating the success of the family care plan, the nurse assesses for the presence of the indicators identified for the chosen outcomes. If the indicators are present, it is likely that the outcome has been achieved. If the indicators or outcomes are partially or not met, all aspects of the family situation must be reexamined: Have the intervention activities been carried out? Are the indicators and outcomes appropriate? Is the nursing diagnosis proper? Has the medical condition or diagnosis changed?

Recognition of individual and family strengths helps to maintain wellness and also directs behavior in crises situations. If a plan of care has to be modified to be more effective, these strengths should be identified and utilized.

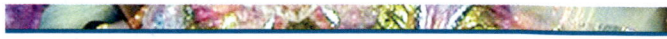

APPLYING THEORETICAL FRAMEWORKS TO INDIVIDUALS AND FAMILIES

A variety of theoretical frameworks provide the nurse with a holistic overview of health promotion for the individual and families across the life span. Major theoretical frameworks that nurses use in promoting the health of the individual and family are needs theories, developmental stage theories, systems theories, and structural–functional theories.

Needs Theories

In needs theories, human needs are ranked on an ascending scale according to how essential the needs are for survival. Abraham Maslow (1970), perhaps the most renowned needs theorist, ranks human needs on five levels (see Figure 12–5 ■ and Box 12–3). The five levels in ascending order are as follows:

- *Physiologic needs.* Needs such as air, food, water, shelter, rest, sleep, activity, and temperature maintenance are crucial for survival.

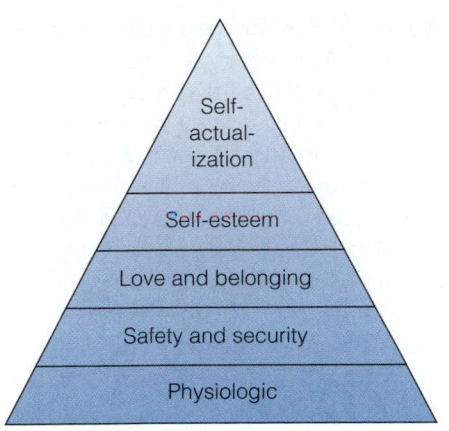

Maslow's hierarchy of needs

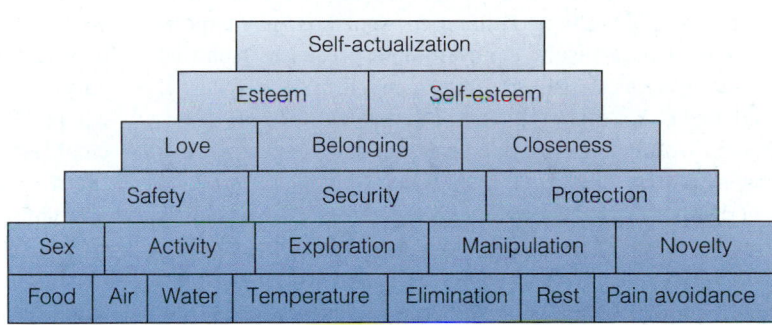

Maslow's hierarchy of needs, as adapted by Kalish

Figure 12–5 ■ Maslow's needs. (From *Psychology of Human Behavior,* 5th ed. by Kalish, copyright 1983. Reprinted with permission of Wadsworth, a division of Thomson Learning: *www.thomsonrights.com.* Fax 800-730-2215.)

- *Safety and security needs.* The need for safety has both physical and psychologic aspects. The person needs to feel safe, both in the physical environment and in relationships.
- *Love and belonging needs.* The third level of needs includes giving and receiving affection, attaining a place in a group, and maintaining the feeling of belonging.
- *Self-esteem needs.* The individual needs both self-esteem (i.e., feelings of independence, competence, and self-respect) and esteem from others (i.e., recognition, respect, and appreciation).
- *Self-actualization.* When the need for self-esteem is satisfied, the individual strives for self-actualization, the innate need to develop one's maximum potential and realize one's abilities and qualities.

Kalish's Hierarchy of Needs

Richard Kalish (1983) has adapted Maslow's hierarchy of needs into six levels rather than five. He suggests an additional category between the physiologic needs and the safety and security needs. This category, referred to as *stimulation needs,* in-cludes sex, activity, exploration, manipulation, and novelty (see Figure 12–5). Kalish emphasizes that children need to explore and manipulate their environments to achieve optimal growth and development. He notes that adults, too, often seek novel adventures or stimulating experiences before considering their safety or security needs.

Characteristics of Basic Needs

All people have the same basic needs; however, each person's needs and the ways in which they react to those needs are influenced by the culture with which the person identifies. For example, professional achievement, independent functioning, and privacy may be important in one culture or subculture and unimportant in another.

- People meet their own needs relative to their own priorities. For example, a poor mother might give up her share of food so that her child might have sufficient food to live.
- Although basic needs generally must be met, some needs can be deferred. An example is the need for independence, which an ill person can defer until well.

BOX 12–3 ■ Maslow's Characteristics of a Self-Actualized Person

- Is realistic, sees life clearly, and is objective about his or her observations
- Judges people correctly
- Has superior perception, is more decisive
- Has clear notion of right and wrong
- Is usually accurate in predicting future events
- Understands art, music, politics, and philosophy
- Possesses humility, listens to others carefully
- Is dedicated to some work, task, duty, or vocation
- Is highly creative, flexible, spontaneous, courageous, and willing to make mistakes
- Is open to new ideas

- Is self-confident and has self-respect
- Has low degree of self-conflict; personality is integrated
- Respects self, does not need fame, possesses a feeling of self-control
- Is highly independent, desires privacy
- Can appear remote and detached
- Is friendly, loving, and governed more by inner directives than by society
- Can make decisions contrary to popular opinion
- Is problem centered rather than self-centered
- Accepts the world for what it is

Note: From Toward a Psychology of Being, 2nd ed., by A. H. Maslow, copyright 1968, NY: Van Nostrand Reinhold. This material is used by permission of John Wiley & Sons, Inc.

- Failure to meet needs results in one or more homeostatic imbalances, which can eventually result in illness.
- A need can make itself felt by either external or internal stimuli. An example is the need for food. A person may experience hunger as a result of physiologic processes (internal stimulation) or as a result of seeing a beautiful cake (external stimulation).
- A person who perceives a need can respond in several ways to meet it. The choice of response is largely a result of learned experiences, lifestyle, and the values of the culture. For example, one woman who comes home from work feeling tired may meet the need for relaxation by walking around the park while another takes a quick nap. Many people's food choices at mealtimes and snack times are based on past experiences, lifestyle, and culture.
- Needs are interrelated. Some needs cannot be met unless related needs are also met. The need for hydration can be influenced by the need for elimination of urine. Likewise, the need for security can be markedly altered if the need for oxygen is threatened by a respiratory obstruction.

Needs can be satisfied in healthy and unhealthy ways. Ways of meeting basic needs are considered healthy when they are not harmful to others or to self, conform to the individual's sociocultural values, and are within the law. Conversely, unhealthy behavior may be harmful to others or to self, does not conform to the individual's sociocultural values, or is not within the law. People who satisfy their basic needs appropriately are healthier, happier, and more effective than those whose needs are frustrated.

Throughout their lifetime, individuals strive to meet needs. A person's perception of a need and his or her response to satisfy a need may be influenced by ethnocultural standards, by external and internal stimuli (e.g., hunger), and by self-determined priorities (e.g., stopping smoking). Positive factors that affect the satisfying of needs are an individual's healthy position on the wellness–illness continuum, the presence of supportive relationships, a good self-concept, and the satisfactory achievement of developmental stages. For example, if an infant achieves the developmental task of learning to trust, then the basic needs of feeling loved and secure are readily resolved.

Knowledge of the theoretical bases of human needs assists nurses in responding therapeutically to a client's behaviors and in understanding themselves and their own responses to needs. Human needs serve as a framework for assessing behaviors, assigning priorities to desired outcomes, and planning nursing interventions. For example, an adult with poor self-esteem would have difficulty accomplishing self-actualization. Therefore, nursing interventions would focus on increasing the client's self-esteem.

Developmental Stage Theories

Developmental stage theories related to individuals categorize a person's behaviors or tasks into approximate age ranges or in terms that describe the features of an age group. The age ranges of the stages do not take into account individual differences;

however, the categories do describe characteristics associated with the majority of individuals at periods when distinctive developmental changes occur and with the specific tasks that must be accomplished. Because human development is highly complex and multifaceted, developmental stage theories describe only one aspect of development, such as cognitive, psychosexual, psychosocial, moral, and faith development. Stage theories emphasize a definite, predictable sequence of development that is orderly and continuous. Each stage is affected by those stages preceding it and affects those stages that follow. For example, an adolescent who is unable to establish a stable sense of personal identity may have difficulty in later developmental stages with adult roles and career aspirations. See Chapter 21 for further information about developmental stages.

Developmental stage theories allow nurses to describe typical behaviors of an individual within a certain age group, explain the significance of those behaviors, predict behaviors that might occur in a given situation, and provide a rationale to control behavioral manifestations. Individuals can be compared with a representative group of people at the same point in time or compared at different points in time. During care, the nurse's knowledge of stage theories can be used in parental and client education, counseling, and anticipatory guidance.

Developmental stage theories view families as ever changing and growing. Crucial, yet predictable, tasks occur at each level or stage of development. Achievement of tasks appropriate at one level is a prerequisite for successfully achieving the tasks expected at the next level. A major task of the family, from a developmental perspective, is to create an environment where the family can master critical developmental tasks. This ensures orderly progression through the stages of the family life cycle.

Systems Theories

The basic concepts of general systems theory were proposed in the 1950s. One of its major proponents, Ludwig von Bertalanffy (1969) introduced systems theory as a universal theory that could be applied to many fields of study. Nurses are increasingly using systems theory to understand not only biologic systems but also systems in families, communities, and nursing and health care. General systems theory provides a way of examining interrelationships and deriving principles.

Systems may be complex and the systems components are often studied as **subsystems.** For family systems, the subsystems would be individuals. Looking back up the hierarchy, the systems above other systems are referred to as **suprasystems**—the family is the suprasystem of the individual. See Figure 12–6 ■ for a hierarchy of the human system.

The biologic system can be subdivided into the neurologic, musculoskeletal, respiratory, circulatory, gastrointestinal, and urinary subsystems, among others. Each subsystem can in turn be subdivided. For example, the urinary system consists of the kidneys, the ureters, and the bladder; the circulatory system consists of the heart and the blood vessels; the neurologic system consists of the brain, the spinal cord, and the nerves. The biologic system can also be subdivided into categories of needs

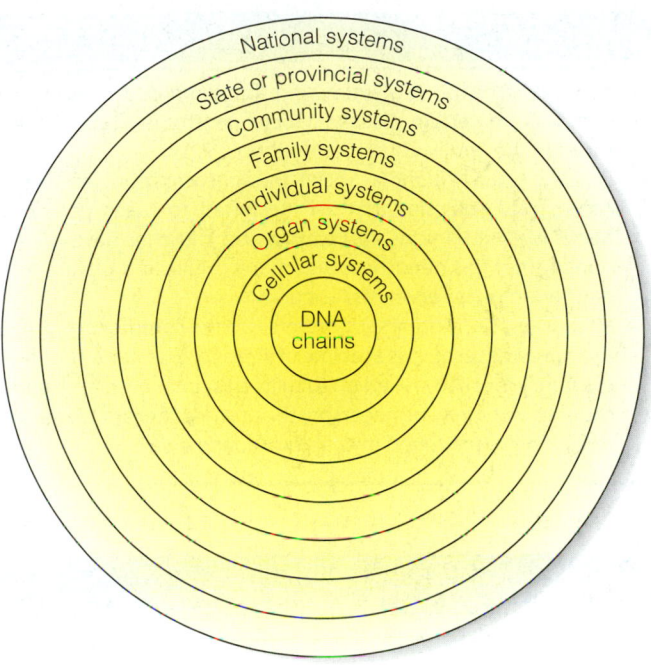

Figure 12–6 ■ A common system hierarchy.

or functional health patterns or activities of daily living, such as nutrition and hydration, sleep/rest, activity/exercise, elimination, and so on.

The psychologic and social systems consist of subsystems that include thinking, feeling, and interaction patterns. Names of the psychologic and social subsystems vary considerably according to individual nurse theorists. For example, Dorothy Johnson (1980), who describes the human system in terms of behaviors, lists the psychologic subsystems of attachment-affiliative, dependence, achievement, and aggressive.

The interrelatedness of all the parts of a system is the basis for nursing's holistic view of the client. A tumor of the liver affects the whole individual, that is, the person may be nauseated, tired, anxious, and so on. A psychologic problem such as stress or anxiety may also manifest itself by physiologic symptoms, such as sleeplessness, nausea, or changes in cardiac function.

The family unit can also be viewed as a system. Its members are interdependent, working toward specific purposes and goals. Families, as open systems, are continually interacting with and influenced by other systems in the community. Boundaries regulate the input from other systems that interact with the family system; they also regulate output from the family system to the community or to society. Boundaries protect the family from the demands and influences of other systems. Families are likely to welcome input from without, encourage individual members to adapt beliefs and practices to meet the changing demands of society, seek out health care information, and use community resources.

Structural–Functional Theory

The structural–functional theory, as the name implies, focuses on family structure and function. The structural component of the the-

ory addresses the membership of the family and the relationships among family members. Intrafamily relationships are complex because of the numerous relationships that exist within the family structure—mother–daughter, brother–sister, spouse–partner, and so on. These relationships are constantly evolving as children mature and leave the family nest and adults age and become more dependent on others to meet their daily needs.

The functional aspect of the theory examines the effects of intrafamily relationships on the family system, as well as their effects on other systems. Some of the main functions of the family include developing a sense of family purpose and affiliation, adding and socializing new members, and providing and distributing care and services to members. A healthy family organizes its members and resources in meeting family goals; it functions in harmony, working toward shared goals.

Nurses generally use a combination of theoretical frameworks in promoting the health of individuals and families. For example, the nurse may provide education for the mother of a toddler who is struggling to accomplish the developmental stage of autonomy described by Erikson (1963). Simultaneously, the nurse may provide guidance for the same family in its stressful transition period between developmental stages as their older school-age child becomes an adolescent.

COMMUNITY HEALTH

A **community** is a collection of people who share some attribute of their lives. It may be that they live in the same locale, attend a particular church, or even share a particular interest such as painting. Groups that constitute a community because of common member interests are often referred to as a *community of interest* (e.g., religious and cultural groups). A community can also be defined as a social system in which the members interact formally or informally and form networks that operate for the benefit of all people in the community. Five of the main functions of a community are described in Box 12–4. In community health, the community may be viewed as having a common health problem, such as a high incidence of infant mortality or of tuberculosis, HIV infection, or another communicable disease. Box 12–5 lists the characteristics of a healthy community. **Community health nursing** focuses on promoting and preserving the health of population groups.

NURSING MANAGEMENT

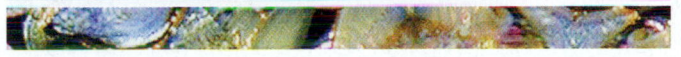

ASSESSING

Several community assessment frameworks have been devised. In one, Anderson and McFarlane (2000) identify eight subsystems of the community for analysis. The subsystems are illustrated around a core, which consists of the people and their characteristics, values, history, and beliefs. The first stage in assessment is to learn about the people in the community. Figure 12–7 ■ shows some of the major components

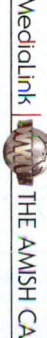

1. *Production, distribution, and consumption of goods and services.* These are the means by which the community provides for the economic needs of its members. This function includes not only the supplying of food and clothing but also the provision of water, electricity, and police and fire protection and the disposal of refuse.
2. *Socialization.* Socialization refers to the process of transmitting values, knowledge, culture, and skills to others. Communities usually contain a number of established institutions for socialization: families, churches, schools, media, voluntary and social organizations, and so on.
3. *Social control.* Social control refers to the way in which order is maintained in a community. Laws are enforced by the police; public health regulations are implemented to protect people from certain diseases. Social control is also exerted through the family, church, and schools.
4. *Social interparticipation.* Social interparticipation refers to community activities that are designed to meet people's needs for companionship. Families and churches have traditionally met this need; however, many public and private organizations also serve this function.
5. *Mutual support.* Mutual support refers to the community's ability to provide resources at a time of illness or disaster. Although the family is usually relied on to fulfill this function, health and social services may be necessary to augment the family's assistance if help is required over an extended period.

A Healthy Community

- Is one in which members have a high degree of awareness of being a community
- Uses its natural resources while taking steps to conserve them for future generations
- Openly recognizes the existence of subgroups and welcomes their participation in community affairs
- Is prepared to meet crises
- Is a problem-solving community; it identifies, analyzes, and organizes to meet its own needs
- Possesses open channels of communication that allow information to flow among all subgroups of citizens in all directions
- Seeks to make each of its systems' resources available to all members
- Has legitimate and effective ways to settle disputes that arise within the community
- Encourages maximum citizen participation in decision making
- Promotes a high level of wellness among all its members

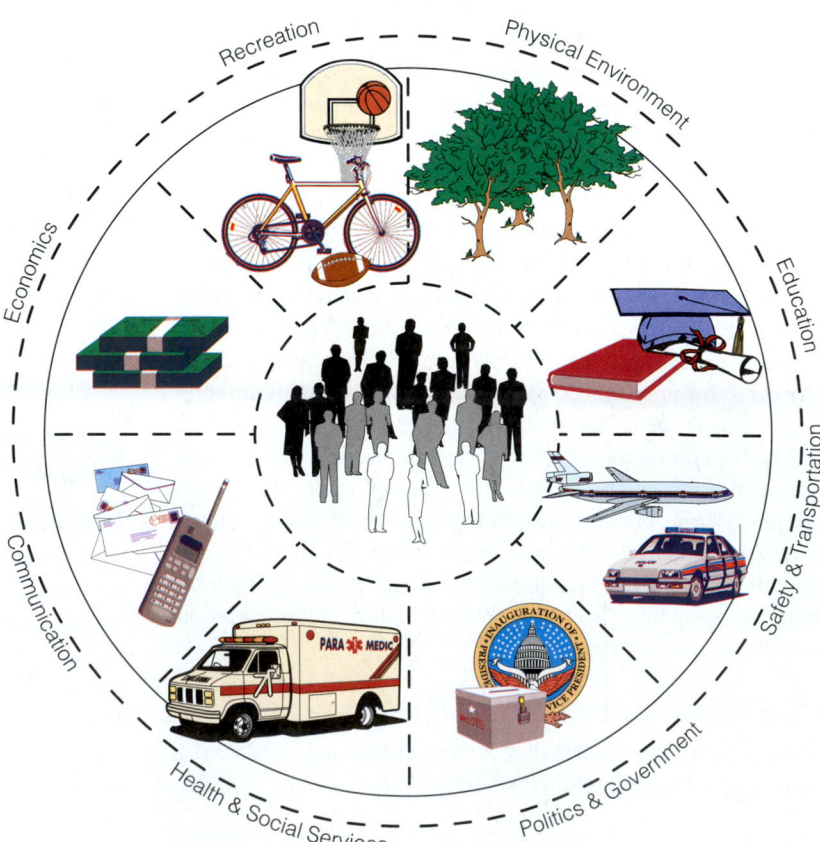

Figure 12–7 ■ The community assessment wheel, the assessment segment of the community-as-partner model. *(Note:* From *Community as Partner: Theory and Practice in Nursing,* 3rd ed. (p. 166), by E. T. Anderson and J. McFarlane, 2000, Philadelphia: Lippincott Williams & Wilkins.)

BOX 12–6   ■ Major Aspects of a Community Assessment

Physical Environment

Consider the natural boundaries, size, and population density; types of dwellings; and incidence of crime, vandalism, and substance abuse.

Education

Consider educational facilities; existing school health facilities; type and amount of health services handled by the school; school lunch programs; extracurricular sports, libraries, and counseling services; continuing education or extended education programs; and extent of parental involvement in the schools.

Safety and Transportation

Consider fire, police, and sanitation services; sources of water and its treatment; quality of the air; garbage disposal service; availability and safety of public transportation; and availability of ambulance services.

Politics and Government

Consider kind of government; organizations active in the community; influential people in the community; issues that have recently appeared on local ballots; and the average election turnout.

Health and Social Services

Consider existing hospitals, health care facilities, and health care services; number, type, and routine caseloads of community

health professionals; geographic, economic, and cultural accessibility to health care services; sources of health information; level of immunization among children and adults; life expectancy in the community; availability of home health care and long-term care services; availability of transportation service to all major health facilities.

Communication

Consider local newspapers; radio and TV stations, postal services, Internet access, and telephone services; frequency of public forums; and presence of informal bulletin boards.

Economics

Consider the main industries and occupations; percentage of the population employed or attending school; income levels and quality and type of housing; occupational health programs; major employers in the community.

Recreation

Consider recreational facilities in the community and outside the community; theaters and movie houses; number and types of church and religious services; number and utilization of playgrounds, pools, parks, and sports facilities; level of participation in various church programs; number and types of social committees, organizations, and clubs available.

Note: From *Community as Partner: Theory and Practice in Nursing,* 3rd ed. (pp. 168–170), by E.T. Anderson and J. McFarlane, 2000, Philadelphia: Lippincott Williams & Wilkins. Adapted with permission.

BOX 12–7   ■ Sources of Community Assessment Data

- City maps to locate community boundaries, roads, churches, schools, parks, hospitals, and so on
- State census data for population composition and characteristics
- Chamber of commerce for employment statistics, major industries, and primary occupations
- County or state health departments for location of health facilities, occupational health programs, numbers of health professionals, numbers of welfare recipients, and so on
- City or regional health planning boards for health needs and practices
- Telephone book for location of social, recreational, and health organizations, committees, and facilities
- Public and university libraries for district social and cultural research reports

- Health facility administrators for information about employee caseloads, prevalent types of problems, and dominant needs
- Recreational directors for programs provided and participation levels
- Police department for incidence of crime, vandalism, and drug addiction
- Teachers and school nurses for incidence of children's health problems and information on facilities and services to maintain and promote health
- Local newspapers for community activities related to health and wellness, such as health lectures or health fairs
- Online computer services that may provide access to public documents related to community health

---

of the community core. Surrounding the core are the eight subsystems. Box 12–6 shows major aspects of a community assessment and Box 12–7 shows sources of community data.

DIAGNOSING

After assessing, validating, and summarizing data, the nurse identifies nursing diagnoses for the community. Here are three community-focused North American Nursing Diagnosis Association (NANDA International, 2003) nursing diagnoses:

- *Ineffective Community Coping:* Pattern of community activities (for adaptation and problem solving) that is unsatisfactory for meeting the demands or needs of the community
- *Readiness for Enhanced Community Coping:* Pattern of community activities for adaptation and problem solving that is satisfactory for meeting the demands or needs of the community but can be improved for management of current and future problems/stressors.
- *Ineffective Community Therapeutic Regimen Management:* Pattern of regulating and integrating into community

processes programs for treatment of illness and the sequelae (consequences) of illness that are unsatisfactory for meeting health-related goals.

PLANNING AND IMPLEMENTING

Planning community health may be oriented toward improved crisis management, disease prevention, health maintenance, or health promotion. The responsibility for planning at the community level is usually broadly based. The exact resources and skills of members of the community often depend on the size of the community. A broadly based planning group is most likely to create a plan that is acceptable to members of the community. Also, people who are involved in planning become educated about the problems, the resources, and the interrelationships within the system.

When setting priorities, health planners must work with consumers, interest groups, or other involved persons to prioritize health problems. It is important to take into consideration the values and interests of community members, the severity of the problems, and the resources available to identify and act on the problems. Because any plan is likely to result in change, members of the planning group should understand and use planned change theory.

EVALUATING

In community health, evaluation determines whether the planned interventions have led to the achievement of the established goals and objectives; for example, was the immunization rate of preschool children improved? Because community health is usually a collaborative process between health providers, community leaders, politicians, and consumers, all may be involved in the evaluation process. Often the community health nurse is the agent of evaluation, collecting and assessing the data that determine the effectiveness of implemented programs.

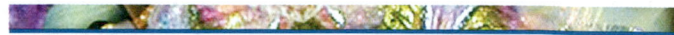

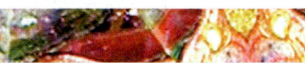

Lifespan Considerations

Elders

Homeostasis mechanisms in the body work to keep body processes stable and constant. In elders, these mechanisms are much slower to respond to changes. An example is if an older person has had an increase in heart rate, it may take hours for it to return to normal. In a younger healthy person, this would occur in a few minutes. These slower self-regulatory and compensatory mechanisms often result in increased risk for complications and slower healing when an elder has a physical stressor, such as surgery, influenza, or pneumonia.

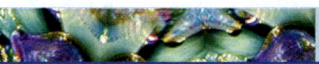

Focus on Critical Thinking

Linda is a young mother of three children who has developed a severe arthritic condition that has affected her ability to work and adequately care for her family. Her illness has created a financial hardship for the family and has strained their roles. Linda and her husband have custody of their children from previous marriages as well as a daughter of their own. They are reluctant to seek assistance from outside sources because they fear interference from their ex-spouses with regard to their children.

1. What aspects of Linda's physical problem must the nurse be concerned about as they relate to the other issues occurring in Linda's life?

2. Explain why Linda's family is considered to be in a health crisis when only Linda is experiencing an illness.
3. What are the advantages or disadvantages of facing illness as a member of a family as opposed to individually?
4. Describe Linda's family from the perspective of general systems theory.
5. Explain why a home health nurse may be better able to assist Linda and her family than a community health nurse.

See Critical Thinking Possibilities in Appendix A.

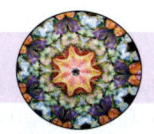 | Chapter Review

Explore MediaLink

NCLEX review questions, case studies, MediaLink applications, and other interactive resources for this chapter can be found on the Companion Website at www.prenhall.com/kozier. Click on Chapter 12 to select the activities for this chapter. For more NCLEX review questions, and an audio glossary, access the Student CD-ROM accompanying this textbook.

Chapter Highlights

- Nursing involves viewing the client as an individual and in a holistic way.
- To ensure holistic health care, the nurse considers all components of health (health promotion, health maintenance, health education and illness prevention, and restorative-rehabilitative care) and recognizes that disturbance in one part of a person affects the whole being.
- Homeostasis is the tendency of the body to maintain a state of relative balance or constancy in response to a changing internal and external environment.
- Physiologic homeostasis is maintained by coordinated functioning of the autonomic nervous, endocrine, respiratory, cardiovascular, renal, and gastrointestinal systems.
- Homeostatic mechanisms regulate hormone secretion, fluid and electrolyte levels, the functions of body viscera, and metabolic processes that provide energy for the body.
- Psychologic homeostasis, or emotional well-being, is acquired or learned through the experience of living and interacting with others.
- Although each individual has unique characteristics, certain needs are common to all people.
- The family is the basic unit of society.
- The family plays an important role in forming the health beliefs and practices of its members.
- Family-centered nursing addresses the health of the family as a unit, as well as the health of family members.
- In today's society, many types of families exist: traditional, two-career, single-parent, those headed by one or more adolescent parents, foster, blended, intragenerational, cohabiting, and gay and lesbian. In addition, many single adults live alone.
- The purpose of family assessment is to determine the level of family functioning, to clarify family interaction patterns, to identify family strengths and weaknesses, and to describe the health status of the family and its individual members.
- Families at risk for health problems may be considered on the basis of family maturity level, presence of hereditary factors, sex or race, lifestyle practices, and sociologic factors such as poverty.
- Nursing diagnoses that relate to family health needs and problems include *Interrupted Family Processes; Readiness for Enhanced Family Coping: Disabled Family Coping: Impaired Parenting; Impaired Home Maintenance;* and *Caregiver Role Strain.*
- Nurses must examine their own values about family, health, illness, and death to be effective in supporting families in crisis.
- A variety of social, psychologic, and nursing theoretical frameworks provide the nurse with a holistic overview of health promotion of individuals and families across the life span.
- Maslow's hierarchy of human needs consists of five categories: physiologic (survival) needs, safety needs, love and belonging needs, self-esteem needs, and self-actualization needs.
- People vary in how they rank their needs at any given moment.
- Needs satisfaction can be altered by illness, significant relationships, self-concept, and developmental levels.
- A community is a collection of people who share some attribute of their lives.
- For community assessment, eight subsystems proposed by Anderson and McFarlane (2000) can be used: physical environment, education, safety and transportation, politics and government, health and social services, communication, economics, and recreation.

Review Questions

12–1. A client has just been told that she will require chemotherapy for her cancer. In applying the concept of holism, the nurse would
  a. offer to come to the client's home to provide needed physical care.
  b. contact the client's spiritual adviser.
  c. inquire how the client thinks this will affect other aspects of her life.
  d. provide the client with information about how to join a support group.

12–2. When a father prepares to leave for work in the morning, his 3-year-old son starts to cry and scream. The father picks him up and delays leaving for a while. The child's behavior most reflects which part of a system?
  a. input
  b. throughput
  c. output
  d. feedback

12–3. A client who identifies his family as "two college roommates, a dog and a cat" is completing a family health history form. The nurse advises the client to
  a. include all information about blood relatives and the animals and roommates that might influence his health.
  b. include only information about genetic/hereditary and environmental illnesses of blood relatives.
  c. leave the area blank since he doesn't live with blood relatives.
  d. use his own judgment in completing the area since the physical exam is more important than the history.

12–4. A client is very worried about how his business is doing while he is hospitalized. He spends much time on the phone and with colleagues instead of resting. The nurse recognizes that, in this case,
  a. this higher level need cannot be met unless the lower level physiologic need is met.

b. his lower level physiologic needs are being deferred while higher needs are addressed.

c. the higher need takes precedence and the lower need no longer must be met.

d. it is necessary for someone else to meet his higher level needs so he can focus on the lower level need.

12–5. There has been a large disaster in a community. Many family homes were destroyed and many individuals in-jured. There is a role for both the community health nurse and the home health nurse. The home health nurse would be responsible for

a. providing for a safe water supply.

b. monitoring for communicable diseases.

c. establishing communication and support systems.

d. assessing and treating individuals' injuries.

Readings and References

Suggested Readings

Cashman, S. B., Bushnell, F. K. L., & Fulmer, H. S. (2001). Community-oriented primary care: A model for public health nursing. *Journal of Health Politics, Policy, and Law, 26,* 617–634.
In 1982, the Institute of Medicine recommended that primary care and community health care be integrated. The resulting community-oriented primary care (COPC) model involves the multidisciplinary work of physicians, nurses, and other health care professionals in planning, implementing, and evaluating care that considers both the individual and the population. In this article, the authors describe one fellowship program that prepares nurses to function in a COPC framework.

Pittman, K. P., Wold, J. L., Wilson, A. H., Huff, C., & Williams, S. (2000). Community connections: Promoting family health. *Family and Community Health, 23,* 72–78.
The authors describe a partnership in which a college of health and human sciences collaborated with an inner-city middle school to meet the health needs of the students and their families. Issues of poverty, substance abuse, violence, and family disintegration contributed to the high-risk nature of the population. Several key "lessons learned" are described, including the need for trust, emphasis on health, and multiple sites for broad and synchronized services.

Related Research

Denham, S. A. (1999). Part I: The definition and practice of family health. *Journal of Family Nursing, 5,* 133–159.

Doornbos, M. M. (2000). King's systems framework and family health: The derivation and testing of a theory. *Journal of Theory Construction and Testing, 4,* 20–26.

Weeks, S. K., O'Connor, P. C., & Enterlante, T. M. (2000). Family health and functional outcomes in rehabilitation. *Rehabilitation Nursing, 25,* 220–230.

References

Anderson, E. T., & McFarlane, J. (2000). *Community as partner: Theory and practice in nursing* (3rd ed.). Philadelphia: Lippincott Williams & Wilkins.

Cannon, W. B. (1939). *The wisdom of the body* (2nd ed.). New York: Norton.

Erikson, E. (1963). *Childhood and society* (2nd ed.). New York: Norton.

Johnson, D. E. (1980). The behavioral system model for nursing. In J. P. Riehl, & C. Roy (Eds.), *Conceptual models for nursing practice* (2nd ed., pp. 207–216). New York: Appleton-Century-Crofts.

Johnson, M., Maas, M., & Moorhead, S. (Eds.). (2000). *Nursing outcomes classification (NOC)* (2nd ed.). St. Louis, MO: Mosby.

Kalish, R. A. (1983). *The psychology of human behavior* (5th ed.). Monterey, CA: Brooks/Cole.

Maslow, A. H. (1998). *Toward a psychology of being* (3rd ed.). New York: John Wiley & Sons.

Maslow, A. H. (1970). *Motivation and personality* (2nd ed.). New York: Harper & Row.

McCloskey, J. C., & Bulechek, G. B. (Eds.). (2000). *Nursing interventions classification (NIC)* (3rd ed.). St. Louis, MO: Mosby.

NANDA International. (2003). NANDA *nursing diagnoses: Definitions and classification 2003–2004.* Philadelphia: Author.

Simmons, T., & O'Neill, G. (2001). *Households and families: 2000.* U.S. Census Bureau, U.S. Department of Commerce, Economics, and Statistics Administration. Retrieved February 19, 2003, from http://www.census.gov/prod/2001pubs/c2kbr01-8.pdf

von Bertalanffy, L. (1969). *General system theory.* New York: George Braziller.

Selected Bibliography

Allender, J. A., & Spradley, B. W. (2000). *Community health nursing: Concepts and practice* (5th ed.). Philadelphia: Lippincott Williams and Wilkins.

Eshleman, J., & Davidhizar, R. (2000). Community assessment: An RN-BSN partnership with community. *Association of Black Nursing Faculty Journal, 11*(2), 28–31.

Plescia, M., Koontz, S., & Laurent, S. (2001). Community assessment in a vertically integrated health care system. *American Journal of Public Health, 91,* 811–814.

Stanhope, M., & Lancaster, J. (1999). *Community and public health nursing* (5th ed.). St. Louis, MO: Mosby.

Stanhope, M., & Lancaster, J. (2001). *Foundations of community health nursing: Community-oriented practice.* Philadelphia: Lippincott Williams and Wilkins.

Williams, R. L., & Yanoshik, K. (2001). Can you do a community assessment without talking to the community? *Journal of Community Health, 26,* 233–247.

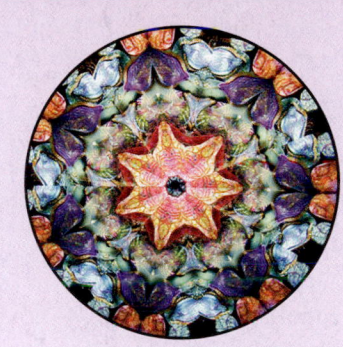

CHAPTER 13

CULTURE AND HERITAGE

LEARNING OUTCOMES

After completing this chapter, you will be able to:

- Describe the rationale for the *National Standards for Culturally and Linguistically Appropriate Services in Health Care.*

- Discuss the components of CulturalCare nursing, heritage consistency, and HEALTH traditions.

- Differentiate biomedical care from folk healing.

- Describe examples of the different health views of culturally diverse people.

- Identify factors related to communication with culturally diverse patients and colleagues.

- Identify methods of heritage assessment.

- Plan culturally sensitive, appropriate, and competent nursing interventions.

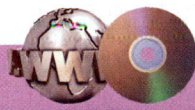

www.prenhall.com/kozier

Additional resources for this chapter can be found on the Student CD-ROM accompanying this textbook, and on the Companion Website at www.prenhall.com/kozier. Click on Chapter 13 to select the activities for this chapter.

CD-ROM
- Audio Glossary
- NCLEX Review

Companion Website
- Additional NCLEX Review
- Case Study: Conveying Cultural Sensitivity
- MediaLink Application:
  Chinese Childbearing Beliefs
- Links to Resources

To provide quality care, nurses must become informed about and sensitive to the culturally diverse subjective meanings of **HEALTH** (defined in this chapter as the balance of the person, both within one's being, physical, mental, and spiritual—and in the outside world—natural, communal, and metaphysical), illness, caring, and healing practices.

Culture can be defined as the nonphysical traits, such as values, beliefs, attitudes, and customs, that are shared by a group of people and passed from one generation to the next (Spector, 2000). Culture also defines how health is perceived; how health care information is received; how rights and protections are exercised; what is considered to be a health problem, and how symptoms and concerns about the health problem are expressed; who should provide treatment and how; and what kind of treatment should be given. **CulturalCare** nursing is a concept that describes the provision of nursing care across cultural boundaries and that takes into account the context in which the client lives and the situations in which the client's health problems arise. It is comprised of both content and process and is essential to the delivery of quality health care to all clients.

Nurses must be aware that, although people from a given group share certain beliefs, values, and experiences, often there is also widespread intra-group diversity. Major differences within groups may be due to such factors as age, gender, level of education, socioeconomic status, and area of origin in the home country (rural or urban). Such factors influence the client's beliefs about health and illness, practices, help-seeking behaviors, and expectations of nurses. For these reasons, effort must be made and care taken to avoid the stereotyping of people from a specific group.

The purpose of this chapter is to present an overview of CulturalCare nursing and to describe the following:

- The rationale for CulturalCare nursing within the larger scope of nursing
- Selected examples of the necessary CulturalCare content
- An introduction to the process of CulturalCare nursing.

> **CLINICAL ALERT** *Culture and language are vital factors in how nursing care is delivered and received and there is the expectation that the diverse cultural needs of clients must be met.* ∎

NATIONAL STANDARDS FOR CULTURALLY AND LINGUISTICALLY APPROPRIATE SERVICES IN HEALTH CARE

The composition of the population of the United States has changed during the past 30 years. Given the ongoing changes in the population, *National Standards for Culturally and Linguistically Appropriate Services in Health Care* (CLAS) have been created (Office of Minority Health [OMH], 2001). Culture and language have a considerable impact on how clients access and respond to health care services. Furthermore, to ensure equal access to quality health care by diverse populations, health care organizations and nurses should "promote and support the attitudes, behaviors, knowledge, and skills necessary for staff to work respectfully and effectively with clients and each other in a culturally diverse work environment" (OMH, 2001, p. 7). The standards have been based on an analytical review of key laws, regulations, contracts, and standards currently in use by federal and state agencies and other national organizations to evaluate the cultural quality of care.

The United States has many cultural groups. It has been called a "melting pot" of peoples. However, the term *cultural mosaic* may be a more accurate description of the way in which many people of different cultures maintain the cultural values, beliefs, traditions, and practices of their **heritage** (things passed down from previous generations) for many generations. In addition to the indigenous peoples (Native Americans and Native Alaskans), much diversity is seen in the long-term resident populations and immigrant groups in North America. In fact, as the population of the United States becomes more diverse, nurses are caring for an increasing number of clients from many different cultural and linguistic backgrounds. There are two major reasons for this: One is the demographic change in the overall population and the other is the enormous amount of immigration that has occurred since the 1990s.

Demographic Change

The American census of 2000 indicates that the White, non-Hispanic majority is now 75.1% of the population, whereas it was 80.3% in 1990, and 83% in 1980 (U. S. Census Bureau, 2001). Thus, people of color now represent about 25% of the population and are growing. In fact, by the year 2020, it is predicted that there will be more people of color than Whites in the United States. Table 13–1 compares the distribution of the U.S. populations of 1980, 1990, and 2000 by ethnic groups (Hobbs & Stoops, 2002). Nurses are predominantly White, and in percentage disproportionate to the demographic profile of the United States. Table 13–2 compares the percentages of American Indian, Asian/Pacific Islander, Black Non-Hispanic, Hispanic, and White Non-Hispanic nurses in 2000 (Spratley, Johnson, Sochalski, Fritz, & Spencer, 2002).

TABLE 13–1 Percentages of American Indians, Asian/Pacific Islanders, Blacks, Whites, and Hispanics in the United States: 1980, 1990, and 2000

Population	1980	1990	2000
American Indian/ Alaska Native	0.6	0.8	0.9
Asian/Pacific Islander	1.5	2.9	3.8
Black	11.7	12.1	12.3
White	83.1	80.3	75.1
Other (or multiple)	3.0	3.9	7.9
Hispanic (of any race)	6.4	9.0	12.5

Note: From *Demographic Trends in the 20th Century* (pp. 77–78) by F. Hobbs and N. Stoops, 2002, Washington, DC: U.S. Government Printing Office.

TABLE 13-2 Percentages of American Indian, Asian/Pacific Islander, Black Non-Hispanic, Hispanic, and White Non-Hispanic Nurses in 2000

Population	Percent
American Indian/ Alaska Native	0.5
Asian/Pacific Islander and other	3.5
Black non-Hispanic	4.9
Hispanic	2.0
White non-Hispanic	86.6

Note: From "The Registered Nurse Population, March 2000: Findings from the National Sample Survey of Registered Nurses," by E. Spratley, A. Johnson, J. Sochalski, M. Fritz, & W. Spencer, 2002, U.S. Department of Health and Human Services Health Resources and Service Administration Bureau of Health Professions, Division of Nursing. Retrieved November 1, 2002, from http://bhpr.hrsa.gov/healthworkforce/rnsurvey/mss1.htm#T1

Immigration

Millions of immigrants were admitted to the United States during the 1990s. The foreign-born population of the United States has grown from 8% in 1990 to 10% in 2000, the highest rate since 1930. The 28.4 million foreign-born population consists of 14.5 million people from Latin America, 7.2 million people from Asian countries, and 4.4 million people from Europe (Bernstein, 2002).

CULTURALCARE NURSING

CulturalCare is professional nursing care that is culturally sensitive, culturally appropriate, and culturally competent. CulturalCare nursing is critical to meeting the complex nursing care needs of a given person, family, and community. It is the provision of nursing care across cultural boundaries and takes into account the context in which the client lives as well as the situations in which the client's health problems arise.

- **Culturally sensitive** implies that the nurse possesses some basic knowledge of and constructive attitudes toward the health traditions observed among the diverse cultural groups found in the setting in which they are practicing.
- **Culturally appropriate** implies that the nurse applies the underlying background knowledge that must be possessed to provide a given client with the best possible health care.
- **Culturally competent** implies that within the delivered care the nurse understands and attends to the total context of the client's situation and uses a complex combination of knowledge, attitudes, and skills.

CulturalCare is inherent in the development of nursing practice to meet the mandates of the CLAS standards. Countless conflicts in the health care delivery arenas are predicated on cultural misunderstandings. Although many of these misunderstandings are related to universal situations, such as verbal and nonverbal language misunderstandings, the conventions of courtesy, sequencing of interactions, phasing of interactions, objectivity, and so forth, many cultural misunderstandings are unique to the delivery of nursing care. CulturalCare is essential and it demands that nurses be able to assess and interpret a given client's health beliefs and practices and cultural needs. CulturalCare alters the perspective of nursing care delivery because it enables the nurse to understand, from a cultural perspective, the manifestations of the client's health care beliefs and practices.

CONCEPTS RELATED TO CULTURALCARE NURSING

All groups of people face issues in adapting to their environment: providing nutrition and shelter, caring for and educating children, dividing labor, developing social organization, controlling disease, and maintaining health. Humans adapt to varying environments by developing cultural solutions to meet these needs. Culture is a universal experience, but no two cultures are exactly alike. Cultural patterns are learned, and it is important for nurses to note that members of a particular group may not share identical cultural experiences. Thus, each member of a cultural group will be somewhat different from his or her own cultural counterparts. For example, third-generation Japanese Americans (Sansei) will differ in cultural understandings from first-generation Japanese (Issei).

Subculture

Large cultural groups often have cultural subgroups or subsystems. A **subculture** is usually composed of people who have a distinct identity and yet are related to a larger cultural group. A subcultural group generally shares ethnic origin, occupation, or physical characteristics with the larger cultural group. Examples of cultural subgroups include occupational groups (e.g., nurses), societal groups (e.g., feminists), and ethnic groups (e.g., Cajuns, who are descendants of French Acadians—17th-century settlers in Canadian Nova Scotia, New Brunswick, and Prince Edward Island).

Bicultural

Bicultural is used to describe a person who crosses two cultures, lifestyles, and sets of values (Giger & Davidhizar, 1999). For example, a young man whose father is Cherokee and whose mother is European American may honor his traditional Cherokee heritage while also being influenced by his mother's cultural values.

Diversity

Diversity refers to the fact or state of being different. Many factors account for diversity: race, gender, sexual orientation, culture, ethnicity, socioeconomic status, educational attainment, religious affiliation, and so on. Diversity therefore occurs not only between cultural groups but also within a cultural group.

Acculturation

While becoming a participant in the dominant culture, a member of a nondominant cultural group is always identified as a member of the culture from which they originate. People immigrating to the United States from any country will be associated with their native countries for many years, if not for all of their lives. The involuntary process of **acculturation** occurs when people adapt to or borrow traits from another culture. The member of the non-dominant cultural group is often forced to learn the new culture to survive. Acculturation can also be defined as the changes of one's cultural patterns to those of the host society (Spector, 2000).

Assimilation

Assimilation is the process by which an individual develops a new cultural identity. Assimilation means becoming like the members of the dominant culture. The process of assimilation encompasses various aspects, such as behavioral, marital, identification, and civic. The underlying assumption is that the person from a given cultural group loses his or her original cultural identity to acquire the new one. In fact, because this is a conscious effort, it is not always possible, and the process may cause severe stress and anxiety. Assimilation can also be described as a collection of subprocesses: a process of inclusion through which a person gradually ceases to conform to any standard of life that differs from the dominant group standards and, at the same time, a process through which the person learns to conform to all the dominant group standards. The process of assimilation is considered complete when the foreigner is fully merged into the dominant cultural group (McLemore, Romo, & Baker, 2001).

The concepts of assimilation and acculturation are complex and sensitive. The dominant society expects that all immigrants are in the process of acculturation and assimilation and that the world view that we share as nurses is commonly shared by our clients. Because we live in a society with many cultures, however, many variations of health beliefs and practices exist. Several other factors for cultural consideration include race, prejudice, stereotyping, discrimination, and culture shock.

Race

Race is the classification of people according to shared biologic characteristics, genetic markers, or features. People of the same race have common characteristics such as skin color, bone structure, facial features, hair texture, and blood type. Different ethnic groups can belong to the same race, and different cultures can be found within one ethnic group. For example, the terms *Caucasian* and *European American* describe the race of people whose origins are in Europe. Whereas British Americans are a subgroup of European Americans, Scottish Americans (an ethnic subgroup of British Americans) may share different cultural practices than other British Americans. It is important to understand that not all people of the same race have the same culture. Culture should not be confused with either race or ethnic group.

Prejudice

Prejudice is a negative belief or preference that is generalized about a group and that leads to "prejudgment." Prejudice occurs because either the person making the judgment does not understand the given person or his or her heritage, or the person making the judgment generalizes an experience of one individual from a culture to all members of that group.

Stereotyping

Stereotyping is assuming that all members of a culture or ethnic group are alike. For example, a nurse may assume that all Italians verbally express pain loudly or that all Chinese people like rice. Stereotyping may be based on generalizations founded in research, or it may be unrelated to reality. For example, research indicates that most Italians are likely to express pain verbally; however, a specific Italian client may not do so. Stereotyping that is unrelated to reality is frequently an outcome of racism or discrimination. Nurses need to realize that not all people of a specific group have the same health beliefs, practices, and values. It is therefore essential to identify a specific client's beliefs, needs, and values rather than assuming they are the same as those attributable to the larger group.

Discrimination

Discrimination, the differential treatment of individuals or groups based on categories such as race, ethnicity, gender, social class, or exceptionality, occurs when a person acts on prejudice and denies another person one or more of the fundamental rights.

Culture Shock

Culture shock is a disorder that occurs in response to transition from one cultural setting to another. A person's former behavior patterns are ineffective in such a setting, and basic cues for social behavior are absent (Spector, 2000). This phenomena may occur when one moves from one geographic location to another or when a person immigrates to a new country. It may occur when a person is admitted into a hospital and has to adapt to a foreign situation. Expressions of culture shock may range from silence and immobility to agitation, rage, or fury.

HERITAGE CONSISTENCY

Heritage consistency is a concept developed by Zitzow and Estes (1981; D. Zitzow, personal communication, September 26, 2002) to describe "the degree to which one's lifestyle reflects his or her respective tribal culture." The concept has been expanded in an attempt to study the degree to which a person's lifestyle reflects his or her traditional culture, whether European, Asian, African, or Hispanic. The values indicating heritage consistency exist on a continuum, and a person can possess characteristics of both heritage consistency (**traditional**), that is, observance of the beliefs and practices of one's traditional cultural belief system; and **heritage inconsistency,** the observance of the beliefs and practices of one's acculturated (or **modern**) belief system. The model of heritage consistency has four overlapping components: culture, ethnicity, religion, and socialization.

Culture

There is no single definition of culture, and all too often definitions tend to omit salient aspects of culture or to be too general to have any real meaning. One of the most common definitions of culture is the combination of nonphysical traits, such as values, beliefs, attitudes, and customs, that are shared by a group of people and passed from one generation to the next. The following are additional examples of definitions of this elusive term:

1. Culture is the thoughts, communications, actions, beliefs, values, and institutions of racial, ethnic, religious, or social groups (OMH, 2001, p. 4).
2. Culture is the sum total of socially inherited characteristics of a human group that comprises everything which one generation can tell, convey, or hand down to the next.
3. Culture is the luggage that each of us carries around for our lifetime. It is the sum of beliefs, practices, habits, likes, dislikes, norms, customs, rituals, and so forth that we learned from our families. In turn, we transmit cultural luggage to our children (Spector, 2000, p. 78).
4. Culture is a "metacommunication system," wherein not only the spoken words have meaning, but everything else as well (Matsumoto & Matsumoto, 1989, p. 14).

Culture is a complex whole in which each part is related to every other part. It is learned, and the capacity to learn culture is genetic, but the subject matter is not genetic and must be learned by each person in his or her family and social community. Culture also depends on an underlying social matrix, including knowledge, belief, art, law, morals, and custom (Bohannan, 1992).

Ethnicity

Cultural background is a fundamental component of one's **ethnic** background or ethnicity, a group within the social system that claims to posses variable traits such as a common religion or language. The term *ethnic* has for some time aroused strongly negative feelings and often is rejected by the general population. One can speculate that the upsurge in the use of the term stems from the recent interest of people in discovering their personal backgrounds, a fact used by some politicians who overtly court "the ethnics." Paradoxically, in a nation as large as the United States and comprising as many different peoples as it does—with the American Indians being the only true native population—we find ourselves still reluctant to speak of ethnicity and ethnic differences. This stance stems from the fact that most foreign groups that came to this land often shed the ways of the "old country" and quickly attempted to assimilate themselves into the mainstream, or the so-called melting pot.

There are at least 106 groups in the United States that meet many of the characteristics of an ethnic group. People from every country in the world have immigrated to this country. Among the foreign-born peoples of the United States represented in the 2000 census, the largest numbers of Latin American immigrants have come from Cuba, El Salvador, and Mexico; African immigrants from Egypt, Ghana, and Nigeria; Asian immigrants from China, India, and the Philippines; and European immigrants from the British Isles, Germany, and the former Soviet Union. The percent of the total numbers coming from a specific area have remained relatively constant during the past 15 years for some groups (e.g., Europe and the Caribbean), while others have experienced greater increases (e.g., Africa) (U.S. Census Bureau, 2001).

Religion

The third major component of a person's heritage is religion. Although the word has many definitions, **religion** may be considered a system of beliefs, practices, and ethical values about divine or superhuman power or powers worshipped as the creator(s) and ruler(s) of the universe. The practice of religion is revealed in numerous cults, sects, denominations, and churches. Ethnicity and religion are clearly related, and one's religion quite often is determined by one's ethnic group. Religion gives a person a frame of reference and a perspective with which to organize information. Religious teachings vis-á-vis health help to present a meaningful philosophy and system of practices within a system of social controls having specific values, norms, and ethics. These are related to health in that adherence to a religious code is conducive to spiritual harmony. Illness is sometimes seen as the punishment for the violation of religious codes and morals. It is not possible to isolate the aspects of culture, religion, and ethnicity that shape a person's worldview. Each is part of the other, and all three are united within the person.

Socialization

Socialization is the process of being raised within a culture and acquiring the characteristics of that group. Education—be it elementary school, high school, college, or nursing—is a form of socialization. For many people who have been socialized within the boundaries of a traditional culture or a nonmodern culture (usually associated with the East or third and fourth world nations), modern "American," or Western, first world culture becomes a second cultural identity. Those who immigrate here, legally or illegally, from non-Western or nonmodern countries may find socialization into the American culture to be an extremely difficult and painful process. As time passes, many people experience biculturalism and divided loyalties. In addition, many people who have been socialized in cultures wherein traditional health care resources are used may prefer to use this type of care even when residing within a cultural setting with modern health care resources available.

HEALTH TRADITIONS

The HEALTH traditions model is predicated on the concept of holistic HEALTH and describes what people do from a traditional perspective to maintain, protect, and restore HEALTH.

Imagine HEALTH as a complex, interrelated, threefold phenomenon, that is, the balance of all aspects of the person—the body, mind, and spirit.

Interrelated Aspects

- The body includes all physical aspects, such as genetic inheritance, body chemistry, gender, age, nutrition, and physical condition.
- The mind includes cognitive processes, such as thoughts, memories, and knowledge of such emotional processes as feelings, defenses, and self-esteem.
- The spiritual facet includes both positive and negative learned spiritual practices and teachings, dreams, symbols, stories; protecting forces; and metaphysical or native forces.

These aspects are in constant flux and change over time, yet each is completely related to the others and also related to the context of the person. The context includes the person's family, culture, work, community, history, and environment (Spector, 2000).

The HEALTH traditions model, Table 13–3, consists of nine interrelated facets, represented by the following:

1. *Traditional methods of maintaining HEALTH*—physical, mental, and spiritual—include following a proper diet and wearing proper clothing, concentrating and using the mind, and practicing one's religion.
2. *Traditional methods of protecting HEALTH*—physical, mental, and spiritual—include wearing protective objects, such as amulets, avoiding people who may cause trouble, and placing religious objects in the home.
3. *Traditional methods of restoring HEALTH*—physical, mental, and spiritual—include the use of herbal remedies, exorcism, and healing rituals.

TABLE 13–3 The Nine Interrelated Facets of Health (Physical, Mental, and Spiritual) and Personal Methods of Maintaining Health, Protecting Health, and Restoring Health

	Physical	Mental	Spiritual
MAINTAIN HEALTH	Proper clothing Proper diet Exercise/Rest	Concentration Social and family support systems Hobbies	Religious worship Prayer Meditation
PROTECT HEALTH	Special foods and food combination Symbolic clothing	Avoid certain people who can cause illness Family activities	Religious customs Superstitions Wearing amulets and other symbolic objects to prevent the "Evil Eye" or defray other sources of harm
RESTORE HEALTH	Homeopathic remedies lineaments Herbal teas Special foods Massage Acupuncture/moxibustion	Relaxation Exorcism Curanderos and other traditional healers Nerve teas	Religious rituals, special prayers Meditation Traditional healings Exorcism

Note: From Cultural Diversity in Health and Illness, 5th ed. (p. 100) by R. E. Spector, 2000, Upper Saddle River, NJ: Prentice Hall.

Symbolic Examples

Figure 13–1 ■ depicts symbolic, HEALTH-related images that may be used to maintain, protect, or restore physical, mental, or spiritual HEALTH by people of different heritages.

1. Thousand-year-old eggs, from China, represent traditional foods that may be eaten daily to maintain physical HEALTH.
2. The enjoyment of nature, the natural environment, may be a universal way of maintaining mental HEALTH.
3. The Islamic prayer, from East Jerusalem, represents prayer, a way of maintaining spiritual HEALTH.
4. Red string, from the Tomb of Rachel in Bethlehem, Israel, may be worn to protect physical HEALTH.
5. The eye, from Cuba, represents the plethora of eye-related objects that may be worn or hung in the home to protect the mental HEALTH of people by shielding them from the envy and bad wishes of others.
6. The thunderbird, from the Hopi nation, may be worn for spiritual protection and good luck.
7. The herbal remedy from Africa represents aromatic plants that may be used by people from all ethnocultural traditional backgrounds as one method of restoring physical HEALTH.
8. Tiger balm, from Singapore, represents substances that are used in massage therapy as a way of restoring mental HEALTH.
9. Rosary beads, from Italy, symbolize prayer and meditation methods used in the spiritual restoration of HEALTH.

There are an infinite number of examples one could present. A major aspect of conducting the heritage assessment of a client is to determine what items are used by a specific person and its meaning to the person.

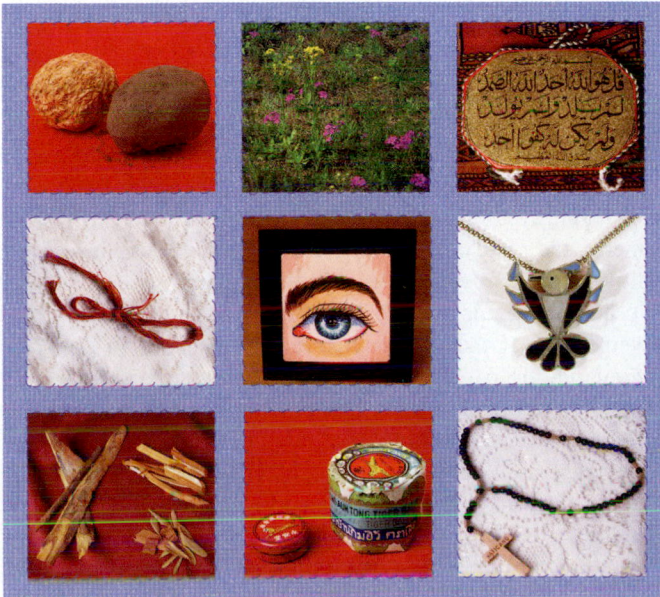

Figure 13–1 ■ Symbols of the HEALTH traditions model and themes. (From *Cultural Diversity in Health and Illness*, 5th ed. by R. E. Spector, 2000, Upper Saddle River, NJ: Prentice Hall.)

SELECTED PARAMETERS FOR CULTURALCARE NURSING

This section outlines selected CulturalCare phenomena of significance to CulturalCare nursing. Information about cultural aspects of death and dying are found in Chapter 41 ⬅ and about pain management in Chapter 44. ⬅

Health Beliefs and Practices

Andrews and Boyle (2002) describe three views of health beliefs: magico-religious, scientific, and holistic. In the **magico-religious health belief view,** health and illness are controlled by supernatural forces. The client may believe that illness is the result of "being bad" or opposing God's will. Getting well is also viewed as dependent on God's will. The client may make statements such as "If it is God's will, I will recover" or "What did I do wrong to be punished with cancer?" Some cultures believe that magic can cause illness. A sorcerer or witch may put a spell or hex on the client. Some people view illness as possession by an evil spirit. Although these beliefs are not supported by empirical evidence, clients who believe that such things can cause illness may in fact become ill as a result. Such illnesses may require magical treatments in addition to scientific treatments. For example, a man who experiences gastric distress, headaches, and hypertension after being told that a spell has been placed on him may recover only if the spell is removed by the culture's healer.

The **scientific** or **biomedical health belief** is based on the belief that life and life processes are controlled by physical and biochemical processes that can be manipulated by humans (Andrews & Boyle, 2002). The client with this view will believe that illness is caused by germs, viruses, bacteria, or a breakdown of the human machine, the body. This client will expect a pill, or treatment, or surgery to cure health problems.

The **holistic health belief** holds that the forces of nature must be maintained in balance or harmony. Human life is one aspect of nature that must be in harmony with the rest of nature. When the natural balance or harmony is disturbed, illness results. The medicine wheel is an ancient symbol used by Native Americans of North and South America to express many concepts. For health and wellness, the medicine wheel teaches the four aspects of the individual's nature: the physical, the mental, the emotional, and the spiritual. The four dimensions must be in balance to be healthy. The medicine wheel can also be used to express the individual's relationship with the environment as a dimension of wellness.

The concept of yin and yang in the Chinese culture and the hot–cold theory of illness in many Spanish cultures are examples of holistic health beliefs. When a Chinese client has a yin illness or a "cold" illness, the treatment may include a yang or "hot" food (e.g., hot tea). For example, a Chinese client who has been diagnosed with cancer, a yin disease, will want to eat cultural foods that have yang properties.

What is considered hot or cold varies considerably across cultures. In many cultures, the mother who has just delivered a baby should be offered warm or hot foods and kept warm with blankets because childbirth is seen as a "cold" condition. Conventional scientific thought recommends cooling the body to reduce a fever. The physician may order liquids for the client and cool compresses to be applied to the forehead, the axillae, or the groin. Galanti (1997) states that many cultures believe that the best way to treat a fever is to "sweat it out." Clients from these cultures may want to cover up with several blankets, take hot baths, and drink hot beverages. The nurse must keep in mind that a treatment strategy that is consistent with the client's beliefs may have a better chance of being successful. For example, the Latino client who avoids "hot" foods when experiencing a stomach disturbance may be eating foods consistent with the bland diet that is normally prescribed by physicians.

Sociocultural forces, such as politics, economics, geography, religion, and the predominant health care system, influence the client's health status and health care behavior. For example, people who have limited access to scientific health care may turn to folk medicine or folk healing. **Folk medicine** is defined as those beliefs and practices relating to illness prevention and healing that derive from cultural traditions rather than from modern medicine's scientific base. Many students can recall special teas or "cures" used by older family members to prevent or treat colds, fevers, indigestion, and other common health problems. People also continue to use chicken soup as a treatment for influenza (the "flu").

Why do individuals use these nontraditional folk healing methods? Folk medicine, in contrast to biomedical health care, is thought to be more humanistic. The consultation and treatment takes place in the community of the recipient, frequently in the home of the healer. It is less expensive than scientific or biomedical care because the health problem is identified primarily through conversation with the client and the family. The healer often prepares the treatments, for example, teas to be ingested, poultices to be applied, or charms or amulets to be worn. A frequent component of treatment is some ritual practice on the part of the healer or the client to cause healing to occur. Because folk healing is more culturally based, it is often more comfortable and less frightening for the client.

> **CLINICAL ALERT** *Treatments once considered to be folk treatments, including acupuncture, therapeutic touch, and massage, are now being investigated for their therapeutic effect.* ■

It is important for the nurse to obtain information about folk or family healing practices that may have been used before the client decided to seek Western medical treatment. Often clients are reluctant to share home remedies with health care professionals for fear of being laughed at or rebuked.

Family Patterns

The family is the basic unit of society. Cultural values can determine communication within the family group, the norm for family size, and the roles of specific family members. In some families, the man is considered the provider and decision maker. The woman may need to consult her husband before making decisions about her medical treatment or the treatment of her children. Some families are matriarchal; that is, the mother or grandmother is viewed as the leader of the family and is usually the decision maker. The nurse needs to identify who has the "authority" to make decisions in a client's family. If the decision maker is someone other than the client, the nurse needs to include that person in health care discussions.

The value placed on children and elders within a society is culturally derived. In some cultures, children are not disciplined by spanking or other forms of physical punishment. Rather, children are allowed to interact with their environment while caregivers provide subtle direction to prevent harm or injury. In other cultures, elderly people are considered the holders of the culture's wisdom and are therefore highly respected. Responsibility for caring for older relatives is determined by cultural practices. In many cultures, older relatives who cannot live independently often live with a married son or daughter and family.

Cultural gender-role behavior may also affect nurse–client interactions. In some countries, men dominate and women have little status. Men from these countries may not accept instruction from a female nurse or physician but will be receptive to the same instruction given by a male physician or nurse. Some cultures have a prevailing concept of machismo, or male superiority. The positive aspects of machismo require that the adult man provide for and protect his family, including extended family members. The woman is expected to maintain the home and raise the children.

Cultural family values may also dictate the extent of the family's involvement in the hospitalized client's care. In some cultures, the nuclear and the extended family will want to visit for long periods and participate in care. In other cultures, the entire clan may want to visit and participate in the client's care. This can cause concern on nursing units with strict visiting policies. The nurse should evaluate the positive benefits of family participation in the client's care and modify visiting policies as appropriate.

Cultures that value the needs of the extended family as much as those of the individual may hold the belief that personal and family information must stay within the family. Some cultural groups are very reluctant to disclose family information to outsiders, including health care professionals. This attitude can present difficulties for health care professionals who require knowledge of family interaction patterns to help clients with emotional problems.

Naming systems in many cultures differ from those in North America. In some cultures (e.g., Japanese and Vietnamese), the family name comes first and the given name second. One or two names may or may not be added between the family and given names. Other nomenclature may be used to delineate sexual, child, or adult status. For example, in traditional Japanese culture, adults address other adults by their surname followed by *san,* meaning *Mr., Mrs.,* or *Miss.* An example is Maurakami san. The children are referred to by their first names followed by *kun* for boys and *chan* for girls. Sikhs and Hindus traditionally have three names. Hindus have a personal name, a complimentary name, and then a family name. Sikhs have a personal name, then the title *Singh* for men and *Kaur* for women, and lastly the family name. Names by marriage also vary. In Central America, a woman who marries retains her father's name and takes her husband's. For example, if Louisa

Viccario marries Carlos Gonzales she becomes Louisa Viccario de Gonzales. The connecting *de* means "belonging to." Their son is Pedro Gonzales Viccario. Nurses need to become familiar with appropriate ways to address clients.

Communication Style

Communication and culture are closely interconnected. Through communication, the culture is transmitted from one generation to the next, and knowledge about the culture is transmitted within the group and to those outside the group. Communicating with clients of various ethnic and cultural backgrounds is critical to providing culturally competent nursing care. There can be cultural variations in both verbal and nonverbal communication.

Verbal Communication

The most obvious cultural difference is in verbal communication: vocabulary, grammatical structure, voice qualities, intonation, rhythm, speed, pronunciation, and silence. In North America, the dominant language is English; however, immigrant groups who speak English still encounter language differences because English words can have different meanings in different English-speaking cultures. For example, in the United States, a *boot* is a type of footwear that comes to the ankle or higher; in England, a boot can also be the trunk of a car. Spanish is spoken by people in several regions of the world: Spain, South America, Central America, Mexico, the Caribbean, and the Philippines, for example. It is the second most commonly spoken language in the United States. Nevertheless, each cultural group that speaks Spanish may use different vocabulary, apply rules of grammar differently, and use different pronunciation, so that often two people of different Latino cultures, speaking Spanish together, may not completely understand each other.

Initiating verbal communication may be influenced by cultural values. The busy nurse may want to complete nursing admission assessments quickly. The client, however, may be offended when the nurse immediately asks personal questions. In some cultures, it is believed that social courtesies should be established before business or personal topics are discussed. Discussing general topics can convey that the nurse is interested in the client and has time for the client. This enables the nurse to develop a rapport with the client before progressing to discussion that is more personal.

Verbal communication becomes even more difficult when an interaction involves people who speak different languages. Both clients and health professionals experience frustration when they are unable to communicate verbally with each other. Techniques for therapeutic communication with persons who have limited English are shown in the accompanying Practice Guidelines.

For the client whose language is not the same as that of the health care provider, an intermediary may be necessary. A **translator** converts written material (such as patient education pamphlets) from one language into another. An **interpreter** is "an individual who mediates spoken communication between people speaking different languages without adding, omitting, or distorting meaning or editorializing. The objective of the professional interpreter is for the complete transfer of the

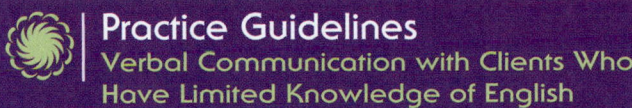

Practice Guidelines
Verbal Communication with Clients Who Have Limited Knowledge of English

- Avoid slang words, medical terminology, and abbreviations.
- Augment spoken conversation with gestures or pictures to increase the client's understanding.
- Speak slowly, in a respectful manner, and at a normal volume. Speaking loudly does not help the client understand and may be offensive.
- Frequently validate the client's understanding of what is being communicated. Be wary of interpreting a client's smiling and nodding to mean that the client understands; the client may only be trying to please the nurse and not understand what is being said.

thought behind the utterance in one language into an utterance in a second language" (California Healthcare Interpreters Association, 2002, p. 64). Thus, a true interpreter has demonstrated ethical and interpreting skills and the knowledge and expertise required to function in a health care situation. In some states, mandates require hospitals to have certified interpreters available for clients who require them. Many institutions that are located in culturally diverse communities have translators available on staff or maintain a list of employees who are fluent in other languages. Embassies, consulates, ethnic churches (e.g., Russian Orthodox, Greek Orthodox), ethnic clubs (e.g., Polish American Club, Italian American Club), or telephone companies may also be able to provide interpreters. However, asking a family member or other nonprofessional to interpret can create difficulties. Cultural rules often dictate who can discuss what with whom. Guidelines for using an interpreter are shown in the Practice Guidelines on page 214.

> **CLINICAL ALERT**   *Nurses who speak a second language may be asked to interpret for others. Nursing schools and health care institutions may not permit nursing students to interpret for a procedure consent because a lack of knowledge about the procedure may lead the student to give inaccurate information. Check the institution's policy before agreeing to interpret for institutional staff and physicians.* ■

Nurses and other health care providers must remember that clients for whom English is a second language may lose command of their English when they are in stressful situations. Clients who have used English comfortably for years in social and business communication may forget and revert back to their primary language when they are ill or distressed. It is important for the nurse to assure the client that this is normal and to promote behaviors to facilitate verbal communication.

Nonverbal Communication

To communicate effectively with culturally diverse clients, the nurse needs to be aware of two aspects of nonverbal communication behaviors: what nonverbal behaviors mean to the client

Practice Guidelines
Using an Interpreter

- Avoid asking a member of the client's family, especially a child or spouse, to act as interpreter. The client, not wishing family members to know about his or her problem, may not provide complete or accurate information.
- Be aware of gender and age differences; it is preferable to use an interpreter of the same gender as the client to avoid embarrassment and faulty translation of sexual matters.
- Avoid an interpreter who is politically or socially incompatible with the client. For example, a Bosnian Serb may not be the best interpreter for a Muslim, even if he speaks the language.
- Address the questions to the client, not to the interpreter.
- Ask the interpreter to translate as closely as possible the words used by the nurse.
- Speak slowly and distinctly. Do not use metaphors, for example, "Does it swell like a grapefruit?" or "Is the pain stabbing like a knife?"
- Observe the facial expressions and body language that the client assumes when listening and talking to the interpreter.

and what specific nonverbal behaviors mean in the client's culture. Before assigning meaning to nonverbal behavior, the nurse must consider the possibility that the behavior may have a different meaning for the client and the family. To provide safe and effective care, nurses who work with specific cultural groups should learn more about cultural behavior and communication patterns within these cultures.

Nonverbal communication can include the use of silence, touch, eye movement, facial expressions, and body posture. Some cultures are quite comfortable with long periods of silence, whereas others consider it appropriate to speak before the other person has finished talking. Many people value silence and view it as essential to understanding a person's needs or use silence to preserve privacy. Some cultures view silence as a sign of respect, whereas to other people silence may indicate agreement.

Touching involves learned behaviors that can have both positive and negative meanings. In the American culture, a firm handshake is a recognized form of greeting that conveys character and strength. In some European cultures, greetings may include a kiss on one or both cheeks. In some societies, touch is considered magical and because of the belief that the soul can leave the body on physical contact, casual touching is forbidden. In some Asian cultures (e.g., people from India, Sri Lanka, Thailand, and Laos), only certain elders are permitted to touch the head of others, and children are never patted on the head. Nurses should therefore touch a client's head only with permission.

Cultures dictate what forms of touch are appropriate for individuals of the same sex and opposite sex. In many cultures, for example, a kiss is not appropriate for a public greeting between persons of the opposite sex, even those who are family members; however, a kiss on the cheek is acceptable as a greeting among individuals of the same sex. The nurse should watch interaction among clients and families for cues to the appropriate degree of touch in that culture. The nurse can also assess the client's re-

sponse to touch when providing nursing care, for example, by noting the client's reaction to the physical examination or the bath.

Facial expression can also vary between cultures. Giger and Davidhizar (1999) state that Italian, Jewish, African American, and Spanish-speaking persons are more likely to smile readily and use facial expression to communicate feelings, whereas Irish, English, and Northern European people tend to have less facial expression and are less open in their response, especially to strangers. Facial expressions can also convey a meaning opposite to what is felt or understood.

Eye movement during communication has cultural foundations. In Western cultures, direct eye contact is regarded as important and generally shows that the other is attentive and listening. It conveys self-confidence, openness, interest, and honesty. Lack of eye contact may be interpreted as secretiveness, shyness, guilt, lack of interest, or even a sign of mental illness. However, other cultures may view eye contact as impolite or an invasion of privacy. In the Hmong culture, continuous direct eye contact is considered rude, but intermittent eye contact is acceptable. The nurse should not misinterpret the character of the client who avoids eye contact.

Body posture and hand gestures are also culturally learned. For example, the V sign means victory in some cultures, but it is an offensive gesture in other cultures. Tapping the index finger on one's temple may mean someone is intelligent in the United States but crazy in Holland.

Communication is an essential part of establishing a relationship with a client and his or her family. It is also important for developing effective working relationships with health care colleagues. To enhance their practice, nurses can observe the communication patterns of clients and colleagues and be aware of their own communication behaviors.

Space Orientation

Space is a relative concept that includes the individual, the body, the surrounding environment, and objects within that environment. The relationship between the individual's own body and objects and persons within space is learned and is influenced by culture. For example, in nomadic societies, space is not owned; it is occupied temporarily until the tribe moves on. In Western societies people tend to be more territorial, as reflected in phrases such as "This is my space" or "Get out of my space." In Western cultures, spatial distances are defined as the intimate zone, the personal zone, and the social and public zones. The size of these areas may vary with the specific culture. Nurses move through all three zones as they provide care for clients. The nurse needs to be aware of the client's response to movement toward the client. The client may physically withdraw or back away if the nurse is perceived as being too close. The nurse will need to explain to the client why there is a need to be close to the client. To assess the lungs with a stethoscope, for example, the nurse needs to move into the client's intimate space. The nurse should first explain the procedure and await permission to continue.

Clients who reside in long-term care facilities, or who are hospitalized for an extended time, may want to personalize their space. They may want to arrange their room differently or control the placement of objects on their bedside cabinet or over-bed table. The nurse should be responsive to clients' needs to have some control over their space. When there are no medical contraindications, clients should be permitted and encouraged to have objects of personal significance. Having personal and cultural items in one's environment can increase self-esteem by promoting not only one's individuality but also one's cultural identity. Of course, the nurse should caution the client about responsibility for loss of personal items.

Time Orientation

Time orientation refers to an individual's focus on the past, the present, or the future. Most cultures include all three time orientations, but one orientation is more likely to dominate. The American focus on time tends to be directed to the future, emphasizing time and schedules. Nursing students know what times they "must" be in class or clinical. They know what courses they will take in future semesters. European Americans often plan for next week, their vacation, or their retirement. Other cultures may have a different concept of time. For example, the Navajo Indians do not have a word for "late" and a Navajo mother may not become upset if her child does not achieve a specific developmental milestone, such as walking or toileting, on schedule.

The culture of nursing and health care values time. Appointments are scheduled, and treatments are prescribed with time parameters (e.g., changing a dressing once a day). Medication orders include how often the medicine is to be taken and when (e.g., digoxin 0.25 mg, once a day, in the morning). Nurses need to be aware of the meaning of time for clients. When caring for clients who are "present oriented," it is important to avoid fixed schedules. The nurse can offer a time range for activities and treatments. For example, instead of telling the client to take digoxin every day at 10:00 AM, the nurse might tell the client to take it every day in the morning or every day after getting out of bed.

Nutritional Patterns

Most cultures have staple foods, that is, foods that are plentiful or readily accessible in the environment. For example, the staple food for Asians is rice; of Italians, pasta; and of Eastern Europeans, wheat. Even clients who have been in the United States or Canada for several generations often continue to eat the foods of their cultural homeland.

The way food is prepared and served is also related to cultural practices. For example, in the United States a traditional food served for the Thanksgiving holiday is stuffed turkey; however, in different regions of the country the contents of the stuffing may vary. In Southern states, the stuffing may be made of cornbread; in New England, of seasoned bread and chestnuts.

The way in which staple foods are prepared also varies. For example, some Asian cultures prefer steamed rice; others prefer boiled rice. Southern Asians from India prepare unleavened bread from wheat flour rather than the leavened bread of European Americans.

Food-related cultural behaviors can include whether to breastfeed or bottle-feed infants, and when to introduce solid foods to them. Food can also be considered part of the remedy for illness. Foods classified as "hot" foods or foods that are hot in temperature may be used to treat illnesses that are classified as "cold" illnesses. For example, corn meal (a "hot" food) may be used to treat arthritis (a "cold" illness). Each culture group defines what it considers to be hot and cold entities.

Religious practice associated with specific cultures also affects diet. Some Roman Catholics avoid meat on certain days, such as Ash Wednesday and Good Friday, and some Protestant faiths prohibit meat, tea, coffee, or alcohol. Both Orthodox Judaism and Islam prohibit the ingestion of pork or pork products. Orthodox Jews observe kosher customs, eating certain foods only if they have been inspected by a rabbi and prepared according to dietary laws. For example, the eating of milk products and meat products at the same meal is prohibited. Some Buddhists, Hindus, and Sikhs are strict vegetarians. The nurse must be sensitive to such religious dietary practices.

PROVIDING CULTURALCARE

All phases of the nursing process are affected by the client's and the nurse's cultural values, beliefs, and behaviors. As the client's culture and the nurse's culture come together in the nurse–client relationship, a unique cultural environment is created that can improve or impair the client's outcome. Self-awareness of personal biases can enable nurses to develop modifying behaviors or (if they are unable to do so) to remove themselves from situations where care may be compromised. Nurses can become more aware of their own culture through values clarification (see Chapter 5). ⊘ The nurse must also consider the cultural values dominant in the health care setting because those, too, may influence the client's outcome. Box 13–1 lists texts authored by nurses that may be helpful in developing cultural knowledge.

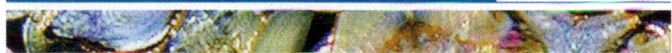

NURSING MANAGEMENT

ASSESSING

The Assessment Interview on page 217 depicts the questions to ask when conducting a heritage assessment. The tool is a way of interviewing and facilitating communication with clients and their families. It is designed to enhance the process in order to determine if clients are identifying with their traditional cultural heritage (heritage consistent) or if they have acculturated into the dominant culture of the modern society they reside in (heritage inconsistent). The tool may be used in any setting and both facilitates conversation and helps in the planning of CulturalCare. Once a conversation begins and the person describes aspects of cultural heritage, it becomes possible to develop an understanding of the person's unique health and illness beliefs, practices, and cultural needs.

Examples of Heritage Consistency

The following factors and examples indicative of heritage consistency can be explored to determine the depth to which

BOX 13–1   ■ Selected Nurse Authored Texts

Andrews, M. M., & Boyle, J. S. (2002). *Transcultural concepts in nursing care* (4th ed.). Philadelphia: Lippincott Williams & Wilkins.

D'Avanzo, C., & Geissler, E. M. (2003). *Pocket guide to cultural health assessment* (3rd ed.). St. Louis, MO: Mosby.

Ferguson, V. D. (1999). *Case studies in cultural diversity: A workbook.* New York: National League for Nursing Press/Jones & Bartlett.

Johnson, R. W. (1999). *African American voices: African American health educators speak out.* New York: National League for Nursing Press/Jones & Bartlett.

Kelley, M. L., & Fitzsimons, V. M. (2000). *Understanding cultural diversity: Culture, curriculum, and community.* New York: National League for Nursing Press/Jones & Bartlett.

Leininger, M., & McFarland, M. R. (Eds.). (2002). *Transcultural nursing: Concepts, theories, research, and practice* (3rd ed.). New York: McGraw Hill.

Purnell, L. D., & Paulanka, B. J. (1998). *Transcultural health care.* Philadelphia: F. A. Davis.

Smith-Stoner, M. (2002). *Transcultural nursing secrets.* Philadelphia: Lippincott Williams & Wilkins.

Spector, R. E. (2000). *Cultural diversity in health and illness* (5th ed.). Upper Saddle River, NJ: Prentice Hall Health.

Spector, R. E. (2000). *CulturalCare: Guides to heritage assessment and HEALTH traditions.* Upper Saddle River, NJ: Prentice Hall Health.

Torres, S. (1999). *Hispanic voices: Hispanic health educators speak out.* New York: National League for Nursing Press/Jones & Bartlett.

Zhan, L. (1999). *Asian voices: Asian and Asian-American health educators speak out.* New York: National League for Nursing Press/Jones & Bartlett.

a person identifies with his or her traditional heritage, that is, the cultural beliefs and practices of his or her family heritage:

1. The person's childhood development occurred in the person's country of origin or in an immigrant neighborhood of like ethnic group in the United States. For example, the person was raised in a specific ethnic neighborhood, such as an Italian, Black, Hispanic, or Jewish one, in a given part of a city and was exposed only to the culture, language, foods, and customs of that particular group.

2. Extended family members encouraged participation in traditional religious and cultural activities. For example, the parents sent the person to religious (parochial) school, and most social activities were church related.

3. The individual engages in frequent visits to the country of origin or returns to the "old neighborhood" in the United States. The desire to return to the old country or to the old neighborhood is prevalent in many people; however, many people, for various reasons, cannot return. The people who came here to escape religious persecution or whose families were killed during World War II, during the Holocaust, in the killing fields of Cambodia, or in other recent massacres may not want to return to their homelands. Other reasons why people may not return to their native country include political conditions in the homeland or lack of relatives or friends in that land.

4. The individual's family home is within the ethnic community of which he or she is a member. As adults, persons elect to live with their families in the ethnic neighborhood wherein the people are from a similar heritage.

5. The individual participates in ethnic cultural events, such as religious festivals or national holidays, sometimes with singing, dancing, and costumes. For example, the person is active in social and cultural groups and participates in family festivities.

6. The individual was raised in an extended family setting. For example, when the person was growing up, grandparents or aunts and uncles may have been living in the same house or close by. The person's social frame of reference was the family.

7. The individual maintains regular contact with the extended family. For example, the person maintains close ties with family members of the same generation, the surviving members of the older generation, and members of the younger generation.

8. The individual's name has not been Americanized. For example, the person has restored the family name to its original if it had been changed by immigration authorities at the time the family immigrated or if the family changed the name at a later time in an attempt to assimilate to the dominant culture more fully.

9. The individual was educated in a parochial (nonpublic) school with a religious or ethnic philosophy similar to the family's background. The person's education plays an enormous role in socialization, and the major purpose of education is to socialize a given person into the dominant culture. Children learn English and the customs and norms of American life in the schools. In the parochial or private schools, they not only learn English but also are socialized in the culture and norms of the particular religious or ethnic group that is sponsoring the school.

10. The individual engages in social activities primarily with others of the same religious or ethnic background. For example, the major portion of the person's personal time is spent attending meetings and events sponsored by those with whom they identify.

11. The individual has knowledge of the culture and language of origin. For example, the person has been socialized in the traditional ways of the family and expresses this as a central theme of life.

12. The individual expresses pride in his or her heritage. For example, the person may identify him- or herself as ethnic American and display flags, wear clothing, or participate in ethnic activities to a great extent.

Conveying Cultural Sensitivity

The process of heritage and HEALTH traditions assessment is important. How and when questions are asked requires sensitivity and clinical judgment. The timing and phrasing of ques-

Assessment Interview

HERITAGE ASSESSMENT TOOL

This set of questions is to be used to describe a given client's—or your own—ethnic, cultural, and religious background. In performing a *heritage assessment* it is helpful to determine how deeply a given person identifies with his or her traditional heritage. This tool is most useful in setting the stage for assessing and understanding a person's traditional health and illness beliefs and practices and in helping to determine the community resources that will be appropriate to target for support when necessary. The greater the number of positive responses, the greater the degree to which the person may identify with his or her traditional heritage. The one exception to positive answers is the question about whether or not a person's name was changed.

1. Where was your mother born? _____
2. Where was your father born? _____
3. Where were your grandparents born? _____
   a. Your mother's mother? _____
   b. Your mother's father? _____
   c. Your father's mother? _____
   d. Your father's father? _____
4. How many brothers _____ and sisters _____ do you have?
5. What setting did you grow up in? Urban _____ Rural _____
6. What country did your parents grow up in?
   Father _____
   Mother _____
7. How old were you when you came to the United States? _____
8. How old were your parents when they came to the United States?
   Mother _____
   Father _____
9. When you were growing up, who lived with you?
   _____
10. Have you maintained contact with
    a. Aunts, uncles, cousins?   (1) Yes _____   (2) No _____
    b. Brothers and sisters?   (1) Yes _____   (2) No _____
    c. Parents?   (1) Yes _____   (2) No _____
    d. Your own children?   (1) Yes _____   (2) No _____
11. Did most of your aunts, uncles, cousins live near your home?
    (1) Yes _____ (2) No _____
12. Approximately how often did you visit family members who lived outside of your home?
    (1) Daily _____ (2) Weekly _____ (3) Monthly _____
    (4) Once a year or less _____ (5) Never _____

13. Was your original family name changed?
    (1) Yes _____ (2) No _____
14. What is your religious preference?
    (1) Catholic _____ (2) Jewish _____
    (2) Protestant _____ Denomination _____
    (4) Other _____ (5) None _____
15. Is your spouse the same religion as you?
    (1) Yes _____ (2) No _____
16. Is your spouse the same ethnic background as you?
    (1) Yes _____ (2) No _____
17. What kind of school did you go to?
    (1) Public _____ (2) Private _____ (3) Parochial _____
18. As an adult, do you live in a neighborhood where the neighbors are the same religion and ethnic background as yourself?
    (1) Yes _____ (2) No _____
19. Do you belong to a religious institution?
    (1) Yes _____ (2) No _____
20. Would you describe yourself as an active member?
    (1) Yes _____ (2) No _____
21. How often do you attend your religious institution?
    (1) More than once a week _____ (2) Weekly _____
    (3) Monthly _____
    (4) Special holidays only _____ (5) Never _____
22. Do you practice your religion in your home?
    (1) Yes _____ (2) No _____ (if yes, please specify)
    (3) Praying _____ (4) Bible reading _____ (5) Diet _____
    (6) Celebrating religious holidays _____
23. Do you prepare foods special to your ethnic background?
    (1) Yes _____ (2) No _____
24. Do you participate in ethnic activities?
    (1) Yes _____ (2) No _____ (if yes, please specify)
    (3) Singing _____ (4) Holiday celebrations _____
    (5) Dancing _____ (6) Festivals _____
    (7) Costumes _____ (8) Other _____
25. Are your friends from the same religious background as you?
    (1) Yes _____ (2) No _____
26. Are your friends from the same ethnic background as you?
    (1) Yes _____ (2) No _____
27. What is your native language? _____
28. Do you speak this language?
    (1) Prefer _____ (2) Occasionally _____ (3) Rarely _____
29. Do you read your native language?
    (1) Yes _____ (2) No _____

Note: From *Cultural Diversity in Health & Illness*, 5th ed. (pp. 295–297), by R. E. Spector, 2000, Upper Saddle River, NJ: Prentice Hall.

tions need to be adapted to the individual. Timing is important in introducing questions. Sensitivity is needed in phrasing questions. Trust must be established before clients can be expected to volunteer and share sensitive information. The nurse therefore needs to spend time with clients, introduce some social conversation, and convey a genuine desire to understand their values and beliefs.

Before a heritage assessment begins, determine what language the client speaks and the client's degree of fluency in the English language. It is also important to learn about the client's communications patterns and space orientation. This is accomplished by observing both verbal and nonverbal communication. For example, does the client do the speaking or defer to another? What nonverbal communication behaviors does the client exhibit (e.g., touching, eye contact)? What significance do these behaviors have for the nurse–client interaction? What is the client's proximity to other people and objects within the environment? How does the client react to the nurse's movement toward the client? What cultural objects within the environment have importance for health promotion or health maintenance?

It is vital for nurses to be culturally sensitive and to convey this sensitivity to clients, support people, and other health care personnel. Some ways to do so follow:

- Always address clients, support people, and other health care personnel by their last names (e.g., Mrs. Aylia, Dr. Rush) until they give you permission to use other names. In some cultures, the more formal style of address is a sign of respect, whereas the informal use of first names may be considered disrespect. It is important to ask people how they wish to be addressed.
- When meeting a person for the first time, introduce yourself by your full name, and then explain your role (e.g., "My name is Alicia Bernett and I am a student nurse at Nightingale School of Nursing.") This helps establish a relationship and provides an opportunity for clients, others, and nurses to learn the pronunciation of one another's names and their roles.
- Be authentic with people, and be honest about the knowledge you lack about their culture. When you do not understand a person's actions, politely and respectfully seek information.
- Use language that is culturally sensitive; for example, say "gay," "lesbian," or "bisexual" rather than "homosexual"; do not use "man" or "mankind" when referring to a woman. Ask if the person prefers to be referred to as an "Hispanic" or "Latino"; as an "African American" or "Black."
- Find out what the client thinks about his or her health problems, illness, and treatments. Assess whether this information is congruent with the dominant health care culture. If the beliefs and practices are incongruent, establish whether this will have a negative effect on the client's health.
- Do not make any assumptions about the client, and always ask about anything you do not understand.
- Show respect for the client's values, beliefs, and practices, even if they differ from your own or from those of the dominant culture. If you do not agree with them, it is important to respect the client's right to hold these beliefs.
- Show respect for the client's support people. In some cultures, men in the family make decisions affecting the client, while in other cultures women make the decisions.
- Make a concerted effort to obtain the client's trust, but do not be surprised if it develops slowly or not at all. The heritage assessment takes time and usually needs to extend over several meetings.

DIAGNOSING

The nursing diagnoses developed by NANDA are focused on nursing care provided in the United States and Canada and are based on Western cultural beliefs. "Never has this work been portrayed or disseminated as relevant to other cultures" (Carpenito, 2002, p. 81). However, nurses must still provide appropriate care to clients of any culture. This is accomplished through developing cultural sensitivity and considering how a client's culture influences their responses to health conditions, much as the nurse considers how clients' age or gender influence a nursing diagnosis, plan, and delivery of nursing care.

Research Note
What Is the Nature of a Cross-Cultural Team's Experience of Caring for Children of Cambodian Refugee Families?

Various traditional health beliefs, such as the description of symptoms as "bad wind" and the practice of "dermabrasion" influence the nursing care of Cambodian immigrants. The purpose of research by Tellep, Chim, Murphy, and Cureton (2001) was to explore the experience of the school district staff in providing care for Cambodian refugee children. Data for this descriptive study were collected by interviewing school nurses and Cambodian liaisons in a large school district. Using Dobson's conceptual framework of transcultural health visiting, the data were analyzed. Several themes, including intracultural reciprocity, transcultural reciprocity, intergenerational conflict, and spiritual healing emerged and are being used to provide guidance to future team approaches.

Implications: When nurses are providing care to new immigrants, such as people from Cambodia, they need to be aware of any health beliefs and practices that are different than those of the Western health care system. Nurses are in need of comprehensive studies of the status of Cambodian refugees' health that use Cambodian explanatory models. Cambodian nurses, teachers, and outreach workers are vital to expediting the research process.

Note: From "Great Suffering, Great Compassion: A Transcultural Opportunity for School Nurses Caring for Cambodian Children," by T. L. Tellep, M. Chim, S. Murphy, and V. Y. Cureton, 2001, *Journal of Transcultural Nursing, 12,* pp. 261–274.

PLANNING

"Cultural competence is about delivering care while attending to the total situation for the patient and family" (Leonard, 2001, *Cultural Competence section, para. 6*). There are several steps involved in the process that lead to the development of cultural competency. The knowledge and skills necessary to incorporate CulturalCare into standard nursing require the acquisition of a broad base of knowledge about the different heritages and social structures a given client comes from. It is an ongoing process and the skills and knowledge base grow over time. As one's knowledge base grows, the ability to convey cultural sensitivity also grows (see Box 13–2).

The following are examples of the necessary steps:

1. Become aware of one's own cultural heritage. Where were your parents, grandparents born? What are examples of their traditional health and illness beliefs and practices? Do they value stoic behavior in relation to pain, or is it permissible to state that you are in pain? Are the rights of the individual valued over and above the rights of the family? Only by knowing one's own culture (values, practices, and beliefs) can a person be ready to learn about another's.

2. Become aware of the client's heritage and HEALTH traditions as described by the client. It is important to avoid assuming that all people of the same ethnic background have the same cultural beliefs and values. When the nurse has

BOX 13–2 ■ Health-Related Practices of Asian, African American, and Hispanic Peoples

Asian
- Coining and cupping are traditional medical practices, not forms of abuse.
- Fevers are treated by wrapping the ill person in warm blankets and having him or her drink warm liquids.
- Do not provide ice water unless requested. May prefer hot liquids, such as tea.
- Rich tradition of herbal remedies. Health care providers should be sure to discuss the use of home or herbal remedies to avoid potential drug interactions.
- Instruct on the use of Western medication because traditional Chinese medicine is taken differently. Explain the importance of taking pills as prescribed, even after symptoms have disappeared.

African American
- Menstruation is believed to rid the body of dirty and excess blood. With too little flow, they may fear bad blood is staying in the body; too much flow can weaken the body. Influences views of birth control.

- Have rich tradition of herbal remedies. Health care providers should be sure to discuss the use of home or herbal remedies to avoid potential drug interactions.
- May avoid dairy products due to high incidence of lactose intolerance. Check for family history.
- Focus on present time may interfere with use of preventive medicine and follow-up care.

Hispanic
- Certain foods or medications upset hot–cold body balance. Try offering alternative foods or liquids for medications.
- Do not provide ice water unless requested.
- Respect postpartum prescriptions for rest.
- Sponge baths may be preferred after giving birth.
- Allow family members to spend as much time with the patient as possible and provide nontechnical care.
- Strong beliefs in fate and external control over events may lead to less adherence to medical regimens.

knowledge of the client's culture, mutual respect between client and nurse is more likely to develop.

3. Become aware of adaptations the client made to live in a North American culture. During this part of the interview, a nurse can also identify the client's preferences in health practices, diet, hygiene, and so on.

4. Form a CulturalCare nursing plan with the client that incorporates his or her cultural beliefs regarding the maintenance, protection, and restoration of health. In this way, cultural values, practices, and beliefs can be incorporated with the necessary nursing care.

IMPLEMENTING

The implementation of CulturalCare nursing includes (a) cultural preservation and maintenance and (b) cultural accommodation and negotiation. Cultural preservation may involve the use of cultural health care practices, such as giving herbal tea, chicken soup, or "hot foods" to the ill client. Accommodation of the client's viewpoint and negotiating appropriate care requires expert communication skills, such as responding empathetically, validating information, and effectively summarizing content. Negotiation is a collaborative process. It acknowledges that the nurse–client relationship is reciprocal and that differences exist between the parties about notions of health, illness, and treatment. The nurse attempts to bridge the gap between the nurse's (scientific) and the client's (cultural) perspectives. During the negotiation process, the client's views are first explored and acknowledged. Relevant scientific information is then provided. If the client's views reveal that certain behaviors would not affect the client's condition adversely, then they are incorporated in planning care. If the client's views can lead to harmful behavior or outcomes, then an attempt is made to shift the client's perspectives to the scientific view.

Negotiation occurs when cultural treatment practices conflict with those of the health care system. It must be determined precisely how the client is managing the illness, what practices could be harmful, and which practices can be safely combined with Western medicine. For example, reducing dosages of an antihypertensive medication or replacing insulin therapy with herbal measures may be detrimental. Some herbal remedies are synergistic with Western medicines and others are antagonistic; therefore, it is necessary to fully inform the client about the possible outcomes. Consider these examples of potential conflicts between cultural beliefs or practices and the dominant American health care system:

- Native American women value ample body size and may be resistant to weight control.
- The decision to circumcise male infants is often made based on cultural and family beliefs and can occasionally conflict with medical advice.
- An Hispanic or Asian client may be unable to obtain hospice care if the family will not permit the patient to be informed of the diagnosis or prognosis.
- Members of the Jehovah's Witness faith do not accept blood transfusions even in life-threatening situations.
- Orthodox Sikhs do not cut their hair. This can conflict with the need to shave the skin for medical procedures.

When a client chooses to follow only cultural practices and declines all prescribed medical or nursing interventions, the nurse and client must adjust the client goals. Monitoring the client's condition to identify changes in health and to recognize impending crises before they become irreversible may be all that is realistically achievable. At a time of crisis, the opportunity may arise to renegotiate care.

CulturalCare nursing is challenging. It requires discovery of the meaning of the client's behavior, flexibility, creativity, and knowledge to adapt nursing interventions. An effort must be made to learn from each experience. This knowledge will improve the delivery of culture-specific care to future clients. The accompanying box offers suggestions for providing CulturalCare to clients and families.

EVALUATING

Evaluating nursing care of clients that incorporates the concepts of heritage and ethnicity is performed in the same way as with any client. Client outcomes are compared with the goals and expected outcomes established following comprehensive assessment that includes sensitivity to cultural diversity. However, if the outcomes are not achieved, and the client and nurse are from different cultures, the nurse should be especially careful to consider whether the client's belief system has been adequately included as an influencing factor.

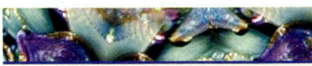

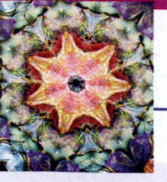

Providing Culturally Competent Care

FAMILIES

- Learn the rituals, customs, and practices of the major cultural groups with whom you come into contact. Learn to appreciate the richness of diversity and consider it an asset rather than a hindrance in your practice.
- Identify personal biases, attitudes, prejudices, and stereotypes.
- Include cultural assessment of the client and family as part of overall assessment.
- Recognize that it is the client's (or family's) right to make their own health care choices.
- Convey respect and cooperate with traditional helpers and caregivers.

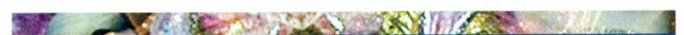

Focus on Critical Thinking

Rachel was born to a Jewish couple and lists her religion as Jewish. Her father died when she was 10 years old and her mother remarried 3 years later. Rachel was legally adopted by her Italian stepfather, who was a devout Catholic. Although the family participated in Catholic–Italian traditions, Rachel's mother taught her many Jewish traditions as well, so that her heritage would be preserved. Rachel is now 58 years old, practices traditions from both her Jewish and Italian upbringing, and is dying of cancer. You are the nurse caring for Rachel during her final days.

1. Differentiate between Rachel's culture, ethnicity, and race.
2. How might Rachel's mixed cultural background pose a dilemma for you as her nurse or for her family?

3. How might Rachel's culture affect her approach to death and the care of her body following her death?
4. Of what benefit would a cultural assessment be to Rachel or her family since she is dying?
5. How could nurses' race, culture, or religion influence their care of clients who are racially or culturally different?

See Critical Thinking Possibilities in Appendix A.

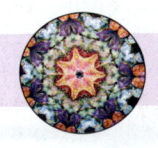

Chapter Review

EXPLORE MediaLink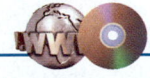

NCLEX review questions, case studies, MediaLink applications, and other interactive resources for this chapter can be found on the Companion Website at www.prenhall.com/kozier. Click on Chapter 13 to select the activities for this chapter.

For more NCLEX review questions, and an audio glossary, access the Student CD-ROM accompanying this textbook.

Chapter Highlights

- People in the United States come from a variety of backgrounds, and many retain at least some of their traditional values, including health beliefs and practices.

- People may live within their traditional heritage or, they may embrace both their original ethnocultural traditional heritage(s) and the modern culture of the United States.

- An individual's heritage and cultural background can influence health beliefs and practices.
- Through acculturation, most groups in the United States modify some of their traditional cultural characteristics.
- Personal characteristics also modify an individual's cultural values, beliefs, and practices.

- Health beliefs and practices, family patterns, communication style, space and time orientation, and nutritional patterns may influence the relationship between the nurse and the client who have different cultural backgrounds.
- When assessing a client, the nurse considers the client's cultural values, beliefs, and practices related to health and health care.

Review Questions

13–1. The major factor contributing to the need for CulturalCare is
   a. an increasing birth rate.
   b. limited access to health care services.
   c. demographic change.
   d. a decreasing rate of immigration.

13–2. The term *culturally sensitive* implies that the nurse
   a. is prepared in transcultural nursing.
   b. possesses knowledge of the traditions of diverse peoples.
   c. applies underlying knowledge to providing nursing care.
   d. understands the context of the client's situation.

13–3. In initiating care for a client of a different culture than the nurse, which of the following would be an appropriate statement?
   a. "Since, in your culture, people don't drink ice water, I will bring you hot tea."
   b. "Do you have any books I could read about people of your culture?"

   c. "Please let me know if I do anything that is not acceptable in your culture."
   d. "You will need to set aside your usual customs and practices while you are in the hospital."

13–4. The term *culturally competent* implies that the nurse
   a. is prepared in transcultural nursing.
   b. possesses knowledge of the traditions of diverse peoples.
   c. applies underlying knowledge to providing nursing care.
   d. understands the context of the client's situation.

13–5. Culture is the
   a. classification of human beings into groups based on particular physical characteristics.
   b. condition of belonging to a group whose members share a unique heritage.
   c. socially inherited characteristics of a human group.
   d. learned behavior by a particular person.

Readings and References

Suggested Readings

Morgan, J. D. (Ed.). (1999). *Meeting the needs of our clients creatively: The impact of art and culture on caregiving.* Amityville, NY: Baywood Publishing.
   This book focuses on how nurses can help themselves and their clients grieve using artistic and cultural perspectives. Twenty-one contributors present how death has been viewed and presented by our different cultures. The text also presents practical applications of creative caregiving with grieving clients of diverse cultures.

Schloman, B. F. (2000, June). Breaking through the foreign language barrier: Resources on the Web. *Online Journal of Issues in Nursing, 5*(4). Retrieved September 28, 2002, from http://www.nursingworld.org/ojin/infocol/info_4.htm
   This article describes some of the many Internet resources for nurses in the areas of translation, foreign language dictionaries, language tutors, and patient education materials in various languages.

Related Research

Brooks, N., Magee, P., Bhatti, G., Briggs, C., Buckley, S., Guthrie, S., et al. (2000). Asian pa-

tients' perspectives on the communication facilities provided in a large inner city hospital. *Journal of Clinical Nursing, 9,* 706–712.

Taylor, G. A. J. (2002). Effects of a culturally sensitive breast self examination intervention. *Outcomes Management, 6*(2), 73–79.

References

Andrews, M. M., & Boyle, J. S. (2002). *Transcultural concepts in nursing care* (4th ed.). Philadelphia: Lippincott Williams & Wilkins.

Bernstein, R. (2002). *Census brief: Current population survey coming to America: A profile of the nation's foreign born (2000 update).* Washington, DC: U. S. Department of Commerce.

Bohannan, P. (1992). *We, the alien: An introduction to cultural anthropology.* Prospect Heights, IL: Waveland Press.

California Healthcare Interpreters Association. (2002). *California standards for healthcare interpreters: Ethical principles, protocols, and guidance on roles and interventions.* Los Angeles: Author.

Carpenito, L. J. (2002). *Nursing diagnosis: Application to clinical practice* (9th ed.). Philadelphia, Lippincott.

Galanti, G. (1997). *Caring for patients from different cultures: Case studies from American hospitals* (2nd ed.). Philadelphia: University of Pennsylvania Press.

Giger, J. N., & Davidhizar, R. (1999). *Transcultural nursing: Assessment and intervention* (3rd ed.). St. Louis, MO: Mosby.

Leonard, B. J. (2001, May 3). Quality nursing care celebrates diversity. *Online Journal of Issues in Nursing, 6*(2), Article 3. Retrieved September 29, 2002, from http://www.nursingworld.org/ojin/topic15/tpc15_3.htm

Matsumoto, M., & Matsumoto, M. (1989). *The unspoken way Haragei: Silence in Japanese business and society.* Tokyo: Kodahsha International.

McLemore, S. D., Romo, H. D., & Baker, S. G. (2001). *Racial and ethnic relations in America* (6th ed.). Boston: Allyn & Bacon.

Office of Minority Health. (2001). *National standards for culturally and linguistically appropriate services in health care.* Washington, DC: U. S. Department of Health and Human Services.

Spector, R. E. (2000). *Cultural diversity in health and illness* (5th ed.). Upper Saddle River, NJ: Prentice Hall.

Spratley, E., Johnson, A., Sochalski, M., Fritz, W., & Spencer, W. (2002). *The registered nurse population March 2000: Findings from the national sample survey of registered nurses.* Retrieved November 1, 2002, from the U.S. Department of Health and Human Services Health Resources and Service Administration Bureau of Health Professions Division of Nursing website: http://bhpr.hrsa.gov/healthworkforce/rnsurvey/rnss1.htm#T1

Tellep, T. L., Chim, M., Murphy, S., & Cureton, V. Y. (2001). Great suffering, great compassion: A transcultural opportunity for school nurses caring for Cambodian children. *Journal of Transcultural Nursing, 12,* 261–274.

U.S. Census Bureau. (2001). *Profiles of general demographic characteristics 2000.* Washington, DC: U.S. Department of Commerce.

Zitzow, D., & Estes, G. (1981). The heritage consistency continuum in counseling Native American students. In *Contemporary American Indian issues in higher education.* Los Angeles: American Indian Studies Center, University of California.

Selected Bibliography

Bhimani, R., & Acorn, S. (1998). Managing within a culturally diverse environment. *Canadian Nurse, 94,* 32–36.

Cohen, M. Z., & Palos, G. (2001). Culturally competent care. *Seminars in Oncology Nursing, 17,* 153–158.

Doswell, W. M., & Erlen, J. A. (1998). Multicultural issues and ethical concerns in the delivery of nursing care interventions. *Nursing Clinics of North America, 33,* 353–361.

Duffy, M. M., & Alexander, A. (1999). Overcoming language barriers for non-English speaking patients. *ANNA Journal, 26,* 507–510, 528.

George, M. (2001). The challenge of culturally competent health care: Applications for asthma. *Heart and Lung, The Journal of Acute and Critical Care, 30,* 392–400.

Giger, J. N., & Davidhizar, R. (2002). The Giger and Davidhizar Transcultural Assessment Model. *Journal of Transcultural Nursing, 13,* 185–188.

Johnson, R.A., & Tripp-Reimer, T. (2001). Aging, ethnicity, & social support: A review, part 1. *Journal of Gerontological Nursing, 27*(6), 15–21.

Kim-Godwin, Y. S., Clarke, P. N., & Barton, L. (2001). A model for the delivery of culturally competent community care. *Journal of Advanced Nursing, 35,* 918–925.

Labun, E. (2001). Cultural discovery in nursing practice with Vietnamese clients. *Journal of Advanced Nursing, 35,* 874–881.

Laviola, Y., & Twomey, T. C. (2002). Cultural competence: Bridging the gap with Hispanic clients. *Rehabilitation Nursing, 27*(1), 5–6.

MacAvoy, S., & Lippman, D. T. (2001). Teaching culturally competent care: Nursing students experience rural Appalachia. *Journal of Transcultural Nursing, 12,* 221–227.

Papadopoulos, I., & Lees, S. (2002). Developing culturally competent researchers. *Journal of Advanced Nursing, 37,* 258–264.

Phillips, J., & Weekes, D. (2002). Incorporating multiculturalism into oncology nursing research: The last decade. *Oncology Nursing Forum, 29,* 807–816.

Wong, F. K. Y. (1998). The integration of traditional Chinese health practices in nursing. *Reflections, 24*(2), 20–21.

CHAPTER 14

COMPLEMENTARY AND ALTERNATIVE HEALING MODALITIES

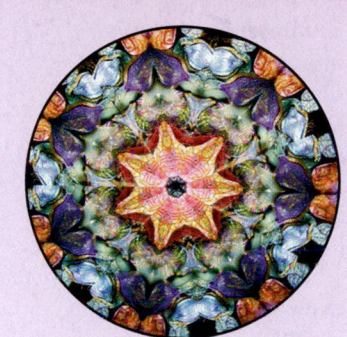

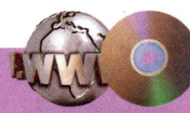

MediaLink

www.prenhall.com/kozier

Additional resources for this chapter can be found on the Student CD-ROM accompanying this textbook, and on the Companion Website at www.prenhall.com/kozier. Click on Chapter 14 to select the activities for this chapter.

CD-ROM
• Audio Glossary
• NCLEX Review

Companion Website
• Additional NCLEX Review
• Case Study: Complementary Alternative Medicine
• MediaLink Application:
    Support for Alternative Therapies
• Links to Resources

LEARNING OUTCOMES

After completing this chapter, you will be able to:

- Explain the Office of Alternative Medicine's definition of complementary and alternative (CAM) medicine as a social process.

- Describe the evidence suggesting a role for nurses in promoting better communication between physicians and patients using CAM.

- Explain the concepts of holism and the goal of holistic nursing.

- Identify four common forms of touch therapy.

- Describe what happens during a biofeedback session.

- Describe the goals that yoga and meditative practices have in common.

- Differentiate between the purposes and the effects of meditation.

- Define disease from the perspective of traditional Chinese medicine.

- Define health from the perspective of chiropractic.

- Discuss the strengths and weaknesses of the homeopathic theory "like cures like."

Although nurses have always been concerned with the whole person, they are increasingly embracing ideas about health and healing that are very different from those that inform the health care delivery system. Conceptualizations of health, disease, pain, and death vary widely from culture to culture. The same is true for the therapies or practices designed to promote health, cure disease, ease pain and suffering, and give meaning and dignity to death. Nurses are progressively incorporating ideas and therapies from other cultures and traditions into their practice. These therapies include massage, imagery, meditation, acupressure, art and music therapy, breathing exercises, biofeedback, reflexology, tai chi and chi gong exercises, therapeutic touch, prayer, and spiritual work.

CULTURE AND THE EVOLUTION OF TERMS

A number of terms have been used for the therapies just mentioned, including *nonorthodox, unconventional, alternative,* and *complementary.* The medical subject headings (MeSH) of the National Library of Medicine refer to **complementary therapies,** defined as "Therapeutic practices which are not currently considered an integral part of conventional allopathic medical practice. They may lack biomedical explanations but as they become better researched some (PHYSICAL THERAPY; DIET; ACUPUNCTURE) become widely accepted whereas others (humors, radium therapy) quietly fade away, yet are important historical footnotes. Therapies are termed as Complementary when used in addition to conventional treatments and as Alternative when used instead of conventional treatment." (National Library of Medicine, 2003, scope note).

Prior to the creation of the above complementary therapies definition, the MeSH definition referred to **alternative medicine** as "an unrelated group of non-orthodox practices, often with explanatory systems that do not follow conventional biomedical explanations" (Pavek, 1996, p. 25). This previous definition reflects difficulties associated with transferring complex understandings and practices from one culture to another. Therapies can appear to be unrelated when transported from one culture to another and studied in piecemeal fashion. Both Asia and Europe have developed sophisticated medical theories and have long histories of empirically documented experience and traditions that are markedly different from those of North Americans. Alternative medicine implies a perspective that is "standard." Coward and Ratanakul (1999) published a cross-cultural study on ethical problems in health care and reported that we often forget that Western scientific understandings and medical practices are cultural phenomena with their own sets of strengths and weaknesses. Conventional Western medicine is not necessarily a standard against which other practices can be reasonably judged.

The term **complementary and alternative medicine (CAM)** was first articulated at the national level in 1996: "Complementary and alternative medicine is defined through a social process as those practices that do not form part of the dominant system for managing health and disease" (Jonas, 1996, p. 1). Anthropologists have described this social process as a struggle, not simply to manage health and disease, but also to determine what is true about health and disease (MacIntyre, Holzemer, & Philippek, 1997).

Modern scientific medicine has numerous strengths, including a preference for evidence-based practice. Fishman (2000) argues that a major shortcoming of scientific medicine is an "inadequate appreciation of cultural diversity in determining the efficacy of health care" (p. 31). An interdisciplinary team of Canadian and Thai researchers who studied the ethics of health care across cultures reports that Western biomedicine is also a culture. "Nothing is wrong with this biomedical culture in and of itself, so long as it does not make itself God—sees itself as embodying the absolute truth (modern medical science) to which all other cultures must unquestioningly submit" (Coward & Ratanakul, 1999, p. 3).

CAM USE IN THE UNITED STATES

Federal legislation established the Office of Alternative Medicine (OAM) within the National Institutes of Health (NIH) in 1991 with the charge to investigate and evaluate promising unconventional medical practices. Eisenberg et al. (1993) published a seminal study reporting that 34% of adults in the United States used one or more of what he called "unconventional therapies" in the previous year. Although exercise and prayer were the two most frequently reported unconventional modalities, these were excluded from the overall 34% result. Eisenberg et al. concluded that persons with poorer health used more unconventional medicine than did those with better health. Eighty-three percent of those using alternative therapies for serious medical conditions also sought treatment from a physician; however, nearly three-fourths of those using alternative therapies did not inform their physician that they did so. Nurses have an opportunity to play a major role in facilitating better communication between patients and physicians as well as providing healing interventions that complement both Western medical and CAM practices.

In 1998, the OAM was elevated to become the National Center for Complementary and Alternative Medicine (NCCAM) and its work broadened to include research, research training, educational grants and contracts, and outreach mechanisms to disseminate information to the public. This was, in part, a response to the increase in use of CAM from 427 million visits in 1990 to approximately 630 million CAM visits costing over $21 billion in 1997 (NCCAM, 2000).

There is a direct relationship between the use of CAM and insurance coverage for the services (Wolsko, Eisenberg, Davis, Ettner, & Phillips, 2002). Although statistics vary, the March 2002 final report of the White House Commission on Complementary and Alternative Medicine Policy reported that 70% of insurance plans cover chiropractic, 17% cover acupuncture, and 12% cover massage therapy. The commission recommended that insurers and purchasers of insurance evaluate health benefit plans that incorporate safe and effective CAM interventions.

CONCEPTS OF HOLISM AND HOLISTIC NURSING

The term **holism** was coined by Jan Smuts, a South African statesman, in his book *Holism and Evolution* (1926). Smuts theorized that nature tends to bring things together to form whole organisms and that the determining factors in nature and evolution are wholes, not their constituent parts. The concept attracted further interest in the 1940s and 1950s, when Dunbar (1945), a pioneer in psychosomatic medicine, published studies that related stress and personality type to physical illness, and Hans Selye (1956) published his theory about the psychophysiology of stress. Nurse theorist Martha Rogers (1970) introduced her philosophy of the *Science of Unitary Human Beings*—landmark work that set the stage for such holistic nursing theories as those of Parse (1981), Newman (1986), and Watson (1988).

In holistic theory, all living organisms are seen as interacting, unified wholes that are more than the mere sum of their parts. Viewed in this light, any disturbance in one part is a disturbance of the whole system; in other words, the disturbance affects the whole being. Thus, the nurse must keep the whole person in mind when assessing one part of an individual and consider how that part relates to all others. The nurse must also consider how the individual interacts with and relates to the external environment and to others.

Holistic theories maintain that health requires that the forces of nature be kept in balance or harmony. Human life is one as-

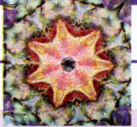

Assessment Interview
CAM

- Have you ever used teas, herbs, or other natural products to improve your health?
- What traditional or folk remedies are used in your family?
- Do you meditate, pray, or use relaxation techniques for healing purposes?
- Have you ever had a massage, seen a chiropractor, or had acupuncture? If so, what do you think about those treatments?

pect of nature that must be in harmony with the rest of nature. When the natural balance or harmony is disturbed, illness results. Many cultures have held the holistic health belief view for centuries. **Holistic health,** then, involves the total person: the whole of the person's being and the overall quality of lifestyle. **Holistic health care** includes health education, health promotion, health maintenance, illness prevention, and restorative-rehabilitative care. The identification of patient needs, and the planning, implementation, and evaluation of holistic care require sensitivity to individual, family, and cultural values. The Assessment Interview box contains suggested questions that may be used to elicit information about the client's perspectives on CAM while taking the health history.

The goal of **holistic nursing** as described by the American Holistic Nurses' Association (AHNA) is to enhance healing of the whole person from birth to death (Frisch, Dossey, Guzzetta, & Quinn, 2000). Holistic nurses recognize the biopsychosocial and spiritual dimensions of persons. They also recognize that individuals are unitary wholes whose lives are intertwined with family, community, culture, and environment. The AHNA *Standards of Holistic Nursing Practice* center around five core values: holistic philosophy and education; holistic ethics, theories, and research; holistic nurse self-care; holistic communication, therapeutic environment, and cultural diversity; and holistic caring process (Dossey, Keegan, & Guzzetta, 2000). As such, CAM is only one part of the practice of holistic nursing.

Holistic health practitioners focus on whole-brain thinking, a blending of linear thought processes regulated by the left hemisphere of the brain and intuitive thought processes regulated by the right hemisphere. The left brain has consistently been referred to as the dominant hemisphere and valued by Western medicine because it regulates reason, logic, and verbal, mathematical, and calculative aspects of thinking. Intuitive processes, or right-brain functions, regulate creativity, artistry, poetry, and "knowing-without-knowing-why" aspects of cognition.

> ➤ **CLINICAL ALERT**   *What constitutes traditional, alternative, complementary, or holistic to one person may be considered mainstream to another. Do not assume anything about the client's belief system—be sure to assess.* ■

CONCEPTS OF HEALING

Healing is less understood than pathophysiology. Until recently, the idea of curing rather than healing has dominated the Western mode of health care, with emphasis on technology, power, analysis, and the repair of damaged parts. Curing also implies that the person who offers the cure is active, and the person who receives the cure is passive.

Dossey's Eras of Medicine

Two important practitioners in the field of CAM are Larry and Barbara Dossey. Larry Dossey, MD, executive editor of *Alternative Therapies in Health and Medicine* established in 1995, categorized three different eras of medicine according to their approach to health, illness, and healing (Dossey, 1993).

Era I refers to "physical" medicine, which originated in the late 1860s and remains influential and effective today. It focuses on the effects of "things" on the body and includes Western medical therapies such as drugs, surgery, radiation, and so on. Era I is guided by classical laws of matter and energy; the universe and body are viewed as a vast clocklike mechanism that function according to causal, deterministic principles.

Era II refers to "mind–body" medicine, which arose in the mid-1950s and is still developing. Dossey (1993) marks the mid-1950s as the beginning of Era II medicine because it was then that mind–body approaches first began to spark attention among researchers. Perceptions, thoughts, emotions, attitudes, and images were found to affect the body profoundly and gained recognition as being therapeutic and important to healing. Mind–body therapies focus on helping individuals to use their minds to heal their own bodies and include relaxation techniques, most types of imagery therapies, biofeedback, hypnosis, and counseling.

Era III refers to "nonlocal" or "transpersonal" medicine. Dossey differentiates Era III therapies from Era II therapies as follows: Era I and Era II therapies are "local" in emphasis. They adhere to a classical time–space framework in which the mind is seen as localized to points in space (that is, the brain) and time (the present moment). In contrast, Era III medicine does not regard the "mind" or "consciousness" as localized within the individual brain and confined to the present moment; rather it claims that the mind can move through time and space. Thus, Era III medicine is seen as nonlocal and transpersonal; the mind is seen as a factor that can effect healing between persons. Era III therapies always involve a sender, or healer, and a receiver, or person being healed. Therapies include noncontact therapeutic touch, intercessory prayer, transpersonal imagery, some types of shamanic healing, and all forms of distant healing. Noncontact therapeutic touch and intercessory prayer are discussed later in this chapter.

The Bodymind or Minded Body

Barbara Dossey, PhD, RN, has been an educator, consultant, researcher, and author in the area of holistic nursing since the early 1980s. Dr. Dossey and her colleagues use the term **bodymind** to refer to a state of integration that includes body, mind, and spirit (Bartol & Courts, 2000). Traditionally, the mind was believed to be located within the anatomic structure of the brain; others propose, however, that memories, thoughts, and behavior processes are stored throughout the body. This author prefers the term **minded body,** to emphasize that the qualities we associate with the mind (including knowledge, emotions, and consciousness) are distributed throughout the body. The difficulty with this language comes because the body is part of our everyday experience while the mind and spirit are abstract concepts. According to Benner and Wrubel (1989), persons are not minds or spirits *in* bodies (the proverbial ghost in the machine), but rather embodied wholes. Benner takes issue with holistic thinkers who see bodies as mere vehicles for the development or expression of minds, souls, and spirits and insists that the minded, conscious, knowing body is a sacred whole.

The limbic-hypothalamic system, centered in the brain and biochemically interconnected with all other parts of the body, facilitates the integration of thoughts, emotions, and sensations at the physiologic and cellular levels. Theoretical bases for bodymind healing are complex; they include but are not limited to information transduction, and modulation of the autonomic, endocrine, immune, and neuropeptide systems (Bartol & Courts, 2000).

Information transduction is the conversion or transformation of information or energy from one form to another. The mind is seen as nature's way of receiving, generating, and transducing information. Information (an idea or event) that is novel—challenging, intriguing, or mysterious—has the highest information value. Such information evokes changes in the body and mind that prompt neural pathways and consciousness to connect to bring about information transduction. Two examples of transduction are the use of relaxation techniques and imagery. Relaxation techniques can effect decreases in blood pressure, heart rate, respiratory rate, and pain. Imagery transforms images or ideas into an act of relaxation and physiologic healing.

Mind modulation refers to the process by which the brain converts neural messages (thoughts, attitudes, feelings, and emotions) into neurohormonal messenger molecules and communicates them to all body systems that evoke states of health or illness (Bartol & Courts, 2000). The mind modulates cellular biochemical activities within all major organ systems, that is, the autonomic nervous system, endocrine system, immune system, and the neuropeptide system. All of these systems are closely related; none is separate from the other. The activity of any one of these systems can modulate the activity of the other systems.

Mind modulation through the autonomic nervous system is used in holistic therapies such as relaxation, imagery, meditation, and music therapy. These therapies encourage bodymind healing by decreasing a person's sympathetic response to stress, thus enabling the calming effect of the parasympathetic system to dominate (see Table 14–1).

Mind modulation via the immune system involves receptor sites on the surface of T and B lymphocytes that are able to activate, direct, and modify immune function. Research has revealed a direct correlation between relaxation, imagery, and the function of the immune system.

TABLE 14-1 Effects of the Autonomic Nervous System

Parasympathetic Branch (Relaxation)	Sympathetic Branch (Activation)
Decreased pupil size	Increased pupil size
Decreased lacrimal secretion	Increased lacrimal gland secretion
Increased salivary flow	Decreased salivary flow
Decreased heart rate	Increased heart rate
Vasodilation	Vasoconstriction
Bronchoconstriction	Bronchodilation
Increased gastric motility and secretion	Decreased gastric motility and secretion
Increased pancreatic secretion	Decreased pancreatic secretion
	Increased adrenal secretions (epinephrine and cortisol)*
Increased intestinal motility	Decreased intestinal motility

Increased adrenal secretions bring about the fight-or-flight response or the general adaptation syndrome.

Neuropeptides, amino acid messenger molecules produced at various sites throughout the body, are another key to understanding bodymind interconnections. When a neuropeptide attaches to a receptor site, it either facilitates or blocks a cellular response. Neuropeptides are "messenger molecules" that are responsible for connecting the body and emotions. The autonomic, endocrine, and immune systems are the vehicles for the neuropeptides.

Another area of study in mind–body research is **psychoneuroimmunology,** which focuses on the relationships among stress, the immune system, and health outcomes (DeAngelis, 2002). Many studies have shown links between emotional and social conditions and physiological function. Although research has yet to demonstrate absolute effects, there is also evidence of the reverse: that activity in the body affects the brain. Future work will include attempts to identify which interventions (such as stress management) modify the person's psychological state in efforts to influence their physiologic functioning.

HEALING MODALITIES

Nurses with a holistic orientation often use a variety of self-care practices in their own lives. The relative health and well-being of the nurse constitutes a vital force in the healing process. Box 14–1 lists methods that can be particularly useful to nurses working to foster their own health and well-being.

This chapter presents four major groups of healing modalities: touch, mind–body, aroma, and transpersonal therapies. Any nurse can use some of these with clients, while other modalities require advanced training. In addition to having the requisite skill, nurses also must be familiar with the legal scope of nursing under which they practice. In the United States in 2001, 25 state boards of nursing included aspects of CAM in their practice acts and another 6 states were in the process of discussing the topic. For example, in California, all nurses can use complementary and alternative techniques for reducing pain such as focused breathing and relaxation, massage, guided imagery, music, humor, and distraction, as well as medication therapy for reducing pain (conventional therapy).

The more complex complementary and alternative therapies become part of advanced education and nursing practice, frequently in the context of continuing education workshops or seminars; examples include acupressure, aromatherapy, massage, yoga, and reflexology. Acupuncture and chiropractic require licenses to practice in California. Applied kinesiology, herbal therapy, homeopathy, and Ayurveda usually require formal education preparation and practice, and in some instances these therapies have private certification. (Sparber, 2001, California section, para. 3–4)

Touch Therapies

Healing through touch goes back to early civilization. One of the earliest written documents on this subject originated in Asia 5,000 years ago. Hippocrates wrote about the effects of therapeutic massage and manipulation when Greek civilization was at its height. Although most cultures have developed some type of touch therapy, attitudes toward touch vary widely from culture to culture. Touch may stimulate the production of healing-promoting chemicals by the immune or limbic system. Common touch therapies are described next.

Massage

Over the centuries, nurses have provided back massage. Massage was thought to improve the circulation of the blood and assist in relaxation. More recently, the benefits have been more precisely identified and categorized as physical, mental-emotional, and spiritual.

Physically, massage relaxes muscles and releases lactic acid that accumulates during exercise. It can also improve the flow of blood and lymph, stretch joints, and relieve pain and congestion. Massage is also thought to release body toxins and stimulate the immune system, thereby helping the body combat disease.

In the mental-emotional area, massage can relieve anxiety and provide a sense of relaxation and well-being. Spiritually, it

BOX 14-1   ■ Self-Healing Methods for Nurses

■ *Clarify values and beliefs.* Identify those things that are important, meaningful, and valuable to you, and assess whether your actions are consistent with your beliefs. For example, do you value time spent with your children and time reading or listening to music?

■ *Set realistic goals.* Identify long-term goals and then short-term goals that will help you meet the long-term goals. For example, a long-term goal might be to experience an increase in emotional and physical comfort and a short-term goal to take a 30-minute walk each evening.

■ *Challenge the belief that others always come first.* Overinvolvement with clients leads to overwork and overly solicitous helping that neglects the client's responsibilities, autonomy, and resources. It leaves little time for fulfillment of personal needs. Identify behaviors that indicate overinvolvement, such as saying yes much too often, a tendency to avoid conflict whenever possible, feeling selfish when not responding to someone else's needs, and always listening to others who need emotional support but seldom asking anyone to pay attention to your emotional needs. Assess whether you need to adjust your perspective and behavior. Learn to ask for what you need, acknowledge that you are doing the best you can, and affirm that you can meet your own needs as well as care for others.

■ *Learn to manage stress.* Stress management requires the following:
  • Acknowledge the mind–body connection, that is, the relationship among thoughts, feelings, behaviors, and the physiologic response to stress.
  • Monitor stress warning signals and invoke the relaxation response on a regular basis such as once a day for 20 minutes or twice a day for 10 minutes. "Mini-relaxations" (e.g., taking several deep breaths and thinking about something pleasant such as your favorite pet) throughout the day can also be used to counter the tension and anxiety associated with stress.
  • Develop the skill of personal presence (physically "being there" and psychologically "being with" a client or other person). To be available to others in this way requires practicing the skill of being present to yourself. Avoid allowing yourself to be hurried, distracted, or fragmented. Focus full attention on the activity you are doing at the moment.

■ *Maintain and enhance physical health.* Eat healthy, balanced meals, exercise regularly, and obtain adequate rest.

■ *Develop a support network.* Fellow nurses can often provide perspectives and insights to help cope with commonly shared experiences.

Note: From "Awakening the Healer Within," by C. L. Wells-Federman, 1996, *Holistic Nursing Practice, 10,* pp. 13–29. Adapted with permission.

---

provides a sense of harmony and balance. The individuals receiving a massage may enter a meditative state, thus relaxing and expanding their awareness.

A variety of massage strokes or movements may be used singly or in combination, depending on the outcome desired. These include effleurage (stroking), friction, pressure, and pétrissage (kneading or large, quick pinches of the skin, subcutaneous tissue, and muscle). See Figure 14–1 ■. For back massage techniques, see procedure 43-1 in Chapter 43. ∞

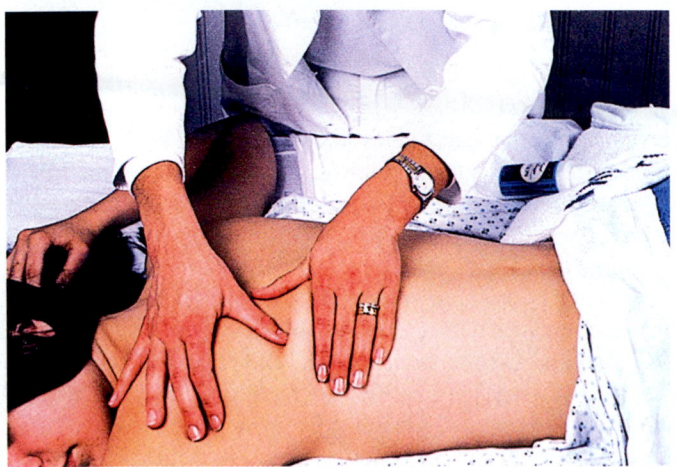

Figure 14-1 ■ Pétrissage is used over the shoulders and back.

Foot Reflexology

Reflexology is based on the principle that the hands and feet are mirrors of the body and that they have reflex points that correspond to each of the body's glands, structures, and organs. When a reflex area is massaged, it stimulates the corresponding organs in that zone. The actual massage technique varies depending on the purpose of the treatment.

Reflexology, also called zone therapy, can trace its origins to ancient Egypt. Modern foot reflexology is attributed to William H. Fitzgerald, who developed the theory in the early 1900s. His main contribution was his theory that there are 10 equal longitudinal zones that run the length of the body from the top of the head to the tips of the toes and 5 closely associated zones on each arm. Each great toe is the start of a line that runs up the medial aspect of the body through the center of the face ending at the top of the head. Each zone (five on each side of the body) has a reflex area on the hand and the foot. According to the precepts of reflexology, more than 72,000 nerves in the body terminate in the feet (see Figure 14–2 ■). When the flow of energy is blocked or becomes congested, massaging the reflex points can release the tension. Blockages in any part of the zone can affect the entire zone.

In the 1930s, Eunice Ingham asserted that the feet are more responsive to reflexology treatments than the fingers. The main goal of foot reflexology is to provide relaxation by maintaining or restoring a state of health and relieving congestion or tension in the zone.

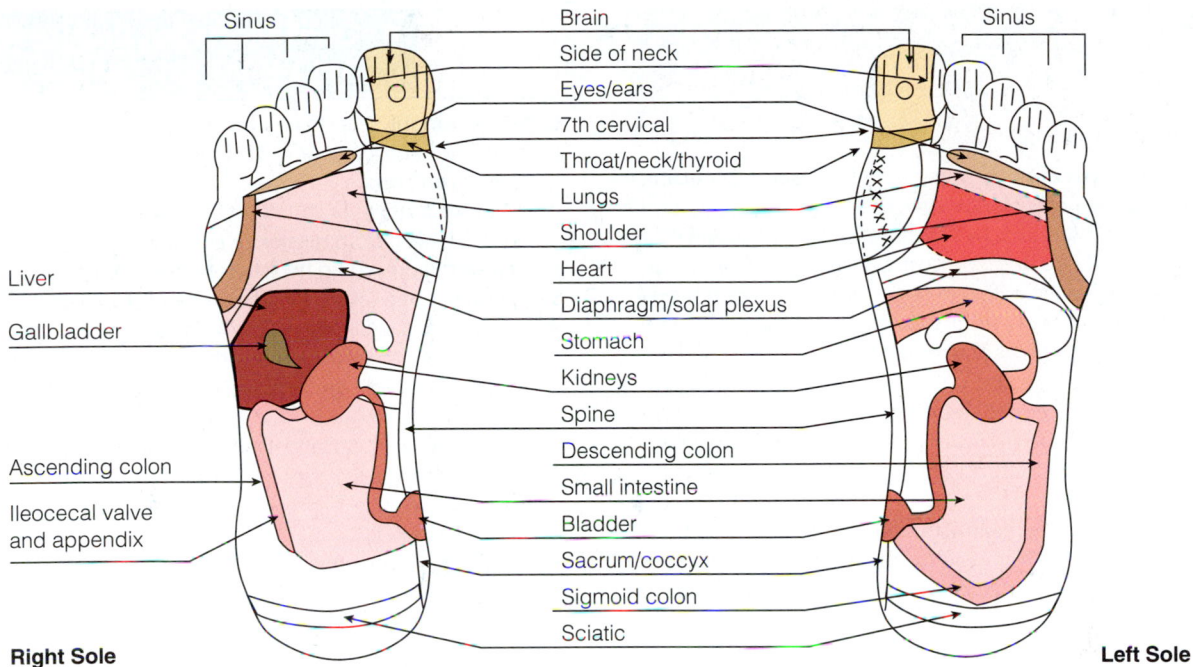

Figure 14–2 ■ Foot reflex areas.

At this time, no research has validated the theory of the healing properties of foot reflexology. However, it is believed that foot reflexology, like other massages of the feet, can stimulate relaxation, which affects the autonomic response, which in turn affects the endocrine and immune systems and neuropeptides. Although reflexology is a relatively safe procedure, experienced reflexologists need to be consulted when the client has circulatory disorders of the extremities are experienced.

Acupressure

Acupressure is a form of healing in which the therapist exerts finger pressure on specific sites. According to the theory that underlies acupressure, 657 designated points can be massaged. These points are similar to those used in acupuncture and shiatsu massage. The points run along 12 pathways or meridians that connect the points on each half of the body. The application of finger or thumb pressure is thought to restore balance in the flow of energy, and when energy can flow freely, the body can heal itself.

Acupressure is used both to diagnose and to treat ailments. With the application of acupressure, the body is theoretically kept in harmony, thus terminating many minor ailments and preventing them from becoming major diseases. In shiatsu, pressure is applied to the same spots using the points of the thumbs and fingers and also the heel of the hand. Shiatsu's main purpose is to maintain health rather than treat illness.

Reiki

Reiki (pronounced *ray-key*) is a Japanese word meaning universal life-force-energy. In this therapy, the practitioner places the hands on the client and energy flows from one to the other. The amount and effectiveness of the energy is said to depend on the openness and the need of the recipient rather than the direction of flow by the practitioner. Although usually performed using direct contact between the practitioner and the client, Reiki can also be performed from a distance.

There are three degrees of Reiki training. The First Degree, which can be taught in a weekend, focuses on the hand positions. The Second Degree, which can be learned in one day, emphasizes the use of Reiki on a client at a distance. The Third Degree, the master level, prepares the practitioner to teach (Nield-Anderson & Ameling, 2000).

Mind–Body Therapies

In mind–body therapies, individuals focus on realigning or creating balance in mental processes to bring about healing. Advocates of these therapies need to avoid promoting the notion of the mind healing the body through conscious "control." It is easy to slip into a mind-*over*-matter mentality that is not consistent with holistic care. A failure to achieve the desired healing can also promote guilt. The focus of mind–body therapies is on bringing balance to thoughts, emotions, or the breath for its own sake. Because people are integrated wholes this can help restore peace and balance throughout, but an instrumental approach (practicing yoga to fight cancer as opposed to practicing yoga for the health that yoga brings) may be less effective. Mind–body therapies include progressive relaxation, biofeedback, imagery, yoga, meditation, prayer, music therapy, humor and laughter, and hypnosis.

Progressive Relaxation

Relaxation techniques have been used extensively to reduce high levels of stress and chronic pain. Relaxation techniques enable

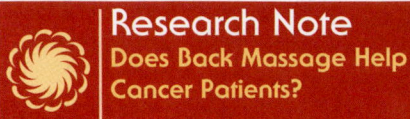

Research Note
Does Back Massage Help Cancer Patients?

In previous years, back massage was a routine aspect of nursing care of hospitalized clients. However, this is no longer as common as in the past. Research by Smith, Kemp, Hemphill, and Vojir (2002) compared the pretest and post-test ratings of pain, symptom distress, sleep, and anxiety in patients who received therapeutic massage and those who did not. For the experimental group, 20 cancer patients received massage consisting of 15 to 30 minutes of effleurage and pétrissage three times over one week. In an effort to reduce the effect of just having focused nursing attention, the control group received 20 minutes of focused communication that included teaching, relaxation techniques, and discussion.

Results showed that mean scores of pain and symptom distress were significantly improved for the massage group. Sleep quality ratings were not significantly improved for the massage group but significantly worsened in the control group. There were no statistically significant changes in anxiety score for either group. The authors acknowledge some limitations in generalizing the findings to other cancer or noncancer patients: The patients were not randomly assigned to the groups nor did they experience both treatments, and the vast majority of the patients were white men. In addition, the overall number of patients studied was rather small.

Implications: In spite of the limitations in this research study, it does provide support for the effectiveness of massage. No negative impact of the treatment was found. The study findings are consistent with those of other research that has shown positive effects of massage on pain and symptom distress. More research is needed to demonstrate if massage can have positive effects on other subjective experiences for cancer patients.

Note: From "Outcomes of Therapeutic Massage for Hospitalized Cancer Patients," by M. C. Smith, J. Kemp, L. Hemphill, and C. P. Vojir, 2002, *Journal of Nursing Scholarship, 34,* pp. 257–262.

BOX 14–2 ■ Guidelines for Progressive Relaxation

- Sit comfortably in a chair, with your feet flat on the ground.
- Tense and tighten your right fist. Focus on the feeling of tension as you do so.
- Allow the muscles in your right fist to relax. Contrast the difference in feeling from tension to relaxation.
- Repeat the preceding two steps for the left fist.
- Now tense and relax both your left and right fists.
- Focus on and relish the feeling of relaxation.
- Now tighten the muscles in both fists and both arms. Feel the tension, fully relax the muscles, and again focus on the sensation of relaxation.
- Progressively tighten and relax each muscle group in the body: toes, ankles, knees, buttocks and groin, stomach and lower back muscles, chest and upper back muscles, shoulders, forehead, jaw muscles.
- Couple deep breathing with progressive relaxation. While relaxing your muscles, inhale deeply, send the breath to the fist (or other muscle group), and exhale.

The entire exercise should last a minimum of 10 minutes.

---

the client to exert control over the body's responses to tension and anxiety. For many years, nurses on maternity units have encouraged women in labor to relax and breathe rhythmically.

Progressive relaxation requires that the client tense and then relax successive muscle groups, and focus attention on discriminating between the feelings experienced when the muscle group is relaxed and when it was tense. Jacobsen (1938), the originator of the progressive relaxation technique, found that tension of a muscle group before its relaxation actually achieves a greater degree of relaxation than simply commanding oneself to relax. This technique can result in decreased oxygen consumption, metabolism, respiratory rate, cardiac rate, muscle tension, and systolic and diastolic blood pressures.

Three requisites to relaxation are correct posture, a mind at rest, and a quiet environment. The client must be positioned comfortably, with all body parts supported, joints slightly flexed, and no strain or pull on muscles (e.g., arms and legs

should not be crossed). To rest the mind, the client is asked to gaze slowly around the room (e.g., across the ceiling, down the wall, along a window curtain, around the fabric pattern, and back up the wall). This exercise focuses the mind outside of the body and creates a second center of concentration.

Procedures for teaching progressive relaxation vary. The method for relaxing muscle groups, the specific muscle groups to be relaxed, the number of sessions involved, and the role of the instructor (taped versus live instructions) may differ. Tension of muscle groups is often maintained for 5 to 7 seconds and followed by relaxation of the muscle group at a predetermined cue. To achieve maximum relaxation, various positive and affirmative phrases are used, such as "Let all the tension go" and "Enjoy the feelings as your muscles become relaxed and loose." Guidelines for progressive relaxation are outlined in Box 14–2.

Biofeedback

Biofeedback is a technique that teaches various forms of relaxation by providing a response from physiologic processes. Biofeedback is often described as a technique to bring bodily processes under conscious control, and that is why physicians often prescribe it. However, the intent of the treatment and its mechanism are different. While the intent and motivation may be to increase the patient's blood flow, the focus is teaching the client to relax. Subtle feedback from temperature meters or an electromyogram helps clients learn to identify when they are more relaxed and when they are more tense. Specifically, biofeedback teaches clients to achieve a generalized state of relaxation characterized by parasympathetic dominance and to reduce the pattern of physiologic arousal manifested in stress-related disorders.

Imagery

Imagery has been defined as "application of the conscious use of the power of the imagination with the intention of activating biological, psychological, or spiritual healing" (Schaub & Dossey, 2000, p. 541). People respond powerfully to images that can produce physical, mental, emotional, and spiritual changes. Most images are unconscious, and these produce changes as well. Conscious imagery involves creating mental pictures of what is desired and can be evoked from memories, dreams, fantasies, and hopes. Although imagery is often thought of as visualization, imagery can employ all the senses—seeing, hearing, feeling, touching, or even tasting the created image.

Images can be either concrete or symbolic. A concrete image is one that is biologically correct; for example, a concrete image of body cells would resemble the way cells appear under a microscope. A person can also form symbolic images, which often replace concrete images. For example, a person receiving chemotherapy may visualize a dragon (representing the chemotherapeutic agent) traveling throughout the bloodstream eating cancer cells.

Table 14–2 describes several types of imagery that can be performed independently by clients or with the assistance of a skilled helper. When imagery is assisted, it is referred to as *guided imagery.*

> ► **CLINICAL ALERT** *Although relaxation, biofeedback, and imagery are different techniques, all three involve the process of physical resting and rhythmic breathing.* ■

Yoga

The word **yoga,** derived from the Sanskrit root *yug* meaning "to bind" or "to yoke," is the uniting of all the powers of the body, mind, and spirit. Yoga is an approach to living a balanced life based on ancient teachings found in Hindu spiritual treatises (the Upanishads) written in 800–400 BC. The great yogi Patanjali (500 BC) classified the teachings of the Upanishads into eight ways of being, referred to as *Ashtanga yoga,* meaning integrated or eight-limbed yoga. The first two stages are the foundation of yoga. If a person does not practice them, the following six stages become meaningless. The remaining six stages set out practices that help a person to master the first two stages. The eight stages follow.

1. *Yama* (universal moral commandments). This refers to improvement in social behavior and is achieved by five noble practices: nonviolence (both physical and psychologic), truthfulness, refraining from stealing, self-restraint in every sphere of life, and refraining from hoarding.
2. *Niyama* (rules for daily conduct). These refer to improvement in personal behavior and are achieved by maintaining a purity of body and mind, developing a habit of contentment, practicing austerity in every sphere of life, studying relevant literature, and practicing dedication to God daily.
3. *Asanas* (physical postures). These consist of a series of 84 main postures (e.g., cobra posture and plough posture) intended to improve body health. The bending, stretching, and holding properties of the postures are designed to relax and tone the muscles and improve the function of various organs of the endocrine and nervous systems. People may assume 10 to 15 yogic postures, including stationary exercises, for all parts of the body for a period of about 15 minutes daily.
4. *Pranayama* (breath control). This stage includes eight main breath control techniques. Through the practice of various exercises, an individual learns not only to control breathing but also to restrain and quiet the flow of life force

TABLE 14–2 Selected Types of Imagery

Type	Description	Example
Body–mind	The conscious formation of an image that is directed to a body part or activity that requires attention or increased energy	A client visualizes a construction worker building new tissues and structure to heal a wound.
Correct biologic	Images that are biologically correct and appear as they do in real life as they would under a microscope	A client visualizes white blood cells engulfing bacteria or having normal blood flow to the hands and feet.
End-state	Images of a final healed state	A client who has an injured shoulder visualizes playing tennis.
Generalized healing	Image of an event, light, sense of unity, universal power, or spirit	A client describes being bathed with the warmth of the sun, or a white light penetrating the core of his being, or "an angel hovering over me."
Spontaneous	Images that enter the conscious mind but are not deliberately created; unexpected reception of an image	A client describes feelings of tension in the back of the neck as a huge knot.
Transpersonal	Images connecting persons to higher levels of consciousness	A client imagines self as a river and feels becoming flowing and flexible.

Note: From "Imagery: Awakening the Inner Healer" by B. Schaub and B. M. Dossey in *Holistic Nursing: A Handbook for Practice,* 3rd ed. (pp. 539–581), B. M. Dossey, L. Keegan, and C. E. Guzzetta, Eds., 2000, Gaithersburg, MD: Aspen.

energy (*prana*). According to yogic philosophy, there is a direct relationship between life force activity and the rate of breathing. When the life force is operating smoothly, the breath is calm and regular, but when it is excited, breathing becomes erratic. Breath control is designed to still the mind and achieve transcendental awareness by controlling the life force. This is done by regulating and harmonizing the breath in particular patterns.

5. *Pratyahara* (controlling the senses). This aspect of yoga involves restraining the activities of the sense organs with the ultimate goal of restraining the mind. It is achieved by minimizing the stimulation of the sense organs and leading as simple a life as possible.

6. *Dharana* (concentration of the mind on one point). Learning to avoid all distractions and concentrate on an object of one's choice involves tremendous perseverance and willpower. The concentration helps to calm mental excitement and to induce tranquillity and serenity of the mind.

7. *Dhayana* (meditation). This stage refers to meditation that occurs when a person's concentration has become one pointed, enabling the person to unify consciousness completely and experience a state of transcendental awareness.

8. *Samadhi* (supraconsciousness). This stage refers to extension of conscious control over successively deeper realms of consciousness.

There are two basic types of yoga, both based on the Ashtanga principles. These are Jnana yoga and Hatha yoga. The goal of both forms is enlightenment or union with God through mastery of the self. Jnana yoga is an attempt to reach enlightenment through the study of ancient scriptures and knowledge. Hatha yoga is an attempt to reach enlightenment by quieting the mind and purifying the body.

Popular yoga classes of the 21st century are based on various forms of Hatha yoga, a series of gentle stretching exercises using specific *asanas* and *pranayama*. Translated, *Ha-Tha* means "sun/moon," a symbolic representation of the male and female energies in the body. Hatha yoga seeks to attain a balance between the sun and the moon, the masculine and the feminine, the sympathetic and the parasympathetic, the day and the night, and the warm and the cool. Modern Ashtanga yoga tends to emphasize aerobic fitness with flowing rhythmic movement from one posture to another. Individuals interested in beginning yoga are advised to explore the specific program offered to ensure that it includes the techniques most suited to their needs.

Meditation

Meditation is a technique used to quiet the mind and focus it in the present and to release fears, worries, anxieties, and doubts concerning the past and the future. It produces a state of deep peace and rest combined with mental alertness. Originally, meditation was viewed as a religious practice and is still practiced by many as a form of prayer. However, one does not need to be religious to meditate or to receive the benefits of meditation.

Meditation involves both relaxation and focused attention. Skill in meditation is enhanced when the person first masters the skills of breathing, progressive relaxation, and imagery.

Because many types of meditation exist, the techniques used to achieve the desired outcome vary widely. In one type of meditation, referred to as *concentrative meditation,* the person visualizes and focuses attention on one particular object (e.g., a candle or a flower) or repeats the words of a mantra so that all other objects and stimuli in the environment are excluded. The Sanskrit word *om* or *aum,* meaning "one," is a commonly used mantra. Hindus believe that *om* is the universal sound, and that its vibrational sound quality enhances a feeling of peace and deep meditation. People may, however, choose a word or phrase meaningful to them such as *shalom, peace,* or "I am at one with God."

In another type of meditation, referred to as *opening up* or *mindfulness meditation,* the person attempts to remain open to all stimuli. Various types of meditation integrate elements of both techniques. For example, a person may focus on a breathing pattern (Zen meditation) or on a mantra (transcendental meditation) but be willing to allow other thoughts to "come up," watch those thoughts, and then return to the original focus.

Guidelines for meditation:

1. Create a special time and place for meditation. Ideally, choose the early morning or evening, and wait at least 2 hours after eating so that complete energy is devoted to meditation rather than to digestive demands. A quiet, comfortable place, devoid of distractions, is helpful.

2. Sit either cross-legged on the floor or upright in a straight-backed chair, keeping the spine straight and the body relaxed. Avoid a lying position; this increases the tendency to fall asleep.

3. Support the palms on the thighs, and close the eyes.

4. Follow deep-breathing or progressive relaxation exercises.

5. Focus attention completely on either breathing or a chosen mental image. If using a mantra, repeat the word or phrase either aloud or silently while exhaling. When distracting thoughts appear, allow them to drift into and out of your mind without giving them undue attention; then refocus on your breathing or your mantra.

6. Practice this process daily for 10- to 20-minute periods.

Prayer

Prayer is similar to meditation but is intended to be communication with God, a saint, or some other being who answers the prayer. Prayer may be conducted individually or in groups and may even be conducted at a distance by individuals unknown to the person for whom the prayers of healing are made. (See the discussion of intercessory prayer later in this chapter.)

Music Therapy

Music therapy may be defined as "the behavioral science concerned with the systematic application of music to produce relaxation and desired changes in emotions, behavior, and physiology" (Guzetta, 2000, p. 585). The human body has a fundamental vibrating pattern, according to music therapists. Thus musical vibrations that closely relate to the body's fundamental frequency or vibrating pattern can have a profound healing effect on the entire human body, mind, and spirit, bringing about changes in emotions, organs, hormones, enzymes, cells, and atoms. Theoretically, carefully selected music helps to restore regulatory functions that are out of tune during times of stress and illness. Music aligns the body, mind, and spirit with its own fundamental frequency.

Music therapy consists of listening, rhythm, body movement, and singing. It is used for a variety of reasons. Music can serve as a vehicle for altering ordinary levels of consciousness to achieve the mind's fullest potential. Individuals can move through various stages of consciousness: normal waking, expanded sensory threshold, daydreaming, trance, and meditative states.

Using music therapy, people can also shift their perception of time from actual time of hours, minutes, and seconds (which is perceived in the left cerebral hemisphere) to experiential time—that which is perceived through memory. Listeners can actually lose track of time for extended periods, enabling them to reduce anxiety, fear, and pain. Because music is nonverbal in nature, it appeals to the right cerebral hemisphere, which regulates the intuitive, creative, imaging way of processing information. The right brain recognizes pitch, rhythm, style, and melody. Music does not need logic or analysis from the left brain. However, as a person's knowledge of music increases, left-brain functioning may dominate; musicians, for example, analyze compositional techniques and other features of the music. To benefit from music therapy, a person needs to learn to let go of conditioned responses to integrate the functioning of both hemispheres of the brain.

Music therapy can be used in a variety of practice settings. Quiet, soothing music without words is often used to induce relaxation (see Figure 14–3 ■). Musical selections without words are preferred so that clients do not concentrate on the messages and meaning of words rather than allowing themselves to flow with the music. Music recordings are often used to relax and distract clients in perioperative holding areas, cardiac care units, birthing rooms, counseling rooms, rehabilitation and physical therapy units, and sleep induction units.

For individualized therapy, the nurse needs knowledge of the effects that particular types of music produce. Therapeutic music can include mood, choral, classical, romantic, impressionist, country, soft rock-and-roll, opera, or New Age music. To select appropriate music, the nurse needs to consider the client's preferences as well as the goals of therapy. Additionally, the nurse must consider appropriate times for use and length of therapy sessions. For example, some people may wish to have a music session after a morning shower to balance the body–mind for the day's events. The usual duration of a session is about 20 minutes. Clients are encouraged to let the body respond to the music as it wishes; that is, to relax the muscles, lie down, hum, clap, or dance. Some clients may wish to make their own recording of musical selections they find appealing. The healing capabilities of music are intimately bound with personal experience and what can achieve inner quietness or other desired qualities within that person.

Humor and Laughter

Health care professionals recently have focused on the positive effects of humor and laughter on health and disease. Humor involves the ability to discover, express, or appreciate the comical or absurdly incongruous, to be amused by one's own imperfections or the whimsical aspects of life, and to see the funny side of an otherwise serious situation. Humor in nursing is defined as helping the client "to perceive, appreciate, and express what is funny, amusing, or ludicrous in order to establish relationships, relieve tension, release anger, facilitate learning, or cope with painful feeling" (McCloskey & Bulechek, 2000, p. 380). Elaboration of these functions of humor in nursing situations follows:

- *Establishing relationships.* Humor decreases the social distance between persons and assists in putting persons at ease. When tension is decreased, people can focus on the message and on other people rather than on their own feelings. Use of humor helps the nurse establish rapport with clients, an important factor in achieving success in nursing interventions.
- *Relieving tension and anxiety.* Freud in 1905 stated that laughter releases psychic energy previously used to block expression of socially or personally unacceptable impulses. The effective use of humor relieves the tension of emotionally charged events. The personal nature of humor, for example, helps clients deal with the impersonal nature of wearing a hospital gown and numbered ID band and with embarrassing questions and uncomfortable tests. People can also use humor prophylactically to decrease stress.
- *Releasing anger and aggression.* Humor helps individuals act out impulses or feelings in a safe and nonthreatening manner. It dissipates feelings of anger and aggression by focusing on the comic elements of a situation.
- *Facilitating learning.* Many lectures and presentations begin with a joke or cartoon. Humor not only reduces the presenter's

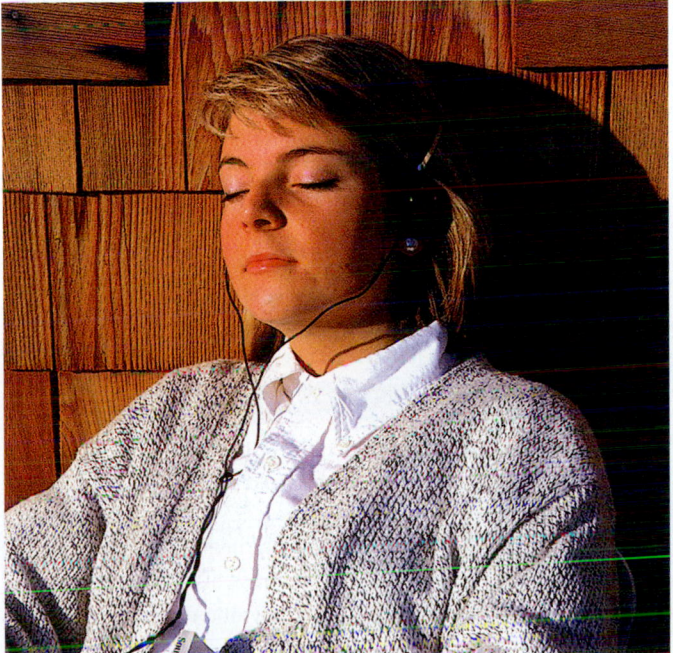

Figure 14–3 ■ Listening to music can provide a variety of therapeutic benefits.

anxiety but also gains the audience's attention. People learn more when humor is used and anxiety levels are reduced. People also recall more information when they associate information with a joke. Use of humor in instruction, however, needs to be carefully planned so that it will contribute to learning.

- *Coping with painful feelings.* People may use humor to blunt the immediate effect of situations that are too painful, such as the effect of a threatening diagnosis or treatment. Humor diminishes anxiety and fear and reduces tension, thus enabling the person to confront and deal with the situation.

Humor also has physiologic benefits that involve alternating states of stimulation and relaxation. Laughter stimulates increases in respiratory rate, heart rate, muscular tension, and oxygen exchange. A state of relaxation follows laughter, during which heart rate, blood pressure, respiration, and muscle tension decrease. Humor stimulates the production of catecholamines and hormones. It also releases endorphins, thereby increasing pain tolerance.

Humor brings out and integrates people's positive emotions: hope, faith, will to live, festivity, purpose, and determination. It therefore has healing properties.

To use humor effectively, nurses need to be aware of their own feelings as well as the feelings of others and cultural variations in what people consider humorous.

Many health care settings are now interested in providing humor as a caring skill and have recognized that "laughter is the best medicine." "Humor" rooms are being created for clients and staff that are supplied with games, funny audiotapes and videotapes, humorous books, collections of cartoons, and so on.

Hypnosis

Hypnosis is an altered state of consciousness in which an individual's concentration is focused and distraction is minimized. Hypnosis can be used to control pain, alter body functions, and change lifestyle habits. Scientists do not understand exactly how hypnosis relieves pain; however, one theory is that it prevents pain stimuli in the brain from penetrating the conscious mind. Another theory is that hypnosis works by activating nerve pathways in the brain that cause the release of natural morphinelike substances called enkephalins and endorphins. These opioids modify behavior and the perception of pain.

Hypnosis requires a client's active participation; clients can even learn to invoke their own hypnotic state. Hypnosis does not take away a person's self-control; in fact, people under hypnosis cannot be made to do anything that they consider immoral or dangerous. In a hypnotic trance, the client does not fall asleep but does become so sharply focused that minor distractions are ignored. A number of hypnosis techniques are used, depending on the type of pain and the preference of the client and the therapist. One of the most commonly used is symptom suppression, in which the client's awareness of the symptom (i.e., pain) is blocked and the client is distanced from it. The effectiveness of this type of hypnosis depends on the severity of the symptom and the client's ability to concentrate.

Aromatherapy

Buckle (2002) defines **clinical aromatherapy** as the controlled use of essential oils for specific measurable outcomes. The early Egyptians used aromatherapy to relieve pain, and in the 19th century, rosemary leaves were burned in hospitals for fumigation. Today aromatherapists use essential oils to promote a number of positive health outcomes including the improvement of mood, edema, acne, allergies, bruising, and stress.

The essential oils that are used in aromatherapy are distilled from flowers, roots, bark, leaves, wood resins, and lemon or orange rinds. Oils can be massaged into the body, applied as hot or cold compresses, added to bath water, or inhaled. When essential oils are inhaled, aromas are detected by the olfactory receptor cells in the nares. The stimuli travel along the olfactory nerve (cranial nerve I) to the olfactory bulb and then to the brain where they are thought to play a role in emotions, memory, and a variety of body functions including heart rate, blood pressure, breathing, and immune response. About 300 essential oils are currently used in aromatherapy. Examples are shown in Table 14–3.

Nurses should caution people who are considering aromatherapy to be aware that aromatic oils vary in quality, their production is not regulated, and some may be toxic when inhaled (e.g., bitter almond, birch, camphor, wintergreen). The skin should always be tested for allergies by applying a very small amount of the diluted oil before a whole treatment is tried. Essential oils should not be used near the eyes and should always be diluted in a suitable oil or water before application to the skin. These oils are not for internal use and should be stored in dark-colored glass bottles and kept away from sunlight and heat. Many oils are listed in popular publications as a contraindication in pregnancy because they have a reputation of being emmenagogic (bring on menstruation). In contrast, there are many reports that aromatherapy can be useful in pregnancy and delivery. If the client is pregnant, she should be advised to discuss this in depth with her health care provider before using essential oils.

> **CLINICAL ALERT** *CAM modalities may be combined, for example, music played while being massaged with essential oils.* ■

TABLE 14–3 Selected Essential Oils and Some of Their Uses

Oil	Use
Cinnamon	Constipation, exhaustion, flatulence
Eucalyptus	Arthritis, bronchitis, cold sores, colds, coughing, fever, sinusitis
Geranium	Mood modifier, antidiarrheal agent
Lavender	Relief for headache, stress, and insomnia
Peppermint	Relief for nausea, antipyretic, respiratory aid
Sandalwood	Bronchitis, chapped skin, depression, dry skin, laryngitis, stress

Transpersonal Therapies

Transpersonal therapies are therapies that effect healing between persons. Two therapies are discussed in this chapter: noncontact therapeutic touch and intercessory prayer.

Noncontact Therapeutic Touch

Noncontact **therapeutic touch (TT)** is a process by which practitioners believe they can transmit energy to a person who is ill or injured to potentiate the healing process. It is derived from, but not the same as, the "laying on of hands" associated with some religious philosophies. Delores Krieger (1979), who coined the term *therapeutic touch,* refers to TT as a healing meditation.

Basic to therapeutic touch are the concepts that the human being is an energy field, known as a human field, and that energy can be intentionally channeled from one person to another. The human field extends beyond the level of the skin and is perceptible to the trained sense (primarily touch) of a healer. This energy field can be most clearly "felt" within several feet of the body. An everyday experience that may demonstrate this field phenomenon is the feeling of having one's space invaded when someone stands too close in a crowded elevator, even though there is no physical contact.

The body and the environment are considered open systems that constantly exchange energy and matter. The pattern and organization of the human field are constantly affected by the flow of energy to and from the environment. In a healthy person, equilibrium exists between the inward and outward flow of energy. In situations of disease, illness, or pain, the pattern and organization of the field are disrupted; there may be a loss of energy, a disruption in the flow, an accumulation, or a blockage of energy flow.

Therapeutic touch is NIC intervention 5465 and is defined as "Attuning to the universal healing field, seeking to act as an instrument for healing influence, and using the natural sensitivity of the hands to gently focus and direct the healing process" (McCloskey & Bulechek, 2000, p. 665). The activities include these:

1. Centering is the process of focusing attention inward to achieve a sense of detachment, sensitivity, and balance.
2. Assessing is a head-to-toe scanning process in which the nurse holds the palms of both hands one to two inches over the client's skin surface. The purpose of the assessment is to detect asymmetric differences in the client's energy flow, such as heat, cold, tingling, congestion, pressure, emptiness, or other sensations.
3. Move the hands (palms facing the client) in a sweeping motion from the area where pressure was perceived down along the long bones of the body.
4. Highly skilled nurses may also transfer energy from the nurse to the client. The nurse must know which form of energy to use, how to modulate energy, and where to apply energy. This assists clients to repattern their energy. The form of energy has different effects and is related to col-

ors: Blue energy is sedating; yellow energy is stimulating and energizing; and green energy is harmonizing. The nurse modulates these energy forms by mentally visualizing the color, for example, by visualizing light through a blue stained-glass window. The nurse may apply energy directly over an identified area of congestion or to one of the *chakras* (special channels that serve as entry areas for energy from the environment, located in the thoracic or solar plexus). Energy transference helps restore the balance of the energy field and provides additional energy to promote self-healing.

To date, the energy fields and energy flow of TT have not been susceptible to measurement. No one has been able to demonstrate that real energy passes between the therapist and the client. These findings lead some to believe that the real power of TT is in the considerable psychologic boost of receiving a therapy that the practitioner honestly and persuasively believes can heal, and in the personal connection that TT offers.

Intercessory Prayer

Intercessory prayer refers to prayer offered in favor of another. The praying people are referred to as *intercessors.* Research demonstrates inconclusive evidence on the impact of intercessory prayer on the well-being of others. In a review of 59 randomized clinical trials examining the efficacy of alternative therapies, two major rigorous studies were found that showed significant benefit of intercessory prayer on cardiac patients (Abbot, 2000). However, another large study of 799 cardiac patients showed no such positive effect (Aviles et al., 2001). Clearly, more research is needed, although an intervention such as prayer that has no adverse effects should not be withheld pending the findings.

ALTERNATIVE MEDICAL THERAPIES

Interest in CAM is rapidly increasing as the public demands more choice in and takes more responsibility for its own health care. Some people choose CAM as their first treatment for problems such as back pain; others choose CAM when their health care needs have not been met through traditional medicine. Some physicians provide CAM treatments as a part of their practice but patients should be aware that physicians who include CAM in their practice are not all equally qualified to do so.

Acupuncture and Oriental Medicine

Traditional Chinese medicine (TCM) has been evolving for thousands of years and has a long history throughout Asia. TCM is grounded in a sophisticated system that incorporates medical and philosophical theories and a long history of empirically documented experience and tradition. The theory and practice of TCM has evolved differently throughout Asia and Europe, but this is consistent with the underlying philosophical premise that health and environment are interrelated. Treatment modalities in TCM include acupuncture, herbs, exercise, diet, and massage.

Traditional Chinese medicine is based on the premise that the body's vital energy or **qi** (pronounced *chee*) circulates through pathways or meridians and can be accessed and manipulated through specific anatomical points along the surface of the body. Disease is described as an imbalance or interruption in the flow of qi. The focus of acupuncture treatment is to restore balance and free flow of qi in order to help the body to heal itself. This is achieved by the insertion of fine, sterile needles into specific points along meridians, in various areas of the body (see Figure 14–4 ■). Once inserted, the needles may be heated, stimulated by a mild electrical current, or manipulated manually. Sometimes the herb "moxa" is burned over particular acupuncture points to facilitate the flow of qi.

Acupuncture was introduced in the United States in the 1970s after President Nixon's historic and high-profile visit to China. In 1997, the NIH issued a statement endorsing acupuncture. "There is sufficient evidence of acupuncture's value to expand its use into conventional medicine and to encourage further studies of its physiology and clinical value" (Acupuncture, 1997). As a result, more health professionals are considering integrating acupuncture with conventional treatment.

Research has shown that acupuncture is effective in relieving postoperative pain and nausea associated with pregnancy and chemotherapy (Acupuncture, 1997). Acupuncture appears to be effective in a wide variety of conditions including stroke, headache, chronic low back pain, menstrual cramps, muscle pain, carpal tunnel syndrome, addiction, asthma, and pregnancy-associated nausea. Acupuncture treatment may also result in a reduction in the amount of pain medication or anesthesia that may be required. With few exceptions, most acupuncturists in the United States are educated at the master's level in single-purpose institutions that have not met the regional accreditation standards required of the colleges and universities that house nursing and other allied health programs. However, this is a relatively new profession in the United States, and a handful of programs are already housed in regionally accredited institutions.

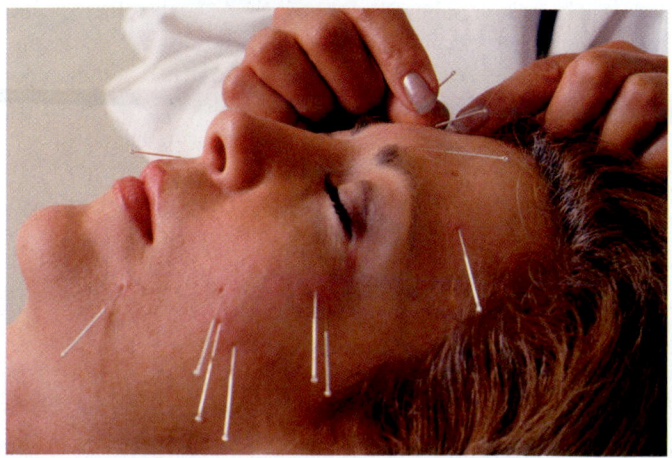

Figure 14–4 ■ Acupuncture involves the insertion of thin, sterile needles. (Yoav Levy/Phototake NYC.)

Chiropractic

Chiropractic, from the Greek meaning "done by hand," involves adjustments of the spine and joints (Cassileth, 1998) and is grounded in the assumption that maintaining the alignment of the spine and joints facilitates the flow of energy throughout the body, including the nervous, circulatory, respiratory, gastrointestinal, and limbic systems. Chiropractors are concerned with maintaining the self-regulatory systems of the body and focus on helping the body to heal itself. Spinal manipulation has been used for centuries in Europe, Asia, and ancient Egypt to maintain and restore health.

D. D. Palmer introduced modern chiropractic education in 1895, at a time when spinal manipulation was central to the ways osteopaths practiced medicine. Chiropractic is currently the most widely accepted and commonly used CAM treatment in the United States. Chiropractors may use x-rays, visual inspection, muscular strengths and weaknesses, range of motion, and posture to assess the spine for misaligned vertebrae.

Despite years of tremendous resistance from organized medicine, chiropractic is widely accepted throughout the world and by many in the medical community. Increasing numbers of chiropractors are appointed to hospital staffs, state regulatory boards, and commissioned as health care providers in the armed forces (Goldberg, Anderson, & Trivieri, 2002). In several states, chiropractors have the authority to serve as "gatekeepers" for managed care plans (Cooper & McKee, 2000). Cooper and McKee cite outcome studies showing that the relief of low back pain is attributed to spinal adjustments. However, efficacy is the same whether the treatment was performed by a chiropractor, an allopathic or osteopathic physician, or a physical therapist (Andersson et al., 1999; Cherkin, Deyo, Bettie, Street, & Barlow, 1998).

While low back pain treated by spinal manipulation constitutes the major focus of chiropractic practice, more than half of U.S. states allow chiropractors to perform acupuncture and at least 20 permit them to practice homeopathy (Cooper & McKee, 2000). Again, whether physicians or chiropractors, not all practitioners licensed to perform CAM treatments are equally educated or qualified to do so. Most chiropractors are prepared in professional doctoral programs offered by single-purpose institutions. The isolation of chiropractic education from other disciplines in allied health has helped the profession develop autonomy, but the development of integrated theories of holistic health and appropriate research methods for alternative medicine suffer when faculty and students from different disciplines work in isolation from each other.

Herbal Medicine

Herbs have been used since antiquity for the prevention and treatment of illness. Herbs are defined as plants that are valued for their medicinal properties, flavors, and scents. Americans continue to show increased interest in the use of herbs and herbal tonics in search of a more natural way of life or dissatisfaction with the treatment offered by the medical profession.

Difficult to measure accurately, Americans purchase $4 to $7 billion worth of herbs annually, and this number increases each year. However, not all herbs—although natural—are safe when ingested. Most herbs are consumed without untoward reactions when they are taken in small amounts. The determination of the safety and efficacy of herbal products is difficult because the Food and Drug Administration (FDA), manufacturers, and herbal experts disagree on how to interpret the varying evidence available for many types of herbal remedies. See the accompanying Practice Guidelines for cautions regarding some commonly used herbs.

The Dietary Supplement Health and Education Act, passed in 1994, ruled that herbs can be labeled with information on their effects on the structure and function of the body. These labels must be accompanied by a disclaimer stating that the FDA has not reviewed the herb and it is not intended to be used as a drug. Canadians attempted to regulate herbs and encountered a number of cross-cultural difficulties (Coward & Ratanakul, 1999). Many herbs used in TCM are toxic when used alone, but practitioners prescribe them as part of formulas that include other herbs to counter the toxic effects. Regulating single herbs used in TCM would be almost impossible because, unlike Western medicine, the practice of TCM is not organized around single herbal medicines. No government standards currently exist for the quality of herbal products sold in the United States.

Herbs may be sold to manufacturers as whole plants, plant parts, cut pieces, or finely ground particles. The only definitive way to truly know the purity and concentration of a particular product is to perform assays. However, herbal manufacturers have little incentive to do potentially costly assays since there is no pressure from the government for quality control.

Although a healthy lifestyle is the primary promoter of good health, and conventional medicine may be the best therapy for many problems, selected herbal therapies may have a place among options for health and illness management. With the current proliferation of lay literature on herbal remedies and the wide availability of such products in health food stores, more people are relying on herbal and other less conventional therapies for a wide variety of problems.

Whether ingested as "teas, or substance or supplements," the study of herbs is best approached through a nutritional framework and epidemiological studies rather than through separate clinical trials (Arab, 2000). Despite the cultural problems noted by Coward and Ratanakul (1999) at the beginning of this chapter, Arab argues against separating conventional pharmaceutical and alternative herbal therapies in the medical curriculum and advocates for studying them side by side. Health care professionals should include questions about herbal teas and supplements when taking a patient's history.

Homeopathy

Until the late 18th century, conventional Western medicine was characterized by such practices as bloodletting (using leeches) and toxic mercury-based purgatives. From 1790 to 1810, a German physician and chemist, Samuel Hahnemann, performed a series of experiments and concluded that medicinal substances produced a similar set of symptoms in healthy people (Micozzi, 2000). His observations led him to develop a the-

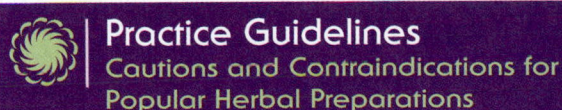

Practice Guidelines
Cautions and Contraindications for Popular Herbal Preparations

- *Comfrey:* hepatotoxic and carcinogenic (Chavez & Chavez, 2000)
- *Echinacea:* loses effectiveness if taken for more than 14 to 21 days at a time; not to be used with progressive systemic disorders such as tuberculosis, leukosis, collagenosis, multiple sclerosis, AIDS, HIV infection, and other autoimmune disorders (Blumenthal, 1998)
- *Gingko biloba:* increases microcirculation (Blumenthal, 1998); caution with anticoagulant medication, bleeding disorders, and surgery (Ang-Lee, Moss, & Yuan, 2001)
- *Ginseng:* many different types; adverse effects include headache, insomnia, palpitations, hypertension, hypotension (Chavez & Chavez, 2000); "GI symptoms, nervousness, confusion, depression and neonatal effects have been reported" (Arab, 2000, p. 215)
- *Kava (kava-kava):* use associated with liver failure (Hepatic Toxicity, 2002)
- *Milk thistle:* mild laxative effect that subsides after 2 to 3 days (Chavez & Chavez, 2000)
- *St. John's wort:* contraindicated with MAO inhibitors, anticoagulants, and protease inhibitors (Schulz, 2001)

ory of **homeopathy,** a term derived from the Greek words *homoios* (meaning "similar") and *pathos* (meaning "suffering"). According to homeopathic theory, the right medicinal substance for a particular set of symptoms is the one that naturally produces those symptoms in healthy people, commonly referred to as "like cures like."

Typically, homeopathic remedies consist of plant, animal, or mineral substances that are diluted in water or alcohol and vigorously shaken. The dilution and shaking process can be repeated several times until no chemical trace of the original substance can be detected. Paradoxically, the greater the dilution, the more powerful the medication. "Homeopaths explain this seeming contradiction by asserting that the water or alcohol contains 'trace memories' in the form of electromagnetic frequencies of the active ingredient it once contained" (Cassileth, 1998, p. 37). Cassileth critiques this explanation, while Goldberg et al. (2002) points to nuclear magnetic resonance imaging studies that report distinctive readings of subatomic activity in several homeopathic remedies. The Cassileth argument uses chemistry-based reasoning to critique homeopathy, while Goldberg et al. use arguments related to quantum physics and the emerging field of energy medicine.

As of 2002, only three U.S. states licensed homeopathic providers although nurse practitioners, physician assistants, dentists, veterinarians, chiropractors, licensed acupuncturists, nurse midwives, podiatrists, and naturopaths can practice homeopathy if their state practice acts permit. Homeopathy is even more popular in Europe. In the United States, the FDA regulates the manufacture, labeling, and dispensing of homeopathic medicines, most of which are available over the counter.

Naturopathy

Naturopathic medicine developed in Europe during the 18th and 19th centuries and flourished in the United States from the mid-19th century until the 1930s when conventional medicine almost replaced it. Unlike the Indian Ayurvedic medical system of body, mind, senses, and the soul or TCM, naturopathic medicine is not grounded in theoretical understandings that are substantially different from those of conventional Western medicine (Cassileth, 1998). However, naturopaths avoid pharmaceutical drugs and ground their practice in six principles (Downey, 2000):

1. The healing power of nature
2. Treat the whole person
3. First do no harm
4. Identify and treat the cause
5. Prevention
6. The physician as teacher.

The practice of **naturopathy** focuses on nutrition, herbs, homeopathy, acupuncture, hydrotherapy (including spas, colonic irrigation, hot–cold therapies, and wraps), physical medicine (including massage, exercise, and manipulation), counseling, and minor surgical interventions. Naturopathic physicians complete a baccalaureate degree and 4 years of graduate study that leads to a doctorate in naturopathic medicine (N.D.). At the end of 2002, the American Association of Naturopathic Physicians estimated that there were 4,000 to 5,000 graduates of accredited American and Canadian naturopathic colleges, and naturopaths are licensed by 12 states (with licensure laws pending in at least 7 others) and four Canadian provinces, but their scope of practice is more limited than that of a traditional medical doctor.

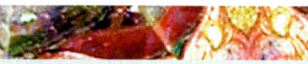

Lifespan Considerations

Elders

Practices that use meditation and movement such as tai chi, yoga, and qi gong are very beneficial to elders. They can be easily adapted if the person has a disability. Benefits include

- Improved flexibility and mobility
- Improved cardiovascular tone
- Improved balance
- Increased muscle strength
- Increased socialization if done in a group setting.

The creative arts such as music, drawing, and journaling often encourage reflections of the past and the present and help keep the imagination alive. This is beneficial in maintaining wellness and in coping with the changes associated with aging.

Two of the most common alternative therapies used by elders, chiropractic and herbs, pose safety concerns and should be given attention by nurses when taking histories and doing assessments. The safety of spinal manipulations for low back pain in elders has not been established. Herbal therapies may cause adverse herb–drug interactions and may place the elder at higher risk due to chronic health conditions and kidney and liver inefficiency related to aging changes (Foster, Philips, Hamei, & Eisenberg, 2000).

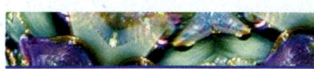

Focus on Critical Thinking

Tim Le is a 68-year-old accountant who has been diagnosed with gastric cancer. He lost a great deal of weight before the diagnosis and during treatment with chemotherapy and radiation. He is now admitted to the hospital with pain and weakness preventing him from working or performing many activities of daily living. His wife, Susan Carter, stays with him the majority of the day. His elderly parents visit often and bring him homemade food and drink. They do not speak English. In the process of placing bathing items in Tim's bedside stand, the nurse notes several plastic bags of a tea-like product in the drawer.

1. What aspects of this case suggest that it would be appropriate for the nurse to discuss the use of alternative therapies with the client or family?

2. Which alternative therapies might be most useful for this client and are in keeping with the principle of "do no harm"?
3. How should the nurse respond to finding the bags in the client's drawer? What options should be considered and what are the likely results of each?
4. How might the nurse's own belief system influence his or her interactions with the client and family regarding CAM?

See Critical Thinking Possibilities in Appendix A.

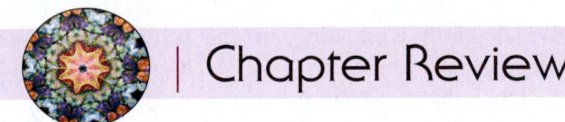 | Chapter Review

EXPLORE MediaLink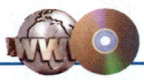

NCLEX review questions, case studies, MediaLink applications, and other interactive resources for this chapter can be found on the Companion Website at www.prenhall.com/kozier. Click on Chapter 14 to select the activities for this chapter.

For more NCLEX review questions, and an audio glossary, access the Student CD-ROM accompanying this textbook.

Chapter Highlights

- "Complementary and alternative medicine is defined through a social process as those practices that do not form part of the dominant system for managing health and disease" (Jonas, 1996, p. 1).
- Eighty-three percent of those using alternative therapies for serious medical conditions also sought treatment from a physician; however, nearly three-fourths of those using alternative therapies did not inform their physician that they were doing so.
- The goal of holistic nursing as described by the American Holistic Nurses' Association is to enhance healing of the whole person from birth to death.
- Holistic thinkers propose that knowledge, thoughts, memories, emotions, consciousness, and behavior processes are distributed throughout the body.
- The limbic-hypothalamic system, centered in the brain and biochemically interconnected with all other parts of the body, facilitates the integration of thoughts, emotions, and sensations at the physiologic and cellular levels.
- Four of the most common touch therapies are therapeutic massage, foot reflexology, acupressure, and Reiki. For nurses to become skilled in these therapies, special courses of study may be required.
- In mind–body therapies, individuals focus on realigning or creating balance in mental processes to bring about healing,

but advocates of these therapies need to avoid promoting the nonholistic notion of mind-*over*-matter.
- Biofeedback uses temperature meters or an electromyogram to help clients learn to modulate and reduce the physiologic arousal manifested in stress-related disorders.
- The goal of yoga is enlightenment or union with God through self mastery/unification of the body, mind, and spirit.
- Meditation is used to quiet the mind, focus on the present and release fears, worries, anxieties, and doubts about the past and the future. Not surprisingly, physiologic processes associated with arousal and stress tend to decrease during meditation.
- Acupuncture and TCM theory are based on the premise that the body's vital energy or qi (pronounced *chee*) circulates through pathways or meridians and can be accessed and manipulated through specific anatomical points along the surface of the body. Disease is described as an imbalance or interruption in the flow of qi.
- Chiropractic is grounded in the assumption that maintaining the alignment of the spine and joints facilitates the flow of energy throughout the body.
- Homeopathic theory maintains that the right medicinal substance for a particular set of symptoms is the one that naturally produces those symptoms in healthy people, commonly referred to as "like cures like."

Review Questions

14–1. Which of the following statements best describes complementary and alternative medicine (CAM)?
  a. CAM is an unrelated group of nonorthodox healing practices imported from several cultures
  b. CAM is defined through a social process as those practices that do not form part of the dominant system for managing health and disease.
  c. CAM therapies include chiropractic, traditional Chinese medicine, touch therapies, naturopathy, and homeopathy.
  d. CAM may be used to augment Western medicine but should never substitute for scientifically tested and approved treatments.

14–2. The most important reason nurses should ask about CAM use during the history is because
  a. the majority of people using CAM do not notify their physicians.
  b. the nurse can provide support to patients who fear that physicians will be unsupportive of their CAM choices.
  c. the CAM treatment may prove more beneficial than the Western treatment.
  d. some herbal and pharmaceutical combinations are contraindicated.

14–3. Which of the following best describes what happens during a biofeedback session?

a. Bodily processes such as blood flow to cardiac arteries are brought under conscious control through physiologic feedback.

b. Clients develop conscious control over sympathetic responses and increase parasympathetic dominance through physiologic feedback.

c. Physiologic feedback helps clients learn to modulate and reduce the physiologic arousal manifested in stress-related disorders.

d. Physiologic feedback helps clients learn to slow their respirations and heart rate and lower their blood pressure

14–4. Which of the following are the primary purposes of meditation?

a. Quiet the mind and focus it in the present.

b. Slow the breath and achieve peace.

c. Promote healing and relaxation.

d. Release fears, anxieties, and doubts.

14–5. Which of the following defines disease from the perspective of traditional Chinese medicine (TCM)?

a. an imbalance between yin and yang

b. an imbalance or interruption in the flow of qi

c. an imbalance or disruption in key social relationships

d. an imbalance or disruption in thoughts or emotions

Readings and References

Suggested Readings

Research reviews. (2002). *Acupuncture in Medicine, 20,*(1), 41–48.
   The Research Review section of this journal summarizes research in acupuncture and oriental medicine and provides complete citations for further reading. This particular issue includes a review of a study on the effects of deep needling at location PC6 for hyperemesis gravidarum (the condition of excessive vomiting sometimes experienced by pregnant women).

Related Research

Astin, J. A. (1998). Why patients use alternative medicine: Results of a national survey. *Journal of the American Medical Association, 279,* 1548–1553.

Freeman, L. W., & Lawlis, G. F. (2001). *Mosby's complementary and alternative medicine: A research-based approach.* St. Louis, MO: Mosby.

References

Abbot, N. C. (2000). Healing as a therapy for human disease: A systematic review. *Journal of Alternative and Complementary Medicine,* 6(2), 159–169.

Acupuncture [Electronic version]. (1997). *NIH Consensus Statement Online* 15(5): 1–34. Retrieved April 7, 2003, from http://consensus.nih.gov/cons/107/107_statement.htm.

Andersson, G. B. J., Lucente, T., Davis, A. M., Kappler, R. E., Lipton, J. A., & Leurgans, S. (1999). A comparison of osteopathic spinal manipulation with standard care for patients with low back pain. *New England Journal of Medicine, 341,* 1465–1468.

Ang-Lee, M. K., Moss, J., & Yuan, C. S. (2001). Herbal medicines and perioperative care. *Journal of the American Medical Association, 286,* 208–216.

Arab, L. (2000). What physicians need to know about medicinal herbs. In M. Hager (Ed.), *Education of health professionals in complementary/alternative medicine.* New York: Josiah Macy Jr. Foundation.

Aviles, J. M., Whelan, E., Hernke, D. A., Williams, B. A., Kenny, K. E., O'Fallon, W. M., et al.

(2001). Intercessory prayer and cardiovascular disease progression in a coronary care unit population: A randomized controlled trial. *Mayo Clinic Proceedings, 76,* 1192–1198.

Bartol, G. M., & Courts, N. F. (2000). The psychophysiology of bodymind healing. In B. M. Dossey, L. Keegan, & C. E. Guzzetta (Eds.), *Holistic nursing: A handbook for practice* (3rd ed., pp. 69–88). Gaithersburg, MD: Aspen.

Benner, P., & Wrubel, J. (1989). *The primacy of caring: Stress and coping in health and illness.* New York: Addison-Wesley.

Blumenthal, M. (Ed.). (1998). *The complete German Commission E monographs: Therapeutic guide to herbal medicines.* Boston: Integrative Medicine Communications.

Buckle, J. (2002). *Clinical aromatherapy in nursing.* Don Mills, Ontario, Canada: Oxford University Press Canada.

Cassileth, B. R. (1998). *The alternative medicine handbook: The complete reference guide to alternative and complementary therapies.* New York: W. W. Norton.

Chavez, M. L., & Chavez, P. I. (2000). Herbal medicine. In D. W. Novey (Ed.), *Clinician's complete reference to complementary and alternative medicine* (pp. 545–565). St. Louis, MO: Mosby.

Cherkin, D., Deyo, R. A., Battie, M., Street, J., & Barlow, W. (1998). A comparison of physical therapy, chiropractic manipulation, and provision of an educational booklet for the treatment of patients with low back pain. *New England Journal of Medicine, 339,* 1021–1029.

Cooper, R. A., & McKee, H. J. (2000). Who is practicing? In M. Hager (Ed.), *Education of health professionals in complementary/alternative medicine.* New York: Josiah Macy Jr. Foundation.

Coward, H., & Ratanakul, P. (Eds.). (1999). *A cross-cultural dialogue on health care ethics.* Waterloo, Ontario: Wilfrid Laurier University Press.

DeAngelis, T. (2002). A bright future for PNI [Electronic version]. *Monitor on Psychology,* 33(6). Retrieved April 7, 2003, From http://www.apa.org/monitor/jun02/brightfuture.html

Dossey, L. (1993). *Healing words: The power of prayer and the practice of medicine.* San Francisco: Harper.

Dossey, B. M., Keegan, L., & Guzetta, C. E. (Eds.). (2000). *Holistic nursing: A handbook for practice* (3rd ed.). Gaithersburg, MD: Aspen.

Downey, C. (2000). Naturopathic medicine. In D. W. Novey (Ed.), *Clinician's complete reference to complementary and alternative medicine* (pp. 274–282). St. Louis, MO: Mosby.

Dunbar, F. (1945). *Psychosomatic diagnosis.* New York: Paul B. Haebar.

Eisenberg, D. M., Kessler, R. C., Foster, C., Norlock, F. E., Calkins, D. R., & Delbanco, T. L. (1993). Unconventional medicine in the United Sates. *New England Journal of Medicine, 328,* 246–252.

Fishman, A. P. (2000). State of the art. In M. Hager (Ed.). *Education of health professionals in complementary/alternative medicine.* New York: Josiah Macy Jr. Foundation.

Foster, D. F., Philips, R. S., Hamei, M. B., & Eisenberg, D. M. (2000). Alternative medicine use in older Americans. *Journal of the American Geriatrics Society, 48,* 1560–1565.

Frisch, N. C., Dossey, B. M., Guzzetta, C. E., & Quinn, J. A. (2000). *AHNA standards of holistic nursing practice: Guidelines for caring and healing.* New York: Aspen.

Goldberg, B., Anderson, J. W., & Trivieri, L. (2002). *Alternative medicine: The definitive guide* (2nd ed.). Berkeley, CA: Ten Speed Press.

Guzzetta, C. E. (2000). Music therapy: Hearing the melody of the soul. In B. M. Dossey, L. Keegan, & C. E. Guzzetta (Eds.), *Holistic nursing: A handbook for practice* (3rd ed., pp. 585–610). Gaithersburg, MD: Aspen.

Hepatic toxicity possibly associated with kava-containing products—United States, Germany, and Switzerland, 1999—2002. (2002). *Morbidity and Mortality Weekly Report 51*(47), 1065–1067.

Jacobsen, E. (1938). *Progressive relaxation.* Chicago: University of Chicago Press.

Jonas, W. (1996). Dr. Jonas addresses advisory council. *Complementary and Alternative Medicine at the NIH, 3*(1). Bethesda, MD: Office of Alternative Medicine at the National Institutes of Health.

Krieger, D. (1979). *The therapeutic touch: How to use your hands to help or heal.* Englewood Cliffs, NJ: Prentice Hall.

MacIntyre, R. C., Holzemer, W. L., & Philippek, M. (1997). Complementary and alternative medicine in HIV/AIDS part I: Issues and context. *Journal of the Association of Nurses in AIDS Care, 8*(1), 23–31.

McCloskey, J. C., & Bulechek, G. M. (Eds.). (2000). *Nursing interventions classification (NIC)* (3rd ed.), St. Louis, MO: Mosby.

Micozzi, M. S. (2000). A taxonomy of complementary and alternative medicine. In M. Hager (Ed.), *Education of health professionals in complementary/alternative medicine.* New York: Josiah Macy Jr. Foundation.

National Council for Complementary and Alternative Medicine. (2000). *Expanding horizons for healthcare: Five-year strategic plan 2001–2005.* Bethesda, MD: Author.

National Library of Medicine. (2003). *Medical subject headings: Complementary therapies.* Retrieved Febrary 24, 2003 from http://www.nlm.nih.gov/cgi/mesh/2003/MB_cgi

Newman, M. A. (1986). *Health as expanding consciousness.* St. Louis, MO: Mosby.

Nield-Anderson, L., & Ameling, A. (2000). Reiki: A complementary therapy for nursing practice. *Journal of Psychosocial Nursing & Mental Health Services, 39*(4), 42–49.

Parse, R. R. (1981). *Man–living–health: Theory of nursing.* New York: Wiley.

Pavek, R. R. (1996). New MeSH terms add accessibility to alternative medicine literature. *Alternative Therapies in Health and Medicine, 2*(2), 25–28.

Rogers, M. E. (1970). *An introduction to the theoretical basis of nursing.* Philadelphia: F. A. Davis.

Schaub, B. G., & Dossey, B. M. (2000). Imagery: Awakening the inner healer. In B. M. Dossey, L. Keegan, & C. E. Guzzetta (Eds.), *Holistic nursing: A handbook for practice* (3rd ed., pp. 539–581). Gaithersburg, MD: Aspen.

Schulz, V. (2001). Incidence and clinical relevance of the interactions and side effects of Hypericum preparations. *Phytomedicine, 8*(2), 152–60.

Selye, H. (1956). *The stress of life.* New York: McGraw-Hill.

Smith, M. C., Kemp, J., Hemphill, L., & Vojir, C. P. (2002). Outcomes of therapeutic massage for hospitalized cancer patients. *Journal of Nursing Scholarship, 34,* 257–262.

Smuts, J. (1926). *Holism and evolution.* New York: Macmillan.

Sparber, A. (2001, August 31). State boards of nursing and scope of practice of registered nurses performing complementary therapies. *Online Journal of Issues in Nursing, 6*(3), Article 10. Retrieved June 2, 2003, from http://www.nursingworld.org/ojin/topic15/tpc15_6.htm

Watson, J. (1988). *Nursing: Human science and human care.* New York: National League for Nursing.

Wells-Federman, C. L. (1996). Awakening the healer within. *Holistic Nursing Practice, 10,* 13–29.

White House Commission on Complementary and Alternative Medicine Policy. (2002). *Final report.* Washington, DC: Author.

Wolsko, P. M., Eisenberg, D. M., Davis, R. B., Ettner, S. L., & Phillips, R. S. (2002). Insurance coverage, medical conditions, and visits to alternative medicine providers: Results of a national survey. *Archives of Internal Medicine,162,* 281–287.

Selected Bibliography

Alspach, G. (1998). Alternative and complementary therapies: Treading tentatively out of the mainstream. *Critical Care Nurse, 18*(5), 13–16.

Bauer-Wu, S. M. (2002). Integrated care. Psychoneuroimmunology part I: Physiology. *Clinical Journal of Oncology Nursing, 6,* 167–170.

Bauer-Wu, S. M. (2002). Integrated care. Psychoneuroimmunology part II: mind–body interventions. *Clinical Journal of Oncology Nursing, 6,* 243–246.

Boykin, A., & Schoenhofer, S. O. (2000). Nursing as caring: An overview of a general theory of nursing. In M. E. Parker (Ed.), *Nursing theories and nursing practice.* Philadelphia: F. A. Davis.

Cohen, M. H. (1998). *Complementary & alternative medicine: Legal boundaries and regulatory perspectives.* Baltimore, MD: Johns Hopkins University Press.

Donley, R. (1998). The alternative health care revolution. *Nursing Economics, 16,* 298–302.

Ernst, E., & White, A. (1999). *Acupuncture: A scientific approach.* Oxford: Butterworth-Heinemann.

Festrow, C. W. (1999). *Professional's handbook of complementary & alternative medicines.* Springhouse, PA: Springhouse Publishers.

Freeman, E. M., & MacIntyre, R. C. (1999). Evaluating alternative medicine and HIV disease. *Nursing Clinics of North America, 34*(1), 147–162.

Frisch, N. (2001, May 31). Standards for holistic nursing practice: A way to think about our care that includes complementary and alternative modalities. *Online Journal of Issues in Nursing, 6*(2), article 4. Retrieved June 2, 2003, from http://www.nursingworld.org/ojin/topic15/tpc15_4.htm

Guzzetta, C. (1998). *Essential readings in holistic nursing.* New York: Aspen Publishers.

Huebscher, R. (1998). Alternative and complementary therapies. *Nurse Practitioner Forum, 9,* 200–255.

Huebscher, R. (1998). Quality in natural/alternative/complementary health care practice. *Nurse Practitioner Forum, 9,* 119–120.

Jobst, K. A. (1999). Obstacles to healing in medicine and science: The interplay of science, paradigm, and culture. *Journal of Alternative and Complementary Medicine, 5,* 391–394.

Jonas, W. B., & Levin, J. S. (Eds.). (2000). *Essentials of complementary and alternative medicine.* Philadelphia, PA: Lippincott.

Milton, D. (1999). *Complementary & alternative therapies: An implementation guide to integrative health care.* Chicago, IL: American Hospital Association.

Snyder, M., & Lindquist, R. (2001, May 31). Issues in complementary therapy: How we got to where we are. *Online Journal of Issues in Nursing, 6*(2), article 1. Retrieved June 2, 2003, from http://www.nursingworld.org/ojin/topic15/tpc15_1.htm

Taylor, A. G. (1998). A nurse-directed interdisciplinary center for the study of complementary therapies. *Journal of Emergency Nursing, 24,* 486–487.

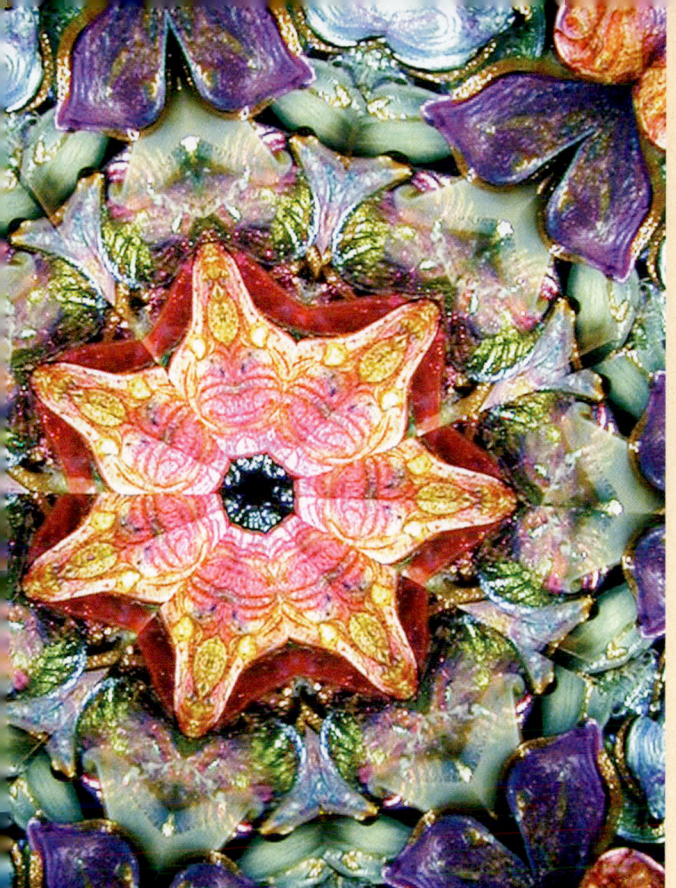

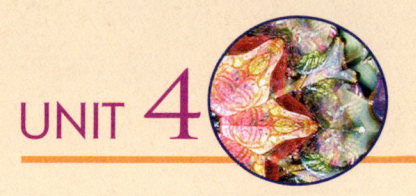

THE NURSING PROCESS

The nursing process is a systematic, client-centered method for structuring the delivery of nursing care. The nursing process entails gathering and analyzing data in order to identify client strengths and potential or actual health problems and developing and continually reviewing a plan of nursing interventions to achieve mutually agreed outcomes. At every stage of the process, the nurse works closely with the client to individualize care and build a relationship of mutual regard and trust.

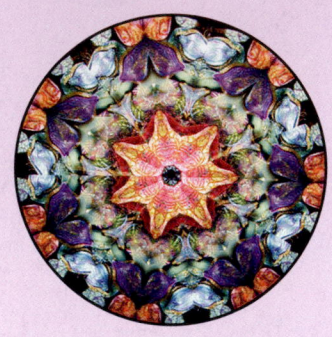

CHAPTER 15

CRITICAL THINKING AND THE NURSING PROCESS

LEARNING OUTCOMES

After completing this chapter, you will be able to:

- Discuss the skills and attitudes of critical thinking.

- Identify the elements of critical thinking.

- Discuss the relationships among the nursing process, critical thinking, the problem-solving process, and the decision-making process.

- Explore ways of demonstrating critical thinking.

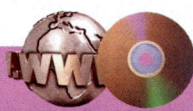

MediaLink

www.prenhall.com/kozier

Additional resources for this chapter can be found on the Student CD-ROM accompanying this textbook, and on the Companion Website at www.prenhall.com/kozier. Click on Chapter 15 to select the activities for this chapter.

CD-ROM
- Audio Glossary
- NCLEX Review

• Companion Website
- Additional NCLEX Review
- Case Study: Increased Pressure Ulcers
- MediaLink Application:
  Practice Critical Thinking
- Links to Resources

Critical thinking is "the intellectually disciplined process of actively and skillfully conceptualizing, applying, analyzing, synthesizing, and/or evaluating information gathered from, or generated by, observation, experience, reflection, reasoning, or communication, as a guide to belief and action" (Scriven & Paul, n.d., ¶1). Nurses are expected to use critical thinking to solve client problems and make better decisions. Thus critical thinking, problem solving, and decision making are interrelated processes, with creativity enhancing the result.

CRITICAL THINKING

Critical thinking is essential to safe, competent, skillful nursing practice. The amount of knowledge that nurses must use and the continuing rapid growth of this knowledge prevent nurses from being effective practitioners if they attempt to function with only the information acquired in school or outlined in books. Decisions that nurses must make about client care and about the distribution of limited resources force them to think and act in areas where there are neither clear answers nor standard procedures and where conflicting forces turn decision making into a complex process. Nurses therefore need to embrace the attitudes that promote critical thinking and master critical-thinking skills in order to process and evaluate both previously learned and new information.

Nurses use critical-thinking skills in a variety of ways:

- *Nurses use knowledge from other subjects and fields.* Because nurses deal holistically with human responses, they must draw meaningful information from other subject areas (i.e., make interdisciplinary connections) in order to understand the meaning of client data and to plan effective interventions. Nursing students take courses in the biologic and social sciences and in the humanities so that they can acquire a strong foundation on which to build their nursing knowledge and skill. For example, the nurse might use knowledge from nutrition, physiology, and physics to promote wound healing and prevent further injury to a client with a pressure ulcer.
- *Nurses deal with change in stressful environments.* Nurses work in rapidly changing situations. Treatments, medications, and technology change constantly, and a client's condition may change from minute to minute. Routine actions may therefore not be adequate to deal with the situation at hand. Familiarity with the routine for giving medications, for example, does not help the nurse deal with a client who is frightened of injections or with one who does not wish to take a medication. When unexpected situations arise, critical thinking enables the nurse to recognize important cues, respond quickly, and adapt interventions to meet specific client needs.
- *Nurses make important decisions.* During the course of a workday, nurses make vital decisions of many kinds. These decisions often determine the well-being of clients and even their very survival, so it is important that the decisions be sound. Nurses use critical thinking to collect and interpret the information needed to make decisions. Nurses must, for example, use good judgment to decide which observations must be reported to the physician immediately and which can be noted in the client record for the physician to address later, during a routine visit with the client.

Creativity is a major component of critical thinking. When nurses incorporate creativity into their thinking, they are able to find unique solutions to unique problems. **Creativity** is thinking that results in the development of new ideas and products. Creativity in problem solving and decision making is the ability to develop and implement new and better solutions.

Creativity is required when the nurse encounters a new situation or a client situation in which traditional interventions are not effective. For example, Ned Rodriguez, a pediatric home health nurse, is caring for 9-year-old Pauline, who has ineffective respirations following abdominal surgery. The physician has ordered incentive spirometry (a treatment device that promotes alveolar expansion). Pauline is frightened by the equipment and tires quickly during the treatments. Ned offers Pauline a bottle of blow bubbles and a blowing wand. Pauline is delighted with blowing bubbles. Ned knows that the respiratory effort in blowing bubbles will promote alveolar expansion and suggests that Pauline blow bubbles between incentive spirometry treatments.

Creative thinkers must have knowledge of the problem. They must have assessed the present problem and be knowledgeable about the underlying facts and principles that apply. For example, in the previous situation, Ned knows the anatomy and physiology of respiratory function and is aware of the purpose of incentive spirometry. He also understands pediatric growth and

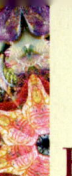

development. In trying to assist Pauline, he builds on his knowledge and comes up with a creative solution. Using creativity, nurses

- Generate many ideas rapidly
- Are generally flexible and natural; that is, they are able to change viewpoints or directions in thinking rapidly and easily
- Create original solutions to problems
- Tend to be independent and self-confident, even when under pressure
- Demonstrate individuality.

SKILLS IN CRITICAL THINKING

Complex mental processes such as analysis, problem solving, and decision making require the use of cognitive critical-thinking skills. These skills include critical analysis, inductive and deductive reasoning, making valid inferences, differentiating facts from opinions, evaluating the credibility of information sources, clarifying concepts, and recognizing assumptions.

Critical analysis is the application of a set of questions to a particular situation or idea to determine essential information and ideas and discard superfluous information and ideas. The questions are not sequential steps; rather, they are a set of criteria for judging an idea. Not all questions will need to be applied to every situation, but one should be aware of all the questions in order to choose those questions appropriate to a given situation. Socrates (born about 470 BC) was a Greek philosopher who developed the Socratic method of posing a question and seeking an answer. Box 15–1 lists Socratic questions to use in critical analysis. **Socratic questioning** is a technique one can use to look beneath the surface, recognize and examine assumptions, search for inconsistencies, examine multiple points of view, and differentiate what one knows from what one merely believes. Nurses should employ Socratic questioning when listening to an end-of-shift report, reviewing a history or progress notes, planning care, or discussing a client's care with colleagues.

Two other critical thinking skills are inductive and deductive reasoning. In **inductive reasoning,** generalizations are formed from a set of facts or observations. When viewed together, certain bits of information suggest a particular interpretation. For example, the nurse who observes that a client has dry skin, poor turgor, sunken eyes, and dark amber urine may make the generalization that the client appears dehydrated. **Deductive reasoning,** by contrast, is reasoning from the general to the specific. The nurse starts with a conceptual framework—for example, Maslow's hierarchy of needs or a self-care framework—and makes descriptive interpretations of the client's condition in relation to that framework. For example, the nurse who uses the needs framework might categorize data and define the client's problem in terms of elimination, nutrition, or protection needs.

In a more simplistic example, inductive reasoning is like looking at the pieces of a jigsaw puzzle and attempting to describe the whole (without seeing a picture of the completed puzzle). As the puzzler puts more and more pieces together, the whole picture becomes clearer. In deductive reasoning, the puzzler sees the whole picture (from the box cover) and puts the puzzle together by organizing the pieces into border pieces, or colors, or some other grouping.

In critical thinking, the nurse also differentiates statements of fact, inference, judgment, and opinion. Table 15–1 shows how these may be applied to a client. Evaluating the credibility of information sources is an important step in critical thinking. Unfortunately, we cannot always believe what we read or are told. The nurse may need to ascertain the accuracy of information by checking other documents or with other informants.

Concepts are ideas or views representing things in the real world and their meanings. Each person has developed their conceptualizations based on experience, input from others, study, and other activities. To clearly comprehend a client situation, the nurse and the client must agree on the meaning of concept terms. For example, if the client says to the nurse "I think I have a tumor," the nurse needs to clarify what this word means to the client—the medical definition of tumor (a solid mass) or the common lay meaning of cancer—before responding.

Persons also live their lives under certain assumptions. Some people view humans as having a basically generous na-

---

BOX 15–1 ■ Socratic Questions

Questions about the Question (or Problem)
- Is this question clear, understandable, and correctly identified?
- Is this question important?
- Could this question be broken down into smaller parts?
- How might _____ state this question?

Questions about Assumptions
- You seem to be assuming _____; is that so?
- What could you assume instead? Why?
- Does this assumption always hold true?

Questions about Point of View
- You seem to be using the perspective of _____. Why?
- What would someone who disagrees with your perspective say?
- Can you see this any other way?

Questions about Evidence and Reasons
- What evidence do you have for that?
- Is there any reason to doubt that evidence?
- How do you know?
- What would change your mind?

Questions about Implications and Consequences
- What effect would that have?
- What is the probability that will actually happen?
- What are the alternatives?
- What are the implications of that?

TABLE 15–1 Differentiating Types of Statements

Statement	Description	Example
Facts	Can be verified through investigation	Blood pressure is affected by blood volume.
Inferences	Conclusions drawn from the facts, going beyond facts to make a statement about something not currently known	If blood volume is decreased (e.g., in hemorrhagic shock), the blood pressure will drop.
Judgments	Evaluation of facts or information that reflect values or other criteria; a type of opinion	It is harmful to the client's health if the blood pressure drops too low.
Opinions	Beliefs formed over time and include judgments that may fit facts or be in error	Nursing intervention can assist in maintaining the client's blood pressure within normal limits.

ture while others believe that the human tendency is to act in their own best interest. The nurse may believe that life should be considered worth living no matter what the condition while the client believes that quality of life is more important than quantity of life. If they recognize that they make choices based on these assumptions, they can still work together toward an acceptable plan of care. Difficulty arises when people do not take the time to consider what assumptions underlie their beliefs and actions.

ATTITUDES THAT FOSTER CRITICAL THINKING

Certain attitudes are crucial to critical thinking. These attitudes are based on the assumption that a rational person is motivated to develop, learn, and grow. A critical thinker works to develop the following attitudes or traits: independence of thought, fair-mindedness, insight into egocentricity and sociocentricity, intellectual humility and suspension of judgment, intellectual courage, integrity, perseverance, confidence in reason, interest in exploring both thoughts underlying feeling and feelings underlying thoughts, and curiosity (Paul, 1995).

Independence of Thought

Critical thinking requires that individuals think for themselves. People acquire many beliefs as children, not necessarily based on reason but in order to have an explanation they comprehend. As they mature and acquire knowledge and experience, critical thinkers examine their beliefs in the light of new evidence. Critical thinkers consider seriously a wide range of ideas, learn from them, and then make their own judgments about them. Nurses are open minded about considering different methods of performing technical skills—not just the single way they may have been taught in school.

Fair-Mindedness

Critical thinkers are fair-minded, assessing all viewpoints with the same standards and not basing their judgments on personal or group bias or prejudice. Fair-mindedness helps one to consider opposing points of view and to try to understand new ideas fully before rejecting or accepting them. Critical thinkers strive to be open to the possibility that new evidence could

change their minds. The nurse listens to opinions of all the members of a family, young and old.

Insight into Egocentricity and Sociocentricity

Critical thinkers are open to the possibility that their personal biases or social pressures and customs could unduly affect their thinking. They actively try to examine their own biases and bring them to awareness each time they think or make a decision. For example, a nurse spends extensive time trying to teach a client how to prevent a future recurrence of some problem but is mystified when the client appears uninterested and does not follow the nurse's advice. The nurse's egocentric tendency to assume that all clients are motivated and interested in preventive care (just because the nurse is) resulted in an inaccurate assessment of the client's desire to learn; both the nurse's and the client's time was wasted. Had the nurse assessed the client's background and beliefs about the problem (that is, had the nurse collected sufficient evidence), the nurse might have identified a problem more relevant to the client's priorities and, thus, developed a better care plan.

Intellectual Humility and Suspension of Judgment

Intellectual humility means having an awareness of the limits of one's own knowledge. Critical thinkers are willing to admit what they do not know; they are willing to seek new information and to rethink their conclusions in light of new knowledge. They never assume that what everybody believes to be right will always be right, because new evidence may emerge. A hospital nurse might be unable to imagine how the elderly wife will care for her husband who has recently had a stroke. However, the nurse also recognizes that it is not possible to really know what the couple can achieve.

Intellectual Courage

With an attitude of courage, one is willing to consider and examine fairly one's own ideas or views, especially those to which one may have a strongly negative reaction. This type of courage comes from recognizing that beliefs are sometimes false or misleading. Values and beliefs are not always acquired rationally. Rational beliefs are those that have been examined and found to be supported by solid reasons and data. After such examination, it is inevitable that some beliefs previously held to be true will be found to contain questionable elements and that some truth will emerge from ideas considered dangerous or false. Courage is needed to be true to new thinking in such cases, especially if social penalties for nonconformity are severe. As an example, previously many nurses believed that allowing family members to observe an emergency (such as CPR) would be psychologically harmful to the family and that members would get in the health care team's way. Others felt that blanket exclusion of family members was unnecessary and extremely stressful for some of them. As a result, nurses initiated research that has demonstrated that family presence can be accomplished without detrimental effects to the nurse, the patient, or the family.

Research Note
Can We Achieve an International Definition of Critical Thinking?

The Delphi technique is an iterative research method that uses groups of qualified respondents to identify characteristics of the concept under study. In a project reported on by Scheffer and Rubenfeld (2000), 55 nurses from nine countries responded to five rounds of mailings. In the initial mailing, the nurses generated characteristics of critical thinking in nurses. Researchers clustered the responses and in subsequent rounds, the nurses defined and refined the clusters resulting in habits of mind and skills. Finally, the clusters were given names, subskills were identified, and participants voted on agreement with the consensus statement. The final 10 habits of mind were (in alphabetical order) confidence, contextual perspective, creativity, flexibility, inquisitiveness, intellectual integrity, intuition, open-mindedness, perseverance, and reflection. The final 7 skills were analyzing, applying standards, discriminating, information seeking, logical reasoning, predicting, and transforming knowledge.

Implications: The purpose of this study was to generate language around critical thinking that was (a) directly for practicing nurses and (b) international. It has yet to be shown how the descriptions of these skills and habits of mind will be received by others in the field. The participating nurses represented only 23 states in the United States plus seven other countries: Brazil, Canada, England, Iceland, Japan, Korea, and the Netherlands. In some of these countries, English is widely spoken while in others it is not. Most of the countries would be considered "Western," although there were two Asian countries. Of course, many other perspectives and cultures are not represented.

Future research is indicated. The authors generate their own questions about how these habits and skills relate to the nursing process, problem solving, diagnostic reasoning, and other related processes. However, this is an excellent beginning and the collaborative and international perspective should continue.

Note: From "A Consensus Statement on Critical Thinking in Nursing," by B. K. Scheffer and M. G. Rubenfeld, 2000, *Journal of Nursing Education, 39,* pp. 352–359.

Integrity

Intellectual integrity requires that individuals apply the same rigorous standards of proof to their own knowledge and beliefs as they apply to the knowledge and beliefs of others. Critical thinkers question their own knowledge and beliefs as quickly and thoroughly as they challenge those of another. They are readily able to admit and evaluate inconsistencies within their own beliefs and between their own beliefs and those of another. A nurse might believe that wound care always requires sterile technique. Reading a new article on the use and outcomes of clean technique for some wounds leads the critically thinking nurse to reconsider.

Perseverance

Nurses who are critical thinkers show perseverance in finding effective solutions to client and nursing problems. This determination enables them to clarify concepts and sort out related issues, in spite of difficulties and frustrations. Confusion and frustration are uncomfortable, but critical thinkers resist the temptation to find a quick and easy answer. Important questions tend to be complex and confusing and therefore often require a great deal of thought and research to arrive at an answer. The nurse needs to stick to the issue until it is resolved. For example, the nurses on a unit have tried to establish a policy for selected clients to leave the hospital on a pass rather than have to be discharged and readmitted in the same day. The need for involvement of nursing, medical, administrative, and accounting staff gradually generates solutions to stumbling blocks. The development of the policy moves forward, although very slowly.

Confidence in Reason

Critical thinkers believe that well-reasoned thinking will lead to trustworthy conclusions. Therefore, they cultivate an attitude of confidence in the reasoning process and examine emotion-laden arguments using the standards for evaluating thought, by asking questions such as these: Is that argument fair? Is it based on sufficient evidence? Consider nurses attempting to determine the best way to allocate holiday time off for staff. Should they use seniority, random selection (lottery), give preference to those who have children, use "first-come, first-served," or another method?

The critical thinker develops skill in both inductive reasoning and deductive reasoning. As the nurse gains greater awareness of the thinking process and more experience in improving such thinking, confidence in the process will grow. This nurse will not be afraid of disagreement and indeed will be concerned when others agree too quickly. Such a nurse can serve as a role model to colleagues, inspiring and encouraging them to think critically as well.

Interest in Exploring Both Thoughts and Feelings

A critical thinker knows that emotions can influence thinking and that often feelings underlie thoughts. The rational, critical thinker adopts the attitude that feelings are real and need to be acknowledged. However, feelings need to be explored to determine whether they are based on reality or interpretations, memories, or fears. Nurses need to identify, examine, and control or modify feelings that are interfering with clear critical thinking. As one example, if a client is injured by a piece of equipment that the nurse reported was malfunctioning but had not yet been repaired, the nurse may feel anger, guilt, and frustration. Although the nurse may initially think the client should sue for the injury, to deal with strong negative emotion the nurse can take these steps:

1. Limit action for a while to avoid hasty conclusions and impulsive decisions.
2. Discuss negative feelings with a confidant.
3. Expend some of the energy generated by the emotion by, for example, walking or exercising.
4. Reflect on the situation and determine whether the emotional response was appropriate.

After the strong emotion is dissipated, the nurse can then objectively move toward needed conclusions or make required decisions.

Curiosity

The internal conversation going on within the mind of a critical thinker is filled with questions: Why do we believe this? What causes that? Does it have to be this way? Could something else work? What would happen if we did it another way? Who says that is so? The curious nurse may value tradition but is not afraid to examine traditions to be sure they are still valid. The nurse may, for example, apply these questions to the issue of moving responsibility for a procedure such as the drawing of arterial blood samples among the nursing, respiratory therapy, or laboratory department staff.

STANDARDS AND ELEMENTS OF CRITICAL THINKING

How can one know whether one's thinking is critical thinking? Paul (1995) proposes that thinkers can use universal standards, shown in Table 15–2. Explicitly stating the standards for critical thinking promotes the reliability and validity of the thinking and thus makes appropriate action more likely. The standards are applied by asking questions to check one's reasoning about the problem. The standards are applied to the elements of thought (Figure 15–1 ■). These elements may be considered in any order and therefore are presented in a circular scheme.

APPLYING CRITICAL THINKING TO NURSING PRACTICE

Nurses function effectively some part of every day without thinking critically. Many small decisions are based primarily on habit with minimal thinking involved; examples include selecting what uniform to wear, choosing which route to take to work, and deciding what to eat for lunch. Psychomotor skills in

TABLE 15–2 Universal Intellectual Standards	
Standard	**Sample Question**
Clarity	What is an example of this?
Accuracy	How can I find out if that is true?
Relevance	How does that help me with the issue?
Logicalness	Does that follow from the evidence?
Breadth	Do I need to consider another point of view?
Precision	Can I be more specific?
Significance	Which of these facts is most important?
Completeness	Have I missed any important aspects?
Fairness	Am I considering the thinking of others?
Depth	What makes this a difficult problem?

Note: From *The Miniature Guide to Critical Thinking: Concepts and Tools* (pp. 7–9), by R. Paul & L. Elder, 1999, Santa Rosa: CA, Foundation for Critical Thinking. Adapted with permission.

nursing often involve minimal thinking, such as operating a familiar piece of equipment. But the higher order skills of critical thinking are put into play as soon as a new idea is encountered or a less-than-routine decision must be made.

The **nursing process** is a systematic, rational method of planning and providing individualized nursing care. The phases of the nursing process—assessing, diagnosing, planning, implementing, and evaluating—are discussed in detail in the chapters that follow. The relationship of Paul and

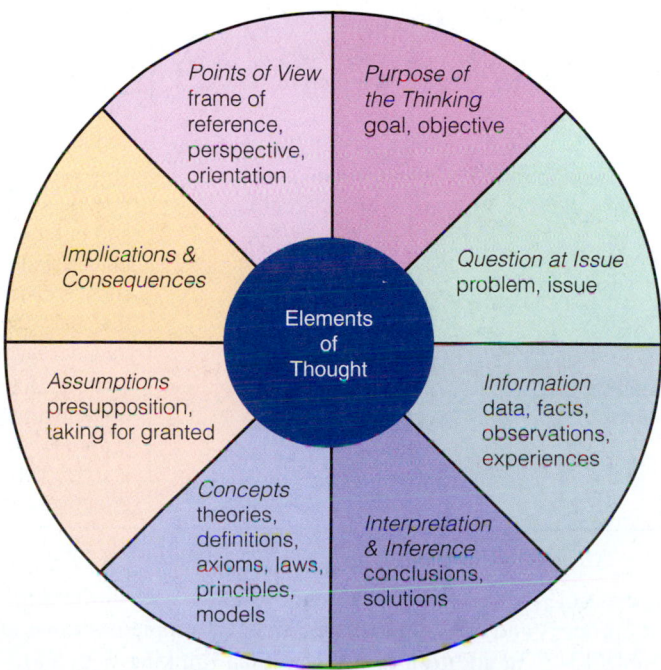

Figure 15–1 ■ The elements of thought. (Note: From *The Miniature Guide to Critical Thinking: Concepts and Tools* (p. 2), by R. Paul and L. Elder, 1999, Santa Rosa, CA: Foundation for Critical Thinking. Adapted with permission.)

TABLE 15–3 Relationship of Paul and Elder's Elements of Thought to the Nursing Process

Paul's Elements of Thought	Parallels to the Nursing Process	Clinical Application
Information	Assessing	*Data:* A 45-year-old male Latino complains of severe headache; 20 lb overweight; blood pressure 180/95 mm Hg. States he has been taking high blood pressure pills only when he has a headache. Is self-employed as a gardener; lives with wife, mother-in-law, and four children.
		Given these data, a critical thinker is aware that more data must be obtained about the client's cultural health values and reasons for stated behavior. Failure to think critically and to obtain additional data leads to inaccurate goals, diagnosis, and interventions.
Purpose of thinking	Goal setting	*Goal:* To increase compliance with medication regimen in order to relieve headaches and prevent a cerebrovascular accident (CVA). Thinking critically, a nurse will try to determine the client's goals and to agree to mutual goals.
Question at issue	Diagnosing	A critical thinker will defer identifying the client's diagnosis until more data are obtained and the client's priorities are known. This prevents a premature diagnosis based on insufficient data.
Points of view	Diagnosing	As a critical thinker, the nurse is aware that the client's point of view may differ from the nurse's. Although the nurse may support the Western medical belief system that puts high priority on preventing disease, the critical thinker is also aware that the client may hold diverse views of health and illness, therapy, and preventive measures.
Interpretation and inference (conclusions and recommendations)	Diagnosing	The critical thinker recognizes that the client's erratic use of the prescribed medication may have multiple causes (e.g., troublesome side effects, or belief that illness is due to God's will and is not preventable) and will not infer a diagnosis with etiology until more data are obtained. Failure to think critically can lead to interpretations that are irrelevant, inadequate, and superficial (e.g., an erroneous interpretation that the client's problem is lack of sufficient knowledge).
Assumptions (presuppositions)	Diagnosing	The critical thinker makes assumptions in accordance with a broad, unbiased database and mutually set client goals. The critical thinker avoids making unverified assumptions, such as that an increase in knowledge will increase this client's compliance or that this client is motivated to prevent a CVA.
Concepts (theories, laws, principles, models)	Diagnosing Planning	The critical thinker uses concepts about motivation, change theory, and multicultural nursing to understand the client's behavior and motivation to change. Failure to think critically can lead to exclusive reliance on a simplistic concept, such as "knowledge creates change."
Implications and consequences	Planning Implementing	The critical thinker considers the implications and consequences of selected nursing strategies before implementing plans of care. Plans of care, including goals and outcomes, are based on ongoing assessment of the client's cultural values, beliefs, and needs. Failure to think critically may lead to ineffective interventions, such as client teaching that focuses only on resolving a knowledge deficit about the prescribed medication. The critical thinker recognizes that a knowledge deficit may or may not be one of several problems.
Interpretation and inference	Evaluating	The critical thinker bases evaluation of client outcomes and the effectiveness of nursing interventions on well-developed, measurable criteria and considers rationally whether outcomes have been validated. Failure to think critically may lead to client noncompliance and an inference that the client did not learn effectively and needs further instruction.

Elder's (1995) elements of thought to the phases of the nursing process and application to a clinical example is shown in Table 15–3. In addition to using critical thinking with an individual client, when setting priorities for the day, a nurse employs critical thinking. When analyzing a situation and planning strategies for conflict resolution or change, the nurse manager uses critical-thinking attitudes and skills. The nurse clinician and nurse manager seek to be aware of their thinking while they are thinking, as they apply standards for thinking, and as their thinking progresses.

Problem Solving

In **problem solving,** the nurse obtains information that clarifies the nature of the problem and suggests possible solutions. The nurse then carefully evaluates the possible solutions and chooses the best one to implement. The situation is carefully monitored over time to ensure its initial and continued effectiveness. The nurse does not discard the other solutions but holds them in reserve in the event that the first solution is not effective. The nurse may also encounter a similar problem in a different client situation where an alternative solution is determined to be the most effective. Therefore, problem solving for one situation contributes to the nurse's body of knowledge for problem solving in similar situations.

There are various approaches to problem solving. Commonly used are trial and error, intuition, the research process, and the scientific/modified scientific method.

Trial and Error

One way to solve problems is through trial and error, in which a number of approaches are tried until a solution is found. However, without considering alternatives systematically, one cannot know why the solution works. Trial-and-error methods in nursing care can be dangerous because the client might suffer harm if an approach is inappropriate. However, nurses often use trial and error in the home setting where, due to logistics, equipment, and patient lifestyle, hospital procedures cannot work as effectively (e.g., there may be no pole from which to hang an IV bag or no electricity to plug in a device).

Intuition

Intuition is the understanding or learning of things without the conscious use of reasoning. It is also known as sixth sense, hunch, instinct, feeling, or suspicion. As a problem-solving approach, intuition is viewed by some people as a form of guessing and, as such, an inappropriate basis for nursing decisions. However, others view intuition as an essential and legitimate aspect of clinical judgment acquired through knowledge and experience. The nurse must first have the knowledge base necessary to practice in the clinical area and then use that knowledge in clinical practice. Clinical experience allows the nurse to recognize cues and patterns and begin to reach correct conclusions.

Experience is important in improving intuition because the rapidity of the judgment depends on the nurse having seen similar client situations many times before. Sometimes nurses use the words "I had a feeling" to describe the critical-thinking element of considering evidence. These nurses are able to judge quickly which evidence is most important and to act on that limited evidence. Nurses in critical care often pay closer attention than usual to a client when they sense that the client's condition could change suddenly.

Although the intuitive method of problem solving is gaining recognition as part of nursing practice, it is not recommended for novices or students, however, because they usually lack the knowledge base and clinical experience on which to make a valid judgment.

Research Process and Scientific/Modified Scientific Method

The research process, discussed in Chapter 2 ⊂⊃ , is a formalized, logical, systematic approach to solving problems. The classic scientific method is most useful when the researcher is working in a controlled situation. Health professionals, often working with people in uncontrolled situations, require a modified approach to the scientific method for solving problems. For example, unlike experiments with animals, the effects of diet on health are complicated by a person's race, lifestyle, and personal preferences.

Table 15–4 compares the research process or scientific method with the modified scientific method. Critical thinking is important in all problem-solving processes as the nurse evaluates all potential solutions to a given problem and makes a decision to select the most appropriate solution for that situation.

Decision Making

Nurses make decisions in the course of solving problems, for example, in each step of the nursing process. Decision making, however, is also used in situations that do not involve problem solving. Nurses make value decisions (e.g., to keep client information confidential); time management decisions (e.g., taking clean linens to the client's room at the same time as the medication in order to save steps); scheduling decisions (e.g., to bathe the client before visiting hours); and priority decisions (e.g., which interventions are most urgent and which can be delegated).

TABLE 15–4 Comparison between the Research Process and the Modified Scientific Method

Research Process (Scientific Method)	Modified Scientific Method
State a research question or problem.	Define the problem.
Define the purpose of or the rationale for the study.	
Review related literature.	Gather information.
Formulate hypotheses and defining variables.	Analyze the information.
Select a method to test hypotheses.	Develop solutions.
Select a population, sample, and setting.	
Conduct a pilot study.	Make a decision.
Collect the data.	Implement the decision.
Analyze the data.	Evaluate the decision.
Communicate conclusions and implications.	

Decision making is a critical-thinking process for choosing the best actions to meet a desired goal. Decisions must be made whenever several mutually exclusive choices are available or when there is an option to act or not. For example, the individual who wishes to become a nurse in the United States has several possible courses of action: a diploma program, an associate degree program, or a baccalaureate program. Prospective students must choose. Therefore, they must evaluate the different types of programs, as well as personal circumstances, to make a decision appropriate to their situations.

Nurses must make decisions and assist clients to make decisions. When faced with several client needs at the same time, the nurse must prioritize and decide which client to assist first. The nurse may (a) look at advantages and disadvantages of each option, (b) apply Maslow's hierarchy of needs, (c) consider which tasks can be delegated to others, or (d) use another priority-setting framework. When a client is trying to make a decision about what course of treatment to follow, the nurse may need to provide information or resources the client can use in making a decision. Nurses must make decisions in their own personal and professional lives. For example, the nurse must decide whether to work in a hospital or community setting, whether to join a professional association, and whether to carry professional liability insurance.

Here are sequential steps to the decision-making process:

1. *Identify the purpose.* The nurse identifies why a decision is needed and what needs to be determined.
2. *Set the criteria.* When the nurse sets the criteria for decision making, three questions must be answered: What is the desired outcome, what needs to be preserved, and what needs to be avoided? For example, for a client with pain, the criteria would be as follows:
   a. What needs to be achieved? Relief of pain.
   b. What needs to be preserved? Physical functioning, cognitive functioning, psychologic functioning, client comfort.
   c. What needs to be avoided? Central nervous system depression, respiratory depression, nausea.
3. *Weight the criteria.* In this step, the decision maker sets priorities or ranks activities or services in order of importance from least important to most important as they relate to the specific situation. Because the weighting is specific to the situation, an activity may be ranked as most important in one situation and of less importance in another situation. For example, if a client with the pain has terminal cancer, pain relief may be more important than avoiding the side effects of the pain medication.
4. *Seek alternatives.* The decision maker identifies all possible ways to meet the criteria. In clinical situations, the alternatives may be selected from a range of nursing interventions or client care strategies. Pain may be treated with oral or injectable medications, as needed (PRN) or on a schedule, or without pharmacologic intervention at all, instead using complementary alternative modalities (CAM).
5. *Examine alternatives.* The nurse analyzes the alternatives to ensure that there is an objective rationale in relation to the established criteria for choosing one strategy over another. For pain that results from a procedure (such as removal of

a foreign object), CAM may not be strong enough relief and oral medication may be effective but act too slowly, so an intravenous narcotic might be the better choice.
6. *Project.* The nurse applies creative thinking and skepticism to determine what might go wrong as a result of a decision and develops plans to prevent, minimize, or overcome any problems. If the intravenous narcotic is selected, what safety procedures need to be in place, for example, a narcotic antidote and supplemental oxygen?
7. *Implement.* The decision plan is placed into action. The pain treatment is begun.
8. *Evaluate the outcome.* As with all nursing care, in evaluating, the nurse determines the effectiveness of the plan and whether the initial purpose was achieved. How does the client rate the level of pain following the procedure?

The decision-making process and the nursing process share similarities and the nurse uses decision making in all steps of the nursing process. Table 15–5 compares these processes.

DEVELOPING CRITICAL-THINKING ATTITUDES AND SKILLS

After gaining an idea of what it means to think critically, solve problems, and make decisions, nurses need to become aware of their own thinking style and abilities. Acquiring critical-thinking skills and a critical attitude then becomes a matter of practice. Critical thinking is not an "either-or" phenomenon; people develop and use it more or less effectively along a continuum. Some people make better evaluations than others; some people believe information from nearly any source; and still others seldom believe anything without carefully evaluating the credibility of the information. Critical thinking is not easy. Solving problems and making decisions is risky. Sometimes the outcome is not what was desired. With effort, however, everyone can achieve some level of critical thinking to become an effective problem solver and decision maker.

TABLE 15–5 Comparison between the Nursing Process and the Decision-Making Process

Nursing Process	Decision-Making Process*
Assess	Identify the purpose
Diagnose	
Plan	Set the criteria
	Weight the criteria
	Seek alternatives
	Examine alternatives
	Project
Implement	Implement
Evaluate	Evaluate the outcome

*The decision-making process parallels the nursing process but is also used during each step of the process.

Self-Assessment

The nurse should reflect on some of the attitudes discussed earlier that facilitate critical thinking, attitudes such as curiosity, fair-mindedness, humility, courage, and perseverance. A nurse might benefit from a rigorous personal assessment to determine which attitudes he or she already possesses and which need to be cultivated. This could also be done with a partner or as a group. The nurse first determines which attitudes are held strongly and form a base for thinking and which are held minimally or not at all. The nurse also needs to reflect on situations where he or she made decisions that were later regretted and analyzes thinking processes and attitudes or asks a trusted colleague to assess them. Identifying weak or vulnerable skills and attitudes is also important.

Tolerating Dissonance and Ambiguity

The nurse needs to take deliberate efforts to cultivate critical-thinking attitudes. For example, to develop fair-mindedness, one could deliberately seek out information that is in opposition to one's own views; this provides practice in understanding and learning to be open to other viewpoints. It is a human tendency to seek out information that corresponds to one's previously held beliefs and to ignore evidence that may contradict cherished ideas. This perspective is true for both the nurse and the client. Elders may have great difficulty accepting the pervasiveness of technology or that people don't stay in the hospital as long as they did in the 1970s or that having a diagnosis of cancer doesn't always mean that one is going to die. On the other hand, elders have a wealth of knowledge and experience and often know better than the health care provider what will work well and be acceptable to them. Nurses should increase their tolerance for ideas that contradict previously held beliefs, and they should practice suspending judgment.

Suspending judgment means tolerating ambiguity for a time. If an issue is complex, it may not be resolved quickly or neatly, and judgment should be postponed. For a while, the nurse will need to say, "I don't know" and be comfortable with that answer until more is known. Although postponing judgment may not be feasible in emergency situations where fast action is required, it is usually feasible in other situations.

Seeking Situations Where Good Thinking Is Practiced

Nurses will find it valuable to attend conferences in clinical or educational settings that support open examination of all sides of issues and respect for opposing viewpoints. Cultivating a questioning attitude, using either Socratic questioning or another technique, is vital. Nurses need to review the standards for evaluating thinking and apply them to their own thinking. If nurses are aware of their own thinking—while they are doing the thinking—they can detect thinking errors.

Creating Environments that Support Critical Thinking

A nurse cannot develop or maintain critical-thinking attitudes in a vacuum. Nurses in leadership positions must be particularly aware of the climate for thinking that they establish, and they must actively create a stimulating environment that encourages differences of opinion and fair examination of ideas and options. Nurses must embrace exploration of the perspectives of persons from different ages, cultures, religions, socioeconomic levels, and family structures. As leaders, nurses should encourage colleagues to examine evidence carefully before they come to conclusions, and to avoid "group think," the tendency to defer unthinkingly to the will of the group.

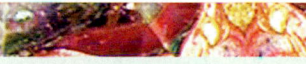
Lifespan Considerations

Elders

While it is important to include clients in decision making and planning nursing care, it is especially difficult to do this when working with elders with impaired cognitive abilities, such as Alzheimer's disease. The goal should be to allow them to have as much control and input as possible, while keeping things simple and direct so they may be understood. Elders with impactments are usually unable to perform multiple tasks or even to think of more than one step at a time. Presenting and discussing issues at their level helps to maintain respect and dignity and allows them to participate in their own care for as long as possible.

Focus on Critical Thinking

Mr. W. is a 53-year-old recently retired engineer with a history of irritable bowel syndrome that causes frequent diarrhea and rectal bleeding. His wife is a schoolteacher. It is mid-December when he comes to your clinic complaining about "not feeling good." You conclude he is having a reoccurrence of his intestinal problem.

1. What questions would you ask yourself to check this assumption?
2. How would you demonstrate that you are using the critical-thinking attitude of "confidence in reasoning"?

3. Socrates might ask you about the consequences of your conclusion by posing the question "What are the implications of your thinking?" How would you answer? Consider the implications if you are correct and if you are incorrect in your assumption.
4. Critical thinkers look for subtle cues. Which cues in this situation require follow-up?

See Critical Thinking Possibilities in Appendix A.

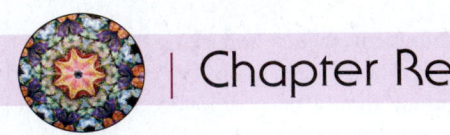 | ## Chapter Review

EXPLORE MediaLink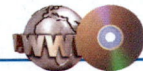

NCLEX review questions, case studies, MediaLink applications, and other interactive resources for this chapter can be found on the Companion Website at www.prenhall.com/kozier. Click on Chapter 15 to select the activities for this chapter.

For more NCLEX review questions, and an audio glossary, access the Student CD-ROM accompanying this textbook.

Chapter Highlights

- Nurses need critical-thinking skills and attitudes to be safe, competent, skillful practitioners.
- Critical thinking is a purposeful mental activity that guides beliefs and actions.
- Nurses use critical thinking as they apply knowledge from other subjects and fields to nursing practice, deal with change in stressful environments, and make important decisions related to client care. When nurses incorporate creativity into their thinking, they are able to find unique solutions to unique problems.
- Creativity enhances critical thinking. Creative nurses generate many ideas rapidly, are flexible and natural, create original solutions to problems, tend to be independent and self-confident, and demonstrate individuality.
- Critical thinking skills include the ability to do critical analysis, inductive and deductive reasoning, make valid inferences, differentiate facts from opinions, evaluate the credibility of information sources, clarify concepts, and recognize assumptions.
- Critical thinkers have certain attitudes: independence of thought, fair-mindedness, insight into egocentricity and sociocentricity, intellectual humility and suspension of judgment, intellectual courage, integrity, perseverance, confidence in reason, interest in exploring both thoughts underlying feeling and feelings underlying thoughts, and curiosity.
- Critical thinking consists of high-level cognitive processes that include problem solving and decision making. There are

several problem-solving methods: trial and error, intuition, the nursing process, the scientific method, and the modified scientific method. Nurses use the scientific method or research process when they participate in nursing and health research.

- Elements of thought, according to Paul, include purpose of thinking, question at issue, information, interpretation and inference, concepts, assumptions, implications and consequences, and points of view. Critical thinkers consider these elements when solving problems and making decisions.
- The nursing process and critical thinking are interrelated and interdependent, but they are not identical. Both involve problem solving, decision making, and creativity.
- Nurses must make decisions in both their personal and professional lives. The steps of the decision-making process include identifying the purpose of the decision, setting the criteria, weighting the criteria, seeking alternatives, examining alternatives, projecting, implementing, and evaluating the action.
- Everyone has at least some level of critical-thinking skill, and that skill can be developed with practice. Some guidelines to enhance critical-thinking skills and attitudes include performing a self-assessment, tolerating dissonance and ambiguity, seeking situations where good thinking is productive, and creating environments that support critical thinking.

Review Questions

15–1. A client who has diarrhea also has a physician's order for a bulk laxative daily. The nurse, not realizing that bulk laxatives can help solidify certain types of diarrhea, concludes "The physician does not know the client has diarrhea." This statement is an example of:
   a. a fact.
   b. an inference.
   c. a judgment.
   d. an opinion.
15–2. Although the client states he is hungry, he continuously declines to eat the food served to him in the hospital. Using critical thinking skills, the nurse would
   a. clarify with the client any assumptions the nurse has about why he doesn't eat.

   b. continue to leave the food at the beside until the client is hungry enough to eat.
   c. notify the physician that tube feeding may be indicated soon.
   d. believe the client is not really hungry.
15–3. The nurse has concerns that the holiday work schedule has not been formulated fairly. When asked, the nurse manager states that it is the same type of schedule used in the past and other nurses have found it acceptable. Which response by the nurse demonstrates an attitude of critical thinking in this situation?
   a. accepting the preferences of the majority.
   b. rethinking to see where the nurse has made a false conclusion

c. considering going to a higher authority

d. continuing the inquiry until the nurse is comfortable with the explanation

15–4. The client who is short of breath benefits from the head of the bed being elevated. However, extended use of this position can cause skin breakdown in the sacral area. In solving this problem, the nurse determines that the best approach would be to study the amount of sacral pressure found in various other positions. This approach is an example of

a. the scientific method.

b. the trial-and-error method.

c. intuition.

d. the nursing process.

15–5. In the decision-making process, after the nurse sets and weights the criteria and examines alternatives, but before implementing the plan, the nurse should

a. reexamine the purpose for making the decision.

b. consult the client and family members to determine their view of the criteria.

c. identify and consider various means for reaching the outcomes.

d. determine the logical course of action should intervening problems arise.

Readings and References

Suggested Readings

Ignatavicius, D. D. (2001). Six critical thinking skills for at-the-bedside success. *Dimensions of Critical Care Nursing, 20*(2), 30–33.
The author defines critical thinking and describes the six cognitive skills necessary to become an expert critical thinker: interpretation, analysis, evaluation, inference, explanation, and self-regulation. Although the article is aimed at nurses in a position to promote these skills in other staff, its message is appropriate for students and practicing nurses.

Raingruber, B., & Haffer, A. (2001). *Using your head to land on your feet: A beginning nurse's guide to critical thinking.* Philadelphia: F. A. Davis.
Textbook/workbook presents chapters with 10 to 12 scenarios written by students, describing situations faced in the clinical setting. After scenarios are questions to help the reader identify and evaluate decision points. Includes mind maps and a decision-making model on a pocket-sized card for use in clinical practice.

Related Research

Botes, A. (2000). Critical thinking by nurses on ethical issues like the termination of pregnancies. *Curationis: South African Journal of Nursing, 23*(3), 26–31.

Di Vito, T. P. (2000). Identifying critical thinking behaviors in clinical judgments. *Journal for Nurses in Staff Development, 15,* 174–180.

References

Paul, R. W. (1995). *Critical thinking: How to prepare students for a rapidly changing world.* Santa Rosa, CA: Foundation for Critical Thinking.

Paul, R., & Elder, L. (1999). *The miniature guide to critical thinking: Concepts and tools.* Santa Rosa, CA: Foundation for Critical Thinking.

Scheffer, B. K., & Rubenfeld, M. G. (2000). A consensus statement on critical thinking in nursing. *Journal of Nursing Education, 39,* 352–359.

Scriven, M., & Paul, R. (n.d.). *Defining critical thinking.* Retrieved February 23, 2003, from http://www.criticalthinking.org/University/univclass/Defining.html

Selected Bibliography

Alfaro-LeFevre, R. (1999). *Critical thinking in nursing: A practical approach* (2nd ed.). Philadelphia: W. B. Saunders.

Bandman, E. L., & Bandman, G. (1998). *Critical thinking in nursing.* East Norwalk, CT: Appleton & Lange.

Benner, P. E., Hooper-Kyriakidis, P. L., & Stannard, D. (1999). *Clinical wisdom and interventions in critical care: A thinking-in-action approach.* Philadelphia: W. B. Saunders.

Facione, P. (1990). *Critical thinking: A statement of expert consensus for purposes of educational assessment and instruction.* Millbrae, CA: California Academic Press.

Facione, P. (1998). *Critical thinking: What it is and why it counts.* Millbrae, CA: California Academic Press.

Foundation for Critical Thinking. (2001). *Critical thinking: Basic theory and instructional structure.* Dillon Beach, CA: Author.

Green, C. J. (2000). *Critical thinking in nursing: Case studies across the curriculum.* Upper Saddle River, NJ: Prentice Hall Health.

Locsin, R. C. (2001). The dilemma of decision-making processing thinking critical to nursing. *Holistic Nursing Practice, 15*(3), 1–3.

Lunney M. (Ed.). (2001). *Critical thinking & nursing diagnoses: Case studies & analyses.* Philadelphia: North American Nursing Diagnosis Association.

Nicoteri, J. A. (1998). Critical thinking skills. *American Journal of Nursing, 98*(10), 62, 64.

Oermann, M. H. (1999). Critical thinking, critical practice. *Nursing Management, 30*(4), 40C–D, 40F, 40H–I.

Paul, R., & Elder, L. (2000). *Critical thinking: Tools for taking charge of your learning and your life.* Upper Saddle River, NJ: Prentice Hall.

Pesut, D. J., & Herman, J. (1999). *Clinical reasoning: The art and science of critical and creative thinking.* Albany, NY: Delmar.

Schuster, P. M. (2002). *Concept mapping: A critical-thinking approach to care planning.* Philadelphia: F. A. Davis.

Wilkinson, J. M. (2001). *Nursing process and critical thinking* (3rd ed.). Upper Saddle River, NJ: Prentice Hall Health.

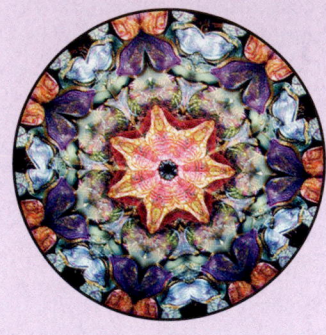

CHAPTER | 16

ASSESSING

LEARNING OUTCOMES

After completing this chapter, you will be able to:

- Describe the phases of the nursing process.
- Identify major characteristics of the nursing process.
- Identify the four major activities associated with the assessment process.
- Identify the purpose of assessing.
- Differentiate objective and subjective data and primary and secondary data.
- Identify three methods of data collection, and give examples of how each is useful.
- Compare directive and nondirective approaches to interviewing.
- Compare closed and open-ended questions, providing examples and listing advantages and disadvantages of each.
- Describe important aspects of the interview setting.
- Contrast various frameworks used for nursing assessment.

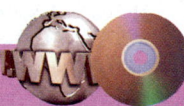

MediaLink

www.prenhall.com/kozier

Additional resources for this chapter can be found on the Student CD-ROM accompanying this textbook, and on the Companion Website at www.prenhall.com/kozier. Click on Chapter 16 to select the activities for this chapter.

CD-ROM
- Audio Glossary
- NCLEX Review
- Animations:
    Anatomical Landmarks
    Introduction to Body Systems
    Lymphatic Systems
    A & P Review:
        Anterior View
        Posterior View
        Body Cavity
        Lymphatic System
        Body Organization

- **Companion Website**
- Additional NCLEX Review
- Case Study: Down's Syndrome Client
- MediaLink Application:
    Researching Community Resources
- Links to Resources

Hall originated the term *nursing process* in 1955, and Johnson (1959), Orlando (1961), and Wiedenbach (1963) were among the first to use it to refer to a series of phases describing the process of nursing. Since then, various nurses have described the process of nursing and organized the phases in different ways.

The purpose of the nursing process is to identify a client's health status and actual or potential health care problems or needs, to establish plans to meet the identified needs, and to deliver specific nursing interventions to meet those needs. The client may be an individual, a family, or a group.

OVERVIEW OF THE NURSING PROCESS

The use of the nursing process in clinical practice gained additional legitimacy in 1973 when the phases were included in the American Nurses Association (ANA) *Standards of Clinical Nursing Practice.* The Standards of Care within the most current *Standards of Clinical Nursing Practice* (see Box 1–1 on page 10 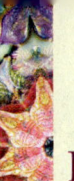) include the five phases of the nursing process: assessment, diagnosis, planning, implementation, and evaluation (ANA, 1998). Most states have since revised their nurse practice acts to reflect the nursing process. See Figure 16–1 ■ for an illustration of the nursing process in action.

Phases of the Nursing Process

Although nursing theorists may use different terms to describe the phases of the nursing process, the activities of the nurse using the process are similar. For example, *diagnosing* may also be called *analysis,* and *implementing* may be called *intervention* or *intervening.*

An overview of the five-phase nursing process is shown in Table 16–1 on page 260. Each of the five phases is discussed in depth in this and subsequent chapters of this unit. The phases of the nursing process are not discrete entities but overlapping, continuing subprocesses (see Figure 16–2 ■ on page 261). For example, assessing, which may be considered the first phase of the nursing process, is also carried out during the implementing and evaluating phases. This occurs, for instance, when, while actually administering medications (implementing), the nurse continuously notes the client's skin color, level of consciousness, and so on.

Each phase of the nursing process affects the others; they are closely interrelated. For example, if inadequate data are obtained during assessing, the nursing diagnoses will be incomplete or incorrect; inaccuracy will also be reflected in the planning, implementing, and evaluating phases.

Characteristics of the Nursing Process

The nursing process has unique characteristics that enable responsiveness to the changing health status of the client. These characteristics include its cyclic and dynamic nature, client centeredness, focus on problem solving and decision making, interpersonal and collaborative style, universal applicability, and use of critical thinking.

- Data from each phase provides input into the next phase. Findings from evaluating feed back into assessing. Hence, the nursing process is a regularly repeated event or sequence of events (a cycle) that are continuously changing (dynamic) rather than staying the same (static).
- The nursing process is client centered. The nurse organizes the plan of care according to client problems rather than nursing goals. In the assessment phase, the nurse collects data to determine the client's habits, routines, and needs, enabling the nurse to incorporate client routines into the care plan as much as possible.
- The nursing process is an adaptation of problem solving (see Chapter 15 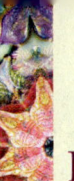) and systems theory (see Chapter 12). 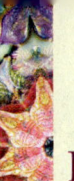 It can be viewed as parallel to but separate from the process used by physicians (the medical process). Both processes (a) begin with data gathering and analysis, (b) base action (intervention or treatment) on a problem statement (nursing diagnosis or medical diagnosis), and (c) include an evaluative component. However, the medical process focuses on physiologic systems and the disease process, whereas the nursing process is directed toward a client's responses to disease and illness.
- Decision making is involved in every phase of the nursing process. Nurses can be highly creative in determining when and how to use data to make decisions. They are not bound by standard responses and may apply their repertoire of skills and knowledge to assist clients. This facilitates the individualization of the nurse's plan of care.

The nursing process is a systematic, rational method of planning and providing nursing care. Its goal is to identify a client's healthcare status, and actual or potential health problems, to establish plans to meet the identified needs, and to deliver specific nursing interventions to address those needs. The nursing process is cyclical; that is, its components follow a logical sequence, but more than one component may be involved at one time. At the end of the first cycle, care may be terminated if goals are achieved, or the cycle may continue with reassessment, or the plan of care may be modified.

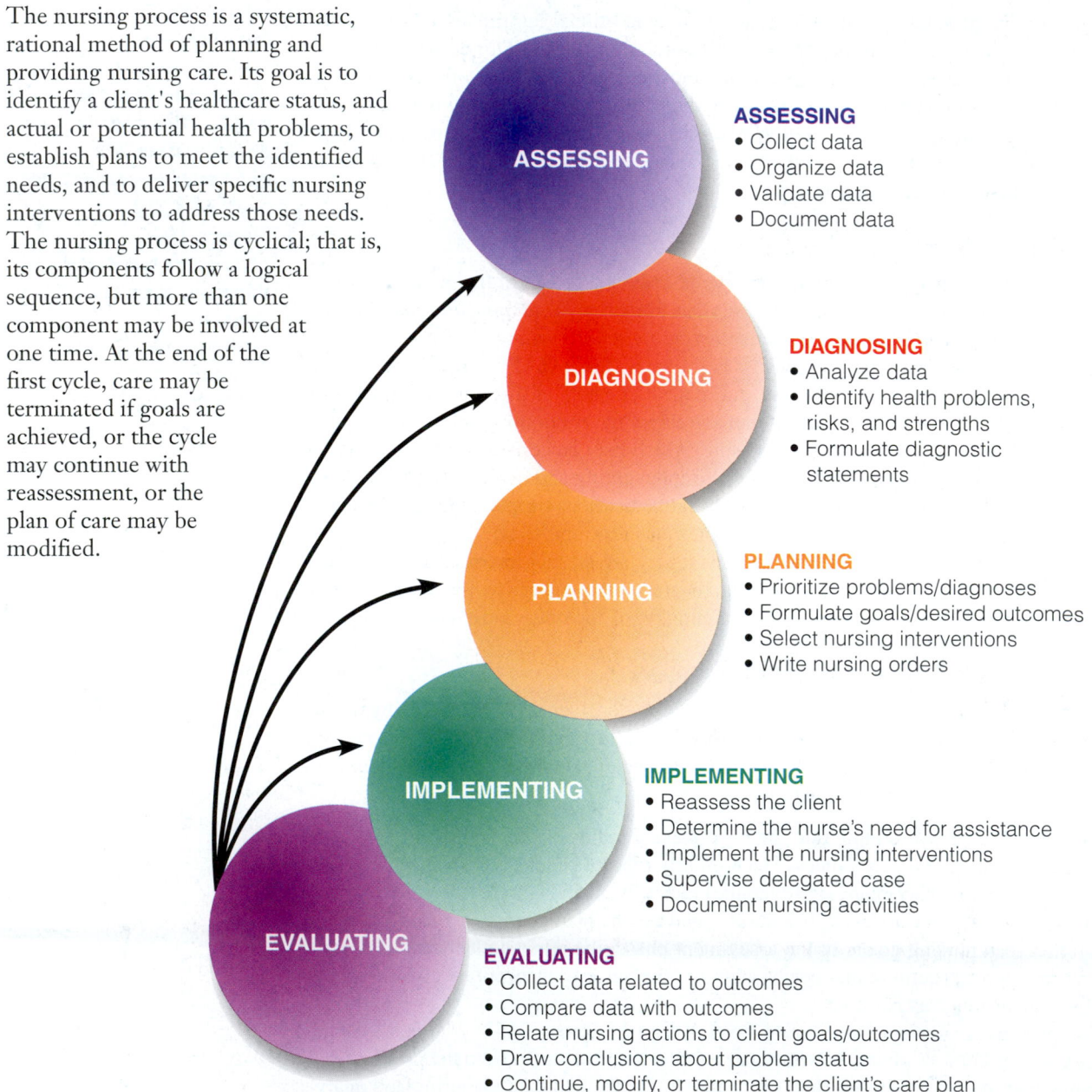

ASSESSING
- Collect data
- Organize data
- Validate data
- Document data

DIAGNOSING
- Analyze data
- Identify health problems, risks, and strengths
- Formulate diagnostic statements

PLANNING
- Prioritize problems/diagnoses
- Formulate goals/desired outcomes
- Select nursing interventions
- Write nursing orders

IMPLEMENTING
- Reassess the client
- Determine the nurse's need for assistance
- Implement the nursing interventions
- Supervise delegated case
- Document nursing activities

EVALUATING
- Collect data related to outcomes
- Compare data with outcomes
- Relate nursing actions to client goals/outcomes
- Draw conclusions about problem status
- Continue, modify, or terminate the client's care plan

Figure 16–1 ■ The nursing process in action.

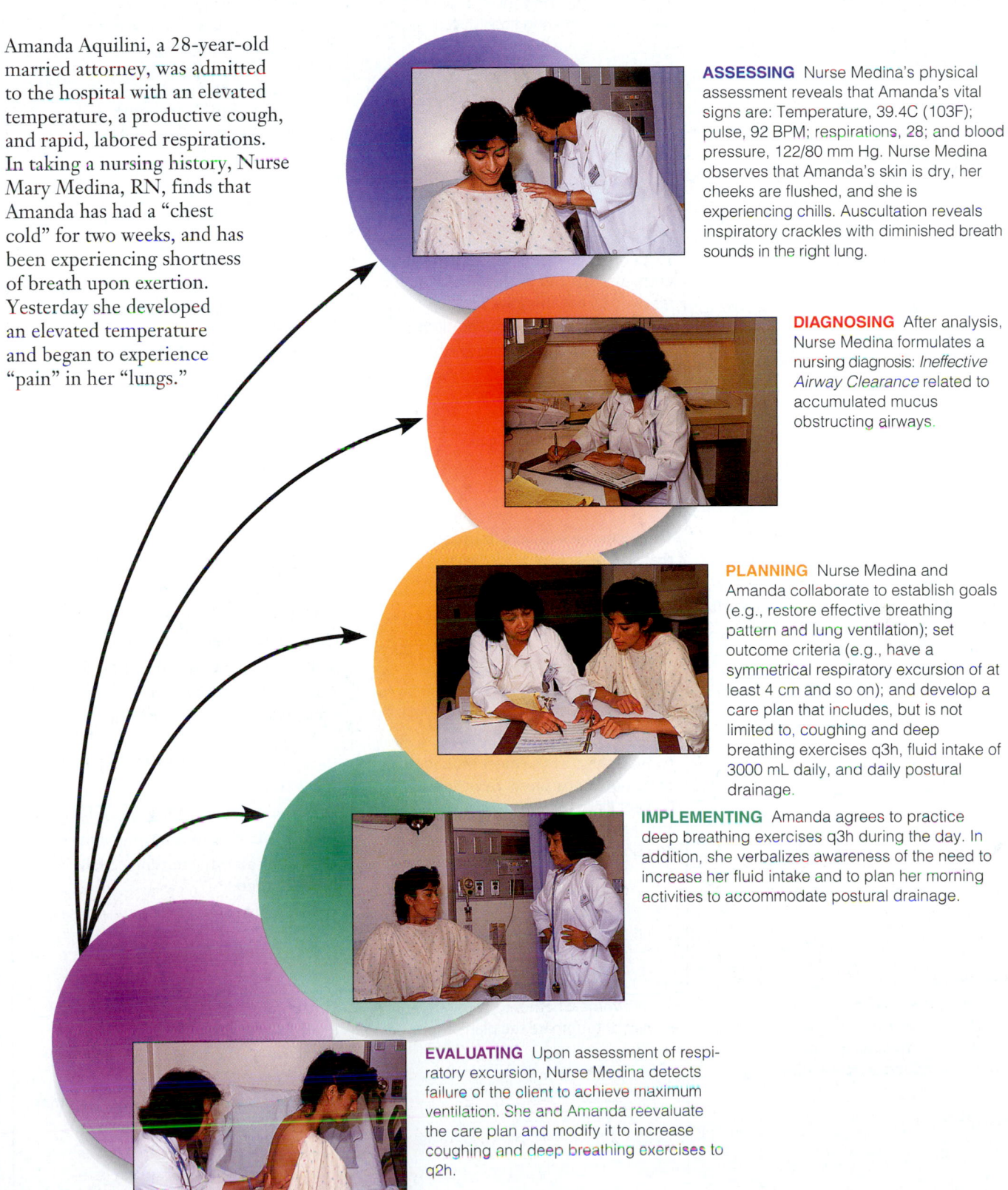

Amanda Aquilini, a 28-year-old married attorney, was admitted to the hospital with an elevated temperature, a productive cough, and rapid, labored respirations. In taking a nursing history, Nurse Mary Medina, RN, finds that Amanda has had a "chest cold" for two weeks, and has been experiencing shortness of breath upon exertion. Yesterday she developed an elevated temperature and began to experience "pain" in her "lungs."

ASSESSING Nurse Medina's physical assessment reveals that Amanda's vital signs are: Temperature, 39.4C (103F); pulse, 92 BPM; respirations, 28; and blood pressure, 122/80 mm Hg. Nurse Medina observes that Amanda's skin is dry, her cheeks are flushed, and she is experiencing chills. Auscultation reveals inspiratory crackles with diminished breath sounds in the right lung.

DIAGNOSING After analysis, Nurse Medina formulates a nursing diagnosis: *Ineffective Airway Clearance* related to accumulated mucus obstructing airways.

PLANNING Nurse Medina and Amanda collaborate to establish goals (e.g., restore effective breathing pattern and lung ventilation); set outcome criteria (e.g., have a symmetrical respiratory excursion of at least 4 cm and so on); and develop a care plan that includes, but is not limited to, coughing and deep breathing exercises q3h, fluid intake of 3000 mL daily, and daily postural drainage.

IMPLEMENTING Amanda agrees to practice deep breathing exercises q3h during the day. In addition, she verbalizes awareness of the need to increase her fluid intake and to plan her morning activities to accommodate postural drainage.

EVALUATING Upon assessment of respiratory excursion, Nurse Medina detects failure of the client to achieve maximum ventilation. She and Amanda reevaluate the care plan and modify it to increase coughing and deep breathing exercises to q2h.

TABLE 16–1 Overview of the Nursing Process

Phase and Description	Purpose	Activities
Assessing Collecting, organizing, validating, and documenting client data	To establish a database about the client's response to health concerns or illness and the ability to manage health care needs	Establish a database: • Obtain a nursing health history. • Conduct a physical assessment. • Review client records. • Review nursing literature. • Consult support persons. • Consult health professionals. Update data as needed. Organize data. Validate data. Communicate/document data.
Diagnosing Analyzing and synthesizing data	To identify client strengths and health problems that can be prevented or resolved by collaborative and independent nursing interventions To develop a list of nursing and collaborative problems	Interpret and analyze data. • Compare data against standards. • Cluster or group data (generate tentative hypotheses). • Identify gaps and inconsistencies. Determine client's strengths, risks, diagnoses, and problems. Formulate nursing diagnoses and collaborative problem statements. Document nursing diagnoses on the care plan.
Planning Determining how to prevent, reduce, or resolve the identified client problems; how to support client strengths; and how to implement nursing interventions in an organized, individualized, and goal-directed manner	To develop an individualized care plan that specifies client goals/desired outcomes, and related nursing interventions	Set priorities and goals/outcomes in collaboration with client. Write goals/desired outcomes. Select nursing strategies/interventions. Consult other health professionals. Write nursing orders and nursing care plan. Communicate care plan to relevant health care providers.
Implementing Carrying out the planned nursing interventions	To assist the client to meet desired goals/outcomes; promote wellness; prevent illness and disease; restore health; and facilitate coping with altered functioning	Reassess the client to update the database. Determine need for nursing assistance. Perform planned nursing interventions. Communicate what nursing actions were implemented. • Document care and client responses to care. • Give verbal reports as necessary.
Evaluating Measuring the degree to which goals/outcomes have been achieved and identifying factors that positively or negatively influence goal achievement	To determine whether to continue, modify, or terminate the plan of care	Collaborate with client and collect data related to desired outcomes. Judge whether goals/outcomes have been achieved. Relate nursing actions to client outcomes. Make decisions about problem status. Review and modify the care plan as indicated or terminate nursing care. Document achievement of outcomes and modification of the care plan.

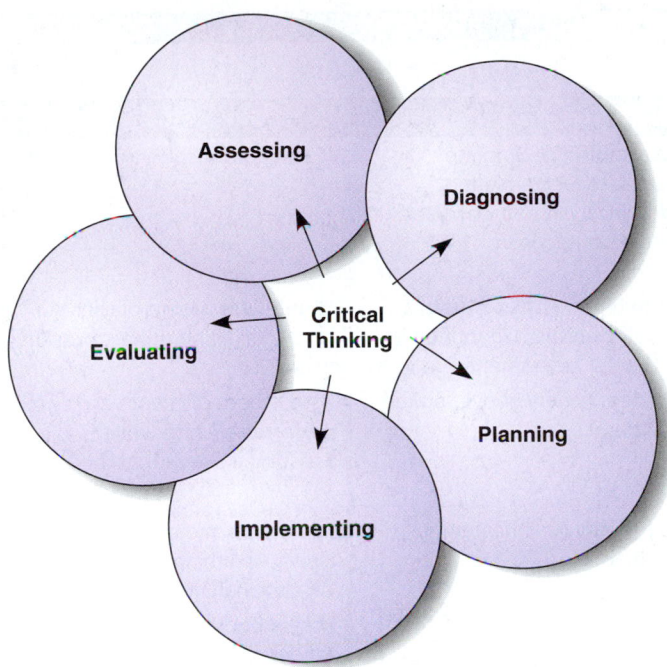

Figure 16–2 ■ The five overlapping phases of the nursing process. Each phase depends on the accuracy of the preceding phase. Each phase involves critical thinking.

Nursing Process Phase	Critical-Thinking Activities
Assessing	Making reliable observations
	Distinguishing relevant from irrelevant data
	Distinguishing important from unimportant data
	Validating data
	Organizing data
	Categorizing data according to a framework
	Recognizing assumptions
Diagnosing	Finding patterns and relationships among cues
	Identifying gaps in the data
	Making inferences
	Suspending judgment when lacking data
	Making interdisciplinary connections
	Stating the problem
	Examining assumptions
	Comparing patterns with norms
	Identifying factors contributing to the problem
Planning	Forming valid generalizations
	Transferring knowledge from one situation to another
	Developing evaluative criteria
	Hypothesizing
	Making interdisciplinary connections
	Prioritizing client problems
	Generalizing principles from other sciences
Implementing	Applying knowledge to perform interventions
	Testing hypotheses
Evaluating	Deciding whether hypotheses are correct
	Making criterion-based evaluations

TABLE 16–2 Examples of Critical Thinking in the Nursing Process

Note: From *Nursing Process & Critical Thinking*, 3rd ed. (pp. 65–66), by J. M. Wilkinson, 2001, Upper Saddle River, NJ: Pearson Education Nursing. Adapted with permission.

- The nursing process is interpersonal and collaborative. It requires the nurse to communicate directly and consistently with clients and families to meet their needs. It also requires that nurses collaborate, as members of the health care team, in a joint effort to provide quality client care.
- The universally applicable characteristic of the nursing process means that it is used as a framework for nursing care in all types of health care settings, with clients of all age groups.
- Nurses must use a variety of critical-thinking skills to carry out the nursing process. Table 16–2 provides examples of critical thinking in the nursing process.

ASSESSING

Assessing is the systematic and continuous collection, organization, validation, and documentation of **data** (information). In effect, assessing is a continuous process carried out during all phases of the nursing process. For example, in the evaluation phase, assessment is done to determine the outcomes of the nursing strategies and to evaluate goal achievement. All phases of the nursing process depend on the accurate and complete collection of data.

There are four different types of assessments: initial assessment, problem-focused assessment, emergency assessment, and time-lapsed reassessment (see Table 16–3). Assessments vary according to their purpose, timing, time available, and client status.

Nursing assessments focus on a client's responses to a health problem. A nursing assessment should include the client's perceived needs, health problems, related experience, health practices, values, and lifestyles. To be most useful, the data collected should be relevant to a particular health problem. Therefore, nurses should think critically about what to assess. The Joint

Commission on Accreditation of Healthcare Organizations (2001) requires that each patient have an initial assessment consisting of a history and physical performed and documented within 24 hours of admission as an inpatient.

The assessment process involves four closely related activities: collecting data, organizing data, validating data, and documenting data (see Figure 16–3 ■).

COLLECTING DATA

Data collection is the process of gathering information about a client's health status. It must be both systematic and continuous to prevent the omission of significant data and reflect a client's changing health status.

TABLE 16–3 Types of Assessment

Type	Time Performed	Purpose	Example
Initial assessment	Performed within specified time after admission to a health care agency	To establish a complete database for problem identification, reference, and future comparison	Nursing admission assessment
Problem-focused assessment	Ongoing process integrated with nursing care	To determine the status of a specific problem identified in an earlier assessment	Hourly assessment of client's fluid intake and urinary output in an ICU
		To identify new or overlooked problems	Assessment of client's ability to perform self-care while assisting a client to bathe
Emergency assessment	During any physiologic or psychologic crisis of the client	To identify life-threatening problems	Rapid assessment of a person's airway, breathing status, and circulation during a cardiac arrest
			Assessment of suicidal tendencies or potential for violence
Time-lapsed reassessment	Several months after initial assessment	To compare the client's current status to baseline data previously obtained	Reassessment of a client's functional health patterns in a home care or outpatient setting or, in a hospital, at shift change

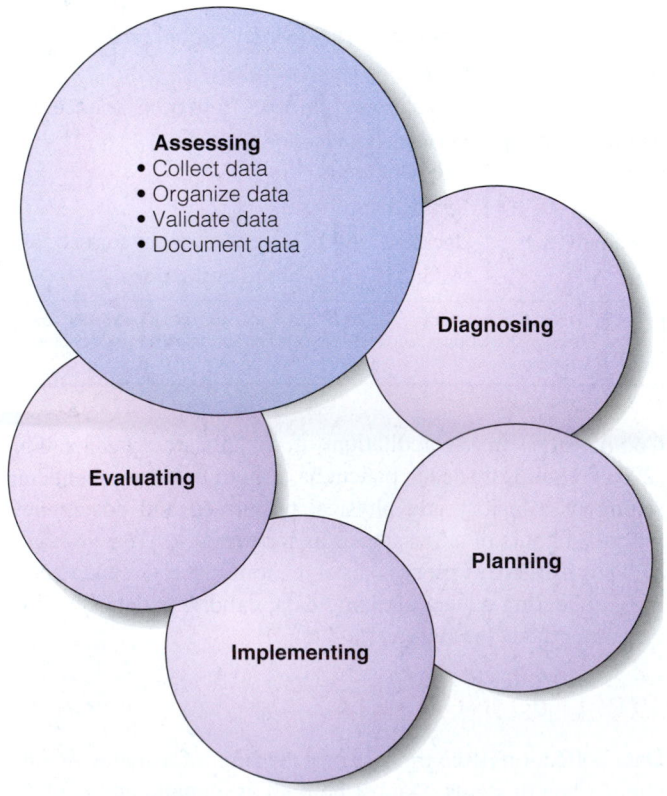

Figure 16–3 ■ Assessing. The assessment process involves four closely related activities.

A **database** is all the information about a client; it includes the nursing health history (see Box 16–1), physical assessment, the physician's history and physical examination, results of laboratory and diagnostic tests, and material contributed by other health personnel.

Client data should include past history as well as current problems. For example, a history of an allergic reaction to penicillin is a vital piece of historical data. Past surgical procedures, folk healing practices, and chronic diseases are also examples of historical data. Current data relate to present circumstances, such as pain, nausea, sleep patterns, and religious practices. To collect data accurately, both the client and nurse must actively participate.

Types of Data

Data can be subjective or objective. **Subjective data,** also referred to as **symptoms** or **covert data,** are apparent only to the person affected and can be described or verified only by that person. Itching, pain, and feelings of worry are examples of subjective data. Subjective data include the client's sensations, feelings, values, beliefs, attitudes, and perception of personal health status and life situation.

Objective data, also referred to as **signs** or **overt data,** are detectable by an observer or can be measured or tested against an accepted standard. They can be seen, heard, felt, or smelled, and they are obtained by observation or physical examination. For example, a discoloration of the skin or a blood pressure

BOX 16–1 ■ Components of a Nursing Health History

Biographic Data

Client's name, address, age, sex, marital status, occupation, religious preference, health care financing, and usual source of medical care.

Chief Complaint or Reason for Visit

The answer given to the question "What is troubling you?" or "What brought you to the hospital or clinic?" The chief complaint should be recorded in the client's own words.

History of Present Illness

- When the symptoms started
- Whether the onset of symptoms was sudden or gradual
- How often the problem occurs
- Exact location of the distress
- Character of the complaint (e.g., intensity of pain or quality of sputum, emesis, or discharge)
- Activity in which the client was involved when the problem occurred
- Phenomena or symptoms associated with the chief complaint
- Factors that aggravate or alleviate the problem

Past History

- *Childhood illnesses,* such as chickenpox, mumps, measles, rubella (German measles), rubeola (red measles), streptococcal infections, scarlet fever, rheumatic fever, and other significant illnesses
- *Childhood immunizations* and the date of the last tetanus shot
- *Allergies* to drugs, animals, insects, or other environmental agents and the type of reaction that occurs
- *Accidents and injuries:* how, when, and where the incident occurred, type of injury, treatment received, and any complications
- *Hospitalization for serious illnesses:* reasons for the hospitalization, dates, surgery performed, course of recovery, and any complications
- *Medications:* all currently used prescription and over-the-counter medications, such as aspirin, nasal spray, vitamins, or laxatives

Family History of Illness

To ascertain risk factors for certain diseases, the ages of siblings, parents, and grandparents and their current state of health or, if they are deceased, the cause of death are obtained. Particular attention should be given to disorders such as heart disease, cancer, diabetes, hypertension, obesity, allergies, arthritis, tuberculosis, bleeding, alcoholism, and any mental health disorders.

Lifestyle

- *Personal habits:* the amount, frequency, and duration of substance use (tobacco, alcohol, coffee, cola, tea, and illicit or recreational drugs)
- *Diet:* description of a typical diet on a normal day or any special diet, number of meals and snacks per day, who cooks and shops for food, ethnically distinct food patterns, and allergies
- *Sleep/rest patterns:* usual daily sleep/wake times, difficulties sleeping, and remedies used for difficulties

- *Activities of daily living (ADLs):* any difficulties experienced in the basic activities of eating, grooming, dressing, elimination, and locomotion
- *Instrumental activities of daily living:* any difficulties experienced in food preparation, shopping, transportation, housekeeping, laundry, and ability to use the telephone, handle finances, and manage medications
- *Recreation/hobbies:* exercise activity and tolerance, hobbies and other interests, and vacations

Social Data

- *Family relationships/friendships:* The client's support system in times of stress (who helps in time of need?), what effect the client's illness has on the family, and whether any family problems are affecting the client. See also the discussion of family assessment in Chapter 12. ⚭
- *Ethnic affiliation:* Health customs and beliefs; cultural practices that may affect health care and recovery. See also detailed ethnic/cultural assessment guide in Chapter 13. ⚭
- *Educational history:* Data about the client's highest level of education attained and any past difficulties with learning.
- *Occupational history:* Current employment status, the number of days missed from work because of illness, any history of accidents on the job, any occupational hazards with a potential for future disease or accident, the client's need to change jobs because of past illness, the employment status of spouses or partners and the way child care is handled, and the client's overall satisfaction with the work.
- *Economic status:* Information about how the client is paying for medical care (including what kind of medical and hospitalization coverage the client has), and whether the client's illness presents financial concerns.
- *Home and neighborhood conditions:* Home safety measures and adjustments in physical facilities that may be required to help the client manage a physical disability, activity intolerance, and activities of daily living; the availability of neighborhood and community services to meet the client's needs.

Psychologic Data

- *Major stressors* experienced and the client's perception of them
- *Usual coping pattern* with a serious problem or a high level of stress
- *Communication style:* ability to verbalize appropriate emotion; nonverbal communication—such as eye movements, gestures, use of touch, and posture; interactions with support persons; and the congruence of nonverbal behavior and verbal expression

Patterns of Health Care

All health care resources the client is currently using and has used in the past. These include the family physician, specialists (e.g., ophthalmologist or gynecologist), dentist, folk practitioners (e.g., herbalist or curandero), health clinic, or health center; whether the client considers the care being provided adequate; and whether access to health care is a problem.

TABLE 16–4 Examples of Subjective and Objective Data

Subjective	Objective
"I feel weak all over when I exert myself."	Blood pressure 90/50
	Apical pulse 104
	Skin pale and diaphoretic
Client states he has a cramping pain in his abdomen. States, "I feel sick to my stomach."	Vomited 100 mL green-tinged fluid
	Abdomen firm and slightly distended
	Active bowel sounds auscultated in all four quadrants
"I'm short of breath."	Lung sounds clear bilaterally; diminished in right lower lobe
Wife states: "He doesn't seem so sad today"	Client cried during interview
"I would like to see the chaplain before surgery."	Holding open Bible
	Has small silver cross on bedside table

reading is objective data. During the physical examination, the nurse obtains objective data to validate subjective data and to complete the assessment phase of the nursing process. Information supplied by family members, significant others, or other health professionals is considered subjective if it is not based on fact. If the client's daughter says, "Dad is very confused today," that is subjective data. However, if she says, "Dad couldn't remember his address or phone number today," that is objective data.

A complete database of both subjective and objective data provides a baseline for comparing the client's responses to nursing and medical interventions. Examples of subjective and objective data are shown in Table 16–4.

Sources of Data

Sources of data are primary or secondary. The client is the primary source of data. Family members or other support persons, other health professionals, records and reports, laboratory and diagnostic analyses, and relevant literature are secondary or indirect sources. In fact, all sources other than the client are considered secondary sources.

Client

The best source of data is usually the client, unless the client is too ill, young, or confused to communicate clearly. The client can provide subjective data that no one else can offer.

Support People

Family members, friends, and caregivers who know the client well often can supplement or verify information provided by the client. They might convey information about the client's response to illness, the stresses the client was experiencing before the illness, family attitudes on illness and health, and the client's home environment.

Support people are an especially important source of data for a client who is very young, unconscious, or confused. In some cases—a client who is physically or emotionally abused, for example—the person giving information may wish to re-

main anonymous. Before eliciting data from support people, the nurse should ensure that the client, if mentally able, accepts such input. The nurse should also indicate on the nursing history that the data were obtained from a support person.

Client Records

Client records include information documented by various health care professionals. Client records also contain data regarding the client's occupation, religion, and marital status. By reviewing such records before interviewing the client, the nurse can avoid asking questions for which answers have already been supplied. Repeated questioning can be stressful and annoying to clients and cause concern about the lack of communication among health professionals. Types of client records include medical records, records of therapies, and laboratory records.

Medical records (e.g., medical history, physical examination, operative report, progress notes, and consultations done by physicians) are often a source of a client's present and past health and illness patterns. These records can provide nurses with information about the client's coping behaviors, health practices, previous illnesses, and allergies.

Records of therapies provided by other health professionals, such as social workers, nutritionists, dietitians, or physical therapists, help the nurse obtain relevant data not expressed by the client. For example, a social agency's report on a client's living conditions or a home health care agency's report on a client's coping at home can also be helpful to the nurse conducting an assessment.

Laboratory records also provide pertinent health information. For example, the determination of blood glucose level allows health professionals to monitor the administration of oral hypoglycemic medications. Any laboratory data about a client must be compared to the agency or performing laboratory's norms for that particular test and for the client's age, sex, and so on. Diagnostic studies commonly ordered are discussed in Chapter 32.

The nurse must always consider the information in client records in light of the present situation. For example, if the most recent medical record is 10 years old, the client's health practices and coping behaviors are likely to have changed. Older clients may have numerous previous records. These are very useful and contribute to a full understanding of the health history, especially if the client's memory is impaired.

Health Care Professionals

Because assessment is an ongoing process, verbal reports from other health care professionals serve as other potential sources of information about a client's health. Nurses, social workers, physicians, and physiotherapists, for example, may have information from either previous or current contact with the client. Sharing of information among professionals is especially important to ensure continuity of care when clients are transferred to and from home and health care agencies.

Literature

The review of nursing and related literature, such as professional journals and reference texts, can provide additional information for the database. A literature review includes but is not limited to the following information:

- Standards or norms against which to compare findings (e.g., height and weight tables, normal developmental tasks for an age group)
- Cultural and social health practices
- Spiritual beliefs
- Assessment data needed for specific client conditions
- Nursing interventions and evaluation criteria relevant to a client's health problems
- Information about medical diagnoses, treatment, and prognoses

Data Collection Methods

The primary methods used to collect data are observing, interviewing, and examining. Observation occurs whenever the nurse is in contact with the client or support persons. Interviewing is used mainly while taking the nursing health history. Examining is the major method used in the physical health assessment.

In reality, the nurse uses all three methods simultaneously when assessing clients. For example, during the client interview the nurse observes, listens, asks questions, and mentally retains information to explore in the physical examination.

Observing

To *observe* is to gather data by using the senses. Observation is a conscious, deliberate skill that is developed through effort and with an organized approach. Although nurses observe mainly through sight, most of the senses are engaged during careful observations. Examples of client data observed through the senses are shown in Table 16–5.

Observation has two aspects: (a) noticing the data and (b) selecting, organizing, and interpreting the data. A nurse who observes that a client's face is flushed must relate that observation to, for example, body temperature, activity, environmental tem-

TABLE 16–5 Using the Senses to Observe Client Data

Sense	Example of Client Data
Vision	Overall appearance (e.g., body size, general weight, posture, grooming); signs of distress or discomfort; facial and body gestures; skin color and lesions; abnormalities of movement; nonverbal demeanor (e.g., signs of anger or anxiety); religious or cultural artifacts (e.g., books, icons, candles, beads)
Smell	Body or breath odors
Hearing	Lung and heart sounds; bowel sounds; ability to communicate; language spoken; ability to initiate conversation; ability to respond when spoken to; orientation to time, person, and place; thoughts and feelings about self, others, and health status
Touch	Skin temperature and moisture; muscle strength (e.g., hand grip); pulse rate, rhythm, and volume; palpatory lesions (e.g., lumps, masses, nodules)

perature, and blood pressure. Errors can occur in selecting, organizing, and interpreting data. For example, a nurse might not notice certain signs, either because they are unexpected or because they do not conform to preconceptions about a client's illness. Nurses often need to focus on specific data in order not to be overwhelmed by a multitude of data. Observing, therefore, involves discriminating among data, that is, distinguishing data in a meaningful manner. For example, nurses caring for newborns learn to ignore the usual sounds of machines in the nursery but respond quickly to an infant's cry or movement.

The experienced nurse is often able to attend to an intervention (e.g., give a bed bath or monitor an intravenous infusion) and at the same time make important observations (e.g., note a change in respiratory status or skin color). The beginning student must learn to make observations and complete tasks simultaneously.

Nursing observations must be organized so that nothing significant is missed. Most nurses develop a particular sequence for observing events, usually focusing on the client first. For example, a nurse walks into a client's room and observes, in the following order:

1. Clinical signs of client distress (e.g., pallor or flushing, labored breathing, and behavior indicating pain or emotional distress)
2. Threats to the client's safety, real or anticipated (e.g., a lowered side rail)
3. The presence and functioning of associated equipment (e.g., intravenous equipment and oxygen)
4. The immediate environment, including the people in it

Interviewing

An **interview** is a planned communication or a conversation with a purpose, for example, to get or give information, identify problems of mutual concern, evaluate change, teach, provide support, or provide counseling or therapy. One example of the interview is the nursing health history, which is a part of the nursing admission assessment.

There are two approaches to interviewing: directive and nondirective. The **directive interview** is highly structured and elicits specific information. The nurse establishes the purpose of the interview and controls the interview, at least at the outset. The client responds to questions but may have limited opportunity to ask questions or discuss concerns. Nurses frequently use directive interviews to gather and to give information when time is limited (e.g., in an emergency situation).

During a **nondirective interview,** or rapport-building interview, by contrast, the nurse allows the client to control the purpose, subject matter, and pacing. **Rapport** is an understanding between two or more people.

A combination of directive and nondirective approaches is usually appropriate during the information-gathering interview. The nurse begins by determining areas of concern for the client. If, for example, a client expresses worry about surgery, the nurse pauses to explore the client's worry and to provide support. Simply noting the worry, without dealing with it, can leave the impression that the nurse does not care about the client's concerns or dismisses them as unimportant.

TYPES OF INTERVIEW QUESTIONS. Questions are often classified as closed or open ended, and neutral or leading. **Closed questions,** used in the directive interview, are restrictive and generally require only "yes" or "no" or short factual answers giving specific information. Closed questions often begin with "when," "where," "who," "what," "do (did, does)," or "is (are, was)." Examples of closed questions are "What medication did you take?" "Are you having pain now? Show me where it is." "How old are you?" "When did you fall?" The highly stressed person and the person who has difficulty communicating will find closed questions easier to answer than open-ended questions.

Open-ended questions, associated with the nondirective interview, invite clients to discover and explore, elaborate, clarify, or illustrate their thoughts or feelings. An open-ended question specifies only the broad topic to be discussed, and invites answers longer than one or two words. Such questions give clients the freedom to divulge only the information that they are ready to disclose. The open-ended question is useful at the beginning of an interview or to change topics and to elicit attitudes.

Open-ended questions may begin with "what" or "how." Examples of open-ended questions are "How have you been feeling lately?" "What brought you to the hospital?" "How did you feel in that situation?" "Would you describe more about how you relate to your child?" "What would you like to talk about today?"

The type of question a nurse chooses depends on the needs of the client at the time. Nurses often find it necessary to use a combination of closed and open-ended questions throughout an interview to accomplish the goals of the interview and obtain needed information. See Box 16–2 for advantages and disadvantages of open-ended and closed questions.

A **neutral question** is a question the client can answer without direction or pressure from the nurse, is open ended, and is used in nondirective interviews. Examples are "How do you feel about that?" "Why do you think you had the operation?" A **leading question,** by contrast, is usually closed, used in a directive interview, and thus directs the client's answer. Examples are "You're stressed about surgery tomorrow, aren't you?" "You will take your medicine, won't you?" The leading question gives the client less opportunity to decide whether the answer is true or not. Leading questions create problems if the client, in an effort to please the nurse, gives inaccurate responses. This can result in inaccurate data.

PLANNING THE INTERVIEW AND SETTING. Before beginning an interview, the nurse reviews available information, for example, the operative report, information about the current illness, or literature about the client's health problem. The nurse also reviews the agency's data-collection form to identify which data must be collected and which data are within the nurse's discretion to collect based on the specific client. If a form is not available, most nurses prepare an interview guide to help them remember areas of information and determine what questions to ask. The guide includes a list of topics and subtopics rather than a series of questions.

Each interview is influenced by time, place, seating arrangement or distance, and language.

Time. Nurses need to plan interviews with hospitalized clients when the client is physically comfortable and free of pain, and when interruptions by friends, family, and other health professionals are minimal. Nurses should schedule interviews with clients in their homes at a time selected by the client. The client should be made to feel comfortable and unhurried.

Place. A well-lighted, well-ventilated, moderate-sized room that is relatively free of noise, movements, and interruptions encourages communication. In addition, a place where others cannot overhear or see the client is desirable.

Seating arrangement. A seating arrangement with the nurse behind a desk and the client seated across creates a formal setting that suggests a business meeting between a superior and a subordinate. In contrast, a seating arrangement in which the parties sit on two chairs placed at right angles to a desk or table or a few feet apart, with no table between, creates a less formal atmosphere, and the nurse and client tend to feel on equal terms. In groups, a horseshoe or circular chair arrangement can avoid a superior or head-of-the-table position.

By standing and looking down at a client who is in bed or in a chair, the nurse risks intimidating the client, who may perceive the nurse as having greater status. When a client is in bed, the nurse can sit at a 45-degree angle to the bed. This position is less formal than sitting behind a table or standing at the foot of the bed. During an initial admission interview, a client may feel less confronted if there is an overbed table between the client and the nurse. Sitting on a client's bed hems the client in and makes staring difficult to avoid.

Distance. The distance between the interviewer and interviewee should be neither too small nor too great, because people feel

BOX 16–2 ■ Selected Advantages and Disadvantages of Open-Ended and Closed Questions

Open-Ended Questions

Advantages
1. They let the interviewee do the talking.
2. The interviewer is able to listen and observe.
3. They are easy to answer and nonthreatening.
4. They reveal what the interviewee thinks is important.
5. They may reveal the interviewee's lack of information, misunderstanding of words, frame of reference, prejudices, or stereotypes.
6. They can provide information the interviewer may not ask for.
7. They can reveal the interviewee's degree of feeling about an issue.
8. They can convey interest and trust because of the freedom they provide.

Disadvantages
1. They take more time.
2. Only brief answers may be given.
3. Valuable information may be withheld.
4. They often elicit more information than necessary.
5. Responses are difficult to document and require skill in recording.
6. The interviewer requires skill in controlling an open-ended interview.
7. Responses require psychologic insight and sensitivity from the interviewer.

Closed Questions

Advantages
1. Questions and answers can be controlled more effectively.
2. They require less effort from the interviewee.
3. They may be less threatening, since they do not require explanations or justifications.
4. They take less time.
5. Information can be asked for sooner than it would be volunteered.
6. Responses are easily documented.
7. Questions are easy to use and can be handled by unskilled interviewers.

Disadvantages
1. They may provide too little information and require follow-up questions.
2. They may not reveal how the interviewee feels.
3. They do not allow the interviewee to volunteer possibly valuable information.
4. They may inhibit communication and convey lack of interest by the interviewer.
5. The interviewer may dominate the interview with questions.

Note: From *Interviewing: Principles and Practices,* 10th ed. (pp. 55–60), by C. J. Stewart and W. B. Cash, Jr., 2002, New York: McGraw-Hill. All rights reserved. Adapted with permission.

---

uncomfortable when talking to someone who is too close or too far away. Most people feel comfortable maintaining a distance of 2 to 3 feet during an interview. Some clients require more or less personal space, depending on their cultural and personal needs. See Box 16–3. For additional information, see Chapter 24.

Language. Failure to communicate in language the client can understand is a form of discrimination. The nurse must convert complicated medical terminology into common English usage, and interpreters or translators are needed if the client and the nurse do not speak the same language. Translating medical terminology is a specialized skill because not all persons fluent in the conversational form of the language are familiar with anatomic or other health terms. Interpreters, however, may make judgments about precise wording but also about subtle meanings that require additional explanation or clarification according to the specific language and ethnicity. They may edit the original source to make the meaning clearer or more culturally appropriate.

BOX 16–3 ■ Personal Space Variables

- Accepted distance between individuals in conversation varies with ethnicity. It is about 8 to 12 inches in Arab countries, 18 inches in the United States, 24 inches in Britain, and 36 inches in Japan.
- Men of all cultures usually require more space than women.
- Anxiety increases the need for space.
- Direct eye contact increases the need for space. " In East Asian and Scandinavian countries, direct eye contact is considered disrespectful" (O'Carroll, 2001, ¶7).
- Physical contact is used only if it has a therapeutic purpose. Touch, even a simple hand on the shoulder, can be misinterpreted—especially between persons of opposite gender.

Note: From *"Getting Too Close (or Too Far) for Comfort,"* by E. O'Carroll, March 1, 2001. Retrieved February 23, 2003, from http://travel.boston.com/columns/sl/030502_close.html. Reprinted with permission from Smarter Living (www.smarterliving.com).

If giving written documents to clients, the nurse must determine that the client can read in his or her native language. Live translation is preferred since the client can then ask questions for clarification. Nurses must be cautious when asking family members, client visitors, or agency nonprofessional staff to assist with translation. Issues of confidentiality or gender mismatch can interfere with effective communication. Services such as AT&T Language Line are available 24 hours a day in about 140 languages, for a fee paid by the health care provider. Many large agencies are establishing their own on-call translator services for the languages commonly spoken in their geographical regions.

Even among clients who speak English, there may be differences in understanding terminology. Clients from different parts of the country may have strong accents or clients less well educated and teen clients may ascribe different meanings to words. For example, "cool" may imply something good to one client and something not warm to another. The nurse must always confirm accurate understandings.

STAGES OF AN INTERVIEW. An interview has three major stages: the opening or introduction, the body or development, and the closing.

The opening. The opening can be the most important part of the interview because what is said and done at that time sets the tone for the remainder of the interview. The purposes of the opening are to establish rapport and orient the interviewee.

Establishing rapport is a process of creating goodwill and trust. It can begin with a greeting ("Good morning, Mr. Johnson") or a self-introduction ("Good morning. I'm Becky James, a nursing student") accompanied by nonverbal gestures such as a smile, a handshake, and a friendly manner. The nurse must be careful not to overdo this stage; too much superficial talk can arouse anxiety about what is to follow and may appear insincere.

In orientation, the nurse explains the purpose and nature of the interview, for example, what information is needed, how long it will take, and what is expected of the client. The nurse tells the client how the information will be used and usually states that the client has the right not to provide data.

The following is an example of an interview introduction:

Step 1—Establish Rapport
Nurse: Hello, Ms. Goodwin, I'm Ms. Fellows. I'm a nursing student, and I'll be assisting with your care here.

Client: Hi. Are you a student from the college?

Nurse: Yes, I'm in my final year. Are you familiar with the campus?

Client: Oh, yes! I'm an avid football fan. My nephew graduated in 2000, and I often attend football games with him.

Nurse: That's great! Sounds like fun.

Client: Yes, I enjoy it very much.

Step 2—Orientation
Nurse: May I sit down with you here for about 10 minutes to talk about how I can help you while you're here?

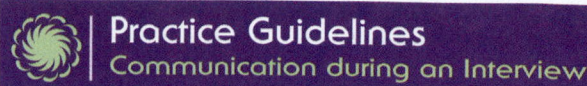

Practice Guidelines
Communication during an Interview

- Listen attentively, using all your senses, and speak slowly and clearly.
- Use language the client understands, and clarify points that are not understood.
- Plan questions to follow a logical sequence.
- Ask only one question at a time. Double questions limit the client to one choice and may confuse both the nurse and the client.
- Allow the client the opportunity to look at things the way they appear to him or her and not the way they appear to the nurse or someone else.
- Do not impose your own values on the client.
- Avoid using personal examples, such as saying, "If I were you . . . ."
- Nonverbally convey respect, concern, interest, and acceptance.
- Use and accept silence to help the client search for more thoughts or to organize them.
- Use eye contact and be calm, unhurried, and sympathetic.

Client: All right. What do you want to know?

Nurse: Well, to plan your care after your operation, I'd like to get some information about your normal daily activities and what you expect here in the hospital. I'll take notes while we talk to get the important points and have them available to the other staff who will also look after you.

Client: OK. That's all right with me.

Nurse: If there is anything you don't want to talk about, please feel free to say so, and if there is anything you would rather I didn't write down, just tell me.

Client: Sure, that will be fine.

The body. In the body of the interview, the client communicates what he or she thinks, feels, knows, and perceives in response to questions from the nurse. Effective development of the interview demands that the nurse use communication techniques that make both parties feel comfortable and serve the purpose of the interview (see Chapter 24). For communicating during an interview, see Practice Guidelines.

The closing. The nurse terminates the interview when the needed information has been obtained. In some cases, however, a client terminates it, for example, when deciding not to give any more information or when unable to offer more information for some other reason—fatigue, for example. The closing is important for maintaining the rapport and trust and for facilitating future interactions. The following techniques are commonly used to close an interview:

1. Offer to answer questions: "Do you have any questions?" "I would be glad to answer any questions you have." Be sure to allow time for the person to answer, or the offer will be regarded as insincere.

2. Conclude by saying "Well, that's all I need to know for now" or "Well, those are all the questions I have for now." Preceding a remark with the word "well" generally signals that the end of the interaction is near.

3. Thank the client. "Thank you for your time and help. The questions you have answered will be helpful in planning your nursing care."

4. Express concern for the person's welfare and future: "Take care of yourself." "I hope all goes well for you."

5. Plan for the next meeting, if there is to be one, or state what will happen next. Include the day, time, place, topic, and purpose: "Let's get together again here on the fifteenth at 9:00 AM to see how you are managing then." Or "Ms. Goodwin, I will be responsible for giving you care three mornings per week while you are here. I will be in to see you each Monday, Tuesday, and Wednesday between eight o'clock and noon. At those times, we can adjust your care if we need to."

6. Provide a summary to verify accuracy and agreement. Summarizing serves several purposes: It helps to terminate the interview, it reassures the client that the nurse has listened, it checks the accuracy of the nurse's perceptions, it clears the way for new ideas, and it helps the client to note progress and forward direction. "Let's review what we covered in this interview." Summaries are particularly helpful for clients who are anxious or who have difficulty staying with the topic. "Well, it seems to me that you are especially worried about your hospitalization and chest pain because your father died of a heart attack five years ago. Is that correct? . . . I'll discuss this with you again tomorrow, and we'll decide what plans need to be made to help you."

Examining

The physical examination or physical assessment is a systematic data-collection method that uses observation (i.e., the senses of sight, hearing, smell, and touch) to detect health problems. To conduct the examination the nurse uses techniques of inspection, auscultation, palpation, and percussion (see Chapter 28).

The physical examination is carried out systematically. It may be organized according to the examiner's preference, in a head-to-toe approach or a body systems approach. Usually, the nurse first records a general impression about the client's overall appearance and health status, for example, age, body size, mental and nutritional status, speech, and behavior. Then the nurse takes such measurements as vital signs, height, and weight. The **cephalocaudal** or head-to-toe approach begins the examination at the head, progresses to the neck, thorax, abdomen, and extremities, and ends at the toes. The nurse using a body systems approach investigates each system individually, that is, the respiratory system, the circulatory system, the nervous system, and so on. During the physical examination, the nurse assesses all body parts and compares findings on each side of the body (e.g., lungs). These techniques are discussed in detail in Chapters 27 and 28.

Instead of giving a complete examination, the nurse may focus on a specific problem area noted from the nursing assessment, such as the inability to urinate. On occasion, the nurse may find it necessary to resolve a client complaint or problem (e.g., shortness of breath) before completing the examination. Alternatively, the nurse may perform a screening examination. A **screening examination,** also called a **review of systems,** is a brief review of essential functioning of various body parts or systems. An example of a screening examination is the nursing admission assessment form shown in Figure 16–4 ■. Data obtained from this examination are measured against norms or standards, such as ideal height and weight standards or norms for body temperature or blood pressure levels.

ORGANIZING DATA

The nurse uses a written (or computerized) format that organizes the assessment data systematically. This is often referred to as a nursing health history, nursing assessment, or nursing database form. The format may be modified according to the client's physical status such as one focused on musculoskeletal data for orthopedic clients.

Nursing Conceptual Models

Most schools of nursing and health care agencies have developed their own structured assessment format. Many of these are based on selected nursing theories (see Chapter 3). Three examples are Gordon's functional health pattern framework, Orem's self-care model, and Roy's adaptation model.

Gordon (2000) provides a framework of 11 functional health patterns (see Box 16–4 on page 272). Gordon uses the word *pattern* to signify a sequence of recurring behavior. The nurse collects data about dysfunctional as well as functional behavior. Thus, by using Gordon's framework to organize data, nurses are able to discern emerging patterns.

Orem, Taylor, and Renpenning (2000) delineate eight universal self-care requisites of humans (see Box 16–5 on page 272). Roy and Andrews (1998) outline the data to be collected according to the Roy adaptation model and classify observable behavior into four categories: physiologic, self-concept, role function, and interdependence (see Box 16–6 on page 272).

Figure 16–4 is a concise data-collection tool that is organized according to body systems and specific nursing concerns (e.g., screening for falls and allergies); it does not use one particular nursing model. In Box 16–7 on page 273, the Amanda Aquilini data from Figure 16–4 is shown after being organized according to the 11 functional health patterns. Note how the categories in the box differ from those in Figure 16–4. As a rule, the nurse organizes the data using the same model on which the data-collection tool is based. However, different models are provided here to demonstrate differences in organizing frameworks, and to show that the nurse is not limited to the framework provided by the data-collection tool.

ADMISSION DATA

Date 4-16-03 Time 3:15 p.m Primary Language English
Arrived Via: ☐ Wheelchair ☐ Stretcher ☒ Ambulatory
From: ☐ Admitting ☐ ER ☒ Home ☐ Nursing Home ☐ Other
Admitting M.D. R. Katz Time Notified 5 p.m.

ORIENTATION TO UNIT

	YES	NO		YES	NO
Arm Band Correct	☒	☐	Visiting Hours	☒	☐
Allergy Band	☒	☐	Smoking Policy	☒	☐
Telephone	☒	☐	TV, Lights, Bed Controls,		
Electrical Policy	☒	☐	Call Lights, Side Rails	☒	☐
Educational Mat©l	☒	☐	Nurses Station	☒	☐
(TV Brochure)	☒	☐			

Family M.D. R. Katz
Weight 125 lb. Height 5ft. 2in. BP:R — L 122/80
Temp. 103F Pulse 92, weak Resp 28, shallow
Source Providing Information ☒ Patient ☐ Other
Unable to Obtain History ☐
Reason for Admission (Onset, Duration, Pt.'s Perception) ("Chest cold" X2 weeks S.O.B on exertion. "Lung pain, fever," "Dr. says I have pneumonia.")

ALLERGIES & REACTIONS

Drugs Penicillin
Food/Other
Signs & Symptoms rash, nausea
Blood Reaction ☐ Yes ☒ No Dyes/Shellfish ☐ Yes ☒ No

MEDICATIONS

Current Meds	Dose/Freq.	Last Dose
Synthroid	0.1 mg. daily	4-16, 8 a.m.

Disposition of Meds: ☒ Home ☐ Pharmacy ☐ Safe *At Bedside

MEDICAL HISTORY

☒ No Major Problems ☐ Gastro
☐ Cardiac ☐ Arthritis
☐ Hyper/Hypotension ☐ Stroke
☐ Diabetes ☐ Seizures
☐ Cancer ☐ Glaucoma
☐ Respiratory ☒ Other Childbirth-2000

Surgery/Procedures	Date
Appendectomy	1981
Partial thyroidectomy	1995

SPECIAL ASSISTIVE DEVICES

☐ Wheelchair ☐ Contacts ☐ Venous ☐ Dentures
☐ Braces ☐ Hearing Aid Access ☐ Partial
☐ Cane/Crutches ☐ Prosthesis Device ☐ Upper
☐ Walker ☐ Glasses ☐ Epidural Catheter ☐ Lower
☐ Other None

VALUABLES

Patient informed Hospital not responsible for personal belongings.
Valuables Disposition: ☐ Patient ☐ Safe ☐ Given to
Patient/SO Signature None

PSYCHOSOCIAL HISTORY

Recent Stress None
Coping Mechanism Not assessed because of fatigue
Support System Husband, coworkers, friends
Calm: ☒ Yes ☐ No
Anxious: ☐ Yes ☐ No Facial muscles tense; trembling
Religion Catholic. Would want Last Rites
Tobacco Use: ☐ Yes ☒ No
Alcohol Use: ☐ Yes ☒ No
Drug Use: ☐ Yes ☒ No

NEUROLOGICAL

Oriented: ☒ Person ☒ Place ☒ Time ☐ Confused ☐ Sedated
☐ Alert ☐ Restless ☒ Lethargic ☐ Comatose
Pupils: ☒ Equal ☐ Unequal ☒ Reactive ☐ Sluggish
☐ Other 3mm.
Extremity Strength: ☒ Equal ☐ Unequal
Speech: ☒ Clear ☐ Slurred ☐ Other

MUSCULO-SKELETAL

Normal ROM of Extremities ☒ Yes ☐ No
☒ Weakness ☐ Paralysis ☐ Contractures ☐ Joint Swelling ☒ Pain
☐ Other ↓ related to fatigue when coughing ↙

RESPIRATORY

Pattern: ☐ Even ☐ Uneven ☒ Shallow ☒ Dyspnea
☒ Other diminished breath sounds
Breathing Sounds: ☐ Clear ☒ Other inspiratory crackles
Secretions: ☐ None ☒ Other pink, thick sputum
Cough: ☐ None ☒ Productive ☐ Nonproductive

CARDIOVASCULAR

Pulses: Apical Rate 92-W ☒ Reg. ☐ Irregular ☐ Pacemaker
S = Strong W = Weak A = Absent D = Doppler
Radial R 92 L — Pedal R — L —
Edema: ☒ Absent ☐ Present Site
Perfusion: ☐ Warm ☐ Dry ☒ Diaphoretic ☐ Cool (Hot)

GASTROINTESTINAL

Oral Mucosa ☐ Normal ☒ Other pale and dry
Bowel Sounds: ☒ Normal ☐ Other Abd. soft
Wt. Change: ☐ ☒ N/V Stool Frequency/Character 1/day; soft
Last B/M 4-15-03 ☐ Ostomy (type)
Equip.

GENITOURINARY

Urine: Last Voided This morning
☐ Normal ☐ Anuria ☐ Hematuria ☐ Dysuri ☐ Incontinent
☒ Other ↓ amount & frequency since ill
☐ Catheter (type) Other
LMP 4-1-03 ☐ Vaginal/Penile Discharge
Other

SELF CARE

Need Assist with: ☐ Ambulating ☐ Elimination
☐ Meals ☒ Hygiene ☐ Dressing
While fatigued

Amanda Aquilini [F. age 28]
#4637651

✳ NORTH BROWARD HOSPITAL DISTRICT
NURSING ADMINISTRATION ASSESSMENT

Figure 16–4 ■ Assessment for Amanda Aquilini. (Nursing assessment tool courtesy of North Broward Hospital District, Broward County, Florida. Reprinted with permission.)

NUTRITION

General Appearance: ☑ Well Nourished ☐ Emaciated ☐ Other _____

Appetite: ☐ Good ☐ Fair ☑ Poor -x 2 days

Diet _Liquid_ **Meal Pattern** _3/day_

☐ Feeds Self ☐ Assist ☐ Total Feed

SKIN ASSESSMENT

Color: ☐ Normal ☐ Flushed ☑ Pale ☐ Dusky ☐ Cyanotic ☐ Jaundiced ☑ Other _Cheeks flushed, hot_

General Description _Surgical scars:_ _RLQ abdomen; anterior neck_

_____
_____
_____
_____

Note Cultures Obtained _____
_____
_____
_____

PRESSURE SORE ™AT RISKʃ SCREENING CRITERIA

OVERALL SKIN CONDITION

Grade

☐ 0	Turgor (elasticity adequate, skin warm and moist)
☑ 1	Poor turgor, skin cold & dry
☐ 2	Areas mottled, red or denuded
☐ 3	Existing skin ulcer/lesions

BOWEL AND BLADDER CONTROL

Grade

☑ 0	Always able to ask for bedpan
☐ 1	Incontinence of urine
☐ 2	Incontinence of feces
☐ 3	Totally incontinent Confined to bed

REHABILITATIVE STATE

Grade

☐ 0	Fully ambulatory
☑ 1	Ambulated with assistance
☐ 2	Chair to bed ambulation only
☐ 3	Confined to bed
☐ 4	Immobile in bed

NUTRITIONAL STATE

Grade

☐ 0	Eats all
☑ 1	Eats very little
☐ 2	Refuses food often
☐ 3	Tube feeding
☐ 4	Intravenous feeding

MENTAL STATE

Grade

☑ 0	Alert and clear
☐ 1	Confused
☐ 2	Disoriented/senile
☐ 3	Stuporous
☐ 4	Unconcious

CHRONIC DISEASE STATUS (i.e. COPD, ASCVD. Peripheral Vascular Disease, Diabetes, or Renal Disease, Cancer, Motor or Sensory Deficits, Elderly, Other)

Grade

☑ 0	Absent
☐ 1	One Present
☐ 2	Two Present
☐ 3	Three or more Present

TOTAL _____ Refer to Skin Care Protocol

FALLS SCREENING

If one or more of the following are checked institute fall precautions/plan of care

☐ History of Falls ☐ Unsteady Gait ☐ Confusion/Disorientation ☐ Dizziness

If two or more of the following are checked institute fall precautions/plan of care

☐ Age over 80 ☐ Utilizes cane, walker, w/c ☐ Sleeplessness

☐ Impaired vision ☐ Urgency/frequency in elimination

☐ Multiple Diagnoses ☐ Impaired hearing

☐ Inability to understand or follow directions ☐ Medication/Sedative /Diuretic etc.

NURSE SIGNATURE/TITLE	DATE	TIME
Mary Medina, RN	_4-16-03_	_3:30pm_
NURSE SIGNATURE/TITLE	DATE	TIME

EDUCATION/DISCHARGE PLANNING

1. What do you know about your present illness? _"Dr. says I have pneumonia." "I will have an I.V."_

2. What information do you want or need about your illness? _____

3. Would you like family/SO involved in your care? _Husband, Michael_

4. How long do you expect to be in the hospital? _"1-2 days"_

5. What concerns do you have about leaving the hospital? _____

CHECK APPROPRIATE BOX

Will patient need post discharge assistance with ADLs/physical functioning? ☐ Yes ☑ No ☐ Unknown

Does patient have family capable of and willing to provide assistance post discharge?

☑ Yes ☐ No ☐ Unknown ☐ No family

Is assistance needed beyond that which family can provide?

☐ Yes ☑ No ☐ Unknown

Previous admission in the last six months?

☐ Yes ☑ No ☐ Unknown

Patient lives with _Husband and 1 child_

Planned discharge to _Home_

Comments: _Fatigue and anxiety may have interfered with learning. Re-teach anything covered at admission, later._

Social Services Notified ☐ Yes ☑ No

NARRATIVE NOTES

S--c/o sharp chest pain when coughing and dyspnea on exertion. States unable to carry out regular daily exercise for past week. Coughing relieved "if I sit up and sit still." Nausea associated with coughing. Having occasional "chills." Occasionally becomes frightened, stating, "I can't breathe." Well groomed but "too tired to put on make-up." O--Chest expansion < 3cm, no nasal flaring or use of accessory muscles. Breath sounds and insp. crackles in ® upper and lower chest. Assesses own supports as "good" (eg, relationship c̄ husband). Is "worried" about daughter. States husband will be out of town until tomorrow. Left 3-year-old daughter with neighbor. Concerned too about her work (is attorney). "I'll never get caught up." Had water at noon—no food today. Agrees to save urine for 24 hr. specimen. IV D₅W LR 1000 mL started in ® arm, 100 mL/hr. Slow capillary refill. Keeping head of bed↑ to facilitate breathing.

✸✸ **NORTH BROWARD HOSPITAL DISTRICT**
NURSING ADMINISTRATION ASSESSMENT

Figure 16–4 ■ (continued)

BOX 16–4 ■ Gordon's Typology of 11 Functional Health Patterns

- *Health-perception/health-management pattern.* Describes the client's perceived pattern of health and well-being and how health is managed.
- *Nutritional/metabolic pattern.* Describes the client's pattern of food and fluid consumption relative to metabolic need and pattern indicators of local nutrient supply.
- *Elimination pattern.* Describes the patterns of excretory function (bowel, bladder, and skin).
- *Activity/exercise pattern.* Describes the pattern of exercise, activity, leisure, and recreation.
- *Sleep-rest pattern.* Describes patterns of sleep, rest, and relaxation.
- *Cognitive/perceptual pattern.* Describes sensory-perceptual and cognitive patterns.
- *Self-perception/self-concept pattern.* Describes the client's self-concept pattern and perceptions of self (e.g., self-conception/worth, comfort, body image, feeling state).
- *Role/relationship pattern.* Describes the client's pattern of role participation and relationships.
- *Sexuality/reproductive pattern.* Describes the client's patterns of satisfaction and dissatisfaction with sexuality pattern; describes reproductive patterns.
- *Coping/stress-tolerance pattern.* Describes the client's general coping pattern and the effectiveness of the pattern in terms of stress tolerance.
- *Value/belief pattern.* Describes the patterns of values, beliefs (including spiritual), and goals that guide the client's choices or decisions.

Note: From Manual of Nursing Diagnosis, 10th ed. (pp. 2–5), by M. Gordon, © 2002, St. Louis, MO: Mosby, with permission from Elsevier Science.

BOX 16–5 ■ Orem's Self-Care Model

Universal Self-Care Requisites

1. The maintenance of a sufficient intake of air.
2. The maintenance of a sufficient intake of water.
3. The maintenance of a sufficient intake of food.
4. The provision of care associated with elimination processes and excrement.
5. The maintenance of a balance between activity and rest.
6. The maintenance of a balance between solitude and social interaction.
7. The prevention of hazards to human life, human functioning, and human well-being.
8. The promotion of human functioning and development within social groups in accord with human potential, known human limitations, and human desire to be normal. (Normalcy is used in the sense of that which is essentially human and that which is in accord with the genetic and constitutional characteristics and the talents of individuals.)

Note: From Nursing Concepts of Practice, 6th ed. (p. 225), by D. E. Orem, S. G. Taylor, and K. M. Renpenning, 2000, St. Louis, MO: Mosby, with permission from Elsevier Science.

BOX 16–6 ■ Roy's Adaptation Model

Adaptive Modes

1. Physiologic needs
   - Activity and rest
   - Nutrition
   - Elimination
   - Fluid and electrolytes
   - Oxygenation
   - Protection
   - Regulation: temperature
   - Regulation: the senses
   - Regulation: endocrine system
2. Self-concept
   - Physical self
   - Personal self
3. Role function
4. Interdependence

Note: From The Roy Adaptation Model: The Definitive Statement, 2nd ed., by C. Roy and H. A. Andrews, 1999, Upper Saddle River, NJ: Prentice-Hall. Reprinted with permission.

Wellness Models

Nurses use wellness models to assist clients to identify health risks and to explore lifestyle habits and health behaviors, beliefs, values, and attitudes that influence levels of wellness. Such models generally include the following:

- Health history
- Physical fitness evaluation
- Nutritional assessment
- Life-stress analysis
- Lifestyle and health habits
- Health beliefs
- Sexual health
- Spiritual health
- Relationships
- Health risk appraisal.

See Chapter 11 ∞ for details.

Nonnursing Models

Frameworks and models from other disciplines may also be helpful for organizing data. These frameworks are narrower than the model required in nursing; therefore, the nurse usually needs to combine these with other approaches to obtain a complete history.

Body Systems Model

The body systems model focuses on abnormalities of the following anatomic systems:

- Integumentary system
- Respiratory system
- Cardiovascular system
- Nervous system
- Musculoskeletal system
- Gastrointestinal system

BOX 16–7 ■ Data for Amanda Aquilini, Organized According to Functional Health Patterns

Health Perception/Health Management
- Aware/understands medical diagnosis
- Gives thorough history of illnesses and surgeries
- Complies with Synthroid regimen
- Relates progression of illness in detail
- Expects to have antibiotic therapy and "go home in a day or two"
- States usual eating pattern "3 meals a day"

Nutritional/Metabolic
- 158 cm (5 ft, 2 in) tall; weighs 56 kg (125 lb)
- Usual eating pattern "3 meals a day"
- "No appetite" since having "cold"
- Has not eaten today; last fluids at noon
- Nauseated
- Oral temp 39.4C (103F)
- Decreased skin turgor

Elimination
- Usually no problem
- Decreased urinary frequency and amount × 2 days
- Last bowel movement yesterday, formed, states was "normal"

Activity/Exercise
- No musculoskeletal impairment
- Difficulty sleeping because of cough
- "Can't breathe lying down"
- States "I feel weak"
- Short of breath on exertion
- Exercises daily

Cognitive/Perceptual
- No sensory deficits
- Pupils 3 mm, equal, brisk reaction
- Oriented to time, place, and person
- Responsive, but fatigued
- Responds appropriately to verbal and physical stimuli
- Recent and remote memory intact
- States "short of breath" on exertion
- Reports "pain in lungs," especially when coughing
- Experiencing chills
- Reports nausea

Roles/Relationships
- Lives with husband and 3-year-old daughter
- Husband out of town; will be back tomorrow afternoon
- Child with neighbor until husband returns
- States "good" relationships with friends and coworkers
- Working mother, attorney

Self-Perception/Self-Concept
- Expresses "concern" and "worry" over leaving daughter with neighbors until husband returns
- Well-groomed, says, "Too tired to put on makeup"

Coping/Stress
- Anxious: "I can't breathe"
- Facial muscles tense; trembling
- Expresses concerns about work: "I'll never get caught up"

Value/Belief
- Catholic
- No special practices desired except anointing of the sick
- Middle-class, professional orientation
- No wish to see chaplain or priest at present

Medication/History
- Synthroid 0.1 mg per day
- Client has history of appendectomy, partial thyroidectomy

Nursing Physical Assessment
- 28 years old
- Height 158 cm (5 ft, 2 in); weight 56 kg (125 lb)
- TPR 39.4C, 92, 28
- Radial pulses weak, regular
- Blood pressure 122/80 sitting
- Skin hot and pale, cheeks flushed
- Mucous membranes dry and pale
- Respirations shallow; chest expansion < 3 cm
- Cough productive of small amounts of pale pink sputum
- Inspiratory crackles auscultated throughout right upper and lower chest
- Diminished breath sounds on right side
- Abdomen soft, not distended
- Old surgical scars: anterior neck, RLQ abdomen
- Diaphoretic

- Genitourinary system
- Reproductive system
- Immune system.

Maslow's Hierarchy of Needs

Maslow's hierarchy of needs clusters data pertaining to the following:

- Physiologic needs (survival needs)
- Safety and security needs
- Love and belonging needs
- Self-esteem needs
- Self-actualization needs.

See Chapter 12 ⚭ for details.

Developmental Theories

Several physical, psychosocial, cognitive, and moral developmental theories may be used by the nurse in specific situations. Examples include the following:

- Havighurst's age periods and developmental tasks
- Freud's five stages of development
- Erikson's eight stages of development
- Piaget's phases of cognitive development
- Kohlberg's stages of moral development.

See Chapter 21 ⚭ for additional information.

TABLE 16–6 Validating Assessment Data

Guidelines	Example
Compare subjective and objective data to verify the client's statements with your observations.	Client's perceptions of "feeling hot" need to be compared with measurement of the body temperature.
Clarify any ambiguous or vague statements.	*Client:* "I've felt sick on and off for 6 weeks."
	Nurse: "Describe what your sickness is like. Tell me what you mean by 'on and off'."
Be sure your data consist of cues and not inferences.	*Observation:* Dry skin and reduced tissue turgor
	Inference: Dehydration
	Action: Collect additional data that are needed to make the inference in the diagnosing phase. For example, determine the client's fluid intake, amount and appearance of urine, and blood pressure.
Double-check data that are extremely abnormal.	*Observation:* A resting pulse of 30 beats per minute or a blood pressure of 210/95
	Action: Repeat the measurement. Use another piece of equipment as needed to confirm abnormalities, or ask someone else to collect the same data.
Determine the presence of factors that may interfere with accurate measurement.	A crying infant will have an abnormal respiratory rate and will need quieting before accurate assessment can be made.
Use references (textbooks, journals, research reports) to explain phenomena.	A nurse considers tiny purple or bluish-black swollen areas under the tongue of an elderly client to be abnormal until reading about physical changes of aging. Such varicosities are common.

VALIDATING DATA

The information gathered during the assessment phase must be complete, factual, and accurate because the nursing diagnoses and interventions are based on this information. **Validation** is the act of "double-checking" or verifying data to confirm that it is accurate and factual. Validating data helps the nurse complete these tasks:

- Ensure that assessment information is complete.
- Ensure that objective and related subjective data agree.
- Obtain additional information that may have been overlooked.
- Differentiate between cues and inferences. **Cues** are subjective or objective data that can be directly observed by the nurse; that is, what the client says or what the nurse can see, hear, feel, smell, or measure. **Inferences** are the nurse's interpretation or conclusions made based on the cues (e.g., a nurse observes the cues that an incision is red, hot, and swollen; the nurse makes the inference that the incision is infected).
- Avoid jumping to conclusions and focusing in the wrong direction to identify problems.

Not all data require validation. For example, data such as height, weight, birth date, and most laboratory studies that can be measured with an accurate scale can be accepted as factual. As a rule, the nurse validates data when there are discrepancies between data obtained in the nursing interview (subjective data) and the physical examination (objective data), or when the client's statements differ at different times in the assessment. Guidelines for validating data are shown in Table 16–6.

To collect data accurately, nurses need to be aware of their own biases, values, and beliefs and to separate fact from inference, interpretation, and assumption (see Chapter 15). 🔗 For example, a nurse seeing a man holding his arm to his chest might assume that he is experiencing chest pain, when in fact he has a painful hand.

To build an accurate database, nurses must validate assumptions regarding the client's physical or emotional behavior. In the previous example, the nurse should ask the client why he is holding his arm to his chest. The client's response may validate the nurse's assumptions or prompt further questioning. Figure 16–4 indicates that the nurse auscultated Amanda Aquilini's heart and lungs to validate her statement that she had "lung pain" and "shortness of breath" on exertion. Failure to validate assumptions can lead to an inaccurate or incomplete nursing assessment.

DOCUMENTING DATA

To complete the assessment phase, the nurse records client data. Accurate documentation is essential and should include all data collected about the client's health status. Data are recorded in a factual manner and not interpreted by the nurse. For example, the nurse records the client's breakfast intake (objective data) as "coffee 240 mL, juice 120 mL, 1 egg, and 1 slice of toast," rather than as "appetite good" (a judgment). A judgment or conclusion such as "appetite good" or "normal appetite" may have different meanings for different people. To increase accuracy, the nurse records subjective data in the client's own words. Restating in other words what someone says increases the chance of changing the original meaning (see Chapter 20). 🔗

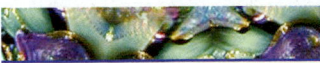

Focus on Critical Thinking

Eighty-two-year-old Ms. T. is in the hospital for hip replacement surgery.

1. What are the key areas of information to obtain regarding her past history?
2. Which physiologic systems are the most important for data collection before her surgery?

3. What exactly would you say to her to determine if someone will be at home to assist her after discharge?
4. Which other sources of data might be appropriate to access in her case?

See Critical Thinking Possibilities in Appendix A.

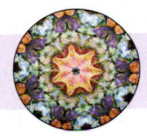 # Chapter Review

EXPLORE MediaLink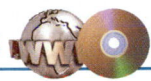

NCLEX review questions, case studies, MediaLink applications, and other interactive resources for this chapter can be found on the Companion Website at www.prenhall.com/kozier. Click on Chapter 16 to select the activities for this chapter.

For animations, more NCLEX review questions, and an audio glossary, access the Student CD-ROM accompanying this textbook.

Chapter Highlights

- The nursing process is a systematic, rational method of planning and providing individualized nursing care for individuals, families, groups, and communities.
- The goals of the nursing process are to identify a client's actual or potential health care needs, to establish plans to meet the identified needs, and to deliver and evaluate specific nursing interventions to meet those needs.
- The nursing process can be used in all health care settings; it is cyclic and dynamic, client centered, interpersonal and collaborative, universally applicable, and focuses on problem solving and decision making.
- The nursing process is organized into five interrelated, interdependent phases: assessing, diagnosing, planning, implementing, and evaluating.
- Assessing involves collecting, organizing, validating, and recording data.
- Diagnosing is the process of making a clinical judgment (nursing diagnosis) about a client's potential or actual health problems.
- Planning involves setting priorities, writing goals/desired outcomes, and establishing a written plan for nursing interventions.
- Implementing is carrying out the nursing interventions. It incorporates all the activities performed to promote health, prevent complications, treat present problems, and facilitate the client's coping with chronic alterations in health status.
- Evaluating is the process of comparing client responses to preselected outcomes to determine whether goals have been met. It includes review and modification of the care plan.

- Assessment involves active participation by the client and nurse in obtaining subjective and objective data about the client's health status.
- The client is the primary source of data. Secondary sources are family, friends, health team members, the health record, and pertinent literature.
- Subjective data are the client's personal perceptions, often gathered during the nursing health history.
- Objective data (e.g., data observed and collected during the physical examination) are detectable by an observer.
- The primary methods of data collection are observing, interviewing, and examining.
- Observation is a conscious, deliberate skill involving use of the senses.
- The nurse uses a combination of directive and nondirective interviewing (including closed and open-ended questions) to obtain the nursing health history.
- Nursing models provide formats for collecting and organizing client data.
- The nursing assessment must be complete and accurate because nursing diagnoses and interventions are based on this information.
- Some data must be validated. Subjective data can be used to validate objective data, and vice versa. Primary and secondary data can also be used to validate each other.
- Data must be recorded in a factual manner, without interpretation or inferences.

Review Questions

16–1 The phase of the nursing process known as *nursing diagnosis* or *diagnosing* may also be referred to as
   a. analysis
   b. defining
   c. interpreting
   d. determination

16–2 During the assessment phase of the nursing process, the nurse would
   a. propose hypotheses
   b. generate desired outcomes
   c. validate data
   d. document care

16–3 Which of the following is secondary subjective data?
   a. The nurse measures a weight loss of 10 pounds since the last clinic visit.
   b. Spouse states the client has lost all appetite.
   c. The nurse palpates edema in lower extremities.
   d. Client states severe pain when walking up stairs.

16–4 The nurse wishes to determine the client's feelings about a recent diagnosis. Which interview question is most likely to elicit this information?
   a. "What did the doctor tell you about your diagnosis?"
   b. "Are you worried about your diagnosis?"
   c. "Tell me how you are reacting to the diagnosis."
   d. "How has your family taken the diagnosis?"

16–5 Use of a conceptual or theoretical framework for collecting and organizing assessment data helps to ensure that the nurse
   a. can correlate the data with other members of the health care team.
   b. can demonstrate cost-effective care.
   c. can use creativity and intuition in creating a plan of care.
   d. includes all necessary information for a thorough appraisal.

Readings and References

Suggested Readings

Carroll-Johnson, R. M. (2001). Learning to think. *Nursing Diagnosis, 12*(2), 43–44.
   This article describes the author's view of the importance of critical thinking in the nursing process as it relates to the formulation of accurate nursing diagnoses.

Cameron, J. I. (2000). Facilitating data collection in stroke patients and elderly—response. *Stroke, 31,* 3081–3082.
   In this letter to the editor regarding an article previously published on the assessment of quality of life following stroke, the author presents the viewpoint that the original authors failed to adequately describe how best to collect data from this unique group of clients. Specific suggestions on ways to enhance the chances of obtaining the desired data are presented.

Related Research

Brooks, N., Magee, P., Bhatti, G., Briggs, C., Buckley, S., Guthrie, et al. (2000). Asian patients' perspective on the communication facilities provided in a large inner city hospital. *Journal of Clinical Nursing, 9,* 706–712.

References

American Nurses Association. (1998). *Standards of clinical nursing practice* (2nd ed.). Kansas City, MO: Author.

Gordon, M. (2002). *Manual of nursing diagnosis* (10th ed.). St. Louis, MO: Mosby.

Hall, L. (1955, June). Quality of nursing care. *Public Health News.* Newark, NJ: State Department of Health.

Johnson, D. E. (1959). A philosophy of nursing. *Nursing Outlook, 7,* 198–200.

Joint Commission on Accreditation of Healthcare Organizations. (2001). *Accreditation manual for hospitals.* Chicago: Author.

O'Carroll, E. (2001, March 1). Getting too close (or too far) for comfort. Retrieved February 23, 2003, from http://travel.boston.com.columns/sl/030502_close.html

Orem, D. E., Taylor, S. G., & Renpenning, K. M. (2000). *Nursing: Concepts of practice* (6th ed.). St. Louis, MO: Mosby.

Orlando, I. (1961). *The dynamic nurse–patient relationship.* New York: Putnam.

Roy, C., & Andrews, H. A. (1999). *The Roy adaptation model: The definitive statement* (2nd ed.). Upper Saddle River, NJ: Prentice Hall.

Stewart, C. J., & Cash, W. B., Jr. (2002). *Interviewing principles and practices* (10th ed.). New York: McGraw-Hill.

Wiedenbach, E. (1963). The helping art of nursing. *American Journal of Nursing, 63*(11), 54.

Wilkinson, J. M. (2001). *Nursing process & critical thinking* (3rd ed.). Upper Saddle River, NJ: Prentice Hall.

Selected Bibliography

Ackley, B. J., & Ladwig, G. B. (2002). *Nursing diagnosis handbook: A guide to planning care* (5th ed.). St. Louis, MO: Mosby.

Alfaro-LeFevre. (2001). *Applying the nursing process: Promoting collaborative care* (5th ed.). Philadelphia: Lippincott Williams & Wilkins.

Duffy, M. M., & Alexander, A. (1999). Overcoming language barriers for non-English speaking patients. *ANNA Journal, 26,* 507–510, 528.

Gardner, P. (2002). *Nursing process.* Albany, NY: Delmar.

Johnson, M., Maas, M., & Moorhead, S. (Eds.). (2000). *Nursing outcomes classification (NOC)* (2nd ed.). St. Louis, MO: Mosby.

McCloskey, J. C., Bulechek, G. B. (Eds.). (2000). *Nursing interventions classification (NIC)* (3rd ed.). St. Louis: Mosby.

McCloskey, J. C., Bulechek, G. B., Dochterman, J., & Maas, M. (Eds.). (2000). *Nursing diagnoses, outcomes, and interventions: NANDA, NOC and NIC linkages.* St. Louis, MO: Mosby.

NANDA International. (2003). NANDA *nursing diagnoses: Definitions and classification 2003-2004.* Philadelphia: Author.

Pakieser, R. A., & McNamee, M. (1999). How to work with an interpreter. *Journal of Continuing Education in Nursing, 30,* 71–74.

Sparks, S. M., & Taylor, C. M. (2001). *Nursing diagnostic reference manual* (5th ed.). Springhouse, PA: Springhouse.

Wilkinson, J. M. (2000). *Nursing diagnosis handbook with NIC interventions and NOC outcomes* (7th ed.). Upper Saddle River, NJ: Prentice Hall Health.

CHAPTER 17

DIAGNOSING

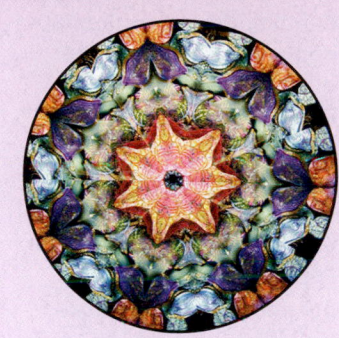

LEARNING OUTCOMES

After completing this chapter, you will be able to:

- Differentiate various types of nursing diagnoses.
- Identify the components of a nursing diagnosis.
- Compare nursing diagnoses, medical diagnoses, and collaborative problems.
- Identify basic steps in the diagnostic process.
- Describe various formats for writing nursing diagnoses.
- Describe the characteristics of a nursing diagnosis.
- List common errors in writing diagnostic statements.
- Describe the evolution of the nursing diagnosis movement, including work currently in progress.
- List advantages of a taxonomy of nursing diagnoses.

MediaLink

www.prenhall.com/kozier

Additional resources for this chapter can be found on the Student CD-ROM accompanying this textbook, and on the Companion Website at www.prenhall.com/kozier. Click on Chapter 17 to select the activities for this chapter.

CD-ROM
- Audio Glossary
- NCLEX Review

Companion Website
- Additional NCLEX Review
- Case Study:
    Selecting Nursing Diagnoses for Client with Pneumonia
- MediaLink Application:
    Resources for a Chronically Ill Child
- Links to Resources

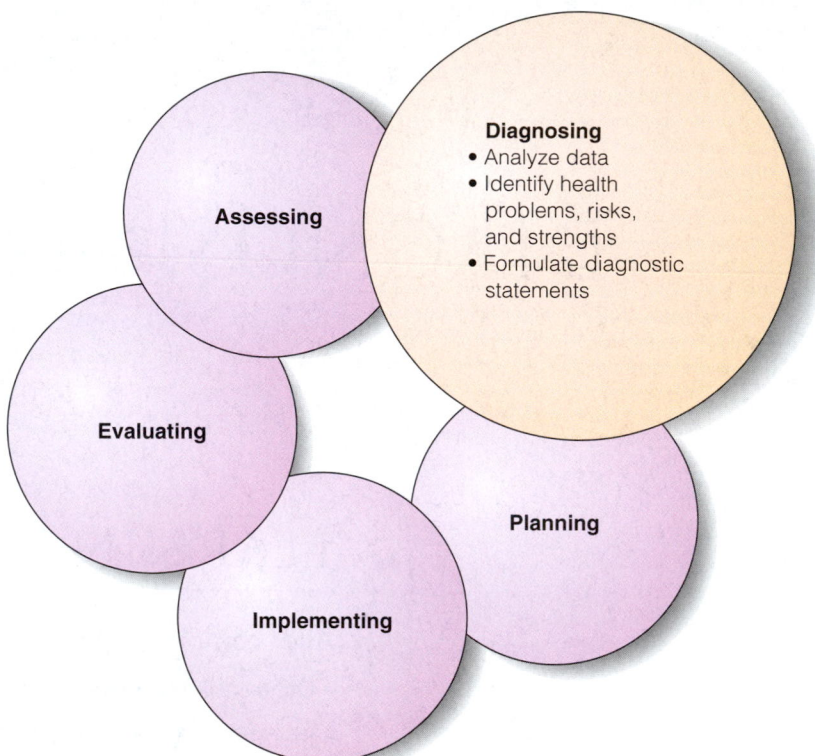

Figure 17–1 ■ Diagnosing. The pivotal second phase of the nursing process, in which the nurse interprets assessment data, identifies client strengths and health problems, and formulates diagnostic statements.

Diagnosing is the second phase of the nursing process. In this phase, nurses use critical-thinking skills to interpret assessment data and identify client strengths and problems. Diagnosing is a pivotal step in the nursing process. All activities preceding this phase are directed toward formulating the nursing diagnoses; all the care-planning activities following this phase are based on the nursing diagnoses (see Figure 17–1 ■).

The identification and development of nursing diagnoses began formally in 1973, when two faculty members of Saint Louis University, Kristine Gebbie and Mary Ann Lavin, perceived a need to identify nurses' roles in an ambulatory care setting. The First National Conference to identify nursing diagnoses was sponsored by the Saint Louis University School of Nursing and Allied Health Professions in 1973. Subsequent national conferences occurred in 1975, 1980, and every 2 years thereafter.

International recognition came with the First Canadian Conference in Toronto in 1977 and the International Nursing Conference in May 1987 in Calgary, Alberta, Canada. In 1982, the conference group accepted the name North American Nursing Diagnosis Association (NANDA), recognizing the participation and contributions of nurses in the United States and Canada.

The purpose of NANDA is to define, refine, and promote a taxonomy of nursing diagnostic terminology of general use to professional nurses. A **taxonomy** is a classification system or set of categories arranged on the basis of a single principle or set of principles. The members of NANDA include staff nurses, clinical specialists, faculty, directors of nursing, deans, theorists, and researchers. The group has currently approved more than 150 nursing diagnosis labels for clinical use and testing. In 2000, Taxonomy I was revised and is now referred to as Taxonomy II (see the list in Appendix D on page 1445).

NANDA NURSING DIAGNOSES

To use the concept of nursing diagnoses effectively in generating and completing a nursing care plan, the nurse must be familiar with the definitions of terms used, the types, and the components of nursing diagnoses.

Definitions

The term *diagnosing* refers to the reasoning process, whereas the term **diagnosis** is a statement or conclusion regarding the nature of a phenomenon. The standardized NANDA names for the diagnoses are called **diagnostic labels;** and the client's problem statement, consisting of the diagnostic label plus **etiology** (causal relationship between a problem and its related or risk factors), is called a **nursing diagnosis.**

In 1990, NANDA adopted an official working definition of nursing diagnosis: "... a clinical judgment about individual, family, or community responses to actual and potential health problems/life processes. Nursing diagnoses provide the basis for selection of nursing interventions to achieve outcomes for which the nurse is accountable" (as cited in NANDA International, 2003, p. 251). This definition implies the following:

- Professional nurses (registered nurses) are responsible for making nursing diagnoses, even though other nursing personnel may contribute data to the process of diagnosing and may implement specified nursing care. The American Nurses Association *Standards of Clinical Nursing Practice* (1998) states that nurses are accountable for this phase of the nursing process. The Joint Commission on Accreditation of Healthcare Organizations (JCAHO) requires evidence of nursing diagnoses in clients' medical records as well (JCAHO, 2001).
- The domain of nursing diagnosis includes only those health states that nurses are educated and licensed to treat. For example, nurses are not educated to diagnose or treat diseases such as diabetes mellitus; this task is defined legally as within the practice of medicine. Yet nurses can diagnose and treat *Deficient Knowledge, Ineffective Coping,* or *Imbalanced Nutrition,* all of which may accompany diabetes mellitus.
- A nursing diagnosis is a judgment made only after thorough, systematic data collection.
- Nursing diagnoses describe a continuum of health states: deviations from health, presence of risk factors, and areas of enhanced personal growth.

Types of Nursing Diagnoses

The five types of nursing diagnoses are actual, risk, wellness, possible, and syndrome.

1. An *actual diagnosis* is a client problem that is present at the time of the nursing assessment. Examples are *Ineffective Breathing Pattern* and *Anxiety.* An actual nursing diagnosis is based on the presence of associated signs and symptoms.
2. A **risk nursing diagnosis** is a clinical judgment that a problem does not exist, but the presence of **risk factors** indicates that a problem is likely to develop unless nurses intervene. For example, all people admitted to a hospital have some possibility of acquiring an infection; however, a client with diabetes or a compromised immune system is at higher risk than others. Therefore, the nurse would ap-

propriately use the label *Risk for Infection* to describe the client's health status.

3. A **wellness diagnosis** "Describes human responses to levels of wellness in an individual, family or community that have a readiness for enhancement" (NANDA International, 2003, p. 263). Examples of wellness diagnosis would be *Readiness for Enhanced Spiritual Well-Being* or *Readiness for Enhanced Family Coping.*
4. A **possible nursing diagnosis** is one in which evidence about a health problem is incomplete or unclear. A possible diagnosis requires more data either to support or to refute it. For example, an elderly widow who lives alone is admitted to the hospital. The nurse notices that she has no visitors and is pleased with attention and conversation from the nursing staff. Until more data are collected, the nurse may write a nursing diagnosis of *Possible Social Isolation* related to unknown etiology.
5. A **syndrome diagnosis** is a diagnosis that is associated with a cluster of other diagnoses (Alfaro-LeFevre, 1998). Currently six syndrome diagnoses are on the NANDA International list. *Risk for Disuse Syndrome,* for example, may be experienced by long-term bedridden clients. Clusters of diagnoses associated with this syndrome include *Impaired Physical Mobility, Risk for Impaired Tissue Integrity, Risk for Activity Intolerance, Risk for Constipation, Risk for Infection, Risk for Injury, Risk for Powerlessness, Impaired Gas Exchange,* and so on.

Components of a NANDA Nursing Diagnosis

A nursing diagnosis has three components: (1) the problem and its definition, (2) the etiology, and (3) the defining characteristics. Each component serves a specific purpose.

Problem (Diagnostic Label) and Definition

The problem statement, or diagnostic label, describes the client's health problem or response for which nursing therapy is given. It describes the client's health status clearly and concisely in a few words. The purpose of the diagnostic label is to direct the formation of client goals and desired outcomes. It may also suggest some nursing interventions.

To be clinically useful, diagnostic labels need to be specific; when the word *Specify* follows a NANDA label, the nurse states the area in which the problem occurs, for example, *Deficient Knowledge (Medications)* or *Deficient Knowledge (Dietary Adjustments).*

Qualifiers are words that have been added to some NANDA labels to give additional meaning to the diagnostic statement; for example:

- *Deficient* (inadequate in amount, quality, or degree; not sufficient; incomplete)
- *Impaired* (made worse, weakened, damaged, reduced, deteriorated)
- *Decreased* (lesser in size, amount, or degree)

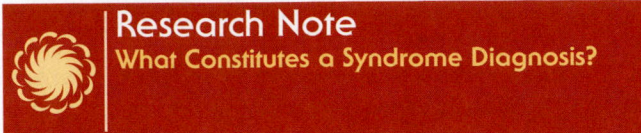

Research Note
What Constitutes a Syndrome Diagnosis?

Only a few of the nursing diagnoses approved by NANDA are termed *syndromes*. The authors of a descriptive study (Cruz & Pimenta, 2001) aimed to establish chronic pain as a syndrome rather than as a single nursing diagnosis. One of the elements of a syndrome is that it embodies a group of diagnoses. In their study, the authors interviewed and examined 114 patients with pain that had lasted at least 3 months, 60% of whom experienced cancer pain and 40% noncancer pain. Based on the data, the authors determined the presence of nursing diagnoses. There were a total of 544 diagnoses for the entire group. A diagnosis was considered part of the syndrome if of high enough frequency (over the 75th percentile) and present in both cancer and noncancer groups. The six diagnoses that met the final criteria were constipation/risk for constipation, disturbed sleep pattern, impaired physical mobility, deficient knowledge, anxiety/fear, and activity intolerance. The authors recognize some significant limitations in this study, especially the difficulties associated with researching very subjective concepts.

Implications: If nursing diagnosis is to become standardized and accepted means of describing client conditions and communicating with other members of the health care team, research must be done to assist in the testing and documentation of the diagnoses. This research project takes a significant step forward in examining the reliability and validity of nursing diagnoses and additionally contributes an international perspective since the work was conducted in Brazil. It also points out some of the great difficulties in studying diagnoses such as pain that rely on client report much more than on objective signs of the sensation. The authors appropriately recommend that the research be replicated and suggest that another study using acute rather than chronic pain may also inform the examination of pain syndrome diagnoses.

Note: From "Chronic Pain: Nursing Diagnosis or Syndrome?" by D. A. L. M. Cruz and C. A. M. Pimenta, 2001, *Nursing Diagnosis, 12,* pp. 117–127.

- *Ineffective* (not producing the desired effect)
- *Compromised* (to make vulnerable to threat).

Each diagnostic label approved by NANDA carries a definition that clarifies its meaning. For example, the definition of the diagnostic label *Activity Intolerance* is shown in Table 17–1.

Etiology (Related Factors and Risk Factors)

The etiology component of a nursing diagnosis identifies one or more probable causes of the health problem, gives direction to the required nursing therapy, and enables the nurse to individualize the client's care. As shown in Table 17–1, the probable causes of *Activity Intolerance* include sedentary lifestyle, generalized weakness, and so on. Differentiating among possible causes in the nursing diagnosis is essential because each may require different nursing interventions. Table 17–2 provides examples of problems that have different etiologies and therefore require different interventions.

Defining Characteristics

Defining characteristics are the cluster of signs and symptoms that indicate the presence of a particular diagnostic label. For actual nursing diagnoses, the defining characteristics are the client's signs and symptoms. For risk nursing diagnoses, no subjective and objective signs are present. Thus the factors that cause the client to be more than "normally" vulnerable to the problem form the etiology of a risk nursing diagnosis.

The NANDA lists of defining characteristics are still being developed and refined. Characteristics are listed separately according to whether they are subjective or objective in nature.

Differentiating Nursing Diagnoses from Medical Diagnoses

A nursing diagnosis is a statement of nursing judgment and refers to a condition that nurses are licensed to treat. A medical diagnosis is made by a physician and refers to a condition that only a physician can treat. Medical diagnoses refer to disease

TABLE 17–1 Components of a Nursing Diagnosis Label

Diagnosis and Definition	Etiology/Related Factors	Defining Characteristics
Activity Intolerance: Insufficient physiological or psychological energy to endure or complete required or desired daily activities	Bedrest or immobility Generalized weakness Imbalance between oxygen supply/demand Sedentary life style	Verbal report of fatigue or weakness Abnormal heart rate or blood pressure response to activity Electrocardiographic changes reflecting arrhythmias or ischemia Exertional discomfort or dyspnea

Note: From *NANDA Nursing Diagnoses: Definitions and Classification, 2003–2004* (p. 3), by NANDA International, 2003, Philadelphia: Author. Reprinted with permission.

TABLE 17–2 Examples of Nursing Interventions to Address Different Etiologies

Diagnostic Label (Problem)	Client	Etiology	Example of Nursing Interventions
Constipation	Al Martinez	Long-term laxative use	Work with Mr. Martinez to develop a plan for gradual withdrawal from the laxatives; teach components of a high-fiber diet.
	Jerry Wong	Inactivity and insufficient fluid intake	Help Mr. Wong develop an exercise regimen that he can follow at home; obtain information about his daily schedule and types of fluids he likes; help Mr. Wong develop a plan for including sufficient amounts of fluids in his diet.
Ineffective Breastfeeding	Zoe James	Breast engorgement	Teach Ms. James to massage her breasts before feeding; use hot packs or hot shower before nursing infant.
	Jenny King	Inexperience and lack of knowledge	Teach Ms. King to feed infant on demand; show her how to be sure infant is sucking and swallowing; and demonstrate different holding positions for feedings.

processes—specific pathophysiologic responses that are fairly uniform from one client to another. In contrast, nursing diagnoses describe a client's physical, sociocultural, psychologic, and spiritual responses to an illness or a health problem. See how these responses vary among individuals:

> Seventy-year-old Mary Cain and 20-year-old Kristi Vidan both have rheumatoid arthritis. Their disease processes are much the same. X-ray studies show that in both clients, the extent of inflammation and the number of joints involved are similar, and both clients experience almost constant pain. Ms. Cain views her condition as part of the aging process and is responding with acceptance. Ms. Vidan, however, is responding with anger and hostility because she views her disease as a threat to her personal identity, role performance, and self-esteem.

A client's medical diagnosis remains the same for as long as the disease process is present, but nursing diagnoses change as the client's responses change. Ms. Vidan's response to her illness may change over time to become more similar to that of Ms. Cain.

Nurses have responsibilities related to both medical and nursing diagnoses. Nursing diagnoses relate to the nurse's **independent functions,** that is, the areas of health care that are unique to nursing and separate and distinct from medical management.

Nurses may not prescribe all the care for a nursing diagnosis, but if the problem is a nursing diagnosis, the nurse can prescribe most of the interventions needed for prevention or resolution. For example, most clients with a nursing diagnosis of *Pain* have medical orders for analgesics, but many independent nursing interventions can also alleviate pain (e.g., guided imagery or teaching a client to "splint" an incision). With regard to medical diagnoses, nurses are obligated to carry out physician-prescribed therapies and treatments, that is, **dependent functions.** See Chapter 18 ⊂⊃ for a discussion of independent and dependent nursing interventions.

Differentiating Nursing Diagnoses from Collaborative Problems

A collaborative problem is a type of potential problem that nurses manage using both independent and physician-prescribed interventions. Independent nursing interventions for a collaborative problem focus mainly on monitoring the client's condition and preventing development of the potential complication. Definitive treatment of the condition requires both medical and nursing interventions.

Collaborative problems tend to be present when a particular disease or treatment is present; that is, each disease or treatment has specific complications that are always associated with it. For example, a statement of collaborative problems is "Potential complication of pneumonia: atelectasis, respiratory failure, pleural effusion, pericarditis, and meningitis."

Nursing diagnoses, by contrast, involve human responses, which vary greatly from one person to the next. Therefore, the same set of nursing diagnoses cannot be expected to occur with a particular disease or condition; moreover, a single nursing diagnosis may occur as a response to any number of diseases. For example, all postpartum clients have similar collaborative problems, such as "Potential complication of childbearing: postpartum hemorrhage," but not all new mothers have the same nursing diagnoses. Some might experience *Impaired Parenting* (delayed bonding), but most will not; some might have a *Deficient Knowledge* problem whereas others will not. Table 17–3 provides a comparison of nursing diagnoses, medical problems, and collaborative problems.

THE DIAGNOSTIC PROCESS

The diagnostic process uses the critical-thinking skills of analysis and synthesis. Critical thinking is a cognitive process during which a person reviews data and considers explanations

TABLE 17–3 Comparison of Nursing Diagnoses, Medical Diagnoses, and Collaborative Problems

Category	Nursing Diagnoses	Medical Diagnoses	Collaborative Problems
Example	*Activity Intolerance* related to decreased cardiac output	Myocardial infarction	Potential complication of myocardial infarction: congestive heart failure
Description	Describe human responses to disease process or health problem; consist of a one-, two-, or three-part statement, usually including problem and etiology	Describe disease and pathology; do not consider other human responses; usually consist of not more than three words	Involve human responses—mainly physiologic complications of disease, tests, or treatments; consist of a two-part statement of situation/pathophysiology and the potential complication
Orientation and responsibility for diagnosing	Oriented to the individual; nurses responsible for diagnosing	Oriented to pathology; physician responsible for diagnosing; diagnosis not within the scope of nursing practice	Oriented to pathophysiology; nurses responsible for diagnosing
Treatment orders	Nurse orders most interventions to prevent and treat	Physician orders primary interventions to prevent and treat	Nurse collaborates with physician and other health care professionals to prevent and treat (require medical orders) for definitive treatment
Nursing focus	Treat and prevent	Implement medical orders for treatment and monitor status of condition	Prevent and monitor for onset or status of condition
Nursing actions	Independent	Dependent (primarily)	Some independent actions, but primarily for monitoring and preventing
Duration	Can change frequently	Remains the same while disease is present	Present when disease or situation is present
Classification system	Classification system is developed and being used but is not universally accepted	Well-developed classification system accepted by the medical profession	No universally accepted classification system

before forming an opinion. Analysis is the separation into components, that is, the breaking down of the whole into its parts. Synthesis is the opposite, that is, the putting together of parts into the whole.

The diagnostic process is used continuously by most nurses. An experienced nurse may enter a client's room and immediately observe significant data and draw conclusions about the client. As a result of attaining knowledge, skill, and expertise in the practice setting, the expert nurse may seem to perform these mental processes automatically. Novice nurses, however, need guidelines to understand and formulate nursing diagnoses. The diagnostic process has three steps:

- Analyzing data
- Identifying health problems, risks, and strengths
- Formulating diagnostic statements.

Analyzing Data

In the diagnostic process, analyzing involves the following steps:

1. Compare data against standards (identify significant cues).
2. Cluster cues (generate tentative hypotheses).
3. Identify gaps and inconsistencies.

For experienced nurses, these activities occur continuously rather than sequentially.

Comparing Data with Standards

Nurses draw on knowledge and experience to compare client data to standards and norms and identify significant and relevant cues. A **standard** or **norm** is a generally accepted measure, rule, model, or pattern. The nurse uses a wide range of standards, such as growth and development patterns, normal vital signs, and laboratory values. A cue is considered significant if it does any of the following (Gordon, 2002):

- Points to negative or positive change in a client's health status or pattern. These may be positive or negative. For example, the client states: "I have recently experienced shortness of breath while climbing stairs" or "I have not smoked for 3 months."
- Varies from norms of the client population. The client's pattern may fit within cultural norms but vary from norms of the general society. The client may consider a pattern—for example, eating very small meals and having little appetite—to be normal. This pattern, however, may not be productive and may require further exploration.
- Indicates a developmental delay. To identify significant cues, the nurse must be aware of the normal patterns and changes that occur as the person grows and develops. For example, by age 9 months an infant is usually able to sit alone without support. The infant who has not accomplished this task needs further assessment for possible developmental delays.

TABLE 17–4   Comparing Cues to Standards and Norms

Type of Cue	Client Cues	Standard/Norm
Deviation from population norms	Height is 158 cm (5 ft., 2 in.). Woman with small frame. Weighs 109 kg (240 lbs).	Height and weight tables indicate that the "ideal" weight for a woman 158 cm (5 ft, 2 in.) with a small frame is 49–53 kg (108–121 lbs).
Developmental delay	Child is 17 months old. Parents state child has not yet attempted to speak. Child laughs aloud and makes cooing sounds.	Children usually speak their first word by 10 to 12 months of age.
Changes in client's usual health status	States, "I'm just not hungry these days." Ate only 15% of food on breakfast tray. Has lost 13 kg (30 lbs) in past 3 months.	Client usually eats three balanced meals per day. Adults typically maintain stable weight.
Dysfunctional behavior	Amy's mother reports that Amy has not left her room for 2 days. Amy is age 16. Amy has stopped attending school and has withdrawn from social contact.	Adolescents usually like to be with their peers; social group very important. Functional behavior includes school attendance.
Changes in client's usual behavior	Mrs. Stuart reports that lately her husband angers easily. "Yesterday he even yelled at the dog." "He just seems so tense."	Mr. Stuart is usually relaxed and easygoing. He is friendly and kind to animals.

Table 17–4 lists specific examples of client cues and norms to which they may be compared.

Clustering Cues

Data clustering or grouping cues is a process of determining the relatedness of facts and determining whether any patterns are present, whether the data represent isolated incidents, and whether the data are significant. This is the beginning of synthesis.

The nurse may cluster data inductively (as in Table 17–5) by combining data from different assessment areas to form a pattern. Or the nurse may begin with a framework, such as Gordon's functional health patterns, and cluster the subjective and objective data into the appropriate categories (see Box 16–4, page 272). The latter is a deductive approach to data clustering, or pattern formation.

Experienced nurses may cluster data as they collect and interpret it, as evidenced in remarks or thoughts such as "I'm getting a picture of. . . " or "This cue doesn't fit the picture." The novice nurse does not have the knowledge base or the clinical experience that aids in recognizing cues. Thus the novice must take careful assessment notes, search data for abnormal cues, and use textbook resources for comparing the client's cues with the defining characteristics and etiologic factors of the accepted nursing diagnoses.

Data clustering involves making inferences about the data. The nurse interprets the possible meaning of the cues and labels the cue clusters with tentative diagnostic hypotheses. Data clustering or grouping for Amanda Aquilini is illustrated in Table 17–5, in which data are clustered according to standardized diagnosis labels.

Identifying Gaps and Inconsistencies in Data

Skillful assessment minimizes gaps and inconsistencies in data. However, data analysis should include a final check to ensure that data are complete and correct.

Inconsistencies are conflicting data. Possible sources of conflicting data include measurement error, expectations, and inconsistent or unreliable reports. For example, a nurse may learn from the nursing history that the client reports not having seen a doctor in 15 years, yet during the physical health examination he states, "My doctor takes my blood pressure every year." All inconsistencies must be clarified before a valid pattern can be established. See "Validating Data" in Chapter 16. ∞

Identifying Health Problems, Risks, and Strengths

After data are analyzed, the nurse and client can together identify strengths and problems. This is primarily a decision-making process (see Chapter 15). ∞

Determining Problems and Risks

After grouping and clustering the data, the nurse and client together identify problems that support tentative actual, risk, and possible diagnoses. In addition the nurse must determine whether the client's problem is a nursing diagnosis, medical diagnosis, or collaborative problem. See Figure 17–2 ∎ and Table 17–3.

Significant cues and data clusters for Amanda Aquilini that were extracted from Figure 16–4 on page 270 and Box 16–7 on page 273 ∞ are shown in Table 17–5. In this example, the nurse and client identified eight tentative problems: *Imbalanced*

TABLE 17–5 Formulating Nursing Diagnoses for Amanda Aquilini

Functional Health Pattern	Client Cue Clusters	Inferences (Tentative Identification of Problems)	Formulating Diagnostic Statements
Health perception/ health management			No problem *Strength:* Shows healthy lifestyle, understanding of and compliance with treatment regimens
Nutritional/ metabolic (includes hydration)	"No appetite" since having "cold" Has not eaten today; last fluids at noon today Nauseated × 2 days	*Imbalanced Nutrition: Less than Body Requirements*	*Imbalanced Nutrition: Less than Body Requirements* related to decreased appetite and nausea and increased metabolism (secondary to disease process) *Strength:* Normal weight for height
	Last fluids at noon today Oral temp 39.4C (103F) Skin hot and pale, cheeks flushed Mucous membranes dry Poor skin turgor *Cues from elimination pattern:* Decreased urinary frequency and amount × 2 days	*Deficient Fluid Volume*	*Deficient Fluid Volume* related to intake insufficient to replace fluid loss secondary to fever, diaphoresis, anorexia
Elimination	Decreased urinary frequency and amount × 2 days	Cues consist of elimination data but are actually symptoms of a fluid volume problem in the nutritional/ metabolic functional health pattern	No elimination problem
Activity/exercise	Difficulty sleeping because of cough "Can't breathe lying down"	*Disturbed Sleep Pattern*	*Disturbed Sleep Pattern* related to cough, pain, orthopnea, fever, and diaphoresis
	States "I feel weak" Short of breath on exertion *Cues from cognitive/perceptual pattern:* Responsive but fatigued "I can think OK, just weak" *Cues from cardiovascular pattern:* Radial pulses weak, regular Pulse rate 92	*Activity Intolerance*	*Activity Intolerance* related to general weakness, imbalance between oxygen supply/demand *Strength:* No musculoskeletal impairment, normal energy level is satisfactory, exercises regularly
Cognitive/ perceptual	Reports pain in chest, especially when coughing	*Acute Pain*	*Acute Pain (Chest)* related to cough secondary to pneumonia *Strength:* No cognitive or sensory deficits
	Responsive but fatigued "I can think OK, just weak"	These are cognitive/ perceptual data, but they reflect symptoms of problems in the activity/exercise pattern	
Roles/ relationships	Husband out of town; will be back tomorrow afternoon Child with neighbor until husband returns	*Interrupted Family Processes* related to mother's illness and temporary unavailability of father to provide child care Cues also related to a problem in the coping/ stress pattern	*Risk for Interrupted Family Processes* related to mother's illness and temporary unavailability of father to provide child care *Strength:* Neighbors available and willing to help
Self-perception/ self-concept	Expresses "concern" and "worry" over leaving daughter with neighbors until husband returns	Cue is a symptom of a problem in the coping/ stress pattern	No self- perception/self-concept problem

TABLE 17–5 Formulating Nursing Diagnoses for Amanda Aquilini (continued)

Functional Health Pattern	Client Cue Clusters	Inferences (Tentative Identification of Problems)	Formulating Diagnostic Statements
Coping/stress	Anxious: "I can't breathe" Facial muscles tense; trembling Expresses concerns about work: "I'll never get caught up" *Cues from role/relationship pattern:* Husband out of town; will be back tomorrow afternoon Child with neighbor until husband returns *Cues from self-perception/self-concept patterns:* Expresses "concern" and "worry" over leaving daughter with neighbors	*Anxiety* related to difficulty breathing, inability to work, and child care	*Anxiety* related to difficulty breathing and concerns over work and parenting roles
Medication/history	No significant cues	No problem	No problem
Physical assessment			
• Cardiovascular	Radial pulses weak, regular Pulse rate 92	Cues are symptoms only; symptoms of exercise/rest and oxygenation problems	No cardiovascular problem
• Oxygenation	Skin hot, pale, and moist Respirations shallow; chest expansion, 3 cm Cough productive of small amounts of thick pale pink sputum Inspiratory crackles auscultated throughout right upper and lower lungs Diminished breath sounds on right side Mucous membranes pale, dry	*Ineffective Airway Clearance* related to disease process	*Ineffective Airway Clearance* related to viscous secretions and shallow chest expansion secondary to pain, fluid volume deficit, and fatigue
• Skin	Old surgical scars, anterior neck, RLQ abdomen	No problem now	Old problems; resolved

Nutrition: Less than Body Requirements; Deficient Fluid Volume; Disturbed Sleep Pattern; Activity Intolerance; Acute Pain (Chest); Interrupted Family Processes; Anxiety; and *Ineffective Airway Clearance.*

Note that some data may indicate a possible problem but when clustered with other data, the possible problem disappears. For example, the following data for Amanda Aquilini, "Decreased urinary frequency and amount × 2 days," suggests a possible urinary elimination problem. However, when these data are considered along with data associated with *Deficient Fluid Volume,* the nurse eliminates urinary elimination as a problem.

Determining Strengths

At this stage, the nurse and client also establish the client's strengths, resources, and abilities to cope. Most people have a clearer perception of their problems or weaknesses than of their strengths and assets, which they often take for granted. By taking an inventory of strengths, the client can develop a more well-rounded self-concept and self-image. Strengths can be an aid to mobilizing health and regenerative processes.

A client's strength might be weight that is within the normal range for age and height, thus enabling the client to cope better

with surgery. In another instance, a client's strengths might be absence of allergies and being a nonsmoker.

A client's strengths can be found in the nursing assessment record (health, home life, education, recreation, exercise, work, family and friends, religious beliefs, and sense of humor, for example), the health examination, and the client's records. See Table 17–5 for the strengths identified for Amanda Aquilini.

Formulating Diagnostic Statements

Most nursing diagnoses are written as two-part or three-part statements, but there are variations of these.

Basic Two-Part Statements

The basic two-part statement includes the following:

1. *Problem (P):* statement of the client's response (NANDA label)
2. *Etiology (E):* factors contributing to or probable causes of the responses.

The two parts are joined by the words *related to* rather than *due to.* The phrase *due to* implies that one part causes or is responsible for the other part. By contrast, the phrase *related to*

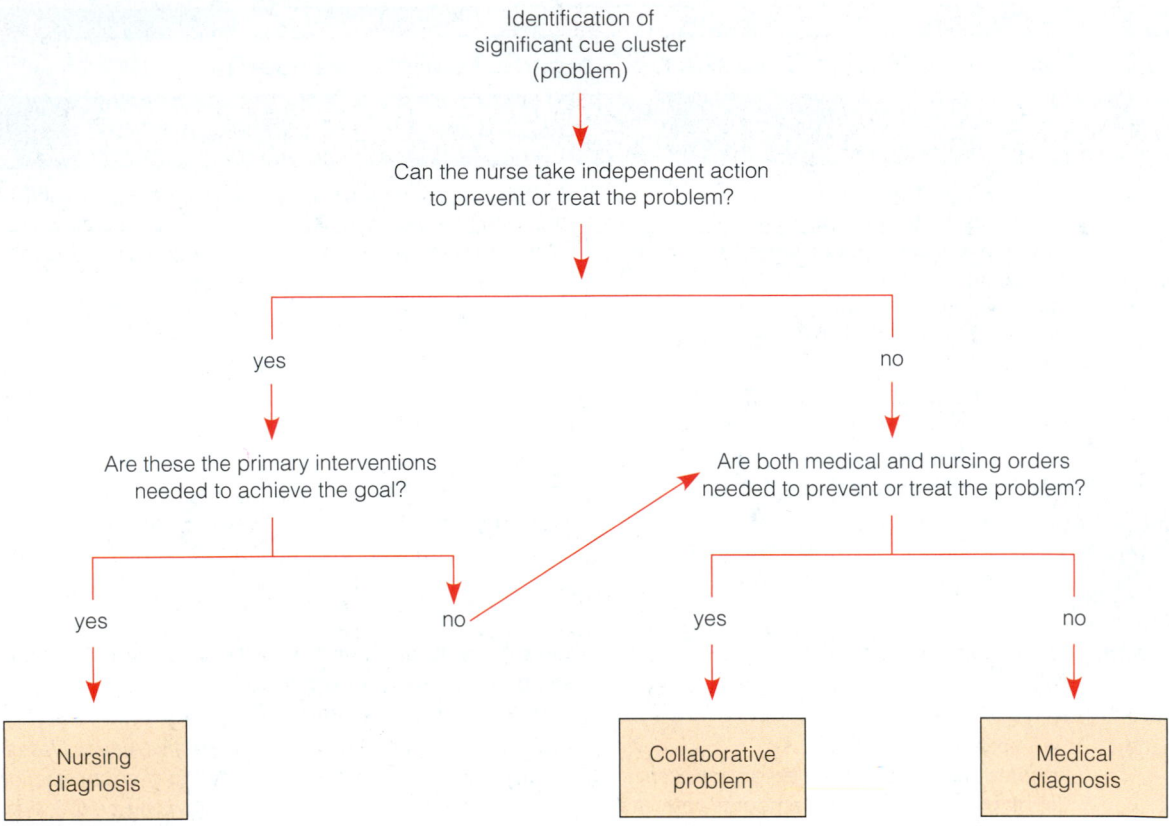

Figure 17–2 ■ Decision tree for differentiating among nursing diagnoses, collaborative problems, and medical diagnoses.

BOX 17–1	■ Basic Two-Part Diagnostic Statement		
Problem	**Related to**	**Etiology**	
Constipation	related to	prolonged laxative use	
Ineffective Breastfeeding	related to	breast engorgement	

merely implies a relationship. Some examples of two-part nursing diagnoses are shown in Box 17–1.

Some NANDA labels contain the word *Specify*. For these, the nurse must add words to indicate the problem more specifically. The format is still a two-part statement, for example, *Noncompliance (Specify). Noncompliance (Diabetic Diet)* related to denial of having disease. For ease in alphabetizing, many NANDA lists are arranged with qualifying words after the main word (e.g., *Infection, Risk for*). Avoid writing diagnostic

statements in that manner; instead, write them as they would be stated in normal conversation (e.g., *Risk for Infection*).

Basic Three-Part Statements

The basic three-part nursing diagnosis statement is called the **PES format** and includes the following:

1. *Problem (P):* statement of the client's response (NANDA label)
2. *Etiology (E):* factors contributing to or probable causes of the response
3. *Signs and symptoms (S):* defining characteristics manifested by the client.

Actual nursing diagnoses can be documented by using the three-part statement (see Box 17–2) because the signs and symptoms have been identified. This format cannot be used for

BOX 17–2	■ Basic Three-Part Diagnostic Statement			
Problem	**Related to**	**Etiology**	**As Manifested by**	**Signs and Symptoms**
Situational Low Self-Esteem	related to (r/t)	rejection by husband	as manifested by (a.m.b.)	hypersensitivity to criticism; states "I don't know if I can manage by myself" and rejects positive feedback

Nutrition and Metabolic Patterns with Related Nursing Diagnoses

HEALTH PERCEPTION HEALTH MANAGEMENT
- Perceived health status
- Perceived health management
- Health care behaviors: health promotion and illness prevention activities, medical treatments, follow-up care

VALUE-BELIEF
- Values, goals, or beliefs (including spirituality) that guide choices or decisions
- Perceived conflicts in values, beliefs, or expectations that are health related

COPING-STRESS-TOLERANCE
- Capacity to resist challenges to self-integrity
- Methods of handling stress
- Support systems
- Perceived ability to control and manage situations

NUTRITIONAL-METABOLIC
- Daily consumption of food and fluids
- Favorite foods
- Use of dietary supplements
- Skin lesions and ability to heal
- Condition of the integument
- Weight, height, temperature

NANDA Nursing Diagnoses
- Risk for Aspiration
- Risk for Imbalanced Body Temperature
- Impaired Dentition
- Feeding Self-Care Deficit
- Fluid Volume Deficit
- Fluid Volume Excess
- Risk for Deficient Fluid Volume
- Hyperthermia
- Hypothermia
- Risk for Infection
- Impaired Oral Mucous Membranes
- Nausea
- Imbalanced Nutrition: Less than Body Requirements
- Imbalanced Nutrition: More than Body Requirements
- Impaired Skin Integrity
- Risk for Impaired Skin Integrity
- Impaired Swallowing
- Ineffective Thermoregulation
- Impaired Tissue Integrity
- Risk For Trauma
- Adult Failure to Thrive

SEXUALITY-REPRODUCTIVE
- Satisfaction with sexuality or sexual relationships
- Reproductive pattern
- Female menstrual and perimeno-pausal history

ELIMINATION
- Patterns of bowel and urinary excretion
- Perceived regularity or irregularity of elimination
- Use of laxatives or routines
- Changes in time, modes, quality or quantity of excretions
- Use of devices for control

ROLE-RELATIONSHIP
- Perception of major roles, relationships, and responsibilities in current life situation
- Satisfaction with or disturbances in roles and relationships

ACTIVITY-EXERCISE
- Patterns of personally relevant exercise, activity, leisure, and recreation
- ADLs which require energy expenditure
- Factors that interfere with the desired pattern (e.g., illness or injury)

SELF-PERCEPTION–SELF-CONCEPT
- Attitudes about self
- Perceived abilities, worth, self-image, emotions
- Body posture and movement, eye contact, voice and speech patterns

SLEEP-REST
- Patterns of sleep and rest-/relaxation in a 24-hr period
- Perceptions of quality and quantity of sleep and rest
- Use of sleep aids and routines

COGNITIVE-PERCEPTUAL
- Adequacy of vision, hearing, taste, touch, smell
- Pain perception and management
- Language, judgment, memory, decisions

Cognitive Perceptual Patterns with Related Nursing Diagnoses

HEALTH PERCEPTION HEALTH MANAGEMENT
- Perceived health status
- Perceived health management
- Health care behaviors: health promotion and illness prevention activities, medical treatments, follow-up care

VALUE-BELIEF
- Values, goals, or beliefs (including spirituality) that guide choices or decisions
- Perceived conflicts in values, beliefs, or expectations that are health related

COPING-STRESS-TOLERANCE
- Capacity to resist challenges to self-integrity
- Methods of handling stress
- Support systems
- Perceived ability to control and manage situations

NUTRITIONAL-METABOLIC
- Daily consumption of food and fluids
- Favorite foods
- Use of dietary supplements
- Skin lesions and ability to heal
- Condition of the integument
- Weight, height, temperature

NANDA Nursing Diagnoses

- Acute Confusion
- Decreased Intracranial Adaptive Capacity
- Autonomic Dysreflexia
- Risk for Autonomic Dysreflexia
- Chronic Confusion
- Impaired Verbal Communication
- Acute Pain
- Chronic Pain
- Impaired Memory
- Unilateral Neglect
- Risk for Peripheral Neurovascular Dysfunction
- Risk for Post-Trauma Syndrome
- Ineffective Protection
- Disturbed Sensory Perception
- Disturbed Thought Processes
- Decisional Conflict
- Risk for Trauma
- Wandering
- Unilateral Neglect
- Impaired Environmental Interpretation Syndrome

SEXUALITY-REPRODUCTIVE
- Satisfaction with sexuality or sexual relationships
- Reproductive pattern
- Female menstrual and perimeno-pausal history

ELIMINATION
- Patterns of bowel and urinary excretion
- Perceived regularity or irregularity of elimination
- Use of laxatives or routines
- Changes in time, modes, quality or quantity of excretions
- Use of devices for control

ROLE-RELATIONSHIP
- Perception of major roles, relationships, and responsibilities in current life situation
- Satisfaction with or disturbances in roles and relationships

ACTIVITY-EXERCISE
- Patterns of personally relevant exercise, activity, leisure, and recreation
- ADLs which require energy expenditure
- Factors that interfere with the desired pattern (e.g., illness or injury)

SELF-PERCEPTION–SELF-CONCEPT
- Attitudes about self
- Perceived abilities, worth, self-image, emotions
- Body posture and movement, eye contact, voice and speech patterns

SLEEP-REST
- Patterns of sleep and rest-/relaxation in a 24-hr period
- Perceptions of quality and quantity of sleep and rest
- Use of sleep aids and routines

COGNITIVE-PERCEPTUAL
- Adequacy of vision, hearing, taste, touch, smell
- Pain perception and management
- Language, judgment, memory, decisions

Activity and Exercise Patterns with Related Nursing Diagnoses

HEALTH PERCEPTION HEALTH MANAGEMENT
- Perceived health status
- Perceived health management
- Health care behaviors: health promotion and illness prevention activities, medical treatments, follow-up care

VALUE-BELIEF
- Values, goals, or beliefs (including spirituality) that guide choices or decisions
- Perceived conflicts in values, beliefs, or expectations that are health related

COPING-STRESS-TOLERANCE
- Capacity to resist challenges to self-integrity
- Methods of handling stress
- Support systems
- Perceived ability to control and manage situations

NUTRITIONAL-METABOLIC
- Daily consumption of food and fluids
- Favorite foods
- Use of dietary supplements
- Skin lesions and ability to heal
- Condition of the integument
- Weight, height, temperature

NANDA Nursing Diagnoses
- Activity Intolerance
- Risk for Activity Intolerance
- Bathing/Hygiene Self-Care Deficit
- Dressing/Grooming Self-Care Deficit
- Impaired Bed Mobility
- Risk for Disuse Syndrome
- Deficient Diversional Activity
- Fatigue
- Risk for Falls
- Impaired Home Maintenance
- Impaired Physical Mobility
- Impaired Wheelchair Mobility
- Impaired Transfer Ability
- Impaired Walking
- Delayed Surgical Recovery
- Decreased Cardiac Output
- Ineffective Breathing Pattern
- Ineffective Airway Clearance
- Impaired Gas Exchange
- Risk for Peripheral Neurovascular Dysfunction
- Impaired Tissue Perfusion
- Ineffective Tissue Perfusion
- Impaired Spontaneous Ventilation
- Dysfunctional Ventilatory Weaning Response

SEXUALITY-REPRODUCTIVE
- Satisfaction with sexuality or sexual relationships
- Reproductive pattern
- Female menstrual and perimenopausal history

ELIMINATION
- Patterns of bowel and urinary excretion
- Perceived regularity or irregularity of elimination
- Use of laxatives or routines
- Changes in time, modes, quality or quantity of excretions
- Use of devices for control

ROLE-RELATIONSHIP
- Perception of major roles, relationships, and responsibilities in current life situation
- Satisfaction with or disturbances in roles and relationships

ACTIVITY-EXERCISE
- Patterns of personally relevant exercise, activity, leisure, and recreation
- ADLs which require energy expenditure
- Factors that interfere with the desired pattern (e.g., illness or injury)

SELF-PERCEPTION–SELF-CONCEPT
- Attitudes about self
- Perceived abilities, worth, self-image, emotions
- Body posture and movement, eye contact, voice and speech patterns

SLEEP-REST
- Patterns of sleep and rest-/relaxation in a 24-hr period
- Perceptions of quality and quantity of sleep and rest
- Use of sleep aids and routines

COGNITIVE-PERCEPTUAL
- Adequacy of vision, hearing, taste, touch, smell
- Pain perception and management
- Language, judgment, memory, decisions

Elimination Patterns with Related Nursing Diagnoses

HEALTH PERCEPTION HEALTH MANAGEMENT
- Perceived health status
- Perceived health management
- Health care behaviors: health promotion and illness prevention activities, medical treatments, follow-up care

VALUE-BELIEF
- Values, goals, or beliefs (including spirituality) that guide choices or decisions
- Perceived conflicts in values, beliefs, or expectations that are health related

COPING-STRESS-TOLERANCE
- Capacity to resist challenges to self-integrity
- Methods of handling stress
- Support systems
- Perceived ability to control and manage situations

NUTRITIONAL-METABOLIC
- Daily consumption of food and fluids
- Favorite foods
- Use of dietary supplements
- Skin lesions and ability to heal
- Condition of the integument
- Weight, height, temperature

NANDA Nursing Diagnoses
- Bowel Incontinence
- Constipation
- Perceived Constipation
- Risk for Constipation
- Diarrhea
- Impaired Urinary Elimination
- Functional Urinary Incontinence
- Reflex Urinary Incontinence
- Stress Urinary Incontinence
- Total Urinary Incontinence
- Urge Urinary Incontinence
- Risk for Urge Urinary Incontinence
- Perceived Constipation
- Urinary Retention
- Self-care Deficit: Toileting

SEXUALITY-REPRODUCTIVE
- Satisfaction with sexuality or sexual relationships
- Reproductive pattern
- Female menstrual and perimeno-pausal history

ELIMINATION
- Patterns of bowel and urinary excretion
- Perceived regularity or irregularity of elimination
- Use of laxatives or routines
- Changes in time, modes, quality or quantity of excretions
- Use of devices for control

ROLE-RELATIONSHIP
- Perception of major roles, relationships, and responsibilities in current life situation
- Satisfaction with or disturbances in roles and relationships

ACTIVITY-EXERCISE
- Patterns of personally relevant exercise, activity, leisure, and recreation
- ADLs which require energy expenditure
- Factors that interfere with the desired pattern (e.g., illness or injury)

SELF-PERCEPTION–SELF-CONCEPT
- Attitudes about self
- Perceived abilities, worth, self-image, emotions
- Body posture and movement, eye contact, voice and speech patterns

SLEEP-REST
- Patterns of sleep and rest-/relaxation in a 24-hr period
- Perceptions of quality and quantity of sleep and rest
- Use of sleep aids and routines

COGNITIVE-PERCEPTUAL
- Adequacy of vision, hearing, taste, touch, smell
- Pain perception and management
- Language, judgment, memory, decisions

Sexuality-Reproductive Patterns with Related Nursing Diagnoses

HEALTH PERCEPTION HEALTH MANAGEMENT
- Perceived health status
- Perceived health management
- Health care behaviors: health promotion and illness prevention activities, medical treatments, follow-up care

VALUE-BELIEF
- Values, goals, or beliefs (including spirituality) that guide choices or decisions
- Perceived conflicts in values, beliefs, or expectations that are health related

COPING-STRESS-TOLERANCE
- Capacity to resist challenges to self-integrity
- Methods of handling stress
- Support systems
- Perceived ability to control and manage situations

NUTRITIONAL-METABOLIC
- Daily consumption of food and fluids
- Favorite foods
- Use of dietary supplements
- Skin lesions and ability to heal
- Condition of the integument
- Weight, height, temperature

NANDA Nursing Diagnoses
- Rape-Trauma Syndrome
- Sexual Dysfunction
- Ineffective Sexuality Patterns

SEXUALITY-REPRODUCTIVE
- Satisfaction with sexuality or sexual relationships
- Reproductive pattern
- Female menstrual and perimeno-pausal history

ELIMINATION
- Patterns of bowel and urinary excretion
- Perceived regularity or irregularity of elimination
- Use of laxatives or routines
- Changes in time, modes, quality or quantity of excretions
- Use of devices for control

ROLE-RELATIONSHIP
- Perception of major roles, relationships, and responsibilities in current life situation
- Satisfaction with or disturbances in roles and relationships

ACTIVITY-EXERCISE
- Patterns of personally relevant exercise, activity, leisure, and recreation
- ADLs which require energy expenditure
- Factors that interfere with the desired pattern (e.g., illness or injury)

SELF-PERCEPTION–SELF-CONCEPT
- Attitudes about self
- Perceived abilities, worth, self-image, emotions
- Body posture and movement, eye contact, voice and speech patterns

SLEEP-REST
- Patterns of sleep and rest-/relaxation in a 24-hr period
- Perceptions of quality and quantity of sleep and rest
- Use of sleep aids and routines

COGNITIVE-PERCEPTUAL
- Adequacy of vision, hearing, taste, touch, smell
- Pain perception and management
- Language, judgment, memory, decisions

FUNCTIONAL HEALTH PATTERNS CONCEPT MAPS

Functional Health Patterns with Related Nursing Diagnoses

HEALTH PERCEPTION HEALTH MANAGEMENT
- Perceived health status
- Perceived health management
- Health care behaviors: health promotion and illness prevention activities, medical treatments, follow-up care

VALUE-BELIEF
- Values, goals, or beliefs (including spirituality) that guide choices or decisions
- Perceived conflicts in values, beliefs, or expectations that are health related

COPING-STRESS-TOLERANCE
- Capacity to resist challenges to self-integrity
- Methods of handling stress
- Support systems
- Perceived ability to control and manage situations

NUTRITIONAL-METABOLIC
- Daily consumption of food and fluids
- Favorite foods
- Use of dietary supplements
- Skin lesions and ability to heal
- Condition of the integument
- Weight, height, temperature

- Latex Allergy Response
- Caregiver Role Strain
- Chronic Sorrow
- Compromised Family Coping
- Death Anxiety
- Anxiety
- Decisional Conflict
- Disturbed Body Image
- Fatigue
- Fear
- Deficient Fluid Volume
- Excess Fluid Volume
- Ineffective Health Maintenance
- Health-seeking Behaviors
- Risk for Infection
- Deficient Knowledge
- Nausea
- Acute Pain
- Chronic Pain
- Risk for Injury
- Powerlessness
- Disturbed Personal Identity
- Ineffective Protection
- Delayed Surgical Recovery
- Self-Care Deficit
- Low Self-esteem
- Disturbed Sleep Pattern
- Ineffective Therapeutic Regimen Management
- Disturbed Thought Process
- Risk for Violence

SEXUALITY-REPRODUCTIVE
- Satisfaction with sexuality or sexual relationships
- Reproductive pattern
- Female menstrual and perimeno-pausal history

ELIMINATION
- Patterns of bowel and urinary excretion
- Perceived regularity or irregularity of elimination
- Use of laxatives or routines
- Changes in time, modes, quality or quantity of excretions
- Use of devices for control

ROLE-RELATIONSHIP
- Perception of major roles, relationships, and responsibilities in current life situation
- Satisfaction with or disturbances in roles and relationships

ACTIVITY-EXERCISE
- Patterns of personally relevant exercise, activity, leisure, and recreation
- ADLs which require energy expenditure
- Factors that interfere with the desired pattern (e.g., illness or injury)

SELF-PERCEPTION–SELF-CONCEPT
- Attitudes about self
- Perceived abilities, worth, self-image, emotions
- Body posture and movement, eye contact, voice and speech patterns

SLEEP-REST
- Patterns of sleep and rest-/relaxation in a 24-hr period
- Perceptions of quality and quantity of sleep and rest
- Use of sleep aids and routines

COGNITIVE-PERCEPTUAL
- Adequacy of vision, hearing, taste, touch, smell
- Pain perception and management
- Language, judgment, memory, decisions

risk diagnoses because the client does not have signs and symptoms of the diagnosis.

The PES format is especially recommended for beginning diagnosticians because the signs and symptoms validate why the diagnosis was chosen and make the problem statement more descriptive.

The disadvantage of the PES format is that it can create very long problem statements, thereby making the problem and etiology unclear. However, because the signs and symptoms can be helpful in planning nursing interventions, they should be easily accessible. To promote access without long problem statements, the nurse can record the signs and symptoms in the nursing notes instead of on the care plan. Another possibility, recommended for students, is to list the signs and symptoms on the care plan below the nursing diagnosis, grouping the subjective (S) and objective (O) data. The signs and symptoms are easily accessible, and the problem and etiology stand out clearly. For example:

Noncompliance (*Diabetic Diet*) related to unresolved anger about diagnosis as manifested by

S— "I forget to take my pills."
 "I can't live without sugar in my food."
O—Weight 98 kg (215 lbs) [gain of 4.5 kg (10 lbs)]
 Blood pressure 190/100

One-Part Statements

Some diagnostic statements, such as wellness diagnoses and syndrome nursing diagnoses, consist of a NANDA label only. As the diagnostic labels are refined they tend to become more specific, so that nursing interventions can be derived from the label itself. Therefore, an etiology may not be needed. For example, adding an etiology to the label *Rape-Trauma Syndrome* does not make the label any more descriptive or useful.

NANDA has specified that any new wellness diagnoses will be developed as one-part statements beginning with the words *Readiness for Enhanced* followed by the desired higher level wellness (for example, *Readiness for Enhanced Parenting*).

Currently the NANDA list includes several wellness diagnoses. Some of these are *Spiritual Well-Being, Effective Breastfeeding, Health-Seeking Behaviors,* and *Anticipatory Grieving.* These are usually accepted as one-part statements but may be made more explicit by adding a descriptor, for example, *Health-Seeking Behaviors* (*Low-Fat Diet*).

Variations of Basic Formats

Variations of the basic one-, two-, and three-part statements include the following:

1. Writing *unknown etiology* when the defining characteristics are present but the nurse does not know the cause or contributing factors. One example is *Noncompliance* (*Medication Regimen*) related to unknown etiology.
2. Using the phrase *complex factors* when there are too many etiologic factors or when they are too complex to state in a brief phrase. The actual causes of chronic low self-esteem, for instance, may be long term and complex, as in the fol-

lowing nursing diagnosis: *Chronic Low Self-Esteem* related to complex factors.
3. Using the word *possible* to describe either the problem or the etiology. When the nurse believes more data are needed about the client's problem or the etiology, the word *possible* is inserted. Examples are *Possible Low Self-Esteem* related to loss of job and rejection by family; *Altered Thought Processes* possibly related to unfamiliar surroundings.
4. Using *secondary to* to divide the etiology into two parts, thereby making the statement more descriptive and useful. The part following *secondary to* is often a pathophysiologic or disease process, as in *Risk for Impaired Skin Integrity* related to decreased peripheral circulation secondary to diabetes.
5. Adding a second part to the general response or NANDA label to make it more precise. For example, the diagnosis *Impaired Skin Integrity* does not indicate the location of the problem. To make this label more specific, the nurse can add a descriptor as follows: *Impaired Skin Integrity* (*Left Lateral Ankle*) related to decreased peripheral circulation.

Collaborative Problems

Carpenito (1997) suggests that all collaborative (multidisciplinary) problems begin with the diagnostic label *Potential Complication* (PC). Nurses should include in the diagnostic statement both the possible complication they are monitoring and the disease or treatment that is present to produce it. For example, if the client has a head injury and could develop increased intracranial pressure, the nurses should write the following:

Potential Complication of Head Injury:
Increased intracranial pressure

When monitoring for a group of complications associated with a disease or pathology, the nurse states the disease and follows it with a list of the complications:

Potential Complication of Pregnancy-Induced Hypertension:
seizures, fetal distress, pulmonary edema, hepatic/renal failure, premature labor, CNS hemorrhage

In some situations an etiology might be helpful in suggesting interventions. Nurses should write the etiology when (a) it clarifies the problem statement, (b) it can be concisely stated, and (c) it helps to suggest nursing actions. See the examples in Box 17–3.

Evaluating the Quality of the Diagnostic Statement

In addition to using the correct format, nurses must consider the content of their diagnostic statements. The statements should, for example, be accurate, concise, descriptive, and specific. The nurse must always validate the diagnostic statements with the client and compare the client's signs and symptoms to the NANDA defining characteristics. For risk problems, the nurse compares the client's risk factors to NANDA risk factors. After writing nursing diagnoses, the nurse checks them against the criteria in Table 17–6.

BOX 17–3 ■ Collaborative Problems			
Disease/Situation	**Complication**	**Related to**	**Etiology**
Potential complication of childbirth:	hemorrhage	related to	uterine atony retained placental fragments bladder distention
Potential complication of diuretic therapy:	arrhythmia	related to	low serum potassium

Avoiding Errors in Diagnostic Reasoning

Some error is inherent in any human undertaking, and diagnosis is no exception. However, it is important that nurses make nursing diagnoses with a high level of accuracy. Nurses can avoid some common errors of reasoning by recognizing them and applying the appropriate critical-thinking skills. Error can occur at any point in the diagnostic process: data collection, data interpretation, and data clustering.

The following suggestions help to minimize diagnostic error:

- *Verify.* Hypothesize possible explanations of the data, but realize that all diagnoses are only tentative until they are verified. Begin and end the diagnostic process by talking with the client and family. When collecting data, ask them what their health problems are and what they believe the causes to be. At the end of the process, ask them to verify your diagnoses.

- *Build a good knowledge base and acquire clinical experience.* Nurses must apply knowledge from many different areas to recognize significant cues and patterns and generate hypotheses about the data. To name only a few, principles from chemistry, anatomy, and pharmacology each help the nurse understand client data in a different way.

- *Have a working knowledge of what is normal.* Nurses need to know the population norms for vital signs, laboratory tests, speech development, breath sounds, and so on. In addition, nurses must determine what is normal for a particular person, taking into account age, physical makeup, lifestyle, culture, and the person's own perception of what is normal. For example, normal blood pressure for adults is in the range of 110/60 to 140/80. However, a nurse might obtain a reading of 90/50 that is perfectly normal for a particular client. The nurse should compare findings to the client's baseline when possible.

TABLE 17–6 Guidelines for Writing a Nursing Diagnostic Statement

Guideline	Correct Statement	Incorrect or Ambiguous Statement
1. State in terms of a problem, not a need.	*Deficient Fluid Volume* (problem) related to fever	*Fluid Replacement* (need) related to fever
2. Word the statement so that it is legally advisable.	*Impaired Skin Integrity* related to immobility (legally acceptable)	*Impaired Skin Integrity* related to improper positioning (implies legal liability)
3. Use nonjudgmental statements.	*Spiritual Distress* related to inability to attend church services secondary to immobility (nonjudgmental)	*Spiritual Distress* related to strict rules necessitating church attendance (judgmental)
4. Make sure that both elements of the statement do not say the same thing.	*Risk for Impaired Skin Integrity* related to immobility	*Impaired Skin Integrity* related to ulceration of sacral area (response and probable cause are the same)
5. Be sure that cause and effect are correctly stated (i.e., the etiology causes the problem or puts the client at risk for the problem).	*Pain: Severe Headache* related to fear of addiction to narcotics	*Pain* related to severe headache
6. Word the diagnosis specifically and precisely to provide direction for planning nursing intervention.	*Impaired Oral Mucous Membrane* related to decreased salivation secondary to radiation of neck (specific)	*Impaired Oral Mucous Membrane* related to noxious agent (vague)
7. Use nursing terminology rather than medical terminology to describe the client's response.	*Risk for Ineffective Airway Clearance* related to accumulation of secretions in lungs (nursing terminology)	*Risk for Pneumonia* (medical terminology)
8. Use nursing terminology rather than medical terminology to describe the probable cause of the client's response.	*Risk for Ineffective Airway Clearance* related to accumulation of secretions in lungs (nursing terminology)	*Risk for Ineffective Airway Clearance* related to emphysema (medical terminology)

- *Consult resources.* Both novices and experienced nurses should consult appropriate resources whenever in doubt about a diagnosis. Professional literature, nursing colleagues, and other professionals are all appropriate resources. The nurse should use a nursing diagnosis handbook to determine whether the client's signs and symptoms truly fit the NANDA label chosen.

- *Base diagnoses on patterns—that is, on behavior over time—rather than on an isolated incident.* For example, even though Amanda Aquilini is concerned today about needing to leave her child with a neighbor, it is likely that this concern will be resolved without intervention by the next day. Therefore, the admitting nurse should not diagnose *Interrupted Family Processes.*

- *Improve critical-thinking skills.* These skills help the nurse to be aware of and avoid errors in thinking, such as overgeneralizing, stereotyping, making unwarranted assumptions, and so on. See Chapter 15. 🔗

ONGOING DEVELOPMENT OF NURSING DIAGNOSES

The first taxonomy of nursing diagnoses was alphabetical. This ordering was considered unscientific by some, and a hierarchic structure was sought. In 1982, NANDA accepted the "nine patterns of unitary man" as an organizing principle. In 1984 NANDA renamed the "patterns of unitary man" as "human response patterns" (Kim, McFarland, & McLane, 1984), as listed in Box 17–4.

Having undergone refinements, revisions, and acceptance of new diagnoses, the taxonomy is now called Taxonomy II (NANDA International, 2003). The diagnoses are no longer grouped by Gordon's patterns but by seven axes: diagnostic concept, time, unit of care, age, health status, descriptor, and topology (see Box 17–5). In addition, diagnoses are now listed alphabetically by concept, not by first word.

Review and refinement of diagnostic labels continue as new and modified labels are discussed at each biannual conference.

BOX 17–4	■ Human Response Patterns

1. *Exchanging:* mutual giving and receiving
2. *Communicating:* sending messages
3. *Relating:* establishing bonds
4. *Valuing:* assigning relative worth
5. *Choosing:* selection of alternatives
6. *Moving:* activity
7. *Perceiving:* reception of information
8. *Knowing:* meaning associated with information
9. *Feeling:* subjective awareness of information

Nurses submit diagnoses to the Diagnostic Review Committee, which reviews and "stages" the diagnosis according to how well developed and supported it is. The NANDA board of directors gives final approval for incorporation of the diagnosis into the official list of labels. Diagnoses on the NANDA list are not finished products but are approved for clinical use and further study. Many on the list have been studied only minimally. For example, many of the diagnoses added in 1994 are still in the early stages of development.

In 1997, NANDA changed the name of its official journal from *Nursing Diagnosis* to *Nursing Diagnosis: The International Journal of Nursing Language and Classification.* The subtitle emphasizes that nursing diagnosis is part of a larger, developing system of standardized nursing language. This system includes classifications of nursing interventions (NIC) and nursing outcomes (NOC) that are being developed by other research groups and linked to the NANDA diagnostic labels. NIC and NOC are discussed in greater detail in Chapter 18. 🔗

Research groups are examining what nurses do from these three different perspectives (diagnoses, interventions, and outcomes) to clarify and communicate the role nurses play in the health care system. A standardized language will also enable nurses to implement a Nursing Minimum Data Set needed for computerized client records.

BOX 17–5	■ Taxonomy II

Axis	Dimension of the Human Response	Values	Examples
1	Diagnostic concept	$N = 99$	Anxiety, falls, nutrition, walking
2	Time	$N = 4$	Acute, chronic, intermittent, continuous
3	Unit of care	$N = 4$	Individual, family, group, community
4	Age	$N = 12$	Infant, adolescent, young old adult
5	Health status	$N = 3$	Wellness, risk, actual
6	Descriptor	$N = 26$	Anticipatory, deficient, imbalanced, perceived
7	Topology	$N = 17$ body parts/regions	Cerebral, gustatory, renal, visual

Note: From *NANDA Nursing Diagnoses: Definitions and Classification, 2003–2004* by NANDA International, 2003, Philadelphia: Author. Adapted with permission.

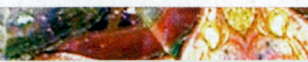

Lifespan Considerations

Elders

Elders tend to have multiple problems with complex physical and psychosocial needs when they are ill. If the nurse has done a thorough, accurate assessment, nursing diagnoses can be selected to cover all problems and, at the same time, prioritize the special needs. For example, if a client is admitted with severe congestive heart failure, prompt attention will be focused on *Decreased Cardiac Output* and *Excess Fluid Volume,* with interventions selected to improve these areas quickly. As these conditions improve, then other nursing diagnoses, such as *Activity Intolerance* and *Deficient Knowledge* related to a new medication regime, might require more attention. They are all part of the same medical problem of congestive heart failure, but each nursing diagnosis has specific expected outcomes and nursing interventions. The client's strengths should be an essential consideration in all phases of the nursing process.

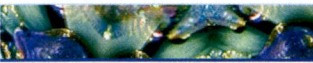

Focus on Critical Thinking

Mr. H. has recently been diagnosed with lung cancer. Someone has written the nursing diagnosis of *Anxiety* on his care plan.

1. What data/defining characteristics would support this nursing diagnosis?
2. Which related factors might exist in his situation?
3. Which other nursing diagnosis might you expect to find in Mr. H.'s case?

4. Another nursing diagnosis on the care plan reads "Lung cancer related to smoking." Is this diagnosis written in an acceptable format? If not, why not?

See Critical Thinking Possibilities in Appendix A.

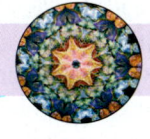 Chapter Review

EXPLORE MediaLink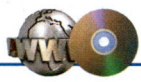

NCLEX review questions, case studies, MediaLink applications, and other interactive resources for this chapter can be found on the Companion Website at www.prenhall.com/kozier. Click on Chapter 17 to select the activities for this chapter.

For more NCLEX review questions, and an audio glossary, access the Student CD-ROM accompanying this textbook.

Chapter Highlights

- The purpose of the North American Nursing Diagnosis Association is to define, refine, and promote a taxonomy of nursing diagnostic terminology.
- Diagnosis is a reasoning process that uses critical thinking.
- Professional standards of care hold that registered nurses are responsible for making nursing diagnoses, even though others may contribute data or implement care.
- A nursing diagnosis is a clinical judgment about the client's responses to actual and potential health problems or life processes.
- A nursing diagnosis provides the basis for selecting independent nursing interventions to achieve outcomes for which the nurse is accountable.
- There are various types of nursing diagnoses: actual, risk, wellness, possible, and syndrome.
- A nursing diagnosis has three components: the problem (and its definition), the etiology, and the defining characteristics. Each component serves a specific purpose.

- Nursing diagnoses differ from medical diagnoses and collaborative problems in orientation, duration, and nursing focus.
- A collaborative problem is a type of potential problem that nurses manage using both independent and physician-prescribed interventions.
- The three phases of the diagnostic process are data analysis; identification of the client's health problems, health risks, and strengths; and formulation of diagnostic statements.
- In data analysis and processing, the nurse compares data against standards to identify significant cues, clusters the data, and identifies gaps and inconsistencies.
- Significant cues are those that (a) point to change in a client's health status or pattern, (b) vary from norms of the client population, or (c) indicate a developmental delay.
- It is important to identify client strengths as well as problems.
- The basic format for a nursing diagnostic statement is "*Problem* related to *etiology.*" However, there are several variations on this format.

- The development of a taxonomy of nursing diagnosis labels is an ongoing process.
- The organizing principles for the NANDA Taxonomy II are the seven axes: diagnostic concept, time, unit of care, age, potentiality, descriptor, and topology.
- Work is progressing on a unified standardized nursing language that includes NANDA nursing diagnoses, a nursing interventions classification, and a nursing outcomes classification.

Review Questions

17–1. In the nursing process phase of diagnosing, between the actions of analyzing data and formulating the diagnostic statement, the nurse must
   a. assess the client's needs.
   b. delineate client problems and strengths.
   c. determine which interventions are most likely to succeed.
   d. estimate the cost of several different approaches.

17–2. For the diagnostic statement "hypothermia," the etiology (related and risk factors) could be
   a. pallor.
   b. hypertension.
   c. malnutrition.
   d. tachycardia.

17–3. In which one of the following is the nursing diagnostic statement properly worded?
   a. Risk for caregiver role strain related to unpredictable illness course.

   b. Risk for falls related to tendency to collapse.
   c. Emesis due to nausea.
   d. Sleep deprivation secondary to fatigue.

17–4. An advantage to using a three-part diagnostic statement in the PES format is that such a statement
   a. is always more accurate.
   b. is shorter.
   c. applies to risk and wellness diagnoses also.
   d. documents the indicators of the problem.

17–5. A collaborative (multidisciplinary) problem is indicated instead of a nursing or medical diagnosis when
   a. both medical and nursing interventions are required to treat the problem.
   b. the nurse cannot take independent action to treat the problem.
   c. nursing interventions are the primary actions required to treat the problem.
   d. no medical diagnosis (disease) can be determined.

Readings and References

Suggested Readings

Christensen, R. A., & Taylor, C. M. (2000). What's your diagnosis? *Nursing, 30*(1), 32HN1–32HN4. Considers very different perspectives on nursing diagnosis: Do they help, do they hurt, or do they matter?

Rantz, M. J. (2001). The value of a standard language. *Nursing Diagnosis, 12,* 107–108. Rantz responds to the viewpoint printed in a previous issue of the journal in which the discussion centered on the differences between nursing diagnoses and patient problems. Rantz asserts that the terminology associated with nursing diagnosis contributes to the important goal of assisting nurses to convey the essence of nursing care in a multidisciplinary world.

Related Research

Delaney, C., Herr, K., Maas, M., & Specht, J. (2000). Reliability of nursing diagnoses documented in a computerized nursing information system. *Nursing Diagnosis, 11,* 121–134.

Fu, M., LeMone, P., McDaniel, R. W., & Bausler, C. (2001). A multivariate validation of the defining characteristics of fatigue. *Nursing Diagnosis, 12,* 15–27.

References

Alfaro-LeFevre, R. (1998). *Applying the nursing process. A step-by-step guide* (4th ed.). Philadelphia/New York: Lippincott.

American Nurses Association. (1998). *Standards of clinical nursing practice* (2nd ed). Kansas City, MO: Author.

Carpenito, L. J. (1997). *Nursing diagnosis: Application to clinical practice* (7th ed.). Philadelphia: Lippincott-Raven.

Cruz, D. A. L. M., & Pimenta, C. A. M. (2001). Chronic pain: Nursing diagnosis or syndrome? *Nursing Diagnosis, 12,* 117–127.

Gordon, M. (2002). *Manual of nursing diagnosis* (10th ed.). St. Louis, MO: Mosby.

Joint Commission on Accreditation of Healthcare Organizations. (2001). *Accreditation manual for hospitals.* Chicago: Author.

Kim, M. J., McFarland, G. K., & McLane, A. M. (Eds.). (1984). *Classification of nursing diagnoses: Proceedings of the fifth national conference.* St. Louis, MO: Mosby.

NANDA International. (2003). *NANDA nursing diagnoses: Definitions and classification 2003-2004.* Philadelphia: Author.

Selected Bibliography

Gebbie, K. M. (1976). *Classification of nursing diagnoses: Summary of the second national conference.* St. Louis, MO: Mosby.

Gordon, M. (1982). Historical perspective: The National Group for Classification of Nursing Diagnoses. In M. J. Kim & D. A. Moritz (Eds.), *Classification of nursing diagnoses: Proceedings of the fourth national conference.* New York: McGraw-Hill.

Johnson, M., Maas, M., & Moorhead, S. (Eds.). (2000). *Nursing outcomes classification (NOC)* (2nd ed.). St. Louis, MO: Mosby.

McCloskey, J.C., & Bulechek, G. M. (Eds.). (2000). *Nursing interventions classification (NIC)* (3rd ed.). St. Louis, MO: Mosby.

McCloskey, J. C., Bulechek, G. M., Dochterman, J., & Maas, M. (Eds.). (2000). *Nursing diagnoses, outcomes, and interventions: NANDA, NOC and NIC linkages.* St. Louis, MO: Mosby.

What's in a name? [Editorial]. (1997). *Nursing Diagnosis: The Journal of Nursing Language and Classification, 8*(1), 3.

Whitley, G. G. (1996). Barriers to the use of nursing diagnosis language in clinical settings. *Nursing Diagnosis, 7*(1), 25–32.

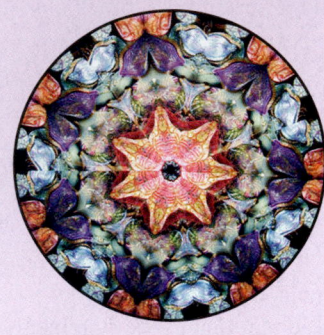

CHAPTER 18

PLANNING

LEARNING OUTCOMES

After completing this chapter, you will be able to:

- Compare and contrast initial planning, ongoing planning, and discharge planning.

- Identify activities that occur in the planning process.

- Explain how standards of care and preprinted care plans can be individualized and used in creating a comprehensive nursing care plan.

- Identify essential guidelines for writing nursing care plans.

- Identify factors that the nurse must consider when setting priorities.

- State the purposes of establishing client goals/desired outcomes.

- Describe the relationship of goals/desired outcomes to the nursing diagnoses.

- Identify guidelines for writing goals/desired outcomes.

- Discuss the Nursing Outcomes Classification, including an explanation of how to use the outcomes and indicators in care planning.

- Describe the process of generating and choosing nursing interventions.

- List the five components of a nursing order.

- Discuss the Nursing Interventions Classification, including an explanation of how to use the interventions and activities in care planning.

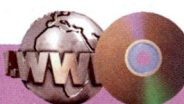

MediaLink

www.prenhall.com/kozier

Additional resources for this chapter can be found on the Student CD-ROM accompanying this textbook, and on the Companion Website at www.prenhall.com/ kozier. Click on Chapter 18 to select the activities for this chapter.

CD-ROM
- Audio Glossary
- NCLEX Review

Companion Website
- Additional NCLEX Review
- Case Study:
    Client Who had a Bicycle Accident
- MediaLink Application:
    Client with Peptic Ulcers

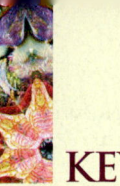

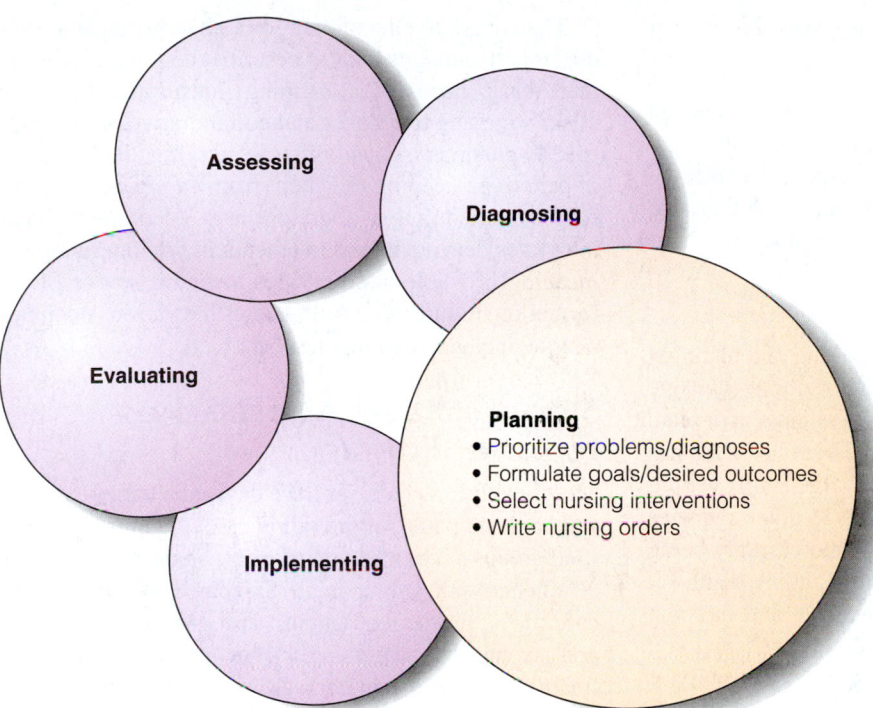

Figure 18–1 ■ **Planning.** The third phase of the nursing process, in which the nurse and client develop client goals/desired outcomes and nursing interventions to prevent, reduce, or alleviate the client's health problems.

Planning is a deliberative, systematic phase of the nursing process that involves decision making and problem solving. In planning, the nurse refers to the client's assessment data and diagnostic statements for direction in formulating client goals and designing the nursing interventions required to prevent, reduce, or eliminate the client's health problems (see Figure 18–1 ■). A **nursing intervention** is "any treatment, based upon clinical judgment and knowledge, that a nurse performs to enhance patient/client outcomes" (McCloskey & Bulechek, 2000, p. xix). The product of the planning phase is a client care plan.

Although planning is basically the nurse's responsibility, input from the client and support persons is essential if a plan is to be effective. Nurses do not plan for the client, but encourage the client to participate actively to the extent possible. In a home setting, the client's support people and caregivers are the ones who implement the plan of care; thus, its effectiveness depends largely on them.

TYPES OF PLANNING

Planning begins with the first client contact and continues until the nurse–client relationship ends, usually when the client is discharged from the health care agency.

Initial Planning

The nurse who performs the admission assessment usually develops the initial comprehensive plan of care. This nurse has the benefit of the client's body language as well as some intuitive kinds of information that are not available solely from the written database. Planning should be initiated as soon as possible after the initial assessment, especially because of the trend toward shorter hospital stays.

Ongoing Planning

Ongoing planning is done by all nurses who work with the client. As nurses obtain new information and evaluate the client's responses to care, they can individualize the initial care plan further. Ongoing planning also occurs at the beginning of a shift as the nurse plans the care to be given that day. Using ongoing assessment data, the nurse carries out daily planning for the following purposes

1. To determine whether the client's health status has changed
2. To set priorities for the client's care during the shift
3. To decide which problems to focus on during the shift
4. To coordinate the nurse's activities so that more than one problem can be addressed at each client contact.

Discharge Planning

Discharge planning, the process of anticipating and planning for needs after discharge, is a crucial part of comprehensive health care and should be addressed in each client's care plan. Because the average stay of clients in acute care hospitals has become shorter, people are sometimes discharged still needing care. Although many clients are discharged to other agencies (e.g., long-term care facilities), such care is increasingly being delivered in the home. Effective discharge planning begins at first client contact and involves comprehensive and ongoing assessment to obtain information about the client's ongoing needs. For details about discharge planning see "Continuity of Care" in Chapter 7. 🔗

DEVELOPING NURSING CARE PLANS

The end product of the planning phase of the nursing process is a formal or informal plan of care. An **informal nursing care plan** is a strategy for action that exists in the nurse's mind. For example, the nurse may think, "Mrs. Phan is very tired. I will need to reinforce her teaching after she is rested." A **formal nursing care plan** is a written or computerized guide that organizes information about the client's care. The most obvious benefit of a formal written care plan is that it provides for continuity of care.

A **standardized care plan** is a formal plan that specifies the nursing care for groups of clients with common needs (e.g., all clients with myocardial infarction). An **individualized care plan** is tailored to meet the unique needs of a specific client—needs that are not addressed by the standardized plan. It is important that all caregivers work toward the same outcomes and, if available, use approaches shown to be effective with a particular client. Nurses also use the formal care plan for direction about what needs to be documented in client progress notes and as a guide for delegating and assigning staff to care for clients. When nurses use the client's nursing diagnoses to develop goals and nursing interventions, the result is a holistic, individualized plan of care that will meet the client's unique needs.

Care plans include the actions nurses must take to address the client's nursing diagnoses and produce the desired outcomes. The nurse begins the plan when the client is admitted to the agency and constantly updates it throughout the client's stay in response to changes in the client's condition and evaluations of goal achievement. During the planning phase the nurse must (a) decide which of the client's problems need individualized plans and which problems can be addressed by standardized plans and routine care, and (b) write individualized desired outcomes and nursing orders for client problems that require nursing attention beyond preplanned, routine care.

The complete plan of care for a client is made up of several different documents that (a) describe the routine care needed to meet basic needs (e.g., bathing, nutrition), (b) address the client's nursing diagnoses and collaborative problems, and (c) specify nursing responsibilities in carrying out the medical plan of care (e.g., keeping the client from eating or drinking before surgery; scheduling a laboratory test). A complete plan of care integrates dependent and independent nursing functions into a meaningful whole and provides a central source of client information. Figure 18–2 ■ illustrates the various documents that may be included in a nursing care plan.

Standardized Approaches to Care Planning

Most health care agencies have devised a variety of preprinted, standardized plans for providing essential nursing care to specified groups of clients who have certain needs in common (e.g., all clients with pneumonia). Standards of care, standardized care plans, protocols, policies, and procedures are developed and accepted by the nursing staff in order to (a) ensure that minimally acceptable standards are met and (b) promote efficient use of nurses' time by removing the need to author common activities that are done over and over for many of the clients on a nursing unit.

Standards of care describe nursing actions for clients with similar medical conditions rather than individuals, and they describe achievable rather than ideal nursing care. They define the interventions for which nurses are held accountable; they do not contain medical interventions. Standards of care are usually agency records and not part of the client's care plan, but they may be referred to in the plan (e.g., a nurse might write "See unit standards of care for cardiac catheterization"). Standards of care may or may not be organized according to problems or nursing diagnoses. They are written from the perspective of the nurse's responsibilities. Figure 18–3 ■ shows unit standards of care for the client with thrombophlebitis.

Standardized care plans are preprinted guides for the nursing care of a client who has a need that arises frequently in the agency (e.g., a specific nursing diagnosis or all nursing diagnoses associated with a particular medical condition). They are written from the perspective of what care the client can expect. They should not be confused with standards of care. Although the two have some similarities, they have important differences. Figure 18–4 ■ shows a standardized care plan for *Deficient Fluid Volume*. Standardized care plans:

- Are kept with the client's individualized care plan on the nursing unit. When the client is discharged, they become part of the permanent medical record.
- Provide detailed interventions and contain additions or deletions from the standards of care of the agency.
- Typically are written in the nursing process format:

  Problem ⇒ Goals/Desired Outcomes ⇒
  Nursing Interventions ⇒ Evaluation

- Frequently include checklists, blank lines, or empty spaces to allow the nurse to individualize goals and nursing interventions.

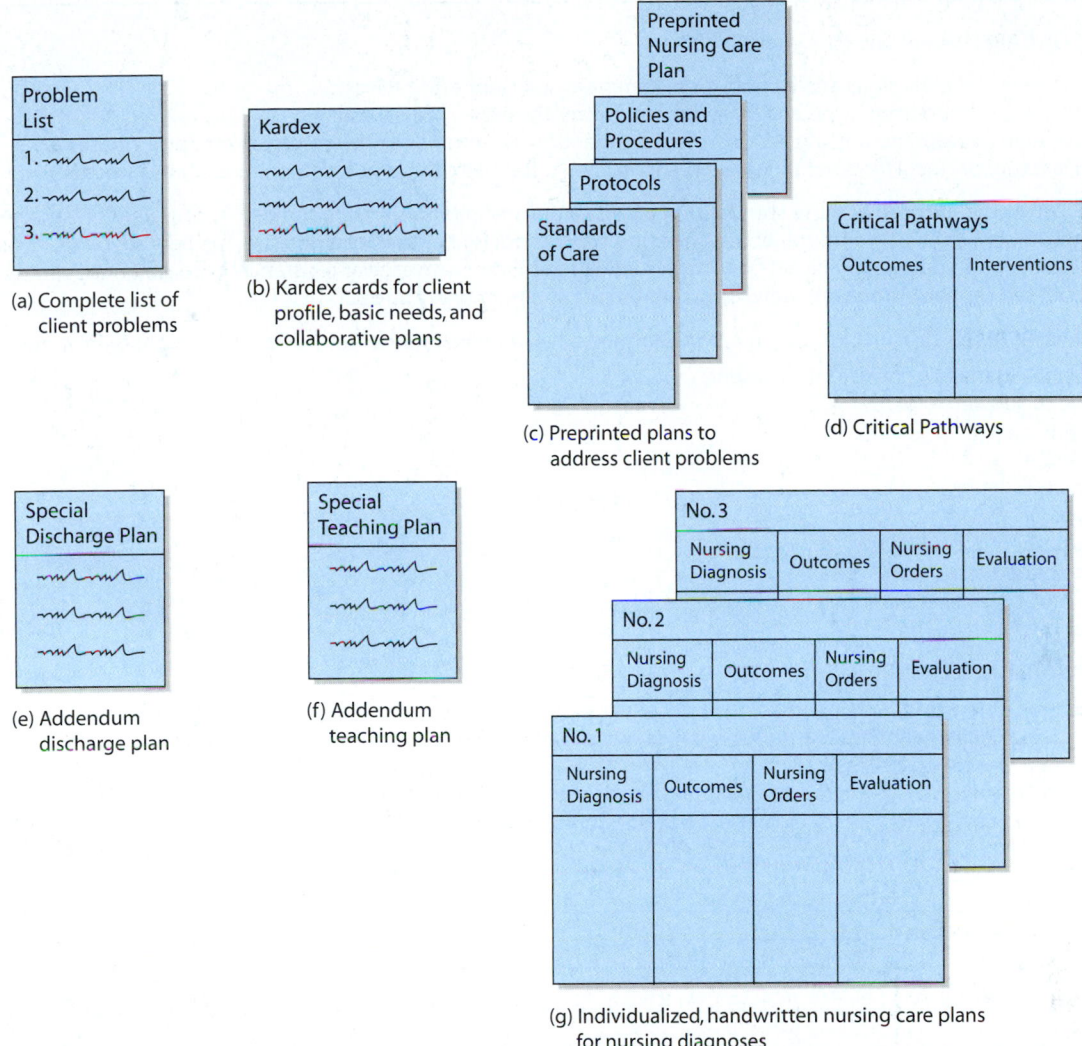

(a) Complete list of client problems

(b) Kardex cards for client profile, basic needs, and collaborative plans

(c) Preprinted plans to address client problems

(d) Critical Pathways

(e) Addendum discharge plan

(f) Addendum teaching plan

(g) Individualized, handwritten nursing care plans for nursing diagnoses

Figure 18–2 ■ Documents that may be included in a complete client care plan. (*Note:* From *Nursing Process & Critical Thinking*, 3rd ed. (p. 436), by J. M. Wilkinson, 2001, Upper Saddle River, NJ: Prentice Hall. Reprinted with permission.)

The use of standardized care plans is supported by the Joint Commission on Accreditation of Healthcare Organizations standards for nursing care, which no longer require a handwritten care plan for every client.

Like standards of care and standardized care plans, **protocols** are preprinted to indicate the actions commonly required for a particular group of clients. For example, an agency may have a protocol for admitting a client to the intensive care unit, for administering magnesium sulfate to a client with preeclampsia, or for caring for a client receiving continuous epidural analgesia. Protocols may include both physician's orders and nursing interventions. Depending on the agency, protocols may or may not be included in the client's permanent record.

Policies and **procedures** are developed to govern the handling of frequently occurring situations. For example, a hospital may have a policy specifying the number of visitors a client may have. Some policies and procedures are similar to protocols and specify what is to be done, for example, in the case of cardiac arrest. If a policy covers a situation pertinent to client

care, it is usually noted on the care plan (e.g., "Make Social Service referral according to Policy Manual"). Policies are institutional records and do not become a part of the care plan or permanent record.

A **standing order** is a written document about policies, rules, regulations, or orders regarding client care. Standing orders give nurses the authority to carry out specific actions under certain circumstances, often when a physician is not immediately available. In a hospital critical care unit, a common example is the administration of emergency antiarrhythmic medications when a client's cardiac monitoring pattern changes. In a home care setting, a physician may write a standing order for the nurse to obtain blood tests for a client who has been on a certain therapy for a prescribed amount of time.

Regardless of whether care plans are handwritten, computerized, or standardized, nursing care must be individualized to fit the unique needs of each client. In practice, a care plan usually consists of both preprinted and handwritten sections. The nurse uses standardized care plans for predictable, commonly

STANDARDS OF CARE: Patient with Thrombophlebitis

Goal: 1. To monitor for early signs and symptoms of compromised respiratory status.
2. To report any abnormal signs and/or symptoms promptly to the medical staff.
3. To initiate appropriate nursing actions when signs and/or symptoms of compromised respiratory status occur.
4. To institute protocol for emergency intervention should the client develop cardiopulmonary dysfunction.

SUPPORTIVE DATA: The purpose of these standards of care is to prevent, monitor, report, and record the client's response to a diagnosis of thrombophlebitis. Thrombophlebitis places the client at risk for pulmonary embolism. The hemodynamic consequences of embolic obstruction to pulmonary blood flow involve increased pulmonary vascular resistance, increased right ventricular workload, decreased cardiac output, and development of shock and pulmonary arrest.

CLINICAL MANIFESTATIONS: Nursing assessments performed q3–4h should monitor for the following signs/symptoms:

- Dyspnea (generally consistently present)
- Sudden substernal pain
- Rapid/weak pulse
- Syncope
- Anxiety
- Fever
- Cough/hemoptysis
- Accelerated respiratory rate
- Pleuritic type chest pain
- Cyanosis

PREVENTIVE NURSING MEASURES:

- Encourage increased fluid intake to prevent dehydration.
- Maintain anticoagulant intravenous therapy as prescribed (See Protocol for Anticoagulant Administration).
- Maintain prescribed bedrest.
- Prevent venous stasis from improperly fitting elastic stockings; check q3–4h.
- Encourage dorsiflexion exercises of the lower extremities while on bedrest.

INDIVIDUALIZED PLANS/ADDITIONAL NURSING/MEDICAL ORDERS

Do not massage lower extremities.
Intake and output q8h.

Initiated by: _S. Ibarra, RN_   Date: _4-9-05_

Figure 18–3 ■ Standards of care for thrombophlebitis. (*Note:* From *Nursing Process & Critical Thinking*, 3rd ed. (p. 445), by J. M. Wilkinson, 2001, Upper Saddle River, NJ: Prentice Hall. Reprinted with permission.)

occurring problems and handwrites an individual plan for unusual problems or problems needing special attention. For example, a standardized care plan for all "clients with a medical diagnosis of pneumonia" would probably include a nursing diagnosis of *Deficient Fluid Volume* and direct the nurse to assess the client's hydration status. On a respiratory or medical unit this would be a common nursing diagnosis; therefore, Amanda Aquilini's nurse was able to obtain a standardized plan directing care commonly needed by clients with *Deficient Fluid Volume* (see Figure 18–4). However, the nursing diagnosis *Risk for Interrupted Family Processes* would not be common to all clients with pneumonia; it is specific to Amanda. Therefore, the goals and nursing interventions for that diagnosis would need to be handwritten by the nurse.

Formats for Nursing Care Plans

Although formats differ from agency to agency, the care plan is often organized into four columns or categories: (a) nursing diagnoses, (b) goals/desired outcomes, (c) nursing orders, and (d) evaluation. Some agencies use a three-column plan in which evaluation is done in the goals column or in the nurses' notes; others have a five-column plan that adds a column for assessment data preceding the nursing diagnosis column.

Student Care Plans

Because student care plans are a learning activity as well as a plan of care, they may be more lengthy and detailed than care plans used by working nurses. To help students learn to write care plans, educators may require that more of the plan be handwritten. They may also modify the three-, four-, or five-column plan by adding a column for "Rationale" after the nursing orders column. A **rationale** is the scientific principle given as the reason for selecting a particular nursing intervention. Students may also be required to cite supporting literature for their stated rationale. Another method of organizing and representing care plan information is the use of a concept map. For an example of a Nursing Care Plan, see pages 310–311.

A **concept map** is a visual tool in which ideas or data are enclosed in circles or boxes of some shape and relationships between these are indicated by connecting lines or arrows.

Etiology	Desired Outcomes	Nursing Order (Identify Frequency)
✓ Decreased oral intake	✓ Urinary output > 30 mL/hr	✓ Monitor intake and output q _1_ h
✓ Nausea	✓ Urine specific gravity 1.005–1.025	✓ Weigh daily
__ Depression	✓ Serum Na⁺ normal	✓ Monitor serum electrolyte levels X 1 or _until normal_
✓ Fatigue, weakness	✓ Mucous membranes moist	✓ Check skin turgor and mucous membranes q _8_ h
__ Difficulty swallowing	✓ Skin turgor good	✓ Monitor temperature q _4_ h
__ Other:_____	✓ No weight loss	✓ Administer prescribed IV therapy (Monitor according to protocol for Intravenous Therapy) _1000 mL D₅ LR at 100 mL/hr_
✓ Excess fluid loss	✓ 8-hour intake =	✓ Offer oral liquids q _1_ h
✓ Fever or increased metabolic rate	_400 mL oral_	Type _clear, cold_____
✓ Diaphoresis	Other:	✓ Instruct client regarding amount, type, and schedule of fluid intake.
✓ Vomiting		✓ Assess understanding of type of fluid loss; teach accordingly
__ Diarrhea		✓ Mouth care prn with _mouthwash_
__ Burns		✓ Institute measures to reduce fever (eg, lower room temperature, remove bed covers, offer cold liquids.)
__ Other_____		Other Nursing Orders:_____
		Monitor urine specific gravity
Defining Characteristics		_q shift_
✓ Insufficient intake		_____
✓ Negative balance of intake and output		_____
✓ Dry mucous membranes		_____
✓ Poor skin turgor		_____
__ Concentrated urine		_____
__ Hypernatremia		
✓ Rapid, weak pulse		
__ Falling B/P		
__ Weight loss		

Plan initiated by: _M. Medina RN_____ **Date** _4-15-05_____

Plan/outcomes evaluated_____ **Date**_____

Plan/outcomes evaluated_____ **Date**_____

Client: _Amanda Aquilini_____

Figure 18–4 ■ A standardized care plan for the nursing diagnosis of *Deficient Fluid Volume.*

Concept maps are creative endeavors. They can take many different forms and encompass various categories of data, according to the creator's interpretation of the client or health condition. The concept map for Amanda Aquilini in this chapter includes unique boxes that enclose assessment, nursing diagnosis, outcomes, and interventions and the arrows represent the flow of the phases of the nursing process. (See Concept Map on page 312.)

Computerized Care Plans

Computers are increasingly being used to create and store nursing care plans. The computer can generate both standardized and individualized care plans. Nurses access the client's stored care plan from a centrally located terminal at the nurses' station or from terminals in client rooms. For an individualized plan the nurse chooses the appropriate diagnoses from a menu suggested by the computer. The computer then lists possible goals and nursing interventions for those diagnoses; the nurse chooses those appropriate for the client and types in any additional goals and interventions or nursing actions not listed on the menu. The nurse can read the plan on the computer screen or print out an updated working copy.

Multidisciplinary (Collaborative) Care Plans

A **multidisciplinary care plan** is a standardized plan that outlines the care required for clients with common, predictable—usually medical—conditions. Such plans, also referred to as **collaborative care plans** and **critical pathways,** sequence the care that must be given on each day during the projected length of stay for the specific type of condition. Like the traditional nursing care plan, a multidisciplinary care plan can specify outcomes and nursing interventions to address client problems (including nursing diagnoses). However, it includes medical treatments to be performed by other health care providers as well.

The plan is usually organized with a column for each day, listing the interventions that should be carried out and the client outcomes that should be achieved on that day. There are as many columns on the multidisciplinary care plan as the preset number of days allowed for the client's diagnosis-related group (DRG). For further information see Chapter 6. ⚭ Multidisciplinary care plans do not include detailed nursing activities. They should be drawn from but do not replace standards of care and standardized care plans.

Guidelines for Writing Nursing Care Plans

The nurse should use the following guidelines when writing nursing care plans:

1. *Date and sign the plan.* The date the plan is written is essential for evaluation, review, and future planning. The nurse's signature demonstrates accountability to the client and to the nursing profession, since the effectiveness of nursing actions can be evaluated.

2. *Use category headings:* "Nursing Diagnoses," "Goals/Desired Outcomes," "Nursing Interventions,"and "Evaluation." Include a date for the evaluation of each goal.

3. *Use standardized medical or English symbols and key words rather than complete sentences to communicate your ideas.* For example, write "Turn and reposition q2h" rather than "Turn and reposition the client every two hours." Or write "Clean wound c̄ H_2O_2 bid" rather than "Clean the client's wound with hydrogen peroxide twice a day, morning and evening." See Table 20–4 ⚭ on page 343 for a list of standard medical abbreviations.

4. *Be specific.* Because nurses are now working shifts of different lengths, some working 12-hour shifts, and some working 8-hour shifts, it is even more important to be specific about expected timing of an intervention. If the order reads "change incisional dressing q shift," it could mean either twice in 24 hours, or three times in 24 hours, depending on the shift time. This miscommunication becomes even more serious when medications are ordered to be given "q shift." Writing down specific times during the 24-hour period will help clarify.

5. *Refer to procedure books or other sources of information rather than including all the steps on a written plan.* For example, write "See unit procedure book for tracheostomy care," or attach a standard nursing plan about such procedures as radiation-implantation care and preoperative or postoperative care.

6. *Tailor the plan to the unique characteristics of the client by ensuring that the client's choices, such as preferences about the times of care and the methods used, are included.* This reinforces the client's individuality and sense of control. For example, the written nursing intervention "Provide prune juice at breakfast rather than other juice" indicates that the client was given a choice of beverages.

7. *Ensure that the nursing plan incorporates preventive and health maintenance aspects as well as restorative ones.* For example, carrying out the order "Provide active-assistance ROM (range-of-motion) exercises to affected limbs q2h" prevents joint contractures and maintains muscle strength and joint mobility.

8. *Ensure that the plan contains interventions for ongoing assessment of the client* (e.g., "Inspect incision q8h").

9. *Include collaborative and coordination activities in the plan.* For example, the nurse may write orders to ask a nutritionist or physical therapist about specific aspects of the client's care.

10. *Include plans for the client's discharge and home care needs.* It is often necessary to consult and make arrangements with the community health nurse, social worker, and specific agencies that supply client information and needed equipment. Add teaching and discharge plans as addenda if they are lengthy and complex.

THE PLANNING PROCESS

In the process of developing client care plans, the nurse engages in the following activities:

- Setting priorities
- Establishing client goals/desired outcomes
- Selecting nursing interventions
- Writing nursing orders.

Setting Priorities

Priority setting is the process of establishing a preferential sequence for addressing nursing diagnoses and interventions. The nurse and client begin planning by deciding which nursing diagnosis requires attention first, which second, and so on. Instead of rank-ordering diagnoses, nurses can group them as having high, medium, or low priority. Life-threatening problems, such as loss of respiratory or cardiac function, are designated as high priority. Health-threatening problems, such as acute illness and decreased coping ability, are assigned medium priority because they may result in delayed development or cause destructive physical or emotional changes. A low-priority problem is one that arises from normal developmental needs or that requires only minimal nursing support.

Nurses frequently use Maslow's hierarchy of needs when setting priorities (see Figure 12–5 on page 197). 🔗 In Maslow's hierarchy, physiologic needs such as air, food, and water are basic to life and receive higher priority than the need for security or activity. Growth needs, such as self-esteem, are not perceived as "basic" in this framework. Thus nursing diagnoses such as *Ineffective Airway Clearance* and *Impaired Gas Exchange* would take priority over nursing diagnoses such as *Anxiety* or *Ineffective Coping*.

It is not necessary to resolve all high-priority diagnoses before addressing others. The nurse may partially address a high-priority diagnosis and then deal with a diagnosis of lesser priority. Furthermore, because clients usually have several problems, the nurse often deals with more than one diagnosis at a time. Table 18–1 lists the priorities assigned to Amanda Aquilini's nursing diagnoses, which were identified in Chapter 17. 🔗

Priorities change as the client's responses, problems, and therapies change. The nurse must consider a variety of factors when assigning priorities, including the following:

1. *Client's health values and beliefs:* Values concerning health may be more important to the nurse than to the client. For example, a client may believe being home for the children to be more urgent than a health problem. When there is such a difference of opinion, the client and nurse should discuss it openly to resolve any conflict. However, in a life-threatening situation the nurse usually must take the initiative.

2. *Client's priorities:* Involving the client in prioritizing and care planning enhances cooperation. Sometimes, however, the client's perception of what is important conflicts with the nurse's knowledge of potential problems or complications. For example, an elderly client may not regard turning and repositioning in bed as important, preferring to be undisturbed. The nurse, however, aware of the potential complications of prolonged bed rest (e.g., muscle weakness and pressure sores), needs to inform the client and carry out these necessary interventions.

3. *Resources available to the nurse and client:* If money, equipment, or personnel are scarce in a health care agency, then a problem may be given a lower priority than usual. Nurses in a home setting, for example, do not have the resources of a hospital. If the necessary resources are not available, the solution of that problem might need to be postponed, or the client may need a referral. Client resources, such as finances or coping ability, may also influence the setting of priorities. For example, a client who is unemployed may defer dental treatment; a client whose husband is terminally ill and dependent on her may feel unable to cope with nutritional guidance directed toward losing weight.

4. *Urgency of the health problem:* Regardless of the framework used, life-threatening situations require that the nurse assign them high priority. For example, in Table 18–1, although Amanda Aquilini is anxious about child care, her *Ineffective Airway Clearance* has higher priority. Situations that affect the integrity of the client, that is, those that could have a negative or destructive effect on the client, also have high priority. Such health problems as drug abuse and radical alteration of self-concept due to amputation can be destructive both to the individual and to the family.

5. *Medical treatment plan:* The priorities for treating health problems must be congruent with treatment by other health professionals. For example, a high priority for the client might be to become ambulatory; however, if the physician's therapeutic regimen calls for extended bed rest, then ambulation must assume a lower priority in the nursing care plan. The nurse can provide or teach exercises to facilitate ambulation later, provided the client's health permits. The nursing diagnosis related to ambulation is not ignored; it is merely deferred.

Establishing Client Goals/Desired Outcomes

After establishing priorities, the nurse and client set goals for each nursing diagnosis (see Figure 18–5 ■). On a care plan the **goals/desired outcomes** describe, in terms of observable client responses, what the nurse hopes to achieve by implementing the nursing interventions. The terms *goal* and *desired outcome* are used interchangeably in this text, except when discussing and using standardized language. Some references also use the terms *expected outcome, predicted outcome, outcome criterion,* and *objective.*

Some nursing literature differentiates the terms by defining goals as broad statements about the client's status and desired outcomes as the more specific, observable criteria used to evaluate whether the goals have been met. For example:

Goal (broad):   Improved nutritional status.
Desired outcome (specific):   Gain 5 lb by April 25.

TABLE 18–1   Assigning Priorities to Nursing Diagnoses for Amanda Aquilini

Nursing Diagnosis	Priority	Rationale
Ineffective Airway Clearance related to (1) viscous secretions secondary to *Deficient Fluid Volume* and (2) shallow chest expansion secondary to pain and fatigue	High priority	Loss of respiratory functioning is a life-threatening problem. The nurse's primary concern must be to promote Amanda's oxygenation by addressing the etiologies of this problem.
Deficient Fluid Volume: intake insufficient to replace fluid loss related to fever and diaphoresis	High priority	Severe *Deficient Fluid Volume* is life threatening. Although not that severe for Amanda, it is a high-priority problem because it is also a contributing factor for *Ineffective Airway Clearance.* Collaborative efforts to improve her hydration have already begun (intravenous fluids). The nurse must immediately and continuously assess and promote Amanda's hydration.
Anxiety related to (1) difficulty breathing and (2) concerns over work and parenting roles	Medium priority	Although Amanda is concerned about work and parenting roles, these are not a threat to life. Also, treatment of her high-priority problem, *Ineffective Airway Clearance,* will relieve one of the etiologies of this problem (dyspnea). Meanwhile, the nurse must provide symptomatic relief of Amanda's anxiety during periods of dyspnea because extreme anxiety could further compromise her oxygenation by causing her to breathe ineffectively and increase the rate at which she uses oxygen.
Risk for Interrupted Family Processes related to mother's illness and potential temporary unavailability of father to provide child care	Low priority	Amanda's child is currently being cared for. If Amanda's husband returns as planned, this problem will not develop into an actual problem. No interventions are needed at present, except for continued assessment and reassurance.
Impaired Nutrition: Less than Body Requirements related to decreased appetite, nausea, and increased metabolism secondary to disease process	Low priority	This problem is not currently health threatening, but it could be if it were to persist. It will almost certainly resolve in a day or two as the medical problem is treated. If the medical problem does not resolve quickly, this will change to a medium priority.
Bathing/Hygiene Self-Care Deficit, related to weakness secondary to ineffective airway clearance and sleep pattern disturbance	Low priority	This problem is caused by the other higher priority problems; therefore, it will resolve as they resolve. Meanwhile, the nurse merely needs to assist Amanda with bathing and so on to support and conserve her energy until she is strong enough to resume her own care.
Sleep Pattern Disturbance related to cough, pain, orthopnea, fever, and diaphoresis	Low priority	Lack of sleep is health threatening. But for the moment (until night) the nurse does not need to address this problem. *Sleep Pattern Disturbance* does contribute to Amanda's *Ineffective Airway Clearance,* but it is not the main cause. Therefore, measures to promote sleep will be low priority until evening. After the nurse has attended to Amanda's oxygenation and hydration needs, this problem priority will change.
Acute Pain (Chest) related to cough secondary to pneumonia	Not on care plan	The nurse did not write *Pain* as a problem on the care plan because *Pain* is to be addressed as the etiology of *Sleep Pattern Disturbance* and *Ineffective Airway Clearance.* The pain etiologies (cough and pneumonia) will be treated by medications (collaborative interventions). Independent nursing actions would address the problem rather than the etiology and would be the same as the nursing actions for *Ineffective Airway Clearance.*

When goals are stated broadly, as in this example, the care plan must include both goals and desired outcomes. They are sometimes combined into one statement linked by the words as evidenced by, as follows:

Improved nutritional status as evidenced by weight gain of 5 lb by April 25.

Writing the broad, general goal first may help students to think of the specific outcomes that are needed, but the broad goal is just a starting point for planning. It is the specific, observable outcomes that must be written on the care plan and used to evaluate client progress. Table 18–2 shows both broad goals and specific outcomes.

The Nursing Outcomes Classification

Standardized nursing language is required in all phases of the nursing process if nursing data are to be included in computerized databases that are analyzed and used in nursing practice.

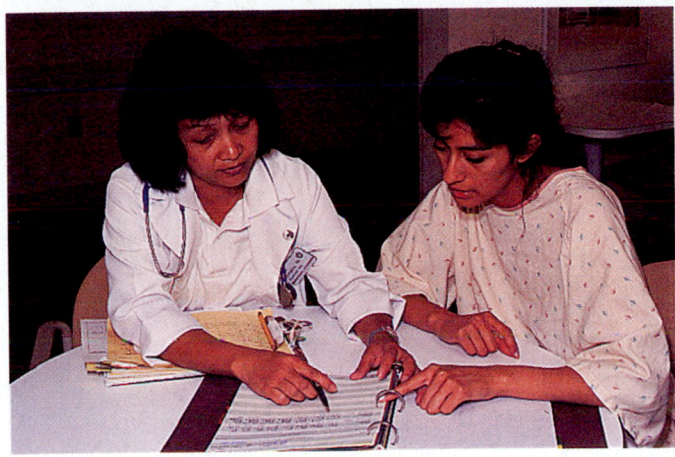

Figure 18–5 ■ Nurse Medina and Amanda collaborate to set goals and outcome criteria and develop a care plan.

Working toward this end, researchers have developed a taxonomy, the **Nursing Outcomes Classification (NOC),** for describing client outcomes that respond to nursing interventions (Johnson, Maas, & Moorhead, 2000). In the taxonomy, outcomes belong to one of seven domains (e.g., physiologic health or family health) and a class within the domain (e.g., nutrition under physiologic health or family well-being under family health). Each NOC outcome is assigned a four-digit identifier, indicated in this text by square brackets, and a definition. Table 18–3 shows a NOC outcome associated with movement.

A NOC outcome is similar to a goal in traditional language. It is "a measurable patient or family caregiver state, behavior, or perception that is conceptualized as a variable and is largely influenced by and sensitive to nursing interventions" (Johnson et al., 2000, p. 25). The NOC outcomes are broadly stated and conceptual. To be measured, an outcome must be made more specific by identifying the specific indicators that apply to a client. An **indicator** is concrete, an "observable patient state, behavior, or self-reported perception or evaluation" (Johnson et al., 2000, p. 25) and is similar to desired outcomes in traditional language. Indicators are also stated in neutral terms, but each outcome includes a five-point scale (a measure) that is used to rate the client's status on each indicator. (See Appendix B). 🔗 When using the NOC taxonomy to write a desired outcome on a care plan, the nurse writes the label, the indicators that apply to the particular client, and the location on the measuring scale that is

desired for each indicator. For example, using the NOC outcome in Table 18–3 for the client diagnosed in Table 18–2, the individualized desired outcomes would read as follows:

Mobility Level:
  Transfer performance (5, completely independent)
  Ambulation: walking (4, independent with assistive device)

Stated in traditional language, that goal would read: "Client will have improved mobility, as evidenced by ability to transfer independently and walk with assistive device (walker)."

Purpose of Desired Outcomes/Goals

Desired outcomes/goals serve the following purposes:

1. Provide direction for planning nursing interventions. Ideas for interventions come more easily if the desired outcomes state clearly and specifically what the nurse hopes to achieve.
2. Serve as criteria for evaluating client progress. Although developed in the planning step of the nursing process, desired outcomes serve as the criteria for judging the effectiveness of nursing interventions and client progress in the evaluation step (see Chapter 19). 🔗
3. Enable the client and nurse to determine when the problem has been resolved.
4. Help motivate the client and nurse by providing a sense of achievement. As goals are met, both client and nurse can see that their efforts have been worthwhile. This provides motivation to continue following the plan, especially when difficult lifestyle changes need to be made.

Long-Term and Short-Term Goals

Goals may be short term or long term. A short-term goal might be "Client will raise right arm to shoulder height by Friday." In the same context, a long-term goal might be "Client will regain full use of right arm in 6 weeks." Short-term goals are useful (a) for clients who require health care for a short time and (b) for those who are frustrated by long-term goals that seem difficult to attain and who need the satisfaction of achieving a short-term goal. In an acute care setting, much of the nurse's time is spent on the client's immediate needs, so most goals are short term. However, clients in acute care settings also need long-term goals to guide planning for their discharge to long-term agencies or home care, especially in a managed care environment. Long-term goals are

TABLE 18–2 Deriving Desired Outcomes from Nursing Diagnoses		
Nursing Diagnosis	**Opposite Healthy Responses (Goals)**	**Desired Outcomes**
Impaired Physical Mobility: inability to bear weight on left leg, related to inflammation of knee joint	Improved mobility Ability to bear weight on left leg	Ambulate with crutches by end of the week. Stand without assistance by end of the month.
Ineffective Airway Clearance related to poor cough effort, secondary to incision pain and fear of damaging sutures	Effective airway clearance	Lungs clear to auscultation during entire postoperative period. No skin pallor or cyanosis by 12 hours postoperation. Within 24 hours after surgery, will demonstrate good cough effort.

TABLE 18–3 Example of a Standardized Client Outcome (NOC)

Domain I: Functional Health
Class C: Mobility
Outcome: Mobility Level [0208]
Definition: Ability to move purposefully

Mobility level	Dependent, Does Not Participate	Requires Assistive Person and Device	Requires Assistive Person	Independent with Assistive Device	Completely Independent
Indicators					
Balance performance	1	2	3	4	5
Body positioning performance	1	2	3	4	5
Muscle movement	1	2	3	4	5
Joint movement	1	2	3	4	5
Transfer performance	1	2	3	4	5
Ambulation: walking	1	2	3	4	5
Ambulation: wheelchair	1	2	3	4	5
Other: (specify)	1	2	3	4	5

Note: From Nursing Outcomes Classification (NOC) (p. 203), by M. Johnson, M. Maas, and S. Moorhead, Eds., 2000, St. Louis, MO: Mosby. Reprinted with permission.

often used for clients who live at home and have chronic health problems and for clients in nursing homes, extended care facilities, and rehabilitation centers.

Relationship of Desired Outcomes/Goals to Nursing Diagnoses

Goals are derived from the client's nursing diagnoses—primarily from the first clause (problem). The problem clause contains the unhealthy response; it states what should change. Therefore, the essential client goals are derived from the problem clause. For example, if the nursing diagnosis is *Risk for Deficient Fluid Volume* related to diarrhea and inadequate intake secondary to nausea, the essential goal statement might be

Maintain fluid balance, as evidenced by urinary and stool output in balance with fluid intake, normal skin turgor, and moist mucous membranes.

In this example, a general goal (fluid balance) is stated as the opposite of the problem (*Deficient Fluid Volume*) and then followed by a list of observable desired outcomes. If achieved, the outcomes would be evidence that the problem, *Deficient Fluid Volume,* has been prevented. See Table 18–2 for additional goals and desired outcomes from nursing diagnoses.

For every nursing diagnosis, the nurse must write at least one desired outcome that, when achieved, directly demonstrates resolution of the problem clause. When developing goals/desired outcomes, ask the following questions:

1. What is the problem clause?
2. What is the opposite, healthy response?
3. How will the client look or behave if the healthy response is achieved? (What will I be able to see, hear, measure, palpate, smell, or otherwise observe with my senses?)
4. What must the client do and how well must the client do it to demonstrate problem resolution or to demonstrate the capability of resolving the problem?

Components of Goal/Desired Outcome Statements

Goal/desired outcome statements should usually have the following four components:

1. *Subject.* The subject, a noun, is the client, any part of the client, or some attribute of the client, such as the client's pulse or urinary output. The subject is often omitted in goals; it is assumed that the subject is the client unless indicated otherwise.
2. *Verb.* The verb specifies an action the client is to perform, for example, what the client is to do, learn, or experience. Verbs that denote directly observable behaviors, such as *administer, show, walk,* must be used. See Box 18–1 for some examples.
3. *Conditions or modifiers.* Conditions or modifiers may be added to the verb to explain the circumstances under which the behavior is to be performed. They explain what, where, when, or how. For example:

Walks with the help of a cane (how).
After attending two group diabetes classes, lists signs and symptoms of diabetes (when).

BOX 18–1 ■ Examples of Action Verbs

Apply	Drink	Select
Assemble	Explain	Share
Breathe	Help	Sit
Choose	Identify	Sleep
Compare	Inject	State
Define	List	Talk
Demonstrate	Move	Transfer
Describe	Name	Turn
Differentiate	Prepare	Verbalize
Discuss	Report	

When at home, maintains weight at existing level (where).

Discusses *food pyramid and recommended daily servings* (what).

Conditions need not be included if the criterion of performance clearly indicates what is expected.

4. *Criterion of desired performance.* The criterion indicates the standard by which a performance is evaluated or the level at which the client will perform the specified behavior. These criteria may specify time or speed, accuracy, distance, and quality. To establish a time-achievement criterion, the nurse needs to ask "How long?" To establish an accuracy criterion, the nurse asks "How well?" Similarly, the nurse asks "How far?" and "What is the expected standard?" to establish distance and quality criteria, respectively. Examples are:

Weighs 75 kg *by April* (time).
Lists *five out of six* signs of diabetes (accuracy).
Walks *one block per day* (time and distance).
Administers insulin *using aseptic technique* (quality).

Table 18–4 illustrates the format that should be used to write outcomes. Table 18–5 lists desired outcomes that were developed for Amanda Aquilini.

Guidelines for Writing Goals/Desired Outcomes

The following guidelines can help nurses write useful goals and desired outcomes:

1. Write goals and outcomes in terms of client responses, not nurse activities. Beginning each goal statement with *the client will* may help focus the goal on client behaviors and responses. Avoid statements that start with *enable, facilitate, allow, let, permit,* or similar verbs followed by the word *client.* These verbs indicate what the nurse hopes to accomplish, not what the client will do.

   Correct: Client will drink 100 cc of water per hour (client behavior)
   Incorrect: Maintain client hydration (nursing action)

2. Be sure that desired outcomes are realistic for the client's capabilities, limitations, and designated time span, if it is indicated. Limitations refers to finances, equipment, family support, social services, physical and mental condition, and time. For example, the outcome "Measures insulin accurately" may be unrealistic for a client who has poor vision due to cataracts.

3. Ensure that the goals and desired outcomes are compatible with the therapies of other professionals. For example, the outcome "Will increase the time spent out of bed by 15 minutes each day" is not compatible with a physician's prescribed therapy of bed rest.

4. Make sure that each goal is derived from only one nursing diagnosis. For example, the goal "The client will increase the amount of nutrients ingested and show progress in the ability to feed self" is derived from two nursing diagnoses: *Feeding Self-Care Deficit* and *Impaired Nutrition: Less than Body Requirements.* Keeping the goal statement related to only one diagnosis facilitates evaluation of care by ensuring that planned nursing interventions are clearly related to the diagnosis.

5. Use observable, measurable terms for outcomes. Avoid words that are vague and require interpretation or judgment

TABLE 18–4　Components of Goals/Desired Outcomes

Subject	Verb	Conditions/ Modifiers	Criterion of Desired Performance
Client	drinks	2500 mL of fluid	daily (time)
Client	administers	correct insulin dose	using aseptic technique (quality standard)
Client	lists	three hazards of smoking (after reading literature)	(accuracy indicated by "three hazards")
Client	recalls	five symptoms of diabetes before discharge	(accuracy indicated by "five symptoms")
Client	walks	the length of the hall without a cane	by date of discharge (time)
Client's ankle	measures	less than 10 inches in circumference	in 48 hours (time)
Client	performs	leg ROM exercises as taught	every 8 hours (time)
Client	identifies	foods high in salt from a prepared list	before discharge (time)
Client	states	the purposes of his medications	before discharge (time)

TABLE 18–5   Desired Outcomes for Amanda Aquilini

Nursing Diagnosis*	Goal Statements [NOC#]/Desired Outcomes
Ineffective Airway Clearance related to viscous secretions and shallow chest expansion secondary to fluid volume deficit, pain, and fatigue	Respiratory Status: Gas exchange [0402], as evidenced by • Absence of pallor and cyanosis (skin and mucous membranes) • Use of correct breathing/coughing technique after instruction • Productive cough • Symmetric chest excursion of at least 4 cm Within 48–72 hours: • Lungs clear to auscultation • Respirations 12–22/min, pulse <100 beats/min • Inhales normal volume of air on incentive spirometer
Deficient Fluid Volume: intake insufficient to replace fluid loss related to vomiting, fever, and diaphoresis	Fluid balance [0601], as evidenced by • Urine output greater than 30 mL/h • Urine specific gravity 1.005–1.025 • Good skin turgor • Moist mucous membranes • Stating the need for oral fluid intake
Anxiety related to difficulty breathing and concerns about work and parenting roles	Anxiety control [1402], as evidenced by • Listening to and following instructions for correct breathing and coughing technique, even during periods of dyspnea • Verbalizing understanding of condition, diagnostic tests, and treatments (by end of day) • Decrease in reports of fear and anxiety; none within 12 h • Voice steady, not shaky • Respiratory rate of 12–22/min • Freely expressing concerns and possible solutions about work and parenting roles
Risk for Interrupted Family Processes related to mother's illness and temporary unavailability of father to provide child care	Family coping [2600], as evidenced by • Report of satisfactory child care arrangements having been made • Client and husband communicating effectively and working together to solve problems • Family members expressing feelings and providing mutual support
Imbalanced Nutrition: Less than Body Requirements related to decreased appetite, nausea, and increased metabolism secondary to disease process	Nutritional status: Nutrient intake [1009], as evidenced by • Eating at least 85% of each meal • Maintaining present weight • Verbalizing importance of adequate nutrition • Verbalizing improved appetite
Bathing/Hygiene Self-Care Deficit related to activity intolerance secondary to airway clearance and sleep pattern disturbance	Self-care: Activities of daily living [0300], as evidenced by • Ambulates to bathroom without dyspnea, fatigue, ineffective or shortness of breath • Within 24 hours, bathes with assistance in bed; within 48 hours, bathes with assistance at sink; within 72 hours, bathes in shower without dyspnea • Reports satisfaction and comfort with hygiene needs
Disturbed Sleep Pattern related to cough, pain, orthopnea, and diaphoresis	Sleep [0004], as evidenced by • Observed sleeping at night rounds • Reports feeling rested • Does not experience orthopnea

The nursing diagnoses are listed in priority order.

by the observer. For example, phrases such as *increase daily exercise* and *improve knowledge of nutrition* can mean different things to different people. If used in outcomes, these phrases can lead to disagreements about whether the outcome was met. These phrases may be suitable for a broad client goal but are not sufficiently clear and specific to guide the nurse when evaluating client responses.

6. Make sure the client considers the goals/desired outcomes important and values them. Some outcomes, such as those for problems related to self-esteem, parenting, and com-

munication, involve choices that are best made by the client or in collaboration with the client.

Some clients may know what they wish to accomplish with regard to their health problem; others may not know all the outcome possibilities. The nurse must actively listen to the client to determine personal values, goals, and desired outcomes in relation to current health concerns. Clients are usually motivated and expend the necessary energy to reach goals they consider important.

See the Nursing Care Plan on pages 310–311 for three of Amanda Aquilini's nursing diagnoses.

Selecting Nursing Interventions and Activities

Nursing interventions and activities are the actions that a nurse performs to achieve client goals. The specific interventions chosen should focus on eliminating or reducing the etiology of the nursing diagnosis, which is the second clause of the diagnostic statement.

When it is not possible to change the etiologic factors, the nurse chooses interventions to treat the signs and symptoms or the defining characteristics in NANDA terminology. Examples of this situation would be *Pain* related to surgical incision and *Anxiety* related to unknown etiology.

Interventions for risk nursing diagnoses should focus on measures to reduce the client's risk factors, which are also found in the second clause.

Correct identification of the etiology during the diagnosing phase provides the framework for choosing successful nursing interventions. For example, the diagnostic label *Activity Intolerance* may have several etiologies: pain, weakness, sedentary lifestyle, anxiety, or cardiac arrhythmias. Interventions will vary according to the cause of the problem.

Types of Nursing Interventions

Nursing interventions are identified and written during the planning step of the nursing process; however, they are actually performed during the implementing step. Nursing interventions include both direct and indirect care, as well as nurse-initiated, physician-initiated, and other provider-initiated treatments. Direct care is an intervention performed through interaction with the client. Indirect care is an intervention performed away from but on behalf of the client such as interdisciplinary collaboration or management of the care environment.

Independent interventions are those activities that nurses are licensed to initiate on the basis of their knowledge and skills. They include physical care, ongoing assessment, emotional support and comfort, teaching, counseling, environmental management, and making referrals to other health care professionals. Recall from Chapter 17 👓 that nursing diagnoses are client problems that can be treated primarily by independent nursing interventions. McCloskey and Bulechek (2000) refer to these as *nurse-initiated treatments.* In performing an autonomous activity, the nurse determines that the client requires certain nursing interventions, either carries these out or delegates them to other nursing personnel, and is accountable or answerable for the decision and the actions. An example of an independent action is planning and providing special mouth care for a client after diagnosing *Impaired Oral Mucous Membranes.*

Dependent interventions are activities carried out under the physician's orders or supervision, or according to specified routines. McCloskey and Bulechek (2000) call these *physician-initiated treatments.* Physicians' orders commonly include orders for medications, intravenous therapy, diagnostic tests, treatments, diet, and activity. The nurse is responsible for explaining, assessing the need for, and administering the medical orders. Nursing interventions may be written to individualize the medical order based on the client's status. For example, for a medical order of "Progressive ambulation, as tolerated," a nurse might write the following:

1. Dangle for 5 min, 12 h postop.
2. Stand at bedside 24 h postop; observe for pallor, dizziness, and weakness.
3. Check pulse before and after ambulating. Do not progress if pulse > 110.

Collaborative interventions are actions the nurse carries out in collaboration with other health team members, such as physical therapists, social workers, dietitians, and physicians. Collaborative nursing activities reflect the overlapping responsibilities of, and collegial relationships between, health personnel. For example, the physician might order physical therapy to teach the client crutch-walking. The nurse would be responsible for informing the physical therapy department and for coordinating the client's care to include the physical therapy sessions. When the client returns to the nursing unit, the nurse would assist with crutch-walking and collaborate with the physical therapist to evaluate the client's progress.

The amount of time the nurse spends in an independent versus a collaborative or dependent role varies according to the clinical area, type of institution, and specific position of the nurse.

Considering the Consequences of Each Intervention

Usually several possible interventions can be identified for each nursing goal. The nurse's task is to choose those that are most likely to achieve the desired client outcomes. The nurse begins by considering the risks and benefits of each intervention. An intervention may have more than one consequence. For example, "Provide accurate information" could result in the following client behaviors:

- Increased anxiety
- Decreased anxiety
- Wish to talk with the physician
- Desire to leave the hospital
- Relaxation.

Determining the consequences of each intervention requires nursing knowledge and experience. For example, the nurse's experience may suggest that providing information the night before the client's surgery may increase the client's worry and tension, whereas maintaining the usual rituals before sleep is more effective. The nurse might then consider providing information several days before surgery.

Criteria for Choosing Nursing Interventions

After considering the consequences of the alternative nursing interventions, the nurse chooses one or more that are likely to be most effective. Although the nurse bases this decision on knowledge and experience, the client's input is important.

The following criteria can help the nurse choose the best nursing interventions. The plan must be

- Safe and appropriate for the individual's age, health, and condition.
- Achievable with the resources available. For example, a home care nurse might wish to include a nursing order for an elderly client to "Check blood glucose daily"; but in order for that to occur, either the client must have intact sight, cognition, and memory to carry this out independently, or daily visits from a home care nurse must be available and affordable.
- Congruent with the client's values, beliefs, and culture.
- Congruent with other therapies (e.g., if the client is not permitted food, the strategy of an evening snack must be deferred until health permits).
- Based on nursing knowledge and experience or knowledge from relevant sciences (i.e., based on a rationale). For examples of rationales, refer to the Nursing Care Plan for Amanda Aquilini on pages 310–311.
- Within established standards of care as determined by state laws, professional associations (American Nurses Association), and the policies of the institution. Many agencies have policies to guide the activities of health professionals and to safeguard clients. Rules for visiting hours and procedures to follow when a client has cardiac arrest are examples. If a policy does not benefit clients, nurses have a responsibility to bring this to the attention of the appropriate people.

Writing Nursing Orders

After choosing the appropriate nursing interventions, the nurse writes them on the care plan as nursing orders. **Nursing orders** are instructions for the specific individualized activities the nurse performs to help the client meet established health care goals. The term *order* connotes a sense of accountability for the nurse who gives the order and for the nurse who carries it out. See examples of nursing orders for Amanda Aquilini in the Nursing Care Plan on pages 310–311. The degree of detail included in the nursing orders depends to some degree on the health personnel who will carry out the order. For examples of the components of a nursing order, see Table 18–6.

Date

Nursing orders are dated when they are written and reviewed regularly at intervals that depend on the individual's needs. In an intensive care unit, for example, the plan of care will be continually monitored and revised. In a community clinic, weekly or biweekly reviews may be indicated.

Action Verb

The action verb starts the order and must be precise. For example, "Explain (to the client) the actions of insulin" is a more precise statement than "Teach (the client) about insulin." "Measure and record ankle circumference daily at 0900 h" is more precise than "Assess edema of left ankle daily." Sometimes a modifier for the verb can make the nursing order more precise. For example, "Apply spiral bandage firmly to left lower leg" is more precise than "Apply spiral bandage to left leg."

Content Area

The content is the what and the where of the order. In the preceding order, "spiral bandage" and "left leg" state the what and where of the order. The content area in this example may also clarify whether the foot or toes are to be left exposed.

Time Element

The time element answers when, how long, or how often the nursing action is to occur. Examples are "Assist client with tub bath at 0700 daily" and "Administer analgesic 30 minutes prior to physical therapy."

TABLE 18–6   Components of Nursing Orders

Date	Action Verb	Content Area	Time Element	Signature
4/14/03	Monitor	for verbalization of interest in group activities	with each client contact	J. Jonas, RN
4/14/03	Instruct	(client) to avoid drinking liquids with meals if nausea occurs	evening shift, 4/14/03	J. Jonas, RN
4/14/03	Pad	side rails	during periods of restlessness and confusion	C. Van, RN
4/14/03	Discuss	(with family) their need for help with client's care at home	on Friday	L. Chung, RN
4/14/03	Palpate	uterine fundus for firmness	hourly ×2, then q4h × 24h	C. Patti, RN

Signature

The signature of the nurse prescribing the order shows the nurse's accountability and has legal significance.

Relationship of Nursing Orders to Problem Status

Depending on the type of client problem, the nurse writes orders for observation, prevention, treatment, and health promotion.

Observation orders include assessments made to determine whether a complication is developing, as well as observation of the client's responses to nursing and other therapies. The nurse should write observation orders for both real problems and those for which the client is at risk. Some examples are "Auscultate lungs q8h," "Observe for redness over sacrum q2h," and "Record intake and output hourly."

Prevention orders prescribe the care needed to prevent complications or reduce risk factors. They are needed mainly for potential nursing diagnoses and collaborative problems. Examples of prevention orders are "Turn, cough, and deep breathe q2h" (prevents respiratory complications) and "If fundus is boggy, massage until firm" (prevents postpartum hemorrhage).

Treatment orders include teaching, referrals, physical care, and other care needed to treat an actual nursing diagnosis. Some orders may accomplish either prevention or treatment functions, depending on the status of the problem. In the preceding examples, the order "Turn, cough, and deep breathe q2h" can also be intended to treat an existing respiratory problem and the order "If fundus is boggy, massage until firm" can also be intended to treat an actual postpartum hemorrhage.

Health promotion orders are appropriate when the client has no health problems or when the nurse makes a wellness nursing diagnosis. Such nursing interventions focus on helping the client identify areas for improvement that will lead to a higher level of wellness and actualize the client's overall health potential. Examples are "Discuss the importance of daily exercise" and "Explore infant-stimulation techniques."

Delegating Implementation

Delegating is another activity that occurs during the planning phase of the nursing process. While choosing nursing interventions and writing nursing orders on the client's care plan, the nurse must also determine who should actually perform the activity. The American Nurses Association defines **delegation** as "the transfer of responsibility for the performance of an activity from one person to another while retaining accountability for the outcome." This differs from **assignment** which is a "downward or lateral transfer of both the responsibility *and accountability* [emphasis added] of an activity from one individual to another" (ANA, 1992, Attachment I, #5–6). The ability to delegate client care and assign tasks is a vital skill for registered nurses because many health care institutions use assistive personnel (e.g., licensed practical nurses and unlicensed nursing assistants). To delegate appropriately, the nurse must match the needs of the client and family with the skills and knowledge of the available caregivers. This requires knowing the background, experience, knowledge, skills, and strengths of each person, and understanding which tasks are and are not within their legal scope of practice.

The nurse has two responsibilities in delegating and assigning: (1) appropriate delegation of duties (that is, giving people duties within their scope of practice) and (2) adequate supervision of personnel to whom work is delegated or assigned. The RN can delegate certain tasks to an unlicensed person but cannot assign responsibility for total nursing care. The RN is responsible for seeing that delegated tasks are carried out properly. Assistive personnel may perform tasks such as measuring intake and output, but the RN is still responsible for analyzing data, planning care, and evaluating outcomes. Because there are no universal standards for the training of unlicensed personnel, nurses often must assume responsibility for supplementing the training those staff members have received (see also Chapter 26). ∞

THE NURSING INTERVENTIONS CLASSIFICATION

Chapter 17 ∞ described the efforts of the North American Nursing Diagnosis Association (NANDA) to standardize the language for describing problems that require nursing care and to create a taxonomy of standardized client outcome labels. A group of nurse researchers also recognized the need for a standardized language to describe the interventions that nurses perform. A taxonomy of nursing interventions referred to as the **Nursing Interventions Classification (NIC)** taxonomy has been developed by the Iowa Intervention Project (McCloskey & Bulechek, 2000). This taxonomy consists of three levels: (a) level 1, domains; (b) level 2, classes; and (c) level 3, interventions. Table 18–7 shows the seven domains and 30 classes of interventions within the taxonomy.

More than 486 interventions (level 3) have been developed. Similar to NANDA diagnoses, each broadly stated intervention includes a label (name), a definition, and a list of activities that outline the key actions of nurses in carrying out the intervention (see Box 18–2). The level 3 intervention Touch is one of several interventions developed within the Behavioral domain and its class entitled Coping Assistance.

All NIC interventions have been linked to NANDA nursing diagnostic labels. The nurse can look up a client's nursing diagnosis to see which nursing interventions are suggested. However, each nursing diagnosis contains suggestions for several interventions, so nurses need to select the appropriate interventions based on their judgment and knowledge of the client. For example, the nursing diagnostic label *Sleep Pattern Disturbance* has 10 NIC interventions listed for problem resolution and 18 additional optional interventions (see Box 18–3).

When planning and documenting care in an agency that uses the NIC taxonomy, the nurse chooses from the computer (or writes, if using a manual system) the broad intervention label (e.g., Touch). Not all activities suggested for the intervention

TABLE 18–7 NIC Taxonomy

Level 1: Domains	Level 2: Classes (lettered for cross-referencing)
Domain 1 *Physiological: Basic* Care that supports physical functioning	A. Activity and Exercise Management: Interventions to organize or assist with physical activity and energy conservation and expenditure B. Elimination Management: Interventions to establish and maintain regular bowel and urinary elimination patterns and manage complications due to altered patterns C. Immobility Management: Interventions to manage restricted body movement and the sequelae D. Nutrition Support: Interventions to modify or maintain nutritional status E. Physical Comfort Promotion: Interventions to promote comfort using physical techniques F. Self-Care Facilitation: Interventions to provide or assist with routine activities of daily living
Domain 2 *Physiological: Complex* Care that supports homeostatic regulation	G. Electrolyte and Acid–Base Management: Interventions to regulate electrolyte/acid–base balance and prevent complications H. Drug Management: Interventions to facilitate desired effects of pharmacological agents I. Neurologic Management: Interventions to optimize neurologic functions J. Perioperative Care: Interventions to provide care before, during, and immediately after surgery K. Respiratory Management: Interventions to promote airway patency and gas exchange L. Skin/Wound Management: Interventions to maintain or restore tissue integrity M. Thermoregulation: Interventions to maintain body temperature within a normal range N. Tissue Perfusion Management: Interventions to optimize circulation of blood and fluids to the tissue
Domain 3 *Behavioral* Care that supports psychosocial functioning and facilitates lifestyle changes	O. Behavior Therapy: Interventions to reinforce or promote desirable behaviors or alter undesirable behaviors P. Cognitive Therapy: Interventions to reinforce or promote desirable cognitive functioning or alter undesirable cognitive functioning Q. Communication Enhancement: Interventions to facilitate delivering and receiving verbal and nonverbal messages R. Coping Assistance: Interventions to assist another to build on own strengths, to adapt to a change in function, or to achieve a higher level of function S. Patient Education: Interventions to facilitate learning T. Psychological Comfort Promotion: Interventions to promote comforts using psychological techniques
Domain 4 *Safety* Care that supports protection against harm	U. Crisis Management: Interventions to provide immediate short-term help in both psychological and physiological crises V. Risk Management: Interventions to initiate risk-reduction activities and continue monitoring risks over time
Domain 5 *Family* Care that supports the family unit	W. Childbearing Care: Interventions to assist in understanding and coping with the psychological and physiological changes during the childbearing period Z. Childrearing Care: Interventions to assist in child rearing X. Lifespan Care: Interventions to facilitate family unit functioning and promote the health and welfare of family members throughout the lifespan
Domain 6 *Health System* Care that supports effective use of the health care delivery system	Y. Health System Mediation: Interventions to facilitate the interface between patient/family and the health care system a. Health System Management: Interventions to provide and enhance support services for the delivery of care b. Information Management: Interventions to facilitate communication among health care providers
Domain 7 *Community* Care that supports the health of the community	c. Community Health Promotion: Interventions that promote the health of the whole community. d. Community Risk Management: Interventions that assist in detecting or preventing health risks to the whole community

Note: From *Nursing Interventions Classification (NIC),* 3rd ed. (pp. 90–91), by J. C. McCloskey and G. M. Bulechek, Eds., 2000, St. Louis, MO: Mosby. Reprinted with permission.

would be needed for every client, so the nurse chooses the activities appropriate for the client and individualizes them to fit the supplies, equipment, and other resources available in the agency.

When writing individualized nursing orders on a care plan, the nurse should record the activities rather than the broad intervention labels. However, when the NIC taxonomy becomes more widely used it may be possible to write only the intervention labels and assume that all nurses would know the activities to carry them out.

The NIC taxonomy provides many benefits to nurse practitioners, nurse educators, nurse administrators, and the nursing profession as a whole (see Box 18–4).

BOX 18–2 ■ Example of a NIC Nursing Intervention Label

Intervention: Touch
DEFINITION: Providing comfort and communication through purposeful tactile contact
ACTIVITIES:
- Observe cultural taboos about touch.
- Give a reassuring hug, as appropriate.
- Put arm around patient's shoulders, as appropriate.
- Hold patient's hand to provide emotional support.
- Apply gentle pressure at wrist, hand, or shoulder of seriously ill patient.
- Rub back in synchrony with patient's breathing, as appropriate.
- Stroke body part in slow, rhythmical fashion, as appropriate.
- Massage around painful area, as appropriate.
- Elicit from parents common actions used to soothe and calm their child.

- Hold infant or child firmly and snugly.
- Encourage parents to touch newborn or ill child.
- Surround premature infant with blanket rolls (nesting).
- Swaddle infant snugly in a blanket to keep arms and legs close to the body.
- Place infant on mother's body immediately after birth.
- Encourage mother to hold, touch, and examine the infant while umbilical cord is being severed.
- Encourage parents to hold infant.
- Encourage parents to massage infant.
- Demonstrate quieting techniques for infants.
- Provide appropriate pacifier for nonnutritional sucking in newborns.
- Provide oral stimulation exercises before tube feedings in premature infants.

Note: From *Nursing Interventions Classification (NIC)* 3rd ed. (p. 669), by J. C. McCloskey and G. M. Bulechek, Eds., 2000, St. Louis, MO: Mosby. Reprinted with permission.

BOX 18–3 ■ Examples of NIC Interventions Linked to the NANDA Nursing Diagnosis of Disturbed Sleep Pattern

Disturbed Sleep Pattern
Definition: Time limited disruption of sleep (natural, periodic suspension of consciousness) amount and quality

Suggested Nursing Interventions for Problem Resolution

Dementia Management	Medication Prescribing
Environmental Management	Security Enhancement
Environmental Management: Comfort	Simple Relaxation Therapy
Medication Administration	Sleep Enhancement
Medication Management	Touch

Additional Optional Interventions

Anxiety Reduction	Music Therapy
Autogenic Training	Nutrition Management
Bathing	Pain Management
Calming Technique	Positioning
Coping Enhancement	Progressive Muscle
Energy Management	Relaxation
Exercise Promotion	Self-Care Assistance: Toileting
Exercise Therapy: Ambulation	Simple Massage
Kangaroo Care	Urinary Incontinence Care: Enuresis
Meditation	

Note: From *Nursing Interventions Classification (NIC)* 3rd ed. (p. 781), by J. C. McCloskey and G. M. Bulechek, Eds., 2000, St. Louis, MO: Mosby. Reprinted with permission.

- Helps demonstrate the impact that nurses have on the health care delivery system.
- Standardizes and defines the knowledge base for nursing curricula and practice.
- Facilitates the appropriate selection of a nursing intervention.
- Facilitates communication of nursing treatments to other nurses and other providers.
- Enables researchers to examine the effectiveness and cost of nursing care.
- Assists educators to develop curricula that better articulate with clinical practice.
- Facilitates the teaching of clinical decision making to novice nurses.
- Assists administrators in planning more effectively for staff and equipment needs.
- Promotes the development of a reimbursement system for nursing services.
- Facilitates the development and use of nursing information systems.
- Communicates the nature of nursing to the public.

Note: From *Nursing Interventions Classification (NIC)* 3rd ed. (p. xi), by J. C. McCloskey and G. M. Bulechek, Eds., 2000, St. Louis, MO: Mosby. Reprinted with permission.

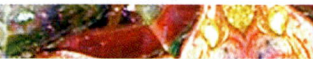

Lifespan Considerations

Elders

When a client is in an extended care facility or a long-term care facility, interventions and medications often remain the same day after day. It is important to review the care plan on a regular basis, because changes in the condition of elders may be subtle and go unnoticed. This applies to both changes of improvement or deterioration. Either one should receive attention so that appropriate revisions can be made in expected outcomes and interventions. Outcomes need to be realistic with consideration given to the client's physical condition, emotional condition, support systems, and mental status. Outcomes often have to be stated and expected to be completed in very small steps. For instance, a client who has had a cerebrovascular accident may spend weeks learning to brush her own teeth or dress herself. When these small steps are successfully completed, it gives the client a sense of accomplishment and motivation to continue working toward increasing self-care. This particular example also demonstrates the need to work collaboratively with other departments, such as physical and occupational therapy, to develop the nursing care plan.

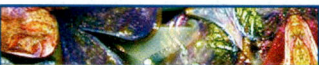

NURSING CARE PLAN FOR AMANDA AQUILINI

NURSING DIAGNOSIS: INEFFECTIVE AIRWAY CLEARANCE RELATED TO VISCOUS SECRETIONS AND SHALLOW CHEST EXPANSION SECONDARY TO FLUID VOLUME DEFICIT, PAIN, AND FATIGUE

DESIRED OUTCOMES [NOC#]/INDICATORS	NURSING ORDERS	RATIONALE
Respiratory Status: Gas exchange [0402], as evidenced by • Absence of pallor and cyanosis (skin and mucous membranes) • Use of correct breathing/coughing technique after instruction • Productive cough • Symmetric chest excursion of at least 4 cm	Monitor respiratory status q4h: rate, depth, effort, skin color, mucous membranes, amount and color of sputum. Monitor results of blood gases, chest x-ray studies, and incentive spirometer volume as available. Monitor level of consciousness. Auscultate lungs q4h. Vital signs q4h (TPR, BP, pulse oximetry).	To identify progress toward or deviations from goal. *Ineffective Airway Clearance* leads to poor oxygenation, as evidenced by pallor, cyanosis, lethargy, and drowsiness. Inadequate oxygenation causes increased pulse rate. Respiratory rate may be decreased by narcotic analgesics. Shallow breathing further compromises oxygenation.
Within 48–72 hours • Lungs clear to auscultation • Respirations 12–22/min; pulse, 100 beats/min • Inhales normal volume of air on incentive spirometer	Instruct in breathing and coughing techniques. Remind to perform, and assist q3h. Administer prescribed expectorant; schedule for maximum effectiveness.	To enable client to cough up secretions. May need encouragement and support because of fatigue and pain. Helps loosen secretions so they can be coughed up and expelled.

NURSING CARE PLAN FOR AMANDA AQUILINI *continued*

DESIRED OUTCOMES [NOC#]/INDICATORS	NURSING ORDERS	RATIONALE
	Maintain Fowler's or semi-Fowler's position.	Gravity allows for fuller lung expansion by decreasing pressure of abdomen on diaphragm.
	Administer prescribed analgesics. Notify physician if pain not relieved.	Controls pleuritic pain by blocking pain pathways and altering perception of pain, enabling client to increase thoracic expansion. Unrelieved pain may signal impending complication.
	Administer oxygen by nasal cannula as prescribed. Provide portable oxygen if client goes off unit (e.g., for x-ray examination).	Supplemental oxygen makes more oxygen available to the cells, even though less air is being moved by the client, thereby reducing the work of breathing.
	Assist with postural drainage daily at 0930. Administer prescribed antibiotic to maintain constant blood level. Observe for rash and GI or other side effects.	Gravity facilitates movement of secretions upward through the respiratory passage. Resolves infection by bacteriostatic or bactericidal effect, depending on type of antibiotic used. Constant level required to prevent pathogens from multiplying. Allergies to antibiotics are common.

NURSING DIAGNOSIS: DEFICIENT FLUID VOLUME: INTAKE INSUFFICIENT TO REPLACE FLUID LOSS (SEE STANDARDIZED CARE PLAN FOR DEFICIENT FLUID VOLUME, FIGURE 18–4).

NURSING DIAGNOSIS: ANXIETY RELATED TO DIFFICULTY BREATHING AND CONCERN ABOUT WORK AND PARENTING ROLES.

DESIRED OUTCOMES [NOC#]/INDICATORS	NURSING ORDERS	RATIONALE
Anxiety control [1402], as evidenced by • Listening to and following instructions for correct breathing and coughing technique, even during periods of dyspnea	When client is dyspneic, stay with her; reassure her you will stay.	Presence of a competent caregiver reduces fear of being unable to breathe. Control of anxiety will help client to maintain effective breathing pattern.
• Verbalizing understanding of condition, diagnostic tests, and treatments (by end of day)	Remain calm; appear confident. Encourage slow, deep breathing.	Reassures client the nurse can help her. Focusing on breathing may help client feel in control and decrease anxiety.
• Decrease in reports of fear and anxiety • Voice steady, not shaky • Respiratory rate of 12–22/min	When client is dyspneic, give brief explanations of treatments and procedures. When acute episode is over, give detailed information about nature of condition, treatments, and tests.	Anxiety and pain interfere with learning. Knowing what to expect reduces anxiety.
• Freely expressing concerns and possible solutions about work and parenting roles Explore alternatives as needed. Note whether husband returns as scheduled. If not, institute care plan for actual *Interrupted Family Processes*	As client can tolerate, encourage to express and expand on her concerns about her child and her work.	Awareness of source of anxiety enables client to gain control over it. Husband's continued absence would constitute a defining characteristic for this nursing diagnosis.

continued on page 312

NURSING CARE PLAN FOR AMANDA AQUILINI *continued*

Applying Critical Thinking

1. What assumptions does the nurse make when deciding that using a standardized care plan for *Deficient Fluid Volume* is appropriate for this client?

2. Identify an outcome in the care plan and its nursing order that contribute to discharge care planning. What evidence supports your choice?

3. Consider how the nurse shares the development of the care plan and outcomes with the client.

4. Not every order has a time frame or interval specified. It may be implied. Under what circumstances is this acceptable practice?

5. In Table 18–1, *Ineffective Airway Clearance* is Amanda's highest priority nursing diagnosis. Under what conditions might this diagnosis be of only moderate priority in Amanda's case?

See Critical Thinking Possibilities in Appendix A.

CONCEPT MAP   Ineffective Airway Clearance (Gas Exchange)

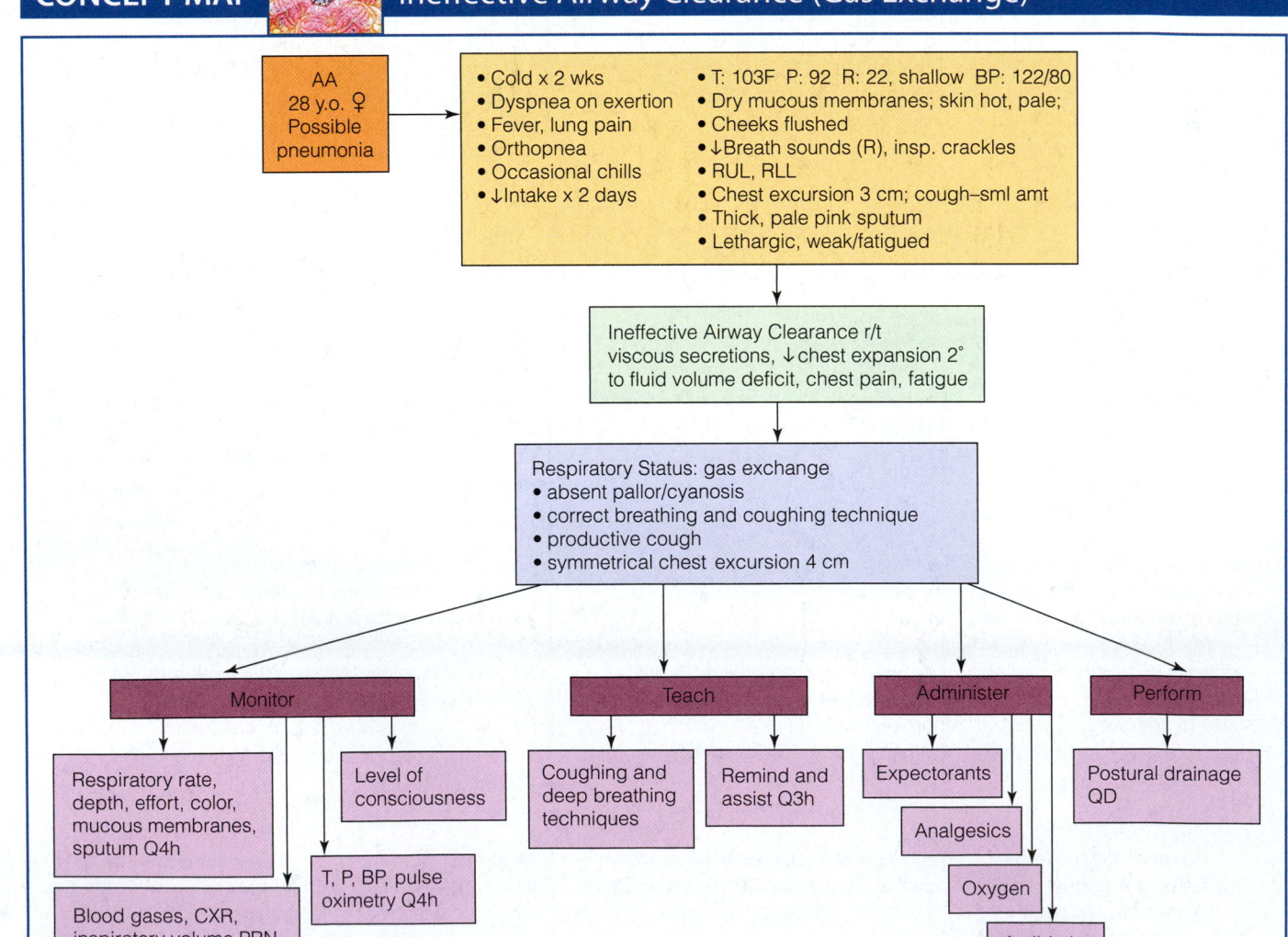

AA
28 y.o. ♀
Possible
pneumonia

- Cold x 2 wks
- Dyspnea on exertion
- Fever, lung pain
- Orthopnea
- Occasional chills
- ↓Intake x 2 days

- T: 103F P: 92 R: 22, shallow BP: 122/80
- Dry mucous membranes; skin hot, pale;
- Cheeks flushed
- ↓Breath sounds (R), insp. crackles
- RUL, RLL
- Chest excursion 3 cm; cough–sml amt
- Thick, pale pink sputum
- Lethargic, weak/fatigued

Ineffective Airway Clearance r/t viscous secretions, ↓chest expansion 2° to fluid volume deficit, chest pain, fatigue

Respiratory Status: gas exchange
- absent pallor/cyanosis
- correct breathing and coughing technique
- productive cough
- symmetrical chest excursion 4 cm

Monitor
- Respiratory rate, depth, effort, color, mucous membranes, sputum Q4h
- T, P, BP, pulse oximetry Q4h
- Blood gases, CXR, inspiratory volume PRN
- Level of consciousness

Teach
- Coughing and deep breathing techniques
- Remind and assist Q3h

Administer
- Expectorants
- Analgesics
- Oxygen
- Antibiotics

Perform
- Postural drainage QD

Legend: Assessment ☐   Nursing Diagnosis ☐   Outcomes ☐   Nursing Interventions ☐   Activities ☐

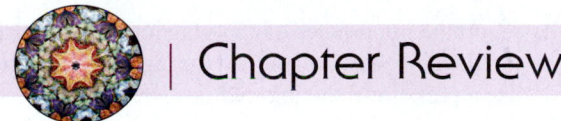

Chapter Review

EXPLORE MediaLink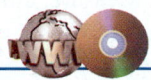

NCLEX review questions, case studies, MediaLink applications, and other interactive resources for this chapter can be found on the Companion Website at www.prenhall.com/kozier. Click on Chapter 18 to select the activities for this chapter.

For more NCLEX review questions, and an audio glossary, access the Student CD-ROM accompanying this textbook.

Chapter Highlights

- Planning is the process of designing nursing activities required to prevent, reduce, or eliminate a client's health problems.
- Planning involves the nurse, the client, support persons, and other caregivers.
- Shorter acute care hospitalization necessitates careful discharge planning.
- Standardized care plans should be adapted and used with individualized plans to meet individual client needs.
- The nursing care plan provides direction for individualized care of the client.
- The planning process includes setting diagnostic priorities, establishing client goals/desired outcomes, selecting nursing interventions, writing nursing orders, and developing a nursing care plan.
- The nurse consults with other nurses or health professionals to verify information, implement changes, or obtain additional knowledge to aid in client goals.
- Nursing diagnoses are assigned high, medium, and low priorities in consultation with the client, if health permits.
- Client goals/desired outcomes are used to plan nursing interventions that will achieve anticipated changes in the client.
- A taxonomy of nursing outcome statements, the Nursing Outcomes Classification (NOC) has been developed to describe measurable states, behaviors, or perceptions that re-

spond to nursing interventions. Each has a definition, measuring scale, and indicators.
- Desired outcomes describe specific and measurable client responses and help the nurse evaluate the effectiveness of the nursing interventions.
- Client goals/desired outcomes are derived from the first clause of the nursing diagnosis.
- Goal statements and desired outcomes are written in terms of the client's behavior.
- Nursing interventions and activities are focused on the etiology or second clause of the nursing diagnosis.
- Nursing activities are the specific actions taken by the nurse to help the client meet health care goals.
- Independent nursing interventions are those the nurse is licensed to prescribe or delegate.
- Projecting the consequences of each nursing strategy requires nursing knowledge and experience.
- A taxonomy of nursing interventions referred to as the Nursing Interventions Classification (NIC) taxonomy has been developed. These interventions have been linked to the NANDA nursing diagnostic labels. Similar to NANDA diagnoses, each broadly stated intervention includes a label (name), a definition, and a list of activities that outline the key actions of nurses in carrying out the intervention.

Review Questions

You are assigned to care for a 75-year-old man who has had elective surgery to replace an arthritic hip. The client was admitted directly to the surgery unit and is now back in his room on the orthopedic floor several hours after being discharged from the postanesthesia recovery unit.

18–1. Which type(s) of planning will be performed during this first postoperative shift?
   a. initial
   b. ongoing
   c. discharge
   d. all of the above

18–2. The client requests that his family members be allowed to stay overnight with him in his room. To determine whether this request can be honored, the nurse may need to consult
   a. hospital policies.
   b. standardized care plans.
   c. orthopedic protocols.
   d. standards of care.

18–3. Assessment reveals that the client is drowsy when not aroused, states his pain is 4 on a scale of 0 to 10, VS are within preoperative range, extremities are warm with

good pulses but very dry skin, declines oral fluids due to nausea, reports no bowel movement in the past 2 days, hip dressing is dry with drains intact. Which of the following most likely would be considered of high priority for a change in the current care plan?
a. pain
b. nausea
c. constipation
d. potential for wound infection

18–4. Another nurse establishes a nursing diagnosis of *Risk for Impaired Skin Integrity* related to immobility, dry skin, and surgical incision. Which of the following represents a properly stated outcome/goal? The client will
a. turn in bed q2h.

b. report the importance of applying lotion to skin daily.
c. not develop skin breakdown during hospitalization.
d. use a pressure-reducing mattress.

18–5. The care plan reveals a nursing order stated, in full, as "4/2/03 Measure client's fluid intake and output. F. Jenkins, RN." What element of a proper nursing order has been omitted?
a. action verb
b. content
c. time
d. none

Readings and References

Suggested Readings

NIC/NOC letter–published twice a year in February and August, available online at http://www.nursing.uiowa.edu/centers/cncce/nicnocnews.htm

Thomassy, C. S., & McShea, C. S. (2001). Shifting gears: Jump-start interdisciplinary patient care. *Nursing Management, 32*(5), 40–44. Fragmented and potentially inconsistent care can result when each discipline creates its own recording tools for assessing clients, planning, and documenting care. This hospital created a three-part form—essential assessments, care and education planning, and transition care planning—to be used by all disciplines. Although issues of change and cooperation are not necessarily easily overcome, the improvements in interdisciplinary collaboration and quality care are considered to be much worth the effort.

Related Research

Determining cost of nursing interventions: A beginning. . . . Iowa Intervention Project. (2001). *Nursing Economics, 19,* 146–160.

O'Connor, N. A., Kershaw, T., & Hameister, A. D. (2001). Documenting patterns of nursing interventions using cluster analysis. *Journal of Nursing Measurement, 9*(1), 73–90.

References

American Nurses Association. (1992). *The American Nurses Association position state-

ment on registered nurse utilization of unlicensed personnel.* Kansas City, MO: Author.

Johnson, M., Maas, M., & Moorhead, S. (Eds.). (2000). *Nursing outcomes classification (NOC)* (2nd ed.). St. Louis, MO: Mosby.

McCloskey, J. C., & Bulechek, G. M. (Eds.). (2000). *Nursing interventions classification (NIC)* (3rd ed.). St. Louis, MO: Mosby.

Wilkinson, J. M. (2001). *Nursing process & critical thinking* (3rd ed.). Upper Saddle River, NJ: Prentice Hall Health.

Selected Bibliography

Alfaro-LeFevre, R. (1998). *Applying the nursing process. A step-by-step guide* (4th ed.). Philadelphia: Lippincott.

American Nurses Association. (1998). *Standards of clinical nursing practice* (2nd ed.). Washington, DC: Author.

Aquilino, M. L., & Keenan, G. (2000). Having our say: Nursing's standardized nomenclatures. *American Journal of Nursing, 100*(7), 33–38.

Carpenito, L. J. (2001). *Nursing diagnosis: Application to clinical practice* (9th ed.). Philadelphia: Lippincott Williams &Wilkins.

Gardner, P. (2002). *Nursing process.* Albany, NY: Delmar.

Johnson, M., & Maas, M. (1999). Nursing-sensitive patient outcomes: Development and importance for use in assessing health care effectiveness. In E. Cohen & V. DeBack (Eds.), *The outcomes mandate: Case management in health care today* (pp. 37–48). St. Louis, MO: Mosby.

LaDuke, S. (2000). NIC puts nursing into words. *Nursing Management, 31*(2), 43–44.

Maas, M., Moorhead, S., Specht, J., Schoenfelder, D., Swanson, E. A., & Johnson, M. (2000). Concept development of nursing-sensitive patient outcomes. In B. Rogers & K. Knafl (Eds.), *Concept analysis in nursing research* (pp. 387–400). New York: Springer.

McCloskey, J. C., Bulechek, G. M., Dochterman, J., & Maas, M. (Eds.). (2000). *Nursing diagnoses, outcomes, and interventions: NANDA, NOC and NIC linkages.* St. Louis, MO: Mosby.

NANDA International. (2003). *NANDA nursing diagnoses: Definitions & classification 2003–2004.* Philadelphia: Author.

Payne, J. (2000). The Nursing interventions classification: A language to define nursing. *Oncology Nursing Forum, 27,* 99–103.

Schoenfelder, D., Swanson, E., Specht, J., Johnson, M., & Maas, M. (2000). Outcome indicators for direct and indirect caregiving. *Clinical Nursing Research, 9*(1), 47–69.

Sparks, S. M., & Taylor, C. M. (2001). *Nursing diagnostic reference manual* (5th ed.). Springhouse, PA: Springhouse.

Wilkinson, J. M. (2000). *Nursing diagnosis handbook with NIC interventions and NOC outcomes* (7th ed.). Upper Saddle River, NJ: Prentice Hall Health.

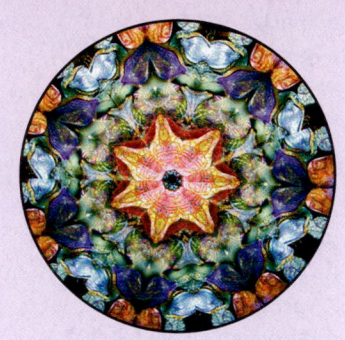

CHAPTER 19

IMPLEMENTING AND EVALUATING

LEARNING OUTCOMES

After completing this chapter, you will be able to:

- Explain how implementing relates to other phases of the nursing process.

- Describe three categories of skills used to implement nursing interventions.

- Discuss the five activities of the implementing phase.

- Identify guidelines for implementing nursing interventions.

- Explain how evaluating relates to other phases of the nursing process.

- Describe five components of the evaluation process.

- Describe the steps involved in reviewing and modifying the client's care plan.

- Name the two components of an evaluation statement.

- Differentiate quality improvement from quality assurance.

- Describe three components of quality evaluation: structure, process, and outcomes.

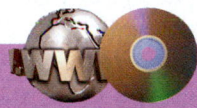

MediaLink

www.prenhall.com/kozier

Additional resources for this chapter can be found on the Student CD-ROM accompanying this textbook, and on the Companion Website at www.prenhall. com/kozier. Click on Chapter 19 to select the activities for this chapter.

CD-ROM
- Audio Glossary
- NCLEX Review

Companion Website
- Additional NCLEX Review
- Case Study: Treating a Client for Pain
- MediaLink Application:
  Analyzing Effective Quality Assurance
- Links to Resources

The nursing process is action oriented, client centered, and outcome directed. After developing a plan of care based on the assessing and diagnosing phases, the nurse implements the interventions and evaluates the desired outcomes. On the basis of this evaluation, the plan of care is either continued, modified, or terminated. As in all phases of the nursing process, clients and support persons are encouraged to participate as much as possible.

IMPLEMENTING

In the nursing process, implementing is the phase in which the nurse implements the nursing interventions. Using NIC terminology, **implementing** consists of doing and documenting the **activities** that are the specific nursing actions needed to carry out the interventions (or nursing orders). The nurse performs or delegates the nursing activities for the interventions that were developed in the planning step and then concludes the implementing step by recording nursing activities and the resulting client responses.

Although the nurse may act on the client's behalf (e.g., referring the client to a community health nurse for home care), professional standards support client and family participation, as in all phases of the nursing process. The degree of participation depends on the client's health status. For example, an unconscious man is unable to participate in his care and therefore needs to have care given to him. By contrast, an ambulatory client may require very little care from the nurse and carry out health care activities independently.

Relationship of Implementing to Other Nursing Process Phases

The first three nursing process phases—assessing, diagnosing, and planning—provide the basis for the nursing actions performed during the implementing step. In turn, the implementing phase provides the actual nursing activities and client responses that are examined in the final phase, the evaluating phase. Using data acquired during assessment, the nurse can individualize the care given in the implementing phase, tailoring the interventions to fit a specific client rather than applying them routinely to categories of clients (e.g., all clients with pneumonia).

While implementing nursing orders, the nurse continues to reassess the client at every contact, gathering data about the client's responses to the nursing activities and about any new problems that may develop. A nursing activity on the client's care plan for the NIC intervention *Airway Management* might read "Auscultate lungs q4h." When performing this activity, the nurse is both carrying out the intervention (implementing) and performing an assessment.

Not every nursing action is directed by an intervention that follows from a nursing diagnosis. Some routine nursing activities are, themselves, assessments. For example, all clients require hygiene, nutrition, and elimination. When assisting the client with these, nurses carry out actions that may involve assessment. For example, while bathing an elderly client, the nurse observes a reddened area on the client's sacrum. Or, when emptying a urinary catheter bag, the nurse measures 200 mL of strong-smelling, brown urine.

Implementing Skills

To implement the care plan successfully, nurses need cognitive, interpersonal, and technical skills. These skills are distinct from one another; in practice, however, nurses use them in various combinations and with different emphasis, depending on the activity. For instance, when inserting a urinary catheter the nurse needs cognitive knowledge of the principles and steps of the procedure, interpersonal skills to inform and reassure the client, and technical skill in draping the client and manipulating the equipment.

The **cognitive skills** (intellectual skills) include problem solving, decision making, critical thinking, and creativity. They are crucial to safe, intelligent nursing care (see Chapter 15). 🔗

Interpersonal skills are all of the activities, verbal and nonverbal, people use when interacting directly with one another. The effectiveness of a nursing action often depends largely on the nurse's ability to communicate with others. The nurse uses therapeutic communication to understand the client and in turn be understood. A nurse also needs to work effectively with others as a member of the health care team.

Interpersonal skills are necessary for all nursing activities: caring, comforting, advocating, referring, counseling, and supporting are just a few. Interpersonal skills include conveying knowledge, attitudes, feelings, interest, and appreciation of the client's cultural values and lifestyle. Before nurses can be highly skilled in interpersonal relations, they must have self-awareness and sensitivity to others (see Chapters 24 and 37).

Technical skills are "hands-on" skills such as manipulating equipment, giving injections and bandaging, moving, lifting, and repositioning clients. These skills are also called tasks, procedures, or psychomotor skills. The term *psychomotor* includes the interpersonal component, for example, the need to communicate with the client.

Technical skills require knowledge and, frequently, manual dexterity. The number of technical skills expected of a nurse has greatly increased in recent years because of the increased use of technology, especially in acute care hospitals.

Process of Implementing

The process of implementing (see Figure 19–1 ■) normally includes

- Reassessing the client
- Determining the nurse's need for assistance
- Implementing the nursing interventions
- Supervising the delegated care
- Documenting nursing activities.

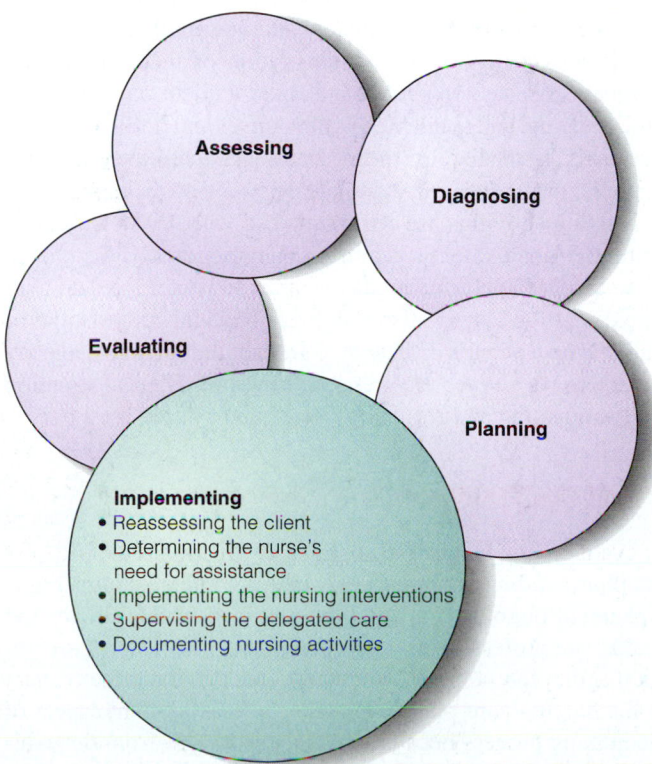

Figure 19–1 ■ **Implementing.** The fourth phase of the nursing process, in which the nurse implements the nursing interventions and documents the care provided.

Reassessing the Client

Just before implementing an intervention, the nurse must reassess the client to make sure the intervention is still needed. Even though an order is written on the care plan, the client's condition may have changed. For example, Gayle Fischer has a nursing diagnosis of *Disturbed Sleep Pattern* related to anxiety and unfamiliar surroundings. During rounds, the nurse discovers that Gayle is sleeping and therefore defers the back massage that had been planned as a relaxation strategy.

New data may indicate a need to change the priorities of care or the nursing activities. For example, a nurse begins to teach Ms. Eves, who has diabetes, how to give herself insulin injections. Shortly after beginning the teaching, the nurse realizes that Ms. Eves is not concentrating on the lesson. Subsequent discussion reveals that she is worried about her eyesight and fears she is going blind. Realizing that the client's level of stress is interfering with her learning, the nurse ends the lesson and makes arrangements for a physician to examine the client's eyes. The nurse also provides supportive communication to help alleviate the client's stress.

Determining the Nurse's Need for Assistance

When implementing some nursing interventions, the nurse may require assistance for one of the following reasons:

- The nurse is unable to implement the nursing activity safely alone (e.g., ambulating an unsteady obese client).
- Assistance would reduce stress on the client (e.g., turning a person who experiences acute pain when moved).
- The nurse lacks the knowledge or skills to implement a particular nursing activity (e.g., a nurse who is not familiar with a particular model of traction equipment needs assistance the first time it is applied).

Implementing the Nursing Interventions

It is important to explain to the client what interventions will be done, what sensations to expect, what the client is expected to do, and what the expected outcome is. For many nursing activities it is also important to ensure the client's privacy, for example by closing doors, pulling curtains, or draping the client. The number and kind of direct nursing interventions is almost unlimited. Nurses also coordinate client care. This activity involves scheduling client contacts with other departments (e.g., laboratory and x-ray technicians, physical and respiratory therapists) and serving as a liaison among the members of the health care team.

When implementing interventions, nurses should follow these guidelines:

- Base nursing interventions on scientific knowledge, nursing research, and professional standards of care (evidence-based practice) whenever possible. The nurse must be aware of the scientific rationale, as well as possible side effects or complications, of all interventions. For example, a client prefers to take an oral medication after meals; however, this medication is not absorbed well in the presence of food. Therefore, the nurse will need to explain why this preference cannot be honored.

- Clearly understand the orders to be implemented and question any that are not understood. The nurse is responsible for intelligent implementation of medical and nursing plans of care. This requires knowledge of each intervention, its purpose in the client's plan of care, any contraindications (e.g., allergies), and changes in the client's condition that may affect the order.

- Adapt activities to the individual client. A client's beliefs, values, age, health status, and environment are factors that can affect the success of a nursing action. For example, the nurse determines that a client chokes when swallowing pills, so consults with the physician to change the order to a liquid form of the medication.

- Implement safe care. For example, when changing a sterile dressing, the nurse practices sterile technique to prevent infection; when giving a medication, the nurse administers the correct dosage by the ordered route.

- Provide teaching, support, and comfort. These independent nursing activities enhance the effectiveness of nursing care plans (see Figure 19–2 ■).

- Be holistic. The nurse must always view the client as a whole and consider the client's responses in that context.

- Respect the dignity of the client and enhance the client's self-esteem. Providing privacy and encouraging clients to make their own decisions are ways of respecting dignity and enhancing self-esteem.

- Encourage clients to participate actively in implementing the nursing interventions. Active participation enhances the client's sense of independence and control. However, clients vary in the degree of participation they desire. Some want total involvement in their care, whereas others prefer little involvement. The amount of desired involvement may be related to the severity of the illness; the client's culture; or the client's fear, understanding of the illness, and understanding of the intervention.

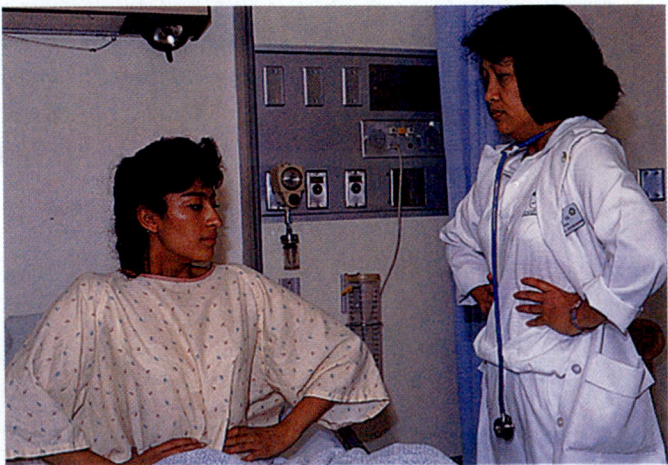

Figure 19–2 ■ Amanda agrees to practice deep-breathing exercises q3h during the day. In addition, she verbalizes awareness of the need to increase her fluid intake and to plan her morning activities to accommodate postural drainage.

Supervising Delegated Care

If care has been delegated to other health care personnel, the nurse responsible for the client's overall care must ensure that the activities have been implemented according to the care plan. Other caregivers may be required to communicate their activities to the nurse by documenting them on the client record, reporting verbally, or filling out a written form. The nurse validates and responds to any adverse findings or client responses. This may involve modifying the nursing care plan.

Documenting Nursing Activities

After carrying out the nursing activities, the nurse completes the implementing phase by recording the interventions and client responses in the nursing progress notes. These are a part of the agency's permanent record for the client. Nursing care must not be recorded in advance because the nurse may determine on reassessment of the client that the intervention should not or cannot be implemented. For example, a nurse is authorized to inject 10 mg of morphine sulfate subcutaneously to a client, but the nurse finds that the client's respiratory rate is 4 breaths per minute. This finding contraindicates the administration of morphine (a respiratory depressant). The nurse withholds the morphine and reports the client's respiratory rate to the nurse in charge and/or physician.

The nurse may record routine or recurring activities (e.g., mouth care) in the client record at the end of a shift. In the meantime, the nurse maintains a personal record of these interventions on a worksheet. In some instances, it is important to record a nursing intervention immediately after it is implemented. This is particularly true of the administration of medications and treatments because recorded data about a client must be up to date, accurate, and available to other nurses and health care professionals. Immediate recording helps safeguard the client, for example, from receiving a duplicate dose of medication.

Nursing activities are communicated verbally as well as in writing. When a client's health is changing rapidly, the charge nurse and/or the physician may want to be kept up to date with verbal reports. Nurses also report client status at a change of shift and on a client's discharge to another unit or health agency in person, via a voice recording, or in writing. For information on documenting and reporting, see Chapter 20. ⌘

EVALUATING

To evaluate is to judge or to appraise. Evaluating is the fifth and last phase of the nursing process. In this context, **evaluating** is a planned, ongoing, purposeful activity in which clients and health care professionals determine (a) the client's progress toward achievement of goals/outcomes and (b) the effectiveness of the nursing care plan. Evaluation is an important aspect of the nursing process because conclusions drawn from the evaluation determine whether the nursing interventions should be terminated, continued, or changed.

Evaluation is continuous. Evaluation done while or immediately after implementing a nursing order enables the nurse to make on-the-spot modifications in an intervention. Evaluation performed at specified intervals (e.g., once a week for the home care client) shows the extent of progress toward goal achievement and enables the nurse to correct any deficiencies and modify the care plan as needed. Evaluation continues until the client achieves the health goals or is discharged from nursing care. Evaluation at discharge includes the status of goal achievement and the client's self-care abilities with regard to follow-up care. Most agencies have a special discharge record for this evaluation.

Through evaluating, nurses demonstrate responsibility and accountability for their actions, indicate interest in the results of the nursing activities, and demonstrate a desire not to perpetuate ineffective actions but to adopt more effective ones.

Relationship of Evaluating to Other Nursing Process Phases

Successful evaluation depends on the effectiveness of the steps that precede it. Assessment data must be accurate and complete so that the nurse can formulate appropriate nursing diagnoses and desired outcomes. The desired outcomes must be stated concretely in behavioral terms if they are to be useful for evaluating client responses. And finally, without the implementing phase in which the plan is put into action, there would be nothing to evaluate.

The evaluating and assessing phases overlap. As previously stated, assessment (data collection) is ongoing and continuous at every client contact. However, data are collected for different purposes at different points in the nursing process. During the assessment phase the nurse collects data for the purpose of making diagnoses. During the evaluation step the nurse collects data for the purpose of comparing it to preselected goals and judging the effectiveness of the nursing care. The act of assessing (data collection) is the same; the differences lie in (a) when the data are collected and (b) how the data are used.

Process of Evaluating Client Responses

Before evaluation, the nurse identifies the desired outcomes (indicators) that will be used to measure client goal achievement. (This is done in the planning step.) Desired outcomes serve two purposes: They establish the kind of evaluative data that need to be collected and provide a standard against which the data are judged. For example, given the following expected outcomes, any nurse caring for the client would know what data to collect:

- Daily fluid intake will not be less than 2500 mL.
- Urinary output will balance with fluid intake.
- Residual urine will be less than 100 mL.

The evaluation process has five components (see Figure 19–3 ■):

- Collecting data related to the desired outcomes (NOC indicators)
- Comparing the data with outcomes
- Relating nursing activities to outcomes
- Drawing conclusions about problem status
- Continuing, modifying, or terminating the nursing care plan.

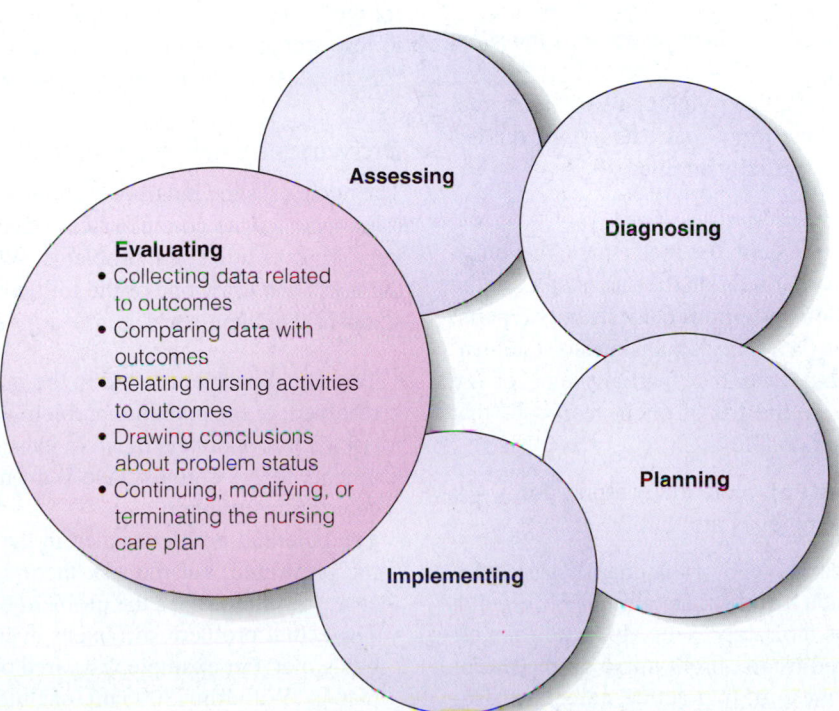

Evaluating
- Collecting data related to outcomes
- Comparing data with outcomes
- Relating nursing activities to outcomes
- Drawing conclusions about problem status
- Continuing, modifying, or terminating the nursing care plan

Assessing

Diagnosing

Planning

Implementing

Figure 19–3 ■ Evaluating. The final phase of the nursing process, in which the nurse determines the client's progress toward goal achievement and the effectiveness of the nursing care plan. The plan may be continued, modified, or terminated.

Collecting Data

Using the clearly stated, precise, and measurable desired outcomes as a guide, the nurse collects data so that conclusions can be drawn about whether goals have been met. It is usually necessary to collect both objective and subjective data.

Some data may require interpretation. Examples of objective data requiring interpretation are the degree of tissue turgor of a dehydrated client or the degree of restlessness of a client with pain. When objective data need interpretation, the nurse may obtain the views of other nurses to substantiate whether change has occurred. Examples of subjective data needing interpretation include complaints of nausea or pain by the client. When interpreting subjective data, the nurse must rely upon either (a) the client's statements (e.g., "My pain is worse now than it was after breakfast") or (b) objective indicators of the subjective data, even though these indicators may require further interpretation (e.g., decreased restlessness, decreased pulse and respiratory rates, and relaxed facial muscles as indicators of pain relief). Data must be recorded concisely and accurately to facilitate the next part of the evaluating process.

Comparing Data with Outcomes

If the first two parts of the evaluation process have been carried out effectively, it is relatively simple to determine whether a desired outcome has been met. Both the nurse and client play an active role in comparing the client's actual responses with the desired outcomes. Did the client drink 3000 mL of fluid in 24 hours? Did the client walk unassisted the specified distance per day? When determining whether a goal has been achieved, the nurse can draw one of three possible conclusions:

1. The goal was met; that is, the client response is the same as the desired outcome.
2. The goal was partially met; that is, either a short-term goal was achieved but the long-term goal was not, or the desired outcome was only partially attained.
3. The goal was not met.

After determining whether a goal has been met, the nurse writes an evaluative statement (either on the care plan or in the nurse's notes). An **evaluation statement** consists of two parts: a conclusion and supporting data. The conclusion is a statement that the goal/desired outcome was met, partially met, or not met. The supporting data are the list of client responses that support the conclusion, for example:

Goal met: Oral intake 300 mL more than output; skin turgor good; mucous membranes moist.

See the nursing care plan at the end of the chapter for evaluation statements for Amanda Aquilini. Data in the Evaluation Statements column on this table represent Ms. Aquilini's responses to care as observed by the night nurse on the morning after her admission to the unit. In practice, care plans usually do not have a column for evaluation statements; rather, these are recorded in the nurse's notes. If NOC indicators are being used with the outcomes, scores on the scales after intervention would be compared with those measured at base-

line to determine improvement. The column explaining rationale for continuing or modifying the plan is included in a student care plan.

Relating Nursing Activities to Outcomes

The fourth aspect of the evaluating process is determining whether the nursing activities had any relation to the outcomes. It should never be assumed that a nursing activity was the cause of or the only factor in meeting, partially meeting, or not meeting a goal.

For example, Mrs. Sophi Ringdale was obese and needed to lose 14 kg (30 lb). When the nurse and client drew up a care plan, one goal was "Lose 1.4 kg (3 lb) by 4/7/03." A nursing strategy in the care plan was "Explain how to plan and prepare a 900-calorie diet." On 4/7/03, the client weighed herself and had lost 1.8 kg (4 lb). The goal had been met—in fact, exceeded. It is easy to assume that the nursing strategy was highly effective. However, it is important to collect more data before drawing that conclusion. On questioning the client, the nurse might find any of the following: (a) The client planned a 900-calorie diet and prepared and ate the food; (b) the client planned a 900-calorie diet but did not prepare the correct food; (c) the client did not understand how to plan a 900-calorie diet, so she did not bother with it.

If the first possibility is found to be true, the nurse can safely judge that the nursing strategy "Explain how to plan and prepare a 900-calorie diet" was effective in helping the client lose weight. However, if the nurse learns that either the second or third possibility actually happened, then it must be assumed that the nursing strategy did not affect the outcome. The next step for the nurse is to collect data about what the client actually did to lose weight. It is important to establish the relationship (or lack thereof) of the nursing actions to the client responses.

Drawing Conclusions about Problem Status

The nurse uses the judgments about goal achievement to determine whether the care plan was effective in resolving, reducing, or preventing client problems. When goals have been met, the nurse can draw one of the following conclusions about the status of the client's problem:

- The actual problem stated in the nursing diagnosis has been resolved; or the potential problem is being prevented and the risk factors no longer exist. In these instances, the nurse documents that the goals have been met and discontinues the care for the problem.
- The potential problem stated in the nursing diagnosis is being prevented, but the risk factors are still present. In this case, the nurse keeps the problem on the care plan.
- The actual problem still exists even though some goals are being met. For example, a desired outcome on a client's care plan is "Will drink 3000 mL of fluid daily." Even though the data may show this outcome has been achieved, other data (dry oral mucous membranes) may indicate that there is *Deficient Fluid Volume*. Therefore, the nursing interventions must be continued even though this one goal was met.

MediaLink | TREATING A CLIENT FOR PAIN CASE STUDY

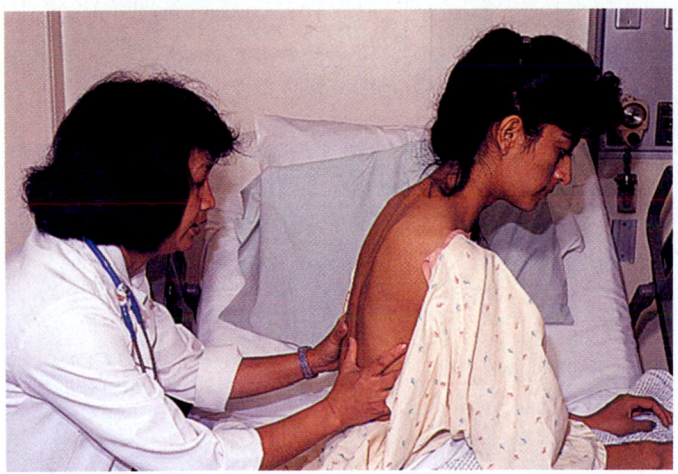

Figure 19–4 ■ Upon assessment of respiratory excursion, Nurse Medina detects failure of the client to achieve maximum ventilation. She and Amanda reevaluate the care plan and modify it to increase coughing and deep-breathing exercises to q2h.

When goals have been partially met or when goals have not been met, two conclusions may be drawn:

• The care plan may need to be revised, since the problem is only partially resolved. The revisions may need to occur during assessing, diagnosing, or planning phases, as well as implementing.

OR

• The care plan does not need revision, because the client merely needs more time to achieve the previously established goal(s). To make this decision, the nurse must assess why the goals are being only partially achieved, including whether the evaluation was conducted too soon.

Continuing, Modifying, and Terminating the Nursing Care Plan

After drawing conclusions about the status of the client's problems, the nurse modifies the care plan as indicated. Depending on the agency, modifications may be made by drawing a line through portions of the care plan, or marking portions using a highlighting pen, or writing "Discontinued" (dc'd) and the date.

Whether or not goals were met, a number of decisions need to be made about continuing, modifying, or terminating nursing care for each problem. Before making individual modifications, the nurse must first determine why the plan as a whole was not completely effective. This requires a review of the entire care plan and a critique of the nursing process steps involved in its development (see Figure 19–4 ■). See Table 19–1 for a checklist to use when reviewing a care plan. Although the checklist uses a closed-ended yes/no format, its only intent is to identify areas that require the nurse's further examination.

ASSESSING. An incomplete or incorrect database influences all subsequent steps of the nursing process and care plan. If data are incomplete, the nurse needs to reassess the client and record the new data. In some instances, new data may indicate the need for new nursing diagnoses, new goals, and new nursing orders.

DIAGNOSING. If the database is incomplete, new diagnostic statements may be required. If the database is complete, the nurse needs to analyze whether the problems were identified correctly and whether the nursing diagnoses are relevant to that database. After making judgments about problem status, the nurse revises or adds new diagnoses as needed to reflect the most recent client data.

PLANNING: DESIRED OUTCOMES. If a nursing diagnosis is inaccurate, obviously the goal statement will need revision. If the nursing diagnosis is appropriate, the nurse then checks that the goals are realistic and attainable. Unrealistic goals require correction. The nurse should also determine whether priorities have changed and whether the client still agrees with the priorities. Goals must also be written for any new nursing diagnoses.

PLANNING: NURSING ORDERS. The nurse investigates whether the nursing interventions were related to goal achievement and whether the best nursing interventions were selected. Even when diagnoses and goals are appropriate, the nursing interventions selected may not have been the best ones to achieve the goal. New nursing orders may reflect changes in the amount of nursing care the client needs, scheduling changes, or rearrangement of nursing activities to group similar activities or to permit longer rest or activity periods for the client. If new nursing diagnoses have been written, then new nursing orders will also be necessary.

IMPLEMENTING. Even if all sections of the care plan appear to be satisfactory, the manner in which the plan was implemented may have interfered with goal achievement. Before selecting new interventions, the nurse should check whether the nursing orders were carried out. Other personnel may not have carried them out, either because the orders were unclear or because they were unreasonable in terms of external constraints such as money, staff, and equipment.

After making the necessary modifications to the care plan, the nurse implements the modified plan and begins the nursing process cycle again. Refer to the Nursing Care Plan at the end of this chapter to see how the plan for Amanda Aquilini was modified after evaluation of goal achievement and review of the nursing process. A line has been drawn through portions the nurse wished to delete; additions to the care plan are shown in italics.

Evaluating the Quality of Nursing Care

In addition to evaluating goal achievement for individual clients, nurses are also involved in evaluating and modifying the overall quality of care given to groups of clients. This is an essential part of professional accountability.

TABLE 19–1 Evaluation Checklist

Assessing	Diagnosing	Planning	Implementing
____ Are data complete, accurate, and validated? ____ Do new data require changes in the care plan?	____ Are nursing diagnoses relevant and accurate? ____ Are nursing diagnoses supported by the data? ____ Has problem status changed (i.e., potential, actual, risk)? ____ Are the diagnoses stated clearly and in correct format? ____ Have any nursing diagnoses been resolved?	**Desired outcomes** ____ Do new nursing diagnoses require new goals? ____ Are goals realistic? ____ Was enough time allowed for goal achievement? ____ Do the goals address all aspects of the problem? ____ Does the client still concur with the goals? ____ Have client priorities changed? **Nursing Orders** ____ Do nursing orders need to be written for new nursing diagnoses or new goals? ____ Do the nursing orders seem to be related to the stated goals? ____ Is there a rationale to justify each nursing order? ____ Are the nursing orders clear, specific, and detailed? ____ Are new resources available? ____ Do the nursing orders address all aspects of the client's goals? ____ Were the nursing orders actually carried out?	____ Was client input obtained at each step of the nursing process? ____ Were goals and nursing interventions acceptable to the client? ____ Did the caregivers have the knowledge and skill to perform the interventions correctly? ____ Were explanations given to the client prior to implementing?

Quality Assurance

A **quality-assurance (QA) program** is an ongoing, systematic process designed to evaluate and promote excellence in the health care provided to clients. Quality assurance frequently refers to evaluation of the level of care provided in a health care agency, but it may be limited to the evaluation of the performance of one nurse or more broadly involve the evaluation of the quality of the care in an agency, or even in a country.

Quality assurance requires evaluation of three components of care: structure, process, and outcome. Each type of evaluation requires different criteria and methods, and each has a different focus.

Structure evaluation focuses on the setting in which care is given. It answers this question: What effect does the setting have on the quality of care? Structural standards describe desirable environmental and organizational characteristics that influence care, such as equipment and staffing.

Process evaluation focuses on how the care was given. It answers questions such as these: Is the care relevant to the client's needs? Is the care appropriate, complete, and timely? Process standards focus on the manner in which the nurse uses the nursing process. Some examples of process criteria are "Checks client's identification band before giving medication" and "Performs and records chest assessment, including auscultation, once per shift."

Outcome evaluation focuses on demonstrable changes in the client's health status as a result of nursing care. Outcome criteria are written in terms of client responses or health status, just as they are for evaluation within the nursing process. For example, "How many clients undergoing hip repairs develop pneumonia?" or "How many clients who have a colostomy experience an infection that delays discharge?"

Quality Improvement

Quality improvement (QI) is also known as continuous quality improvement (CQI), total quality management (TQM), performance improvement (PI), or persistent quality improvement (PQI). According to Schroeder (1994, p. 3), QI is

> the commitment and approach used to continuously improve every process in every part of an organization, with the intent of meeting and exceeding customer expectations and outcomes.

Unlike quality assurance, QI follows client care rather than organizational structure, focuses on process rather than individuals, and uses a systematic approach with the intention of *improving* the quality of care rather than *ensuring* the quality of care. QI studies often focus on identifying and correcting a system's problems, such as duplication of services in a hospital or improving services.

Nursing Audit

An *audit* means the examination or review of records. A *retrospective audit* is the evaluation of a client's record after discharge from an agency. *Retrospective* means "relating to past events." A *concurrent audit* is the evaluation of a client's health care while the client is still receiving care from the agency. These evaluations use interviewing, direct observation of nursing care, and review of clinical records to determine whether specific evaluative criteria have been met.

Another type of evaluation of care is the *peer review*. In nurse peer review, nurses functioning in the same capacity, that is, peers, appraise the quality of care or practice performed by other equally qualified nurses. The peer review is based on preestablished standards or criteria.

There are two types of peer reviews: individual and nursing audits. The individual peer review focuses on the performance of an individual nurse. The nursing audit focuses on evaluating nursing care through the review of records. The success of these audits depends on accurate documentation; auditors assume that if the data have not been recorded, the care has not been given.

Research Note
How Do We Know If Care Plans Are Client Focused?

Kirrane (2001) acknowledged that there are very diverse views on the usefulness of nursing care plans, care pathways, interdisciplinary care maps, and other related tools. She reported on literature supporting evidence of documentation that can speed nursing care and enhance accuracy of documentation. However, no evidence was available to indicate that care plans also were individualized based on client-focused needs. The methodology chosen to evaluate the question in this institution was an audit tool. Five care plans on each of two neurology units were evaluated and, when possible, the client or family was interviewed to determine their perspectives on the care plan. Although detailed results of the audit are not provided in the article, it is clear that the care plans had room for improvement relative to the study question.

Implications: In addition to forming qualitative judgments about the client-focused nature of the care plans, the author used the results of the audit to provide staff development training in writing more objective and specific plans. Staff was strongly supported to author the plans in concert with the client and family. A repeated audit 6 months later showed improvement in the use of appropriate documentation and individualization. In addition, the second audit indicated that clients and families were more aware of the purpose and their role in care planning. The decision was made to have audits become a regular part of care evaluation and to continue to use the results for staff development.

Note: From "An Audit of Care Planning on a Neurology Unit," by C. Kirrane, 2001, *Nursing Standard, 15*(19), pp. 36–39.

Lifespan Considerations

Elders

Evaluation of goals, selected outcomes, and interventions needs to be continuous, with ongoing assessment and reassessment of the situation. Priority needs can change quickly and must be reprioritized when problems occur. Older adults may have conditions that impair communication, such as aphasia from a cerebrovascular accident, dementia, multiple sclerosis, or other neurological conditions. If this is the case, the nurse needs to be even more astute in performing nonverbal assessments and detecting changes or problems. If evaluations are done often and thoroughly, changes can be made (even during the same shift) to improve care and intervene more effectively. Communication and interpersonal skills are as essential in the evaluation phase as they are in the initial assessment.

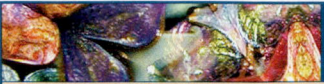

NURSING CARE PLAN FOR AMANDA AQUILINI MODIFIED FOLLOWING IMPLEMENTATION AND EVALUATION

NURSING DIAGNOSIS: INEFFECTIVE AIRWAY CLEARANCE RELATED TO VISCOUS SECRETIONS AND SHALLOW CHEST EXPANSION SECONDARY TO FLUID VOLUME DEFICIT, PAIN, AND FATIGUE.

DESIRED OUTCOMES [NOC#]/INDICATORS	EVALUATION STATEMENTS	NURSING ORDERS	EXPLANATION FOR CONTINUING OR MODIFYING NURSING ORDERS
Respiratory status: gas exchange [0402], as evidenced by		Monitor respiratory status q4h; rate, depth, effort, skin color, mucous membranes, amount and color of sputum.	Retain nursing orders to continue to identify progress. Goal status indicates problem not resolved.
• Absence of pallor and cyanosis (skin and mucous membranes)	Partially met. Skin and mucous membranes not cyanotic, but still pale.	Monitor results of blood gases, chest x-ray studies, pulse oximetry, and incentive spirometer volume as available.	
• Use of correct breathing/ coughing technique after instruction	Partially met. Uses correct technique when pain well controlled by narcotic analgesics.	Monitor level of consciousness.	
• Productive cough	Met. Cough productive of moderate amounts of thick, yellow, pink-tinged sputum.	Auscultate lungs q4h.	
• Symmetric chest excursion of at least 4 cm	Not met. Chest excursion = 3 cm.	Vital signs q4h (TPR, BP, pulse oximetry).	
• Lungs clear to auscultation within 48–72 h	Not met. Scattered inspiratory crackles auscultated throughout right anterior and posterior chest.	Instruct in breathing and coughing techniques. Remind to perform and assist q3h. *Support and encourage. (4/17/03, JW)*	Does not need to be reinstructed as client demonstrates correct techniques. May still need support and encouragement because of fatigue and pain of breathing.
• Respirations 12–22/min, pulse, 100 beats/min	Partially met. Respirations 26/min, pulse 96.	Administer prescribed expectorant; schedule for maximum effectiveness.	
• Inhaling normal volume of air on incentive spirometer	Not met. Tidal volume only 350 mL *(Evaluated 4/17/03, JW)*	Maintain Fowler's or semi-Fowler's position.	
		Administer prescribed analgesics. Notify physician if pain not relieved.	
		Administer oxygen by nasal cannula as prescribed. Provide portable oxygen if client goes off unit (e.g., for x-ray examination).	
		Assist with postural drainage daily at 0930. *On 4/17 teach to continue prn at home. (4/17/03, JW)*	As soon as client is hydrated and fever is controlled, she will probably be discharged to self-care at home.
		Administer prescribed antibiotic to maintain constant blood level. Observe for rash and GI or other side effects.	

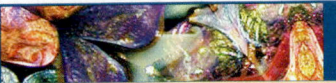
NURSING DIAGNOSIS: ANXIETY RELATED TO DIFFICULTY BREATHING AND CONCERN ABOUT WORK AND PARENTING ROLES.

DESIRED OUTCOMES [NOC#]/INDICATORS	EVALUATION STATEMENTS	NURSING ORDERS	EXPLANATION FOR CONTINUING OR MODIFYING NURSING ORDERS
Anxiety control [1402], as evidenced by • Listening to and following instructions for correct breathing and coughing technique, even during periods of dyspnea	Met. Performed coughing techniques as instructed during periods of dyspnea.	When client is dyspneic, stay with her; reassure her you will stay.	
• Verbalizing understanding of condition, diagnostic tests, and treatments (by end of day)	Met. See nurse's notes for 3–11 shift. Stated, "I know I need to try to breathe deeply even when it hurts." Demonstrated correct use of incentive spirometer and stated understanding of the need to use it. Understands IV is for hydration and antibiotics. *(Evaluated 4/17/03, JW)*	Remain calm, appear confident.	
• Decrease in reports of fear and anxiety	Met. Stated, "I know I can get enough air, but it still hurts to breathe."	Encourage slow, deep breathing.	
• Voice steady, not shaky	Met. Speaks in steady voice.	When client is dyspneic, give brief explanations of treatments and procedures.	
• Respiratory rate of 12–22 min	Not met. Rate 26–36/min.	~~When acute episode is over, give detailed information about nature of condition, treatments, and tests.~~ *Reassess whether client needs any information on condition, treatments, or tests. (4/17/03, JW).*	Detailed information has been given. Because client shows understanding, there is no need to repeat information.
• Freely expresses concerns and possible solutions about work and parenting roles	Partially met. Discussed only briefly on 3–11 shift. Not done on 11–7 shift because of client's need to rest. *(Evaluated 4/17/03, JW)*	As client can tolerate, encourage to express and expand on her concerns about her child and her work. Explore alternatives as needed. Note whether husband returns as scheduled. If he does not, institute care plan for actual *Interrupted Family Process. (Do on 4/17, day shift) (4/17/03, JW)*	It is important that this assessment be made right away, so child care can be arranged if needed.

*In this care plan, a line has been drawn through portions the nurse wished to delete; additions to the care plan are shown in italics.

continued on page 326

Applying Critical Thinking

1. From reviewing Amanda Aquilini's nursing care plan, what general conclusions can you make about the desired outcomes for *Ineffective Airway Clearance* and *Anxiety?*

2. Despite some of the outcomes being only partially met or not met, no new orders were written for several outcomes. What reasons might there be for this?

3. For the nursing diagnosis of *Anxiety,* most of the outcomes are fully met. Would you delete this diagnosis from the care plan at this time?

4. Since the Evaluation Statements column is generally not used on written care plans, where would auditors or persons conducting quality assessments find these data?
See Critical Thinking Possibilities in Appendix A.

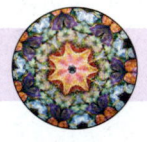 | Chapter Review

EXPLORE MediaLink

NCLEX review questions, case studies, MediaLink applications, and other interactive resources for this chapter can be found on the Companion Website at www.prenhall.com/kozier. Click on Chapter 19 to select the activities for this chapter.

For more NCLEX review questions, and an audio glossary, access the Student CD-ROM accompanying this textbook.

Chapter Highlights

- Implementing is putting planned nursing interventions into action.
- Reassessing occurs simultaneously with the implementing phase of the nursing process.
- Successful implementing and evaluating depend in part on the quality of the preceding phases of assessing, diagnosing, and planning.
- Cognitive, interpersonal, and technical skills are used to implement nursing strategies.
- Before implementing an order, the nurse reassesses the client to be sure that the order is still appropriate.
- The nurse must determine whether assistance is needed to perform a nursing intervention knowledgeably, safely, and comfortably for the client.
- The implementing phase terminates with the documentation of the nursing activities and client responses.
- After the care plan has been implemented, the nurse evaluates the client's health status and the effectiveness of the care plan in achieving client goals.

- The desired outcomes formulated during the planning phase serve as criteria for evaluating client progress and improved health status.
- The desired outcomes determine the data that must be collected to evaluate the client's health status.
- Reexamining the client care plan is a process of making decisions about problem status and critiquing each phase of the nursing process.
- Professional standards of care hold that nurses are responsible and accountable for implementing and evaluating the plan of care.
- Quality assurance evaluation includes consideration of the structures, processes, and outcomes of nursing care.
- Quality improvement is a philosophy and process internal to the institution, and does not rely on inspections by an external agency.

Review Questions

19–1. Of the following, which step of the implementing phase of the nursing process is performed first?
   a. carrying out nursing orders
   b. determining the need for assistance
   c. reassessing the client
   d. documenting interventions

19–2. Under which circumstances is it acceptable practice for the nurse to document a nursing activity *before* it is carried out?
   a. when the activity is routine (e.g., raising the bed rails)
   b. when the activity occurs at regular intervals (e.g., turning the client in bed)

c. when the activity is to be carried out immediately (e.g., a stat medication)

d. it is never acceptable

19–3. The primary purpose of the evaluating phase of the care planning process is to determine whether the

a. desired outcomes have been met.

b. nursing activities were carried out.

c. nursing activities were effective.

d. client's condition has changed.

19–4. The client has a high-priority nursing diagnosis of *Risk for Impaired Skin Integrity* related to the need for several weeks of imposed bedrest. When evaluating the care plan after 1 week, the nurse finds that the client has not developed impaired skin integrity. The most appropriate action with regards to the care plan would be to

a. delete the diagnosis since the problem has not occurred.

b. keep the diagnosis since the risk factors are still present.

c. modify the nursing diagnosis to *Impaired Mobility*.

d. demote the nursing diagnosis to a lower priority.

19–5. The nurse wishes to evaluate the length of time clients must wait for the nurse to respond to the client need reported over the intercom system on each of the different shifts. Which type of quality assessment does this reflect?

a. structure evaluation

b. process evaluation

c. outcome evaluation

d. audit

Readings And References

Suggested Readings

Colton, D. (2000). Quality improvement in health care: Conceptual and historical foundations. *Evaluation & the Health Professions, 23,* 7–42. As indicated by the title of this very comprehensive article, the author reviews the chronological development of the quality improvement movement from originators Deming and Juran in the 1950s to current health organizational behaviorists. It reviews the concepts on which quality improvement is based and compares it to evaluation and similar constructs. Determining cost of nursing interventions: A beginning. . . Iowa Intervention Project. (2001). *Nursing Economics, 19,* 146–60. The investigators of this study sought to determine the amount of education and time needed for each of the 43 interventions of the *Nursing Intervention Classification* taxonomy. Clinical experts were asked to rate the education level by whether a nursing assistant, registered nurse, or registered nurse with additional education or training was required to perform the intervention. The average amount of time needed to perform the intervention was also estimated, classified as requiring 0–15 minutes , 16–30 minutes, 31–45 minutes, 46–60 minutes, or more than 1 hour. A table shows results of these estimations.

Related Research

Rantz, M. J., Popejoy, L., Petroski, G. F., Madsen, R. W., Mehr, D. R., Zwygart-Stauffacher, M., et al. (2001). Randomized clinical trial of a quality improvement intervention in nursing homes. *The Gerontologist, 41,* 525–538.

References

Johnson, M., Maas, M., & Moorhead, S. (Eds.). (2000). *Nursing outcomes classification (NOC)* (2nd ed.). St. Louis, MO: Mosby.

Kirrane, C. (2001). An audit of care planning on a neurology unit. *Nursing Standard, 15*(19), 36–39.

McCloskey, J. C., and Bulechek, G. M. (Eds.). (2000). *Nursing interventions classification (NIC)* (3rd ed.). St. Louis, MO: Mosby.

NANDA International. (2003). NANDA *nursing diagnoses: Definitions & classification 2003-2004.* Philadelphia: Author.

Schroeder, P. (1994). *Improving quality and performance: Concepts, programs and techniques.* St. Louis, MO: Mosby.

Selected Bibliography

Alfaro-LeFevre, R. (2002). *Applying the nursing process. A step-by-step guide* (5th ed.). Philadelphia: Lippincott.

American Nurses Association. (1999). *Nursing quality indicators: Guide for implementation.* Washington, DC: Author.

American Nurses Association. (2000). *Nursing quality indicators beyond acute care: Literature review.* Washington, DC: Author.

Carpenito, L. J. (2002). *Nursing diagnosis: Application to clinical practice* (9th ed.). Philadelphia: Lippincott.

Gardner, P. (2002). *Nursing process.* Albany, NY: Delmar.

LaDuke, S. (2000). NIC puts nursing into words. *Nursing Management, 31*(2), 43–44.

McCloskey, J. C., Bulechek, G. M., Dochterman, J., & Maas, M. (Eds.). (2000). *Nursing diagnoses, outcomes, and interventions: NANDA, NOC and NIC linkages.* St. Louis, MO: Mosby.

Page, C. K. (1999). Performance improvement integration: A whole systems approach. *Journal of Nursing Care Quality, 13*(3), 59–70.

Parsley, K., & Corrigan, P. (1999). *Quality improvement in nursing and health care: Putting evidence into practice.* Cheltenham, UK: Stanley Thornes.

Payne, J. (2000). The nursing interventions classification: A language to define nursing. *Oncology Nursing Forum, 27,* 99–103.

Smith, A. P. (2001). Removing the fluff: The quality in quality improvement. *Nursing Economics, 19,* 183–188.

Wilkinson, J. M. (2000). *Nursing diagnosis handbook with NIC interventions and NOC outcomes* (7th ed.). Upper Saddle River, NJ: Prentice Hall Health.

Wilkinson, J. M. (2001). *Nursing process and critical thinking* (3rd ed.). Upper Saddle River, NJ: Prentice Hall.

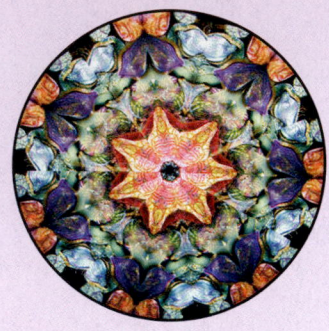

CHAPTER 20

DOCUMENTING AND REPORTING

LEARNING OUTCOMES

After completing this chapter, you will be able to:

- List the measures used to maintain the confidentiality of client records.

- Discuss reasons for keeping client records.

- Compare and contrast different documentation methods: source-oriented and problem-oriented medical records, PIE, focus charting, charting by exception, computerized records, and the case management model.

- Explain how various forms in the client record (e.g., flow sheets, progress notes, care plans, critical pathways, Kardexes, discharge/transfer forms) are used to document steps of the nursing process (assessment, diagnosis, planning, implementation, and evaluation).

- Describe the nurse's role in reporting, conferring, and making referrals.

- Compare and contrast the documentation needed for clients in acute care, home health care, and long-term care settings.

- Identify and discuss guidelines for effective recording that meets legal and ethical standards.

- Identify essential guidelines for reporting client data.

- Identify abbreviations and symbols commonly used for charting.

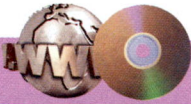

MediaLink

www.prenhall.com/kozier

Additional resources for this chapter can be found on the Student CD-ROM accompanying this textbook, and on the Companion Website at www.prenhall.com/kozier. Click on Chapter 20 to select the activities for this chapter.

CD-ROM
- Audio Glossary
- NCLEX Review

Companion Website
- Additional NCLEX Review
- Case Study:
   Client with Delirium Tremens
- MediaLink Application:
   Establishing a Document System
- Links to Resources

Effective communication among health professionals is vital to the quality of client care. Generally, health personnel communicate through discussion, reports, and records. A **discussion** is an informal oral consideration of a subject by two or more health care personnel to identify a problem or establish strategies to resolve a problem. A **report** is oral, written, or computer-based communication intended to convey information to others. For instance, nurses always report on clients at the end of a hospital work shift. A **record** is written or computer based. The process of making an entry on a client record is called **recording, charting,** or **documenting.**

A clinical record, also called a **chart** or **client record,** is a formal, legal document that provides evidence of a client's care. Although health care organizations use different systems and forms for documentation, all client records have similar information.

Each health care organization has policies about recording and reporting client data, and each nurse is accountable for practicing according to these standards. Agencies also indicate which nursing assessments and interventions can be recorded by RNs and which can be charted by unlicensed personnel. In addition, the Joint Commission on Accreditation of Healthcare Organizations (JCAHO) outlines requirements for client record documentation such as the requirement that charting should be timely, complete, accurate, confidential, and client specific (Smith & Dougherty, 2001).

ETHICAL AND LEGAL CONSIDERATIONS

The American Nurses Association code of ethics (2001) states that ". . . the nurse has a duty to maintain confidentiality of all patient information" (p. 12). The client's record is also protected legally as a private record of the client's care. Access to the record is restricted to health professionals involved in giving care to the client. The institution or agency is the rightful owner of the client's record. This does not, however, exclude the client's rights to the same records. According to Guido (2001), the client has the right to access all information contained within his or her own record and to have a copy of the original record. The hospital may charge a copy fee and may also require certain procedures such as the presence of a hospital representative to answer questions. Competent clients can authorize right of access to their records to others such as insurance carriers and legal representatives (Guido, 2001, p. 186).

> **CLINICAL ALERT** *Take safety measures before faxing confidential information. A fax cover sheet should contain instruction that the faxed material is to be given only to the named recipient. Consent is needed from the client to fax information. Finally, check that the fax number is correct, check the number on the display of the machine after dialing, and check a third time before pressing the "send" button.* ■

For purposes of education and research, most agencies allow student and graduate health professionals access to client records. The records are used in client conferences, clinics, rounds, client studies, and written papers. The student or graduate is bound by a strict ethical code to hold all information in confidence. It is the responsibility of the student or health professional to protect the client's privacy by not using a name or any statements in the notations that would identify the client.

Ensuring Confidentiality of Computer Records

Because of the increased use of computerized client records, health care agencies have developed policies and procedures to ensure the privacy and confidentiality of client information stored in computers. The following are some suggestions for ensuring the confidentiality of computerized records:

1. A personal password is needed to enter and sign off computer files. Do not share this password with anyone, including other health team members.
2. After logging on, never leave a computer terminal unattended.
3. Do not leave client information displayed on the monitor where others may see it.
4. Shred all unneeded computer-generated worksheets.
5. Know the facility's policy and procedure for correcting an entry error.
6. Follow agency procedures for documenting sensitive material, such as a diagnosis of AIDS.

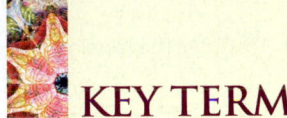

KEY TERMS

change-of-shift report, 344
chart, 329
charting, 329
charting by exception (CBE), 335
client record, 329
discussion, 329
documenting, 329
flow sheet, 333
focus charting, 334
Kardex, 339
narrative charting, 330
PIE, 333
problem-oriented medical record (POMR), 330
problem-oriented record (POR), 330
progress note, 332
record, 329
recording, 329
report, 329
SOAP, 330
source-oriented record, 330
variance, 336

329

PURPOSES OF CLIENT RECORDS

Client records are kept for a number of purposes.

Communication

The record serves as the vehicle by which different health professionals who interact with a client communicate with each other. This prevents fragmentation, repetition, and delays in client care.

Planning Client Care

Each health professional uses data from the client's record to plan care for that client. A physician, for example, may order a specific antibiotic after establishing that the client's temperature is steadily rising and that laboratory tests reveal the presence of a certain microorganism. Nurses use baseline and on-going data to evaluate the effectiveness of the nursing care plan.

Auditing Health Agencies

An audit is a review of client records for quality assurance purposes (see Chapter 19). ⬤ Accrediting agencies such as JC-AHO may review client records to determine if a particular health agency is meeting its stated standards.

Research

The information contained in a record can be a valuable source of data for research. The treatment plans for a number of clients with the same health problems can yield information helpful in treating other clients.

Education

Students in health disciplines often use client records as educational tools. A record can frequently provide a comprehensive view of the client, the illness, effective treatment strategies, and factors that affect the outcome of the illness.

Reimbursement

Documentation also helps a facility receive reimbursement from the federal government. For a facility to obtain payment through Medicare, the client's clinical record must contain the correct diagnosis-related group (DRG) codes and reveal that the appropriate care has been given.

Codable diagnoses, such as DRGs, are supported by accurate, thorough recording by nurses. This not only facilitates reimbursement from the federal government, but also from insurance companies and other third-party payers. If additional care, treatment, or length of stay becomes necessary for the client's welfare, thorough charting will help justify these needs.

Legal Documentation

The client's record is a legal document and is usually admissible in court as evidence. In some jurisdictions, however, the record is considered inadmissible as evidence when the client objects, because information the client gives to the physician is confidential.

Health Care Analysis

Information from records may assist health care planners to identify agency needs, such as overutilized and underutilized hospital services. Records can be used to establish the costs of various services and to identify those services that cost the agency money and those that generate revenue.

DOCUMENTATION SYSTEMS

A number of documentation systems are in current use: the source-oriented record; the problem-oriented medical record; the problems, interventions, evaluation (PIE) model; focus charting, charting by exception (CBE), computerized documentation, and case management.

Source-Oriented Record

The traditional client record is a **source-oriented record.** Each person or department makes notations in a separate section or sections of the client's chart. For example, the admissions department has an admission sheet; the physician has a physician's order sheet, a physician's history sheet, and progress notes; nurses use the nurses' notes; and other departments or personnel have their own records. In this type of record, information about a particular problem is distributed throughout the record. For example, if a client had left hemiplegia (paralysis of the left side of the body), data about this problem might be found in the physician's history sheet, on the physician's order sheet, in the nurses' notes, in the physical therapist's record, and in the social service record. Table 20–1 lists the components of a source-oriented record.

Narrative charting is a traditional part of the source-oriented record. It consists of written notes that include routine care, normal findings, and client problems. There is no right or wrong order to the information, although chronological order is frequently used. Narrative recording is being replaced by other systems, such as charting by exception and focus. However, narrative charting is expedient in emergency situations (see Figure 20–1 ■).

Source-oriented records are convenient because care providers from each discipline can easily locate the forms on which to record data and it is easy to trace the information specific to one's discipline. The disadvantage is that information about a particular client problem is scattered throughout the chart, so it is difficult to find chronological information on a client's problems and progress.

Problem-Oriented Medical Record

In the **problem-oriented medical record (POMR),** or **problem-oriented record (POR),** established by Lawrence Weed in the 1960s, the data are arranged according to the problems the client has rather than the source of the information. Members of the health care team contribute to the problem list, plan of care, and progress notes. Plans for each active or potential problem are drawn up, and progress notes are recorded for each problem.

The advantage of POMR is that (a) it encourages collaboration and (b) the problem list in the front of the chart alerts caregivers

TABLE 20–1   Components of the Source-Oriented Record

Form	Information
Admission (face) sheet	Legal name, birth date, age, gender Social Security number Address Marital status; closest relatives or person to notify in case of emergency Date, time, and admitting diagnosis Food or drug allergies Name of admitting (attending) physician Insurance information Any assigned diagnosis-related group (DRG)
Initial nursing assessment	Findings from the initial nursing history and physical health assessment
Graphic record	Body temperature, pulse rate, respiratory rate, blood pressure, daily weight, and special measurements such as fluid intake and output and oxygen saturation
Daily care record	Activity, diet, bathing, and elimination records
Special flow sheets	Examples: fluid balance record, skin assessment
Medication record	Name, dosage, route, time, date of regularly administered medications Name or initials of person administering the medication
Narrative nurses' notes	Pertinent assessment of client Specific nursing care including teaching and client's responses Client's complaints and how client is coping
Medical history and physical examination	Past and family medical history, present medical problems, differential or current diagnoses, findings of physical examination by the physician
Physician's order sheet	Medical orders for medications, treatments, and so on
Physician's progress notes	Medical observations, treatments, client progress, and so on
Consultation records	Reports by medical and clinical specialists
Diagnostic reports	Examples: laboratory reports, x-ray reports, CT scan reports
Consultation reports	Physical therapy, respiratory therapy
Client discharge plan and referral summary	Started on admission and completed on discharge; includes nursing problems, general information, and referral data

to the client's needs and makes it easier to track the status of each problem. Its disadvantages are that (a) caregivers differ in their ability to use the required charting format, (b) it takes constant vigilance to maintain an up-to-date problem list, and (c) it is somewhat inefficient because assessments and interventions that apply to more than one problem must be repeated.

The POMR has four basic components:

- Database
- Problem list
- Plan of care
- Progress notes.

In addition, flow sheets and discharge notes are added to the record as needed.

Database

The database consists of all information known about the client when the client first enters the health care agency. It includes the nursing assessment, the physician's history, social and family data, and the results of the physical examination and baseline diagnostic tests. Data are constantly updated as the client's health status changes.

Problem List

The problem list (see Figure 20–2 ■) is derived from the database. It is usually kept at the front of the chart and serves as an index to the numbered entries in the progress notes. Problems are listed in the order in which they are identified, and the list is continually updated as new problems are identified and others resolved. All caregivers may contribute to the problem list, which includes the client's physiologic, psychologic, social, cultural, spiritual, developmental, and environmental needs. Physicians write problems as medical diagnoses, surgical procedures, or symptoms; nurses write problems as nursing diagnoses.

As the client's condition changes or more data are obtained, it may be necessary to "redefine" problems. Figure 20–2 illustrates how this has been done for Problems 1B, 1C, and 2. When a problem is resolved, a line is drawn through it and the number is not used again for that client.

Plan of Care

The initial list of orders or plan of care is made with reference to the active problems. Care plans are generated by the person who lists the problems. Physicians write physician's orders or medical care plans; nurses write nursing orders or nursing care

NURSING NOTES

Date	Time	
6/6/03	1400	Passive ROM exercises provided for R arm and leg.
		Active assistive exercises to L arm and leg. Has scratch
		marks on L and R forearms. States, "My skin on my back
		and arms has been itchy for a week." Rash not evident.
		No previous history of pruritus. Is allergic to elastoplast
		but has not been in contact. Dr. J. Wong notified.
		————————————————————— Tom Ritchie RN
	1430	Applied calamine lotion to back and arms. Incontinent
		of urine. Is restless. ——————————— Tom Ritchie RN

Figure 20–1 ■ An example of narrative notes.

plans. The written plan in the record is listed under each problem in the progress notes and is not isolated as a separate list of orders.

Progress Notes

A **progress note** in the POMR is a chart entry made by all health professionals involved in a client's care; they all use the same type of sheet for notes. Progress notes are numbered to correspond to the problems on the problem list and may be lettered for the type of data. For example, the SOAP format is frequently used. **SOAP** is an acronym for subjective data, objective data, assessment, and planning.

S—*Subjective data* consist of information obtained from what the client says. It describes the client's perceptions of and experience with the problem (see Chapter 16). 🔗 When possible, the nurse quotes the client's words; otherwise, they are summarized. Subjective data are included only when it is important and relevant to the problem.

O—*Objective data* consist of information that is measured or observed by use of the senses (e.g., vital signs, laboratory and x-ray results).

A—*Assessment* is the interpretation or conclusions drawn about the subjective and objective data. During the initial assessment, the problem list is created from the database, so the "A" entry should be a statement of

the problem. In all subsequent SOAP notes for that problem, the "A" should describe the client's condition and level of progress rather than merely restating the diagnosis or problem.

P—The *plan* is the plan of care designed to resolve the stated problem. The initial plan is written by the person who enters the problem into the record. All subsequent plans, including revisions, are entered into the progress notes.

Over the years, the SOAP format has been modified. The acronyms *SOAPIE* and *SOAPIER* refer to formats that add interventions, evaluation, and revision.

I—*Intervention* refer to the specific interventions that have actually been performed by the caregiver.

E—*Evaluation* includes client responses to nursing interventions and medical treatments. This is primarily reassessment data.

R—*Revision* reflects care plan modifications suggested by the evaluation. Changes may be made in desired outcomes, interventions, or target dates.

Newer versions of this format eliminate the subjective and objective data and start with *assessment*, which combines the subjective and objective data. The acronym then becomes *AP, APIE,* or *APIER* (Mosby, 1999). See Figure 20–3 ■.

No.	Date Entered	Date Inactive	Client Problem
#1	3/9/03		CVA resulting in Rt hemiplegia and left-sided weakness
#1A	3/9/03		Self-care deficit (hygiene, toileting, grooming, feeding)
#1B	3/9/03		Impaired physical mobility (unable to turn and position self) *Redefined 2/7/04*
#1C	3/9/03		Total urinary incontinence *Redefined 1/17/04*
#1D	3/9/03		Progressive dysphasia
#2	3/9/03		Constipation r/t immobility *Redefined 6/10/03*
#3	3/9/03		History of depression
#4	3/9/03		Essential hypertension
~~#5~~	~~6/6/03~~	~~7/11/03~~	~~Pruritus~~
#2	6/10/03		Risk for constipation r/t insufficient fiber intake
#1C	1/17/04		Urge urinary incontinence at night
#1B	2/7/04		Impaired physical mobility (needs 2-person assistance to transfer and walk)

Figure 20–2 ■ A client's problem list in the POMR. Note that problems 1B, 1C, and 2 were redefined on the dates indicated and listed subsequently.

PIE

The **PIE** documentation model groups information into three categories. PIE is an acronym for problems, interventions, and evaluation of nursing care. This system consists of a client care assessment flow sheet and progress notes. The **flow sheet** uses specific assessment criteria in a particular format, such as human needs or functional health patterns. The time parameters for a flow sheet can vary from minutes to months. In a hospital intensive care unit, for example, a client's blood pressure may be monitored by the minute, whereas in an ambulatory clinic a client's blood glucose level may be recorded once a month.

After the assessment, the nurse establishes and records specific problems on the progress notes, often using North American Nursing Diagnosis Association (NANDA) diagnoses to word the problem. If there is no approved nursing di-

agnosis for a problem, the nurse develops a problem statement using NANDA's three-part format: client's response, contributing or probable causes of the response, and characteristics manifested by the client (see Chapter 17). ⊕ The *problem statement* is labeled "P" and referred to by number (e.g., P #5). The *interventions* employed to manage the problem are labeled "I" and numbered according to the problem (e.g., I #5). The *evaluation* of the effectiveness of the interventions is also labeled and numbered according to the problem (e.g., E #5).

The PIE system eliminates the traditional care plan and incorporates an ongoing care plan into the progress notes. Therefore, the nurse does not have to create and update a separate plan. A disadvantage is that the nurse must review all the nursing notes before giving care to determine which problems are current and which interventions were effective.

SOAP Format	**SOAPIER Format**	**APIE Format**

6/6/03   #5 Generalized pruritus
1400   S— "My skin is itchy on my back and arms, and it's been like this for a week."
O— Skin appears clear—no rash or irritation noted. Marks where client has scratched noted on left and right forearms. Allergic to elastoplast but has not been in contact.
No previous history of pruritus.
A— Altered comfort (pruritus): cause unknown.
P— Instructed not to scratch skin.
— Applied calamine lotion to back and arms at 1430 h.
— Cut fingernails.
— Assess further to determine whether recurrence associated with specific drugs or foods.
— Refer to physician and pharmacist for assessment.
         Tom Ritchie, RN
	6/6/03 #5 Generalized pruritus
	1400 S— "My skin is itchy on my back and arms, and it's been like this for a week."
	O— Skin appears clear—no rash or irritation noted. Marks where client has scratched noted on left and right forearms. Allergic to elastoplast but has not been in contact.
	No previous history of pruritus.
	A— Altered comfort (pruritus): cause unknown.
	P— Instruct to not scratch skin.
	— Apply calamine lotion as necessary.
	— Cut nails to avoid scratches.
	— Assess further to determine whether recurrence associated with specific drugs or foods.
	— Refer to physician and pharmacist for assessment.
	I — Instructed not to scratch skin. Applied calamine lotion to back and arms at 1430 h. Assisted to cut fingernails. Notified physician and pharmacist of problem.
	1600 E— States, "I'm still itchy. That lotion didn't help."
	R— Remove calamine lotion and apply hydrocortisone ungt. as ordered.
	         Tom Ritchie, RN
		6/6/03 A— Generalized pruritus r/t unknown cause
		1400 States, "My skin is itchy on my back and arms, and it's been like this for a week." Skin appears clear. No rash or irritations noted. Marks where client has scratched noted on left and right forearms. Allergic to elastoplast but has not been in contact. No previous history of pruritus.
		P— Instruct to not scratch skin.
		— Apply calamine lotion as necessary.
		— Cut nails to avoid scratches.
		— Assess further to determine whether recurrence associated with specific drugs or foods.
		— Refer to physician and pharmacist for assessment.
		I — Instructed not to scratch skin. Applied calamine lotion to back and arms at 1430 h. Assisted to cut fingernails. Notified physician and pharmacist of problem.
		E— States, "I'm still itchy. That lotion didn't help."
		         Tom Ritchie, RN

Figure 20–3 ■ Examples of nursing progress notes using SOAP, SOAPIER, and APIE formats.

Focus Charting

Focus charting is intended to make the client and client concerns and strengths the focus of care. Three columns for recording are usually used: date and time, focus, and progress notes. The *focus* may be a condition, a nursing diagnosis, a behavior, a sign or symptom, an acute change in the client's condition, or a client strength. The progress notes are organized into (D) data, (A) action, and (R) response, referred to as DAR. The *data* category reflects the assessment phase of the nursing process and consists of observations of client status and behaviors, including data from flow sheets (e.g., vital signs, pupil reactivity). The nurse records both subjective and objective data in this section.

The *action* category reflects planning and implementation and includes immediate and future nursing actions. It may also include any changes to the plan of care. The *response category* reflects the evaluation phase of the nursing process and describes the client's response to any nursing and medical care.

The focus charting system provides a holistic perspective of the client and the client's needs. It also provides a nursing process framework for the progress notes (DAR). The three components do not need to be recorded in order and each note does not need to have all three categories. Flow sheets and checklists are frequently used on the client's chart to record routine nursing tasks and assessment data.

Date/Hour	Focus	Progress Notes
2/11/03 0900	Pain	**D:** Guarding abdominal incision. Facial grimacing. Rates pain at "8" on scale of 0–10. **A:** Administered morphine sulfate 4 mg IV.
0930		**R:** Rates pain at "1." States willing to ambulate.

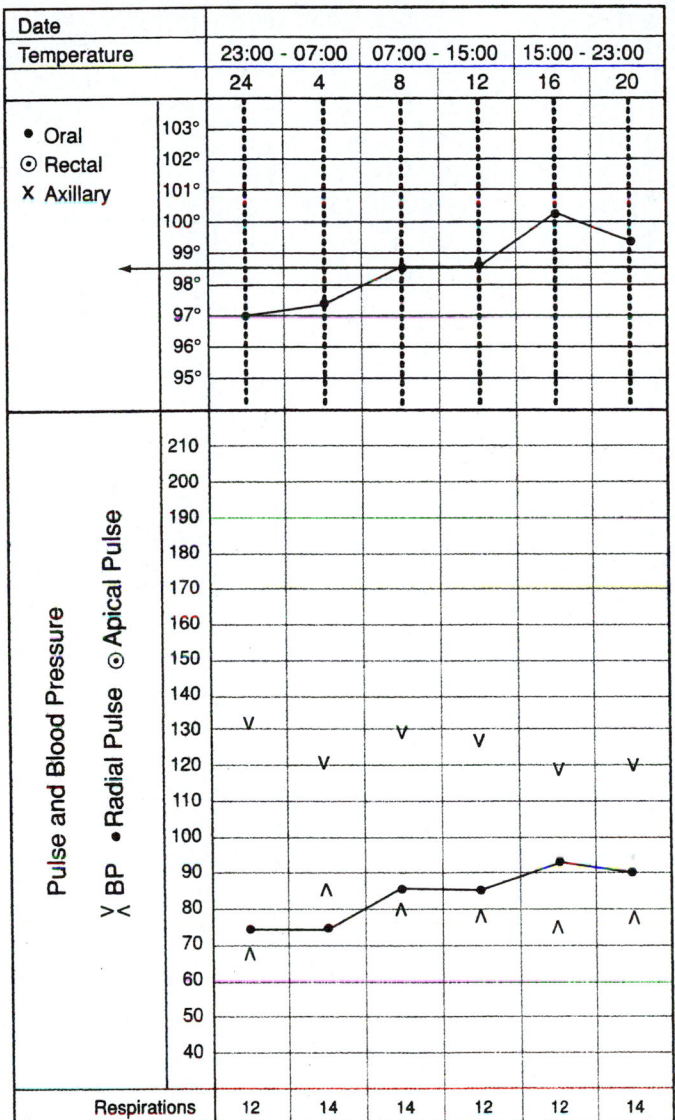

Date						
Temperature		23:00 - 07:00		07:00 - 15:00		15:00 - 23:00
		24	4	8	12	16	20

Figure 20–4 ■ Sample vital signs graphic record.

Charting by Exception

Charting by exception (CBE) is a documentation system in which only abnormal or significant findings or exceptions to norms are recorded. CBE incorporates three key elements (Guido, 2001; Murphy & Burke, 1990):

1. Flow sheets. Examples of flow sheets include a graphic record (Figure 20–4 ■), fluid balance record, daily care record (Figure 20–5 ■), client teaching record, client discharge record, and skin assessment record (Figure 20–6 ■).
2. Standards of nursing care. Documentation by reference to the agency's printed standards of nursing practice eliminates much of the repetitive charting of routine care. An agency using CBE must develop its own specific standards of nursing practice that identify the minimum criteria for client care regardless of clinical area. Some units may also have unit-specific standards unique to their type of client. For example, "The nurse must ensure that the unconscious

client has oral care at least q4h." Documentation of care according to these specified standards involves only a check mark in the routine standards box on the graphic record. If all of the standards are not implemented, an asterisk on the flow sheet is made with reference to the nurses' notes. All exceptions to the standards are fully described in narrative form on the nurses' notes.

3. Bedside access to chart forms. In the CBE system, all flow sheets are kept at the client's bedside to allow immediate recording and to eliminate the need to transcribe data from the nurse's worksheet to the permanent record.

The advantage to this system is the elimination of lengthy, repetitive notes and it makes client changes in condition more obvious. Some authors (Allan & Englebright, 2000), however, believe that CBE may not provide enough information to alert health practioners to potential problems. Burke and Murphy (2000) challenge this position and emphasize the need for the agency to ensure that not only all of the elements of CBE are present, but also all regulatory and accrediting agency requirements are incorporated into the documentation system.

Computerized Documentation

Computerized clinical record systems are being developed as a way to manage the huge volume of information required in contemporary health care. Nurses use computers to store the client's database, add new data, create and revise care plans, and document client progress (see Figure 20–7 ■). Some institutions have a computer terminal at each client's bedside, or nurses carry a small handheld terminal, enabling the nurse to document care immediately after it is given.

Multiple flow sheets are not needed in computerized record systems because information can be easily retrieved in a variety of formats. For example, the nurse can obtain results of a client's blood test, a schedule of all clients on the unit who are to have surgery during the day, a suggested list of interventions for a nursing diagnosis, a graphic chart of a client's vital signs, or a printout of all progress notes for a client. Many systems can generate a work list for the shift, with a list of all treatments, procedures, and medications needed by the client.

Computers make care planning and documentation relatively easy. To record nursing actions and client responses, the nurse either chooses from standardized lists of terms or types narrative information into the computer. Automated speech-recognition technology now allows nurses to enter data by voice for conversion to written documentation.

The computerization of clinical records has made it possible to transmit information from one care setting to another. The Nursing Minimum Data Set (NMDS) is an effort to establish standards for collecting standardized, essential nursing data for inclusion in computer databases. Selected pros and cons of computer documentation are shown in Box 20–1.

Case Management

The case management model emphasizes quality, cost-effective care delivered within an established length of stay. This model

Medical-Surgical
NURSING CARE RECORD

Date: 9/12/2004   0700–1900   Initials: NS   Signature: Nancy Smith RN

Assessment Parameters	Time: 0800 Notes	Time: 1000 Notes	Time: Notes
NEUROMUSCULAR: Alert & oriented to person, place, & time. Behavior appropriate to situation. PERL. MAE with symmetry of strength and no muscle weakness. Ambulates independently and performs self-care. Speech clear. Hears normal conversation. Swallows without difficulty. No c/o numbness or tingling, blurred vision, dizziness, or headache.	✓	✓	☐
CARDIOVASCULAR: Regular apical pulse with no extra sounds. Nail beds pink. Pedal pulses present. No edema. No c/o chest pain.	✓	✓	☐
RESPIRATORY: Respirations regular and unlabored. Breath sounds clear in all fields. No cough or sputum production. No c/o dyspnea.	✱ rales aT bases—clear with coughing. Encouraged C + DB	→	☐
GASTROINTESTINAL: Abdomen soft, non-tender. No distention. Bowel sounds present in all 4 quadrants. No nausea or vomiting. Continent. Soft, brown BMs every 1–2 days.	✱ Bowel sounds absent. N/G Tube patent. Abd. drsg dry and intact.	→	☐
URINARY: Urine clear and yellow to amber. Continent. No c/o discomfort with voiding.	✓	✓	☐

KEY: ✓ = Assessment matches normal assessment parameters
         ✱ = Abnormal finding
         → = No change in abnormal finding since last assessment

Figure 20–5 ■ Sample of a flow sheet to record daily nursing care.

uses a multidisciplinary approach to planning and documenting client care, using *critical pathways*. These forms identify the outcomes that certain groups of clients are expected to achieve on each day of care, along with the interventions necessary for each day. See Figure 20–8 ■ and Chapter 6 ⊙ for more information about critical pathways.

Along with critical pathways, the case management model incorporates graphics and flow sheets. Progress notes typically use some type of charting by exception. For example, if goals are met, no further charting is required. A goal that is not met

is called a **variance.** Variations are deviations to what is planned on the critical pathway—unexpected occurrences that affect the planned care or the client's responses to care. When a variance occurs, the nurse writes a note documenting the unexpected event, the cause, and actions taken to correct the situation or justify the actions taken. See Table 20–2 for an example of how a variance might be documented.

The case management model promotes collaboration and teamwork among caregivers, helps to decrease length of stay, and makes efficient use of time. Because care is goal focused,

SKIN ASSESSMENT FLOW CHART

Date: _____   Assessed by: _____

Number each skin injury/wound on the diagram. Complete information for each skin injury/wound.

Stage 1: Nonblanchable erythema of intact skin
Stage 2: Superficial skin break, shallow crater/blister
Stage 3: Deep tissue involvement/cavity not through fascia
Stage 4: Full thickness skin loss with extensive
          destruction of tissue, tissue necrosis, or damage
          to muscle, bone, or supporting structures

Injury/Wound Types:

Stasis ulcer   Bruise
Pressure ulcer   Skin tear
Arterial ulcer   Rash
Surgical wound   Hematoma
Laceration   Other: specify

Photographs on admission, weekly, and on discharge (note due dates on Kardex).

Site #	Injury/Wound Type (specify)	Stage	Length Width cm	Depth cm	Tunneling Yes/No	Color	Drainage Amt/Type	Odor	Culture Date	Treatments & Comments

Figure 20–6 ■ Sample skin assessment flow sheet.

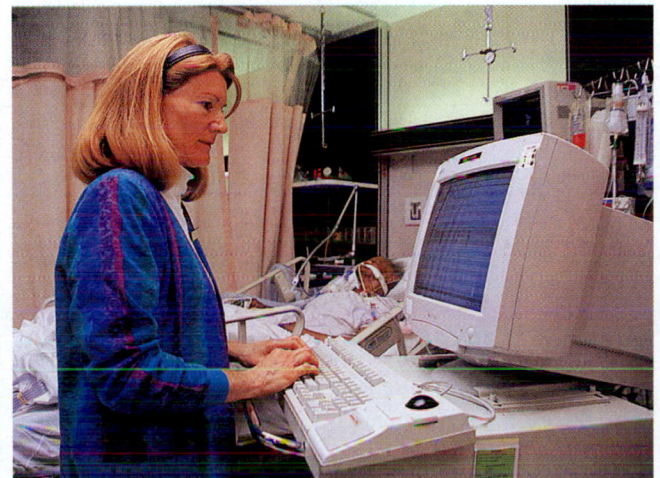

Figure 20–7 ■ A bedside computer. (Mike English/MediChrome.)

the quality may improve. However, critical pathways work best for clients with one or two diagnoses and few individualized needs. Clients with multiple diagnoses (e.g., a client with a hip fracture, pneumonia, diabetes, and pressure sore) or those with an unpredictable course of symptoms (e.g., a neurological client with seizures) are difficult to document on a critical path.

DOCUMENTING NURSING ACTIVITIES

The client record should describe the client's ongoing status and reflect the full range of the nursing process. Regardless of the records system used in an agency, nurses document evidence of the nursing process on a variety of forms throughout the clinical record (Table 20–3).

Admission Nursing Assessment

A comprehensive admission assessment, also referred to as an initial database, nursing history, or nursing assessment, is

BOX 20–1 ■ Selected Pros and Cons of Computer Documentation

Pros

- Computer records can facilitate a focus on client outcomes.
- Bedside terminals can synthesize information from monitoring equipment.
- Allows nurses to use their time more efficiently.
- The system links various sources of client information.
- Client information, requests, and results are sent and received quickly.
- Links to monitors improve accuracy of documentation.
- Bedside terminals eliminate need to take notes on a worksheet before recording.
- Bedside terminals permit the nurse to check an order immediately before administering a treatment or medication.
- Information is legible.
- The system incorporates and reinforces standards of care.
- Standard terminology improves communication.

Cons

- Client's privacy may be infringed on if security measures are not used.
- Breakdowns make information temporarily unavailable.
- System is expensive.
- Extended training periods may be required when a new or updated system is installed.

CRITICAL PATHWAY: TOTAL HIP REPLACEMENT

	DOS/Day 1	Days 2–3
Pain Management	Outcome: • Verbalizes comfort or tolerance of pain Circle: V NV Variance:	Outcome: • Verbalizes comfort with pain control measures Circle: V NV Variance:
Respiratory	Outcomes: • Breath sounds clear to auscultation • Achieves 50% of volume goal on incentive spirometer Circle: V NV Variance:	Outcomes: • Breath sounds clear to auscultation • Achieves 100% of volume goal on incentive spirometer Circle: V NV Variance:
Key: V = Variance	NV = No Variance	
Signature:	Initials:	
Signature:	Initials:	

Figure 20–8 ■ Excerpt from a critical pathway documentation form.

completed when the client is admitted to the nursing unit. As discussed in Chapter 16, 🔗 these forms can be organized according to body systems, functional abilities, health problems and risks, nursing model, or type of health care setting (e.g., labor and delivery, pediatrics, mental health). The nurse generally records ongoing assessments or reassessments on flow sheets or on nursing progress notes.

Nursing Care Plans

According to Smith and Dougherty (2001), JCAHO requires that the clinical record include evidence of client assessments, nursing diagnoses and/or client needs, nursing interventions, client outcomes, and evidence of a current nursing care plan. Depending on the records system being used, the nursing care plan may be separate from the client's chart, recorded in progress notes and other forms in the client record, or incorporated into a multidisciplinary plan of care.

There are two types of nursing care plans: traditional and standardized. The *traditional care plan* is written for each client. The form varies from agency to agency according to the needs of the client and the department. Most forms have three columns: one for nursing diagnoses, a second for ex-

TABLE 20–2 Example of Variance Documentation (Critical Pathway)

A client has had a below-the-knee amputation. On the third postoperative day he has a temperature of 38.8C (102F). Lung sounds are clear and he is not coughing. The nurse notices redness and skin breakdown over the client's sacrum. The critical pathway outcomes specified for Day 3 are "Oral temperature 37.7C (100F)" and "Skin intact over bony prominences." The nurse should chart the following variances:

Date/Time	Variance	Cause	Action Taken/Plans
4/16/03 0900	Elevated temperature	Possible sepsis	4/16—Blood cultures ×3 per order. Monitor temp. q1h. Monitor I&O, hydration, and mental status.
4/16/03 1130	Impaired skin integrity: pressure sore on sacrum	Client does not move about in bed unless reminded	4/16—Positioned on L side. Turn side-to-side q2h while awake. On every client contact, remind client to move about in bed. Apply Duoderm after bath.

TABLE 20–3	Documentation for the Nursing Process
Step*	**Documentation Forms**
Assessment	Initial assessment form, various flow sheets
Nursing diagnosis	Nursing care plan, critical pathway, progress notes, problem list
Planning	Nursing care plan, critical pathway
Implementing	Progress notes, flow sheets
Evaluating	Progress notes

*All steps are recorded on discharge/referral summaries.

pected outcomes, and a third for nursing interventions. See Chapter 18 🔗 for additional information.

Standardized care plans were developed to save documentation time. These plans may be based on an institution's standards of practice, thereby helping to provide a high quality of nursing care. For further information, see Chapter 18. 🔗 Standardized plans must be individualized by the nurse in order to adequately address individual client needs.

Kardexes

The **Kardex** is a widely used, concise method of organizing and recording data about a client, making information quickly accessible to all health professionals. The system consists of a series of cards kept in a portable index file or on computer-generated forms. The card for a particular client can be quickly turned up to reveal specific data. The Kardex may or may not become a part of the client's permanent record. In some organizations it is a temporary worksheet written in pencil for ease in recording frequent changes in details of a client's care. The information on Kardexes may be organized into sections, for example:

• Pertinent information about the client, such as name, room number, age, religion, marital status, admission date, physician's name, diagnosis, type of surgery and date, and next of kin
• List of medications, with the date of order and the times of administration for each
• List of intravenous fluids, with dates of infusions
• List of daily treatments and procedures, such as irrigations, dressing changes, postural drainage, or measurement of vital signs
• List of diagnostic procedures ordered, such as x-ray or laboratory tests
• Allergies
• Specific data on how the client's physical needs are to be met, such as type of diet, assistance needed with feeding, elimination devices, activity, hygienic needs, and safety precautions (e.g., one-person assist)
• A problem list, stated goals, and a list of nursing approaches to meet the goals and relieve the problems.

Although much of the information on the Kardex may be recorded by the nurse in charge or a delegate (e.g., the nursing unit clerk), any nurse who cares for the client plays a key role in initiating the record and keeping the data current. Whether the Kardex is a written paper, or computerized, it is important to have a place on it to record date and initials of the person reviewing or revising it. It is a quick visual guide to ensure that information is current and updated on a regular basis.

Flow Sheets

A flow sheet enables nurses to record nursing data quickly and concisely and provides an easy-to-read record of the client's condition over time.

Graphic Record

This record typically indicates body temperature, pulse, respiratory rate, blood pressure, weight, and, in some agencies, other significant clinical data such as admission or postoperative day, bowel movements, appetite, and activity.

Fluid Balance Record

All routes of fluid intake and all routes of fluid loss or output are measured and recorded on this form. See Chapter 50 🔗 for more information.

Medication Administration Record

Medication flow sheets usually include designated areas for the date of the medication order, the expiration date, the medication name and dose, the frequency of administration and route, and the nurse's signature. Some records also include a place to document the client's allergies (see Chapter 33). 🔗

Skin Assessment Record

A skin or wound assessment is often recorded on a flow sheet such as the one shown in Figure 20–6. These records may include categories related to stage of skin injury, drainage, odor, culture information, and treatments.

Progress Notes

Progress notes made by nurses provide information about the progress a client is making toward achieving desired outcomes. Therefore, in addition to assessment and reassessment data, progress notes include information about client problems and nursing interventions. The format used depends on the documentation system in place in the institution. Various kinds of nursing progress notes are discussed in the "Documentation Systems" section earlier in this chapter. These include narrative nursing notes, SOAP and PIE notes, charting by exception, and focus charting.

Nursing Discharge/Referral Summaries

A discharge note and referral summary are completed when the client is being discharged and transferred to another institution or to a home setting where a visit by a community health nurse is required. See the discussion of discharge planning in

Chapter 7 ↩️ , and the assessment parameters suggested when preparing clients to go home. Many institutions provide forms for these summaries. Some records combine the discharge plan, including instructions for care, and the final progress note. Many are designed with checklists to facilitate data recording.

If the discharge plan is given directly to the client and family, it is imperative that instructions be written in terms that can be readily understood. For example, medications, treatments, and activities should be written in layman's terms, and use of medical abbreviations (such as t.i.d.) should be avoided.

If a client is transferred within the facility or from a long-term facility to a hospital, a report needs to accompany the client to ensure continuity of care in the new area. It should include all components of the discharge instructions, but also describe the condition of the client before the transfer. Any teaching or client instruction that has been done should also be described and recorded.

If the client is being transferred to another institution or to a home setting where a visit by a home health nurse is required, the discharge note takes the form of a referral summary. Regardless of format, discharge and referral summaries usually include some or all of the following:

- Description of client's physical, mental, and emotional status at discharge or transfer
- Resolved health problems
- Unresolved continuing health problems and continuing care needs; may include a review-of-systems checklist that considers integumentary, respiratory, cardiovascular, neurologic, musculoskeletal, gastrointestinal, elimination, and reproductive problems
- Treatments that are to be continued (e.g., wound care, oxygen therapy)
- Current medications
- Restrictions that relate to (a) activity such as lifting, stair climbing, walking, driving, work, (b) diet, and (c) bathing such as sponge bath, tub, or shower
- Functional/self-care abilities in terms of vision, hearing, speech, mobility with or without aids, meal preparation and eating, preparing and administering medications, and so on
- Comfort level
- Support networks including family, significant others, religious adviser, community self-help groups, home care and other community agencies available, and so on
- Client education provided in relation to disease process, activities and exercise, special diet, medications, specialized care or treatments, follow-up appointments, and so on
- Discharge destination (e.g., home, nursing home) and mode of discharge (e.g., walking, wheelchair, ambulance)
- Referral services (e.g., social worker, home health nurse).

LONG-TERM CARE DOCUMENTATION

Long-term facilities usually provide two types of care: skilled or intermediate. Clients needing skilled care require more extensive nursing care and specialized nursing skills. In contrast, an intermediate care focus is needed for clients who usually have chronic illnesses and may only need assistance with activities of daily living (such as bathing and dressing).

Requirements for documentation in long-term care settings are based on professional standards, federal and state regulations, and the policies of the health care agency. Laws influencing the kind and frequency of documentation required are the Health Care Financing Administration and the Omnibus Budget Reconciliation Act (OBRA) of 1987. The OBRA law, for example, requires that (a) a comprehensive assessment (the Minimum Data Set [MDS] for Resident Assessment and Care Screening) be performed within 4 days of a client's admission to a long-term care facility, (b) a formulated plan of care must be completed within 7 days of admission, and (c) the assessment and care screening process must be reviewed every 3 months.

Documentation must also comply with requirements set by Medicare and Medicaid. These requirements vary with the level of service provided and other factors. For example, Medicare provides little reimbursement for services provided in long-term care facilities except for services that require skilled care such as chemotherapy, tube feedings, ventilators, and so on. For such Medicare clients, the nurse must provide daily documentation to verify the need for service and reimbursement.

Nurses need to familiarize themselves with regulations influencing the kind and frequency of documentation required in long-term care facilities. Usually the nurse completes a nursing care *summary* at least once a week for clients requiring skilled care and every 2 weeks for those requiring intermediate care. Summaries should address the following:

- Specific problems noted in the care plan
- Mental status
- Activities of daily living
- Hydration and nutrition status
- Safety measures needed
- Medications

Practice Guidelines
Long-Term Care Documentation

- Complete the assessment and screening forms (MDS) and plan of care within the time period specified by regulatory bodies.
- Keep a record of any visits and of phone calls from family, friends, and others regarding the client.
- Write nursing summaries and progress notes that comply with the frequency and standards required by regulatory bodies.
- Review and revise the plan of care every 3 months or whenever the client's health status changes.
- Document and report any change in the client's condition to the physician and the client's family within 24 hours.
- Document all measures implemented in response to a change in the client's condition.
- Make sure that progress notes address the client's progress in relation to the goals or outcomes defined in the plan of care.

MediaLink   ESTABLISHING A DOCUMENTATION SYSTEM APPLICATION

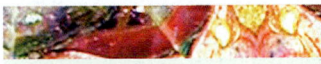

Lifespan Considerations

Elders

Elders in long-term care facilities tend to have chronic conditions and generally experience subtle small changes in their condition. However, when problems do occur, such as a hip fracture, CVA, or pneumonia, they are serious and require prompt attention. This points out the importance of keeping Kardexes and charting in long-term facilities current and up to date in the event that the client needs to be transferred for more skilled care and further treatment. A thorough transfer summary will facilitate communication and promote continuity of care in these situations.

- Treatments
- Preventive measures
- Behavioral modification assessments, if pertinent (if client is taking psychotropic medications or demonstrates behavioral problems)

See the Practice Guidelines on page 340 for documentation in long-term care facilities.

HOME CARE DOCUMENTATION

In 1985 the Health Care Financing Administration, a branch of the U.S. Department of Health and Human Services, mandated that home health care agencies standardize their documentation methods to meet requirements for Medicare and Medicaid and other third-party disbursements. Two records are required: (a) a home health certification and plan of treatment form and (b) a medical update and patient information form. The nurse assigned to the home care client usually completes the forms, which must be signed by both the nurse and the attending physician. See the Practice Guidelines for home health care documentation.

Some home health agencies provide nurses with laptop or handheld computers to make records available in multiple locations. With the use of a modem, the nurse can add new client information to records at the agency without traveling to the office.

GENERAL GUIDELINES FOR RECORDING

Because the client's record is a legal document and may be used to provide evidence in court, many factors are considered in recording. Health care personnel must not only maintain the confidentiality of the client's record but also meet legal standards in the process of recording.

Practice Guidelines
Home Health Care Documentation

- Complete a comprehensive nursing assessment and develop a plan of care to meet Medicare and other third-party payer requirements. Some agencies use the certification and plan of treatment form as the client's official plan of care.
- Write a progress note at each client visit, noting any changes in the client condition; nursing interventions performed (including education and instructional brochures and materials provided to the client and home caregiver); client responses to nursing care; and vital signs as indicated.
- Provide a monthly progress nursing summary to the attending physician and to the reimburser to confirm the need to continue services.
- Keep a copy of the care plan in the client's home and update it as the client's condition changes.
- Report changes in the plan of care to the physician and document that these were reported. Medicare and Medicaid will reimburse only for the skilled services provided that are reported to the physician.
- Encourage the client or home caregiver to record data when appropriate.
- Write a discharge summary for the physician to approve the discharge and to notify the reimbursers that services have been discontinued. Include all services provided, the client's health status at discharge, outcomes achieved, and recommendations for further care.

Practice Guidelines
Documentation

DO	DON'T
■ Chart a change in a client's condition *and* show that follow-up actions were taken.	■ Leave blank space for a colleague to chart later.
■ Read the nurses' notes prior to care to determine if there has been a change in the client's condition.	■ Chart in advance of the event (e.g., procedure, medication).
■ Be timely. A late entry is better than no entry, however, the longer the period of time between actual care and charting, the greater the suspicion.	■ Use vague terms (e.g., "appears to be comfortable," "had a good night").
■ Use objective, specific, and factual descriptions.	■ Chart for someone else.
■ Correct charting errors.	■ Use "patient" or "client" as it is their chart.
■ Chart all teaching.	■ Alter a record even if requested by a superior or a physician.
■ Record the client's actual words by putting quotes around the words.	■ Record assumptions or words reflecting bias (e.g., "complainer," "disagreeable").
■ Chart the client's response to interventions.	
■ Review your notes—are they clear and do they reflect what you want to say?	

Date and Time

Document the date and time of each recording. This is essential not only for legal reasons but also for client safety. Record the time in the conventional manner (e.g., 9:00 AM or 3:20 PM) or according to the 24-hour clock (military clock), which avoids confusion about whether a time was AM or PM (see Figure 20–9 ■).

Timing

Follow the agency's policy about the frequency of documenting, and adjust the frequency as a client's condition indicates; for example, a client whose blood pressure is changing requires more frequent documentation than a client whose blood pressure is constant. As a rule, documenting should be done as soon as possible after an assessment or intervention. No recording should be done *before* providing nursing care.

Legibility

All entries must be legible and easy to read to prevent interpretation errors. Hand printing or easily understood handwriting is usually permissible. Follow the agency's policies about handwritten recording.

Permanence

All entries on the client's record are made in dark ink so that the record is permanent and changes can be identified. Dark ink reproduces well on microfilm and in duplication processes. Follow the agency's policies about the type of pen and ink used for recording.

Accepted Terminology

Use only commonly accepted abbreviations, symbols, and terms that are specified by the agency. Many abbreviations are

standard and used universally; others are used only in certain geographic areas. Many health care facilities are required to supply an approved list of abbreviations to prevent confusion. When in doubt about whether to use an abbreviation, write the term out in full until certain about the abbreviation. Abbreviations can lead to misunderstandings. For example, "D/C" may mean "discharge" or "discontinue"; "od" could mean "once a day" or "right eye"; and "PT" could mean "patient," "physical therapy," or "prothrombin time." The nurse should know and use only the approved list of abbreviations at the facility to avoid putting a client at potential risk. Table 20–4 lists some common abbreviations (except those used for medications, which are described in Chapter 33). Table 20–5 indicates commonly accepted symbols.

Correct Spelling

Correct spelling is essential for accuracy in recording. If unsure how to spell a word, look it up in a dictionary or other resource book. Two decidedly different medications may have similar spellings; for example, digitoxin and digoxin.

> ► CLINICAL ALERT   *Incorrect spelling gives a negative impression to the reader and, thereby, decreases the nurse's credibility.* ■

Signature

Each recording on the nursing notes is signed by the nurse making it. The signature includes the name and title; for example, "Susan J. Green, RN" or "SJ Green, RN." Some agencies have a signature sheet and after signing this signature sheet, the nurse can use their initials. With computerized charting, each nurse has his or her own code, which allows the documentation to be identified.

The following title abbreviations are often used, but nurses need to follow agency policy about how to sign their names.

RN   registered nurse
LVN   licensed vocational nurse
LPN   licensed practical nurse
NA   nursing assistant
NS   nursing student
PCA   patient care associate
SN   student nurse

Accuracy

The client's name and identifying information should be stamped or written on each page of the clinical record. Before making any entry, check that it is the correct chart. Do not identify charts by room number only; check the client's name. Special care is needed when caring for clients with the same last name.

Notations on records must be accurate and correct. Accurate notations consist of facts or observations rather than opinions or interpretations. It is more accurate, for example, to write that the client "refused medication" (fact) than to write that the client "was uncooperative" (opinion); to write that a client "was crying" (observation) is preferable to noting that the client "was de-

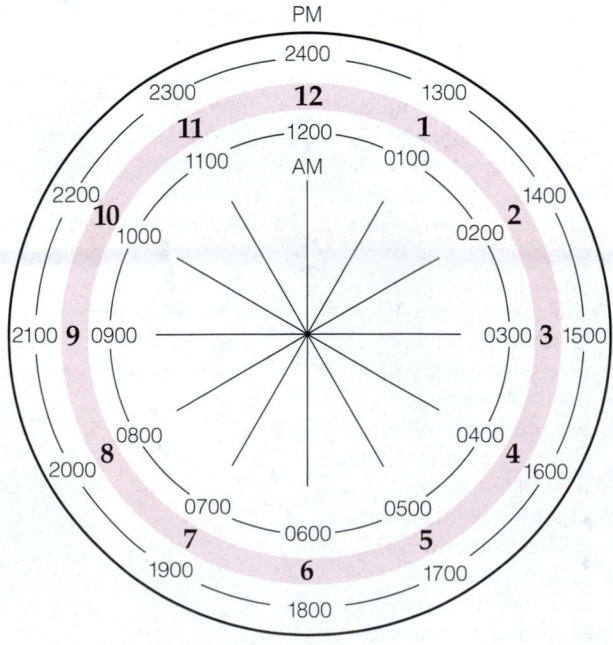

Figure 20–9 ■ The 24-hour clock.

TABLE 20–4 Commonly Used Abbreviations

Abbreviation	Term	Abbreviation	Term
Abd	Abdomen	neg	Negative
ABO	The main blood group system	∅	None
ac	Before meals	#	Number or pounds
ADL	Activities of daily living	NPO (NBM)	Nothing by mouth
ad lib	As desired	NS (N/S)	Normal saline
Adm	Admitted or admission	O_2	Oxygen
AM	Morning	OD	Right eye or overdose
amb	Ambulatory	OOB	Out of bed
amt	Amount	os	Mouth or opening
approx	Approximately	OS	Left eye
bid	Twice daily	pc	After meals
BM (bm)	Bowel movement	PE (PX)	Physical examination
BP	Blood pressure	per	By or through
BRP	Bathroom privileges	PM	Afternoon
c̄	With	po	By mouth
C	Celsius (centigrade)	postop	Postoperatively
CBC	Complete blood count	preop	Preoperatively
c/o	Complains of	prep	Preparation
DAT	Diet as tolerated	prn	When necessary
dc or d/c	Discontinue or discharge	q	Every
drsg	Dressing	qd	Every day
Dx	Diagnosis	qh (q1h)	Every hour
ECG (EKG)	Electrocardiogram	q2h, q3h, etc.	Every 2 hours, 3 hours, etc.
F	Fahrenheit	qhs	Every night at bedtime
fld	Fluid	qid	Four times a day
GI	Gastrointestinal	(R)	Right
gtt	Drop	s̄	Without
h (hr)	Hour	stat	At once, immediately
H_2O	Water	tid	Three times a day
hs	At bedtime	TO	Telephone order
I&O	Intake and output	TPR	Temperature, pulse, respirations
IV	Intravenous	Tr	Tincture
LMP	Last menstrual period	VO	Verbal order
(L)	Left	VS	Vital signs
meds	Medications	WNL	Within normal limits
mL (ml)	Milliliter	wt	Weight
mod	Moderate		

pressed" (interpretation). Similarly, when a client expresses worry about the diagnosis or problem, this should be quoted directly on the record: "Stated: 'I'm worried about my leg.'" When describing something, avoid general words, such as *large*, *good*, or *normal*, which can be interpreted differently. For example, chart specific data such as "2 cm × 3 cm bruise" rather than "large bruise."

When a recording mistake is made, draw a line through it and write the words *mistaken entry* above or next to the original entry, with your initials or name (depending on agency policy). Do not erase, blot out, or use correction fluid. The original entry must remain visible. When using computerized charting, the nurse needs to be aware of the agency's policy and process for correcting documentation mistakes.

TABLE 20–5 Commonly Used Symbols

Symbol	Term	Symbol	Number
>	Greater than	$\bar{o}$	0
<	Less than	$\overline{ss}$	1/2
=	Equal to	$\bar{i}$	1
↑	Increased	$\bar{ii}$	2
↓	Decreased	$\bar{iii}$	3
♀	Female	$\bar{iv}$	4
♂	Male	$\bar{v}$	5
°	Degree	$\bar{vi}$	6
#	Number	$\bar{vii}$	7
ℨ	Dram	$\bar{viii}$	8
℥	Ounce	$\bar{ix}$	9
×	Times	$\bar{x}$	10
@	At		

> ► **CLINICAL ALERT** *Avoid writing the word "error" when a recording mistake has been made. Some believe that the word* error *is a "red flag" for juries and can lead to the assumption that a clinical error has caused a client injury.* ■

Write on every line but never between lines. If a blank appears in a notation, draw a line through the blank space so that no additional information can be recorded at any other time or by any other person, and sign the notation.

Sequence

Document events in the order in which they occur; for example, record assessments, then the nursing interventions, and then the client's responses. Update or delete problems as needed.

Appropriateness

Record only information that pertains to the client's health problems and care. Any other personal information that the client conveys is inappropriate for the record. Recording irrelevant information may be considered an invasion of the client's privacy and/or libelous. A client's disclosure that she was addicted to heroin 20 years ago, for example, would *not* be recorded on the client's medical record unless it had a direct bearing on the client's health problem.

Completeness

Not all data that a nurse obtains about a client can be recorded. However, the information that is recorded needs to be complete and helpful to the client and health care professionals.

Nurses' notes need to reflect the nursing process. Record all assessments, dependent and independent nursing interventions, client problems, client comments and responses to interventions and tests, progress toward goals, and communication with other members of the health team.

Care that is *omitted* because of the client's condition or refusal of treatment must also be recorded. Document what was omitted, why it was omitted, and who was notified.

> ► **CLINICAL ALERT** *Do not assume that the person reading your charting will know that a common intervention (e.g., turning) has occurred because you believe it to be an "obvious" component of care.* ■

Conciseness

Recordings need to be brief as well as complete to save time in communication. The client's name and the word *client* are omitted. For example, write "Perspiring profusely. Respirations shallow, 28/min." End each thought or sentence with a period.

Legal Prudence

Accurate, complete documentation should give legal protection to the nurse, the client's other caregivers, the health care facility, and the client. Admissible in court as a legal document, the clinical record provides proof of the quality of care given to a client. Documentation is usually viewed by juries and attorneys as the best evidence of what really happened to the client (Iyer & Camp, 1999).

> ► **CLINICAL ALERT** *Complete charting, for example, by using the steps of the nursing process as a framework, is the best defense against malpractice.* ■

For the best legal protection, the nurse should not only adhere to professional standards of nursing care but also follow agency policy and procedures for intervention and documentation in all situations—especially high-risk situations. For example:

1100 hours—c/o of feeling dizzy. Raised side rails and instructed to stay in bed and ring call bell if requiring assistance. 1130 hours—found beside bed on floor. Stated, "I climbed over these rails all by myself." When asked about pain, replied, "I feel fine but a little dizzy." Helped into bed. BP 100/60 P90 R24. Dr. RJ Naden notified. _____ RS Woo RN

REPORTING

The purpose of reporting is to communicate specific information to a person or group of people. A report, whether oral or written, should be concise, including pertinent information but no extraneous detail. In addition to change-of-shift reports and telephone reports, reporting can also include the sharing of information or ideas with colleagues and other health professionals about some aspect of a client's care. Examples include the care plan conference and nursing rounds.

Change-of-Shift Reports

A **change-of-shift report** is a report given to all nurses on the next shift. Its purpose is to provide continuity of care for clients

Research Note
Does Nursing Documentation Reflect Actual Work Done by the Nurse?

Using a multiple-cases method of qualitative research, Brooks (1998) conducted a pilot study to investigate nurses' perceptions of the function and value of documentation and barriers to this process. The study consisted of interviewing seven staff nurses using an open-ended questionnaire that focused on their communication about clinical care and their reasoning and decision making for a client they cared for that day. Following the interview, the nurses' comments were compared to the actual documentation on the clients' charts and the nurses were asked to consider the difference between the actual "nurse work" and the documented data.

The data were categorized according to content, which helped identify themes. All of the nurses stated that they valued documentation; however, they felt a hopelessness about the use of the nurses' notes (e.g., "a lot of things we write are not that important"). Barriers to documentation included workload demands and cumbersome charting format. The nurses implied that they did not have the language or motivation to chart about behaviors of nonphysical concerns of the client.

Discrepancies were found between the nursing issues verbalized by the nurses and the documented data. The nurses verbalized how they spent time with their clients on such issues as preoperative anxiety and determining if a client's confusion was new or old. They freely discussed their intuitive judgments and clients' emotions by describing their perceptions of the clients' situations (e.g., "he needs time to talk things out"). The nurses developed strategies that they passed along verbally at the change-of-shift report (e.g., "you need to spend time with him"). The documentation, however, reflected a medical model of primarily physical assessment data. Most of the nurses were surprised by the incongruency between what they said was important and what they documented.

Implications: This pilot study suggests that nurses do not clearly document their knowledge and practice issues. Client behavioral issues were considered important but were verbally communicated rather than documented in the chart. If nursing documentation does not accurately reflect actual work done, nurses are minimizing their contribution to health care. With case-managed health care, it is vitally important that nurses communicate their knowledge and care strategies. Nurses need to present their unique and holistic approach to client care in the client's record.

Note: From "An Analysis of Nursing Documentation as a Reflection of Actual Nurse Work," by J. T. Brooks, 1998, *MEDSURG Nursing, 7*(4), pp. 189–196.

BOX 20–2 ■ Key Elements of a Change-of-Shift Report

- Follow a particular order (e.g., follow room numbers in a hospital).
- Provide basic identifying information for each client (e.g., name, room number, bed designation).
- For new clients, provide the reason for admission or medical diagnosis (or diagnoses), surgery (date), diagnostic tests, and therapies in past 24 hours.
- Include significant changes in client's condition and present information in order (i.e., assessment, nursing diagnoses, interventions, outcomes, and evaluation). For example, "Mr. Ronald Oakes said he had an aching pain in his left calf at 1400 hours. Inspection revealed no other signs. Calf pain is related to altered blood circulation. Rest and elevation of his legs on a footstool for 30 minutes provided relief."
- Provide exact information, such as "Ms. Jessie Jones received morphine 6 mg IV at 2000 hours," not "Ms. Jessie Jones received some morphine during the evening."
- Report clients' need for special emotional support. For example, a client who has just learned that his biopsy results revealed malignancy and who is now scheduled for a laryngectomy needs time to discuss his feelings before preoperative teaching is begun.
- Include current nurse-prescribed and physician-prescribed orders.
- Provide a summary of newly admitted clients, including diagnosis, age, general condition, plan of therapy, and significant information about the client's support people.
- Report on clients who have been transferred or discharged from the unit.
- Clearly state priorities of care and care that is due after the shift begins. For example, in a 7 AM report the nurse might say, "Mr. Li's vital signs are due at 0730, and his IV bag will need to be replaced by 0800." Give this information at the end of that client's report, because memory is best for the first and last information given.
- Be concise. Don't elaborate on background data or routine care (e.g., do not report "Vital signs at 0800 and 1200" when that is the unit standard). Do not report coming and going of visitors unless there is a problem or concern, or visitors are involved in teaching and care. Social support and visits are the norm.

> **CLINICAL ALERT**   *Be aware of where the shift report takes place in order to maintain client confidentiality. An area that is private and free from interruption is best.* ■

---

by providing the new caregivers a quick summary of client needs and details of care to be given.

Change-of-shift reports may be written or given orally, either in a face-to-face exchange or by audiotape recording. The face-to-face report permits the listener to ask questions during the report; written and tape-recorded reports are often briefer and less time consuming. Reports are sometimes given at the bedside, and clients as well as nurses may participate in the exchange of information. Box 20–2 lists key elements of a change-of-shift report.

Telephone Reports

Health professionals frequently report about a client by telephone. Nurses inform physicians about a change in a client's condition; a radiologist reports the results of an x-ray study; a nurse may report to a nurse on another unit about a transferred client.

The nurse receiving a telephone report should document the date and time, the name of the person giving the information, and the subject of the information received and sign the notation. For example:

> 6/6/03 10:35 AM GL Messina, laboratory technician, reported by telephone that Mrs. Sara Ames's hematocrit was 39/100 mL. _____ B. Ireland RN

If there is any doubt about the information given over the telephone, the person receiving the information should repeat it back to the sender to ensure accuracy.

When giving a telephone report to a physician, it is important that the nurse be concise and accurate. Begin with name and relationship to the client (e.g., "This is Jana Gomez, RN; I'm calling about your patient, Dorothy Mendes. I'm her nurse on the 7 PM to 7 AM shift").

Telephone reports usually include the client's name and medical diagnosis, changes in nursing assessment, vital signs related to baseline vital signs, significant laboratory data, and related nursing interventions. The nurse should have the client's chart ready to give the physician any further information.

After reporting, the nurse should document the date, time, and content of the call. For example:

> Dorothy Mendes admitted 12 noon; c/o burning upper right quadrant abdominal pain. BP 120/80, P100, R20 on admission. Demerol 100 mg IM on admission. At 3:15 PM BP 100/40, P120, R30. Pain unchanged. Color pale and diaphoretic. Reported by telephone to Dr. Burns at 2:10 PM. _____ TS Jones RN

Telephone Orders

Physicians often order a therapy (e.g., a medication) for a client by telephone. Most agencies have specific policies about telephone orders. Many agencies allow only registered nurses to take telephone orders.

While the physician gives the order, write it down and repeat it back to the physician to ensure accuracy. Question the physician about any order that is ambiguous, unusual (e.g., an abnormally high dosage of a medication), or contraindicated by the client's condition. Then transcribe the order onto the physician's order sheet, indicating it as a verbal order (VO) or telephone order (TO). See Box 20–3 for selected guidelines.

Once the order is transcribed on the physician's order sheet, the order must be countersigned by the physician within a time period described by agency policy. Many acute care hospitals require that this be done within 24 hours.

Care Plan Conference

A care plan conference is a meeting of a group of nurses to discuss possible solutions to certain problems of a client, such as inability to cope with an event or lack of progress toward goal attainment. The care plan conference allows each nurse an opportunity to offer an opinion about possible solutions to the problem. Other health professionals may be invited to attend the conference to offer their expertise; for example, a social worker may discuss the family problems of a severely burned child, or a dietitian may discuss the dietary problems of a client who has diabetes.

Care plan conferences are most effective when there is a climate of respect—that is, nonjudgmental acceptance of others even though their values, opinions, and beliefs may seem different. Nurses need to accept and respect each person's contributions, listening with an open mind to what others are saying even when there is disagreement.

Nursing Rounds

Nursing rounds are procedures in which two or more nurses visit selected clients at each client's bedside to:

- Obtain information that will help plan nursing care.
- Provide clients the opportunity to discuss their care.
- Evaluate the nursing care the client has received.

During rounds, the nurse assigned to the client provides a brief summary of the client's nursing needs and the interventions being implemented. Nursing rounds offer advantages to both clients and nurses: Clients can participate in the discussions, and nurses can see the client and the equipment being used. To facilitate client participation in nursing rounds, nurses need to use terms that the client can understand. Medical terminology excludes the client from discussion.

BOX 20–3 ■ Guidelines for Telephone Orders

1. Know the state nursing board's position on who can give and accept verbal and phone orders.
2. Know the agency's policy regarding phone orders (e.g., colleague listens on extension and cosigns order sheet).
3. Do not accept an order from a prescriber you do not know.
4. Ask the prescriber to speak slowly and clearly.
5. Ask the prescriber to spell out the medication if you are not familiar with it.
6. Question the drug, dosage, or changes if they seem inappropriate for this client.
7. Read the order back to the prescriber at the end. Use words instead of abbreviations (i.e., three times a day for tid).
8. Write the order on the physician's order sheet. Record date and time and indicate it was a telephone order (TO). Sign name and credentials.
9. When writing a dosage always put a number before a decimal (i.e., 0.3 mL) but never after a decimal (i.e., 6 mgm).
10. Write out units (i.e., 20 units of insulin, not 20 u of insulin).
11. Transcribe the order.
12. Follow agency protocol about the prescriber's protocol for signing telephone orders (i.e., within 24 hours).

Note: From "Taking Orders by Phone," by N. Cirone, 1998, *Nursing, 28*(8), p. 56; and adapted from *Surefire Documentation: How, What, and When Nurses Need to Document* (pp. 271–273) by Mosby, Inc., 1999, St. Louis, MO: Author, with permission from Elsevier Science.

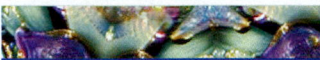

Focus on Critical Thinking

Mr. Anderson, an 80-year-old male, is admitted for back pain. He has a past medical history of hypertension. He told the admitting nurse that he has lost interest in many activities that he normally does because of the constant pain.

You read the following documentation entry by a previous nurse:

8 - Client is a complainer. I listened to him for 20 minutes with no success. BP 210/90 and 180/70. P. 72, R. 18.

    12 - Refused lunch

    2 - Client fell out of bed

1. What guidelines were *not* used in this documentation?
2. The nursing diagnosis for Mr. Anderson is *Acute Pain*. What would you expect to document?
3. Using the following pieces of data for Mr. Anderson, sort them into a SOAP note:
   a. "I didn't sleep last night"

b. positioned on side with pillows behind back
c. continues to need narcotic medication to progress toward goal of pain relief
d. states pain is 8 out of 10
e. "I feel better" (after interventions)
f. last medicated 5 hours previously
g. heating pad applied to lower back
h. BP 210/90, P. 72, R. 18
i. Add to plan of care to offer analgesic around the clock q 4 hours versus PRN
j. 6/6/03 #1 Pain
k. "sharp, stabbing pain in lower back that radiates to left leg"
l. medicated with ordered analgesic

4. Use the same pieces of data and sort them into a DAR note.

See Critical Thinking Possibilities in Appendix A.

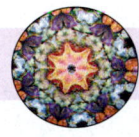 | # Chapter Review

EXPLORE MediaLink

NCLEX review questions, case studies, MediaLink applications, and other interactive resources for this chapter can be found on the Companion Website at www.prenhall.com/kozier. Click on Chapter 20 to select the activities for this chapter.

For more NCLEX review questions, and an audio glossary, access the Student CD-ROM accompanying this textbook.

Chapter Highlights

- Client records are legal documents that provide evidence of a client's care.
- The nurse has a duty to maintain confidentiality of the client's record; this includes special measures to protect client information stored in computers.
- Client records are kept for a number of purposes, including communication, planning client care, auditing health agencies, research, education, reimbursement, legal documentation, and health care analysis.
- In source-oriented clinical records, each health care professional group provides its own record. Recording is oriented around the source of the information.
- In problem-oriented clinical records, recording is organized around client problems.
- Examples of documentation systems include PIE, focus charting, charting by exception (CBE), computerized documentation, and case management.
- Computers make care planning and documentation relatively easy. The use of computer terminals at the bedside allows immediate documentation of nursing actions.

- The case management model emphasizes quality, cost-effective care delivered within an established length of stay.
- The Kardex is used to organize client data making information quick to access for health professionals.
- Nursing progress notes provide information about the progress the client is making toward desired outcomes. The format for the progress note depends on the documentation system at the facility.
- Long-term documentation varies depending on the level of care provided and requirements set by Medicare and Medicaid.
- Home health agencies must standardize their documentation methods to meet requirements for Medicare and Medicaid and other third-party disbursements.
- Legal guidelines for the process of recording in a client record include documenting date and time, legible entries, using dark ink, using correct terminology and spelling, accuracy, appropriateness, completeness, conciseness, and including an appropriate signature.

• The purpose of reporting is to communicate specific information for the goal of improving quality of care. Examples include change-of-shift report, telephone report, telephone orders, care plan conference, and nursing rounds.

Review Questions

20–1. Which of the following actions by a nurse ensures confidentiality of a client's computer record?
  a. The nurse logs on to the client's file and leaves the computer to answer the client's call light.
  b. The nurse shares her computer password.
  c. The nurse closes a client's computer file and logs off.
  d. The nurse leaves client computer worksheets at the computer workstation.

20–2. The case management model using critical pathways would be appropriate for a client with which diagnosis?
  a. myocardial infarction (heart attack)
  b. diabetes, hypertension
  c. myocardial infarction, diabetes, hypertension
  d. diabetes, hypertension, an infected foot ulcer, senile dementia

20–3. Interpret the following order: VO: ii gtts Isopto Atropine OD ac qd
  a. Verify order: two drops Isopto Atropine in left eye before meals every hour.
  b. Verbal order: two drops Isopto Atropine in right eye before meals every day.
  c. Telephone order: two drops Isopto Atropine in right eye after meals every day.
  d. Verbal order: two drops Isopto Atropine in both eyes before meals four times a day.

20–4. Which action should the nurse take when a recording mistake has occurred?
  a. Draw a line through the mistake.
  b. Draw a line through it and write *error* above the entry.
  c. Draw a line through it and write *mistaken entry* above it.
  d. Draw a line through the mistake and write *mistaken entry* and your initials above it.

20–5. Which charting entry would be the most defensible in court?
  a. Client fell out of bed.
  b. Client drunk on admission.
  c. Large bruise on left thigh.
  d. Notified Dr. Jones of BP of 90/40.

Readings and References

Suggested Readings

Frank-Stromborg, M., Christensen, A., & Elmhurst, D. (2001). Nurse documentation: Not done or worse, done the wrong way—part I. *Oncology Nursing Forum, 28*(4), 697–702. The authors focus on nursing documentation and the new technologies (e.g., facsimile, e-mail, computer charting). They stress the importance of nurses knowing the risks, particularly confidentiality and security issues, associated with electronic technology and suggest risk-reduction practices.

Frank-Stromborg, M., Christensen, A., & Elmhurst, D. (2001). Nurse documentation: Not done or worse, done the wrong way—part II. *Oncology Nursing Forum, 28*(5), 841–846. The authors continue to focus on documentation and describe how inadequate nursing documentation can result in a malpractice action. They describe examples of malpractice cases resulting from inadequate or inaccurate documentation. The article provides a clear picture of documentation do's and don'ts.

Staggers, N., Thompson, C. B., & Snyder-Halpern, R. (2001). History and trends in clinical information systems in the United States. *Journal of Nursing Scholarship, 33*(1), 75–81. The authors provide a historical review of clinical information systems and how the changes relate to the changing needs in the health care industry. Hospital information systems used computerized databases to communicate physician orders, to report results from pharmacy and lab, and to implement computerized billing. Support for clinical care and nursing practice, however, was limited. A computer-based patient record (CPR) is needed within managed care networks. The article points out some of the reasons CPR progressed more slowly than expected (e.g., compatibility among computer systems, lengthy system development, need for interdisciplinary focus). Of interest is the predicted future of clinical computing: shift from integration of data within one health network to sharing among networks, which will require resolution of legal, privacy, and security issues. Also, health providers will need to teach consumers how to evaluate the vast amount of health information on the Internet.

Yurkovich, E., & Smyer, T. (1998). Shift report: A time for learning. *Journal of Nursing Education, 37*(9), 401–403. The authors relate that the shift report is a professional socializing process where the language of the working nurse is communicated. The article describes a learning project in which students in one group provided audio-taped shift reports to other students in another clinical group. The students determined the structure of their shift report. They were encouraged to critique the reports of their classmates and to compare them to their own reports. The students learned the importance of focused, concise reports. This required prioritizing the content of the report and including practical, usable information and current client assessments. The project increased the students' confidence in their ability to assume the professional role behavior of presenting a shift report.

Related Research

Getty, M., Ryan, A. S., & Ekins, M. L. (1999). A comparative study of the attitudes of users and non-users towards computerized care planning. *Journal of Clinical Nursing, 8*(4), 431–439.

Lamond, D. (2000). The information content of the nurse change of shift report: A comparative study. *Journal of Advanced Nursing, 31*(4), 794–804.

Larrabee, J. H., Boldreghini, S., Elder-Sorrells, K., Turner, Z. M., Wender, R. G., Hart, J. M., et al. (2001). Evaluation of documentation before and after implementation of a nursing information system in an acute care hospital. *Computers in Nursing, 19*(2), 56–65.

Martin, A., Hinds, C., & Felix, M. (1999). Documentation practices of nurses in long-term care. *Journal of Clinical Nursing, 8*(4), 345–352.

Nahm, R., & Poston, I. (2000). Measurement of the effects of an integrated point-of-care computer system on quality of nursing documentation and patient satisfaction. *Computers in Nursing, 18*(5), 220–229.

Randolph, J. F., Magro, J., Stalmach, D., Cermak, B., & Wilson, B. (1999). A study of the accuracy of telephone orders in nursing homes in Southern California. *Annals of Long-Term Care, 7*(9), 334–338.

References

Allan, J., & Englebright, J. (2000). Patient-centered documentation. *Journal of Nursing Administration, 30*(2), 90–96.

American Nurses Association. (2001). *Code of ethics for nurses with interpretive statements.* Washington, DC: Author.

Brooks, J. T. (1998). An analysis of nursing documentation as a reflection of actual nurse work. *MEDSURG Nursing, 7*(4), 189–196.

Burke, L. J., & Murphy, J. (2000). Letters to the editor: Patient documentation. *Journal of Nursing Administration, 30*(7/8), 342.

Cirone, N. (1998). Taking orders by phone? *Nursing, 28*(8), 56–57.

Guido, G. W. (2001). *Legal and ethical issues in nursing* (3rd ed). Upper Saddle River, NJ: Prentice Hall.

Iyer, P. W., & Camp, N. H. (1999). *Nursing documentation: A nursing process approach* (3rd ed.) St. Louis, MO: Mosby.

Mosby, Inc. (1999). *Surefire documentation: How, what, and when nurses need to document.* St. Louis, MO: Author.

Murphy, J., & Burke, L. J. (1990). Charting by exception: A more efficient way to document. *Nursing, 20*(9), 65, 68–69.

Smith, C. M., & Dougherty, M. (2001). Practice brief: Requirements for the acute care record. *Journal of AHIMA, 72*(3), 56A–56G.

Selected Bibliography

Blachly, B., & Young, H. M. (1998). Reducing the burden of paperwork. Modified charting by exception for medications. *Journal of Gerontological Nursing, 24*(6), 16–20.

Catalano, K., Perlman, K., & Pinney, C. (2001). Critical path network. Improve patient safety to comply with new standards: Demonstrate evidence to JCAHO surveyors. *Hospital Case Management, 9*(7), 103–106.

Celia, L. M. (2002). Legally speaking. Keep electronic records safe! *RN, 65*(6), 69–71.

Feldkamp, J. K. (2002). Legally speaking. The legal landscape of long-term care. *RN, 65*(4), 61–62.

Johnson, T. (2000). Functional health pattern assessment on-line: Lessons learned. *Computers in Nursing, 18*(5), 248–254.

Kibbe, D., & Bard, M. R. (1997, May). How safe are computerized patient records? [Electronic version]. *Family Practice Management.* Retrieved June 5, 2003, from http://www.aafp.org/fpm/970500fm/lead.html

LaDuke, S. (2001). Online nursing documentation: Finding a middle ground. *Journal of Nursing Administration, 31*(6), 283–286.

Meiner, S. E. (1999). *Nursing documentation. Legal focus across practice settings.* Thousand Oaks, CA: Sage Publications.

Raymond, L. (2001). Legally speaking: How to chart for peer review. *RN, 64*(6), 67–70.

Raymond, L. (2002). Documenting for PROs. *Nursing, 32*(3), 50–53.

Smith, L. S. (2000). Charting tips: How to use focus charting. *Nursing, 30*(5), 76.

Smith, L. S. (2000). Charting tips: Safe computer charting. *Nursing, 30*(9), 85.

Springhouse Corp. (1999). *Mastering documentation* (2nd ed.). Springhouse, PA: Author.

Tan, R. S., & Isaacks, S. (1999). Computerized records and quality of care. *Annals of Long-Term Care, 7*(9), 348–353.

Utz, S. W. (1998). Computerized documentation of case management from diagnosis to outcomes. *Nursing Care Management, 3*(6), 247–254.

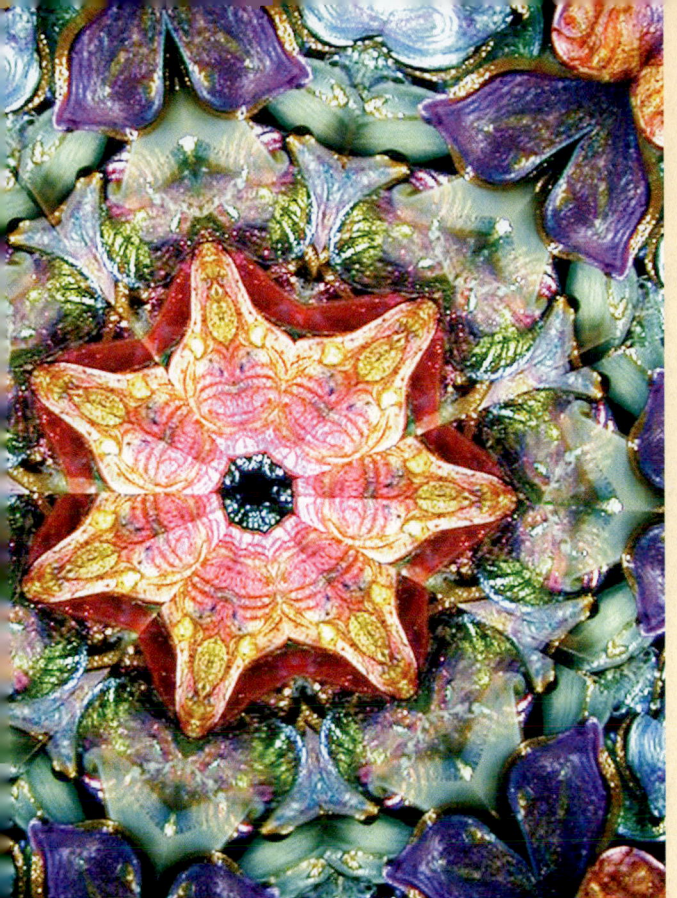

LIFE SPAN DEVELOPMENT

*A*long the intriguing journey from infancy through old age, human beings encounter new and often challenging life changes. An understanding and appreciation of how people develop at various stages of life influences much of nursing practice. The nurse's ability to consider the impact of prevailing life span issues as well as the needs of the individual promotes care that is appropriate, meaningful, and more likely to achieve desired outcomes.

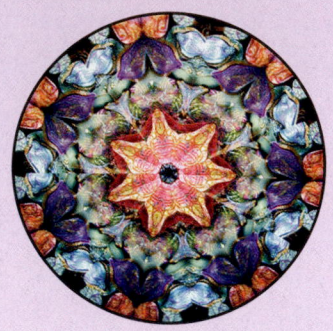

CHAPTER 21

CONCEPTS OF GROWTH AND DEVELOPMENT

LEARNING OUTCOMES

After completing this chapter, you will be able to:

- Differentiate between the terms *growth* and *development*.
- Describe essential principles related to growth and development.
- List factors that influence growth and development.
- Describe the stages of growth and development according to various theorists.
- Identify developmental tasks associated with Havighurst's six age periods.
- Describe characteristics and implications of Freud's five stages of development.
- Identify Erikson's eight stages of development.
- Compare Peck's and Gould's stages of adult development.
- Explain Piaget's theory of cognitive development.
- Compare Kohlberg's and Gilligan's theories of moral development.
- Compare Fowler's and Westerhoff's stages of spiritual development.

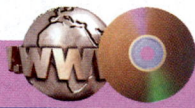

MediaLink

www.prenhall.com/kozier

Additional resources for this chapter can be found on the Student CD-ROM accompanying this textbook, and on the Companion Website at www.prenhall.com/kozier. Click on Chapter 21 to select the activities for this chapter.

CD-ROM
- Audio Glossary
- NCLEX Review

Companion Website
- Additional NCLEX Review
- Case Study: Treating a Six-Year Old Client
- Care Plan Activity:
  Child with Developmental Problems
- MediaLink Application:
  Discharging a Young Client
- Links to Resources

The terms *growth* and *development* both refer to dynamic processes. Often used interchangeably, these terms have different meanings. **Growth** is physical change and increase in size. It can be measured quantitatively. Indicators of growth include height, weight, bone size, and dentition. The pattern of physiologic growth is similar for all people. However, growth rates vary during different stages of growth and development. The growth rate is rapid during the prenatal, neonatal, infancy, and adolescent stages and slows during childhood. Physical growth is minimal during adulthood.

Development is an increase in the complexity of function and skill progression. It is the capacity and skill of a person to adapt to the environment. Development is the behavioral aspect of growth (e.g., a person develops the ability to walk, to talk, and to run).

Growth and development are independent, interrelated processes. For example, an infant's muscles, bones, and nervous system must grow to a certain point before the infant can sit up or walk. Growth generally takes place during the first 20 years of life; development continues after that. Principles of growth and development are shown in Box 21–1.

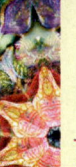

BOX 21–1 ■ Principles of Growth and Development

- Growth and development are continuous, orderly, sequential processes influenced by maturational, environmental, and genetic factors.
- All humans follow the same pattern of growth and development.
- The sequence of each stage is predictable, although the time of onset, the length of the stage, and the effects of each stage vary with the person.
- Learning can either help or hinder the maturational process, depending on what is learned.
- Each developmental stage has its own characteristics. For example, Piaget suggests that in the sensorimotor stage (birth to 2 years) children learn to coordinate simple motor tasks.
- Growth and development occur in a cephalocaudal direction, that is, starting at the head and moving to the trunk, the legs, and the feet (see Figure 21–1 ■). This pattern is particularly obvious at birth, when the head of the infant is disproportionately large.
- Growth and development occur in a proximodistal direction, that is, from the center of the body outward (Figure 21–1). For example, infants can roll over before they can grasp an object with the thumb and second finger.
- Development proceeds from simple to complex, or from single acts to integrated acts. To accomplish the integrated act of drinking and swallowing from a cup, for example, the child must first learn a series of single acts: eye–hand coordination, grasping, hand–mouth coordination, controlled tipping of the cup, and then mouth, lip, and tongue movements to drink and swallow.
- Development becomes increasingly differentiated. Differentiated development begins

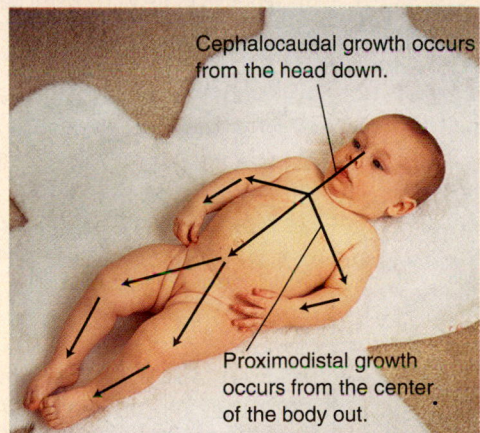

Cephalocaudal growth occurs from the head down.

Proximodistal growth occurs from the center of the body out.

Figure 21–1 ■ Cephalocaudal and proximodistal growth.

with a generalized response and progresses to a skilled specific response. For example, an infant's initial response to a stimulus involves the total body; a 5-year-old child can respond more specifically with laughter or fear.
- Certain stages of growth and development are more critical than others. It is known, for example, that the first 10 to 12 weeks after conception are critical. The incidence of congenital anomalies as a result of exposure to certain viruses, chemicals, or drugs is greater during this stage than others.
- The pace of growth and development is uneven. It is known that growth is greater during infancy than during childhood. Asynchronous development is demonstrated by rapid growth of the head during infancy and the extremities at puberty.

FACTORS INFLUENCING GROWTH AND DEVELOPMENT

The factors that influence growth and development are genetic and environmental. The genetic inheritance of an individual is established at conception. It remains unchanged throughout life and determines such characteristics as gender, physical characteristics (e.g., eye color, potential height), and temperament (e.g., response to stimuli in the environment). Environmental factors include family, religion, climate, culture, school, community, and nutrition. For example, poorly nourished children are more likely to have infections than are well-fed children and may not attain their full height potential.

STAGES OF GROWTH AND DEVELOPMENT

The rate of a person's growth and development is highly individual; however, the sequence of growth and development is predictable. Stages of growth usually correspond to certain developmental changes (see Table 21–1).

TABLE 21–1 Stages of Growth and Development

Stage	Age	Significant Characteristics	Nursing Implications
Neonatal	Birth to 28 days	Behavior is largely reflexive and develops to more purposeful behavior.	Assist parents to identify and meet unmet needs.
Infancy	1 month to 1 year	Physical growth is rapid.	Control the infant's environment so that physical and psychologic needs are met.
Toddlerhood	1 to 3 years	Motor development permits increased physical autonomy. Psychosocial skills increase.	Safety and risk-taking strategies must be balanced to permit growth.
Preschool	3 to 6 years	The preschooler's world is expanding. New experiences and the preschooler's social role are tried during play. Physical growth is slower.	Provide opportunities for play and social activity.
School age	6 to 12 years	Stage includes the preadolescent period (10 to 12 years). Peer group increasingly influences behavior. Physical, cognitive, and social development increases, and communication skills improve.	Allow time and energy for the school-age child to pursue hobbies and school activities. Recognize and support child's achievement.
Adolescence	12 to 20 years	Self-concept changes with biologic development. Values are tested. Physical growth accelerates. Stress increases, especially in face of conflicts.	Assist adolescents to develop coping behaviors. Help adolescents develop strategies for resolving conflicts.
Young adulthood	20 to 40 years	A personal lifestyle develops. Person establishes a relationship with a significant other and a commitment to something.	Accept adult's chosen lifestyle and assist with necessary adjustments relating to health. Recognize the person's commitments. Support change as necessary for health.
Middle adulthood	40 to 65 years	Lifestyle changes due to other changes; for example, children leave home, occupational goals change.	Assist clients to plan for anticipated changes in life, to recognize the risk factors related to health, and to focus on strengths rather than weaknesses.
Older adulthood			
Young-old	65 to 74 years	Adaptation to retirement and changing physical abilities is often necessary. Chronic illness may develop.	Assist clients to keep physically and socially active and to maintain peer group interactions.
Middle-old	75 to 84 years	Adaptation to decline in speed of movement, reaction time, and increasing dependence on others may be necessary.	Assist clients to cope with loss (e.g., hearing, sensory abilities and eyesight, death of loved one). Provide necessary safety measures.
Old-old	85 and over	Increasing physical problems may develop.	Assist clients with self-care as required, and with maintaining as much independence as possible.

Growth and development are commonly thought of as having five major components: physiologic, psychosocial, cognitive, moral, and spiritual. A discussion of some of the major theories relating to these components follows.

GROWTH AND DEVELOPMENT THEORIES

Researchers have advanced several theories about the various stages and aspects of growth and development, particularly with regard to infant and child development.

Developmental Task Theory (Havighurst, 1900–1991)

Robert Havighurst believed that learning is basic to life and that people continue to learn throughout life. He described growth and development as occurring during six stages, each associated with 6 to 10 tasks to be learned (see Table 21–2).

Havighurst promoted the concept of developmental tasks in the 1950s. A **developmental task** is "a task which arises at or about a certain period in the life of an individual, successful achievement of which leads to his happiness and to success with later tasks, while failure leads to unhappiness in the individual, disapproval by society, and difficulty with later tasks" (Havighurst, 1972, p. 2).

Havighurst's developmental tasks provide a framework that the nurse can use to evaluate a person's general accomplishments. However, some nurses find that the broad categories limit its usefulness as a tool in assessing specific accomplishments, particularly those of infancy and childhood.

Psychosocial Theories

Psychosocial development refers to the development of personality. **Personality** is a complex concept that is difficult to define. It can be considered as the outward (interpersonal) expression of the inner (intrapersonal) self. It encompasses a person's temperament, feelings, character traits, independence,

---

TABLE 21–2 Havighurst's Age Periods and Developmental Tasks

Infancy and Early Childhood
1. Learning to walk
2. Learning to take solid foods
3. Learning to talk
4. Learning to control the elimination of body wastes
5. Learning sex differences and sexual modesty
6. Achieving psychologic stability
7. Forming simple concepts of social and physical reality
8. Learning to relate emotionally to parents, siblings, and other people
9. Learning to distinguish right from wrong and developing a conscience

Middle Childhood
1. Learning physical skills necessary for ordinary games
2. Building wholesome attitudes toward oneself as a growing organism
3. Learning to get along with age-mates
4. Learning an appropriate masculine or feminine social role
5. Developing fundamental skills in reading, writing, and calculating
6. Developing concepts necessary for everyday living
7. Developing conscience, morality, and a scale of values
8. Achieving personal independence
9. Developing attitudes toward social groups and institutions

Adolescence
1. Achieving new and more mature relations with age-mates of both sexes
2. Achieving a masculine or feminine social role
3. Accepting one's physique and using the body effectively
4. Achieving emotional independence from parents and other adults
5. Achieving assurance of economic independence
6. Selecting and preparing for an occupation

7. Preparing for marriage and family life
8. Developing intellectual skills and concepts necessary for civic competence
9. Desiring and achieving socially responsible behavior
10. Acquiring a set of values and an ethical system as a guide to behavior

Early Adulthood
1. Selecting a mate
2. Learning to live with a partner
3. Starting a family
4. Rearing children
5. Managing a home
6. Getting started in an occupation
7. Taking on civic responsibility
8. Finding a congenial social group

Middle Age
1. Achieving adult civic and social responsibility
2. Establishing and maintaining an economic standard of living
3. Assisting teenage children to become responsible and happy adults
4. Developing adult leisure-time activities
5. Relating oneself to one's spouse as a person
6. Accepting and adjusting to the physiologic changes of middle age
7. Adjusting to aging parents

Later Maturity
1. Adjusting to decreasing physical strength and health
2. Adjusting to retirement and reduced income
3. Adjusting to death of a spouse
4. Establishing an explicit affiliation with one's age group
5. Meeting social and civil obligations
6. Establishing satisfactory physical living arrangements

Note: From Robert J. Havighurst Developmental Tasks and Education, 3ed. Published by Allyn & Bacon, Boston, MA. Copyright © 1972 by Pearson Education. Reprinted with permission.

MediaLink | DISCHARGING A YOUNG CLIENT APPLICATION

self-esteem, self-concept, behavior, ability to interact with others, and ability to adapt to life changes.

Many theorists attempt to account for psychosocial development in humans. Many of these theories explain the development of a person's personality and the causes of behavior.

Freud (1856–1939)

Sigmund Freud introduced a number of concepts about development that are still used today. The concepts of the unconscious mind, defense mechanisms, and the id, ego, and superego are Freud's. The **unconscious mind** is the part of a person's mental life that the person is unaware of. This concept of the unconscious is one of Freud's major contributions to the field of psychiatry. The **id** resides in the unconscious and, operating on the pleasure principle, seeks immediate pleasure and gratification (Thomas, 2001). The **ego,** operating on the reality principle, balances the gratification demands of the id with the limitations of social and physical circumstances. The methods the ego uses to fulfill the needs of the id in a socially acceptable manner are called defense mechanisms or adaptive mechanisms. **Defense mechanisms,** or **adaptive mechanisms** as they are more commonly called today, are the result of conflicts between the id's impulses and the anxiety that attends these conflicts due to environmental restrictions. The third aspect of

the personality, according to Freud, is the superego. The **superego** contains the conscience and the ego idea. The conscience consists of society's "don'ts" usually as a result of parental and cultural expectations. The ego ideal comprises the standards of perfection toward which the individual strives (Green & Piel, 2002, p. 49). Freud proposes that the underlying motivation to human development is a dynamic, psychic energy, which he calls **libido.**

According to Freud's theory of psychosexual development, the personality develops in five overlapping stages from birth to adulthood. The libido changes its location of emphasis within the body from one stage to another. Therefore, a particular body area has special significance to a client at a particular stage. The first three stages (oral, anal, and phallic) are called *pregenital stages.* The culminating stage is the *genital stage.* Table 21–3 indicates characteristics for each stage.

If the individual does not achieve a satisfactory progression at each stage, the personality becomes fixated at that stage. **Fixation** is immobilization or the inability of the personality to proceed to the next stage because of anxiety. For example, nurses can assist an infant's development by making feeding a pleasurable experience and by making toilet training a positive experience, thereby enhancing the child's feeling of self-control. Freud also emphasizes the importance of infant–parent

TABLE 21–3   Freud's Five Stages of Development

Stage	Age	Characteristics	Implications
Oral	Birth to 1 1/2 year	Mouth is the center of pleasure (major source of gratification and exploration). Security is primary need. Major conflict: weaning	Feeding produces pleasure and sense of comfort and safety. Feeding should be pleasurable and provided when required.
Anal	1 1/2 to 3 years	Anus and bladder are the sources of pleasure (sensual satisfaction, self-control). Major conflict: toilet training	Controlling and expelling feces provide pleasure and sense of control. Toilet training should be a pleasurable experience.
Phallic	4 to 6 years	The child's genitals are the center of pleasure. Masturbation offers pleasure. Other activities can include fantasy, experimentation with peers and questioning of adults about sexual topics. Major conflict: the Oedipus or Electra complex, which resolves when the child identifies with parent of same sex. (The Oedipus complex refers to the male child's attraction for his mother and hostile attitudes toward his father. The Electra complex refers to the female's attraction for her father and hostile attitudes toward her mother.)	The child identifies with the parent of the opposite sex and and later takes on a love relationship outside the family. Encourage identity.
Latency	6 to puberty	Energy is directed to physical and intellectual activities. Sexual impulses tend to be repressed. Develop relationships between peers of the same sex.	Encourage child with physical and intellectual pursuits. Encourage sports and other activities with same sex peers.
Genital	Puberty and after	Energy is directed toward full sexual maturity and function and development of skills needed to cope with the environment.	Encourage separation from parents, achievement of independence, and decision making.

Note: From *Health Promotion Strategies Through the Life Span,* 7th ed., (p. 238), by R. B. Murray and J. P. Zentner, 2001, Upper Saddle River, NJ: Merrill/Prentice Hall. Adapted with permission interaction. Therefore, the nurse as a caregiver should provide a warm, caring atmosphere for an infant and assist parents to do so when the infant returns to their care.

Ideally, an individual progresses through the tasks of each stage and balance is achieved between the id, ego, and superego. Conflict or stress, however, can delay or prolong progression through a stage or cause a person to regress to a previous stage.

Erikson (1902–1996)

Erik H. Erikson (1963, 1964) adapted and expanded Freud's theory of development to include the entire life span, believing that people continue to develop throughout life. He describes eight stages of development (see Table 21–4).

Erikson envisions life as a sequence of levels of achievement. Each stage signals a task that must be achieved. The resolution of the task can be complete, partial, or unsuccessful. Erikson believes that the greater the task achievement, the healthier the personality of the person; failure to achieve a task influences the person's ability to achieve the next task. These

developmental tasks can be viewed as a series of crises, and successful resolution of these crises is supportive to the person's ego. Failure to resolve the crises is damaging to the ego.

Erikson's eight stages reflect both positive and negative aspects of the critical life periods. The resolution of the conflicts at each stage enables the person to function effectively in society. Each phase has its developmental task, and the individual must find a balance between, for example, trust versus mistrust (stage 1) or integrity versus despair (stage 8). See Figures 21–2 ■ and 21–3 ■.

When using Erikson's developmental framework, nurses should be aware of indicators of positive and negative resolution of each stage. It is also important to be aware that the environment is highly influential in development, according to Erikson. Nurses can enhance a client's development by being aware of the person's developmental stage and by helping the person develop coping skills relative to stressors experienced at that level. Nurses can strengthen a client's positive resolution of a developmental task by providing the individual with appropriate opportunities and encouragement. For example, a 10-year-old child

TABLE 21–4   Erikson's Eight Stages of Development

Stage	Age	Central Task	Indicators of Positive Resolution	Indicators of Negative Resolution
Infancy	Birth to 18 months	Trust versus mistrust	Learning to trust others	Mistrust, withdrawal, estrangement
Early childhood	18 months to 3 years	Autonomy versus shame and doubt	Self-control without loss of self-esteem Ability to cooperate and to express oneself	Compulsive self-restraint or compliance Willfulness and defiance
Late childhood	3 to 5 years	Initiative versus guilt	Learning the degree to which assertiveness and purpose influence the environment Beginning ability to evaluate one's own behavior	Lack of self-confidence Pessimism, fear of wrongdoing Overcontrol and overrestriction of own activity
School age	6 to 12 years	Industry versus inferiority	Beginning to create, develop, and manipulate Developing sense of competence and perseverance	Loss of hope, sense of being mediocre Withdrawal from school and peers
Adolescence	12 to 20 years	Identity versus role confusion	Coherent sense of self Plans to actualize one's abilities	Feelings of confusion, indecisiveness, and possible antisocial behavior
Young adulthood	18 to 25 years	Intimacy versus isolation	Intimate relationship with another person Commitment to work and relationships	Impersonal relationships Avoidance of relationship, career, or lifestyle commitments
Adulthood	25 to 65 years	Generativity versus stagnation	Creativity, productivity, concern for others	Self-indulgence, self-concern, lack of interests and commitments
Maturity	65 years to death	Integrity versus despair	Acceptance of worth and uniqueness of one's own life Acceptance of death	Sense of loss, contempt for others

Note: From Childhood and Society, 2nd ed., (pp. 247–274), by E. Erikson, 1963, New York: W. W. Norton. Copyright 1950, © 1963 by W. W. Norton & Company, Inc., renewed © 1978, 1991 by Erik H. Erikson. Reprinted with permission.

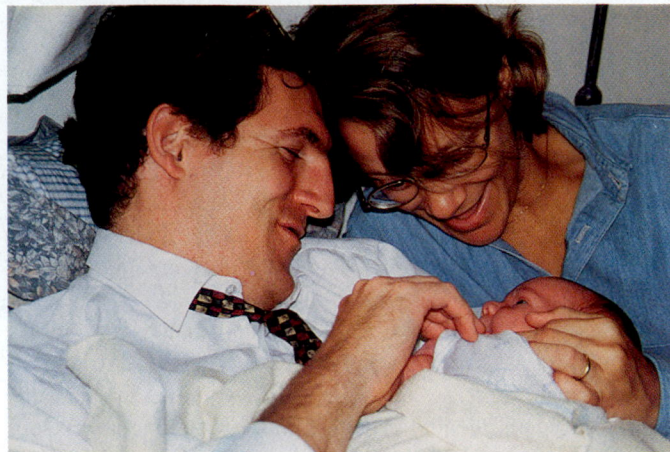

Figure 21–2 ■ Trust is established when the infant's basic needs are met.

can be encouraged to be creative, to finish schoolwork, and to learn how to accomplish these tasks within the limitations imposed by health.

Erikson emphasizes that people must change and adapt their behavior to maintain control over their lives. In his view, no stage in personality development can be bypassed, but people can become fixated at one stage or regress to a previous stage under anxious or stressful conditions. For example, a middle-aged woman who has never satisfactorily accomplished the task of resolving identity versus role confusion might regress to an earlier stage when stressed by an illness with which she cannot cope.

Peck

Theories and models about adult development are relatively recent compared with theories of infant and child development. Research into adult development has been stimulated by a number of factors, including increased longevity and healthier old age. In the past, development was viewed as complete by the time of physical maturity, and aging was considered a decline following maturity. The emphasis was on the decremental aspects rather than the incremental aspects of aging. However, Robert Peck (1968) believes that although physical capabilities and functions decrease with old age, mental and social capacities tend to increase in the latter part of life.

Peck proposes three developmental tasks during old age, in contrast to Erikson's one (integrity versus despair):

1. *Ego differentiation versus work-role preoccupation.* An adult's identity and feelings of worth are highly dependent on that person's work role. On retirement people may experience feelings of worthlessness unless they derive their sense of identity from a number of roles so that one such role can replace the work role or occupation as a source of self-esteem. For example, a man who likes to garden or golf can obtain ego rewards from those activities, replacing rewards formerly obtained from his occupation.

2. *Body transcendence versus body preoccupation.* This task calls for the individual to adjust to decreasing physical ca-

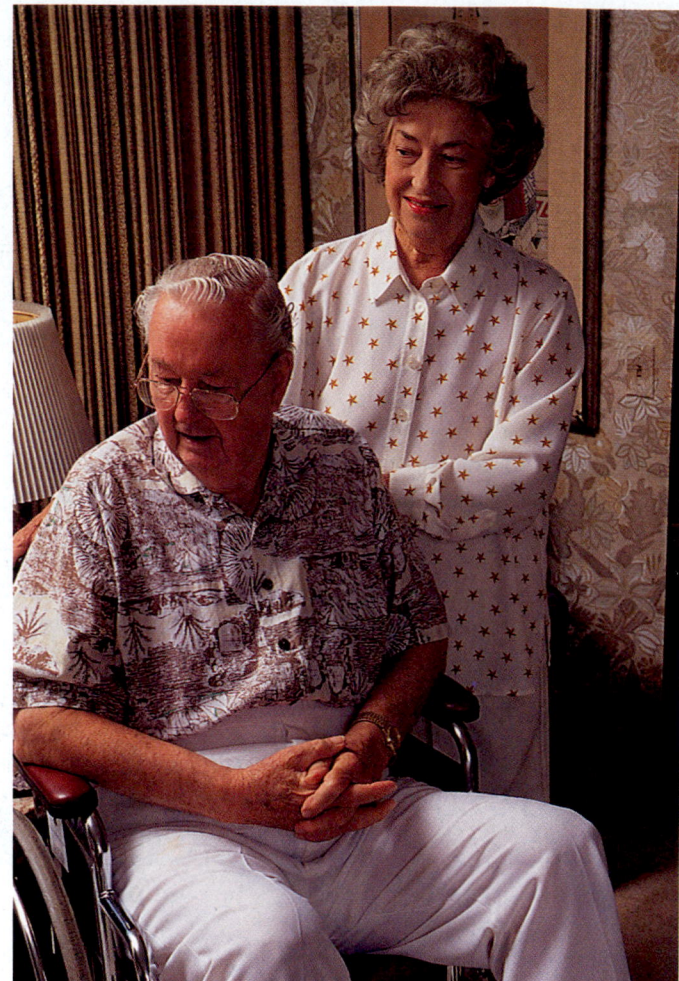

Figure 21–3 ■ Assistive devices help maintain independence and self-esteem, which also helps the older adult's ego integrity to adapt and cope with the reality of aging.

pacities and at the same time maintain feelings of well-being. Preoccupation with declining body functions reduces happiness and satisfaction with life.

3. *Ego transcendence versus ego preoccupation.* Ego transcendence is the acceptance without fear of one's death as inevitable. This acceptance includes being actively involved in one's own future beyond death. Ego preoccupation, by contrast, results in holding onto life and a preoccupation with self-gratification.

Gould

Roger Gould is another theorist who has studied adult development. He believes that transformation is a central theme during adulthood: "Adults continue to change over the period of time considered to be adulthood and... developmental phases may be found during the adult span of life" (Gould, 1972, p. 33). According to Gould, the 20s is the time when a person assumes new roles; in the 30s, role confusion often occurs; in the 40s the person becomes aware of time limitations in relation to accomplishing life's goals; and in the 50s, the acceptance of each stage as a natural progression of life marks the path to adult maturity. Gould's study of 524 men and women led him to describe seven stages of adult development:

- *Stage 1 (ages 16–18).* Individuals consider themselves part of the family rather than individuals and want to separate from their parents.
- *Stage 2 (ages 18–22).* Although the individuals have established autonomy, they feel it is in jeopardy; they feel they could be pulled back into their families.
- *Stage 3 (ages 22–28).* Individuals feel established as adults and autonomous from their families. They see themselves as well-defined but still feel the need to prove themselves to their parents. They see this as the time for growing and building for the future (see Figure 21–4 ■).
- *Stage 4 (ages 29–34).* Marriage and careers are well established. Individuals question what life is all about and wish to be accepted as they are, no longer finding it necessary to prove themselves.
- *Stage 5 (ages 35–43).* This is a period of self-reflection. Individuals question values and life itself. They see time as finite, with little time left to shape the lives of adolescent children.
- *Stage 6 (ages 43–50).* Personalities are seen as set. Time is accepted as finite. Individuals are interested in social activities with friends and spouse and desire both sympathy and affection from spouse.
- *Stage 7 (ages 50–60).* This is a period of transformation, with a realization of mortality and a concern for health. There is an increase in warmth and a decrease in negativism. The spouse is seen as a valuable companion (Gould, 1972, pp. 525–527).

Cognitive Theory (Piaget, 1896–1980)

Cognitive development refers to the manner in which people learn to think, reason, and use language. It involves a person's intelligence, perceptual ability, and ability to process information. Cognitive development represents a progression of mental abilities from illogical to logical thinking, from simple to complex problem solving, and from understanding concrete ideas to understanding abstract concepts.

The most widely known cognitive theorist is Jean Piaget. His theory of cognitive development has contributed to other theories, such as Kohlberg's theory of moral development and Fowler's theory of the development of faith, both discussed in this chapter.

According to Piaget (1966), cognitive development is an orderly, sequential process in which a variety of new experiences (stimuli) must exist before intellectual abilities can develop. Piaget's cognitive developmental process is divided into five major phases: the sensorimotor phase, the preconceptual phase, the intuitive thought phase, the concrete operations phase (see Figure 21–5 ■), and the formal operations phase.

A person develops through each of these phases; each phase has its own unique characteristics (see Table 21–5). In each phase, the person uses three primary abilities: assimilation, accommodation, and adaptation. **Assimilation** is the process through which humans encounter and react to new situations by using the mechanisms they already possess. In this way, people acquire knowledge and skills as well as insights into the world around them. **Accommodation** is a process of change whereby cognitive processes mature sufficiently to allow the person to solve problems that were unsolvable before. This adjustment is possible chiefly because new knowledge has been assimilated. **Adaptation,** or coping behavior, is the ability to handle the demands made by the environment.

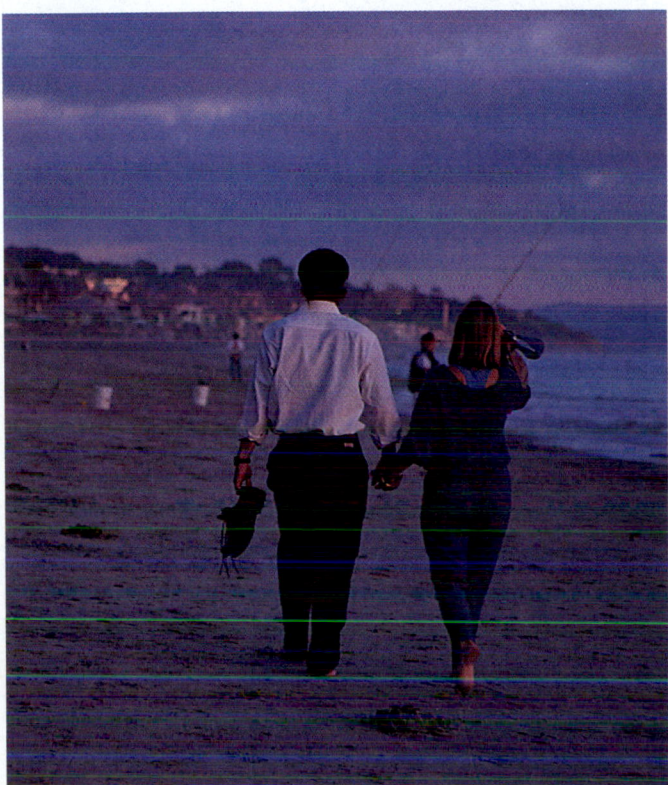

Figure 21–4 ■ Young adults develop meaningful relationships and begin considering a home and family for themselves.

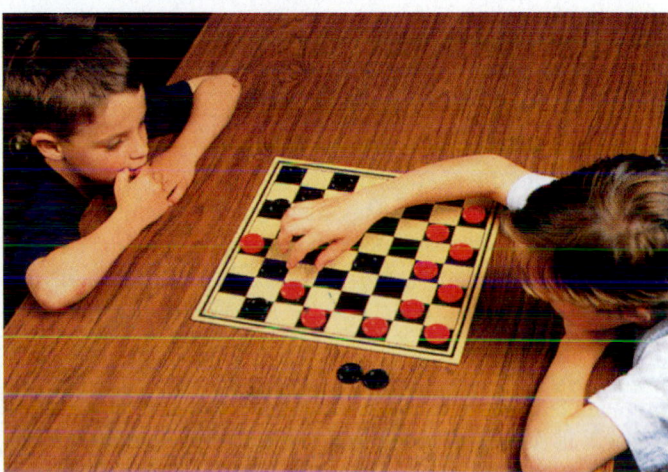

Figure 21–5 ■ School-age (7 to 11 years) children can understand cause-and-effect and concrete relationships or problems.

TABLE 21–5 Piaget's Phases of Cognitive Development

Phases and Stages	Age	Significant Behavior
Sensorimotor phase	Birth to 2 years	
Stage 1 Use of reflexes	Birth to 1 month	Most action is reflexive.
Stage 2 Primary circular reaction	1 to 4 months	Perception of events is centered on the body. Objects are extension of self.
Stage 3 Secondary circular reaction	4 to 8 months	Acknowledges the external environment. Actively makes changes in the environment.
Stage 4 Coordination of secondary schemata	8 to 12 months	Can distinguish a goal from a means of attaining it.
Stage 5 Tertiary circular reaction	12 to 18 months	Tries and discovers new goals and ways to attain goals. Rituals are important.
Stage 6 Inventions of new means	18 to 24 months	Interprets the environment by mental image. Uses make-believe and pretend play.
Preconceptual phase	2 to 4 years	Uses an egocentric approach to accommodate the demands of an environment. Everything is significant and relates to "me." Explores the environment. Language development is rapid. Associates words with objects.
Intuitive thought phase	4 to 7 years	Egocentric thinking diminishes. Thinks of one idea at a time. Includes others in the environment. Words express thoughts.
Concrete operations phase	7 to 11 years	Solves concrete problems. Begins to understand relationships such as size. Understands right and left. Cognizant of viewpoints.
Formal operations phase	11 to 15 years	Uses rational thinking. Reasoning is deductive and futuristic.

Note: From The Origin of Intelligence in Children, by J. Piaget, 1966, International Universities Press, Inc., Copyright © 1966. Adapted with permission.

Nurses can employ Piaget's theory of cognitive development when developing teaching strategies. For example, a nurse can expect a toddler to be egocentric and literal; therefore, explanations to the toddler should focus on the needs of the toddler rather than on the needs of others. A 13-year-old can be expected to use rational thinking and to reason; therefore, when explaining the need for a medication a nurse can outline the consequences of taking and not taking the medication, enabling the adolescent to make a rational decision. Nurses must remember, however, that the range of normal cognitive development is broad, despite the ages arbitrarily associated with each level. When teaching adults, nurses may become aware that some adults are more comfortable with concrete thought and slower to acquire and apply new information than are other adults.

Moral Theories

Moral development, a complex process not fully understood, involves learning what ought to be and what ought not to be done. It is more than imprinting parents' rules and virtues or values on children. The term **moral** means "relating to right and wrong." The terms *morality, moral behavior,* and *moral development* need to be distinguished. **Morality** refers to the requirements necessary for people to live together in society; **moral behavior** is the way a person perceives those requirements and responds to them; **moral development** is the pattern of change in moral behavior with age (see Chapter 5).

Kohlberg (1927–1987)

Lawrence Kohlberg's theory specifically addresses moral development in children and adults (Murray & Zentner, 2001). The morality of an individual's decision was not Kohlberg's concern; rather, he focused on the reasons an individual makes a decision. According to Kohlberg, moral development progresses through three levels and six stages. Levels and stages are not always linked to a certain developmental stage, because some people progress to a higher level of moral development than others.

At Kohlberg's first level, called the *premoral* or *preconventional level,* children are responsive to cultural rules and labels of good and bad, right and wrong. However, children interpret these in terms of the physical consequences of their actions, that is, punishment or reward. At the second level, the *conventional level,* the individual is concerned about maintaining the expectations of the family, group, or nation and sees this as right. The emphasis at this level is conformity and loyalty to one's own expectations as well as society's. Level three is

TABLE 21–6 Kohlberg's Stages of Moral Development

Level	Stage	Average Age
I. Preconventional Person is responsive to cultural rules of labels of good and bad, right or wrong. Externally established rules determine right or wrong actions. Person reasons in terms of punishment, reward, or exchange of favors. **Egocentric focus**	**1. Punishment and Obedient Orientation** Fear of punishment, not respect for authority, is the reason for decisions, behavior, and conformity.	Toddler to 7 years
	2. Instrumental Relativist Orientation Conformity is based on egocentricity and narcissistic needs. There is no feeling of justice, loyalty, or gratitude. "I'll do something if I get something for it or because it pleases you."	Preschooler through school age
II. Conventional Person is concerned with maintaining expectations and rules of the family, group, nation, or society. A sense of guilt has developed and affects behavior. The person values conformity, loyalty, and active maintenance of social order and control. Conformity means good behavior or what pleases or helps another and is approved. **Societal focus**	**3. Interpersonal Concordance Orientation** Decisions and behavior are based on concerns about others' reactions; the person wants others' approval or a reward. An empathic response, based on understanding of how another person feels, is a determinant for decisions and behavior. ("I can put myself in your shoes.")	School age through adulthood (Most American women are in this stage)
	4. Law-and-Order Orientation The person wants established rules from authorities, and the reason for decisions and behavior is that social and sexual rules and traditions demand the response. ("I'll do something because it's the law and my duty.")	Adolescence and adulthood (Most men are in this stage)
III. Postconventional The person lives autonomously and defines moral values and principles that are distinct from personal identification with group values. He or she lives according to principles that are universally agreed on and that the person considers appropriate for life. **Universal focus**	**5. Social Contract Legalistic Orientation** The social rules are not the sole basis for decisions and behavior because the person believes a higher moral principle applies such as equality, justice, or due process.	Middle-age or older adult. Only 20% or less of Americans achieve this stage
	6. Universal Ethical Principle Orientation Decisions and behaviors are based on internalized rules, on conscience rather than social laws, and on self-chosen ethical and abstract principles that are universal, comprehensive, and consistent.	Middle-age or older adult. Few people attain or maintain this stage. Examples of this stage are seen in times of crisis or extreme situations.

Note: From *Health Promotion Strategies Through the Life Span,* 7th ed., (pp. 252–253), by R. B. Murray and J. P. Zentner, 2001, Upper Saddle River, NJ: Merril/Prentice Hall. Adapted with permission.

called the *postconventional, autonomous,* or *principled level.* At this level, people make an effort to define valid values and principles without regard to outside authority or to the expectations of others (see Table 21–6).

Gilligan

After more than 10 years of research with women subjects, Carol Gilligan (1982) reported that women often consider the dilemmas Kohlberg used in his research to be irrelevant.

Women scored consistently lower on his scale of moral development in spite of the fact that they approached moral dilemmas with considerable sophistication. Gilligan believes that most frameworks for research in moral development do not include the concepts of caring and responsibility.

Gilligan found that moral development proceeds through three levels and two transitions, with each level representing a more complex understanding of the relationship of self and others and each transition resulting in a crucial reevaluation of the conflict between selfishness and responsibility (Murray & Zentner, 2001, p. 251).

- *Stage 1: caring for oneself.* In this first stage of development, the person is concerned only with caring for the self. The individual feels isolated, alone, and unconnected to others. There is no concern or conflict with the needs of others because the self is the most important. The focus of this stage is survival. The transition of this stage occurs when the individual begins to view this approach as selfishness and moves toward responsibility. The person begins to realize a need for relationships and connections with other people.
- *Stage 2: caring for others.* During this stage, the individual recognizes the selfishness of earlier behavior and begins to understand the need for caring relationships with others. Caring relationships bring with them responsibility. The definition of responsibility includes self-sacrifice, where "good" is considered to be "caring for others." The individual now approaches relationships with a focus of not hurting others. This approach causes the individual to be more responsive and submissive to others' needs, excluding any thoughts of meeting one's own needs. A transition from goodness to truth occurs when the individual recognizes that this approach can cause difficulties with relationships because of the lack of balance between caring for oneself and caring for others. The woman makes decisions on personal intentions and consequences of actions rather than on how she thinks others will react (Murray & Zentner, 2001, p. 253).
- *Stage 3: caring for self and others.* During this last stage, a person sees the need for a balance between caring for others and caring for the self. The concept of responsibility now includes responsibility for the self and for other people. Care remains the focus on which decisions are made. However, the person recognizes the interconnections between the self and others and realizes that if one's own needs are not met, other people may also suffer.

Gilligan (1982) believes women often see morality in the integrity of relationships and caring, so that the moral problems they encounter are different from those of men. Men tend to consider what is right to be what is just, whereas for women what is right is taking responsibility for others as a self-chosen decision (p. 140). The ethic of justice, or fairness, is based on the idea of equality: Everyone should receive the same treatment. This is the development path usually followed by men and widely accepted by moral theorists. By contrast, the ethic of care is based on the premise of nonviolence: No one should be harmed. This is the path typically followed by women but given little attention in the literature of moral theory.

In the development of maturity, according to Gilligan (1982), both viewpoints blend "in the realization that just as inequality adversely affects both perspectives in an unequal relationship, so too violence is destructive for everyone involved" (p. 174). The blending of these two perspectives could give rise to a new view of human development and a better understanding of human relations.

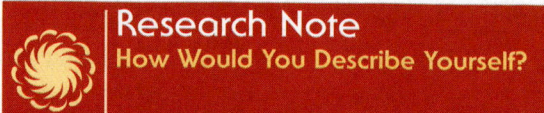

Research Note
How Would You Describe Yourself?

Belknap's (2002) qualitative research study used Gilligan's theory of moral development to extend the body of knowledge on how abused and formerly abused women experience self. The author interviewed 18 women, ranging in age from 18 to 51 years from diverse cultural and ethnic backgrounds, who identified themselves as abused by an intimate male partner. Fourteen were no longer living with the abusive partner and four were currently living with the abusive partner.

The women were first asked to talk about their lives in general, followed by the question "How would you describe yourself to yourself?" Then, the woman was asked to describe a real-life situation and her response to it. From the interpreted interviews, the author identified four distinct voices of separation and connection, which related to Gilligan's stages of moral development. At one end of a continuum, the women described themselves as lonely, angry, with little self-esteem and no connection to others. The other end of the continuum reflected women in the transition period of goodness to truth where they realized the need to care for themselves in addition to caring for and helping others (e.g., children).

The findings indicate that the women who rejected the notion that good equals self-sacrifice (Gilligan's stage 2) progressed to a more positive perception of self and viewed their moral choice as based not on either/or but on a sense of self-worth, and they chose actions that were caring and responsive to both the needs of self and the needs of others. They were in the transitional period: from goodness to truth.

Implications: Nurses who care for women who are experiencing or recovering from abuse need to understand where the woman sees herself in relationship to others and self. More inquiry needs to be accomplished as to how and what strategy nurses can use to facilitate the woman's progress through Gilligan's stages of moral development.

Note: From "Sense of Self: Voices of Separation and Connection in Women Who Have Experienced Abuse," by R. A. Belknap, 2002, *Canadian Journal of Nursing Research, 33*(4), pp. 139–153.

Spiritual Theories

The spiritual component of growth and development refers to individuals' understanding of their relationship with the universe and their perceptions about the direction and meaning of life.

Fowler

James Fowler describes the development of faith as a force that gives meaning to a person's life. He uses the term *faith* as a form of knowing, a way of being in relation to "an ultimate environment." To Fowler, "faith is a relational phenomenon; it is an active 'mode-of-being-in-relation' to another or others in which we invest commitment, belief, love, risk and hope" (Fowler & Keen, 1985, p. 18). Fowler's stages in the development of faith are given in Table 21–7.

TABLE 21–7   Fowler's Stages of Spiritual Development

Stage	Age	Description
0. Undifferentiated	0 to 3 years	Infant unable to formulate concepts about self or the environment
1. Intuitive-projective	4 to 6 years	A combination of images and beliefs given by trusted others, mixed with the child's own experience and imagination
2. Mythic-literal	7 to 12 years	Private world of fantasy and wonder; symbols refer to something specific; dramatic stories and myths used to communicate spiritual meanings
3. Synthetic-conventional	Adolescent or adult	World and ultimate environment structured by the expectations and judgments of others; interpersonal focus
4. Individuating-reflexive	After 18 years	Constructing one's own explicit system; high degree of self-consciousness
5. Paradoxical-consolidative	After 30 years	Awareness of truth from a variety of viewpoints
6. Universalizing	Maybe never	Becoming an incarnation of the principles of love and justice

Note: From *Life Maps: Conversations in the Journey of Faith*, by J. Fowler and S. Keen, 1985, Waco, TX: Word Books; and *How to Help Your Child Have a Spiritual Life: A Parents' Guide to Inner Development*, by A. Hollander, 1980, New York: A and W Publishers. Adapted with permission.

Fowler's theory and developmental stages were influenced by the work of Piaget, Kohlberg, and Erikson. Fowler believes that the development of faith is an interactive process between the person and the environment. In each of Fowler's stages, new patterns of thought, values, and beliefs are added to those already held by the individual; therefore the stages must follow in sequence. Faith stages, according to Fowler, are separate from the cognitive stages of Piaget: They evolve from a combination of knowledge and values.

Westerhoff

Westerhoff describes faith as a way of being and behaving that evolves from an experienced faith guided by parents and others during a person's infancy and childhood to an owned faith that is internalized in adulthood and serves as a directive for personal action (see Table 21–8). For the client who is ill, faith—whether in a higher authority (e.g., God, Allah, Jehovah), in the client's own self, in the health care team, or in a combination of all—provides strength and trust.

TABLE 21–8   Westerhoff's Four Stages of Faith

Stage	Age	Behavior
Experienced faith	Infancy/early adolescence	Experiences faith through interaction with others who are living a particular faith tradition.
Affiliative faith	Late adolescence	Actively participates in activities that characterize a particular faith tradition; experiences awe and wonderment; feels a sense of belonging.
Searching faith	Young adulthood	Through a process of questioning and doubting own faith, acquires a cognitive as well as an affective faith.
Owned faith	Middle adulthood/old age	Puts faith into personal and social action and is willing to stand up for what the individual believes even against the nurturing community.

Note: From *Will Our Children Have Faith?* (pp. 79–103), by J. Westerhoff, 1976, New York: Seabury Press. Adapted with permission.

APPLYING GROWTH AND DEVELOPMENT CONCEPTS TO NURSING PRACTICE

Different theories explain one or more aspects of an individual's growth and development. Typically, theorists examine only one aspect of an individual's development, such as the cognitive, moral, or physical aspects. The area chosen for examination usually reflects the researcher's academic discipline and personal interest. The theorists may also limit the population that is studied to a particular part of the life span, such as infancy, childhood, or adulthood.

Although such theories can be useful, they have limitations. First, the theory chosen may explain only one aspect of the growth and development process. Yet a person does not develop in fragmented sections but rather as a whole human being. Thus the nurse may find it necessary to apply several theories for an adequate understanding of the growth and development of a client.

Another limitation of some theories is the suggestion that certain tasks are performed at a specific age. In most cases, the child

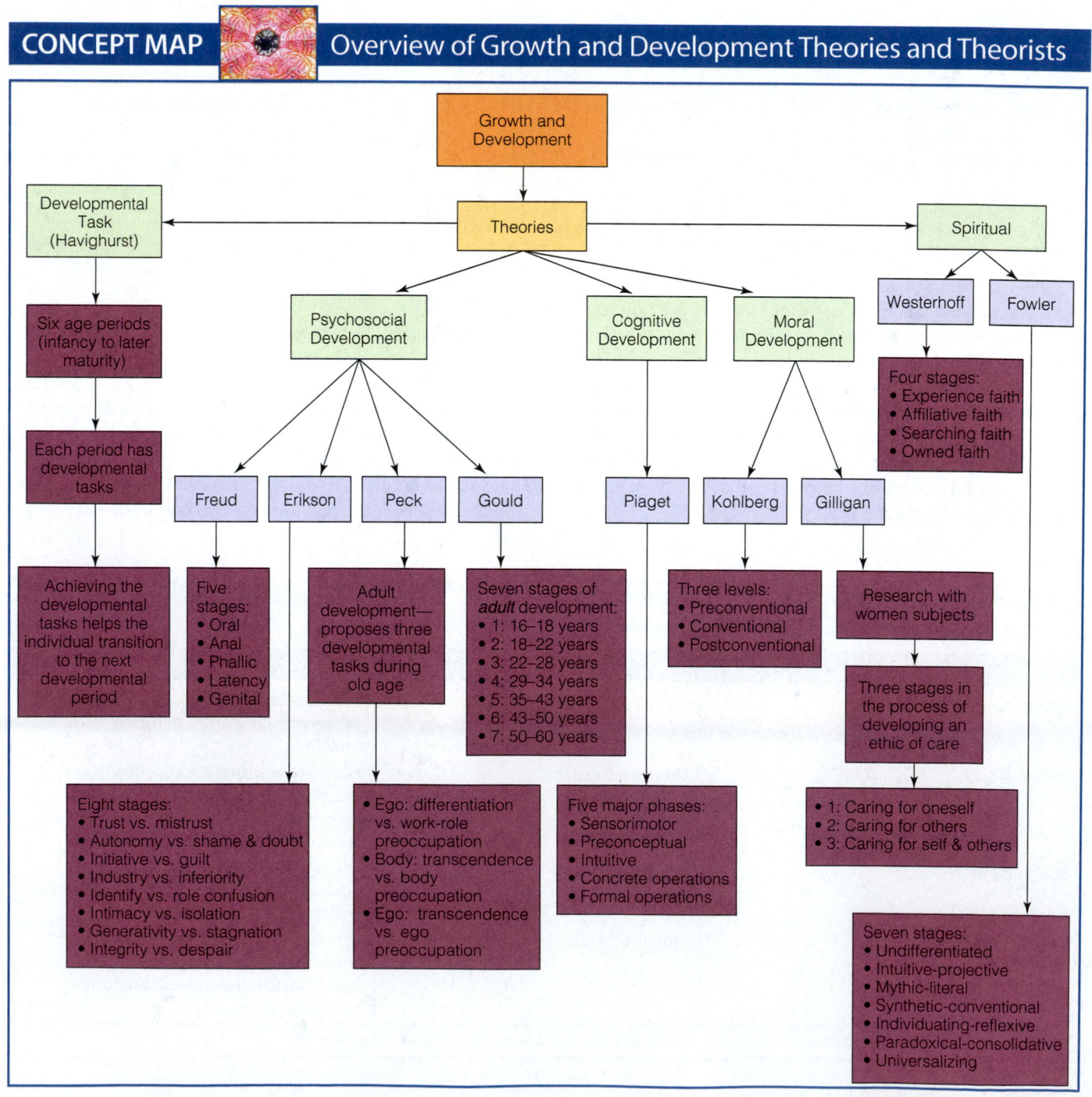

CONCEPT MAP — Overview of Growth and Development Theories and Theorists

or adult does accomplish the task at the time specified by the guidelines. In other cases, however, the nurse may find that an individual does not accomplish the task or meet the milestone at the exact time suggested by the theory. Such individual differences are not easily defined or categorized by a single theory. Human development is a complex synthesis of physiologic, cognitive, psychologic, moral, and spiritual development. Nurses should expect individual variations and take these into consideration when applying these theories about growth and development. In so doing, they will be better able to understand a client's development and plan effective nursing interventions.

In nursing, developmental theories can be useful in guiding assessment, explaining behavior, and providing a direction for nursing interventions. An understanding of a child's intellectual ability helps a nurse to anticipate and explain certain reactions, responses, and needs. Nurses can then encourage client behavior that is appropriate for that particular developmental stage.

Theories are also useful in planning a nursing intervention. For instance, choosing the appropriate toy for a 3-year-old boy requires some knowledge of the physical and cognitive development of the child, as well as a sensitivity for individual preferences.

In adult care, knowledge about the physical, cognitive, and psychologic aspects of the aging process is a fundamental aspect of administering sensitive nursing care. For example, nurses can use their familiarity with the theories of development to help clients understand and anticipate the psychosocial changes that take place after retirement or the physical limitations that come with old age.

Focus on Critical Thinking

Mr. Scott has brought his 2½-year-old son, Brandon, into your clinic for a routine physical. While waiting for the examination to begin, Brandon tries to jump off the exam table, play with the otoscope, and open all of the cupboards in the room. When asked to sit down, Brandon says "no" and runs away from his dad. He is, however, easily distracted with the toys brought from home. Mr. Scott asks, "What can I do to control him?"

1. According to Erikson, what stage of development is Brandon showing?
2. How could knowledge of Piaget's cognitive development direct your answers to Mr. Scott?
3. Using your knowledge of growth and development, what advice would you give Mr. Scott?

See Critical Thinking Possibilities in Appendix A.

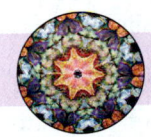

Chapter Review

Explore MediaLink

NCLEX review questions, case studies, care plan activities, MediaLink applications, and other interactive resources for this chapter can be found on the Companion Website at www.prenhall.com/kozier. Click on Chapter 21 to select the activities for this chapter. For more

NCLEX review questions, and an audio glossary, access the Student CD-ROM accompanying this textbook.

Chapter Highlights

- The terms *growth* and *development* represent independent, interrelated, and dynamic processes.
- Growth is physical change and increase in size. The pattern of physiologic growth is similar for all people.
- Development is an increase in the complexity of function and skill progression. It is the capacity and skill of the individual to adapt to the environment.
- Genetics and environment are the primary factors influencing growth and development.
- The rate of a person's growth and development is highly individual, but the sequence of growth and development is predictable.

- Components of growth and development are generally categorized as physiologic, psychosocial, cognitive, moral, and spiritual.
- Robert Havighurst believes that learning is basic to life and that people continue to learn throughout life. His theory describes six age periods with developmental tasks for each period.
- Psychosocial development refers to the development of personality. Psychosocial theorists include Freud, Erickson, Peck, and Gould.
- Cognitive development refers to the manner in which people learn to think, reason, and use language. The most widely known cognitive theorist is Piaget.

- Moral development, a complex process not fully understood, involves learning what ought to be and what ought not to be done. Kohlberg's theory focuses on the reasons an individual makes a decision.
- The spiritual component of growth and development refers to individuals' understanding of their relationship with the universe and their perceptions about the direction and meaning of life. Fowler and Westerhoff are two theorists who describe stages of spiritual development or faith.
- In nursing, developmental theories can be useful in guiding assessment, explaining behavior, and providing a direction for nursing interventions.

Review Questions

21–1. The parents of a 5-month-old infant asks you about the sequence and timing of developmental milestones. This is their second child. The older child is 3 years old. Using your knowledge of growth and development, your best answer would be
  a. "This infant should reach each milestone at exactly the same time as your older child."
  b. "Every child is different and your infant may reach each milestone in a different order than your older child did."
  c. "Although each child is different, the sequence of reaching each milestone should follow the same pattern but may be at a different rate."
  d. "Every child is different. There are no predictable patterns. Enjoy the uniqueness of each child."

21–2. The study of growth and development is exploration of the
  a. physical changes of the growing child.
  b. increasing complexity of function and skill progression of the growing child.
  c. environmental factors such as family, religion, and culture of the growing child.
  d. physical developments and the escalated sophistication of function and skill progression of the growing child.

21–3. Eleven-year-old Samantha is brought by her father for her yearly physical checkup. He expresses concern that she "seems all wrapped up in her soccer team and the friends that she has made and she doesn't have time for her family." Using your knowledge of Havighurst's developmental tasks, what would be your best response?
  a. "This seems to be unusual. Are there problems in your home that you are not telling me about?"

  b. "Although this is normal for 11-year-old girls, this transition can be difficult for families."
  c. "You need to become involved in her life and insist that she stay home with the family."
  d. "This is normal development and you are silly to worry about the time she is spending with her friends."

21–4. A review of which theorist would be helpful before teaching a preschool class of 4- to 5-year-olds about how to brush their teeth?
  a. Fowler
  b. Erikson
  c. Gould
  d. Peck

21–5. A 5-year-old boy is coming for his preadmission workup for surgery. When shown the IV pump that will be used, he becomes afraid that it "will bite me because I have been bad." Using your knowledge of Piaget, Erikson, and Fowler, your best action would be to
  a. reassure the child by letting him touch and explore the machine, and by explaining, in simple terms, how the IV pump works.
  b. understand that his imagination is out of control. Tell him that his fears are silly and that he needs to be a "big boy."
  c. recognize that he is too young to understand and that he needs to be quickly distracted.
  d. Reassure him that if he is a "good boy" the bad machine will not bite him. This action acknowledges his need for fantasy.

Readings and References

Suggested Readings

Paludi, M. A. (2002). *Human development in multicultural contexts. A book of readings.* Upper Saddle River, NJ: Prentice Hall.
  The author focuses on the ways in which culture influences development. Each chapter includes two parts. The first is an overview of cultural influences for the specific life stages from infancy to adulthood. The other part consists of readings that present specific multicultural studies pertaining to the specific stage of development.

Related Research

Abide, M. M., Richards, H. C., & Ramsay, S. G. (2001). Moral reasoning and consistency of belief and behavior: Decisions about substance abuse. *Journal of Drug Education, 31*(4), 367–384.

Alaimo, K., Olson, C. M., & Frongillo, E. A. (2001). Food insufficiency and American school-aged children's cognitive, academic, and psychosocial development. *Pediatrics, 108*(1), 44–51.

Paris, R., & Bradley, C. L. (2001). The challenge of adversity: Three narratives of alcohol de-

pendence, recovery, and adult development. *Qualitative Health Research, 11*(5), 647–667.

Wink, P., & Dillon, M. (2002). Spiritual development across the adult life course: Findings from a longitudinal study. *Journal of Adult Development, 9*(1), 79–94.

References

Belknap, R. A. (2002). Sense of self: Voices of separation and connection in women who have experienced abuse. *Canadian Journal of Nursing Research, 33*(4), 139–153.

Erikson, E. H. (1963). *Childhood and society* (2nd ed.). New York: Norton.

Erikson, E. H. (1964). *Insight and responsibility: Lectures on the ethical implications of psychoanalytic insight.* New York: Norton.

Fowler, J., & Keen, S. (1985). *Life maps: Conversations in the journey of faith.* Waco, TX: Word Books.

Gilligan, C. (1982). *In a different voice: Psychological theory and women's development.* Cambridge, MA: Harvard University Press.

Gould, R. L. (1972). The phases of adult life: A study in developmental psychology. *American Journal of Psychiatry, 129,* 33–43.

Green, M., & Piel, J. A. (2002). *Theories of human development. A comparative approach.* Boston: Allyn & Bacon.

Havighurst, R. J. (1972). *Developmental tasks and education* (3rd ed.). New York: Longman Publishers.

Hollander, A. (1980). *How to help your child have a spiritual life: A parent's guide to inner development.* New York: A and W publishers.

Murray, R. B., & Zentner, J. P. (2001). *Health promotion strategies through the life span* (7th ed.). Upper Saddle River, NJ: Prentice Hall.

Peck, R. (1968). Psychological developments in the second half of life. In B. L. Neugarten (Ed.), *Middle age and aging.* Chicago: University of Chicago Press.

Piaget, J. (1966). *Origins of intelligence in children.* New York: Norton.

Thomas, R. M. (2001). *Recent theories of human development.* Thousand Oaks, CA: Sage Publications.

Westerhoff, J. (1976). *Will our children have faith?* New York: Seabury Press.

Selected Bibliography

Armstrong, T. D., & Crowther, M. R. (2002). Spirituality among older African Americans. *Journal of Adult Development, 9*(1), 3–12.

Erikson, E. H. (1985). *The life cycle completed: A review.* New York: Norton.

Fowler, J. W. (1982). Stages of faith. San Francisco: Harper Collins.

Freud, S. (1923). *The ego and the id.* London: Hogarth Press.

Freud, S. (1961). *The ego and the id and other works* (Vol. 19). Strachey, J., translator. London: Hogarth Press and the Institute of Psychoanalysis.

Mitchell, K. (2002). Women's morality: A test of Carol Gilligan's theory. *Journal of Social Distress and the Homeless, 11*(1), 81–110.

Polan, E., & Taylor, D. (2003). *Journey across the life span. Human development and health promotion* (2nd ed.). Philadelphia: F. A. Davis.

Stuart-Hamilton, I. (2000). *The psychology of ageing. An introduction* (3rd ed.). London and Philadelphia: Jessica Kingsley Publishers.

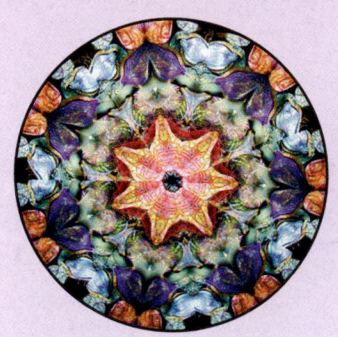

CHAPTER | 22

PROMOTING HEALTH FROM CONCEPTION THROUGH ADOLESCENCE

LEARNING OUTCOMES

After completing this chapter, you will be able to:

- Identify tasks characteristic of different stages of development from infancy through adolescence.

- Describe usual physical development from infancy through adolescence.

- Trace psychosocial development according to Erikson from infancy through adolescence.

- Explain cognitive development according to Piaget from infancy through adolescence.

- Describe moral development according to Kohlberg from childhood through adolescence.

- Describe spiritual development according to Fowler throughout childhood and adolescence.

- Identify assessment activities and expected characteristics from birth through late childhood.

- Identify essential activities of health promotion and protection to meet the needs of infants, toddlers, preschoolers, school-age children, and adolescents.

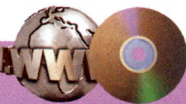

MediaLink

www.prenhall.com/kozier

Additional resources for this chapter can be found on the Student CD-ROM accompanying this textbook, and on the Companion Website at www.prenhall.com/kozier. Click on Chapter 22 to select the activities for this chapter.

CD-ROM
- Audio Glossary
- NCLEX Review
- Animations:
    Oogenesis
    Cell Division
    Conception
    Embryonic Heart Formation
      and Circulation
    Formation of Placenta
    Sperm Production

Companion Website
- Additional NCLEX Review
- Case Study: Motor and Social
    Development in Infancy
- Care Plan Activity: Teen with Lymphocytic
    Leukemia Care Plan Activity
- MediaLink Application: Safety Tips for
    Children
- Links to Resources

A knowledge of growth and development is essential for nurses if they are to identify developmental needs and problems. This chapter applies the concepts of growth and development introduced in Chapter 21 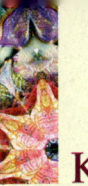 to the prenatal period and to the neonate, infant, toddler, preschooler, school-age child, and adolescent. Each developmental stage includes physical, psychosocial, cognitive, moral, and spiritual aspects. Health assessment and promotion of health and wellness are emphasized.

CONCEPTION AND PRENATAL DEVELOPMENT

Prenatal or intrauterine development lasts approximately 9 calendar months (10 lunar months) or 38 to 40 weeks, depending on the method of calculation. (A lunar month is 28 days.) If the time is calculated from the day of conception, this stage of life is 38 weeks or 9½ lunar months. If the time is calculated from the first day of the last menstrual period, its average length is 10 lunar months or 40 weeks.

Traditionally, pregnancy has been divided into three periods called **trimesters,** each of which lasts about 3 months. Each trimester includes certain landmarks for developmental changes in the mother and the fetus. The two phases of intrauterine life can also be considered in trimestral terms. The embryonic phase is the first trimester, and the fetal phase includes the second and third trimesters.

The **embryonic phase** is the period during which the fertilized ovum develops into an organism with most of the features of the human. This period is considered to encompass the first 8 weeks of pregnancy.

Within the first 3 weeks of life, the embryo tissues differentiate into three layers—the **ectoderm** (outer layer), **mesoderm** (middle layer), and **endoderm** or **entoderm** (inner layer). The ectoderm and endoderm are formed in the second week; the mesoderm forms in the third week. From the beginning of the third week through the eighth week after conception, these layers form the basic structure of all of the body's complex organs and systems. For example, the ectoderm forms the brain and spinal cord, the mesoderm forms the heart, and the endoderm forms the bladder and urethra (Pillitteri, 2003).

Three other events occur concurrently during the first 3 weeks:

1. The embryo is implanted in the endometrium of the uterus.
2. The fetal membranes differentiate into the chorion, precursor to the placenta and the amnion, precursor to the amniotic sac.
3. Placental function starts. The **placenta** is a flat, disc-shaped organ and is highly vascular. It normally forms in the upper segment of the endometrium of the uterus. Its functions are to exchange nutrients and gases between the embryo or fetus and the mother.

The **fetal phase** of development is characterized by a period of rapid growth in the size of the fetus. Both genetic and environmental factors affect its growth.

At the end of the second trimester, or 6 lunar months, the fetus resembles a small baby. Because very little fat is present beneath the skin, the skin appears wrinkled, red, and transparent. Underlying vessels are visible. A protective covering called **vernix caseosa** begins to develop over the skin. This is a white, cheeselike substance that adheres to the skin and can become one-eighth inch thick by birth. **Lanugo,** a fine downy hair, also covers the body. At about 5 months, the mother first perceives movement by the fetus, and the first fetal heartbeat may be heard.

At the end of the third trimester (9½ lunar months), the fetus has developed to approximately 50 cm (20 in.) and 3.2 to 3.4 kg (7.0 to 7.5 lb). The lanugo has disappeared, and the skin is a more normal color and appears less wrinkled. More subcutaneous fat makes the baby look more rotund; the last 2 months *in utero* are largely devoted to accumulating weight. Box 22–1 lists maternal factors that can lead to a higher risk of a low-birth-weight baby.

Health Promotion

During the intrauterine stage of development, the embryo or fetus relies on the maternal blood flow through the placenta to meet its basic survival needs. The health of the mother is essential for proper growth and development.

MediaLink | OOGENESIS AND CELL DIVISION ANIMATIONS

BOX 22–1 ■ Maternal Factors that Contribute to a Higher Risk of Low-Birth-Weight Babies

- Underweight before pregnancy
- Less than 21 pounds gained during pregnancy
- Inadequate prenatal care
- Age of 16 years or younger or 35 years or older
- Low socioeconomic level
- Poor nutrition during pregnancy

- Smoking cigarettes during pregnancy
- Use of addictive drugs or alcohol during pregnancy
- History of abortion
- Complications during pregnancy, poor health status, exposure to infections
- High stress levels, including physical or emotional abuse

Note: From Health Promotion Strategies Through the Life Span, 7th ed. (p. 309), by R. B. Murray and J. P. Zentner, 2001. Reprinted by permission.

MediaLink | CONCEPTION ANIMATION

Oxygen

To meet the fetal demands for oxygen, the pregnant mother gradually increases her normal blood flow by about one-third, peaking at about 8 months; increases her respiratory rate by about 40%; and increases her cardiac output significantly. Initially the heart of the embryo lies outside its body, but it is repositioned in the chest early in the second trimester. Fetal circulation travels from the placenta through two umbilical arteries, which carry blood depleted of oxygen away from the fetus. By 20 weeks the fetal heartbeat is audible through a fetoscope; the heartbeat is audible as early as the 10th week if a Doppler stethoscope with ultrasound is used.

Nutrition and Fluids

The fetus obtains nourishment from the placental circulation and by swallowing amniotic fluid. Nutritional needs are met when the mother eats a well-balanced diet containing sufficient calories to meet both her needs and those of the fetus.

Adequate folic acid, one of the B vitamins, is important in order to prevent neural tube defects (e.g., spina bifida) in the fetus. One of the objectives of *Healthy People 2010* is to increase the proportion of pregnancies begun with an optimum folic acid level (USDHHS, 2000). The neural tube defect occurs in the first few weeks of fetal development. As a result, it is recommended that all women capable of becoming pregnant consume 400 micrograms of folic acid daily. The nurse can teach the client about folic-rich foods (e.g., green leafy vegetables, oranges, dried beans) and suggest she take a vitamin supplement that contains folic acid.

Rest and Activity

The fetus sleeps most of the time but does develop a pattern of sleep and wakefulness that can persist after birth. Fetal activity can be felt by the mother at about the fifth lunar month of pregnancy.

Elimination

Fetal feces are formed in the intestines from swallowed amniotic fluid throughout pregnancy, but are normally not excreted until after birth. Inadequate oxygenation of the fetus during the third trimester can result in relaxation of the anal sphincter and passage of feces into the amniotic fluid. Urine normally is excreted into the amniotic fluid when the kidneys mature (16 to 20 weeks).

Temperature Maintenance

Although amniotic fluid provides a constant temperature for the fetus, significant changes in maternal temperature can alter the temperature of the amniotic fluid and the fetus. Significant temperature increases due to illness, hot whirlpool baths, or saunas may result in birth defects.

Safety

As stated earlier, the body systems form during the embryonic period. As a result, the embryo is particularly vulnerable to damage from a **teratogen,** which is anything that adversely affects normal cellular development in the embryo or fetus (Venes, 2001). It is important for the nurse to inquire about possible pregnancy when giving medications that are known teratogens and to also ask when the woman is scheduled for tests that involve radiography (x-ray).

Smoking and alcohol can impact the environment for the fetus. According to Buchanan (2002), "smoking during pregnancy is considered a cause of low birth weight" and has also been "linked to still births, sudden infant death syndrome, cleft palates, and cleft lips" (p. 245). Curet and Hsi (2002) report that "perinatal alcohol exposure increases the risk of low birth weight, developmental and behavioral abnormalities, spontaneous abortion, and stillbirth" (p. 74).

NEONATES AND INFANTS (BIRTH TO 1 YEAR)

Babies are considered neonates from birth to the end of the first month. Infants are babies from 1 month of age to 1 year.

Physical Development

An infant's basic task is survival, which requires breathing, sleeping, sucking, eating, swallowing, digesting, and eliminating. Because many of the infant's activities and pleasures are mouth centered, this stage in development is often referred to as Freud's oral stage. Infants undergo significant physiologic change in these areas: weight, length, head growth, vision, and motor development.

Weight

At birth, most babies weigh from 2.7 to 3.8 kg (6.0 to 8.5 lb). Just after birth, most infants lose 5% to 10% of their birth weight because of fluid loss. This weight loss is normal, and infants usually regain that weight in about 1 week. After several days babies usually gain weight at the rate of 150 to 210 g (5 to 7 ounces) weekly for 6 months. By 5 months of age infants usually reach twice their birth weight, and by age 12 months, three times their birth weight.

Length

The average length of a European American newborn in the United States is about 50 cm (20 in.). Female babies on the average are smaller than male babies.

Two recumbent lengths are the crown-to-rump length (the sitting length) and the head-to-heel length (from the top of the head to the base of the heels). See Figure 22–1■. Normally the crown-to-rump length is approximately the same as the head circumference. By 6 months infants gain another 13.75 cm (5.5 in.) of height. By 12 months they add another 7.5 cm (3 in.). The rate of increase in height is largely influenced by the baby's size at birth and by nutrition.

Head and Chest Circumference

Assessment of head circumference is of particular importance in infants and children to determine the growth rate of the skull and the brain. An infant's head should be measured at every visit to the physician or nurse until the child is 2 years old (see Figure 22–2 ■). Normal head circumference (**normocephaly**) is often related to chest circumference. At birth the average infant's head circumference is 35 cm (14 in.) and generally varies only 1 or 2 cm (0.5 in.). The chest circumference of the newborn is usually less than the head circumference by about 2.5 cm (1 in.). As the infant grows, the chest circumference becomes larger than the head circumference. At about 9 or 10 months the head and chest circumferences are about the same, and after 1 year of age the chest circumference is larger.

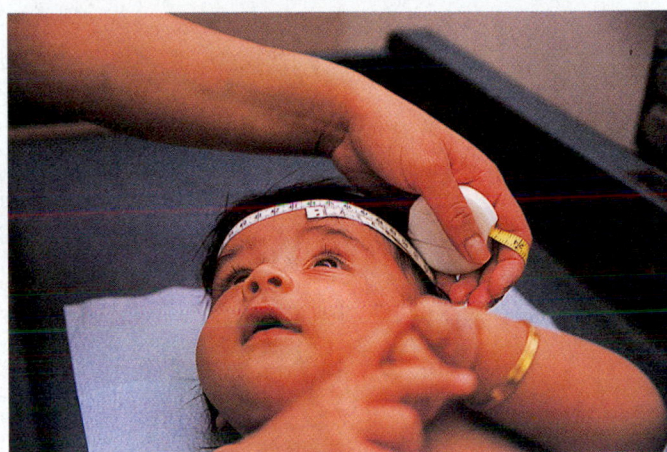

Figure 22–2 ■ An infant's head circumference is measured around the skull, above the eyebrows.

Head Molding

The heads of many newborn babies are misshapen because of the molding of the head that occurs during vaginal deliveries. Molding of the head is made possible by **fontanelles** (unossified membranous gaps) in the bone structure of the skull and by overriding of the **sutures** (junction lines of the skull bones). Within a week, a newborn's head usually regains its symmetry, a fact that reassures parents. The larger anterior fontanelle (4 to 6 cm in diameter and diamond shaped) can increase in size for several months after birth. After 6 months the size gradually decreases until closure occurs between 9 and 18 months. The posterior fontanelle between the parietal bones and the occipital bone closes between 2 and 33 months after birth (see Figure 22–3 ■).

Vision

The newborn can follow large moving objects and blinks in response to bright light and to sound. The pupils of the newborn respond slowly, and the eyes cannot focus on close objects. At 4 months the infant can recognize familiar objects and follow moving ones. By 6 months the infant can perceive colors. After 9 months most can recognize facial characteristics and often smile in response to a familiar face. By 12 months depth perception has developed, and the infant will be able to recognize where a change in level occurs, such as at the edge of the bed.

Hearing

Newborns with intact hearing will react with a startle to a loud noise, a reaction called the *Moro reflex*. Within a few days, they are able to distinguish different sounds. For example, they can tell the difference between their mother's voice and that of another woman. At about 5 months of age, the infant will pause while sucking in order to listen to the mother's voice. A 9-month-old infant is able to locate the source of sounds and recognizes familiar ones. By 1 year, the infant listens to sounds, begins to distinguish words, and responds to simple commands.

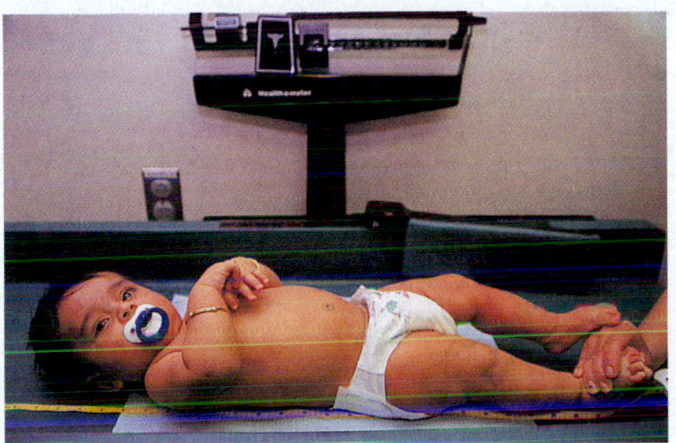

Figure 22–1 ■ Measuring an infant head to heel, from the top of the head to the base of the heels.

MediaLink | EMBRYONIC HEART FORMATION AND CIRCULATION ANIMATION

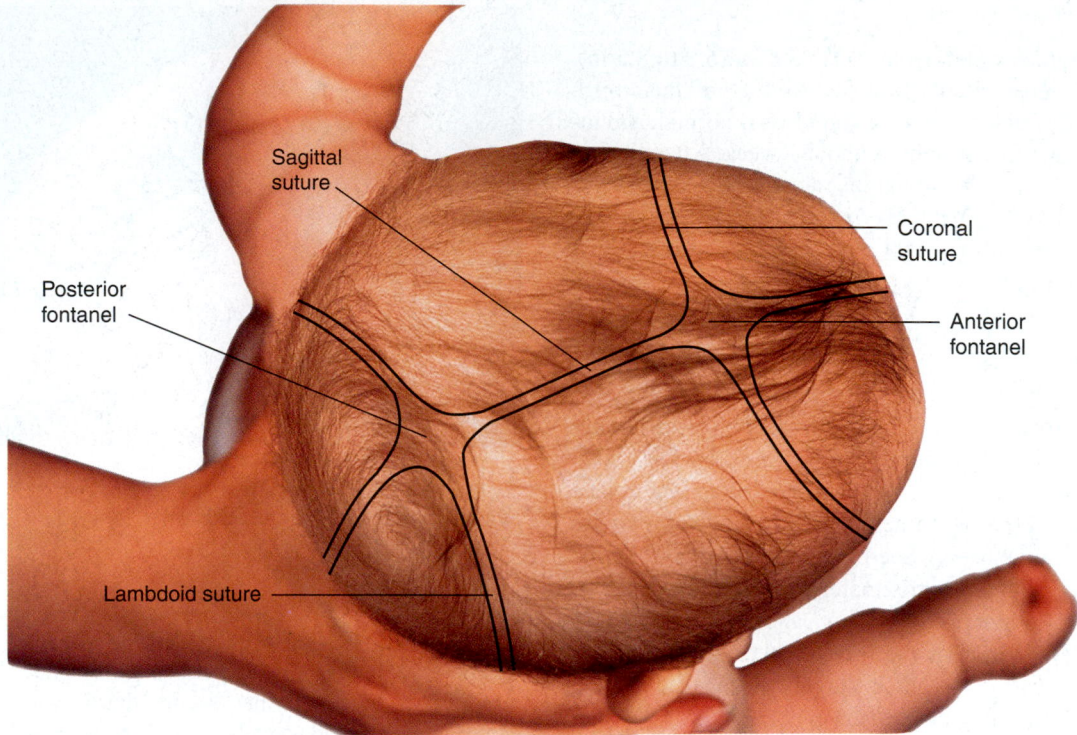

Figure 22–3 ■ The bones of the skull, showing the fontanelles and suture lines.

Smell and Taste

The senses of smell and taste are functional shortly after birth. Newborns prefer sweet tastes and tend to decrease their sucking in response to liquids with a salty content. They are able to recognize the smell of their mother's milk and respond to this smell by turning toward the mother.

Touch

The sense of touch is well developed at birth. Skin-to-skin touching is important for an infant's development. The infant responds positively to the warmth, love, and security it perceives when touched, held, and cuddled. The newborn is also sensitive to temperature extremes and pain; however, babies react diffusely and cannot isolate the discomfort. The pain of an open safety pin in the buttock, for example, is not isolated in the buttock.

Reflexes

The reflexes of the newborn are unconscious, involuntary responses. They are neither learned nor consciously carried out; rather, they are nervous system responses to a number of stimuli. Reflexes normally present at birth are the rooting, sucking, Moro, palmar grasp, plantar, tonic neck, stepping, and Babinski reflexes (see Box 22–2). Infant reflexes disappear during the

---

BOX 22–2   ■ Infant Reflexes

- *Sucking reflex:* A feeding reflex that occurs when the infant's lips are touched. The reflex persists throughout infancy.
- *Rooting reflex:* A feeding reflex elicited by touching the baby's cheek, causing the baby's head to turn to the side that was touched. This reflex usually disappears after 4 months.
- *Moro reflex:* Often assessed to estimate the maturity of the central nervous system. A loud noise, a sudden change in position, or an abrupt jarring of the crib elicits this reflex. The infant reacts by extending both arms and legs outward with the fingers spread, then suddenly retracting the limbs. Often the infant cries at the same time. This reflex disappears after 4 months.
- *Palmar grasp reflex:* Occurs when a small object is placed against the palm of the hand, causing the fingers to curl around it. This reflex disappears after 3 months.

- *Plantar reflex:* Similar to the palmar grasp reflex; an object placed just beneath the toes causes them to curl around it. This reflex disappears after 8 months.
- *Tonic neck reflex (TNR) or fencing reflex:* A postural reflex. When a baby who is lying on its back turns its head to the right side, for example, the left side of the body shows a flexing of the left arm and the left leg. This reflex disappears after 4 months.
- *Stepping reflex (walking or dancing reflex):* Can be elicited by holding the baby upright so that the feet touch a flat surface. The legs then move up and down as if the baby were walking. This reflex usually disappears at about 2 months.
- *Babinski reflex:* When the sole of the foot is stroked, the big toe rises and the other toes fan out. A newborn baby has a positive Babinski. After age 1, the infant exhibits a negative Babinski; that is, the toes curl downward. A positive Babinski after age 1 indicates brain damage.

first year of life. In addition, the abilities to yawn, stretch, sneeze, burp, and hiccup are all present at birth.

Motor Development

Motor development is the development of the baby's abilities to move and to control the body. Initially, body movement is uncoordinated. At 1 month of age the infant lifts the head momentarily when prone, turns the head when prone, and has a head lag when pulled to a sitting position. After 6 months they can sit without support (see Figure 22–4 ■). At 9 months they can reach, grasp a rattle, and transfer it from hand to hand. At 12 months they can turn the pages of a book, put objects into a container, walk with some assistance, and help to dress themselves.

Psychosocial Development

According to Erikson (1963), the central crisis at this stage is trust versus mistrust. Resolution of this stage determines how the person approaches subsequent developmental stages. During the first year of life, infants depend on the parents for all their physiologic and psychologic needs. Fulfillment of these needs is required for the infant to develop a basic sense of trust. Parents can enhance this sense of trust by (a) responding consistently to an infant's needs, (b) providing a predictable environment in which routines are established, and (c) being sensitive to the infant's needs and meeting these needs skillfully and promptly. Mothering or nurturing behavior, such as consistent care, handling, stroking, and cuddling, is essential for healthy psychosocial development. By 8 months, most infants exhibit attachment to their parents and may show displeasure when left with strangers.

The newborn reacts socially to caregivers by paying attention to the face or voice and by cuddling when held. It is able to interact with the environment by responding to various stimuli such as touch and sound. Table 22–1 provides examples of motor and social development.

Infants have no understanding of waiting and no time frame by which to measure waiting. The initial reaction of an infant to stress is crying, and crying is the infant's way of communicating stress. Infants learn gradually to tolerate stress. According to Freud, infants have an oral focus, and they reduce

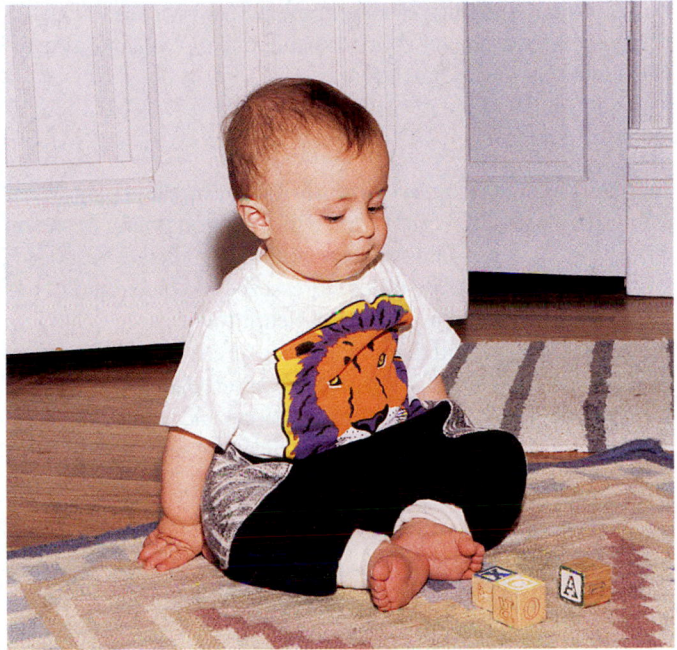

Figure 22–4 ■ An infant sits without support at 6 months of age.

tension by sucking and mouthing objects. Nurses and parents can also reduce the stress of an infant by maintaining the infant's routine as much as possible and limiting the number of strangers interacting with the infant.

Cognitive Development

According to Piaget (1966), cognitive development is a result of interaction between an individual and the environment. Piaget refers to the initial period of cognitive development as the sensorimotor phase. This phase has six stages, three of which take place during the first year. From 4 to 8 months infants begin to have perceptual recognition. By 6 months they respond to new stimuli, and they remember certain objects and look for them for a short time. By 12 months infants have a concept of both space and time. They experiment to reach a goal, such as a toy on a chair.

TABLE 22–1 Examples of Motor and Social Development in Infancy

Age	Motor Development	Social Development
Newborn	Turns head from side to side when in a prone position. Grasps by reflex when object is placed in palm of hand.	Displays displeasure by crying and satisfaction by soft vocalizations. Attends to adult face and voice by eye contact and quieting.
6 months	Lifts chest and shoulders off table when prone, bearing weight on hands. Manipulates small objects.	Starts to imitate sounds. Vocalizes one-syllable sounds: "ma ma," "da da."
9 months	Creeps and crawls. Uses pincer grasp with thumb and forefinger.	Complies with simple verbal commands. Displays fear of being left alone (e.g., going to bed). Waves "bye-bye."
12 months	Walks alone with help. Uses spoon to feed self.	Clings to mother in unfamiliar situations. Demonstrates emotions such as anger and affection.

An infant's cognitive development also proceeds from reflexive ability of the newborn to using one or two actions to attain a goal by the age of 1 year.

Moral Development

Infants associate right and wrong with pleasure and pain. What gives them pleasure is right, since they are too young to reason otherwise. When infants receive abundant positive responses from the parent such as smiles, caresses, and voice tones of approval in these early months, they learn that certain behaviors are wrong or good and that pain or pleasure is the consequence. In later months and years, children can tell easily and quickly by changes in parental facial expressions and voice tones that their behavior is either approved or disapproved.

Health Problems

A number of health problems of neonates and infants require interventions from health care personnel. Safety concerns are of particular importance.

Failure to Thrive

Failure to thrive is a unique syndrome in which an infant falls below the fifth percentile for weight and height on a standard growth chart or is falling in percentiles on a growth chart (Pillitteri, 2003, p. 1700). The two categories for this syndrome are organic causes (e.g., cardiac disease) and inorganic causes, which usually involves the parent–child relationship. Infants deprived of mothering, especially from months 3 to 15, will not learn to form significant relationships or to trust others. Touch, cuddling, and visual and auditory stimulation are all critical for the infant. It is through these mechanisms that the baby comes to know self and the environment. Infants who fail to establish a loving, responsive relationship with a caregiver often fail to develop normally. Infants with inorganic failure to thrive show delayed development without any physical cause. They are often malnourished and fail to gain weight and grow normally.

Infant Colic

Colic is acute abdominal pain caused by periodic contractions of the intestines. It occurs in infants under 3 months of age and for most infants disappears at 3 months of age (Pillitteri, 2003). Although the direct cause is not known, factors such as swallowing air, feeding too rapidly, allergies, taking excessive amounts of carbohydrates, infant emotional distress, and anxiety of the caregiver may be associated with colic.

To help relieve the colic, the nurse can assess the infant during feeding and suggest possible changes. Suggestions may include changing the formula or nipple, increasing the burping frequency, cuddling the infant, and finding the position that provides the infant with the most comfort.

Crying

Crying is often of great concern. When an infant's crying lasts up to 10 to 12 hours a day it is described as colicky (see the pre-

ceding section). A crying or fussy period lasting 1 to 2 hours a day is usually considered normal for infants.

Child Abuse

Reports of child abuse have increased in recent years. It can take various forms including physical abuse, physical neglect, sexual abuse, and emotional abuse and neglect. **Shaken baby syndrome (SBS)** is violent shaking of the infant by the arms or shoulders causing a whiplash, which can lead to severe injury in infants. Cerebral damage, subdural hematoma, neurologic defects, blindness, and spinal cord damage can result. These injuries often occur without external evidence of head injury. Subdural and retinal hemorrhages accompanied by the absence of external signs of trauma are hallmarks of the syndrome. Nurses should teach parents about the dangers in shaking infants.

Sudden Infant Death Syndrome

The sudden and unexpected death of an infant may be a case of **sudden infant death syndrome (SIDS)**. A postmortem examination usually fails to reveal a cause. The highest incidence of SIDS occurs in the second to fourth month of life. *Healthy People 2010* includes an objective to increase the percentage of healthy full-term infants who are put down to sleep on their backs (USDHHS, 2000). Research has shown that sleeping on the side or back, not prone, greatly decreases the risk of SIDS. The back is preferred because the infant may roll onto its stomach from a side-lying position (see Figure 22–5 ■).

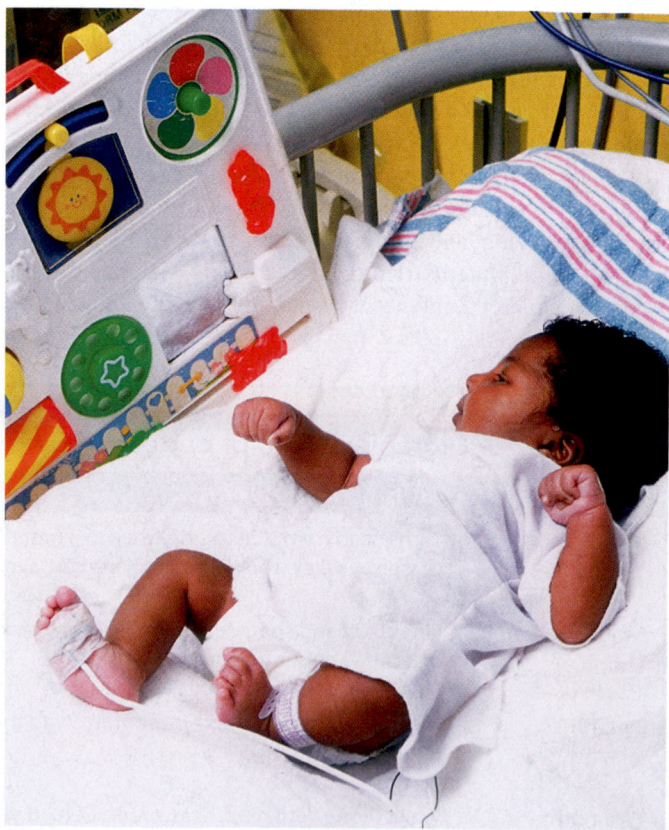

Figure 22–5 ■ Place infant on back for sleeping.

TABLE 22–2 Apgar Scoring System to Assess the Newborn

Sign	Score		
	0	1	2
1. Heart rate	Absent	Slow (below 100 per minute)	Above 100 per minute
2. Respirations	Absent	Slow, irregular	Regular rate, crying
3. Muscle tone	Flaccid	Some flexion of extremities	Active movements
4. Reflex irritability	None	Grimace	Cries
5. Color	Body pale or cyanotic	Body pink (for African American babies, pink mucous membranes), extremities blue	Body completely pink, pink mucous membranes in African American babies

Health Assessment and Promotion

Health assessment occurs immediately on birth and continues for the promotion of wellness.

Apgar Scoring

Newborn babies can be assessed immediately by the **Apgar scoring system.** This provides a numeric indicator of the baby's physiologic capacities to adapt to extrauterine life. Each of five signs is assigned a maximum score of 2, so that the maximum score achievable is 10. A score under 7 suggests that the baby is having difficulty, and a score under 4 indicates that the baby's condition is critical. Apgar scoring is usually carried out 60 seconds after birth and is repeated in 5 minutes. Those with very low scores require special resuscitative measures and care. See Table 22–2.

Developmental Screening Tests

Development can be assessed by observing the infant's behavior and by using standardized tests such as the **Denver Developmental Screening Test (DDST).** The DDST is used to screen children from birth to 6 years of age. The test is intended to estimate the abilities of a child compared to those of an average group of children of the same age. Four main areas of development are screened: personal-social, fine-motor adaptive, language, and gross motor.

Ongoing Nursing Assessments

During ongoing assessments, the nurse examines and observes the infant, taking into account variations that occur with developmental age and activity. For example, the pulse of the baby at birth is affected by the child's activity, rising up to 170 when the infant is crying and falling to as low as 70 during sleep.

In addition, the nurse actively listens to the caregiver for possible problems or areas of concern and reviews with the parent the expected behavior or characteristics for the particular age group. It is important for the caregiver to know that certain behaviors, responses, and activities of the infant are normal and expected. It is also important to discuss the many individual differences that can, quite normally, occur.

The assessment interview is also a time to be supportive of the parent's role, to assess the attachment of the mother to the infant, and to observe the interactions between the infant and parent. Assessment guidelines for the infant are shown in the Developmental Assessment Guidelines.

The first month of life is thought to be critical for physical adjustments to extrauterine life and for the psychosocial adjustment of the parents. From 1 month to 1 year infants experience rapid change, with advances in physical growth and psychosocial development. For a summary of health and wellness promotion, see Box 22–3.

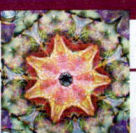

Developmental Assessment Guidelines

THE INFANT

In these five developmental areas, does the infant do the following?

Physical Development
- Demonstrate physical growth (weight, length, head and chest circumference) within the normal range.
- Manifest appropriately sized fontanelles for age.
- Exhibit vital signs within normal range for age.

Motor Development
- Perform gross and fine motor milestones within the normal range for age.
- Exhibit reflexes appropriate for age.

Sensory Development
- Follow a moving object within normal range for age.
- Respond to sounds, such as talking or clapping hands.

Psychosocial Development
- Interact appropriately with parent through body movements and vocalizations.

Development in Activities of Daily Living
- Eat and drink appropriate amounts of breast milk, formula, and/or solid foods.
- Exhibit an elimination pattern within normal range for age.
- Exhibit a rest and sleep pattern appropriate for age.

BOX 22–3 ■ Health Promotion Guidelines for Infants

Health Examinations
- At 2 weeks and at 2, 4, 6, and 12 months

Protective Measures
- Immunizations: diphtheria pertussis-tetanus (DPT), oral poliovirus vaccine (OPV), pneumococcal, measles-mumps-rubella (MMR), *Haemophilus influenzae* type B, hepatitis B, and varicella vaccines as recommended
- Fluoride supplements if there is inadequate water fluoridation (less than 0.7 part per million)
- Screening for tuberculosis
- Screening for phenylketonuria (PKU)
- Prompt attention for illnesses
- Appropriate skin hygiene and clothing

Infant Safety
- Importance of supervision
- Car seat, crib, playpen, bath, and home environment safety measures
- Feeding measures (e.g., avoid propping bottle)
- Providing toys with no small parts or sharp edges

Nutrition
- Breastfeeding and bottle-feeding techniques
- Formula preparation
- Feeding schedule
- Introduction of solid foods
- Need for iron supplements at 4 to 6 months

Elimination
- Characteristics and frequency of stool and urine elimination
- Diarrhea and its effects

Rest/Sleep
- Usual sleep and rest patterns

Sensory Stimulation
- Touch: holding, cuddling, rocking
- Vision: colorful, moving toys
- Hearing: soothing voice tones, music, singing
- Play: toys appropriate for development

TODDLERS (1 TO 3 YEARS)

Toddlers develop from having no voluntary control to being able to walk and speak. They also learn to control their bladder and bowels, and they acquire a wide variety of information about their environment.

Physical Development

Two-year-old children lose the baby look. Toddlers are usually chubby, with relatively short legs and a large head. The face appears small when compared to the skull, but as the toddler grows, the face seems to grow from under the skull and appears better proportioned. Toddlers have a pronounced lumbar lordosis and a protruding abdomen. The abdominal muscles develop gradually with growth, and the abdomen flattens.

Weight

Two-year-olds can be expected to weigh approximately four times their birth weight. The weight gain is about 2 kg (5 lb) between ages 1 and 2 years and about 1 to 2 kg (2 to 5 lb) between 2 and 3 years. The 3-year-old weighs about 13.6 kg (30 lb).

Height

A toddler's height can be measured as height or length. Height is measured while the toddler stands, and length is measured while the toddler is in a recumbent position. Although the measurements differ slightly, nurses must specify which measurement is used to avoid confusion. Between ages 1 and 2 years, the average growth in height is 10 to 12 cm (4 to 5 in.), and between 2 and 3 years it slows to 6 to 8 cm (2½ to 3½ in.).

Head Circumference

The head circumference of the toddler increases about 2.5 cm (1 in.) on average. By 24 months the head is 80% of the average adult size and the brain is 70% of its adult size.

Sensory Abilities

Visual acuity is fairly well established at 1 year; average estimates of acuity for the toddler are 20/70 at 18 months and 20/40 at 2 years of age. Accommodation to near and far objects is fairly well developed by 18 months and continues to mature with age. At 3 years of age, the toddler can look away from a toy prior to reaching out and picking it up. This ability requires the integration of visual and neuromuscular mechanisms.

The senses of hearing, taste, smell, and touch become increasingly developed and associated with each other. Hearing in the 3-year-old is at adult levels. The taste buds of the toddler are sensitive to the natural flavors of food, and the 3-year-old prefers familiar odors and tastes. Touch is a very important sense, and a distressed toddler is often soothed by tactile sensations.

Motor Abilities

Fine muscle coordination and gross motor skills improve during toddlerhood. At the age of 18 months babies can pick up raisins or cereal pieces and place them in a receptacle. They can also hold a spoon and a cup and can walk upstairs with assistance. They will probably crawl down the stairs.

At 2 years, toddlers can hold a spoon and put it into the mouth correctly. They are able to run, their gait is steady, and they can balance on one foot and ride a tricycle (Figure 22–6 ■). By 3 years most children are toilet trained, although they still may have the occasional accident when playing or during the night.

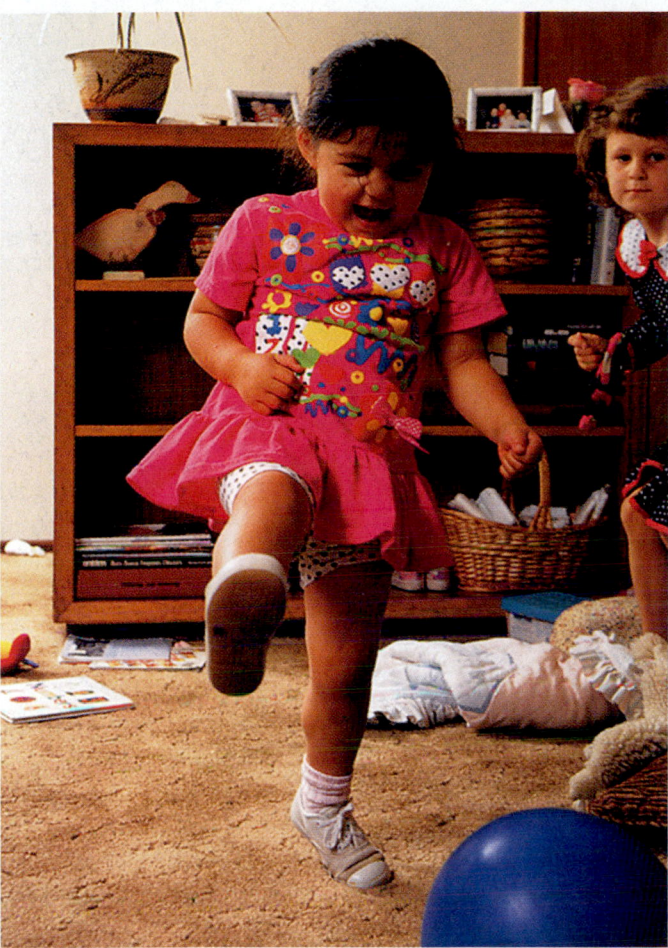

Figure 22–6 ■ A toddler has enough gross and fine motor ability to jump and kick a ball.

Psychosocial Development

According to Freud, the ages of 2 and 3 years represent the anal phase of development, when the rectum and anus are the specially significant areas of the body. Erikson sees the period from 18 months to 3 years as the time when the central developmental task is autonomy versus shame and doubt.

Toddlers begin to develop their sense of autonomy by asserting themselves with the frequent use of the word "no." They are often frustrated by restraints to their behavior and between ages 1 and 3 may have temper tantrums. However, they slowly gain control over their emotions, usually with the guidance of their caregivers. Parents need to have a great deal of patience coupled with an understanding of the importance of this developmental milestone. To be effective, caregivers need to give the child some measure of control and at the same time be consistent in setting limits so that the child learns the results of misbehavior. The nurse can also assist the parents and caregivers in promoting the toddler's development by suggesting the activities summarized in Box 22–4.

Self-concept is made up of body image development, feelings about self, adaptive and defensive mechanisms, reactions from others, and one's perceptions of these reactions, attitudes, values, and many of life's experiences (Murray & Zentner, 2001,

BOX 22–4 ■ Fostering the Toddler's Psychosocial Development

- Provide toys suitable for the toddler, including some toys challenging enough to motivate but not so difficult that the toddler will fail. (Failure will intensify feelings of self-doubt and shame.)
- Make positive suggestions rather than commands. Avoid an emotional climate of negativism, blame, and punishment.
- Give the toddler choices, all of which are safe; however, limit number to two or three.
- When toddler has a temper tantrum, make sure the child is safe, and then leave.
- Help the toddler to develop inner control by setting and enforcing consistent, reasonable limits.
- Praise the toddler's accomplishments.

p. 407). Children learn to develop a sense of self-concept through their immediate social environment, in which their parents play a significant role. If the children's social interactions with their parents are negative (e.g., constant disapproval regarding eating, toilet training, or other behavior), the children may begin to see themselves as bad. This perception is the basis of a negative self-concept. Parents need to give toddlers positive input so that they can develop a positive and healthy self-concept. With a healthy sense of self-esteem and security, the toddler is able to deal with periodic failures later in life without damage to self-esteem.

Although toddlers like to explore the environment, they always need to have a significant person nearby. Parents need to know that young children experience acute **separation anxiety,** the fear and frustration that come with parental absences. Abandonment is their greatest fear. At this age, the child may have difficulty accepting a baby-sitter or strongly resist being left by the parents at a day-care center. For example, toddlers may become highly anxious when separated from their parents and admitted to hospital. **Regression** or reverting to an earlier development stage may be indicated by bed-wetting or using baby talk. Nurses can assist parents by helping them understand that this behavior is normal and indicates that these toddlers are trying to establish their position in the family.

Experience with separation helps the child cope with parental absences. Children need room for exploration and interaction with other children and adults. At the same time, they need to know that the parental bond of a loving and close relationship remains secure.

Toddlers assert their independence by saying "no" or by dawdling. During the toddler stage, receptive and expressive language skills are developing quickly. Children can understand words and follow directions long before they can actually form them into sentences. By 1 year of age, toddlers can recognize their own names.

Cognitive Development

According to Piaget, the toddler completes the fifth and sixth stages of the sensorimotor phase and starts the preconceptual phase at about 2 years of age. In the fifth stage, the toddler solves problems by a trial-and-error process. By stage 6, toddlers can solve problems mentally. For example, when given a new toy the toddler will not immediately handle the toy to see how it works, but will instead look at it carefully to think about how it works.

During Piaget's preconceptual phase, toddlers develop considerable cognitive and intellectual skills. They learn about the sequence of time. They have some symbolic thought; for example, a chair may represent a place of safety, and a blanket may symbolize comfort. Concepts start to form in late toddlerhood. A concept develops when the child learns words to represent classes of objects or thoughts. An example of a concrete concept is *table,* representing a number of articles of furniture that are all different but all tables.

Moral Development

According to Kohlberg, the first level of moral development is the preconventional when children respond to punishment and reward. During the second year of life, children begin to know that some activities elicit affection and approval. They also recognize that certain rituals, such as repeating phrases from prayers, also elicit approval. This provides children with feelings of security. By 2 years of age, toddlers are learning what attitudes their parents hold about moral matters.

Spiritual Development

According to Fowler (1981), the toddler's stage of spiritual development is undifferentiated. Toddlers may be aware of some religious practices, but they are primarily involved in learning knowledge and emotional reactions rather than establishing spiritual beliefs. A toddler may repeat short prayers at bedtime, conforming to a ritual, because praise and affection result. This parental or caregiver response enhances the toddler's sense of security.

Health Problems

Toddlers experience significant health problems due to accidents, visual problems, dental caries, and respiratory and ear infections.

Accidents

Accidents are the leading cause of mortality of toddlers. They are curious and like to feel and taste everything. The most common causes of fatal injuries are automobile accidents, drowning, burns, poisoning, and falls. Parents or other caregivers need to take the appropriate preventive measures to guard against these health threats (Figure 22–7 ■).

Visual Problems

During this period, the toddler should be screened for amblyopia strabismus. **Amblyopia** (reduced visual acuity in one eye) is usually the result of strabismus. The child with amblyopia has straight eyes, whereas the child with **strabismus** (cross-eye) has a deviant eye.

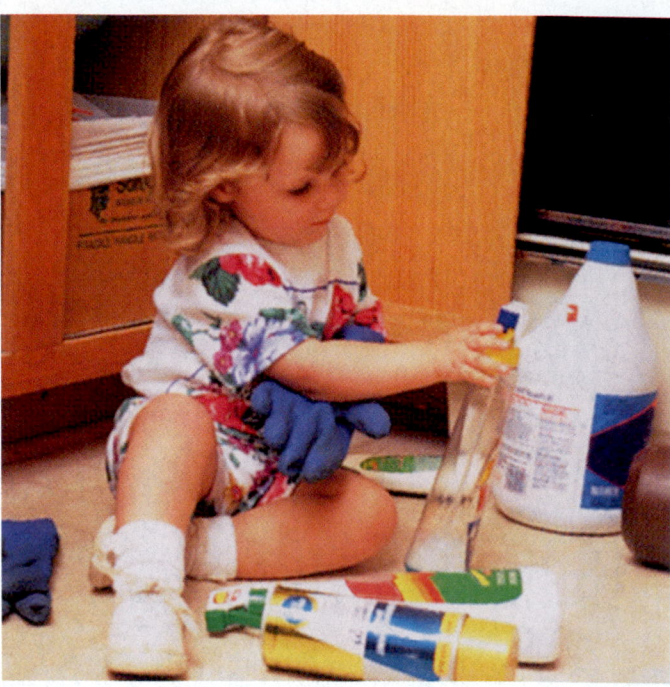

Figure 22–7 ■ Keep medicines and other poisonous materials locked away.

Dental Caries

Dental caries occur frequently during the toddler period, often as a result of the excessive intake of sweets or a prolonged use of the bottle during naps and at bedtime.

Respiratory Tract and Ear Infections

Respiratory and middle ear infections are common during toddlerhood.

Health Assessment and Promotion

Assessment activities for the toddler are similar to those for the infant in terms of measuring weight, length (height), and vital signs (see the Developmental Assessment Guidelines).

Promoting health and wellness includes such areas as accident prevention, toilet training, and good dental hygiene. For a summary of health promotion for toddlers, see Box 22–5.

PRESCHOOLERS (4 AND 5 YEARS)

During the preschool period physical growth slows, but control of the body and coordination increase greatly. Preschoolers' world gets larger as they meet relatives, friends, and neighbors.

Physical Development

By the time children are 4 or 5 years old, they appear taller and thinner than toddlers because children tend to grow more in height than in weight. The preschooler's brain almost reaches its adult size by 5 years. The extremities of the body grow more quickly than the body trunk, making the child's body appear

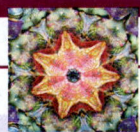

Developmental Assessment Guidelines

THE TODDLER

In these four developmental areas, does the toddler do the following?

Physical Development

- Demonstrate physical growth (weight, height, and head circumference) within normal range.
- Manifest vital signs within normal range for age.
- Exhibit vision and hearing abilities within normal range.

Motor Development

- Perform gross and fine motor milestones within the normal range for age. For example, by 3 years of age is the toddler able to do the following?
  - Walk up steps without assistance.
  - Balance on one foot, jump, and walk on toes.
  - Copy a circle.
  - Build a bridge from blocks.
  - Ride a tricycle.

Psychosocial Development

- Perform psychosocial developmental milestones for age. For example, by 3 years of age is the toddler able to do the following?
  - Express likes and dislikes.
  - Display curiosity and ask questions.
  - Accept separation from mother for short periods of time.
  - Begin to play and communicate with children and others outside the immediate family.
  - Understand words such as *up, down, cold,* and *hungry.*
  - Speak in sentences of three to four words.
  - Imitate religious rituals of the family.

Development in Activities of Daily Living

- Feed self.
- Eat and drink a variety of foods.
- Begin to develop bowel and bladder control.
- Exhibit a rest and sleep pattern appropriate for age.
- Dress self.

---

somewhat out of proportion. The posture of preschoolers gradually changes as the pelvis is straightened and the abdominal muscles become stronger. Thus the preschooler appears slender with erect posture.

Weight

Weight gain in preschool children is generally slow. By 5 years they have added only another 3 to 5 kg (7 to 12 lb) to their 3-year-old weight, increasing it to somewhere between 18 and 20 kg (40 and 45 lb).

Height

Preschool children grow about 5 to 6.25 cm (2.0 to 2.5 in.) each year. Thus by 5 years of age they double the birth length and measure 100 cm (40 in.).

Vision

Preschool children are generally **hyperopic** (farsighted), that is, unable to focus on near objects. As the eye grows in length, it becomes **emmetropic** (it refracts light normally). If the eyes become too long, the child becomes **myopic** (nearsighted), that

---

BOX 22–5 ■ Health Promotion Guidelines for Toddlers

Health Examinations
- At 15 and 18 months and then as recommended by the physician
- Dental visit starting at age 3
- Hearing tests by 18 months or earlier

Protective Measures
- Immunizations: continuing DPT, OPV series, pneumococcal, MMR, *Haemophilus influenzae* type B, and hepatitis B vaccines as recommended
- Screenings for tuberculosis and lead poisoning
- Fluoride supplements if there is inadequate water fluoridation (less than 0.7 part per million)

Toddler Safety
- Importance of supervision and teaching child to obey commands
- Home environment safety measures (e.g., lock medicine cabinet)

- Outdoor safety measures (e.g., close supervision near water)
- Appropriate toys

Nutrition
- Importance of nutritious meals and snacks
- Teaching simple mealtime manners
- Dental care

Elimination
- Toilet training techniques

Rest/Sleep
- Dealing with sleep disturbances

Play
- Providing adequate space and a variety of activities
- Toys that allow "acting on" behaviors and provide motor and sensory stimulation

is, unable to focus on objects that are far away. In severe cases of hyperopia or myopia, glasses may be prescribed. By the end of the preschool years, visual ability has improved; normal vision for the 5-year-old is approximately 20/30. The Snellen E chart can be used to assess the preschooler's vision.

Hearing and Taste

The hearing of the preschool child has reached optimal levels, and the ability to listen (attending to and comprehending what is said) has matured since the toddler age. As for the sense of taste, preschoolers show their preferences by asking for something "yummy," and may refuse something they consider "yucky."

Motor Abilities

By 5 years of age, children are able to wash their hands and face and brush their teeth (see Figure 22–8 ■). They are self-conscious about exposing their bodies and go to the bathroom without telling others. Typically, preschool children run with increasing skill each year. By 5 years of age, they run skillfully and can jump three steps. Preschoolers can balance on their toes and dress themselves without assistance.

Psychosocial Development

Erikson writes that the major developmental crisis of the preschooler is initiative versus guilt. Preschoolers must solve problems in accordance with their consciences. Their personalities develop. Erikson views the crises at this time as important for the development of the individual's self-concept. According to Erikson, preschoolers must learn what they can do. As a result, preschoolers imitate behavior, and their imaginations and creativity become lively.

Parents can enhance the self-concept of the preschooler by providing opportunities for new achievements where the child can learn, repeat, and master. For example, a child obtains a two-wheel bike with safety wheels and quickly learns coordination, balance, use of the brakes, and bicycle safety. Mastery

of these tasks provides the child with a sense of accomplishment. The child is soon ready for the new challenge of mastering the two-wheeler.

The self-concept of the preschooler is also based on gender identification. Preschoolers are aware of the two sexes and identify with the correct one. They often imitate sexual stereotypes and usually begin by identifying with the parent of the same sex. They may mimic the parent's behavior, attitudes, and appearance (see Figure 22–9 ■). Parents need to be aware that preschoolers are curious about their own bodies and sexual functions, as well as those of others, and will often ask questions. Parents should not imply that a question is inappropriate or that a particular subject is bad.

Freud theorizes that the preschooler is in the phallic stage of development. The biologic focus of the child during this stage is the genital area. The phase of close emotional relationships with both parents changes to the phase Freud referred to as the Electra or Oedipus complex. At this time, the child focuses feelings of love chiefly on the parent of the opposite sex, and the parent of the same sex may receive some hostile feelings. The child begins to develop sexual interests and becomes interested in clothes and hair styles.

During the preschool years, four adaptive mechanisms are learned: identification, introjection, imagination, and repression. **Identification** occurs when the child perceives the self as

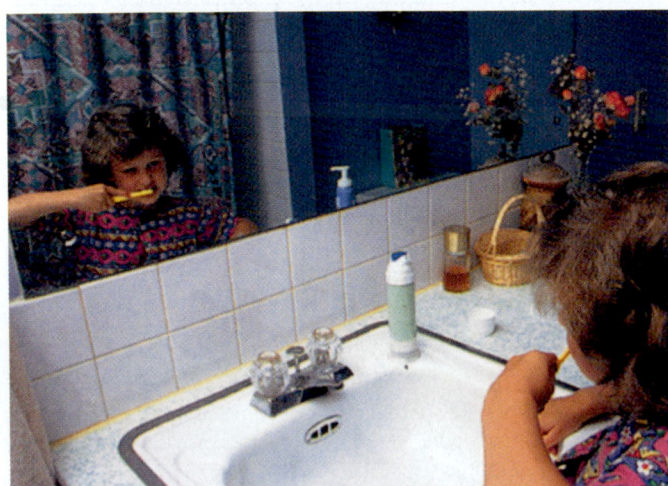

Figure 22–8 ■ A preschooler brushing her teeth.

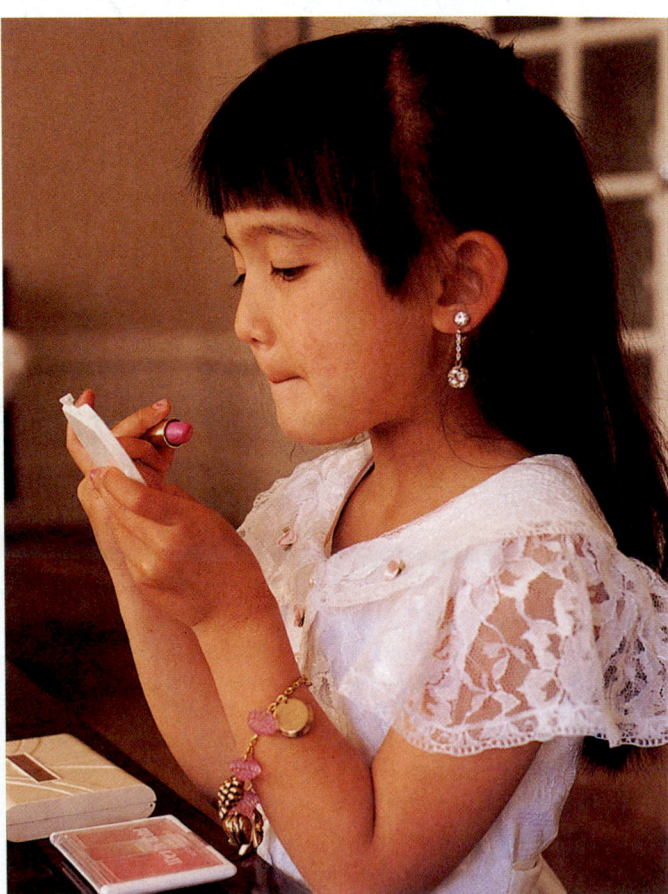

Figure 22–9 ■ Preschoolers often identify with the parent of the same sex and like to mimic behavior.

similar to another person and behaves like that person. For example, a boy may internalize the attitudes and gender behavior of his father. **Introjection** is similar to identification. It is the assimilation of the attributes of others. When preschoolers observe their parents, they assimilate many of their values and attitudes. **Imagination** is an important part of preschoolers' lives. The preschooler has an active imagination and fantasizes in play; for example, a chair becomes a beautiful throne to a girl, and she is the ruler. **Repression** is removing experiences, thoughts, and impulses from awareness. The preschooler generally represses thoughts related to the Oedipus or Electra complex.

Preschool children gradually emerge as social beings. At the age of 3 or 4, they learn to play with a small number of their peers. They gradually learn to play with more people as they grow older. Preschoolers participate more in the family than they did previously. In associations with neighbors, family guests, and baby-sitters, too, they learn about social relationships.

In their speech, children of 4 years are often dogmatic; they tend to believe that what they know is right. Four-year-olds love nonsense words such as "jump-jump" and can string them together much to an adult's exasperation. At 4, children are aggressive in their speech and capable of long conversations, often mixing fact and fiction. By 5 years of age, speaking skills are well developed. Children use words purposefully and ask questions to acquire information. They do not merely practice speaking as 3- and 4-year-olds do, but speak as a means of social interaction. Exaggeration is common among 4- and 5-year-olds.

Preschoolers also become increasingly aware of themselves. They play with their bodies largely out of curiosity. They know where the body begins and ends as well as the correct names for the different parts. By 5 years of age, they are able to draw a person including all the features. Preschoolers also learn about their feelings; they know the words *cry, sad, laugh,* and the feelings related to them. They also begin to learn how to control their feelings and behavior. The preschooler uses the same types of coping mechanisms in response to stress as the toddler does, although protest behavior (kicking, screaming) is less likely to occur in the older preschooler. Preschoolers usually have greater ability to verbalize stress.

Preschoolers need to feel that they are loved and that they are an important part of the family. The child who has to compete with siblings for parental attention will often display jealousy. Parents and caregivers should be aware that preschoolers need time to adjust to a new baby and may need additional attention or special activities to help them through this adjustment period. Preschoolers with older siblings may also experience sibling rivalry. Siblings may fight and argue and become aggressive because of their daily proximity or competition for parental attention. Parents who can plan some special time or activity for each child will help that child to feel loved and may decrease the sibling rivalry.

Guidance and discipline are important parts of the parental role during the preschool years. As children seek independence from adults, they often test limits by refusing to cooperate and by repeatedly ignoring parental requests. These power struggles can sometimes be avoided by encouraging children to be responsible for their own behavior as much as possible and by

setting reasonable expectations and consistent limits. When conflict does occur, parents can employ mutual discussion and compromise.

Cognitive Development

The preschooler's cognitive development, according to Piaget, is the phase of intuitive thought. Children are still egocentric, but egocentrism gradually subsides as they experience their expanding world. Preschoolers learn through trial and error, and they think of only one idea at a time. They do not understand relationships such as those between mother and father or sister and brother. Children start to understand words are associated with objects in late toddlerhood or the early preschool years. Preschoolers become concerned about death as something inevitable, but they do not explain it. They also associate death with others rather than themselves.

Most children at the age of 5 years can count pennies; however, the opportunity to spend money usually does not occur until they attend school. Reading skills also start to develop at this age. Young children like fairy tales and books about animals and other children.

Moral Development

Preschoolers are capable of prosocial behavior, that is, any action that a person takes to benefit someone else. The term *prosocial* is synonymous with *kind* and connotes sharing, helping, protecting, giving aid, befriending, showing affection, and giving encouragement.

At this stage of development, preschoolers do not have a fully formed conscience; however, they do develop some internal controls. Moral behavior is largely learned by modeling, initially after parents and later significant others. The preschooler usually behaves well in social settings.

Children who perceive their parents as strict may become resentful or overly obedient. Preschoolers usually control their behavior because they want love and approval from their parents. Moral behavior to a preschooler may mean taking turns at play or sharing. Nurses can assist parents by discussing moral development and encouraging parents to give preschoolers recognition for actions such as sharing. It is also important for parents to answer preschoolers' "why" questions and discuss values with them.

Spiritual Development

Many preschoolers enroll in Sunday school or faith-oriented classes. The preschooler usually enjoys the social interaction of these classes. According to Fowler, children from the ages of 4 to 6 years are at the intuitive-projective stage of spiritual development. Faith at this stage is primarily a result of the teaching of significant others, such as parents and teachers. Children learn to imitate religious behavior, for example, bowing the head in prayer, although they don't understand the meaning of the behavior. Preschoolers require simple explanations, such as those in picture books, of spiritual matters. Children at this age use their imaginations to envision such ideas as angels or the devil.

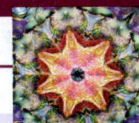

Developmental Assessment Guidelines

THE PRESCHOOLER

In these four developmental areas, does the preschooler do the following?

Physical Development

- Demonstrate physical growth (weight, height) within normal range.
- Manifest vital signs within normal range for age.
- Exhibit vision and hearing abilities within normal range.

Motor Development

- Perform gross and fine motor milestones within the normal range for age. For example, by 5 years of age is the preschooler able to do the following?
  - Jump rope and skip.
  - Climb playground equipment.
  - Ride a bicycle with training wheels.
  - Print letters and numbers.

Psychosocial Development

- Perform psychosocial developmental milestones for age. For example, by 5 years of age is the preschooler able to do the following?

- Separate easily from parents.
- Display imagination and creativity.
- Enjoy playing with peers in cooperative activities.
- Understand right from wrong and respond to others' expectations of behavior.
- Identify four colors.
- Exhibit increasing vocabulary using complete sentences and all parts of speech.
- Cooperate in doing simple chores (e.g., putting away toys).
- Identify with individuals of own sex.

Development in Activities of Daily Living

- Demonstrate development of toilet training.
- Perform simple hygiene measures.
- Dress and undress self.

Health Problems

Preschoolers often have health problems similar to those they had in toddlerhood. Respiratory tract problems and communicable diseases frequently occur as the preschooler interacts with other children at nursery schools and day care. Accidents and dental caries continue to be problems during this age. Congenital abnormalities such as cardiac disorders and hernias are often corrected at this age.

Health Assessment and Promotion

During assessment, the preschooler can often participate in answering questions with assistance from parents or caregivers. For instance, children who attend preschool can describe the typical lunch and how much of it they usually eat. Preschoolers can also describe the types of activities they enjoy. Guidelines for the preschooler are shown in the Developmental Assessment Guidelines.

Promoting health and wellness includes such areas as preventing accidents, dental health, good nutrition, cognitive stimulation, and sufficient sleep. For a summary of health promotion, see Box 22–6.

SCHOOL-AGE CHILDREN (6 TO 12 YEARS)

The school-age period starts when children are about 6 years of age, when the deciduous teeth are shed. This period includes the preadolescent (prepuberty) period. It ends at about 12 years, with the onset of puberty. Puberty is the age when the reproductive organs become functional and secondary sex characteristics develop. Because the average age of onset of puberty is 10 for girls and 12 for boys, some people define the school-age years as 6 to 10 for girls and 6 to 12 for boys. Skills learned during this stage are particularly important in relation to work later in life and willingness to try new tasks. In general, the period from 6 to 12 years is one of rapid and dramatic change.

Physical Development

The school-age child gains weight rapidly and thus appears less thin than previously. Individual differences due to both genetic and environmental factors are obvious at this time.

Weight

At 6 years boys tend to weigh about 21 kg (46 lb), about 1 kg (2 lb) more than girls. The weight gain of schoolchildren from 6 to 12 years of age averages about 3.2 kg (7 lb) per year, but the major weight gains occur from age 10 to 12 for boys and from 9 to 12 for girls. By 12 years of age boys and girls weigh on the average 40 to 42 kg (88 to 95 lb); girls are usually heavier.

Height

At 6 years both boys and girls are about the same height, 115 cm (46 in.). They are about 150 cm (60 in.) by 12 years. Before puberty, children of both sexes have a growth spurt, girls between 10 and 12 years and boys between 12 and 14 years. Thus girls may well be taller than boys at 12 years.

BOX 22–6	■ Health Promotion Guidelines for Preschoolers

Health Examinations
- Every 1 to 2 years

Protective Measures
- Immunizations: continuing DPT, OPV series, MMR, hepatitis, and other immunizations as recommended
- Screenings for tuberculosis
- Vision and hearing screening
- Regular dental screenings and fluoride treatment

Preschooler Safety
- Educating child about simple safety rules (e.g., crossing the street)
- Teaching child to play safely (e.g., bicycle and playground safety)
- Educating to prevent poisoning

Nutrition
- Importance of nutritious meals and snacks

Elimination
- Teaching proper hygiene (e.g., washing hands after using bathroom)

Rest/Sleep
- Dealing with sleep disturbances (e.g., nightmares)

Play
- Providing times for group play activities
- Teaching child simple games that require cooperation and interaction
- Providing toys and dress-ups for role-playing

The extremities tend to grow more quickly than the trunk, thus school-age children's bodies appear somewhat ill proportioned. By 6 years of age the thoracic curvature starts to develop, and the lordosis disappears. Full adult posture is not assumed, however, until after the complete development of the skeletal musculature during the adolescent period.

Vision

The depth and distance perception of children 6 to 8 years of age is accurate. By age 6 children have full binocular vision. The eye muscles are well developed and coordinated, and both eyes can focus on one object at the same time. Because the shape of the eye changes during growth, the farsightedness of the preschool years gradually changes to 20/20 vision during the school-age years; 20/20 vision is usually well established between 9 and 11 years of age.

Hearing and Touch

Auditory perception is fully developed in school-age children, who are able to identify fine differences in voices, both in sound and in pitch. At this stage, children also have a well-developed sense of touch and are able to locate points of heat and cold on all body surfaces. They are also able to identify an unseen object, such as a pencil or a book, simply by touch. This ability is called **stereognosis.**

Prepubertal Changes

Little change takes place in the reproductive and endocrine systems until the prepuberty period. During prepuberty, at about ages 9 to 13, endocrine functions slowly increase. This change in endocrine function can result in increased perspiration and more active sebaceous glands.

Motor Abilities

During the middle years (6 to 10), children perfect their muscular skills and coordination. By 9 years most children are becoming skilled in games of interest, such as football or baseball. These skills are often associated with school, and many of them are learned there. By 9 years most children have sufficient fine motor control for such activities as building models or sewing.

Psychosocial Development

According to Erikson, the central task of school-age children is industry versus inferiority. At this time children begin to create and develop a sense of competence and perseverance. School-age children are motivated by activities that provide a sense of worth. They concentrate on mastering skills that will help them function in the adult world. Although children of this age work hard to succeed, they are always faced with the possibility of failure, which can lead to a sense of inferiority. If children have been successful in previous stages, they are motivated to be industrious and to cooperate with others toward a common goal.

Freud describes the period from 6 through 12 years of age as the latency stage. During this time the focus is on physical and intellectual activities, while sexual tendencies seem to be repressed.

In school, children have the restraints of the school system imposed on their behavior, and they learn to develop controls. Children compare their skills with those of their peers in a number of areas, including motor development, social development, and language. This comparison assists in the development of self-concept.

As they grow older, schoolchildren learn to play with more children at one time. Usually the 6- and 7-year-old is a member of a peer group that is usually informal and transitory with the leadership changing from time to time. During this period of socialization with others, children gradually become less self-concerned and more cooperative and conscious of the group. This group can be a greater influence than the family in teaching attitudes. During middle to late childhood children usually join a more formalized group of peers, which is formed by the children themselves and is often structured around common interests. These groups of later school years usually consist of children of the same gender.

The schoolchild's self-concept continues to mature. Children recognize similarities and differences between themselves and others. School-age children compare themselves with others and obtain feedback from teachers and peers. Children who are successful and receive recognition for their efforts feel competent and in control of themselves and of the environment. Children who feel unaccepted by their peers or who receive negative feedback and little recognition can feel inferior and worthless.

Although the focus of interest for this age group has moved to school, peers, and other activities, the home remains the crucial place for the child's development of high self-esteem.

Cognitive Development

According to Piaget, the ages 7 to 11 years mark the phase of concrete operations. During this stage the child changes from egocentric interactions to cooperative interactions (see Figure 22–10 ■). School-age children also develop an increased understanding of concepts that are associated with specific objects, for example, environmental conservation or wildlife preservation. Children at this time develop logical reasoning from intuitive reasoning. For example, they learn to add and subtract to obtain an answer to a problem. Children also learn about cause-and-effect relationships at this age; for example, they know that a stone will not float because it is heavier than water.

Money is a concept that gains meaning for children when they start school. By the time they are 7 or 8 years old, children usually know the value of most coins. The concept of time is also learned at this age. By 6 years of age children enter school; the schedule in school helps them learn time periods. However, it is not until 9 or 10 years of age that children are able to understand the long periods of time in the past. Knowing the time of day and the day of the week are relatively easy for children because they relate time to routine activities. For example, a girl may go to school Monday through Friday, play on Saturday, go to Sunday school on Sunday morning, and go out with her father Sunday afternoon. Children are beginning to read a clock by the time they are 6 years old.

Reading skills are usually well developed later in childhood, and what a child reads is largely influenced by the family. By 9 years of age most children are self-motivated. They compete with themselves, and they like to plan in advance. By 12 years they are motivated by inner drive rather than by competition with peers. They like to talk, to discuss different subjects, and to debate.

Moral Development

Some school-age children are at Kohlberg's stage 1 of the preconventional level (punishment and obedience); that is, they act to avoid being punished. Some school-age children, however, are at stage 2 (instrumental-relativist orientation). These children do things to benefit themselves. Fairness, that is, everyone getting a fair share or chance, becomes important. Later in childhood, most children progress to the conventional level. This level has two stages: Stage 3 is the "good boy–nice girl" stage, and stage 4 is the law and order orientation. Children usually reach the conventional level between the ages of 10 and 13. The child shifts from the concrete interests of individuals to the interests of groups. The motivation for moral action at this stage is to live up to what significant others think of the child.

Spiritual Development

According to Fowler, the school-age child is at stage 2 in spiritual development, the mythic-literal stage. Children learn to distinguish fantasy from fact. Spiritual facts are those beliefs that are accepted by a religious group, whereas fantasy is thoughts and images formed in the child's mind. Parents and the minister, rabbi, or priest help the child distinguish fact from fantasy. These people still influence the child more than peers in spiritual matters.

When children do not understand such events as the creation of the world, they use fantasy to explain them. The school-age child needs to have concepts such as prayer presented in concrete terms. For example, the child thinks of God as having human qualities, such as a kind old man or a person who punishes when behavior does not meet his standards.

School-age children may ask many questions about God and religion in these years and will generally believe that God is good and always present to help. Just before puberty, children become aware that their prayers are not always answered and become disappointed. At this age, some children reject religion, whereas others continue to accept it. This decision is largely influenced by the parents. If a child continues religious training, the child is ready to apply reason rather than blind belief in most situations.

Health Problems

School-age children continue to have as many communicable diseases, dental caries, and accidents as preschoolers (see Figure 22–11 ■). Another health concern is the increasing num-

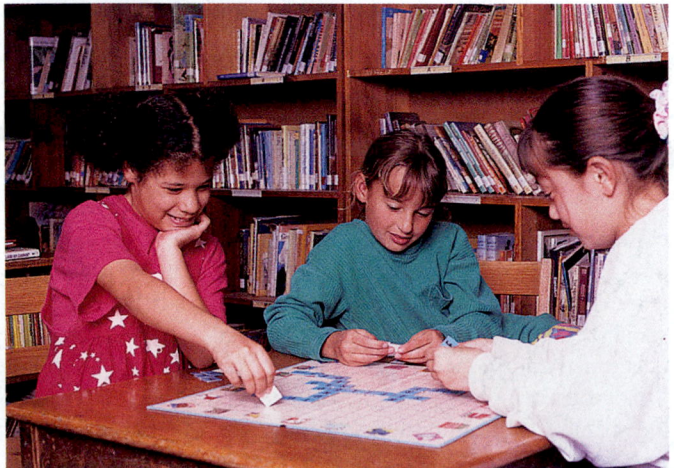

Figure 22–10 ■ Expanding cognitive skills enable school-age children to interact cooperatively in activities of an increasingly complex nature, as shown by the children playing this board game.

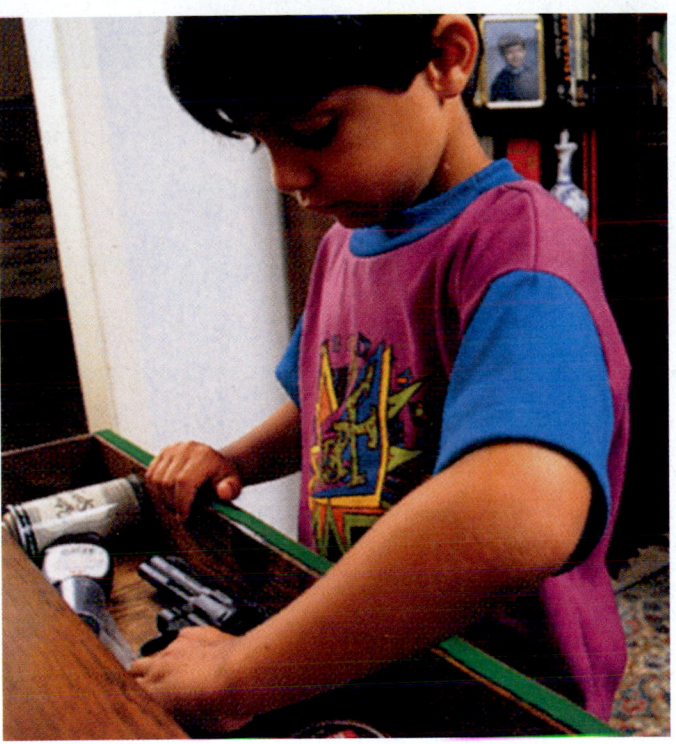

Figure 22–11 ■ Teach children never to touch guns without a parent present.

ber of overweight children. Being overweight, is the most common nutritional problem among children (Broadwater, 2002). Obesity in childhood can often lead to adult obesity and increased risk for diabetes, hypertension, and cardiovascular disease.

Health Assessment and Promotion

During the assessment interview the nurse responds to questions from the parent or other caregiver, gives appropriate feedback, and lends encouragement and support. The nurse also demonstrates interest in the child and enthusiasm for the child's strengths. Guidelines for the school-age child are shown in the Developmental Assessment Guidelines.

Promoting health and wellness includes dental hygiene and regular dental examinations, safety measures to prevent accidents, promoting a healthy diet and physical fitness, supporting autonomy and self-esteem, and hygiene measures to prevent infections. Box 22-7 provides health promotion guidelines for this age group.

ADOLESCENTS (12 TO 18 YEARS)

Adolescence is the period during which the person becomes physically and psychologically mature and acquires a personal identity. At the end of this critical period in development, the person should be ready to enter adulthood and assume its responsibilities. The length of adolescence is culturally determined to some extent. In North America adolescence is longer than in some cultures, extending to 18 or 20 years of age.

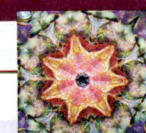

Developmental Assessment Guidelines

THE SCHOOL-AGE CHILD

In these four developmental areas, does the school-age child do the following?

Physical Development
- Demonstrate physical growth (weight, height) within normal range.
- Manifest vital signs within normal range for age.
- Exhibit vision and hearing abilities within normal range.
- Demonstrate male or female prepubertal changes within normal range.

Motor Development
- Possess coordinated motor skills for age. For example, by 12 years of age, is the child able to do the following?
  - Do tricks on a bike, climb a tree, shinny up a rope.
  - Throw and catch a small ball.
  - Play a musical instrument.

Psychosocial Development
- Perform psychosocial developmental milestones for age. For example, by 12 years of age is the child able to do the following?

- Make friends of the same sex and establish a peer group.
- Become less dependent on family and venture away from them.
- Interact well with parents.
- Control strong and impulsive feelings.
- Participate in organized competitions.
- Read, print, and manipulate numbers and letters easily.
- Exhibit a concept of money and make change for small amounts of money.
- Express self in a logical manner and talk through problems.
- Enjoy riddles and read and understand comics.
- Invest in a hobby or collection.
- Like to help others.
- Think of self as likable and healthy.

Development in Activities of Daily Living
- Demonstrate concern for personal cleanliness and appearance.
- Express need for privacy.

BOX 22-7 ■ Health Promotion Guidelines for School-Age Children

Health Examinations
- Annual physical examination or as recommended

Protective Measures
- Immunizations as recommended
- Screening for tuberculosis
- Periodic vision, speech, and hearing screenings
- Regular dental screenings and fluoride treatment
- Providing accurate information about sexual issues (e.g., reproduction, AIDS)

School-Age Child Safety
- Using proper equipment when participating in sports and other physical activities (e.g., helmets, pads)
- Encouraging child to take responsibility for own safety (e.g., participating in bicycle and water safety courses)

Nutrition
- Importance of child not skipping meals and eating a balanced diet
- Experiences with food that may lead to obesity

Elimination
- Utilizing positive approaches for elimination problems (e.g., enuresis)

Play and Social Interactions
- Providing opportunities for a variety of organized group activities
- Accepting realistic expectations of child's abilities
- Acting as role models in acceptance of other persons who may be different
- Providing a home environment that limits TV viewing and video games and encourages completion of homework

---

Puberty is the first stage of adolescence in which sexual organs begin to grow and mature. **Menarche** (onset of menstruation) occurs in girls. **Ejaculation** (expulsion of semen) occurs in boys. For girls, puberty normally starts between 10 and 14 years; for boys, between 12 and 16 years. The adolescent period is often subdivided into three stages: early adolescence lasts from ages 12 to 13; middle adolescence extends from 14 to 16 years; and late adolescence extends from 17 to 18 or 20 years. Late adolescence is a more stable stage than the other two. In the late period, adolescents are involved mostly with planning their future and economic independence.

Physical Development

During puberty, growth is markedly accelerated compared to the slow, steady growth of the child. This period, marked by sudden and dramatic physical changes, is referred to as the **adolescent growth spurt.** In boys, the growth spurt usually begins between ages 12 and 16; in girls, it begins earlier, usually between ages 10 and 14. Because the growth spurt begins earlier in girls, many girls surpass boys in height at this time.

Physical Growth

Physical growth continues throughout adolescence. Growth is fastest for boys at about 14 years, and the maximum height is often reached at about 18 or 19 years. Some men add another 1 or 2 cm to their height during their 20s as the vertebral column gradually continues to grow. During the period of 10 to 18 years of age, the average American male doubles his weight, gaining about 32 kg (72 lb), and grows about 41 cm (16 in.). The fastest rate of growth in girls occurs at about age 12; they reach their maximum height at about 15 to 16 years. During ages 10 to 18, the average American female gains about 25 kg (55 lb) and grows about 24 cm (9 in.).

Physical growth during adolescence is greatly influenced by a number of factors, such as heredity, nutrition, medical care, illness, physical and emotional environment, family size, and culture. Generally, people in the United States have grown taller in recent years. This increase in average height is thought to be due to many of the preceding factors.

Growth is noted first in the musculoskeletal system. This growth follows a sequential pattern: The head, hands, and feet are the first to grow to adult status. Next, the extremities reach their adult size. Because the extremities grow before the trunk, the adolescent looks leggy, awkward, and uncoordinated. After the trunk grows to full size, the shoulders, chest, and hips grow. Skull and facial bones also change proportions: The forehead becomes more prominent, and the jawbones develop.

Glandular Changes

The eccrine and apocrine glands increase their secretions and become fully functional during puberty. The **eccrine glands,** found over most of the body, produce sweat. The **apocrine glands** develop in the axillae, anal and genital areas, external auditory canals, and around the umbilicus and the areola of the breasts. Apocrine sweat is released onto the skin in response to emotional stimuli only. **Sebaceous glands** also become active under the influence of androgens in both males and females. The sebaceous glands, which secrete sebum, become most active on the face, neck, shoulder, upper back, and chest and are often the cause of an increased incidence of acne.

Sexual Characteristics

During puberty, both primary and secondary sex characteristics develop. **Primary sexual characteristics** relate to the organs necessary for reproduction, such as the testes, penis, vagina, and uterus. **Secondary sexual characteristics** differentiate the male from the female but do not relate directly to reproduction.

Examples are pubic hair growth, breast development, and voice changes.

The first noticeable sign that puberty has begun in males is the appearance of pubic hair and the enlargement of the scrotum and testes. The milestone of male puberty is considered to be the first ejaculation, which commonly occurs at about 14 years of age. Fertility follows several months later. Sexual maturity is achieved by age 18.

Often the first noticeable sign of puberty in females is the appearance of the breast bud, although the appearance of hair along the labia may precede this. The milestone of female puberty is the menarche, which occurs about 2 years after the breast bud appears. At first, menstrual periods are scanty and irregular and may occur without ovulation. Ovulation is usually established 1 to 2 years after menarche. Female internal reproductive organs reach adult size about age 18 to 20.

Psychosocial Development

According to Erikson (1963), the psychosocial task of the adolescent is the establishment of identity. The danger of this stage is role confusion. The inability to settle on an occupational identity commonly disturbs the adolescent. Less commonly, doubts about sexual identity arise. Because of the adolescent's dramatic body changes, the development of a stable identity is difficult. Erikson says that adolescents help one another through this identity crisis by forming cliques and a separate youth culture. These cliques often exclude all those who are "different" in skin color, cultural background, aspects of dress, gestures, and tastes.

Adolescents are usually concerned about their body, their appearance, and their physical abilities. Hair styling, skin care, and clothes become very important. In-groupers of an adolescent clique can be excessively clannish and cruel in excluding out-groupers; this intolerance is a temporary defense against identity confusion (Erikson, 1963, p. 236).

In their search for a new identity, adolescents have to refight the battles of many of the previous stages of development. The task of developing trust in self and others is again encountered when adolescents look for ideal persons whom they can trust and with whom they can prove trustworthy. Development of autonomy is restaged in their search for ways to express their right to choose freely. The search for an occupational role that allows expression of an autonomous, freely chosen direction is one example. Free choice and autonomy present conflicts to the adolescent. Conflict arises between behaving well in the eyes of the parents and behaving in a manner that may expose them to the ridicule of their peers. The sense of initiative is also restaged. The adolescent has unlimited imagination and ambition and aspires to great accomplishments. The sense of industry is reenacted when the adolescent chooses a career. The extent to which these tasks were achieved earlier influences the adolescent's ability to achieve a healthy self-concept and self-identity.

The adolescent needs to establish a self-concept that accepts both personal strengths and weaknesses. Faced with dramatic changes in body structure and function and greater expectations to assume responsibilities, many adolescents experience temporary difficulty in developing a positive self-image. Adolescents who are accepted, loved, and valued by family and peers generally tend to gain confidence and feel good about themselves. Adolescents who have difficulty forming relationships or who are perceived by peers as too different and not included in adolescent cliques may develop less favorable self-images and have low self-esteem. Adolescents need to learn to build on their strengths and not be preoccupied by their perceived faults.

Teenagers with physical handicaps or illnesses are particularly vulnerable to peer rejection. Nurses and educators can promote peer understanding and acceptance by discussing the individual's specific problems with the peer group. Adolescents gain self-concepts largely from the impressions that others have of them. If others accept defects—for example, a lost finger—teenagers accept those defects more readily. Establishing groups of peers who have similar problems can provide an opportunity for the individual to develop close relationships with others and feel valued and accepted.

Although sexual identification begins at about 3 or 4 years of age, it is a significant part of adolescence. The adolescent male strives to achieve a masculine sexual identity; the adolescent female, a feminine sexual identity. Because sex roles are becoming less defined in North American society, adopting masculine and feminine roles is increasingly confusing to today's adolescent. Job and family roles are less traditional and sex specific. In forming a sexual identity, adolescents first fantasize the male or female role and then enact various aspects of that imagined role. In response to their own feelings and that of others, aspects of the role are either adopted or rejected. Later, adolescents begin to establish intimacy with a partner or partners. This intimacy lays the groundwork for the commitments of adulthood. Sexual experimentation is not part of true intimacy, but once intimacy is achieved, sexual activity is often included.

Adolescents are sexually active and may engage in masturbation as well as heterosexual and homosexual activity. The 2001 Youth Risk Behavior Surveillance System reported that 45% of high school students had sexual intercourse and 42% of sexually active students had not used a condom at their last sexual intercourse (Grunbaum et al., 2002). These behaviors increase the risk for sexually transmitted disease (STDs) and pregnancy. Almost 4 million of the new cases of STDs each year occur in adolescents and, in addition, about 1 million teenagers become pregnant each year (USDHHS, 2000).

At about the age of 15 years, many adolescents gradually draw away from the family and gain independence. This need for independence combined with the need for family support sometimes creates conflict within the adolescent and between the adolescent and the family. The young person may appear hostile or depressed at times during this painful process. At this age, adolescents prefer to be with their peers rather than their parents and may seek advice from adults other than their parents. Parents sometimes are bewildered by this stage of development; instead

MediaLink | TEEN WITH LYMPHOCYTIC LEUKEMIA CARE PLAN ACTIVITY

Research Note
What Is the Effect of a High-School-Based Child Care Center on Parenting Teens and Their Children?

A descriptive study by William and Sadler (2001) examined the above question through a retrospective record review of 52 low-income, urban adolescent parents enrolled at a child-care center within a high school. Research has shown that adolescent parents usually do not complete school, have less chances for employment, and greater dependence on public assistance. The children of adolescent parents are at risk also. Research has shown that there is less interaction between adolescent mothers and their children, which can lead to increased cognitive and behavioral problems at school age.

The authors examined specific outcomes with the following results: GPA scores increased and absentee rate decreased; no repeat births during the 3 years of the study; 100% school completion rate; and the children were up to date in their physical examinations and immunizations.

Implications: This research supports the growing body of literature on how support services are helpful to adolescent parents and their children. Nurses need to be aware of such programs in their community for referral purposes. It is also important for nurses to participate and collaborate in this type of service that helps promote the health of teens and their children.

Note: From "Effects of an Urban High School-Based Child Care Center on Self-Selected Adolescent Parents and Their Children," by E. G. Williams and L. S. Sadler, 2001, *Journal of School Health, 71*(2), pp. 47–52.

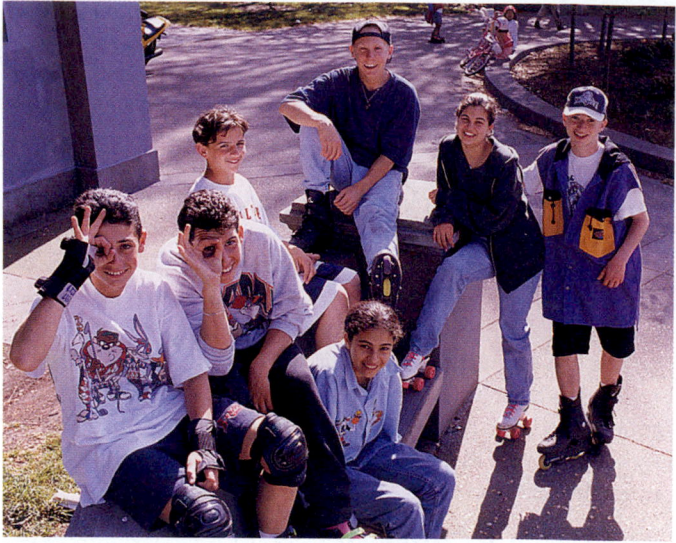

Figure 22–12 ■ Adolescent peer group relationships enhance a sense of belonging, self-esteem, and self-identity.

of reducing controls, they increase them, causing the adolescent to rebel.

Adolescents also have to resolve their ambivalent feelings toward the parent of the opposite sex. As part of the resolution, adolescents may develop brief crushes on adults outside the family—teachers or neighbors, for example. Adolescents sometimes adopt some of the attributes of the adults with whom they are infatuated. This modeling can be helpful in the maturing process.

Some of the discord in the family at this time is due to the generation gap. The values of the adolescent may differ from those of the parents. This difference may be difficult for the parents to understand and to accept. Adolescents still need guidance from their parents, although they appear to neither want it nor need it. However, adolescents need to know that their parents care about them and that their parents still want to help them. Restrictions and guidance need to be presented in a manner that makes adolescents feel loved. They need consistency in guidance and fewer restrictions than previously. They should have the independence they can handle yet know that their parents will assist them when they need help.

During adolescence, **peer groups** assume great importance (see Figure 22–12 ■). The peer group has a number of functions. It provides a sense of belonging, pride, social learning, and sexual roles. Most peer groups have well-

defined, sex-specific modes of acceptable behavior. In adolescence, the peer groups change with age. They start as single-sex groups, evolve to mixed groups, and finally narrow to couples who share activities.

Not all adolescents, however, are heterosexual. For homosexuals, adolescence is a difficult time. Because peer acceptance is crucial to self-acceptance, lesbian and gay adolescents usually conform to the heterosexual codes and behaviors of their peer groups even though these do not feel natural or correct. Conforming may exact a great personal cost. Adolescents who choose to be openly gay or lesbian face not only the ostracism of their peers but also the misunderstanding and hostility of parents, teachers, and other important adults.

Cognitive Development

Cognitive abilities mature during adolescence. Between the ages of 11 and 15, the adolescent begins Piaget's formal operations stage of cognitive development. The main feature of this stage is that people can think beyond the present and beyond the world of reality. Adolescents are highly imaginative and idealistic. They consider things that do not exist but that might be and consider ways things could be or ought to be. This type of thinking requires logic, organization, and consistency.

The adolescent becomes more informed about the world and environment. Adolescents use new information to solve everyday problems and can communicate with adults on most subjects. The adolescent's capacity to absorb and use knowledge is great. Adolescents usually select their own areas for learning; they explore interests from which they may evolve a career plan. Study habits and learning skills developed in adolescence are used throughout life.

Moral Development

According to Kohlberg, the young adolescent is usually at the conventional level of moral development. Most still accept the

Golden Rule and want to abide by social order and existing laws. Adolescents examine their values, standards, and morals. They may discard the values they have adopted from parents in favor of values they consider more suitable.

When adolescents move into the postconventional or principled level, they start to question the rules and laws of society. Right thinking and right action become a matter of personal values and opinions, which may conflict with societal laws. Adolescents consider the possibility of rationally changing the law and emphasize individual rights. Not all adolescents or even adults proceed to this postconventional level. See the discussion about Kohlberg's stages of moral development in Chapter 21. 🔗

Spiritual Development

According to Fowler, the adolescent or young adult reaches the synthetic-conventional stage of spiritual development. As adolescents encounter different groups in society, they are exposed to a wide variety of opinions, beliefs, and behaviors regarding religious matters. The adolescent may reconcile the differences in one of the following ways:

- Deciding any differences are wrong
- Compartmentalizing the differences (For example, a friend may not be able to go to dances on Friday evenings because of religious observances, but the friend can share activities on other days.)
- Obtaining advice from a significant other, such as a parent or a minister.

Often the adolescent believes that various religious beliefs and practices have more similarities than differences. At this stage, the adolescent's focus is on interpersonal rather than conceptual matters.

Nursing activities relative to this stage of spiritual development include

- Presenting an open, accepting attitude to adolescent's questions and statements regarding spiritual matters and their implications for health
- Arranging for adolescents to see a member of their religious faith if so desired, or to talk with members of their church peer group for support
- Providing a comfortable environment in which adolescents can practice the rituals of their faith.

Health Problems

The 2001 Youth Risk Behavior Surveillance System reported the following health-risk behaviors for youth and young adults (Grunbaum et al., 2002): 75% of all deaths in the 10 to 24 age group resulted from four causes:

- Motor-vehicle crashes (see Figure 22-13 ■)
- Homicides
- Suicide
- Other unintentional injuries (e.g., falls, drowning, poisoning).

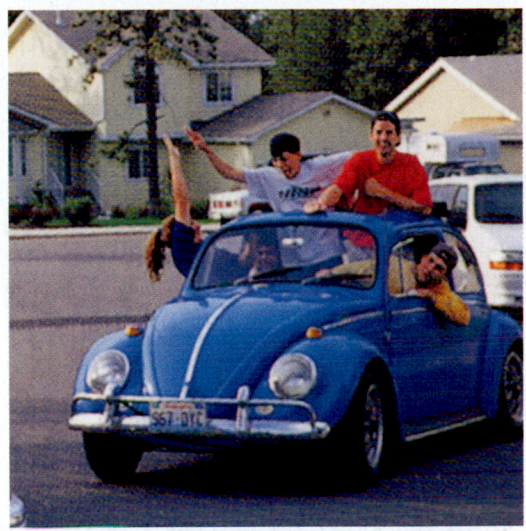

Figure 22–13 ■ To prevent motor vehicle crashes, insist on driver's education classes and enforce rules about safe driving.

During the month prior to the survey, high school students engaged in the following risk behaviors:

- 14% never wore a seat belt
- 30% had ridden with a driver who had been drinking alcohol
- 17% had carried a weapon
- 47% had drunk alcohol
- 24% had used marijuana
- 8.8% had attempted suicide at sometime in the previous 12 months.

Murray and Zentner (2001) report that suicide in adolescents is frequently reported as an accidental death. Motor vehicle accidents, drug and alcohol overdoses, firearm accidents, and even homicides can be disguised suicides. Psychological, social, and physiologic stressors are the apparent causes for the rising number of suicides. Other adolescent health problems are cardiovascular disease, depression, tooth decay, gingivitis, malalignment of teeth, neglect, and abuse.

Health Assessment and Promotion

Guidelines for growth and development of the adolescent are shown in the Developmental Assessment Guidelines.

Adolescents are usually self-directed in meeting their health needs. Because of maturation changes, however, they need teaching and guidance in a number of health care areas.

Promoting health and wellness includes screening for tobacco, alcohol, and drug use and for sexual practices, and checking blood pressure, height, and weight. For a summary of health promotion see Box 22–8.

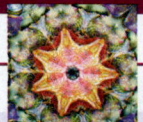

Development Assessment Guidelines

THE ADOLESCENT

In these three developmental areas, does the adolescent do the following?

Physical Development

- Exhibit physical growth (weight, height) within normal range for age and sex.
- Demonstrate male or female sexual development consistent with standards.
- Manifest vital signs within normal range for age and sex.
- Exhibit vision and hearing abilities within normal range.

Psychosocial Development

- Interact well with parents, teachers, peers, siblings, and persons in authority.

- Like self.
- Think and plan for the future, such as college or a career.
- Choose a lifestyle and interests that fit own identity.
- Determine own beliefs and values.
- Begin to establish a sense of identity in the family.
- Seek help from appropriate persons about problems.

Development in Activities of Daily Living

- Demonstrate knowledge of physical development, menstruation, reproduction, and birth control.
- Exhibit healthy lifestyle practices in nutrition, exercise, recreation, sleep patterns, and personal habits.
- Demonstrate concern for personal cleanliness and appearance.

BOX 22–8 ■ Health Promotion Guidelines for Adolescents

Health Examinations
- As recommended by the physician

Protective Measures
- Immunizations as recommended, such as adult tetanus-diphtheria vaccine and hepatitis B vaccine
- Screening for tuberculosis
- Periodic vision and hearing screenings
- Regular dental assessments
- Obtaining and providing accurate information about sexual issues

Adolescent Safety
- Adolescent's taking responsibility for using motor vehicles safely (e.g., completing a driver's education course, wearing seat belt and helmet)
- Making certain that proper precautions are taken during all athletic activities (e.g., medical supervision, proper equipment)

- Parents' keeping lines of communication open and being alert to signs of substance abuse and emotional disturbances in the adolescent

Nutrition and Exercise
- Importance of healthy snacks and appropriate patterns of food intake and exercise
- Factors that may lead to nutritional problems (e.g., obesity, anorexia nervosa, bulimia)
- Balancing sedentary activities with regular exercise

Social Interactions
- Encouraging adolescent to establish relationships that promote discussion of feelings, concerns, and fears
- Parents' encouraging adolescent peer group activities that promote appropriate moral and spiritual values
- Parents' acting as role models for appropriate social interactions
- Parents' providing a comfortable home environment for appropriate adolescent peer group activities

---

Focus on Critical Thinking

Bridget Thomas is 16 years old and is brought to your clinic at the public health district by her 17-year-old boyfriend. They are asking about birth control methods. You notice that she seems to be shy and afraid to talk. In the exam room, she tells you that she thinks that she may already be pregnant but is afraid to tell her boyfriend or her family. She is very thin and needs dental care.

1. According to Erikson, what stage of development is Bridget showing?
2. How could knowledge of Piaget's cognitive development direct your answers?
3. Using your knowledge of growth and development, what health promotion advice would you give Bridget?

See Critical Thinking Possibilities in Appendix A.

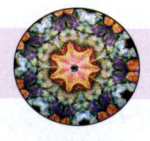 ## | Chapter Review

---

EXPLORE MediaLink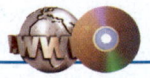

NCLEX review questions, case studies, care plan activities, MediaLink applications, and other interactive resources for this chapter can be found on the Companion Website at www.prenhall.com/kozier.

Click on Chapter 22 to select the activities for this chapter. For animations, more NCLEX review questions, and an audio glossary, access the Student CD-ROM accompanying this textbook.

Chapter Highlights

- Prenatal or intrauterine development lasts about 9 calendar months.
- The embryonic phase is the 8-week period during which the fertilized ovum develops into an organism with most of the features of the human.
- Monitoring the infant's weight, length, head and chest circumferences, fontanelle size and status, vision, hearing, smell and taste, touch, reflexes, and motor development are important indicators to the newborn's growth and health.
- Infants from birth to 12 months reveal marked growth in size and stature with appropriate nutrition and care: Birth weight doubles by 5 months and triples by 12 months.
- During infancy, motor development is notable: At 1 month infants can lift their heads momentarily when prone; at 6 months they can sit unsupported; and at 12 months they can walk with help.
- Fulfillment of the infant's physiologic and psychologic needs is required to develop a basic sense of trust. Parents can enhance this sense of trust by responding consistently to an infant's needs, providing a predictable environment in which routines are established, and being sensitive to the infant's needs and meeting those needs skillfully and promptly.
- Cognitive development, for the infant, is a result of interaction between an indivudal and the environment. The infant needs a variety of sensory and motor stimuli.
- The toddler group, ages 12 months to 3 years, develops from having no voluntary control to being able to walk and speak. They also learn to control their bladders and bowels, and they acquire all kinds of information about their environment.
- During the preschool years, ages 4 to 5, physical growth slows, but control of the body and coordination increase greatly. The preschoolers' world gets larger as they meet relatives, friends, and neighbors.

- The school-age period starts when children are about 6 years of age, when deciduous teeth are shed. In general, this period from 6 to 12 years is one of rapid and dramatic change. Skills learned during this stage are particularly important in relation to work later in life and willingness to try new tasks.
- During psychosocial development, school-age children face Erikson's conflict of industry versus inferiority.
- School-age children begin to understand relationships and change from being egocentric to having cooperative interactions; according to Piaget, they are in the concrete operations phase of cognitive development.
- Most school-age children progress to the conventional level of moral development and to the mythic-literal stage of spiritual development.
- Rapid growth in height, development of secondary sexual characteristics, sexual maturity, and increasing independence from the family are major landmarks of adolescence.
- Peer groups assume great importance during adolescence; they provide a sense of belonging, pride, social learning, and sexual roles.
- Adolescents are at Fowler's synthetic-conventional stage of spiritual development.
- Adolescents between the ages of 11 and 15 begin the formal operations stage of cognitive development; they are able to think logically, rationally, and futuristically and can conceptualize things as they could be rather than as they are.
- The adolescent is at Kohlberg's conventional level of moral development, and some proceed to the postconventional or principled level.
- The four leading causes of adolescent death are motor vehicle crashes, homicide, suicide, and other unintentional injuries.

Review Questions

22–1. You are working the night shift on a postpartum floor. As you walk in to see Mrs. Yee, you notice that she is crying and rubbing her baby's head. She says "Look how lopsided my little Sam's head is. It is all my fault. My mom told me that I should have laid down more instead of sitting. Now, Sam's head is all smashed and funny looking." Your best response would be based on the knowledge that
   a. side-lying is better for the fetus than sitting upright, but it is too late to worry about it at this point.
   b. the heads of many newborn babies are misshapen because of the molding of the head that occurs during labor and delivery.
   c. many well-meaning family members give erroneous information that needs to be corrected immediately.
   d. all babies have misshapen heads but within a week, the newborn's head will regain its symmetry.

22–2. Sally, who is 24 months old, is clinging to her mother and cries every time you try to examine her. From your knowledge of psychosocial development you know that

   a. this is normal toddler development.
   b. this child needs further psychological evaluation.
   c. Sally is manipulative and should be taken from her mother to be examined.
   d. this is normal behavior for a 12-month-old, but Sally is too old for this action and is showing signs of regression.

22–3. Five-year-old Maria is brought to the emergency department with a broken arm from falling off the playground equipment. Her parents want some ideas of how to keep her occupied while wearing the cast. Your suggestions might include which of the following?
   a. There is no need to limit her activities.
   b. Let her watch television or do puzzles, as long as she is sitting.
   c. Encourage her to draw, play games, and do simple chores. Just try to keep her arm supported in a sling.
   d. She can ride a bike, jump rope, watch television, or play games.

22–4. During the school-age phase of concrete operations, children develop logical reasoning from intuitive reasoning. An example of this might be
a. a science-fair project comparing how fast different objects fall from a set height.
b. feeling responsible for wishing that a sibling would go away, and now that sibling is ill and hospitalized.
c. understanding how geometric figures might fit into a futuristic and idealistic world.
d. learning to ride a bike.

22–5. When explaining teenage growth and development the nurse knows that
a. the first noticeable sign of puberty in females is appearance of the breast bud.
b. in boys, the growth spurt usually begins between ages 10 and 14.
c. the apocrine glands, found over most of the body, begin to produce sweat.
d. the leading cause of death in adolescents does not include motor vehicle crashes, suicide, and homicide.

Readings and References

Suggested Readings

Epstein, J. L., & Kiryk, P. D. (Eds.). (2002). Adolescent health. *The Nursing Clinics of North America, 37,* 373–573.
    This issue is devoted to adolescent health. Its comprehensive coverage includes articles relating to adolescent health concerns such as health care needs of homeless adolescents, caring for sexual minority youths, improving the health and well-being of adolescent boys, adolescent drug and alcohol use, sexually transmitted infection, nursing care of adolescents who have been sexually assaulted, effective contraceptive counseling, effective prenatal care for adolescent girls, adolescents with eating disorders, and the chronically ill adolescent.

Murray, R. B., & Zentner, J. P. (2001). *Health assessment and promotion strategies through the life span* (7th ed.). Upper Saddle River, NJ: Prentice Hall.
    Part III of this book, Chapters 7–11, provides a comprehensive discussion of assessment and health promotion for the family and developing person from infancy through adolescence. It includes family development and relationships, physiologic concepts, psychosocial concepts, and health care and nursing applications.

Related Research

Johnson, P. J., & Hellerstedt, W. L. (2002). Current or past physical or sexual abuse as a risk marker for sexually transmitted disease in pregnant women. *Perspectives on Sexual and Reproductive Health, 34*(2), 62–67.

Mims, B., & Biordi, D. L. (2001). Communication patterns in African-American families with adolescent mothers of single or repeat pregnancies. *Journal of National Black Nurses' Association, 12*(1), 34–41.

Pletsch, P. K. (2002). Reduction of primary and secondary smoke exposure for low-income black pregnant women. *The Nursing Clinics of North American, 37,* 315–329.

References

Broadwater, H. R. (2002). Reshaping the future for overweight kids. *RN, 65*(11), 36–41.

Buchanan, L. (2002). Evidence based practice: Implementing a smoking cessation program for pregnant women based on current clinical practice guidelines. *Journal of the American Academy of Nurse Practitioners, 14*(6), 243–250.

Curet, L. B., & Hsi, A. C. (2002). Drug abuse during pregnancy. *Clinical Obstetrics and Gynecology, 45*(1), 73–88.

Erikson, E. H. (1963). *Childhood and society* (2nd ed.). New York: Norton.

Fowler, J. W. (1981). *Stages of faith: The psychology of human development and the quest for meaning.* New York: Harper & Row.

Grunbaum, J. A., Kann, L., Kinchen, S. A., Williams, B., Ross, J. G., Lowry, R., et al. (2002, June 28). Youth risk behavior surveillance—United States, 2001. *Morbidity and Mortality Weekly Report, 51* (55-4) 1–62.

Murray, R. B., & Zentner, J. P. (2001). *Health assessment and promotion strategies through the life span* (7th ed.). Upper Saddle River, NJ: Prentice Hall.

Piaget, J. (1966). *Origins of intelligence in children.* New York: Norton.

Pillitteri, A. (2003). *Maternal & child health nursing: Care of the childbearing & childrearing family* (4th ed.). Philadelphia: Lippincott Williams & Wilkins.

U.S. Department of Health and Human Services. (2000). *Healthy people 2010: Objectives for improving health (Part B: Focus area 16. Maternal, infant, and child health. Understanding and improving health* (2nd ed.) [Electronic version]. Washington, DC: Author. Retrieved March 8, 2003, from http://www.healthypeople.gov/document/html/volume2/16mich.htm

Venes, D. (Ed.). (2001). *Taber's cyclopedic medical dictionary* (19th ed.) [Electronic version]. Philadelphia: F. A. Davis Company. Retrieved November 30, 2002, from http://www. tabers.com

Williams, E. G., & Sadler, L. S. (2001). Effects of an urban high school-based child care center on self-selected adolescent parents and their children. *Journal of School Health, 71*(2), 47–52.

Selected Bibliography

Ball, J. W., & Bindler, R. C. (2003). *Pediatric nursing. Caring for children* (3rd ed.). Upper Saddle River, NJ: Prentice Hall.

Busen, N. H. (2001). Perioperative preparation of the adolescent surgical patient. *AORN Journal, 73,* 337–363.

Carl, D. L., Roux, G., & Matacale, R. (2000). Exploring dental hygiene and perinatal outcomes. Oral health implications for pregnancy and early childhood. *AWHONN Lifelines, 4*(1), 22–27.

Doswell, W. M., & Braxter, B. (2002). Risk-taking behaviors in early adolescent minority women: Implications for research and practice. *Journal of Obstetric Gynecologic and Neonatal Nursing, 31,* 454–461.

Edelman, K. L., & Mandle, C. L. (2002). *Health promotion throughout the lifespan* (5th ed.). St. Louis, MO: Mosby.

Mattson, S. (2000). Providing culturally competent care strategies and approaches for perinatal clients. *AWHONN Lifelines, 4*(5), 37–39.

Murray, S. S., McKinney, E. S., & Gorrie, T. M. (2002). *Foundations of maternal-newborn nursing* (3rd ed.). Philadelphia: W. B. Saunders Company.

Simpson, K. R., & Creehan, P. A. (2001). *Association of women's health, obstetric and neonatal nurses's. Perinatal nursing* (2nd ed.). Philadelphia: Lippincott.

CHAPTER 23

PROMOTING HEALTH IN ADULTS AND OLDER ADULTS

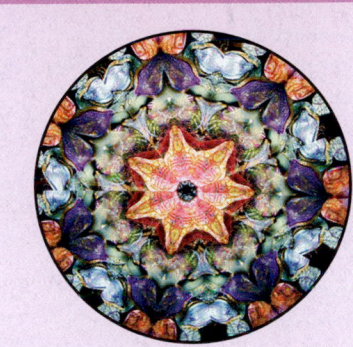

LEARNING OUTCOMES

After completing this chapter, you will be able to:

- Identify characteristic tasks of the different stages of development during young, middle, and older adulthood.

- Describe the usual physical development occurring in young, middle, and older adulthood.

- Compare psychosocial development according to Erikson during the various stages of adulthood.

- Explain changes in cognitive development according to Piaget throughout adulthood.

- Describe moral development according to Kohlberg throughout adulthood.

- Describe spiritual development according to Fowler throughout adulthood.

- Identify selected health problems associated with young, middle-aged, and older adults.

- Identify developmental assessment guidelines for young, middle-aged, and older adults.

- List examples of health promotion topics from young adulthood through older adulthood.

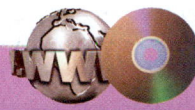

MediaLink

www.prenhall.com/kozier

Additional resources for this chapter can be found on the Student CD-ROM accompanying this textbook, and on the Companion Website at www.prenhall.com/kozier. Click on Chapter 23 to select the activities for this chapter.

CD-ROM
- Audio Glossary
- NCLEX Review

Companion Website
- Additional NCLEX Review
- Case Study: Developmental Phases of Adulthood
- Care Plan Activity: Parenting Responsibilities
- MediaLink Application: Developing a Health Promotion Program
- Links to Resources

The adult phase of development encompasses the years from the end of adolescence to death. Because the developmental tasks of young adults differ from those of older adults, adulthood is often divided into three phases: young adulthood, middle adulthood, and late adulthood. In this book, young adults are defined as people 20 to 40 years old; middle-aged adults, as 40 to 65; and older adults, over 65. This chapter applies the concepts of growth and development introduced in Chapter 21 ⚭ to the young adult, the middle-aged adult, and the older adult. Each developmental stage includes physical, psychosocial, cognitive, moral, and spiritual aspects. Also included are health problems and health assessment and promotion guidelines.

YOUNG ADULTS (20 TO 40 YEARS)

The age at which a person is considered an adult depends on how adulthood is described. Legally, a person in the United States can vote at 18 years. The legal age for alcohol consumption outside the home varies among states from 18 to 21 years. Another criterion of adulthood is financial independence, which is also highly variable. Some adolescents support themselves as early as 16 years of age, usually because of family circumstances. By contrast, some adults are financially dependent on their families for many years, for example, during prolonged periods of education.

Adulthood may also be indicated by moving away from home and establishing one's own living arrangements. Yet this independence also varies greatly. Some adolescents leave home because of family problems. In recent years, however, more young adults have been choosing to remain at home. In addition, many adults under 30 have returned to their parents' homes to live. The factors contributing to this trend include high housing costs, high divorce rates, high unemployment rates, and the many problems resulting from drug abuse. Some young people who are employed full time receive only minimum wage and are unable to earn enough money to be totally self-supporting.

Maturity is the state of maximal function and integration, or the state of being fully developed. Many other characteristics are generally recognized as representative of maturity. Mature individuals are guided by an underlying philosophy of life. They take many perspectives into account and are tolerant of the views of others. A comprehensive philosophy allows a person to make sense out of life and thus helps that person maintain a sense of purpose and hope in the face of human tragedies. Mature persons are open to new experiences and continued growth; they can tolerate ambiguity, are flexible, and can adapt to change. In addition, mature people have the quality of self-acceptance; they are able to be reflective and insightful about life and to see themselves as others see them. Mature persons also assume responsibility for themselves and expect others to do the same. They confront the tasks of life in a realistic and mature manner, make decisions, and accept responsibility for those decisions.

Young adults are typically busy people who face many challenges. They are expected to assume new roles at work, in the home, and in the community, and to develop interests, values, and attitudes related to these roles.

Physical Development

People in their early 20s are in their prime physical years. The musculoskeletal system is well developed and coordinated. This is the period when athletic endeavors reach their peak. All other systems of the body (e.g., cardiovascular, visual, auditory, and reproductive) are also functioning at peak efficiency.

Although physical changes are minimal during this stage, weight and muscle mass may change as a result of diet and exercise. In addition, extensive physical and psychosocial changes occur in pregnant and lactating women. These changes are discussed in maternal/child textbooks.

Psychosocial Development

In contrast to the minimal physical changes, psychosocial development of the young adult is great. Box 23–1 reviews this psychosocial development according to the theories of Freud, Erikson, and Havighurst.

Young adults face a number of new experiences and changes in lifestyle as they progress toward maturity. Choices must be made about education and employment, about whether to marry

<table>
<tr><td>

BOX 23-1 ■ **Psychosocial Development: Young Adult**

The young adult
- Is in the genital stage in which energy is directed toward attaining a mature sexual relationship, according to Freud's theory.
- Is in the intimacy versus isolation phase of Erikson's stages of development.
- Has the following developmental tasks, according to Havighurst:
  - Selecting a mate
  - Learning to live with a partner
  - Starting a family
  - Rearing children
  - Managing a home
  - Getting started in an occupation
  - Taking on civic responsibility
  - Finding a congenial social group.

</td></tr>
</table>

or remain single, about starting a home, and about rearing children. Social responsibilities include forming new friendships and assuming some community activities.

Occupational choice and education are largely inseparable. Education influences occupational opportunities; conversely, an occupation, once chosen, can determine the education needed and sought. Education enhances employment opportunities and usually ensures economic survival. As the role of women has changed, many women now choose to assume active careers and civic roles in society in addition to their roles as mother and/or wife (Figure 23–1 ■).

Remaining single is becoming the lifestyle of more and more young adults. Many people choose to remain single, perhaps to pursue an education and then to have the freedom to pursue their chosen vocation. Some unmarried individuals choose to live with another person of the opposite or same sex and share living arrangements and certain expenses. Some people who are gay or lesbian commit themselves legally to a partner as in marriage.

Although nontraditional lifestyles are becoming more acceptable in society, attitudes toward these various lifestyles can contribute social pressures that lead to stress responses. The multiple roles of adulthood (citizen, worker, taxpayer, homeowner, wife/husband, daughter/son, brother/sister, parent, friend, and so on) may also create stress as a result of role conflict.

Cognitive Development

Piaget believes that cognitive structures are complete during the *formal operations period,* from roughly 11 to 15 years. From that time, formal operations (for example, generating hypotheses) characterize thinking throughout adulthood and are applied to more areas. Egocentrism continues to decline; however, according to Piaget these changes do not involve a change in the structure of thought, only a change in its content and stability.

Recently, researchers in the field of psychology have suggested that Piaget's formal operational stage is not the last stage of human development. Some have proposed a concept of post-formal thought (Stuart-Hamilton, 2000, p. 84). *Postformal thought,* sometimes called the problem finding stage, is characterized by "creative thought in the form of discovered problems, relativistic thinking, the formation of generic problems, the raising of general questions from ill-defined problems, the use of intuition, insight, and hunches, and the development of significant scientific thought" (Murray & Zentner, 2001, p. 633). In addition to the adolescent ability to think in abstract terms, postformal thinkers possess an understanding of the temporary or relative nature of knowledge. They are able to comprehend and balance arguments created by both logic and emotion.

Moral Development

Young adults who have mastered the previous stages of Kohlberg's theory of moral development now enter the postconventional level. At this time, the person is able to separate self from the expectations and rules of others and to define morality in terms of personal principles. When individuals perceive a conflict with society's rules or laws, they judge according to their own principles. For example, a person may intentionally break the law and join a protest group to stop hunters from killing wild animals, believing that the principle of wildlife conservation justifies the protest action. This type of reasoning is called *principled reasoning.* See also Gilligan's ethic of care in Chapter 21. 🔗 Gilligan argues that as individuals approach young adulthood, men and women tend to define moral problems somewhat differently. Men often use an "ethic of justice" and define moral problems in terms of rules and rights. Women, by contrast, often define moral problems in terms of obligation to care and to avoid hurt.

Spiritual Development

According to Fowler, the individual enters the individuating-reflective period sometime after 18 years of age. During this period, the individual focuses on reality. A 27-year-old adult

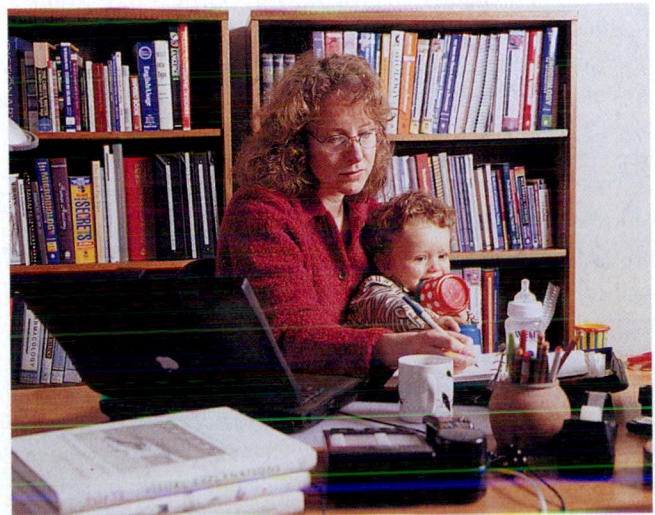

Figure 23–1 ■ Many young women combine active careers with motherhood.

may ask philosophic questions regarding spirituality and may be self-conscious about spiritual matters. The religious teaching that the young adult had as a child may now be accepted or redefined.

Health Problems

Young adulthood is generally a healthy time of life. Health problems that do occur and are common in this age group include accidents, suicide, substance abuse, hypertension, sexually transmitted disease (STD), abuse of women, and certain malignancies. Some of the problems such as accidents, substance abuse, and STDs are related to behaviors that could possibly be prevented through appropriate education and other primary prevention strategies.

Accidents

Healthy People 2010 (USDHHS, 2000) reports that leading causes of death differ among the various population groups. For example, unintentional injuries (primarily motor vehicle crashes) are the fifth leading cause of death for the total population but the leading cause of death for people aged 1 to 44 years (p. 21). Education about safety precautions and accident prevention is a major role of the nurse in promoting the health of young adults. For a further discussion of safety education for young adults, see Chapter 30. 🔗

Suicide

Suicide is the fifth leading cause of death among young adults in the United States (Murray & Zentner, 2001, p. 666). Many suicides may actually be mistaken for accidental death (automobile accidents, combining alcohol and barbiturates, or discharging a gun while cleaning it). Suicide may result from problems with close relationships such as those with marriage partners or parents, or from depression related to perceived occupational, academic, or financial failure. In general, suicide results from the young adult's inability to cope with the pressures, responsibilities, and expectations of adulthood.

The nurse's role in the prevention of suicide includes identifying behaviors that may indicate potential problems: depression; a variety of physical complaints, including weight loss, sleep disturbances, and digestive disorders; and decreased interest in social and work roles along with an increase in isolation. A young adult identified as at risk for suicide should be referred to a mental health professional or a crisis center. Nurses can also reduce the incidence of suicide by participating in educational programs that provide information about the early signs of suicide.

Hypertension

Hypertension is a major problem for young African American adults, particularly men. Many of the causes for this higher incidence of hypertension are unknown. In addition to biologic inheritance, contributing factors may include smoking, obesity, a high-sodium diet, and high stress levels. Hypertension is a major risk factor in the development of chronic heart disease or stroke (cerebrovascular accidents). Blood pressure measurements are usually advised at least every 2 years for young adults to screen for hypertension.

Substance Abuse

Substance abuse is a major threat to the health of young adults. Alcohol, marijuana, amphetamines, and cocaine, for example, can bring about feelings of well-being that may be highly valued by people with adjustment problems. Prolonged use can lead to physical and psychologic dependency and subsequent health problems. For example, drug abuse during pregnancy can lead to fetal damage. Prolonged use of alcohol can lead to such diseases as cirrhosis of the liver and cancer of the esophagus.

Nursing strategies related to drug abuse include teaching about the complications of their use, changing individual attitudes toward drug abuse, and counseling regarding problems that lead to drug abuse.

Smoking is another type of drug abuse that can lead to diseases such as lung cancer and cardiovascular disease. The nurse's role regarding smoking is to (a) serve as a role model by not smoking; (b) provide educational information regarding the dangers of smoking; (c) help make smoking socially unacceptable, for example, by posting No Smoking signs in client lounges and offices; and (d) suggest resources such as hypnosis, lifestyle training, and behavior modification to clients who desire to stop smoking.

Sexually Transmitted Disease

STDs such as genital herpes, AIDS, syphilis, and gonorrhea are common infections in young adults. Nursing functions are largely educational. The use of condoms greatly reduces the transfer of infectious microorganisms from one partner to another. Knowledge about the symptoms of these diseases can help the client obtain early treatment. In dealing with clients with an STD, the nurse must be nonjudgmental and accepting of the client's lifestyle and treat any information obtained as confidential (see Chapter 38). 🔗

Violence

Violence has spread throughout the United States and either claims lives or threatens the well-being of all ages of people. The youth are perpetrators and victims of violence. For example, *Healthy People 2010* (USDHHS, 2000) reports that homicide is the second leading cause of death for young persons aged 15 to 24 years and the leading cause of death for African Americans in this age group (pp. 15-45–15-46). The elderly, females, and children continue to be targets of both physical and sexual assaults.

Abuse of Women

The problem of battering or abuse of women affects families at all socioeconomic levels. Stresses that predispose families to abuse may include financial problems, separation from family and community support, and physical as well as social isolation. A nurse who works with women should (a) have open communication that will encourage them to share their problems; (b) help them to develop self-esteem that will enable them to have the courage to leave the violent situation; (c) provide information about resources, such as welfare and shelters, that will allow them to begin an alternative lifestyle; and (d) continue to support and educate the women so that they can understand the causes and results of abusive and violent behavior.

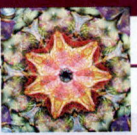

Developmental Assessment Guidelines

THE YOUNG ADULT

In these three developmental areas, does the young adult do the following?

Physical Development

- Exhibit weight within normal range for age and sex.
- Manifest vital signs (e.g., blood pressure) within normal range for age and sex.
- Demonstrate visual and hearing abilities within normal range.
- Exhibit appropriate knowledge (e.g., about sexually transmitted diseases) and attitudes about sexuality.

Psychosocial Development

- Feel independent from parents.
- Have a realistic self-concept.

- Like self and direction life is going.
- Interact well with family.
- Cope with the stresses of change and growth.
- Have well-established bonds with significant others, such as marriage partner or close friends.
- Have a meaningful social life.
- Demonstrate emotional, social, and economic responsibility for own life.
- Have a set of values that guide behavior.

Development in Activities of Daily Living

- Have a healthy lifestyle.

Malignancies

Testicular cancer is the most common neoplasm in men aged 20 to 34 (Barkauskas, Bauman, & Darling-Fisher, 2002). Testicular self-examination, a means of early identification of scrotal cancer, should be conducted monthly. For additional information, see Chapter 38.

Of all cancers among women, cancer of the breast is a leading cause of death. Breast cancer is rare under the age of 25 but the risk increases after the age of 30 (Murray & Zentner, 2001, p. 662). Young women need to form the habit of doing breast self-examinations once a month. For detailed information, see Chapter 38. The earlier a breast lump is discovered, the greater the effectiveness of treatment.

Young adult females should also be screened for cervical cancer by having a routine **Papanicolaou (Pap) test.** A Pap test is done by obtaining and examining cells from the uterine cervical os. The cells are obtained during a pelvic examination. For more information on the vaginal exam, see Chapter 28. The nurse should also screen for high-risk factors for cervical cancer:

sexual activity at an early age, multiple sexual partners, or a history of syphilis, herpes genitalis, or *Trichomonas vaginitis*. Many young adults are reluctant to have these examinations and screenings. Therefore, it is important for nurses to explain the purpose of the test and to encourage all young women to begin this preventive measure by age 20. See cancer screening guidelines in Chapter 28.

Health Assessment and Promotion

Assessment guidelines for the growth and development of the young adult are shown in the accompanying Developmental Assessment Guidelines.

Young adults are usually interested in meeting their health needs. However, because of the many stresses and changes that occur throughout this 20-year period, the nurse needs to offer teaching and guidance in several health care areas. The nurse may wish to discuss some or all of the health promotion topics outlined in Box 23–2. These topics are discussed in detail in subsequent chapters throughout the book.

BOX 23–2 ■ Health Promotion Guidelines for Young Adults

Health Tests and Screenings

- Routine physical examination (every 1 to 3 years for females; every 5 years for males)
- Immunizations as recommended, such as tetanus-diphtheria boosters
- Regular dental assessments (e.g., annually)
- Periodic vision and hearing screenings
- Breast self-examination monthly, 1 week after onset of period
- Professional breast examination every 1 to 3 years
- Papanicolaou smear annually or at onset of sexual activity
- Testicular self-examination every month
- Screening for cardiovascular disease (e.g., cholesterol test every 5 years if results are normal; blood pressure to detect hypertension; baseline electrocardiogram at age 35 for males)
- Tuberculosis skin test every 2 years

Safety

- Motor vehicle safety reinforcement (e.g., using designated drivers when drinking, maintaining brakes and tires)
- Sun protection measures
- Workplace safety measures
- Water safety reinforcement (e.g., no diving in shallow water)

Nutrition and Exercise

- Importance of adequate iron intake in diet
- Nutritional and exercise factors that may lead to cardiovascular disease (e.g., obesity, cholesterol and fat intake, lack of vigorous exercise)

Social Interactions

- Encouraging personal relationships that promote discussion of feelings, concerns, and fears
- Setting short- and long-term goals for work and career choices

MIDDLE-AGED ADULTS (40 TO 65 YEARS)

The middle years, from 40 to 65, have been called the years of stability and consolidation. For most people, it is a time when children have grown and moved away or are moving away from home. Thus partners generally have more time for and with each other and time to pursue interests they may have deferred for years (see Figure 23–2 ■).

Physical Development

A number of changes take place during the middle years. At 40, most adults can function as effectively as they did in their 20s. However, during ages 40 to 65 many physical changes take place. See Table 23–1 for a summary of these changes.

Both men and women experience decreasing hormonal production during the middle years. The **menopause** refers to the so-called "change of life" in women, when menstruation ceases. It is said to have occurred when a woman has not had a menstrual period within a year. The menopause usually occurs anywhere between ages 40 and 55. The average is about 47 years. At this time, ovarian activity declines until ovulation ceases. Common symptoms are hot flashes, chilliness, a tendency of the breasts to become smaller and flabby, and a tendency to gain weight. Insomnia and headaches also occur with relative frequency. Psychologically, the menopause can be an anxiety-producing time, especially if the ability to bear children is an integral part of the woman's self-concept.

The **climacteric** (andropause) refers to the change of life in men, when sexual activity decreases. In men there is no change comparable to the menopause in women. Androgen levels decrease very slowly; however, men can father children even in late life. The psychologic problems that men experience are generally related to the fear of getting old and to retirement, boredom, and finances. See Chapter 38 🔗 for further details about sexual health.

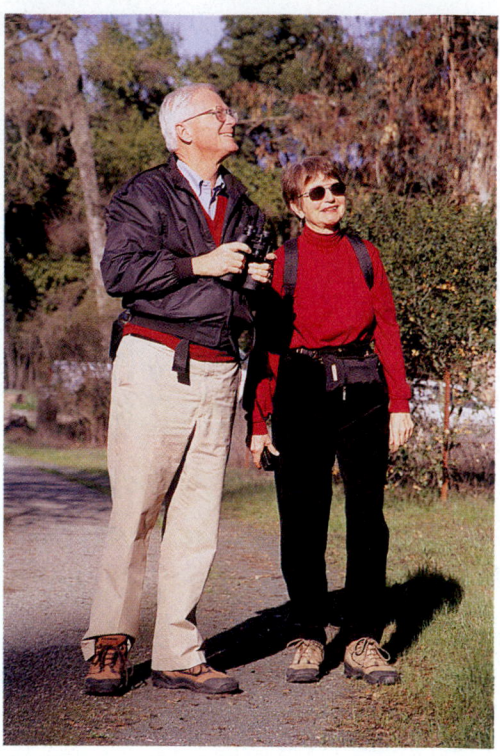

Figure 23–2 ■ Middle-aged adults have time to pursue interests that may have been put aside for child care.

Psychosocial Development

Before the mid-1900s, the developmental tasks of middle-aged adults received little attention. Havighurst outlines seven tasks for this age group (see Box 23–3). Erikson (1963, p. 266) views the developmental choice of the middle-aged adult as generativity versus stagnation. **Generativity** is defined as the concern for establishing and guiding the next generation. In other words, the concern about providing for the welfare of hu-

---

TABLE 23–1 Physical Changes of the Middle-Aged Adult

Category	Description
Appearance	Hair begins to thin, and gray hair appears. Skin turgor and moisture decrease, subcutaneous fat decreases, and wrinkling occurs. Fatty tissue is redistributed, resulting in fat deposits in the abdominal area.
Musculoskeletal system	Skeletal muscle bulk decreases at about age 60. Thinning of the intervertebral discs causes a decrease in height of about 1 inch. Calcium loss from bone tissue is more common among postmenopausal women. Muscle growth continues in proportion to use.
Cardiovascular system	Blood vessels lose elasticity and become thicker.
Sensory perception	Visual acuity declines, often by the late 40s, especially for near vision (presbyopia). Auditory acuity for high-frequency sounds also decreases (presbycusis), particularly in men. Taste sensations also diminish.
Metabolism	Metabolism slows, resulting in weight gain.
Gastrointestinal system	Gradual decrease in tone of large intestine may predispose the individual to constipation.
Urinary system	Nephron units are lost during this time, and glomerular filtration rate decreases.
Sexuality	Hormonal changes take place in both men and women.

BOX 23–3 ■ Psychosocial Development: Middle-Aged Adult

The middle-aged adult

■ Is in the generativity versus stagnation phase of Erikson's stages of development.

■ According to Havighurst, has the following developmental tasks:

• Achieving adult civic and social responsibility
• Establishing and maintaining an economic standard of living
• Assisting teenage children to become responsible and happy adults
• Developing adult leisure-time activities
• Relating oneself to one's spouse as a person
• Accepting and adjusting to the physiologic changes of middle age
• Adjusting to aging parents.

mankind is equal to the concern of providing for self. People in their 20s and 30s tend to be self- and family-centered. In middle age, the self seems more altruistic, and concepts of service to others and love and compassion gain prominence. These concepts motivate charitable and altruistic actions, such as church work, social work, political work, community fundraising drives, and cultural endeavors. Marriage partners have more time for companionship and recreation, thus marriage can be more satisfying in the middle years of life. Partners have time to work together in volunteer activities, and time for one partner to go out for lunch and for the other to go fishing. Generative middle-aged persons are able to feel a sense of comfort in their lifestyle and receive gratification from charitable endeavors.

Erikson believes that people who are unable to expand their interests at this time and who do not assume the responsibilities of middle age suffer a sense of boredom and impoverishment, that is, stagnation. These people have difficulty accepting their aging bodies and become withdrawn and isolated. They are preoccupied with self and unable to give to others. Some may regress to younger patterns of behavior, for example, adolescent behavior.

Robert Peck (1968) believes that although physical capabilities and functions decrease with age, mental and social capacities tend to increase in the latter part of life. Four sets of developmental tasks can be dealt with simultaneously during middle age (see Box 23–4).

The middle-aged person looks older and feels older. People usually accept the fact that they are aging; however, a few try to defy the years by changing their dress and even their actions. Some men and women have extramarital affairs and marry younger partners. A new freedom to be independent and follow one's individual interests arises. Prior to this period, the marriage partner or lover and other persons were crucial to a definition of self. Now the middle-aged person does not make comparisons with others, often no longer fears aging or death, relaxes the sense of competitiveness, and enjoys the independence and freedom of middle age. Other people's opinions become less important, and the earlier habit of trying to please everyone is overcome. The person establishes ethical and moral standards that are independent of the standards of others. The focus shifts from inner self and being to others and doing. Religious and philosophical concerns become important.

Gail Sheehy (1976) suggests that the transition into middle life is as critical as adolescence. She outlines characteristics of the midlife crisis and calls the decade between the ages of 35 to 45 the "deadline decade." According to Sheehy, most women pass through the midlife crisis between 35 and 40; most men, between 40 and 45. This crisis occurs when individuals recognize that they have reached the halfway mark of life. Although people of these ages are reaching their prime, they begin to recognize that time is at a premium and that life is finite. Youthfulness and physical strength can no longer be taken for granted.

Middle age can be viewed by the individual as either a crisis (a major and revolutionary turning point in one's life, involving

BOX 23–4 ■ Tasks of Middle Age

■ *Valuing wisdom versus physical power and attractiveness.* As individuals approach middle age, physical strength and attractiveness decline. It then becomes necessary to gain satisfaction and ego strength through mental and intellectual abilities. Middle-aged persons must learn to rely more on their wisdom and accumulated experiences than on their physical powers.

■ *Socializing versus sexualizing.* In middle age, people should begin to redefine their interpersonal relationships. It is no longer appropriate to relate to the opposite sex in terms of physical attractiveness; other criteria such as friendship, warmth, and understanding should be adopted.

■ *Emotional flexibility versus emotional rigidity.* This task concerns the ability to become flexible, such as being able to shift emotional investment from one person to another and from one task to another. During this phase of life, the children often leave home, and parents may die. Middle-aged adults must be able to develop new roles, socially and emotionally, or they may find themselves isolated.

■ *Mental flexibility versus mental rigidity.* Individuals often become set in their ways as they approach middle age. They may not seek new ideas or accept the novel solutions of others. To cope most effectively, however, middle-aged adults should strive to remain flexible in their thinking. The solutions of the past may not solve today's problems. New ideas and perspectives should be considered.

Note: From *Psychological Aspects of Aging: Proceedings from a Conference on Planning Research* (pp. 44–49), by J. E. Anderson (Ed.), 1965, Washington D.C.: American Psychological Association. Adapted with permission.

changes in commitments to career or spouse and children and accompanied by significant and ongoing emotional turmoil for both the individual and others) or as a transition from youth to later maturity (Murray & Zentner, 2001, p. 733).

Cognitive Development

The middle-aged adult's cognitive and intellectual abilities change very little. Cognitive processes include reaction time, memory, perception, learning, problem solving, and creativity. Reaction time during the middle years stays much the same or diminishes during the later part of the middle years. Memory and problem solving are maintained through middle adulthood. Learning continues and can be enhanced by increased motivation at this time in life.

Middle-aged adults are able to carry out all the strategies described in Piaget's phase of formal operations. Some may use postformal operations strategies to assist them in understanding the contradictions that exist in both personal and physical aspects of reality. The experiences of the professional, social, and personal life of middle-aged persons will be reflected in their cognitive performance. Thus approaches to problem solving and task completion will vary considerably in a middle-aged group. The middle-aged adult can "reflect on the past and current experience and can imagine, anticipate, plan and hope" (Murray & Zentner, 2001, p. 722).

Moral Development

According to Kohlberg, the adult can move beyond the conventional level to the postconventional level (see Chapter 21). Kohlberg believes that extensive experience of personal moral choice and responsibility is required before people can reach the postconventional level. Kohlberg found that few of his subjects achieved the highest level of moral reasoning. To move from stage 4, a law and order orientation, to stage 5, a social contract orientation, requires that the individual move to a stage in which rights of others take precedence. People in stage 5 take steps to support another's rights.

Spiritual Development

Not all adults progress through Fowler's stages to the fifth, called the paradoxical-consolidative stage. At this stage, the individual can view "truth" from a number of viewpoints. Fowler's fifth stage corresponds to Kohlberg's fifth stage of moral development. Fowler believes that only some individuals after the age of 30 years reach this stage.

In middle age, people tend to be less dogmatic about religious beliefs, and religion often offers more comfort to the middle-aged person than it did previously. People in this age group often rely on spiritual beliefs to help them deal with illness, death, and tragedy.

Health Problems

Many middle-aged adults remain healthy; however, the risk of developing a health problem is greater than that of the young adult. Leading causes of death in this age group include motor

vehicle and occupational accidents, chronic disease such as cancer, and cardiovascular disease. Lifestyle patterns in combination with aging, family history, and developmental stressors (e.g., menopause, climacteric) and situational stressors (e.g., divorce) are often related to health problems that do arise. For example, smoking and excessive alcohol consumption place an individual at greater risk of developing chronic respiratory problems, lung cancer, and liver disease. Overeating can result in obesity, diabetes mellitus, atherosclerosis, and its associated risk for hypertension and coronary artery disease. The nurse can play an important role in teaching middle-aged clients about preventive health care to avoid or minimize the risk of such health problems.

Accidents

Changing physiologic factors, as well as concern over personal and work-related responsibilities, may contribute to the accident rate of middle-aged people. Motor vehicle accidents are the most common cause of accidental death in this age group. Decreased reaction times and visual acuity may make the middle-aged adult prone to accidents. Other accidental causes of death for middle-aged adults include falls, fires, burns, poisonings, and drownings. Occupational accidents continue to be a significant safety hazard during the middle years. Safety highlights for the middle-aged adult are presented in Chapter 30.

Cancer

Cancer accounts for considerable mortality and morbidity in both men and women. It is the second leading cause of death among people between the ages of 25 and 64 in the United States. The patterns of cancer types and incidences for men and women have changed during the past several decades. Men have a high incidence of cancer of the lung and bladder. In women, breast cancer is highest in incidence, followed by cancer of the colon and rectum, uterus, and lung. The incidence of lung cancer is increasing in women.

Female clients may need to be reminded to perform monthly breast self-examinations and male clients to perform monthly testicular self-examinations in order to detect growths. Postmenopausal women should report any vaginal bleeding.

Cardiovascular Disease

Coronary heart disease (CHD) is the leading cause of death in the United States. Several factors contribute to risk of CHD. These include smoking, obesity, hypertension, hyperlipidemia, diabetes mellitus, sedentary lifestyle, a family history of myocardial infarction or sudden death in a father less than 55 years old or in a mother less than 65 years old, and the individual's age. Men over 45 years of age and women over 55 years of age are at greater risk of developing CHD than younger adults. Physical inactivity places individuals at greater risk of developing CHD than any other factor (Edelman & Mandle, 2002, p. 323).

Obesity

Middle-aged adults who gain weight may not be aware of some common facts about this age period. Decreased metabolic ac-

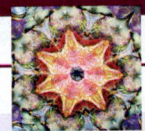

Developmental Assessment Guidelines

THE MIDDLE-AGED ADULT

In these three developmental areas, does the middle-aged adult do the following?

Physical Development

- Exhibit weight within normal range for age and sex.
- Manifest vital signs (e.g., blood pressure) within normal range for age and sex.
- Manifest visual and hearing abilities within normal range.
- Exhibit appropriate knowledge and attitudes about sexuality (e.g., about menopause).
- Verbalize any changes in eating, elimination, or exercise.

Psychosocial Development

- Accept aging body.

- Feel comfortable and respect self.
- Enjoy new freedom to be independent.
- Accept changes in family roles (e.g., having teenaged children and aging parents).
- Interact well and share companionable activities with life partner.
- Expand and renew previous interests.
- Pursue charitable and altruistic activities.
- Have a meaningful philosophy of life.

Development in Activities of Daily Living

- Follow preventive health practice.

---

tivity and decreased physical activity mean a decrease in caloric need. The nurse's role in nutritional health promotion is to counsel clients to prevent obesity by reducing caloric intake and participating in regular exercise. Clients should also be warned that being overweight is a risk factor for many chronic diseases such as diabetes and hypertension and for problems of mobility such as arthritis. Clients should seek medical advice before considering any major changes in their diets.

Alcoholism

The excessive use of alcohol can result in unemployment, disrupted homes, accidents, and diseases. It is estimated that 4 million people in the United States are dependent on alcohol and can be considered alcoholics. Nurses can help clients by providing information about the dangers of excessive alcohol use, by helping the individual clarify values about health, and by referring the client to special groups such as Alcoholics Anonymous.

Mental Health Alterations

Developmental stressors, such as the menopause, the climacteric, aging, and impending retirement, and situational stressors, such as divorce, unemployment, and death of a spouse, can precipitate increased anxiety and depression in middle-aged adults. Clients may benefit from support groups or individual therapy to help them cope with specific crises.

Health Assessment and Promotion

Assessment guidelines for the growth and development of the middle-aged adult are shown in the accompanying Developmental Assessment Guidelines. Middle-aged adults usually take care of their health needs and are interested in maintaining health and preventing the acceleration of the aging process.

The nurse may choose to discuss some or all of the health promotion topics with the middle-aged adult client (see Box 23–5).

These topics are discussed in detail in subsequent chapters throughout the book.

OLDER ADULTS (OVER 65 YEARS)

Older adults are the fastest growing group in the United States today. In 2000, 35 million people 65 and older were counted in the United States, which represents a 12% increase since 1990. The greatest percentage increase occurred in the oldest age group. The 85-year-olds and over increased by 38%. In addition, the percent of people 65 years and older living in nursing homes declined from 5.1% in 1990 to 4.5% in 2000 (Hetzel & Smith, 2001).

Various systems are used to categorize the aging population (see Box 23–6). Another term used to describe the "old-old" or "extreme aged" is *frail elderly*. **Frail elderly,** however, is more likely to be used to describe the elder individual who has significant physiologic and functional impairment, whatever the age.

In the past century, scientists have postulated theories of why people age. More recently, as both the absolute number and the population percentage of elders increase, there is renewed scientific interest in why people age, how people age, and what factors affect the physical, psychologic, and functional status of older persons. Biologic theories of aging are either intrinsic or extrinsic. Extrinsic theory encompasses factors in the environment; intrinsic theory addresses factors within the body. Table 23–2 describes the various biologic theories of aging.

Physical Changes

As the person ages, a number of physical changes occur; some are visible, some are not. In general, lean body mass is reduced and fat tissue increases until around age 60. Bone mass decreases. Extracellular fluid remains constant, however, intracellular fluid decreases and leads to reduced total body fluid.

BOX 23–5	■ Health Promotion Guidelines for Middle-Aged Adults

Health Tests and Screening

- Routine physical examination (annually for females; every 2 to 3 years or as directed by physician for males)
- Immunizations as recommended, such as a tetanus booster every 10 years and influenza and pneumococcal vaccinations
- Regular dental assessments (e.g., yearly)
- Tonometry for signs of glaucoma and other eye diseases every 2 to 3 years or annually if indicated
- Breast self-examination as for young adults and first day of every month after menopause
- Testicular self-examination monthly
- Screenings for cardiovascular disease (e.g., blood pressure measurement; electrocardiogram and cholesterol test as directed by the physician)
- Screenings for colorectal, breast, cervical, uterine, and prostate cancer (see cancer screening guidelines in Chapter 28) 🔗
- Screening for tuberculosis every 2 years

Safety

- Motor vehicle safety reinforcement, especially when driving at night

- Workplace safety measures
- Home safety measures: keeping hallways and stairways lighted and uncluttered, using smoke detectors, using nonskid mats and hand rails in the bathrooms

Nutrition and Exercise

- Importance of adequate protein, calcium, and vitamin D in diet
- Nutritional and exercise factors that may lead to cardiovascular disease (e.g., obesity, cholesterol and fat intake, lack of vigorous exercise)
- An exercise program that emphasizes skill and coordination

Social Interactions

- The possibility of a midlife crisis: encourage discussion of feelings, concerns, and fears
- Providing time to expand and review previous interests
- Retirement planning (financial and possible diversional activities), with partner if appropriate

---

BOX 23–6	■ Categorizing the Aging Population

- Young-old: 65 to 75 years
- Old: 75 to 85 years
- Old-old: 85 to 100 years
- Elite old: Over 100 years

Note: From *Gerontological Nursing,* 5th ed. (p. 14), by C. Eliopoulos, 2001, Philadelphia: Lippincott, Williams & Wilkins. Reprinted with permission.

Thus, elders are at risk for developing dehydration (Eliopoulos, 2001). Table 23–3 on page 404 provides a summary of the normal physical changes associated with aging.

Integument

Obvious changes occur in the integumentary system (skin, hair, nails) with age. The skin becomes drier and more fragile, the hair loses color, the fingernails and toenails become thickened and brittle, and in women over 60, facial hair increases.

Responses to these changes vary among individuals and cultures. For example, one person may feel distinguished with gray hair, whereas another may feel embarrassed or depressed, interpreting gray hair as a sign of losing one's youth.

These integumentary changes accompany progressive losses of subcutaneous fat and muscle tissue, muscle atrophy, and loss of elastic fiber, resulting in a "double" chin, sagging of eyelids and earlobes, and wrinkling of skin, especially in areas exposed to sun. Bony prominences become visible. In older women, the breasts become smaller and may sag; if large and pendulous, they may cause chafing where the skin surfaces touch. Loss of subcutaneous fat also decreases elders tolerance of cold.

Neuromusculoskeletal

With aging comes gradual reduction in the speed and power of skeletal or voluntary muscle contractions and sustained muscular effort. Exercise can strengthen weakened muscles, and up to about age 50 the skeletal muscles can increase in bulk and density. After that time there is a steady decrease in muscle fibers, ultimately leading to the typical wasted appearance of the very old person. Thus elders often complain about their lack of strength and how quickly they tire. Activities can still be carried out, but at a slower pace. Often balance is impaired with age. Prolonged muscle efforts may be sustained by older people provided they take judicious rest pauses and avoid capacity or peak performance.

The person's reaction time slows with age. Reaction time can be delayed further by decreased muscle tone as a result of diminished physical activity. Elders compensate for this reaction difference by being exceptionally cautious, for instance, in their driving habits, which exasperates some impatient young drivers.

Slight loss in overall stature occurs with age. This can be exaggerated by muscular weakness resulting in a stooping posture and **kyphosis** (humpback of the upper spine). **Osteoporosis,** a decrease in bone density, along with increased brittleness of bone make the elders prone to serious fractures, some of which may be spontaneous and are called **pathologic fractures.** Osteoporosis occurs more frequently in people with insufficient intake of dietary calcium, in women after menopause, and in individuals who are immobilized or physically inactive. Often considered a woman's disease, it is important to remember that osteoporosis affects men also (Curry & Hogstel, 2002).

Some degenerative joint changes occur, making movement stiffer and more restricted. Stiffness is aggravated by inactiv-

TABLE 23–2 Common Biologic Theories of Aging

Theory Type	Hypotheses
Wear-and-tear theories	Proposes that humans, like automobiles, have vital parts that run down with time, leading to aging and death.
	Proposes that the faster an organism lives, the quicker it dies.
	Proposes that cells wear out through exposure to internal and external stressors, including trauma, chemicals, and buildup of natural wastes.
Endocrine theory	Proposes that events occurring in the hypothalamus and pituitary are responsible for changes in hormone production and response that result in the organism's decline.
Free-radical theory	Proposes that unstable free radicals (groups of atoms) result from the oxidation of organic materials, such as carbohydrates and proteins. These radicals cause biochemical changes in the cells, and the cells cannot regenerate themselves.
Genetic theories	Proposes that the organism is genetically programmed for a predetermined number of cell divisions, after which the cells/organism dies.
	Proposes that when damage to the protein synthesis occurs, faulty proteins will be synthesized and will gradually accumulate, causing a progressive decline in the organism.
Cross-linking theories	Proposes that the irreversible aging of proteins such as collagen is responsible for the ultimate failure of tissues and organs.
	Proposes that as cells age, chemical reactions create strong bonds, or cross-linkages, between proteins. These bonds cause loss of elasticity, stiffness, and eventual loss of function.
Immune theories	Proposes that the immune system becomes less effective with age, and viruses that have incubated in the body become able to damage body organs.
	Proposes that a decrease in immune function may result in an increase in autoimmune responses, causing the body to produce antibodies that attack itself.

ity; for example, if a person sits too long, the joints become stiff, and the person has difficulty standing and walking. A continual program of physical activity and proper nutrition will slow bone density loss and decrease muscle atrophy and stiffness (see Figure 23–3 ■).

Sensory/Perceptual

Each of the five senses becomes less efficient in older adulthood. Changes in vision associated with aging include the obvious changes around the eye, such as the shrunken appearance of the eyes due to loss of orbital fat, the slowed blink reflex, and the looseness of the eyelids, particularly the lower lid, due to poorer muscle tone. Other changes result in loss of visual acuity, less power of adaptation to darkness and dim light, decrease in accommodation to near and far objects, loss of peripheral vision, and difficulty in discriminating similar colors, especially blues, greens, and purples.

By the age of 80 all elders have some lens opacity **(cataracts)** that reduces visual acuity and causes glare to be a problem. Surgical removal of cataracts is common at this age. Changes in the ciliary muscles, which control the shape of the lens, reduce the power of the lens to adjust to near and far vision. The diameter of the pupil is reduced, and the amount of light entering the eye is thereby restricted. This slows the reaction time to decreases in light or illumination, a problem compounded with driving at night. Diminished retinal function and reduced peripheral vision also occur.

The loss of hearing ability related to aging, called **presbycusis,** affects people over age 65. Gradual loss of hearing is more common among men than women, perhaps because men are more frequently in noisy work environments. Hearing loss is greater in the higher frequencies than the lower. Thus older adults with hearing loss usually hear speakers with low, distinct voices best. Elders may have more difficulty compensating for hearing loss than the young, who pay closer attention to the lip movements of the speaker.

Older people have a poorer sense of taste and smell and are less stimulated by food than the young. This change significantly affects appetite in the older adult, contributing to poor nutrition. Decreased or absent sense of smell and taste also add to the health hazard of increased salt usage and safety issues (e.g., can't smell a gas leak).

Loss of skin receptors takes place gradually, producing an increased threshold for sensations of pain, touch, and temperature. The older person may not be able to distinguish hot from cold or the intensity of heat. Stimuli causing severe pain in a younger person may cause only minor sensation or pressure in elders. This places the older adult at higher risk for burns and other injuries.

Pulmonary

Respiratory efficiency is reduced with age. The person inhales a smaller volume of air because of the musculoskeletal changes in the chest wall that reduce the size of the chest. A greater volume of residual air is left in the lungs after expiration, and the capacity to cough efficiently decreases because of weaker expiratory muscles. Mucous secretions tend to collect more readily in the respiratory tree. Thus susceptibility to

TABLE 23-3 Normal Physical Changes Associated with Aging

Physical Changes	Rationale
Integumentary	
Increased skin dryness	Decrease in sebaceous gland activity and tissue fluid
Increased skin pallor	Decreased vascularity
Increased skin fragility	Reduced thickness and vascularity of the dermis; loss of subcutaneous fat
Progressive wrinkling and sagging of the skin	Loss of skin elasticity, increased dryness, and decreased subcutaneous fat
Brown "age spots" (lentigo senilus) on exposed body parts (e.g., face, hands, arms)	Clustering of melanocytes (pigment-producing cells)
Decreased perspiration	Reduced number and function of sweat glands
Thinning and graying of scalp, pubic, and axillary hair	Progressive loss of pigment cells from the hair bulbs
Slower nail growth and increased thickening with ridges	Increased calcium deposition
Neuromuscular	
Decreased speed and power of skeletal muscle contractions	Decrease in muscle fibers
Slowed reaction time	Diminished conduction speed of nerve fibers and decreased muscle tone
Loss of height (stature)	Atrophy of intervertebral discs
Osteoporosis	Bone demineralization
Joint stiffness	Deterioration of joint cartilage
Impaired balance	Decreased muscle reaction time and coordination
Sensory/perceptual	
Loss of visual acuity	Degeneration leading to lens opacity (cataracts), thickening, and inelasticity (presbyopia)
Increased sensitivity to glare and decreased ability to adjust to darkness	Changes in the ciliary muscles; rigid pupil sphincter; decrease in pupil size
Partial or complete glossy white circle around the periphery of the cornea (arcus senilis)	Fatty deposits
Progressive loss of hearing	Changes in the structures and nerve tissues in the (presbycusis) inner ear; thickening of the eardrum
Decreased sense of taste, especially the sweet sensations at the tip of the tongue	Decreased number of taste buds in the tongue because of tongue atrophy
Decreased sense of smell	Atrophy of the olfactory bulb at the base of the brain (responsible for smell perception)
Increased threshold for sensations of pain, touch, and temperature	Possible nerve conduction and neuron changes
Pulmonary	
Decreased ability to expel foreign or accumulated matter	Decreased elasticity and ciliary activity
Decreased lung expansion, less effective exhalation, reduced vital capacity, and increased residual volume	Weakened thoracic muscles; calcification of costal cartilage, making the rib cage more rigid; dilation from inelasticity of alveoli
Difficult, short, heavy, rapid breathing (dyspnea) following intense exercise	Diminished delivery and diffusion of oxygen to the tissues to repay the normal oxygen debt because of exertion or changes in both respiratory and vascular tissues
Cardiovascular	
Reduced cardiac output and stroke volume, particularly during increased activity or unusual demands; may result in shortness of breath on exertion and pooling of blood in the extremities	Increased rigidity and thickness of heart valves (hence decreased filling/emptying abilities); decreased contractile strength
Reduced elasticity and increased rigidity of arteries	Increased calcium deposits in the muscular layer
Increase in diastolic and systolic blood pressure	Inelasticity of systemic arteries and increased peripheral resistance
Orthostatic hypertension	Reduced sensitivity of the blood pressure–regulating baroreceptors

TABLE 23–3 Normal Physical Changes Associated with Aging (continued)

Physical Changes	Rationale
Gastrointestinal	
Delayed swallowing time	Alterations in the swallowing mechanism
Increased tendency for indigestion	Gradual decrease in digestive enzymes, reduction in gastric pH, and slower absorption rate
Increased tendency for constipation	Decreased muscle tone of the intestines; decreased peristalsis
Urinary	
Reduced filtering ability of the kidney and impaired renal function	Decreased number of functioning nephrons (basic functional units of the kidney) and arteriosclerotic changes in blood flow
Less effective concentration of urine	Decreased tubular function
Urinary urgency and urinary frequency	Enlarged prostate gland in men; weakened muscles supporting the bladder or weakness of the urinary sphincter in women
Tendency for a nocturnal frequency and retention of residual urine	Decreased bladder capacity and tone
Genitals	
Prostate enlargement (benign) in men	Exact mechanism is unclear; possible endocrine changes
Multiple changes in women (shrinkage and atrophy of the vulva, cervix, uterus, fallopian tubes, and ovaries; reduction in secretions; and changes in vaginal flora)	Diminished secretion of female hormones and more alkaline vaginal pH

respiratory infections increases in elders. **Dyspnea** (difficult breathing) occurs frequently with increased activity, such as running for a bus or carrying heavy parcels upstairs.

Cardiovascular

The working capacity of the heart diminishes with age. This is particularly evident when increased demands are made on the heart muscles, such as during periods of exercise or emotional stress. The heart rate at normal rest may decrease with age. However, the heart rate of the older person is slow to respond to stress and slow to return to normal after periods of physical activity.

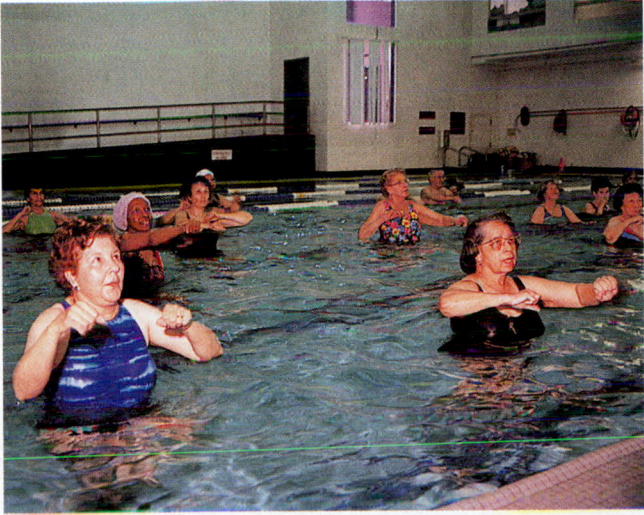

Figure 23–3 ■ A regular program of exercise is important for maintenance of joint mobility and muscle tone and can promote socialization.

Changes in the arteries occur concurrently. Reduced arterial elasticity may result in diminished blood supply to, for instance, the legs and the brain, resulting in pain on exertion in the calf muscles and dizziness, respectively. In addition, there may be a delay in the circulatory adjustments required when a person quickly stands up from a lying position. The delay results in an abrupt drop in systolic blood pressure known as *orthostatic hypotension.*

For blood pressure measurements, it is not unusual to have a slight increase in the systolic pressure while the diastolic pressure remains the same. A significant increase in blood pressure is more the result of other factors such as diet, weight, or stress rather than age (Polan & Taylor, 2003, p. 231).

Gastrointestinal

The digestive system is also impaired by aging. Gradual decreases in digestive enzymes occur; examples are ptyalin in salivary secretions, which converts starch; pepsin and trypsin, which digest protein; and lipase, a fat-splitting enzyme.

There is also a decrease in the number of absorbing cells in the intestinal tract and a reduction in gastric pH. These factors lower the absorption rate, slowing the absorption of nutrients and drugs. The muscle tone of the intestines also decreases, causing a decrease in peristalsis and elimination. These changes in muscle tone, digestive juices, and intestinal activity may lead to indigestion and constipation in the older adult.

Urinary

The excretory function of the kidney diminishes with age, but usually not significantly below normal levels unless a disease process intervenes. The kidney's filtering abilities may also be impaired; thus waste products may be filtered and excreted more slowly.

Research Note
Are There Health Barriers to Physical Activity in the Elderly?

In a recent study, 212 participants, aged 60 to 80, were initiated in a nurse-managed walking program (Cooper, Bilbrew, Dubbert, Karr, & Kirschner, 2001). Self- and interviewer-administered instruments and observations of performance during walking were used to assess potential barriers to physical activity. Results showed that pain, fatigue, mobility problems, and sensory impairments were significant barriers to their participation in walking. Self-perception of their health was high—35.8% described their health as very good and 42.5% as good. Variables not included in this study, but suggested for future studies were life experiences, changes in cognitive function and mental health, and self-perception.

Interventions recommended to help overcome these barriers included the following:

- Organize work and activities to balance rest and activity.
- Exercise on alternate days to give joints and muscles time to rest and recuperate.
- Use assistive devices, such as canes and walkers as needed.
- Walk in a safe and well-lighted area and on a smooth surface.
- Walk with a companion or group.

Implications: Promoting health and fitness in this age group is important to physical health and mental well-being. If the types of barriers can be identified, then appropriate interventions can be implemented to try to overcome these barriers and safely increase physical activity. Maintenance of physical activity decreases the risk for osteoporosis and falls, decreases peripheral resistance and insulin resistance, and helps to maintain mobility.

Note: From "Health Barriers to Walking for Exercise in Elderly Primary Care," by K. Cooper, D. Bilbrew, P. Dubbert, K. Karr, and K. Kirschner, *Geriatric Nursing, 22,* pp. 258–262 © 2001, with permission from Elsevier.

More noticeable changes are those related to the bladder. Complaints of urinary urgency and urinary frequency are common. The capacity of the bladder and its ability to completely empty diminish with age. Many elders need to arise during the night to void (nocturnal frequency) and may experience retention of residual urine, predisposing the elderly adult to bladder infections.

Genitals

Degenerative changes in the gonads are gradual in men. Production of testosterone continues, and the testes can produce sperm well into old age although there is a gradual decrease in the number of sperm produced. In women the degenerative changes in the ovaries are noticed by the abrupt cessation of menses in middle age during the menopause.

Changes in the gonads of older women result from diminished secretion of the ovarian hormones. Some changes, such as the shrinking of the uterus and ovaries, go unnoticed. Other changes are obvious. The breasts atrophy, and lubricating vagi-

nal secretions are reduced. Reduced natural lubrication is the cause of painful intercourse, which often necessitates the use of lubricating jellies.

Psychosocial Development

A number of theories explain psychosocial aging. According to **disengagement theory,** aging involves mutual withdrawal (disengagement) between the older person and others in the elderly person's environment. This withdrawal relieves the older person of some of society's pressures and gradually reduces the number of people with whom the older person interacts. According to **activity theory,** the best way to age is to stay active physically and mentally, and according to **continuity theory,** people maintain their values, habits, and behavior in old age. A person who is accustomed to having people around will continue to do so, and the person who prefers not to be involved with others is more likely to disengage. This theory accounts for the great variety of behavior seen in elderly people (see Figure 23–4 ■).

According to Erikson, the developmental task at this time is ego integrity versus despair. People who attain ego integrity view life with a sense of wholeness and derive satisfaction from past accomplishments. They view death as an acceptable completion of life. According to Erikson (1963), people who develop integrity accept "one's one and only life cycle" (p. 263). By contrast, people who despair often believe they have made poor choices during life and wish they could live life over.

Acknowledging that the "young-old" and "old-old" differ not only in physical characteristics but also in psychosocial responses, many people have difficulty with Erikson's singular developmental task. Peck (1968) proposes the following three developmental tasks of the older adult in contrast to Erikson's task of ego integrity versus despair:

1. Ego differentiation versus work-role preoccupation
2. Body transcendence versus body preoccupation
3. Ego transcendence versus ego preoccupation.

For details about these tasks see Chapter 21. See Box 23–7 for further developmental tasks of the older adult.

Retirement

Today, a majority of the people over age 65 are unemployed. However, many who are healthy continue to work on a full- or part-time basis. Work offers these people a better income, a sense of self-worth, and the chance to continue long-established routines. Some need to work for economic reasons.

Retirement can be a time when projects or recreational activities deferred for a long time can be pursued (see Figure 23–5 ■). Retired people are no longer governed by an alarm clock and can get up when they please. The enjoyment of staying up later is another luxury. Few elders however, spend much time resting or sleeping. Being accustomed to activity most of their lives, most elders find many outlets, including jobs, community projects, travel, volunteer services, intellectual or recreational pursuits, or hobbies (Figure 23–6 ■).

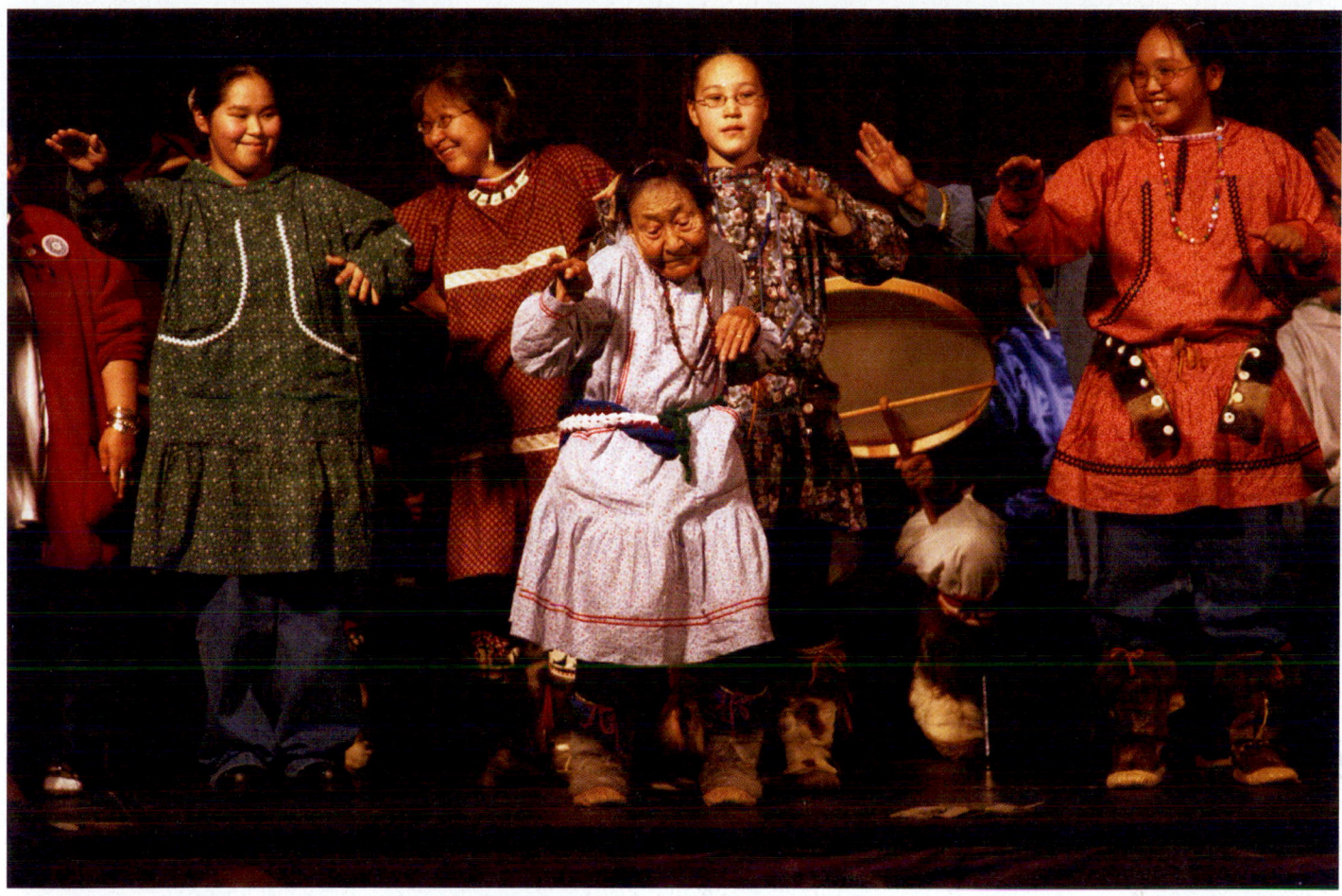

Figure 23–4 ■ Three generations of Alaskan Native American women dancing. The feeling of community provides socialization and support systems for many cultures. (Erik Hill/Anchorage Daily News.)

BOX 23–7	■ Developmental Tasks of the Older Adult

65 to 75 years
- Adjusting to decreasing physical strength and health
- Adjusting to retirement and lower and fixed income
- Adjusting to the death of parents, spouses and friends
- Adjusting to new relationships with adult children
- Adjusting to leisure time
- Adjusting to slower physical and cognitive responses
- Keeping active and involved
- Making satisfying living arrangements as aging progresses

75 years and older
- Adapting to living alone
- Safeguarding physical and mental health
- Adjusting to the possibility of moving into a nursing home
- Remaining in touch with other family members
- Finding meaning in life
- Adjusting to one's own death

Note: From *Readings in Gerontology,* 2nd ed., by M. Brown, 1978, St. Louis, MO: Mosby, *Gerontological Nursing,* 2nd ed., by M. Stanley & P.G. Beare, 1999, Philadelphia: F. A. Davis; *Health Promotion Strategies Through the Life Span,* 7th ed, by R. B. Murray & J. P. Zentner, 2001, Upper Saddle River, NJ: Prentice Hall.

The lifestyle of later years is to a large degree formulated in youth. This fact was recognized by the poet Robert Browning: "Grow old along with me! / The best is yet to be, / The last of life, for which the first was made." People who attempt suddenly to refocus and enrich their lives at retirement usually have difficulty. Those who learned early in life to live well-balanced and fulfilling lives are generally more successful in retirement. The woman who has been concerned only with the accomplishments of her children or the man who has been concerned only with the paycheck and his job status can be left with a feeling of emptiness when children leave and the job no longer exists. The later years can foster a sense of integrity and continuity, or they can be years of despair.

Economic Change

The financial needs of elders vary considerably. Though most need less money for clothing, entertainment, and work, and although some own their homes outright, costs continue to rise, making it difficult for some to manage. Food and medical costs alone are often a financial burden. Adequate financial resources enable the older person to remain independent.

Problems with income are often related to low retirement benefits, lack of pension plans for many workers, and the increased

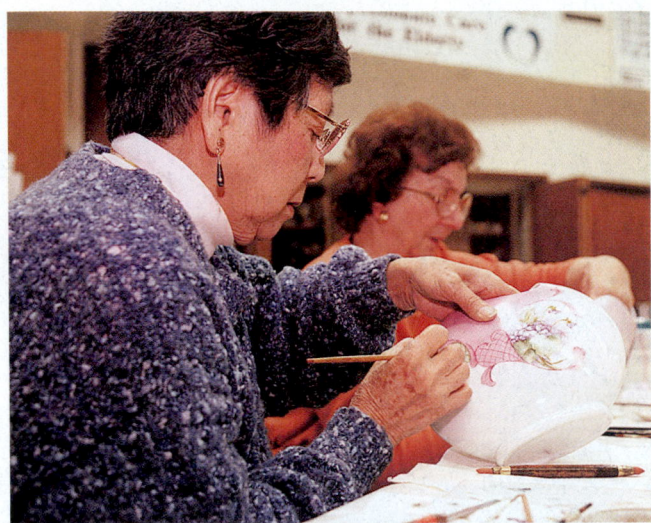

Figure 23–5 ■ Many elders find creative outlets during retirement.

length of the retirement years. Older members of minority groups often have greater financial problems than older whites. Older women of all ages usually have lower incomes than men, and the oldest women may be the poorest.

Nurses should be aware of the costs of health care. For example, while assisting a client to plan a diet, the nurse must consider which foods the client can afford to buy. The nurse or the client can request the physician to order lower priced medications. In addition, the supplies used in a client's care should be as economical as possible.

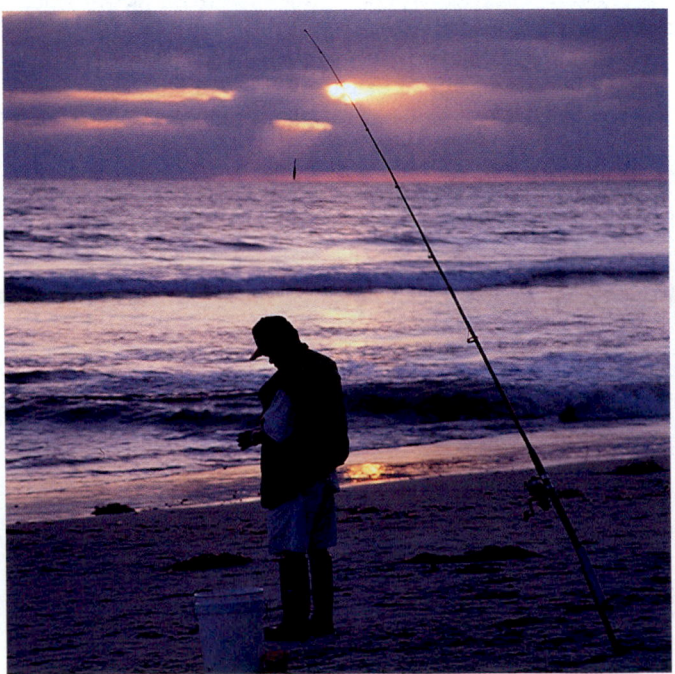

Figure 23–6 ■ Retirement provides time for enjoying hobbies.

Relocation

During late adulthood, many people experience relocation. A variety of factors may lead to this decision. The house or apartment may be too large or too expensive. The work involved in maintaining the house may become burdensome or impossible for the aged person or couple. Some elders with decreased mobility want living arrangements that are all on one floor or need more accessible bathroom facilities.

Making the decision to move is often stressful. The elder may be moving to an apartment, which may mean leaving the comfort of the family home and the neighbors and friends of several decades. Some need to move nearer to their children for general support and supervision. For many, this decision is difficult and stressful. For others, relocation is voluntary. The person may be seeking a more moderate climate with better recreational facilities geared to a more leisurely lifestyle. Adjustment will be much easier for the elder making a voluntary move.

More living choices and options are available for the older adult today. Depending on their needs, examples include:

- *Assisted living.* This is a facility that meets the needs of the older person (e.g., wide doorways, grab bars in the bathroom, a call light). Various degrees of personal care assistance may be provided.
- *Adult day care.* The older adult who lives at home can attend a day-care center that provides health and social services to the older person. While the older adult is at day care, the caregiver has a respite from the daily care.
- *Adult foster care and group homes.* These programs offer services to individuals who can care for themselves but require some form of supervision for safety purposes.

Some elders however, must relocate to long-term care facilities or nursing homes. The decision to enter a nursing home is frequently made when elders can no longer care for themselves, often because of problems of mobility and memory impairment. The facilities in nursing homes differ in many ways and offer varying degrees of independence to the residents. All provide meals but vary in giving other services, such as assistance with hygiene and dressing, physical therapy or exercise, recreational activities, transportation services, and medical and nursing supervision.

Nurses in hospitals should find out whether a client is being discharged to a nursing home or to a private home. Many nursing homes provide nursing services to clients and require appropriate information to provide for continuity of care. Clients returning home, however, may require the assistance of a home care nurse.

Maintaining Independence and Self-Esteem

Most elders thrive on independence. It is important to them to be able to look after themselves even if they have to struggle to do so. Although it may be difficult for younger family members to watch an older person completing tasks in a slow, determined way, aging people need this sense of accomplishment.

Children might notice that the aging father or mother with failing vision cannot keep the kitchen as clean as before. The aging parent may be slower and less meticulous in carpentry tasks or gardening. To maintain the older adult's sense of self-respect, nurses and family members need to encourage them to do as much as possible for themselves, provided that safety is maintained. Many young people err in thinking that they are helpful to older people when they take over for them and do the job much faster and more efficiently.

Aging people need to be recognized for their unique individual characteristics. It can be difficult to recognize these differences because elders have less energy than the young to show how they are different. Perhaps this is one reason elders tend to talk about past accomplishments, jobs, deeds, and experiences.

Nurses need to acknowledge the older client's ability to think, reason, and make decisions. Most elders are willing to listen to suggestions and advice, but they do not want to be ordered around. The nurse can support a decision by an elder even if eventually the decision is reversed because of failing health.

Older people appreciate thoughtfulness, consideration, and acceptance of their waning abilities. For example, having dinner out in a well-lighted restaurant or not expecting grandmother to baby-sit for too many hours, if at all, are actions that recognize the diminished vision and energy of older people. The values and standards held by older people need to be accepted, whether they are related to ethical, religious, or household matters. For example, respect an older person's decision to hang the laundry outside rather than to use a dryer or to cook on a conventional stove rather than in a microwave oven.

Facing Death and Grieving

Well-adjusted aging couples usually thrive on companionship. Many couples rely increasingly on their mates for this company and may have few outside friends. Great bonds of affection and closeness can develop during this period of aging together and nurturing each other. When a mate dies, the remaining partner inevitably experiences feelings of loss, emptiness, and loneliness. Many are capable of living alone and can manage to do so; however, reliance on younger family members increases as age advances and ill health occurs. Some widows and widowers remarry, particularly the latter because most widowers are less inclined than widows to maintain a household.

More women than men face bereavement and solitude because women usually live longer. Older people are often reminded of the brevity of life by the death of friends. It is a time when one's life is reviewed with happiness or regret. Feelings of serenity or guilt and inadequacy can arise. Independence established prior to loss of a mate makes this adjustment period easier. A person who has some meaningful friendships, economic security, ongoing interests in the community, or private hobbies and a peaceful philosophy of life copes more easily with bereavement. Successful relationships with children and grandchildren are also of inestimable value. See Chapter 41 🔗 for a discussion about facing death.

Nurses can sometimes help clients who are alone a great deal to adjust their living arrangements or lifestyle so that they have more companionship. Moving to a retirement home that has other people in similar circumstances and organized social activities is one example. Many communities provide social centers for the elders, for example, drop-in centers or community centers that offer day trips for seniors. Nurses can refer clients to services and encourage them to obtain companionship.

Cognitive Development

Piaget's phases of cognitive development end with the formal operations phase. However, considerable research on cognitive abilities and aging is currently being conducted. Intellectual capacity includes perception, cognitive agility, memory, and learning.

Perception, or the ability to interpret the environment, depends on the acuteness of the senses. If the aging person's senses are impaired, the ability to perceive the environment and react appropriately is diminished. Changes in the nervous system may also affect perceptual capacity.

Changes in the cognitive structures occur as a person ages. It is believed that progressive loss of neurons occurs. In addition, blood flow to the brain decreases, the meninges appear to thicken, and brain metabolism slows. As yet, little is known about the effect of these physical changes on the cognitive functioning of the older adult.

In older adults, changes in cognitive abilities are more often a difference in speed than in ability. Overall the older adult maintains intelligence, problem solving, judgment, creativity, and other well-practiced cognitive skills. Intellectual loss generally reflects a disease process such as atherosclerosis, which causes the blood vessels to narrow and diminishes perfusion of nutrients to the brain. Most older adults do not experience cognitive impairments.

Memory is also a component of intellectual capacity that involves the following steps:

1. Momentary perception of stimuli from the environment referred to as **sensory memory.**
2. Storage in **short-term memory** (information held in the brain for immediate use or what one has in mind at a given moment). An example of this type of memory is when you call information for a telephone number and remember the number only for the brief time needed to dial the number. Short-term memory also deals with activities or the recent past of minutes to a few hours that is often referred to as **recent memory.**
3. Encoding in which the information leaves short-term memory and enters **long-term memory,** the repository for information stored for periods longer than 72 hours and usually weeks and years. Memories of childhood friends, teachers, and events are stored in long-term memory. Older people who remember the flowers in their wedding bouquet or the names of the boys on their dance card are drawing from long-term memory.

In older adults, retrieval of information from long-term memory can be slower, especially if the information is not frequently used. Most age-related differences occur in short-term memory. Older adults tend to forget the recent past. This forgetfulness can be improved by the use of memory aids, making notes or lists, and placing objects in consistent locations.

Older people need additional time for learning, largely because of the problem of retrieving information. Motivation is also important. Older adults have more difficulty than younger ones in learning information they do not consider meaningful. It is suggested that the older person should remain mentally active to maintain cognitive ability at the highest possible level. Lifelong mental activity, particularly verbal activity, helps the older person retain a high level of cognitive function and may help maintain long-term memory. Cognitive impairment that interferes with normal life is not considered part of normal aging. A decline in intellectual abilities that interferes with social or occupational functions should always be regarded as abnormal. Family members should be advised to seek prompt medical evaluation.

Moral Development

According to Kohlberg, moral development is completed in the early adult years. Most old people stay at Kohlberg's conventional level of moral development and some are at the preconventional level. An older person at the preconventional level obeys rules to avoid pain and the displeasure of others. At stage 1, a person defines good and bad in relation to self, whereas older people at stage 2 may act to meet another's needs as well as their own. Older adults at the conventional level follow society's rules of conduct in response to the expectations of others.

The value and belief patterns that are important to older adults may have little or no significance to younger people because they developed during a time that was very different from today. In addition, a large number of today's elders are either foreign-born or first-generation citizens. Cultural background, life experiences, gender, religion, and socioeconomic status all influence one's values. The nurse must identify and consider the specific values of the older client when nursing care is planned.

Spiritual Development

Older adults can contemplate new religious and philosophical views and try to understand ideas missed previously or interpreted differently. The older person also derives a sense of worth by sharing experiences or views. In contrast, the older adult who has not matured spiritually may feel impoverishment or despair as the drive for economic and professional success wanes.

Carson (1989) states that religion "takes on new meaning for the elderly, who may find comfort, solace, and affirmation in religious activities" (pp. 44–45). The older person's knowledge becomes wisdom, an inner resource for dealing with both positive and negative life experiences. Many older people have strong religious convictions and continue to attend religious meetings or services. Involvement in religion often helps the older adult to resolve issues related to the meaning of life, to adversity, or to good fortune. The "old-old" person who cannot attend formal services often continues religious participation in a more private manner. Many older adults watch television evangelists and some, being vulnerable to fund-raising ventures, send these organizations money that they can ill afford to spare.

According to Fowler and Keen (1985), some people enter the sixth stage of spiritual development, universalizing. People whose spiritual development reaches this level think and act in a way that exemplifies love and justice.

Health Problems

Health problems that older adults may experience include accidents, chronic disabling disease, drug abuse and misuse, alcoholism, dementia, and abuse. Leading causes of death in people ages 65 and over are heart disease, cerebrovascular disease (stroke), pneumonia/influenza, obstructive lung disease, and cancer.

Accidents

Accident prevention is a major concern for older people. *Healthy People 2010* (USDHHS, 2000) reports that falls account for 87% of all fractures among adults aged 65 years and older (pp. 13–15). Because vision is limited, reflexes are slowed, and bones are brittle, caution is required in climbing stairs, driving a car, and even walking. Driving, particularly night driving, requires caution because accommodation of the eye to light is impaired and peripheral vision is diminished. Older persons need to learn to turn the head before changing lanes and should not rely on side vision, for example, when crossing a street. Driving in fog or other hazardous conditions should be avoided.

Fires are a hazard for the older adult with a failing memory. The older person may forget that the iron or stove is left on or may not extinguish a cigarette completely. Because of reduced sensitivity to pain and heat, care must be taken to prevent burns when the person bathes or uses heating devices.

Many older adults suffer and die each year from hypothermia. **Hypothermia** is a body temperature below normal. A lowered metabolism and loss of normal insulation from thinning subcutaneous tissue decrease the older client's ability to retain heat.

Because older clients who take analgesics or sedatives may become lethargic or confused, they should be monitored regularly and closely. Other measures to induce sleep should be used whenever possible. Nurses can help older clients make the home environment safe. Specific hazards can be identified and corrected; for example, hand rails can be installed on staircases. The nurse teaches the importance of taking only prescribed medications and contacting a health professional at the first indication of intolerance to them.

Persons with Alzheimer's disease or other types of dementia experience increasing safety needs as their condition deteriorates. Their behavior usually regresses to that of a child and the same safety precautions need to be instituted. Some of these are keeping poisons and medications out of reach (preferably locked up), taking knobs off kitchen stoves to prevent burns and fires, and putting special locks on doors for persons who tend to wander. Attention should be given to these potential problems whether the client lives at home or is in a health facility.

Guidelines for accident prevention for the older adult are detailed in Chapter 30. 🔗

Chronic Disabling Illness

Many older adults function well within the community without impairments; others are afflicted with one or more chronic illnesses that may seriously impair their functioning. Examples of these are arthritis, osteoporosis, heart disease, stroke, obstructive lung disease, hearing and visual alterations, and cognitive dysfunctions. In addition, acute illnesses such as pneumonia, fractures, trauma from falls, motor vehicle accidents, or other incidents may create chronic health problems. Chronic illness brings about many changes to the client and to family members. The client, for example, may need increasing help with the activities of daily living such as ambulation, feeding, hygiene, and so on; health care expenses often escalate and may become an economic concern; family roles may need to be altered; and family members may need to change their lifestyle to meet caregiving needs.

Drug Use and Misuse

Older adults who frequently suffer from one or more chronic diseases often require medication. Episodes of acute illness may require additional medications. Clients may purchase over-the-counter (OTC) drugs to remedy common discomforts related to aging, such as constipation, sleep disturbance, and joint pain. Over the last few years, the use of vitamins, food supplements, and herbal remedies has increased. These agents fall under the category of OTC drugs and are often not reported by the client as part of their medicine regime. An accurate assessment should include a listing of all of these agents. Many of these agents have not had adequate testing for effectiveness, side effects, or interactions with other medications.

The complexities involved in the self-administration of medication may lead to a variety of misuse situations, including taking too much or too little medication, combining alcohol and medication, combining prescribed medications with OTC drugs, taking medications at the wrong time, or taking someone else's medication. Other potential misuse situations occur when more than one physician prescribes medications and the client fails to tell each doctor what has been previously prescribed.

Additionally, the pharmacodynamics of drugs are altered in older adults. The variations in absorption, distribution, metabolism, and excretion of drugs are related to physiologic changes associated with aging. These variations are discussed in Chapter 33. 🔗

Alcoholism

Murray and Zentner (2001) state that approximately 10% to 15% (more than 2 million) older Americans are alcoholics (p. 792). There are two types of older alcoholics: those who began drinking alcohol in their youth and those who began excessive alcohol use later in life to help them cope with the changes and problems of their older years. Many late-onset alcoholics are widowers.

Chronic drinking has major effects on all body systems, causes progressive liver and kidney damage, damages the stomach and related organs, and slows mental response, frequently leading to accidents and death. Alcohol interacts with various drugs, altering the normal effect of the medication on the body. Some medications have an increased effect when taken with alcohol (e.g., anticoagulants and narcotics), whereas the action of other medications (e.g., antibiotics) is inhibited. For the older adult who has a chronic illness and takes many medications, the combination of drugs and alcohol can lead to serious drug overdose.

Clients who are alcoholics should not be stereotyped or prejudged by the nurse. Rather, they should be accepted, listened to, and offered help. The nurse should assess the number and type of alcoholic beverages consumed as well as the pattern and frequency of consumption. It is important that the nurse discuss any medications the client is taking and review the side effects and interaction effects of alcohol and medication. The role of the nurse is to act as a client advocate and facilitate the treatment of the drinking problem in addition to the prevention of possible complications.

Dementia

Dementia is a slow, insidious process that results in progressive loss of cognitive function. It is characterized by changes in memory, judgment, language, mathematic calculation, abstract reasoning, and problem-solving ability and by impulsive behavior, stupor, confusion, and disorientation (Wold, 1999, pp. 252–253). The most common type of dementia is Alzheimer's disease (AD). Its cause is unknown. Alzheimer's disease affects about 3 million people in the United States. In the next 50 years, the prevalence of AD is expected to increase to 1 in every 45 older adults (Brookmeyer, Gray, & Kawas, 1998). The symptoms of AD have been grouped into three or four stages and may vary somewhat from client to client. The most prominent symptoms are cognitive dysfunctions, including decline in memory, learning, attention, judgment, orientation, and language skills. The symptoms are progressive, and all victims experience a steady decline in cognitive and physical abilities, lasting between 7 and 15 years and ending in death. In the last stage, the client requires total assistance, is unable to communicate, is incontinent, and may be unable to walk. There is no cure or specific treatment for AD. Several drugs have been developed, but none has been shown consistently to reverse the progression of the disease.

It is estimated that about 1 million people with AD are cared for in the home. The burden of care is frequently on women—wives and daughters—who are themselves aging. AD is devastating for the families and caregivers of its victims. The caregivers often drive themselves to physical and emotional exhaustion while they render continuous care and experience the anguish of seeing a loved one turned into a person who no longer remembers who he or she is. The nurse's responsibility is to provide supportive nursing care, accurate information, and referral assistance, if placement in a nursing care facility becomes necessary. It is important for the nurse to do an ongoing assessment of both the client and the caregiver, because changes will occur as the client's condition deteriorates. If this is noted, proper resources can be used to help decrease the stress of the caregiver. An example would be to use an adult day-care center or respite care for a few hours a day to provide the caregiver with some time of his/her own.

Elder Abuse

The rate of elder abuse is unknown due to the incidence of cases that are unreported. As the proportion of older adults in the population increases, it is possible that elder abuse will become an even greater problem. Elder abuse may affect either sex; however, the victims most often are women who are over 75 years of age, physically or mentally impaired, and dependent for care on the abuser. The abuse may involve physical, psychologic, or emotional abuse; sexual abuse; financial abuse; violation of human or civil rights; and active or passive neglect.

When elder abuse involves physical neglect, victims may suffer from dehydration, malnutrition, and oversedation. The victim may be deprived of necessary articles, such as glasses, hearing aids, or walkers. Psychologically, the person may suffer verbal assaults, threats, humiliation, or harassment. Abuse may also include failure to provide appropriate medications or medical treatment, isolation, unreasonable confinement, lack of privacy, an unsafe environment, and involuntary servitude. Some are financially exploited by relatives who steal from them or misuse their property or funds. Others are beaten and even raped by family members. Most victims experience two or more forms of abuse.

Elder abuse or neglect may occur in private homes, senior citizens' homes, nursing homes, hospitals, and long-term care facilities. Many of the abusers are either sons or daughters; others include spouses, relatives (grandchildren, siblings, nieces, and nephews), and in some instances health care providers.

Older adults at home may fail to report abuse or neglect for many reasons. They may be ashamed to admit that their children have abused them or fear retaliation if they seek help. They may fear being sent to an institution. They frequently lack financial resources or lack the mental capacity to be aware of abuse or neglect and to report the situation. Examples of crimes are assault and financial abuse of an older person who is physically or mentally incompetent and has no trustworthy friend or relative to help. In some instances, nurses can intervene by educating caregivers about the needs of older adults and resources available to provide increased home support. They should also report the situation to the appropriate person in the health care agency.

Nurses should be familiar with the laws of their particular state regarding the reporting of suspected or known abuse. The legally competent adult cannot be forced, however, to leave the abusive situation and in many cases may decide to stay. If the client is not legally competent, court proceedings to attain guardianship can be initiated.

Health Assessment and Promotion

Assessment guidelines for the development of the older adult are shown in the accompanying Developmental Assessment Guidelines. Assessment activities include measurement of weight, height, and vital signs; observation of the skin for hydration status or presence of lesions; examination of visual acuity using the Snellen chart; examination of hearing acuity using the Weber, and Rinne tests (see Chapter 28); and questions about the following:

- Usual dietary pattern
- Any problems with bowel or urinary elimination
- Activity/exercise and sleep/rest patterns
- Family and social activities and interests
- Any problems with reading, writing, or problem solving
- Adjustment to retirement or loss of partner.

Health care professionals should also be alert for these signs:

- Symptoms of depression
- Risk factors for suicide
- Signs of abnormal bereavement
- Changes in cognitive function
- Medications that increase risk of falls
- Signs of physical abuse or neglect

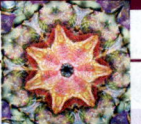

Developmental Assessment Guidelines

THE OLDER ADULT

In these three developmental areas, does the older adult do the following?

Physical Development
- Adjust to physiologic changes (e.g., appearance, sensory/perceptual, musculoskeletal, neurologic, cardiovascular).
- Adapt lifestyle to diminishing energy and ability.
- Maintain vital signs (especially blood pressure) within normal range for age and sex.

Psychosocial Development
- Manage retirement years in a satisfying manner.
- Participate in social and leisure activities.

- Have a social network of friends and support persons.
- View life as worthwhile.
- Have high self-esteem.
- Gain support from value system and/or spiritual philosophy.
- Accept and adjust to the death of significant others.

Development in Activities of Daily Living
- Exhibit healthy practices in nutrition, exercise, recreation, sleep patterns, and personal habits.
- Have the ability to care for self or to secure appropriate help with activities of daily living.
- Have satisfactory living arrangements and income to meet changing needs.

BOX 23–8	■ Health Promotion Guidelines for Older Adults

Health Tests and Screening
- As for middle-aged adults

Safety
- Home safety measures to prevent falls, fire, burns, scalds, and electrocution
- Motor vehicle safety reinforcement, especially when driving at night
- Precautions to prevent pedestrian accidents

Nutrition and Exercise
- Importance of a well-balanced diet with fewer calories to accommodate lower metabolic rate and decreased physical activity
- Importance of sufficient amounts of vitamin D and calcium to prevent osteoporosis

- Nutritional and exercise factors that may lead to cardiovascular disease (e.g., obesity, cholesterol and fat intake, lack of exercise)
- A regular program of moderate exercise to maintain joint mobility, muscle tone, and bone calcification

Elimination
- Importance of adequate roughage in the diet, adequate exercise, and at least six 8-ounce glasses of fluid daily to prevent constipation

Social Interactions
- Encouraging intellectual and recreational pursuits
- Encouraging personal relationships that promote discussion of feelings, concerns, and fears
- Availability of social community centers and programs for seniors

- Skin lesions (malignant and peripheral)
- Tooth decay, gingivitis, loose teeth
- Peripheral arterial disease.

Older persons are usually concerned about their health and are interested in information and behavioral strategies directed toward improving it. The nurse may wish to discuss some or all of the health promotion topics outlined in Box 23–8. These topics are discussed in detail in subsequent chapters throughout the book.

CONSIDERATIONS FOR ADULTS OF ALL AGES

Health promotion is an important nursing function for all clients and includes prevention of disease, maintenance of health and functional status, learning to live with and effectively manage alterations of health, such as having diabetes, and being able to access accurate and understandable health-related information. Cultural and developmental considerations are essential elements in knowing the client well and being able to plan individualized care that will focus on client strengths as well as special needs.

Health Promotion

During the last few years, we have had the greatest increase in available knowledge and information and technological advances in history. This points to the importance of being very specific and focused when presenting health promotion ideas to adults of all ages. Older adults, by virtue of living the longest, have witnessed the largest amount of changes in their lifetimes.

Consideration of health promotion and wellness should include the following: What media is most important for information dissemination (e.g., television, Internet, postal mailings, magazines, newspapers)? What are their family roles (e.g., who makes the health care decisions)? Who are their social supports (e.g., church, senior centers, family and friends)? What are the cultural considerations? Nurses working in hos-

pitals, clinics, and physician's offices have the opportunity to teach and encourage health promotion activities, but they can also play a part in the community network and information dissemination methods mentioned above. It is important that information be valid and accurate. Some sources might be providing "misinformation" to the public. Knowing the client and family well will help the nurse to focus on specific needs more effectively.

Culture

Culture and heritage are discussed in Chapter 13. ⬡ Beare and Stanley (1999) have compiled a table that lists various cultural groups with information specific to their cultures. Information presented includes communication, family roles, high-risk health behaviors, nutrition, death rituals, spirituality, health care practices, and health care practitioners. Increasing knowledge of these factors can be a determining factor in planning and providing more effective nursing care. An example would be that in many cultures the extended family remains very important, so teaching and providing care is truly a "family affair" and should involve all concerned members of the family.

Developmental Nursing Considerations

Developmental tasks and expectations of the young adult, middle-aged adult, and older adult were discussed earlier in this chapter. Why is this an integral part of planning nursing care? The ultimate goal should always be to maximize the potential of the individual. This pertains to all ages of adulthood, but especially to middle-aged and older adults, when they are beginning to experience physical and psychosocial changes and losses. Many of the changes are inevitable changes related to aging. When strengths are capitalized on, it gives them a better attitude and the fortitude to better cope with their special needs and changes.

An example could be a middle-aged man, who served in the Vietnam War while he was in his 20s. Developmentally, this should have been the time for him to learn to develop healthy relationships. During the war, several close friends were killed. In the years that followed, he probably did one of two things—he changed his life values, appreciating things in a very different way, or he became isolated in his relationships, fearing the risk of losing friends as he did during the war. If the task of developing healthy relationships is not resolved, it will continue and present problems throughout his lifetime. It interferes with psychosocial and physical health. Identifying the problem will help nurses be supportive, recommend appropriate resources,

and develop interventions that will capitalize on the client's strengths. Having a good understanding of developmental tasks lays the foundation for planning individualized nursing care. It helps clients be a part of their care and increases their self-concept. Every person has life events that change their world, as they have known it. It is not the event itself that is so vital, but the person's perception and reaction to the event that becomes the key to their attitudes, behaviors, and ultimate outcomes.

Focus on Critical Thinking

Alice Green, a 78-year-old female, has had a bone density scan as part of a regular physical exam and has been told that she has severe osteoporosis. Her physician has ordered a new experimental medication that is supposed to maintain bone mass in clients with osteoporosis. She lives alone in her own home and is able to perform activities of daily living independently.

1. How would you define osteoporosis to Mrs. Green?
2. What risk factors related to osteoporosis should be included in an assessment of Mrs. Green?

3. Which of the risk factors are modifiable or can be altered by a change in lifestyle?
4. What medication teaching is essential when a client is taking medications to increase or maintain bone mass in osteoporosis?
5. What preventive measures should be taught to decrease risks of fractures and to maintain bone mass?

See Critical Thinking Possibilities in Appendix A.

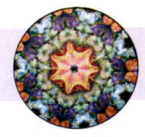 ## | Chapter Review

EXPLORE MediaLink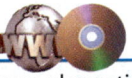

NCLEX review questions, case studies, care plan activities, MediaLink applications, and other interactive resources for this chapter can be found on the Companion Website at www.prenhall.com/kozier.

Click on Chapter 23 to select the activities for this chapter. For more NCLEX review questions, and an audio glossary, access the Student CD-ROM accompanying this textbook.

Chapter Highlights

- Adult development is often divided into three phases: young adults (20 to 40 years), middle-aged adults (40 to 65 years), and older adults (65 years onward). Late adulthood is usually categorized into young-old (65 to 75 years), old (75 to 85 years), old-old (85 to 100 years), and the elite old (over 100 years).
- The young adult is essentially in a stable period physically, but psychological change is great. Choices must be made about education, occupation, marriage or an alternative lifestyle, child rearing, a place to live, civic roles, and so on.
- The middle-aged adult needs to adjust to an aging body, the increasing dependence of parents, and the increasing independence of children; however, new independent interests can be pursued.
- Both middle-aged men and women enter a midlife crisis in which they need to reexamine their purpose and reevaluate ways to use their energies and abilities.

- Older adults experience many physical changes associated with aging. All body systems undergo change: integumentary, neuromuscular, sensory/perceptual, pulmonary, cardiovascular, gastrointestinal, and genitourinary.
- Several theories have been proposed to account for the biologic aging process: wear-and-tear, rate of living, stress, endocrine, free-radical, genetic, programmed senescence, error catastrophe, collagen, cross-linking, immunologic, and autoimmune theories.
- Psychosocial theories about aging include the disengagement, activity, and continuity theories.
- The older adult has to adjust to possible psychosocial changes, including retirement (which necessitates financial and social adjustments), relocation, increasing dependence on others, and coping with losses and death.
- Cognitive development continues during young adulthood and the middle-aged years. Developments may extend be-

yond the formal operations phase of Piaget to one of post-formal operations thinking. The intellectual abilities of the healthy older adult undergo minimal change. In older adults, retrieval of information from long-term memory can be slower. Most changes occur in short-term or recent memory.

- In the realm of moral development, most adults are in either Kohlberg's stage 4 (the law and order orientation) at the conventional level or in stage 5 (the social contract and legalistic orientation) at the postconventional level.
- Spiritual development of young, middle-aged, and older adults continues into Fowler's paradoxical-consolidative stage. Some adults enter the sixth stage of spiritual development, universalizing.
- Health problems of young adults include accidents, suicide, hypertension (in African American males), substance abuse, sexually transmitted disease, abuse of women, and malignancies. Problems of middle-aged adults include accidents, cancer, cardiovascular disease, obesity, alcoholism, and mental health alterations. Health problems of older adults in-

clude accidents, chronic disabling disease, drug use and misuse, alcoholism, dementia, and abuse.

- Health promotion information for all adults needs to include positive health practices that can promote health and wellness. These include (a) recommended physical, visual, hearing, and dental assessments; (b) screenings for cardiovascular disease and tuberculosis; (c) breast and testicular self-examinations; (d) immunizations; (e) Papanicolaou smears for women; (f) safety precautions to prevent accidents; (g) the importance of appropriate nutrition and exercise; and (h) for older adults, the importance of measures to prevent constipation.
- When nurses have a good understanding of developmental tasks, their clients can be assessed more completely, and nurses can help them to maximize their potential and develop interventions that use resources to work on special needs. This becomes crucial in middle-aged and older adults as they experience many inevitable psychosocial and physical losses and changes.

Review Questions

23–1. Cancer is the second leading cause of death in people between the ages of 25 and 64. Which type of cancer is increasing in incidence in women?
   a. cervical cancer
   b. lymphoma
   c. lung cancer
   d. colon cancer

23–2. An older client is seen by the home health nurse weekly. The client's husband died 8 months ago. Which of the following behaviors of the client would cause concern and possibly indicate that the woman is experiencing ineffective coping?
   a. She always shows the nurse photographs of her family.
   b. She is neglecting her personal grooming.
   c. She visits the cemetery and her husband's grave every 2 weeks.
   d. She is Catholic and goes to mass on a regular daily basis.

23–3. A nurse in a long-term care facility is caring for several elders with noticeable hearing losses. Which of the following is true of elderly people with hearing losses?
   a. Elders usually have middle ear changes.
   b. Elders often hear only what they want to hear.
   c. Elders usually respond better to low-pitched tones.
   d. All elders with hearing losses should be fitted with a hearing aid.

23–4. An 85-year-old man goes to an adult day-care center daily. The nurse notices that he frequently tells stories of when he was younger and came from New York City on the "orphan trains" and was adopted by a Swedish family in Nebraska. His stories are told in a very positive manner. How would the nurse assess his behavior?
   a. She would refer him for a geriatric psychiatric evaluation.
   b. She would consider this a normal response for his developmental level.
   c. She would converse with him, but distract him and change the conversation.
   d. She would see this as a need to involve him in more social activities at the day-care center.

23–5. A 70-year-old woman has Alzheimer's disease and becomes agitated every evening, pacing and insisting on leaving to go "home." What is the best intervention to be done to help calm the woman?
   a. Take her to her room, turn the lights out, and leave her alone.
   b. Encourage her to participate in group activities that have just begun.
   c. Turn on the television and encourage her to watch it.
   d. Touch her in a gentle way, such as putting your arm around her waist.

Readings and References

Suggested Readings

Haight, B. K., Barba, B. E., Tesh, A. S., & Courts, N. F. (2002). Thriving: A life span theory. *Journal of Gerontological Nursing, 28*(3), 14–22.

The authors describe the theory of thriving, which is holistic and multidisciplinary with a life span focus.

Johnson, R., Sorofman, B., & Tripp-Reimer, T. (1999). Cultural dimensions in gerontological nursing. In P. Beare & M. Stanley (Eds.),

Gerontological nursing (2nd ed., pp. 21–36). Philadelphia: F. A. Davis.

The authors provide a comprehensive discussion of cultural dimensions in gerontological nursing. Tables are provided that list selected cultural groups and prevailing attitudes specific to each group: communication, family roles, high-risk health behaviors, nutrition, death rituals, spirituality, health care practices, and health care practitioners.

Related Research

Cooper, K., Bilbrew, D., Dubbert, P., Kerr, K., & Kirschner, K. (2001). Health barriers to walking for exercise in elderly primary care. *Geriatric Nursing, 22,* 258–262.

Grando, V. T., Mehr, D., Popejoy, L., Maas, M., Rantz, M., Wipke-Tevis, D. D., et al., (2002). Why older adults with light care needs enter and remain in nursing homes. *Journal of Gerontological Nursing, 28*(7), 47–53.

Hawranik, P., & Pangman, V. (2002). Perceptions of a senior citizens' wellness center. The community's voice. *Journal of Gerontological Nursing, 28*(11), 38–44.

References

Anderson, J. E. (Ed.). (1956). *Psychological aspects of aging: Proceedings from a conference on planning research.* Washington D.C.: American Psychological Association.

Barkauskas, V. H., Bauman, L. C., & Darling-Fisher, C. (2002). *Health and physical assessment* (3rd ed.). St. Louis, MO: Mosby.

Beare, P., & Stanley, M. (Eds.). (1999). *Gerontological nursing* (2nd ed.). Philadelphia: F. A. Davis.

Brookmeyer, R., Gray, S., & Kawas, C. (1998). Projections of Alzheimer's disease in the United States and the public health impact of delaying disease onset. *American Journal of Public Health, 88,* 1337–1342.

Brown M. (1998). *Readings in gerontology* (2nd ed.). St. Louis, MO: CV. Mosby.

Carson, V. B. (1989). *Spiritual dimensions in nursing practice.* Philadelphia: W. B. Saunders.

Cooper, K., Bilbrew, D., Dubbert, P., Karr, K., & Kirschner, K. (2001). Health barriers to walking for exercise in elderly primary care. *Geriatric Nursing, 22,* 258–262.

Curry, L., & Hogstel, M. (2002). Osteoporosis: Education and awareness can make a difference. *American Journal of Nursing, 102*(1), 26–33.

Duvall, E. M. (1977). *Family development* (5th ed.). Philadelphia: Lippincott.

Edelman, C., & Mandle, C. L. (2002). *Health promotion throughout the life span* (5th ed.). St. Louis, MO: Mosby.

Eliopoulos, C. (2001). *Gerontological nursing* (5th ed.). Philadelphia: Lippincott.

Erikson, E. H. (1963). *Childhood and society* (2nd ed.). New York: Norton.

Fowler, J., & Keen, S. (1985). *Life maps: Conversations in the journey of faith.* Waco, TX: Word Books.

Havighurst, R. J. (1972). *Developmental tasks and education* (3rd ed.). New York: Longman.

Hetzel, L., & Smith, A. (2001). *The 65 years and over population: 2000. Census 2000 brief.* Washington, DC: U.S. Census Bureau.

Murray, R. B., & Zentner, J. P. (2001). *Health promotion strategies through the life span* (7th ed.). Upper Saddle River, NJ: Prentice Hall.

Peck, R. (1968). Psychological development in the second half of life. In B. L. Neugarten (Ed.), *Middle age and aging.* Chicago: University of Chicago Press.

Polan, E., & Taylor, D. (2003). *Journey across the life span. Human development and health promotion* (2nd ed.). Philadelphia: F. A. Davis.

Sheehy, G. (1976). *Passages: Predictable crises of adult life.* New York: Dutton.

Stuart-Hamilton, I. (2000). *The psychology of ageing* (3rd ed.). Philadelphia: Jessica Kingley Publishers.

U.S. Department of Health and Human Services. (2000). *Healthy people 2010: Understanding and improving health* (2nd ed.). *Goal 15: Injury and violence prevention.* Washington, DC: Author.

Wold, G. (1999). *Basic geriatric nursing* (2nd ed.). St. Louis, MO: Mosby.

Selected Bibliography

Clark, M. J. (2003). *Community health nursing. Caring for populations* (4th ed.). Upper Saddle River, NJ: Prentice Hall.

Erikson, E. H. (1982). *The life cycle completed: A review.* New York: Norton.

Fowler, J. W. (1981). *Stages of faith: The psychology of human development and the quest for meaning.* New York: Harper & Row.

Freud, S. (1923). *The ego and the id.* London: Hogarth Press.

Gilligan, C. (1982). *In a different voice: Psychological theory and women's development.* Cambridge, MA: Harvard University Press.

Kohlberg, L. (1971). *Recent research in moral development.* New York: Holt, Rinehart & Winston.

Kohlberg, L. (1981). *The psychology of moral development: Moral stages and the idea of justice.* San Francisco: Harper & Row.

Paludi, M. A. (2002). *Human development in multicultural contexts. A book of readings.* Upper Saddle River, NJ: Prentice Hall.

Peck, R. (1955). Psychological developments in the second half of life. In J. Anderson (Ed.), *Psychological aspects of aging.* Washington, DC: American Psychological Association.

Piaget, J. (1966). *Origins of intelligence in children.* New York: Norton.

Sheehy, G. (1995). *New passages. Mapping your life across time.* New York: Ballantine Books.

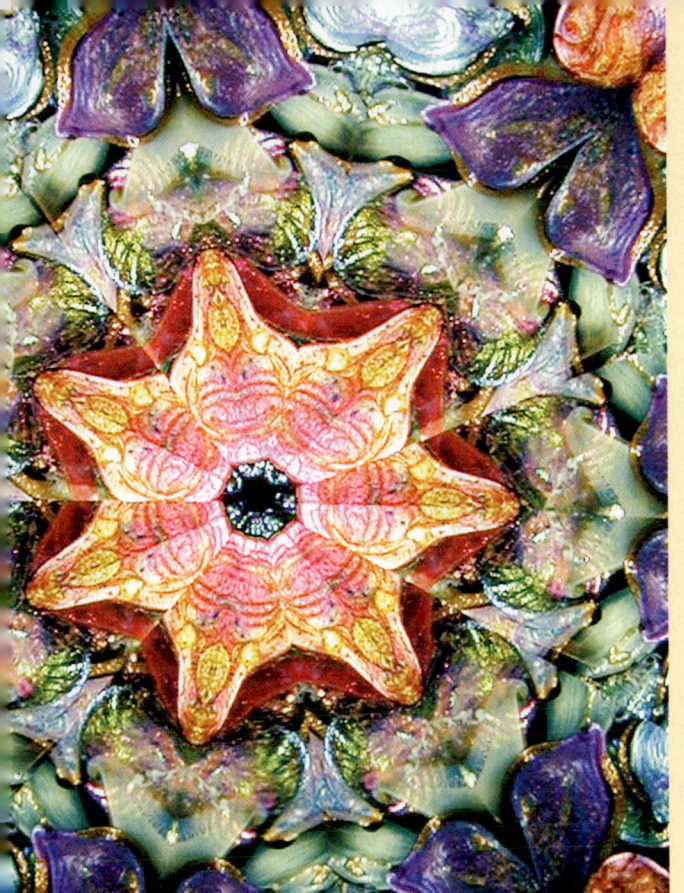

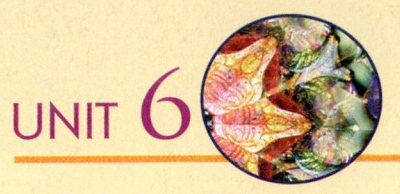

INTEGRAL ASPECTS OF NURSING

*E*ffective communication is an essential element of an optimal nurse–client relationship and of the leader–manager role. Nurses are attuned to all forms of communication, recognizing that gestures, expressions, and other kinds of body language often convey a message more powerfully and accurately than mere words. The nurse responds not only to the factual content of a message but also to the feelings expressed through verbal and nonverbal modes. Establishing client rapport facilitates a vital nursing role—the process of teaching, a structured form of communication designed to produce learning.

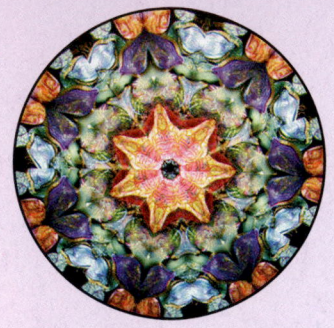

CHAPTER 24

CARING, COMFORTING, AND COMMUNICATING

LEARNING OUTCOMES

After completing this chapter you will be able to:

- Discuss nursing theory related to caring.

- Describe essential aspects of the comforting process.

- Describe factors influencing the communication process.

- Discuss nurse–patient communication as a dynamic process.

- Describe four phases of the helping relationship.

- Identify types of groups helpful in promoting health and comfort.

- Identify features of effective groups.

- Discuss how nurses use communication skills in each phase of the nursing process.

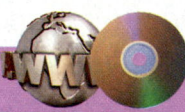

MediaLink

www.prenhall.com/kozier

Additional resources for this chapter can be found on the Student CD-ROM accompanying this textbook, and on the Companion Website at www.prenhall.com/kozier. Click on Chapter 24 to select the activities for this chapter.

CD-ROM
- Audio Glossary
- NCLEX Review

Companion Website
- Additional NCLEX Review
- Case Study: Providing Comfort
- Care Plan Activity: Treating an Immigrant Family
- MediaLink Application: Communication Resources
- Links to Resources

Communication is a critical skill for nursing. It is the process by which humans meet their survival needs, build relationships, and experience joy. In nursing, communication is a dynamic process used to gather assessment data, to teach and persuade, and to express caring and comfort. Comforting is the process by which nurses assist clients and significant others to face the distresses and discomforts they may encounter. In nursing, communication is an integral part of the helping relationship.

CARING

Caring is considered by many nurses to be an essential aspect of nursing. Madeleine Leininger (1984) states that care is the essence of nursing and the dominant, distinctive, and unifying feature of nursing. She says that there can be no cure without caring, but that there may be caring without curing. She emphasizes that human caring, although a universal phenomenon, varies among cultures in its expressions, processes, and patterns.

Leininger (1984) identifies many caring constructs (see Box 24–1). She believes that health care personnel should work toward an understanding of care and the values, health beliefs, and lifestyles of different cultures, which will form the basis for providing culture-specific care.

Jean Watson (1985), who also believes the practice of caring is central to nursing, describes caring as grounded in a set of universal human values (kindness, concern, and love of self and others). Caring is described as the moral ideal of nursing; it involves the will to care, the intent to care, and caring actions. Caring actions include communication, positive regard, support, or physical interventions by the nurse.

Miller (1995) defines caring as "intentional action that conveys physical and emotional security and genuine connectedness with another person or group of people. Caring validates the humanness of both the care giver and the cared for." (p. 32).

According to Gadow (1984) and Noddings (1984), caring may or may not involve action or verbal communication. The most caring act may be nonaction as desired by the client.

The outcomes of caring are varied. Caring can promote self-actualization, promote individual growth, preserve human dignity and worth, augment self-healing, and relieve distress. Conversely, "caring" may not evoke a tangible outcome. It may not be a means to an end; it may be regarded as an end in itself. The goodness of caring is often found in the process itself—that of engagement and connection.

COMFORTING

Comforting is a characteristic unique to nursing and an essential aspect of caring. "Making the client as comfortable as possible" has been a frequent nursing action since the days of Florence Nightingale. Nurses have always provided comfort measures that provide strength, solace, support, encouragement, hope, and assistance.

KEY TERMS

attentive listening, 428
caring, 419
comfort, 420
comforting, 420
communication, 421
congruent communication, 427
decode, 422
empathy, 434
encoding, 421
feedback, 422
group, 435
group dynamics, 435
helping relationships, 429
nonverbal communication, 423
personal space, 426
process recording, 440
proxemics, 426
territoriality, 427
therapeutic communication, 428
verbal communication, 423

BOX 24–1 ■ Leininger's Descriptions of Care and Caring

- Caring includes assistive, supportive, and facilitative acts toward or for another individual or group with evident or anticipated needs.
- Caring serves to ameliorate or to improve human conditions. It emphasizes healthful, enabling activities of individuals and groups that are based on culturally defined, ascribed, or sanctioned helping modes.
- Caring is essential to human development, growth, and survival.

- Caring behaviors include comfort, compassion, concern, coping behavior, empathy, enabling, facilitating, interest, involvement, health consultative acts, health instruction acts, health maintenance acts, helping behaviors, love, nurturance, presence, protective behaviors, restorative behaviors, sharing, stimulating behaviors, stress alleviation, succor, support, surveillance, tenderness, touching, and trust.

The Comforting Process

Comforting is a complex process that "includes discrete, transitory actions, such as touching, or broad, longer lasting interventions such as listening" (Morse, 1996, p. 6). The comforting process is a client-led process because it occurs in response to cues presented by the client. The comforting measures provided, however, are generally nurse controlled in that nurses select the appropriate comfort measures and adjust them according to the needs of the client. Comfort is not merely a passive process on the part of the client, however. Clients are often actively engaged in increasing their personal comfort. In these instances nurses support the clients' own attempts to achieve comfort. Thus the comfort process, whenever possible, involves the cooperative actions of both clients and nurses.

Comfort

The desired outcome or product of comforting is comfort. The origin of the word *comfort* is the Latin word *confortare,* meaning "to strengthen greatly." **Comfort** implies a renewal, an amplification of power or sense of control, an invigorating influence, a positive mind-set, and a readiness for action.

Comfort Needs

Kolcaba (1991, 1995) identifies comfort needs within four contexts: physical, psychospiritual, social, and environmental:

- Physical comfort needs relate to bodily sensations and the physiologic problems associated with the medical diagnosis.
- Psychospiritual comfort needs relate to the internal awareness of self, including esteem, concept, sexuality, and meaning in one's life. They can also include the person's relationship to a higher order or being.
- Social comfort needs relate to interpersonal, family, and social relationships.
- Environmental comfort needs relate to the external background of human experience and can include light, noise, ambience, color, temperature, and natural versus synthetic elements. They may also include culturally specific food and language.

Intensity (Type) of Comfort

Three types of comfort described by Kolcaba are relief, ease, and transcendence. *Relief* from discomfort is the experience of having a specific need met. Relief may be incomplete, partial, or temporary, lasting only a short time until discomfort arises again. It enables the client to return to former functions or a peaceful death. *Ease* refers to a state of calm or peaceful contentment. This state of comfort can exist without a prior state of discomfort or may indicate complete relief from discomforts that are lasting, rather than temporary relief from severe discomforts. This state of comfort enables the client to perform activities efficiently. *Transcendence* refers to the state in which the client rises above problems or pain. This state of comfort differs from the other two states in that the client is invigorated or inspired for extraordinary performance as an end state, rather than ordinary performance, which is the end state for relief and ease. Extraordinary performance requires unusual effort to shed one's preoccupation with pain, disability, or other difficulties. For example, transcendence may be necessary when illness and injury cause a permanent change in the body, such as with clients who have debilitating arthritis and pain or a spinal cord injury.

Comfort Measures

Comfort measures may be provided both directly to the client and indirectly through other personnel, family, or environment. Examples of indirect actions include maintaining a quiet environment, coordinating the activities of other health care personnel, and supporting the client's family members or significant others. Comfort measures are initiated when the nurse perceives client distress or discomfort or the client indicates a specific need for comforting. Because there are such diverse states of discomfort, nurses need to be creative and innovative in providing specific, individualized care. Comfort care may require simple physical actions such as providing a warm blanket, offering a cup of tea, or applying lotion to dry skin. However, it also requires nursing knowledge and skills specific to the client's medical and nursing problems. Examples include interventions for skin breakdown, pain, infection, airway clearance, confusion, and so on. Comfort measures also encompass the client's psychospiritual, social, and environmental realms. Examples of psychospiritual comfort measures are talking in soothing tones, acknowledging and accepting feelings, offering your presence, and encouraging decision making. Social measures may include supporting family and friends and encouraging visits by family and friends. Environmental comfort measures may involve merely opening a window or removing clutter. Table 24–1 provides examples of specific communication strategies that provide comfort.

Because the goal of any comforting measure is enhanced comfort, success in comfort care is evaluated by comparing comfort levels before and after intervention. Absolute or total comfort in a hospital setting is often not possible. Nurses are therefore challenged to encourage and inspire clients to rise above adversities.

COMMUNICATING

The term *communication* has various meanings, depending on the context in which it is used. To some, communication is the interchange of information between two or more people; in other words, the exchange of ideas or thoughts. This kind of communication uses methods such as talking and listening or writing and reading. However, painting, dancing, and storytelling are also methods of communication. In addition, thoughts are conveyed to others not only by spoken or written words but also by gestures or body actions.

Communication may have a more personal connotation than the interchange of ideas or thoughts. It can be a transmission of feelings or a more personal and social interaction between people. Frequently, one member of a couple comments that the other is not communicating. Some teenagers complain about a

TABLE 24–1 Communication Strategies for Providing Comfort

Characteristic	Description	Example of Nurses Response
Empathy	An expression of understanding of "how it is for the client" who is distressed, suffering, or sad. Adversity of situation validated.	"I hear how this is for you." "I understand how hard this is for you." "Your feelings are very normal in this situation."
Positive talk	Nurse has a positive impact by keeping the client informed, encouraged, or coached.	"You are doing really well; this is a very difficult procedure." "Taking these steps is hard, but you are improving. Good work!" "Most families in this situation have these types of feelings and thoughts."
Therapeutic touch	The nurse, when appropriate, maintains physical contact with the client, and reassures and comforts the client.	"How about if I hold your hand during this procedure." "I am just going to rub your shoulder for a minute until the pain medication starts to work."
Competent physical and technical skills	The nurse's level of professionalism and efficiency decreases the anxiety and promotes comfort.	"This will just take a second with a little pin prick to start this IV. You have excellent veins." "We do this procedure frequently. Do you have any questions we haven't answered yet?"
Vigilance	The client trusts that the nurse is involved in his/her care.	"I am back to check on how you are doing." "I will not be gone for more than 30 minutes and if you need me before, use the call light and I will come. Does 30 minutes sound doable to you?"

generation gap—being unable to communicate with understanding or feeling to a parent or authority figure. Sometimes a nurse is said to be efficient but lacking in something called *bedside manner*. For the purpose of this text, **communication** is any means of exchanging information or feelings between two or more people. It is a basic component of human relationships, including nursing.

The intent of any communication is to elicit a response. Thus, communication is a process. It has two main purposes: to influence others and to obtain information. Communication can be described as helpful or unhelpful. The former encourages a sharing of information, thoughts, or feelings between two or more people. The latter hinders or blocks the transfer of information and feelings.

Nurses who communicate effectively are better able to collect assessment data, initiate interventions, evaluate outcomes of interventions, initiate change that promotes health, and prevent legal problems associated with nursing practice. The communication process is built on a trusting relationship with a client and support persons. Effective communication is essential for the establishment of a nurse–client relationship.

Communication can occur on an intrapersonal level within a single individual as well as on interpersonal and group levels. Intrapersonal communication is the communication that you have with yourself; another name is *self-talk*. Both the sender and the receiver of a message usually engage in self-talk. It involves thinking about the message before it is sent, while it is being sent, and after it is sent, and it occurs constantly. Consequently, intrapersonal communication can interfere with a person's ability to hear a message as the sender intended (see Figure 24–1 ■).

The Communication Process

Face-to-face communication involves a sender, a message, a receiver, and a response, or feedback (see Figure 24–2 ■). In its simplest form, communication is a two-way process involving the sending and the receiving of a message. Because the intent of communication is to elicit a response, the process is ongoing; the receiver of the message then becomes the sender of a response, and the original sender then becomes the receiver.

Sender

The *sender*, a person or group who wishes to convey a message to another, can be considered the *source-encoder*. This term suggests that the person or group sending the message must have an idea or reason for communicating (source) and must put the idea or feeling into a form that can be transmitted. **Encoding** involves the selection of specific signs or symbols (codes) to transmit the message, such as which language and words to use, how to arrange the words, and what tone of voice and gestures to use. For example, if the receiver speaks English, the sender usually selects English words. If the message is "Mr. Johnson, you have to wait another hour for your pain medication," the tone of voice selected and a shake of the head can reinforce it. The nurse must not only deal with dialects and foreign languages but also must cope with two language levels—the layperson's and the health professional's.

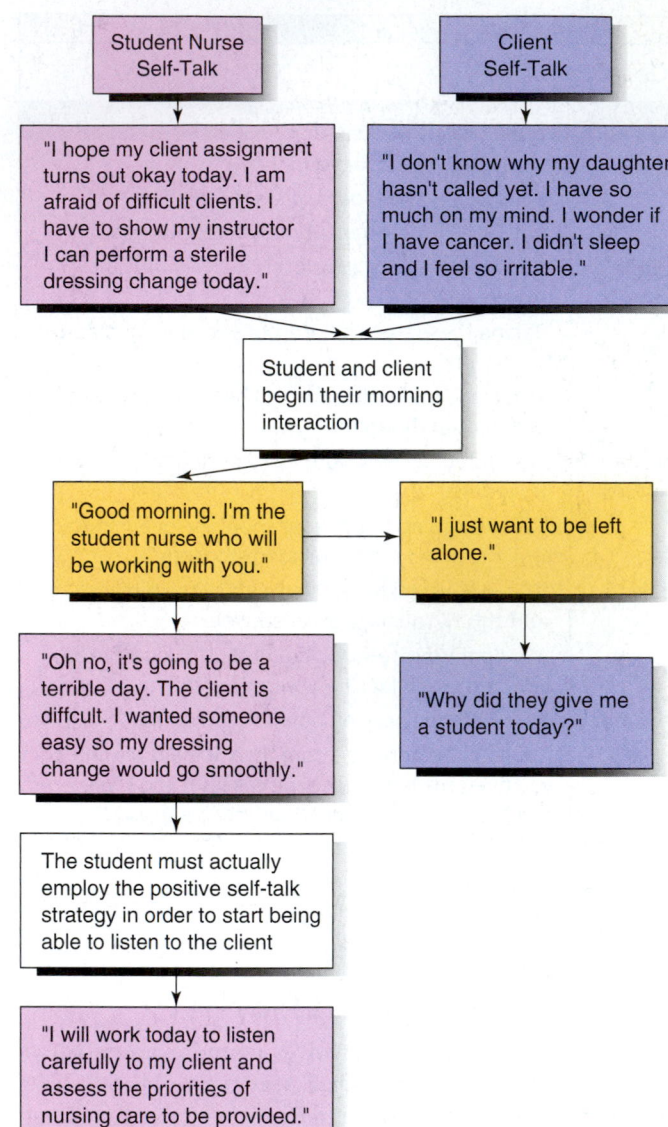

Figure 24–1 ■ Improving student nurse self-talk.

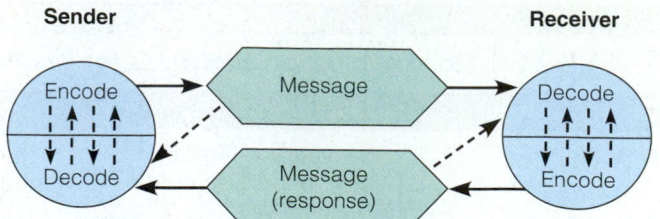

Figure 24–2 ■ The communication process. The dashed arrows indicate intrapersonal communication (self-talk). The solid lines indicate interpersonal communication.

This person is the *decoder,* who must perceive what the sender intended (interpretation). Perception uses all of the senses to receive verbal and nonverbal messages. To **decode** means to relate the message perceived to the receiver's storehouse of knowledge and experience and to sort out the meaning of the message. Whether the message is decoded accurately by the receiver, according to the sender's intent, depends largely on their similarities in knowledge and experience and sociocultural background. If the meaning of the decoded message matches the intent of the sender, then the communication has been effective. Ineffective communication occurs when the message sent is misinterpreted by the receiver. For example, Mr. Johnson may perceive the message accurately—"No pain medication for another hour." However, if experience has taught him that he can receive the pain medication early if a certain nurse is on duty, he will interpret the intent of the message differently.

Response

The fourth component of the communication process, the response, is the message that the receiver returns to the sender. It is also called **feedback.** Feedback can be either verbal, non-

Message

The second component of the communication process is the *message* itself—what is actually said or written, the body language that accompanies the words, and how the message is transmitted. The medium used to convey the message is the channel, and it can target any of the receiver's senses. It is important for the channel to be appropriate for the message and it should help make the intent of the message more clear.

Talking face to face with a person may be more effective in some instances than telephoning or writing a message. Recording messages on tape or communicating by radio or television may be more appropriate for larger audiences. Written communication is often appropriate for long explanations or for a communication that needs to be preserved. The nonverbal channel of touch is often highly effective (see Figure 24–3 ■).

Receiver

The *receiver,* the third component of the communication process, is the listener, who must listen, observe, and attend.

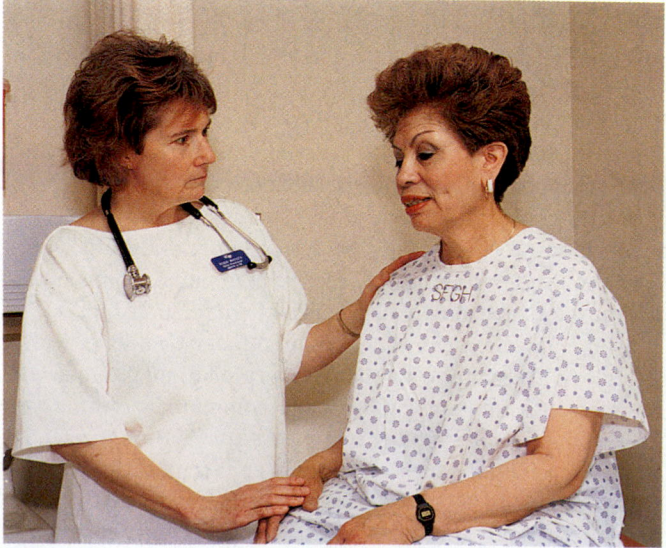

Figure 24–3 ■ Appropriate forms of touch can communicate caring.

verbal, or both. Nonverbal examples are a nod of the head or a yawn. Either way, feedback allows the sender to correct or re-word a message. In the case of Mr. Johnson, the receiver may appear irritated or say, "Well, the nurse on the other shift gives me my pain medication early if I need it." The sender then knows the message was interpreted accurately. However, now the original sender becomes the receiver, who is required to de-code and respond.

Modes of Communication

Communication is generally carried out in two different modes: verbal and nonverbal. **Verbal communication** uses the spoken or written word; **nonverbal communication** uses other forms, such as gestures or facial expressions, and touch. Although both kinds of communication occur concurrently, the majority of communication is nonverbal. Learning about nonverbal communication is important for nurses in develop-ing effective communication patterns and relationships with clients.

Verbal Communication

Verbal communication is largely conscious because people choose the words they use. The words used vary among indi-viduals according to culture, socioeconomic background, age, and education. As a result, countless possibilities exist for the way ideas are exchanged. An abundance of words can be used to form messages. In addition, a wide variety of feelings can be conveyed when people talk.

When choosing words to say or write, nurses need to con-sider (a) pace and intonation, (b) simplicity, (c) clarity and brevity, (d) timing and relevance, (e) adaptability, (f) credibil-ity, and (g) humor.

PACE AND INTONATION. The manner of speech, as in the pace or rhythm and intonation, will modify the feeling and impact of the message. The intonation can express enthusiasm, sadness, anger, or amusement. The pace of speech may indicate interest, anxiety, boredom, or fear. For example, speaking slowly and softly to an excited client may help calm the client.

SIMPLICITY. Simplicity includes the use of commonly under-stood words, brevity, and completeness. Many complex tech-nical terms become natural to nurses. However, laypersons often misunderstand these terms. Words such as vasoconstriction or cholecystectomy are meaningful to the nurse and easy to use but are ill advised when communicating with clients. Nurses need to learn to select appropriate under-standable terms based on the age, knowledge, culture, and education of the client. For example, instead of saying to a client, "The nurses will be catheterizing you tomorrow for a urine analysis," it may be more appropriate and understand-able to say, "Tomorrow we need to get a sample of your urine, so we will collect it by putting a small tube into your bladder." The latter statement is more likely to elicit a response from the client as to why it is needed and whether it will be un-comfortable, because the person understands the message be-ing conveyed by the nurse.

CLARITY AND BREVITY. A message that is direct and simple will be more effective. Clarity is saying precisely what is meant and brevity is using the fewest words necessary. The result is a message that is simple and clear. An aspect of this is congru-ence, or consistency, where the nurse's behavior or nonverbal communication matches the words spoken. When the nurse tells the client, "I am interested in hearing what you have to say," the nonverbal behavior would include the nurse facing the client, making eye contact, and leaning forward. The goal is to communicate clearly so that all aspects of a situation or cir-cumstance are understood. To ensure clarity in communication, nurses also need to speak slowly and enunciate carefully.

TIMING AND RELEVANCE. Nurses need to be aware of both relevance and timing when communicating with clients. No matter how clearly or simply words are stated or written, the timing needs to be appropriate to ensure that words are heard. Moreover, the messages need to relate to the person or to the person's interests and concerns.

This involves sensitivity to the client's needs and concerns. For example, a client who is enmeshed in fear of cancer may not hear the nurse's explanations about the expected proce-dures before and after gallbladder surgery. In this situation it is better for the nurse first to encourage the client to express con-cerns, and then to deal with those concerns. The necessary ex-planations can be provided at another time when the client is able to listen.

Another problem in timing is asking several questions at once. For example, a nurse enters a client's room and says in one breath, "Good morning, Mrs. Brody. How are you this morning? Did you sleep well last night? Your husband is com-ing to see you before your surgery, isn't he?" The client no

Research Note
Is Chat or Social Talk an Effective Communication Technique?

The purpose of this study by Fenwick, Barclay, and Schmeid (2001) was to explore the use of chat or social talk as a commu-nication technique that was helpful in family-centered care in neonatal nurseries. The researchers used grounded theory analysis of over 60 hours of interview data with 28 women, the-matic analysis of 50 hours of interviews with 20 nurses, and con-tent analysis of 398 tape-recorded interactions between nurses and parents. The research found that verbal exchanges that take place between nurse and mother influence a woman's level of confidence, her sense of control, and her feelings of connection to the infant. Chatting facilitated sharing.

Implications: This study confirms that the nurse chatting or using social talk with the mother was a very powerful clinical tool for facilitating rapport. Chat helps put a human face on helping.

Note: From "Chatting: An Important Clinical Tool in Facilitating Mothering in Neonatal Nurseries," by J. Fenwick, L. Barclay, and V. Schmied, 2001, *Journal of Advanced Nursing, 33,* pp. 583–593. Adapted with permission from Blackwell Publishing, Oxford, UK.

doubt wonders which question to answer first, if any. A related pattern of poor timing is to ask a question and then not wait for an answer before making another comment. On the other hand, research shows that by allowing the client to respond to the social talk or chat, the nurse develops a rapport with the client (Fenwick, Barclay, & Schmeid, 2001). This rapport can help facilitate effective therapeutic communication.

ADAPTABILITY. Spoken messages need to be altered in accordance with behavioral cues from the client. This adjustment is referred to as *adaptability*. What the nurse says and how it is said must be individualized and carefully considered. This requires astute assessment and sensitivity on the part of the nurse. For example, a nurse who usually smiles, appears cheerful, and greets his client with an enthusiastic "Hi, Mrs. Brown!" notices that the client is not smiling and appears distressed. It is important for the nurse to then modify his tone of speech and express concern in his facial expression while moving toward the client.

CREDIBILITY. *Credibility* means worthiness of belief, trustworthiness, reliability. Credibility may be the most important criterion of effective communication. Nurses foster credibility by being consistent, dependable, and honest. The nurse needs to be knowledgeable about what is being discussed and to have accurate information. Nurses should convey confidence and certainty in what they are saying, while being able to acknowledge their limitations (e.g., "I don't know the answer to that, but I will find someone who does").

HUMOR. The use of humor can be a positive and powerful tool in the nurse–client relationship, but it must be used with care. Humor can be used to help clients adjust to difficult and painful situations. The physical act of laughter can be both an emotional and physical release, reducing tension by providing a different perspective and promoting a sense of well-being.

Nonverbal Communication

Nonverbal communication is sometimes called *body language*. It includes gestures, body movements, use of touch, and physical appearance, including adornment. Nonverbal communication often tells others more about what a person is feeling than what is actually said, because nonverbal behavior is controlled less consciously than verbal behavior (see Figure 24–4 ■). Nonverbal communication either reinforces or contradicts what is said verbally. For example, if a nurse says to a client, "I'd be happy to sit here and talk to you for a while," yet glances nervously at a watch every few seconds, the actions contradict the verbal message. The client is more likely to believe the nonverbal behavior, which conveys "I am very busy and need to leave."

Observing and interpreting the client's nonverbal behavior is an essential skill for nurses to develop. To observe nonverbal behavior efficiently requires a systematic assessment of the person's overall physical appearance, posture, gait, facial expressions, and gestures. Whatever is observed, the nurse needs to exercise caution in interpretation, always clarifying any observation with the client.

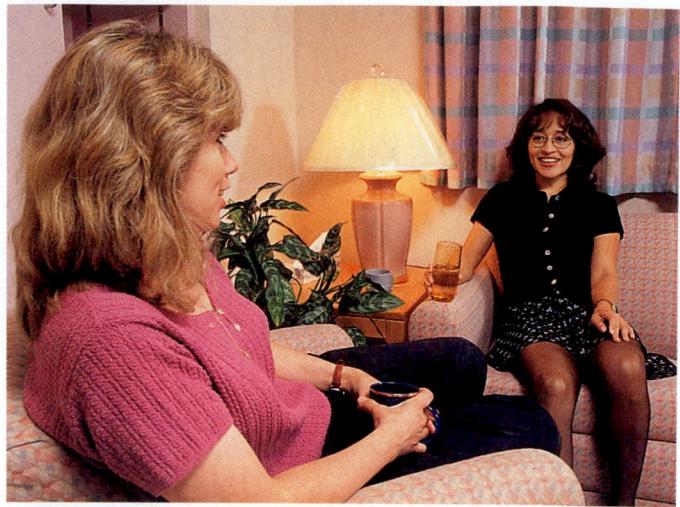

A

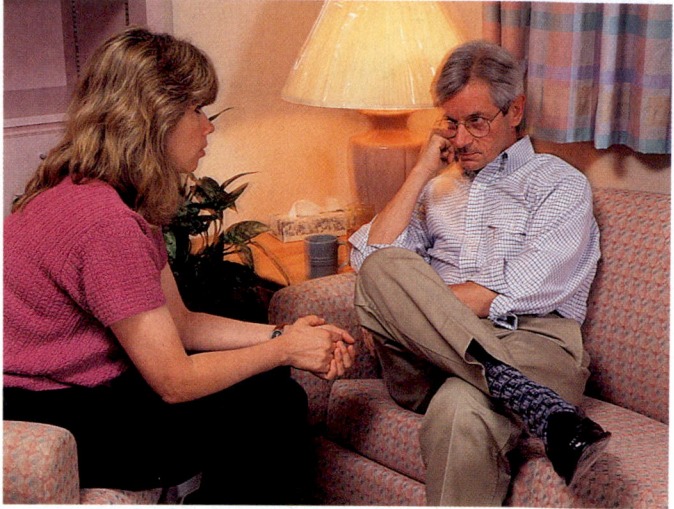

B

Figure 24–4 ■ Nonverbal communication sometimes conveys meaning more effectively than words. *A.* The postures of these women indicate openness to communication. *B.* The listener's posture suggests resistance to communication.

Clients who have altered thought processes, such as in schizophrenia or dementia, may experience times when expressing themselves verbally is difficult or impossible. During these times, the nurse needs to be able to interpret the feeling or emotion that the client is expressing nonverbally. An attentive nurse who clarifies observations very often portrays caring and acceptance to the client. This can be a beginning for establishing a trusting relationship between the nurse and the client, even in clients who have difficulty communicating appropriately.

Transculturally, nonverbal communication varies widely. Even for behaviors such as smiling and handshaking, cultures differ. For example, to many Hispanics smiling and handshaking are an integral part of an interaction and essential to establishing trust. The same behavior might be perceived by a Russian as insolent and frivolous.

The nurse cannot always be sure of the correct interpretation of the feelings expressed nonverbally. The same feeling can be expressed nonverbally in more than one way, even within the same cultural group. For example, anger may be communicated by aggressive or excessive body motion, or it may be communicated by frozen stillness. In some cultures, a smile may be used to conceal anger. Therefore, the interpretation of such observations requires validation with the client. For example, the nurse might say, "You look like you have been crying. Is something upsetting you?"

PERSONAL APPEARANCE. Clothing and adornments can be sources of information about a person. Although choice of apparel is highly personal, it may convey social and financial status, culture, religion, group association, and self-concept. Charms and amulets may be worn for decorative or for health protection purposes. When the symbolic meaning of an object is unfamiliar the nurse can inquire about its significance, which may foster rapport with the client.

How a person dresses is often an indicator of how the person feels. Someone who is tired or ill may not have the energy or the desire to maintain their normal grooming. When a person known for immaculate grooming becomes lax about appearance, the nurse may suspect a loss of self-esteem or a physical illness. The nurse must validate these observed nonverbal data by asking the client. For acutely ill clients in hospital or home care settings, a change in grooming habits may signal that the client is feeling better. A man may request a shave, or a woman may request a shampoo and some makeup.

POSTURE AND GAIT. The ways people walk and carry themselves are often reliable indicators of self-concept, current mood, and health. Erect posture and an active, purposeful stride suggest a feeling of well-being. Slouched posture and a slow, shuffling gait suggest depression or physical discomfort. Tense posture and a rapid, determined gait suggest anxiety or anger. The posture of people when they are sitting or lying can also indicate feelings or mood. Again, the nurse clarifies the meaning of the observed behavior by describing to the client what the nurse sees and then asking what it means or whether the nurse's interpretation is correct. For example, "You look like it really hurts you to move. I'm wondering how your pain is and if you might need something to make you more comfortable?"

FACIAL EXPRESSION. No part of the body is as expressive as the face (see Figure 24–5 ■). Feelings of surprise, fear, anger, disgust, happiness, and sadness can be conveyed by facial expressions. Although the face may express the person's genuine emotions, it is also possible to control these muscles so the emotion expressed does not reflect what the person is feeling. When the message is not clear, it is important to get feedback to be sure of the intent of the expression. Many facial expressions convey a universal meaning. The smile expresses happiness. Contempt is conveyed by the mouth turned down, the head tilted back, and the eyes directed down the nose. No single expression can be interpreted accurately, however, without considering other reinforcing physical cues, the setting in which it occurs, the expression of others in the same setting, and the cultural background of the client.

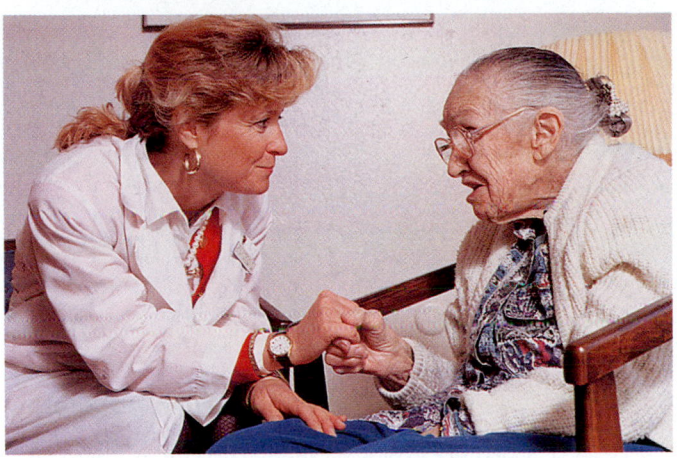

Figure 24–5 ■ The nurse's facial expression communicates warmth and caring.

Nurses need to be aware of their own expressions and what they are communicating to others. Clients are quick to notice the nurse's facial expression, particularly when the client feels unsure or uncomfortable. The client who questions the nurse about a feared diagnostic result will watch whether the nurse maintains eye contact or looks away when answering. The client who has had disfiguring surgery will examine the nurse's face for signs of disgust. It is impossible to control all facial expression, but the nurse must learn to control expressions of feelings such as fear or disgust in some circumstances.

Eye contact is another essential element of facial communication. In many cultures, mutual eye contact acknowledges recognition of the other person and a willingness to maintain communication. Often a person initiates contact with another person with a glance, capturing the person's attention prior to communicating. A person who feels weak or defenseless often averts the eyes or avoids eye contact; the communication received may be too embarrassing or too dominating.

GESTURES. Hand and body gestures may emphasize and clarify the spoken word, or they may occur without words to indicate a particular feeling or to give a sign. A father awaiting information about his daughter in surgery may wring his hands, tap his foot, pick at his nails, or pace back and forth. A gesture may more clearly indicate the size or shape of an object. A wave good-bye and the motioning of a visitor toward a chair are gestures that have relatively universal meanings. Some gestures, however, are culture specific. The Anglo American gesture meaning "shoo" or "go away" means "come here" or "come back" in some Asian cultures. In the Hmong culture it is considered rude to point at something with your toe.

For people with special communication problems, such as the deaf, the hands are invaluable in communication. Many people who are deaf learn sign language. Ill persons who are unable to reply verbally can similarly devise a communication system using the hands. The client may be able to raise an index finger once for "yes" and twice for "no." Other signals can often be devised by the client and the nurse to denote other meanings.

Lifespan Considerations

Communication

Infants
- Infants communicate through their senses. Teach parents about the importance of touch.
- They respond best to a high-pitched, soft or gentle tone of voice and eye contact.

Toddlers and Preschoolers
- Allow time for them to complete verbalizing their thoughts without interruption.
- Provide a simple response to questions because they have short attention spans.
- Drawing a picture can provide another way for the child to communicate.

School-Age Children
- Talk to the child at his or her eye level to help decrease intimidation.
- Include the child in the conversation when communicating with the parents.

Adolescents
- Take time to build rapport with the adolescent.
- Use active listening skills.
- Project a nonjudgmental attitude and nonreactive behaviors, even when the adolescent says disturbing remarks.

Factors Influencing the Communication Process

Many factors influence the communication process. Some of these are development, gender, values and perceptions, personal space, territoriality, roles and relationships, environment, congruence, and attitudes.

Development

Language, psychosocial, and intellectual development moves through stages across the life span. Knowledge of a client's developmental stage will allow the nurse to modify the message accordingly. The use of dolls and games with simple language may help explain a procedure to an 8-year-old. With adolescents who have developed more abstract thinking skills, a more detailed explanation can be given, whereas a well-educated, middle-aged business executive may wish to have detailed technical information provided. Older clients are apt to have had a wider range of experiences with the health care system, which may influence their response or understanding. With aging also come changes in vision and hearing acuity that can affect nurse–client interactions.

Gender

From an early age, females and males communicate differently. Girls tend to use language to seek confirmation, minimize differences, and establish intimacy. Boys use language to establish independence and negotiate status within a group. These differences can continue into adulthood so that the same communication may be interpreted differently by a man and a woman.

Values and Perceptions

Values are the standards that influence behavior, and *perceptions* are the personal view of an event. Because each person has unique personality traits, values, and life experiences, each will perceive and interpret messages and experiences differently. For example, if the nurse draws the curtains around a crying woman and leaves her alone, the woman may interpret this as

"The nurse thinks that I will upset others and that I shouldn't cry" or "The nurse respects my need to be alone." It is important for the nurse to be aware of a client's values and to validate or correct perceptions to avoid creating barriers in the nurse–client relationship.

Personal Space

Personal space is the distance people prefer in interactions with others. **Proxemics** is the study of distance between people in their interactions. Middle-class North Americans use definite distances in various interpersonal relationships, along with specific voice tones and body language. Communication thus alters in accordance with four distances, each with a close and a far phase. Tamparo and Lindh (2000, p. 31) list the following examples:

1. *Intimate:* Touching to 1½ feet
2. *Personal:* 1½ to 4 feet
3. *Social:* 4 to 12 feet
4. *Public:* 12 to 15 feet.

Intimate distance communication is characterized by body contact, heightened sensations of body heat and smell, and vocalizations that are low. Vision is intense, restricted to a small body part, and may be distorted. Intimate distance is frequently used by nurses. Examples include cuddling a baby, touching the sightless client, positioning clients, observing an incision, and restraining a toddler for an injection. It is a natural protective instinct for people to maintain a certain amount of space immediately around them, and the amount varies with individuals and cultures. When someone who wants to communicate steps too close, the receiver automatically steps back a pace or two. In their therapeutic roles, nurses often are required to violate this personal space. However, it is important for them to be aware when this will occur and to forewarn the client. In many instances, the nurse can respect (not come as close as) a person's intimate distance. In other instances, the nurse may come within intimate distance to communicate warmth and caring.

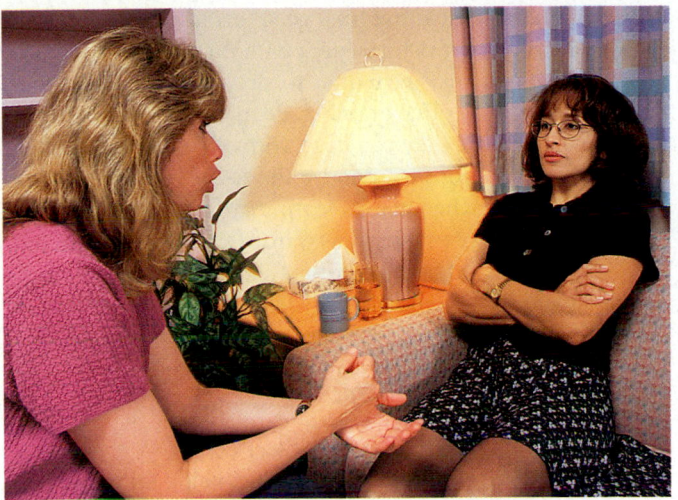

Figure 24–6 ■ Personal space influences communication in social and professional interactions. Encroachment into another individual's personal space creates tension.

Personal distance is less overwhelming than intimate distance. Voice tones are moderate, and body heat and smell are noticed less. Physical contact such as a handshake or touching a shoulder is possible. More of the person is perceived at a personal distance, so that nonverbal behaviors such as body stance or full facial expressions are seen with less distortion. Much communication between nurses and clients occurs at this distance. Examples occur when nurses are sitting with a client, giving medications, or establishing an intravenous infusion. Communication at a close personal distance can convey involvement by facilitating the sharing of thoughts and feelings. On the other hand, it can also create tension if the distance encroaches upon the other's personal space (Figure 24–6 ■). At the outer extreme of 4 feet, however, less involvement is conveyed. Bantering and some social conversations usually take place at this distance.

Social distance is characterized by a clear visual perception of the whole person. Body heat and odor are imperceptible, eye contact is increased, and vocalizations are loud enough to be overheard by others. Communication is therefore more formal and is limited to seeing and hearing. The person is protected and out of reach for touch or personal sharing of thoughts or feelings. Social distance allows more activity and movement back and forth. It is expedient in communicating with several people at the same time or within a short time. Examples occur when nurses make rounds or wave a greeting to someone. Social distance is important in accomplishing the business of the day. However, it is frequently misused. For example, the nurse who stands in the doorway and asks a client, "How are you today?" will receive a more noncommittal reply than the nurse who moves to a personal distance to make the same inquiry.

Public distance requires loud, clear vocalizations with careful enunciation. Although the faces and forms of people are seen at public distance, individuality is lost. Instead, the perception is of the group of people or the community.

Territoriality

Territoriality is a concept of the space and things that an individual considers as belonging to the self. Territories marked off by people may be visible to others. For example, clients in a hospital often consider their territory as bounded by the curtains around the bed unit or by the walls of a private room. This human tendency to claim territory must be recognized by all health care workers. Clients often feel the need to defend their territory when it is invaded by others; for example, when a visitor or nurse removes a chair to use at another bed, the visitor has inadvertently violated the territoriality of the client whose chair was removed. Nurses need to obtain permission from clients to remove, rearrange, or borrow objects in their hospital area.

Roles and Relationships

The roles and the relationships between sender and receiver affect the communication process. Roles such as nursing student and instructor, client and physician, or parent and child affect the content and responses in the communication process. Choice of words, sentence structure, and tone of voice vary considerably from role to role. In addition, the specific relationship between the communicators is significant. The nurse who meets with a client for the first time communicates differently from the nurse who has previously developed a relationship with that client.

Environment

People usually communicate most effectively in a comfortable environment. Temperature extremes, excessive noise, and a poorly ventilated environment can all interfere with communication. Also, lack of privacy may interfere with a client's communication about matters the client considers private. For example, a client who is worried about the ability of his wife to care for him after discharge from hospital may not wish to discuss this concern with a nurse within hearing of other clients in the room. Environmental distraction can impair and distort communication.

Congruence

In **congruent communication,** the verbal and nonverbal aspects of the message match. Clients more readily trust the nurse when they perceive the nurse's communication as congruent. This will also help to prevent miscommunication. Congruence between verbal expression and nonverbal expression is easily seen by the nurse and the client. Nurses are taught to assess clients, but clients are often just as adept at reading a nurse's expression or body language. If there is an incongruence, the body language or nonverbal communication is usually the one with the true meaning. For example, when teaching a client how to care for a colostomy, the nurse might say, "You won't have any problem with this." However, if the nurse looked worried or disgusted while saying this, the client is less likely to trust the nurse's words.

Interpersonal Attitudes

Attitudes convey beliefs, thoughts, and feelings about people and events. Attitudes are communicated convincingly and rapidly to others. Attitudes such as caring, warmth, respect, and acceptance facilitate communication, whereas condescension, lack of interest, and coldness inhibit communication.

Caring and *warmth* convey a feeling of emotional closeness, in contrast to an impersonal approach. Caring is more enduring and intense than warmth. It conveys deep and genuine concern for the person, whereas warmth conveys friendliness and consideration, shown by acts of smiling and attention to physical comforts (Brammer, 1988). Caring involves giving feelings, thoughts, skill, and knowledge. It requires psychologic energy and poses the risk of gaining little in return, yet by caring, people usually reap the benefits of greater communication and understanding.

Respect is an attitude that emphasizes the other person's worth and individuality. It conveys that the person's hopes and feelings are special and unique even though similar to others in many ways. People have a need to be different from—and at the same time similar to—others. Being too different can be isolating and threatening. A nurse conveys respect by listening open mindedly to what the other person is saying, even if the nurse disagrees. Nurses can learn new ways of approaching situations when they conscientiously listen to another person's perspective.

Acceptance emphasizes neither approval nor disapproval. The nurse willingly receives the client's honest feelings. An accepting attitude allows clients to express personal feelings freely and to be themselves. The nurse may need to restrict acceptance in situations where clients' behaviors are harmful to themselves or to others. Helping the client to find appropriate behaviors for feelings is often part of client teaching.

Therapeutic Communication

Therapeutic communication promotes understanding and can help establish a constructive relationship between the nurse and the client. Unlike the social relationship, where there may not be a specific purpose or direction, the therapeutic helping relationship is client and goal directed.

Nurses need to respond not only to the content of a client's verbal message but also to the feelings expressed. It is important to understand how the client views the situation and feels about it before responding. The content of the client's communication is the words or thoughts, as distinct from the feelings. Sometimes people can convey a thought in words while their emotions contradict the words; that is, words and feelings are incongruent. For example, a client says, "I am glad he has left me; he was very cruel." However, the nurse observes that the client has tears in her eyes as she says this. To respond to the client's *words,* the nurse might simply rephrase, saying "You are pleased that he has left you." To respond to the client's *feelings,* the nurse would need to acknowledge the tears in the client's eyes, saying, for example, "You seem saddened by all this." Such a response helps the client to focus on her feelings.

In some instances, the nurse may need to know more about the client and her resources for coping with these feelings.

Sometimes clients need time to deal with their feelings. Strong emotions are often draining. People usually need to deal with feelings before they can cope with other matters, such as learning new skills or planning for the future. This is most evident in hospitals when clients learn that they have a terminal illness. Some require hours, days, or even weeks before they are ready to start other tasks. Some need only time to themselves, others need someone to listen, others need assistance identifying and verbalizing feelings, and others need assistance making decisions about future courses of action.

Attentive Listening

Attentive listening is listening actively, using all the senses, as opposed to listening passively with just the ear. It is probably the most important technique in nursing and is basic to all other techniques. Attentive listening is an active process that requires energy and concentration. It involves paying attention to the total message, both verbal and nonverbal, and noting whether these communications are congruent. Attentive listening means absorbing both the content and the feeling the person is conveying, without selectivity. The listener does not select or listen solely to what the listener wants to hear; the nurse focuses not on the nurse's own needs but rather on the client's needs. Attentive listening conveys an attitude of caring and interest, thereby encouraging the client to talk (see Figure 24–7 ■).

Attentive listening also involves listening for key themes in the communication. The nurse must be careful not to react quickly to the message. The speaker should not be interrupted and the nurse (the responder) should take time to think about the message before responding. As a listener, the nurse also should ask questions either to obtain additional information or to clarify.

Nurses need to be aware of their own biases. A message that reflects different values or beliefs should not be discredited for

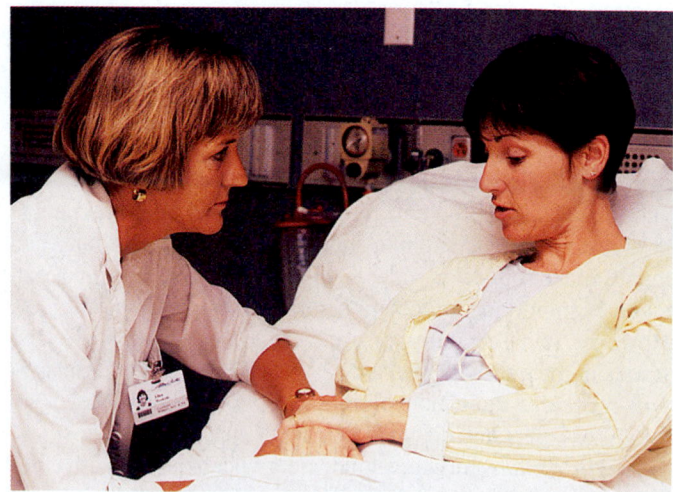

Figure 24–7 ■ The nurse conveys attentive listening through a posture of involvement.

that reason. Rondeau (1992) suggests that the message sender (i.e., the client) should decide when to close a conversation. When the nurse closes the conversation, the client may assume that the nurse considers the message unimportant.

In summary, attentive listening is a highly developed skill, but fortunately it can be learned with practice. A nurse can convey attentiveness in listening to clients in various ways. Common responses are nodding the head, uttering "uh huh" or "mmm," repeating the words that the client has used, or saying "I see what you mean." Each nurse has characteristic ways of responding, and the nurse must take care not to sound insincere or phony.

Physical Attending

Egan (1998) has outlined five specific ways to convey physical attending, which he defines as the manner of being present to another or being with another. Listening, in his frame of reference, is what a person does while attending. The five actions of physical attending, which convey a "posture of involvement," are described in Box 24–2.

Therapeutic communication techniques facilitate communication and focus on the client's concerns (see Table 24–2). Techniques that specifically focus on comforting a client were shown earlier in Table 24–1.

Barriers to Communication

Nurses need to recognize barriers or nontherapeutic responses to effective communication (see Table 24–3 on page 432). Failure to listen, improperly decoding the client's intended message, and placing the nurse's needs above the client's needs are major barriers to communication.

THE HELPING RELATIONSHIP

Nurse–client relationships are referred to by some as *interpersonal relationships,* by others as *therapeutic relationships,* and by still others as **helping relationships.** Helping is a growth-facilitating process that strives to achieve two basic goals (Egan, 1998):

1. Helps clients manage their problems in living more effectively and develop unused or underused opportunities more fully.
2. Helps clients become better at helping themselves in their everyday lives.

A helping relationship may develop over weeks of working with a client, or within minutes. The keys to the helping relationship are (a) the development of trust and acceptance between the nurse and the client and (b) an underlying belief that the nurse cares about and wants to help the client.

The helping relationship is influenced by the personal and professional characteristics of the nurse and the client. Age, sex, appearance, diagnosis, education, values, ethnic and cultural background, personality, expectations, and setting can all affect the development of the nurse–client relationship. Consideration of all of these factors, combined with good communication skills and sincere interest in the client's welfare, will enable the nurse to create a helping relationship. Characteristics of helping relationships are named in Box 24–3 on page 434.

Phases of the Helping Relationship

The helping relationship process can be described in terms of four sequential phases, each characterized by identifiable tasks and skills. The relationship must progress through the stages in succession because each builds on the one before. Nurses can identify the progress of a relationship by understanding these phases: preinteraction phase, introductory phase, working (maintaining) phase, and termination phase. Table 24–4 on page 433 summarizes the tasks and skills required.

Preinteraction Phase

The preinteraction phase is similar to the planning stage before an interview. In most situations, the nurse has information

---

BOX 24–2   ■   Actions of Physical Attending

- Face the other person squarely. This position says, "I am available to you." Moving to the side lessens the degree of involvement.
- Adopt an open posture. The nondefensive position is one in which neither arms nor legs are crossed. It conveys that the person wishes to encourage the passage of communication, as the open door of a home or an office does.
- Lean toward the person. People move naturally toward one another when they want to say or hear something—by moving to the front of a class, by moving a chair nearer a friend, or by leaning across a table with arms propped in front. The nurse conveys involvement by leaning forward, closer to the client.
- Maintain good eye contact. Mutual eye contact, preferably at the same level, recognizes the other person and denotes willingness to maintain communication. Eye contact neither glares at nor stares down another but is natural.

- Try to be relatively relaxed. Total relaxation is not feasible when the nurse is listening with intensity, but the nurse can show relaxation by taking time in responding, allowing pauses as needed, balancing periods of tension with relaxation, and using gestures that are natural.

These five attending postures need to be adapted to the specific needs of clients in a given situation. For example, leaning forward may not be appropriate at the beginning of an interview. It may be reserved until a closer relationship grows between the nurse and the client. The same applies to eye contact, which is generally uninterrupted when the communicators are very involved in the interaction.

TABLE 24-2 Therapeutic Communication Techniques

Technique	Description	Examples
Using silence	Accepting pauses or silences that may extend for several seconds or minutes without interjecting any verbal response.	Sitting quietly (or walking with the client) and waiting attentively until the client is able to put thoughts and feelings into words.
Providing general leads	Using statements or questions that (a) encourage the client to verbalize, (b) choose a topic of conversation, and (c) facilitate continued verbalization.	"Can you tell me how it is for you?" "Perhaps you would like to talk about…". "Would it help to discuss your feelings?" "Where would you like to begin?" "And then what?"
Being specific and tentative	Making statements that are specific rather than general, and tentative rather than absolute.	"Rate your pain on a scale of 0–10" (specific statement) "Are you in pain?" (general statement) "You seem unconcerned about your diabetes." (tentative statement) "You don't care about your diabetes and you never will." (absolute statement)
Using open-ended questions	Asking broad questions that lead or invite the client to explore (elaborate, clarify, describe, compare, or illustrate) thoughts or feelings. Open-ended questions specify only the topic to be discussed and invite answers that are longer than one or two words.	"I'd like to hear more about that." "Tell me about…". "How have you been feeling lately?" "What brought you to the hospital?" "What is your opinion?" "You said you were frightened yesterday. How do you feel now?"
Using touch	Providing appropriate forms of touch to reinforce caring feelings. Because tactile contacts vary considerably among individuals, families, and cultures, the nurse must be sensitive to the differences in attitudes and practices of clients and self.	Putting an arm over the client's shoulder. Placing your hand over the client's hand.
Restating or paraphrasing	Actively listening for the client's basic message and then repeating those thoughts and/or feelings in similar words. This conveys that the nurse has listened and understood the clients basic message and also offers clients a clearer idea of what they have said.	*Client:* "I couldn't manage to eat any dinner last night—not even the dessert." *Nurse:* "You had difficulty eating yesterday." *Client:* "Yes, I was very upset after my family left." *Client:* "I have trouble talking to strangers." *Nurse:* "You find it difficult talking to people you do not know?"
Seeking clarification	A method of making the client's broad overall meaning of the message more understandable. It is used when paraphrasing is difficult or when the communication is rambling or garbled. To clarify the message, the nurse can restate the basic message or confess confusion and ask the client to repeat or restate the message.	"I'm puzzled." "I'm not sure I understand that." "Would you please say that again?" "Would you tell me more?"
	Nurses can also clarify their own message with statements.	"I meant this rather than that." "I'm sorry that wasn't very clear. Let me try to explain another way."
Perception checking or seeking consensual validation	A method similar to clarifying that verifies the meaning of specific words rather than the overall meaning of a message.	*Client:* "My husband never gives me any presents." *Nurse:* "You mean he has never given you a present for your birthday or Christmas?" *Client:* "Well—not never. He does get me something for my birthday and Christmas, but he never thinks of giving me anything at any other time."

TABLE 24-2 Therapeutic Communication Techniques (continued)

Technique	Description	Examples
Offering self	Suggesting one's presence, interest, or wish to understand the client without making any demands or attaching conditions that the client must comply with to receive the nurse's attention.	"I'll stay with you until your daughter arrives." "We can sit here quietly for a while; we don't need to talk unless you would like to." "I'll help you to dress to go home, if you like."
Giving information	Providing, in a simple and direct manner, specific factual information the client may or may not request. When information is not known, the nurse states this and indicates who has it or when the nurse will obtain it.	"Your surgery is scheduled for 11 AM tomorrow." "You will feel a pulling sensation when the tube is removed from your abdomen." "I do not know the answer to that, but I will find out from Mrs. King, the nurse in charge."
Acknowledging	Giving recognition, in a nonjudgmental way, of a change in behavior, an effort the client has made, or a contribution to a communication. Acknowledgment may be with or without understanding, verbal or nonverbal.	"You trimmed your beard and mustache and washed your hair." "I notice you keep squinting your eyes. Are you having difficulty seeing?" "You walked twice as far today with your walker."
Clarifying time or sequence	Helping the client clarify an event, situation, or happening in relationship to time.	Client: "I vomited this morning." Nurse: "Was that after breakfast?" Client: "I feel that I have been asleep for weeks." Nurse: "You had your operation Monday, and today is Tuesday."
Presenting reality	Helping the client to differentiate the real from the unreal.	"That telephone ring came from the program on television." "I see shadows from the window coverings." "Your magazine is here in the drawer. It has not been stolen."
Focusing	Helping the client expand on and develop a topic of importance. It is important for the nurse to wait until the client finishes stating the main concerns before attempting to focus. The focus may be an idea or a feeling; however, the nurse often emphasizes a feeling to help the client recognize an emotion disguised behind words.	Client: "My wife says she will look after me, but I don't think she can, what with the children to take care of, and they're always after her about something—clothes, homework, what's for dinner that night." Nurse: "Sounds like you are worried about how well she can manage."
Reflecting	Directing ideas, feelings, questions, or content back to clients to enable them to explore their own ideas and feelings about a situation.	Client: "What can I do?" Nurse: "What do you think would be helpful?" Client: "Do you think I should tell my husband?" Nurse: "You seem unsure about telling your husband."
Summarizing and planning	Stating the main points of a discussion to clarify the relevant points discussed. This technique is useful at the end of an interview or to review a health teaching session. It often acts as an introduction to future care planning.	"During the past half hour we have talked about...." "Tomorrow afternoon we may explore this further." "In a few days I'll review what you have learned about the actions and effects of your insulin." "Tomorrow, I will look at your feeling journal."

about the client before the first face-to-face meeting. Such information may include the client's name, address, age, medical history, and/or social history. Planning for the initial visit may generate some anxious feelings in the nurse. If the nurse recognizes these feelings and identifies specific information to be discussed, positive outcomes can evolve.

Introductory Phase

The introductory phase, also referred to as the *orientation phase* or the *prehelping phase*, is important because it sets the tone for the rest of the relationship. During this initial encounter, the client and the nurse closely observe each other and form judgments about the other's behavior. The three stages of this introductory phase are opening the relationship, clarifying the problem, and structuring and formulating the contract (Brammer, 1988). Other important tasks of the introductory phase include getting to know each other and developing a degree of trust.

After introductions, the nurse may initially engage in some social interaction to put the client at ease. For example, the

TABLE 24-3 Barriers to Communication

Technique	Description	Examples
Stereotyping	Offering generalized and oversimplified beliefs about groups of people that are based on experiences too limited to be valid. These responses categorize clients and negate their uniqueness as individuals.	"Two-year-olds are brats." "Women are complainers." "Men don't cry." "Most people don't have any pain after this type of surgery."
Agreeing and disagreeing	Akin to judgmental responses, agreeing and disagreeing imply that the client is either right or wrong and that the nurse is in a position to judge this. These responses deter clients from thinking through their position and may cause a client to become defensive.	*Client:* "I don't think Dr. Broad is a very good doctor. He doesn't seem interested in his patients." *Nurse:* "Dr. Broad is head of the Department of Surgery and is an excellent surgeon."
Being defensive	Attempting to protect a person or health care services from negative comments. These responses prevent the client from expressing true concerns. The nurse is saying "You have no right to complain." Defensive responses protect the nurse from admitting weaknesses in the health care services, including personal weaknesses.	*Client:* "Those night nurses must just sit around and talk all night. They didn't answer my light for over an hour." *Nurse:* "I'll have you know we literally run around on nights. You're not the only client, you know."
Challenging	Giving a response that makes clients prove their statement or point of view. These responses indicate that the nurse is failing to consider the client's feelings, making the client feel it necessary to defend a position.	*Client:* "I felt nauseated after that red pill." *Nurse:* "Surely you don't think I gave you the wrong pill?" *Client:* "I feel as if I am dying." *Nurse:* "How can you feel that way when your pulse is 60?" *Client:* "I believe my husband doesn't love me." *Nurse:* "You can't say that; why, he visits you every day."
Probing	Asking for information chiefly out of curiosity rather than with the intent to assist the client. These responses are considered prying and violate the client's privacy. Asking "why" is often probing and places the client in a defensive position.	*Client:* "I was speeding along the street and didn't see the stop sign." *Nurse:* "Why were you speeding?" *Client:* "I didn't ask the doctor when he was here." *Nurse:* "Why didn't you?"
Testing	Asking questions that make the client admit to something. These responses permit the client only limited answers and often meet the nurse's need rather than the client's.	"Who do you think you are?" (forces people to admit their status is only that of client) "Do you think I am not busy?" (forces the client to admit that the nurse really is busy)
Rejecting	Refusing to discuss certain topics with the client. These responses often make clients feel that the nurse is rejecting not only their communication but also the clients themselves.	"I don't want to discuss that. Let's talk about...." "Let's discuss other areas of interest to you rather than the two problems you keep mentioning." "I can't talk now. I'm on my way for coffee break."
Changing topics and subjects	Directing the communication into areas of self-interest rather than considering the client's concerns is often a self-protective response to a topic that causes anxiety. These responses imply that what the nurse considers important will be discussed and that clients should not discuss certain topics.	*Client:* "I'm separated from my wife. Do you think I should have sexual relations with another woman?" *Nurse:* "I see that you're 36 and that you like gardening. This sunshine is good for my roses. I have a beautiful rose garden."
Unwarranted reassurance	Using clichés or comforting statements of advice as a means to reassure the client. These responses block the fears, feelings, and other thoughts of the client.	"You'll feel better soon." "I'm sure everything will turn out all right." "Don't worry."
Passing judgment	Giving opinions and approving or disapproving responses, moralizing, or implying one's own values. These responses imply that the client must think as the nurse thinks, fostering client dependence.	"That's good (bad)." "You shouldn't do that." "That's not good enough." "What you did was wrong (right)."
Giving common advice	Telling the client what to do. These responses deny the client's right to be an equal partner. Note that giving expert rather than common advice is therapeutic.	*Client:* "Should I move from my home to a nursing home?" *Nurse:* "If I were you, I'd go to a nursing home, where you'll get your meals cooked for you."

TABLE 24–4 Tasks and Skills for Each Phase of the Helping Relationship

Phase	Tasks	Skills
Preinteraction Phase	The nurse reviews pertinent assessment data, knowledge, considers potential areas of concern, and develops plans for interaction.	Organized data gathering; recognizing limitations and seeking assistance as required.
Introductory Phase		
1. Opening the relationship	Both client and nurse identify each other by name. When the nurse initiates the relationship, it is important to explain the nurse's role to give the client an idea of what to expect. When the client initiates the relationship, the nurse needs to help the client express concerns and reasons for seeking help. Vague, open-ended questions, such as "What's on your mind today?" are helpful at this stage.	A relaxed, attending attitude to put the client at ease. It is not easy for all clients to receive help.
2. Clarifying the problem	Because the client initially may not see the problem clearly, the nurse's major task is to help clarify the problem.	Attentive listening, paraphrasing, clarifying, and other effective communication techniques discussed in this chapter. A common error at this stage is to ask too many questions of the client. Instead focus on priorities.
3. Structuring and formulating the contract (obligations to be met by both the nurse and client)	Nurse and client develop a degree of trust and verbally agree about (a) location, frequency, and length of meetings, (b) overall purpose of the relationship, (c) how confidential material will be handled, (d) tasks to be accomplished, and (e) duration and indications for termination of the relationship.	Communication skills listed above and ability to overcome resistive behaviors if they occur.
Working Phase	Nurse and client accomplish the tasks outlined in the introductory phase, enhance trust and rapport, and develop caring.	
1. Exploring and understanding thoughts and feelings	The nurse assists the client to explore thoughts and feelings and acquires an understanding of the client. The client explores thoughts and feelings associated with problems, develops the skill of listening, and gains insight into personal behavior.	Listening and attending skills, empathy, respect, genuineness, concreteness, self-disclosure, and confrontation. Skills acquired by the client are nondefensive listening and self-understanding.
2. Facilitating and taking action	The nurse plans programs within the client's capabilities and considers long- and short-term goals. The client needs to learn to take risks (i.e., accept that either failure or success may be the outcome). The nurse needs to reinforce successes and help the client recognize failures realistically.	Decision-making and goal setting skills. Also, for the nurse: reinforcement skills; for the client: risk taking.
Termination Phase	Nurse and client accept feelings of loss. The client accepts the end of the relationship without feelings of anxiety or dependence.	For the nurse: summarizing skills; for the client: ability to handle problems independently.

nurse and client may talk about what a nice day it is and what they would like to do if at home.

During the initial parts of the introductory phase, the client may display some resistive behaviors. *Resistive behaviors* are those that inhibit involvement, cooperation, or change. They may be due to difficulty in acknowledging the need for help and thus a dependent role, fear of exposing and facing feelings, anxiety about the discomfort involved in changing problem-causing behavior patterns, and fear or anxiety in response to the nurse's approach, which may, in the client's opinion, be inappropriate.

Resistive behaviors can be overcome by conveying a caring attitude, genuine interest in the client, and competence. These behaviors of the nurse also foster the development of trust in the relationship. Trust can be described as a reliance on someone without doubt or question, or the belief that the other person is capable of assisting in times of distress and in all likelihood will do so. To trust another person involves risk; clients become vulnerable when they share thoughts, feelings, and attitudes with the nurse. Trust, however, enables the client to express thoughts and feelings openly.

By the end of the introductory phase, clients should begin to

- Develop trust in the nurse.
- View the nurse as a competent professional capable of helping.
- View the nurse as honest, open, and concerned about their welfare.
- Believe the nurse will try to understand and respect their cultural values and beliefs.
- Believe the nurse will respect client confidentiality.
- Feel comfortable talking with the nurse about feelings and other sensitive issues.
- Understand the purpose of the relationship and the roles.
- Feel that they are active participants in developing a mutually agreeable plan of care.

Working Phase

During the working phase of a helping relationship, the nurse and the client begin to view each other as unique individuals. They begin to appreciate this uniqueness and care about each other. Caring is sharing deep and genuine concern about the welfare of another person. Once caring develops, the potential for empathy increases.

The working phase has two major stages: exploring and understanding thoughts and feelings, and facilitating and taking action. The nurse helps the client to explore thoughts, feelings, and actions and helps the client plan a program of action to meet preestablished goals.

EXPLORING AND UNDERSTANDING THOUGHTS AND FEELINGS. The nurse requires the following skills for this phase of the helping relationship:

- *Empathetic listening and responding.* Nurses must listen attentively and communicate (respond) in ways that indicate they have listened to what was said and understand how the client feels. The nurse responds to content or feelings or both, as appropriate. The nurse's nonverbal behaviors are also important. Nonverbal behaviors indicating empathy include moderate head nodding, a steady gaze, moderate gesturing, and little activity or body movement. According to Egan (1998), **empathy** "can be seen as an intellectual process that

involves understanding correctly another person's emotional state and point of view" and also as an emotional response experienced by the helper (p. 73). Empathetic listening focuses on a kind of "being with" clients to develop an understanding of them and their world. This understanding, however, must also be communicated effectively to the client—empathetic response. The end result of empathy is comforting and caring for the client and a helping, healing relationship.

- *Respect.* The nurse must show respect for the client's willingness to be available, desire to work with the client, and a manner that conveys the idea of taking the client's point of view seriously.

- *Genuineness.* Personal statements can be helpful in solidifying the rapport between the nurse and the client. The nurse might offer such comments as "I recall when I was in (a similar situation), and I felt angry about being put down." Egan (1998) outlines five behaviors that are components of genuineness (see Box 24–4). Nurses need to exercise caution when making references about themselves. These statements must be used with discretion. The extreme of matching each of the client's problems with a better story of the nurse's own is of little value to the client.

- *Concreteness.* The nurse must assist the client to be concrete and specific rather than to speak in generalities. When the client says, "I'm stupid and clumsy," the nurse narrows the topic to the specific by pointing out, "You tripped on the rug."

- *Confrontation.* The nurse points out discrepancies between thoughts, feelings, and actions that inhibit the client's self-understanding or exploration of specific areas. This is done empathetically, not judgmentally.

During this first stage of the working phase, the intensity of interaction increases, and feelings such as anger, shame, or self-consciousness may be expressed. If the nurse is skilled in this stage and if the client is willing to pursue self-exploration, the outcome is a beginning understanding on the part of the client about behavior and feelings.

FACILITATING TAKING ACTION. Ultimately the client must make decisions and take action to become more effective. The responsibility for action belongs to the client. The nurse, however, collaborates in these decisions, provides support, and may offer options or information.

Termination Phase

The termination phase of the relationship is often expected to be difficult and filled with ambivalence. However, if the previous phases have evolved effectively, the client generally has a positive outlook and feels able to handle problems independently. On the other hand, because caring attitudes have developed, it is natural to expect some feelings of loss, and each person needs to develop a way of saying good-bye.

Many methods can be used to terminate relationships. Summarizing or reviewing the process can produce a sense of accomplishment. This may include sharing reminiscences of how things were at the beginning of the relationship and comparing them to how they are now. It is also helpful for both the nurse and the client to express their feelings about termination openly and honestly. Thus termination discussions need to start in advance of the termination interview. This allows time for the client to adjust to independence. In some situations referrals are necessary, or it may be appropriate to offer an occasional standby meeting to give support as needed. Follow-up phone calls or e-mails are other interventions that ease the client's transition to independence.

Developing Helping Relationships

Whatever the practice setting, the nurse establishes some type of helping relationship in which mutual goals (outcomes) are set with the client or, if the client is unable to participate, with support persons. Although special training in counseling techniques is advantageous, there are many ways of helping clients that do not require special training.

- Listen actively.
- Help to identify what the person is feeling. Often clients who are troubled are unable to identify or to label their feelings and consequently have difficulty working them out or talking about them. Responses such as "You seem angry about taking orders from your boss" or "You sound as if you've been lonely since your wife died" can help clients recognize what they are feeling and talk about it.
- Put yourself in the other person's shoes (i.e., empathize). Communicate to the client in a way that shows an understanding of the client's feelings and the behavior and experience underlying these feelings.
- Be honest. In effective relationships nurses honestly recognize any lack of knowledge by saying "I don't know the answer to that right now"; openly discuss their own discomfort by saying, for example, "I feel uncomfortable about this discussion"; and admit tactfully that problems do exist, for instance, when a client says "I'm a mess, aren't I?"
- Be genuine and credible. Clients will sense whether or not the nurse is truly concerned.
- Use your ingenuity. There are always many courses of action to consider in handling problems. Whatever course is chosen needs to further the achievement of the client's goals (outcomes), be compatible with the client's value system, and offer the probability of success.
- Be aware of cultural differences that may affect meaning and understanding (see Chapter 13). To facilitate nurse–client

interaction, recognize the language(s) and/or dialect(s) the client uses. Provide a bilingual interpreter as needed for clients limited in the English language.
- Maintain client confidentiality. To maintain the client's right to privacy, share information only with other health care professionals as needed for effective care and treatment.
- Know your role and your limitations. Every person has unique strengths and problems. When you feel unable to handle some problems, the client should be informed and referred to the appropriate health professional. Clarify functions and roles, specifically what is expected of the client, the nurse, and the physician.

GROUP COMMUNICATION

People are born into a group (i.e., a family) and interact with others at all stages of life in various groups: peer groups, work groups, recreational groups, religious groups, and so on. A **group** is two or more people who have shared needs and goals, who take each other into account in their actions, and who thus are held together and set apart from others by virtue of their interactions. Groups exist to help people achieve goals (outcomes) that would be unattainable by individual effort alone. For example, groups can often solve problems more effectively than one person by pooling the ideas and expertise of several individuals; in addition, information can be disseminated to groups more quickly than to individuals.

Group Dynamics

The communication that takes place between members of any group is known as **group dynamics.** The manner of this communication will be determined by a number of interrelated factors and variables. Each member of the group will have an effect on the group dynamics, based on their motivation for participating, their similarity to other group members, the maturity of the group members in expressing their feelings, and the goal of the group.

The unique dynamics of each group will influence its maturation or group process, as well as the effectiveness of the group. Three main functions are required for any group to be effective. It must maintain a degree of group unity or cohesion. It needs to develop and modify its structure to improve its effectiveness. And it must accomplish its goals. The characteristics of an effectively functioning group are shown in Table 24–5.

Types of Health Care Groups

Much of a nurse's professional life is spent in a wide variety of groups, ranging from dyads (two-person groups) to large professional organizations. As a participant in a group, the nurse may be required to fulfill different roles: member or leader, teacher or learner, advisor or advisee, and so on.

Common types of health care groups include task groups, teaching groups, self-help groups, self-awareness/growth groups, therapy groups, and work-related social support groups. There are similarities and differences among the characteristics of these various types of groups and the nurse's role.

TABLE 24-5 Comparative Features of Effective and Ineffective Groups

Factor	Effective Groups	Ineffective Groups
Atmosphere	Comfortable and relaxed; a working atmosphere in which people demonstrate their interest and involvement.	Tense; lacks privacy or voluntary commitment to the group.
Purpose	Goals, tasks, and outcomes are clarified, understood, and modified so that members of the group can commit themselves to purposes through cooperation.	Purposes are unclear, misunderstood, or imposed.
Leadership and member participation	Leadership is democratic with a shift in leadership from time to time depending on knowledge or experience.	Authoritarian; leader may dominate the group, or the members may defer unduly. Member participation is unequal, with some members dominating.
Communication	Open; ideas and feelings are encouraged.	Closed; only idea production is encouraged. Feelings are ignored. Members may have "hidden agendas" (personal goals at cross-purposes with group goals).
Decision making	By the group, although various decision-making procedures appropriate to the situation may be instituted.	By the highest authority in the group, or one or two strong members of the group, with minimal involvement by members. Disagreements are ignored.
Cohesion	Facilitated through valuing other group members, open expression of feelings, trust, and support.	Leader claims full credit for achievements. Comments are critical and focus on personal characteristics.
Conflict tolerance	The reasons for disagreements or conflicts are carefully examined, and the group seeks to resolve them.	Fear of conflict prevents decisions and growth.
Power	Determined by the members' abilities and the information they possess. Power is shared.	Determined by position in the group. Obedience to authority is strong. The issue is who controls, based on individual emotional needs of members.
Problem solving	High; constructive criticism is frequent, frank, relatively comfortable, and oriented toward problem solving.	Low; criticism may be destructive, taking the form of either overt or covert personal attacks.
Creativity	Encouraged.	Discouraged.

Task Groups

The task group is one of the most common types of work-related groups to which nurses belong. Examples are health care planning committees, nursing service committees, nursing team meetings, nursing care conference groups, and hospital staff meetings. The focus of such groups is the completion of a specific task, and the format is defined at the outset by the leader and/or members. The methods vary according to the task to be performed.

The leader of a task group, usually called the chairperson, must be accepted by the members as an appropriate leader and therefore should be an expert in the area of task emphasis. The chairperson's role is to identify the specific task, clarify communication, and assist in expressing opinions and offering solutions. Committee members are generally selected in terms of their individual functional role and employment status, rather than in terms of their personal characteristics. Member participation is determined by the task. A target date for termination of the group is usually set in advance.

Teaching Groups

The major purpose of teaching groups is to impart information to the participants. Examples of teaching groups include con-tinuing education and client health care groups. Numerous subjects are often handled via the group teaching format: childbirth techniques, birth control methods, effective parenting, nutrition, management of chronic illness such as diabetes, exercise for middle-aged and older adults, and instructions to family members about follow-up care for discharged clients. A nurse who leads a group in which the primary purpose is to teach or learn must be skilled in the teaching-learning process (see Chapter 25).

Self-Help Groups

A self-help group is a small, voluntary organization composed of individuals who share a similar health, social, or daily living problem. One of the central beliefs of the self-help movement is that people who experience a particular social or health problem have an understanding of that condition which those without it do not.

Self-help groups are available for a range of problems (e.g., stillbirth, parenting, pregnant adolescents, divorce, drug abuse, cancer, menopause, mental illness, diabetes, AIDS, women's health, caregivers of elderly people, and grief). Alcoholics Anonymous was the first self-help group. Positive aspects of self-help groups are outlined in Box 24–5.

BOX 24–5 ■ Positive Aspects of Self-Help Groups

- Members can experience almost instant kinship because the essence of the group is the idea that "you are not alone."
- Members can talk about their feelings and listen to the concerns of others, knowing they all share this experience.
- The group atmosphere is generally one of acceptance, support, encouragement, and caring.
- Many members act as role models for newer members and can inspire them to attempt tasks they might consider impossible.
- The group provides the opportunity for people to help as well as to be helped—a critical component in restoring self-esteem after significant losses.

The major functions of the nurse's role in self-help groups include the following:

- Help clients form such groups by identifying key people who can act as facilitators.
- Share expertise with clients and help them gain appropriate knowledge and skills.
- Inform clients and support persons about existing self-help groups available to them.
- Participate as a member of a self-help group when this is appropriate. The nurse's role is that of a resource person, that is, of being "on tap, but not on top."
- Help out in times of crisis.

Self-Awareness/Growth Groups

The purpose of self-awareness/growth groups is to develop or use interpersonal strengths. The overall aim is to improve the person's functioning in the group to which they return, whether job, family, or community. From the beginning, broad goals are usually apparent, for example, to study communication patterns, group process, or problem solving. Because the focus of these groups is interpersonal concerns around current situations, the work of the group is oriented to reality testing with a here-and-now emphasis. Members are responsible for correcting inefficient patterns of relating and communicating with each other. They learn group process through participation and involvement and guided exercises.

Therapy Groups

Therapy groups work toward self-understanding, more satisfactory ways of relating or handling stress, and changing patterns of behavior toward health.

Members of the therapy group are referred to as clients or, in some settings, as patients. They are selected by health professionals after extensive selection interviews that consider the pattern of personalities, behaviors, needs, and identification of group therapy as the treatment of choice. Duration of therapy groups is not usually set. A termination date is usually mutually determined by the therapist and members.

Research Note
Will Online Support Help Clients?

The purpose of this article by Perreault-Coursiere (2001) is to look at the role that the emerging frontier of cyberspace might play in the role of today's nurse. Currently it is estimated that the United States has 136 million users of the Internet. The online milieus present an opportunity for nursing to examine this new social support experience. This complex article reviews a theory of online social support in a holistic conceptualization. Research showed that chronically ill seniors would use online services 37 minutes per day. Other researchers have shown that dementia caregivers benefit from online support by decreasing their isolation and enhancing their decision making.

Implications: The graying of America will mean that increasing numbers of nurses will be working with clients who are in the home needing a variety of support systems. Nursing in the technological age will need to have awareness of reliable sources of information and online support networks for client.

Note: From "A Theory of Online Social Support," by S. Perreault-LaCoursiere, 2001, *Advances in Nursing Science, 24,* pp. 60–77.

Work-Related Social Support Groups

Many nurses, for example, hospice, emergency, and acute care nurses, experience high levels of vocational stress. Various types of group support can buffer such stress. Group members who know about the work of others can encourage and challenge members to be more creative and enthusiastic about their work and to achieve more. For example, a nurse may help another team member consider alternative strategies for intervention. Members also can share the joys of success and the frustration of failure through active listening without giving advice or making judgments. This type of social support is best given outside of the work environment.

COMMUNICATION AND THE NURSING PROCESS

Communication is an integral part of the nursing process. Nurses use communication skills in each phase of the nursing process. Communication is also important when caring for clients who have communication problems. Communication skills are even more important when the client has sensory, language, or cognitive deficits.

NURSING MANAGEMENT

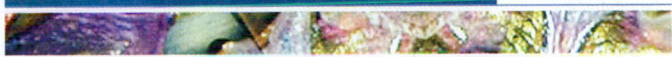

ASSESSING

To assess the client's communication, the nurse determines communication impairments or barriers and communication style. Remember that culture may influence when and how a

Lifespan Considerations

Communication with Elders

Older adults may have physical or cognitive problems that necessitate nursing interventions for improvement of communication skills. Some of the common ones are as follows:

- Sensory deficits, such as vision and hearing
- Cognitive impairment, as in dementia
- Neurological deficits from strokes or other neurological conditions, such as aphasia (expressive and/or receptive) and lack of movement
- Psychosocial problems, such as depression.

Recognition of specific needs and obtaining appropriate resources for clients can greatly increase their socialization and quality of life. Interventions directed toward improving communication in clients with these special needs are as follows:

- Make sure that assistive devices, glasses, and hearing aids are being used and are in good working order.
- Make referrals to appropriate resources, such as speech therapy.

- Make use of communications aids, such as communication boards, computers, or pictures, when possible.
- Keep environmental distractions to a minimum.
- Speak in short, simple sentences, one subject at a time—reinforce or repeat what is said when necessary.
- Always face the person when speaking—coming up behind someone may be frightening.
- Include family and friends in conversation.
- Use reminiscing, either in individual conversations or in groups, to maintain memory connections and to enhance self-identity and self-esteem in the older adult.
- When verbal expression and nonverbal expression are incongruent, believe the nonverbal. Clarification of this and attentiveness to their feelings will help promote a feeling of caring and acceptance
- Find out what has been important and has meaning to the person and try to maintain these things as much as possible. Even simple things such as bedtime rituals become important if they are lost in a hospital or extended care setting.

---

client speaks. Obviously, language varies according to age and development. With children, the nurse observes sounds, gestures, and vocabulary.

Impairments to Communication

Various barriers may alter a client's ability to send, receive, or comprehend messages. These include language deficits, sensory deficits, cognitive impairments, structural deficits, and paralysis. The nurse must assess each to determine their presence.

Language Deficits. Determine the client's primary language for communicating and whether a fluent interpreter is required. Some clients who use English as a second language may have language skills that are inadequate to meet their needs.

Sensory Deficits. The ability to hear, see, feel, and smell are important adjuncts to communication. Deafness can significantly alter the message the client receives; impaired vision alters the ability to observe nonverbal behavior, such as a smile or a gesture; inability to feel and smell can impair the client's capabilities to report injuries or detect the smoke from a fire. For clients with severe hearing impairments, follow these steps:

- Look for a Medic-Alert bracelet (or necklace or tag) indicating hearing loss.
- Determine whether the client wears a hearing aid and whether it is functioning.
- Observe whether the client is attempting to see your face to read lips.
- Observe whether the client is attempting to use hands to communicate with sign language.

Cognitive Impairments. Any disorder that impairs cognitive functioning (e.g., cerebrovascular disease, Alzheimer's disease, and brain tumors or injuries) may affect a client's ability to use and understand language. These clients may develop to-

tal loss of speech, impaired articulation, or the inability to find or name words. Certain medications such as sedatives, antidepressants, and neuroleptics may also impair speech, causing the client to use incomplete sentences or to slur words.

The nurse assesses whether these clients respond when asked a question and, if so, assesses the following: Is the client's speech fluent or hesitant? Does the client use words correctly? Can the client comprehend instructions as evidenced by following directions? Can the client repeat words or phrases? In addition, the nurse assesses the client's ability to understand written words: Can the client follow written directions? Can the client respond correctly by pointing to a written word? Can the client read aloud? Can the client recognize words or letters if unable to read whole sentences? The nurse uses large, clearly written words when trying to establish abilities in this area.

When the client is unconscious, the nurse looks for any indication that suggests comprehension of what is communicated (e.g., tries to arouse the client verbally and through touch). Ask a closed question like "Can you hear me?" and watch for a nonverbal response such as a nod of the head for yes or a shake for no; or ask for a hand squeeze or blink of the eye once for yes or twice for no.

Structural Deficits. Structural deficits of the oral and nasal cavities and respiratory system can alter a person's ability to speak clearly and spontaneously. Examples include cleft palate, artificial airways such as an endotracheal tube or tracheostomy, and laryngectomy (removal of the larynx). Extreme dyspnea (shortness of breath) can also impair speech patterns.

Paralysis. If verbal impairment is combined with paralysis of the upper extremities that impairs the client's ability to write, the nurse should determine whether the client can point, nod, shrug, blink, or squeeze a hand. Any of these could be used to devise a beginning communication system.

Style of Communication

In assessing communication style, the nurse considers both verbal and nonverbal communication. In addition to physical barriers, some psychologic illnesses (e.g., depression or psychosis) influence the ability to communicate. The client may demonstrate constant verbalization of the same words or phrases, a loose association of ideas, or flight of ideas.

Verbal Communication.

When assessing verbal communication, the nurse focuses on three areas: the content of the message, the themes, and verbalized emotions. In addition, the nurse considers the following:

- Whether the communication pattern is slow, rapid, quiet, spontaneous, hesitant, evasive, and so on
- The vocabulary of the individual, particularly any changes from the vocabulary normally used (For example, a person who normally never swears may indicate increased stress or illness by an uncharacteristic use of profanity.)
- The presence of hostility, aggression, assertiveness, reticence, hesitance, anxiety, or loquaciousness (incessant verbalization) in communication
- Difficulties with verbal communication, such as slurring, stuttering, inability to pronounce a particular sound, lack of clarity in enunciation, inability to speak in sentences, loose association of ideas, flight of ideas, or the inability to find or name words or identify objects
- Refusal or inability to speak.

Nonverbal Communication.

Consider nonverbal communication in relation to the client's culture. Pay particular attention to facial expression, gestures, body movements, affect, tone of voice, posture, and eye contact.

DIAGNOSING

Impaired verbal communication may be used as a nursing diagnosis when "an individual experiences a decreased, delayed, or absent ability to receive, process, transmit, and use a system of symbols—anything that has meaning (i.e., transmits meaning)" (Wilkinson, 2000, p. 65). Communication problems may be *receptive* (e.g., difficulty hearing) or *expressive* (e.g., difficulty speaking).

Wilkinson (2000) points out that the *Impaired Verbal Communication* diagnosis may not be useful when an individual's communication problems are caused by a psychiatric illness or a coping problem. In those instances, the diagnoses of *Fear* or *Anxiety* may be more appropriate. Other nursing diagnoses (NANDA International, 2003) used for clients experiencing communication problems that involve impaired verbal communication as the *etiology* could include the following:

- *Anxiety* related to impaired verbal communication
- *Powerlessness* related to impaired verbal communication
- *Situational Low Self-Esteem* related to impaired verbal communication
- *Social Isolation* related to impaired verbal communication
- *Impaired Social Interaction* related to impaired verbal communication.

PLANNING

When a nursing diagnosis related to impaired verbal communication has been made, the nurse and client determine outcomes and begin planning ways to promote effective communication. The overall client outcome for persons with *Impaired Verbal Communication* is to reduce or resolve the factors impairing the communication. Specific nursing interventions will be planned from the stated etiology. Examples of outcome criteria to evaluate the effectiveness of nursing interventions and achievement of client goals follow.

The client

- Communicates that needs are being met.
- Begins to establish a method of communication:
  - Signals yes/no to direct questions using vocalization or agreed-on physical cue (i.e., eye blink, hand squeeze)
  - Uses verbal or nonverbal techniques to indicate needs.
- Perceives the message accurately, as evidenced by appropriate verbal and/or nonverbal responses.
- Communicates effectively:
  - Using dominant language
  - Using translator/interpreter
  - Using sign language
  - Using word board or picture board
  - Using a computer
- Regains maximum communication abilities.
- Expresses minimum fear, anxiety, frustration, and depression.
- Uses resources appropriately.

IMPLEMENTING

Nursing interventions to facilitate communication with clients who have problems with speech or language include manipulating the environment, providing support, employing measures to enhance communication, and educating the client and support person.

Manipulate the Environment

A quiet environment with limited distractions will make the most of the communication efforts of both the client and the nurse and increase the possibility of effective communication. Sufficient light will help in conveying nonverbal messages, which is especially important if visual or auditory acuity is impaired. Initially, the nurse needs to provide a calm, relaxed environment, which will help reduce any anxiety the client may have. Remember that any factor that affects communication can create feelings of frustration, anxiety, depression, or hostility in the client. Communication normally contributes to a client's sense of security and feelings that he or she is not alone, so communication problems may cause some clients to feel isolated and confused. To further reduce these emotions, the nurse should acknowledge and praise the client's attempts at communication.

Provide Support

The nurse should convey encouragement to the client and provide nonverbal reassurance, perhaps by touch if appropriate. If the nurse does not understand, it is critical to let the client know so that he or she can provide clarification with other words or

MediaLink | IMMIGRANT FAMILY CARE PLAN ACTIVITY

through some other means of communication. When speaking with a client who will have difficulty understanding, the nurse should check frequently to determine what the client has heard and understood. Using open-ended questions will assist the nurse in obtaining accurate information about the effectiveness of communication. For example, Maria Perez, who has limited English skills, is being taught about diet related to her Crohn's disease. If the nurse asks, "Do you understand what to eat?" Maria may nod her head yes. However, this does not give the nurse confirmation that the message given has been received. Rather the nurse needs to say, "What do you think will be good for you to eat when you go home?" The nurse's body language (e.g., gestures, posture, facial expression, and eye contact) should convey acceptance and approval.

Employ Measures to Enhance Communication

First determine how the client can best receive messages: by listening, by looking, through touch, or through an interpreter. Ways to help communication include keeping words simple and concrete and discussing topics of interest to the client. It is often helpful to use alternative communication strategies such as word boards, pictures, or paper and pencil.

Often interpreters can assist a client and nurse to communicate when the client lacks fluency in the dominant language. Some hospitals have a list of interpreters for various languages who can assist at the bedside. If the client's support person offers to interpret it is important to ask the client's permission, for the sake of confidentiality. Then instruct the person interpreting to translate as precisely as possible, without interpretation.

Educate the Client and Support Persons

Sometimes clients and support people can be prepared in advance for communication problems, for example, before an intubation or throat surgery. By explaining anticipated problems, the client is often less anxious when problems arise.

EVALUATING

Evaluation is useful for both client and nurse communication.

Client Communication

To establish whether client outcomes have been met in relation to communication, the nurse must listen actively, observe nonverbal cues, and use therapeutic communication skills to determine that communication was effective. Examples of statements indicating outcome achievement include "Using picture board effectively to indicate needs" or "The client stated, 'I listened more closely to my daughter yesterday and found out how she feels about our divorce.'"

Nurse Communication

For nurses to evaluate the effectiveness of their own communication with clients, process recordings are frequently used. A **process recording** is a verbatim (word-for-word) account of a conversation. It can be taped or written and includes all verbal and nonverbal interactions of both the client and nurse.

One method of writing a process recording is to make two columns on a page. The first column lists what the nurse and the client said along with the associated nonverbal behavior. The second column contains an analysis about the nurse's responses. An example of a process recording is found in Table 24–6.

Once a process recording has been completed, it should be analyzed in terms of the content and meaning of the interaction based on communication theory. Each of the nurse's statements is interpreted in terms of the communication skill used, with the rationale for and effectiveness of its use. Any barriers to effective communication can be identified with a possible alternative response noted. The outcome for nurses should be increased awareness and insight regarding their communication strengths, as well as identification of areas for future skills development.

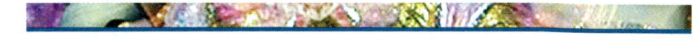

TABLE 24–6 Sample Process Recording

Mary Jane Adams, a nursing aide, reports to Irene Olsen, the staff nurse, that Sandra Barrett, the client in room 815, had finished only her orange juice when Ms. Adams collected the breakfast trays. Mrs. Barrett had been admitted 2 days earlier for diagnostic studies. Concerned about her client, Ms. Olsen walks down the corridor to room 815, knocks, and enters. Mrs. Barrett turns away from the window, tears in her eyes, as Ms. Olsen enters.

Nurse/Client Dialogue	Analysis
NURSE: Good morning, Mrs. Barrett.	Acknowledging.
CLIENT: Hello.	
NURSE: I understand you didn't eat your breakfast.	Making a specific statement but ignoring the nonverbal.
CLIENT: I wasn't hungry.	
NURSE: Is something wrong?	Asking a closed question that fails to facilitate exploration.
CLIENT: No. (Eyes fill with tears.)	
NURSE: You look sad, as if you're about to cry.	Giving feedback.

TABLE 24–6 Sample Process Recording (continued)

Nurse/Client Dialogue	Analysis
CLIENT: (Cries)	
NURSE: I'll sit here awhile with you. (Sits down.)	Offering self.
CLIENT: (Continues to cry.)	
NURSE: (After a 30-second pause) Sometimes it's hard to share the things you're concerned about with someone you don't know well. I'd like to be able to help.	Empathizing. Supporting. Offering self.
CLIENT: (Angrily) You can help me by telling me the truth.	
NURSE: (Leans forward and maintains eye contact.)	Actively listening and demonstrating interest.
CLIENT: Everyone beats around the bush when I ask them what's wrong with me. The nurse manager said, "What do you think is wrong?" That kind of put-off drives me up the wall!	
NURSE: You're angry because you're not getting any answers. It seems as if the staff knows something about your condition and they're keeping it from you.	Paraphrasing.
CLIENT: They all seem to be in cahoots. Nobody tells me anything. (Pause.) (Softly) If the news was good, they wouldn't beat around the bush.	
NURSE: I'm wondering if you're worried that because people haven't answered your question it means that you have a serious illness?	Paraphrasing.
CLIENT: Good news is always easy to give.	
NURSE: Yes, people do seem to be able to deliver good news easier and faster. I also know that we don't have any news—good or bad—to give you because none of the laboratory or x-ray results are back yet. I know that doesn't help answer your questions, but I hope it relieves you a bit from worrying that there is some bad news that's being withheld.	Giving information. Supporting.
CLIENT: Well, when my father-in-law had surgery for a bleeding ulcer, the x-ray and laboratory results were available immediately.	
NURSE: When there's a question of emergency surgery being needed, then test results are asked for immediately. Usually, though, it's preferable to wait for an accurate reading and a thorough written report.	Giving information.
CLIENT: Are you absolutely sure?	
NURSE: You don't sound convinced.	Acknowledging the implied.
CLIENT: Listen, I don't mean to give you a hard time. It's just that … it may not seem like an emergency to my doctor or the lab people, but it sure is to me. I can't stand not knowing. I don't know the results of the tests I had yesterday. I don't know how many more tests I have to have. Will I have to have surgery? When can I go home?	
NURSE: The problem you need help with now is finding out the answers to four questions: What are the results of yesterday's tests? Is your doctor considering any other tests for you and, if so, what are they? Is surgery being planned? And when can you go home? Let's try to figure out how you can get the answers to these questions.	Summarizing. Encouraging problem solving.
CLIENT: Well, I can't call my doctor on the phone. All his receptionist will do is take the message. And, anyway, I'm afraid that he'll be offended if he thinks I'm complaining about him. You won't tell him, will you?	
NURSE: No, not unless you and I decide together that it would be the best solution.	Encouraging collaboration.
CLIENT: I suppose I could try to forget about it and be patient, just like everyone tells me to.	
NURSE: You've tried that, but you're still worried, fearful, and angry. Let's think of some other possibilities.	Encouraging further exploration.
CLIENT: Maybe you could call his office for me! Since you're a nurse, they'll probably put your call right through.	

continued on page 442

TABLE 24-6 Sample Process Recording (continued)

Nurse/Client Dialogue	Analysis
NURSE: So far there are three possible solutions—calling his office yourself, waiting until he comes to visit you later this afternoon, or having me call his office. Are there any other possible solutions that we haven't considered?	Focusing on solutions.
CLIENT: I can't think of any other.	
NURSE: Okay, then, which do you think would be best?	
CLIENT: I guess I'd feel better if you called his office. I just don't want him to think that I'm criticizing him.	
NURSE: You're concerned about what he might think of you because of this phone call. Let's discuss how I should handle the call and what I should say.	Demonstrating respect for the client. Paraphrasing. Encouraging collaboration and problem solving.

Note: From material by Carol Ren Kneisl, RN, MS, APRN, Orange Beach, AL. Adapted with permission.

Focus on Critical Thinking

You are the nursing student assigned to care for Mr. Manasovitz, a 45-year-old man, who will be returning from the recovery room after undergoing the removal of a mass from his abdomen. While you are preparing his room for his return, the nurse and physician arrive to talk with Mrs. Manasovitz about her husband's surgery. The physician explains that the mass was malignant and invasive. Mr. Manasovitz is a candidate for chemotherapy, but his prognosis is guarded because of the extent of the tumor growth. Mrs. Manasovitz looks away, closes her eyes, and only nods her head "yes." As the physician leaves, the nurse approaches Mrs. Manasovitz, sits next to her and puts her arm around Mrs. Manasovitz, who begins to cry. The nurse uses a soothing voice to tell Mrs. Manasovitz that it is okay to cry and assures her she will remain with her. The two of them sit in silence until Mrs. Manasovitz is able to express her feelings. The nurse listens atten-

tively. Later the nurse offers to get a cup of coffee for Mrs. Manasovitz and asks if there is anything she can do to assist Mrs. Manasovitz at this difficult time.

1. Interpret Mrs. Manasovitz's nonverbal behavior in response to the news about her husband's surgery.
2. Evaluate the nurse's response toward Mrs. Manasovitz based on the concepts of caring and comforting.
3. Why is it important for the nurse to effectively communicate with Mrs. Manasovitz at this time?
4. The nurse was described as listening attentively to Mrs. Manasovitz. Cite actions that portray attentive listening.

See Critical Thinking Possibilities in Appendix A.

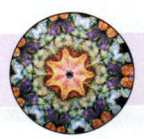 # Chapter Review

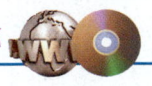 ## EXPLORE MediaLink

NCLEX review questions, case studies, care plan activities, MediaLink applications, and other interactive resources for this chapter can be found on the Companion Website at www.prenhall.com/kozier. Click on Chapter 24 to select the activities for this chapter.

For more NCLEX review questions, and an audio glossary, access the Student CD-ROM accompanying this textbook.

Chapter Highlights

- Communication is a critical nursing skill used to gather assessment data for nursing diagnoses, to teach and persuade, and to express caring and comfort

- Caring is said to be the essence of nursing. Caring is described as the moral ideal of nursing; it involves the will to care, the intent to care, and caring actions

- Caring acts to promote individual growth, preserve human dignity and worth, augment self-healing, and relieve distress.
- Comforting is a characteristic unique to nursing and an essential aspect of caring.
- Comfort needs can be viewed in the framework of physical, psychospiritual, social, and environmental needs. Nurses need to be knowledgeable, skilled, and innovative to individualize comforting strategies.
- Communication is a two-way interpersonal process involving the sender of the message and the receiver of the message. It also involves intrapersonal messages, or self-talk, which can affect the message, the interpretation of the message, and the response.
- Because the sender must encode the message and determine the appropriate channels for conveying it, and because the receiver must perceive the message, decode it, and then respond, the communication process includes four elements: sender, message, receiver, and feedback.
- Verbal communication is effective when the criteria of pace and intonation, simplicity, clarity and brevity, timing, relevance, adaptability, and credibility are met.
- Nonverbal communication often reveals more about a person's thoughts and feelings than verbal communication; it includes personal appearance, posture and gait, facial expressions, and gestures.
- When assessing verbal and nonverbal behaviors, the nurse needs to consider cultural influences and be aware that a single nonverbal expression can indicate any of a variety of feelings and that words can have various meanings.
- When communication is effective, verbal and nonverbal expressions are congruent.

- Many factors influence the communication process: development, gender, values and perceptions, personal space (intimate, personal, social, and public distance), territoriality, roles and relationships, environment, congruence, and attitudes.
- Many techniques facilitate therapeutic communication: using silence, providing general leads, being specific and tentative, using open-ended questions, using touch, restating or paraphrasing, seeking clarification, perception checking or seeking consensual validation, offering self, giving information, acknowledging, clarifying time or sequence, presenting reality, focusing, reflecting, summarizing and planning.
- Techniques that inhibit communication include stereotyping, being defensive, challenging, testing, rejecting, changing topics and subjects, unwarranted reassurance, passing judgment, and giving common advice.
- The effective nurse–client relationship is a helping relationship that facilitates growth of the individual.
- Four phases of the helping relationship include the preinteraction phase, the introductory phase, the working phase, and the termination phase; each has a specific purpose or goal and requires specific skills of the nurse.
- Nurses interact with groups of clients and colleagues in a wide variety of settings. To use groups rationally and effectively, nurses must understand the features of effective groups.
- To help clients with communication problems the nurse manipulates the environment, provides support, employs measures to enhance communication, and educates the client and support persons.
- Process recordings are frequently made by nurses to evaluate their own communication. With them, nurses can analyze both the process and the content of the communication.

Review Questions

24–1. A student nurse is caring for a 72-year-old Alzheimer's patient who is very confused. Her communication tool box should include
   a. written directions for bathing.
   b. speaking very loudly.
   c. gentle touch while guiding ADLs.
   d. flat facial expression.

24–2. Proxemics is
   a. intimate distance communication.
   b. the study of distance between people in interaction.
   c. perceptions that are the personal view of an event.
   d. a constructive relationship between the nurse and client.

24–3. The nurse who develops the skill of attentive listening understands that the skill requires
   a. absorbing both the content and the feeling the person is conveying without selectivity.
   b. assuming what needs the client has.
   c. adopting a closed professional posture.
   d. total relaxation by the listening nurse.

24–4. A nurse points out to a pain client who is struggling with cancer. "It is normal to feel frustrated about the discomfort." What skill in the working phase of the helping relationship is the nurse using?
   a. respect
   b. genuineness
   c. concreteness
   d. confrontation

24–5. A 45-year-old depressed patient has not bathed or dressed in clean clothes today. She is sitting with her menu unable to make a decision about lunch. Which of the following would be the appropriate nursing diagnosis?
   a. *Anxiety*
   b. *Powerlessness*
   c. *Chronic Low Self-Esteem*
   d. *Social Isolation*

Readings and References

Suggested Readings

Deering, C. G. (1999). To speak or not to speak? Self-disclosure with patients. *American Journal of Nursing, 99*(1), 34–38.
A helpful article that assists nurses to evaluate when and what types of self-disclosure are appropriate. It also includes practice guidelines for keeping therapeutic self-disclosure effective.

Deering, C. G., & Cody, D. J. (2002). Communicating with children and adolescents. *American Journal of Nursing, 102*(3), 34–41. The authors focus on communication techniques that work with children and adolescents, according to age, behavior, and the context of the interaction.

Related Research

Atkin, C. K., Smith, S. W., Roberto, A. J., Fediuk, T., & Wagner, T. (2002). Correlates of verbally aggressive communication in adolescents. *Journal of Applied Communication Research, 30*(3), 251–268.

Burgio, L. D., Allen-Burge, R., Roth, D. L., Bourgeois, M. S., Dijkstre, K., Gerstle, J., et al. (2001). Come talk with me: Improving communication between nursing assistants and nursing home residents during care routines. *The Gerontologist, 41,* 449–460.

Engle, V. F., & Graney, M. (2000). Biobehavioral effects of therapeutic touch. *Journal of Nursing Scholarship, 32,* 287–292.

Hemsley, B., Sigafoos, J., Balandin, S., Forbes, R., Taylor, C., Green, V. A., et al. (2001). Nursing the patient with severe communication impairment. *Journal of Advanced Nursing, 35,* 827–835.

Usher, K., & Monkley, D. (2001). Effective communication in an intensive care setting: Nurses' stories. *Contemporary Nurse, 10*(1/2), 91–101.

References

Brammer, L. M. (1988). *The helping relationship: Process and skills* (4th ed.). Upper Saddle River, NJ: Prentice Hall.

Egan, G. (1998). *The skilled helper: A problem-management approach to helping* (6th ed.). Pacific Grove, CA: Brooks/Cole.

Fenwick, J., Barclay, L., & Schmeid, V. (2001). Chatting: An important clinical tool in facilitating mothering in neonatal nurseries. *Advances in Nursing Science, 24,* 34–49.

Gadow, S. (1984). Touch and technology: Two paradigms of patient care. *Journal of Religion and Health, 23*(1), 63–69.

Kolcaba, K. Y. (1991). A taxonomic structure for the concept of comfort. *Image: Journal of Nursing Scholarship, 23,* 237–240.

Kolcaba, K. Y. (1995). Comfort as process and product merged in holistic nursing art. *Journal of Holistic Nursing, 13*(2), 117–131.

Leininger, M. M. (1984). *Care: The essence of nursing and health.* Thorofare, NJ: Charles B. Slack.

Miller, K. L. (1995). Keeping the care in nursing care. Our biggest challenge. *JONA, 25*(11), 29–32.

Morse, J. (1996). The science of comforting. *Reflections, 22*(4), 6–7.

NANDA International. (2003). *NANDA nursing diagnosis: Definitions & classification 2003-2004.* Philadelphia: Author.

Noddings, N. (1984). *Caring: A feminine approach to ethics and moral education.* Berkeley: University of California Press.

Perreault-LaCoursiere, S. (2001). A theory of on-line social support. *Advances in Nursing Science, 24,* 60–77.

Rondeau, K. V. (1992). Effective communication means really listening. *Canadian Journal of Medical Technology, 52*(2), 78–80.

Tamparo, C. T., & Lindh, W. Q. (2000). *Therapeutic communications for health professionals* (2nd ed). Albany, NY: Delmar: Thompson Learning.

Watson, J. (1985). *Nursing: Human science and human care.* Norwalk, CT: Appleton-Century-Crofts.

Wilkinson, J. M. (2000). *Nursing diagnosis handbook with NIC interventions and NOC outcomes* (7th ed) Upper Saddle River, NJ: Prentice Hall Health.

Selected Bibliography

Anonymous. (2002). What makes teams work? *HR Focus Supplement, 79*(4), S1–S4.

Bush, K. (2001). Do you really listen to patients? *RN, 64*(3), 35–37.

Falk-Rafael, A. R. (2001). Watson's philosophy, science and theory of human caring as a conceptual framework for guiding community health nursing. *Advances in Nursing Science, 24,* 34–49.

Hawley, M. P. (2000). Nursing comforting strategies. *Clinical Nursing Research, 9,* 441–458.

Hilgers, J. (2003). Comforting a confused patient. *Nursing, 33*(1), 48–50.

Nelson, M. L. (2001). Helping students to know and respond to human suffering. *Nursing Science Quarterly, 14,* 202–204.

Nuss-Kotecki, C. (2002). Baccalaureate nursing students communication process in the clinical setting. *Journal of Nursing Education, 41,* 61–70.

Olsen, D. P. (2001). Empathetic maturity: Theory of moral point of view in clinical relations. *Advanced Nursing Science, 24*(1), 36–46.

Saewyc, E. (2000). Nursing theories of caring: A paradigm for adolescent nursing practice. *Journal of Holistic Nursing, 18,* 114–128.

Smith, M. C. (1999). Caring and the science of unitary beings. *Advances in Nursing Science, 21,* 14–28.

Viego, A., & Kaplow, R. (2000). Use of nursing resources and comfort of cancer patients with and without do-not-resuscitate orders in the intensive care unit. *American Journal of Critical Care, 9,* 87–95.

Watt-Wattson, J., Garfinkel, P., Gallop, R., Stevens, B., & Streiner, D. (2000). The impact of nurses' empathetic responses on patients' pain management in acute care. *Nursing Research, 49,* 191–200.

TEACHING

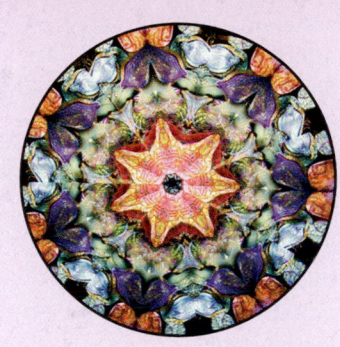

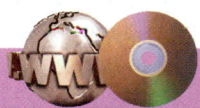
LEARNING OUTCOMES

After completing this chapter, you will be able to:

- Discuss the importance of the teaching role of the nurse.

- Describe the attributes of learning.

- Compare and contrast andragogy, pedagogy, and geragogy.

- Discuss the learning theories of behaviorism, cognitivism, and humanism and how nurses can use each of these theories.

- Describe the three domains of learning.

- Identify factors that affect learning.

- Assess learning needs of learners and the learning environment.

- Identify nursing diagnoses, outcomes, and interventions that reflect the learning needs of clients.

- Describe the essential aspects of a teaching plan.

- Discuss guidelines for effective teaching.

- Discuss strategies to use when teaching clients of different cultures.

- Identify methods to evaluate learning.

- Demonstrate effective documentation of teaching–learning activities.

Teaching client education is a major aspect of nursing practice and an important independent nursing function. In 1992, the American Hospital Association passed *A Patient's Bill of Rights* mandating client education as a right of all clients. In addition, legislation related to nursing frequently has included client teaching as a function of nursing, thereby making teaching a legal and professional responsibility.

Client education is multifaceted, involving promoting, protecting, and maintaining health. It involves teaching about reducing health risk factors, increasing a person's level of wellness, and taking specific protective health measures. Box 25–1 lists specific areas of health teaching.

TEACHING

Teaching is a system of activities intended to produce learning. The teaching process is intentionally designed to produce specific learning.

The teaching–learning process involves dynamic interaction between teacher and learner. Each participant in the process communicates information, emotions, perceptions, and attitudes to the other. The teaching process and the nursing process are much alike (see Table 25–1).

Nurses teach a variety of learners in various settings. They teach clients and their families or significant others in the hospital, the home, or in assisted living and long-term care facilities. Nurses teach large and small groups of learners in community health education programs.

Nurses also teach professional colleagues and other health care personnel in academic institutions such as vocational schools, colleges, and universities, and in health care facilities such as hospitals or nursing homes.

Teaching Clients and Their Families

Nurses may teach individual clients in one-to-one teaching episodes. For example, the nurse may teach about wound care while changing a client's dressing or may teach about diet, exercise, and other lifestyle behaviors that minimize the risk of a heart attack for a client who has a cardiac

---

BOX 25–1 ■ Areas for Client Education

Promotion of Health
- Increasing a person's level of wellness
- Growth and development topics
- Fertility control
- Hygiene
- Nutrition
- Exercise
- Stress management
- Lifestyle modification
- Resources within the community

Prevention of Illness/Injury
- Health screening (e.g., blood glucose levels, blood pressure, blood cholesterol, Pap test, mammograms, vision, hearing, routine physical examinations)
- Reducing health risk factors (e.g., lowering cholesterol level)
- Specific protective health measures (e.g., immunizations, use of condoms, use of sunscreen, use of medication, umbilical cord care)
- First aid
- Safety (e.g., using seat belts, helmets, walkers)

Restoration of Health
- Information about tests, diagnosis, treatment, medications

- Self-care skills or skills needed to care for family member
- Resources within health care setting and community

Adapting to Altered Health and Function
- Adaptations in lifestyle
- Problem-solving skills
- Adaptation to changing health status
- Strategies to deal with current problems (e.g., home IV skills, medications, diet, activity limits, prostheses)
- Strategies to deal with future problems (e.g., fear of pain with terminal cancer, future surgeries, or treatments)
- Information about treatments and likely outcomes
- Referrals to other health care facilities or services
- Facilitation of strong self-image
- Grief and bereavement counseling

TABLE 25–1 Comparison of the Teaching Process and the Nursing Process

Step	Teaching Process	Nursing Process
1	Collect data; analyze client's learning strengths and deficits.	Collect data; analyze client's strengths and deficits.
2	Make educational diagnoses.	Make nursing diagnoses.
3	Prepare teaching plan: • Write learning outcomes. • Select content and time frame. • Select teaching strategies.	Plan nursing goals/desired outcomes and select interventions.
4	Implement teaching plan.	Implement nursing strategies.
5	Evaluate client learning based on achievement of learning outcomes.	Evaluate client outcomes based on achievement of goal criteria.

problem. The nurse may also be involved in teaching family members or other support people who are caring for the client. Nurses working in obstetric and pediatric areas teach parents and sometimes grandparents how to care for children.

Because of decreased length of hospital stays, time constraints on client education may occur. Nurses need to provide client education that will ensure the client's safe transition from one level of care to another and make appropriate plans for follow-up education in the client's home. Discharge plans must include both information about what the client has been taught before transfer or discharge and what remains for the client to learn to perform self-care in the home or other residence (see Chapter 7). 🔗

Teaching in the Community

Nurses are often involved in community health education programs. Such teaching activities may be voluntary as part of the nurse's involvement in an organization such as the Red Cross or Planned Parenthood, or they may be compensated as part of the nurse's work role. Community teaching activities may be aimed at large groups of people who have an interest in some aspect of health, such as nutrition classes, CPR or cardiac risk factor reduction classes, and bicycle or swimming safety programs. Community education programs can also be designed for small groups or individual learners, such as childbirth classes or family planning classes.

Teaching Health Personnel

Nurses are also involved in the instruction of professional colleagues. Nurses in nursing practice settings are often involved in the clinical instruction of nursing students. Experienced nurses may function as preceptors for new graduate nurses or for newly employed nurses. Nurses with specialized knowledge and experience may share that knowledge and experience with nurses who are new to that practice area. Such specialized courses include acute care nursing, perioperative nursing, and quality improvement/quality assurance.

Nurses may also be involved in teaching other health professionals. Nurses may participate in the education of medical students or allied health students. In this capacity, the nurse ed-

ucator is often clarifying the role of the nurse for other health professionals or how the nurse can assist them in their care of the client. The nurse may also teach health care colleagues knowledge or skills that are considered the domain of nursing, such as nonpharmaceutical comfort measures.

LEARNING

Like all people, clients have a variety of learning needs. A **learning need** is a desire or a requirement to know something that is presently unknown to the learner. Learning needs include new intellectual knowledge but can also include a new or different skill or physical ability, or a new behavior or a need to change an old behavior. **Learning** is a change in human disposition or capability that persists and that cannot be solely accounted for by growth. Learning is represented by a change in behavior. See Teaching: Client Care for attributes of learning.

An important aspect of learning is the individual's desire to learn and to act on the learning, referred to as **compliance.** In the health care context, compliance is the extent to which a person's behavior coincides with medical or health advice. Compliance is best illustrated when the person recognizes and accepts the need to learn, and then follows through with the appropriate behaviors that reflect the learning. For example, a person diagnosed as having diabetes willingly learns about the

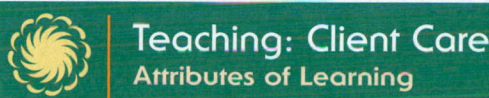

Teaching: Client Care
Attributes of Learning

Learning is
- An experience that occurs inside the learner.
- The discovery of the personal meaning and relevance of ideas.
- A consequence of experience.
- A collaborative and cooperative process.
- An evolutionary process.
- A process that is both intellectual and emotional.

special diet needed and then plans and follows the learned diet. The term *compliance,* however, is viewed in a negative perspective by many people because the term implies the learner is submissive and this is in conflict with the learner's right to determine his or her own health care decisions rather than be told what to do by a health care professional.

Another term that is seen in health care literature is **adherence,** which is commitment or attachment to a regimen. Bastable (2003) explains that both compliance and adherence refer to the "ability to maintain health-promoting regimens, which are determined largely by a health care provider" (p. 169).

Andragogy is the art and science of teaching adults, in contrast to **pedagogy,** the discipline concerned with helping children learn. **Geragogy** is the term used to describe the process involved in stimulating and helping elders to learn (John, 1988).

Nurses can use the following andragogic concepts about adult learners as a guide for client teaching (Knowles, 1984):

- As people mature, they move from dependence to independence.
- An adult's previous experiences can be used as a resource for learning.
- An adult's readiness to learn is often related to a developmental task or social role.
- An adult is more oriented to learning when the material is useful immediately, not sometime in the future.

Learning Theories

Theories about how and why people learn can be traced to the 17th century. Three main theoretical constructs are behaviorism, cognitivism, and humanism.

Behaviorism

Behaviorism was originally advanced by Edward Thorndike, whose major contribution applicable to teaching is that learning should be based on the learner's behavior. In addition to Thorndike, major behaviorist theorists include I. Pavlov, B. F. Skinner, and A. Bandura.

In the behaviorist school of thought, an act is called a *response* when it can be traced to the effects of a stimulus. Behaviorists closely observe responses and then manipulate the environment to bring about the intended change. Thus, to modify a person's attitude and response, a behaviorist would either alter the stimulus condition in the environment or change what happens after a response occurs (Bastable, 2003, p. 45).

Skinner's and Pavlov's work focused on conditioning behavioral responses to a stimulus that causes the response or behavior. To increase the probability of a response, Skinner introduced the importance of **positive reinforcement** (e.g., a pleasant experience such as praise and encouragement) in fostering repetition of an action. Bandura, however, claims that most learning comes from observational learning and instruction rather than from overt trial-and-error behavior. Bandura's research focuses on **imitation,** the process by which individuals copy or reproduce what they have observed, and **modeling,** the process by which a person learns by observing the behavior of others.

Cognitivism

Cognitivism depicts learning as a complex cognitive activity. In other words, learning is largely a mental or intellectual or thinking process. The learner structures and processes information. Perceptions are selectively chosen by the individual and personal characteristics have an impact on how a cue is perceived. Cognitivists also emphasize the importance of social, emotional, and physical contexts in which learning occurs, such as the teacher–learner relationship and environment. Developmental readiness and individual readiness (expressed as motivation) are other key factors associated with cognitive approaches.

Major cognitive theorists include J. Piaget, K. Lewin, and B. Bloom. Piaget's five major phases of cognitive development include the sensorimotor phase, the preconceptual phase, the intuitive phase, the concrete operations phase, and the formal operations phase. Each phase is discussed in Chapter 21. Lewin states that learning involves four different types of changes: change in cognitive structure, change in motivation, change in one's sense of belonging to the group, and gain in voluntary muscle control. His widely known theory of change has three basic stages: unfreezing, moving, and refreezing. These stages are discussed in detail in Chapter 26.

Bloom (1956) has identified three domains or areas of learning: cognitive, affective, and psychomotor. The **cognitive domain,** the "thinking" domain, includes six intellectual abilities and thinking processes beginning with knowing, comprehending, and applying to analysis, synthesis, and evaluation. The **affective domain,** known as the "feeling" domain, is divided into categories that specify the degree of a "person's depth of emotional response to tasks" (Bastable, 2003, p. 330). It includes feelings, emotions, interests, attitudes, and appreciations. The **psychomotor domain,** the "skill" domain, includes motor skills such as giving an injection.

Nurses should include each of Bloom's three domains in client teaching plans. For example, teaching a client how to irrigate a colostomy is in the psychomotor domain. But an important part of a teaching plan for a client with a colostomy is to teach why a specific amount of fluid is used and when the irrigation should be carried out; this is in the cognitive domain. Helping the client accept the colostomy and maintain self-esteem is in the affective domain.

Humanism

Humanistic learning theory focuses on both cognitive and affective qualities of the learner. Prominent members of this school of thought include Abraham Maslow and Carl Rogers. According to humanistic theory, learning is believed to be self-motivated, self-initiated, and self-evaluated. Each individual is viewed as a unique composite of biologic, psychologic, social, cultural, and spiritual factors. Learning focuses on self-development and achieving full potential; it is best when it is relevant to the learner. Autonomy and self-determination are important; the learner identifies the learning needs and takes the initiative to meet these needs. The learner is thus an active participant and takes responsibility for meeting individual learning needs.

Using Learning Theories

The major attributes of the **behaviorist theory** include the careful identification of what is to be taught and the immediate identification of and reward for correct responses. However, the theory is not easily applied to complex learning situations and is limiting in terms of the learner's role in the teaching process. Nurses applying behavioristic theory will

- Provide sufficient practice time and both immediate and repeat testing and redemonstration.
- Provide opportunities for learners to solve problems by trial and error.
- Select teaching strategies that avoid distracting information and that evoke the desired response.
- Praise the learner for correct behavior and provide positive feedback at intervals throughout the learning experience.
- Provide role models of desired behavior.

The major attributes of **cognitive theory** are its recognition of developmental levels of learners and acknowledgments of learners' motivation and environment. However, some or many of the motivational and environmental factors may be beyond the teacher's control. Nurses applying cognitive theory will

- Provide a social, emotional, and physical environment conducive to learning.
- Encourage a positive teacher–learner relationship.
- Select multisensory teaching strategies since perception is influenced by the senses.
- Recognize that personal characteristics have an impact on how cues are perceived and develop appropriate teaching approaches to target different learning styles.
- Assess a person's developmental and individual readiness to learn and adapt teaching strategies to the learner's developmental level.
- Select behavioral objectives and teaching strategies that encompass the cognitive, affective, and psychomotor domains of learning.

The major attributes of **humanism** are its focus on the feelings and attitudes of learners, on the importance of the individual in identifying learning needs and in taking responsibility for them, and on the self-motivation of the learners to work toward self-reliance and independence. Nurses applying humanistic theory will

- Convey empathy in the nurse–client relationship.
- Encourage the learners to establish goals and promote self-directed learning.
- Encourage active learning by serving as a facilitator, mentor, or resource for the learner.
- Expose the learner to new relevant information and ask appropriate questions to encourage the learner to seek answers.

Factors Affecting Learning

Many factors can facilitate or hinder learning by a client. The nurse should be aware of these factors, particularly when available teaching time is limited.

Motivation

Motivation to learn is the desire to learn. It greatly influences how quickly and how much a person learns. Motivation is generally greatest when a person recognizes a need and believes the need will be met through learning. It is not enough for the need to be identified and verbalized by the nurse; it must be experienced by the client. Often the nurse's task is to help the client personally work through the problem and identify the need. Sometimes clients or support people need help identifying information relevant to their situation before they can see a need. For instance, clients with heart disease may need to know the effects of smoking before they recognize the need to stop smoking. Or adolescents may need to know the consequences of an untreated sexually transmitted disease before they see the need for treatment.

Readiness

Readiness to learn is the demonstration of behaviors or cues that reflect the learner's motivation to learn at a specific time. Readiness reflects not only the desire or willingness to learn but also the ability to learn at a specific time. For example, a client may want to learn self-care during a dressing change, but if the client experiences pain or discomfort she may not be able to learn. The nurse can provide pain medication to make the client more comfortable so that she is more able to learn. The nurse's role is often to encourage the development of readiness.

Active Involvement

When the learner is actively involved in the process of learning, learning becomes more meaningful. If the learner actively participates in planning and discussion, learning is faster and retention is better (Figure 25–1 ■). Active learning promotes critical thinking, enabling learners to problem solve more effectively. Clients who are actively involved in learning about their health care may be more able to apply the learning to their own situation. For example, clients who are actively involved

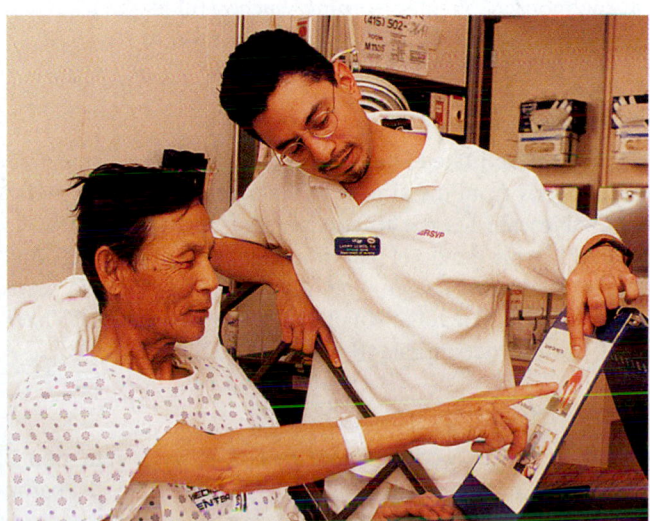

Figure 25–1 ■ Learning is facilitated when the client is interested and actively involved.

in learning about their therapeutic diets may be more able to apply the principles being taught to their cultural food preferences and their usual eating habits. Passive learning, such as listening to a lecture or watching a film, does not foster optimal learning.

Relevance

The knowledge or skill to be learned must be personally relevant to the learner. Clients learn more easily if they can connect the new knowledge to that which they already know or have experienced. For example, if a client is diagnosed with hypertension, is overweight, and has symptoms of headaches and fatigue, he is more likely to understand the need to lose weight if he remembers having more energy when he weighed less. The nurse needs to validate the relevance of learning with the client throughout the learning process.

Feedback

Feedback is information relating a person's performance to a desired goal. It has to be meaningful to the learner. Feedback that accompanies the practice of psychomotor skills helps the person to learn those skills. Support of desired behavior through praise, positively worded corrections, and suggestions of alternative methods are ways of providing positive feedback. Negative feedback such as ridicule, anger, or sarcasm can lead people to withdraw from learning. Such feedback, viewed as a type of punishment, may cause the client to avoid the teacher in order to avoid punishment.

Nonjudgmental Support

People learn best when they believe they are accepted and will not be judged. The person who expects to be judged as a "poor" or "good" client will not learn as well as the person who feels no such threat. Once learners have succeeded in accomplishing a task or understanding a concept, they gain self-confidence in their ability to learn. This reduces their anxiety about failure and can motivate greater learning. Successful learners have increased confidence with which to accept failure.

Simple to Complex

Learning is facilitated by material that is logically organized and proceeds from the simple to the complex. Such organization enables the learner to comprehend new information, assimilate it with previous learning, and form new understandings. Of course, *simple* and *complex* are relative terms, depending on the level at which the person is learning. What is simple for one person may be complex for another.

Repetition

Repetition of key concepts and facts facilitates retention of newly learned material. Practice of psychomotor skills, particularly with feedback from the nurse, improves performance of those skills and facilitates their transfer to another setting.

Timing

People retain information and psychomotor skills best when the time between learning and active use of the learning is short; the longer the time interval, the more learning is forgotten. For example, a woman who is only shown literature and videotapes about administering insulin but is not permitted to administer her own insulin until discharge from the hospital is unlikely to remember what she learned. However, if she is allowed to give her own injections while in the hospital, her learning will be enhanced.

Environment

An optimal learning environment facilitates learning by reducing distraction and providing physical and psychologic comfort. It has adequate lighting that is free from glare, a comfortable room temperature, and good ventilation. Most students know what it is like to try to learn in a hot, stuffy room; the consequent drowsiness interferes with concentration. Noise can also distract the student and interfere with listening and thinking. To facilitate learning in a hospital setting, nurses should choose a time when no visitors are present and interruptions are unlikely.

Privacy is essential for some learning. For example, when a client is learning to irrigate a colostomy, the presence of others can be embarrassing and thus interfere with learning. However, when a client is particularly anxious, having a support person present may give the client confidence.

Many factors inhibit learning. Some of the most common barriers to learning are described next and in Table 25–2.

Emotions

Emotions such as fear, anger, and depression can impede learning. A high level of anxiety resulting in agitation and the inability to focus or concentrate can also inhibit learning. Clients or families who are experiencing extreme emotional states may not hear spoken words or may retain only part of the communication. Emotional responses such as fear and anxiety may be lessened by information that relieves uncertainty. Medications may be prescribed for extremely distraught clients or families to reduce their anxiety and put them in an emotional state in which understanding or learning can occur.

Physiologic Events

Learning can be inhibited by physiologic events such as a critical illness, pain, or sensory deficits. Because the client cannot concentrate and apply energy to learning, the learning itself is impaired. The nurse should try to reduce the physiologic barriers to learning as much as possible before teaching. For example, providing analgesics and rest before teaching is often helpful.

Cultural Aspects

There are also cultural barriers to learning, such as language or values. Obviously the client who does not understand the

TABLE 25-2 Barriers to Learning

Barrier	Explanation	Nursing Implications
Acute illness	Client requires all resources and energy to cope with illness.	Defer teaching until client is less ill.
Pain	Pain decreases ability to concentrate.	Conduct pain assessment before teaching.
Prognosis	Client can be preoccupied with illness and unable to concentrate on new information.	Defer teaching to a better time.
Biorhythms	Mental and physical performances have a circadian rhythm.	Adapt time of teaching to suit client.
Emotion (e.g., anxiety, denial, depression, grief)	Emotions require energy and distract from learning.	Deal with emotions and possible misinformation first.
Language	Client may not be fluent in the nurse's language.	Obtain services of an interpreter or nurse with appropriate language skills.
Age		
• Elders	Vision, hearing, and motor control can be impaired in elders.	Consider sensory and motor deficits and adapt in teaching plan.
• Children	Children have a shorter attention span and vocabulary differences.	Plan shorter and more active learning episodes.
Culture/religion	There may be cultural or religious restrictions on certain types of knowledge, for example, birth control information.	Assess the client's cultural/religious needs when planning learning activities.
Physical disability	Visual, hearing, sensory, or motor impairments may interfere with a client's ability to learn.	Plan teaching activities appropriate to learner's physical abilities. For example, provide audio learning tools for the client who is blind, or large-print materials for the client whose vision is impaired.
Mental disability	Impaired cognitive ability may affect the client's capacity for learning.	Assess client's capacity for learning and plan teaching activities to complement the client's ability while planning more complex learning for the client's caregivers.

nurse's language will learn little. Western medicine may conflict with a client's cultural healing beliefs and practices. To be effective, nurses must deal directly with this conflict; otherwise the client may be partially or totally noncompliant with recommended treatments. Another impediment to learning is differing values held by the client and the health team. For example, a client who comes from a culture that does not value slimness may have difficulty learning about a reducing diet.

Psychomotor Ability

It is important that the nurse be aware of a client's psychomotor skills when planning teaching. Psychomotor skills can be affected by health. For example, an older client who has severe osteoarthritis of the hands may not be able to tie a bandage. The following physical abilities are important for learning psychomotor skills:

1. *Muscle strength.* For example, an older client who cannot rise from a chair because of insufficient leg and muscle strength cannot be expected to learn to lift herself out of a bathtub.

2. *Motor coordination.* Gross motor coordination is required for movements such as walking and fine motor coordination is needed when using utensils such as a fork for eating. For example, a client who has advanced amyotrophic lateral sclerosis (ALS) involving the lower limbs will probably be unable to use a walker.
3. *Energy.* Energy is required for most psychomotor skills, and learning these skills uses more energy. People who are ill or elderly often have limited energy resources; learning and carrying out these skills must be timed for when the client's energy sources are not depleted.
4. *Sensory acuity.* Sight is used for most learning (i.e., walking with crutches, changing a dressing, drawing a medication into a syringe). Clients who have a visual impairment often need the assistance of a support person to carry out such tasks.

NURSE AS EDUCATOR

Being an educator or teacher is an important and primary role for the nurse. Clients and families have the right to health education in order to make informed decisions about their health.

The nurse is in a position to promote healthy lifestyles through the application of health knowledge, the change process, learning theories, and the nursing and teaching process when teaching clients and their families.

NURSING MANAGEMENT

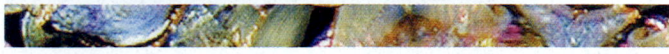

ASSESSING

A comprehensive assessment of learning needs incorporates data from the nursing history and physical assessment and addresses the client's support system. It also considers client characteristics that may influence the learning process: readiness to learn, motivation to learn, and reading and comprehension level, for example. Assessing a person's stage of change and any barriers to change is also important and often overlooked (see Chapter 8).

The nurse's own knowledge of common learning needs required by clients experiencing similar health problems is another source of information. Learning needs change as the client's health status changes, so nurses must constantly reassess them.

Nursing History

Several elements in the nursing history provide clues to learning needs. These elements include (a) age, (b) the client's understanding and perceptions of the health problem, (c) health beliefs and practices, (d) cultural factors, (e) economic factors, (f) learning style, and (g) client's support systems. Examples of interview questions to elicit this information are shown in the accompanying Assessment Interview. Note the number of open-ended questions.

Age. Age provides information on the person's developmental status that may indicate distinctive health teaching content and teaching approaches. Simple questions to school-age children and adolescents will elicit information on what they know. Observing children at play provides information about their motor and intellectual development as well as relationships with other children. For older people, conversation and questioning may reveal slow recall or limited psychomotor skills, sensory deficits, and learning difficulties (see Lifespan Considerations).

Clients' Understanding of Health Problem. Clients' perceptions of their current health problems and concerns may indicate knowledge deficits or misinformation. In addition, the ef-

---

Assessment Interview

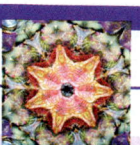

LEARNING NEEDS AND CHARACTERISTICS

Primary Health Problem

- Tell me what you know about your current health problem. What do you think caused it?
- What concerns do you have about it?
- How has the problem affected what you can or cannot do during your usual activities (e.g., work, recreation, shopping, housework)?
- What do you or did you do at home to relieve the problem? How helpful was it?
- How have the treatments you have started helped your problem?
- What, if any, difficulties have the treatments caused you (e.g., inconvenience, cost, discomfort)?
- Tell me about the tests (surgery, treatments) you are going to have.

Health Beliefs

- How would you describe your health generally?
- What things do you usually do to keep healthy?
- What health problems do you think you may be at risk for because of family history, age, diet, occupation, inadequate exercise, or other habits, such as smoking?
- What changes would you be willing to make to decrease your risk for these problems or to improve your health?

Cultural Factors

- What language do you use most often when speaking and writing?

- Do you seek the advice of another health practitioner?
- Do you use herbs or other medications or treatments commonly used in your cultural group?
- Does your current doctor know about these?
- What advice or treatments given previously by your doctor conflicted with values or beliefs you consider important?
- When a conflict arose, what did you do?

Learning Style

- Note the client's age and developmental level.
- What level of education have you received?
- Do you like to read?
- Where do you obtain health information (e.g., physician, nurse, magazines, books, pharmacist, and so on)?
- How do you best learn new things?
  a. By reading about them
  b. By talking about them
  c. By watching a movie or demonstration
  d. By computer
  e. By listening to the teacher
  f. By first being shown how something works and then doing it
  g. On your own or in a group

Client Support System

- Would you like a family member or friend to help you learn about things you need to do to take care of yourself?
- Who do you think would be interested in learning with you?

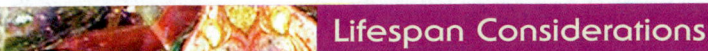

Lifespan Considerations

Elders

Elders often have chronic illnesses that require multiple treatments and/or medications. Health teaching will focus on the same areas as with other ages—health and wellness promotion and prevention of illness and accidents—but often the needs are greatest in learning to live with conditions that they have and to maintain optimal health and functioning. For older adults to be motivated to learn, the material must be practical and have meaning for them individually, especially if the information is new to them. Special considerations in teaching elders are:

- Health promotion is a priority need and should include the following areas:
  - Exercise
  - Nutrition
  - Safety habits
  - Having regular health checkups
  - Understanding medications.
- Set achievable goals—involve the client and family in doing this.

- If using visual aids, use large print and contrasting colors.
- Increase time for teaching and allow for rest periods.
- Repeat information if necessary.
- Use return demonstrations with psychomotor skills, such as teaching someone to learn to do insulin injections.
- Determine where clients obtain most of their health information (newspapers, magazines, television).
- Use examples that they can relate to in their daily lives.
- Be aware of sensory deficits, such as hearing and vision.
- Use the setting with which the individual is most comfortable—either a group or one on one setting.
- If noncompliance is a problem, investigate the cause—it could be due to lack of finances, transportation problems, poor access to medical care, and so on.

Elders come with a lifetime of experiences and learned knowledge of their own. Respect this and always have them use their strengths to work with any problems. Positive reinforcement and ongoing evaluation of what has been taught are important factors in effective health teaching with older adults.

Note: From *Gerontological Nursing,* 2nd ed. (pp. 55–65), by M. Stanley and P. G. Beare, 1999, Philadelphia: F. A. Davis. Adapted with permission.

---

fects of the problem on the client's usual activities can alert the nurse to other areas requiring instruction. For example, people who cannot manage self-care at home often need information about community resources and services.

Health Beliefs and Practices. A client's health beliefs and practices are important to consider in any teaching plan. The health belief model described in Chapter 11 ∞ provides a predictor of preventive health behavior. However, even if a nurse is convinced that a particular client's health beliefs should be changed, doing so may not be possible because so many factors are involved in a person's health beliefs.

Cultural Factors. Many cultural groups have their own folk beliefs and practices with a number of them related to diet, health, illness, and lifestyle. It is therefore important to know how the practices and values held by clients will impact their learning needs. Although the client may readily understand the health care information being taught, this learning may not be implemented in the home where folk medical practices prevail (see Chapter 13). ∞

Economic Factors. Economic factors can also affect a client's learning. For example, a client who cannot afford to obtain a new sterile syringe for each injection of insulin may find it difficult to learn to administer the insulin when the nurse teaches that a new syringe should be used each time.

Learning Style. Considerable research has been done on people's learning styles. The best way to learn varies with the individual. Some people are visual learners and learn best by watching. Other people do not visualize an activity well; they learn best by actually manipulating equipment and discovering how it works. Other people can learn well from reading things

presented in an orderly fashion. Still other people learn best in groups where they can relate to other people. For some, stressing the thinking part of a skill and its logic will promote learning. For other people, stressing the feeling part or interpersonal aspect motivates and promotes learning.

The nurse seldom has the time or skills to assess each learner, identify the person's particular learning style, and then adapt teaching accordingly; what the nurse can do, however, is ask clients how they have learned things best in the past or how they like to learn. Many people know what helps them learn, and the nurse can use this information in planning the teaching. Using a variety of teaching techniques and varying activities during teaching are good ways to match learners with learning styles. One technique will be most effective for some clients, whereas other techniques will be suited to clients with different learning styles.

Client Support System The nurse explores the client's support system to determine the extent to which others may enhance learning and offer support. Family members or a close friend may help the client perform required skills at home and maintain required lifestyle changes.

Physical Examination

The general survey part of the physical examination provides useful clues to the client's learning needs, such as mental status, energy level, and nutritional status. Other parts of the physical examination reveal data about the client's physical capacity to learn and to perform self-care activities. For example, visual ability, hearing ability, and muscle coordination affect the selection of content and approaches to teaching.

Readiness to Learn

Clients who are ready to learn often behave differently from those who are not. A client who is ready may search out information,

Research Note
What Are the Learning Style Preferences of Older Adults?

In a study by VanWynen (2001), the first of its kind, the researcher analyzed the current and previous learning styles of a sample of elders aged 64 to 88, with no cognitive dysfunction and living independently in a residential senior citizen setting. The author points out that research has shown how learning style preferences evolve over time, however, the research extended only from early childhood to 50 years of age. Little research has been conducted to determine if the learning styles of elders changed with the passage of time and life experiences. The results reflected significant differences between current and previous learning styles. The older adults preferred to learn in the late morning with a teacher present and with the opportunity to work with their peers. They preferred a formal learning environment and to listen to a structured presentation by a teacher. Their perceptual preferences were auditory rather than visual.

Implications: Nurses need to remember that a 65-year-old person can be expected to live another 20 years and it is important to provide educational techniques to promote health and wellness of these older adults. This study adds insight into the learning-style patterns of elders. Instead of being told to read a pamphlet, they prefer listening to a personal presentation that allows for interaction that is held in the late morning.

Note: From "A Key to Successful Aging: Learning-Style Patterns of Older Adults," by E. A. VanWynen, 2001, *Journal of Gerontological Nursing, 27*(9), pp. 6–15.

for instance, by asking questions, reading books or articles, talking to others, and generally showing interest. The person who is not ready to learn is more likely to avoid the subject or situation. In addition, the unready client may change the subject when it is brought up by the nurse. For example, the nurse might say, "I was wondering about a good time to show you how to change your dressing," and the client responds, "Oh, my wife will take care of everything."

The nurse assesses for these readiness characteristics:

- *Physical readiness.* Is the client able to focus on things other than physical status, or are pain, fatigue, and immobility using up all of the client's time and energy?
- *Emotional readiness.* Is the client emotionally ready to learn self-care activities? Clients who are extremely anxious, depressed, or grieving over their health status are not ready.
- *Cognitive readiness.* Can the client think clearly at this point? Are the effects of anesthesia and analgesia altering the client's level of consciousness?

Nurses can promote readiness to learn by providing physical and emotional support during the critical stage of recovery. As the client stabilizes physically and emotionally, the nurse can provide opportunities to learn.

Motivation

Motivation relates to whether the client wants to learn and is usually greatest when the client is ready, the learning need is recognized, and the information being offered is meaningful to the client. Assessment of motivation, however, may be difficult. Communication skills used by the nurse can obtain helpful information indicating a readiness for change such as "I'm really ready to lose weight this time." On the other hand, nonverbal behaviors such as disinterest, lack of attention, and missed appointments can indicate a decreased motivation to learn.

Nurses can increase a client's motivation in several ways:

- By relating the learning to something the client values and helping the client see the relevance of the learning
- By helping the client make the learning situation pleasant and nonthreatening
- By encouraging self-direction and independence
- By demonstrating a positive attitude about the client's ability to learn
- By offering continuing support and encouragement as the client attempts to learn (i.e., positive reinforcement)
- By creating a learning situation in which the client is likely to succeed. (Succeeding in small tasks motivates the client to continue learning.)
- By assisting the client to identify the benefits of changing behavior.

Reading Level

Meyer and Rushton (2002) report that millions of adults read at or below the fifth-grade level while most health care literature is written at the seventh- to ninth-grade level or higher. A person with low literacy skill will have a limited vocabulary and difficulty comprehending oral and written information. Low literacy skills are strongly associated with poor health (Schultz, 2002; Winslow, 2001). It is a challenge for the nurse to teach clients with low or no reading and writing skills, however, such teaching is vitally important because clients with low literacy skills also need teaching to improve their health practices.

> **➤ CLINICAL ALERT**   *The literature reflects that the majority of people at the lowest reading levels will report that they "read well."* ■

Identified low literacy risk factors include poverty, unemployment, minority or immigrant status, lack of a high school education, and advanced age (Schultz, 2002, p.46). It is difficult, however, to assess a client's literacy skills because clients may be too embarrassed to admit they can't read. The following client behaviors may cause a nurse to suspect a literacy problem:

- Pattern of noncompliance
- Insisting that they already know the information
- Pattern of excuses for not reading the instructions (e.g., glasses broken, stating will read later).

There are many formulas for assessing reading level of written material. Nurses involved in developing written health teaching materials should write for lower reading levels (see Teaching: Client Care). Winslow (2001) reports that people with good reading skills are not offended by simple reading material and prefer easy-to-read information. Even the simplist written directions, however, won't be helpful for the client with

Teaching: Client Care
Developing Written Teaching Aids

■ Keep language level at or below the fifth-grade level.
■ Use active, not passive, voice.
■ Use easy, common words of one or two syllables (e.g., *use* instead of *utilize* or *give* instead of *administer*).
■ Use a large type size (14 to 16 point).
■ Write short sentences.
■ Place priority information first.
■ Use pictures, drawings, or cartoons, if appropriate.
■ Leave plenty of white space.
■ Obtain feedback from nurses and clients.

Note: From "Writing Easy-to-Read Teaching Aids," by G. G. Mayer, 2002, *Nursing, 32*(3), pp. 48–49; "Research for Practice: Caring for Patients with Limited Literacy," by E. H. Winslow, 1998, *American Journal of Nursing, 98*(7), pp. 55, 57; and *Teaching Patients with Low Literacy Skills,* 2nd ed., by C. C. Doak, L. G. Doak, and J. H. Root, 1996, Philadelphia: J. B. Lippincott.

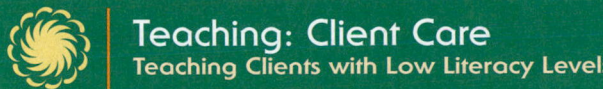

Teaching: Client Care
Teaching Clients with Low Literacy Levels

■ Use multiple teaching methods: Show pictures. Read important information. Small group discussion. Role play. Demonstrate a skill. Hands–on practice.
■ Emphasize key points in simple terms and provide examples.
■ Limit the amount of information in a single teaching session. Instead of one long session with a great deal of information, it is better to have more frequent sessions with a major point at each session.
■ Reinforce information through repetition.
■ Obtain feedback: Ask the client specific questions about the information presented or ask the client to repeat it in his own words.
■ Associate new information with something the client already knows and/or associates with her job or lifestyle.
■ Avoid handouts with many pages and classroom lecture format with a large group.

Note: From "Low-Level Literacy Skills Needn't Hinder Care," by M. Schultz, 2002, *RN, 65*(4), pp. 45–48; "Limited English Proficiency Workers: Health and Safety Education" by O-S Hong, 2001, *AAOHN, 49*(1), pp. 21–26; and *Nurse as Educator: Principles of Teaching and Learning for Nursing Practice* (2nd ed.) (pp. 222–225), by S. B. Bastable, 2003, Sudbury, MA: Jones and Bartlett Publishers.

---

low or no reading skills. See the Teaching: Client Care box for suggestions on how to teach clients with low literacy levels.

DIAGNOSING

Nursing diagnoses for clients with learning needs can be designated in two ways: as the client's primary concern or problem, or as the etiology of a nursing diagnosis associated with the client's response to health alterations or dysfunction (see Identifying Nursing Diagnoses, Outcomes, and Interventions).

Learning Need as the Diagnostic Label

The North American Nursing Diagnostic Association (NANDA) includes the following diagnostic labels appropriate to a client's learning needs when the learning need is the primary concern:

• *Deficient Knowledge:* absence or deficiency of cognitive information related to a specific topic (NANDA, 2003, p. 109).

> ➤ **CLINICAL ALERT**   *The nursing diagnosis Deficient Knowledge was formerly Knowledge Deficit.* ■

Whenever the diagnostic label *Deficient Knowledge* is used, either the client is seeking health information or the nurse has identified a learning need. The area of deficiency should always be included in the diagnosis. Following are examples using the NANDA label *Deficient Knowledge* as the primary concern:

• *Deficient Knowledge (Low-Calorie Diet)* related to inexperience with newly ordered therapy.
• *Deficient Knowledge (Home Safety Hazards)* related to denial of declining health and lack of interest in learning.

Wilkinson (2000) stresses that if *Deficient Knowledge* is used as the primary concern, one client goal must be "client

will acquire knowledge about. . .". The nurse needs to provide the information that will change the client's behavior rather than focus on the behaviors caused by the client's lack of knowledge.

A second nursing diagnostic label where a learning need may be the primary concern is

• *Health Seeking Behavior:* active seeking (by a person in stable health) of ways to alter personal health habits and/or the environment in order to move toward a higher level of health (NANDA, 2003, p. 88).

When this diagnostic label is used, the client is seeking health information; the client may or may not have an altered response or dysfunction at the time but may be seeking information to improve health or prevent illness. This diagnosis is especially appropriate for clients attending community health education programs. The following are examples using the NANDA label *Health Seeking Behavior* as the primary concern:

• *Health Seeking Behavior (Exercise and Activity)* related to desire to improve health behaviors and decrease risk of heart disease. This diagnosis may be appropriate for the client who has identified a personal health risk for a cardiac condition and wants to minimize that risk through exercise.
• *Health Seeking Behavior (Home Safety Hazards)* related to desire to minimize risk of injury. This diagnosis may be appropriate for parents of a toddler who are seeking information to ensure that their home is safe for their child. The diagnosis might also be used when an adult child seeks

IDENTIFYING NURSING DIAGNOSES, OUTCOMES, AND INTERVENTIONS

CLIENTS REQUIRING TEACHING

DATA CLUSTER	NURSING DIAGNOSIS/ DEFINITION	SAMPLE DESIRED OUTCOME [NOC#]/DEFINITION	INDICATORS	SELECTED INTERVENTIONS [NIC#]/DEFINITION	SAMPLE NIC ACTIVITIES
The nurse brings Mr. Steinberg the first dose of a medication ordered by his physician. The nurse asks whether anyone has explained what this medication is and why he is taking it. He says no.	*Deficient Knowledge (Medication Information)* related to lack of exposure to newly prescribed medication/*Absence or deficiency of cognitive information related to specific topic*	Knowledge: Medication [1808]/*Extent of understanding conveyed about the safe use of medication*	Substantial: • Statement of correct medication name • Description of action of medication • Description of side effects of medication • Description of medication precautions	Teaching, Prescribed Medication [5616]/*Preparing a client to safely take prescribed medications and monitor for their effects*	• Inform the client of both the generic and brand names of the medication • Instruct the client on the purpose and action of the medication • Instruct the client on the dosage, route, and duration of the medication • Instruct the client on specific precautions to observe when taking the medication (e.g., no driving) as appropriate
George Evans is a 45-year-old man who has come to the clinic for his annual physical examination. He expresses concern about his family history of heart disease and requests information about activities to decrease his risk of heart disease.	*Health Seeking Behavior (Nutrition, Activity and Exercise Information)* to reduce risk of heart disease/*Active seeking (by a person in stable health) of ways to alter personal health habits and/or the environment in order to move toward a higher level of health*	Adherence Behavior [1600]/*Self-initiated action taken to promote wellness, recovery, and rehabilitation*	Often demonstrated: • Asks questions when appropriate • Seeks health-related information from a variety of sources • Describes strategies to eliminate unhealthy behavior • Reports using strategies to maximize health	Self-Modification Assistance [4470]/*Reinforcement of self-directed change initiated by the client to achieve personally important goals*	• Assist the client in identifying a specific goal for change • Assist the client in identifying target behaviors that need to change to achieve the desired goal • Appraise the client's present knowledge and skill level in relationship to the desired change • Explore with the client potential barriers to change behavior

continued on page 457

IDENTIFYING NURSING DIAGNOSES, OUTCOMES, AND INTERVENTIONS *continued*

CLIENTS REQUIRING TEACHING

DATA CLUSTER	NURSING DIAGNOSIS/ DEFINITION	SAMPLE DESIRED OUTCOME [NOC#]/DEFINITION	INDICATORS	SELECTED INTERVENTIONS [NIC#]/DEFINITION	SAMPLE NIC ACTIVITIES
Mildred Cumming is a 74-year-old widow with a history of hypertension. Her blood pressure is 150/96. She is on daily antihypertensive therapy. When asked if she is taking her medication as prescribed, she tells the nurse that she is taking her medication every other day because it is expensive and she cannot afford to take it every day.	*Noncompliance (With Medication Plan)* related to insufficient finances/*Behavior of person and/or caregiver that fails to coincide with a health-promoting or therapeutic plan agreed on by the person (and/or family and/or community) and health-care professional. In the presence of an agreed-on, health-promoting or therapeutic plan, person's or caregiver's behavior is fully or partially nonadherent and may lead to clinically ineffective or partially ineffective outcomes*	Compliance Behavior [1601]/*Activities taken on the basis of professional advice to promote wellness, recovery, and rehabilitation*	Consistently demonstrated: • Reports following prescribed regimen • Modifies regimen as directed by a health professional	Financial Resource Assistance [7380]/ *Assisting an individual/family to secure and manage finances to meet health care needs*	• Determine if client is eligible for waiver programs • Inform client of available resources and assist in accessing resources (e.g., medication assistance program)

information to ensure that the home of an elderly parent is free of risk factors for falls or other injuries common to the elderly.

A third nursing diagnostic label where a learning need may be the primary concern is

• *Noncompliance:* behavior of person and/or caregiver that fails to coincide with a health-promoting or therapeutic plan agreed on by the person (and/or family and/or community) and health-care professional. In the presence of an agreed-on, health-promoting or therapeutic plan, person's or caregiver's behavior is fully or partially nonadherent and may lead to clinically ineffective or partially ineffective outcomes (NANDA, 2003, p. 120).

The diagnostic label *Noncompliance* should be used with caution. In general, the diagnosis *Noncompliance* is associated with the *intent* to comply but situational factors make it difficult (Wilkinson, 2000, p. 289). Factors that influence a client's compliance with health teaching include understanding or comprehension of the teaching, the experienced negative side effects of the treatment, financial inability to carry out the treatment plan,

language barriers, or poor teaching on the part of the health care team. *Noncompliance* should *not* be used for a client who is unable to follow instructions (e.g., cognitive disability) or for a client who makes an informed decision to refuse or not follow the medical treatment (Wilkinson, 2000, p. 290).

> **CLINICAL ALERT**   *The term* noncompliance *is often perceived as a negative label. Be sure to state the etiology in neutral, nonjudgmental words.* ■

Deficient Knowledge as the Etiology

Another way to deal with identified learning needs of clients is to write deficient knowledge as the etiology, or second part, of the diagnosis statement. Such nursing diagnoses are written in the following format:

• *Risk for (Specify)* related to deficient knowledge (specify).

Examples include the following:

• *Risk for Impaired Parenting* related to deficient knowledge (skills in infant care and feeding).

- *Risk for Infection* related to deficient knowledge (sexually transmitted diseases and their prevention).
- *Anxiety* related to deficient knowledge (bone marrow aspiration).

Other nursing diagnoses in which a knowledge deficit can be the etiology follow:

- *Risk for Injury*
- *Ineffective Breastfeeding*
- *Impaired Adjustment*
- *Ineffective Coping*
- *Ineffective Health Maintenance.*

Note also that most NANDA-approved nursing diagnoses imply a teaching–learning need. For example, the nursing diagnosis *Constipation* suggests the need for a review of bowel hygiene practices including diet, hydration, and exercise/activity.

PLANNING

Developing a teaching plan is accomplished in a series of steps. Involving the client at this time promotes the formation of a meaningful plan and stimulates client motivation. The client who helps formulate the teaching plan is more likely to achieve the desired outcomes (see Teaching: Client Care on the next page).

> ➤ **CLINICAL ALERT** *Knowing the client's stage of change helps determine which interventions will be useful to help the client change.* ∎

Determining Teaching Priorities

The client's learning needs must be ranked according to priority. The client and the nurse should do this together, with the client's priorities always being considered. Once a client's priorities have been addressed, the client is generally more motivated to concentrate on other identified learning needs. For example, a man who wants to know all about coronary artery disease may not be ready to learn how to change his lifestyle until he meets his own need to learn more about the disease. Nurses can also use theoretical frameworks, such as Maslow's hierarchy of needs, to establish priorities (see Chapter 12). ⌖

Setting Learning Outcomes

Learning outcomes can be considered the same as desired outcomes for other nursing diagnoses. They are written in the same way. Like client outcomes, learning outcomes

- State the client (learner) behavior or performance, not nurse behavior. For example, "Identify personal risk factors for heart disease" (client behavior), *not* "Teach the client about cardiac risk factors" (nurse behavior).
- Reflect an observable, measurable activity. The performance may be visible (e.g., walking) or invisible (e.g., adding a column of figures). It is necessary, however, to be able to deduce whether an unobservable activity has been mastered from some performance that represents the activity. For example, the performance of an outcome might be written: "Selects

BOX 25–2	∎ Examples of Verbs for Writing Learning Outcomes	
Cognitive Domain	**Affective Domain**	**Psychomotor Domain**
Compares	Accepts	Assembles
Describes	Attends	Calculates
Evaluates	Chooses	Changes
Explains	Discusses	Demonstrates
Identifies	Displays	Measures
Labels	Initiates	Moves
Lists	Joins	Organizes
Names	Participates	Shows
Plans	Shares	
Selects	Uses	
States		
Writes		

low-fat foods from a menu" (observable), *not* "understands low-fat diet" (unobservable). Examples of measurable verbs used for learning outcomes are shown in Box 25–2. Avoid using words such as *knows, understands, believes,* and *appreciates* because they are neither observable nor measurable.

- May add conditions or modifiers as required to clarify what, where, when, or how the behavior will be performed. Examples are "Demonstrates four-point crutch gait *correctly*" (condition), "Irrigates his colostomy *independently* (condition) as taught," or "States *three* (condition) factors that affect blood sugar level."
- Include criteria specifying the time by which learning should have occurred. For example, "The client will state three things that affect blood sugar level *by end of second diabetic class.*"

Learning outcomes can reflect the learner's command of simple to complex concepts. For example, the learning outcome "The client will list cardiac risk factors" is a low-level knowledge outcome that simply requires the learner to identify all cardiac risk factors; it does not suggest application of the knowledge to the learner's own behaviors. The learning outcome "The client will list personal cardiac risk factors" requires that the learner not only know cardiac risk factors in general but also know his own behaviors that place him at risk for cardiac disease.

In writing learning outcomes, the nurse must be specific about what behaviors and knowledge (cognitive, psychomotor, and affective) the learner must have to be able to positively influence her health state. In most cases, the learning needs are more complex than simple acquisition of knowledge and include the application of that knowledge to oneself (see Identifying Nursing Diagnoses, Outcomes, and Interventions on page 456).

Choosing Content

The content, or what is to be taught, is determined by learning outcomes. For instance, "Identify appropriate sites for insulin injection" means the nurse must include content about the body sites suitable for insulin injections. Nurses can select among many sources of information including books, nursing jour-

Teaching: Client Care
Sample Teaching Plan for Wound Care

Assessment of learner: A 24-year-old male college student suffered a 7-cm (2.5-inch) laceration on the left lower anterior leg during a hockey game. The laceration was cleaned, sutured, and bandaged. The client was given an appointment to return to the health clinic in 10 days for suture removal. Client states that he lives in the college dormitory and is able to do wound care if given instructions. Client is able to understand and read English. Assessed to be in the "preparation" and "action" stages of change.

Nursing Diagnosis: Deficient Knowledge (Care of Sutured Wound) related to no prior experience.

Long-Term Goal: Client's wound will heal completely without infection or other complications.
Intermediate Goal: At clinic appointment, client's wound will be healing without signs of infection, loss of function, or other complication.
Short-Term Goal: Client will respond to questions regarding wound care and perform return demonstration of wound cleansing and bandaging.

Learning Outcomes	Content Outline	Teaching Methods
Upon completion of the instructional session, the client will 1. Describe normal wound healing.	I. Normal wound healing	Describe normal wound healing with the use of audiovisuals.
2. Describe signs and symptoms of wound infection.	II. Infection Signs and symptoms include wound warm to touch, malalignment of wound edges, and purulent wound drainage. Signs of systemic infection include fever and malaise.	Discuss the mechanism of wound infection. Use audiovisuals to demonstrate infected wound appearance. Provide handout describing signs and symptoms of wound infection.
3. Identify equipment needed for wound care.	III. Wound care equipment a. Cleansing solution as prescribed by physician (e.g., clear water, mild soap and water, or antimicrobial solution) b. Bandaging material: Telfa, gauze wrap, adhesive tape.	Demonstrate equipment needed for cleansing and bandaging wound. Provide handout listing equipment needed.
4. Demonstrate wound cleansing and bandaging.	IV. Demonstration of wound cleansing and bandaging on the client's wound or a mannequin	Demonstrate wound cleansing and bandaging on the client's wound or a mannequin. Provide handout describing procedure for cleansing and bandaging wound.
5. Describe appropriate action if questions or complications arise.	V. Resources available for client questions include health clinic, emergency department.	Discuss available resources. Provide handout listing available resources and follow-up treatment plan.
6. Identify date, time, and location of follow-up appointment for suture removal.	VI. Follow-up treatment plan; where and when	Provide written instructions.

Evaluation: The client will
1. Respond to questions regarding self-care of wound.
2. Return demonstration of wound cleansing and bandaging.
3. State contact person and telephone number to obtain assistance.
4. State date, time, and location of follow-up appointment.

nals, and other nurses and physicians. Whatever sources the nurse chooses, content should be

- Accurate
- Current
- Based on learning outcomes
- Adjusted for the learner's age, culture, and ability
- Consistent with information the nurse is teaching

- Selected with consideration of how much time and what resources are available for teaching.

Selecting Teaching Strategies
The method of teaching that the nurse chooses should be suited to the individual and to the material to be learned (Figure 25–2 ■). For example, the person who cannot read

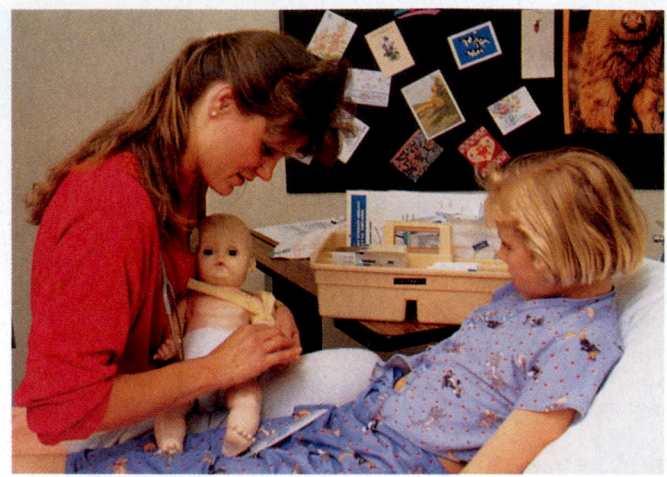

Figure 25–2 ■ Teaching materials and strategies should be suited to the client's age and learning abilities.

needs material presented in other ways; a discussion is usually not the best strategy for teaching how to give an injection; and a nurse using group discussion for teaching should be a competent group leader. As stated earlier, some people are visually oriented and learn best through seeing; others learn best through hearing and having the skill explained. Table 25–3 lists selected teaching strategies.

Organizing Learning Experiences

To save nurses time in constructing their own teaching guides, some health agencies have developed teaching guides for teaching sessions that nurses commonly give. These guides standardize content and teaching methods and make it easier for the nurse to plan and implement client teaching. Standardized teaching plans also ensure consistency of content for the learner, thereby decreasing the risk of confusion if different practices are taught. For example, when teaching infant bathing, the nurse on the unit should be consistent about which soaps are appropriate for the infant's bath and distinguish those which are not. Whether the nurse is implementing a plan devised by another or developing an individualized teaching plan, some guidelines can help the nurse sequence the learning experience:

- Start with something the learner is concerned about; for example, before learning how to administer insulin to himself, an adolescent wants to know how to adjust his lifestyle and yet still play football.

> **CLINICAL ALERT** *Leave a note pad and pen at the client's bedside and encourage him to write down his questions for the nurse or the doctor.* ■

- Cover what the learner knows, and then proceed to the unknown. This gives the learner confidence. Sometimes you will not know the client's knowledge or skill base and will need to elicit this information either by asking questions or by having the client fill out a form, such as a pretest.

- Address early on any area that is causing the client anxiety. A high level of anxiety can impair concentration in other areas. For example, a woman highly anxious about turning her husband in bed might not be able to learn about bathing him until she has successfully learned to turn him.

- Teach the basics before proceeding to the variations or adjustments (e.g., simple to complex). It is confusing to learners to have to consider possible adjustments and variations before they master the basic concepts. For example, when teaching a female client how to insert a retention catheter, it is best to teach the basic procedure before teaching any adjustments that might be needed if the catheter stops draining after insertion.

- Schedule time for review of content and questions the learner(s) may have to clarify information.

> **CLINICAL ALERT** *If the client has no questions, you can help introduce questions by saying, "A few frequently asked questions are. . . ."* ■

IMPLEMENTING

The nurse needs to be flexible in implementing any teaching plan because the plan may need revising. The client may tire sooner than anticipated or be faced with too much information too quickly, the client's needs may change, or external factors may intervene. For instance, the nurse and the client, Mr. Brown, plan to irrigate his colostomy at 10 AM, but when the time comes, Mr. Brown wants additional information before actually doing it himself.

> **CLINICAL ALERT** *Many nurses find that they teach while performing nursing care (e.g., giving medication). Remember to document this informal teaching also.* ■

In this case, the nurse alters the teaching plan and discusses the desired information, provides written information, and defers teaching the psychomotor skill until the next day. It is also important for nurses to use teaching techniques that enhance learning and reduce or eliminate any barrier to learning such as pain or fatigue (see Table 25–2 earlier in this chapter).

Guidelines for Teaching

Knowledge alone is not enough to motivate a person to change a behavior. Do not assume that providing information will automatically result in clients changing their behavior. Learning what needs to be done to change behavior and acting on that knowledge are two different processes (Saarmann, Daugherty, & Riegel, 2000, p. 281). The stages of change, the person's willingness and perceived need to change, and barriers to change are important elements to reflect on when implementing a teaching plan (see Chapter 8). When a client is ready to change a health behavior and when implementing a teaching plan, the nurse may find the following guidelines helpful:

- Rapport between teacher and learner is essential. A relationship that is both accepting and constructive will best assist

TABLE 25–3 Selected Teaching Strategies

Strategy	Major Type of Learning	Characteristics
Explanation or description (e.g., lecture)	Cognitive	Teacher controls content and pace. Learner is passive; therefore retains less information than when actively participating. Feedback is determined by teacher. May be given to individual or group.
One-to-one discussion	Affective, cognitive	Encourages participation by learner. Permits reinforcement and repetition at learner's level. Permits introduction of sensitive subjects.
Answering questions	Cognitive	Teacher controls most of content and pace. Teacher must understand question and what it means to learner. Learner may need to overcome cultural perception that asking questions is impolite and may embarrass the teacher. Can be used with individuals and groups. Teacher sometimes needs to confirm whether question has been answered by asking learner, for example, "Does that answer your question?"
Demonstration	Psychomotor	Often used with explanation. Can be used with individuals, small or large groups. Does not permit use of equipment by learner; learner is passive.
Discovery	Cognitive, affective	Teacher guides problem-solving situation. Learner is active participant; therefore, retention of information is high.
Group discussions	Affective, cognitive	Learner can obtain assistance from supportive group. Group members learn from one another. Teacher needs to keep the discussion focused and prevent monopolization by one or two learners.
Practice	Psychomotor	Allows repetition and immediate feedback. Permits hands-on experience.
Printed and audiovisual materials	Cognitive	Forms include books, pamphlets, films, programmed instruction, and computer learning. Learners can proceed at their own speed. Nurse can act as resource person, need not be present during learning. Potentially ineffective if reading level is too high. Teacher needs to select language of materials that meets learner needs if English is a second language (e.g., Spanish).
Role-playing	Affective, cognitive	Permits expression of attitudes, values, and emotions. Can assist in development of communication skills. Involves active participation by learner. Teacher must create supportive, safe environment for learners to minimize anxiety.
Modeling	Affective, psychomotor	Nurse sets example by attitude, psychomotor skill.
Computer-assisted learning programs	All types of learning	Learner is active. Learner controls pace. Provides immediate reinforcement and review. Use with individuals or groups.

learning. Knowing the learners and the previously described factors that affect learning should be established before planning the teaching.

- The teacher who uses the client's previous learning in the present situation encourages the client and facilitates learning new skills. For instance, a person who already knows how to cook can use this knowledge when learning to prepare food for a special diet.
- The optimal time for each session depends largely on the learner. Whenever possible, ask the client for help to choose the best time, for example, when she feels most rested or when no other activities are scheduled.
- The nurse teacher must be able to communicate clearly and concisely. The words used need to have the same meaning to the learner as to the teacher. A client who is taught not to put water on an area of skin may think a wet washcloth is permissible for washing the area. In effect, the nurse needs to explain that no water or moisture should touch the area.
- Using a layperson's vocabulary enhances communication. Often nurses use terms and abbreviations that have meaning to other health professionals but make little sense to clients. Even words such as *urine* or *feces* may be unfamiliar to clients, and abbreviations such as RR (recovery room) or PAR (postanesthesia room) are often misunderstood.
- The pace of each teaching session also affects learning. Nurses should be sensitive to any signs that the pace is too fast or too slow. A client who appears confused or does not comprehend material when questioned may be finding the pace too fast. When the client appears bored and loses interest, the pace may be too slow, the learning period may be too long, or the client may be tired.
- An environment can detract from or assist learning; for example, noise or interruptions usually interfere with concentration, whereas a comfortable environment promotes learning. If possible, the client should be out of bed for learning activities. Most people associate their bed with rest and sleep, not with learning. Placing the client in a position and location associated with activity or learning may influence the amount of learning that takes place. For instance, a client who is shown a videotape while in bed may be more likely to become drowsy during instruction than a client who is sitting in a bedside chair.
- Teaching aids can foster learning and help focus a learner's attention. To ensure the transfer of learning, the nurse should use the type of supplies or equipment the client will eventually use. Before the teaching session, the nurse needs to assemble all equipment and visual aids and ensure that all audiovisual equipment is functioning effectively. See Teaching: Client Care for teaching tools for children.
- Teaching that involves a number of the learner's senses often enhances learning. For instance, when teaching about changing a surgical dressing, the nurse can tell the client about the procedure (hearing), show how to change the dressing (sight), and show how to manipulate the equipment (touch).
- Learning is more effective when the learners discover the content for themselves. Ways to increase learning include stimulating motivation and self-direction, for example, (a) by pro-

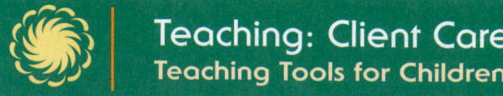

Teaching: Client Care
Teaching Tools for Children

- *Visits.* Visiting the hospital and treatment rooms; seeing people dressed in uniforms, scrub suits, protective gear.
- *Dress-up.* Touching and dressing up in the clothing they will see and wear.
- *Coloring books.* Using coloring books to prepare for treatments, surgery, or hospitalization; shows what rooms, people, and equipment will look like.
- *Story books.* Story books describe how the child will feel, what will be done, and what the place will look like. Parents can read these stories to children several times before the experience. Younger children like this repetition.
- *Dolls.* Practicing procedures on dolls or teddy bears that they will later experience; gives a sense of mastery of the situation. Custom dolls are often available for inserting tubes and giving injections, for example.
- *Puppet play.* Puppets can be used in role-play situations to provide information and show the child what the experience will be like; they help the child express emotions.
- *Health fairs.* Health fairs can educate children about their bodies and ways to stay healthy. Fairs can focus on high-risk problems children face, such as accident prevention, poison control, and other topics identified in the community as a concern.

viding specific, realistic, achievable outcomes; (b) by giving feedback; and (c) by helping the learner derive satisfaction from learning. The nurse may also encourage self-directed independent learning by encouraging the client to explore sources of information required. If certain activities do not assist the learner to attain outcomes, these need to be reassessed; perhaps other activities can replace them. Explanation alone may not be able to teach a client to handle a syringe. Actually handling the syringe may be more effective (Figure 25–3 ■).

- Repetition reinforces learning. Summarizing content, rephrasing (using other words), and approaching the material from another point of view are ways of repeating and clarifying content. For instance, after discussing the kinds of foods that can be included in a diet, the nurse describes the foods again, but in the context of the three meals eaten during one day.
- It is helpful to employ "organizers" to introduce material to be learned. Advanced organizers provide a means of connecting unknown material to known material and generating logical relationships. The following statement can be an advanced organizer: "You understand how urine flows down a catheter from the bladder. Now I will show you how to inject fluid so that it flows up the catheter into the bladder." The details that follow are then seen within a framework that adds meaning.
- The anticipated behavioral changes that indicate learning has taken place must always be within the context of the client's

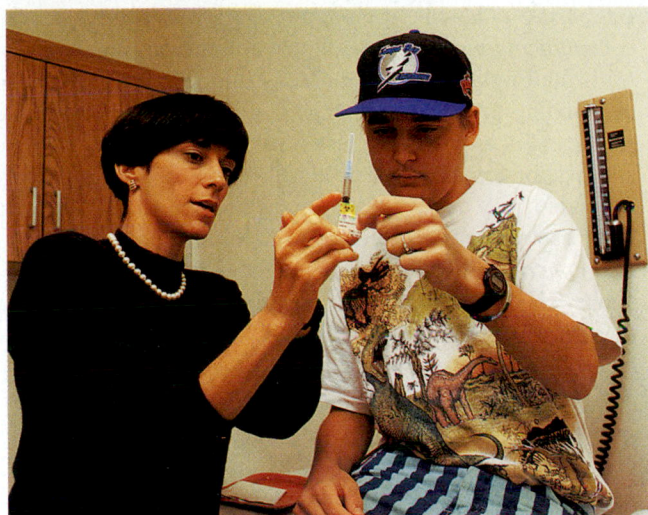

Figure 25–3 ■ Teaching activities may need to include hands-on client participation.

lifestyle and resources. It would be unreasonable to expect a woman to soak in a tub of hot water four times a day if she did not have a bathtub or had to heat water on a stove.

Special Teaching Strategies

One-on-one discussion is the most common method of teaching used by nurses. However, nurses can choose from a number of special teaching strategies: client contracting, group teaching, computer-assisted instruction, discovery/problem solving, and behavior modification. Any strategy the nurse selects must be appropriate for the learner and the learning objectives.

Client Contracting. Client contracting involves establishing a learning contract with a client that specifies certain outcomes and when they are to be met. Here is an example of a self-contract:

> I, Amy Martin, will exercise strenuously for 20 minutes three times per week for a period of 2 weeks and will then buy myself six yellow roses.
>
> Amy Martin   A. Ward, RN
> July 30, 2003   July 30, 2003

The contract, drawn up and signed by the client and the nurse, may specify the learning outcomes, the responsibilities of the client and the nurse, and the methods of follow-up and evaluation. The contract can be changed in two ways: If the client meets the contract outcomes and wants to negotiate new learning outcomes, and if the client decides that he is unable to meet the existing learning outcomes and wants to revise them (Rankin & Stallings, 1996, pp. 162–163). The learning contract allows for freedom, mutual respect, and mutual responsibility.

Group Teaching. Group instruction is economical, and it provides members with an opportunity to share with and learn from others. A small group allows for discussion in which everyone can participate. A large group often necessitates a lecture technique or use of films, videos, slides, or role-playing by teachers.

It is important that all members involved in group instruction have a common need (e.g., prenatal health or preoperative instruction). It is also important that sociocultural factors be considered in the formation of a group.

Computer-Assisted Instruction (CAI). Computer-assisted instruction is popular. Initially, the primary use of computer educational methods was cognitive learning of facts. Now, however, computers can also be used to teach the following:

- Application of information (e.g., answering questions after reading the information about a health subject)
- Psychomotor skills (e.g., filling a syringe on the computer screen to the correct dosage line on the syringe)
- Complex problem-solving skills (e.g., responding to questions based on a client situation).

Computers can be used in a variety of ways:

- Individual health care professionals or clients using one computer
- Families or small groups of three to five clients gathered around one computer taking turns running the program and answering questions together
- Large groups with the computer display screen projected onto an overhead screen and a teacher or one learner using the keyboard
- Individuals or small groups at computers using programs through shared network platforms or through Internet websites. Internet sources for health education are numerous and can be accessed through home computers with a modem.

Individuals using a computer are able to set the pace that meets their particular learning needs. Small groups are less able to do this, and large groups progress through the program at a pace that may be too slow for some learners and too fast for others. It is therefore helpful to group together learners of similar needs and abilities. Whether using the computer alone or in large groups, learners read and view informational material, answer questions, and receive immediate feedback. The correct answer is usually indicated by the use of colors, flashing signs, or written praise. When the learner selects an incorrect answer, the computer may respond with an explanation of why that was not the best answer and encouragement to try again. Many programs ask learners whether they want to review material on which the question and answer were based. Some computer programs feature simulated situations that allow learners to manipulate objects on the screen to learn psychomotor skills. When used to teach such skills, CAI must be followed up with practice on actual equipment supervised by the teacher.

Some clients may have a negative attitude about computers that could act as a barrier to learning. The nurse helps these clients by explaining the steps to start and run the program, to turn the computer on and off, and where and when to insert the computer disk so that the client can use the program when the nurse is not present. Written instructions are also helpful. Most media catalogs, professional journals, and health care libraries contain information about computer programs available to the nurse for client education. The media specialist or librarian in

MediaLink | CLIENT ADMITTED TO THE HOSPITAL FOR THE FIRST TIME CARE PLAN ACTIVITY a health care facility or college is an excellent resource to help the nurse locate appropriate computer programs. Computer educational material is also available for clients with different language needs, for clients with special visual needs, and for clients at different growth and development levels.

Discovery/Problem Solving. In using the discovery/problem-solving technique, the nurse presents some initial information and then asks the learners a question or presents a situation related to the information. The learner applies the new information to the situation and decides what to do. Learners can work alone or in groups. This technique is well suited to family learning. The teacher guides the learners through the thinking process necessary to reach the best solution to the question or the best action to take in the situation. This may also be referred to as *anticipatory problem solving.* For example, the nurse educator might present information on diabetes and glucose management. Then the nurse might ask the learners how they think their insulin and/or diet should be adjusted if their morning glucose was too low. In this way, clients learn what critical components they need to consider to reach the best solution to the problem.

Behavior Modification. The behavior modification system for changing behavior has as its basic assumptions (a) that human behaviors are learned and can be selectively strengthened, weakened, eliminated, or replaced; and (b) that a person's behavior is under conscious control. Under this system, desirable behavior is regarded and undesirable behavior is ignored. The client's response is the key to behavior change. For example, clients trying to quit smoking are not criticized when they smoke, but they are praised or rewarded when they go without a cigarette for a certain period of time. For some people, a learning contract is combined with behavior modification, and includes the following pertinent features:

- Positive reinforcement (e.g., praise) is used.
- The client participates in the development of the learning plan.
- Undesirable behavior is ignored, not criticized.
- The expectation of the client and the nurse is that the task will be mastered (i.e., the behavior will change).

Transcultural Teaching

The nurse and clients of different cultural and ethnic backgrounds have additional barriers to overcome in the teaching–learning process. These barriers include language and communication problems, differing concepts of time, conflicting cultural healing practices, beliefs that may positively or negatively influence compliance with health teaching, and unique high-risk or high-frequency health problems that can be addressed with health-promotion instruction (see Chapter 13). Nurses should consider the following guidelines when teaching clients from various ethnic backgrounds:

- *Obtain teaching materials, pamphlets, and instructions in languages used by clients.* Nurses who are unable to read the foreign language material for themselves can have the translator read the material to them. The nurse can then evaluate the quality of the information and update it with the translator's help as needed.

- *Use visual aids, such as pictures, charts, or diagrams, to communicate meaning.* Audiovisual material may be helpful if the English is spoken clearly and slowly. Even if understanding the verbal message is a problem for the client, seeing a skill or procedure may be helpful. In some instances, a translator can be asked to clarify the video. Alternatively the video may be available in several languages, and the nurse can request the necessary version from the company.

- *Use concrete rather than abstract words.* Use simple language (short sentences, short words), and present only one idea at a time.

- *Allow time for questions.* This helps the client mentally separate one idea or skill from another.

- *Avoid the use of medical terminology or health care language,* such as "taking your vital signs" or "apical pulse." Rather, nurses should say they are going to take a blood pressure or listen to the client's heart.

- *If understanding another's pronunciation is a problem, validate brief information in writing.* For example, during assessments, write down numbers, words, or phrases and have the client read them to verify accuracy.

- *Use humor very cautiously.* Meaning can change in the translation process.

- *Do not use slang words or colloquialisms.* These may be interpreted literally.

- *Do not assume that a client who nods, uses eye contact, or smiles is indicating an understanding of what is being taught.* These responses may simply be the client's way of indicating respect. The client may feel that asking the nurse questions or stating a lack of understanding is inappropriate because it might embarrass the nurse or cause the nurse to "lose face."

- *Invite and encourage questions during teaching.* Let clients know they are urged to ask questions and be involved in making information clearer. When asking questions to evaluate client understanding, avoid asking negative questions. These can be interpreted differently by people for whom English is a second language. "Do you understand how far you can bend your hip after surgery?" is better than the negative question "You don't understand how far you can bend your hip after surgery, do you?" With particularly difficult information or skills teaching, the nurse might say, "Most people have some trouble with this. May I please help you go through this one more time?" In some cultures, expressing a need is not appropriate, and expressing confusion or asking to be shown something again is considered rude.

- *When explaining procedures or functioning related to personal areas of the body, it may be appropriate to have a nurse of the same sex do the teaching.* Because of modesty concerns in many cultures and beliefs about what is considered appropriate and inappropriate male–female interaction, it is wise to have a female nurse teach a female client about personal care, birth control, sexually transmitted diseases, and other potentially sensitive areas. If a translator is needed during explanation of procedures or teaching, the translator should also be female.

- *Include the family in planning and teaching.* This promotes trust and mutual respect. Identify the authoritative family member and incorporate that person into the planning and teaching to promote compliance and support of health teaching. In some cultures, the male head of household is the critical family member to include in health teaching; in other cultures, it is the eldest female member.

- *Consider the client's time orientation.* The client may be more oriented to the present than the nurse. Cultures with a predominant orientation to the present include the Mexican American, Navajo Native American, Appalachian, Eskimo, and Filipino American cultures. Preventing future problems may be less significant for these clients than for others, so teaching prevention may be more difficult. For example, teaching a client why and when to take medications may be more difficult if the client is oriented to the present. In such instances, the nurse can emphasize preventing short-term problems rather than long-term problems. Failure to keep clinic appointments or to arrive on time is common in clients who have a present-time orientation. The nurse can help by arranging transportation and by accommodating these clients when they do arrive rather than rescheduling an appointment that they probably will not keep.

Schedules may be very flexible in present-oriented societies, with sleeping and eating patterns varying greatly. Teaching clients to take medications at bedtime or with a meal does not necessarily mean that these activities will occur at the same time each day. For this reason, the nurse should assess the client's daily routine before teaching the client to pair a treatment or medication with an event the nurse assumes occurs at the same time every day. When teaching a client when to take medication, the nurse should determine whether a clock or watch is available to the client and whether the client can tell time.

- *Identify cultural health practices and beliefs.* Noncompliance with health teaching may be related to conflict with folk medicine beliefs. Noncompliance may also be related to lack of understanding or a fatalism, a belief system in which life events are held to be predestined or fixed in advance and the individual is powerless to change them. To encourage compliance, the nurse may need to involve the client in learning about the causes and preventability of certain health problems.

The nurse should treat the client's cultural healing beliefs with respect and try to identify whether any are in agreement or in conflict with what is being taught. The nurse can then focus on the ones in agreement to promote the integration of new learning with familiar health practices. The client will need an explanation of why certain folk healing practices are harmful and how the recommended health practices will improve health.

EVALUATING

Evaluating is both an ongoing and a final process in which the client, the nurse, and often the support people determine what has been learned.

Evaluating Learning

The process of evaluating learning is the same as evaluating client achievement of desired outcomes for other nursing diagnoses. Learning is measured against the predetermined learning outcomes selected in the planning phase of the teaching process. Thus the outcomes serve not only to direct the teaching plan but also to provide outcome criteria for evaluation. For example, the outcome "Selects foods that are low in carbohydrates" can be evaluated by asking the client to name such foods or to select low-carbohydrate foods from a list.

The best method for evaluating depends on the type of learning. In *cognitive learning,* the client demonstrates acquisition of knowledge. Examples of the evaluation tools for cognitive learning include the following:

- Direct observation of behavior (e.g., observing the client selecting the solution to a problem using the new knowledge)
- Written measurements (e.g., tests)
- Oral questioning (e.g., asking the client to restate information or correct verbal responses to questions)
- Self-reports and self-monitoring. These can be useful during follow-up phone calls and home visits. Evaluating individual self-paced learning, as might occur with computer-assisted instruction, often incorporates self-monitoring.

The acquisition of *psychomotor skills* is best evaluated by observing how well the client carries out a procedure such as changing a dressing or carrying out a urinary self-catheterization.

Affective learning is more difficult to evaluate. Whether attitudes or values have been learned may be inferred by listening to the client's responses to questions, noting how the client speaks about relevant subjects, and by observing the client's behavior that expresses feelings and values. For example, have parents learned to value health sufficiently to have their children immunized? Do clients who state that they value health actually use condoms every time they have sex with a new partner?

Following evaluation, the nurse may find it necessary to modify or repeat the teaching plan if the objectives have not been met or have been met only partially. Follow-up teaching in the home or by phone may be needed for the client discharged from a health facility.

Behavior change does not always take place immediately after learning. Often individuals accept change intellectually first and then change their behavior only periodically (for example, Mrs. Green, who knows that she must lose weight, diets and exercises off and on). If the new behavior is to replace the old behavior, it must emerge gradually; otherwise, the old behavior may prevail. The nurse can assist clients with behavior change by allowing for client vacillation and by providing encouragement.

Evaluating Teaching

It is important for nurses to evaluate their own teaching and the content of the teaching program, just as they evaluate the effectiveness of nursing interventions for other nursing diagnoses. Evaluation should include a consideration of all factors—the timing, the teaching strategies, the amount of information, whether the teaching was helpful, and so on. The nurse may find, for example, that the client was overwhelmed with too much information, was bored, or was motivated to learn more.

Both the client and the nurse should evaluate the learning experience. The client may tell the nurse what was helpful, interesting, and so on. Feedback questionnaires and videotapes of the learning sessions can also be helpful.

The nurse should not feel ineffective as a teacher if the client forgets some of what is taught. Forgetting is normal and should be anticipated. Having the client write down information, repeating it during teaching, giving handouts on the information, and having the client be active in the learning process all promote retention.

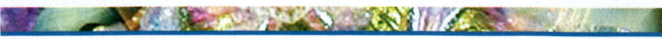

Documenting

Documentation of the teaching process is essential because it provides a legal record that the teaching took place and communicates the teaching to other health professionals. If teaching is not documented, legally it did not occur.

It is also important to document the responses of the client and support people to teaching activities. What did the client or support person say or do to indicate that learning occurred? Has the client demonstrated mastery of a skill or the acquisition of knowledge? The nurse records this in the client's chart as evidence of learning. Many agencies have multiple-copy client teaching forms that include the medical and nursing diagnoses,

the treatment plan, and the client education. After the teaching session is completed, the client and the nurse sign the form and a copy of the form is given to the client as a record of teaching and as reinforcement of the content taught. A second copy of the completed and signed form is placed in the client's chart. The parts of the teaching process that should be documented in the client's chart include the following:

- Diagnosed learning needs
- Learning outcomes
- Topics taught
- Client outcomes
- Need for additional teaching
- Resources provided.

The written teaching plan that the nurse uses as a resource to guide future teaching sessions might also include these elements:

- Actual information and skills taught
- Teaching strategies used
- Time framework and content for each class
- Teaching outcomes and methods of evaluation.

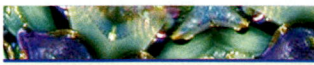 **Focus On Critical Thinking**

Mrs. Yorty is a 59-year-old African American bank vice president who is heavily relied on by her boss and coworkers. Three days ago she was admitted to the hospital with complaints of shortness of breath and mild chest pain. A diagnostic evaluation indicates that she has significant coronary artery disease but has not yet suffered a heart attack. Her physician has indicated that Mrs. Yorty will need to make significant lifestyle changes to reduce her heart attack risk. As her nurse, you have been requested to teach Mrs. Yorty about her disease process, diet, exercise, and stress reduction. As you begin teaching Mrs. Yorty, you note that she is very pleasant and frequently nods her head, but she also seems preoccupied and is readily distracted.

1. How would you evaluate Mrs. Yorty's readiness to learn?
2. Of what benefit would a learning needs assessment be inasmuch as Mrs. Yorty is obviously a well-educated client?
3. You recognize that you have a great deal of information to deliver to Mrs. Yorty and you are concerned that you will not be able to teach it all. What can you do to help Mrs. Yorty and still feel that you have accomplished your teaching goals?
4. How will you know if your teaching is effective?
5. How might your teaching differ if you were teaching Mrs. Yorty at home rather than in a hospital or acute care setting?

See Critical Thinking Possibilities in Appendix A.

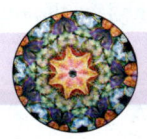 | # Chapter Review

EXPLORE MediaLink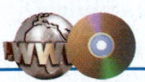

NCLEX review questions, case studies, MediaLink applications, and other interactive resources for this chapter can be found on the Companion Website at www.prenhall.com/kozier. Click on Chapter 25 to select the activities for this chapter.

For more NCLEX review questions, and an audio glossary, access the Student CD-ROM accompanying this textbook.

Chapter Highlights

- Teaching clients and families about their health needs is a major role of the nurse. Nurses also teach colleagues, subor-

dinates, nursing and other health care students, and groups in community education programs.

- Learning is represented by a change in behavior.
- Three main theories of learning are behaviorism, cognitivism, and humanism.
- Bloom has identified three learning domains: cognitive, affective, and psychomotor.
- A number of factors affect learning, including motivation, readiness, active involvement, relevance, feedback, nonjudgmental support, repetition, timing, environment, emotions, physiologic events, psychomotor ability, and cultural aspects.
- Teaching, like the nursing process, consists of six activities: assessing the learner, diagnosing learning needs, developing a teaching plan, implementing the plan, evaluating learning outcomes and teaching effectiveness, and documenting instructional activities.

- Teaching strategies chosen by the nurse should be suited to the client and to the material to be learned.
- A teaching plan is a written plan consisting of learning outcomes, content to teach, and strategies to use in teaching the content. The plan must be revised when the client's needs change or the teaching strategies prove ineffective.
- Evaluating the teaching–learning process is both an ongoing and a final process in which the client, nurse, and support people determine what has been learned.
- Documentation of client teaching is essential to communicate the teaching to other health professionals and to provide a record for legal and accreditation purposes.

Review Questions

25–1. Which of the following activities would be classified under Bloom's affective domain of learning?
   a. teaching how to irrigate a colostomy
   b. learning to accept the loss of a limb
   c. learning to insert a catheter
   d. teaching how to read
25–2. A newly diagnosed diabetic client needs to learn about her diet. Which teaching strategy would promote the best retention of the material?
   a. Give her a videotape about diabetic diets.
   b. Ask a nutritionist to visit the client to present information and handouts about the diabetic diet.
   c. Ask the client to make a list of her favorite foods and how to work them into her diet.
   d. Have the client attend a group meeting for diabetic clients to discuss their adaptation to this chronic health condition.
25–3. In which situation is the client ready to learn?
   a. a 45-year-old man whose doctor just informed him that he has cancer

   b. a 3-year-old child whose parents are reading a story book about going to the hospital
   c. a 60-year-old female who received medication 5 minutes ago for relief of abdominal pain
   d. a 70-year-old man, recovering from a stroke, who has returned from physical therapy
25–4. How can the nurse best assess a client's style of learning?
   a. Ask the client how he learns best.
   b. Perform the REALM test.
   c. Observe the client's interactions with others.
   d. Ask family members.
25–5. A 74-year-old client who takes multiple medications tells the nurse, "I have no idea what that little yellow pill is for." What is the best nursing diagnosis for this client?
   a. *Knowledge Deficit*
   b. *Health-Seeking Behavior*
   c. *Deficient Knowledge (Medication Information)*
   d. *Noncompliance*

Readings and References

Suggested Readings

Davidhizar, R. E., & Brownson, K. (1999). Literacy, cultural diversity, and client education. *Health Care Manager, 18*(1), 39–47. The challenges of client education include low literacy levels of clients and the high reading level of printed materials. The authors also describe cultural barriers that may obstruct effective client education such as elements of communications (e.g., language, dialect, voice volume, use of touch, gestures, eye contact).

Winslow, E. H. (2001). Patient education materials. Can patients read them, or are they ending up in the trash? *American Journal of Nursing, 101*(10), 33–38. The author reviews the relationship between literacy and health and points out the mismatch between a client's reading level and client education materials. The article provides information on how to assess a client's reading level and important points to remember when developing client education materials.

Related Research

Conlin, K. K., & Schumann, L. (2002). Research. Literacy in the health care system: A study on open heart surgery patients. *Journal of the American Academy of Nurse Practitioners, 14*(1), 38–42.

Murphy, P. W., Chesson, A. L., Berman, S. A., Arnold, C. L., & Galloway, G. (2001). Neurology patient education materials: Do our educational aids fit our patients' needs? *Journal of Neuroscience Nursing, 33*(2), 99–104.

Schrecengost, A. (2001). Do humorous preoperative teaching strategies work? *AORN Journal, 74,* 683–689.

References

Bastable, S. (2003). *Nurse as educator: Principles of teaching and learning for nursing practice* (2nd ed.). Boston: Jones and Bartlett.

Bloom, B. S. (Ed.). (1956). *Taxonomy of education objectives. Book 1, Cognitive domain.* New York: Longman.

Doak, C. C., Doak, L. G., & Root, J. H. (1996). *Teaching patients with low literacy skills* (2nd ed.). Philadelphia: J. B. Lippincott.

Hong, O. S. (2001). Limited English proficiency workers: Health and safety education. *AAOHN Journal, 49*(1), 21–25.

John, M. T. (1988), *Geragogy: A theory for teaching the elderly.* New York: Haworth Press.

Johnson, M., Maas, M., & Moorhead, S. (2000). *Nursing outcomes classification (NOC)* (2nd ed.). St. Louis, MO: Mosby.

Knowles, M. S. (1984). *Andragogy in action.* San Francisco: Jossey-Bass.

Mayer, G. G., & Rushton, N. (2002). Writing easy-to-read teaching aids. *Nursing, 32*(3), 48–49.

McCloskey, J. C., & Bulechek, G. M. (2000). *Nursing interventions classification (NIC)* (3rd ed.). St. Louis, MO: Mosby.

NANDA International. (2003). *NANDA nursing diagnoses: Definitions and classification 2003–2004.* Philadelphia: Author.

Rankin, S. H., & Stallings, K. D. (1996). *Patient education: Issues, principles, practices* (3rd ed.). Philadelphia: J. B. Lippincott.

Saarmann, L., Daugherty, J., & Riegel, B. (2000). Patient teaching to promote behavioral change. *Nursing Outlook, 48,* 281–287.

Schultz, M. (2002). Low literacy skills needn't hinder care. *RN, 65*(4), 45–48.

Stanley, M., & Beare, P. G. (1999). *Gerontological nursing* (2nd ed.). Philadelphia: F. A. Davis.

VanWynen, E. A. (2001). Healthy people 2010. A key to successful aging: Learning-style patterns of older adults. *Journal of Gerontological Nursing, 27*(9), 6–15.

Wilkinson, J. M. (2000). *Nursing diagnosis handbook with NIC interventions and NOC outcomes* (7th ed.). Upper Saddle River, NJ: Prentice Hall Health.

Winslow, E. H. (1998). Research for practice: Caring for patients with limited literacy. *American Journal of Nursing, 98*(7), 55, 57.

Winslow, E. H. (2001). Patient education materials: Can patients read them, or are they ending up in the trash? *American Journal of Nursing, 101*(10), 33–38.

Selected Bibliography

Bandura, A. (1971). Analysis of modeling processes. In A. Bandura (Ed.), *Psychological modeling.* Chicago: Aldine.

Binder, S., & Ratzan, S. (2001). Take a tip from educators: Gear message to audience. *Case Management Advisor, 12*(9), 143–144.

Bruccoliere, T. (2000). How to make patient teaching stick. *RN, 63*(2), 34–38.

Davidhizar, R. E., & Brownson, K. (1999). Literacy, cultural diversity, and client education. *Health Care Manager, 18*(1), 39–47.

Gravely, S. (2001). When your patient speaks Spanish—and you don't. *RN, 64*(5), 65–67.

Hansen, M., & Fisher, J. C. (1998). Patient teaching: Patient-centered teaching from theory to practice. *American Journal of Nursing, 98*(1), 56–60.

Lewin, K. (1951). *Field theory in social science.* New York: Harper and Row.

MacDonald, D. (1998). Meeting special learning needs. *RN, 61*(4), 33–34.

Magee, B., Mathews, P. A., Phelps, R. L., & Szczepanik, M. (2001). Gaps in teaching due to staff shortages? Try more efficient methods. *Patient Education Management, 8*(11), 121–124.

Maslow, A. H. (1970). *Motivation and personality.* New York: Harper and Row.

Murphy, V. (2000). Accreditation alert: Meeting JCAHO standards of patient and family education. *Inside Ambulatory Care, 6*(10), 12.

Pavlov, I. P. (1927). *Conditioned reflexes* (G. V. Anrep, trans.). London: Oxford University Press.

Piaget, J. (1966). *Origins of intelligence in children.* New York: Norton.

Rhodes, R. S., & Carlson, J. H. (2001). Patient teaching tips for acute care nurse practitioners. *Nurse Practitioner Forum, 12*(2), 86–91.

Rogers, C. R. (1961). *On becoming a person.* Boston: Houghton-Mifflin.

Rogers, C. R. (1969). *Freedom to learn.* Columbus, Ohio: Chas. E. Merrill.

Skinner, B. F. (1953). *Science and human behavior.* New York: Macmillan.

Tankel, K. (2001). Therapeutic interactions in a medication education group using the psychopharmacology race. *Journal of Psychosocial Nursing and Mental Health Services, 39*(6), 23–31.

The National Work Group on Literacy and Health (1998). Communicating with patients who have limited literacy skills. *The Journal of Family Practice, 46*(2), 169–175.

Treacy, J. T., & Mayer, D. K. (2000). Perspectives on cancer patient education. *Seminars in Oncology Nursing, 16*(1), 47–56.

Weissman, M. A., & Jasovsky, D. A. (1998). Discharge teaching for today's times. *RN, 61*(6), 38–40.

CHAPTER 26

DELEGATING, MANAGING, AND LEADING

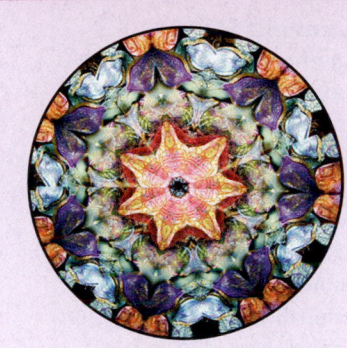

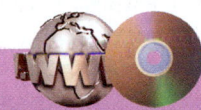

MediaLink

www.prenhall.com/kozier

Additional resources for this chapter can be found on the Student CD-ROM accompanying this textbook, and on the Companion Website at www.prenhall.com/kozier. Click on Chapter 26 to select the activities for this chapter.

CD-ROM
• Audio Glossary
• NCLEX Review

Companion Website
• Additional NCLEX Review
• Case Study: Nurse as Manager and Delegator
• MediaLink Application: Go to Nursing World
• Links to Resources

LEARNING OUTCOMES

After completing this chapter, you will be able to:

- Describe the characteristics of tasks appropriate to delegate to unlicensed and licensed assistive personnel.

- List the five rights of delegation.

- Compare and contrast leadership and management.

- Differentiate formal from informal leaders.

- Compare and contrast different leadership styles.

- Identify characteristics of an effective leader.

- Compare and contrast the levels of management.

- Describe the four functions of management.

- Discuss the roles and functions of nurse managers.

- Identify the skills and competencies needed by a nurse manager.

- Describe the role of the leader/manager in planning for and implementing change.

THE NURSE AS DELEGATOR

Delegation is the transference of responsibility and authority for the performance of an activity to a competent individual. The delegate assumes responsibility for the actual performance of the task or procedure. The delegator retains accountability for the outcome. Delegation is a tool that allows the manager to devote more time to tasks that cannot be delegated. It also enhances the skills and abilities of the delegate, which builds self-esteem, promotes morale, and enhances teamwork and attainment of the organization's goals. In nursing, delegation refers to indirect care—the intended outcome is achieved through the work of someone supervised by the nurse—and involves defining the task, determining who can perform the task, describing the expectation, seeking agreement, monitoring performance, and providing feedback to the delegate regarding performance.

Registered nurses increasingly delegate components of nursing care to other health care workers, especially with the increased use of unlicensed assistive personnel (UAP). An RN who delegates a task to another health care worker is accountable for selecting an appropriately skilled caregiver and for continued evaluation of the client's care. These "nurse extenders" may be persons identified as certified nursing aides/assistants, home health aides, patient care technicians, orderlies, surgical technicians, or a variety of other titles. They have had diverse degrees of training and experience. They are employees and do not include family members or friends who provide some client care.

Each state nurse practice act specifies which actions constitute the legal practice of nursing, which actions are the purview only of nurses, and which may be delegated to others. However, the National Council of State Boards of Nursing (NCSBN) published five "rights" of delegation: The nurse delegates the *right task,* under the *right circumstances,* to the *right person,* with the *right direction and communication,* and the *right supervision and evaluation* (1995).

It is not possible to generate an exhaustive list of exactly which actions may or may not be delegated to unlicensed personnel. Examples of tasks that may and may not be delegated are given in Box 26–1. A statement regarding delegation is included with the steps for each procedure in this book.

The unlicensed person may not delegate tasks to another person. Principles guiding the nurse's decision to delegate ensure the safety and quality of outcomes. These principles are listed in Box 26–2. Even if the task is one that may legally be delegated, the individual nurse must still determine if the task can be delegated to a particular UAP for a specific client. The NCSBN has created a grid to assist in this decision (see Figure 26–1 ■ on page 472). Once the decision has been made to delegate, the nurse must communicate clearly to the UAP and verify that the UAP understands:

- The specific tasks to be done for each client.
- When each task is to be done.

BOX 26–1	■ Examples of Tasks that May and May Not be Delegated to Unlicensed Assistive Personnel

Tasks that **May** Be Delegated to Unlicensed Assistive Personnel	Tasks that **May Not** Be Delegated to Unlicensed Assistive Personnel
■ Taking of vital signs	■ Assessment
■ Measuring and recording intake and output	■ Interpretation of data
■ Patient transfers and ambulation	■ Making a nursing diagnosis
■ Postmortem care	■ Creation of a nursing care plan
■ Bathing	■ Evaluation of care effectiveness
■ Feeding	■ Care of invasive lines
■ Clean catheterization	■ Administering parenteral medications
■ Gastrostomy feedings in established systems	■ Performing venipuncture
■ Attending to safety	■ Insertion of nasogastric tubes
■ Weighing	■ Client education
■ Performing simple dressing changes	■ Performing triage
■ Suctioning of chronic tracheostomies	■ Giving telephone advice
■ Performing basic life support (CPR)	■ Performing sterile procedures

| BOX 26–2 | ■ Principles Used by the Nurse to Determine Delegation to Unlicensed Assistive Personnel |

1. The nurse must assess the individual client prior to delegating tasks.
2. The client must be medically stable or in a chronic condition and not fragile.
3. The task must be considered routine for this client.
4. The task must not require a substantial amount of scientific knowledge or technical skill.
5. The task must be considered safe for this client.
6. The task must have a predictable outcome.
7. Learn the agency's procedures and policies about delegation.
8. Know the scope of practice and the customary knowledge, skills, and job description for each health care discipline represented on your team.
9. Be aware of individual variations in work abilities. Along with different categories of caregivers are individual variations. Each individual has different experiences and may not be capable of performing every task cited in the job description.
10. When unsure about an assistant's abilities to perform a task, observe while the person performs it, or demonstrate it to the person and get a return demonstration before allowing the person to perform it independently.
11. Clarify reporting expectations to ensure the task is accomplished.
12. Create an atmosphere that fosters communication, teaching, and learning. For example, encourage staff to ask questions, listen carefully to their concerns, and make use of every opportunity to teach.

- The expected outcomes for each task including parameters outside of which the unlicensed person must immediately report to the nurse (and any action that must urgently be taken).
- Who is available to serve as a resource if needed.
- When and in what format (written or verbal) a report on the tasks is expected.

A specific task that can be delegated to one UAP may not be appropriate for a different UAP, depending on each UAP's experience and individual skill sets. Also, a task that is appropriate for the UAP to perform with one client may not be appropriate with a different client or the same client under altered circumstances. For example, the taking of routine vital signs may be delegated to the UAP for a client in stable condition but would not be delegated for the same client who has become unstable.

> **CLINICAL ALERT** *Each nurse or other licensed or unlicensed health care provider is responsible for his or her own actions. Anyone who feels unqualified to perform a delegated task must decline to perform it.* ■

It is important to note that the nurse is not held legally responsible for the acts of the unlicensed person, but is accountable for the quality of the act of delegation and has ultimate responsibility to ensure that proper care is provided. Delegation can be an extremely useful strategy in providing thorough and effective nursing care. Skill in delegation, however, must be learned and developed over time. The nurse should not hesitate to consult with others regarding the appropriateness of delegation.

THE NURSE AS LEADER AND MANAGER

The professional nurse frequently assumes the roles of leader and manager. These two roles are linked; that is, managers must have leadership abilities, and leaders often manage, but the two roles differ.

A **leader** influences others to work together to accomplish a specific goal. Leaders are often visionary; they are informed, articulate, confident, and self-aware. Leaders also usually have excellent interpersonal skills and are excellent listeners and communicators. They have initiative and the ability and confidence to innovate change, motivate, facilitate, and mentor others. They may be employed in a variety of positions—from shift team leader to institutional president. Leaders may also hold volunteer positions such as chairperson of a professional organization or a community board of directors.

A **manager** is an employee of an organization who is given authority, power, and responsibility for planning, organizing, coordinating, and directing the work of others, and for establishing and evaluating standards. Managers understand organizational structure and culture. They control human, financial, and material resources. Managers set goals, make decisions, and solve problems. They initiate and implement change.

The purposes of **nursing leadership** vary according to the level of application and include (a) improving the health status of individuals or families, (b) increasing the effectiveness and level of satisfaction among professional colleagues, and (c) improving the attitudes of citizens and legislators toward the nursing profession and their expectations of it.

As managers, nurses are responsible for managing client care and some nurses assume a management position within the organization as nurse manager, supervisor, or executive. As a manager, the nurse is responsible for (a) efficiently accomplishing the goals of the organization, (b) efficiently using the organization's resources, (c) ensuring effective client care, and (d) ensuring compliance with institutional, professional, regulatory, and governmental standards of care. Managers are also responsible for development of licensed and unlicensed personnel within their work group. Table 26–1 further compares the leader and manager roles. Figure 26–2 ■ on page 474 illustrates some of the leading and managing roles.

Elements for Review		client A	client B	client C	client D
Activity/task	Describe activity/task:				
Level of Client Stability	Score the client's level of stability: 0. client condition is chronic/stable/predictable 1. client condition has minimal potential for change 2. client condition has moderate potential for change 3. client condition is unstable/acute/strong potential for change				
Level of UAP Competence	Score the UAP competence in completing delegated nursing care activities in the defined client population: 0. UAP - expert in activities to be delegated, in defined population 1. UAP - experienced in activities to be delegated, in defined population 2. UAP - experienced in activities but not in defined population 3. UAP - novice in performing activities and in defined population				
Level of Licensed Nurse Competence	Score the licensed nurse's competence in relation to both knowledge of providing nursing care to a defined population and competence in implementation of the delegation process: 0. Expert in the knowledge of nursing needs/activities of defined client population *and* expert in the delegation process 1. Either expert in knowledge of needs/activities of defined client population and competent in delegation *or* experienced in the needs/activities of defined client population and expert in the delegation process 2. Experienced in the knowledge of needs/activities of defined client population *and* competent in the delegation process 3. Either experienced in the knowledge of needs/activities of defined client population *or* competent in the delegation process 4. Novice in knowledge of defined population *and* novice in delegation				
Potential for Harm	Score the potential level of risk the nursing care activity has for the client *(risk is probability of suffering harm:)* 0. None 1. Low 2. Medium 3. High				
Frequency	Score based on how often the UAP has performed the specific nursing care activity: 0. Performed at least daily 1. Performed at least weekly 2. Performed at least monthly 3. Performed less than monthly 4. Never performed				
Level of Decision-making	Score the decision-making needed, related to the specific nursing care activity, client (both cognitive and physical status) and client situation: 0. Does not require decision making 1. Minimal level of decision making 2. Moderate level of decision making 3. High level of decision making				
Ability for Self Care	Score the client's level of assistance needed for self-care activities: 0. No assistance 1. Limited assistance 2. Extensive assistance 3. Total care or constant attendance				
	TOTAL SCORE				

Figure 26–1 ■ Delegation Decision-Making Grid (*Note:* From *Delegation Decision-Making Grid,* by National Council of State Board Nursing, 1997, Chicago: Author. Reprinted with permission.)

TABLE 26–1 Comparison of Leader and Manager Roles

Leaders	Managers
May or may not have official appointment to the position	Are appointed officially to the position
Have power and authority to enforce decisions only as long as followers are willing to be led	Have power and authority to enforce decisions
Influence others toward goal setting, either formally or informally	Carry out predetermined policies, rules, and regulations
Are interested in risk taking and exploring new ideas	Maintain an orderly, controlled, rational, and equitable structure
Relate to people personally in an intuitive and empathetic manner	Relate to people according to their roles
Feel rewarded by personal achievements	Feel rewarded when fulfilling organizational mission or goals
May or may not be successful as managers	Are managers as long as the appointment holds

Note: From *The Effective Nurse: Leader and Manager,* 4th ed. (p. 6), by L. M. Douglass, 1995, St. Louis, MO: Mosby. Reprinted with permission.

LEADERSHIP

Leadership may be formal or informal. The **formal leader,** or appointed leader, is selected by an organization and given official authority to make decisions and act. An **informal leader** is not officially appointed to direct the activities of others, but because of seniority, age, or special abilities, is selected by the group as its leader and plays an important role in influencing colleagues, coworkers, or other group members to achieve the group's goals.

Leadership Theory

Early leadership theories focused on what leaders are (trait theories), what leaders do (behavioral theories), and how leaders adapt their leadership style according to the situation (contingency theories). Theories about **leadership style** describe traits, behaviors, motivations, and choices used by individuals to effectively influence others.

Classic Leadership Theories

The trait theorists found that leaders often possess specific traits and abilities including good judgment, decisiveness, knowledge, adaptability, integrity, tact, popularity, nonconformity, and cooperativeness. The behaviorists believed that through education, training, and life experiences, effective leaders develop a particular leadership style. These styles have been characterized as autocratic, democratic, laissez-faire, and bureaucratic.

An **autocratic (authoritarian) leader** makes decisions for the group. The leader believes individuals are externally motivated (their driving force is extrinsic, they desire rewards from others) and incapable of independent decision making. Likened to a dictator, the autocratic leader determines policies, giving orders and directions to the group. Under this leadership style, the group may feel secure because procedures are well defined and activities are predictable. Productivity may also be high. However, the group's needs for creativity, autonomy, and self-motivation are not met, and the degree of openness and trust between the leader and the group members is minimal or absent. Members are often dissatisfied with this leadership style; however, at times an autocratic style is the most effective. When urgent decisions are necessary (e.g., a cardiac arrest, a unit fire, or a mass casualty event), one person must assume the responsibility for making decisions without being challenged by other team members. When group members are unable or do not wish to participate in making a decision, the authoritarian style solves the problem and enables the individual or group to move on. This style can also be effective when a project must be completed quickly and efficiently.

A **democratic (participative, consultative) leader** encourages group discussion and decision making. This type of leader acts as a catalyst or facilitator, actively guiding the group toward achieving the group goals. Group productivity and satisfaction are high as group members contribute to the work effort. The democratic leader assumes individuals are internally motivated (their driving force is intrinsic, they desire self-satisfaction), capable of making decisions, and value independence. Providing constructive criticism, offering information, making suggestions, and asking questions become the focus of the participative leader. This leadership style demands that the leader have faith in the group members to accomplish the goals. Although democratic leadership has been shown to be less efficient and more cumbersome than authoritarian leadership, it allows more self-motivation and more creativity among group members. It also calls for a great deal of cooperation and coordination among group members. This leadership style can be extremely effective in the health care setting.

The **laissez-faire (nondirective, permissive) leader** recognizes the group's need for autonomy and self-regulation. The leader assumes a "hands-off" approach. The leader presupposes the group is internally motivated. However, group members may act independently and at cross purposes because of a lack of cooperation and coordination. A laissez-faire style is most effective for groups whose members have both personal and professional maturity, so that once the group has made a

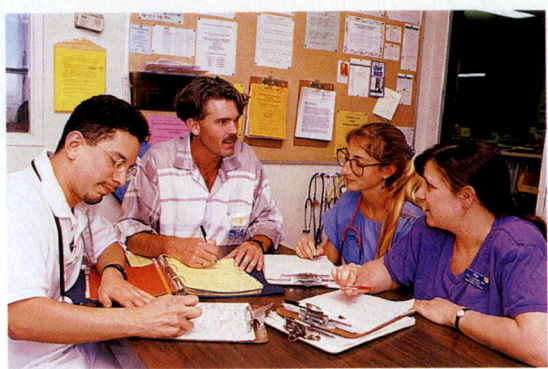

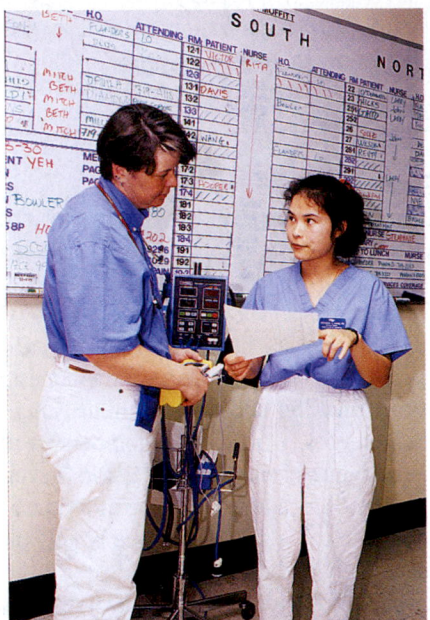

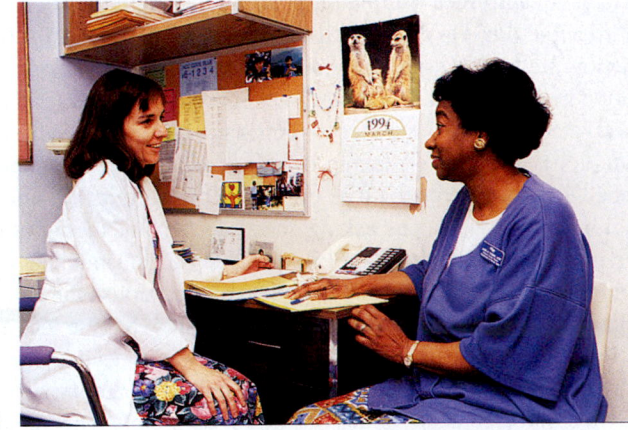

Figure 26–2 ■ Nurses as leaders and managers: *A,* The nurse manager discusses work assignments during change-of-shift report. *B,* The nurse delegates basic client care activities to the nursing assistant. *C,* The nurse consults the social worker during discharge planning.

decision, the members become committed to it and have the required expertise to implement it. Individual group members then perform tasks in their area of expertise while the leader acts as resource person. Table 26–2 compares the authoritarian, democratic, and laissez-faire leadership styles.

The **bureaucratic leader** does not trust self or others to make decisions and instead relies on the organization's rules, policies, and procedures to direct the group's work efforts. Group members are usually dissatisfied with the leader's inflexibility and impersonal relations with them.

According to contingency theorists, effective leaders adapt their leadership style to the situation. A popular contingency theory describes the situational leader. Important attributes of the **situational leader** are (a) recognition of the task behaviors and relationship behaviors of the leader, (b) consideration of the staff members' abilities, (c) knowledge of the nature of the task to be done, and (d) sensitivity to the context or environment in which the task takes place. The task-oriented leadership style is concerned with getting the work done and therefore focuses on activities that encourage group productivity. The relationship-oriented leadership style is concerned with interpersonal relationships and therefore focuses on activities that meet group members' needs. Unlike the singular style of authoritarian, democratic, and laissez-faire leadership styles, situational leaders adapt their leadership style to the readiness and willingness of the individual or group to perform the assigned task.

When employees are insecure or unable or unwilling to perform the task, the leader uses a highly directive leadership style in which specific instructions and close supervision are provided. If the group is motivated and willing but unable to perform the task, the leader again uses a highly directive selling style, but in this case, the leader explains decisions and provides the opportunity for clarification. When the group is able but unwilling or lacking in confidence, a participative high-relationship/low-task leadership style is used. With this style the leader shares ideas and facilitates decision making. The final style, delegating, a low-task and low-relationship style, is used for a group that is willing, able, and confident to perform the task. A delegating leader turns responsibility for decision making and implementation over to the group.

Contemporary Leadership Theories

Contemporary theorists have described charismatic leaders, transactional leaders, transformational leaders, and shared leadership.

A **charismatic leader** is rare and is characterized by an emotional relationship between the leader and the group members. The charming personality of the leader evokes strong feelings of commitment to both the leader and the leader's cause and beliefs. The followers of a charismatic leader often overcome extreme hardship to achieve the group's goals because of faith in the leader.

The **transactional leader** has a relationship with followers based on an exchange for some resource valued by the follower. These incentives are used to promote loyalty and performance. For example, in order to ensure adequate staffing on the night shift, the nurse manager entices a staff nurse to work the night shift in exchange for a weekend shift off. The transactional leader represents the traditional manager, focused on the day-to-day tasks of achieving organizational goals, and understands and meets the needs of the group.

TABLE 26–2 Comparison of Authoritarian, Democratic, and Laissez-Faire Leadership Styles

	Authoritarian	Democratic	Laissez-Faire
Degree of freedom	Little freedom	Moderate freedom	Much freedom
Degree of control	High control	Moderate control	No control
Leader activity level	High	High	Minimal
Assumption of responsibility	Primarily the leader	Shared	Abdicated
Output of the group	High quantity, good quality	Creative, high quality	Variable, may be of poor quality
Efficiency	Very efficient	Less efficient than authoritarian	Inefficient

Note: From *Nursing Leadership and Management: Concepts and Practice*, 4th ed. (p. 82), by R. M. Tappen, 2000, Philadelphia: F. A. Davis. Reprinted with permission.

In contrast, a **transformational leader** fosters creativity, risk taking, commitment, and collaboration by empowering the group to share in the organization's vision. The leader inspires others with a clear, attractive, and attainable goal and enlists them to participate in attaining the goal. Through shared values, honesty, trust, and continual learning the leader empowers the group. Independence, individual growth, and change are facilitated.

Shared leadership recognizes that a professional workforce is made up of many leaders. No one person is considered to have knowledge or ability beyond that of other members of the work group. Appropriate leadership is thought to emerge in relation to the challenges that confront the work group. Examples of shared leadership in nursing are self-directed work teams, coleadership, and shared governance. **Shared governance** is a method that aims to distribute decision making among a group of people

Effective Leadership

Much has been written about effective leadership and style; some descriptive statements about effective leaders are listed in Box 26–3. Leadership is a learned process. To be an effective leader requires an understanding of factors such as needs, goals, and rewards that motivate people; knowledge of leadership skills and of the group's activities; and possession of the interpersonal skills to influence others. Principles of effective leadership include vision, influence, and power.

Vision is a mental image of a possible and desirable future state. Leaders transform visions into realistic goals and communicate their visions to others who accept them as their own.

Influence is an informal strategy used to gain the cooperation of others without exercising formal authority. Influence is exercised through persuasion and excellent communication skills; it is based on a trusting relationship with the followers.

Power is the capacity to influence. It is the ability to exert actions that result in the change in behavior or attitudes of an individual or group. In classic work, French and Raven (as cited in Andrews & Baird, 2000) described five types of power: reward, coercive, legitimate, expert, and referent. **Reward power** is based on the incentives the leader can offer the followers for their cooperation. **Coercive power** is based on the fear of retribution or withholding of rewards. **Legitimate power** is related to the authority associated with a specific position or role. **Expert power** pertains to the respect others have for one's personal abilities, knowledge, or skills. **Referent power** is associated with the admiration and respect for the leader because of the leader's charisma and success.

An effective leader needs to show sensitivity to being a positive role model, demonstrating caring toward coworkers and clients. As is appropriate for any health and caring profession, leadership can also be humanistic, that is, acting in a way that stresses individuals' dignity and worth. Strategies for humanistic leadership are identified in Box 26–4.

> ► **CLINICAL ALERT** *Nurses generally move from first- to middle- to upper-level management positions through promotion. In addition, master of science in nursing administration graduate academic programs are available at many nursing schools.* ■

Medialink GO TO NURSING WORLD APPLICATION

BOX 26–3 ■ **Characteristics of Effective Leaders**

Effective leaders
- Use a leadership style that is natural to them.
- Use a leadership style appropriate to the task and the members.
- Assess the effects of their behavior on others and the effects of others' behavior on themselves.
- Are sensitive to forces acting for and against change.
- Express an optimistic view about human nature.
- Are energetic.
- Are open and encourage openness, so that real issues are confronted.

- Facilitate personal relationships.
- Plan and organize activities of the group.
- Are consistent in behavior toward group members.
- Delegate tasks and responsibilities to develop members' abilities, not merely to get tasks performed.
- Involve members in all decisions.
- Value and use group members' contributions.
- Encourage creativity.
- Encourage feedback about their leadership style.

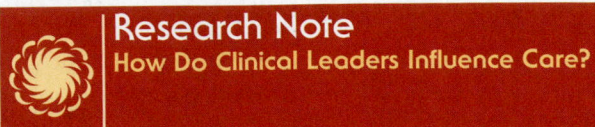

Research Note
How Do Clinical Leaders Influence Care?

An article by Cook (2001) describes exploratory research conducted to examine the role of the leader in the clinical setting. Data from interviews with British clinical nurse leaders and observations in the United States of America and Australia were analyzed with the goal of increasing our understanding of the role of the clinical leader. The researcher concluded that study of leaders' skills, traits, and attitudes will be less productive than emphasis on examination of the preparation of leaders and their impact on client outcomes. A model for examining leadership style and another model of power in the clinical setting are included.

Implications: The work site of nurse leaders varies and the importance of those who function primarily at the clinical bedside must not be underestimated. In an era of evidence-based practice, research on the relationship between leadership and outcomes is much needed.

Note: From "The Renaissance of Clinical Leadership," by M. J. Cook, 2001, *International Nursing Review, 48,* pp. 38–46.

MANAGEMENT

The manager's job is to accomplish the work of the organization. To this end, managers perform roles and functions that vary with the type of organization and the level of management.

Levels of Management

Traditional management is divided into three levels of responsibility. **First-level managers** are responsible for managing the work of nonmanagerial personnel and the day-to-day activities of a specific work group or groups. Their primary responsibility is to motivate staff to achieve the organization's goals. This level of manager represents staff in reports to upper administration and vice versa. Titles may include primary care nurse, team leader, nurse case manager, or charge nurse.

Middle-level managers supervise a number of first-level managers and are responsible for the activities in the depart-

ments they supervise. Middle-level managers serve as liaisons between first-level managers and upper-level managers. They may be called supervisors, nurse managers, or head nurses.

Upper-level (top-level) managers are organizational executives who are primarily responsible for establishing goals and developing strategic plans. Nurse executives are registered nurses who are responsible for the management of nursing within the organization and the practice of nursing. Some nurse executives are also responsible for auxiliary units such as the pharmacy, laboratory, and dietary departments. Nurses in these positions may be called vice president for patient care services, vice president for nursing, director of nursing, or chief nurse.

Management Functions

Four management functions are planning, organizing, directing, and coordinating. These four functions help to achieve the broad goal of quality client care.

Planning

Planning is an ongoing process that involves (a) assessing a situation, (b) establishing goals and objectives based on assessment of a situation or future trends, and (c) developing a plan of action that identifies priorities, delineates who is responsible, determines deadlines, and describes how the intended outcome is to be achieved and evaluated. In short, it involves deciding what, when, where, and how to do it, by whom, and with what resources. Distribution of money, personnel, equipment, and physical space are included in resource allocation. An upper-level manager spends considerable time planning the department's goals and services, determining numbers and types of nurses and other personnel needed to provide these services. On the other hand, a first-level manager such as a staff nurse spends less time planning but manages each client by use of the nursing process.

An example of the planning function is **risk management,** having in place a system to reduce danger to clients and staff. The steps of risk management include anticipating and seeking sources of risk; analyzing, classifying, and prioritizing risks; developing a plan to avoid and manage risk; gathering data that indicate success at avoiding or minimizing risk; and evaluating and modifying risk reduction programs. Central to the process of risk management is communication among all involved persons.

BOX 26–4	■ Strategies for Putting Humanistic Leadership into Action

- Praise or positively recognize staff and colleagues.
- Think good thoughts about yourself and others.
- Give before you get—give colleagues and staff a reason for doing whatever it is that you are asking of them.
- Smile often—it generates enthusiasm and goodwill.
- Remember the names of the people you work with.
- Think, act, and look successful.
- Greet others with a positive, affirmative statement.

- Write informal appreciation notes; this shows appreciation and reinforces positive performance.
- Get out of the nurse's station or office; make a point of circulating among those who work in your circle of influence.
- Talk less and listen more; encourage communication and the sharing of ideas and information.
- Don't condemn, criticize, or complain; instead, work on ways to improve the situation or solve the problem.

Note: From "Empowering Nurses through Enlightened Leadership," by T. K. Glennon, 1992, *Revolution: The Journal of Nurse Empowerment, 2,* pp. 40–44. Adapted with permission.

Organizing

Organizing is also an ongoing process. After identifying the work and evaluating human and material resources, the manager arranges the work into smaller units. Organizing involves determining responsibilities, communicating expectations, and establishing the chain of command for authority and communication. Although upper-level managers delegate much of the work and responsibility and accountability for the work to others, they need to ensure that department objectives, priorities, job descriptions, lines of communication, nursing standards, procedures, and policies clearly describe the expectations.

Directing

Directing is the process of getting the organization's work accomplished. Directing involves assigning and communicating expectations about the task to be completed, providing instruction and guidance, and ongoing decision making. Upper-level managers devote less time to directing than to planning, organizing, and controlling. Directing at this level of management generally involves supervision of the next level of managers such as those in middle management. Unit managers (charge nurses) and staff nurses devote more time directing. For example, charge nurses direct shift work by assigning clients and scheduling meal and break times. Staff nurses direct the care of clients by ordering nursing care, communicating care in written care plans and shift reports, and supervising care that is given by others.

Coordinating

Coordinating is the process of ensuring that plans are carried out and evaluating outcomes. It includes evaluating staff. The manager measures results or actions against standards or desired outcomes and then reinforces effective actions or changes ineffective ones. For example, an upper-level manager evaluates the effectiveness of recruitment, staff turnover, and budget performance. The charge nurse appraises staff performance. The staff nurse determines whether nursing interventions have helped the client achieve desired outcomes.

Principles of Management

A manager has authority, accountability, and responsibility. **Authority** is defined as the legitimate right to direct the work of others. It is an integral component of managing. Authority is conveyed through leadership actions; it is determined largely by the situation, and it is always associated with responsibility and accountability. The manager must feel worthy of the authority granted; authority can be undermined by self-doubt.

Accountability is the ability and willingness to assume responsibility for one's actions and to accept the consequences of one's behavior. Accountability can be viewed as hierarchic, starting at the individual level, then the institutional or professional level, and then the societal level. At the individual or client level, accountability is reflected in the nurse's ethical integrity. At the institutional level, it is reflected in the statement of philosophy and objectives of the nursing department and nursing audits. At the professional level, it is reflected in standards of practice developed by national or provincial nursing associations. At the societal level, it is reflected in legislated nurse practice acts.

Responsibility is an obligation to complete a task. Managers are responsible for utilization of resources, communication to subordinates, and implementation of organizational goals and objectives.

Skills and Competencies of Nurse Managers

To be effective managers, nurses need to be able to think critically, communicate well, manage resources effectively and efficiently, enhance employee performance, build and manage teams, manage conflict, manage time, and initiate and manage change.

Critical Thinking

Critical thinking is a creative cognitive process that includes problem solving and decision making. The nurse manager reasons with logic, exploring assumptions, alternatives, and the consequences of actions. See Chapter 15 ⬯ for further discussion of critical thinking.

Communicating

Managers report spending much of their day communicating. Good communication is essential and often determines the manager's success as a leader. Managers use both verbal and written communication. Effective managers communicate assertively, expressing their ideas clearly, accurately, and honestly.

Managers use **networking,** a process whereby professional links are established through which people can share ideas, knowledge, and information, offer support and direction to each other, and facilitate accomplishment of professional goals.

Managing Resources

One of the greatest responsibilities of managers is their accountability for human, fiscal, and material resources. Budgeting and determining variances between the actual and budgeted expenses are crucial skills for any manager.

Enhancing Employee Performance

Several ways of enhancing employee performance are available to managers. Managers are responsible for ensuring that employees develop through appropriate learning opportunities, whether through in-service education sessions or facilitating attendance at professional workshops and conventions. The nurse manager who empowers the staff by providing information, support, resources, and opportunities to participate will find that employees have greater commitment to the institution, are more effective in their role, have increased self-esteem, and are better able to meet their goals.

In addition, the manager may provide day-to-day coaching or serve as a mentor or preceptor. **Mentors** "give their time, energy, and material support to teach, guide, assist, counsel, and inspire a younger nurse. It is a nurturing relationship . . . " (Tomey, 2000, p. 313). Having a mentor is recognized as important for career development.

In the clinical area, the term **preceptor** is used to describe relationships in which the experienced nurse assists the "new" nurse in improving clinical nursing skill and judgment. The preceptor also instills understanding of the routines, policies, and procedures of the institution and the unit.

Building and Managing Teams

In addition to personnel development, the manager is responsible for building and managing the work team. Familiarity with group processes facilitates the manager's ability to lead the group and enhances development of the group into a work team. Groups develop in stages, during which roles and relationships are established. The purposes of the team as a whole and the role of each member must be clear. Each member must feel that the manager and the other members recognize his or her contributions. In health care, the team may consist of any health care providers: nurses, therapists, unlicensed personnel, clergy, and so on. All members of the team need to use effective communication skills.

Evaluating the group's work is another responsibility of the manager. Effectiveness, efficiency, and productivity are three outcome measures that are frequently used. In health care, **effectiveness** is a measure of the quality or quantity of services provided. **Efficiency** is a measure of the resources used in the provision of nursing services. In nursing, **productivity** is a performance measure of both the effectiveness and efficiency of nursing care. Productivity is frequently measured by the amount of nursing resources used per client or in terms of required versus actual hours of care provided.

CHANGE

Change is the process of making something different from what it was. Change can involve gaining new knowledge or adapting what is currently known in the light of new information. It can also involve obtaining new skills. Change is an integral aspect of nursing, and nurses are often **change agents,** that is, individuals who initiate, motivate, and implement change. Change agents

- Have excellent communication and interpersonal skills with individuals, groups, administration, and all levels of the organization involved in change.
- Project expertise.
- Have knowledge of available resources and how to use them: people, time, money, facilities, information.
- Are skilled in problem solving.
- Are skilled in teaching.

- Are respected by those involved in the change.
- Have the ability to encourage and nurture those going through change.
- Are self-confident, are able to take risks, and can inspire trust in themselves and others.
- Are able to make decisions.
- Have a broad base of knowledge.
- Have a good sense of timing.

> **CLINICAL ALERT**   *Change that is viewed as a threat by one nurse may be viewed as an opportunity by another nurse.* ■

Types of Change

Planned change is an intended, purposive attempt by an individual, group, organization, or larger social system to influence its own status quo or that of another organism or a situation. Problem-solving skills, decision-making skills, and interpersonal skills are important factors in planned change.

Change may also be considered covert or overt. A covert change is hidden or occurs without the individual's awareness. An example is the gradual, subtle increase in the severity of an illness. Overt change is change of which a person is aware. An example might be that a piece of equipment will no longer be available since the agency has changed vendors. People who experience overt change may also experience anxiety. Overt change often necessitates behavioral changes that are at variance with the person's needs or goals.

Unplanned change is an alteration imposed by external events or persons, it occurs when unexpected events force a reaction. It is usually haphazard, and the results can be unpredictable. Drift is a type of unplanned change in which change occurs without effort on anyone's part. Situational, or natural, change also may be considered unplanned and occurs without any control by the person or group impacted. An example is the change that occurs because of a war or a natural disaster. Not all situational changes are negative. For example, as agencies open or close units, the nurse may have the opportunity to change to a new workplace.

Models of Change

In his classic work, Lewin (1951) describes that change involves three stages: unfreezing, moving, and refreezing. During the unfreezing stage, the need for change is recognized, driving and restraining forces are identified, alternative solutions are generated, and participants are motivated to change. In the second stage, moving, participants agree the status quo is undesirable and the actual change is planned in detail and implemented. In the final stage, refreezing, the change is integrated and stabilized. Table 26–3 compares Lewin's theory of change with those of other classic theorists: Lippitt, Havelock, and Rogers.

TABLE 26–3 Classic Theories of Change

Lewin (1951)	Lippitt (1958)	Havelock (1973)	Rogers (1983)
1. Unfreezing	1. Development of a need for change	1. Building a relationship	1. *Knowledge.* The individual, called the decision-making unit, is introduced to change and begins to comprehend it.
	2. Establishment of a change relationship	2. Diagnosing the problem	
	3. Change problem established and defined		
2. Moving	4. Alternative possibilities are examined; goals or intentions are established	3. Acquiring relevant resources	2. *Permission.* The individual develops an attitude toward the change that may be favorable or unfavorable.
	5. Change efforts in the "reality Situation" are attempted	4. Choosing the solution	3. *Decision.* The person makes a choice to adopt or not to adopt the change.
	6. Change is generalized and stabilized	5. Gaining acceptance	4. *Implementation.* The person acts on the choice. At this time, alterations may take place.
3. Refreezing	7. Helping relationship ends or a different type of continuing relationship is defined.	6. Stabilization and generating self-renewal	5. *Confirmation.* The individual looks for confirmation that the choice was right. If the person encounters mixed messages, the choice may be changed.

Note: From *Field Theory in Social Science,* by K. Lewin, 1951, New York: Harper and Row; *The Dynamics of Planned Change,* by R. Lippitt, J. Watson, and B. Westley, 1958, New York: Harcourt Brace; *The Change Agent's Guide to Innovations in Education,* by R. Havelock, 1973, Englewood Cliffs, NJ: Educational Technology Publications; and *Diffusion of Innovations,* 4th ed., by E. Rogers, 1995, New York: Free-Press. Adapted with permission.

An important aspect of planning change is establishing the likelihood of the acceptance of the change and then determining the criteria by which that acceptance can be identified. Accepting change often takes time, particularly when it does not fit into a person's attitudinal framework. The course of acceptance is easier for people if they are involved in the process. If possible, change should be instituted on a small or pilot scale before full implementation. To facilitate acceptance of the change, the change agent needs to identify common driving and restraining forces (see Box 26–5). Guidelines for dealing with resistance to change are found in Box 26–6.

All nurses are affected by change; nobody can avoid it. Nurses knowledgeable about the historical and current trends in nursing and present political, social, technologic, and economic issues make rational plans to deal with opportunities to initiate and guide needed change and to respond to change that affects them in the workplace, government, organizations, and the community.

BOX 26–5   ■ Common Driving and Restraining Forces

Driving Forces
- Perception that the change is challenging
- Economic gain
- Perception that the change will improve the situation
- Visualization of the future impact of change
- Potential for self-growth, recognition, achievement, and improved relationships

Restraining Forces
- Fear that something of personal value will be lost (e.g., threat to job security or self-esteem)

- Misunderstanding of the change and its implications
- Low tolerance for change related to intellectual or emotional insecurity
- Perception that the change will not achieve goals; failure to see the big picture
- Lack of time or energy
- Perceived loss of freedom to engage in particular behaviors

BOX 26-6   ■ Guidelines for Dealing with Resistance to Change

1. Communicate with those who oppose the change. Get to the root of their reasons for opposition.
2. Clarify information and provide accurate information.
3. Be open to revisions but clear about what must remain.
4. Present the negative consequences of resistance (threats to organizational survival, compromised client care, and so on).
5. Emphasize the positive consequences of the change and how the individual or group will benefit. However, do not spend too much energy on rational analysis of why the change is good and why the arguments against it do not hold up. People's resistance frequently flows from feelings that are not rational.
6. Keep resisters involved in face-to-face contact with supporters. Encourage proponents to empathize with opponents, recognize valid objections, and relieve unnecessary fears.
7. Maintain a climate of trust, support, and confidence.
8. Divert attention by creating a different "disturbance." Energy can shift to a "more important" problem inside the system, thereby redirecting resistance. Alternatively, attention can be brought to an external threat to create a "bully phenome-

non." When members perceive a greater environmental threat (such as competition or restrictive governmental policies), they tend to unify internally.
9. Follow the "politics of change." (a) Analyze the organizational chart; know the formal lines of authority. Identify informal lines as well. (b) Identify key persons who will be affected by the change. Pay attention to those immediately above and below the point of change. (c) Find out as much as possible about these key people. What interests them, gets them excited, turns them off? What is on their personal and organizational agendas? Who typically aligns with whom on important decisions? (d) Begin to build a coalition of support before you start the change process. Identify the key people who will most likely support your idea and those who are most likely to be persuaded easily. Talk informally with them to flush out possible objections to your idea and potential opponents. What will the costs and benefits be to them—especially in political terms? Can your idea be modified in ways that retain your objectives but appeal to more key people?

Note: From Effective Leadership and Management in Nursing, *5th ed., by E. J. Sullivan, P. J. Decker, and P. Jamerson, 2001, Upper Saddle River, NJ: Prentice Hall. Adapted with permission.*

Focus on Critical Thinking

You have just interviewed for two nursing positions and are trying to decide which job to pursue. During your first interview for a team member position, the nurse manager, Mr. Caruso, was cheerful, spoke highly of his current staff and complimented them for their ability to set goals and participate in decision making, listened to your ideas, and explored ways in which you could contribute to this team's effectiveness. The second nurse manager, Mrs. Turner, was also cheerful and talkative. She provided you with a job description as a primary nurse caregiver, explained her expectations of you as a new employee, and spoke of new programs she was attempting to implement. Both nurse managers talked about changes taking place in their facilities and the need for employees to remain flexible.

1. Based on the brief data provided, speculate about the leadership style of each of these nurse managers.
2. Think about managers (or leaders) you have known and admired. What characteristics did they have that you would like to integrate into your own management style should you become a nurse manager?
3. Both nurse managers spoke of changes that were taking place in their facility. As a nurse, how can you assist your peers who are unhappy and seem to resist change even when it is positive?
4. How might the delegation of tasks to other nurses or UAPs be different in the two settings?

See Critical Thinking Possibilities in Appendix A.

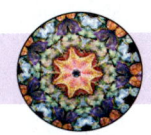 | ## Chapter Review

EXPLORE MediaLink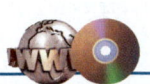

NCLEX review questions, case studies, MediaLink applications, and other interactive resources for this chapter can be found on the Companion Website at www.prenhall.com/kozier. Click on Chapter 26 to select the activities for this chapter.

For more NCLEX review questions, and an audio glossary, access the Student CD-ROM accompanying this textbook.

Chapter Highlights

- Delegation is a tool that a nurse can use to improve productivity. The nurse transfers responsibility and authority to another but retains accountability for the task.
- The professional nurse frequently assumes the roles of leader and manager. Leaders, as employees or volunteers, influence others to accomplish a specific goal, whereas managers have responsibility and accountability for accomplishing the tasks of an organization.
- Managers plan, organize, direct, and coordinate in order to accomplish the work of the organization.
- Several leadership styles have been described, including autocratic, democratic, laissez-faire, and bureaucratic. These styles are often blended to fit the situation. Nurses need to know which style is most consistent with their behavior and learn to incorporate aspects of other styles into their practice.
- Nurse managers work in the organizational framework of the employing agency. Principles of management include authority, accountability, and responsibility.
- As a manager, the nurse is responsible for (a) efficiently accomplishing the goals of the organization, (b) efficiently using the organization's resources, (c) ensuring effective client care, and (d) ensuring compliance with institutional, professional, regulatory, and governmental standards of care. Managers are also responsible for development of licensed and unlicensed personnel within their work group

Review Questions

26–1. The nurse leader informs the staff of a local emergency that she requires them to stay at the hospital and prepare for major casualties. The staff react with great anxiety and disorganization. In this case, a leadership style that will most likely be effective is
  a. authoritarian.
  b. democratic.
  c. laissez-faire.
  d. bureaucratic.

26–2. Which of the following approaches demonstrates transformational leadership?
  a. The leader stimulates group interest in establishing unit goals that contribute to agency mission.
  b. The leader forms subgroups or task forces to create possible solutions to unit problems.
  c. The leader provides funding for continuing education conferences to staff who have not used any sick leave.
  d. The leader adjusts his/her strategies to fit the current situation.

26–3. In which of the following examples might a nurse manager feel he or she has accountability but not authority for the unit.
  a. The manager is told by administration to tell the staff that they must reduce overtime as a means to reduce budgetary costs.
  b. The manager must evaluate the unit staff but is not allowed to hire or fire staff.

  c. The manager is asked to recommend a new staffing procedure to the overall institutional nurse manager group.
  d. The manager prepares a monthly budget variance report that includes plans to correct overspending.

26–4. Although an unlicensed assistive person has performed patient transfers (bed to chair) on many occasions in the past successfully, it would not be acceptable to delegate this unsupervised task to the UAP if
  a. the unit had a new wheelchair.
  b. this was an elderly client.
  c. it was the client's first time out of bed after surgery.
  d. the UAP has just returned from an extended leave of absence for family reasons.

26–5. The nurse manager wishes to implement a new way of determining the vacation schedule for staff. Senior staff oppose the change while newer staff seem more accepting of the change. An effective strategy for resolving this difference in acceptance would be to
  a. provide extensive and detailed rationale for the proposed change.
  b. explain that the change will occur as designed, regardless of the staff's preference.
  c. tell the staff that if they really don't want the change, it will not be implemented.
  d. encourage each side to share their views with each other.

Readings and References

Suggested Readings

Fisher, M. (1999). Do your nurses delegate effectively? *Nursing Management, 30*(5), 23–26. This article outlines the key aspects of delegation used by nurse managers: knowledge of the NCSBN's five rights of delegation, issues of accountability for delegated tasks, knowledge of the state nurse practice act regulations on delegation, and education of all staff regarding elements of effective delegation.

Related Research

Lesh, S. G., Russell, A., Jackson, J., & Sabet, B. (2001). Perceptions of change in the health care industry. *Journal of Allied Health, 30*(1), 11–19.
Lindholm, M., Sivberg, B., & Uden, G. (2000). Leadership styles among nurse managers in

changing organizations. *Journal of Nursing Management, 8,* 327–335.

References

Andrews, P. H., & Baird, J. E. (2000). *Communication for business and the professions* (7th ed.). New York: McGraw-Hill.

Cook, M. J. (2001). The renaissance of clinical leadership, *International Nursing Review, 48,* 38–46.

Douglass, L. M. (1995). *The effective nurse: Leader and manager* (4th ed.). St. Louis, MO: Mosby.

Glennon, T. K. (1992). Empowering nurses through enlightened leadership. *Revolution: The Journal of Nurse Empowerment, 2,* 40–44.

Havelock, R. (1973). *The change agent's guide to innovations in education.* Englewood Cliffs, NJ: Educational Technology Publications.

Lewin, K. (1951). *Field theory in social science.* New York: Harper and Row.

Lippitt, R., Watson, J., & Westley, B. (1958). *The dynamics of planned change.* New York: Harcourt Brace.

National Council of State Boards of Nursing. (1995). *Delegation: Concepts and decision-making process.* Chicago: Author.

National Council of State Boards of Nursing. (1997). *Delegation decision-making grid.* Chicago: National Council of State Boards of Nursing. Retrieved March 17, 2003, from http://www.ncsbn.org/public/res/uap/delegationgrid.pdf

Rogers, E. (1995). *Diffusion of innovations* (4th ed.). New York: Free Press.

Sullivan, E. J., Decker, P. J., & Jamerson, P. (2000). *Effective leadership and management in nursing* (5th ed.). Upper Saddle River, NJ: Prentice Hall.

Tappen, R. M. (2000). *Nursing leadership and management: Concepts and practice* (4th ed.). Philadelphia: F. A. Davis.

Tomey, A. M. (2000). *Guide to nursing management and leadership* (6th ed.). St. Louis, MO: Mosby.

Selected Bibliography

Boucher, M. A. (1998). Delegation alert! *American Journal of Nursing, 98*(2), 26–32.

Bower, F. (2000). *Nurses taking the lead: Personal qualities of effective leadership.* St. Louis, MO: Mosby.

Clegg, A. (2000). Leadership: Improving the quality of patient care. *Nursing Standard, 14*(30), 43–45.

Hansten, R., & Washburn, R. (1998). *Clinical delegation skills: A handbook for professional practice* (2nd ed.). Gaithersburg, MD: Aspen.

Hansten, R., & Washburn, R. (2001, January 29). Delegating to UAPs: Making it work. *NurseWeek, 14*(4), 16–17.

Johnston, B. (1999). Managing change in health care redesign: A model to assist staff in promoting healthy change. *Nursing Economics, 16*(1), 12–17.

Keeling, B., Adair, J., Seider, D., & Kirksey, G. (2000). Appropriate delegation. *American Journal of Nursing, 100*(12), 24A, 24C–D.

Kido, V. J. (2001). The UAP dilemma. *Nursing Management, 32*(11), 27–29.

Lancaster, J. (1999). *Nursing issues in leading and managing change.* St. Louis, MO: Mosby.

Laschinger, H. K. S., & Wong, C. (1999). Staff nurse empowerment and collective accountability: Effect on perceived productivity and self-rated work effectiveness. *Nursing Economics, 17,* 308–316.

Marquis, B. L., & Huston, C. J. (2000). *Leading roles and management functions in nursing* (3rd ed.). Philadelphia: Lippincott.

Perra, B. M. (2000). Leadership: The key to quality outcomes. *Nursing Administration Quarterly, 24*(2), 56–61.

Sullivan, E. J., & Decker, P. J. (2001). *Effective leadership and management in nursing* (5th ed.). Upper Saddle River, NJ: Prentice Hall.

Tappen, R. M., Weiss, S. A., & Whitehead, D. K. (2001). *Essentials of nursing leadership and management* (2nd ed.). Philadelphia: F. A. Davis.

Whetten, D. A., & Cameron, K. S. (1998). *Developing management skills.* Reading, MA: Addison-Wesley.

Wolper, L. F. (1999). *Health care administration: Planning, implementing, and managing organized delivery systems* (3rd ed.). Gaithersburg, MD: Aspen.

Yoder-Wise, P. S. (1999). *Leading and managing in nursing.* St. Louis, MO: Mosby.

Zimmerman, P. G. (1997). Delegating to unlicensed assistive personnel. *Nursing, 27*(5), 71.

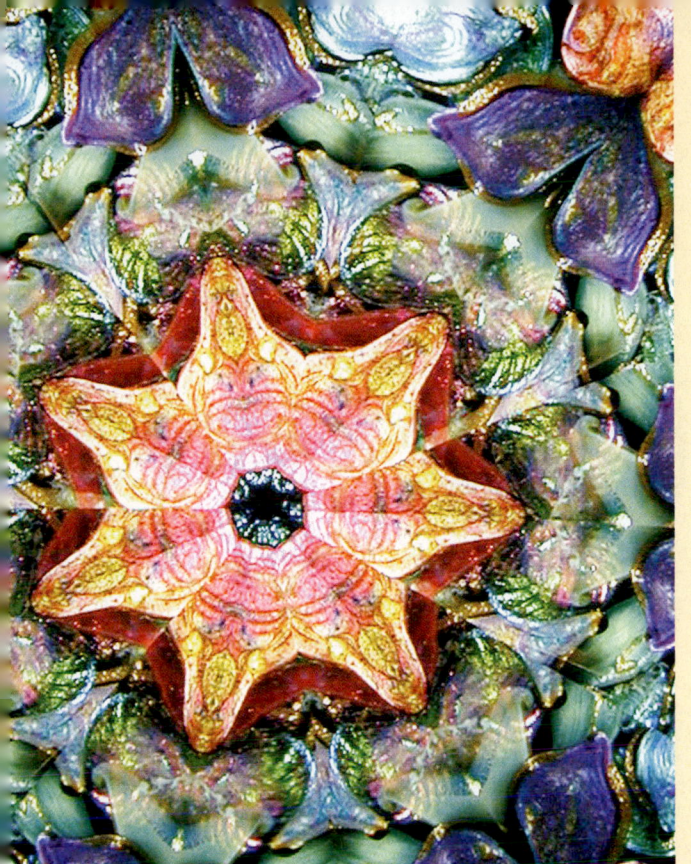

ASSESSING HEALTH

Assessment is an interactive process of information gathering and analysis that nurses carry out to identify client strengths and actual and potential health problems and to evaluate effectiveness of care. A comprehensive assessment includes data about a client's psychosocial, spiritual, cultural, environmental, and developmental status as well as physiologic health. Nurses also regularly perform focused assessments as indicated by client needs.

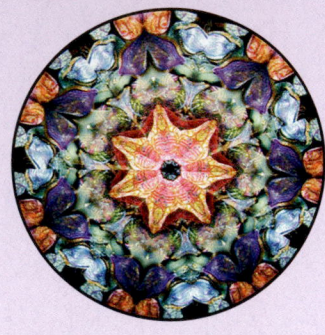

CHAPTER 27

VITAL SIGNS

LEARNING OUTCOMES

After completing this chapter you will be able to:

- Describe factors that affect the vital signs and accurate measurement of them.

- Identify the normal ranges for each vital sign.

- Identify the variations in normal body temperature, pulse, respirations, and blood pressure that occur from infancy to old age.

- Describe factors influencing the body's heat production and loss.

- Compare oral, tympanic, rectal, and axillary methods of measuring body temperature.

- Describe appropriate nursing care for alterations in body temperature.

- Identify nine sites used to assess the pulse and state the reasons for their use.

- List the characteristics that should be included when assessing pulses.

- Explain how to measure the apical pulse and the apical-radial pulse.

- Describe the mechanics of breathing and the mechanisms that control respirations.

- Identify the components of a respiratory assessment.

- Differentiate systolic from diastolic blood pressure.

- Describe five phases of Korotkoff's sounds.

- Describe various methods and sites used to measure blood pressure.

- Discuss measurement of blood oxygenation using pulse oximetry.

- Identify when it is appropriate to delegate measurement of vital signs to unlicensed assistive personnel.

MediaLink

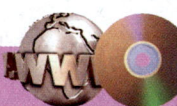

www.prenhall.com/kozier

Additional resources for this chapter can be found on the Student CD-ROM accompanying this textbook, and on the Companion Website at www.prenhall.com/kozier. Click on Chapter 27 to select the activities for this chapter.

CD-ROM
- Audio Glossary
- NCLEX Review

Companion Website
- Additional NCLEX Review
- Case Study: Assessing Vital Signs
- Care Plan Activity: Client with Pneumonia
- MediaLink Application: Joanna Briggs Institute
- Links to Resources

TABLE 27-1 Variations in Normal Vital Signs by Age

Age	Oral Temperature in Degrees Celsius (Fahrenheit)	Pulse (Average and Ranges)	Respirations (Average and Ranges)	Blood Pressure (mm Hg)
Newborns	36.8 (98.2) (axillary)	130 (80–180)	35 (30–80)	73/55
1 year	36.8 (98.2) (axillary)	120 (80–140)	30 (20–40)	90/55
5–8 years	37 (98.6)	100 (75–120)	20 (15–25)	95/57
10 years	37 (98.6)	70 (50–90)	19 (15–25)	102/62
Teen	37 (98.6)	75 (50–90)	18 (15–20)	120/80
Adult	37 (98.6)	80 (60–100)	16 (12–20)	120/80
Older adult (> 70 years)	37 (98.6)	70 (60–100)	16 (15–20)	Possible increased diastolic

The **vital** or **cardinal signs** are body temperature, pulse, respirations, and blood pressure. Recently, many agencies such as the Veterans Administration have designated pain as a fifth vital sign, to be assessed at the same time as each of the other four. Pain assessment is covered in Chapter 44. Pulse oximetry is also commonly measured on the same time as the traditional vital signs. These signs, which should be looked at in total, are checked to monitor the functions of the body. The signs reflect changes in function that otherwise might not be observed. Monitoring a client's vital signs should not be an automatic or routine procedure; it should be a thoughtful, scientific assessment. Vital signs, which should be evaluated with reference to the client's present and prior health status, are compared to the client's usual (if known) and accepted normal standards (see Table 27–1).

When and how often to assess a specific client's vital signs are chiefly nursing judgments, depending on the client's health status. Some agencies have policies about taking clients' vital signs, and physicians may specifically order a vital sign (e.g., "Blood pressure q2h"). Ordered assessments, however, should be considered the minimum; a nurse should measure vital signs more often if the client's health status requires it. Examples of times to assess vital signs are listed in Box 27–1.

Often, someone other than the nurse may measure the client's vital signs. The nurse must recall, however, that prior to delegating this task to unlicensed assistive personnel (UAP), the nurse must have assessed the individual client and determined that the client is medically stable or in a chronic condition and not fragile and that the vital sign measurement is considered routine for this client. Under those circumstances, the UAP may measure, record, and report vital signs but interpretation of the measurements rests with the nurse.

BODY TEMPERATURE

Body temperature reflects the balance between the heat produced and the heat lost from the body, measured in heat units called *degrees*. There are two kinds of body temperature: core temperature and surface temperature. **Core temperature** is the temperature of the deep tissues of the body, such as the abdominal cavity and pelvic cavity. It remains relatively constant. The normal

BOX 27-1 ■ Times to Assess Vital Signs

- On admission to a health care agency to obtain baseline data
- When a client has a change in health status or reports symptoms such as chest pain or feeling hot or faint
- Before and after surgery or an invasive procedure
- Before and/or after the administration of a medication that could affect the respiratory or cardiovascular systems, for example, before giving a digitalis preparation
- Before and after any nursing intervention that could affect the vital signs (e.g., ambulating a client who has been on bed rest)

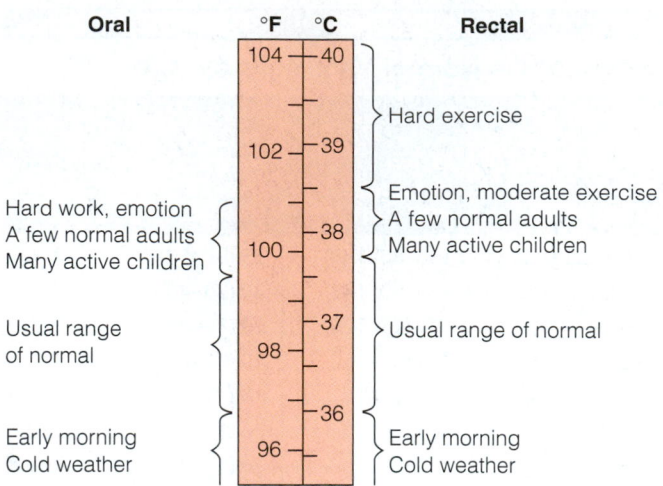

Figure 27–1 ■ Estimated ranges of body temperatures in normal persons. (*Note:* From *Fever and the Regulation of Body Temperature,* by E. F. DuBois, 1948, Springfield, IL: Charles C. Thomas. Reprinted with permission.)

core body temperature is a range of temperatures (Figure 27–1 ■). The **surface temperature** is the temperature of the skin, the subcutaneous tissue, and fat. It, by contrast, rises and falls in response to the environment.

The body continually produces heat as a by-product of metabolism. When the amount of heat produced by the body equals the amount of heat lost, the person is in **heat balance** (Figure 27–2 ■).

A number of factors affect the body's heat production. The most important are these five:

1. *Basal metabolic rate (BMR).* The **basal metabolic rate (BMR)** is the rate of energy utilization in the body required to maintain essential activities such as breathing. Metabolic rates decrease with age. In general, the younger the person, the higher the BMR (Marieb, 1998, p. 952).
2. *Muscle activity.* Muscle activity, including shivering, increases the metabolic rate.

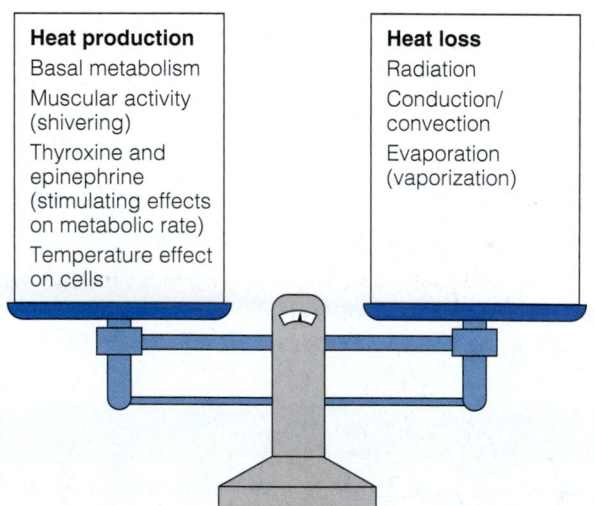

Figure 27–2 ■ As long as heat production and heat loss are properly balanced, body temperature remains constant. Factors contributing to heat production (and temperature rise) are shown on the left side of the scale; those contributing to heat loss (and temperature fall) are shown on the right side of the scale. (*Note:* From *Human Anatomy and Physiology,* 4th ed. (p. 953), by E. N. Marieb, 1998, Menlo Park, CA: Benjamin/Cummings. Adapted with permission.)

3. *Thyroxine output.* Increased thyroxine output increases the rate of cellular metabolism throughout the body. This effect is called **chemical thermogenesis,** the stimulation of heat production in the body through increased cellular metabolism.
4. *Epinephrine, norepinephrine, and sympathetic stimulation.* These hormones immediately increase the rate of cellular metabolism in many body tissues. Epinephrine and norepinephrine directly affect liver and muscle cells, thereby increasing cellular metabolism.
5. *Fever.* Fever increases the cellular metabolic rate and thus increases the body's temperature further.

Heat is lost from the body through radiation, conduction, convection, and vaporization. **Radiation** is the transfer of heat from the surface of one object to the surface of another without contact between the two objects, mostly in the form of infrared rays. For example, radiation accounts for 60% of the heat lost by a nude person standing in a room at normal room temperature (Guyton, 1996, p. 912).

Conduction is the transfer of heat from one molecule to a molecule of lower temperature. Conductive transfer cannot take place without contact between the molecules and normally accounts for minimal heat loss except, for example, when a body is immersed in cold water. The amount of heat transferred depends on the temperature difference and the amount and duration of the contact.

Convection is the dispersion of heat by air currents. The body usually has a small amount of warm air adjacent to it. This warm air rises and is replaced by cooler air, and so people always lose a small amount of heat through convection.

Vaporization is continuous evaporation of moisture from the respiratory tract and from the mucosa of the mouth and from the skin. This continuous and unnoticed water loss is called **insensible water loss,** and the accompanying heat loss is called **insensible heat loss.** Insensible heat loss accounts for about 10% of basal heat loss. When the body temperature increases, vaporization accounts for greater heat loss.

Regulation of Body Temperature

The system that regulates body temperature has three main parts: sensors in the shell and in the core, an integrator in the hypothalamus, and an effector system that adjusts the production and loss of heat. Most sensors or sensory receptors are in the skin. The skin has more receptors for cold than warmth. Therefore, skin sensors detect cold more efficiently than warmth.

When the skin becomes chilled over the entire body, three physiologic processes to increase the body temperature take place:

1. Shivering increases heat production.
2. Sweating is inhibited to decrease heat loss.
3. Vasoconstriction decreases heat loss.

The **hypothalamic integrator,** the center that controls the core temperature, is located in the preoptic area of the hypothalamus. When the sensors in the hypothalamus detect heat, they send out signals intended to reduce the temperature, that is, to decrease heat production, and increase heat loss. When the cold sensors are stimulated, signals are sent out to increase heat production and decrease heat loss.

The signals from the cold-sensitive receptors of the hypothalamus initiate effectors, such as vasoconstriction, shivering, and the release of epinephrine, which increases cellular metabolism and hence heat production. When the warmth-sensitive receptors in the hypothalamus are stimulated, the effector system sends out signals that initiate sweating and peripheral vasodilatation. Also, when this system is stimulated, the person consciously makes appropriate adjustments, such as putting on additional clothing in response to cold or turning on a fan in response to heat.

Factors Affecting Body Temperature

Nurses should be aware of the factors that can affect a client's body temperature so that they can recognize normal temperature variations and understand the significance of body temperature measurements that deviate from normal. Among the factors that affect body temperature are the following:

1. *Age.* The infant is greatly influenced by the temperature of the environment and must be protected from extreme changes. Children's temperatures continue to be more variable than those of adults until puberty. Many older people, particularly those over 75 years old, are at risk of hypothermia (temperatures below 36C, or 96.8F) for a variety of reasons, such as inadequate diet, loss of subcutaneous fat, lack of activity, and reduced thermoregulatory efficiency. Older people are also particularly sensitive to extremes in the environmental temperature due to decreased thermoregulatory controls.
2. *Diurnal variations (circadian rhythms).* Body temperatures normally change throughout the day, varying as much as 1.0C (1.8F) between the early morning and the late afternoon. The point of highest body temperature is usually reached between 2000 and 2400 hours (8:00 PM and midnight), and the lowest point is reached during sleep between 0400 and 0600 hours (4:00 and 6:00 AM). (See Figure 27–3 ■).
3. *Exercise.* Hard work or strenuous exercise can increase body temperature to as high as 38.3 to 40C (101 to 104F) measured rectally.

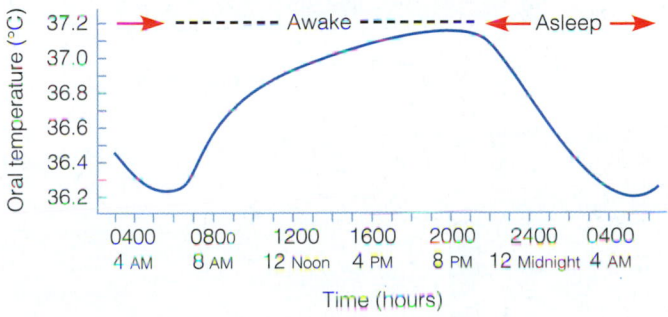

Figure 27–3 ■ Range of oral temperatures during 24 hours for a healthy young adult.

4. *Hormones.* Women usually experience more hormone fluctuations than men. In women, progesterone secretion at the time of ovulation raises body temperature by about 0.3 to 0.6C (0.5 to 1.0F) above basal temperature (Ladewig, London, & Olds, 1998).

5. *Stress.* Stimulation of the sympathetic nervous system can increase the production of epinephrine and norepinephrine, thereby increasing metabolic activity and heat production. Nurses may anticipate that a highly stressed or anxious client could have an elevated body temperature for that reason.

6. *Environment.* Extremes in environmental temperatures can affect a person's temperature regulatory systems. If the temperature is assessed in a very warm room and the body temperature cannot be modified by convection, conduction, or radiation, the temperature will be elevated. Similarly, if the client has been outside in extremely cold weather without suitable clothing, the body temperature may be low.

Alterations in Body Temperature

There are two primary alterations in body temperature: pyrexia and hypothermia.

Pyrexia

A body temperature above the usual range is called **pyrexia, hyperthermia,** or (in lay terms) **fever.** A very high fever, such as 41C (105.8F), is called **hyperpyrexia** (Figure 27–4 ■). The

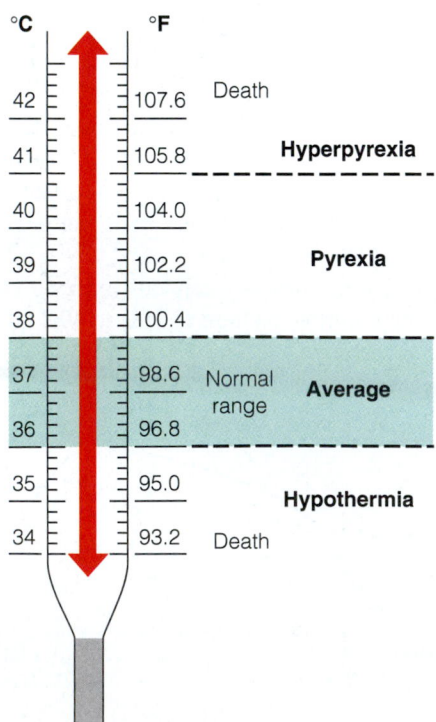

Figure 27–4 ■ Terms used to describe alterations in body temperature (oral measurements) and ranges in Celsius (centigrade) and Fahrenheit scales.

client who has a fever is referred to as **febrile;** the one who has not is **afebrile.**

Four common types of fevers are intermittent, remittent, relapsing, and constant. During an **intermittent fever,** the body temperature alternates at regular intervals between periods of fever and periods of normal or subnormal temperatures. During a **remittent fever,** a wide range of temperature fluctuations (more than 2C [3.6F]) occurs over the 24-hour period, all of which are above normal. In a **relapsing fever,** short febrile periods of a few days are interspersed with periods of 1 or 2 days of normal temperature. During a **constant fever,** the body temperature fluctuates minimally but always remains above normal. A temperature that rises to fever level rapidly following a normal temperature and then returns to normal within a few hours is called a **fever spike.**

The clinical signs of fever vary with the onset, course, and abatement stages of the fever (see Box 27–2). These signs occur as a result of changes in the set point of the temperature control mechanism regulated by the hypothalamus. Under normal conditions, whenever the core temperature rises above 37C (98.6F), the rate of heat *loss* is increased, resulting in a fall in temperature toward the set-point level. Conversely, when the core temperature falls below 37C (98.6F), the rate of heat *production* is increased, resulting in a rise in temperature toward the set point.

In a fever, however, the set point of the hypothalamic thermostat changes suddenly from the normal level to a higher than normal value (e.g., 39.5C [103.1F]) as a result of the effects of tissue destruction, pyrogenic substances, or dehydration on the hypothalamus. Although the set point changes rapidly, the core body temperature (i.e., the blood temperature) reaches this new set point only after several hours. During this interval, the usual heat production responses that cause elevation of the body temperature occur: chills, feeling of coldness, cold skin due to vasoconstriction, and shivering.

When the core temperature reaches the new set point, the person feels neither cold nor hot and no longer experiences chills. Depending on the degree of temperature elevation, other signs may occur during the course of the fever. Very high temperatures, such as 41 to 42C (106 to 108F), damage the parenchyma of cells throughout the body, particularly in the brain where destruction of neuronal cells is irreversible. Damage to the liver, kidneys, and other body organs can also be great enough to disrupt functioning and eventually cause death.

When the cause of the high temperature is suddenly removed, the set point of the hypothalamic thermostat is suddenly reduced to a lower value, perhaps even back to the original normal level. In this instance, the hypothalamus now attempts to lower the temperature to 37C (98.6F), and the usual heat loss responses causing a reduction of the body temperature occur: excessive sweating and a hot, flushed skin due to sudden vasodilatation. This sudden change of events is known as the *crisis,* the *flush,* or the *defervescent (abatement) stage* of a pyrexic condition.

Nursing interventions for a client who has a fever are designed to support the body's normal physiologic processes, provide comfort, and prevent complications. During the course of fever, the nurse needs to monitor the client's vital signs closely.

Nursing measures during the chill phase are designed to help the client decrease heat loss. At this time, the body's phys-

BOX 27-2 ■ Clinical Signs of Fever

Onset (Cold or Chill Stage)
- Increased heart rate
- Increased respiratory rate and depth
- Shivering
- Pallid, cold skin
- Complaints of feeling cold
- Cyanotic nail beds
- "Gooseflesh" appearance of the skin
- Cessation of sweating

Course
- Absence of chills
- Skin that feels warm
- Photosensitivity

- Glassy-eyed appearance
- Increased pulse and respiratory rates
- Increased thirst
- Mild to severe dehydration
- Drowsiness, restlessness, delirium, or convulsions
- Herpetic lesions of the mouth
- Loss of appetite (if the fever is prolonged)
- Malaise, weakness, and aching muscles

Defervescence (fever abatement)
- Skin that appears flushed and feels warm
- Sweating
- Decreased shivering
- Possible dehydration

iologic processes are attempting to raise the core temperature to the new set-point temperature. During the flush or crisis phase, the body processes are attempting to lower the core temperature to the reduced or normal set-point temperature. At this time, the nurse takes measures to increase heat loss and decrease heat production. Nursing interventions for a client with fever are shown Box 27-3.

Hypothermia

Hypothermia is a core body temperature below the lower limit of normal. The three physiologic mechanisms of hypothermia are (a) excessive heat loss, (b) inadequate heat production to counteract heat loss, and (c) impaired hypothalamic thermoregulation. The clinical signs of hypothermia are listed in Box 27-4.

BOX 27-3 ■ Nursing Interventions for Clients with Fever

- Monitor vital signs.
- Assess skin color and temperature.
- Monitor white blood cell count, hematocrit value, and other pertinent laboratory reports for indications of infection or dehydration.
- Remove excess blankets when the client feels warm, but provide extra warmth when the client feels chilled.
- Provide adequate nutrition and fluids (e.g., 2,500–3,000 mL per day) to meet the increased metabolic demands and prevent dehydration.
- Measure intake and output.
- Reduce physical activity to limit heat production, especially during the flush stage.
- Administer antipyretics (drugs that reduce the level of fever) as ordered.
- Provide oral hygiene to keep the mucous membranes moist.
- Provide a tepid sponge bath to increase heat loss through conduction.
- Provide dry clothing and bed linens.

BOX 27-4 ■ Clinical Signs of Hypothermia

- Decreased body temperature, pulse, and respirations
- Severe shivering (initially)
- Feelings of cold and chills
- Pale, cool, waxy skin
- Hypotension
- Decreased urinary output
- Lack of muscle coordination
- Disorientation
- Drowsiness progressing to coma

Hypothermia may be accidental or induced. Accidental hypothermia can occur as a result of (a) exposure to a cold environment, (b) immersion in cold water, and (c) lack of adequate clothing, shelter, or heat. In older people the problem can be compounded by a decreased metabolic rate and the use of sedatives.

Managing hypothermia involves removing the client from the cold and rewarming the client's body. For the client with mild hypothermia, the body is rewarmed by applying blankets; for the client with severe hypothermia, a hyperthermia blanket (an electronically controlled blanket that provides a specified temperature) is applied, and warm intravenous fluids are given. Wet clothing, which increases heat loss because of the high conductivity of water, should be replaced with dry clothing. See Box 27-5 for nursing interventions for clients who have hypothermia.

BOX 27-5 ■ Nursing Interventions for Clients with Hypothermia

- Provide a warm environment.
- Provide dry clothing.
- Apply warm blankets.
- Keep limbs close to body.
- Cover the client's scalp with a cap or turban.
- Supply warm oral or intravenous fluids.
- Apply warming pads.

Induced hypothermia is the deliberate lowering of the body temperature to decrease the need for oxygen by the body tissues. Induced hypothermia can involve the whole body or a body part. It is sometimes indicated prior to surgery (e.g., cardiac and brain surgery). See Identifying Nursing Diagnoses, Outcomes, and Interventions for examples of applying the nursing process to clients with temperature alterations.

Assessing Body Temperature

The four most common sites for measuring body temperature are oral, rectal, axillary, and the tympanic membrane. Each of the sites has advantages and disadvantages (see Table 27–2).

The body temperature is frequently measured *orally*. This method reflects changing body temperature more quickly than the rectal method. If a client has been taking cold or hot food or fluids or smoking, the nurse should wait 30 minutes before taking the temperature orally to ensure that the temperature of the mouth is not affected by the temperature of the food, fluid, or warm smoke.

Rectal temperature readings are considered to be very accurate. In some agencies, taking temperatures rectally is contraindicated for clients with myocardial infarction. It is believed that inserting a rectal thermometer can produce vagal stimulation, which in turn can cause myocardial damage. However, not all authorities share this belief. Rectal temperatures are contraindicated for clients who are undergoing rectal surgery, have diarrhea or diseases of the rectum, are

immunosuppressed, have a clotting disorder, or have significant hemorrhoids.

The axilla is the preferred site for measuring temperature in newborns because it is accessible and offers no possibility of rectal perforation. However, some research indicates that the axillary method is inaccurate when assessing a fever (Bindler, Ball & 2003). Nurses should check agency protocol when taking the temperature of newborns, infants, toddlers, and children. Adult clients for whom the axillary method of temperature assessment is appropriate include those with oral inflammation or wired jaws, clients recovering from oral surgery, clients who cannot breathe through their noses, irrational clients, and clients for whom other temperature sites are contraindicated.

The *tympanic membrane,* or nearby tissue in the ear canal, is another site for core body temperature. Like the sublingual oral site, the tympanic membrane has an abundant arterial blood supply, primarily from branches of the external carotid artery. Because temperature sensors applied directly to the tympanic membrane can be uncomfortable and involve risk of membrane injury or perforation, noninvasive infrared thermometers are now used. Electronic tympanic thermometers are found extensively in both inpatient and ambulatory care settings.

In addition to the four common sites for measuring temperature, the forehead may also be used using a chemical thermometer. Forehead temperature measurements are most useful for infants and children where a more invasive measurement is not necessary. If the forehead indicates a temperature elevation, a glass or electronic thermometer should be used to obtain a more accurate measurement.

IDENTIFYING NURSING DIAGNOSES, OUTCOMES, AND INTERVENTIONS

IMBALANCED BODY TEMPERATURE

NURSING DIAGNOSIS/ DEFINITION	SAMPLE DESIRED OUTCOMES [NOC#]/DEFINITION	INDICATORS	SELECTED INTERVENTIONS [NIC#]/DEFINITION	SAMPLE ACTIVITIES [NIC] (ALSO SEE BOXES 27–3 & 27–5)
Risk for Imbalanced Body Temperature/At risk for failure to maintain body temperature within normal range	Hydration [0602]/ *Amount of water in the intracellular and extracellular compartments of the body*	[†]• Moist mucous membranes • Fever not present	Temperature Regulation [3900]/ *Attaining and/or maintaining body temperature within a normal range*	Monitor temperature every 2 hours, as appropriate Promote adequate fluid and nutritional intake
Hyperthermia/*Body temperature elevated above normal range*	Thermoregulation [0800]/*Balance among heat production, heat gain, and heat loss*	[†]• Skin temperature IER (in expected range) • Body temperature IER (in expected range) • Sweating when hot	Fever Treatment [3740]*/ *Management of a patient with hyperpyrexia caused by nonenvironmental factors*	Monitor intake and output Apply ice bag covered with a towel to groin Cover the patient with only a sheet

[*] *Note:* Thermoregulation is a Level 2 Class (M) under the NIC Level 1 Domain of *Physiological Complex:* Interventions to maintain body temperature within a normal range (see Table 18–7).

[†] The measurement scale ranges from Extremely compromised (1) to Not compromised (5). See Appendix B. 🔗

TABLE 27–2 Advantages and Disadvantages of Four Sites for Body Temperature Measurement

Site	Advantages	Disadvantages
Oral	Accessible and convenient	Glass thermometers can break if bitten.
		Inaccurate if client has just ingested hot or cold food or fluid or smoked.
		Could injure the mouth following oral surgery.
Rectal	Reliable measurement	Inconvenient and more unpleasant for clients; difficult for client who cannot turn to the side.
		Could injure the rectum following rectal surgery.
		A rectal glass thermometer does not respond to changes in arterial temperatures as quickly as an oral thermometer, a fact that may be potentially dangerous for febrile clients because misleading information may be acquired.
		Presence of stool may interfere with thermometer placement. If the stool is soft, the thermometer may be embedded in stool rather than against the wall of the rectum.
Axillary	Safe and noninvasive	The thermometer must be left in place a long time to obtain an accurate measurement.
Tympanic membrane	Readily accessible; reflects the core temperature. Very fast.	Can be uncomfortable and involves risk of injuring the membrane if the probe is inserted too far.
		Repeated measurements may vary. Right and left measurements can differ.
		Presence of cerumen can affect the reading.

Types of Thermometers

Traditionally, body temperatures were measured using *mercury-in-glass thermometers*. Glass thermometers can be hazardous, however, due to exposure to mercury, which is toxic to humans, and broken glass should the thermometer crack or break. In 1998, the U.S. Environmental Protection Agency and the American Hospital Association agreed to the goal of eliminating mercury from health care environments. Some hospitals no longer use mercury-in-glass thermometers, and several cities have banned the sale and manufacture of them. In some cases, plastics have replaced glass and safer chemicals have replaced mercury in modern versions of the thermometer. Thus, the nurse may still encounter this type of thermometer and must be well versed in its safe use.

Although the amount of mercury in a thermometer (or in a flourescent light bulb) is minimal, should it break, cleanup involves several "dos and don'ts." Unsealed mercury slowly vaporizes into the air and these mercury vapors are toxic. Keep children and pets away from the area. Wearing rubber gloves, wipe mercury beads off clothing, skin, or other disposable items with a paper towel placed immediately into a plastic bag. Discard the item. If the spill is on a porous material that cannot be discarded (e.g., carpet), a contractor trained in mercury disposal may be needed. If the mercury is on a hard surface, use folded stiff cardboard to slowly gather the beads and pour them into a wide-mouthed container. Use a flashlight to search for the beads since the light will reflect off the mercury. Dispose of all items used in the cleanup in a plastic bag that is sealed with tape. Shower or wash well. Keep the area well ventilated for several days. Do not use any type of vacuum cleaner or broom since these will disperse the mercury and be contaminated. Do not pour the mercury down a toilet or drain and do not wash or reuse contaminated materials.

> ► CLINICAL ALERT   *Whenever mercury-in-glass thermometers are encountered, the nurse should recommend their immediate replacement with less hazardous thermometers and their safe disposal.* ■

Oral thermometers may have long, short, slender, or rounded tips (Figure 27–5 ■). A rounded thermometer can be used at the rectal as well as other sites. In some agencies, thermometer ends may be color coded; for example, red thermometers may be used for rectal temperatures and blue ones for oral and axillary temperatures.

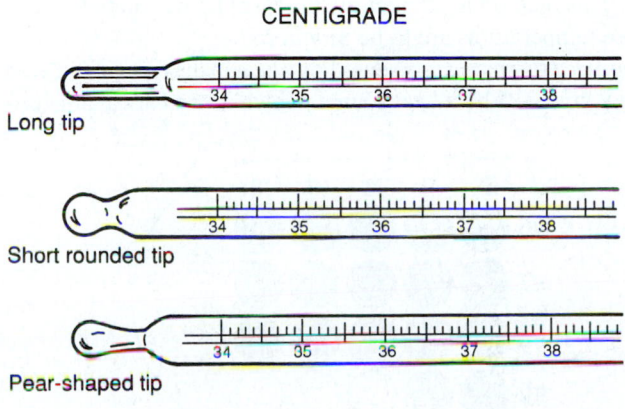

CENTIGRADE

Long tip

Short rounded tip

Pear-shaped tip

Three types of thermometer tips (Centigrade scale).

Figure 27–5 ■ Three types of thermometer tips (centigrade scale).

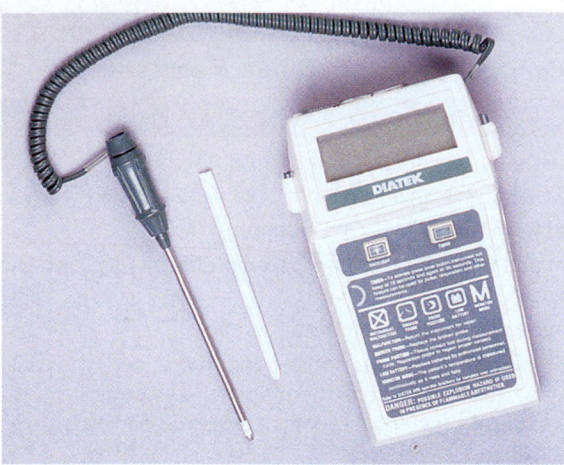

Figure 27–6 ■ An electronic thermometer. Note the probe and probe cover.

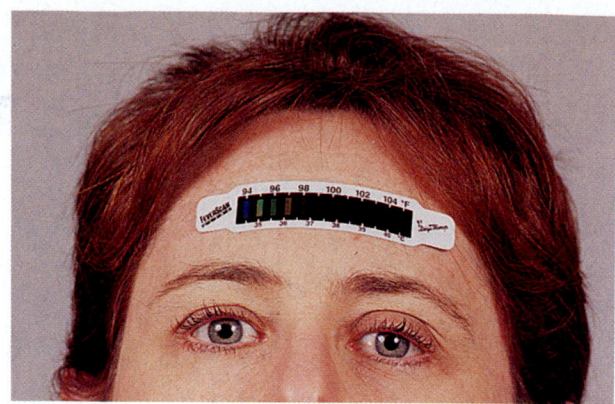

Figure 27–8 ■ A temperature-sensitive skin tape.

Electronic thermometers offer another method of assessing body temperatures. They can provide a reading in only 2 to 60 seconds, depending on the model. The equipment consists of a battery-operated portable electronic unit, a probe that the nurse attaches to the unit, and a probe cover, which is usually disposable (Figure 27–6 ■). Some models have a different circuit and probe for each method of measurement.

Chemical disposable thermometers are also used to measure body temperatures. Chemical thermometers using liquid crystal dots or bars or heat-sensitive tape or patches applied to the forehead change color to indicate temperature. Some of these are single use and others may be reused several times. One type that has small chemical dots at one end is shown in Figure 27–7 ■. To read the temperature, the nurse notes the highest reading among the dots that have changed color.

Temperature-sensitive tape may also be used to obtain a general indication of body surface temperature. It does not indicate the core temperature. The tape contains liquid crystals that change color according to temperature. When applied to the skin, usually of the forehead or abdomen, the temperature digits on the tape respond by changing color (Figure 27–8 ■). The skin area should be dry. After the length of time specified by the manufacturer (e.g., 15 seconds), a color appears on the tape. This method is particularly useful at home and for infants whose temperatures are to be monitored.

Infrared thermometers sense body heat in the form of infrared energy given off by a heat source, which in the ear canal is pri-

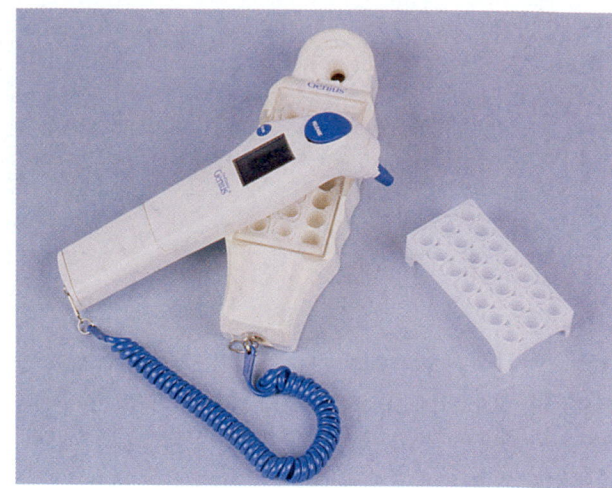

Figure 27–9 ■ An infrared (tympanic) thermometer used to measure the tympanic membrane temperature.

marily the tympanic membrane. (Figure 27–9 ■). The infrared thermometer makes no contact with the tympanic membrane.

Temperature Scales

The body temperature is measured in degrees on two scales: Celsius (centigrade) and Fahrenheit. Sometimes a nurse needs to convert a Celsius reading to Fahrenheit, or vice versa. To convert from Fahrenheit to Celsius, deduct 32 from the Fahrenheit reading and then multiply by the fraction 5/9; that is:

$$C = (\text{Fahrenheit temperature} - 32) \times 5/9$$

For example, when the Fahrenheit reading is 100:

$$C = (100 - 32) \times 5/9 = (68) \times 5/9 = 37.7$$

To convert from Celsius to Fahrenheit, multiply the Celsius reading by the fraction 9/5 and then add 32; that is:

$$F = (\text{Celsius temperature} \times 9/5) + 32$$

For example, when the Celsius reading is 40:

$$F = (40 \times 9/5) + 32 = (72) + 32 = 104$$

Procedure 27–1 explains how to measure body temperature.

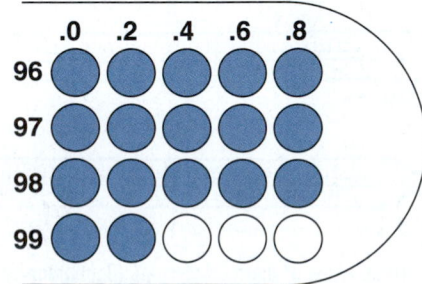

Figure 27–7 ■ A chemical thermometer showing a reading of 99.2F.

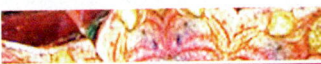

Procedure 27-1 Assessing Body Temperature

Purposes

- To establish baseline data for subsequent evaluation
- To identify whether the core temperature is within normal range
- To determine changes in the core temperature in response to specific therapies (e.g., antipyretic medication, immunosuppressive therapy, invasive procedure)
- To monitor clients at risk for imbalanced body temperature (e.g., clients at risk for infection or diagnosis of infection; those who have been exposed to temperature extremes)

ASSESSMENT

Assess

- Clinical signs of fever
- Clinical signs of hypothermia
- Site most appropriate for measurement
- Factors that may alter core body temperature

PLANNING

Delegation

Routine measurement of the client's temperature can be delegated to UAP or family members/caregivers. The nurse must inform the UAP of the appropriate type of thermometer and site to be used and ensure that the UAP knows when to report an abnormal temperature and how to record the finding. The interpretation of an abnormal temperature and determination of appropriate responses are done by the nurse.

Equipment

- Thermometer
- Thermometer sheath or cover
- Water-soluble lubricant for a rectal temperature
- Disposable gloves
- Towel for axillary temperature
- Tissues/wipes

IMPLEMENTATION

Preparation

Check that all equipment is functioning normally. If necessary, shake a glass thermometer down to below 35C (95F). *The indicator fluid will not fall below the starting level if the client's temperature is less than that. Beginning with the thermometer on a very low temperature allows the nurse to note that the indicator fluid has risen to the client's actual temperature.*

Performance

1. Explain to the client what you are going to do, why it is necessary, and how he or she can cooperate. Discuss how the results will be used in planning further care or treatments.
2. Wash hands and observe appropriate infection control procedures. Don gloves if performing a rectal temperature.
3. Provide for client privacy.
4. Place the client in the appropriate position (e.g., lateral or Sim's position for inserting a rectal thermometer).
5. Place the thermometer (see Box 27–6 on page 495).
   - Apply a protective sheath or probe cover if appropriate.
   - Lubricate a rectal thermometer.
6. Wait the appropriate amount of time: 2 to 3 minutes for an oral or rectal temperature using a glass thermometer, 6 to 9 minutes for an axillary temperature with a glass thermometer. Electronic and tympanic thermometers will indicate that the

reading is complete through a light or tone. Check package instructions for length of time to wait prior to reading chemical dot or tape thermometers.

> ► **CLINICAL ALERT**   *Be sure to record the temperature from an electronic thermometer before replacing the probe into the charging unit. With many models, replacing the probe erases the temperature from the display.* ■

7. Remove the thermometer and discard the cover or wipe with a tissue if necessary.
8. Read the temperature and record it on your worksheet. If the temperature is obviously too high, too low, or inconsistent with the client's condition, recheck it with a thermometer known to be functioning properly.
9. Wash the thermometer if necessary and return it to the storage location.
10. Document the temperature in the client record (Figure 27–10 ■, see page 494). A rectal temperature may be recorded with an "R" next to the value or with the mark on a graphic sheet circled. An axillary temperature may be recorded with "AX" or marked on a graphic sheet with an X.

EVALUATION

- Compare the temperature measurement to baseline data, normal range for age of client, and client's previous temperatures. Analyze considering time of day and any additional influencing factors and other vital signs.
- Conduct appropriate follow-up such as notifying the physician, giving a medication, or altering the client's environment. This includes teaching the client how to lower an elevated temperature through actions such as increasing fluid intake, coughing and deep breathing, or removing heavy coverings.

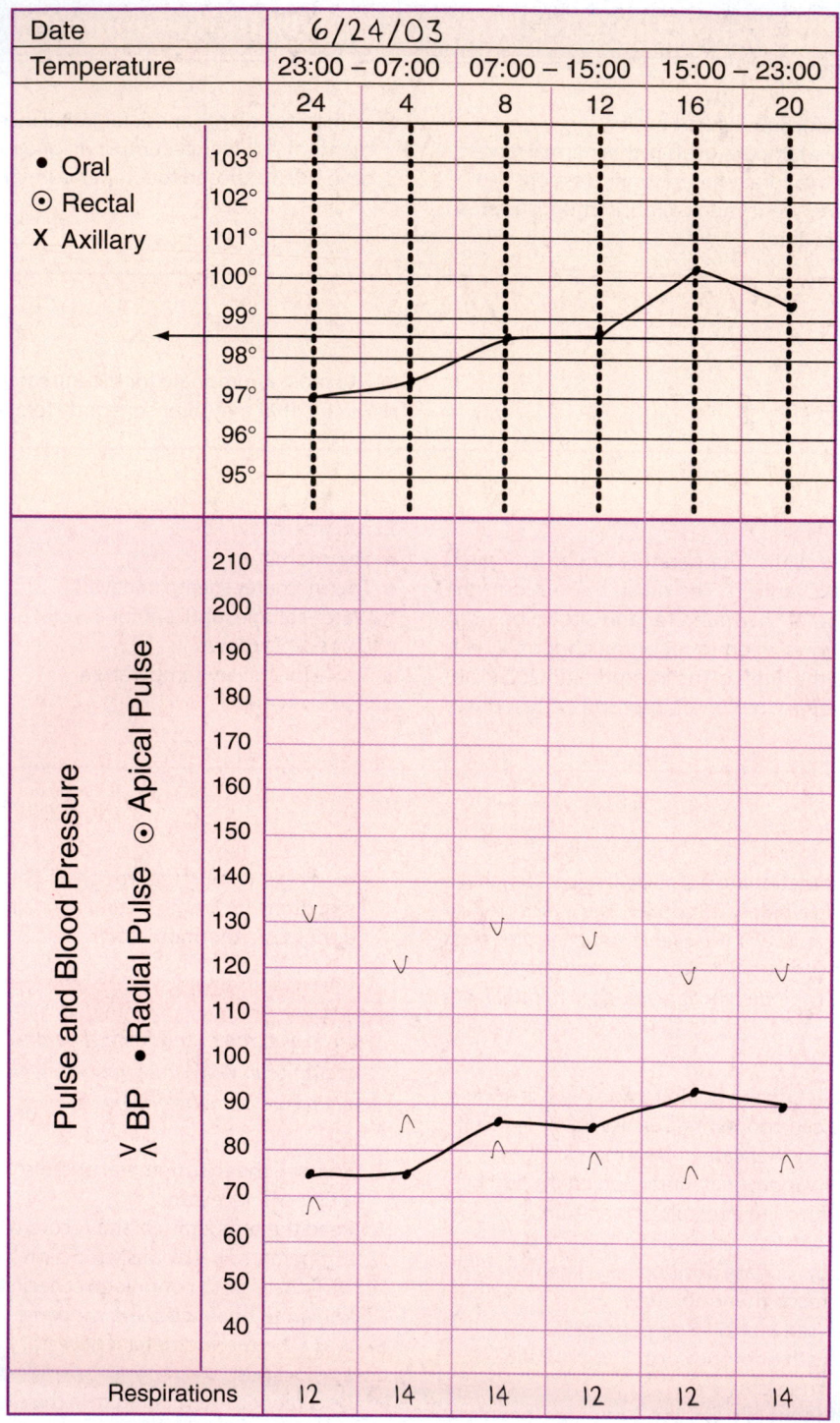

Figure 27–10 ■ Vital signs graphic record.

494

BOX 27–6 ■ Thermometer Placement

Oral   Place the bulb on either side of the frenulum. (Figure 27–11 ■)

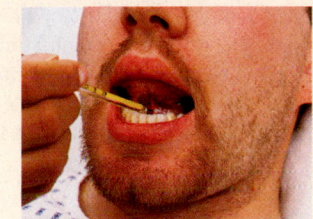

Figure 27–11 ■ Oral thermometer placement.

Rectal   Apply clean gloves.
Instruct the client to take a slow deep breath during insertion. (Figure 27–12 ■)
Never force the thermometer if resistance is felt.
Insert 3.5 cm (1½ in.) in adults.

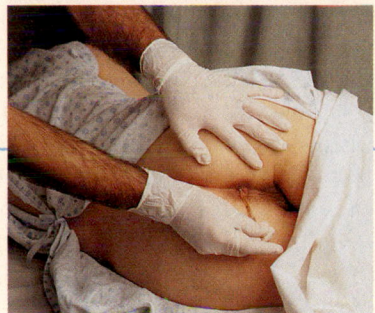

Figure 27–12 ■ Inserting a rectal thermometer.

Axillary   Pat the axilla dry if very moist.
The bulb is placed in the center of the axilla (Figure 27–13 ■)

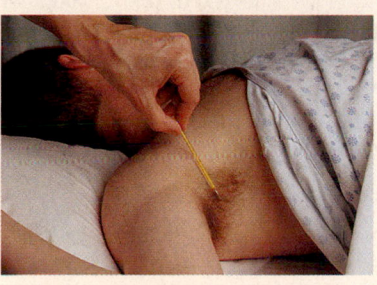

Figure 27–13 ■ Placing the bulb of the thermometer in the center of the axilla.

Tympanic   Pull the pinna slightly upward and backward. (Figure 27–14 ■)
Point the probe slightly anteriorly, toward the eardrum. Insert the probe slowly using a circular motion until snug.

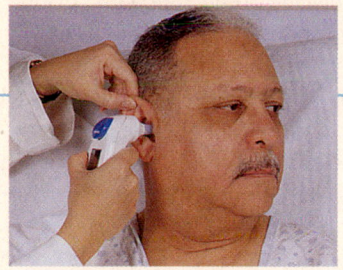

Figure 27–14 ■ Pull the pinna of the ear up and back while inserting the tympanic thermometer.

Lifespan Considerations

Temperature

Infants

- Using the axillary site, you may need to hold the infant's arm against the chest (see Figure 27–15 ■).
- Axillary route may not be as accurate as other routes for detecting fevers in children (Bindler & Ball, 2003).
- The tympanic route is fast and convenient. Place infant supine and stabilize the head. Pull the pinna straight back and slightly downward. Direct the probe tip anteriorly and insert far enough to seal the canal.
- Avoid the tympanic route in a child with active ear infections or tympanic membrane drainage tubes.
- The rectal route is least desirable in infants.

Children

- Tympanic or axillary sites are commonly preferred.
- For the tympanic route, have the child held on an adult's lap with the child's head held gently against the adult for support. Pull the pinna straight back and upward for children over age 3 (see Figure 27–16 ■).
- Avoid the tympanic route in a child with active ear infections or tympanic membrane drainage tubes.
- The oral route may be used for children over age three but nonbreakable, electronic thermometers are recommended.
- For a rectal temperature place the child prone across your lap or in a side-lying position with the knees flexed. Insert the thermometer 1 inch into the rectum.

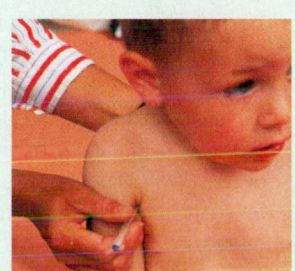

Figure 27–15 ■ Axillary thermometer placement

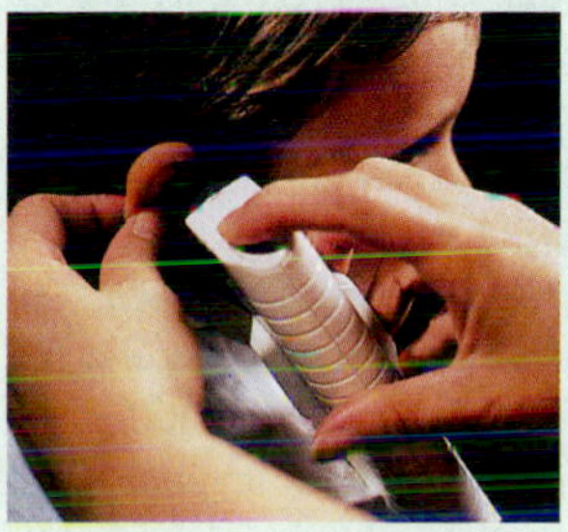

Figure 27–16 ■ Pull the pinna of the ear back and up for placement of a tympanic thermometer in a child over 3 years of age, back and down for children under age 3.

continued on page 496

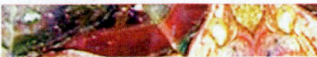

Lifespan Considerations continued

Elders

- Elders' temperatures tend to be lower than those of middle-age adults.
- Elders' temperatures are strongly influenced by both environmental and internal temperature changes. Their thermoregulation control processes are not as efficient as when they are younger and they are at higher risk for both hypothermia and hyperthermia.
- Elders can develop significant buildup of ear cerumen that may interfere with tympanic thermometer readings.

- Elders are more likely to have hemorrhoids. Inspect the anus before taking a rectal temperature.
- Elders' temperatures may not be a valid indication of the seriousness of the pathology of a disease. They may have pneumonia or a urinary tract infection and have only a slight temperature elevation. Other symptoms, such as confusion and restlessness, may be displayed and need follow-up to determine if there is an underlying process.

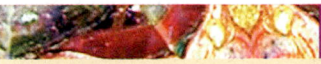

Home Care Considerations

Temperature

- Teach the client accurate use and reading of the type of thermometer to be used. Examine the thermometer used by the client in the home for safety and proper functioning. Observe the client/caregiver taking and reading a temperature. Reinforce the importance of reporting the site and type of thermometer used and the value of using one consistently.
- Discuss means of keeping the thermometer clean, such as warm water and soap, and avoiding cross-contamination.
- Ensure that the client has water-soluble lubricant if using a rectal thermometer.

- Instruct the client or family member to notify the health care provider if the temperature is 37.7C (100F) or higher.
- When making a home visit, take a thermometer with you in case the clients do not have a functional thermometer of their own.
- Check that the client knows how to record the temperature. Provide a recording chart/table if indicated.

Discuss environmental control modifications that should be taken during illness or extreme climate conditions, (e.g., heating, air conditioning, appropriate clothing and bedding).

PULSE

The **pulse** is a wave of blood created by contraction of the left ventricle of the heart. Generally the pulse wave represents the stroke volume output and the amount of blood that enters the arteries with each ventricular contraction. **Compliance** of the arteries is their ability to contract and expand. When a person's arteries lose their distensibility, as can happen in old age, greater pressure is required to pump the blood into the arteries.

Cardiac output is the volume of blood pumped into the arteries by the heart and equals the result of the stroke volume (SV) times the heart rate (HR) per minute. For example, 65 mL × 70 beats per minute = 4.55 L per minute. When an adult is resting, the heart pumps about 5 liters of blood each minute.

In a healthy person, the pulse reflects the heartbeat; that is, the pulse rate is the same as the rate of the ventricular contractions of the heart. However, in some types of cardiovascular disease, the heartbeat and pulse rates can differ. For example, a client's heart may produce very weak or small pulse waves that are not detectable in a peripheral pulse far from the heart. In these instances, the nurse should assess the heartbeat and the peripheral pulse. A **peripheral pulse** is a pulse located away from the heart, for example, in the foot, wrist, or neck. The **apical pulse,** in contrast, is a central pulse; that is, it is located at the apex of the heart.

Factors Affecting the Pulse

The rate of the pulse is expressed in beats per minute (BPM). A pulse rate varies according to a number of factors. The nurse should consider each of the following factors when assessing a client's pulse:

- *Age.* As age increases, the pulse rate gradually decreases. See Table 27–1 for specific variations in pulse rates from birth to adulthood.
- *Gender.* After puberty, the average male's pulse rate is slightly lower than the female's.
- *Exercise.* The pulse rate normally increases with activity. The rate of increase in the professional athlete is often less than in the average person because of greater cardiac size, strength, and efficiency.
- *Fever.* The pulse rate increases (a) in response to the lowered blood pressure that results from peripheral vasodilatation associated with elevated body temperature and (b) because of the increased metabolic rate.
- *Medications.* Some medications decrease the pulse rate, and others increase it. For example, cardiotonics (e.g., digitalis preparations) decrease the heart rate, whereas epinephrine increases it.
- *Hypovolemia.* Loss of blood from the vascular system normally increases pulse rate. In adults the loss of circulating

volume results in an adjustment of the heart rate to increase blood pressure as the body compensates for the lost blood volume. Adults can usually lose up to 10% of their normal circulating volume without adverse effects.

- *Stress.* In response to stress, sympathetic nervous stimulation increases the overall activity of the heart. Stress increases the rate as well as the force of the heartbeat. Fear and anxiety as well as the perception of severe pain stimulate the sympathetic system.
- *Position changes.* When a person is sitting or standing, blood usually pools in dependent vessels of the venous system. Pooling results in a transient decrease in the venous blood return to the heart and a subsequent reduction in blood pressure and increase in heart rate.
- *Pathology.* Certain diseases such as some heart conditions or those that impair oxygenation can alter the resting pulse rate.

Pulse Sites

A pulse may be measured in nine sites (see Figure 27–17 ■).

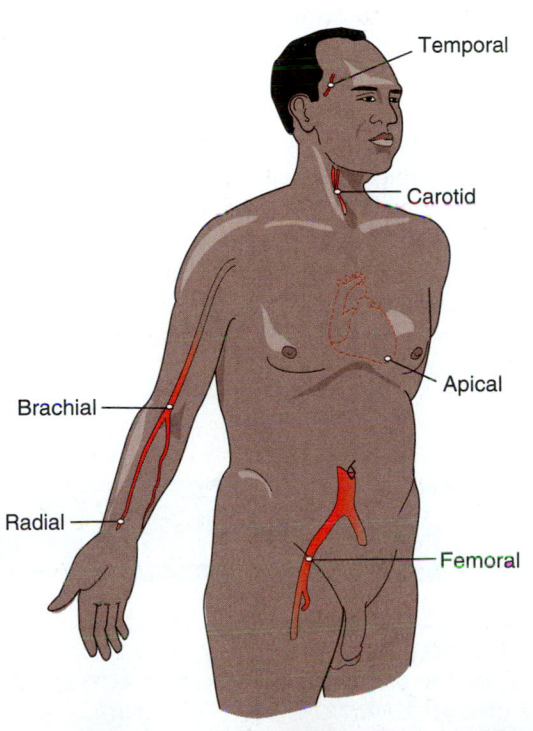

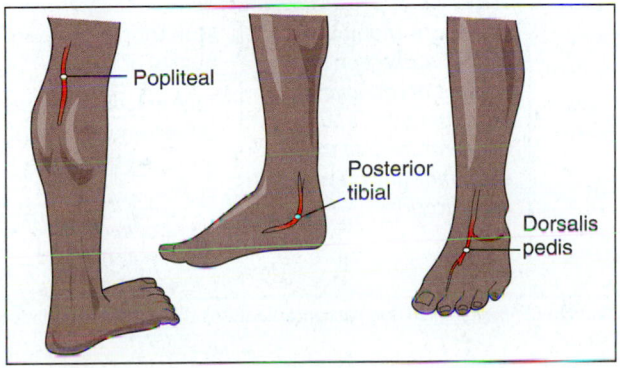

Figure 27–17 ■ Nine sites for assessing pulse.

1. Temporal, where the temporal artery passes over the temporal bone of the head. The site is superior (above) and lateral to (away from the midline of) the eye.
2. Carotid, at the side of the neck where the carotid artery runs between the trachea and the sternocleidomastoid muscle.

> ► **CLINIC AL ALERT** *Never press both carotids at the same time because this can cause a reflex drop in blood pressure or pulse rate.* ■

3. Apical, at the apex of the heart. In an adult this is located on the left side of the chest, about 8 cm (3 in.) to the left of the sternum (breastbone) and at the fourth, fifth, or sixth intercostal space (area between the ribs). For a child 7 to 9 years of age, the apical pulse is located at the fourth or fifth intercostal spaces. Before 4 years of age it is left of the midclavicular line (MCL); between 4 and 6 years, it is at the MCL (see Figure 27–18 ■).
4. Brachial, at the inner aspect of the biceps muscle of the arm or medially in the antecubital space.
5. Radial, where the radial artery runs along the radial bone, on the thumb side of the inner aspect of the wrist.
6. Femoral, where the femoral artery passes alongside the inguinal ligament.
7. Popliteal, where the popliteal artery passes behind the knee.
8. Posterior tibial, on the medial surface of the ankle where the posterior tibial artery passes behind the medial malleolus.
9. Pedal (dorsalis pedis), where the dorsalis pedis artery passes over the bones of the foot, on an imaginary line drawn from the middle of the ankle to the space between the big and second toes. The radial site is most commonly used in adults. It is easily found in most people and readily accessible. Some reasons for use of each site are given in Table 27–3.

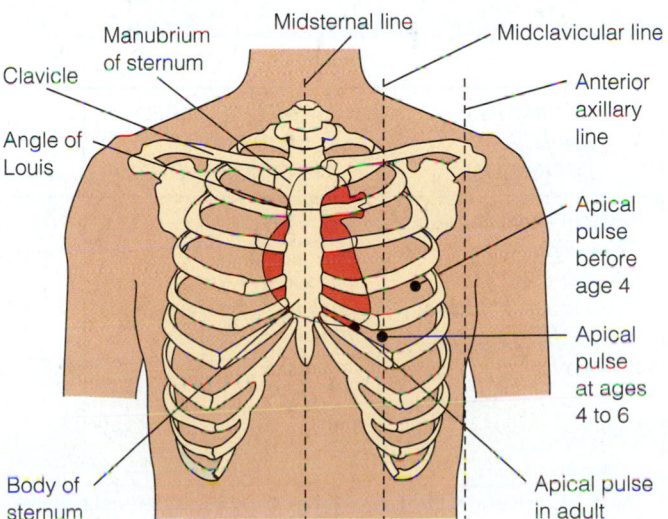

Figure 27–18 ■ Location of the apical pulse for a child under 4 years, a child 4 to 6 years, and an adult.

TABLE 27–3 Reasons for Using Specific Pulse Site

Pulse Site	Reasons for Use
Radial	Readily accessible
Temporal	Used when radial pulse is not accessible
Carotid	Used in cases of cardiac arrest
	Used to determine circulation to the brain
Apical	Routinely used for infants and children up to 3 years of age
	Used to determine discrepancies with radial pulse
	Used in conjunction with some medications
Brachial	Used to measure blood pressure
	Used during cardiac arrest for infants
Femoral	Used in cases of cardiac arrest
	Used for infants and children
	Used to determine circulation to a leg
Popliteal	Used to determine circulation to the lower leg
Posterior tibial	Used to determine circulation to the foot
Pedal	Used to determine circulation to the foot

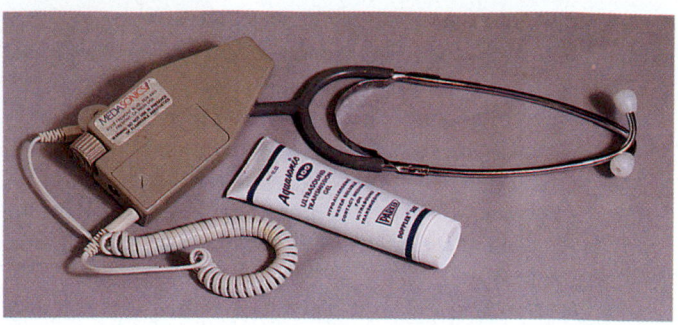

Figure 27–19 ■ A Doppler ultrasound stethoscope (DUS).

See Identifying Nursing Diagnoses, Outcomes, and Interventions below for examples of applying the nursing process to clients with pulse alterations.

Assessing the Pulse

A pulse is commonly assessed by palpation (feeling) or auscultation (hearing). The middle three fingertips are used for palpating all pulse sites except the apex of the heart. A stethoscope is used for assessing apical pulses and fetal heart tones. A Doppler ultrasound stethoscope (DUS; see Figure 27–19 ■) is used for pulses that are difficult to assess. The DUS headset has earpieces similar to standard stethoscope earpieces, but it has a long cord attached to a volume-controlled audio unit and an ultrasound transducer. The DUS detects movement of red blood cells through a blood vessel. In contrast to the conventional stethoscope, it excludes environmental sounds.

A pulse is normally palpated by applying moderate pressure with the three middle fingers of the hand. The pads on the most distal aspects of the finger are the most sensitive areas for detecting a pulse. With excessive pressure one can obliterate a pulse, whereas with too little pressure one may not be able to detect it. Before the nurse assesses the resting pulse, the client should assume a comfortable position. The nurse should also be aware of the following:

IDENTIFYING NURSING DIAGNOSES, OUTCOMES, AND INTERVENTIONS

INEFFECTIVE PERIPHERAL TISSUE PERFUSION

NURSING DIAGNOSIS/ DEFINITION	SAMPLE DESIRED OUTCOMES [NOC#]/DEFINITION	INDICATORS	SELECTED INTERVENTIONS [NIC#]/DEFINITION	SAMPLE ACTIVITIES [NIC]
Ineffective Peripheral Tissue Perfusion/ Decrease in oxygen resulting in the failure to nourish the tissues at the capillary level	Tissue Perfusion [0407]/*Extent to which blood flows through the small vessels of the extremities and maintains tissue function*	†•Distal peripheral pulses strong • Distal peripheral pulses symmetrical	Vital Signs Monitoring [6680]*/*Collection and analysis of cardiovascular, respiratory, and body temperature data to determine and prevent complications*	Monitor presence and quality of pulses Take apical and radial pulses simultaneously and note the difference Monitor cardiac rhythm and rate

* *Note:* Tissue Perfusion Management is a Level 2 Class (M) under the NIC Level 1 Domain of *Physiological Complex:* Interventions to optimize circulation of blood and fluids to the tissue (see Table 18–7).
† The measurement scale ranges from Extremely compromised (1) to Not compromised (5). See Appendix B.

- Any medication that could affect the heart rate.
- Whether the client has been physically active. If so, wait 10 to 15 minutes until the client has rested and the pulse has slowed to its usual rate.
- Any baseline data about the normal heart rate for the client. For example, a physically fit athlete may have a heart rate below 60 BPM.
- Whether the client should assume a particular position (e.g., sitting). In some clients, the rate changes with the position because of changes in blood flow volume and autonomic nervous system activity.

When assessing the pulse, the nurse collects the following data: the rate, rhythm, volume, arterial wall elasticity, and presence or absence of bilateral equality. An excessively fast heart rate (e.g., over 100 BPM in an adult) is referred to as **tachycardia.** A heart rate in an adult of 60 BPM or less is called **bradycardia.** If a client has either tachycardia or bradycardia, the apical pulse should be assessed.

The **pulse rhythm** is the pattern of the beats and the intervals between the beats. Equal time elapses between beats of a normal pulse. A pulse with an irregular rhythm is referred to as a **dysrhythmia** or **arrhythmia.** It may consist of random, irregular beats or a predictable pattern of irregular beats. When a dysrhythmia is detected, the apical pulse should be assessed. An electrocardiogram (ECG or EKG) is necessary to define the dysrhythmia further.

Pulse volume, also called the pulse strength or amplitude, refers to the force of blood with each beat. Usually, the pulse volume is the same with each beat. It can range from absent to bounding. A normal pulse can be felt with moderate pressure of the fingers and can be obliterated with greater pressure. A forceful or full blood volume that is obliterated only with difficulty is called a full or bounding pulse. A pulse that is readily obliterated with pressure from the fingers is referred to as weak, feeble, or thready.

The **elasticity of the arterial wall** reflects its expansibility or its deformities. A healthy, normal artery feels straight, smooth, soft, and pliable. Older people often have inelastic arteries that feel twisted (tortuous) and irregular upon palpation.

When assessing a peripheral pulse to determine the adequacy of blood flow to a particular area of the body, the nurse should also assess the corresponding pulse on the other side of the body. The second assessment gives the nurse data with which to compare the pulses. For example, when assessing the blood flow to the right foot, the nurse assesses the right dorsalis pedis pulse and then the left dorsalis pedis pulse. If the client's right and left pulses are the same, the client's dorsalis pedis pulses are bilaterally equal.

Procedure 27–2 provides guidelines for assessing a peripheral pulse.

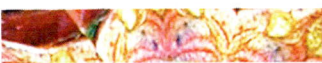

Procedure 27-2 Assessing a Peripheral Pulse

Purposes

- To establish baseline data for subsequent evaluation
- To identify whether the pulse rate is within normal range
- To determine whether the pulse rhythm is regular and the pulse volume is appropriate
- To compare the equality of corresponding peripheral pulses on each side of the body
- To monitor and assess changes in the client's health status
- To monitor clients at risk for pulse alterations (e.g., those with a history of heart disease or experiencing cardiac arrhythmias, hemorrhage, acute pain, infusion of large volumes of fluids, fever)

ASSESSMENT

Assess

- Clinical signs of cardiovascular alterations, other than pulse rate, rhythm, or volume (e.g., dyspnea [difficult respirations], fatigue, pallor, cyanosis [bluish discoloration of skin and mucous membranes], palpitations, syncope [fainting], impaired peripheral tissue perfusion as evidenced by skin discoloration and cool temperature)
- Factors that may alter pulse rate (e.g., emotional status and activity level)
- Site most appropriate for assessment

PLANNING

Delegation

Measurement of the client's radial pulse can be delegated to UAP or family members/caregivers. Reports of abnormal pulse rates or rhythms require reassessment by the nurse, who also determines appropriate action if the abnormality is confirmed. Due to the skill required in locating and interpreting peripheral pulses other than the radial artery and in using Doppler ultrasound devices, UAPs are generally not delegated these techniques.

Equipment

- Watch with a second hand or indicator
- If using a DUS, the transducer probe, the stethoscope headset, transmission gel, and tissues/wipes

continued on page 500

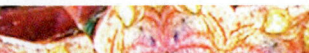

Procedure 27-2 Assessing a Peripheral Pulse *continued*

IMPLEMENTATION

Preparation

If using a DUS, check that the equipment is functioning normally.

Performance

1. Explain to the client what you are going to do, why it is necessary, and how he or she can cooperate. Discuss how the results will be used in planning further care or treatments.
2. Wash hands and observe appropriate infection control procedures.
3. Provide for client privacy.

4. Select the pulse point. Normally, the radial pulse is taken, unless it cannot be exposed or circulation to another body area is to be assessed.
5. Assist the client to a comfortable resting position. When the radial pulse is assessed, with the palm facing downward, the client's arm can rest alongside the body or the forearm can rest at a 90-degree angle across the chest. For the client who can sit, the forearm can rest across the thigh, with the palm of the hand facing downward or inward.

6. Palpate and count the pulse. Place two or three middle fingertips lightly and squarely over the pulse point (Figure 27–20 ■). *Using the thumb is contraindicated because the thumb has a pulse that the nurse could mistake for the client's pulse.*
   - Count for 15 seconds and multiply by 4. Record the pulse in beats per minute on your worksheet. If taking a client's pulse for the first time, when obtaining baseline data, or if the pulse is irregular, count for a full minute. An irregular pulse also requires taking the apical pulse.

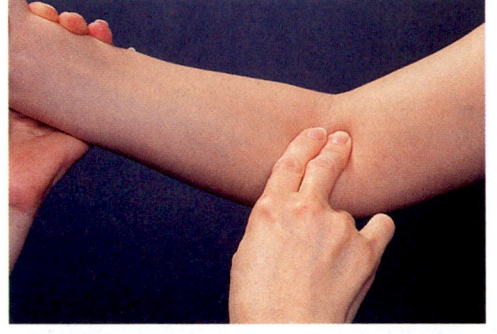

A

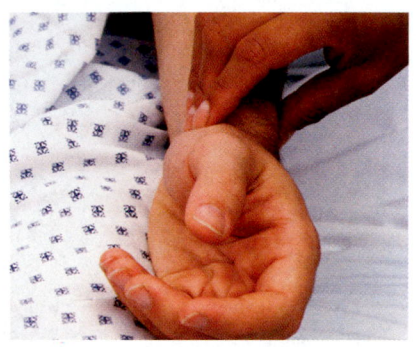

B

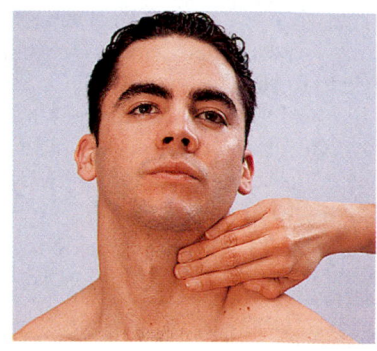

C

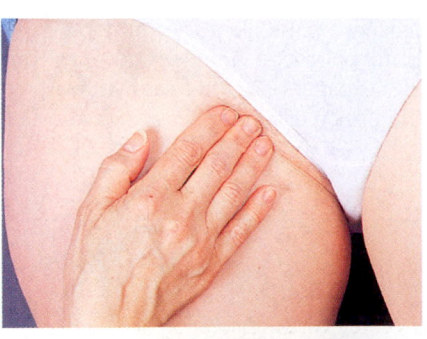

D

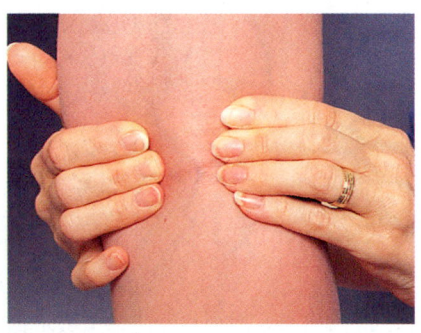

E

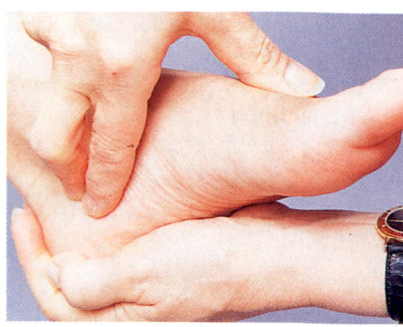

F

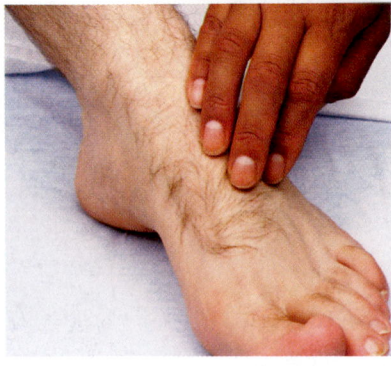

G

Figure 27–20 ■ Assessing the pulses: *A,* brachial; *B,* radial; *C,* carotid; *D,* femoral; *E,* popliteal; *F,* posterior tibial; and *G,* pedal (dorsalis pedis).

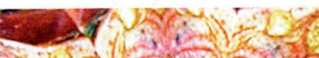

Procedure 27-2 Assessing a Peripheral Pulse *continued*

IMPLEMENTATION *continued*

7. Assess the pulse rhythm and volume.
   - Assess the pulse rhythm by noting the pattern of the intervals between the beats. A normal pulse has equal time periods between beats. If this is an initial assessment, assess for 1 minute.
   - Assess the pulse volume. A normal pulse can be felt with moderate pressure, and the pressure is equal with each beat. A forceful pulse volume is full; an easily obliterated pulse is weak. Record the rhythm and volume on your worksheet.
8. Document the pulse rate, rhythm, and volume and your actions in the client record (see Figure 27–10 in Procedure 27–1). Also record pertinent related data such as variation in pulse rate compared to normal for the client and abnormal skin color and skin temperature in the nurse's notes.

VARIATION: USING A DUS
- If used, plug the stethoscope headset into one of the two output jacks located next to the volume control. DUS units

may have two jacks so that a second person can listen to the signals (see Figure 27–19).
- Apply transmission gel either to the probe at the narrow end of the plastic case housing the transducer, or to the client's skin. *Ultrasound beams do not travel well through air. The gel makes an airtight seal, which then promotes optimal ultrasound wave transmission.*
- Press the "on" button.
- Hold the probe against the skin over the pulse site. Use a light pressure, and keep the probe in contact with the skin (Figure 27–21 ■). *Too much pressure can stop the blood flow and obliterate the signal.*
- Adjust the volume if necessary. Distinguish artery sounds from vein sounds. The artery sound (signal) is distinctively pulsating and has a pumping quality. The venous sound is intermittent and varies with respirations. Both artery and vein sounds are heard simultaneously through the DUS because major arteries and veins are situated close

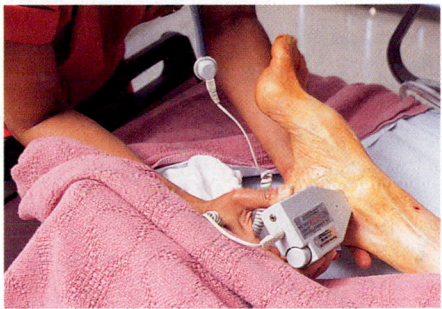

Figure 27–21 ■ Using a (Doppler) ultrasound stethoscope to assess the posterior tibial pulse.

together throughout the body. If arterial sounds cannot be easily heard, then reposition the probe.
- After assessing the pulse, remove all gel from the probe to prevent damage to its surface. Clean the transducer with aqueous solutions. *Alcohol or other disinfectants may damage the face of the transducer.* Remove all gel from the client.

EVALUATION
- Compare the pulse rate to baseline data or normal range for age of client.
- Relate pulse rate and volume to other vital signs; pulse rhythm and volume to baseline data and health status.
- If assessing peripheral pulses, evaluate equality, rate, and volume in corresponding extremities.
- Conduct appropriate follow-up such as notifying the physician or giving medication.

Apical Pulse Assessment

Assessment of the apical pulse is indicated for clients whose peripheral pulse is irregular or unavailable as well as for clients with known cardiovascular, pulmonary, and renal diseases. It is commonly assessed prior to administering medications that affect heart rate. The apical site is also used to assess the pulse for newborns, infants, and children up to 2 to 3 years old. Procedure 27–3 presents guidelines for assessing the apical pulse.

Procedure 27-3 Assessing an Apical Pulse

Purposes
- To obtain the heart rate of newborns, infants, and children 2 to 3 years old or of an adult with an irregular peripheral pulse
- To establish baseline data for subsequent evaluation
- To determine whether the cardiac rate is within normal range and the rhythm is regular
- To monitor clients with cardiac disease and those receiving medications to improve heart action

ASSESSMENT
Assess
- Clinical signs of cardiovascular alterations, other than pulse rate, rhythm, or volume (e.g., dyspnea, fatigue, pallor, cyanosis, syncope)
- Factors that may alter pulse rate (e.g., emotional status, activity level, and medications that affect heart rate such as digoxin, beta blockers, or calcium channel blockers)

continued on page 502

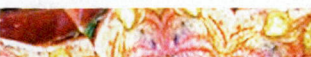

Procedure 27-3 Assessing an Apical Pulse *continued*

PLANNING

Delegation

Due to the degree of skill and knowledge required, UAP are generally not responsible for assessing apical pulses.

Equipment

■ Watch with a second hand or indicator
■ Stethoscope

■ Antiseptic wipes
■ If using a DUS, the transducer probe, the stethoscope headset, transmission gel, and tissues/wipes

IMPLEMENTATION

Preparation

If using a DUS, check that the equipment is functioning normally.

Performance

1. Explain to the client what you are going to do, why it is necessary, and how he or she can cooperate. Discuss how the results will be used in planning further care or treatments.
2. Observe appropriate infection control procedures.
3. Provide for client privacy.
4. Position the client appropriately in a comfortable supine position or in a sitting position. Expose the area of the chest over the apex of the heart.
5. Locate the apical impulse. This is the point over the apex of the heart where the apical pulse can be most clearly heard. It is also referred to as the **point of maximal impulse (PMI).**
   • Palpate the angle of Louis (the angle between the manubrium, the top of the sternum, and the body of the sternum). It is palpated just below the suprasternal notch and is felt as a prominence (see Figure 27–18).
   • Slide your index finger just to the left of the client's sternum, and palpate the second intercostal space.
   • Place your middle or next finger in the third intercostal space, and continue palpating downward until you locate the fifth intercostal space.
   • Move your index finger laterally along the fifth intercostal space toward the MCL. Normally, the apical impulse is palpable at or just medial to the MCL (Figure 27–18).
6. Auscultate and count heartbeats.
   • Use antiseptic wipes to clean the earpieces and diaphragm of the stethoscope if their cleanliness is in doubt. *The diaphragm needs to be cleaned and disinfected if soiled with body substances.*

   • Warm the diaphragm of the stethoscope by holding it in the palm of the hand for a moment. *The metal of the diaphragm is usually cold and can startle the client when placed immediately on the chest.*
   • Insert the earpieces of the stethoscope into your ears in the direction of the ear canals, or slightly forward, *to facilitate hearing.*
   • Tap your finger lightly on the diaphragm *to be sure it is the active side of the head.* If necessary, rotate the head to select the diaphragm side (Figure 27–22 ■).

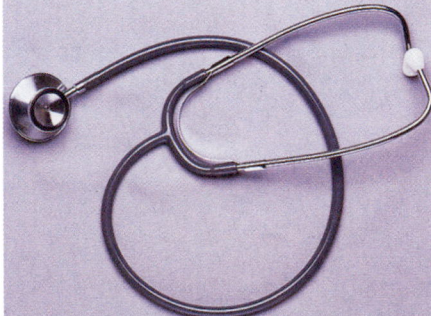

A

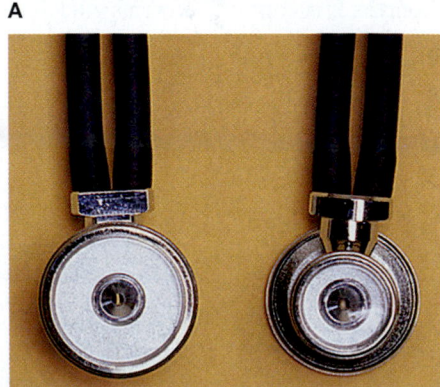

B

Figure 27–22 ■ *A,* stethoscope with both a bell-shaped and flat-disc amplifier. *B,* Close-up of a flat-disc amplifier (left) and a bell amplifier (right).

   • Place the diaphragm of the stethoscope over the apical impulse and listen for the normal S1, and S2 heart sounds, which are heard as "lub-dub" (see Figure 27–23 ■). *The heartbeat is normally loudest over the apex of the heart. Each lub-dub is counted as one heartbeat. The two heart sounds are produced by closure of the valves of the heart. The S1, heart sound (lub) occurs when the atrioventricular valves close after the ventricles have been sufficiently filled. The S2 hear sound (dub) occurs when the semilunar valves close after the ventricles empty.*

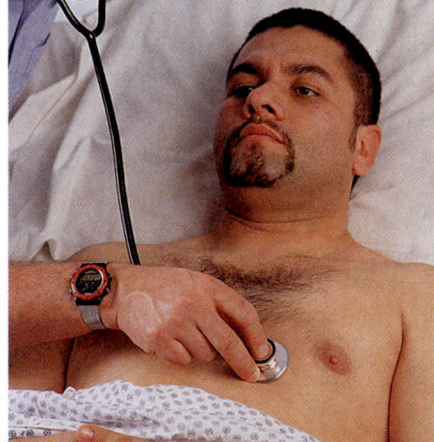

Figure 27–23 ■ Taking an apical pulse using the flat disc of the stethoscope. Note how the amplifier is held against the chest.

   • If the rhythm is regular, count the heartbeats for 30 seconds and multiply by 2. If the rhythm is irregular, count the beats for 60 seconds. A 60-second count provides a more accurate assessment of an irregular pulse than a 30-second count.

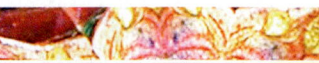

Procedure 27-3 Assessing an Apical Pulse *continued*

IMPLEMENTATION *continued*

7. Assess the rhythm and the strength of the heartbeat.
   - Assess the rhythm of the heartbeat by noting the pattern of intervals between the beats. A normal pulse has equal time periods between beats.

- Assess the strengths (volume) of the heartbeat. Normally, the heartbeats are equal in strength and can be described as strong or weak.
8. Document the pulse site, rate, rhythm, and volume and your actions in the client record. Also record pertinent re-

lated data such as variation in pulse rate compared to normal for the client and abnormal skin color and skin temperature.

EVALUATION

- Relate pulse rate to other vital signs; pulse rhythm to baseline data and health status.
- Report to the physician any abnormal findings such as irregular rhythm, and reduced ability to hear the heartbeat, pallor, cyanosis, dyspnea, tachycardia, or bradycardia.

- Conduct appropriate follow-up such as administering medication ordered based on apical heart rate.

Apical-Radial Pulse Assessment

An **apical-radial pulse** may need to be assessed for clients with certain cardiovascular disorders. Normally, the apical and radial rates are identical. An apical pulse rate greater than a radial pulse rate can indicate that the thrust of the blood from the heart is too feeble for the wave to be felt at the peripheral pulse site, or it can indicate that vascular disease is preventing impulses from being

transmitted. Any discrepancy between the two pulse rates is called a **pulse deficit** and needs to be reported promptly. In no instance is the radial pulse greater than the apical pulse.

An apical-radial pulse can be taken by two nurses or one nurse, although the two-nurse technique may be more accurate. Procedure 27–4 outlines the steps for assessing an apical-radial pulse.

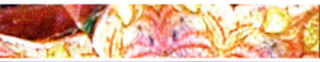

Procedure 27-4 Assessing an Apical-Radial Pulse

Purpose

- To determine adequacy of peripheral circulation or presence of pulse deficit

ASSESSMENT

Assess

- Clinical signs of hypovolemic shock (hypotension, pallor, cyanosis, and cold, clammy skin)

PLANNING

Delegation
UAP are generally not responsible for assessing apical-radial pulses using the one-nurse technique. UAP may perform the radial pulse count for the two-nurse technique.

Equipment
- Watch with a second hand or indicator
- Stethoscope
- Antiseptic wipes

IMPLEMENTATION

Preparation
If using the two-nurse technique, ensure that the other nurse is available at this time.

Performance
1. Explain to the client what you are going to do, why it is necessary, and how

he or she can cooperate. Discuss how the results will be used in planning further care or treatments.
2. Observe appropriate infection control procedures.
3. Provide for client privacy.

4. Position the client appropriately. Assist the client to assume the position described for taking the apical pulse. Position the client appropriately in a comfortable supine position or to a sitting position. Expose the

continued on page 504

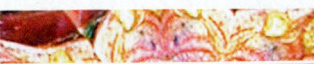

Procedure 27-4 Assessing an Apical-Radial Pulse *continued*

IMPLEMENTATION *continued*

area of the chest over the apex of the heart. If previous measurements were taken, determine what position the client assumed, and use the same position. *This ensures an accurate comparative measurement.*

5. Locate the apical and radial pulse sites. In the two-nurse technique, one nurse locates the apical impulse by palpation or with the stethoscope while the other nurse palpates the radial pulse site. (see Procedures 27–2 and 27–3.)

6. Count the apical and radial pulse rates.

TWO-NURSE TECHNIQUE

- Place the watch where both nurses can see it. The nurse who is taking the radial pulse may hold the watch.

- Decide on a time to begin counting. A time when the second hand is on 12, 3, 6, or 9 or an even number on digital clocks is usually selected. The nurse taking the radial pulse says "Start" at the same time. *This ensures that simultaneous counts are taken.*

- Each nurse counts the pulse rate for 60 seconds. Both nurses end the count when the nurse taking the radial pulse says "Stop." *A full 60-second count is necessary for accurate assessment of any discrepancies between the two pulse sites.*

- The nurse who assesses the apical rate also assesses the apical pulse rhythm and volume (i.e., whether the heartbeat is strong or weak). If the pulse is irregular, note whether the irregular beats come at random or at predictable times.

- The nurse assessing the radial pulse rate also assesses the radial pulse rhythm and volume.

ONE-NURSE TECHNIQUE

- Assess the apical pulse for 60 seconds.
- Assess the radial pulse for 60 seconds.

7. Document the apical and radial (AR) pulse rates, rhythm, volume, and any pulse deficit in the client record. Also record related data such as variation in pulse rate compared to normal for the client and other pertinent observations, such as pallor, cyanosis, or dyspnea.

EVALUATION

- Relate pulse rate and rhythm to other vital signs, to baseline data, and to general health status.
- Report to the physician any changes from previous measurements or any discrepancy between the two pulses.

- Conduct appropriate follow-up such as administering medication or other actions to be taken for a discrepancy in the AR pulse rates.

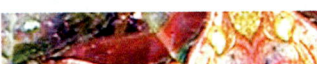

Lifespan Considerations

Pulse

Infants

- Use the apical pulse for the heart rate of newborns, infants, and children 2 to 3 years old to establish baseline data for subsequent evaluation, to determine whether the cardiac rate is within normal range, and to determine if the rhythm is regular.
- Place a baby in a supine position, and offer a pacifier if the baby is crying or restless. Crying and physical activity will increase the pulse rate. For this reason, take the apical pulse rate of infants and small children before assessing body temperatures.
- Locate the apical pulse in the fourth intercostal space, lateral to the midclavicular line during infancy.
- Brachial, popliteal, and femoral pulses may be palpated. Due to a normally low blood pressure and rapid heart rate, infants' other distal pulses may be hard to feel.

Children

- To take a peripheral pulse, position the child comfortably in the adult's arms, or have the adult remain close by. This may decrease anxiety and yield more accurate results.

- To assess the apical pulse, assist a young child to a comfortable supine or sitting position.
- Demonstrate the procedure to the child using a stuffed animal or doll, and allow the child to handle the stethoscope before beginning the procedure. This will decrease anxiety and promote cooperation.
- The apex of the heart is normally located in the fourth intercostal space in young children; fifth intercostal space in children 7 years of age and over.
- Locate the apical impulse along the fourth intercostal space, between the MCL and the anterior axillary line (see Figure 27–18).

Elders

- If the client has severe hand or arm tremors, the radial pulse may be difficult to count.
- Cardiac changes in elders, such as decrease in cardiac output, sclerotic changes to heart valves, and dysrhythmias often indicate that obtaining an apical pulse will be more accurate.
- Elders often have decreased peripheral circulation so that pedal pulses should also be checked for regularity, volume, and symmetry.

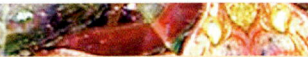

Home Care Considerations

Pulse

- Assist in obtaining and using an electronic pulse device if indicated.

- Teach the client to monitor the pulse prior to taking medications that affect the heart rate. Tell the client to report any notable changes in heart rate or rhythm (regularity) to the health care provider.

RESPIRATIONS

Respiration is the act of breathing. **External respiration** refers to the interchange of oxygen and carbon dioxide between the alveoli of the lungs and the pulmonary blood. **Internal respiration,** by contrast, takes place throughout the body; it is the interchange of these same gases between the circulating blood and the cells of the body tissues.

Inhalation or **inspiration** refers to the intake of air into the lungs. **Exhalation** or **expiration** refers to breathing out or the movement of gases from the lungs to the atmosphere. **Ventilation** is also used to refer to the movement of air in and out of the lungs.

There are basically two types of breathing: **costal (thoracic) breathing** and **diaphragmatic (abdominal) breathing.** Costal breathing involves the external intercostal muscles and other accessory muscles, such as the sternocleidomastoid muscles. It can be observed by the movement of the chest upward and outward. By contrast, diaphragmatic breathing involves the contraction and relaxation of the diaphragm, and it is observed by the movement of the abdomen, which occurs as a result of the diaphragm's contraction and downward movement.

Mechanics and Regulation of Breathing

During *inhalation,* the following processes normally occur (Figure 27–24 ■): The diaphragm contracts (flattens), the ribs move upward and outward, and the sternum moves outward, thus enlarging the thorax and permitting the lungs to expand. During *exhalation* (Figure 27–25 ■), the diaphragm relaxes, the ribs move downward and inward, and the sternum moves inward, thus decreasing the size of the thorax as the lungs are compressed. Normally breathing is carried out automatically and effortlessly. A normal adult inspiration lasts 1 to 1.5 seconds, and an expiration lasts 2 to 3 seconds.

Respiration is controlled by (a) respiratory centers in the medulla oblongata and the pons of the brain and (b) by chemoreceptors located centrally in the medulla and peripherally in the carotid and aortic bodies. These centers and receptors respond to changes in the concentrations of oxygen (O_2), carbon dioxide (CO_2), and hydrogen (H^+) in the arterial blood. See Chapter 48 ⏣ for details.

Assessing Respirations

Resting respirations should be assessed when the client is relaxed because exercise affects respirations, increasing their rate and depth. Anxiety is likely to affect respiratory rate and depth as well. Respirations may also need to be assessed after exercise to identify the client's tolerance to activity. Before assessing a client's respirations, a nurse should be aware of the following:

- The client's normal breathing pattern
- The influence of the client's health problems on respirations
- Any medications or therapies that might affect respirations
- The relationship of the client's respirations to cardiovascular function.

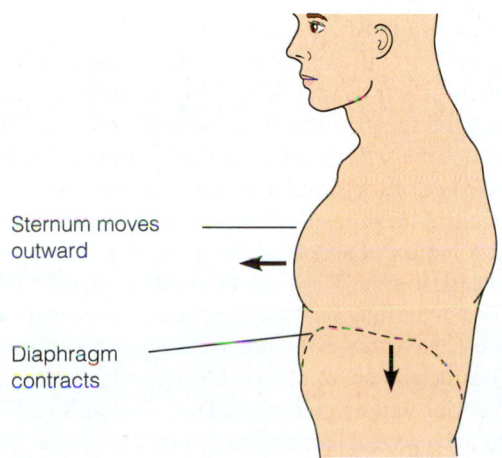

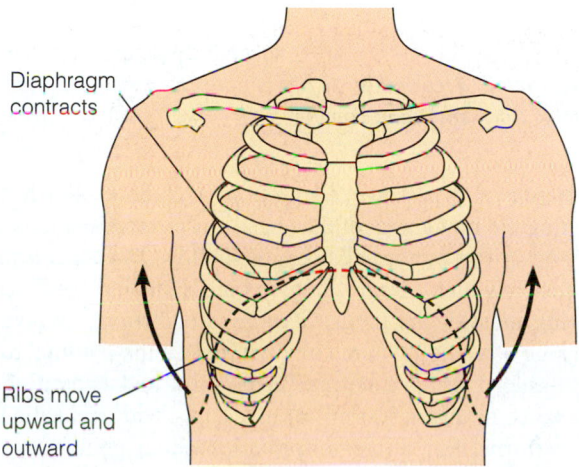

Sternum moves outward

Diaphragm contracts

Diaphragm contracts

Ribs move upward and outward

Figure 27–24 ■ Respiratory inhalation, *Left:* lateral view; *Right:* anterior view.

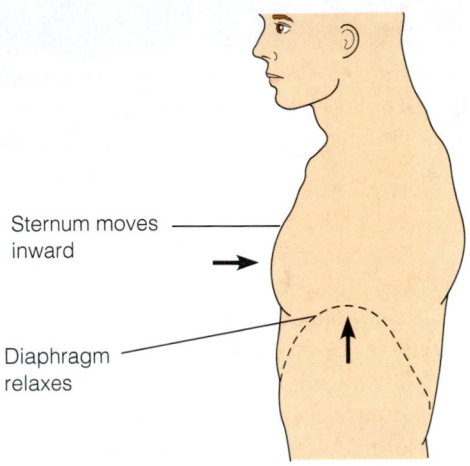

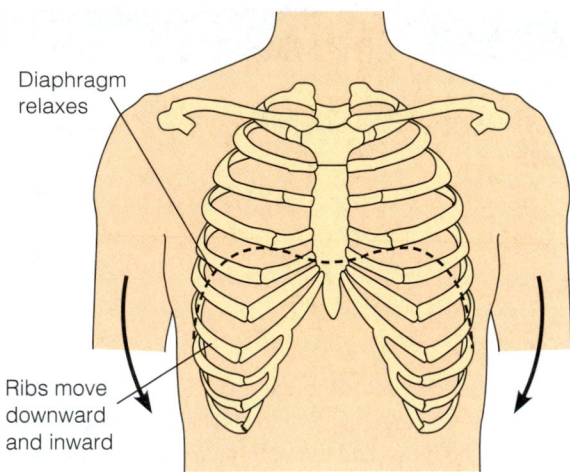

Figure 27–25 ■ Respiratory exhalation. *Left:* lateral view; *Right:* anterior view.

The rate, depth, rhythm, and quality and effectiveness of respirations should be assessed.

The *respiratory rate* is normally described in breaths per minute. Breathing that is normal in rate and depth is called **eupnea.** Abnormally slow respirations are referred to as **bradypnea,** and abnormally fast respirations are called **tachypnea** or **polypnea. Apnea** is the absence of breathing. For the respiratory rates for different age groups, see Table 27–1 on page 485.

Factors Affecting Respirations

Several factors influence respiratory rate. Those that increase the rate include exercise (increases metabolism), stress (readies the body for "fight or flight"), increased environmental temperature, and lowered oxygen concentration at increased altitudes. Factors that may decrease the respiratory rate include decreased environmental temperature, certain medications (e.g., narcotics), and increased intracranial pressure.

> ➤ CLINICAL ALERT   *An adult sleeping client's respirations can fall to fewer than 10 per minute. Use other vital signs to validate the client's condition.* ■

The *depth* of a person's respirations can be established by watching the movement of the chest. Respiratory depth is generally described as normal, deep, or shallow. *Deep respirations* are those in which a large volume of air is inhaled and exhaled, inflating most of the lungs. *Shallow respirations* involve the exchange of a small volume of air and often the minimal use of lung tissue. During a normal inspiration and expiration, an adult takes in about 500 mL of air. This volume is called the **tidal volume.** For further information about pulmonary volumes and pulmonary capacities, see Chapter 48. 🔗

Body position also affects the amount of air that can be inhaled. People in a supine position experience two physiologic processes that suppress respiration: an increase in the volume of blood inside the thoracic cavity and compression of the chest. Consequently, clients lying on their back have poorer lung aeration, which predisposes them to the stasis of fluids and subsequent infection. Certain medications also affect the respiratory depth. For example, narcotics such as morphine and large doses of barbiturates such as secobarbital sodium depress the respiratory centers in the brain, thereby depressing the respiratory rate and depth. **Hyperventilation** refers to very deep, rapid respirations; **hypoventilation** refers to very shallow respirations.

Respiratory rhythm refers to the regularity of the expirations and the inspirations. Normally, respirations are evenly spaced. Respiratory rhythm can be described as *regular* or *irregular.* An infant's respiratory rhythm may be less regular than an adult's. See Chapter 48 🔗 for details about abnormal respiratory rhythms.

Respiratory quality or **character** refers to those aspects of breathing that are different from normal, effortless breathing. Two of these are the amount of effort a client must exert to breathe and the sound of breathing. Usually, breathing does not require noticeable effort; some clients, however, breathe only with decided effort, referred to as *labored breathing.*

The *sound* of breathing is also significant. Normal breathing is silent, but a number of abnormal sounds such as a wheeze are obvious to the nurse's ear. Many sounds occur as a result of the presence of fluid in the lungs and are most clearly heard with a stethoscope. See Chapter 28 🔗 for methods used to assess lung sounds. For details about altered breathing patterns and terms used to describe various patterns and sounds, see Box 27–7.

The effectiveness of respirations is measured in part by the uptake of oxygen from the air into the blood and the release of car-

BOX 27–7 ■ Altered Breathing Patterns and Sounds

Breathing Patterns

Rate
- *Tachypnea*—quick, shallow breaths
- *Bradypnea*—abnormally slow breathing
- *Apnea*—cessation of breathing

Volume
- *Hyperventilation*—overexpansion of the lungs characterized by rapid and deep breaths
- *Hypoventilation*—underexpansion of the lungs, characterized by shallow respirations

Rhythm
- *Cheyne-Stokes breathing*—rhythmic waxing and waning of respirations, from very deep to very shallow breathing and temporary apnea

Ease or Effort
- *Dyspnea*—difficult and labored breathing during which the individual has a persistent, unsatisfied need for air and feels distressed
- *Orthopnea*—ability to breathe only in upright sitting or standing positions

Breath Sounds

Audible without Amplification
- *Stridor*—a shrill, harsh sound heard during inspiration with laryngeal obstruction
- *Stertor*—snoring or sonorous respiration, usually due to a partial obstruction of the upper airway
- *Wheeze*—continuous, high-pitched musical squeak or whistling sound occurring on expiration and sometimes on inspiration when air moves through a narrowed or partially obstructed airway
- *Bubbling*—gurgling sounds heard as air passes through moist secretions in the respiratory tract

Chest Movements
- *Intercostal retraction*—indrawing between the ribs
- *Substernal retraction*—indrawing beneath the breastbone
- *Suprasternal retraction*—indrawing above the clavicles

Secretions and Coughing
- *Hemoptysis*—the presence of blood in the sputum
- *Productive cough*—a cough accompanied by expectorated secretions
- *Nonproductive cough*—a dry, harsh cough without secretions

IDENTIFYING NURSING DIAGNOSES, OUTCOMES, AND INTERVENTIONS

INEFFECTIVE BREATHING PATTERN

NURSING DIAGNOSIS/ DEFINITION	SAMPLE DESIRED OUTCOMES [NOC#]/DEFINITION	INDICATORS	SELECTED INTERVENTIONS [NIC#]/DEFINITION	SAMPLE ACTIVITIES [NIC]
Ineffective Breathing Pattern/Inspiration and/or expiration that does not provide adequate ventilation	Respiratory Status: Ventilation [0403]/*Movement of air in and out of the lungs*	†• Respiratory rate IER (in expected range) • Ease of breathing	Respiratory Monitoring [3350]*/ *Collection and analysis of respiratory data to ensure airway patency and adequate gas exchange*	• Monitor for noisy respirations such as snoring • Monitor rate, rhythm, depth, and effort of respirations

* Note: Respiratory Management is a Level 2 Class (K) under the NIC Level 1 Domain of *Physiological Complex:* Interventions to promote airway patency and gas exchange. See Table 18-7.
†The measurement scale ranges from Extermely compromised (1) to Not compromised (5). See Appendix B.

bon dioxide from the blood into expired air. The amount of hemoglobin in arterial blood that is saturated with oxygen can be measured indirectly through pulse oximetry. Using a pulse oximeter monitor applied to the client's finger, toe, or other site provides a digital readout of both the client's pulse rate and the oxygen saturation (see Procedure 27–7). See the Identifying Nursing Diagnoses, Outcomes, and Interventions box above for an example of applying the nursing process to a client with a breathing disorder.

Procedure 27–5 outlines the steps for assessing respirations.

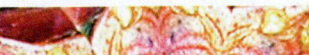

Procedure 27–5 Assessing Respirations

Purposes

- To acquire baseline data against which future measurements can be compared
- To monitor abnormal respirations and respiratory patterns and identify changes
- To assess respirations before the administration of a medication such as morphine (an abnormally slow respiratory rate may warrant withholding the medication)
- To monitor respirations following the administration of a general anesthetic or any medication that influences respirations
- To monitor clients at risk for respiratory alterations (e.g., those with fever, pain, acute anxiety, chronic obstructive pulmonary disease, respiratory infection, pulmonary edema or emboli, chest trauma or constriction, brain stem injury)

ASSESSMENT

Assess

- Skin and mucous membrane color (e.g., cyanosis or pallor)
- Position assumed for breathing (e.g., use of orthopneic position)
- Signs of cerebral anoxia (e.g., irritability, restlessness, drowsiness, or loss of consciousness)
- Chest movements (e.g., retractions between the ribs or above or below the sternum)
- Activity tolerance
- Chest pain
- Dyspnea
- Medications affecting respiratory rate

PLANNING

Delegation

Counting and observing respirations may be delegated to UAP. The follow-up assessment, interpretation of abnormal respirations, and determination of appropriate responses are done by the nurse.

Equipment

- Watch with a second hand or indicator

IMPLEMENTATION

Preparation

For a routine assessment of respirations, determine the client's activity schedule and choose a suitable time to monitor the respirations. A client who has been exercising will need to rest for a few minutes to permit the accelerated respiratory rate to return to normal.

Performance

1. Explain to the client what you are going to do, why it is necessary, and how he or she can cooperate. Discuss how the results will be used in planning further care or treatments.
2. Observe appropriate infection control procedures.
3. Provide for client privacy.

4. Observe or palpate and count the respiratory rate.
   - The client's awareness that you are counting the respiratory rate could cause the client voluntarily to alter the respiratory pattern. If you anticipate this, place a hand against the client's chest to feel the chest movements with breathing, or place the client's arm across the chest and observe the chest movements while supposedly taking the radial pulse.
   - Count the respiratory rate for 30 seconds if the respirations are regular. Count for 60 seconds if they are irregular. An inhalation and an exhalation count as one respiration.

5. Observe the depth, rhythm, and character of respirations.
   - Observe the respirations for depth by watching the movement of the chest. *During deep respirations a large volume of air is exchanged; during shallow respirations a small volume is exchanged.*
   - Observe the respirations for regular or irregular rhythm. *Normally, respirations are evenly spaced.*
   - Observe the character of respirations—the sound they produce and the effort they require. *Normally, respirations are silent and effortless.*
6. Document the respiratory rate, depth, rhythm, and character on the appropriate record (see Figure 27–10 ■).

EVALUATION

- Relate respiratory rate to other vital signs, in particular pulse rate; respiratory rhythm and depth to baseline data and health status.
- Report to the physician respiratory rate significantly above or below the normal range and any notable change in respirations from previous assessments; irregular respiratory rhythm; inadequate respiratory depth; abnormal character of breathing—
- orthopnea, wheezing, stridor, or bubbling; and any complaints of dyspnea.
- Conduct appropriate follow-up such as administering appropriate medications or treatments, positioning the client to ease breathing, and requesting involvement of other members of the health care team such as the respiratory therapist.

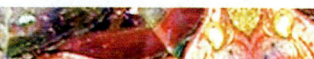
Lifespan Considerations

Respirations

Infants
- An infant or child who is crying will have an abnormal respiratory rate and will need quieting before respirations can be accurately assessed.
- If necessary, place your hand gently on the infant's abdomen to feel the rapid rise and fall during respirations.

Children
- Because young children are diaphragmatic breathers, observe the rise and fall of the abdomen. If necessary, place your hand gently on the abdomen to feel the rapid rise and fall during respirations.

Elders
- Ask the client to remain quiet or count respirations after taking the pulse.
- Elders experience anatomic and physiologic changes that cause the respiratory system to be less efficient. Any changes in rate or type of breathing should be reported immediately.

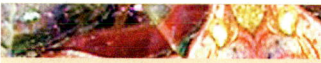
Home Care Considerations

Respirations
- Monitor respiratory rate following the administration of respiratory depressants such as morphine.
- Assess the home setting for factors that could interfere with breathing such as exhaust, gas, or paint fumes or persons who smoke.
- If the client has just come in from another room, allow the client to rest a minute or two before counting respirations.
- Have an adult hold a child gently to reduce movement while counting respirations.

BLOOD PRESSURE

Arterial blood pressure is a measure of the pressure exerted by the blood as it flows through the arteries. Because the blood moves in waves, there are two blood pressure measures: the **systolic pressure,** which is the pressure of the blood as a result of contraction of the ventricles, that is, the pressure of the height of the blood wave; and the **diastolic pressure,** which is the pressure when the ventricles are at rest. Diastolic pressure, then, is the lower pressure, present at all times within the arteries. The difference between the diastolic and the systolic pressures is called the **pulse pressure.**

Blood pressure is measured in millimeters of mercury (mm Hg) and recorded as a fraction. The systolic pressure is written over the diastolic pressure. The average blood pressure of a healthy adult is 120/80 mm Hg. A number of conditions are reflected by changes in blood pressure. Because blood pressure can vary considerably among individuals, it is important for the nurse to know a specific client's baseline blood pressure. For example, if a client's usual blood pressure is 180/100 mm Hg, and it is assessed following surgery to be 120/80 mm Hg, this significant drop in pressure must be reported to the physician.

Determinants of Blood Pressure

Arterial blood pressure is the result of several factors: the pumping action of the heart, the peripheral vascular resistance (the resistance supplied by the blood vessels through which the blood flows), and the blood volume and viscosity.

Pumping Action of the Heart

When the pumping action of the heart is weak, less blood is pumped into arteries (lower cardiac output), and the blood pressure decreases. When the heart's pumping action is strong and the volume of blood pumped into the circulation increases (higher cardiac output), the blood pressure increases.

Peripheral Vascular Resistance

Peripheral resistance can increase blood pressure. The diastolic pressure especially is affected. Some factors that create resistance in the arterial system are the capacity of the arterioles and capillaries, the compliance of the arteries, and the viscosity of the blood.

The internal diameter or capacity of the arterioles and the capillaries determines in great part the peripheral resistance to the blood in the body. The smaller the space within a vessel, the greater the resistance. Normally, the arterioles are in a state of partial constriction. Increased vasoconstriction raises the blood pressure, whereas decreased vasoconstriction lowers the blood pressure.

If the elastic and muscular tissues of the arteries are replaced with fibrous tissue, the arteries lose much of their ability to constrict and dilate. This condition, most common in middle-aged and elderly adults, is known as **arteriosclerosis.**

Blood Volume

When the blood volume decreases (for example, as a result of a hemorrhage or dehydration), the blood pressure decreases because of decreased fluid in the arteries. Conversely, when the volume increases (for example, as a result of a rapid intravenous infusion), the blood pressure increases because of the greater fluid volume within the circulatory system.

Blood Viscosity

Blood pressure is higher when the blood is highly **viscous** (thick), that is, when the proportion of red blood cells to the blood plasma is high. This proportion is referred to as the **hematocrit.** The viscosity increases markedly when the hematocrit is more than 60% to 65%.

Factors Affecting Blood Pressure

Among the factors influencing blood pressure are age, exercise, stress, race, obesity, sex, medications, diurnal variations, and disease processes.

- *Age.* Newborns have a mean systolic pressure of about 75 mm Hg. The pressure rises with age, reaching a peak at the onset of puberty, and then tends to decline somewhat. In older people, elasticity of the arteries is decreased—the arteries are more rigid and less yielding to the pressure of the blood. This produces an elevated systolic pressure. Because the walls no longer retract as flexibly with decreased pressure, the diastolic pressure is also high (see Table 27–1 on page 485.)
- *Exercise.* Physical activity increases the cardiac output and hence the blood pressure; thus 20 to 30 minutes of rest following exercise is indicated before the resting blood pressure can be reliably assessed.
- *Stress.* Stimulation of the sympathetic nervous system increases cardiac output and vasoconstriction of the arterioles, thus increasing the blood pressure reading; however, severe pain can decrease blood pressure greatly by inhibiting the vasomotor center and producing vasodilatation.
- *Race.* African American males over 35 years have higher blood pressures than European American males of the same age.
- *Gender.* After puberty, females usually have lower blood pressures than males of the same age; this difference is thought to be due to hormonal variations. After menopause, women generally have higher blood pressures than before.
- *Medications.* Many medications may increase or decrease the blood pressure.
- *Obesity.* Both childhood and adult obesity predispose to hypertension.
- *Diurnal variations.* Pressure is usually lowest early in the morning, when the metabolic rate is lowest, then rises throughout the day and peaks in the late afternoon or early evening.
- *Disease process.* Any condition affecting the cardiac output, blood volume, blood viscosity, and/or compliance of the arteries has a direct effect on the blood pressure.

Hypertension

A blood pressure that is persistently above normal is called **hypertension.** It is usually asymptomatic and is often a contributing factor to myocardial infarctions (heart attacks). An elevated blood pressure of unknown cause is called *primary hypertension.* An elevated blood pressure of known cause is called *secondary hypertension.* Hypertension is a widespread health problem. Individuals with diastolic blood pressures of 80–89 mm Hg or systolic blood pressures of 120–139 mm Hg should be considered prehypertensive and, without intervention, may develop cardiac disease. Stage 1 hypertension is when the diastolic blood pressure is 90 mm Hg or higher or when the systolic blood pressure is higher than 140 mm Hg (see Table 27–4). Factors associated with hypertension include thickening of the arterial walls, which reduces the size of the arterial lumen, and inelasticity of the arteries as well as such lifestyle factors as cigarette smoking, obesity, heavy alcohol consumption, lack of physical exercise, high blood cholesterol levels, and continued exposure to stress. Follow-up care should include lifestyle changes conducive to lowering the blood pressure as well as monitoring the pressure itself.

TABLE 27–4 Recommendations for Follow-up Based on Initial Set of Blood Pressure Measurements for Adults Age 18 Years and Older

Initial Screening Blood Pressure (mm Hg)*		Follow-up Recommended†
Systolic	Diastolic	
< 130	< 85	Recheck in 2 years.
130–139	85–89	Recheck in 1 year.‡
140–159	90–99	Confirm within 2 months.
160–179	100–109	Evaluate or refer to source of care within 1 month.
180–209	110–119	Evaluate or refer to source of care within 1 week.
≥210	≥120	Evaluate or refer to source of care immediately.

*If the systolic and diastolic categories are different, follow recommendation for the shorter time to follow up (e.g., 160/85 mm Hg should be evaluated or referred to source of care within 1 month).
†The scheduling of follow-up should be modified by reliable information about past blood pressure measurements, other cardiovascular risk factors, or target-organ disease.
‡Consider providing advice about lifestyle modifications.
Note: From the "Sixth Report of the Joint National Committee for the Detection, Evaluation, and Treatment of High Blood Pressure," by National Institutes of Health, National Heart, Lung, and Blood Institute, 1997.

Hypotension

Hypotension is a blood pressure that is below normal, that is, a systolic reading consistently between 85 and 110 mm Hg in an adult whose normal pressure is higher than this. **Orthostatic hypotension** is a blood pressure that falls when the client sits or stands. It is usually the result of peripheral vasodilatation in which blood leaves the central body organs, especially the brain, and moves to the periphery, often causing the person to feel faint. Hypotension can also be caused by analgesics such as meperidine hydrochloride (Demerol), bleeding, severe burns, and dehydration. It is important to monitor hypotensive clients carefully to prevent falls. When assessing for orthostatic hypotension:

- Place the client in a supine position for 2 to 3 minutes.
- Record the client's pulse and blood pressure.
- Assist the client to slowly sit or stand. Support the client in case of faintness.
- After 1 minute in the upright position, recheck the pulse and blood pressure in the same sites as previously.
- Record the results. A rise in pulse of 40 beats per minute or a drop in blood pressure of 30 mm Hg indicates abnormal orthostatic vital signs.

Research Note
How Long Should a Patient Lie and Stand When Taking Orthostatic Blood Pressures?

Lack of agreement within the research literature and in their own institution regarding the technique for measuring orthostatic blood pressures led these authors (Lance et al., 2000) to conduct this study. Thirty-five normal participants exercised, had their pulse and blood pressure measured when rested, then had pulse, blood pressure, and dizziness measured when standing. The variables were the length of time required for resting to produce baseline values and the minimum time standing to return indications of blood pressure drop or dizziness.

The results of the study showed that 10 minutes of resting were needed for baseline values. This was longer than the 5-minute departmental standard and shorter than the 15-minute nursing unit practice. Pulse, blood pressure, and dizziness readings taken immediately upon standing and at 2 minutes were sufficient. Measurements taken after longer periods of standing did not show significant differences from the 2-minute readings.

Implications: The authors acknowledged that their results could not be easily extrapolated to the broader population since their participants were healthy, young (under 25 years old) adults. However, they felt secure enough with their results to implement the standard in their institution while recommending further study on clients with higher risk of orthostatic variations. The article is clear and well written and would easily permit replication of the research. Nurses should pursue the investigation of similar clinical practices that are unstudied or have conflicting results in the published literature.

Note: From "Comparison of Different Methods of Obtaining Orthostatic Vital Signs," by R. Lance et al., 2000, *Clinical Nursing Research, 9,* pp. 479–491.

Assessing Blood Pressure

Blood pressure is measured with a *blood pressure cuff,* a *sphygmomanometer,* and a *stethoscope.* The blood pressure cuff consists of a rubber bag that can be inflated with air. It is called the *bladder* (Figure 27–26 ■). It is covered with cloth and has two tubes attached to it. One tube connects to a rubber bulb that inflates the bladder. When turned counterclockwise, a small valve on the side of this bulb releases the air in the bladder. When the valve is tightened (turned clockwise), air pumped into the bladder remains there.

The other tube is attached to a sphygmomanometer. The sphygmomanometer indicates the pressure of the air within the bladder. There are two types of sphygmomanometers: *aneroid* and *mercury* (Figure 27–27 ■). The aneroid sphygmomanometer is a calibrated dial with a needle that points to the calibrations.

The mercury sphygmomanometer is a calibrated cylinder filled with mercury. The pressure is indicated at the point to which the rounded curve of the **meniscus** (the crescent-shaped dome) rises (Figure 27–28 ■). The blood pressure reading should be made with the eye at the level of the rounded curve in order to be accurate.

Some agencies use *electronic sphygmomanometers* (Figure 27–29 ■), which eliminate the need to listen to the sounds of the client's systolic and diastolic blood pressures through a stethoscope. Electronic blood pressure devices should be calibrated periodically to check accuracy.

Doppler ultrasound stethoscopes are also used to assess blood pressure (see Figure 27–19 earlier in the chapter). These are of particular value when blood pressure sounds are difficult to hear, such as in infants, obese clients, and clients in shock. Systolic pressure may be the only blood pressure obtainable with some ultrasound models.

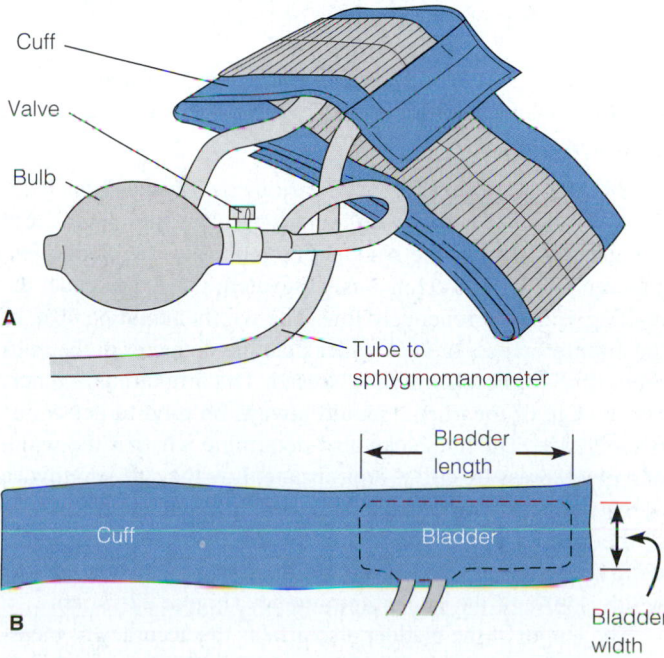

Figure 27–26 ■ *A,* A blood pressure cuff and bulb; *B,* the bladder inside the cuff.

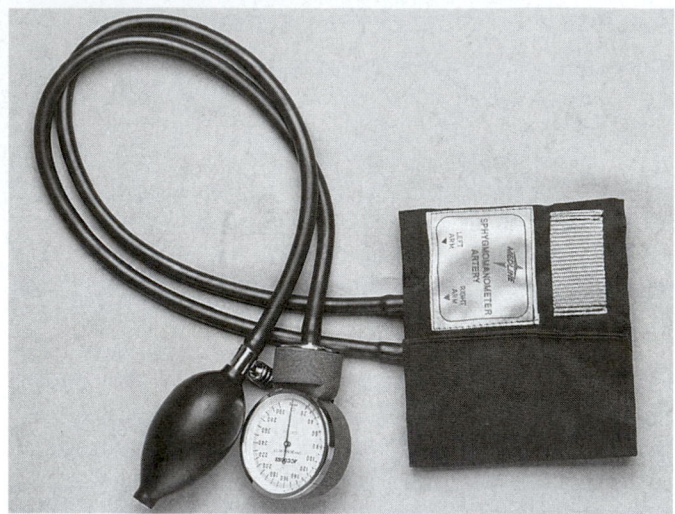

A

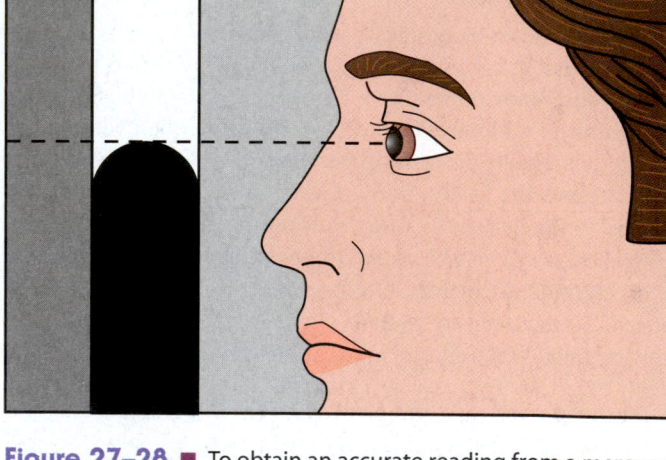

Figure 27–28 ■ To obtain an accurate reading from a mercury manometer, position the meniscus at eye level.

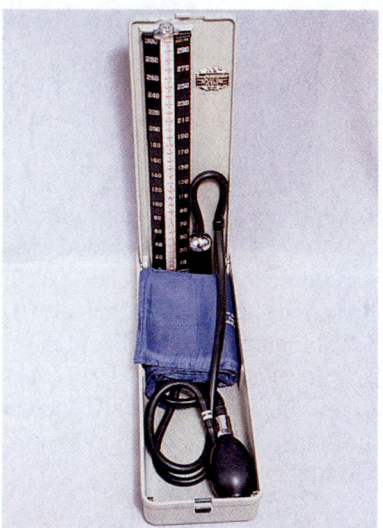

B

Figure 27–27 ■ Blood pressure equipment: *A,* an aneroid manometer and cuff; *B,* a mercury manometer and cuff.

Blood pressure cuffs come in various sizes because the bladder must be the correct width and length for the client's arm (Figure 27–30 ■). If the bladder is too narrow, the blood pressure reading will be erroneously elevated; if it is too wide, the reading will be erroneously low. The width should be 40% of the circumference, or 20% wider than the diameter of the midpoint of the limb on which it is used. The arm circumference, not the age of the client, should always be used to determine bladder size. The nurse can also determine whether the width of a blood pressure cuff is appropriate: Lay the cuff lengthwise at the midpoint of the upper arm, and hold the outermost side of the bladder edge laterally on the arm. With the other hand, wrap the width of the cuff around the arm, and ensure that the width is 40% of the arm circumference (Figure 27–31 ■).

The length of the bladder also affects the accuracy of measurement. The bladder should be sufficiently long to cover at least two-thirds of the limb's circumference.

Blood pressure cuffs are made of nondistensible material so that an even pressure is exerted around the limb. Most cuffs are

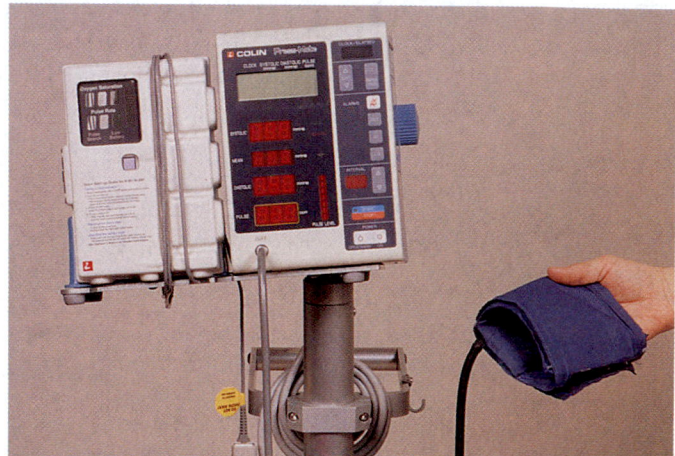

Figure 27–29 ■ Automatic blood pressure monitors register systolic, diastolic, and mean blood pressures.

held in place by hooks, snaps, or Velcro. Others have a cloth bandage that is long enough to encircle the limb several times; this type is closed by tucking the end of the bandage into one of the bandage folds.

Blood Pressure Sites

The blood pressure is usually assessed in the client's arm using the brachial artery and a standard stethoscope. Assessing the blood pressure on a client's thigh is usually indicated in these situations:

- The blood pressure cannot be measured on either arm (e.g., because of burns or other trauma).
- The blood pressure in one thigh is to be compared with the blood pressure in the other thigh.

Blood pressure is not measured on a client's arm or thigh in the following situations:

- The shoulder, arm, or hand (or the hip, knee, or ankle) is injured or diseased.
- A cast or bulky bandage is on any part of the limb.

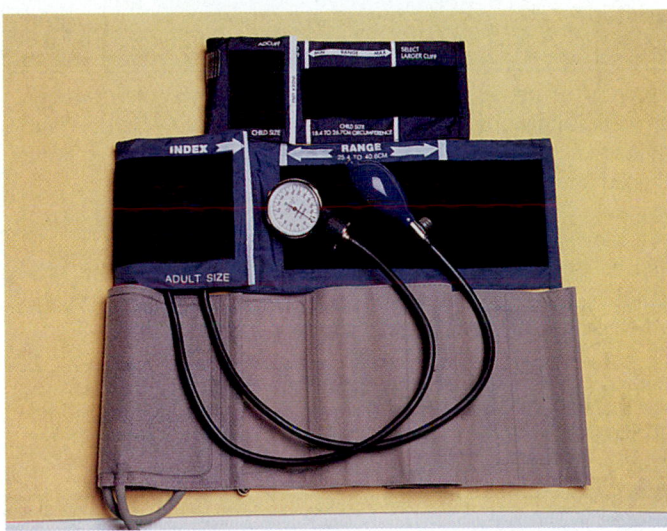

Figure 27–30 ■ Three standard cuff sizes: a small cuff for an infant, small child, or frail adult; a normal adult-size cuff; and a large cuff for measuring the blood pressure on the leg or on the arm of an obese adult.

- The client has had removal of axilla (or hip) lymph nodes on that side.
- The client has an intravenous infusion in that limb.
- The client has an arteriovenous fistula (e.g., for renal dialysis) in that limb.

Methods

Blood pressure can be assessed directly or indirectly. *Direct (invasive monitoring) measurement* involves the insertion of a catheter into the brachial, radial, or femoral artery. Arterial pressure is represented as wavelike forms displayed on an oscilloscope. With correct placement, this pressure reading is highly accurate.

Two *noninvasive indirect methods* of measuring blood pressure are the *auscultatory* and *palpatory* methods. The *auscultatory method* is most commonly used in hospitals, clinics, and homes. Required equipment is a sphygmomanometer, a cuff, and a stethoscope. When carried out correctly, the auscultatory method is relatively accurate.

When taking a blood pressure using a stethoscope, the nurse identifies five phases in the series of sounds called **Korotkoff's sounds** (Figure 27–32 ■). First the nurse pumps the cuff up to about 30 mm Hg above the point where the pulse is no longer

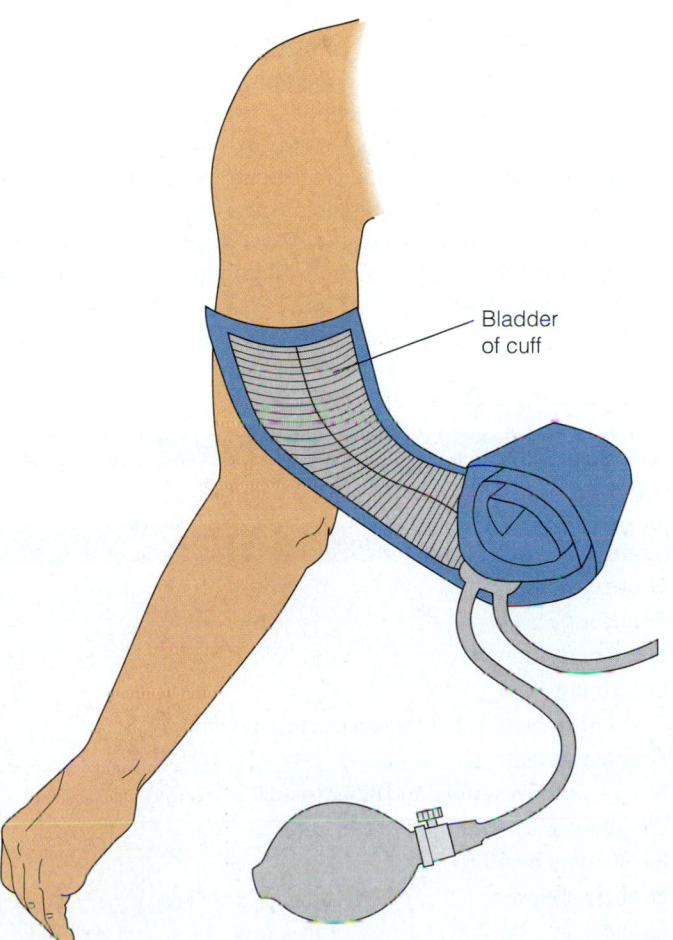

Bladder of cuff

Figure 27–31 ■ Determining that the bladder of a blood pressure cuff is 40% of the arm circumference or 20% wider than the diameter of the midpoint of the limb.

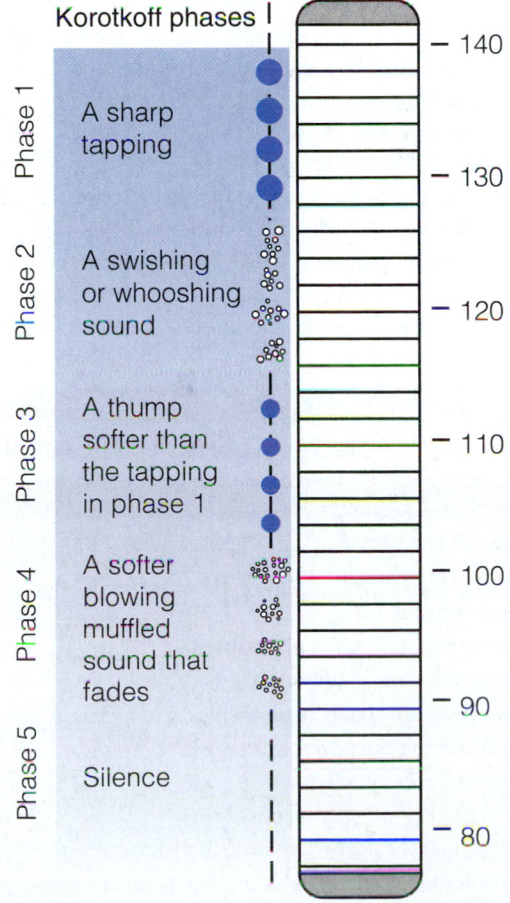

Figure 27–32 ■ Korotkoff's sounds can be differentiated into five phases. In the illustration the blood pressure is 138/90 or 138/102/90.

BOX 27–8   ■ Korotkoff's Sounds

Phase 1 The pressure level at which the first faint, clear tapping or thumping sounds are heard. These sounds gradually become more intense. To ensure that they are not extraneous sounds, the nurse should identify at least two consecutive tapping sounds. The first tapping sound heard during deflation of the cuff is the systolic blood pressure.

Phase 2 The period during deflation when the sounds have a muffled, whooshing, or swishing quality.

Phase 3 The period during which the blood flows freely through an increasingly open artery and the sounds become crisper and more intense and again assume a thumping quality but softer than in phase 1.

Phase 4 The time when the sounds become muffled and have a soft, blowing quality.

Phase 5 The pressure level when the last sound is heard. This is followed by a period of silence. The pressure at which the last sound is heard is the diastolic blood pressure in adults.[*]

---

[*]In agencies where the fourth phase is considered the diastolic pressure, three measures are recommended (systolic pressure, diastolic pressure, and phase 5). These may be referred to as systolic, first diastolic, and second diastolic pressures. The phase 5 (second diastolic pressure) reading may be zero; that is, the muffled sounds are heard even when there is no air pressure in the blood pressure cuff. In some instances, muffled sounds are never heard, in which case a dash is inserted where the reading would normally be recorded (e.g., 190/–/110).

felt; that is the point when the blood flow in the artery is stopped. Then the pressure is released slowly (2 to 3 mm Hg per sound) while the nurse observes the readings on the manometer and relates them to the sounds heard through the stethoscope. Five phases occur but may not always be audible (see Box 27–8).

The *palpatory method* is sometimes used when Korotkoff's sounds cannot be heard and electronic equipment to amplify the sounds is not available, or to prevent misdirection from the presence of an auscultatory gap occurs. An **auscultatory gap,** which occurs particularly in hypertensive clients, is the temporary disappearance of sounds normally heard over the brachial artery when the cuff pressure is high followed by the reappearance of the sounds at a lower level. This temporary disappearance of sounds occurs in the latter part of phase 1 and phase 2 and may cover a range of 40 mm Hg. If a palpated estimation of the systolic pressure is not made prior to auscultation, the nurse may begin listening in the middle of this range and underestimate the systolic pressure. In the palpatory method of blood pressure determination, instead of listening for the blood flow sounds, using light to moderate pressure the nurse palpates the pulsations of the artery as the pressure in the cuff is released. The pressure is read from the sphygmomanometer when the first pulsation is felt.

Common Errors in Assessing Blood Pressure

The importance of the accuracy of blood pressure assessments cannot be overemphasized. Many judgments about a client's health are made on the basis of blood pressure. It is an important indicator of the client's condition and is used extensively as a basis for nursing interventions. Two possible reasons for blood pressure errors are haste on the part of the nurse and subconscious bias. For example, a nurse may be influenced by the client's previous blood pressure measurements or diagnosis and "hear" a value consonant with the practitioner's expectations. Some reasons for erroneous blood pressure readings are given in Table 27–5.

Procedure 27–6 provides guidelines for assessing blood pressure.

TABLE 27–5   Selected Sources of Error in Blood Pressure Assessment

Error	Effect
Bladder cuff too narrow	Erroneously high
Bladder cuff too wide	Erroneously low
Arm unsupported	Erroneously high
Insufficient rest before the assessment	Erroneously high
Repeating assessment too quickly	Erroneously high systolic or low diastolic readings
Cuff wrapped too loosely or unevenly	Erroneously high
Deflating cuff too quickly	Erroneously low systolic and high diastolic readings
Deflating cuff too slowly	Erroneously high diastolic reading
Failure to use the same arm consistently	Inconsistent measurements
Arm above level of the heart	Erroneously low
Assessing immediately after a meal or while client smokes or has pain	Erroneously high
Failure to identify auscultatory gap	Erroneously low systolic pressure and erroneously low diastolic pressure

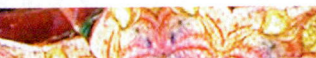

Procedure 27–6 Assessing Blood Pressure

Purposes

- To obtain a baseline measure of arterial blood pressure for subsequent evaluation
- To determine the client's hemodynamic status (e.g., stroke volume of the heart and blood vessel resistance)
- To identify and monitor changes in blood pressure resulting from a disease process and medical therapy (e.g., presence or history of cardiovascular disease, renal disease, circulatory shock, or acute pain; rapid infusion of fluids or blood products)

ASSESSMENT

Assess

- Signs and symptoms of hypertension (e.g., headache, ringing in the ears, flushing of face, nosebleeds, fatigue)
- Signs and symptoms of hypotension (e.g., tachycardia, dizziness, mental confusion, restlessness, cool and clammy skin, pale or cyanotic skin)
- Factors affecting blood pressure (e.g., activity, emotional stress, pain, and time the client last smoked or ingested caffeine)

PLANNING

Delegation

Blood pressure measurement may be delegated to UAP. The interpretation of abnormal blood pressure readings and determination of appropriate responses are done by the nurse.

Equipment

- Stethoscope or DUS
- Blood pressure cuff of the appropriate size
- Sphygmomanometer

IMPLEMENTATION

Preparation

1. Ensure that the equipment is intact and functioning properly. Check for leaks in the rubber tubing of the sphygmomanometer.
2. Make sure that the client has not smoked or ingested caffeine within 30 minutes prior to measurement.

Performance

1. Explain to the client what you are going to do, why it is necessary, and how he or she can cooperate. Discuss how the results will be used in planning further care or treatments.
2. Observe appropriate infection control procedures.
3. Provide for client privacy.
4. Position the client appropriately.
   - The adult client should be sitting unless otherwise specified. Both feet should be flat on the floor *since legs crossed at the knee result in elevated systolic and diastolic blood pressures* (Foster-Fitzpatrick, Ortiz, Sibilano, Marcantonio, & Braun, 1999).
   - The elbow should be slightly flexed with the palm of the hand facing up and the forearm supported at heart level. Readings in any other position should be specified. The blood pressure is normally similar in sitting, standing, and lying positions, but it can vary significantly by position in certain persons. *The blood pressure*

increases when the arm is below heart level and decreases when the arm is above heart level.
   - Expose the upper arm.
5. Wrap the deflated cuff evenly around the upper arm. Locate the brachial artery (Figure 27–20 earlier). Apply the center of the bladder directly over the artery. *The bladder inside the cuff must be directly over the artery to be compressed if the reading is to be accurate.*
   - For an adult, place the lower border of the cuff approximately 2.5 cm (1 in.) above the antecubital space.
6. If this is the client's initial examination, perform a preliminary palpatory determination of systolic pressure. *The initial estimate tells the nurse the maximal pressure to which the manometer needs to be elevated in subsequent determinations. It also prevents underestimation of the systolic pressure or overestimation of the diastolic pressure should an auscultatory gap occur.*
   - Palpate the brachial artery with the fingertips.
   - Close the valve on the pump by turning the knob clockwise.
   - Pump up the cuff until you no longer feel the brachial pulse. At that pressure the blood cannot flow through the artery. Note the pressure on the sphygmomanometer at

which pulse is no longer felt. *This gives an estimate of the maximum pressure required to measure the systolic pressure.*
   - Release the pressure completely in the cuff, and wait 1 to 2 minutes before making further measurements. *A waiting period gives the blood trapped in the veins time to be released. Otherwise, false high systolic readings will occur.*
7. Position the stethoscope appropriately.
   - Cleanse the earpieces with alcohol or recommended disinfectant.
   - Insert the ear attachments of the stethoscope in your ears so that they tilt slightly forward. *Sounds are heard more clearly when the ear attachments follow the direction of the ear canal.*
   - Ensure that the stethoscope hangs freely from the ears to the diaphragm. *Rubbing the stethoscope against an object can obliterate the sounds of the blood within an artery.*
   - Place the bell side of the amplifier of the stethoscope over the brachial pulse. *Because the blood pressure is a low-frequency sound, it is best heard with the bell-shaped diaphragm.* Hold the diaphragm with the thumb and index finger.

continued on page 516

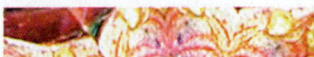

Procedure 27–6 Assessing Blood Pressure *continued*

IMPLEMENTATION *continued*

8. Auscultate the client's blood pressure.
   - Pump up the cuff until the sphygmomanometer reads 30 mm Hg above the point where the brachial pulse disappeared.
   - Release the valve on the cuff carefully so that the pressure decreases at the rate of 2 to 3 mm Hg per second. *If the rate is faster or slower an error in measurement may occur.*
   - As the pressure falls, identify the manometer reading at each of the five phases, if possible.
   - Deflate the cuff rapidly and completely.
   - Wait 1 to 2 minutes before making further determinations. *This permits blood trapped in the veins to be released.*
   - Repeat the above steps once or twice as necessary to confirm the accuracy of the reading.
9. If this is the client's initial examination, repeat the procedure on the client's other arm. There should be a difference of no more than 10 mm Hg between the arms. The arm found to have the higher pressure should be used for subsequent examinations.

VARIATION: OBTAINING A BLOOD PRESSURE BY THE PALPATION METHOD

If it is not possible to use a stethoscope to obtain the blood pressure or if the Korotkoff sounds cannot be heard, palpate the radial or brachial pulse site as the cuff pressure is released. The manometer reading at the point where the pulse reappears represents a blood pressure between what would be auscultated systolic and diastolic values.

VARIATION: TAKING A THIGH BLOOD PRESSURE

- Help the client to assume a prone position. If the client cannot assume this position, measure the blood pressure while the client is in a supine position with the knee slightly flexed. Slight flexing of the knee will facilitate placing the stethoscope on the popliteal space (Figure 27–33 ■).
- Expose the thigh, taking care not to expose the client unduly.
- Locate the popliteal artery (Figure 27–17).
- Wrap the cuff evenly around the midthigh with the compression bladder over the posterior aspect of the thigh and the bottom edge above the knee. *The bladder must be directly over the posterior popliteal artery if the reading is to be accurate.*
- If this is the client's initial examination, perform a preliminary palpatory determination of systolic pressure by palpating the popliteal artery.
- In adults, the systolic pressure in the popliteal artery is usually 20 to 30 mm Hg higher than that in the brachial artery because of use of a larger bladder; the diastolic pressure is usually the same.

VARIATION: USING AN ELECTRONIC INDIRECT BLOOD PRESSURE MONITORING DEVICE (FIGURE 27–29).

- Place the blood pressure cuff on the extremity according to the manufacturer's guidelines.

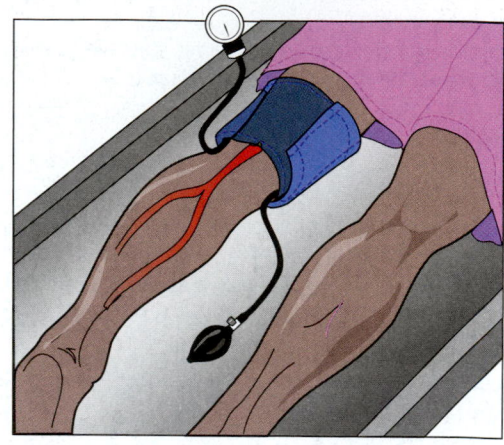

Figure 27–33 ■ Measuring blood pressure in the client's thigh—location of the popliteal artery and application of the cuff.

- Turn on the blood pressure switch.
- If appropriate, set the device for the desired number of minutes between blood pressure determinations.
- When the device has determined the blood pressure reading, note the digital results.

> ► **CLINICAL ALERT** *Electronic/automatic blood pressure cuffs can be left in place for many hours. Remove the cuff and check skin condition periodically.* ■

10. Remove the cuff.
11. Wipe the cuff with an approved disinfectant. *Cuffs can become significantly contaminated.* Many institutions use disposable blood pressure cuffs. The client uses it for the length of stay and then it is discarded. This decreases the risk of spreading infection through sharing of cuffs.
12. Document and report pertinent assessment data according to agency policy. Record two pressures in the form "130/80" where "130" is the systolic (phase 1) and "80" is the diastolic (phase 5) pressure. Record three pressures in the form "130/110/90," where "130" is the systolic, "110" is the first diastolic (phase 4), and "90" is the second diastolic (phase 5) pressure. Use the abbreviations *RA* or *RL* for right arm or right leg and *LA* or *LL* for left arm or left leg. Record a difference of greater than 10 mm Hg between the two arms or legs.

EVALUATION

- Relate blood pressure to other vital signs, to baseline data, and health status.
- Report any significant change in the client's blood pressure. Also report these findings:
  - Systolic blood pressure (of an adult) above 140 mm Hg
  - Diastolic blood pressure (of an adult) above 90 mm Hg
  - Systolic blood pressure (of an adult) below 100 mm Hg
- Conduct appropriate follow-up such as administration of medication. If the blood pressure is significantly higher or lower than usual, implement appropriate safety precautions.

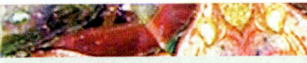

Lifespan Considerations

Blood Pressure

Infants

- Use a pediatric stethoscope with small diaphragm.
- The lower edge of the blood pressure cuff can be closer to the antecubital space of an infant.
- Use the palpation method if auscultation with a stethoscope or DUS is unsuccessful.
- Arm and thigh pressures are equivalent in children under 1 year of age.
- One quick way to determine the normal systolic blood pressure of a child is to use the following formula:

$$\text{Normal systolic BP} = 80 + (2 \times \text{child's age in years})$$

Children

- Explain each step of the process and what it will feel like. Demonstrate on a doll.
- Use the palpation technique for children under 3 years old.
- Cuff bladder *width* should be 40% and *length* should be 80% to 100% of the arm circumference (Figure 27–34 ■).
- Take the blood pressure prior to other uncomfortable procedures so that the blood pressure is not artificially elevated by the discomfort.
- In children, the diastolic pressure is considered to be the onset of phase 4, where the sounds become muffled.
- In children, the thigh pressure is about 10 mm Hg higher than the arm.

Elders

- Skin may be very fragile. Do not allow cuff pressure to remain high any longer than necessary.

- Determine if the client is taking antihypertensives and, if so, when the last dose was taken.
- Medications that cause vasodilation (antihypertensive medications) along with the loss of baroreceptor efficiency in the elderly place them at increased risk for having orthostatic hypotension. Measuring blood pressure while the client is in the lying, sitting, and standing positions, and noting any changes can determine this.
- If the client has arm contractures, assess the blood pressure by palpation, with the arm in a relaxed position. If this is not possible, take a thigh blood pressure.

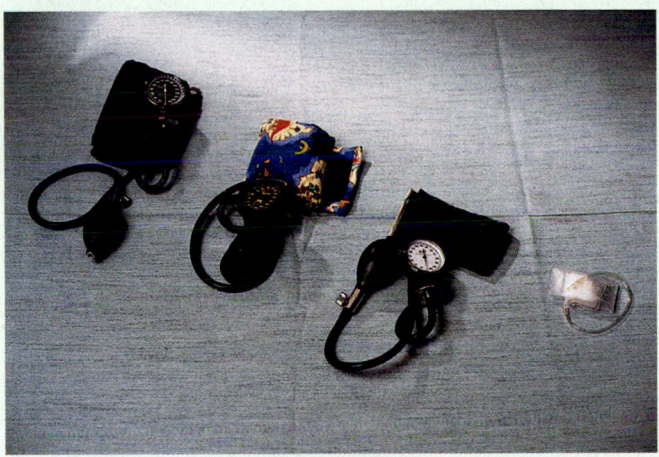

Figure 27–34 ■ Pediatric blood pressure cuffs (with manometers).

MediaLink | JOANNE BRIGGS INSTITUTE APPLICATION

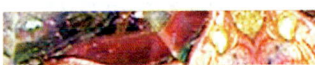

Home Care Considerations

Blood Pressure

- If the client takes blood pressure readings at home, use the same equipment or calibrate it against a system known to be accurate.
- Observe the client or family member taking the blood pressure and provide feedback if further instruction is needed.

- If the client is in a chair or low bed, position yourself so that you maintain the client's arm at heart level and you can read the sphygmomanometer at eye level.

OXYGEN SATURATION

A **pulse oximeter** is a noninvasive device that measures a client's arterial blood oxygen saturation (SaO_2) by means of a sensor attached to the client's finger (Figure 27–35 ■), toe, nose, earlobe, or forehead (or around the hand or foot of a neonate). The pulse oximeter can detect hypoxemia before clinical signs and symptoms, such as dusky skin color and dusky nailbeds color develop.

The pulse oximeter's *sensor* has two parts: (a) two light-emitting diodes (LEDs)—one red, the other infrared—that transmit light through nails, tissue, venous blood, and arterial blood; and (b) a photodetector placed directly opposite the LEDs (e.g., the other side of the finger, toe, or nose). The photodetector measures the amount of red and infrared light absorbed by oxygenated and deoxygenated hemoglobin in arterial blood and reports it as SaO_2. Normal SaO_2 is 95% to 100% and an SaO_2 below 70% is life threatening.

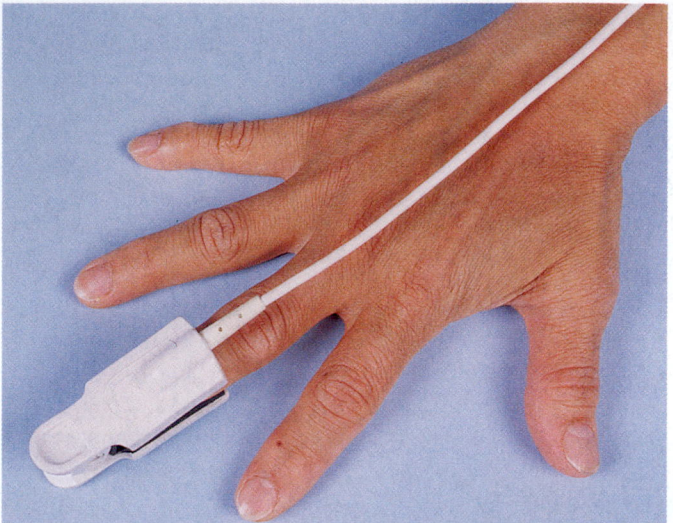

Figure 27–35 ■ Finger tip oximeter sensor (adult).

Pulse oximeters with various types of sensors are available from several manufacturers. The *oximeter unit* consists of an inlet connection for the sensor cable, a faceplate that indicates (a) the oxygen saturation measurement (expressed as a percentage) and (b) the pulse rate. Cordless units are also available (Figure 27–36 ■). A preset alarm system signals high and low SaO_2 measurements and a high and low pulse rate. The high and low SaO_2 levels are generally preset at 100% and 85%, respectively, for adults. The high and low pulse rate alarms are usually preset at 140 and 50 BPM for adults. These alarm limits can, however, be changed according to the manufacturer's directions.

Factors Affecting Oxygen Saturation Readings

- *Hemoglobin.* If the hemoglobin is fully saturated with oxygen, the SaO_2 will appear normal even if the total hemoglo-

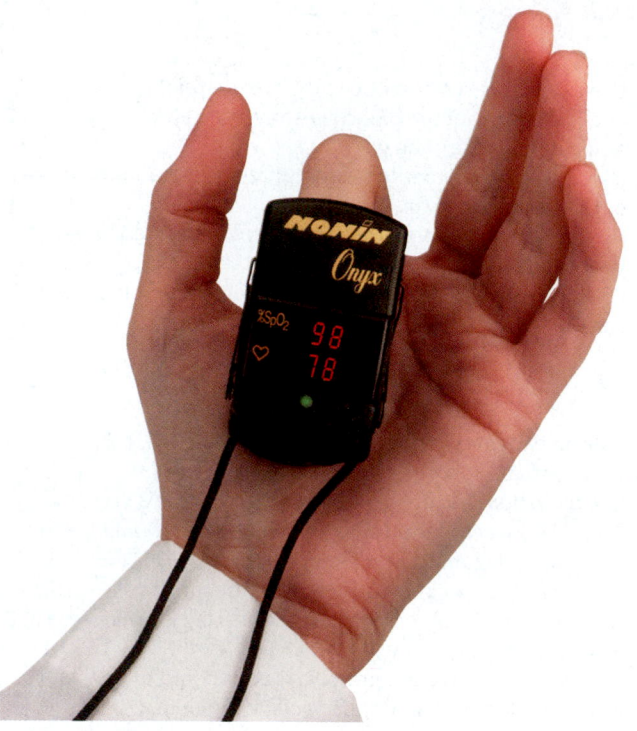

Figure 27–36 ■ Finger tip oximeter sensor (cordless). (Courtesy of Nonin Medical, Inc.).

bin level is low. Thus, the client could be severely anemic and have inadequate oxygen to supply the tissues but the pulse oximeter would return a normal value.
- *Circulation.* The oximeter will not return an accurate reading if the area under the sensor has impaired circulation.
- *Activity.* Shivering or excessive movement of the sensor site may interfere with accurate readings.

Procedure 27–7 outlines the steps in measuring oxygen saturation.

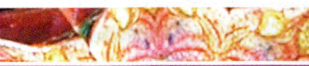 **Procedure 27–7 Measuring Oxygen Saturation**

Purposes

- To measure the arterial blood oxygen saturation (SaO_2)
- To detect the presence of hypoemia before visible signs develop

ASSESSMENT

Assess

- The best location for a pulse oximeter sensor based on the client's age and physical condition
- The client's overall condition including risk factors for development of hypoxemia (e.g., respiratory or cardiac disease) and hemoglobin level

- Vital signs, skin and nail bed color, and tissue perfusion of extremities as baseline data
- Adhesive allergy

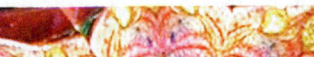

Procedure 27–7 Measuring Oxygen Saturation *continued*

PLANNING

Many hospitals and clinics have pulse oximeters readily available for use with other vital signs equipment (or even as an integrated part of the electronic blood pressure device). Other facilities may have a limited supply of oximeters and the nurse may need to request it from the central supply department.

Delegation

Application of the pulse oximeter sensor and recording of the SaO_2 value may be delegated to UAP. The interpretation of the oxygen saturation value and determination of appropriate responses are done by the nurse.

Equipment
- Nail polish remover as needed
- Alcohol wipe
- Sheet or towel
- Pulse oximeter

IMPLEMENTATION

Preparation

Check that the oximeter equipment is functioning normally.

Performance

1. Explain to the client what you are going to do, why it is necessary, and how he or she can cooperate. Discuss how the results will be used in planning further care or treatments.
2. Observe appropriate infection control procedures.
3. Provide for client privacy.
4. Choose a sensor appropriate for the client's weight, size, and desired location. Because weight limits of sensors overlap, a pediatric sensor could be used for a small adult.
   - If the client is allergic to adhesive, use a clip or sensor without adhesive. If using an extremity, assess the proximal pulse and capillary refill at the point closest to the site.
   - If the client has low tissue perfusion due to peripheral vascular disease or therapy using vasoconstrictive medications, use a nasal sensor or a reflectance sensor on the forehead. Avoid using lower extremities that have a compromised circulation and extremities that are used for infusions or other invasive monitoring.
5. Prepare the site.
   - Clean the site with an alcohol wipe before applying the sensor.

   - It may be necessary to remove a female client's nail polish or acrylic nails *since they can interfere with accurate measurements*.
6. Apply the sensor, and connect it to the pulse oximeter.
   - Make sure the LED and photodetector are accurately aligned, that is, opposite each other on either side of the finger, toe, nose, or earlobe. Many sensors have markings to facilitate correct alignment of the LEDs and photodetector.
   - Attach the sensor cable to the connection outlet on the oximeter. Turn on the machine according to the manufacturer's directions. Appropriate connection will be confirmed by an audible beep indicating each arterial pulsation. Some devices have a wheel that can be turned clockwise to increase the pulse volume and counterclockwise to decrease it.
   - Ensure that the bar of light or waveform on the face of the oximeter fluctuates with each pulsation and reflects the pulse volume or strength.
7. Set and turn on the alarm.
   - Check the preset alarm limits for high and low oxygen saturation and high and low pulse rates. Change

   these alarm limits according to the manufacturer's directions as indicated. Ensure that the audio and visual alarms are on before you leave the client. A tone will be heard and a number will blink on the faceplate.
8. Ensure client safety.
   - Inspect and/or move or change the location of an adhesive toe or finger sensor every 4 hours and a spring-tension sensor every 2 hours.
   - Inspect the sensor site tissues for irritation from adhesive sensors.
9. Ensure the accuracy of measurement.
   - Minimize motion artifacts by using an adhesive sensor, or immobilize the client's monitoring site. *Movement of the client's finger or toe may be misinterpreted by the oximeter as arterial pulsations.*
   - If indicated, cover the sensor with a sheet or towel to block large amounts of light from external sources (e.g., sunlight, procedure lamps, or bilirubin lights in the nursery). *Large amounts of outside light may be sensed by the photodetector and alter the SaO_2 value.*
10. Document the oxygen saturation on the appropriate record at designated intervals.

EVALUATION

- Compare the oxygen saturation to the client's previous oxygen saturation level. Relate to pulse rate and other vital signs.
- Conduct appropriate follow-up such as notifying the physician, adjusting oxygen therapy, or providing breathing treatments.

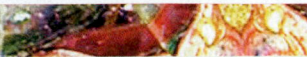

Lifespan Considerations

Pulse Oximetry

Infants

- If an appropriate-sized finger or toe sensor (Figure 27–37 ■) is not available, consider using an earlobe or forehead sensor.
- The high and low SaO_2 levels are generally preset at 95% and 80% for neonates.
- The high and low pulse rate alarms are usually preset at 200 and 100 for neonates.

Children

- Instruct the child that the sensor does not hurt. Disconnect the probe whenever possible to allow for movement.

Elders

- Use of vasoconstrictive medications, poor circulation, or thickened nails may make finger or toe sensors inaccurate.

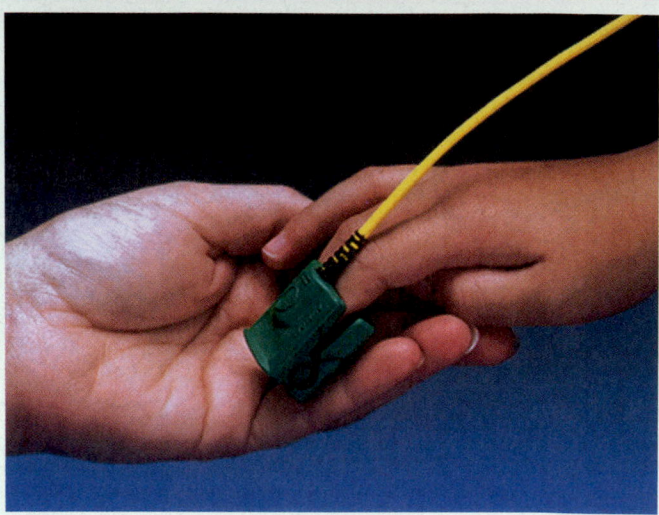

Figure 27–37 ■ Finger tip oximeter sensor-child. (Courtesy of Nonin Medical, Inc.).

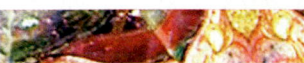

Home Care Considerations

Pulse Oximetry

- Pulse oximetry is a quick, inexpensive, noninvasive method of assessing oxygenation. Like an automatic blood pressure cuff, it also provides a pulse rate reading. Use in the ambulatory or home setting whenever indicated.

- If the client requires frequent or continuous home monitoring, teach the client and family how to apply and maintain the equipment. Remind them to rotate the site periodically and assess for skin trauma.

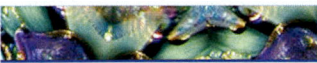

Focus on Critical Thinking

When you approach your elderly client to take her blood pressure, she tells you she doesn't want you to take it.
1. What questions will you ask the client at this time?

After much exploration, the client agrees to let you take the blood pressure. After pumping up the cuff, you are unable to hear any sounds during release of the valve.
1. What would you say to her?

Once you are able to measure the blood pressure, your reading is 180/110.

1. Before taking any action on this blood pressure, what do you need to know?
2. The pulse oximeter on the client's finger reads 85%. Her skin is warm and has normal color; she is awake and oriented, temperature is 37.1C (98.8F), apical pulse 78. What would be your next actions and why?

See Critical Thinking Possibilities in Appendix A.

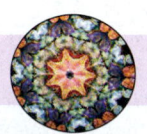

| Chapter Review

EXPLORE MediaLink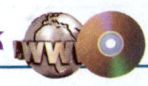

NCLEX review questions, case studies, care plan activities, MediaLink applications, and other interactive resources for this chapter can be found on the Companion Website at www.prenhall.com/kozier. Click on Chapter 27 to select the activities for this chapter.

For more NCLEX review questions, and an audio glossary, access the Student CD-ROM accompanying this textbook.

Chapter Highlights

- Vital signs reflect changes in body function that otherwise might not be observed.
- Body temperature is the balance between heat produced by the body and heat lost from the body.
- Factors affecting body temperature include age, diurnal variations, exercise, hormones, stress, and environmental temperatures.
- Four common types of fever are intermittent, remittent, relapsing, and constant. Clinical signs of fever vary during the onset, course, and abatement stages.
- During a fever, the set point of the hypothalamic thermostat changes suddenly from the normal level to a higher than normal level, but several hours elapse before the core temperature reaches the new set point.
- Hypothermia involves three mechanisms: excessive heat loss, inadequate heat production by body cells, and increasing impairment of hypothalamic thermoregulation.
- Body temperature can be measured orally, tympanically, rectally, or by axilla. The nurse selects the most appropriate site according to the client's age and condition.
- Pulse rate and volume reflect the stroke volume output, the compliance of the client's arteries, and the adequacy of blood flow.
- Normally a peripheral pulse reflects the client's heartbeat, but it may differ from the heartbeat in clients with certain cardiovascular diseases; in these instances, the nurse takes an apical pulse and compares it to the peripheral pulse.
- Many factors may affect a person's pulse rate: age, gender, exercise, presence of fever, certain medications, hypovolemia, stress, (in some situations) position changes, and pathology.
- Although the radial pulse is the site most commonly used, eight other sites may be used in certain situations.
- The difference between the apical and radial pulses is called pulse deficit.
- Respirations are normally quiet, effortless, and automatic and are assessed by observing respiratory rate, depth, rhythm, quality and effectiveness.
- Blood pressure reflects cardiac output, peripheral vascular resistance, blood volume, and blood viscosity.
- Among the factors influencing blood pressure are age, exercise, stress, race, gender, medications, obesity, diurnal variations, and disease processes.
- Orthostatic hypotension occurs when the blood pressure falls as the client assumes an upright position.
- A blood pressure cuff too large or too small will give false readings.
- During blood pressure measurement, the artery must be held at heart level.
- A pulse oximeter measures the percent of hemoglobin saturated with oxygen. A normal result is 95% to 100%.
- Pulse oximeter sensors may be placed on the finger, hand, foot, or nose.

Review Questions

27–1. When you take your client's temperature at 8:00 AM using an oral electronic thermometer, the result is 36.1C (97.2F). All other vital signs are within normal range. What would you do next?
   a. Wait 15 minutes and retake it.
   b. Check what the client's temperature was the last time.
   c. Retake it using a different thermometer.
   d. Chart the temperature; it is normal.

27–2. For which of the following clients would you take an apical pulse rather than a radial pulse?
   a. a client in shock
   b. to check a client's response to changing from a lying to a sitting position
   c. a client with an arrhythmia
   d. a client less than 24 hours postoperative

27–3. As a part of preparing a client for a test, you are to take vital signs. However, the client is on the phone. How would you handle taking the client's respiratory rate?
   a. Count the respirations during the time that the client is listening (rather than talking) on the phone.
   b. Tell the client that it is important to end the phone call now and resume it at a later time.

   c. Wait at the client's bedside until the phone call is completed and then count respirations.
   d. Record the measurement as "deferred" since the talking client is clearly not in respiratory distress and take it later.

27–4. For a client with a previous blood pressure of 138/74 and pulse of 64, approximately how long should the nurse take to release the blood pressure cuff in order to obtain an accurate reading?
   a. 10–20 seconds
   b. 30–45 seconds
   c. 1–1.5 minutes
   d. 3–3.5 minutes

27–5. In which of the following situations would it be most appropriate to delegate the taking of vital signs to a UAP?
   a. A patient being admitted for elective facial surgery and a history of stable hypertension.
   b. A patient receiving a blood transfusion with a history of transfusion reactions.
   c. A client recently started on a new antiarrhythmic agent
   d. A patient who is admitted frequently with asthma attacks.

Readings And References

Suggested Readings

Latman, N. S., Hans, P., Nicholson, L., DeLee-Zint, S., Lewis, K., & Shirey, A. (2001). Evaluation of clinical thermometers for accuracy and reliability. *Biomedical Instrumentation and Technology, 35,* 259–265. The authors of this study wanted to know if the new electronic, digital, infrared tympanic, and liquid crystal thermometers that have become so prevalent were as "good" as glass thermometers. They said it best: "All of the test instruments significantly underestimated higher temperatures and overestimated lower temperatures. This study indicated that the improvements in safety, speed, and ease of use of the newer clinical thermometers have been offset by a loss in accuracy and reliability. It also indicated that the current generation of electronic, digital clinical thermometers, in general, may not be sufficiently accurate or reliable to replace the traditional glass/mercury thermometers." Since safety concerns have all but eliminated mercury, is it possible to increase the accuracy of more modern thermometers? Food for thought.

Related Research

Hwu, Y., Coates, V. E., & Lin, F. (2000). A study of the effectiveness of different measuring times and counting methods of human radial pulse rates. *Journal of Clinical Nursing, 9,* 146–52.

Lanham, D. M., Walker, B., Klocke, E., & Jennings, M. (1999). Accuracy of tympanic temperature readings in children under 6 years of age. *Pediatric Nursing, 25*(1), 39–42.

Lee, V. K., McKenzie, N. E., & Cathcart, M. (1999). Ear and oral temperatures under usual practice conditions. *Research for Nursing Practice, 1*(1). Retrieved March 18, 2003, from http://www.graduateresearch.com/lee.htm

References

Bindler, R. C. & Ball, J. W., (2003). *Clinical skills manual for pediatric nursing: Caring for children* (3rd ed.). Upper Saddle River, NJ: Prentice Hall Health.

DuBois, E. F. (1948). *Fever and the Regulation of Body Temperature.* Springfield, IL: Charles C. Thomas.

Foster-Fitzpatrick, L., Ortiz, A., Sibilano, H., Marcantonio, R., & Braun, L. T. (1999). The effects of crossed leg on blood pressure measurement. *Nursing Research, 48,* 105–108.

Guyton, A. C. (1996). *Textbook of medical physiology* (9th ed.). Philadelphia: W. B. Saunders.

Johnson, M., Maas, M., & Moorhead, S. (Eds.). (2000). *Nursing outcomes classification (NOC)* (2nd ed.). St. Louis, MO: Mosby.

Ladewig, P. W., London, M. L., & Olds, S. B. (1998). *Maternal–newborn nursing care: The nurse, the family, and the community* (4th ed.). Menlo Park, CA: Addison Wesley Longman.

Lance, R., Link, M. E., Padua, M., Clavell, L. E., Johnson, G., & Knebel, E. (2000). Comparison of different methods of obtaining orthostatic vital signs. *Clinical Nursing Research, 9,* 479–491.

Marieb, E. N. (1998). *Human anatomy and physiology* (4th ed.). Menlo Park, CA: Benjamin/Cummings.

McCloskey, J. C., & Bulechek, G. M. (Eds.). (2000). *Nursing interventions classification (NIC)* (3rd ed.). St. Louis, MO: Mosby.

National Institutes of Health, National Heart, Lung, and Blood Institute. (1997). *The sixth report of the Joint National Committee on Prevention, Detection, Evaluation, and Treatment of High Blood Pressure* (NIH Publication #98-4080). Retrieved December 26, 2002, from http://www.nhlbi.nih.gov/guidelines/hypertension/jnc6.pdf

NANDA International. (2003). NANDA *nursing diagnoses: Definitions and classification 2003-2004.* Philadelphia: Author.

Selected Bibliography

Braun, S. K., Preston, P., & Smith, R. N. (1998). Getting a better read on thermometry. *RN, 61*(3), 57–60.

Bushey, P., Chulay, M., & Holland, S. (1997). Correlation of indirect blood pressure measurements and systemic blood pressure. *Critical Care Nurse, 17,* 12.

Carroll, M. (2000). An evaluation of temperature measurement. *Nursing Standard, 14*(44), 39–43.

Consult stat. (2000). Tips for getting more reliable O_2 saturation reading. *RN, 63*(2), 73.

Cowan, T. (1997). Product review: Ambulatory blood pressure monitors. *Professional Nurse, 12,* 373–376.

Faria, S. H. (1999). Assessment of vital signs in the child. *Home Care Provider, 4,* 222–223.

Faria, S. H. (1999). Patient assessment: Assessment of peripheral arterial pulses. *Home Care Provider, 4,* 140–141.

Graves, J. W. (1999). The clinical utility of out-of-office self-measurement of blood pressure. *Home Healthcare Consultant, 6*(11), 26–29.

Howell, M. (2002). Professional nurse study. The correct use of pulse oximetry in measuring oxygen status. *Professional Nurse, 17,* 416–418.

Jevon, P., Ewens, B., & Lowe, R. (2001). Practical procedures for nurses: Measuring apex and radial pulse. *Nursing Times, 96*(50), 43–44.

Karch, A. M., & Karch, F. E. (2000). Practice errors: When a blood pressure isn't routine. *American Journal of Nursing, 100*(3), 23.

McConnell, E. A. (1999). Do's & don'ts: Performing pulse oximetry. *Nursing, 29*(11), 17.

McConnell, E. A. (2000). Do's & don'ts: Using a Doppler device. *Nursing, 30*(7), 17.

Nicholls, P. H. (1997). Consult stat. Wrist and finger BP monitors offer accurate alternatives. *RN, 60,* 64.

Nicoll, L. H. (2002). Heat in motion: Evaluating and managing temperature. *Nursing, 32*(5 Supp.), 1–10.

O'Toole, S. (1998). Temperature measurement devices. *Professional Nurse, 13,* 779–782.

Schiff, L. (2000). Pulse oximeters. *RN 63*(8), 65–66, 68.

Torrance, C., & Elley, K. (1997). Practical procedures for nurses: Assessing pulse—2. *Nursing Times, 93*(42), insert 2.

Torrance, C., & Semple, M. (1997). Practical procedures for nurses: Assessing pulse—1. *Nursing Times, 93*(41), insert 2.

Weiss, M. E., Sitzer, V., Clarke, M., Haley, K., Richards, M., Sanchez, A., et al. (1998). A comparison of temperature measurements using three ear thermometers. *Applied Nursing Research, 11,* 158–166.

Woo, E. K. (1998). Device errors: Infant skin temperature probes: Follow these safety tips for use. *Nursing, 27*(7), 31.

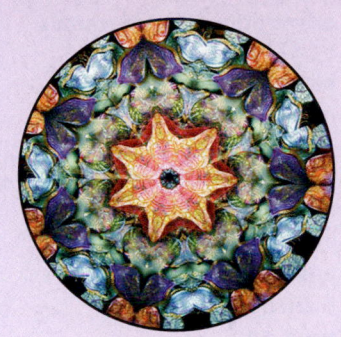

CHAPTER 28

HEALTH ASSESSMENT

LEARNING OUTCOMES

- Identify the purposes of the physical health examination.
- Explain the four methods of examining.
- Explain the significance of selected physical findings.
- Identify expected outcomes of health assessment.
- Identify the steps in selected examination procedures.
- Describe suggested sequencing to conduct a physical health examination in an orderly fashion.
- Discuss variations in examination techniques appropriate for clients of different ages.

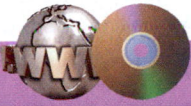

MediaLink

www.prenhall.com/kozier

Additional resources for this chapter can be found on the Student CD-ROM accompanying this textbook, and on the Companion Website at www.prenhall.com/kozier. Click on Chapter 28 to select the activities for this chapter.

CD-ROM
- Audio Glossary
- NCLEX Review
- Animations:
     Otoscope Examination
     Middle Ear Dynamics
     Ear Abnormalities
     Mouth and Throat

Companion Website
- Additional NCLEX Review
- Case Study: Performing Physical Assessments
- MediaLink Applications: Physical Exam
- Links to Resources

Assessing a client's health status is a major component of nursing care and has two aspects: (1) the nursing health history discussed in Chapter 16 ∞ and (2) the physical examination discussed in this chapter. A physical examination can be any of three types: (a) a complete assessment (e.g., when a client is admitted to a health care agency); (b) examination of a body system (e.g., the cardiovascular system); (c) examination of a body area (e.g., the lungs, when difficulty with breathing is observed). *Note:* Some nurses consider *assessment* to be the broad term used in applying the nursing process to health data and *examination* to be the physical process used to gather the data. In this text, the terms *assessment* and *examination* are sometimes used interchangeably—both referring to a critical investigation and evaluation of client status.

PHYSICAL HEALTH ASSESSMENT

A complete health assessment may be conducted starting at the head and proceeding in a systematic manner downward (head-to-toe assessment). However, the procedure can vary according to the age of the individual, the severity of the illness, the preferences of the nurse, the location of the examination, and the agency's priorities and procedures. The order of head-to-toe assessment is given in Box 28–1. Regardless of the procedure used, the client's energy and time need to be considered. The health assessment is therefore conducted in a systematic and efficient manner that results in the fewest position changes for the client.

Frequently, nurses assess a specific body area instead of the entire body. These specific assessments are made in relation to client complaints, the nurse's own observation of problems, the client's presenting problem, nursing interventions provided, and medical therapies. Examples of these situations and assessments are provided in Table 28–1.

These are some of the purposes of the physical examination:

- To obtain baseline data about the client's functional abilities
- To supplement, confirm, or refute data obtained in the nursing history
- To obtain data that will help establish nursing diagnoses and plan of care
- To evaluate the physiologic outcomes of health care and thus the progress of a client's health problem

---

BOX 28–1 ■ Head-to-Toe Framework

- General survey
- Vital signs
- Head
  - Hair, scalp, cranium, face
  - Eyes and vision
  - Ears and hearing
  - Nose and sinuses
  - Mouth and oropharynx
  - Cranial nerves
- Neck
  - Muscles
  - Lymph nodes
  - Trachea
  - Thyroid gland
  - Carotid arteries
  - Neck veins
- Upper extremities
  - Skin and nails
  - Muscle strength and tone
  - Joint range of motion
  - Brachial and radial pulses
  - Biceps tendon reflexes
  - Tendon reflexes
  - Sensation

- Chest and back
  - Skin
  - Chest shape and size
  - Lungs
  - Heart
  - Spinal column
  - Breasts and axillae
- Abdomen
  - Skin
  - Abdominal sounds
  - Specific organs (e.g., liver, bladder)
  - Femoral pulses
- Genitals
  - Testicles
  - Vagina
  - Urethra
- Anus and rectum
- Lower extremities
  - Skin and toenails
  - Gait and balance
  - Joint range of motion
  - Popliteal, posterior tibial, and pedal pulses
  - Tendon and plantar reflexes

TABLE 28–1 Nursing Assessments Addressing Selected Client Situations

Situation	Physical Assessment
Client complains of abdominal pain.	Inspect, auscultate, and palpate the abdomen; assess vital signs.
Client is admitted with a head injury.	Assess level of consciousness using Glasgow Coma Scale (see Table 28–10 later in this chapter); assess pupils for reaction to light and accommodation; assess vital signs.
The nurse prepares to administer a cardiotonic drug to a client.	Assess apical pulse and compare with baseline data.
The client has just had a cast applied to the lower leg.	Assess peripheral perfusion of toes, capillary blanch test, pedal pulse if able, and vital signs.
The client's fluid intake is minimal.	Assess tissue turgor, fluid intake and output, and vital signs.

- To make clinical judgments about a client's health status
- To identify areas for health promotion and disease prevention.

When screening for cancer, nurses should keep in mind the American Cancer Society's guidelines for early detection (see Box 28–2).

Preparing the Client

Most people need an explanation of the physical examination. The nurse should explain when and where it will take place, why it is important, and what will happen during the examination. Health

---

BOX 28–2 ■ Cancer Screening Guidelines for Asymptomatic People

Colorectal Cancer (Males and Females)
- Digital rectal examination annually beginning at age 40
- Fecal occult blood test annually beginning at age 50
- Sigmoidoscopy every 5 years beginning at age 50
- Colonoscopy every 10 years or double contrast barium enema every 5 to 10 years

Breast Cancer (Females)
- Monthly breast self-examination beginning at age 20
- Clinical breast examination every 3 years from age 20 to 40, and then annually beginning at age 40
- Mammogram annually at age 40 and over

Cervical and Uterine Cancer (Females)
- Papanicolaou (Pap) smear annually for all women who are or who have been sexually active or have reached age 18 (After a woman has had three or more consecutive satisfactory normal annual examinations, the Pap test may be performed less frequently at the discretion of her physician.)
- Pelvic examination every 1 to 3 years with Pap test beginning at age 18 to age 40, and annually for women over 40
- Endometrial tissue sample at menopause and if at high risk and thereafter at the discretion of the physician

Prostate Cancer (Males)
- Prostate-specific antigen (PSA) and digital rectal examination annually beginning at age 50 for men who have at least a 10-year life expectancy and for younger men who are at high risk

Health Counseling and Cancer Checkup (Males and Females)
- Examination for cancers of the thyroid, testicles, ovaries, lymph nodes, oral region, and skin every 3 years over age 20 and annually over age 40

Note: From "American Cancer Society Recommendations for Early Detection of Cancer," by R. A. Smith, et al., 2002, *CA: A Cancer Journal for Clinicians, 52,* pp. 8–22.

BOX 28–3	■ Health Assessment of the Adult

- Be aware of normal physiologic changes that occur with age.
- Be aware of stiffness of muscles and joints from aging changes or history of orthopedic surgery. The client may need modification of the usual positioning necessary for examination and assessment.
- Expose only areas of the body to be examined in order to avoid chilling.
- Permit ample time for the client to answer your questions and assume the required positions.
- Be aware of cultural differences. The client may want a family member present during disrobing.
- Arrange for an interpreter if the client's language differs from that of the nurse.
- Ask clients how they wish to be addressed, such as Mrs. or Miss.
- Adapt assessment techniques to any sensory impairment; for example, make sure eyeglasses or hearing aids are nearby.

examinations are usually painless; however, it is important to determine in advance any positions that are contraindicated for a particular client. The nurse assists the client as needed to undress and put on a gown.

Clients should empty their bladders before the examination. Doing so helps them feel more relaxed and facilitates palpation of the abdomen and pubic area. If a urinalysis is required, the urine should be collected in a container for that purpose.

When assessing adults it is important to recognize that people of the same age differ markedly. Box 28–3 provides special considerations for assessing adults, especially elders.

If clients are elderly and/or frail it is wise to plan several assessment times in order to not overtire them. Often clients are anxious about what the nurse will find. They can be reassured during the examination by explanations at each step.

The sequence of the assessment differs with children and adults. With children, always proceed from the least invasive or uncomfortable to the more invasive. Examination of the head and neck, heart and lungs, and range of motion can be done early in the process, while the ears, mouth, abdomen, and genitals should be left for the end of the exam.

Preparing the Environment

It is important to prepare the environment before starting the assessment. The time for the physical assessment should be convenient to both the client and the nurse. The environment needs to be well lighted and the equipment should be organized for use.

Providing privacy is important. Most people are embarrassed if their bodies are exposed or if others can overhear or view them during the assessment. Family and friends should not be present unless the client asks for someone.

A client who is physically relaxed will usually experience little discomfort. The room should be warm enough to be comfortable for the client.

Positioning

Several positions are frequently required during the physical assessment. It is important to consider the client's ability to assume a position. The client's physical condition, energy level, and age should also be taken into consideration. Some positions are embarrassing and uncomfortable and therefore should not be maintained for long. The assessment is organized so that several body areas can be assessed in one position, thus minimizing the number of position changes needed (see Table 28–2).

Draping

Drapes should be arranged so that the area to be assessed is exposed and other body areas are covered. Exposure of the body is frequently embarrassing to clients. Drapes provide not only a degree of privacy but also warmth. Drapes are made of paper, cloth, or bed linen.

Instrumentation

All equipment required for the health assessment should be clean, in good working order, and readily accessible. Equipment is frequently set up on trays, ready for use.

Various instruments are shown in Table 28–3.

Methods of Examining

Four primary techniques are used in the physical examination: inspection, palpation, percussion, and auscultation. These techniques are discussed throughout this chapter as they apply to each body system.

Inspection

Inspection is the visual examination, that is, assessing by using the sense of sight. It should be deliberate, purposeful, and systematic. The nurse inspects with the naked eye and with a lighted instrument such as an otoscope (used to view the ear). In addition to visual observations, olfactory (smell) and auditory (hearing) cues are noted. Nurses frequently use visual inspection to assess moisture, color, and texture of body surfaces, as well as shape, position, size, color, and symmetry of the body. Lighting must be sufficient for the nurse to see clearly; either natural or artificial light can be used. When using the auditory senses it is important to have a quiet environment for accurate hearing. Observation can be combined with the other assessment techniques.

Palpation

Palpation is the examination of the body using the sense of touch. The pads of the fingers are used because their concentration of nerve endings makes them highly sensitive to tactile discrimination. Palpation is used to determine (a) texture (e.g., of the hair); (b) temperature (e.g., of a skin area); (c) vibration (e.g., of a joint); (d) position, size, consistency, and mobility of organs or masses; (e) distention (e.g., of the urinary bladder); (f) pulsation; and (g) the presence of pain upon pressure.

TABLE 28–2 Client Positions and Body Areas Assessed

Position	Description	Areas Assessed	Cautions
Dorsal recumbent	Back-lying position with knees flexed and hips externally rotated; small pillow under the head; soles of feet on the surface	Head and neck, axillae, anterior thorax, lungs, breasts, heart, extremities, peripheral pulses, vital signs, and vagina	May be contraindicated for clients who have cardio-pulmonary problems. Not used for abdominal assessment because of the increased tension of abdominal muscles.
Supine (Horizontal recumbent)	Back-lying position with legs extended; with or without pillow under the head	Head, neck, axillae, anterior thorax, lungs, breasts, heart, abdomen, extremities, peripheral pulses	Tolerated poorly by clients with cardiovascular and respiratory problems.
Sitting	A seated position, back unsupported and legs hanging freely	Head, neck, posterior and anterior thorax, lungs, breasts, axillae, heart, vital signs, upper and lower extremities, reflexes	Elderly and weak clients may require support.
Lithotomy	Back-lying position with feet supported in stirrups; the hips should be in line with the edge of the table.	Female genitals, rectum, and female reproductive tract	May be uncomfortable and tiring for elderly people and often embarrassing.
Sims'	Side-lying position with lowermost arm behind the body, uppermost leg flexed at hip and knee, upper arm flexed at shoulder and elbow	Rectum, vagina	Difficult for the elderly and people with limited joint movement.
Prone	Lies on abdomen with head turned to the side, with or without a small pillow	Posterior thorax, hip joint movement	Often not tolerated by the elderly and people with cardiovascular and respiratory problems.

There are two types of palpation: light and deep. *Light (superficial) palpation* should always precede *deep palpation* because heavy pressure on the fingertips can dull the sense of touch. For light palpation, the nurse extends the dominant hand's fingers parallel to the skin surface and presses gently while moving the hand in a circle (see Figure 28–1 ■ on page 529). With light palpation, the skin is slightly depressed. If it is necessary to determine the details of a mass, the nurse presses lightly several times rather than holding the pressure. See Box 28–4 on page 529 for the characteristics of masses.

Deep palpation is done with two hands (bimanually) or one hand. In deep bimanual palpation, the nurse extends the dominant hand as for light palpation, then places the fingerpads of

the nondominant hand on the dorsal surface of the distal interphalangeal joint of the middle three fingers of the dominant hand (Figure 28–2 ■). The top hand applies pressure while the lower hand remains relaxed to perceive the tactile sensations. For deep palpation using one hand, the fingerpads of the dominant hand press over the area to be palpated. Often the other hand is used to support a mass or organ from below (Figure 28–3 ■). *Deep palpation is done with extreme caution because pressure can damage internal organs. It is usually not indicated in clients who have acute abdominal pain or pain that is not yet diagnosed.*

To test skin temperature, it is best to use the dorsum or back of the hand and fingers, where the skin is thinnest. To test for

TABLE 28-3 Equipment and Supplies Used for a Health Examination

Supplies		Purpose
Flashlight or penlight		To assist viewing of the pharynx and cervix or to determine the reactions of the pupils of the eye
Laryngeal or dental mirror		To observe the pharynx and oral cavity
Nasal speculum		To permit visualization of the lower and middle turbinates; usually, a penlight is used for illumination
Ophthalmoscope		A lighted instrument to visualize the interior of the eye
Otoscope		A lighted instrument to visualize the eardrum and external auditory canal (a nasal speculum may be attached to the otoscope to inspect the nasal cavities)
Percussion (reflex) hammer		An instrument with a rubber head to test reflexes
Tuning fork		A two-pronged metal instrument used to test hearing acuity and vibratory sense
Vaginal speculum		To assess the cervix and the vagina
Cotton applicators		To obtain specimens
Disposable pads		To absorb liquid
Gloves		To protect the nurse
Lubricant		To ease insertion of instruments (e.g., vaginal speculum)
Tongue blades (depressors)		To depress the tongue during assessment of the mouth and pharynx

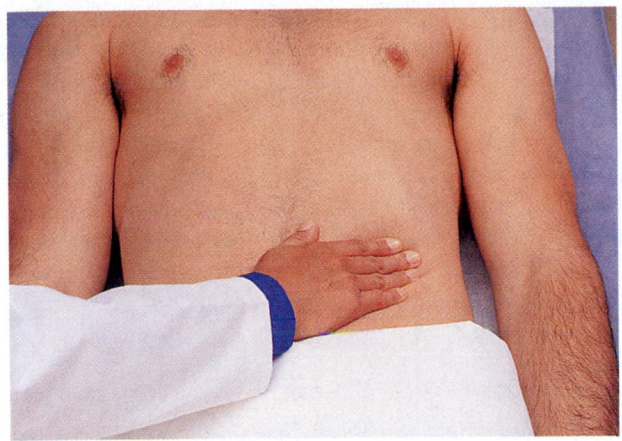

Figure 28–1 ■ The position of the hand for light palpation.

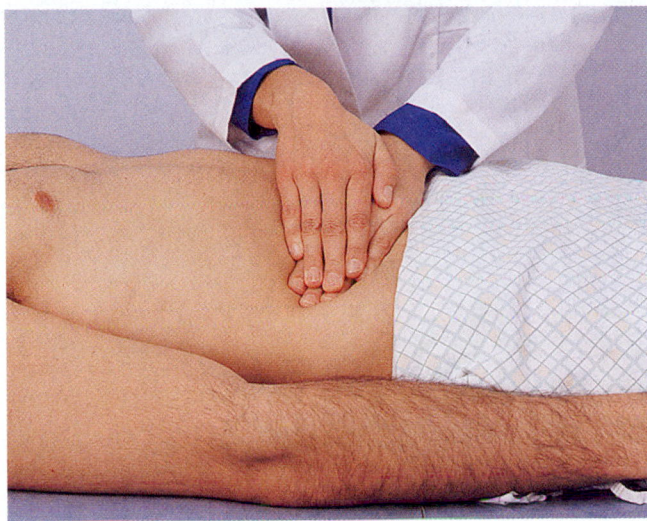

Figure 28–2 ■ The position of the hands for deep bimanual palpation.

vibration, the nurse should use the palmar surface of the hand. General guidelines for palpation include the following:

- The nurse's hands should be clean and warm, and the fingernails short.
- Areas of tenderness should be palpated last.
- Deep palpation should be done after superficial palpation.

The effectiveness of palpation depends largely on the client's relaxation. Nurses can assist a client to relax by (a) gowning and/or draping the client appropriately, (b) positioning the client comfortably, and (c) ensuring that their own hands are warm before beginning. During palpation, the nurse should be sensitive to the client's verbal and facial expressions indicating discomfort.

Percussion

Percussion is the act of striking the body surface to elicit sounds that can be heard or vibrations that can be felt. There are two types of percussion: direct and indirect. In *direct percussion,* the nurse strikes the area to be percussed directly with the pads of two, three, or four fingers or with the pad of the middle finger. The strikes are rapid, and the movement is from the wrist (see Figure 28–4 ■). This technique is not generally used to percuss the thorax but is useful in percussing an adult's sinuses.

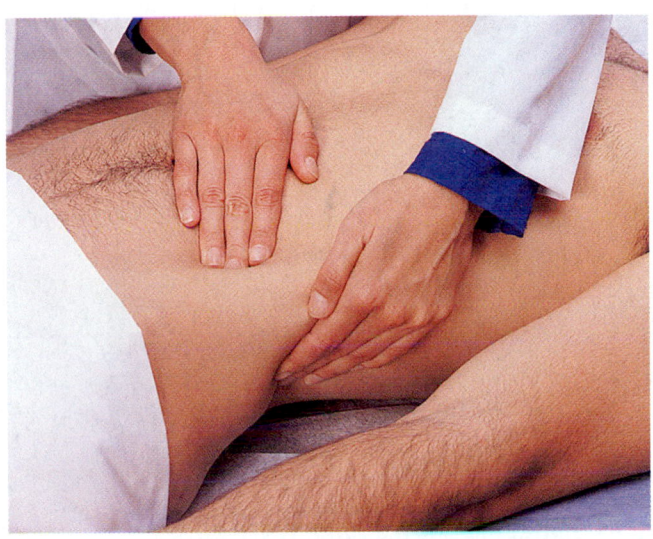

Figure 28–3 ■ Deep palpation using the lower hand to support the body while the upper hand palpates the organ.

Indirect percussion is the striking of an object (e.g., a finger) held against the body area to be examined. In this technique, the middle finger of the nondominant hand, referred to as the **pleximeter,** is placed firmly on the client's skin. Only the distal phalanx and joint of this finger should be in contact with the skin. Using the tip of the flexed middle finger of the other hand, called the **plexor,** the nurse strikes the pleximeter, usually at the distal interphalangeal joint (see Figure 28–5 ■). Some nurses may find a point between the distal and proximal joints to be a more comfortable pleximeter point. The motion comes from the wrist; the forearm remains stationary. The angle between the plexor and the pleximeter should be 90 degrees, and the blows must be firm, rapid, and short to obtain a clear sound.

Percussion is used to determine the size and shape of internal organs by establishing their borders. It indicates

---

BOX 28–4   ■ Characteristics of Masses

Location—Site on the body, dorsal/ventral surface
Size—Length and width in centimeters
Shape—Oval, round, elongated, irregular
Consistency—Soft, firm, hard
Surface—Smooth, nodular
Mobility—Fixed, mobile
Pulsatility—Present or absent
Tenderness—Degree of tenderness to palpation

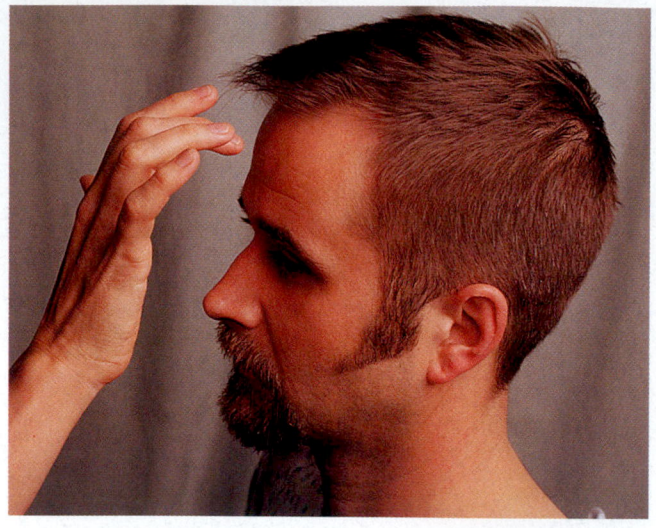

Figure 28-4 ■ Direct percussion. Using one hand to strike the surface of the body.

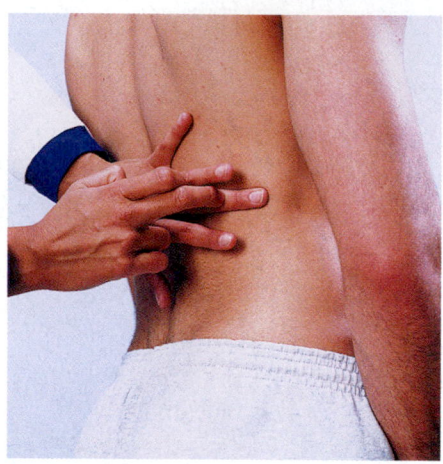

Figure 28-5 ■ Indirect percussion. Using the finger of one hand to tap the finger of the other hand.

whether tissue is fluid filled, air filled, or solid. Percussion elicits five types of sound: flatness, dullness, resonance, hyperresonance, and tympany. **Flatness** is an extremely dull sound produced by very dense tissue, such as muscle or bone. **Dullness** is a thudlike sound produced by dense tissue

such as the liver, spleen, or heart. **Resonance** is a hollow sound such as that produced by lungs filled with air. **Hyperresonance** is not produced in the normal body. It is described as booming and can be heard over an emphysematous lung. **Tympany** is a musical or drumlike sound produced from an air-filled stomach. On a continuum, flatness reflects the most dense tissue (the least amount of air) and tympany the least dense tissue (the greatest amount of air). A percussion sound is described according to its intensity, pitch, duration, and quality (see Table 28-4).

Auscultation

Auscultation is the process of listening to sounds produced within the body. Auscultation may be direct or indirect. *Direct auscultation* is the use of the unaided ear, for example, to listen to a respiration wheeze or the grating of a moving joint. *Indirect auscultation* is the use of a stethoscope, which transmits the sounds to the nurse's ears. A stethoscope is used primarily to listen to sounds from within the body, such as bowel sounds or valve sounds of the heart and blood pressure.

The stethoscope should be 30 to 35 cm (12 to 14 in.) long, with an internal diameter of about 0.3 cm (1/8 in.). It should have both a flat-disc and a bell-shaped diaphragm (see Figure 27-22 on page 502). The flat-disc diaphragm best transmits high-pitched sounds (e.g., bronchial sounds) and the bell-shaped diaphragm best transmits low-pitched sounds, such as some heart sounds. The earpieces of the stethoscope should fit comfortably into the nurse's ears with the earpieces facing forward. The diaphragm of the stethoscope is placed firmly but lightly against the client's skin. If a client is very hairy, it may be necessary to dampen the hairs with a moist cloth so that they will lie flat against the skin and not cause scratching sounds.

Auscultated sounds are described according to their pitch, intensity, duration, and quality. The **pitch** is the frequency of the vibrations (the number of vibrations per second). Low-pitched sounds, such as some heart sounds, have fewer vibrations per second than high-pitched sounds, such as bronchial sounds. The **intensity** (amplitude) refers to the loudness or softness of a sound. Some body sounds are loud, for example, bronchial sounds heard from the trachea; others are soft, for example, normal breath sounds heard in the lungs. The **duration** of a sound is its length (long or short). The **quality** of sound is

TABLE 28-4 Percussion Sounds and Tones					
Sound	**Intensity**	**Pitch**	**Duration**	**Quality**	**Example of Location**
Flatness	Soft	High	Short	Extremely dull	Muscle, bone
Dullness	Medium	Medium	Moderate	Thudlike	Liver, heart
Resonance	Loud	Low	Long	Hollow	Normal lung
Hyperresonance	Very loud	Very low	Very long	Booming	Emphysematous lung
Tympany	Loud	High (distinguished mainly by musical timbre)	Moderate	Musical	Stomach filled with gas (air)

a subjective description of a sound, for example, whistling, gurgling, or snapping.

GENERAL SURVEY

Health assessment begins with a general survey that involves observation of the client's general appearance and mental status, and measurement of vital signs, height, and weight. Many components of the general survey are assessed while taking the client's health history, such as the client's body build, posture, hygiene, and mental status.

Appearance and Mental Status

The general appearance and behavior of an individual must be assessed in relationship to culture, educational level, socioeconomic status, and current circumstances. For example, an individual who has recently experienced a personal loss may appropriately appear depressed. Also, the client's age, sex, and race are useful factors in interpreting findings that suggest increased risk for known conditions. Procedure 28–1 describes how to assess general appearance and mental status.

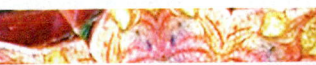 **Procedure 28-1 Assessing Appearance and Mental Status**

PLANNING

Delegation

Due to the substantial knowledge and skill required, assessment of general appearance and mental status is not delegated to unlicensed assistive personnel. However, many aspects are observed during usual care and may be recorded by persons other than the nurse. Abnormal findings must be validated and interpreted by the nurse.

Equipment
None

IMPLEMENTATION

Performance

1. Explain to the client what you are going to do, why it is necessary, and how he or she can cooperate. Discuss how the results will be used in planning further care or treatments.

2. Wash hands and observe appropriate infection control procedures.
3. Provide for client privacy.

Assessment	Normal Findings	Deviations from Normal
4. Observe body build, height, and weight in relation to the client's age, lifestyle, and health.	Proportionate, varies with lifestyle	Excessively thin or obese
5. Observe the client's posture and gait, standing, sitting, and walking.	Relaxed, erect posture; coordinated movement	Tense, slouched, bent posture; uncoordinated movement; tremors
6. Observe the client's overall hygiene and grooming. Relate these to the person's activities prior to the assessment.	Clean, neat	Dirty, unkempt
7. Note body and breath odor in relation to activity level.	No body odor or minor body odor relative to work or exercise; no breath odor	Foul body odor; ammonia odor; acetone breath odor; foul breath
8. Observe for signs of distress in posture or facial expression.	No distress noted.	Bending over because of abdominal pain, wincing, or labored breathing
9. Note obvious signs of health or illness (e.g., in skin color or breathing).	Healthy appearance	Pallor; weakness; obvious illness
10. Assess the client's attitude.	Cooperative	Negative, hostile, withdrawn
11. Note the client's affect/mood; assess the appropriateness of the client's responses.	Appropriate to situation	Inappropriate to situation
12. Listen for quantity of speech (amount and pace), quality (loudness, clarity, inflection), and organization (coherence of thought, overgeneralization, vagueness).	Understandable, moderate pace; exhibits thought association	Rapid or slow pace; uses generalizations; lacks association; exhibits confabulation
13. Listen for relevance and organization of thoughts.	Logical sequence; makes sense; has sense of reality	Illogical sequence; flight of ideas; confusion

14. Document findings in the client record using forms or checklists supplemented by narrative notes when appropriate (see Figure 28–6 ■).

continued on page 532

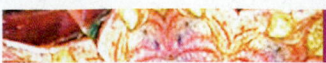

ADMISSION DATA

Date 4-16-03 Time 3:15p.m. Primary Language English

Arrived Via: ☐ Wheelchair ☐ Stretcher ☑ Ambulatory

From: ☐ Admitting ☐ ER ☑ Home ☐ Nursing Home ☐ Other

Admitting M.D. R. Katz   Time Notified 5 p.m.

ORIENTATION TO UNIT

	YES	NO		YES	NO
Arm Band Correct	☑	☐	Visiting Hours	☑	☐
Allergy Band	☑	☐	Smoking Policy	☑	☐
Telephone	☑	☐	TV, Lights, Bed Controls,		
Electrical Policy	☑	☐	Call Lights, Side Rails	☑	☐
Educational Mat'l	☑	☐	Nurses Station	☑	☐
(TV Brochure)	☑	☐			

Family M.D. R. Katz

Weight 125 lb. Height 5ft. 2in.   BP:R — L 122/80

Temp. 103F Pulse 92, weak Resp 28, shallow

Source Providing Information ☑ Patient ☐ Other

Unable to Obtain History ☐

Reason for Admission (Onset, Duration, Pt.'s Perception) "Chest cold" X2 weeks S.O.B on exertion. "Lung pain, fever," "Dr. says I have pneumonia."

ALLERGIES & REACTIONS

Drugs Penicillin

Food/Other

Signs & Symptoms rash, nausea

Blood Reaction ☐ Yes ☑ No Dyes/Shellfish ☐ Yes ☑ No

MEDICATIONS

Current Meds	Dose/Freq.	Last Dose
Synthroid	0.1 mg. daily	4-16, 8 a.m.

Disposition of Meds: ☑ Home ☐ Pharmacy ☐ Safe *At Bedside

MEDICAL HISTORY

☑ No Major Problems   ☐ Gastro

☐ Cardiac   ☐ Arthritis

☐ Hyper/Hypotension   ☐ Stroke

☐ Diabetes   ☐ Seizures

☐ Cancer   ☐ Glaucoma

☐ Respiratory   ☑ Other Childbirth-1998

Surgery/Procedures	Date
Appendectomy	1989
Partial thyroidectomy	1996

SPECIAL ASSISTIVE DEVICES

☐ Wheelchair ☐ Contacts ☐ Venous ☐ Dentures
☐ Braces ☐ Hearing Aid   Access ☐ Partial
☐ Cane/Crutches ☐ Prosthesis Device ☐ Upper
☐ Walker ☐ Glasses ☐ Epidural Catheter ☐ Lower
☐ Other None

VALUABLES

Patient informed Hospital not responsible for personal belongings.

Valuables Disposition: ☐ Patient ☐ Safe ☐ Given to

Patient/SO Signature None

PSYCHOSOCIAL HISTORY

Recent Stress None

Coping Mechanism Not assessed because of fatigue

Support System Husband, coworkers, friends

Calm: ☑ Yes ☐ No

Anxious: ☐ Yes ☐ No Facial muscles tense; trembling

Religion Catholic. Would want Last Rites

Tobacco Use: ☐ Yes ☑ No

Alcohol Use: ☐ Yes ☑ No

Drug Use: ☐ Yes ☑ No

NEUROLOGICAL

Oriented: ☑ Person ☑ Place ☑ Time ☐ Confused ☐ Sedated
☐ Alert ☐ Restless ☑ Lethargic ☐ Comatose

Pupils: ☑ Equal ☐ Unequal ☑ Reactive ☐ Sluggish
☐ Other 3mm.

Extremity Strength: ☑ Equal ☐ Unequal

Speech: ☑ Clear ☐ Slurred ☐ Other

MUSCULO-SKELETAL

Normal ROM of Extremities ☑ Yes ☐ No

☑ Weakness ☐ Paralysis ☐ Contractures ☐ Joint Swelling ☑ Pain
☐ Other ↓ related to fatigue   when coughing

RESPIRATORY

Pattern: ☐ Even ☐ Uneven ☑ Shallow ☑ Dyspnea
☑ Other diminished breath sounds

Breathing Sounds: ☐ Clear ☑ Other inspiratory crackles

Secretions: ☐ None ☑ Other pink, thick sputum

Cough: ☐ None ☑ Productive ☐ Nonproductive

CARDIOVASCULAR

Pulses: Apical Rate 92-W ☑ Reg. ☐ Irregular ☐ Pacemaker
S = Strong W = Weak A = Absent D = Doppler

Radial R 92 L — Pedal R — L —

Edema: ☑ Absent ☐ Present Site

Perfusion: ☐ Warm ☐ Dry ☑ Diaphoretic ☐ Cool (Hot)

GASTROINTESTINAL

Oral Mucosa ☐ Normal ☑ Other pale and dry

Bowel Sounds: ☑ Normal ☐ Other Abd. soft

Wt. Change: ☐ ☑ N/V Stool Frequency/Character 1/day; soft

Last B/M 4-15-0 ☐ Ostomy (type)

Equip.

GENITOURINARY

Urine: Last Voided This morning

☐ Normal ☐ Anuria ☐ Hematuria ☐ Dysuri ☐ Incontinent

☑ Other ↓ amount & frequency since ill

☐ Catheter (type) Other

LMP 4-1-03 ☐ Vaginal/Penile Discharge

Other

SELF CARE

Need Assist with: ☐ Ambulating ☐ Elimination
☐ Meals ☑ Hygiene ☐ Dressing
While fatigued

Amanda Aquilini [F. age 28]
#4637651   DOB 11-02-74

⚹⚹ NORTH BROWARD HOSPITAL DISTRICT
NURSING ADMINISTRATION ASSESSMENT

Figure 28–6 ■ Nursing assessment form.

NUTRITION

General Appearance: ☑ Well Nourished ☐ Emaciated
☐ Other _____
Appetite: ☐ Good ☐ Fair ☑ Poor -×2 days
Diet __Liquid__ Meal Pattern __3/day__
☐ Feeds Self ☐ Assist ☐ Total Feed

SKIN ASSESSMENT

Color: ☐ Normal ☐ Flushed ☑ Pale ☐ Dusky ☐ Cyanotic
☐ Jaundiced ☑ Other __Cheeks flushed, hot__
General Description __Surgical scars:__
__RLQ abdomen; anterior neck__
_____
_____

Note Cultures Obtained _____
_____

PRESSURE SORE ™AT RISK∫ SCREENING CRITERIA

OVERALL SKIN CONDITION
Grade
	0	Turgor (elasticity adequate, skin warm and moist)
✓	1	Poor turgor, skin cold & dry
	2	Areas mottled, red or denuded
	3	Existing skin ulcer/lesions

BOWEL AND BLADDER CONTROL
Grade
✓	0	Always able to ask for bedpan
	1	Incontinence of urine
	2	Incontinence of feces
	3	Totally incontinent Confined to bed

REHABILITATIVE STATE
Grade
	0	Fully ambulatory
✓	1	Ambulated with assistance
	2	Chair to bed ambulation only
	3	Confined to bed
	4	Immobile in bed

NUTRITIONAL STATE
Grade
	0	Eats all
✓	1	Eats very little
	2	Refuses food often
	3	Tube feeding
	4	Intravenous feeding

MENTAL STATE
Grade
✓	0	Alert and clear
	1	Confused
	2	Disoriented/senile
	3	Stuporous
	4	Unconcious

CHRONIC DISEASE STATUS (i.e. COPD, ASCVD. Peripheral Vascular Disease, Diabetes, or Renal Disease, Cancer, Motor or Sensory Deficits, Elderly, Other)
Grade
✓	0	Absent
	1	One Present
	2	Two Present
	3	Three or more Present

TOTAL _____ Refer to Skin Care Protocol

FALLS SCREENING

If one or more of the following are checked institute fall precautions/plan of care
☐ History of Falls ☐ Unsteady Gait ☐ Confusion/Disorientation ☐ Dizziness

If two or more of the following are checked institute fall precautions/plan of care
☐ Age over 80 ☐ Utilizes cane, walker, w/c ☐ Sleeplessness
☐ Impaired vision ☐ Urgency/frequency in elimination
☐ Multiple Diagnoses ☐ Impaired hearing
☐ Inability to understand or follow directions ☐ Medication/Sedative /Diuretic etc.

NURSE SIGNATURE/TITLE	DATE	TIME
Mary Medina, RN	4-16-03	3:30pm
NURSE SIGNATURE/TITLE	DATE	TIME

EDUCATION/DISCHARGE PLANNING

1. What do you know about your present illness? __"Dr. says I have pneumonia." "I will have an I.V."__
2. What information do you want or need about your illness? _____
3. Would you like family/SO involved in your care? __Husband, Michael__
4. How long do you expect to be in the hospital? __"1-2 days"__
5. What concerns do you have about leaving the hospital? _____

CHECK APPROPRIATE BOX

Will patient need post discharge assistance with ADLs/physical functioning? ☐ Yes ☑ No ☐ Unknown
Does patient have family capable of and willing to provide assistance post discharge?
☑ Yes ☐ No ☐ Unknown ☐ No family
Is assistance needed beyond that which family can provide?
☐ Yes ☑ No ☐ Unknown
Previous admission in the last six months?
☐ Yes ☑ No ☐ Unknown
Patient lives with __Husband and 1 child__
Planned discharge to __Home__
Comments: __Fatigue and anxiety may have interfered with learning. Re-teach anything covered at admission, later.__

Social Services Notified ☐ Yes ☑ No

NARRATIVE NOTES

S--c/O sharp chest pain when coughing and dyspnea on exertion. States unable to carry out regular daily exercise for past week. Coughing relieved "if I sit up and sit still." Nausea associated with coughing. Having occasional "chills." Occasionally becomes frightened, stating, "I can't breathe." Well groomed but "too tired to put on make-up."

O--Chest expansion < 3cm, no nasal flaring or use of accessory muscles. Breath sounds and insp. crackles in ® upper and lower chest.
Assesses own supports as "good" (eg, relationship c̄ husband). Is "worried" about daughter. States husband will be out of town until tomorrow. Left 3-year-old daughter with neighbor. Concerned too about her work (is attorney). "I'll never get caught up." Had water at noon—no food today. Informed of need to save urine for 24 hr. specimen. IV D₅W LR 1000 mL started in ®arm, 100 mL/hr. Slow capillary refill. Keeping head of bed↑ to facilitate breathing.

❋❋ **NORTH BROWARD HOSPITAL DISTRICT NURSING ADMINISTRATION ASSESSMENT**

Figure 28-6 ■ *(continued)*

continued on page 534

Procedure 28-1 Assessing Appearance and Mental Status *continued*

EVALUATION

- Perform a detailed follow-up examination of other individual systems based on findings that deviated from expected or normal for the client. Relate findings to previous assessment data if available.

- Report significant deviations from normal to the physician.

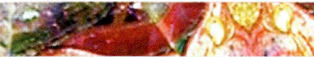

Lifespan Considerations

General Survey

Infants
- Measure height of children under age 2 in the supine position with knees fully extended.
- Weigh without clothing.
- Include measurement of head circumference until age 2.

Children
- Weigh in underwear only.

Elders
- Allow extra time for clients to answer questions.
- Adapt questioning techniques as appropriate for clients with hearing or visual limitations.
- Older adults with osteoporosis can lose several inches in height. Be sure to document height and ask if they are aware of becoming shorter in height.
- When asking about weight loss, be specific about amount and time frame, e.g., "Have you lost more than five pounds in the last two months?"

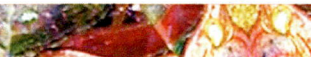

Home Care Considerations

General Survey
- Assess the client in private whenever possible. If a family member is needed to assist with recall of events or translation, obtain the client's permission to have the family member present.

- Use your own equipment when possible in measuring vital signs. Bring a tape measure for measuring height. Recognize that the client's home scale for measuring weight may not be accurate.

> ► **CLINICAL ALERT** *Review the agency charting form before beginning your assessment to ensure that you have all of the equipment you need and know how to perform the assessment in a systematic approach.* ■

Vital Signs

Vital signs are measured (a) to establish baseline data against which to compare future measurements and (b) to detect actual and potential health problems. See Chapter 27 ⊂⊃ for measurements of temperature, pulse, respirations, blood pressure, and oxygen saturation. See Chapter 44 ⊂⊃ for pain assessment.

Height and Weight

In adults, the ratio of weight to height provides a general measure of health. By asking clients about their height and weight before actually measuring them, the nurse obtains some idea of the person's self-image. Excessive discrepancies between the client's responses and the measurements may provide clues to actual or potential problems in self-concept. It is also important that the nurse and client be aware of any significant unintentional weight gain or loss.

The nurse measures height with a measuring stick attached to weight scales or to a wall. The client removes the shoes and stands erect, with heels together, and the heels, buttocks, and back of the head against the measuring stick; eyes should be looking straight ahead. The nurse raises the L-shaped sliding arm on the weight scale until it rests on top of the client's head, or places a small flat object such as a ruler or book on the client's head. The edge of the flat object should abut the measuring guide.

Weight is usually measured when a client is admitted to a health agency and often regularly, for example, each morning before breakfast. When accuracy is essential, the nurse should use the same scale each time (because every scale weighs differently), take the measurements at the same time each day, and make sure the client wears the same kind of clothing and no shoes. The client stands on a platform, and the weight is read from a digital display panel or a balancing arm. Clients who cannot stand are weighed on chair (Figure 28–7 ■) or bed scales. The bed scales (Figure 28–8 ■) have canvas straps or a stretcherlike apparatus. A machine lifts the client above the bed, and the weight is reflected either on a digital display panel or on a balance arm like that of a standing scale.

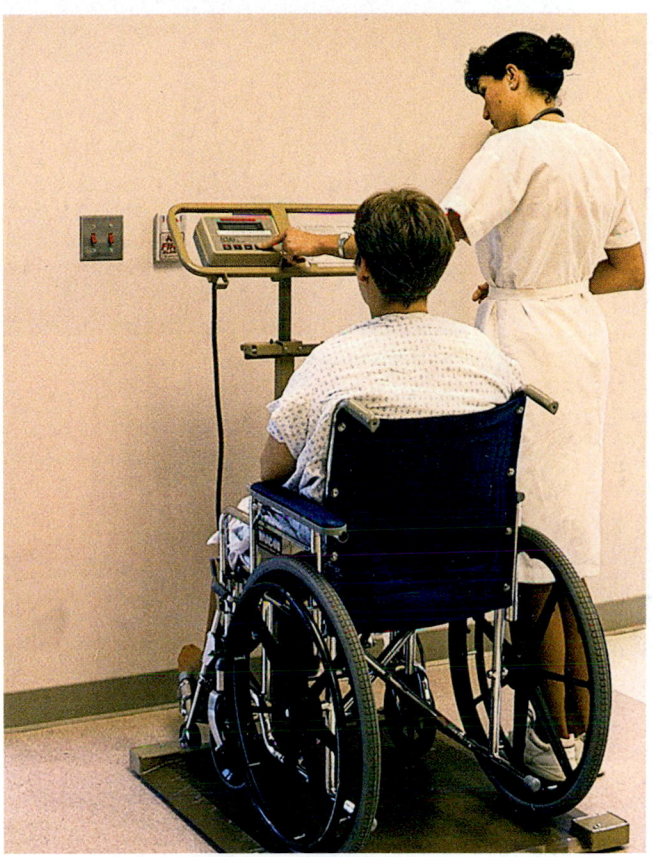

Figure 28–7 ■ Chair scale.

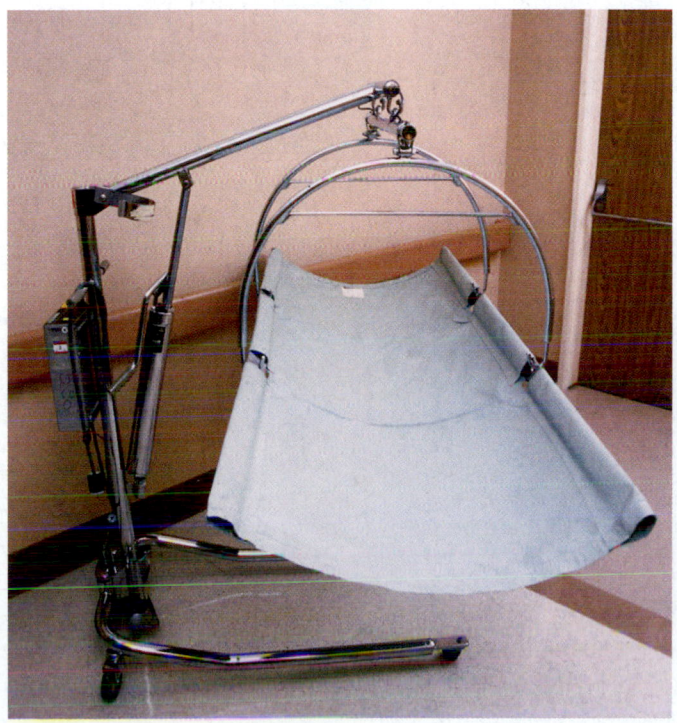

Figure 28–8 ■ Bed scale.

THE INTEGUMENT

The integument includes the skin, hair, and nails. The examination begins with a generalized inspection using a good source of lighting, preferably indirect natural daylight.

Skin

Assessment of the skin involves inspection and palpation. The entire skin surface may be assessed at one time or as each aspect of the body is assessed. In some instances, the nurse may also need to use the olfactory sense to detect unusual skin odors; these are usually most evident in the skinfolds or in the axillae. Pungent body odor is frequently related to poor hygiene, hyperhidrosis (excessive perspiration), or bromhidrosis (foul-smelling perspiration).

Pallor is the result of inadequate circulating blood or hemoglobin and subsequent reduction in tissue oxygenation. It may be difficult to determine in clients with dark skin. It is usually characterized by the absence of underlying red tones in the skin and may be most readily seen in the buccal mucosa. In brown-skinned clients, pallor may appear as a yellowish brown tinge; in black-skinned clients, the skin may appear ashen gray. Pallor in all people is usually most evident in areas with the least pigmentation such as the conjunctiva, oral mucous membranes, nail beds, palms of the hand, and soles of the feet.

Cyanosis (a bluish tinge) is most evident in the nail beds, lips, and buccal mucosa. In dark-skinned clients, close inspection of the palpebral conjunctiva (the lining of the eyelids) and palms and soles may also show evidence of cyanosis. **Jaundice** (a yellowish tinge) may first be evident in the sclera of the eyes and then in the mucous membranes and the skin. Nurses should take care not to confuse jaundice with the normal yellow pigmentation in the sclera of a dark-skinned or Black client. If jaundice is suspected, the posterior part of the hard palate should also be inspected for a yellowish color tone. **Erythema** is a redness associated with a variety of rashes.

Dark-skinned clients have areas of lighter pigmentation, such as the palms, lips, and nail beds. Localized areas of hyperpigmentation (increased pigmentation) and hypopigmentation (decreased pigmentation) may also occur as a result of changes in the distribution of melanin (the dark pigment) or in the function of the melanocytes in the epidermis. An example of hyperpigmentation in a defined area is a birthmark; an example of hypopigmentation is vitiligo. **Vitiligo,** seen as patches of hypopigmented skin, is caused by the destruction of melanocytes in the area. Albinism is the complete or partial lack of melanin in the skin, hair, and eyes. Other localized color changes may indicate a problem such as edema or a localized infection. **Edema** is the presence of excess interstitial fluid. An area of edema appears swollen, shiny, and taut and tends to blanch the skin color or, if accompanied by inflammation, may redden the skin. Generalized edema is most often an indication of impaired venous circulation and in some cases reflects cardiac dysfunction or vein abnormalities.

A skin lesion is an alteration in a client's normal skin appearance. Primary skin lesions are those that appear initially in response to some change in the external or internal environment of the skin (see Figure 28–9 ■, A–H). Secondary skin

A. Macule, Patch Flat, unelevated change in color. Macules are 1 mm to 1 cm in size and circumscribed. Examples: freckles, measles, petechiae, flat moles. Patches are larger than 1 cm and may have an irregular shape. Examples: port wine birthmark, vitiligo (white patches), rubella.

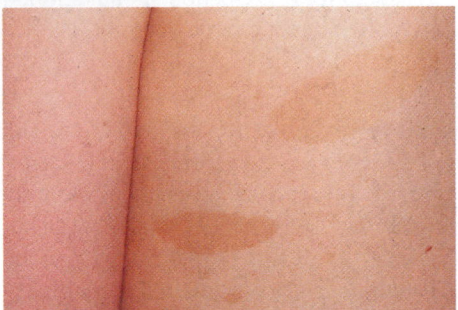

Multiple café-au-lait macules

D. Nodule, Tumor Elevated, solid, hard mass that extends deeper into the dermis than a papule. Nodules have a circumscribed border and are 0.5 to 2 cm. Examples: squamous cell carcinoma, fibroma. Tumors are larger than 2 cm and may have an irregular border. Examples: malignant melanoma, hemangioma.

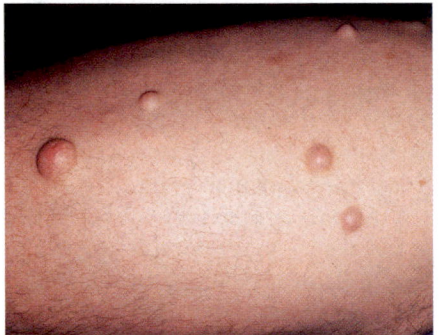

Peripheral neurofibromas

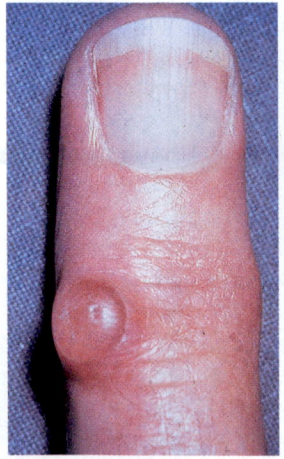

Digital mucous cycst

B. Papule Circumscribed, solid elevation of skin. Papules are less than 1 cm. Examples: warts, acne, pimples, elevated moles.

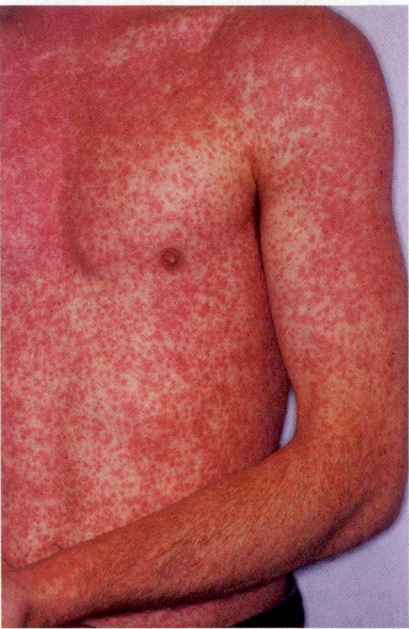

Papular drug eruption (Courtesy Scott D. Bennion, MD.)

E. Pustule Vesicle or bulla filled with pus. Examples: acne vulgaris, impetigo.

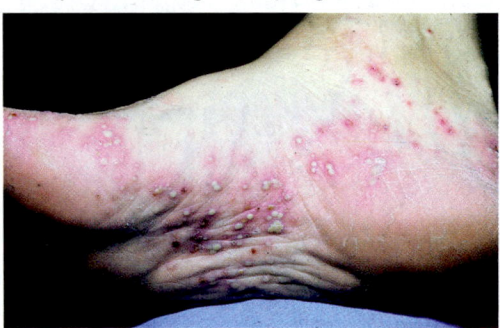

Chronic pustular psoriasis

G. Cyst A 1-cm or larger, elevated, encapsulated, fluid-filled or semisolid mass arising from the subcutaneous tissue or dermis. Examples: sebaceous and epidermoid cysts, chalazion of the eyelid.

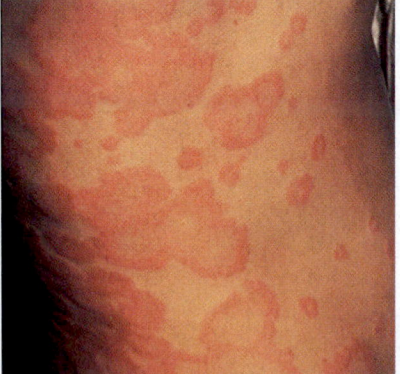

Allergic wheals, urticaria

C. Plaque Plaques are larger than 1 cm. Examples: psoriasis, rubeola.

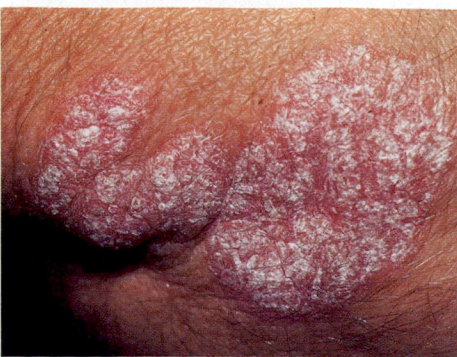

Psoriasis vulgaris

F. Vesicle, Bulla A circumscribed, round or oval, thin translucent mass filled with serous fluid or blood. Vesicles are less than 0.5 cm. Examples: herpes simplex, early chicken pox, small burn blister. Bullae are larger than 0.5 cm. Examples: large blister, second-degree burn, herpes simplex.

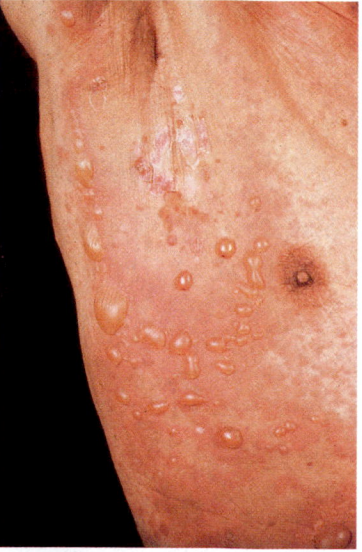

Bullous pemphigoid

H. Wheal A reddened, localized collection of edema fluid; irregular in shape. Size varies. Examples: hives, mosquito bites.

Figure 28–9 ■ Primary Skin Lesions (*Note: (A-G) from Dermatology Secrets in Color,* 2nd ed., by J. E. Fitzpatrick and J. L. Aeling, 2001, Philadelphia: Hanley & Belfus, Inc.; *(H)* Reprinted with permission from the American Academy of Dermatology. All rights reserved.)

536

TABLE 28–5 Secondary Skin Lesions

Atrophy

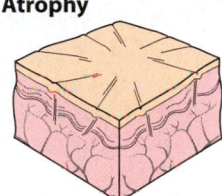

A translucent, dry, paperlike, sometimes wrinkled skin surface resulting from thinning or wasting of the skin due to loss of collagen and elastin.

Examples Striae, aged skin.

Erosion

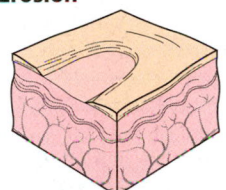

Wearing away of the superficial epidermis causing a moist, shallow depression. Because erosions do not extend into the dermis, they heal without scarring.

Examples Scratch marks, ruptured vesicles.

Lichenification

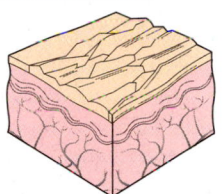

Rough, thickened, hardened area of epidermis resulting from chronic irritation such as scratching or rubbing.

Example Chronic dermatitis.

Scales

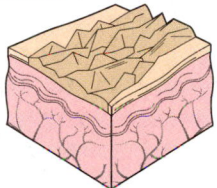

Shedding flakes of greasy, keratinized skin tissue. Color may be white, gray, or silver. Texture may vary from fine to thick.

Examples Dry skin, dandruff, psoriasis, and eczema.

Crust

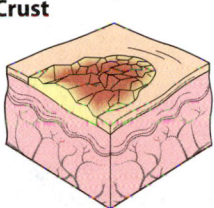

Dry blood, serum, or pus left on the skin surface when vesicles or pustules burst. Can be red-brown, orange, or yellow. Large crusts that adhere to the skin surface are called scabs.

Examples Eczema, impetigo, herpes, or scabs following abrasion.

Ulcer

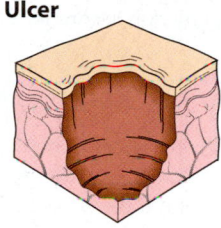

Deep, irregularly shaped area of skin loss extending into the dermis or subcutaneous tissue. May bleed. May leave scar.

Examples Decubitus ulcers (pressure sores), stasis ulcers, chancres.

Fissure

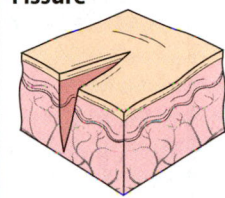

Linear crack with sharp edges, extending into the dermis.

Examples Cracks at the corners of the mouth or in the hands, athlete's foot.

Scar

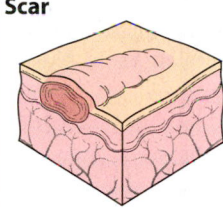

Flat, irregular area of connective tissue left after a lesion or wound has healed. New scars may be red or purple; older scars may be silvery or white.

Examples Healed surgical wound or injury, healed acne.

Keloid

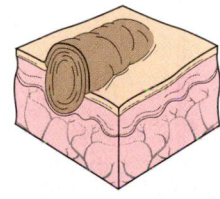

Elevated, irregular, darkened area of excess scar tissue caused by excessive collagen formation during healing. Extends beyond the site of the original injury. Higher incidence in people of African descent.

Examples Keloid from ear piercing or surgery.

Excoriation

Linear erosion induced by scratching.

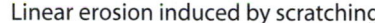
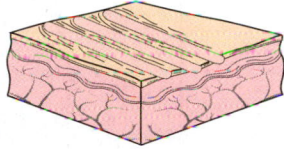

lesions are those that do not appear initially but result from modifications such as chronicity, trauma, or infection of the primary lesion. For example, a vesicle or blister (primary lesion) may rupture and cause an erosion (secondary lesion). Table 28–5 illustrates secondary lesions. Nurses are responsible for describing skin lesions accurately in terms of location (e.g., face), distribution (i.e., body regions involved), and configuration (the arrangement or position of several lesions)

as well as color, shape, size, firmness, texture, and characteristics of individual lesions.

Procedure 28–2 describes how to assess the skin.

> **CLINICAL ALERT** *If possible and the client agrees, take a digital or instant photograph of significant skin lesions for the client record. Include a measuring guide (ruler or tape) in the picture to demonstrate lesion size.*

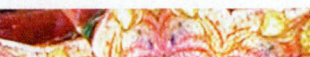

Procedure 28-2 Assessing the Skin

PLANNING

- Review characteristics of primary and secondary skin lesions if necessary (see Figure 28–9 and Table 28–5).
- Ensure that adequate lighting is available.

Delegation

Due to the substantial knowledge and skill required, assessment of the skin is not delegated to unlicensed assistive personnel. However, the skin is observed during usual care and these persons should record their findings. Abnormal findings must be validated and interpreted by the nurse.

Equipment

- Millimeter ruler
- Examination gloves
- Magnifying glass

IMPLEMENTATION

Performance

1. Explain to the client what you are going to do, why it is necessary, and how he or she can cooperate. Discuss how the results will be used in planning further care or treatments.
2. Wash hands and observe appropriate infection control procedures.
3. Provide for client privacy.
4. Inquire if the client has any history of the following: pain or itching; presence and spread of any lesions, bruises, abrasions, pigmented spots; previous experience with skin problems; associated clinical signs; family history; presence of problems in other family members; related systemic conditions; use of medications, lotions, home remedies; excessively dry or moist feel to the skin; tendency to bruise easily; any association of the problem to season of year, stress, occupation, medications, recent travel, housing, personal contact, and so on; any recent contact with allergens, e.g., metal paint.

Assessment	Normal Findings	Deviations from Normal
5. Inspect skin color (best assessed under natural light and on areas not exposed to the sun).	Varies from light to deep brown; from ruddy pink to light pink; from yellow overtones to olive	Pallor, cyanosis, jaundice, erythema
6. Inspect uniformity of skin color.	Generally uniform except in areas exposed to the sun; areas of lighter pigmentation (palms, lips, nail beds) in dark-skinned people	Areas of either hyperpigmentation or hypopigmentation
7. Assess edema, if present (i.e., location, color, temperature, shape, and the degree to which the skin remains indented or pitted when pressed by a finger). See Box 28–5.	No edema	Edema

---

BOX 28–5 ■ Scale for Edema

Scale for Describing Edema

1+ Barely detectable (2 mm)

2+ Indentation of 2–4 mm

3+ Indentation of 5–7 mm

4+ Indentation of more than 7 mm

---

8. Inspect, palpate, and describe skin lesions. Apply gloves if lesions are open or draining. Palpate lesions to determine shape and texture. Describe lesions according to location, distribution, color, configuration, size, shape, type, or structure (see Box 28–6).	Freckles, some birthmarks, some flat and raised nevi; no abrasions or other lesions	Various interruptions in skin integrity

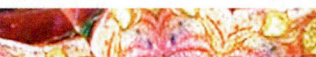

Procedure 28-2 Assessing the Skin *continued*

IMPLEMENTATION *continued*

BOX 28–6 ■ Describing Skin Lesions

- *Type or structure.* Skin lesions are classified as *primary* (those that appear initially in response to some change in the external or internal environment of the skin) and *secondary* (those that do not appear initially but result from modifications such as chronicity, trauma, or infection of the primary lesion). For example, a vesicle (primary lesion) may rupture and cause an erosion (secondary lesion).
- *Size, shape, and texture.* Note size in millimeters and whether the lesion is circumscribed or irregular; round or oval shaped; flat, elevated, or depressed; solid, soft, or hard; rough or thickened; fluid filled or has flakes.
- *Color.* There may be no discoloration, one discrete color (e.g., red, brown, or black), several colors, as with *ecchymosis* (a bruise),

in which an initial dark red or blue color fades to a yellow color. When color changes are limited to the edges of a lesion, they are described as *circumscribed;* when spread over a large area, they are described as *diffuse.*
- *Distribution.* Distribution is described according to the location of the lesions on the body and symmetry or asymmetry of findings in comparable body areas.
- *Configuration.* Configuration refers to the arrangement of lesions in relation to each other. Configurations of lesions may be annular (arranged in a circle), clustered together or grouped, linear (arranged in a line), arc or bow shaped, merged together or indiscrete, follow the course of coetaneous nerves, or meshed in the form of a network.

Assessment	Normal Findings	Deviations from Normal
9. Observe and palpate skin moisture.	Moisture in skin folds and the axillae (varies with environmental temperature and humidity, body temperature, and activity)	Excessive moisture (e.g., in hyperthermia); excessive dryness (e.g., in dehydration)
10. Palpate skin temperature. Compare the two feet and the two hands, using the backs of your fingers.	Uniform; within normal range	Generalized hyperthermia (e.g., in fever); generalized hypothermia (e.g., in shock); localized hyperthermia (e.g., in infection); localized hypothermia (e.g., in arteriosclerosis)
11. Note skin turgor (fullness or elasticity) by lifting and pinching the skin on an extremity.	When pinched, skin springs back to previous state	Skins stays pinched or tented or moves back slowly (e.g., in dehydration)

12. Document findings in the client record using forms or checklists supplemented by narrative notes when appropriate. Draw location of skin lesions on body surface diagrams (see Figure 28–10 ■).

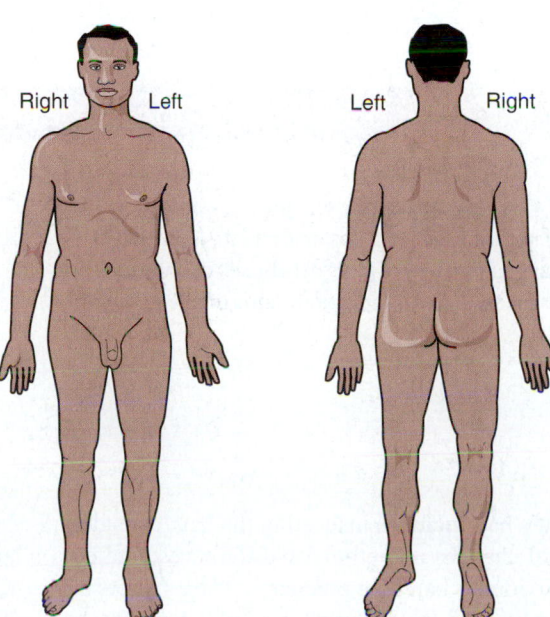

Figure 28–10 ■ Diagram for charting skin lesions.

continued on page 540

Procedure 28-2 Assessing the Skin *continued*

EVALUATION

- Compare findings to previous skin assessment data if available to determine if lesions or abnormalities are changing.
- Report significant deviations from normal to the physician.

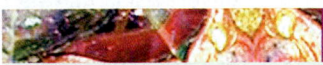

Lifespan Considerations

Assessing the Skin

Infants

- Newborns may be jaundiced for several weeks after birth.
- Newborns may have milia (whiteheads), small white nodules over the nose and face, and vernix caseosa (white cheesy, greasy material on the skin).
- In dark-skinned races, areas of hyperpigmentation may be found in the sacral area.
- If a rash is present, inquire in detail about immunization history.
- Assess skin turgor by pinching the skin on the abdomen.

Children

- In dark-skinned races, areas of hyperpigmentation may be found in the sacral area.
- As puberty approaches, skin may change in oiliness and acne may appear.
- If a rash is present, inquire in detail about immunization history.

Elders

- Changes in white skin occur at an earlier age than in black skin.
- The skin loses its elasticity and wrinkles. Wrinkles first appear on the skin of the face and neck, which are abundant in collagen and elastic fibers.
- The skin appears thin and translucent because of loss of dermis and subcutaneous fat.
- The skin is dry and flaky because sebaceous and sweat glands are less active. Dry skin is more prominent over the extremities.

- The skin takes longer to return to its natural shape after being tented between the thumb and finger.
- Due to the normal loss of peripheral skin turgor in elders, assess for hydration by checking skin turgor over the sternum or clavicle.
- Flat tan to brown-colored macules, referred to as *senile lentigines* or *melanotic freckles,* are normally apparent on the back of the hand and other skin areas that are exposed to the sun. These macules may be as large as 1 to 2 cm.
- Warty lesions (*seborrheic keratosis*) with irregularly shaped borders and a scaly surface often occur on the face, shoulders, and trunk. These benign lesions begin as yellowish to tan and progress to a dark brown or black.
- *Vitiligo* tends to increase with age and is thought to result from an autoimmune response.
- Cutaneous tags (*acrochordons*) are most commonly seen in the neck and axillary regions. These skin lesions vary in size and are soft, often flesh colored, and pedicled.
- Visible, bright red, fine dilated blood vessels (*telangiectasias*) commonly occur as a result of the thinning of the dermis and the loss of support for the blood vessel walls.
- Pink to slightly red lesions with indistinct borders (*actinic keratoses*) may appear at about age 50, often on the face, ears, backs of the hands, and arms. They may become malignant if untreated.

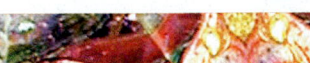

Home Care Considerations

Assessing the Skin

- When making a home visit, take a penlight or examination lamp with you in case the home has inadequate lighting.
- If skin lesions are suggestive of physical abuse, follow state regulations for follow-up and reporting. Signs of abuse may include a pattern of bruises, unusual location of burns, or lesions that are not easily explainable. If lesions are present in adults or verbal-age children, conduct the interview and assessment in private.

Hair

Assessing a client's hair includes inspecting the hair, considering developmental changes and ethnicity differences, and determining the individual's hair care practices and the factors influencing them. Much of the information about hair can be obtained by questioning the client.

Normal hair is resilient and evenly distributed. In people with severe protein deficiency (kwashiorkor), the hair color is faded and appears reddish or bleached, and the texture is coarse and dry. Some therapies cause **alopecia** (hair loss), and some disease conditions affect the coarseness of hair. For example, hypothyroidism can cause very thin and brittle hair.

Procedure 28–3 describes how to assess the hair.

Procedure 28-3 Assessing the Hair

PLANNING

Delegation
Assessment of the hair is not delegated to unlicensed assistive personnel. However, many aspects are observed during usual care and may be recorded by persons other than the nurse. Abnormal findings must be validated and interpreted by the nurse.

Equipment
■ Examination gloves

IMPLEMENTATION

Performance

1. Explain to the client what you are going to do, why it is necessary, and how he or she can cooperate. Discuss how the results will be used in planning further care or treatments.
2. Wash hands, apply gloves, and observe other appropriate infection control procedures.
3. Provide for client privacy.

4. Inquire if the client has any history of the following: recent use of hair dyes, rinses, or curling or straightening preparations; recent chemotherapy (if alopecia is present); presence of disease, such as hypothyroidism, which can be associated with dry, brittle hair.

Assessment	Normal Findings	Deviations from Normal
5. Inspect the evenness of growth over the scalp.	Evenly distributed hair	Patches of hair loss (i.e., alopecia)
6. Inspect hair thickness or thinness.	Thick hair	Very thin hair (e.g., in hypothyroidism)
7. Inspect hair texture and oiliness.	Silky, resilient hair	Brittle hair (e.g., hypothyroidism); excessively oily or dry hair
8. Note presence of infections or infestations by parting the hair in several areas, checking behind the ears and along the hairline at the neck.	No infection or infestation	Flaking, sores, lice, nits (louse eggs), and ringworm
9. Inspect amount of body hair.	Variable	Hirsutism (abnormal hairiness) in women

10. Document findings in the client record using forms or checklists supplemented by narrative notes when appropriate.

EVALUATION
■ Report significant deviations from normal to the physician.

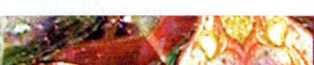

Lifespan Considerations

Assessing the Hair

Infants
■ It is normal for infants to have either very little or a great deal of body and scalp hair.

Children
■ As puberty approaches, axillary and pubic hair will appear.

Elders
■ There may be loss of scalp, pubic, and axillary hair.
■ In women, the hair of the eyebrows and some facial hair become coarse.
■ Hairs of the eyebrows, ears, and nostrils become bristle-like and coarse.

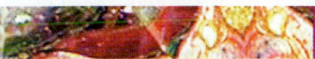

Home Care Considerations

Assessing the Hair
■ When making a home visit, ask to see the products the client usually uses on the hair. Assist the client to determine if the products are appropriate for the client's type of hair and scalp, e.g., for dry or oily hair. Provide education regarding hygiene of the hair and scalp.

■ When making a home visit, examine the equipment that the client uses on the hair. Provide client teaching regarding appropriate combs and brushes and regarding safety in using electric hair styling appliances such as hair dryers.

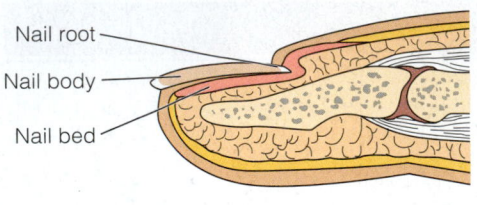
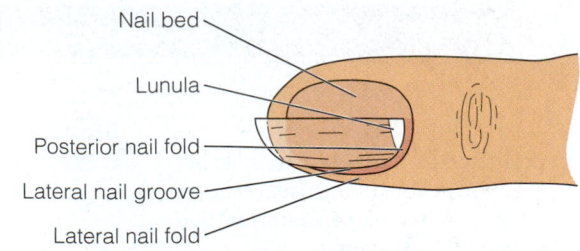

Figure 28–11 ■ The parts of a nail.

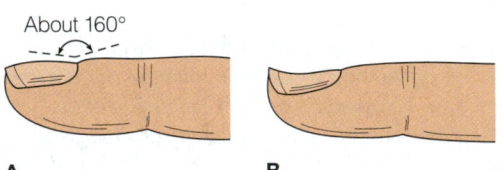
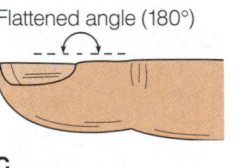
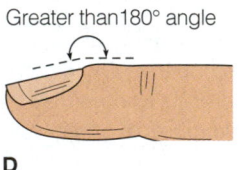
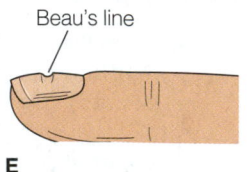

About 160°   Flattened angle (180°)   Greater than 180° angle   Beau's line

A   B   C   D   E

Figure 28–12 ■ *A,* A normal nail, showing the convex shape and the nail plate angle of about 160 degrees; *B,* a spoon-shaped nail, which may be seen in clients with iron deficiency anemia; *C,* early clubbing; *D,* late clubbing (may be caused by long-term oxygen lack); *E,* Beau's line on nail (may result from severe injury or illness).

Nails

Nails are inspected for nail plate shape, angle between the nail and the nail bed, nail texture, nail bed color, and the intactness of the tissues around the nails. The parts of the nail are shown in Figure 28–11 ■.

The nail plate is normally colorless and a convex curve. The angle between the nail and the nail bed is normally 160 degrees (Figure 28–12 ■, *A*). One nail abnormality is the spoon shape, in which the nail curves upward from the nail bed (Figure 28–12 ■, *B*). This condition, called koilonychia, may be seen in clients with iron deficiency anemia. **Clubbing** is a condition in which the angle between the nail and the nail bed is 180 degrees or greater (Figure 28–12 ■, *C* and ■ *D*). Clubbing may be caused by a long-term lack of oxygen.

Nail texture is normally smooth. Excessively thick nails can appear in the elderly, in the presence of poor circulation, or in relation to a chronic fungal infection. Excessively thin nails or the presence of grooves or furrows can reflect prolonged iron deficiency anemia. Beau's lines are horizontal depressions in the nail that can result from injury or severe illness (Figure 28–12 ■, *E*).

The nail bed is highly vascular, a characteristic that accounts for its pink color in white people. A bluish or purplish tint to the nail bed may reflect cyanosis, and pallor may reflect poor arterial circulation.

The tissue surrounding the nails is normally intact epidermis. Paronychia is an inflammation of the tissues surrounding a nail (often referred to as an "ingrown nail"). The tissues appear inflamed and swollen and tenderness is usually present. A **blanch test** can be carried out to test the capillary refill, that is, peripheral circulation. Normal nail bed capillaries blanch when pressed but quickly turn pink or their usual color when pressure is released. A slow rate of capillary refill may indicate circulatory problems.

Procedure 28–4 describes how to assess the nails.

Procedure 28-4 Assessing the Nails

PLANNING

Delegation
Assessment of the nails is not delegated to unlicensed assistive personnel. However, many aspects are observed during usual care and may be recorded by persons other than the nurse. Abnormal findings must be validated and interpreted by the nurse.

Equipment
None

IMPLEMENTATION

Performance

1. Explain to the client what you are going to do, why it is necessary, and how he or she can cooperate. Discuss how the results will be used in planning further care or treatments.
2. Observe appropriate infection control procedures.
3. Provide for client privacy.
4. Inquire if the client has any history of the following: presence of diabetes mellitus, peripheral circulatory disease, previous injury, or severe illness.

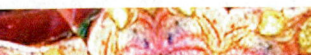

Procedure 28-4 Assessing the Nails *continued*

IMPLEMENTATION *continued*

Assessment	Normal Findings	Deviations from Normal
5. Inspect fingernail plate shape to determine its curvature and angle.	Convex curvature; angle of nail plate about 160° (Figure 28–12, *A*).	Spoon nail (Figure 28–12, *B*); clubbing (180 or greater) (Figure 28–12, *C* and *D*).
6. Inspect fingernail and toenail texture.	Smooth texture	Excessive thickness or thinness or presence of grooves or furrows; Beau's lines (Figure 28–12, *E*)
7. Inspect fingernail and toenail bed color.	Highly vascular and pink in light-skinned clients; dark-skinned clients may have brown or black pigmentation in longitudinal streaks	Bluish or purplish tint (may reflect cyanosis); pallor (may reflect poor arterial circulation)
8. Inspect tissues surrounding nails.	Intact epidermis	Hangnails; paronychia (inflammation)
9. Perform blanch test of capillary refill. Press two or more nails between your thumb and index finger; look for blanching and return of pink color to nail bed.	Prompt return of pink or usual color (generally less than 4 seconds)	Delayed return of pink or usual color (may indicate circulatory impairment)

10. Document findings in the client record using forms or checklists supplemented by narrative notes when appropriate.

EVALUATION

■ Perform a detailed follow-up examination of other individual systems based on findings that deviated from expected or normal for the client. Relate findings to previous assessment data if available.

■ Report significant deviations from normal to the physician.

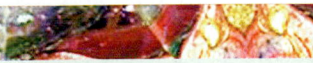

Lifespan Considerations

Assessing the Nails

Infants
■ Newborns nails grow very quickly, are extremely thin, and tear easily.

Children
■ Bent, bruised, or ingrown toenails may indicate shoes that are too tight.
■ Nail biting should be discussed with a family member.

Elders
■ The nails grow more slowly and thicken.
■ Longitudinal bands commonly develop, and the nails tend to split.
■ Bands across the nails may indicate protein deficiency; white spots, zinc deficiency; and spoon-shaped nails, iron deficiency.

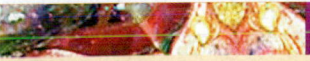

Home Care Considerations

Assessing the Nails

■ If indicated, teach the client or family member about proper nail care including how to trim and shape the nails to avoid paronychia.

THE HEAD

During assessment of the head, the nurse inspects and palpates simultaneously and also auscultates. The nurse examines the skull, face, eyes, ears, nose, sinuses, mouth, and pharynx.

Skull and Face

There is a large range of normal shapes of skulls. A normal head size is referred to as **normocephalic.** Names of areas of the head are derived from names of the underlying bones: frontal, parietal, occipital, mastoid process, mandible, maxilla, and zygomatic (Figure 28–13 ■).

Many disorders cause a change in facial shape or condition. Kidney or cardiac disease can cause edema of the eyelids. Hyperthyroidism can cause **exophthalmos,** a protrusion of the eyeballs with elevation of the upper eyelids, resulting in a startled or staring expression. Hypothyroidism, or myxedema, can cause a dry, puffy face with dry skin and coarse features and thinning of scalp hair and eyebrows. Increased adrenal hormone production or administration can cause a round face with reddened cheeks, referred to as *moon face,* and excessive hair growth on the upper lips, chin, and sideburn areas. Prolonged

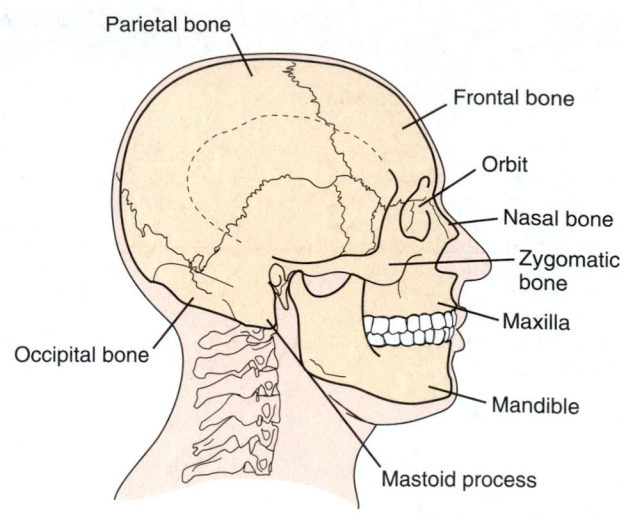

Figure 28–13 ■ Bones of the head.

illness, starvation, and dehydration can result in sunken eyes, cheeks, and temples. Procedure 28–5 describes how to assess the skull and face.

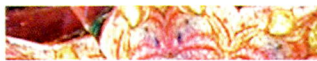

Procedure 28-5 Assessing the Skull and Face

PLANNING

Delegation

Assessment of the skull and face is not delegated to unlicensed assistive personnel. However, many aspects are observed during usual care and may be recorded by persons other than the nurse. Abnormal findings must be validated and interpreted by the nurse.

Equipment

None

IMPLEMENTATION

Performance

1. Explain to the client what you are going to do, why it is necessary, and how he or she can cooperate. Discuss how the results will be used in planning further care or treatments.
2. Observe appropriate infection control procedures.
3. Provide for client privacy.

4. Inquire if the client has any history of the following: any past problems with lumps or bumps, itching, scaling, or dandruff; any history of loss of consciousness, dizziness, seizures, headache, facial pain, or injury; when and how any lumps occurred; length of time any other problem existed; any known cause of problem; associated symptoms, treatment, and recurrences.

Assessment	Normal Findings	Deviations from Normal
5. Inspect the skull for size, shape, and symmetry.	Rounded (normocephalic and symmetrical, with frontal, parietal, and occipital prominences); smooth skull contour	Lack of symmetry; increased skull size with more prominent nose and forehead; longer mandible (may indicate excessive growth hormone or increased bone thickness)
6. Palpate the skull for nodules or masses and depressions. Use a gentle rotating motion with the fingertips. Begin at the front and palpate down the midline, then palpate each side of the head.	Smooth, uniform consistency; absence of nodules or masses	Sebaceous cysts; local deformities from trauma

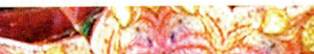

Procedure 28-5 Assessing the Skull and Face *continued*

IMPLEMENTATION *continued*

Assessment	Normal Findings	Deviations from Normal
7. Inspect the facial features (e.g., symmetry of structures and of the distribution of hair).	Symmetric or slightly asymmetric facial features; palpebral fissures equal in size; symmetric nasolabial folds	Increased facial hair; thinning of eyebrows; asymmetric features; exophthalmos; myxedema facies; moon face
8. Inspect the eyes for edema and hollowness.		Periorbital edema; sunken eyes
9. Note symmetry of facial movements. Ask the client to elevate the eyebrows, frown, or lower the eyebrows, close the eyes tightly, puff the cheeks, and smile and show the teeth. See Procedure 28–17, Assessing the Neurologic system on page 604.	Symmetric facial movements.	Asymmetric facial movements (e.g., eye on affected side cannot close completely); drooping of lower eyelid and mouth; involuntary facial movements (i.e., tics or tremors)

10. Document findings in the client record using forms or checklists supplemented by narrative notes when appropriate.

Evaluation

■ Perform a detailed follow-up examination of other systems based on findings that deviated from expected or normal for the client. Relate findings to previous assessment data if available.

■ Report significant deviations from normal to the physician.

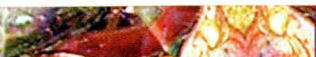

Lifespan Considerations

Assessing the Skull and Face

Infants

■ Most newborns' heads are shaped according to the method of delivery for the first week.

■ The posterior fontanel (soft spot) usually closes by 8 weeks but the anterior fontanel may remain up to 18 months.
■ Voluntary head control should be present by about 6 months of age.

The Eyes and Vision

Many people consider vision the most important sense because it allows them to interact freely with their environment and enjoy the beauty of life around them. To maintain optimum vision, people need to have their eyes examined regularly throughout life. It is recommended that people under age 40 have their eyes tested every 3 to 5 years, or more frequently if there is a family history of diabetes, hypertension, blood dyscrasia, or eye disease (e.g., glaucoma). After age 40, an eye examination is recommended every 2 years to rule out the possibility of glaucoma.

An eye assessment should be carried out as part of the client's initial physical examination; periodic reassessments need to be made for clients in long-term care. Examination of the eyes includes assessment of **visual acuity** (the degree of detail the eye can discern in an image), ocular movement, **visual fields** (the area an individual can see when looking straight ahead), and external structures. Most eye assessment procedures involve inspection. Consideration is also given to developmental changes and to individual hygiene practices, if the client wears contact lenses or an artificial eye. For the anatomical structures of the eye, see Figures 28–14 ■ and 28–15 ■.

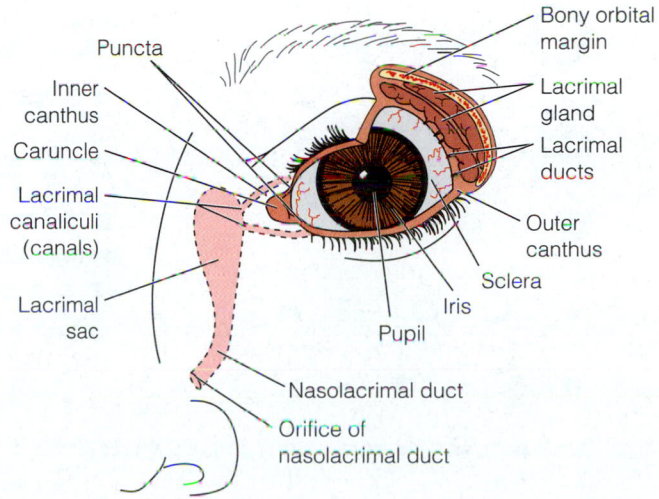

Figure 28–14 ■ The external structures and lacrimal apparatus of the left eye.

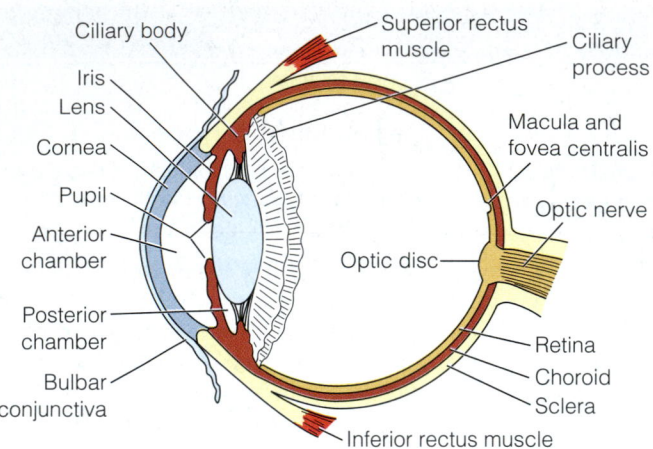
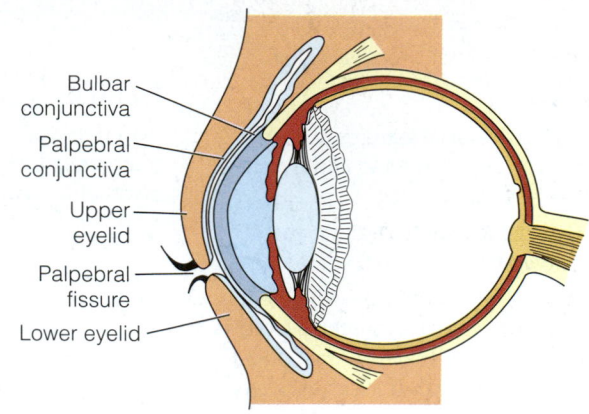

Figure 28–15 ■ Anatomic structures of the right eye, lateral view.

Many people wear eyeglasses or contact lenses to correct common refractive errors of the lens of the eye. These errors include **myopia** (nearsightedness), **hyperopia** (farsightedness), and **presbyopia** (loss of elasticity of the lens and thus loss of ability to see close objects). Presbyopia begins at about 45 years of age. People notice that they have difficulty reading newsprint. Often two corrective lenses (bifocals) are required—one for near vision or reading, the other for far vision. **Astigmatism,** an uneven curvature of the cornea that prevents horizontal and vertical rays from focusing on the retina, is a common problem that may occur in conjunction with myopia and hyperopia.

Three types of eye charts are available to test visual acuity (see Figure 28–16 ■). The child acquires normal 20/20 vision by 6 years of age. People with denominators of 40 or more on the Snellen chart with or without corrective lenses need to be referred to an ophthalmologist.

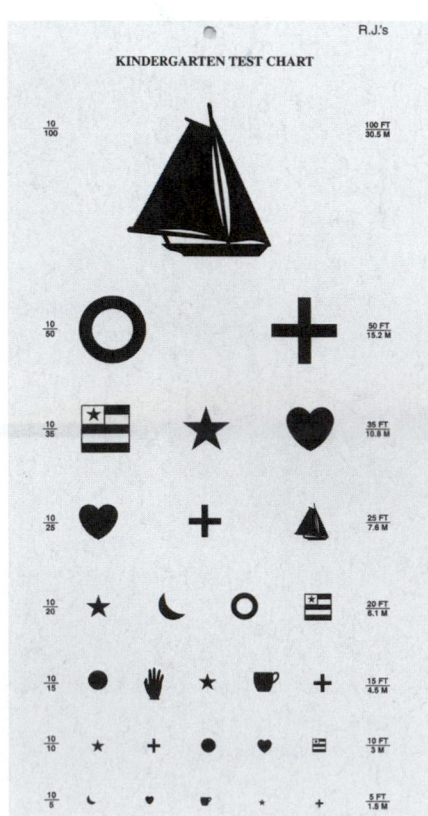
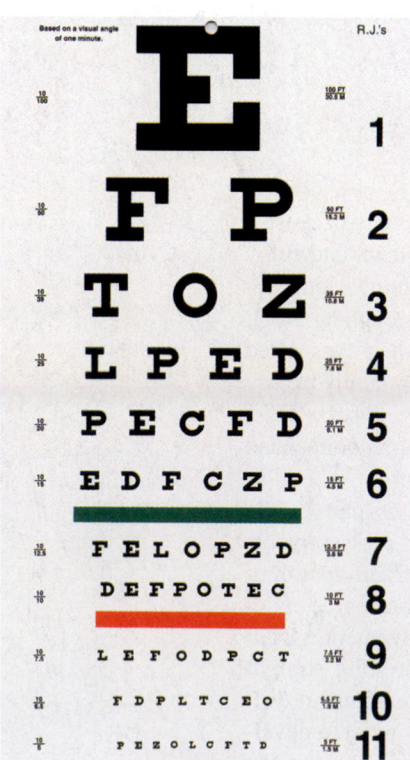
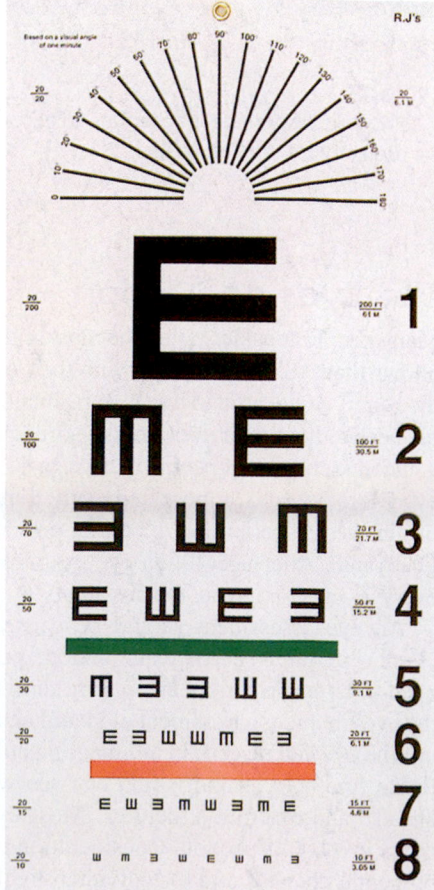

Figure 28–16 ■ Three types of eye charts; the preschool children's chart (*left*), Snellen standard chart (*center*), and the Snellen E chart for clients unable to read (*right*).

Common inflammatory visual problems that nurses may encounter in clients include conjunctivitis, dacryocystitis, hordeolum, iritis, and contusions or hematomas of the eyelids and surrounding structures. **Conjunctivitis** (inflammation of the bulbar and palpebral conjunctiva) may result from foreign bodies, chemicals, allergenic agents, bacteria, or viruses. Redness, itching, tearing, and mucopurulent discharge occur. During sleep, the eyelids may become encrusted and matted together. **Dacryocystitis** (inflammation of the lacrimal sac) is manifested by tearing and a discharge from the nasolacrimal duct. **Hordeolum (sty)** is a redness, swelling, and tenderness of the hair follicle and glands that empty at the edge of the eyelids. *Iritis* (inflammation of the iris) may be caused by local or systemic infections and results in pain, tearing, and photophobia (sensitivity to light). Contusions or hematomas are "black eyes" resulting from injury.

Cataracts tend to occur in those over 65 years old. This opacity of the lens or its capsule, which blocks light rays, is frequently removed and replaced by a lens implant. Cataracts may also occur in infants due to a malformation of the lens if the mother contracted rubella in the first trimester of pregnancy. **Glaucoma** (a disturbance in the circulation of aqueous fluid, which causes an increase in intraocular pressure) is the most frequent cause of blindness in people over 40. It can be controlled if diagnosed early. Danger signs of glaucoma include blurred or foggy vision, loss of peripheral vision, difficulty focusing on close objects, difficulty adjusting to dark rooms, and seeing rainbow-colored rings around lights.

Eyelids that lie at or below the pupil margin are referred to as ptosis and are usually associated with aging, edema from drug allergy or systemic disease (e.g., kidney disease), congenital lid muscle dysfunction, neuromuscular disease (e.g., myasthenia gravis), and third cranial nerve impairment. Eversion, an outturning of the eyelid, is called ectropion; inversion, an inturning of the lid, is called entropion. These abnormalities are often associated with scarring injuries or the aging process.

Pupils are normally black, are equal in size (about 3 to 7 mm in diameter), and have round, smooth borders. Cloudy pupils are often indicative of cataracts. Enlarged pupils (**mydriasis**) may indicate injury or glaucoma, or result from certain drugs (e.g., atropine). Constricted pupils (**miosis**) may indicate an inflammation of the iris or result from such drugs as morphine or pilocarpine. It is also an age-related change in older adults. Unequal pupils (anisocoria) may result from a central nervous system disorder; however, slight variations may be normal. The iris is normally flat and round. A bulging toward the cornea can indicate increased intraocular pressure.

Procedure 28–6 describes how to assess a client's eye structures and visual acuity.

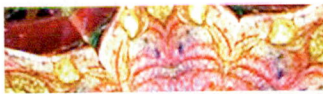

Procedure 28-6 Assessing the Eye Structures and Visual Acuity

PLANNING

Place the client in an appropriate room for assessing the eyes and vision. The nurse must be able to control natural and overhead lighting during some portions of the examination.

Delegation
Due to the substantial knowledge and skill required, assessment of the eyes and vision are not delegated to unlicensed assistive personnel. However, many aspects are observed during usual care and may be recorded by persons other than the nurse. Abnormal findings must be validated and interpreted by the nurse.

Equipment
- Cotton tip applicator
- Gauze square
- Examination gloves
- Millimeter ruler
- Penlight
- Snellen's or E chart
- Opaque card

IMPLEMENTATION

Performance

1. Explain to the client what you are going to do, why it is necessary, and how he or she can cooperate. Discuss how the results will be used in planning further care or treatments.
2. Wash hands, apply gloves, and observe appropriate infection control procedures.
3. Provide for client privacy.
4. Inquire if the client has any history of the following: family history of diabetes, hypertension, blood dyscrasia, or eye disease, injury, or surgery; client's last visit to an ophthalmologist; current use of eye medications; use of contact lenses or eyeglasses; hygienic practices for corrective lenses; current symptoms of eye problems (e.g., changes in visual acuity, blurring of vision, tearing, spots, photophobia, itching, or pain).

continued on page 548

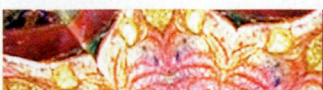

Procedure 28-6 Assessing the Eye Structures and Visual Acuity *continued*

IMPLEMENTATION *continued*

Assessment	Normal Findings	Deviations from Normal
EXTERNAL EYE STRUCTURES		
5. Inspect the eyebrows for hair distribution and alignment and skin quality and movement (ask client to raise and lower the eyebrows).	Hair evenly distributed; skin intact Eyebrows symmetrically aligned; equal movement	Loss of hair; scaling and flakiness of skin Unequal alignment and movement of eyebrows
6. Inspect the eyelashes for evenness of distribution and direction of curl.	Equally distributed; curled slightly outward	Turned inward (see inversion of eyelid, below)
7. Inspect the eyelids for surface characteristics (e.g., skin quality and texture), position in relation to the cornea, ability to blink, and frequency of blinking. For proper visual examination of the upper eyelids, elevate the eyebrows with your thumb and index fingers, and have the client close the eyes (Figure 28–17 ■). Inspect the lower eyelids while the client's eyes are closed.	Skin intact; no discharge; no discoloration Lids close symmetrically Approximately 15 to 20 involuntary blinks per minute; bilateral blinking When lids open, no visible sclera above corneas, and upper and lower borders of cornea are slightly covered	Redness, swelling, flaking, crusting, plaques, discharge, nodules, lesions Lids close asymmetrically, incompletely, or painfully Rapid, monocular, absent, or infrequent blinking Ptosis, ectropion, or entropion; rim of sclera visible between lid and iris

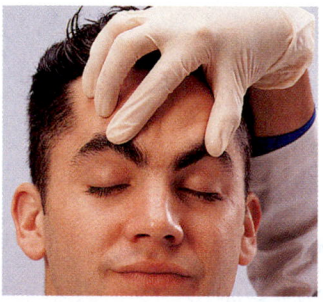

Figure 28–17 ■ Inspecting the upper eyelids.

Assessment	Normal Findings	Deviations from Normal
8. Inspect the bulbar conjunctiva (that lying over the sclera) for color, texture, and the presence of lesions. Retract the eyelids with your thumb and index finger, exerting pressure over the upper and lower bony orbits, and ask the client to look up, down, and from side to side.	Transparent; capillaries sometimes evident; sclera appears white (yellowish in dark-skinned clients)	Jaundiced sclera (e.g., in liver disease); excessively pale sclera (e.g., in anemia); reddened sclera; lesions or nodules (may indicate damage by mechanical, chemical, allergenic, or bacterial agents)
9. Inspect the palpebral conjunctiva (that lining the eyelids) by everting the lids. Note color, texture, and the presence of lesions. Evert both lower lids, and ask the client to look up. Then gently retract the lower lids with the index fingers.	Shiny, smooth, and pink or red	Extremely pale (possible anemia); extremely red (inflammation); nodules or other lesions
10. Evert the upper lids if a problem is suspected (see Box 28–7).		

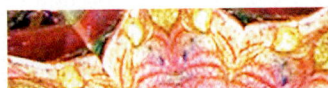

Procedure 28-6 Assessing the Eye Structures and Visual Acuity continued

IMPLEMENTATION continued

BOX 28–7 ■ Everting the Upper Eyelid

- Ask the client to look down while keeping the eyes slightly open. Closing the eyelids contracts the orbicular muscle, which prevents lid eversion.
- Gently grasp the client's eyelashes with the thumb and index finger. Pull the lashes gently downward. Upward or outward pulling on the eyelashes causes muscle contraction.
- Place a cotton-tipped applicator stick about 1 cm above the lid margin, and push it gently downward while holding the eyelashes (see Figure 28–18 ■). These actions evert the lid, that is, flip the lower part of the lid over on top of itself.

- Hold the margin of the everted lid or the eyelashes against the ridge of the upper bony orbit with the applicator stick or the thumb (see Figure 28–19 ■).
- Inspect the conjunctiva for color, texture, lesions, and foreign bodies.
- To return the lid to its normal position, gently pull the lashes forward, and ask the client to look up and blink.

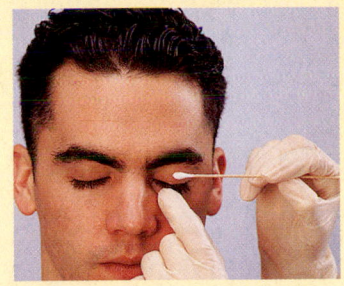

Figure 28–18 ■ Everting the upper eyelid.

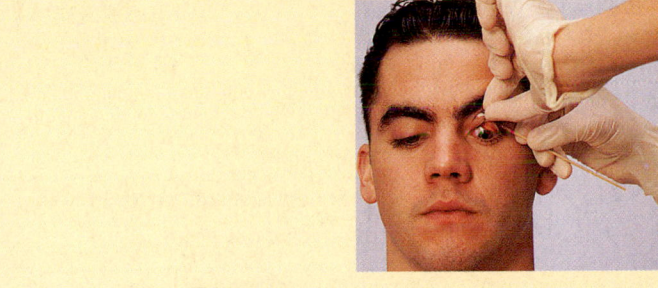

Figure 28–19 ■ Holding the margin of the everted upper eyelid.

Assessment	Normal Findings	Deviations from Normal
11. Inspect and palpate the lacrimal gland (see Box 28–8).	No edema or tenderness over lacrimal gland	Swelling or tenderness over lacrimal gland

BOX 28–8 ■ Palpating the Lacrimal Gland, Lacrimal Sac, and Nasolacrimal Duct

- Using the tip of your index finger, palpate the lacrimal gland (see Figure 28–20 ■).
- Observe for edema between the lower lid and the nose.

- Observe for evidence of increased tearing.
- Using the tip of your index finger, palpate inside the lower orbital rim near the inner canthus (see Figure 28–21 ■).

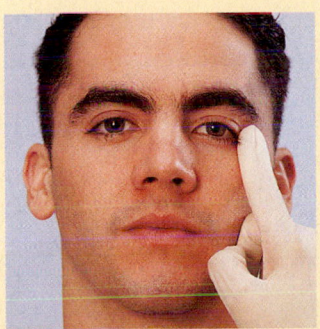

Figure 28–20 ■ Palpating the lacrimal gland.

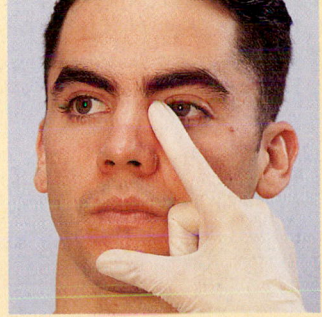

Figure 28–21 ■ Palpating the lacrimal sac and the nasolacrimal duct.

continued on page 550

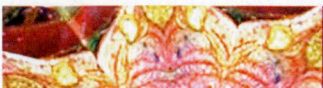

Procedure 28-6 Assessing the Eye Structures and Visual Acuity *continued*

IMPLEMENTATION *continued*

Assessment	Normal Findings	Deviations from Normal
12. Inspect and palpate the lacrimal sac and nasolacrimal duct (see Box 28–8).	No edema or tearing	Evidence of increased tearing; regurgitation of fluid on palpation of lacrimal sac
13. Inspect the cornea for clarity and texture. Ask the client to look straight ahead. Hold a penlight at an oblique angle to the eye, and move the light slowly across the corneal surface.	Transparent, shiny, and smooth; details of the iris are visible In older people, a thin, grayish white ring around the margin, called arcus senilis, may be evident	Opaque; surface not smooth (may be the result of trauma or abrasion) Arcus senilis in clients under age 40 is abnormal
14. Perform the corneal sensitivity (reflex) test to determine the function of the fifth (trigeminal) cranial nerve. Ask the client to keep both eyes open and look straight ahead. Approach from behind and beside the client, and lightly touch the cornea with a corner of the gauze.	Client blinks when the cornea is touched, indicating that the trigeminal nerve is intact	One or both eyelids fail to respond
15. Inspect the anterior chamber for transparency and depth. Use the same oblique lighting as used to test the cornea.	Transparent No shadows of light on iris Depth of about 3 mm	Cloudy Crescent-shaped shadows on far side of iris Shallow chamber (possible glaucoma)
16. Inspect the pupils for color, shape, and symmetry of size. Pupil charts are available in some agencies. See Figure 28–22 ■ for variations in pupil diameters.	Black in color; equal in size; normally 3 to 7 mm in diameter; round, smooth border, iris flat and round	Cloudiness, mydriasis, miosis, anisocoria; bulging of iris toward cornea

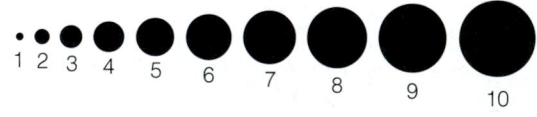

1 2 3 4 5 6 7 8 9 10

Figure 28–22 ■ Variations in pupil diameters in millimeters.

Assessment	Normal Findings	Deviations from Normal
17. Assess each pupil's direct and consensual reaction to light to determine the function of the third (oculomotor) and fourth (trochlear) cranial nerves (see Box 28–9).	Illuminated pupil constricts (direct response) Nonilluminated pupil constricts (consensual response)	Neither pupil constricts Unequal responses Absent responses
18. Assess each pupil's reaction to accommodation (Box 28–9).	Pupils constrict when looking at near object; pupils dilate when looking at far object; pupils converge when near object is moved toward nose	One or both pupils fail to constrict, dilate, or converge

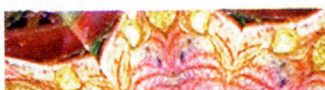

Procedure 28-6 Assessing the Eye Structures and Visual Acuity *continued*

IMPLEMENTATION *continued*

BOX 28–9 ■ Assessing Pupil Reactions

Direct and Consensual Reaction to Light
- Partially darken the room.
- Ask the client to look straight ahead.
- Using a penlight or flashlight and approaching from the side, shine a light on the pupil.
- Observe the response of the illuminated pupil. It should constrict (direct response).
- Shine the light on the pupil again, and observe the response of the other pupil. It should also constrict (consensual response).

Reaction to Accommodation
- Hold an object (a penlight or pencil) about 10 cm (4 in.) from the bridge of the client's nose.

- Ask the client to look first at the top of the object and then at a distant object (e.g., the far wall) behind the penlight. Alternate the gaze from the near to the far object.
- Observe the pupil response. The pupils should constrict when looking at the near object and dilate when looking at the far object.
- Next, move the penlight or pencil toward the client's nose. The pupils should converge. To record normal assessment of the pupils, use the abbreviation PERRLA (pupils equally round and react to light and accommodation).

Assessment	Normal Findings	Deviations from Normal
VISUAL FIELDS 19. Assess peripheral visual fields to determine function of the retina and neuronal visual pathways to the brain and second (optic) cranial nerve (see Box 28–10).	When looking straight ahead, client can see objects in the periphery	Visual field smaller than normal (possible glaucoma); one-half vision in one or both eyes (indicates nerve damage)

BOX 28–10 ■ Assessing Peripheral Visual Fields

- Have the client sit directly facing you at a distance of 60 to 90 cm (2 to 3 ft).
- Ask the client to cover the right eye with a card and look directly at your nose.
- Cover or close your eye directly opposite the client's covered eye (i.e., your left eye), and look directly at the client's nose.
- Hold an object (e.g., a penlight or pencil) in your fingers, extend your arm, and move the object into the visual field from various points in the periphery (see Figure 28–23 ■). The object should be at an equal distance from the client and yourself. Ask the client to tell you when the moving object is first spotted.
  a. To test the temporal field of the left eye, extend and move your right arm in from the client's right periphery. Temporally, peripheral objects can be seen at right angles (90 degrees) to the central point of vision.
  b. To test the upward field of the left eye, extend and move the right arm down from the upward periphery. The upward field of vision is normally 50 degrees because the orbital ridge is in the way.
  c. To test the downward field of the left eye, extend and move the right arm up from the lower periphery. The downward field of vision is normally 70 degrees because the cheekbone is in the way.

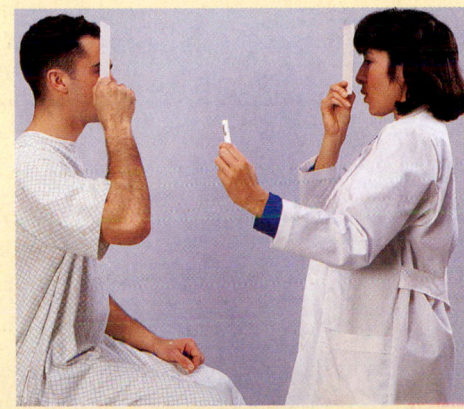

Figure 28–23 ■ Assessing the client's left peripheral visual field.

  d. To test the nasal field of the left eye, extend and move your left arm in from the periphery. The nasal field of vision is normally 50 degrees away from the central point of vision because the nose is in the way.
- Repeat the above steps for the right eye, reversing the process.

continued on page 552

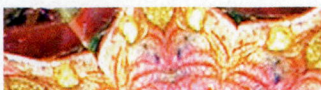

Procedure 28-6 Assessing the Eye Structures and Visual Acuity *continued*

IMPLEMENTATION *continued*

Assessment	Normal Findings	Deviations from Normal
EXTRAOCULAR MUSCLE TESTS 20. Assess six ocular movements to determine eye alignment and coordination. These can be performed on clients over 6 months of age (see Box 28–11).	Both eyes coordinated, move in unison, with parallel alignment	Eye movements not coordinated or parallel; one or both eyes fail to follow a penlight in specific directions, e.g., strabismus (cross-eye or squint) Nystagmus other than end point (may indicate neurologic impairment)

BOX 28–11 ■ Assessing the Six Ocular Movements

- Stand directly in front of the client and hold the penlight at a comfortable distance, such as 30 cm (1 ft) in front of the client's eyes.
- Ask the client to hold the head in a fixed position facing you and to follow the movements of the penlight with the eyes only.
- Move the penlight in a slow, orderly manner through the six cardinal fields of gaze, that is, from the center of the eye along the lines of the arrows in Figure 28–24 ■ and back to the center.
- Stop the movement of the penlight periodically so that nystagmus can be detected.

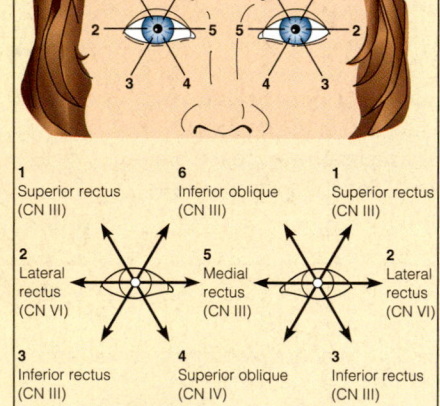

Figure 28–24 ■ The six muscles that govern eye movement.

Assessment	Normal Findings	Deviations from Normal
VISUAL ACUITY 21. Assess near vision by providing adequate lighting and asking the client to read from a magazine or newspaper held at a distance of 36 cm (14 in.). If the client normally wears corrective lenses, the glasses or lenses should be worn during the test.	Able to read newsprint	Difficulty reading newsprint unless due to aging process
22. Assess distance vision by asking the client to wear corrective lenses, unless they are used for reading only, i.e., for distances of only 36 cm (12 to 14 in.). See Box 28–12.	20/20 vision on Snellen chart	Denominator of 40 or more on Snellen chart with corrective lenses

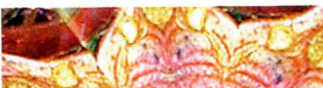

Procedure 28-6 Assessing the Eye Structures and Visual Acuity *continued*

IMPLEMENTATION *continued*

BOX 28–12 ■ Assessing Distance Vision

- Ask the client to stand or sit 6 m (20 ft) from a Snellen or character chart (see Figure 28–25 ■), cover the eye not being tested, and identify the letters or characters on the chart.
- Take three readings: right eye, left eye, both eyes.
- Record the readings of each eye and both eyes, i.e., the smallest line from which the person is able to read one-half or more of the letters.

At the end of each line of the Snellen chart are standardized numbers (fractions). The top line is 20/200. The numerator (top number) is always 20, the distance the person stands from the chart. The denominator (bottom number) is the distance from which the normal eye can read the chart. Therefore, a person who has 20/40 vision, can see at 20 feet from the chart what a normal-sighted person can see at 40 feet from the chart. Visual acuity is recorded as "s̄c" (without correction), or "c̄c" (with correction). You can also indicate how many letters were misread in the line, e.g., "visual acuity 20/40 − 2 c̄c" indicates that two letters were misread in the 20/40 line by a client wearing corrective lenses.

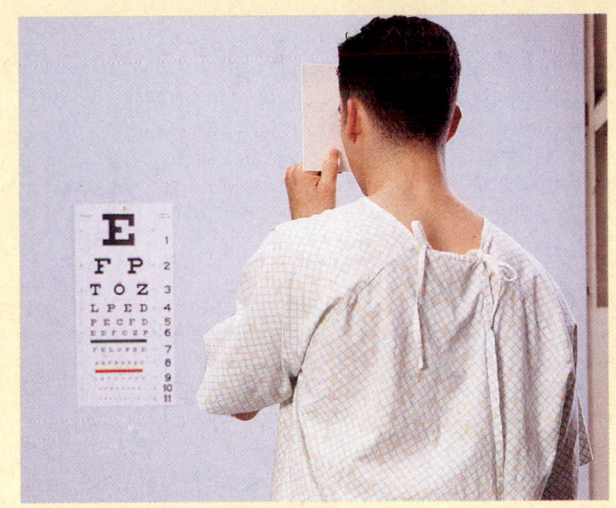

Figure 28–25 ■ Testing distance vision.

Assessment	Normal Findings	Deviations from Normal
23. Perform functional vision tests if the client is unable to see the top line (20/200) of the Snellen chart (see Box 28–13).		Functional vision only (e.g., light perception, hand movements, counting fingers at 1 ft)

BOX 28–13 ■ Performing Functional Vision Tests

Light Perception
Shine a penlight into the client's eye from a lateral position, and then turn the light off. Ask the client to tell you when the light is on or off. If the client knows when the light is on or off, the client has light perception, and the vision is recorded as "LP."

Hand Movements (H/M)
Hold your hand 30 cm (1 ft) from the client's face and move it slowly back and forth, stopping it periodically. Ask the client to tell you when your hand stops moving. If the client knows when your hand stops moving, record the vision as "H/M 1 ft."

Counting Fingers (C/F)
Hold up some of your fingers 30 cm (1 ft) from the client's face, and ask the client to count your fingers. If the client can do so, note on the vision record "C/F 1 ft."

24. Document findings in the client record using forms or checklists supplemented by narrative notes when appropriate.

EVALUATION

- Perform a detailed follow-up examination of other systems based on findings that deviated from expected or normal for the client. Relate findings to previous assessment data if available.
- Report significant deviations from normal to the physician. Persons with denominators of 40 or more on the Snellen or character chart, with or without corrective lenses, need to be referred to an ophthalmologist.

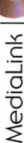

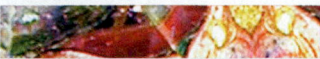

Lifespan Considerations

Assessing the Eyes and Vision

Infants
- Infants 4 weeks of age should gaze at and follow objects.
- Ability to focus with both eyes should be present by 6 months of age.

Children
- Epicanthal folds, common in Asian cultures, may cover the medial canthus and cause eyes to appear misaligned.
- Dark-skinned children's sclerae may be darker and have small brown macules.
- Preschool children's acuity can be checked with picture cards or the E chart. Acuity should approach 20/20 by 6 years of age.

Elders

Visual Acuity
- Visual acuity decreases as the lens of the eye ages and becomes more opaque and loses elasticity.
- The ability of the iris to accommodate to darkness and dim light diminishes.
- Peripheral vision diminishes.
- The adaptation to light (glare) and dark decreases.
- Accommodation to far objects often improves, but accommodation to near objects decreases.
- Color vision declines; older people are less able to perceive purple colors and to discriminate pastel colors.

- Many elders wear corrective lenses; they are most likely to have hyperopia. Visual changes are due to loss of elasticity (presbyopia) and transparency of the lens.

External Eye Structures
- The skin around the orbit of the eye may darken.
- The eyeball may appear sunken because of the decrease in orbital fat.
- Skin folds of the upper lids may seem more prominent, and the lower lids may sag.
- The eyes may appear dry and lusterless because of the decrease in tear production from the lacrimal glands.
- A thin, grayish white arc or ring (*arcus senilis*) appears around part or all of the cornea. It results from an accumulation of a lipid substance on the cornea. The cornea tends to cloud with age.
- The iris may appear pale with brown discolorations as a result of pigment degeneration.
- The conjunctiva of the eye may appear paler than that of younger adults and may take on a slightly yellow appearance because of the deposition of fat.
- Pupil reaction to light and accommodation is normally symmetrically equal but may be less brisk.
- The pupils can appear smaller in size, unequal, and irregular in shape because of sclerotic changes in the iris.

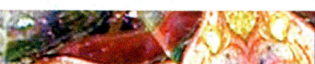

Home Care Considerations

Assessing the Eyes and Vision
- When making a home visit, take your equipment and charts with you. Also include a tape measure to lay out the 20 feet for distance vision testing.
- Use the assessment as an opportunity to reinforce proper eye care and need for regular vision testing.

> **► CLINICAL ALERT**   *A Rosenbaum eye chart may be used to test near vision. It consists of paragraphs of text or characters in different sizes on a 3.5- by 6.5-in. card. Be sure the client has a literacy level appropriate for the text used.* ■

The Ears and Hearing

Assessment of the ear includes direct inspection and palpation of the external ear, inspection of the remaining parts of the ear by an **otoscope,** and determination of auditory acuity. The ear is usually assessed during an initial physical examination; periodic reassessments may be necessary for long-term clients or those with hearing problems.

The ear is divided into three parts: external ear, middle ear, and inner ear. Most of the structures mentioned next are illustrated in Figure 28–26 ■. The external ear includes the **auricle** or **pinna,** the external auditory canal, and the **tympanic membrane,** or eardrum. Landmarks of the auricle include the **lobule**

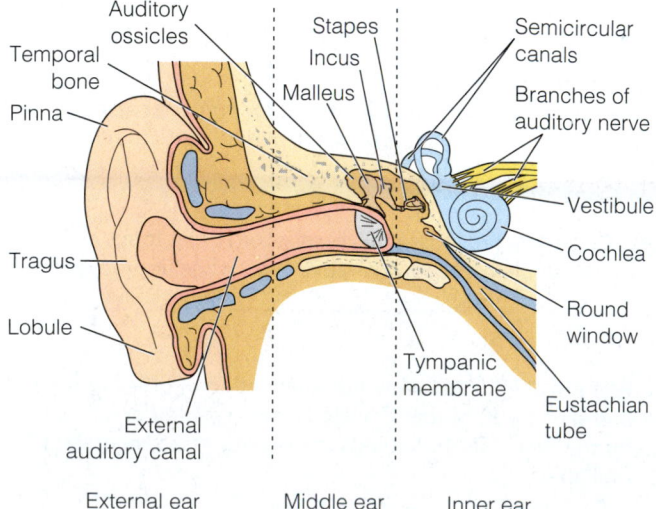

Figure 28–26 ■ Anatomic structures of the external, middle, and inner ear.

(earlobe), **helix** (the posterior curve of the auricle's upper aspect), **antihelix** (the anterior curve of the auricle's upper aspect), **tragus** (the cartilaginous protrusion at the entrance to the ear canal), **triangular fossa** (a depression of the antihelix), and **external auditory meatus** (the entrance to the ear canal). Although not part of the ear, the **mastoid,** a bony prominence behind the ear, is another important landmark. The external ear canal is curved, is about 2.5 cm (1 in) long in the adult, and ends at the tympanic membrane. It is covered with skin that has many fine hairs, glands, and nerve endings. The glands secrete **cerumen** (earwax), which lubricates and protects the canal.

The curvature of the external ear canal differs with age. In the infant and toddler, the canal has an upward curvature. By age 3, the ear canal assumes the more downward curvature of adulthood.

The middle ear is an air-filled cavity that starts at the tympanic membrane and contains three **ossicles** (bones of sound transmission): the **malleus** (hammer), which is the most easily seen, the **incus** (anvil), and the **stapes** (stirrups). The **Eustachian tube,** another part of the middle ear, connects the middle ear to the nasopharynx. The tube stabilizes the air pressure between the external atmosphere and the middle ear, thus preventing rupture of the tympanic membrane and discomfort produced by marked pressure differences.

The inner ear contains the **cochlea,** a seashell-shaped structure essential for sound transmission and hearing, and the **vestibule** and **semicircular canals,** which contain the organs of equilibrium.

Sound transmission and hearing are complex processes. In brief, sound can be transmitted by air conduction or bone conduction. Air-conducted transmission occurs by this process:

1. A sound stimulus enters the external canal and reaches the tympanic membrane.
2. The sound waves vibrate the tympanic membrane and reach the ossicles.
3. The sound waves travel from the ossicles to the opening in the inner ear (oval window).
4. The cochlea receives the sound vibrations.
5. The stimulus travels to the auditory nerve (the eighth cranial nerve) and the cerebral cortex.

Bone-conducted sound transmission occurs when skull bones transport the sound directly to the auditory nerve.

Audiometric evaluations, which measure hearing at various decibels, are recommended for children and elders. A common hearing deficit with age is loss of ability to hear high frequency sounds, such as *f, s, sh,* and *ph.* This neurosensory hearing deficit does not respond well to use of a hearing aid.

In some practice settings, the nurse does not perform otoscopic examinations. The examination is limited to inspection of the external ear canal and the color of the tympanic membrane.

Conduction hearing loss is the result of interrupted transmission of sound waves through the outer and middle ear structures. Possible causes are a tear in the tympanic membrane or an obstruction, due to swelling or other causes, in the auditory canal. **Sensorineural hearing loss** is the result of damage to the inner ear, the auditory nerve, or the hearing center in the brain. **Mixed hearing loss** is a combination of conduction and sensorineural loss. Procedure 28–7 describes how to assess the ears and hearing.

MediaLink | MIDDLE EAR DYNAMICS ANIMATION

Procedure 28-7 Assessing the Ears and Hearing

PLANNING

It is important to conduct the ear and hearing examination in an area that is quiet. In addition, the location should allow the client to be positioned sitting or standing at the same level as the nurse.

Delegation
Assessment of the ears and hearing is not delegated to unlicensed assistive personnel. However, many aspects are observed during usual care and may be recorded by persons other than the nurse. Abnormal findings must be validated and interpreted by the nurse.

Equipment
■ Otoscope with several sizes or ear specula

IMPLEMENTATION

Performance

1. Explain to the client what you are going to do, why it is necessary, and how he or she can cooperate. Discuss how the results will be used in planning further care or treatments.
2. Wash hands and observe appropriate infection control procedures.
3. Provide for client privacy.
4. Inquire if the client has any history of the following: family history of hearing problems or loss; presence of any ear problems; medication history, especially if there are complaints of ringing in ears; any hearing difficulty: its onset, factors contributing to it, and how it interferes with activities of daily living; use of a corrective hearing device: when and from whom it was obtained.
5. Position the client comfortably, seated if possible.

continued on page 556

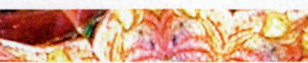

Procedure 28-7 Assessing the Ears and Hearing *continued*

IMPLEMENTATION *continued*

Assessment	Normal Findings	Deviations from Normal
AURICLES 6. Inspect the auricles for color, symmetry of size, and position. To inspect position, note the level at which the superior aspect of the auricle attaches to the head in relation to the eye.	Color same as facial skin Symmetrical Auricle aligned with outer canthus of eye, about 10° from vertical (see Figure 28–27 ■).	Bluish color of earlobes (e.g., cyanosis); pallor (e.g., frostbite); excessive redness (inflammation or fever) Asymmetry Low-set ears (associated with a congenital abnormality, such as Down syndrome)

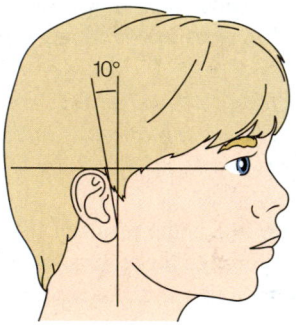

Normal alignment

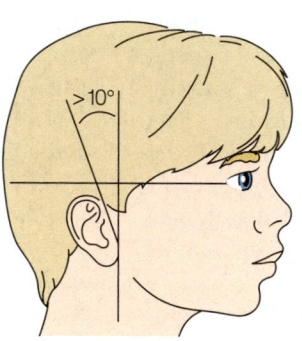

Low-set ears and deviation in alignment

Figure 28–27 ■ Alignment of ears.

Assessment	Normal Findings	Deviations from Normal
7. Palpate the auricles for texture, elasticity, and areas of tenderness. • Gently pull the auricle upward, downward, and backward. • Fold the pinna forward (it should recoil). • Push in on the tragus. • Apply pressure to the mastoid process.	Mobile, firm, and not tender; pinna recoils after it is folded	Lesions (e.g., cysts); flaky, scaly skin (e.g., seborrhea); tenderness when moved or pressed (may indicate inflammation or infection of external ear)
EXTERNAL EAR CANAL AND TYMPANIC MEMBRANE 8. Using an otoscope, inspect the external ear canal for cerumen, skin lesions, pus, and blood (see Box 28–14).	Distal third contains hair follicles and glands Dry cerumen, grayish-tan color; or sticky, wet cerumen in various shades of brown	Redness and discharge Scaling Excessive cerumen obstructing canal

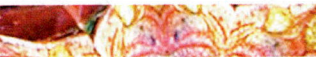

Procedure 28-7 Assessing the Ears and Hearing *continued*

IMPLEMENTATION *continued*

BOX 28–14 ■ Inspecting the ears with an otoscope

■ Attach a speculum to the otoscope. Use the largest diameter that will fit the ear canal without causing discomfort. This achieves maximum vision of the entire ear canal and tympanic membrane.

■ Tip the client's head away from you, and straighten the ear canal. For an adult, straighten the ear canal by pulling the pinna up and back (see Figure 28–28 ■). Straightening the ear canal facilitates vision of the ear canal and the tympanic membrane.

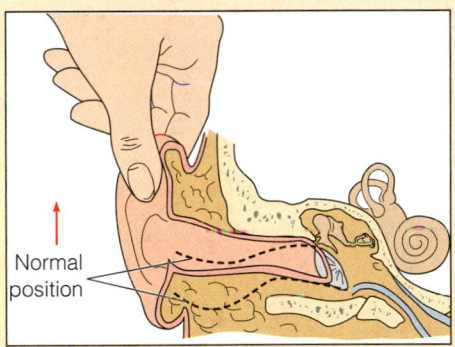

Figure 28–28 ■ Straightening the ear canal of an adult by pulling the pinna up and back.

■ Hold the otoscope either (a) right side up, with your fingers between the otoscope handle and the client's head or (b) upside down, with your fingers and the ulnar surface of your hand against the client's head (see Figure 28–29 ■). This stabilizes the head and protects the eardrum and canal from injury if a quick head movement occurs.

■ Gently insert the tip of the otoscope into the ear canal, avoiding pressure by the speculum against either side of the ear canal. The inner two-thirds of the ear canal is bony; if the speculum is pressed against either side, the client will experience discomfort.

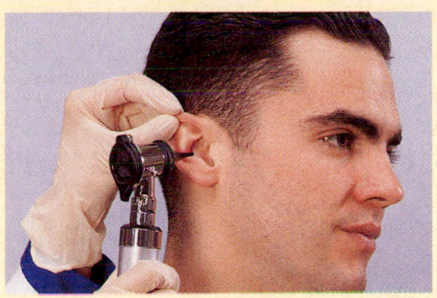

Figure 28–29 ■ Inserting an otoscope.

Assessment	Normal Findings	Deviations from Normal
9. Inspect the tympanic membrane for color and gloss.	Pearly gray color, semitransparent (Figure 28–30 ■)	Pink to red, some opacity Yellow-amber White Blue or deep red Dull surface

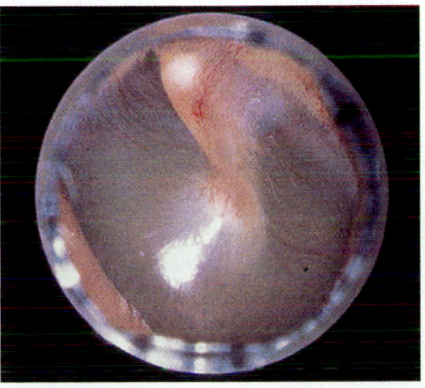

Figure 28–30 ■ Normal tympanic membrane.

continued on page 558

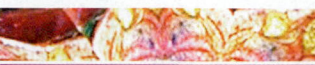

Procedure 28-7 Assessing the Ears and Hearing *continued*

IMPLEMENTATION *continued*

Assessment	Normal Findings	Deviations from Normal
GROSS HEARING ACUITY TESTS		
10. Assess client's response to normal voice tones. If client has difficulty hearing the normal voice, proceed with the following tests.	Normal voice tones audible	Normal voice tones not audible (e.g., requests nurse to repeat words or statements, leans toward the speaker, turns the head, cups the ears, or speaks in loud tone of voice)
10A. Perform the watch tick test. The ticking of a watch has a higher pitch than the human voice. • Have the client occlude one ear. Out of the client's sight, place a ticking watch 2 to 3 cm (1 to 2 in.) from the unoccluded ear. • Ask what the client can hear. Repeat with the other ear.	Able to hear ticking in both ears	Unable to hear ticking in one or both ears
10B. *Tuning Fork Tests* Perform Weber's test to assess bone conduction (see Box 28–15).	Sound is heard in both ears or is localized at the center of the head (Weber negative)	Sound is heard better in impaired ear, indicating a bone-conductive hearing loss or sound is heard better in ear without a problem, indicating a sensorineural disturbance (Weber positive)
Conduct the Rinne test to compare air conduction to bone conduction (see Box 28–15).	Air-conducted (AC) hearing is greater than bone-conducted (BC) hearing, i.e., AC > BC (positive Rinne)	Bone conduction time is equal to or longer than the air conduction time, i.e., BC > AC or BC = AC (negative Rinne; indicates a conductive hearing loss)

BOX 28–15 ■ Performing Tuning Fork Tests

Weber's Test
This test assesses bone conduction by testing the lateralization (sideward transmission) of sounds.
■ Hold the tuning fork at its base. Activate it by tapping the fork gently against the back of your hand near the knuckles or by stroking the fork between your thumb and index fingers. It should be made to ring softly.
■ Place the base of the vibrating fork on top of the client's head (see Figure 28–31 ■) and ask where the client hears the noise.

Rinne Test
This test compares air conduction to bone conduction.

■ Ask the client to block the hearing in one ear intermittently by moving a fingertip in and out of the ear canal.
■ Hold the handle of the activated tuning fork on the mastoid process of one ear (see Figure 28–32 ■, *A*) until the client states that the vibration can no longer be heard.
■ Immediately hold the still vibrating fork prongs in front of the client's ear canal (see Figure 28–32 ■, *B*). Push aside the client's hair if necessary. Ask whether the client now hears the sound. Sound conducted by air is heard more readily than sound conducted by bone. The tuning fork vibrations conducted by air are normally heard longer.

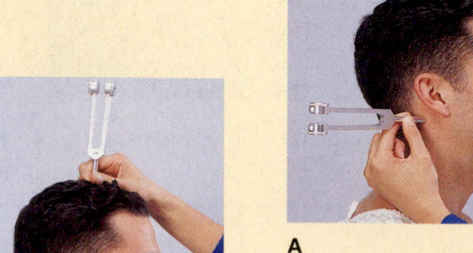

Figure 28–31 ■ Placing the base of a tuning fork on the client's skull (Weber's test).

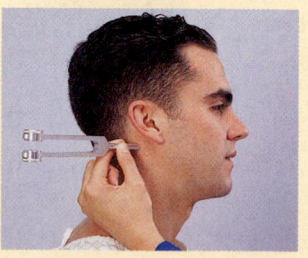

A

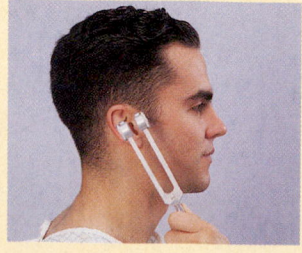

B

Figure 28–32 ■ Rinne test–tuning fork placement. *A,* base of the tuning fork on the mastoid process; *B,* tuning fork prongs placed in front of the client's ear.

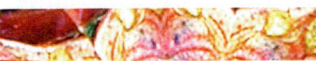

Procedure 28-7 Assessing the Ears and Hearing *continued*

IMPLEMENTATION *continued*

11. Document findings in the client record using forms or check-lists supplemented by narrative notes when appropriate.

EVALUATION

- Perform a detailed follow-up examination of the neurologic system based on findings that deviated from expected or normal for the client. Relate findings to previous assessment data if available.

- Report significant deviations from normal to the physician.

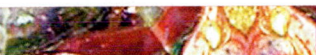

Lifespan Considerations

Assessing the Ears and Hearing

Infants
- To assess gross hearing, ring a bell from behind the infant or have the parent call the child's name to check for a response. At 3-4 months of age, the child will turn head and eyes toward the sound.

Children
- To inspect the external canal and tympanic membrane in children less than 3 years old, pull the pinna down and back. Insert the speculum only ¼ to ½ inch.

Elders
- The skin of the ear may appear dry and be less resilient because of the loss of connective tissue.

- Increased coarse and wire-like hair growth occurs along the helix, antihelix, and tragus.
- The pinna increases in both width and length, and the earlobe elongates.
- Earwax is drier.
- The tympanic membrane is more translucent and less flexible. The intensity of the light reflex may diminish slightly.
- Sensorineural hearing loss occurs.
- Generalized hearing loss (presbycusis) occurs in all frequencies, although the first symptom is the loss of high-frequency sounds: the *f, s, sh,* and *ph* sounds. To such persons, conversation can be distorted and result in what appears to be inappropriate or confused behavior.

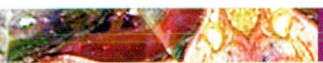

Home Care Considerations

Assessing the Ears and Hearing
- Ensure that the examination is conducted in a quiet place. In particular, elders will have difficulty accurately reporting results of hearing tests if there is excessive outside noise.

- If necessary, ask the adult present with an infant or child to assist in holding the child still during the examination.

Nose and Sinuses

A nurse can inspect the nasal passages very simply with a flashlight. However, a nasal *speculum* and a penlight or an otoscope with a nasal attachment facilitates examination of the nasal attachment.

Assessment of the nose includes inspection and palpation of the external nose (the upper third of the nose is bone; the remainder is cartilage); patency of the nasal cavities; and inspection of the nasal cavities.

If the client reports difficulty or abnormality in smell, the nurse may test the client's olfactory sense by asking the client to identify common odors such as coffee or mint. This is done by asking the client to close the eyes and placing vials containing the scent under the client's nose.

The nurse also inspects and palpates the facial sinuses (Figure 28–33 ■). Procedure 28–8 describes how to assess the nose and sinuses.

MediaLink

EAR ABNORMALITIES ANIMATION

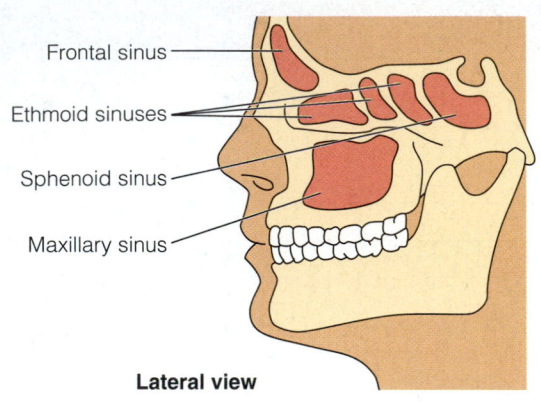
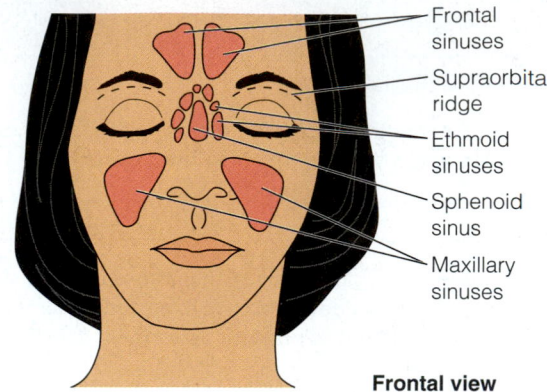

Lateral view

Frontal view

Figure 28–33 ■ The facial sinuses.

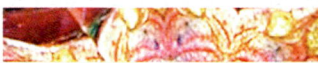

Procedure 28-8 Assessing the Nose and Sinuses

PLANNING

Delegation

Assessment of the nose and sinuses is not delegated to unlicensed assistive personnel. However, many aspects are observed during usual care and may be recorded by persons other than the nurse. Abnormal findings must be validated and interpreted by the nurse.

Equipment

■ Nasal speculum
■ Flashlight/penlight

IMPLEMENTATION

Performance

1. Explain to the client what you are going to do, why it is necessary, and how he or she can cooperate. Discuss how the results will be used in planning further care or treatments.
2. Observe appropriate infection control procedures.
3. Provide for client privacy.

4. Inquire if the client has any history of the following: allergies, difficulty breathing through the nose, sinus infections, injuries to nose or face, nosebleeds; any medications taken; any changes in sense of smell.
5. Position the client comfortably, seated if possible.

Assessment	Normal Findings	Deviations from Normal
NOSE		
6. Inspect the external nose for any deviations in shape, size, or color and flaring or discharge from the nares.	Symmetric and straight No discharge or flaring Uniform color	Asymmetric Discharge from nares Localized areas of redness or presence of skin lesions
7. Lightly palpate the external nose to determine any areas of tenderness, masses, and displacements of bone and cartilage.	Not tender; no lesions	Tenderness on palpation; presence of lesions
8. Determine patency of both nasal cavities. Ask the client to close the mouth, exert pressure on one naris, and breathe through the opposite naris. Repeat the procedure to assess patency of the opposite naris.	Air moves freely as the client breathes through the nares	Air movement is restricted in one or both nares
9. Inspect the nasal cavities using a flashlight or a nasal speculum (see Box 28–16).		

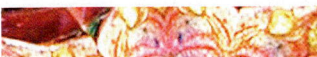

Procedure 28-8 Assessing the Nose and Sinuses *continued*

IMPLEMENTATION *continued*

BOX 28–16 ■ Using a nasal speculum

- Hold the speculum in your right hand to inspect the client's left nostril and your left hand to inspect the client's right nostril.
- Tip the client's head back.
- Facing the client, insert the tip of the closed speculum (blades together) about 1 cm or up to the point at which the blade widens. Care must be taken to avoid pressure on the sensitive nasal septum (see Figure 28–34 ■).
- Stabilize the speculum with your index finger against the side of the nose. Use the other hand to position the head and then to hold the light.

- Open the speculum as much as possible and inspect the floor of the nose (vestibule), the anterior portion of the septum, the middle meatus, and the middle turbinates. The posterior turbinate is rarely visualized because of its position (see Figure 28–35 ■).
- Inspect the lining of the nares and the integrity and the position of the nasal septum.

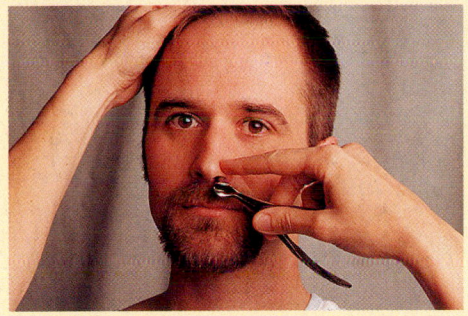

Figure 28–34 ■ Using a nasal speculum to inspect the nasal passages.

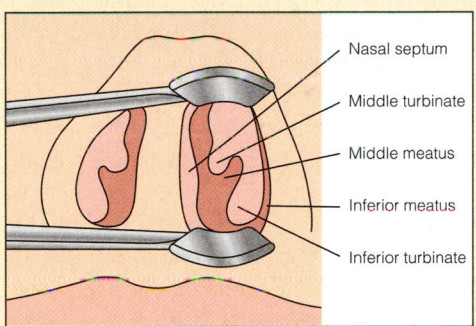

Nasal septum
Middle turbinate
Middle meatus
Inferior meatus
Inferior turbinate

Figure 28–35 ■ The inferior and middle turbinates of the nasal passage.

Assessment	Normal Findings	Deviations from Normal
10. Observe for the presence of redness, swelling, growths, and discharge.	Mucosa pink	Mucosa red, edematous
	Clear, watery discharge	Abnormal discharge (e.g., purulent)
	No lesions	Presence of lesions (e.g., polyps)
11. Inspect the nasal septum between the nasal chambers.	Nasal septum intact and in midline	Septum deviated to the right or to the left.
FACIAL SINUSES		
12. Palpate the maxillary and frontal sinuses for tenderness.	Not tender	Tenderness in one or more sinuses
13. Document findings in the client record using forms or checklists supplemented by narrative notes when appropriate.		

EVALUATION

- Perform a detailed follow-up examination of other systems based on findings that deviated from expected or normal for the client. Relate findings to previous assessment data if available.
- Report significant deviations from normal to the physician.

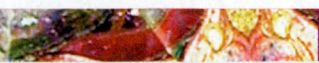

Lifespan Considerations

Assessing the Nose and Sinuses

Infants
- A speculum is usually not necessary to examine the septum, turbinates, and vestibule. Instead, push the tip of the nose upward with the thumb and shine a light into the nares.

Children
- A speculum is usually not necessary to examine the septum, turbinates, and vestibule. It might cause the child to be apprehensive. Instead, push the tip of the nose upward with the thumb and shine a light into the nares.

- Ethmoid sinuses develop by age 6. Sinus problems in children under this age are rare.

Elders
- The sense of smell markedly diminishes because of a decrease in the number of olfactory nerve fibers and atrophy of the remaining fibers. Elders are less able to identify and discriminate odors.
- Nosebleeds may result from hypertensive disease or other arterial vessel changes.

Mouth and Oropharynx

The mouth and pharynx are composed of a number of structures: lips, inner and buccal mucosa, the tongue and floor of the mouth, teeth and gums, hard and soft palate, uvula, salivary glands, tonsillar pillars, and tonsils. Anatomic structures of the mouth are shown in Figure 28–36 ■.

By age 25, most people have all their permanent teeth. For information about structures of the teeth, see Chapter 31. ⌾

Normally, three pairs of salivary glands empty into the oral cavity: the parotid, submandibular, and sublingual glands. The *parotid gland* is the largest and empties through the Stensen's duct opposite the second molar. The *submandibular gland* empties through Wharton's duct, which is situated at the side of the frenulum on the floor of the mouth. The *sublingual salivary gland* lies in the floor of the mouth and has numerous openings.

Dental **caries** (cavities) and **periodontal disease** (**pyorrhea**) are the two problems that most frequently affect the teeth. Both problems are commonly associated with plaque and tartar deposits. **Plaque** is an invisible soft film that adheres to the enamel surface of teeth; it consists of bacteria, molecules of saliva, and remnants of epithelial cells and leukocytes. When plaque is unchecked, tartar (dental calculus) forms. **Tartar** is a visible, hard deposit of plaque and dead bacteria that forms at the gum lines. Tartar buildup can alter the fibers that attach the teeth to the gum and eventually disrupt bone tissue. Periodontal disease is characterized by **gingivitis** (red, swollen gingiva, i.e., gum), bleeding, receding gum lines, and the formation of pockets between the teeth and gums. In advanced periodontal

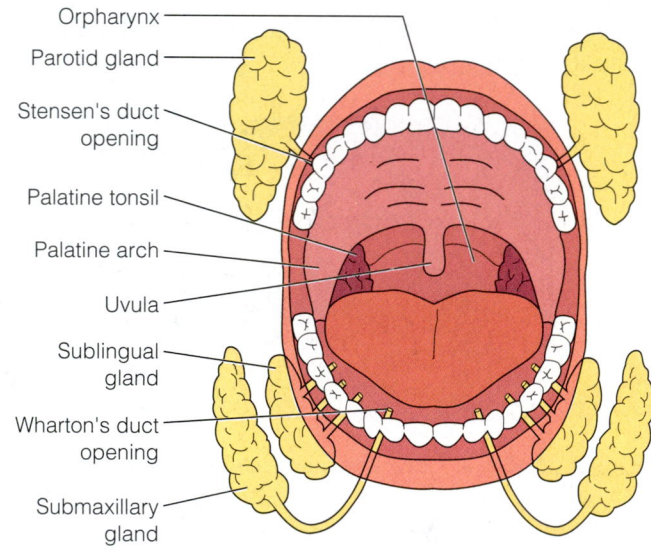

Figure 28–36 ■ Anatomic structures of the mouth.

disease, the teeth are loose and pus is evident when the gums are pressed.

Other problems nurses may see are **glossitis** (inflammation of the tongue), stomatitis (inflammation of the oral mucosa), and **parotitis** (inflammation of the parotid salivary gland). The accumulation of foul matter (food, microorganisms, and epithelial elements) on the teeth and gums is referred to as **sordes.**

Procedure 28–9 describes assessment of the mouth and oropharynx.

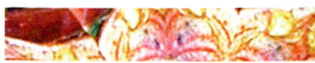

Procedure 28-9 Assessing the Mouth and Oropharynx

PLANNING

If possible, arrange for the client to sit with the head against a firm surface such as a headrest or examination table. This makes it easier for the client to hold the head still during the examination.

Delegation
Assessment of the mouth and oropharynx is not delegated to unlicensed assistive personnel. However, many aspects are observed during usual care and may be recorded by persons other than the

nurse. Abnormal findings must be validated and interpreted by the nurse.

Equipment
- Examination gloves
- Tongue depressor
- 2×2 gauze pads
- Flashlight or penlight

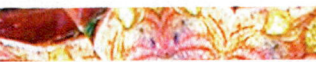 **Procedure 28-9 Assessing the Mouth and Oropharynx** *continued*

IMPLEMENTATION

Performance

1. Explain to the client what you are going to do, why it is necessary, and how he or she can cooperate. Discuss how the results will be used in planning further care or treatments.
2. Observe appropriate infection control procedures.
3. Provide for client privacy.
4. Inquire if the client has any history of the following: routine pattern of dental care, last visit to dentist; length of time ulcers or other lesions have been present; any denture discomfort; any medications client is receiving.
5. Position the client comfortably, seated if possible.

Assessment	Normal Findings	Deviations from Normal
LIPS AND BUCCAL MUCOSA		
6. Inspect the outer lips for symmetry of contour, color, and texture. Ask the client to purse the lips as if to whistle.	Uniform pink color (darker, e.g., bluish hue, in Mediterranean groups and dark-skinned clients) Soft, moist, smooth texture Symmetry of contour Ability to purse lips	Pallor; cyanosis Blisters; generalized or localized swelling; fissures, crusts, or scales (may result from excessive moisture, nutritional deficiency, or fluid deficit) Inability to purse lips (indicative of facial nerve damage)
7. Inspect and palpate the inner lips and buccal mucosa for color, moisture, texture, and the presence of lesions. See Box 28–17.	Uniform pink color (freckled brown pigmentation in dark-skinned clients) Moist, smooth, soft, glistening, and elastic texture (drier oral mucosa in elderly due to decreased salivation)	Pallor; white patches (leukoplakia) Excessive dryness Mucosal cysts; irritations from dentures; abrasions, ulcerations; nodules

---

BOX 28–17 ■ Inspecting and Palpating the Lip, Mucosa, Teeth, Gums

Inner Lip and Front Teeth
- Apply examination gloves.
- Ask the client to relax the mouth, and, for better visualization, pull the lip outward and away from the teeth.
- Grasp the lip on each side between the thumb and index finger (see Figure 28–37 ■).
- Palpate any lesions for size, tenderness, and consistency.
- Inspect the front teeth and gums.

Buccal Mucosa and Back Teeth
- Ask the client to open the mouth. Using a tongue depressor, retract the cheek (see Figure 28–38 ■). View the surface buccal mucosa from top to bottom and back to front. A flashlight or penlight will help illuminate the surface. Repeat the procedure for the other side.

- Ask the client to open the mouth again. Using a penlight to assist visualization, move a finger along the inside cheek. Another finger may be moved outside the cheek.
- Examine the back teeth. For proper vision of the molars, use the index fingers of both hands to retract the cheek (see Figure 28–39 ■). Ask the client to relax the lips and first close, then open, the jaw. Closing the jaw assists in observation of tooth alignment and loss of teeth; opening the jaw assists in observation of dental fillings and caries. Observe the number of teeth, tooth color, the state of fillings, dental caries, and tartar along the base of the teeth. Note the presence and fit of partial or complete dentures.

Gums
- Inspect the gums around the molars. Observe for bleeding, color, retraction (pulling away from the teeth), edema, and lesions.
- Assess the texture of the gums by gently pressing the gum tissue with a tongue depressor.

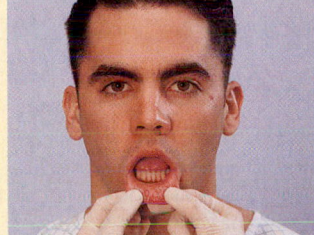

Figure 28–37 ■ Inspecting the mucosa of the lower lip.

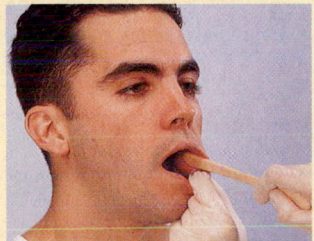

Figure 28–38 ■ Inspecting the buccal mucosa using a tongue depressor.

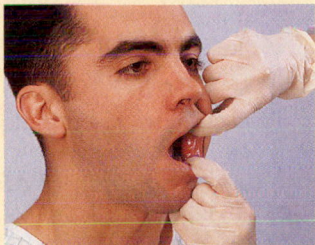

Figure 28–39 ■ Inspecting the back teeth.

continued on page 564

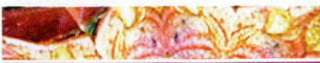

Procedure 28-9 Assessing the Mouth and Oropharynx *continued*

IMPLEMENTATION *continued*

Assessment	Normal Findings	Deviations from Normal
TEETH AND GUMS		
8. Inspect the teeth and gums while examining the inner lips and buccal mucosa (see Box 28–17).	32 adult teeth	Missing teeth; ill-fitting dentures
	Smooth, white, shiny tooth enamel	Brown or black discoloration of the enamel (may indicate staining or the presence of caries)
	Pink gums (bluish or dark patches in dark-skinned clients)	Excessively red gums
	Moist, firm texture to gums	Spongy texture; bleeding; tenderness (may indicate periodontal disease)
	No retraction of gums (pulling away from the teeth)	Receding, atrophied gums; swelling that partially covers the teeth
9. Inspect the dentures. Ask the client to remove complete or partial dentures. Inspect their condition, noting in particular broken or worn areas.	Smooth, intact dentures	Ill-fitting dentures; irritated and excoriated area under dentures
TONGUE/FLOOR OF THE MOUTH		
10. Inspect the surface of the tongue for position, color, and texture. Ask the client to protrude the tongue.	Central position	Deviated from center [may indicate damage to hypoglossal (twelfth cranial) nerve]; excessive trembling
	Pink color (some brown pigmentation on tongue borders in dark-skinned clients); moist; slightly rough; thin whitish coating	Smooth red tongue (may indicate iron, vitamin B_{12}, or vitamin B_3 deficiency)
	Smooth, lateral margins; no lesions	Dry, furry tongue (associated with fluid deficit)
	Raised papillae (taste buds)	Nodes, ulcerations, discolorations (white or red areas); areas of tenderness
11. Inspect tongue movement. Ask the client to roll the tongue upward and move it from side to side.	Moves freely; no tenderness	Restricted mobility
12. Inspect the base of the tongue, the mouth floor, and the frenulum. Ask the client to place the tip of the tongue against the roof of the mouth.	Smooth tongue base with prominent veins	Swelling, ulceration
13. Palpate the tongue and floor of the mouth for any nodules, lumps, or excoriated areas. To palpate the tongue, use a piece of gauze to grasp its tip (stabilize it), and with the index finger of your other hand, palpate the back of the tongue, its borders, and its base (see Figure 28–40 ■).	Smooth with no palpable nodules	Swelling, nodules

To assess function of the glossopharyngeal and hypoglossal nerves, see the neurologic assessment, later in this chapter.

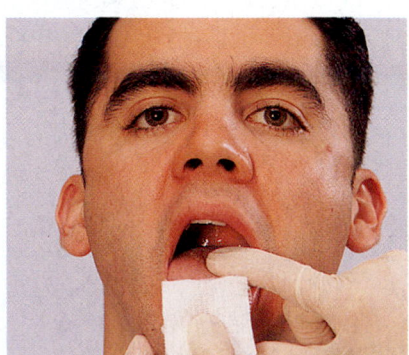

Figure 28–40 ■ Palpating the tongue.

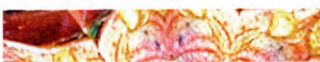

Procedure 28-9 Assessing the Mouth and Oropharynx *continued*

IMPLEMENTATION *continued*

Assessment	Normal Findings	Deviations from Normal
SALIVARY GLANDS		
14. Inspect salivary duct openings for any swelling or redness. See Figure 28–36.	Same as color of buccal mucosa and floor of mouth	Inflammation (redness and swelling)
PALATES AND UVULA		
15. Inspect the hard and soft palate for color, shape, texture, and the presence of bony prominences. Ask the client to open the mouth wide and tilt the head backward. Then, depress tongue with a tongue blade as necessary, and use a penlight for appropriate visualization.	Light pink, smooth, soft palate Lighter pink hard palate, more irregular texture	Discoloration (e.g., jaundice or pallor) Palates the same color Irritations Bony growths (exostoses) growing from the hard palate
16. Inspect the uvula for position and mobility while examining the palates. To observe the uvula, ask the client to say "ah" so that the soft palate rises.	Positioned in midline of soft palate	Deviation to one side from tumor or trauma; immobility [may indicate damage to trigeminal (fifth cranial) nerve or vagus (tenth cranial) nerve]
OROPHARYNX AND TONSILS		
17. Inspect the oropharynx for color and texture. Inspect one side at a time to avoid eliciting the gag reflex. To expose one side of the oropharynx, press a tongue blade against the tongue on the same side about halfway back while the client tilts the head back and opens the mouth wide. Use a penlight for illumination, if needed.	Pink and smooth posterior wall	Reddened or edematous; presence of lesions, plaques, or drainage
18. Inspect the tonsils (behind the fauces) for color, discharge, and size.	Pink and smooth No discharge Of normal size (see Box 28–18 for a grading system to describe the size of tonsils) or not visible	Inflamed Presence of discharge Swollen

---

BOX 28–18 ■ Grading System to Describe Size of Tonsils

- *Grade 1 (normal):* The tonsils are behind the tonsillar pillars (the soft structures supporting the soft palate).
- *Grade 2:* The tonsils are between the pillars and the uvula.
- *Grade 3:* The tonsils touch the uvula.
- *Grade 4:* One or both tonsils extend to the midline of the oropharynx.

---

19. Elicit the gag reflex by pressing the posterior tongue with a tongue blade.	Present	Absent (may indicate problems with glossopharyngeal or vagus nerves)
20. Document findings in the client record using forms or checklists supplemented by narrative notes when appropriate.		

EVALUATION

- Perform a detailed follow-up examination of neurological and other systems based on findings that deviated from expected or normal for the client. Relate findings to previous assessment data if available.
- Report significant deviations from normal to the physician.

Lifespan Considerations

Assessing the Mouth and Oropharynx

Infants
■ Inspect the palate for a cleft.

Children
■ Tooth development should be appropriate for age.
■ White spots on the teeth may indicate excessive fluoride ingestion.
■ Drooling is common up to 2 years of age.
■ The tonsils are normally larger in children than in adults and commonly extend beyond the palatine arch until the age of 11 or 12 years.

Elders
■ The oral mucosa may be drier than that of younger persons because of decreased salivary gland activity. Decreased salivation occurs only in elderly people taking prescribed medications such as antidepressants, antihistamines, decongestants, diuretics, antihypertensives, tranquilizers, antispasmodics, and antineoplastics. Extreme dryness is associated with dehydration.
■ Some receding of the gums occurs, giving an appearance of increased toothiness.

■ There may be a brownish pigmentation to the gums, especially in Black persons.
■ Taste sensations diminish. Sweet and salty tastes are lost first. Elderly persons may add more salt and sugar to food than they did when they were younger. Diminished taste sensation is due to atrophy of the taste buds and a decreased sense of smell. It indicates diminished function of the fifth and seventh cranial nerves.
■ Tiny purple or bluish black swollen areas (varicosities) under the tongue, known as *caviar spots,* are not uncommon.
■ The teeth may show signs of staining, erosion, chipping, and abrasions due to loss of dentin.
■ Tooth loss occurs as a result of dental disease but is preventable with good dental hygiene.
■ The gag reflex may be slightly sluggish.
■ Elders who are homebound or are in long-term care facilities often have teeth or dentures in need or repair, due to the difficulty of obtaining dental care in these situations. Do a thorough assessment of missing teeth and those in need of repair, whether they are natural teeth or dentures.

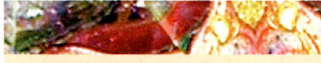

Home Care Considerations

Assessing the Mouth and Oropharynx
■ Although clients may be sensitive to discussion of their personal hygiene practices, use the assessment as an opportunity to provide teaching regarding appropriate oral and dental care for the entire family. Refer clients to a dentist if indicated.

NECK

Examination of the neck includes the muscles, lymph nodes, trachea, thyroid gland, carotid arteries, and jugular veins. Areas of the neck are defined by the sternocleidomastoid muscles, which divide each side of the neck into two triangles: the anterior and posterior (Figure 28–41 ■). The trachea, thyroid gland, anterior cervical nodes, and carotid artery lie within the anterior triangle (Figure 28–42 ■); the carotid artery runs parallel and anterior to the sternocleidomastoid muscle. The posterior lymph nodes lie within the posterior triangle (Figure 28–43 ■).

Each sternocleidomastoid muscle extends from the upper sternum and the medial third of the clavicle to the mastoid process of the temporal bone behind the ear. These muscles turn and laterally flex the head. Each trapezius muscle extends from the occipital bone of the skull to the lateral third of the clavicle. These muscles draw the head to the side and back, elevate the chin, and elevate the shoulders to shrug them.

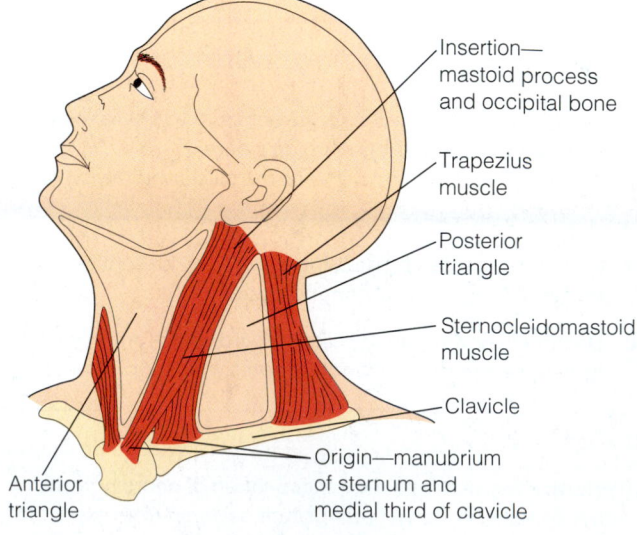

Figure 28–41 ■ Major muscles of the neck.

Lymph nodes in the neck that collect lymph from the head and neck structures are grouped serially and referred to as *chains*. See Figure 28–43 and Table 28–6. The deep cervical chain is not shown in Figure 28–43 because it lies beneath the sternocleidomastoid muscle.

Procedure 28–10 describes how to assess the neck.

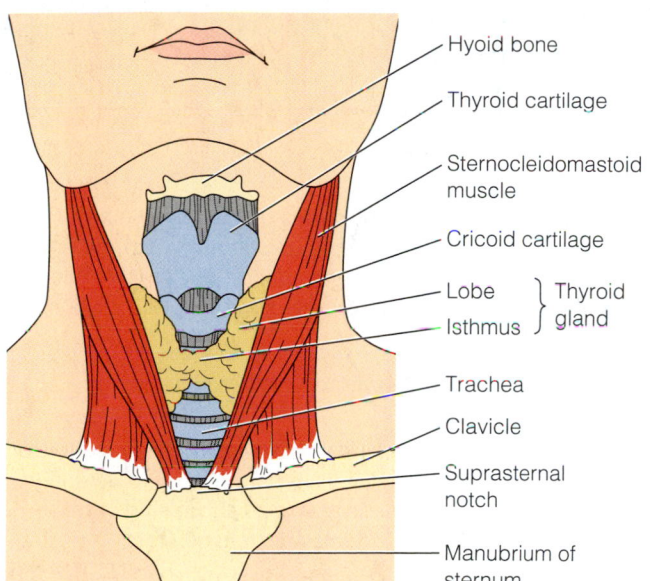

Figure 28–42 ■ Structures of the neck.

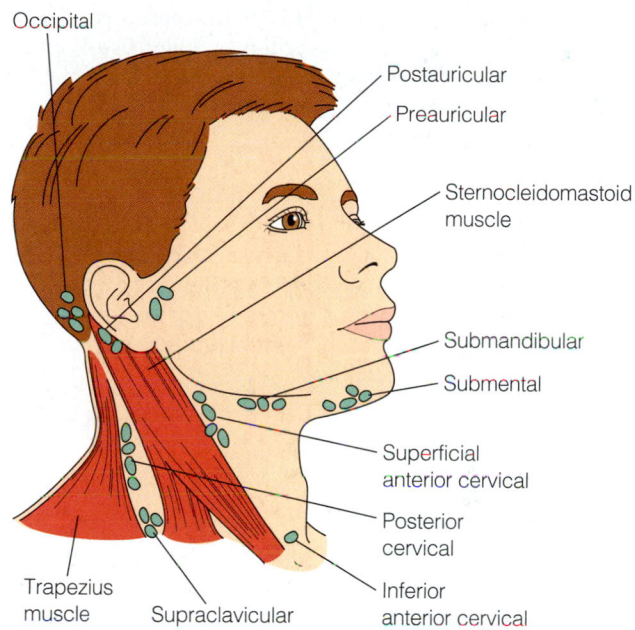

Figure 28–43 ■ Lymph nodes of the neck.

TABLE 28–6 Lymph Nodes of the Head and Neck

Node Center	Location	Area Drained
Head		
Occipital	At the posterior base of the skull	The occipital region of the scalp and the deep structures of the back of the neck
Postauricular (mastoid)	Behind the auricle of the ear or in front of the mastoid process	The parietal region of the head and part of the ear
Preauricular	In front of the tragus of the ear	The forehead and upper face
Floor of Mouth		
Submandibular (submaxillary)	Along the medial border of the lower jaw, halfway between the angle of the jaw and the chin	The chin, upper lip, cheek, nose, teeth, eyelids, part of the tongue and of the floor of the mouth
Submental	Behind the tip of the, mandible in the midline, under the chin	The anterior third of the tongue, gums, and floor of the mouth
Neck		
Superficial (anterior) cervical chain	Along the anterior to the sternocleidomastoid muscle	The skin and neck
Posterior cervical chain	Along the anterior aspect of the trapezius muscle	The posterior and lateral regions of the neck, occiput, and mastoid
Deep cervical chain	Under the sternocleidomastoid muscle	The larynx, thyroid gland, trachea, and upper part of the esophagus
Supraclavicular	Above the clavicle, in the angle between the clavicle and the sternocleidomastoid muscle	The lateral regions of the neck and lungs

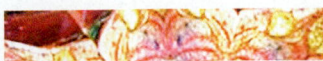

Procedure 28-10 Assessing the Neck

PLANNING

Delegation

Assessment of the neck is not delegated to unlicensed assistive personnel. However, many aspects are observed during usual care and may be recorded by persons other than the nurse. Abnormal findings must be validated and interpreted by the nurse.

Equipment

None

IMPLEMENTATION

Performance

1. Explain to the client what you are going to do, why it is necessary, and how he or she can cooperate. Discuss how the results will be used in planning further care or treatments.
2. Observe appropriate infection control procedures.
3. Provide for client privacy.
4. Inquire if the client has any history of the following: any problems with neck lumps; neck pain or stiffness; when and how any lumps occurred; any previous diagnoses of thyroid problems; and any other treatments provided (e.g., surgery, radiation).

Assessment	Normal Findings	Deviations from Normal
NECK MUSCLES		
5. Inspect the neck muscles (sternocleidomastoid and trapezius) for abnormal swellings or masses. Ask the client to hold the head erect.	Muscles equal in size; head centered	Unilateral neck swelling; head tilted to one side (indicates presence of masses, injury, muscle weakness, shortening of sternocleidomastoid muscle, scars)
6. Observe head movement. Ask client to	Coordinated, smooth movements with no discomfort	Muscle tremor, spasm, or stiffness
● Move the chin to the chest (determines function of the sternocleidomastoid muscle).	Head flexes 45°	Limited range of motion; painful movements; involuntary movements (e.g., up-and-down nodding movements associated with Parkinson's disease)
● Move the head back so that the chin points upward (determines function of the trapezius muscle).	Head hyperextends 60°	Head hyperextends less than 60°
● Move the head so that the ear is moved toward the shoulder on each side (determines function of the sternocleidomastoid muscle).	Head laterally flexes 40°	Head laterally flexes less than 40°
● Turn the head to the right and to the left (determines function of the sternocleidomastoid muscle).	Head laterally rotates 70°	Head laterally rotates less than 70°
7. Assess muscle strength.		
● Ask the client to turn the head to one side against the resistance of your hand. Repeat with the other side (determines the strength of the sternocleidomastoid muscle).	Equal strength	Unequal strength
● Shrug the shoulders against the resistance of your hands (determines the strength of the trapezius muscles).	Equal strength	Unequal strength
LYMPH NODES		
8. Palpate the entire neck for enlarged lymph nodes, using the guidelines shown in Box 28–19.	Not palpable	Enlarged, palpable, possibly tender (associated with infection and tumors)

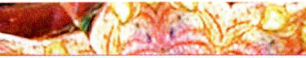

Procedure 28-10 Assessing the Neck *continued*

IMPLEMENTATION *continued*

BOX 28–19 ■ Palpating Neck Lymph Nodes

- Face the client, and bend the client's head forward slightly or toward the side being examined to relax the soft tissue and muscles.
- Palpate the nodes using the pads of the fingers. Move the fingertips in a gentle rotating motion.
- When examining the submental and submandibular nodes, place the fingertips under the mandible on the side nearest the palpating hand, and pull the skin and subcutaneous tissue laterally over the mandibular surface so that the tissue rolls over the nodes.
- When palpating the supraclavicular nodes, have the client bend the head forward to relax the tissues of the anterior neck and to relax the shoulders so that the clavicles drop. Use your hand nearest the side to be examined when facing the client, i.e., your left hand for the client's right nodes. Use your free hand to flex the client's head forward if necessary. Hook your index and third fingers over the clavicle lateral to the sternocleidomastoid muscle (see Figure 28–44 ■).
- When palpating the anterior cervical nodes and posterior cervical nodes, move your fingertips slowly in a forward circular motion against the sternocleidomastoid and trapezius muscles, respectively.
- To palpate the deep cervical nodes, bend or hook your fingers around the sternocleidomastoid muscle.

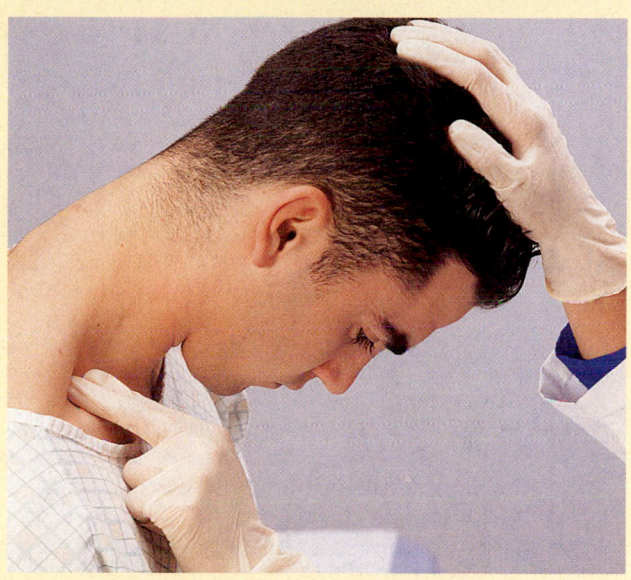

Figure 28–44 ■ Palpating the supraclavicular lymph nodes.

Assessment	Normal Findings	Deviations from Normal
TRACHEA		
9. Palpate the trachea for lateral deviation. Place your fingertip or thumb on the trachea in the suprasternal notch (see Figure 28–43, earlier), and then move your finger laterally to the left and the right in spaces bordered by the clavicle, the anterior aspect of the sternocleidomastoid muscle, and the trachea.	Central placement in midline of neck; spaces are equal on both sides	Deviation to one side, indicating possible neck tumor; thyroid enlargement; enlarged lymph nodes
THYROID GLAND		
10. Inspect the thyroid gland.		
● Stand in front of the client.		
● Observe the lower half of the neck overlying the thyroid gland for symmetry and visible masses.	Not visible on inspection	Visible diffuseness or local enlargement
● Ask the client to hyperextend the head and swallow. If necessary, offer a glass of water to make it easier for the client to swallow. This action determines how the thyroid and cricoid cartilages move and whether swallowing causes a bulging of the gland.	Gland ascends during swallowing but is not visible	Gland is not fully movable with swallowing

continued on page 570

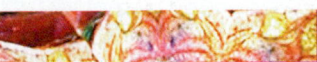

Procedure 28-10 Assessing the Neck *continued*

IMPLEMENTATION *continued*

Assessment	Normal Findings	Deviations from Normal
11. Palpate the thyroid gland for smoothness. Note any areas of enlargement, masses, or nodules. See Box 28–20 for palpation methods.	Lobes may not be palpated If palpated, lobes are small, smooth, centrally located, painless, and rise freely with swallowing	Solitary nodules

---

BOX 28–20 ■ Palpating the Thyroid Gland

Stand in front of or behind the client, and ask the client to lower the chin slightly. Lowering the chin relaxes the neck muscles, facilitating palpation.

Posterior Approach

■ Place your hands around the client's neck, with your fingertips on the lower half of the neck over the trachea (see Figure 28–45 ■).

■ Ask the client to swallow (taking a sip of water, if necessary), and feel for any enlargement of the thyroid isthmus as it rises. The isthmus lies across the trachea, below the cricoid cartilage. See Figure 28–42, earlier.

■ To examine the right thyroid lobe, have the client lower the chin slightly and turn the head slightly to the right (the side being examined). With your left fingers, displace the trachea slightly to the right. With your right fingers, palpate the right thyroid lobe. Have the client swallow while you are palpating.

■ Repeat the last step, in reverse, to examine the left thyroid lobe.

Anterior Approach

■ Place the tips of your index and middle fingers over the trachea, and palpate the thyroid isthmus as the client swallows.

■ To examine the right thyroid lobe, have the client lower the chin slightly and turn the head slightly to the right. With your right fingers, displace the trachea slightly to the client's right (your left). With your left fingers, palpate the right thyroid lobe (see Figure 28–46 ■).

■ To examine the left thyroid lobe, repeat the above step in reverse.

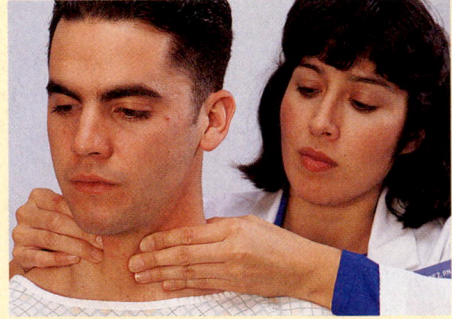

Figure 28–45 ■ Placement of the fingertips over the trachea to begin palpation of the thyroid gland (posterior approach).

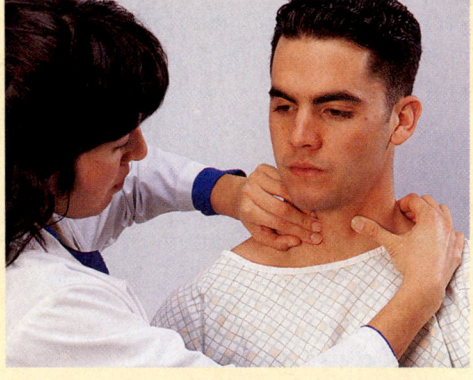

Figure 28–46 ■ Palpating the thyroid (anterior approach).

12. If enlargement of the gland is suspected, auscultate over the thyroid area for a bruit (a soft rushing sound created by turbulent blood flow). Use the bell-shaped diaphragm of the stethoscope.	Absence of bruit	Presence of bruit
13. Document findings in the client record using forms or checklists supplemented by narrative notes when appropriate.		

EVALUATION

■ Perform a detailed follow-up examination of other systems based on findings that deviated from expected or normal for the client. Relate findings to previous assessment data if available.

■ Report significant deviations from normal to the physician.

Lifespan Considerations

Assessing the Neck

Infants and Children

- Examine the neck while the infant or child is lying supine. Lift the head and turn it from side to side to determine neck mobility.

- An infant's neck is normally short, lengthening by about age 3 years. This makes palpation of the trachea difficult.

THORAX AND LUNGS

Assessing the thorax and lungs is frequently critical to assessing the client's aeration status. Changes in the respiratory system can come about slowly or quickly. In clients with chronic obstructive pulmonary disease (COPD), such as chronic bronchitis, emphysema, and asthma, changes are frequently gradual.

The client's posture is important. Some people with chronic respiratory problems tend to bend forward or even prop their arms on a support to elevate their clavicles. This posture is an attempt to expand the chest fully and thus breathe with less effort.

Chest Landmarks

Before beginning the assessment, the nurse must be familiar with a series of imaginary lines on the chest wall and be able to locate the position of each rib and some spinous processes. These landmarks help the nurse to identify the position of underlying organs (e.g., lobes of the lung) and to record abnormal assessment findings. Figure 28–47 ■ shows the anterior, lateral, and posterior series of lines. The midsternal line is a vertical line running through the center of the sternum. The midclavicular lines (right and left) are vertical lines from the midpoints of the clavicles. The anterior axillary lines (right and left) are vertical lines from the anterior axillary folds (Figure 28–47, A). Figure 28–47, B, shows the three imaginary lines of the lateral chest. The posterior axillary line is a vertical line from the posterior axillary fold. The midaxillary line is a vertical line from the apex of the axilla. Figure 28–47, C, shows the

posterior chest landmarks. The vertebral line is a vertical line along the spinous processes. The scapular lines (right and left) are vertical lines from the inferior angles of the scapulae.

Locating the position of each rib and certain spinous processes is essential for identifying underlying lobes of the lung. Figure 28–48 ■, A, shows an anterior view of the chest and underlying lungs; Figure 28–48, B, a posterior view; and Figure 28–48, C, right and left lateral views. Each lung is first divided into the upper and lower lobes by an oblique fissure that runs from the level of the spinous process of the third thoracic vertebra (T-3) to the level of the sixth rib at the midclavicular line. The right upper lobe is abbreviated RUL; the right lower lobe, RLL. Similarly, the left upper lobe is abbreviated LUL; the left lower lobe, LLL. The right lung is further divided by a minor fissure into the right upper lobe and right middle lobe (RML). This fissure runs anteriorly from the right midaxillary line at the level of the fifth rib to the level of the fourth rib.

These specific landmarks, that is, T-3 and the fourth, fifth, and sixth ribs, are located as follows. The starting point for locating the ribs anteriorly is the **angle of Louis,** the junction between the body of the **sternum** (breastbone) and the **manubrium** (the handlelike superior part of the sternum that joins with the clavicles). The superior border of the second rib attaches to the sternum at this manubriosternal junction (Figure 28–49 ■). The nurse can identify the manubrium by first palpating the clavicle and following its course to its attachment at the manubrium. The nurse then palpates and counts distal ribs and intercostal spaces (ICSs) from the second rib. It is important

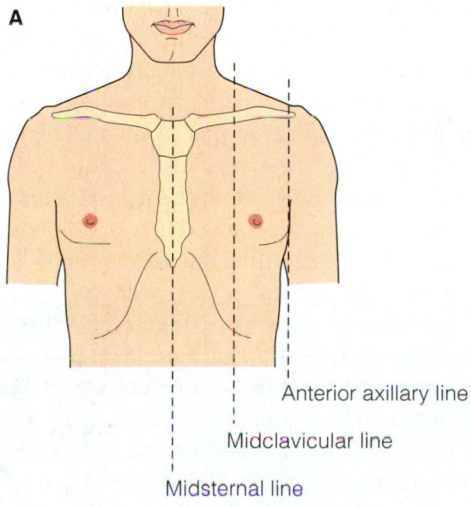

Anterior axillary line

Midclavicular line

Midsternal line

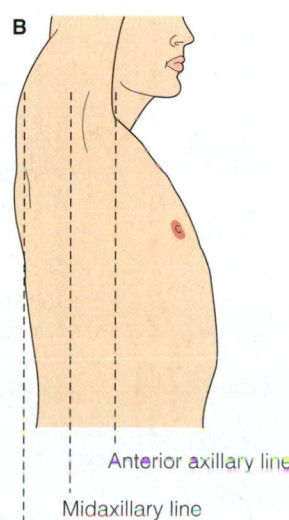

Anterior axillary line

Midaxillary line

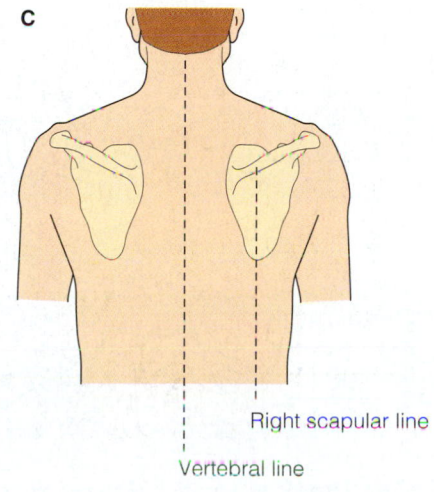

Right scapular line

Vertebral line

Figure 28–47 ■ Chest wall landmarks: A, anterior chest; B, lateral chest; C, posterior chest.

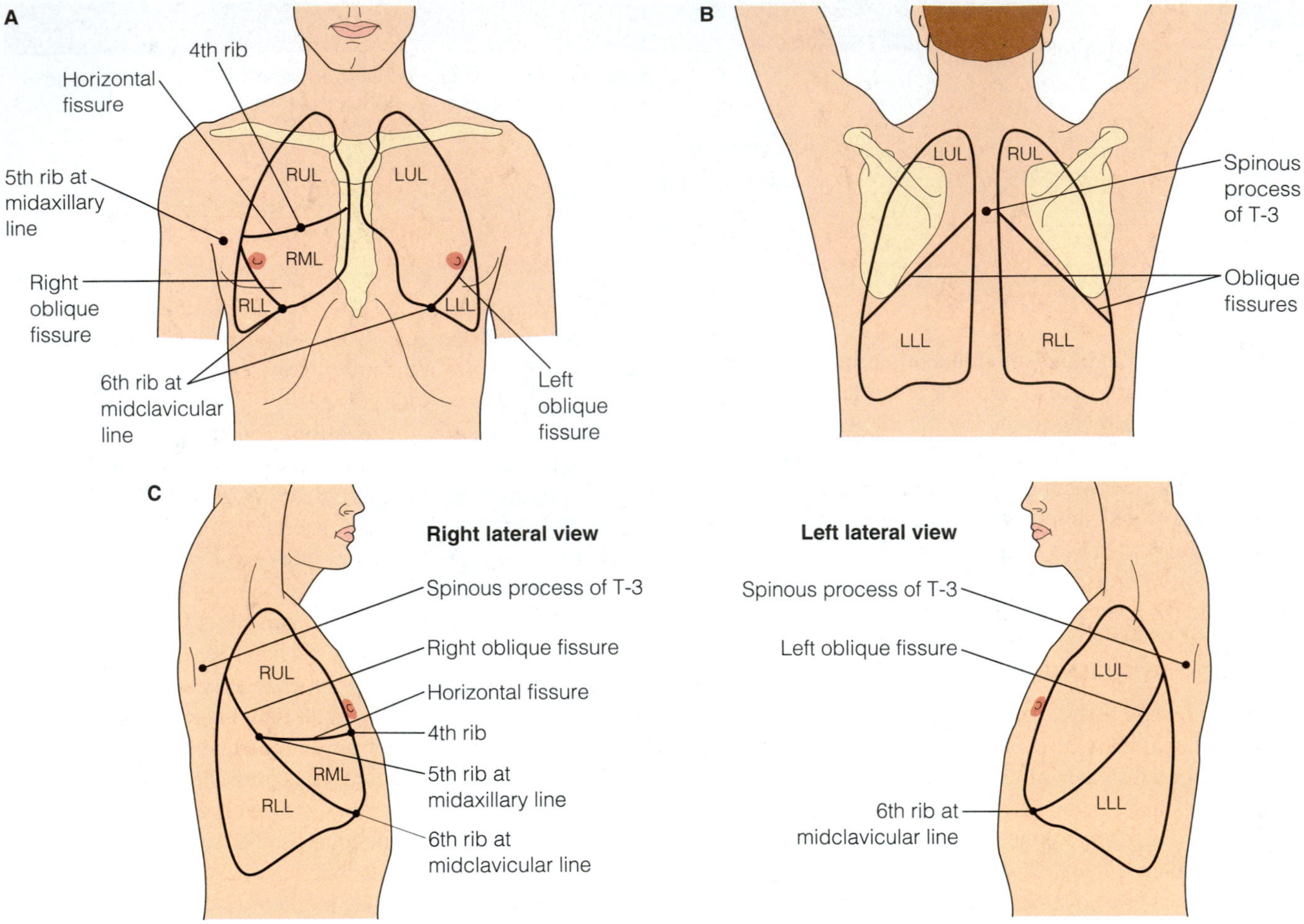

A

4th rib

Horizontal
fissure

5th rib at
midaxillary
line

Right
oblique
fissure

6th rib at
midclavicular
line

RUL   LUL

RML

RLL   LLL

Left
oblique
fissure

B

LUL   RUL

LLL   RLL

Spinous
process
of T-3

Oblique
fissures

C

Right lateral view

Spinous process of T-3

Right oblique fissure

Horizontal fissure

4th rib

5th rib at
midaxillary line

6th rib at
midclavicular line

RUL

RML

RLL

Left lateral view

Spinous process of T-3

Left oblique fissure

6th rib at
midclavicular line

LUL

LLL

Figure 28–48 ■ Chest landmarks: *A,* anterior chest landmarks and underlying lungs; *B,* posterior chest landmarks and underlying lungs; *C,* lateral chest landmarks and underlying lungs.

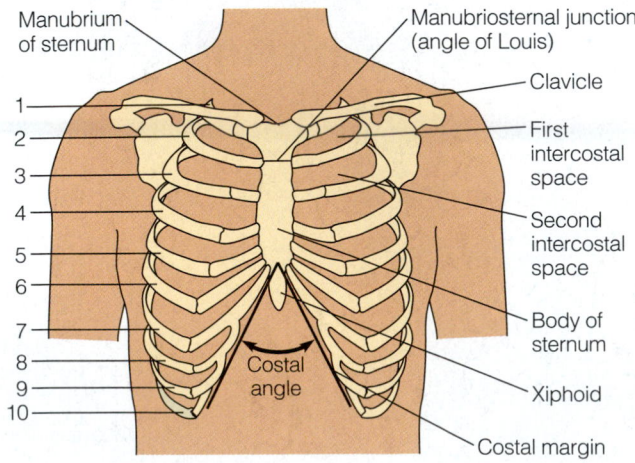

Manubrium
of sternum

Manubriosternal junction
(angle of Louis)

Clavicle

First
intercostal
space

Second
intercostal
space

Body of
sternum

Xiphoid

Costal margin

Costal
angle

1
2
3
4
5
6
7
8
9
10

Figure 28–49 ■ Location of the anterior ribs, angle of Louis, and the sternum.

to note that an ICS is numbered according to the number of the rib immediately *above* the space. When palpating for rib identification, the nurse should palpate along the midclavicular line rather than the sternal border because the rib cartilages are very close at the sternum. Only the first seven ribs attach directly to the sternum.

The counting of ribs is more difficult on the posterior than on the anterior thorax. For identifying underlying lung lobes, the pertinent landmark is T-3. The starting point for locating T-3 is the spinous process of the seventh cervical vertebra (C-7), also referred to as the *vertebra prominens* (Figure 28–50 ■). When the client flexes the neck anteriorly, a prominent process can be observed and palpated. This is the spinous process of the seventh cervical vertebra. If two spinous processes are observed, the superior one is C-7, and the inferior one is the spinous process of the first thoracic vertebra (T-1). The nurse then palpates and counts the spinous processes from C-7 to T-3.

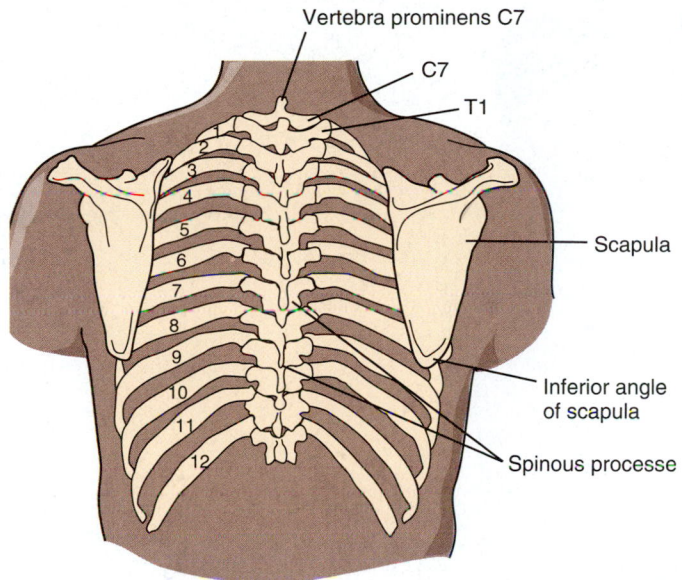

Figure 28–50 ■ Location of the posterior ribs in relation to the spinous processes.

Each spinous process up to T-4 is adjacent to the corresponding rib number; e.g., T-3 is adjacent to the third rib. After T-4, however, the spinous processes project obliquely, causing the spinous process of the vertebra to lie, not over its correspondingly numbered rib, but over the rib below. Thus, the spinous process of T-5 lies over the body of T-6 and is adjacent to the sixth rib.

Chest Shape and Size

In adults, the thorax is oval. Its anteroposterior diameter is half its transverse diameter (Figure 28–51 ■). The overall shape of the thorax is elliptical; that is, its diameter is smaller at the top than at the base. In older adults, kyphosis and osteoporosis alter the size of the chest cavity as the ribs move downward and forward.

There are several deformities of the chest (Figure 28–52 ■). Pigeon chest (*pectus carinatum*), a permanent deformity, may be caused by rickets. A narrow transverse diameter, an increased anteroposterior diameter, and a protruding sternum characterize pigeon chest. A funnel chest (*pectus excavatum*), a congenital defect, is the opposite of pigeon chest in that the sternum is depressed, narrowing the anteroposterior diameter. Because the sternum points posteriorly in clients with a funnel chest, abnormal pressure on the heart may result in altered function. A barrel chest, in which the ratio of the anteroposterior to transverse diameter is 1 to 1, is seen in clients with thoracic kyphosis (excessive convex curvature of the thoracic spine) and emphysema (chronic pulmonary condition in which the air sacs, or alveoli, are dilated and distended). Scoliosis is a lateral deviation of the spine.

Breath Sounds

Abnormal breath sounds, called **adventitious breath sounds,** occur when air passes through narrowed airways or airways filled with fluid or mucus, or when pleural linings are inflamed. Table 28–7 describes normal breath sounds. Adventitious sounds are often superimposed over normal sounds. The four types of adventitious sounds—crackles (referred to as rales or **crepitations**), gurgles, pleural friction rubs, and wheezes—are described in Table 28–8. Absence of breath sounds over some lung areas is also a significant finding that is associated with collapsed and surgically removed lobes.

Assessment of the lungs and thorax includes all methods of examination: inspection, palpation, percussion, and auscultation. Procedure 28–11 describes how to assess the thorax and lungs.

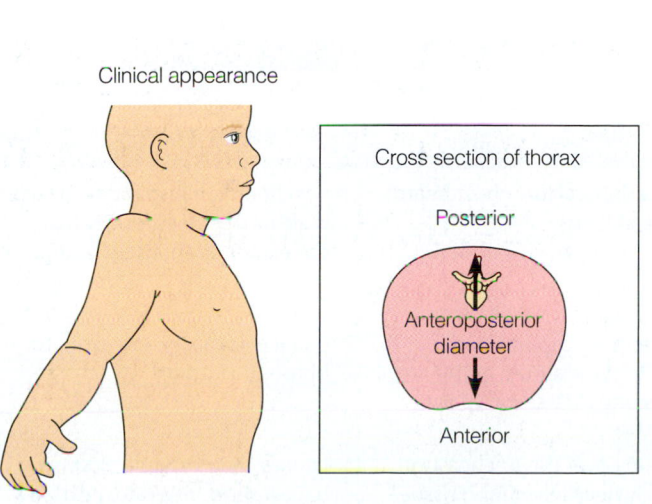
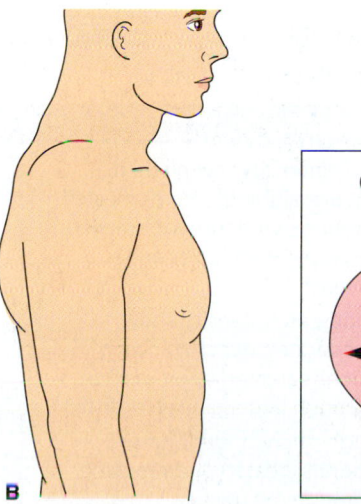
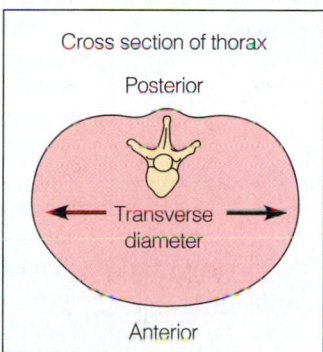

Figure 28–51 ■ Configurations of the thorax showing anteroposterior diameter and transverse diameter: *A*, infant; *B*, adult.

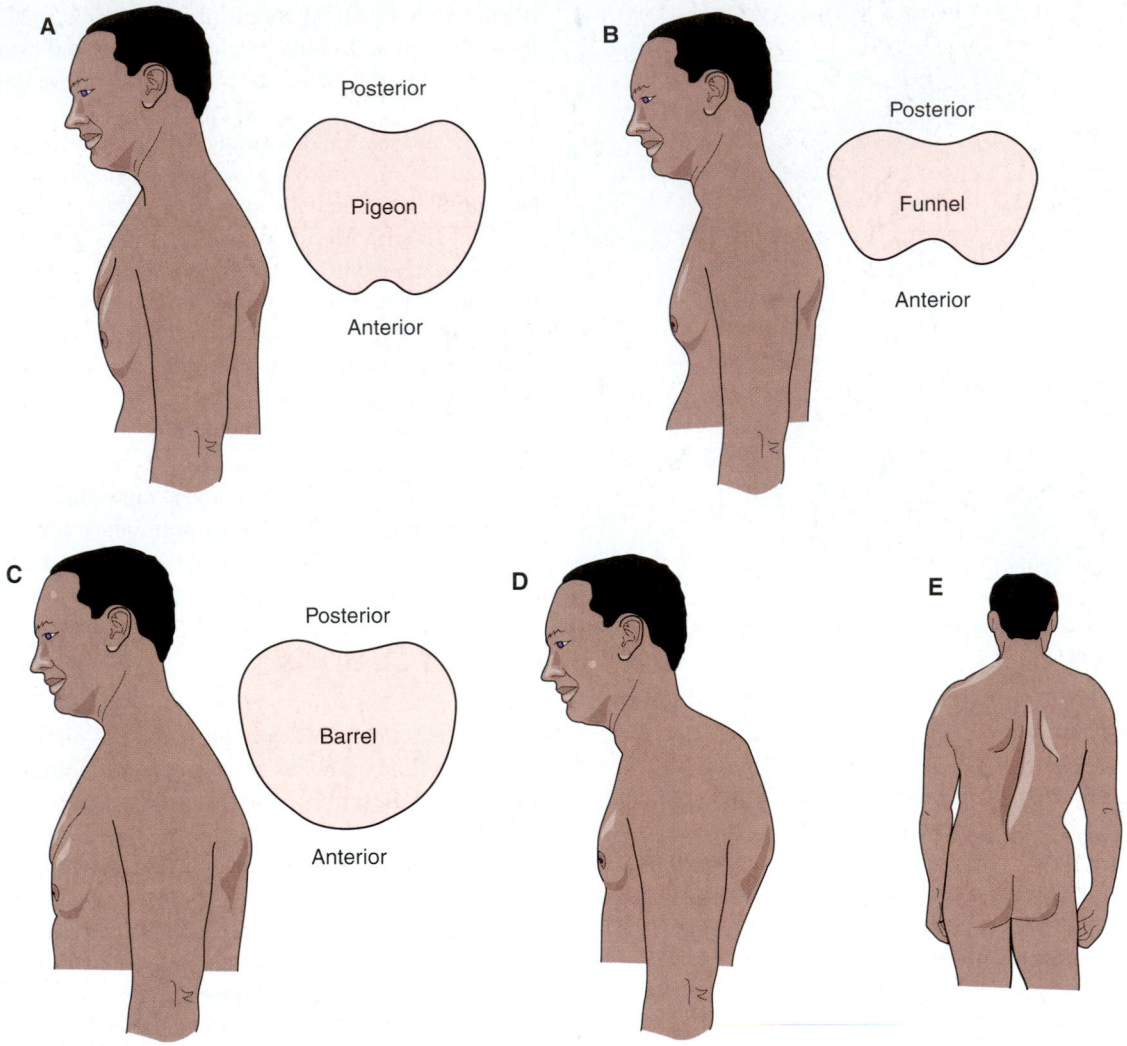

Figure 28–52 ■ Chest deformities. *A,* pigeon chest; *B,* funnel chest; *C,* barrel chest; *D,* kyphosis; *E,* scoliosis.

TABLE 28–7 Normal Breath Sounds

Type	Description	Location	Characteristics
Vesicular	Soft-intensity, low-pitched, "gentle sighing" sounds created by air moving through smaller airways (bronchioles and alveoli)	Over peripheral lung; best heard at base of lungs	Best heard on inspiration, which is about 2.5 times longer than the expiratory phase (5:2 ratio)
Broncho-vesicular	Moderate-intensity and moderate-pitched "blowing" sounds created by air moving through larger airway (bronchi)	Between the scapulae and lateral to the sternum at the first and second intercostal spaces	Equal inspiratory and expiratory phases (1:1 ratio)
Bronchial (tubular)	High-pitched, loud, "harsh" sounds created by air moving through the trachea	Anteriorly over the trachea; not normally heard over lung tissue	Louder than vesicular sounds; have a short inspiratory phase and long expiratory phase (1:2 ratio)

TABLE 28-8 Adventitious Breath Sounds

Name	Description	Cause	Location
Crackles (rales)	Fine, short, interrupted crackling sounds; alveolar rales are high pitched. Sound can be simulated by rolling a lock of hair near the ear. Best heard on inspiration but can be heard on both inspiration and expiration. May not be cleared by coughing.	Air passing through fluid or mucus in any air passage	Most commonly heard in the bases of the lower lung lobes
Gurgles (rhonchi)	Continuous, low-pitched, coarse, gurgling, harsh, louder sounds with a moaning or snoring quality. Best heard on expiration but can be heard on both inspiration and expiration. May be altered by coughing.	Air passing through narrowed air passages as a result of secretions, swelling, tumors	Loud sounds can be heard over most lung areas but predominate over the trachea and bronchi
Friction rub	Superficial grating or creaking sounds heard during inspiration and expiration. Not relieved by coughing.	Rubbing together of inflamed pleural surfaces	Heard most often in areas of greatest thoracic expansion (e.g., lower anterior and lateral chest)
Wheeze	Continuous, high-pitched, squeaky musical sounds. Best heard on expiration. Not usually altered by coughing.	Air passing through a constricted bronchus as a result of secretions, swelling, tumors	Heard over all lung fields

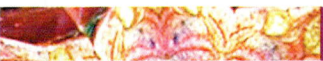

Procedure 28-11 Assessing the Thorax and Lungs

PLANNING

For efficiency, the nurse usually examines the posterior chest first, then the anterior chest. For posterior and lateral chest examinations, the client is uncovered to the waist and in a sitting position. A sitting or lying position may be used for anterior chest examination. The sitting position is preferred because it maximizes chest expansion. Good lighting is essential, especially for chest inspection.

Delegation

Assessment of the thorax and lungs is not delegated to unlicensed assistive personnel. However, many aspects of breathing are observed during usual care and may be recorded by persons other than the nurse. Abnormal findings must be validated and interpreted by the nurse.

Equipment
- Stethoscope
- Skin marker/pencil
- Centimeter ruler

IMPLEMENTATION

Performance

1. Explain to the client what you are going to do, why it is necessary, and how he or she can cooperate. Discuss how the results will be used in planning further care or treatments.
2. Wash hands and observe appropriate infection control procedures.
3. Provide for client privacy. In women, drape the anterior chest when it is not being examined.
4. Inquire if the client has any history of the following: family history of illness, including cancer, allergies, tuberculosis; lifestyle habits such as smoking and occupational hazards (e.g., inhaling fumes); any medications being taken; current problems (e.g., swellings, coughs, wheezing, pain).

continued on page 576

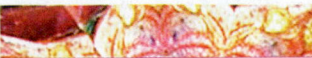

Procedure 28-11 Assessing the Thorax and Lungs *continued*

IMPLEMENTATION *continued*

Assessment	Normal Findings	Deviations from Normal
POSTERIOR THORAX		
5. Inspect the shape and symmetry of the thorax from posterior and lateral views. Compare the anteroposterior diameter to the transverse diameter.	Anteroposterior to transverse diameter in ratio of 1:2 Chest symmetric	Barrel chest; increased anteroposterior to transverse diameter Chest asymmetric
6. Inspect the spinal alignment for deformities. Have the client stand. From a lateral position, observe the three normal curvatures: cervical, thoracic, and lumbar.	Spine vertically aligned	Exaggerated spinal curvatures (kyphosis, lordosis)
● To assess for lateral deviation of spine (scoliosis), observe the standing client from the rear. Have the client bend forward at the waist and observe from behind.	Spinal column is straight, right and left shoulders and hips are at same height.	Spinal column deviates to one side, often accentuated when bending over. Shoulders or hips not even.
7. Palpate the posterior thorax.		
● For clients who have no respiratory complaints, rapidly assess the temperature and integrity of all chest skin.	Skin intact; uniform temperature	Skin lesions; areas of hyperthermia
● For clients who do have respiratory complaints, palpate all chest areas for bulges, tenderness, or abnormal movements. Avoid deep palpation for painful areas, especially if a fractured rib is suspected. In such a case, deep palpation could lead to displacement of the bone fragment against the lungs.	Chest wall intact; no tenderness; no masses	Lumps, bulges; depressions; areas of tenderness; movable structures (e.g., rib)
8. Palpate the posterior chest for respiratory excursion (thoracic expansion). Place the palms of both your hands over the lower thorax with your thumbs adjacent to the spine and your fingers stretched laterally (Figure 28–53 ■). Ask the client to take a deep breath while you observe the movement of your hands and any lag in movement.	Full and symmetric chest expansion [i.e., when the client takes a deep breath, your thumbs should move apart an equal distance and at the same time; normally the thumbs separate 3 to 5 cm (1½ to 2 in.) during deep inspiration]	Asymmetric and/or decreased chest expansion

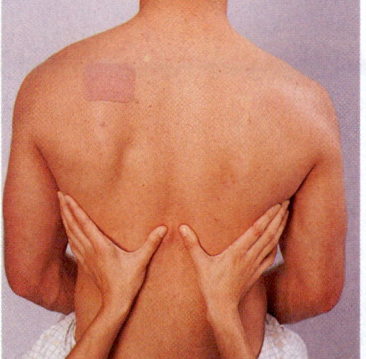

Figure 28–53 ■ Position of the nurse's hands when assessing respiratory excursion on the posterior thorax.

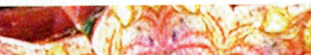

Procedure 28-11 Assessing the Thorax and Lungs *continued*

IMPLEMENTATION *continued*

Assessment	Normal Findings	Deviations from Normal
9. Palpate the chest for vocal (tactile) fremitus, the faintly perceptible vibration felt through the chest wall when the client speaks.	Bilateral symmetry of vocal fremitus	Decreased or absent fremitus (associated with pneumothorax)
● Place the palmar surfaces of your fingertips or the ulnar aspect of your hand or closed fist on the posterior chest, starting near the apex of the lungs (see Figure 28–54 ■, position A).	Fremitus is heard most clearly at the apex of the lungs	Increased fremitus (associated with consolidated lung tissue, as in pneumonia)
● Ask the client to repeat such words as "blue moon" or "one, two, three."	Low-pitched voices of males are more readily palpated than higher pitched voices of females	

● Repeat the two steps, moving your hands sequentially to the base of the lungs, through positions B–E in Figure 28–54 ■.

● Compare the fremitus on both lungs and between the apex and the base of each lung, using either one hand and moving it from one side of the client to the corresponding area on the other side

    or

using two hands that are placed simultaneously on the corresponding areas of each side of the chest.

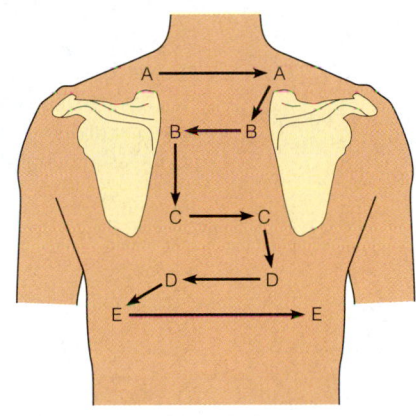

Figure 28–54 ■ Areas and sequence for palpating tactile fremitus on the posterior chest.

10. Percuss the thorax (see Box 28–21).	Percussion notes resonate, except over scapula	Asymmetry in percussion
	Lowest point of resonance is at the diaphragm (i.e., at the level of the 8th to 10th rib posteriorly)	Areas of dullness or flatness over lung tissue (associated with consolidation of lung tissue or a mass)
	Note: percussion on a rib normally elicits dullness	
11. Percuss for diaphragmatic excursion (movement of the diaphragm during maximal inspiration and expiration). See Box 28–21.	Excursion is 3 to 5 cm (1½ to 2 in.) bilaterally in women and 5 to 6 cm (2 to 3 in.) in men	Restricted excursion (associated with lung disorder)
	Diaphragm is usually slightly higher on the right side	
12. Auscultate the chest using the flat-disc diaphragm of the stethoscope (best for transmitting the high-pitched breath sounds).	Vesicular and bronchovesicular breath sounds (see Table 28–7)	Adventitious breath sounds (e.g., crackles, rhonchi, wheeze, friction rub; see Table 28–8)
● Use the systematic zigzag procedure used in percussion (Figure 28–55 ■).		Absence of breath sounds (associated with collapsed and surgically removed lung lobes)

● Ask the client to take slow, deep breaths through the mouth. Listen at each point to the breath sounds during a complete inspiration and expiration.

● Compare findings at each point with the corresponding point on the opposite side of the chest.

continued on page 578

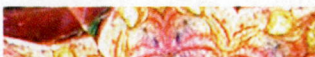

Procedure 28-11 Assessing the Thorax and Lungs *continued*

IMPLEMENTATION *continued*

BOX 28–21 ■ Percussing the Thorax

Percussing for Normal Thorax Sounds

Percussion of the thorax is performed to determine whether underlying lung tissue is filled with air, liquid, or solid material and to determine the positions and boundaries of certain organs. Because percussion penetrates to a depth of 5 to 7 cm (2 to 3 in.), it detects superficial rather than deep lesions. Percussion sounds and tones are described in Table 28–4, earlier.

- Ask the client to bend the head and fold the arms forward across the chest. This separates the scapula and exposes more lung tissue to percussion.
- Percuss in the intercostal spaces at about 5 cm (2 in) intervals in a systematic sequence (see Figure 28–55 ■). Figure 28–56 ■ shows normal percussion sounds in the posterior chest.
- Compare one side of the lung with the other.

- Percuss the lateral thorax every few inches, starting at the axilla and working down to the eighth rib.

Percussing for Diaphragmatic Excursion

- Ask the client to take a deep breath and hold it while you percuss downward along the scapular line until dullness is produced at the level of the diaphragm. Mark this point with a marking pencil, and repeat the procedure on the other side of the chest.
- Ask the client to take a few normal breaths and then expel the last breath completely and hold it while you percuss upward from the marked point to assess and mark the diaphragmatic excursion during deep expiration on each side.
- Measure the distance between the two marks.

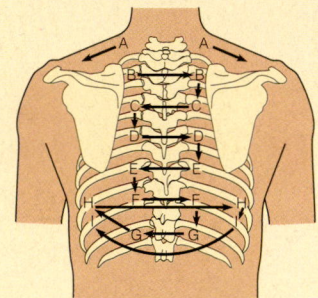

Figure 28–55 ■ Sequence for posterior chest percussion.

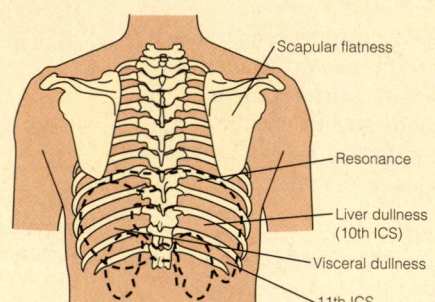

Figure 28–56 ■ Normal percussion sounds on the posterior chest.

Assessment	Normal Findings	Deviations from Normal
ANTERIOR THORAX		
13. Inspect breathing patterns (e.g., respiratory rate and rhythm).	Quiet, rhythmic, and effortless respirations (see Chapter 27, ∞ page 505)	See Chapter 27, Box 27–7 ∞ , on page 507 for abnormal breathing patterns and sounds
14. Inspect the costal angle (angle formed by the intersection of the costal margins) and the angle at which the ribs enter the spine.	Costal angle is less than 90°, and the ribs insert into the spine at approximately a 45° angle (see Figure 28–48, earlier)	Costal angle is widened (associated with chronic obstructive pulmonary disease)
15. Palpate the anterior chest (see posterior chest palpation).		
16. Palpate the anterior chest for respiratory excursion.	Full symmetric excursion; thumbs normally separate 3 to 5 cm (1½ to 2 in.)	Asymmetric and/or decreased respiratory excursion

- Place the palms of both your hands on the lower thorax, with your fingers laterally along the lower rib cage and your thumbs along the costal margins (see Figure 28–57 ■).
- Ask the client to take a deep breath while you observe the movement of your hands.

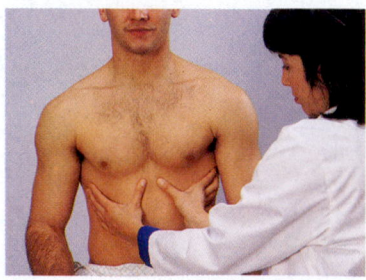

Figure 28–57 ■ Position of nurse's hands when assessing respiratory excursion on the anterior thorax.

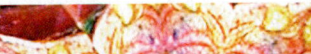

Procedure 28-11 Assessing the Thorax and Lungs *continued*

IMPLEMENTATION *continued*

Assessment	Normal Findings	Deviations from Normal
17. Palpate tactile fremitus in the same manner as for the posterior chest and using the sequence shown in Figure 28–58 ■. If the breasts are large and cannot be retracted adequately for palpation, this part of the examination is usually omitted.	Same as posterior vocal fremitus; fremitus is normally decreased over heart and breast tissue	Same as posterior fremitus

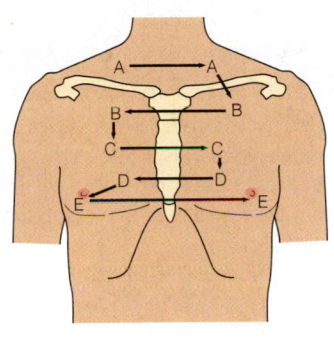

Figure 28–58 ■ Areas and sequence for palpating tactile fremitus on the anterior chest.

Assessment	Normal Findings	Deviations from Normal
18. Percuss the anterior chest systematically. ● Begin above the clavicles in the supraclavicular space, and proceed downward to the diaphragm (Figure 28–59 ■). ● Compare one side of the lung to the other. ● Displace female breasts for proper examination.	Percussion notes resonate down to the sixth rib at the level of the diaphragm but are flat over areas of heavy muscle and bone, dull on areas over the heart and the liver, and tympanic over the underlying stomach (Figure 28–60 ■).	Asymmetry in percussion notes Areas of dullness or flatness over lung tissue

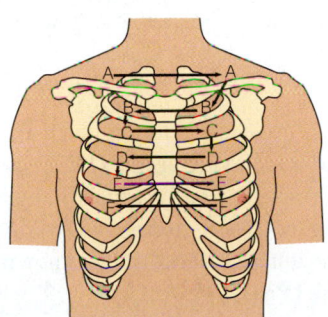

Figure 28–59 ■ Sequence for anterior chest percussion.

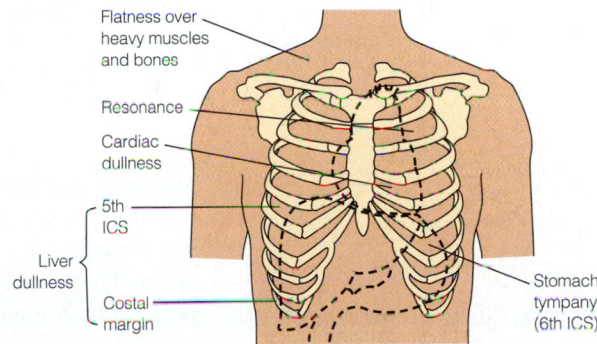

Flatness over heavy muscles and bones
Resonance
Cardiac dullness
5th ICS
Liver dullness
Costal margin
Stomach tympany (6th ICS)

Figure 28–60 ■ Normal percussion sounds on the anterior chest.

Assessment	Normal Findings	Deviations from Normal
19. Auscultate the trachea.	Bronchial and tubular breath sounds (see Table 28–7 on page 574)	Adventitious breath sounds (see Table 28–8 on page 575)
20. Auscultate the anterior chest. Use the sequence used in percussion (see Figure 28–59), beginning over the bronchi between the sternum and the clavicles.	Bronchovesicular and vesicular breath sounds (see Table 28–7)	Adventitious breath sounds (see Table 28–8)

continued on page 580

Procedure 28-11 Assessing the Thorax and Lungs *continued*

IMPLEMENTATION *continued*

21. Document findings in the client record using forms or check-lists supplemented by narrative notes when appropriate.

EVALUATION

■ Relate findings to previous assessment data if available.
Report significant deviations from normal to the physician.

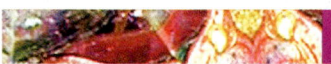

Lifespan Considerations

Assessing the Thorax and Lungs

Infants

■ The thorax is rounded; that is, the diameter from the front to the back (anteroposterior) is equal to the transverse diameter. It is also cylindrical, having a nearly equal diameter at the top and the base.
■ To assess tactile fremitus, place the hand over the crying infant's chest.
■ Auscultated sounds will be louder and harsher.
■ Infants tend to breathe more abdominally than thoracically.

Children

■ By 6 years of age, the anteroposterior diameter has decreased in proportion to the transverse one.
■ Children tend to breathe more abdominally than thoracically up to age 6.

Elders

■ The thoracic curvature may be accentuated (kyphosis) because of osteoporosis and changes in cartilage, resulting in collapse of the vertebrae. This can also compromise and decrease normal respiratory effort.
■ Kyphosis and osteoporosis alter the size of the chest cavity as the ribs move downward and forward.

■ The anteroposterior diameter of the chest widens, giving the person a barrel-chested appearance. This is due to loss of skeletal muscle strength in the thorax and diaphragm and constant lung inflation from excessive expiratory pressure on the alveoli.
■ Breathing rate and rhythm are unchanged at rest; the rate normally increases with exercise but may take longer to return to the preexercise rate.
■ Inspiratory muscles become less powerful, and the inspiration reserve volume decreases. A decrease in depth of respiration is therefore apparent.
■ Expiration may require the use of accessory muscles. The expiratory reserve volume significantly increases because of the increased amount of air remaining in the lungs at the end of a normal breath.
■ Deflation of the lung is incomplete.
■ Small airways lose their cartilaginous support and elastic recoil; as a result, they tend to close, particularly in basal or dependent portions of the lung.
■ Elastic tissue of the alveoli loses its stretchability and changes to fibrous tissue. Exertional capacity decreases.
■ Cilia in the airways decrease in number and are less effective in removing mucus; elderly clients are therefore at greater risk for pulmonary infections.

CARDIOVASCULAR AND PERIPHERAL VASCULAR SYSTEMS

Heart

Nurses assess the heart through observations (inspection), palpation, and auscultation, in that sequence. Auscultation is more meaningful when other data are obtained first. The heart is usually assessed during an initial physical assessment; periodic reassessments may be necessary for long-term or at-risk clients or those with cardiac problems. Heart examinations are usually performed while the client is in a semireclined position.

In the average adult, most of the heart lies behind and to the left of the sternum. A small portion (the right atrium) extends to the right of the sternum. The upper portion of the heart (both atria), referred to as its *base,* lies toward the back. The lower portion (the ventricles), referred to as its *apex,* points anteriorly. The apex of the left ventricle actually touches the chest wall at or medial to the left midclavicular line (MCL) and at or near the fifth left intercostal space (LICS), which is slightly below the left nipple (see Figure 27–18 on page 497). This point where the apex touches the anterior chest wall is known as the **point of maximal impulse (PMI).**

> ► CLINICAL ALERT *Remember that the base of the lungs is the lower (inferior) portion, and the base of the heart is the upper (superior) portion.* ■

The **precordium,** the area of the chest overlying the heart, is inspected and palpated for the presence of abnormal pulsations or lifts or heaves. The terms **lift** and heave, often used interchangeably, refer to a rising along the sternal border with each heartbeat. A lift occurs when cardiac action is very forceful. It should be confirmed by palpation with the palm of the hand.

Enlargement or overactivity of the left ventricle produces a heave lateral to the apex, whereas enlargement of the right ventricle produces a heave at or near the sternum.

Heart sounds can be heard by auscultation. The normal first two heart sounds are produced by closure of the valves of the heart. The first heart sound, S_1, occurs when the atrioventricular (A-V) valves close. These valves close when the ventricles have been sufficiently filled. Although the right and left A-V valves do not close simultaneously, the closures occur closely enough to be heard as one sound, a dull, low-pitched sound described as "lub." After the ventricles empty their blood into the aorta and pulmonary arteries, the semilunar valves close, producing the second heart sound, S_2, described as "dub." S_2 has a higher pitch than S_1 and is also shorter. These two sounds, S_1 and S_2 ("lub-dub"), occur within 1 second or less, depending on the heart rate.

The two heart sounds are audible anywhere on the precordial area, but they are best heard over the aortic, pulmonic, tricuspid, and apical areas (see Figure 28–61 ■). Each area is associated with the closure of heart valves: the aortic area with the aortic valve (inside the aorta as it arises from the left ventricle); the pulmonic area with the pulmonic valve (inside the pulmonary artery as it arises from the right ventricle); the tricuspid area with the tricuspid valve (between the right atrium and ventricle); and the apical area with the mitral valve (between the left atrium and ventricle).

Associated with these sounds are systole and diastole. **Systole** is the period in which the ventricles contract. It begins with S_1 and ends at S_2. Systole is normally shorter than diastole. **Diastole** is the period in which the ventricles relax. It starts with S_2 and ends at the subsequent S_1. Normally no sounds are audible during these periods (see Figure 28–62 ■). The experienced nurse, however, may perceive extra heart sounds (S_3 and S_4) during diastole. Both sounds are low in pitch and heard best at the apical site, with the bell of the stethoscope, and with the client lying on the left side. S_3 occurs early in diastole right after S_2 and sounds like "lub-dub-*ee*" (S_1, S_2, S_3) or "Kentuc-*ky*." It often disappears when the client sits up.

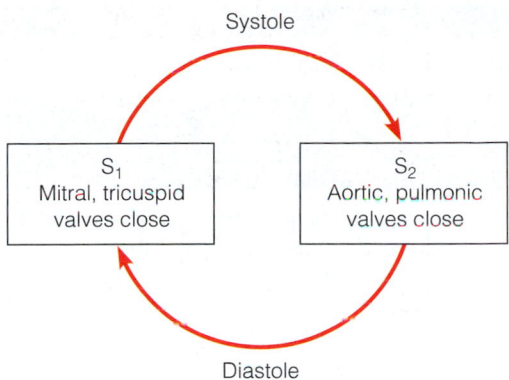

Figure 28–62 ■ Relationship of heart sounds to systole and diastole.

S_3 is normal in children and young adults. In older adults, it may indicate heart failure. It occurs near the very end of diastole just before S_1 and creates the sound of "*dee*-lub-dub" (S_4, S_1, S_2) or "*Ten*-nessee." S_4 is rarely heard in healthy young adults. S_4 may be heard in many elderly clients and can be a sign of hypertension.

Normal heart sounds are summarized in Table 28–9.

Central Vessels

The carotid arteries supply oxygenated blood to the head and neck (see Figure 28–63 ■). Because they are the only source of blood to the brain, prolonged occlusion of these arteries can result in serious brain damage. The carotid pulses correlate with central aortic pressure, thus reflecting cardiac function better than the peripheral pulses. When cardiac output is diminished, the peripheral pulses may be difficult or impossible to feel, but the carotid pulse should be felt easily.

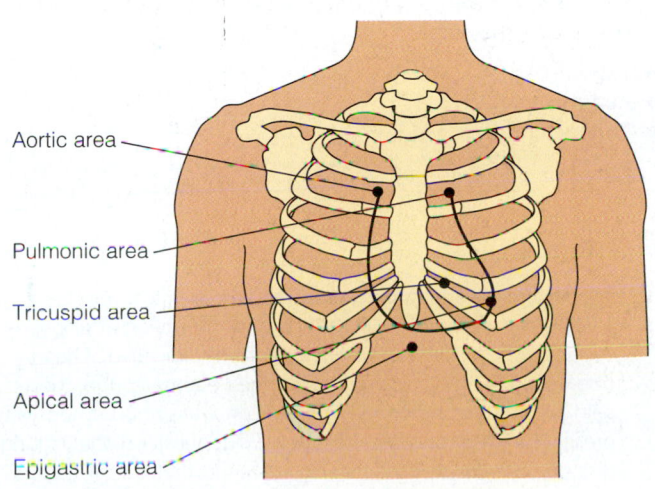

Figure 28–61 ■ Anatomic sites of the precordium.

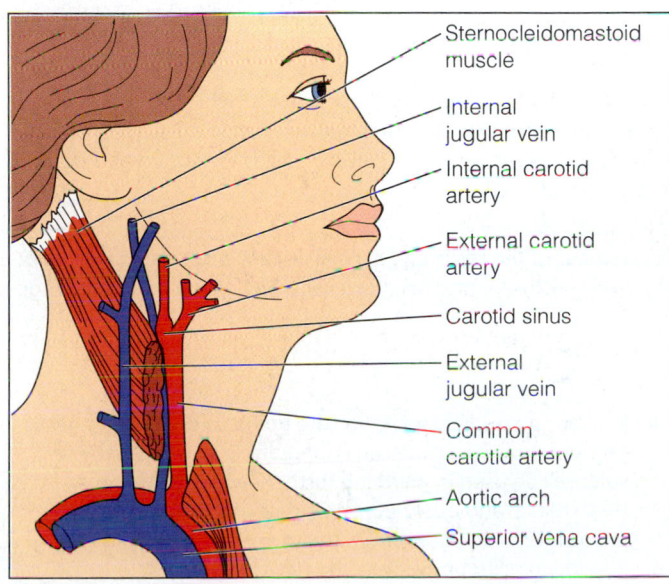

Figure 28–63 ■ Arteries and veins of the right side of the neck.

TABLE 28-9 Normal Heart Sounds

Sound or Phase	Description	Area			
		Aortic	Pulmonic	Tricuspid	Apical
S_1	Dull, low pitched, and longer than S_2; sounds like "lub"	Less intensity than S_2	Less intensity than S_2	Louder than or equal to S_2	Louder than or equal to S_2
Systole	Normally silent interval between S_1 and S_2				
S_2	Higher pitch than S_1; sounds like "dub"	Louder than S_1	Louder than S_1; abnormal if louder than the aortic S_2 in adults over 40 years of age	Less intensity than or equal to S_1	Less intensity than or equal to S_1
Diastole	Normally silent interval between S_2 and next S_1				

The carotid is also auscultated for a bruit, and if a bruit is found, the carotid artery is then palpated for a thrill. A **bruit** (a blowing or swishing sound) is created by turbulence of blood flow due either to a narrowed arterial lumen (a common development in older people) or to a condition, such as anemia or hyperthyroidism, which elevates cardiac output. A **thrill,** which frequently accompanies a bruit, is a vibrating sensation like the purring of a cat or water running through a hose. It, too, indicates turbulent blood flow due to arterial obstruction.

The jugular veins drain blood from the head and neck directly into the superior vena cava and right side of the heart. The external jugular veins are superficial and may be visible above the clavicle. The internal jugular veins lie deeper along the carotid artery and may transmit pulsations onto the skin of the neck. Normally, external neck veins are distended and visible when a person lies down; they are flat and not as visible when a person stands up, because gravity encourages venous drainage. By inspecting the jugular veins for pulsations and distention, the nurse can assess the adequacy of function of the right side of the heart and venous pressure. Bilateral jugular vein distention (JVD) may indicate right-sided heart failure.

Procedure 28–12 describes how to assess the heart and central vessels.

Procedure 28-12 Assessing the Heart and Central Vessels

PLANNING

Heart examinations are usually performed while the client is in a semireclined position. The practitioner stands at the client's right side, where palpation of the cardiac area is facilitated and optimal inspection allowed.

Delegation
Assessment of the heart and central vessels is not delegated to unlicensed assistive personnel. However, many aspects of cardiac function are observed during usual care and may be recorded by persons other than the nurse. Abnormal findings must be validated and interpreted by the nurse.

Equipment
- Stethoscope
- Centimeter ruler

IMPLEMENTATION

Performance

1. Explain to the client what you are going to do, why it is necessary, and how he or she can cooperate. Discuss how the results will be used in planning further care or treatments.
2. Wash hands and observe appropriate infection control procedures.
3. Provide for client privacy.
4. Inquire if the client has any history of the following: family history of incidence and age of heart disease, high cholesterol levels, high blood pressure, stroke, obesity, congenital heart disease, arterial disease, and hypertension, and rheumatic fever; client's past history of rheumatic fever, heart murmur, heart attack, varicosities, or heart failure; present symptoms indicative of heart disease, e.g., fatigue, dyspnea, orthopnea, edema, cough, chest pain, palpitations, syncope, hypertension, wheezing, hemoptysis; presence of diseases that affect heart, e.g., obesity, diabetes, lung disease, endocrine disorders; lifestyle habits that are risk factors for cardiac disease, e.g., smoking, alcohol intake, eating and exercise patterns, areas and degree of stress perceived.

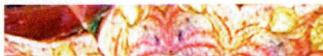

Procedure 28-12 Assessing the Heart and Central Vessels *continued*

IMPLEMENTATION *continued*

Assessment	Normal Findings	Deviations from Normal
5. Simultaneously inspect and palpate the precordium for the presence of abnormal pulsations, lifts, or heaves. To locate the valve areas of the heart, see Box 28–22.		
● Inspect and palpate the aortic and pulmonic areas, observing them at an angle and to the side, to note the presence or absence of pulsations. Observing these areas at an angle increases the likelihood of seeing pulsations.	No pulsations	Pulsations
● Inspect and palpate the tricuspid area for pulsations and heaves or lifts.	No pulsations No lift or heave	Pulsations Diffuse lift or heave, indicating enlarged or overactive right ventricle
● Inspect and palpate the apical area for pulsation, noting its specific location (it may be displaced laterally or lower) and diameter. If displaced laterally, record the distance between the apex and the MCL in centimeters.	Pulsations visible in 50% of adults and palpable in most PMI in fifth LICS at or medial to MCL Diameter of 1 to 2 cm (1/3 to 1/2 in.) No lift or heave	PMI displaced laterally or lower (indicates enlarged heart) Diameter over 2 cm (indicates enlarged heart or aneurysm) Diffuse lift or heave lateral to apex (indicates enlargement or overactivity of left ventricle)
● Inspect and palpate the epigastric area at the base of the sternum for abdominal aortic pulsations.	Aortic pulsations	Bounding abdominal pulsations (e.g., aortic aneurysm)

BOX 28–22 ■ Locating the Aortic, Pulmonic, Tricuspid, and Apical Areas of the Precordium

- Locate the angle of Louis. It is felt as a prominence on the sternum.
- Move your fingertips down each side of the angle until you can feel the second intercostal spaces. The client's right second intercostal space is the aortic area, and the left second intercostal space is the pulmonic area.
- From the pulmonic area, move your fingertips down three left intercostal spaces along the side of the sternum. The left fifth intercostal space close to the sternum is the tricuspid or right ventricular area.
- From the tricuspid area, move your fingertips laterally 5 to 7 cm (2 to 3 in.) to the left midclavicular line (LMCL). This is the apical or mitral area, or point of maximal impulse (PMI). If you have difficulty locating the PMI, have the client roll onto the left side to move the apex closer to the chest wall.

---

6. Auscultate the heart in all four anatomic sites: aortic, pulmonic, tricuspid, and apical (mitral). Auscultation need not be limited to these areas; however, the nurse may need to move the stethoscope to find the most audible sounds for each client. Box 28–23 describes the steps involved in auscultating the heart.	S_1: Usually heard at all sites Usually louder at apical area S_2: Usually heard at all sites Usually louder at base of heart Systole: silent interval; slightly shorter duration than diastole at normal heart rate (60 to 90 beats/min) Diastole: silent interval; slightly longer duration than systole at normal heart rates S_3 in children and young adults S_4 in many older adults	Increased or decreased intensity Varying intensity with different beats Increased intensity at aortic area Increased intensity at pulmonic area Sharp-sounding ejection clicks S_3 in older adults S_4 may be a sign of hypertension

continued on page 584

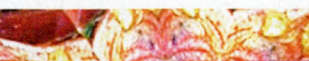

Procedure 28-12 Assessing the Heart and Central Vessels *continued*

IMPLEMENTATION *continued*

BOX 28–23 ■ Auscultating the Heart

- Eliminate all sources of room noise. Heart sounds are of low intensity, and other noise hinders the nurse's ability to hear them.
- Keep the client in a supine position with head elevated 30° to 45°.
- Use both the flat-disc diaphragm and the bell-shaped diaphragm to listen to all areas.
- In every area of auscultation, distinguish both S_1 and S_2 sounds.

- When auscultating, concentrate on one particular sound at a time in each area: the first heart sound, followed by systole, then the second heart sound, then diastole. Systole and diastole are normally silent intervals.
- Later, reexamine the heart while the client is in the upright sitting position. Certain sounds are more audible in certain positions.

Assessment	Normal Findings	Deviations from Normal
CAROTID ARTERIES		
7. Palpate the carotid artery, using extreme caution (see Box 28–24).	Symmetric pulse volumes	Asymmetric volumes (possible stenosis or thrombosis)
	Full pulsations, thrusting quality	Decreased pulsations (may indicate impaired left cardiac output)
	Quality remains same when client breathes, turns head, and changes from sitting to supine position	Increased pulsations
	Elastic arterial wall	Thickening, hard, rigid, beaded, inelastic walls (indicate arteriosclerosis)

BOX 28–24 ■ Palpating and Auscultating the Carotid Artery

Palpation
- Palpate only one carotid artery at a time. This ensures adequate cerebral blood flow through the other and thus prevents possible ischemia. Ischemia is a deficiency of blood in a body part due to constriction or obstruction of a blood vessel.
- Avoid exerting too much pressure and massaging the area. Pressure can occlude the artery and carotid sinus massage can precipitate bradycardia. The carotid sinus is a small dilation at the beginning of the internal carotid artery just above the bifurcation of the common carotid artery, in the upper third of the neck.

- Ask the client to turn the head slightly toward the side being examined. This makes the carotid artery more accessible.

Auscultation
- Turn the client's head slightly away from the side being examined. This facilitates the placement of the stethoscope.
- Auscultate the carotid artery on one side and then the other.
- Listen for the presence of a bruit.
- If you hear a bruit, gently palpate the artery to determine the presence of a thrill.

---

8. Auscultate the carotid artery to determine the presence of a bruit (see Box 28–24).	No sound heard on auscultation	Presence of bruit in one or both arteries (suggests occlusive artery disease)
JUGULAR VEINS		
9. Inspect the jugular veins for distention while the client is placed in a semi-Fowler's position (30° to 45° angle), with the head supported on a small pillow.	Veins not visible (indicating right side of heart is functioning normally)	Veins visibly distended (indicating advanced cardiopulmonary disease)

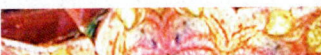

Procedure 28-12 Assessing the Heart and Central Vessels *continued*

IMPLEMENTATION *continued*

Assessment	Normal Findings	Deviations from Normal
10. If jugular distention is present, assess the jugular venous pressure (JVP).		Bilateral measurements above 3 to 4 cm are considered elevated (may indicate right-sided heart failure)
		Unilateral distention (may be caused by local obstruction)

10. If jugular distention is present, assess the jugular venous pressure (JVP).

- Locate the highest visible point of distention of the internal jugular vein. Although either the internal or the external jugular vein can be used, the internal jugular vein is more reliable. The external jugular vein is more easily affected by obstruction or kinking at the base of the neck.
- Measure the vertical height of this point in centimeters from the sternal angle, the point at which the clavicles meet (see Figure 28–64 ■).
- Repeat the preceding steps on the other side.

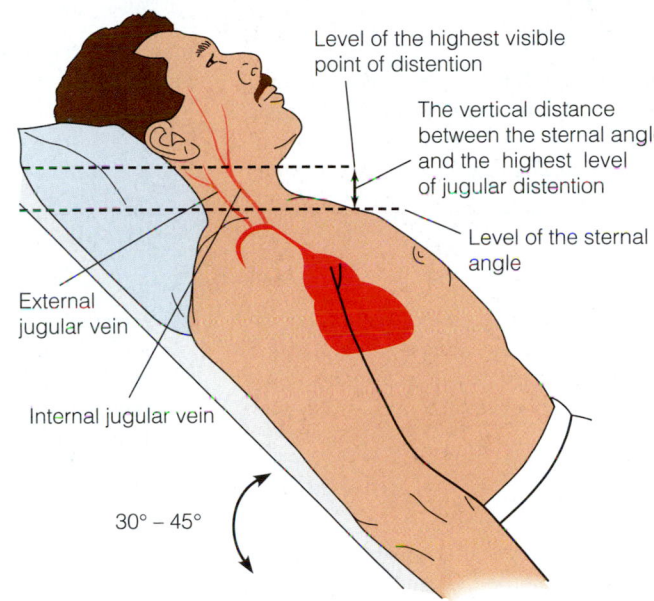

Level of the highest visible point of distention

The vertical distance between the sternal angle and the highest level of jugular distention

Level of the sternal angle

External jugular vein

Internal jugular vein

30° – 45°

Figure 28–64 ■ Assessing the highest point of distention of the jugular vein.

11. Document findings in the client record using forms or checklists supplemented by narrative notes when appropriate.

EVALUATION

- Perform a detailed follow-up examination based on findings that deviated from expected or normal for the client. Relate findings to previous assessment data if available.

- Report significant deviations from normal to the physician.

Lifespan Considerations

Assessing the Heart and Central Vessels

Infants
- Physiologic splitting of the second heart sound may be heard when the child takes a deep breath and the aortic valve closes a split second before the pulmonic valve. If splitting is heard during normal respirations, it is abnormal and may indicate an atrial-septal defect.

Children
- Heart sounds are louder because of the thinner chest wall.
- A third heart sound, best heard at the apex, is present in about one-third of all children.
- The PMI is higher and more medial in children under 8 years old.

Elders
- If no disease is present, heart size remains the same size throughout life.
- Cardiac output and strength of contraction decrease, thus lessening the older person's activity tolerance.
- The heart rate returns to its resting rate more slowly after exertion than it did when the individual was younger.
- S_4 heart sound is considered normal in older adults.
- Extra systoles commonly occur. Ten or more systoles per minute are considered abnormal.
- Sudden emotional and physical stresses may result in cardiac arrhythmias and heart failure.

Peripheral Vascular System

Assessing the peripheral vascular system includes measuring the blood pressure, palpating peripheral pulses, and inspecting the skin and tissues to determine **perfusion** (blood supply to an area) to the extremities. Certain aspects of peripheral vascular assessment are often incorporated into other parts of the assessment procedure. For example, blood pressure is usually measured at the beginning of the physical examination (see the section on assessing blood pressure in Chapter 27). ⚭ Pulse sites and pulse assessments are described in Chapter 27. ⚭

Procedure 28–13 describes how to assess the peripheral vascular system.

Procedure 28-13 Assessing the Peripheral Vascular System

PLANNING

Delegation
Due to the substantial knowledge and skill required, assessment of the peripheral vascular system is not delegated to unlicensed assistive personnel. However, many aspects of the vascular system are observed during usual care and may be recorded by persons other than the nurse. Abnormal findings must be validated and interpreted by the nurse.

Equipment
None

IMPLEMENTATION

Performance

1. Explain to the client what you are going to do, why it is necessary, and how he or she can cooperate. Discuss how the results will be used in planning further care or treatments.
2. Wash hands and observe appropriate infection control procedures.
3. Provide for client privacy.
4. Inquire if the client has any history of the following: past history of heart disorders, varicosities, arterial disease, and hypertension; lifestyle habits such as exercise patterns, activity patterns and tolerance, smoking, and use of alcohol.

Assessment	Normal Findings	Deviations from Normal
PERIPHERAL PULSES		
5. Palpate the peripheral pulses (except the carotid pulse) on both sides of the client's body individually, simultaneously, and systematically to determine the symmetry of pulse volume. If you have difficulty palpating some of the peripheral pulses, use a Doppler ultrasound probe.	Symmetric pulse volumes Full pulsations	Asymmetric volumes (indicate impaired circulation) Absence of pulsation (indicates arterial spasm or occlusion) Decreased, weak, thready pulsations (indicate impaired cardiac output) Increased pulse volume (may indicate hypertension, high cardiac output, or circulatory overload)
PERIPHERAL VEINS		
6. Inspect the peripheral veins in the arms and legs for the presence and/or appearance of superficial veins when limbs are dependent and when limbs are elevated.	In dependent position, presence of distention and nodular bulges at calves When limbs elevated, veins collapse (veins may appear tortuous or distended in older people)	Distended veins in the thigh and/or lower leg or on posterolateral part of calf from knee to ankle
7. Assess the peripheral leg veins for signs of phlebitis (see Box 28–25).	Limbs not tender Symmetric in size	Tenderness on palpation Pain in calf muscles with forceful dorsiflexion of the foot (positive Homans') Warmth and redness over vein Swelling of one calf or leg

---

BOX 28-25 ■ Assessing Peripheral Leg Veins for Signs of Phlebitis

■ Inspect the calves for redness and swelling over vein sites.
■ Palpate the calves for firmness or tension of the muscles, the presence of edema over the dorsum of the foot, and areas of localized warmth. Palpation augments inspection findings, particularly in greater pigmented people in whom redness may not be visible.

■ Push the calves from side to side to test for tenderness.
■ Firmly dorsiflex the client's foot while supporting the entire leg in extension (Homans' test), or have the person stand or walk.

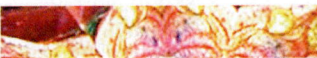

Procedure 28-13 Assessing the Peripheral Vascular System *continued*

IMPLEMENTATION *continued*

Assessment	Normal Findings	Deviations from Normal
PERIPHERAL PERFUSION		
8. Inspect the skin of the hands and feet for color, temperature, edema, and skin changes.	Skin color pink	Cyanotic (venous insufficiency)
		Pallor that increases with limb elevation
		Dusky red color when limb is lowered (arterial insufficiency)
		Brown pigmentation around ankles (arterial or chronic venous insufficiency)
	Skin temperature not excessively warm or cold	Skin cool (arterial insufficiency)
	No edema	Marked edema (venous insufficiency)
	Skin texture resilient and moist	Mild edema (arterial insufficiency)
		Skin thin and shiny or thick, waxy, shiny, and fragile, with reduced hair and ulceration (venous or arterial insufficiency)
9. Assess the adequacy of arterial flow if arterial insufficiency is suspected (See Box 28–26).	Buerger's test: Original color returns in 10 seconds; veins in feet or hands fill in about 15 seconds	Delayed color return or mottled appearance; delayed venous filling; marked redness of arms or legs (indicates arterial insufficiency)
	Capillary refill test: Immediate return of color	Delayed return of color (arterial insufficiency)

BOX 28–26 ■ Assessing the Adequacy of Arterial Blood Flow

Buerger's Test (Arterial Adequacy Test)

■ Assist the client to a supine position. Ask the client to raise one leg or one arm about 30 cm (1 ft) above heart level, move the foot or hand briskly up and down for about 1 minute, and then sit up and dangle the leg or arm.

■ Observe the time elapsed until return of original color and vein filling. Original color normally returns in 10 seconds, and the veins fill in about 15 seconds.

Capillary Refill Test

■ Squeeze the client's fingernail and toenail between your fingers sufficiently to cause blanching.

■ Release the pressure, and observe how quickly normal color returns. Color normally returns immediately.

Other Assessments

■ Inspect the fingernails for changes indicative of circulatory impairment. See the section on assessment of nails, earlier in this chapter.

■ See also peripheral pulse assessment, earlier.

---

10. Document findings in the client record using forms or checklists supplemented by narrative notes when appropriate.

EVALUATION

■ Perform a detailed follow-up examination of the heart or central vessels, integument, or other systems based on findings that deviated from expected or normal for the client. Relate findings to previous assessment data if available.

■ Report significant deviations from normal to the physician.

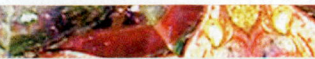

Lifespan Considerations

Assessing the Peripheral Vascular System

Infants
- Palpation of the pulses in the lower extremities (particularly the femoral pulses) is essential to screen for coarctation of the aorta.

Elders
- The overall effectiveness of blood vessels decreases as smooth muscle cells are replaced by connective tissue. The lower extremities are more likely to show signs of arterial and venous impairment because of the more distal and dependent position.
- Peripheral vascular assessment should always include upper and lower extremities' temperature, color, pulses, edema, skin integrity, and sensation. Any differences in symmetry of these findings should be noted.
- Proximal arteries become thinner and dilate.

- Peripheral arteries become thicker and dilate less effectively because of arteriosclerotic changes in the vessel walls.
- Blood vessels lengthen and become more tortuous and prominent. Varicosities occur more frequently.
- In some instances, arteries may be palpated more easily because of the loss of supportive surrounding tissues. Often, however, the most distal pulses of the lower extremities are more difficult to palpate because of decreased arterial perfusion.
- Systolic and diastolic blood pressures increase, but the increase in the systolic pressure is greater. As a result, the pulse pressure widens. Any client with a blood pressure reading above 140/90 should be referred for follow-up assessments.
- Peripheral edema is frequently observed and is most commonly the result of chronic venous insufficiency or low protein levels in the blood (hypoproteinemia).

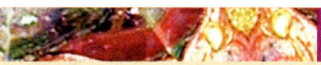

Home Care Considerations

Assessing the Peripheral Vascular System
- Use the assessment as an opportunity to provide teaching regarding appropriate care of the extremities in those at high risk for or with actual vascular impairment. Educate clients and families regarding skin and nail care, exercise, and positioning to promote circulation.

BREASTS AND AXILLAE

The breasts of men and women need to be inspected and palpated. Men have some glandular tissue beneath each nipple, a potential site for malignancy, whereas mature women have glandular tissue throughout the breast. In females, the largest portion of glandular breast tissue is located in the upper outer quadrant of each breast. From this quadrant, there is a projection of breast tissue into the axilla, called the *axillary tail of Spence* (see Figure 28–65 ■). The majority of breast tumors are located in this upper outer breast quadrant and in the tail of Spence. During assessment, the nurse can localize specific findings by using this division of the breast into quadrants and the axillary tail.

Clients need to be instructed to do a breast self-examination (BSE) once a month. Clients also need to be informed about breast health guidelines (see Box 28–27).

Procedure 28–14 describes a nursing assessment of the breasts and axillae.

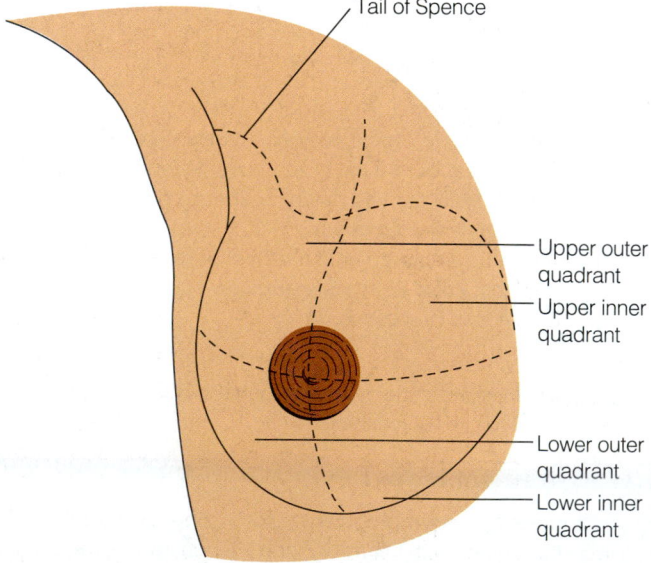

Figure 28–65 ■ Four breast quadrants and the axillary tail of Spence.

BOX 28–27 ■ Breast Health Guidelines

Women Ages 20 to 39
- Monthly breast self-exam
- Clinical breast exam by a health professional every 3 years

Women Ages 40 and Older
- Monthly breast self-exam
- Clinical breast exam by a health professional every year
- Screening mammogram every year

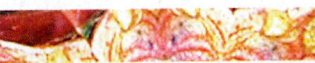

Procedure 28-14 Assessing the Breasts and Axillae

PLANNING

Delegation

Assessment of the breasts and axillae is not delegated to unlicensed assistive personnel. However, persons other than the nurse may record aspects observed during usual care. Abnormal findings must be validated and interpreted by the nurse.

Equipment

- Centimeter ruler

IMPLEMENTATION

Performance

1. Explain to the client what you are going to do, why it is necessary, and how he or she can cooperate. Inquire whether the client has ever had a clinical breast exam previously. Discuss how the results will be used in planning further care or treatments.
2. Observe appropriate infection control procedures.
3. Provide for client privacy.
4. Inquire if the client has any history of the following: breast self-examination; technique used and when performed in relation to the menstrual cycle; history of breast masses and what was done about them; any pain or tenderness in the breasts and relation to the woman's menstrual cycle; any discharge from the nipple; medication history (some medications, e.g., oral contraceptives, steroids, digitalis, and diuretics, may cause nipple discharge; estrogen replacement therapy may be associated with the development of cysts or cancer); risk factors that may be associated with development of breast cancer (e.g., mother, sister, aunt with breast cancer; alcohol consumption, high-fat diet, obesity, use of oral contraceptives, menarche before age 12, menopause after age 55, age 30 or more at first pregnancy).

Assessment	Normal Findings	Deviations from Normal
5. Inspect the breasts for size, symmetry, and contour or shape while the client is in a sitting position.	*Females:* Rounded shape; slightly unequal in size; generally symmetric *Males:* Breasts even with the chest wall; if obese, may be similar in shape to female breasts	Recent change in breast size; swellings; marked asymmetry
6. Inspect the skin of the breast for localized discolorations or hyperpigmentation, retraction or dimpling, localized hypervascular areas, swelling or edema (see Figure 28–66 ■).	Skin uniform in color (same in appearance as skin of abdomen or back) Skin smooth and intact Diffuse symmetric horizontal or vertical vascular pattern in light-skinned people Striae (stretch marks); moles and nevi	Localized discolorations or hyperpigmentation Retraction or dimpling (result of scar tissue or an invasive tumor) Unilateral, localized hypervascular areas (associated with increased blood flow) Swelling or edema appearing as pig skin or orange peel due to exaggeration of the pores

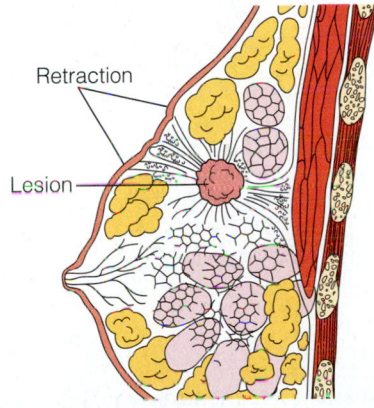

Figure 28–66 ■ A lesion causing retraction of the skin.

7. Emphasize any retraction by having the client
   - Raise the arms above the head.
   - Push the hands together, with elbows flexed (Figure 28–67 ■).
   - Press the hands down on the hips (Figure 28–68 ■).

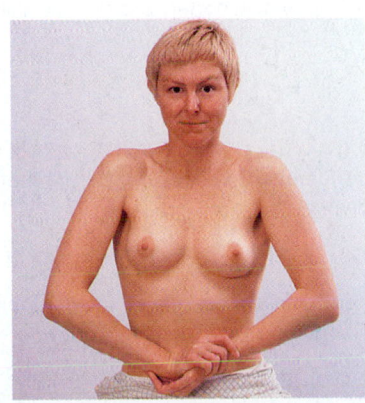

Figure 28–67 ■ Pushing the hands together to accentuate retraction of breast tissues.

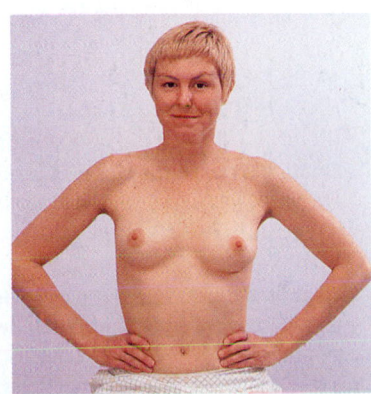

Figure 28–68 ■ Pressing the hands down on the hips to accentuate retraction of breast tissue.

continued on page 590

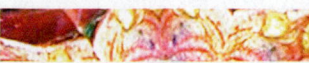

Procedure 28-14 Assessing the Breasts and Axillae *continued*

IMPLEMENTATION *continued*

Assessment	Normal Findings	Deviations from Normal
8. Inspect the areola area for size, shape, symmetry, color, surface characteristics, and any masses or lesions.	Round or oval and bilaterally the same	Any asymmetry, mass, or lesion
	Color varies widely, from light pink to dark brown	
	Irregular placement of sebaceous glands on the surface of the areola (Montgomery's tubercles)	
9. Inspect the nipples for size, shape, position, color, discharge, and lesions.	Round, everted, and equal in size; similar in color; soft and smooth; both nipples point in same direction	Asymmetrical size and color
	No discharge, except from pregnant or breast-feeding females	Presence of discharge, crusts, or cracks
	Inversion of one or both nipples that is present from puberty	Recent inversion of one or both nipples
10. Palpate the axillary, subclavicular, and supraclavicular lymph nodes (Figure 28–69 ■) while the client sits with the arms abducted and supported on the nurse's forearm. For palpation of clavicular lymph nodes, see page 569. Use the flat surfaces of all fingertips to palpate the four areas of the axilla: • the edge of the greater pectoral muscle (musculus pectoralis major) along the anterior axillary line • the thoracic wall in the midaxillary area • the upper part of the humerus, and • the anterior edge of the latissimus dorsi muscle along the posterior axillary line.	No tenderness, masses, or nodules	Tenderness, masses, or nodules

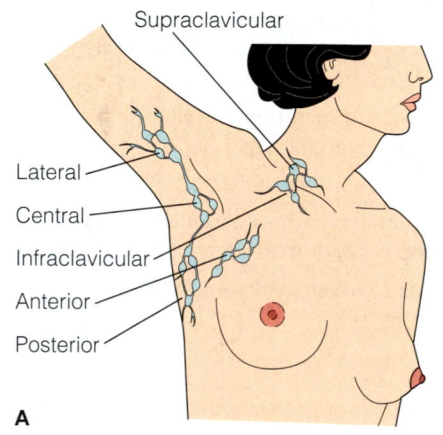
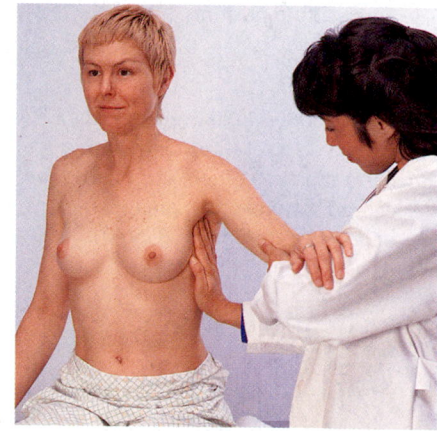

Figure 28–69 ■ Location and palpation of the lymph nodes that drain the lateral breast. *A,* Lymph nodes; *B,* palpating the axilla.

Assessment	Normal Findings	Deviations from Normal
11. Palpate the breast for masses, tenderness, and any discharge from the nipples. See Box 28–28 for palpation methods.	No tenderness, masses, nodules, or nipple discharge	Tenderness, masses, nodules, or nipple discharge
12. Palpate the areola and the nipples for masses. Compress each nipple to determine the presence of any discharge. If discharge is present, milk the breast along its radius to identify the discharge-producing lobe. Assess any discharge for amount, color, consistency, and odor. Note also any tenderness on palpation.	No tenderness, masses, nodules, or nipple discharge	Tenderness, masses, nodules, or nipple discharge

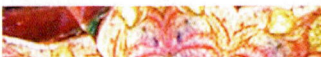

Procedure 28-14 Assessing the Breasts and Axillae *continued*

IMPLEMENTATION *continued*

BOX 28–28 ■ Palpating a Client's Breast

Palpation of the breast is generally performed while the client is supine. In the supine position, the breasts flatten evenly against the chest wall, facilitating palpation. For clients who have a past history of breast masses, who are at high risk for breast cancer, or who have pendulous breasts, examination in both a supine and a sitting position is recommended.

■ If the client reports a breast lump, start with the "normal" breast to obtain baseline data that will serve as a comparison to the reportedly involved breast.

■ To enhance flattening of the breast, instruct the client to abduct the arm and place her hand behind her head. Then place a small pillow or rolled towel under the client's shoulder.

■ For palpation, use the palmar surface of the middle three fingertips (held together) and make a gentle rotary motion on the breast.

■ Choose one of three patterns for palpation:
   a. Hands-of-the-clock or spokes-on-a-wheel (see Figure 28–70 ■)
   b. Concentric circles (see Figure 28–71 ■)
   c. Vertical strips pattern (see Figure 28–72 ■)

■ Start at one point for palpation, and move systematically to the end point to ensure that all breast surfaces are assessed.

■ Pay particular attention to the upper outer quadrant area and the tail of Spence.

■ If you detect a mass, record the following data:
   a. *Location:* the exact location relative to the quadrants and axillary tail, or the clock (as in Figure 28–70) and the distance from the nipple in centimeters

   b. *Size:* the length, width, and thickness of the mass in centimeters. If you are able to determine the discrete edges, record this fact.
   c. *Shape:* whether the mass is round, oval, lobulated, indistinct, or irregular.
   d. *Consistency:* whether the mass is hard or soft.
   e. *Mobility:* whether the mass is movable or fixed.
   f. *Skin over the lump:* whether it is reddened, dimpled, or retracted.
   g. *Nipple:* whether it is displaced or retracted.
   h. *Tenderness:* whether palpation is painful.

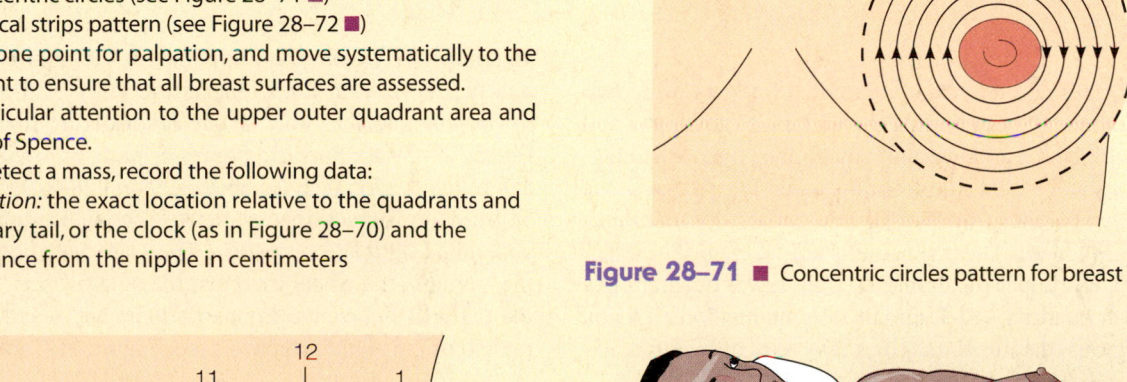

Figure 28–71 ■ Concentric circles pattern for breast palpation.

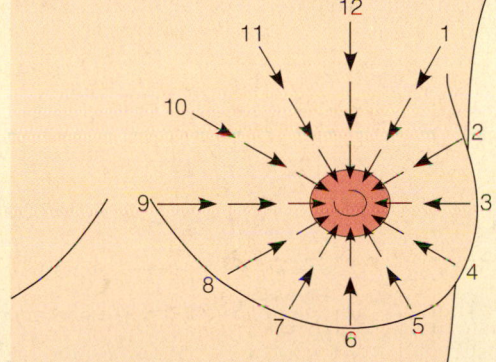

Figure 28–70 ■ Hands-of-the-clock or spokes-on-a-wheel pattern of breast palpation.

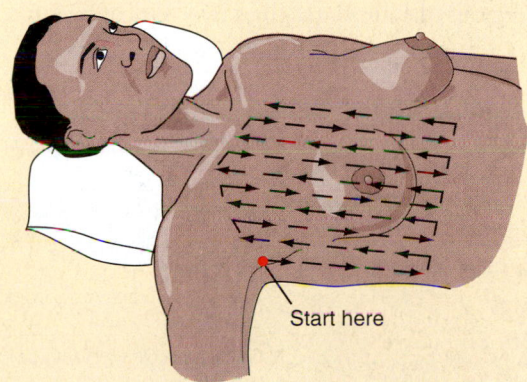

Figure 28–72 ■ Vertical strips pattern of breast palpation.

13. Teach the client the technique of breast self-examination (see Chapter 38).

14. Document findings in the client record using forms or checklists supplemented by narrative notes when appropriate.

EVALUATION

■ Perform a detailed follow-up examination based on findings that deviated from expected or normal for the client. Relate findings to previous assessment data if available.

■ Report significant deviations from normal to the physician.

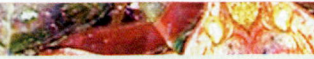

Lifespan Considerations

Assessing the Breasts and Axillae

Infants

■ Newborns up to 2 weeks of age may have breast enlargement and white discharge from the nipples (witch's milk).

Children

■ Female breast development begins between 12 and 13 years of age and occurs in five stages. One breast may develop more rapidly than the other.

Stage 1   Elevation of the nipple
Stage 2   Enlargement of the areola
Stage 3   Enlargement of the breast
Stage 4   Projection of the areola and nipple
Stage 5   Recession of the areola by about age 14 or 15, leaving only the nipple projecting.

■ Boys may have some breast development in early adolescence. The 2-year transient breast growth reaches only the second stage.
■ Gynecomastia, enlargement of breast tissue in males, can occur during puberty and may affect only one breast.

Pregnant Females

■ Breast, areola, and nipple size increase.
■ The areolae and nipples darken; nipples may become more erect; areolae contain small, scattered, elevated Montgomery's glands.
■ Superficial veins become more prominent and jagged linear stretch marks may develop.
■ A thick yellow fluid (colostrum) may be expressed from the nipples after the first trimester.

Elders

■ In the postmenopausal female, breasts change in shape and often appear pendulous or flaccid; they lack the firmness they had in younger years.
■ The presence of breast lesions may be detected more readily because of the decrease in connective tissue.
■ General breast size remains the same. Although glandular tissue atrophies, the amount of fat in breasts (predominantly in the lower quadrants) increases in most women.

ABDOMEN

The nurse locates and describes abdominal findings using two common methods of subdividing the abdomen: quadrants and regions. To divide the abdomen into quadrants, the nurse imagines two lines: a vertical line from the xiphoid process to the pubic symphysis, and a horizontal line across the umbilicus (see Figure 28–73 ■). These quadrants are labeled right upper quadrant (*1*), left upper quadrant (*2*), right lower quadrant (*3*), and left lower quadrant (*4*). Using the second method, division into nine regions, the nurse imagines two vertical lines that ex-

tend superiorly from the midpoints of the inguinal ligaments, and two horizontal lines, one at the level of the edge of the lower ribs and the other at the level of the iliac crests (see Figure 28–74 ■). Specific organs or parts of organs lie in each abdominal region (see Boxes 28–29 and 28–30).

In addition, practitioners often use certain landmarks to locate abdominal signs and symptoms. These are the xiphoid process of the sternum, the costal margins, the anterosuperior iliac spine, the inguinal ligaments (Poupart's ligaments), and the superior margin of the pubic symphysis (see Figure 28–75 ■).

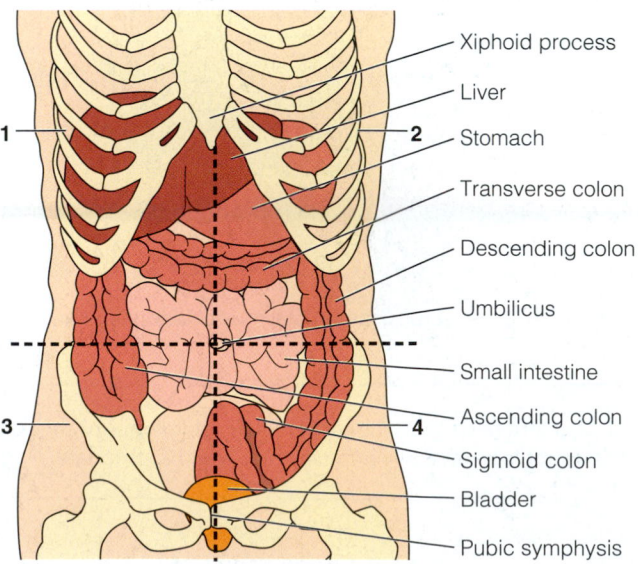

Figure 28–73 ■ The four abdominal quadrants and the underlying organs: *1*, right upper quadrant; *2*, left upper quadrant; *3*, right lower quadrant; *4*, left lower quadrant.

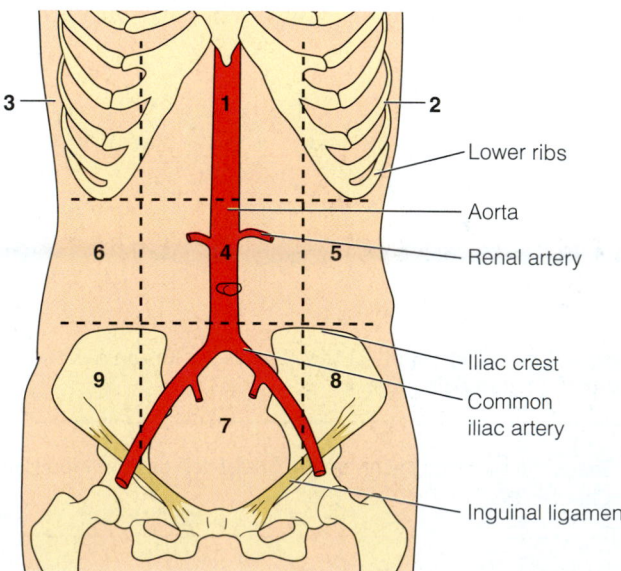

Figure 28–74 ■ The nine abdominal regions: *1*, epigastric; *2*, *3*, left and right hypochondriac; *4*, umbilical; *5*, *6*, left and right lumbar; *7*, suprapubic and hypogastric; *8*, *9*, left and right inguinal or iliac.

BOX 28–29 ■ Organs in the Four Abdominal Quadrants

Right Upper Quadrant
Liver
Gallbladder
Duodenum
Head of pancreas
Right adrenal gland
Upper lobe of right kidney
Hepatic flexure of colon
Section of ascending colon
Section of transverse colon

Left Upper Quadrant
Left lobe of liver
Stomach
Spleen
Upper lobe of left kidney
Pancreas
Left adrenal gland
Splenic flexure of colon
Section of transverse colon
Section of descending colon

Right Lower Quadrant
Lower lobe of right kidney
Cecum
Appendix
Section of ascending colon
Right ovary
Right fallopian tube
Right ureter
Right spermatic cord
Part of uterus

Left Lower Quadrant
Lower lobe of left kidney
Sigmoid colon
Section of descending colon
Left ovary
Left fallopian tube
Left ureter
Left spermatic cord
Part of uterus

BOX 28–30 ■ Organs in the Nine Abdominal Regions

Right Hypochondriac
Right lobe of liver
Gallbladder
Part of duodenum
Hepatic flexure of colon
Upper half of right kidney
Suprarenal gland

Right Lumbar
Ascending colon
Lower half of right kidney
Part of duodenum and jejunum

Right Inguinal
Cecum
Appendix
Lower end of ileum
Right ureter
Right spermatic cord
Right ovary

Epigastric
Aorta
Pyloric end of stomach
Part of duodenum
Pancreas
Part of liver

Umbilical
Omentum
Mesentery
Lower part of duodenum
Part of jejunum and ileum

Hypogastric (Pubic)
Ileum
Bladder
Uterus

Left Hypochondriac
Stomach
Spleen
Tail of pancreas
Splenic flexure of colon
Upper half of left kidney
Suprarenal gland

Left Lumbar
Descending colon
Lower half of left kidney
Part of jejunum and ileum

Left Inguinal
Sigmoid colon
Left ureter
Left spermatic cord
Left ovary

- Xiphoid process
- Costal margins
- Midline
- Anterior superior iliac spines
- Umbilicus
- Inguinal (Poupart's) ligaments
- Superior margin of pubic bone

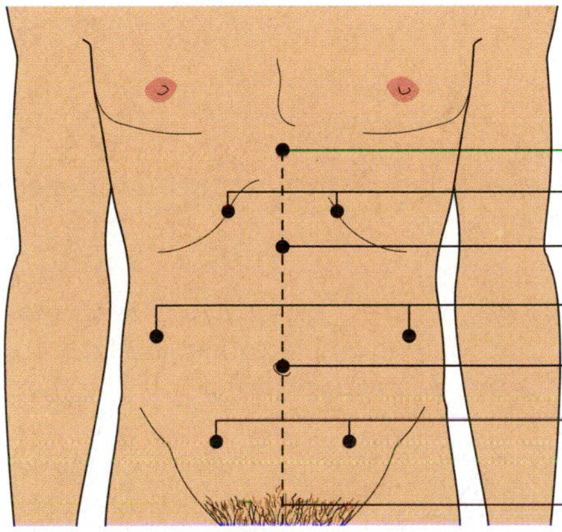

Figure 28–75 ■ Landmarks commonly used to identify abdominal areas.

Assessment of the abdomen involves all four methods of examination (inspection, auscultation, palpation, and percussion). When assessing the abdomen, the nurse performs inspection first, followed by auscultation, percussion, and/or palpation. Auscultation is done before palpation and percussion because palpation and percussion cause movement or stimulation of the bowel, which can increase bowel motility and thus heighten bowel sounds, creating false results. Procedure 28–15 describes how to assess the abdomen.

Procedure 28-15 Assessing the Abdomen

PLANNING

- Ask the client to urinate since an empty bladder makes the assessment more comfortable.
- Ensure that the room is warm since the client will be exposed.

Delegation

Assessment of the abdomen is not delegated to unlicensed assistive personnel. However, signs and symptoms of problems may be observed during usual care and should be recorded by those per-

sons. Abnormal findings must be validated and interpreted by the nurse.

Equipment

- Examining light
- Tape measure (metal or unstretchable cloth)
- Water-soluble skin-marking pencil
- Stethoscope

continued on page 594

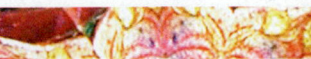

Procedure 28-15 Assessing the Abdomen *continued*

IMPLEMENTATION

Performance

1. Explain to the client what you are going to do, why it is necessary, and how he or she can cooperate. Discuss how the results will be used in planning further care or treatments.
2. Observe appropriate infection control procedures.
3. Provide for client privacy.
4. Inquire if the client has any history of the following: incidence of abdominal pain: its location, onset, sequence, and chronology; its quality (description); its frequency; associated symptoms (e.g., nausea, vomiting, diarrhea); bowel habits; incidence of constipation or diarrhea (have client describe what client means by these terms); change in appetite, food intolerances, and foods ingested in last 24 hours; specific signs and symptoms [e.g., heartburn, flatulence and/or belching, difficulty swallowing, hematemesis (vomiting blood), blood or mucus in stools, and aggravating and alleviating factors]; previous problems and treatment (e.g., stomach ulcer, gallbladder surgery, history of jaundice).
5. Assist the client to a supine position, with the arms placed comfortably at the sides. Place small pillows beneath the knees and the head to reduce tension in the abdominal muscles. Expose only the client's abdomen from chest line to the pubic area to avoid chilling and shivering, which can tense the abdominal muscles.

Assessment	Normal Findings	Deviations from Normal
INSPECTION OF THE ABDOMEN		
6. Inspect the abdomen for skin integrity (refer to the discussion of skin assessment, earlier in this chapter).	Unblemished skin	Presence of rash or other lesions
	Uniform color	Tense, glistening skin (may indicate ascites, edema)
	Silver-white striae (stretch marks) or surgical scars	Purple striae (associated with Cushing's disease)
7. Inspect the abdomen for contour and symmetry:		
• Observe the abdominal contour (profile line from the rib margin to the pubic bone) while standing at the client's side when the client is supine.	Flat, rounded (convex), or scaphoid (concave)	Distended
• Ask the client to take a deep breath and to hold it *(makes an enlarged liver or spleen more obvious)*.	No evidence of enlargement of liver or spleen	Evidence of enlargement of liver or spleen
• Assess the symmetry of contour while standing at the foot of the bed.	Symmetric contour	Asymmetric contour, e.g., localized protrusions around umbilicus, inguinal ligaments, or scars (possible hernia or tumor)
• If distention is present, measure the abdominal girth by placing a tape around the abdomen at the level of the umbilicus (Figure 28–76 ■).		

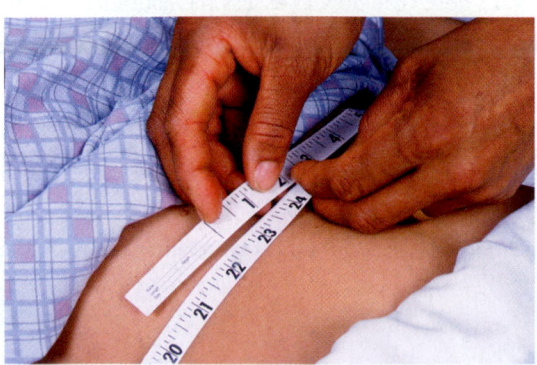

Figure 28–76 ■ Measuring abdominal girth.

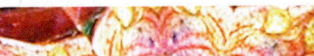

Procedure 28-15 Assessing the Abdomen *continued*

IMPLEMENTATION *continued*

Assessment	Normal Findings	Deviations from Normal
8. Observe abdominal movements associated with respiration, peristalsis, or aortic pulsations.	Symmetric movements caused by respiration Visible peristalsis in very lean people Aortic pulsations in thin persons at epigastric area	Limited movement due to pain or disease process Visible peristalsis in nonlean clients (with bowel obstruction) Marked aortic pulsations
9. Observe the vascular pattern.	No visible vascular pattern	Visible venous pattern (dilated veins) is associated with liver disease, ascites, and venocaval obstruction
AUSCULTATION OF THE ABDOMEN 10. Auscultate the abdomen for bowel sounds, vascular sounds, and peritoneal friction rubs. The auscultation procedure is shown in Box 28–31.	Audible bowel sounds Absence of arterial bruits Absence of friction rub	Absent, hypoactive, or hyperactive bowel sounds Loud bruit over aortic area (possible aneurysm) Bruit over renal or iliac arteries

---

BOX 28–31   Auscultating the Abdomen

Warm the hands and the stethoscope diaphragms. Cold hands and a cold stethoscope may cause the client to contract the abdominal muscles, and these contractions may be heard during auscultation.

For Bowel Sounds

■ Use the flat-disc diaphragm. Intestinal sounds are relatively high pitched and best accentuated by the flat-disc diaphragm. Light pressure with the stethoscope is adequate.

■ Ask when the client last ate. Shortly after or long after eating, bowel sounds may normally increase. They are loudest when a meal is long overdue. Four to 7 hours after a meal, bowel sounds may be heard continuously over the ileocecal valve area while the digestive contents from the small intestine empty through the valve into the large intestine.

■ Place the flat-disc diaphragm of the stethoscope in each of the four quadrants of the abdomen over all of the auscultatory sites shown in Figure 28–77 ■.

■ Listen for active bowel sounds—irregular gurgling noises occurring about every 5 to 20 seconds. The duration of a single sound may range from less than a second to more than several seconds.

■ Normal bowel sounds are described as audible. Alterations in sounds are described as absent, hypoactive, i.e., extremely soft and infrequent (e.g., one per minute), or hyperactive/increased, i.e., high-pitched, loud, rushing sounds that occur frequently (e.g., every 3 seconds) also known as borborygmi. True absence

of sounds (none heard in 3 to 5 minutes) indicates a cessation of intestinal motility. Hypoactive sounds indicate decreased motility and are usually associated with manipulation of the bowel during surgery, inflammation, paralytic ileus, or late bowel obstruction. Hyperactive sounds indicate increased intestinal motility and are usually associated with diarrhea, an early bowel obstruction, or the use of laxatives.

For Vascular Sounds

■ Use the bell of the stethoscope over the aorta, renal arteries, iliac arteries, and femoral arteries (see Figure 28–78 ■).

■ Listen for bruits (blowing sound due to restricted blood flow through narrowed vessels).

Peritoneal Friction Rubs

■ Peritoneal friction rubs are rough, grating sounds like two pieces of leather rubbing together. Friction rubs may be caused by inflammation, infectious, or abnormal growths.

■ To auscultate the splenic site, place the stethoscope over the left lower rib cage in the anterior axillary line, and ask the client to take a deep breath. A deep breath may accentuate the sound of a friction rub area.

■ To auscultate the liver site, place the stethoscope over the lower right rib cage.

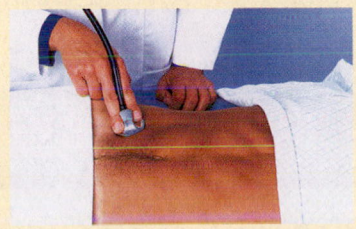

Figure 28–77 ■ Auscultating the abdomen for bowel sounds.

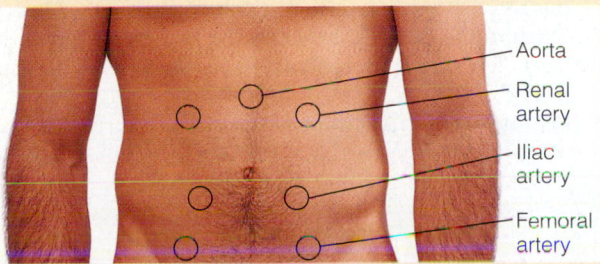

Aorta
Renal artery
Iliac artery
Femoral artery

Figure 28–78 ■ Sites for auscultating the abdomen.

---

continued on page 594

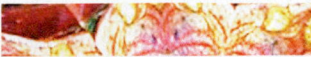

Procedure 28-15 Assessing the Abdomen *continued*

IMPLEMENTATION *continued*

Assessment	Normal Findings	Deviations from Normal
PERCUSSION OF THE ABDOMEN		
11. Percuss several areas in each of the four quadrants to determine presence of tympany (gas in stomach and intestines) and dullness (decrease, absence, or flatness of resonance over solid masses or fluid). Use a systematic pattern: Begin in the lower left quadrant, proceed to the lower right quadrant, the upper right quadrant, and the upper left quadrant (Figure 28–79 ■).	Tympany over the stomach and gas-filled bowels; dullness, especially over the liver and spleen, or a full bladder	Large dull areas (associated with presence of fluid or a tumor)

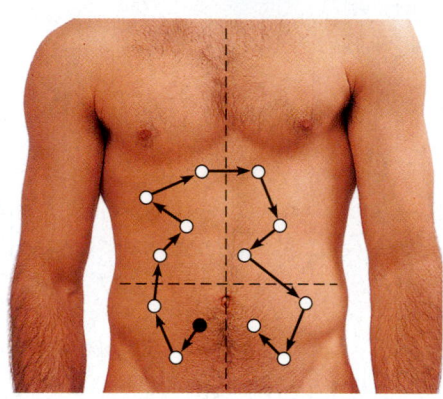

Figure 28–79 ■ Systematic percussion sites for all four quadrants.

Assessment	Normal Findings	Deviations from Normal
PERCUSSION OF THE LIVER		
12. Percuss the liver to determine its size (see Box 28–32).	6 to 12 cm (2½ to 3½ in.) in the midclavicular line; 4 to 8 cm (1½ to 3 in.) at the midsternal line	Enlarged size (associated with liver disease)

BOX 28–32 ■ Percussing the Liver

Percussion to determine liver size begins in the right midclavicular line below the level of the umbilicus and proceeds as follows:

1. Percuss upward over tympanic areas until a dull percussion sound indicates the lower liver border. Mark the site with a skin-marking pencil (see Figure 28–80 ■).
2. Then percuss downward at the right midclavicular line, beginning from an area of lung resonance and progressing downward until a dull percussion sound indicates the upper liver border (usually at the fifth to seventh interspace). Mark this site.
3. Measure the distance between the two marks (upper and lower liver border) in centimeters to establish the liver span or size.
4. Repeat steps 1 to 3 at the midsternal line.

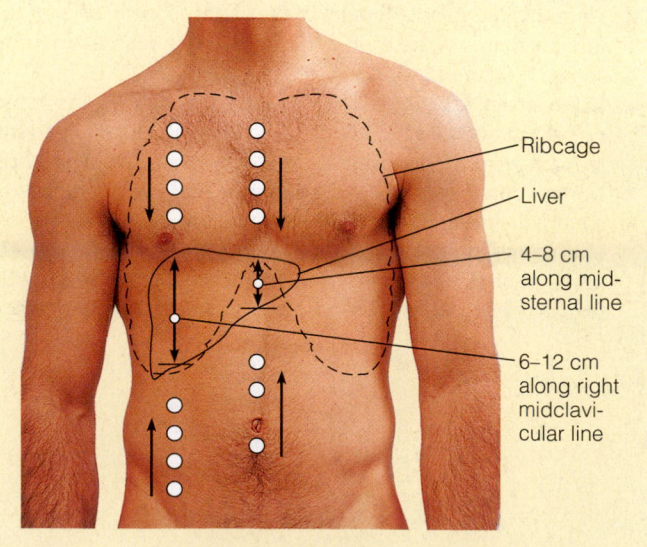

Ribcage

Liver

4–8 cm along midsternal line

6–12 cm along right midclavicular line

Figure 28–80 ■ Percussion pattern to determine liver size.

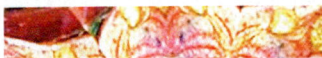

Procedure 28-15 Assessing the Abdomen *continued*

IMPLEMENTATION *continued*

Assessment	Normal Findings	Deviations from Normal
PALPATION OF THE ABDOMEN		
13. Perform light palpation first to detect areas of tenderness and/or muscle guarding. Systematically explore all four quadrants. See Box 28–33 for palpation technique.	No tenderness; relaxed abdomen with smooth, consistent tension	Tenderness and hypersensitivity Superficial masses Localized areas of increased tension
14. Perform deep palpation over all four quadrants. See Box 28–33.	Tenderness may be present near xiphoid process, over cecum, and over sigmoid colon	Generalized or localized areas of tenderness Mobile or fixed masses

---

BOX 28–33 ■ Palpating the Abdomen

Palpation is used to detect tenderness, the presence of masses or distention, and the outline and position of abdominal organs (e.g., the liver, spleen, and kidneys). Before palpation, (a) ensure that the client's position is appropriate for relaxation of the abdominal muscles, and (b) warm the hands. Cold hands can elicit muscle tension and thus impede palpatory evaluation.

Light Palpation
- Hold the palm of your hand slightly above the client's abdomen, with your fingers parallel to the abdomen.
- Depress the abdominal wall lightly, about 1 cm or to the depth of the subcutaneous tissue, with the pads of your fingers (see Figure 28–81 ■).
- Move the finger pads in a slight circular motion.
- Note areas of tenderness or superficial pain, masses, and muscle guarding. To determine areas of tenderness, ask the client to tell you about them and watch for changes in the client's facial expressions.
- If the client is excessively ticklish, begin by pressing your hand on top of the client's hand while pressing lightly. Then slide your hand off the client's and onto the abdomen to continue the examination.

Deep Palpation
- Palpate sensitive areas last.
- Press the distal half of the palmar surface of the fingers of one hand into the abdominal wall.
  or
  Use the bimanual method of palpation discussed earlier in this chapter, page 529.
- Depress the abdominal wall about 4 to 5 cm (1½ to 2 in.) (see Figure 28–82 ■).
- Note masses and the structure of underlying contents. If a mass is present, determine its size, location, mobility, contour, consistency, and tenderness. Normal abdominal structures that may be mistaken for masses include the lateral borders of the rectus abdominis muscles, the feces-filled colon, the aorta, and the uterus.
- Check for rebound tenderness in areas where the client complains of pain. With one hand, press slowly and deeply over the area indicated and then lift the hand quickly. If the client does not complain of pain during the deep pressure but indicates pain at the release of the pressure, rebound tenderness is present. This can indicate peritoneal inflammation and should be reported to the physician immediately.

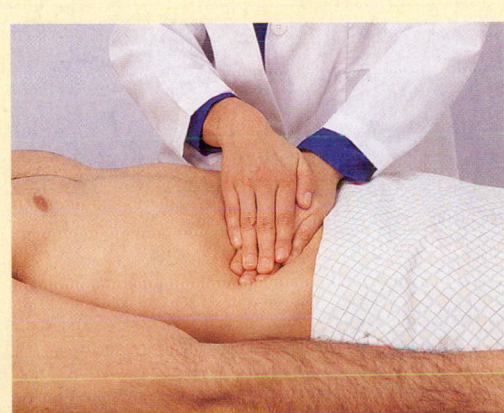

Figure 28–81 ■ Light palpation of the abdomen.

Figure 28–82 ■ Deep palpation of the abdomen.

continued on page 598

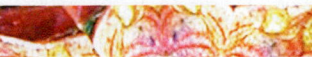

Procedure 28-15 Assessing the Abdomen *continued*

IMPLEMENTATION *continued*

Assessment	Normal Findings	Deviations from Normal
PALPATION OF THE LIVER		
15. Palpate the liver to detect enlargement and tenderness. See palpation methods in Box 28–34.	May not be palpable Border feels smooth	Enlarged (abnormal finding, even if liver is smooth and not tender) Smooth but tender; nodular or hard

---

BOX 28–34 ■ Palpating the Liver

Two bimanual approaches are used in palpation of the liver. In using the first method, place one hand along the anterior rib cage and the other hand on the posterior rib cage.

- Stand on the client's right side.
- Place your left hand on the posterior thorax at about the 11th or 12th rib. This hand is used to push upward and provide support of underlying structures for the subsequent anterior palpation.
- Place your right hand along the rib cage at about a 45° angle to the right of the rectus abdominis muscle or parallel to the rectus muscle with the fingers pointing toward the rib cage (see Figure 28–83 ■).
- While the client exhales, exert a gradual and gentle downward and forward pressure beneath the costal margin until you reach a depth of 4 to 5 cm (1½ to 2 in.). During expiration, the abdominal wall relaxes, facilitating deep palpation.
- Maintain your hand position, and ask the client to inhale deeply. This makes the liver border descend and moves the liver into a palpable position.
- While the client inhales, feel the liver border move against your hand. It should feel firm and have a regular contour. If you do not palpate the liver initially, ask the client to take two or three more deep breaths while you maintain or apply slightly more palpation pressure. Livers are harder to palpate in obese, tense, or very physically fit people.

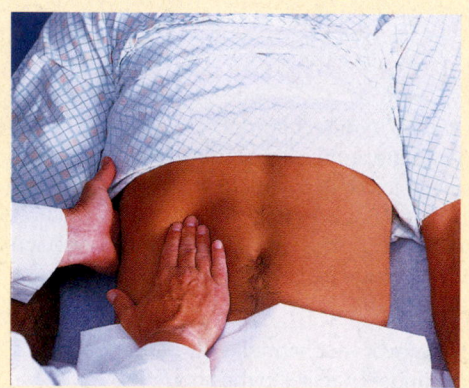

Figure 28–83 ■ Palpating the liver.

- If the liver is enlarged (i.e., palpable below the costal margin), measure the number of centimeters it extends below the costal region.

A second method is the bimanual palpation method discussed on page 529, in which one hand is superimposed on the other (Figure 28–2, earlier). The techniques and principles used for palpating the liver with one hand apply to the two-hand method as well.

Assessment	Normal Findings	Deviations from Normal
PALPATION OF THE BLADDER		
16. Palpate the area above the pubic symphysis if the client's history indicates possible urinary retention (see Figure 28–84 ■).	Not palpable	Distended and palpable as smooth, round, tense mass (indicates urinary retention)

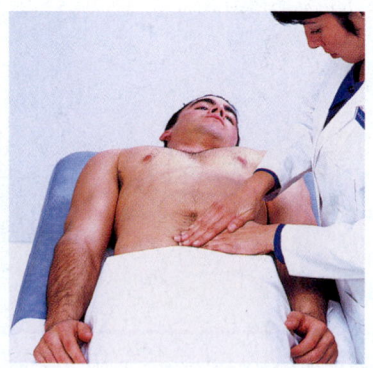

Figure 28–84 ■ Palpating the bladder.

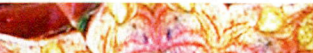

Procedure 28-15 Assessing the Abdomen *continued*

IMPLEMENTATION *continued*

17. Document findings in the client record using forms or check-lists supplemented by narrative notes when appropriate.

EVALUATION

■ Perform a detailed follow-up examination of other systems based on findings that deviated from expected or normal for the client. Relate findings to previous assessment data if available.

■ Report significant deviations from normal to the physician.

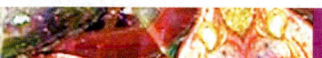

Lifespan Considerations

Assessing the Abdomen

Infants
■ The abdomen of the newborn and infant is round.

Children
■ Toddlers have a characteristic "pot belly" appearance, which persists until about the fifth year.
■ Peristaltic waves are usually more visible than in adults.
■ Children may not be able to pinpoint areas of tenderness; by observing facial expressions the examiner can determine areas of maximum tenderness.
■ The liver is relatively larger than in adults. It can be palpated 1 to 2 cm below the right costal margin.
■ If the child is ticklish, guarding, or fearful, use a task that requires concentration (such as squeezing the hands together) to distract the child's attention.

Elders
■ The rounded abdomens of elders are due to an increase in adipose tissue and a decrease in muscle tone.
■ The abdominal wall is slacker and thinner, making palpation easier and more accurate than in younger clients. Muscle wasting and loss of fibroconnective tissue occur.
■ The pain threshold in elders is often higher; major abdominal problems such as appendicitis or other acute emergencies may therefore go undetected.

■ Gastrointestinal pain needs to be differentiated from cardiac pain. Gastrointestinal pain may be located in the chest or abdomen, whereas cardiac pain is usually located in the chest. Factors aggravating gastrointestinal pain are usually related to either ingestion or lack of food intake; gastrointestinal pain is usually relieved by antacids, food, or assuming an upright position. Common factors that can aggravate cardiac pain are activity or anxiety; rest or nitroglycerin relieves cardiac pain.
■ Stool passes through the intestines at a slower rate in elderly clients, and the perception of stimuli that produce the urge to defecate often diminishes.
■ Fecal incontinence may occur in confused or neurologically impaired older adults.
■ Many older persons erroneously believe that the absence of a daily bowel movement signifies constipation. When assessing for constipation, the nurse must consider the client's diet, activity, medications, and characteristics and ease of passage of feces as well as the frequency of bowel movements.
■ The incidence of colon cancer is higher among older adults than younger adults. Symptoms include a change in bowel function, rectal bleeding, and weight loss. Changes in bowel function, however, are associated with many factors, such as diet, exercise, and medications.
■ Decreased absorption of oral medications often occurs with aging.
■ In the liver, impaired metabolism of some drugs may occur with aging.

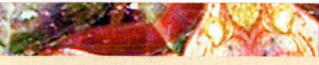

Home Care Considerations

Assessing the Abdomen

■ Be sure you have the required equipment on a home visit, including a tape measure and skin-marking pen.
■ Examining the client in the home may be facilitated since the setting is familiar. Use pillows to position the client.

■ A complete abdominal examination may not be necessary. Focus the assessment on areas indicated by the history and present complaint.

MUSCULOSKELETAL SYSTEM

The musculoskeletal system encompasses the muscles, bones, and joints. The completeness of an assessment of this system depends largely on the needs and problems of the individual client. The nurse usually assesses the musculoskeletal system for muscle strength, tone, size, and symmetry of muscle development, and fasciculations and tremors. A **fasciculation** is an abnormal contraction (shortening) of a bundle of muscle fibers. A **tremor** is an involuntary trembling of a limb or body part.

Tremors may involve large groups of muscle fibers or small bundles of muscle fibers. An **intention tremor** becomes more apparent when an individual attempts a voluntary movement, such as holding a cup of coffee. A **resting tremor** is more apparent when the client is at rest and diminishes with activity.

Bones are assessed for normal form. Joints are assessed for tenderness, swelling, thickening, crepitation (the sound of bone grating on bone), presence of nodules, and range of motion. Body posture is assessed for normal standing and sitting positions. For information about body posture, see Chapter 42.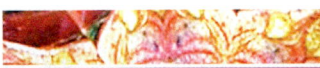

Procedure 28–16 describes how to assess the musculoskeletal system.

Procedure 28-16 Assessing the Musculoskeletal System

PLANNING

Delegation

Assessment of the musculoskeletal system is not delegated to unlicensed assistive personnel. However, many aspects of its functioning are observed during usual care and may be recorded by persons other than the nurse. Abnormal findings must be validated and interpreted by the nurse.

Equipment
- Goniometer

IMPLEMENTATION

Performance

1. Explain to the client what you are going to do, why it is necessary, and how he or she can cooperate. Discuss how the results will be used in planning further care or treatments.
2. Wash hands and observe appropriate infection control procedures.
3. Provide for client privacy.
4. Inquire if the client has any history of the following: presence of muscle pain: onset, location, character, associated phenomena (e.g., redness and swelling of joints), and aggravating and alleviating factors; any limitations to movement or inability to perform activities of daily living; previous sports injuries; any loss of function without pain.

Assessment	Normal Findings	Deviations from Normal
MUSCLES		
5. Inspect the muscles for size. Compare the muscles on one side of the body (e.g., of the arm, thigh, and calf) to the same muscle on the other side. For any discrepancies, measure the muscles with a tape.	Equal size on both sides of body	Atrophy (a decrease in size) or hypertrophy (an increase in size)
6. Inspect the muscles and tendons for contractures (shortening).	No contractures	Malposition of body part, e.g., foot drop (foot flexed downward)
7. Inspect the muscles for fasciculations and tremors. Inspect any tremors of the hands and arms by having the client hold the arms out in front of the body.	No fasciculation or tremors	Presence of fasciculation or tremor
8. Palpate muscles at rest to determine muscle tonicity (the normal condition of tension, or tone, of a muscle at rest).	Normally firm	Atonic (lacking tone)
9. Palpate muscles while the client is active and passive for flaccidity, spasticity, and smoothness of movement.	Smooth coordinated movements	Flaccidity (weakness or laxness) or spasticity (sudden involuntary muscle contraction)
10. Test muscle strength. See tests in Box 28–35. Compare the right side with the left side.	Equal strength on each body side	25% or less of normal strength

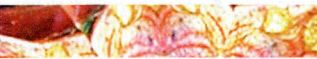

Procedure 28-16 Assessing the Musculoskeletal System *continued*

IMPLEMENTATION *continued*

BOX 28–35 ■ Testing and Grading Muscle Strength

Muscle/Activity

Sternocleidomastoid: Client turns the head to one side against the resistance of your hand. Repeat with the other side.

Trapezius: Client shrugs the shoulders against the resistance of your hands.

Deltoid: Client holds arm up and resists while you try to push it down.

Biceps: Client fully extends each arm and tries to flex it while you attempt to hold arm in extension.

Triceps: Client flexes each arm and then tries to extend it against your attempt to keep arm in flexion.

Wrist and finger muscles: Client spreads the fingers and resists as you attempt to push the fingers together.

Grip strength: Client grasps your index and middle fingers while the you try to pull the fingers out.

Hip muscles: Client is supine, both legs extended; client raises one leg at a time while you attempt to hold it down.

Hip abduction: Client is supine, both legs extended. Place your hands on the lateral surface of each knee; client spreads the legs apart against your resistance.

Hip adduction: Client is in same position as for hip abduction. Place your hands between the knees; client brings the legs together against your resistance.

Hamstrings: Client is supine, both knees bent. Client resists while you attempt to straighten the legs.

Quadriceps: Client is supine, knee partially extended; client resists while you attempt to flex the knee.

Muscles of the ankles and feet: Client resists while you attempt to dorsiflex the foot and again resists while you attempt to flex the foot.

Grading Muscle Strength

0: 0% of normal strength; complete paralysis

1: 10% of normal strength; no movement, contraction of muscle is palpable or visible

2: 25% of normal strength; full muscle movement against gravity, with support

3: 50% of normal strength; normal movement against gravity

4: 75% of normal strength; normal full movement against gravity and against minimal resistance

5: 100% of normal strength; normal full movement against gravity and against full resistance.

Assessment	Normal Findings	Deviations from Normal
BONES		
11. Inspect the skeleton for normal structure and deformities.	No deformities	Bones misaligned
12. Palpate the bones to locate any areas of edema or tenderness.	No tenderness or swelling	Presence of tenderness or swelling (may indicate fracture, neoplasms, or osteoporosis)
JOINTS		
13. Inspect the joint for swelling. Palpate each joint for tenderness, smoothness of movement, swelling, crepitation, and presence of nodules.	No swelling No tenderness, swelling, crepitation, or nodules Joints move smoothly	One or more swollen joints Presence of tenderness, swelling, crepitation, or nodules
14. Assess joint range of motion. See Chapter 42 🔗 for the types of joint movements. ● Ask the client to move selected body parts. The amount of joint movement can be measured by a **goniometer,** a device that measures the angle of the joint in degrees. (Figure 28–85 ■).	Varies to some degree in accordance with person's genetic makeup and degree of physical activity	Limited range of motion in one or more joints

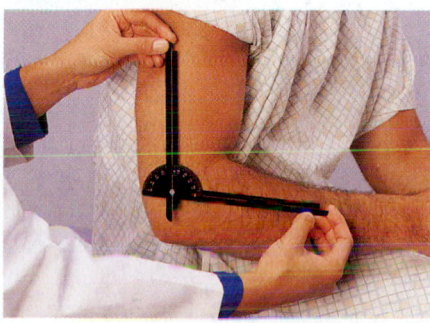

Figure 28–85 ■ A goniometer is used to measure joint range of motion.

continued on page 602

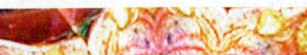

Procedure 28-16 Assessing the Musculoskeletal System *continued*

IMPLEMENTATION *continued*

15. Document findings in the client record using forms or checklists supplemented by narrative notes when appropriate.

EVALUATION

■ Perform a detailed follow-up examination of other systems based on findings that deviated from expected or normal for the client. Relate findings to previous assessment data if available.

■ Report significant deviations from normal to the physician.

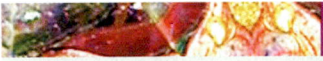

Lifespan Considerations

Assessing the Musculoskeletal System

Infants
■ Palpate the clavicles of newborns. A mass and crepitus may indicate a fracture experienced during vaginal delivery.
■ Newborns naturally return their arms and legs to the fetal position when extended and released.
■ Check muscle strength by holding the infant lightly under the arms. The infant should not fall through the hands if normal muscle strength is present.
■ Check infants for developmental dysplasia of the hip (congenital dislocation) by examining for asymmetric gluteal folds, asymmetric abduction of the legs, or apparent shortening of the femur.

Children
■ Should be able to sit without support by 8 months of age.
■ Pronation of the feet is common in children between 12 and 30 months of age.

■ Genu varum (bowleg) is normal in children for 1 year after beginning to walk.
■ Lordosis (swayback) is common in children before age 5.
■ Observe the child in normal activities to determine motor function.

Elders
■ Muscle mass decreases progressively with age, but there are wide variations among different individuals.
■ The decrease in speed, strength, resistance to fatigue, reaction time, and coordination in the older person is due to a decrease in nerve conduction and muscle tone.
■ The bones become more fragile and osteoporosis leads to a loss of total bone mass. As a result, elderly people are predisposed to fractures and compressed vertebrae.
■ In most elderly people, osteoarthritic changes in the joints can be observed.
■ Note any surgical scars from joint replacement surgeries.

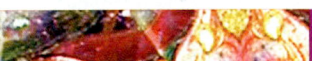

Home Care Considerations

Assessing the Musculoskeletal System
■ When making a home visit, observe the client in natural movement around the living area. To assess children, have them remove their clothes down to the underwear.

■ A complete examination of joints, bone, and muscles may not be necessary. Focus the assessment on areas indicated by the history and present complaint.

NEUROLOGIC SYSTEM

A thorough neurologic examination may take 1 to 3 hours; however, routine screening tests are usually done first. If the results of these tests raise questions, more extensive evaluations are made. Three major considerations determine the extent of a neurologic exam: (a) the client's chief complaints, (b) the client's physical condition (i.e., level of consciousness and ability to ambulate), because many parts of the examination require movement and coordination of the extremities, and (c) the client's willingness to participate and cooperate.

Examination of the neurologic system includes assessment of (a) mental status including level of consciousness, (b) the cranial nerves, (c) reflexes, (d) motor function, and (e) sensory function. Parts of the neurologic assessment are performed throughout the health examination. For example, the nurse performs a large part of the mental status assessment during the taking of the history and when observing the client's general appearance. Also, the nurse assesses the function of many cranial nerves. Cranial nerves II, III, IV, V, and VI (ophthalmic branch) are assessed with the eyes and vision, and cranial nerve VIII (cochlear branch) is assessed with the ears and hearing.

Mental Status

Assessment of mental status reveals the client's general cerebral function. These functions include intellectual (cognitive) as well as emotional (affective) functions.

If problems with use of language, memory, concentration, or thought processes are noted during the nursing history, a more extensive examination is required during neurologic assessment. Major areas of mental status assessment include language, orientation, memory, and attention span and calculation.

Language

Any defects in or loss of the power to express oneself by speech, writing, or signs, or to comprehend spoken or written language due to disease or injury of the cerebral cortex, is called **aphasia.** Aphasias can be categorized as sensory or receptive aphasia and motor or expressive aphasia.

Sensory or receptive aphasia is the loss of the ability to comprehend written or spoken words. Two types of sensory aphasia are auditory (or acoustic) aphasia and visual aphasia. Clients with auditory aphasia have lost the ability to understand the symbolic content associated with sounds. Clients with visual aphasia have lost the ability to understand printed or written figures.

Motor or expressive aphasia involves loss of the power to express oneself by writing, making signs, of speaking. Clients may find that even though they can recall words, they have lost the ability to combine speech sounds into words.

Orientation

This aspect of the assessment determines the client's ability to recognize other persons (*person*), awareness of when and where they presently are (*time* and *place*), and who they, themselves, are (*self*).

Memory

The nurse assesses the client's recall of information presented seconds previously (immediate recall), events or information from earlier in the day or examination (recent memory), and knowledge recalled from months or years ago (remote or long-term memory).

Attention Span and Calculation

This component determines the client's ability to focus on a mental task that is expected to be able to be performed by persons of normal intelligence.

Level of Consciousness

Level of consciousness (LOC) can lie anywhere along a continuum from a state of alertness to coma. A fully alert client responds to questions spontaneously; a comatose client may not respond to verbal stimuli. The Glasgow Coma Scale was originally developed to predict recovery from a head injury; however, it is used by many professionals to assess LOC. It tests in three major areas: eye response, motor response, and verbal response. An assessment totaling 15 points indicates the client is alert and completely oriented. A comatose client scores 7 or less.

Cranial Nerves

The nurse needs to be aware of specific nerve functions and assessment methods for each cranial nerve to detect abnormalities. In some cases, each nerve is assessed; in other cases only selected nerve functions are evaluated.

Reflexes

A **reflex** is an automatic response of the body to a stimulus. It is not voluntarily learned or conscious. The deep tendon reflex (DTR) is activated when a tendon is stimulated (tapped) and its associated muscle contracts. The quality of a reflex response varies among individuals and by age. As a person ages, reflex responses may become less intense.

Reflexes are tested using a percussion hammer. The response is described on a scale of 0 to 14. Experience is necessary to determine appropriate scoring for an individual. Several reflexes are normally tested during the physical examination: (a) the biceps reflex, (b) the triceps reflex, (c) the brachioradialis reflex, (d) the patellar reflex, (e) the Achilles reflex, and (f) the plantar (Babinski) reflex.

Motor Function

Neurologic assessment of the motor system evaluates proprioception and cerebellar function. Structures involved in proprioception are the proprioceptors, the posterior columns of the spinal cord, the cerebellum, and the vestibular apparatus (which is innervated by cranial nerve VIII) in the labyrinth of the internal ear.

Proprioceptors are sensory nerve terminals, occurring chiefly in the muscles, tendons, joints, and the internal ear, that give information about movements and the position of the body. Stimuli from the proprioceptors travel through the posterior columns of the spinal cord. Deficits of function of the posterior columns of the spinal cord result in impairment of muscle and position sense. Clients with such an impairment often must watch their own arm and leg movements to ascertain the position of the limbs.

The cerebellum (a) helps to control posture, (b) acts with the cerebral cortex to make body movements smooth and coordinated, and (c) controls skeletal muscles to maintain equilibrium.

Sensory Function

Sensory functions include touch, pain, temperature, position, and tactile discrimination. The first three are routinely tested. Generally, the face, arms, legs, hands, and feet are tested for touch and pain, although all parts of the body can be tested. If the client complains of numbness, peculiar sensations, or paralysis, the practitioner should check sensation more carefully over flexor and extensor surfaces of limbs, mapping out clearly any abnormality of touch or pain by examining responses in the area about every 2 cm (1 in.). This is a lengthy procedure. Abnormal responses to touch stimuli include loss of sensation (anesthesia); more than normal sensation (hyperesthesia); less than normal sensation (hypoesthesia); or an abnormal sensation such as burning, pain, or an electric shock (paresthesia).

A variety of common health conditions including diabetes and arteriosclerotic heart disease result in loss of the protective sensation in the lower extremities. This loss can lead to unrecognized tissue damage and eventually the need for amputation. In efforts to identify clients at increased risk for damage to the feet, the Bureau of Primary Health Care of the U.S. government has established the Lower Extremity Amputation Prevention (LEAP) program. The most important aspect of LEAP is assessment of sensation using a special monofilament that delivers 10 grams of force. Health care providers should perform an initial foot screen on all patients with diabetes and at least annually thereafter. Patients who are at risk should have their feet and shoes evaluated at least four times a year to help prevent foot problems from occurring. More information about the program and how to obtain and use the filament are available at http://www.bphc.hrsa.gov/leap.

A more detailed neurologic examination includes position sense, temperature sense, and tactile discrimination. Three types of tactile discrimination are generally tested: **one-**and **two-point discrimination,** the ability to sense whether one or two areas of the skin are being stimulated by pressure; **stereognosis,** the act of recognizing objects by touching and manipulating them; and **extinction,** the failure to perceive touch on one side of the body when two symmetric areas of the body are touched simultaneously.

Procedure 28–17 describes how to assess the neurologic system.

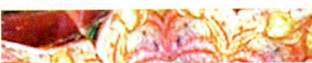 Procedure 28-17 Assessing the Neurologic System

PLANNING

If possible, determine whether a screening or full neurologic examination is indicated. This will impact preparation of the client, equipment, and timing.

Delegation

Due to the substantial knowledge and skill required, assessment of the neurologic system is not delegated to unlicensed assistive personnel. However, many aspects of neurologic behavior are observed during usual care and may be recorded by persons other than the nurse. Abnormal findings must be validated and interpreted by the nurse.

Equipment (Depending on Components of Examination)

- Percussion hammer
- Tongue depressors (one broken diagonally for testing pain sensation)
- Wisps of cotton to assess light-touch sensation
- Test tubes of hot and cold water for skin temperature assessment (optional)

IMPLEMENTATION

Performance

1. Explain to the client what you are going to do, why it is necessary, and how he or she can cooperate. Discuss how the results will be used in planning further care or treatments.
2. Wash hands and observe appropriate infection control procedures.
3. Provide for client privacy.
4. Inquire if the client has any history of the following: presence of pain in the head, back, or extremities, as well as onset and aggravating and alleviating factors; disorientation to time, place, or person; speech disorder; any history of loss of consciousness, fainting, convulsions, trauma, tingling or numbness, tremors or tics, limping, paralysis, uncontrolled muscle movements, loss of memory, mood swings, or problems with smell, vision, taste, touch, or hearing.

LANGUAGE

5. Any defects in or loss of the power to express oneself by speech, writing, or signs or to comprehend spoken or written language due to disease or injury of the cerebral cortex is called aphasia. If the client displays difficulty speaking,
   - Point to common objects, and ask the client to name them.
   - Ask the client to read some words and to match the printed and written words with pictures.
   - Ask the client to respond to simple verbal and written commands, e.g., "point to your toes" or "raise your left arm."

ORIENTATION

6. Determine the client's orientation to *time, place* and *person* by tactful questioning. Ask the client the city and state or residence, time of day, date, day of the week, duration of illness, and names of family members. More direct questioning may be necessary for some people, e.g., "Where are you now?" "What day is it today?" Most people readily accept these questions if initially the nurse asks, "Do you get confused at times?" If the client cannot answer these questions accurately, also include assessment of the *self* by asking the client to state his or her full name.

MEMORY

7. Listen for lapses in memory. Ask the client about difficulty with memory. If problems are apparent, three categories of memory are tested: immediate recall, recent memory, and remote memory.
   To assess immediate recall:
   - Ask the client to repeat a series of three digits, e.g., 7–4–3, spoken slowly.
   - Gradually increase the number of digits, e.g., 7–4–3–5, 7–4–3–5–6, and 7–4–3–5–6–7–2, until the client fails to repeat the series correctly.
   - Start again with a series of three digits, but this time ask the client to repeat them backward. The average person can repeat a series of

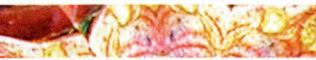

Procedure 28-17 Assessing the Neurologic System *continued*

IMPLEMENTATION *continued*

five to eight digits in sequence and four to six digits in reverse order.
To assess recent memory:

- Ask the client to recall the recent events of the day, such as how the client got to the clinic. This information must be validated, however.
- Ask the client to recall information given early in the interview, e.g., the name of a doctor.
- Provide the client with three facts to recall, e.g., a color, an object, an address, or a three-digit number, and ask the client to repeat all three. Later in the interview, ask the client to recall all three items.

To assess remote memory, ask the client to describe a previous illness or surgery, e.g., 5 years ago, or a birthday or anniversary.

ATTENTION SPAN AND CALCULATION

8. Test the ability to concentrate or *attention span* by asking the client to recite the alphabet or to count backward from 100. Test the ability to calculate by asking the client to subtract 7 or 3 progressively from 100, i.e., 100, 93, 86, 79, or 100, 97, 94, 91 (referred to as *serial sevens* or *serial threes*). Normally, an adult can complete serial sevens test in about 90 seconds with three or fewer errors. Because educational level and language or cultural differences affect calculating ability, this test may be inappropriate for some people.

LEVEL OF CONSCIOUSNESS

9. Apply the Glasgow Coma Scale: eye response, motor response, and verbal response. An assessment totaling 15 points indicates the client is alert and completely oriented. A comatose client scores 7 or less (see Table 28–10 on page 613).

CRANIAL NERVES

10. For the specific functions and assessment methods of each cranial nerve, see Table 28–11 on page 614. The names and order of the cranial nerves can be recalled by a mnemonic device: "On old Olympus's treeless top, a Finn and German viewed a hop." The first letter of each word in the sentence is the same as the first letter of the name of the cranial nerve, in order. Test each nerve not already being

evaluated in another component of the health assessment.

REFLEXES

11. Test reflexes using a percussion hammer, comparing one side of the body with the other to evaluate the symmetry of response. The response is described on a scale of 0 to +4. See Box 28–36 for a scale describing reflex responses.

BICEPS REFLEX The biceps reflex tests the spinal cord level C-5, C-6.

- Partially flex the client's arm at the elbow, and rest the forearm over the thighs, placing the palm of the hand down.
- Place the thumb of your nondominant hand horizontally over the biceps tendon.
- Deliver a blow (slight downward thrust) with the percussion hammer to your thumb.
- Observe the normal slight flexion of the elbow, and feel the bicep's contraction through your thumb (see Figure 28–86 ■, A).

TRICEPS REFLEX The triceps reflex tests the spinal cord level C-7, C-8.

- Flex the client's arm at the elbow, and support it in the palm of your nondominant hand.
- Palpate the triceps tendon about 2 to 5 cm (1 to 2 in.) above the elbow.
- Deliver a blow with the percussion hammer directly to the tendon (see Figure 28–86 ■, B).

BRACHIORADIALIS REFLEX The brachioradialis reflex tests the spinal cord level C-3, C-6.

- Rest the client's arm in a relaxed position on your forearm or on the client's own leg.
- Deliver a blow with the percussion hammer directly on the radius 2 to 5 cm (1 to 2 in.) above the wrist or the styloid process, the bony prominence on the thumb side of the wrist (see Figure 28–86 ■, C).
- Observe the normal flexion and supination of the forearm. The fingers of the hand may also extend slightly.

PATELLAR REFLEX The patellar reflex tests the spinal cord level L-2, L-3, L-4.

- Ask the client to sit on the edge of the examining table so that the legs hang freely.
- Locate the patellar tendon directly below the patella (kneecap).
- Deliver a blow with the percussion hammer directly to the tendon (see Figure 28–86 ■, D).
- Observe the normal extension or kicking out of the leg as the quadriceps muscle contracts.
- If no response occurs and you suspect the client is not relaxed, ask the client to interlock the fingers and pull. *This action often enhances relaxation so that a more accurate response is obtained.*

ACHILLES REFLEX The Achilles reflex tests the spinal cord level S-1, S-2.

- Observe the normal slight extension of the elbow.

> **► CLINICAL ALERT** *All questions and tests used in a neurologic examination must be age, language, education level, and culturally appropriate. Individualize questions and tests before using them. ■*

BOX 28–36 ■ Scale for Grading Reflex Responses

0	No reflex response
+1	Minimal activity (hypoactive)
+2	Normal response
+3	More active than normal
+4	Maximal activity (hyperactive)

continued on page 606

MediaLink | PERFORMING PHYSICAL ASSESSMENTS CASE STUDY

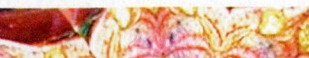

Procedure 28-17 Assessing the Neurologic System *continued*

IMPLEMENTATION *continued*

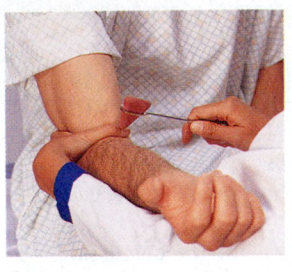

A

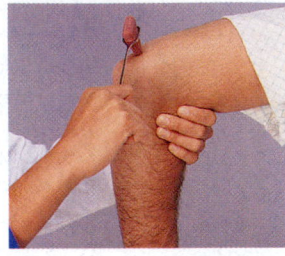

B

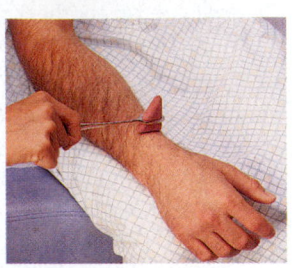

C

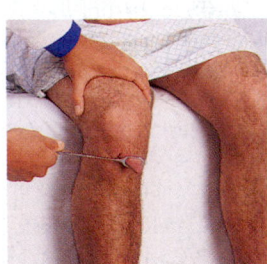

D

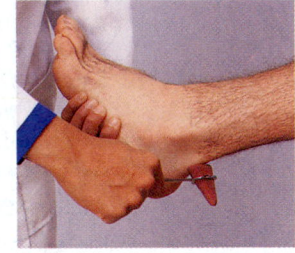

E

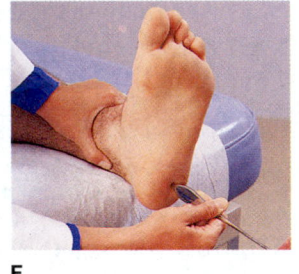

F

Figure 28–86 ■ Testing reflexes: *A,* the biceps reflex; *B,* the triceps reflex; *C,* the brachioradialis reflex; *D,* the patellar reflex; *E,* the Achilles reflex; *F,* the plantar (Babinski) reflex.

■ With the client in the same position as for the patellar reflex, slightly dorsiflex the client's ankle by supporting the foot lightly in the hand.

■ Deliver a blow with the percussion hammer directly to the Achilles tendon just above the heel (see Figure 28–86 ■, *E*).

■ Observe and feel the normal plantar flexion (downward jerk) of the foot.

PLANTAR (BABINSKI) REFLEX The planter, or Babinski, reflex is superficial. It may be absent in adults without pathology or overridden by voluntary control.

■ Use a moderately sharp object, such as the handle of the percussion hammer, a key, or the dull end of a pin or applicator stick.

■ Stroke the lateral border of the sole of the client's foot, starting at the heel, con-tinuing to the ball of the foot, and then proceeding across the ball of the foot to-ward the big toe (see Figure 28–86 ■, *F*).

■ Observe the response. Normally, all five toes bend downward; this reaction is negative Babinski. In an abnormal Babinski response the toes spread out-ward and the big toe moves upward.

MOTOR FUNCTION

Assessment	Normal Findings	Deviations from Normal
12. *Gross Motor and Balance Tests* Generally, the Romberg test and one other gross motor function and bal-ance tests are used.		
WALKING GAIT Ask the client to walk across the room and back, and assess the client's gait.	Has upright posture and steady gait with opposing arm swing; walks unaided, main-taining balance	Has poor postrue and unsteady, irregular, staggering gait with wide stance; bends legs only from hips; has rigid or no arm movements
ROMBERG TEST Ask the client to stand with feet together and arms resting at the sides, first with eyes open, then closed. Stand close during this test *to prevent the client from falling.*	*Negative Romberg:* may sway slightly but is able to maintain upright posture and foot stance	Positive Romberg: cannot maintain food stance; moves the feet apart to maintain stance
		If client cannot maintain balance with the eyes shut, client may have sensory ataxia
		If balance cannot be maintained whether the eyes are open or shut, client may have cerebellar ataxia

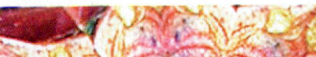

Procedure 28-17 Assessing the Neurologic System *continued*

IMPLEMENTATION *continued*

Assessment	Normal Findings	Deviations from Normal
STANDING ON ONE FOOT WITH EYES CLOSED Ask the client to close the eyes and stand on one foot and then the other. Stand close to the client during this test.	Maintains stance for at least 5 seconds	Cannot maintain stance for 5 seconds
HEEL-TOE WALKING Ask the client to walk a straight line, placing the heel of one foot directly in front of the toes of the other foot.	Maintains heel-toe walking along a straight line (see Figure 28–87 n)	Assumes a wider foot gait to stay upright

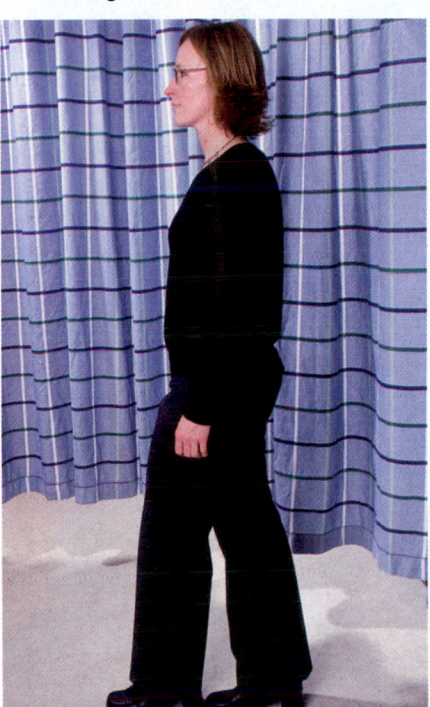

Figure 28–87 ■ Heel-toe walking test.

Assessment	Normal Findings	Deviations from Normal
TOE OR HEEL WALKING Ask the client to walk several steps on the toes and then on the heels.	Able to walk several steps on toes or heels	Cannot maintain balance on toes or heels
13. *Fine Motor Tests for the Upper Extremities*		
FINGER-TO-NOSE TEST Ask the client to abduct and extend the arms at shoulder height and rapidly touch the nose alternately with one index finger and then the other. The client repeats the test with the eyes closed if the test is performed easily.	Repeatedly and rhythmically touches the nose (see Figure 28–88 ■)	Misses the nose or gives lazy response

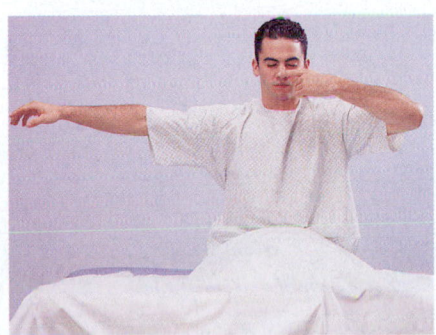

Figure 28–88 ■ Finger-to-nose test.

continued on page 608

Procedure 28-17 Assessing the Neurologic System *continued*

IMPLEMENTATION *continued*

Assessment	Normal Findings	Deviations from Normal
ALTERNATING SUPINATION AND PRONATION OF HANDS ON KNEES Ask the client to pat both knees with the palms of both hands and then with the backs of the hands alternately at an ever-increasing rate.	Can alternately supinate and pronate hands at rapid pace (see Figure 28–89 ■)	Performs with slow, clumsy movements and irregular timing; has difficulty alternating from supination to pronation

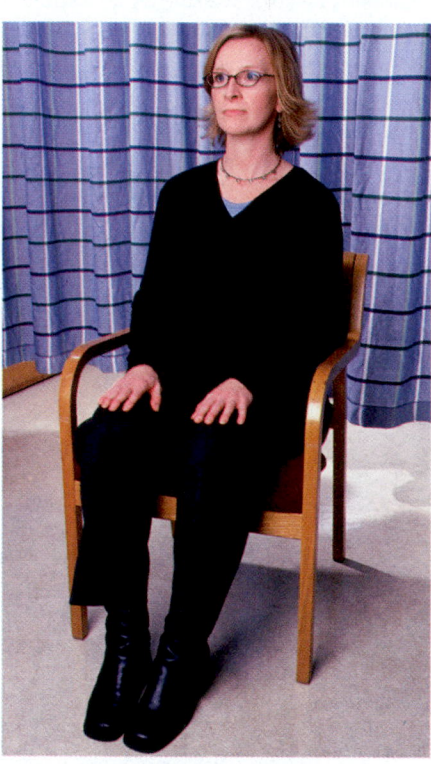
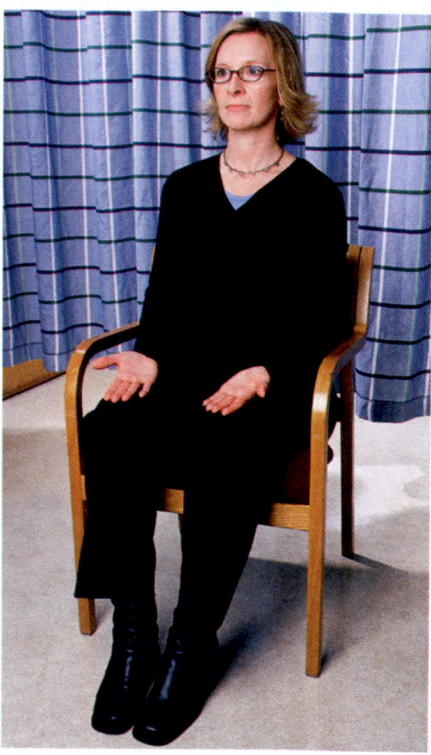

Figure 28–89 ■ Alternating supination and pronation of hands on knees test.

FINGER TO NOSE AND TO THE NURSE'S FINGER Ask the client to touch the nose and then your index finger, held at a distance at about 45 cm (18 in.), at a rapid and increasing rate.	Performs with coordination and rapidity (see Figure 28–90 ■)	Misses the finger and moves slowly

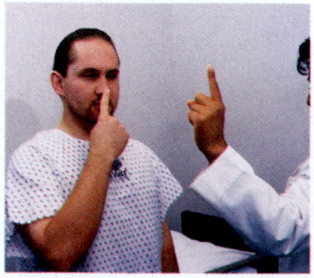
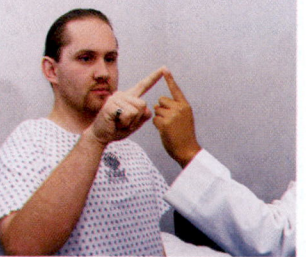

Figure 28–90 ■ Finger to nose and to the nurse's finger test.

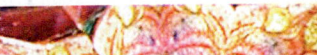

Procedure 28-17 Assessing the Neurologic System *continued*

IMPLEMENTATION *continued*

Assessment	Normal Findings	Deviations from Normal
FINGERS TO FINGERS Ask the client to spread the arms broadly at shoulder height and then bring the fingers together at the midline, first with the eyes open and then closed, first slowly and then rapidly.	Performs with accuracy and rapidity (see Figure 28–91 ■)	Moves slowly and is unable to touch fingers consistently

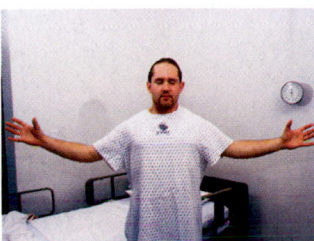
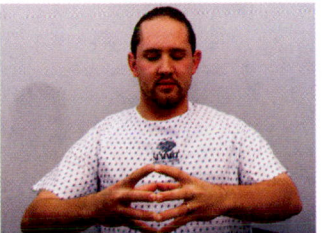

Figure 28–91 ■ Fingers-to-fingers test.

| **FINGERS TO THUMB (SAME HAND)**
Ask the client to touch each finger of one hand to the thumb of the same hand as rapidly as possible | Rapidly touches each finger to thumb with each hand (see Figure 28–92 ■). | Cannot coordinate this fine discrete movement with either one or both hands |

14. Fine Motor Tests for the Lower Extremities
    Ask the client to lie supine and to perform these tests.

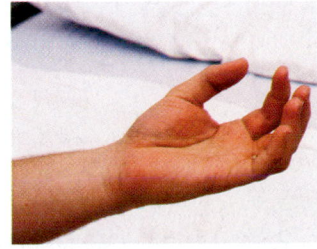
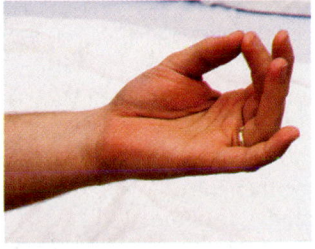

Figure 28–92 ■ Fingers-to-thumb (same hand) test.

| **HEEL DOWN OPPOSITE SHIN**
Ask the client to place the heel of one foot just below the opposite knee and run the heel down the shin to the foot. Repeat with the other foot. The client may also use a sitting position for this test. | Demonstrates bilateral equal coordination (see Figure 28–93 ■). | Has tremors or is awkward; heel moves off shin |

Figure 28–93 ■ Heel down opposite shin test.

continued on page 610

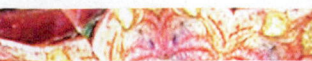

Procedure 28-17 Assessing the Neurologic System *continued*

IMPLEMENTATION *continued*

Assessment	Normal Findings	Deviations from Normal
TOE OR BALL OF FOOT TO THE NURSE'S FINGER Ask the client to touch your finger with the large toe of each foot.	Moves smoothly, with coordination (see Figure 28–94 ■).	Misses your finger; cannot coordinate movement

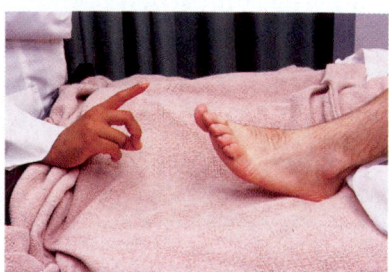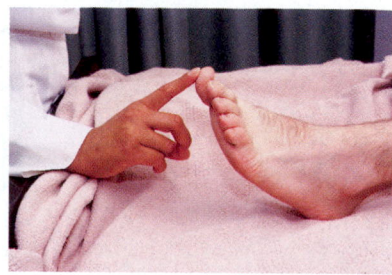

Figure 28–94 ■ Toe or ball of foot to the nurse's finger test.

15. Light-Touch Sensation

Compare the light-touch sensation of symmetric areas of the body. *Sensitivity to touch varies among different skin areas.*

- Ask the client to close the eyes and to respond by saying "yes" or "now" whenever the client feels the cotton wisp touching the skin.

- With a wisp of cotton, lightly touch one specific spot and then the same spot on the other side of the body (see Figure 28–95 ■).

- Test areas on the forehead, cheek, hand, lower arm, abdomen, foot, and lower leg. Check a specific area of the limb first (i.e., the hand before the arm and the foot before the leg), *because the sensory nerve may be assumed to be intact if sensation is felt at its most peripheral part.*

- Ask the client to point to the spot where the touch was felt. *This demonstrates whether the client is able to determine tactile location (point localization), i.e., can accurately perceive where the client was touched.*

- If areas of sensory dysfunction are found, determine the boundaries of sensation by testing responses about every 2.5 cm (1 in.) in the area. Make a sketch of the sensory loss area for recording purposes.

Light tickling or touch sensation

Anesthesia, hyperesthesia, hypoesthesia, and paresthesia

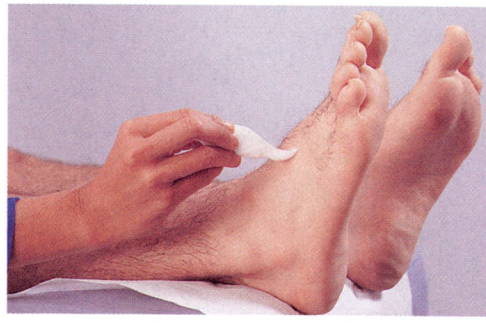

Figure 28–95 ■ Assessing light-touch sensation.

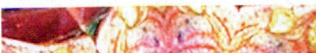

Procedure 28-17 Assessing the Neurologic System *continued*

IMPLEMENTATION *continued*

Assessment	Normal Findings	Deviations from Normal
16. Pain Sensation Assess pain sensation as follows: • Ask the client to close the eyes and to say "sharp," "dull," or "don't know" when the sharp or dull end of the broken tongue depressor is felt. • Alternately, use the sharp and dull end of a sterile pin or needle to lightly prick designated anatomic areas at random, e.g., hand, forearm, foot, lower leg, abdomen (see Figure 28–96 ■). The face is not tested in this manner. *Alternating the sharp and dull ends of the instrument more accurately evaluates the client's response.* • Allow at least 2 seconds between each test to prevent summation effects of stimuli, i.e., several successive stimuli perceived as one stimulus.	Able to discriminate "sharp" and "dull" sensations 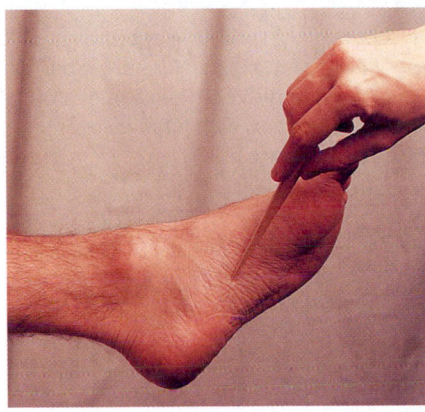 **Figure 28–96** ■ Assessing pain sensation using a broken tongue depressor.	Areas of reduced, heightened, or absent sensation (map them out for recording purposes)
17. Temperature Sensation Temperature sensation is not routinely tested if pain sensation is found to be within normal limits. If pain sensation is not normal or is absent, testing sensitivity to temperature may prove more reliable. • Touch skin areas with test tubes filled with hot or cold water. • Have the client respond by saying "hot," "cold," or "don't know."	Able to discriminate between "hot" and "cold" sensations	Areas of dulled or lost sensation (when sensations of pain are dulled, temperature sense is usually also impaired because distribution of these nerves over the body is similar)
18. Position or Kinesthetic Sensation Commonly, the middle fingers and the large toes are tested for the kinesthetic sensation (sense of position). • To test the fingers, support the client's arm with one hand, and hold the client's palm in the other. To test the toes, place the client's heels on the examining table. • Ask the client to close the eyes. • Grasp a middle finger or a big toe firmly between your thumb and index finger, and exert the same pressure on both sides of the finger or toe while moving it. • Move the finger or toe until it is up, down, or straight out, and ask the client to identify the position. • Use a series of brisk up-and-down movements before bringing the finger or toe suddenly to rest in one of the three positions.	Can readily determine the position of fingers and toes	Unable to determine the position of one or more fingers or toes

continued on page 612

Procedure 28-17 Assessing the Neurologic System *continued*

IMPLEMENTATION *continued*

Assessment	Normal Findings	Deviations from Normal
19. Tactile Discrimination For all tests, the client's eyes need to be closed.		

ONE- AND TWO-POINT DISCRIMINATION
Alternately stimulate the skin with two pins simultaneously and then with one pin. Ask whether the client feels one or two pinpricks.
	Perception varies widely in adults over different parts of the body. Normally, a person can distinguish between a one- and two-point stimulus within the following minimum distances:
	
	  Fingertips, 2.8 mm
	  Palms of hands, 8–12 mm
	  Chest, forearm, 40 mm
	  Back, 50–70 mm
	  Upper arm, thigh, 75 mm
	  Toes, 3–8 mm
		Unable to sense whether one or two areas of the skin are being stimulated by pressure

STEREOGNOSIS (ABILITY TO RECOGNIZE OBJECTS BY TOUCHING THEM) Place familiar objects, such as a key, paper clip, or coin, in the client's hand, and ask the client to identify them.	Recognizes common objects	Unable recognize common objects
If the client has a motor impairment of the hand and is unable to manipulate an object, write a number or letter on the client's palm, using a blunt instrument, and ask the client to identify it.	Able to identify numbers or letters written on palm	Unable to identify numbers or letters written on palm
EXTINCTION PHENOMENON Simultaneously stimulate two symmetric areas of the body, such as the thighs, the cheeks, or the hands.	Both points of stimulus are felt	Failure to perceive touch on one side of the body when two symmetric areas of the body are touched simultaneously (frequently noted in clients with lesions of the sensory cortex)
20. Document findings in the client record using forms or checklists supplemented by narrative notes when appropriate. Describe any abnormal findings in objective terms, e.g., "When		asked to count backwards by threes, client made seven errors and completed the task in 4 minutes."

EVALUATION

- Perform a detailed follow-up examination of other systems based on findings that deviated from expected or normal for the client. Relate findings to previous assessment data if available.
- Report significant deviations from normal to the physician.

Assessing the Neurologic System

Infants

- Reflexes commonly tested in newborns include the rooting reflex—when the baby's cheek is touched, the head turns toward that side; palmar grasp—baby's fingers curl around an object; tonic neck reflex—when the baby is supine and the head is turned to one side, the arm and leg on that side extend while those on the opposite side flex (fencing position). Most of these disappear by 6 months of age.

Children

- Present the procedures as games whenever possible.
- Positive Babinski reflex is abnormal after the child ambulates or at age 2.
- For children under age 5, the Denver Developmental Screening Test II provides a comprehensive neurologic evaluation—particularly for motor function.
- Note the child's ability to understand and follow directions.
- Assess immediate recall or recent memory by using names of cartoon characters. Normal recall in children is one less than age in years.
- Assess for signs of hyperactivity or abnormally short attention span.
- Should be able to walk backward by age 2, balance on one foot for 5 seconds by age 4, heel-toe walk by age 5, and heel-toe walk backward by age 6.
- Romberg test is appropriate over age 3.

Elders

- A full neurologic assessment can be lengthy. Conduct in several sessions if indicated and cease the tests if the client is noticeably fatigued.
- A decline in mental status is not a normal result of aging. Changes are more the result of physical or psychologic disorders (e.g., fever, fluid and electrolyte imbalances, medications). Acute, abrupt-onset mental status changes are usually caused by delirium. These changes are often reversible with treatment. Chronic subtle insidious mental health changes are usually caused by dementia and are usually irreversible.
- Intelligence and learning ability are unaltered with age. Many factors, however, inhibit learning (e.g., anxiety, illness, pain, cultural barrier).
- Short-term memory is often less efficient. Long-term memory is usually unaltered.
- Because old age is often associated with loss of support persons, depression is a common disorder. Mood changes, weight loss, anorexia, constipation, and early morning awakening may manifest it.
- The stress of being in unfamiliar situations can cause confusion in the elderly person.
- As a person ages, reflex responses may become less intense.
- Because older clients tire more easily than younger clients, a total neurologic assessment is often done at a different time than the other parts of the physical assessment.
- Although there is a progressive decrease in the number of functioning neurons in the central nervous system and in the sense organs, the older client usually functions well because of the abundant reserves in the number of brain cells.
- Impulse transmission and reaction to stimuli are slower.
- Many elderly clients have some impairment of hearing, vision, smell, temperature and pain sensation, memory, and mental endurance.
- Coordination changes, including a reduced speed of fine finger movements. Standing balance remains intact, and Romberg's test remains negative.
- Reflex responses may slightly increase or decrease. Many show loss of Achilles reflex, and the plantar reflex may be difficult to elicit.
- When testing sensory function, the nurse needs to give the older client time to respond. Normally, older clients have unaltered perception of light touch and superficial pain, decreased perception of deep pain, and decreased perception of temperature stimuli. Many also reveal a decrease or absence of position sense in the large toes.

TABLE 28–10 Levels of Consciousness: Glasgow Coma Scale

Faculty Measured	Response	Score
Eye opening	Spontaneous	4
	To verbal command	3
	To pain	2
	No response	1
Motor response	To verbal command	6
	To localized pain	5
	Flexes and withdraws	4
	Flexes abnormally	3
	Extends abnormally	2
	No response	1
Verbal response	Oriented, converses	5
	Disoriented, converses	4
	Uses inappropriate words	3
	Makes incomprehensible sounds	2
	No response	1

TABLE 28-11 Cranial Nerve Functions and Assessment Methods

Cranial Nerve	Name	Type	Function	Assessment Method
I	Olfactory	Sensory	Smell	Ask client to close eyes and identify different mild aromas, such as coffee, vanilla, peanut butter, orange, lemon, lime, chocolate.
II	Optic	Sensory	Vision and visual fields	Ask client to read Snellen chart; check visual fields by confrontation; and conduct an ophthalmoscopic examination.
III	Oculomotor	Motor	Extraocular eye movement (EOM); movement of sphincter of pupil; movement of ciliary muscles of lens	Assess six ocular movements and pupil reaction.
IV	Trochlear	Motor	EOM; specifically, moves eyeball downward and laterally	Assess six ocular movements.
V	Trigeminal Ophthalmic branch	Sensory	Sensation of cornea, skin of face, and nasal mucosa	While client looks upward, lightly touch lateral sclera of eye to elicit blink reflex. To test light sensation, have client close eyes, wipe a wisp of cotton over client's forehead and paranasal sinuses. To test deep sensation, use alternating blunt and sharp ends of a safety pin over same areas.
	Maxillary branch	Sensory	Sensation of skin of face and anterior oral cavity (tongue and teeth)	Assess skin sensation as for ophthalmic branch above.
	Mandibular branch	Motor and sensory	Muscles of mastication; sensation of skin of face	Ask client to clench teeth.
VI	Abducens	Motor	EOM; moves eyeball laterally	Assess directions of gaze.
VII	Facial	Motor and sensory	Facial expression; taste (anterior two-thirds of tongue)	Ask client to smile, raise the eyebrows, frown, puff out cheeks, close eyes tightly. Ask client to identify various tastes placed on tip and sides of tongue: sugar (sweet), salt, lemon juice (sour), and quinine (bitter); identify areas of taste.
VIII	Auditory Vestibular branch	Sensory	Equilibrium	Assessment methods are discussed with cerebellar functions (in next section).
	Cochlear branch	Sensory	Hearing	Assess client's ability to hear spoken word and vibrations of tuning fork.
IX	Glossopharyngeal	Motor and sensory	Swallowing ability, tongue movement, taste (posterior tongue)	Apply tastes on posterior tongue for identification. Ask client to move tongue from side to side and up and down.
X	Vagus	Motor and sensory	Sensation of pharynx and larynx; swallowing; vocal cord movement	Assessed with cranial nerve IX; assess client's speech for hoarseness.
XI	Accessory	Motor	Head movement; shrugging of shoulders	Ask client to shrug shoulders against resistance from your hands and turn head to side against resistance from your hand (repeat for other side).
XII	Hypoglossal	Motor	Protrusion of tongue; moves tongue up and down and side to side	Ask client to protrude tongue at midline, then move it side to side.

FEMALE GENITALS AND INGUINAL AREA

The examination of the genitals and reproductive tract of women includes assessment of the inguinal lymph nodes and inspection and palpation of the external genitals. Completeness of the assessment of the genitals and reproductive tract depends on the needs and problems of the individual client. In most practice settings, generalist nurses perform only inspection of the external genitals and palpation of the inguinal lymph nodes.

For sexually active adolescent and adult women, a Papanicolaou test (Pap test) is used to detect cancer of the cervix. If there is an increased or abnormal vaginal discharge, specimens should be taken to check for sexually transmitted disease.

Examination of the genitals usually creates uncertainty and apprehension in women, and the lithotomy position required can cause embarrassment. The nurse must explain each part of the examination in advance and perform the examination in an objective and efficient manner.

Procedure 28–18 describes how to assess the female genitals and inguinal area.

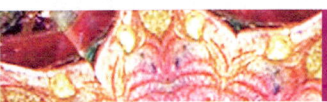

Procedure 28-18 Assessing the Female Genitals and Inguinal Area

PLANNING

Delegation

Due to the substantial knowledge and skill required, assessment of the female genitals and inguinal lymph nodes is not delegated to unlicensed assistive personnel. However, persons other than the nurse may record any aspect that is observed during usual care. Abnormal findings must be validated and interpreted by the nurse.

Equipment

- Examination gloves
- Drape
- Supplemental lighting, if needed

IMPLEMENTATION

Performance

1. Explain to the client what you are going to do, why it is necessary, and how she can cooperate. Discuss how the results will be used in planning further care or treatments.
2. Wash hands, apply gloves, and observe appropriate infection control procedures.
3. Provide for client privacy.
4. Inquire if the client has any history of the following: age of onset of menstruation, last menstrual period (LMP), regularity of cycle, duration, amount of daily flow, and whether menstrua-tion is painful; incidence of pain during intercourse; vaginal discharge; number of pregnancies, number of live births, labor or delivery complications; urgency and frequency of urination at night; blood in urine, painful urination, incontinence; history of sexually transmitted disease, past and present.
5. Position the client supine with feet elevated on the stirrups of an examination table. Alternately, assist the client into the dorsal recumbent position with knees flexed and thighs externally rotated.

Assessment	Normal Findings	Deviations from Normal
6. Inspect the distribution, amount, and characteristics of pubic hair.	There are wide variations; generally kinky in the menstruating adult, thinner and straighter after menopause Distributed in the shape of an inverse triangle	Scant pubic hair (may indicate hormonal problem) Hair growth should not extend over the abdomen
7. Inspect the skin of the pubic area for parasites, inflammation, swelling, and lesions. To assess pubic skin adequately, separate the labia majora and labia minora.	Pubic skin intact, no lesions Skin of vulva area slightly darker than the rest of the body Labia round, full, and relatively symmetric in adult females	Lice, lesions, scars, fissures, swelling, erythema, excoriations, scars from episiotomies, varicosities, or leukoplakia
8. Inspect the clitoris, urethral orifice, and vaginal orifice when separating the labia minora.	Clitoris does not exceed 1 cm in width and 2 cm in length Urethral orifice appears as a small slit and is the same color as surrounding tissues No inflammation, swelling, or discharge	Presence of lesions Presence of inflammation, swelling, or discharge

continued on page 616

MediaLink | PHYSICAL EXAM APPLICATION

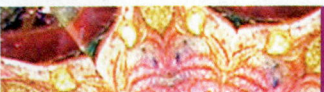

Procedure 28-18 Assessing the Female Genitals and Inguinal Area *continued*

IMPLEMENTATION *continued*

Assessment	Normal Findings	Deviations from Normal
9. Palpate the inguinal lymph nodes (see Figure 28–97 ■). Use the pads of the fingers in a rotary motion, noting any enlargement or tenderness.	No enlargement or tenderness	Enlargement and tenderness

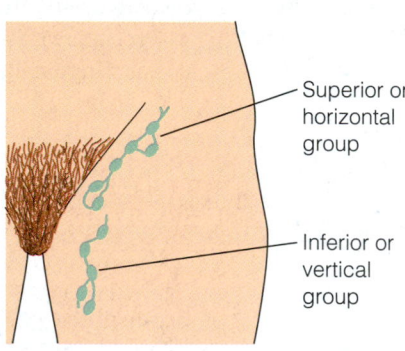

Superior or horizontal group

Inferior or vertical group

Figure 28–97 ■ Lymph nodes of the groin area.

10. Document findings in the client record using forms or checklists supplemented by narrative notes when appropriate.

EVALUATION

- Perform a detailed follow-up examination based on findings that deviated from expected or normal for the client. Relate findings to previous assessment data if available.

- Report significant deviations from normal to the physician or nurse practitioner qualified to perform an internal vaginal examination.

In many agencies only nurse practitioners examine the internal genitals. However, generalist nurses often assist with this examination and need to be familiar with the procedure. Examination of the internal genitals involves (a) palpating Skene's and Bartholin's glands, (b) assessing the pelvic musculature, (c) inserting a vaginal speculum to inspect the cervix and vagina, and (d) obtaining a Papanicolaou smear.

The speculum examination of the vagina involves the insertion of a plastic or metal speculum that consists of two blades and an adjustable thumb screw (Figure 28–98 ■). Various sizes are available (small, medium, and large); the appropriate size

needs to be selected for each client. A virgin or a sexually inactive older woman will probably require a small speculum; otherwise the size of the speculum depends on the individual's sexual and obstetric history. The speculum may be lubricated with water-soluble lubricant if specimens are not being collected. Most examiners lubricate the speculum with warm water. After visualizing the cervix, the examiner takes smear specimens from one or more of the sites.

The nurse's responsibilities when assisting with an examination of the internal female genitals include the following:

1. *Assembling equipment.* These include drapes, gloves, vaginal speculum of correct size, warm water or lubricant, and supplies for cytology and culture studies.
2. *Preparing the client.* Advise the client not to douche prior to the procedure. Explain the procedure. It should take only 5 minutes and is normally not painful. Assist the client to a lithotomy position as needed, and drape her appropriately.
3. *Supporting the client during the procedure.* This involves explaining the procedure as needed, and encouraging the client to take deep breaths that will help the pelvic muscles relax.
4. *Monitoring and assisting the client after the procedure.* Assist the client from the lithotomy position and with per-

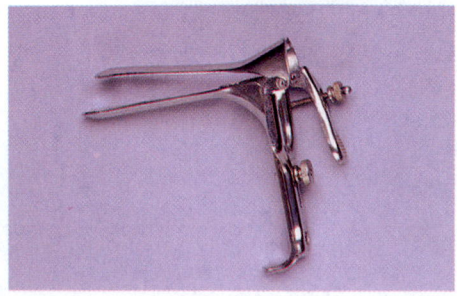

Figure 28–98 ■ A vaginal speculum.

ineal care as needed. Observe any discharge from the vagina. Normally characteristics of cervical mucus vary throughout the menstrual cycle from clear to white and from thin to thick, even stringy. Three common types of vaginal infections produce characteristic discharge: Monilial or yeast infections produce a thick, white, curdy, patchy discharge; trichomonal infections produce a profuse, watery, gray or green, frothy, odorous discharge; bacterial infections produce an odorous discharge.

5. *Documenting the procedure.* Include the date and time it was performed, the name of the examiner, and any nursing assessments and interventions.

Lifespan Considerations

Assessing the Female Genitals and Inguinal Lymph Nodes

Infants

- Infants can be held in a supine position on the mother's lap with the knees supported in a flexed position and separated.
- In newborns, in response to maternal estrogen, the labia and clitoris may be edematous and enlarged, and there may be a white vaginal discharge.

Children

- Ensure that you have the parent or guardian's approval to perform the examination and then tell the child what you are going to do. Preschool children are taught to resist touching of their "private parts."
- Assessment of adolescent girls is limited to inspection of the external genitals, unless the girl is sexually active. If so, and the girl has an increased or abnormal vaginal discharge, specimens should be taken to check for sexually transmitted disease. Box 28–37 shows the five stages of pubic hair development during puberty.
- The clitoris is a common site for syphilitic chancres in younger females.

Elders

- Labia are atrophied and flatter in older females.
- The clitoris is a common site for cancerous lesions in older females.
- The vulva atrophies as a result of a reduction in vascularity, elasticity, adipose tissue, and estrogen levels. Because the vulva is more fragile, it is more easily irritated.
- The vaginal environment becomes drier and more alkaline, resulting in an alteration of the type of flora present and a predisposition to vaginitis. Dyspareunia (difficult or painful coitus) is also a common occurrence.
- The cervix and uterus decrease in size.
- The fallopian tubes and ovaries atrophy.
- Ovulation and estrogen production cease.
- Vaginal bleeding unrelated to estrogen therapy is abnormal in older women.
- Prolapse of the uterus occurs in older females, especially those who have had multiple pregnancies.
- Older females may be arthritic and find the examination position uncomfortable.

BOX 28–37 ■ Five Stages of Pubic Hair Development in Females

Stage 1   Preadolescence. No pubic hair except for fine body hair.

Stage 2   Usually occurs at ages 11 and 12. Sparse, long, slightly pigmented curly hair develops along the labia.

Stage 3   Usually occurs at ages 12 and 13. Hair becomes darker in color and curlier and develops over the pubic symphysis.

Stage 4   Usually occurs between ages 13 and 14. Hair assumes the texture and curl of the adult but is not as thick and does not appear on the thighs.

Stage 5   Sexual maturity. Hair assumes adult appearance and appears on the inner aspect of the upper thighs (see Figure 28–99 ■).

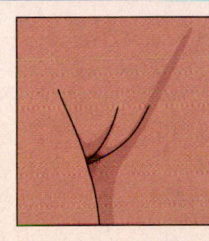
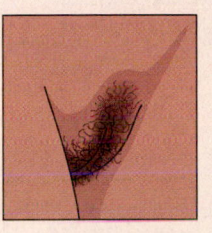
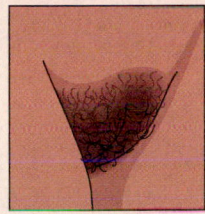
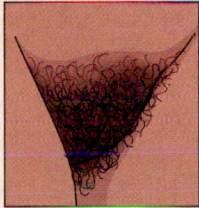

1   2

3   4   5

Figure 28–99 ■ Stages of female pubic hair development.

MALE GENITALS AND INGUINAL AREA

In adult men, complete examination should include assessment of the external genitals, the presence of any hernias, and the prostate gland. As with women, nurses in some practice settings performing routine assessment of clients may assess only the external genitals. The male reproductive and urinary systems (see Figure 28–100 ■) share the urethra, which is the passageway for both urine and semen. Therefore, in physical assessment of the male these two systems are frequently assessed together.

Examination of the male genitals by a female practitioner is becoming increasingly common. Most male clients accept examination by a female, especially if she is emotionally comfortable herself about performing it and does so in a matter-of-fact and competent manner. If the female nurse does not feel comfortable about this part of the examination or if the client is

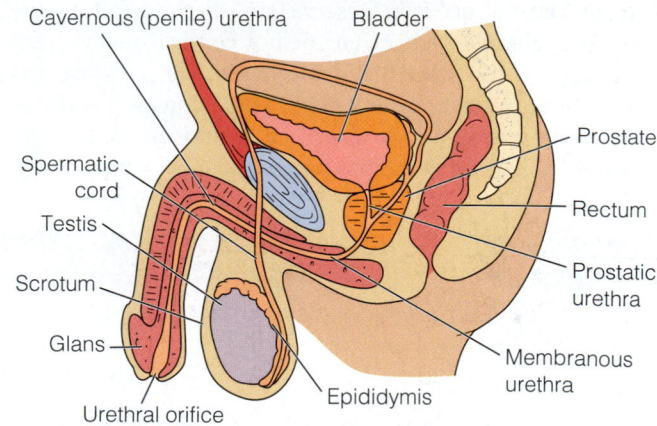

Figure 28–100 ■ The male urogenital tract.

TABLE 28–12 Stages of Male Pubic Hair and External Genital Development (12 to 16 Years)

Stage	Pubic Hair	Penis	Testes/Scrotum
1 (preadolescent)	None, except for body hair like that on the abdomen	Size is relative to body size, as in childhood	Size is relative to body size, as in childhood
2	Scant, long, slightly pigmented at base of penis	Slight enlargement occurs	Becomes reddened in color and enlarged
3	Darker, begins to curl and becomes more coarse; extends over pubic symphysis	Elongation occurs	Continuing enlargement
4	Continues to darken and thicken; extends on the sides, above and below	Increase in both breadth and length; glans develops	Continuing enlargement; color darkens
5	Adult distribution that extends to inner thighs, umbilicus, and anus	Adult appearance	Adult appearance

reluctant to be examined by a woman, the nurse should refer this part of the examination to a male practitioner.

Development of secondary sex characteristics is assessed in relationship to the client's age. See Table 28–12 for the five stages of the development of pubic hair, the penis, and the testes and scrotum during puberty.

All male clients should be screened for the presence of inguinal or femoral hernias. A **hernia** is a protrusion of the intestine through the inguinal wall or canal. The loop of bowel may even extend down to the scrotum. An indirect inguinal hernia is a loop of bowel that enters the internal inguinal ring. It may stay in the canal, exit through the external ring, or pass into the scrotum. A direct inguinal hernia enters the inguinal canal directly through a weakness in the abdominal wall just behind the external inguinal ring. It does not pass through the inguinal canal. A femoral hernia is lower and more lateral than an inguinal hernia and may look like an enlarged lymph node.

Cancer of the prostate gland is the most common cancer in adult men and occurs primarily in men over age 50. Examination of the prostate gland is performed with the examination of the rectum and anus (see Procedure 28–20).

Testicular cancer is much rarer than prostate cancer and occurs primarily in young men ages 15 to 35. Testicular cancer is most commonly found on the anterior and lateral surfaces of the testes. Testicular self-examination should be conducted monthly (see Chapter 38).

The techniques of inspection and palpation are used to examine the male genitals. Procedure 28–19 describes how the nurse can conduct an assessment of the male genitals and inguinal area.

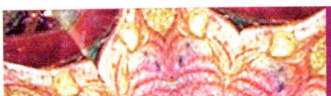 ## Procedure 28-19 Assessing the Male Genitals and Inguinal Area

PLANNING

Delegation
Due to the substantial knowledge and skill required, assessment of the male genitals and inguinal area is not delegated to unlicensed assistive personnel. However, persons other than the nurse may record any aspect that is observed during usual care. Abnormal findings must be validated and interpreted by the nurse.

Equipment
- Examination gloves

IMPLEMENTATION

Performance

1. Explain to the client what you are going to do, why it is necessary, and how he can cooperate. Discuss how the results will be used in planning further care or treatments.
2. Wash hands, apply gloves, and observe appropriate infection control procedures.
3. Provide for client privacy.
4. Inquire if the client has any history of the following: Usual voiding patterns and any changes, bladder control, urinary incontinence, frequency, urgency, abdominal pain; any symptoms of sexually transmitted disease; any swellings that could indicate presence of hernia; family history of nephritis, malignancy of the prostate, or malignancy of the kidney.

Assessment	Normal Findings	Deviations from Normal
PUBIC HAIR 5. Inspect the distribution, amount, and characteristics of pubic hair.	Triangular distribution, often spreading up the abdomen	Scant amount or absence of hair
PENIS 6. Inspect the penile shaft and glans penis for lesions, nodules, swellings, and inflammation.	Penile skin intact	Presence of lesions, nodules, swellings, or inflammation
	Appears slightly wrinkled and varies in color as widely as other body skin	
	Foreskin easily retractable from the glans penis	
	Small amount of thick white smegma between the glans and foreskin	
7. Inspect the urethral meatus for swelling, inflammation, and discharge. • Compress or ask the client to compress the glans slightly to open the urethral meatus to inspect it for discharge.	Pink and slitlike appearance Positioned at the tip of the penis	Inflammation; discharge Variation in meatal locations (e.g., hypospadias, on the underside of the penile shaft, and epispadias, on the upper side of the penile shaft)

continued on page 620

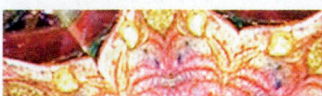

Procedure 28-19 Assessing the Male Genitals and Inguinal Area *continued*

IMPLEMENTATION *continued*

Assessment	Normal Findings	Deviations from Normal
• If the client has reported a discharge, instruct the client to strip the penis from the base to the urethra (i.e., grasp the base of the penis, with the thumb at the front and fingers behind, and while applying moderate pressure, move the thumb and fingers slowly down the shaft of the penis.		
8. Palpate the penis for tenderness, thickening, and nodules. Use your thumb and first two fingers.	Smooth and semifirm Is slightly movable over the underlying structures	Presence of tenderness, thickening, or nodules Immobility

SCROTUM

Assessment	Normal Findings	Deviations from Normal
9. Inspect the scrotum for appearance, general size, and symmetry.	Scrotal skin is darker in color than that of the rest of the body and is loose	Discolorations; any tightening of skin (may indicate edema or mass)
• To facilitate inspection of the scrotum during a physical examination, ask the client to hold the penis out of the way.	Size varies with temperature changes (the dartos muscles contract when the area is cold and relax when the area is warm)	Marked asymmetry in size
• Inspect all skin surfaces by spreading the rugated surface skin and lifting the scrotum as needed to observe posterior surfaces.	Scrotum appears asymmetric (left testis is usually lower than right testis)	
10. Palpate the scrotum to assess status of underlying testes, epididymis, and spermatic cord. Palpate both testes simultaneously for comparative purposes. The palpation procedure is outlined in Box 28–38.	Testicles are rubbery, smooth, and free of nodules and masses Testis is about 2 × 4 cm (0.7 × 1.5 in.) Epididymis is resilient, normally tender, and softer than the spermatic cord Spermatic cord is firm	Testicles are enlarged, with uneven surface (possible tumor) Epididymis is nonresilient and painful

---

BOX 28–38 ■ Palpating the Scrotum

■ Using your first two fingers and thumb, palpate each testis for size, consistency, shape, smoothness, and presence of masses. During assessment of male adolescents, establish the descent of the testicles into the scrotum; note undescended testes.

■ Palpate the epididymis between your thumb and index finger. It is located at the top of the testis and extends behind it.

■ Palpate the spermatic cord between thumb and index finger. It is usually found at the top lateral portion of the scrotum and feels firm.

■ If swelling, irregularities, or nodules are detected during the scrotal examination, attempt to transilluminate the lesion. This is done by darkening the room and shining a flashlight behind the scrotum through the mass. Serous fluid causes the light to show with a red glow; tissue or blood does not transilluminate.

■ Describe all scrotal masses in terms of their size, shape, placement, consistency, tenderness, and presence of transillumination.

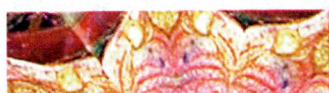

Procedure 28-19 Assessing the Male Genitals and Inguinal Area *continued*

IMPLEMENTATION *continued*

Assessment	Normal Findings	Deviations from Normal
INGUINAL AREA		
11. Inspect both inguinal areas for bulges while the client is standing, if possible.	No swelling or bulges	Swelling or bulge (possible inguinal or femoral hernia)
● First, have the client remain at rest.		
● Next, have the client hold his breath and strain or bear down as though having a bowel movement. Bearing down may make the hernia more visible.		
12. Palpate hernias as described in Box 28–39.	No palpable bulge	Palpable bulge in the area

---

BOX 28–39 ■ Palpating a Hernia

Direct Hernia
- Using your right hand for the client's right side or left hand for the client's left side, advance your index finger into the loose scrotal skin and over the external inguinal ring.
- Instruct the client to bear down.
- If a hernia is present, a palpable bulge will appear in the area.

Indirect Hernia
- Attempt to move the index or little finger into the path of the inguinal canal while the client flexes the knee on the same side.

- When your finger has moved as far as possible, ask the client to bear down.
- If a hernia is present, it will be felt as a mass of tissue touching the finger and withdrawing from it.

Femoral Hernia
- Palpate the inguinal area directly again, first while the client is at rest and then while the client bears down.
- If a hernia is present, a bulge will be felt most prominently when the client bears down.

---

13. Document findings in the client record using forms or checklists supplemented by narrative notes when appropriate.

EVALUATION

- Perform a detailed follow-up examination based on findings that deviated from expected or normal for the client. Relate findings to previous assessment data if available.

- Report significant deviations from normal to the physician.

Lifespan Considerations

Assessing the Male Genitals and Inguinal Area

Infants
- The foreskin of the uncircumcised infant is normally tight the first 2 or 3 months of life and is not readily retractable.

Children
- The scrotum is usually palpated to determine whether testes are descended.
- Ensure that you have the parent or guardian's approval to perform the examination and then tell the child what you are going to do. Preschool children are taught to resist touching of their "private parts."
- In young boys, the cremasteric reflex can cause the testes to ascend into the inguinal canal. If possible have the boy sit cross-legged, which stretches the muscle and decreases the reflex.

- Table 28–12 shows the five stages of development of public hair, penis, and testes/scrotum.

Elders
- The penis decreases in size with age; the size and firmness of the testes decrease.
- Testosterone is produced in smaller amounts.
- More time and direct physical stimulation are required for an older man to achieve an erection, but he can maintain the erection for a longer period before ejaculation than he could at a younger age.
- Seminal fluid is reduced in amount and viscosity.
- Urinary frequency, nocturia, dribbling, and problems with beginning and ending the stream are usually the result of prostatic enlargement.

RECTUM AND ANUS

Rectal examination, an essential part of every comprehensive physical examination, involves inspection and palpation (digital examination). The extent of the assessment of the rectum and anus depends on the rectal problems stated by the client in the nursing history. In many practice settings, the nurse performs only inspection of the anus.

Procedure 28–20 describes how to assess the rectum and anus.

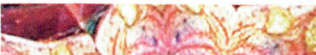 **Procedure 28-20 Assessing the Rectum and Anus**

PLANNING

Delegation
Assessment of the rectum and anus is not delegated to unlicensed assistive personnel. However, many aspects are observed during usual care and may be recorded by persons other than the nurse. Abnormal findings must be validated and interpreted by the nurse.

Equipment
- Examination gloves
- Water-soluble lubricant

IMPLEMENTATION

Performance

1. Explain to the client what you are going to do, why it is necessary, and how he or she can cooperate. Discuss how the results will be used in planning further care or treatments. Because digital examination can cause apprehension and embarrassment in the client, it is important that the nurse help the client relax by encouraging the client to take slow, deep breaths (tension can cause spasms of the anal sphincters, making the examination uncomfortable) and inform the client about potential sensations such as feelings of defecation or passing gas.
2. Wash hands, apply gloves, and observe appropriate infection control procedures for all rectal examinations.
3. Provide for client privacy. Drape the client appropriately to prevent undue exposure of body parts.
4. Inquire if the client has any history of the following: bright blood in stools, tarry black stools, diarrhea, constipation, abdominal pain, excessive gas, hemorrhoids, or rectal pain; family history of colorectal cancer; when last stool specimen for occult blood was performed and the results; and for males, if not obtained during the genitourinary examination, any signs or symptoms of prostate enlargement (e.g., slow urinary stream, hesitance, frequency, dribbling, and nocturia).
5. Position the client. In adults, a left lateral or Sims' position with the upper leg acutely flexed is required for the examination. For females, a dorsal recumbent position with hips externally rotated and knees flexed or a lithotomy position may be used (see Figure 28–101 ■). For males, a standing position while the client bends over the examining table may also be used. This position is commonly used to examine the prostate gland.

Position	Description
Sims'	Side-lying position with **lowermost arm behind the body**, **uppermost leg flexed at hip and knee**, upper arm flexed at shoulder and elbow.
Lithotomy	Back-lying position with **feet supported in stirrups**; the hips should be in line with the edge of the table.
Dorsal recumbent	Back-lying position with knees flexed and hips **externally rotated**; small pillow under the head; soles of feet on the surface.

Figure 28–101 ■ Left Sims' lithotomy, and dorsal recumbent positions.

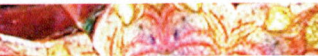

Procedure 28-20 Assessing the Rectum and Anus *continued*

IMPLEMENTATION *continued*

Assessment	Normal Findings	Deviations from Normal
6. Inspect the anus and surrounding tissue for color, integrity, and skin lesions. Then, ask the client to bear down as though defecating. Bearing down creates slight pressure on the skin that may accentuate rectal fissures, rectal prolapse, polyps, or internal hemorrhoids. Describe the location of all abnormal findings in terms of a clock, with the 12 o'clock position toward the pubic symphysis.	Intact perianal skin; usually slightly more pigmented than the skin of the buttocks Anal skin is normally more pigmented, coarser, and moister than perianal skin and is usually hairless	Presence of fissures (cracks), ulcers, excoriations, inflammations, abscesses, protruding hemorrhoids (dilated veins seen as reddened protrusions of the skin), lumps or tumors, fistula openings, or rectal prolapse (varying degrees of protrusion of the rectal mucous membrane through the anus)
7. Palpate the rectum for anal sphincter tonicity, nodules, masses, and tenderness. See Box 28–40 for palpation technique.	Anal sphincter has good tone	Hypertonicity of the anal sphincter (may occur in the presence of an anal fissure or other lesion that causes contraction) Hypotonicity of anal sphincter (may occur after rectal surgery or result from a neurologic deficiency)
	Rectal wall is smooth and not tender	Rectal wall is tender and nodular

BOX 28–40 ■ Palpating the Rectum

- Lubricate your gloved index finger, and instruct the client to bear downward as though having a bowel movement. This relaxes the anal sphincter.
- Slowly insert your finger into the anus and into the rectum in the direction of the umbilicus. The anal canal (distance from the anal opening to the anorectal junction) is short (less than 3 cm [about 1 in.]). The posterior wall of the rectum follows the curve of the coccyx and sacrum. The nurse's finger is usually able to palpate a distance of 6 to 10 cm (2 to 4 in.).

- Never force digital insertion. If lesions are painful or bleeding occurs, discontinue the examination.
- Ask the client to tighten the anal sphincter around your finger, and note the tone of the anal sphincter.
- Rotate the pad of the index finger along the anal and the rectal walls, feeling for nodules, masses, and tenderness.
- Note the location of any abnormalities of the rectum (e.g., "anterior wall, 2 cm proximal to the internal anal sphincter").

Assessment	Normal Findings	Deviations from Normal
8. On withdrawing the finger from the rectum and anus, observe it for feces.	Brown color	Presence of mucus, blood, or black tarry stool
9. Document findings in the client record using forms or checklists supplemented by narrative notes when appropriate.		

EVALUATION

- Perform a detailed follow-up examination based on findings that deviated from expected or normal for the client. Relate findings to previous assessment data if available.

- Report significant deviations from normal to the physician.

Lifespan Considerations

Assessing the Rectum and Anus

Infants
- Lightly touching the anus should result in a brief anal contraction.
- A rectal examination is not routinely performed on children.

Children
- Erythema and scratch marks around the anus may indicate a pinworm parasite.
- A rectal examination is not routinely performed on children.

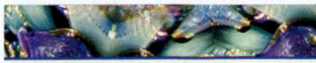

Focus on Critical Thinking

A 75-year-old woman is admitted to your unit for evaluation after being found in her apartment unconscious on the floor. She is now awake but moving slowly. Her vital signs are within normal limits.

1. In the hospital, it is unrealistic to expect to be able to spend an uninterrupted 30 to 60 minutes with a single client performing an admission assessment. Which three systems would have top priority for her initial assessment and why?
2. While gathering relevant history data, what should you do if the client answers with simple one-word answers or gestures?

3. Because the client may be in significant discomfort from her fall, it is not easy for her to move about for the examination. How might you organize your assessment to minimize her need to change positions frequently?
4. If the client is unable to provide a detailed recent history, what other sources of these data could you consider?

See Critical Thinking Possibilities in Appendix A.

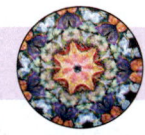 | # Chapter Review

EXPLORE MediaLink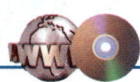

NCLEX review questions, case studies, MediaLink applications, and other interactive resources for this chapter can be found on the Companion Website at www.prenhall.com/kozier. Click on Chapter 28 to select the activities for this chapter.

For animations, more NCLEX review questions, and an audio glossary, access the Student CD-ROM accompanying this textbook.

Chapter Highlights

- The health examination is conducted to assess the function and integrity of the client's body parts.
- The health examination may entail a complete head-to-toe assessment or individual assessment of a body system or body part.
- The health assessment is conducted in a systematic manner that requires the fewest position changes for the client.
- Aspects of the physical assessment procedures should be incorporated in the assessment, intervention, and evaluation phases of the nursing process.
- Data obtained in the physical health examination supplement, confirm, or refute data obtained during the nursing history.
- Nursing history data help the nurse focus on specific aspects of the physical health examination.

- Data obtained in the physical health examination help the nurse establish nursing diagnoses, plan the client's care, and evaluate the outcomes of nursing care.
- Initial assessment findings provide baseline data about the client's functional abilities against which subsequent assessment findings are compared.
- Skills in inspection, palpation, percussion, and auscultation are required for the physical health examination; these skills are used in that order throughout the examination except during abdominal assessment, when auscultation follows inspection and precedes percussion and palpation.
- Knowledge of the normal structure and function of body parts and systems is an essential requisite to conducting physical assessment.

Review Questions

28–1. Which of the following sounds would the nurse expect to find on auscultation of normal lung?
  a. tympany over the right upper lobe
  b. resonance over the left upper lobe
  c. hyperresonnance over the left lower lobe
  d. dullness above the left 10th intercostal space

28–2. The client should be sitting upright during palpation of which of the following areas?
  a. abdomen
  b. heart
  c. breast
  d. head and neck

28–3. Upon auscultating the abdomen, which finding should be reported to the physician?
  a. bruit over the aorta
  b. absence of bowel sounds for 60 seconds
  c. continuous bowel sounds over the ileocecal valve
  d. a completely irregular pattern of bowel sounds

28–4. The nurse is unable to locate the client's popliteal pulse during a routine examination. What would be the appropriate next step?
  a. Check for a pedal pulse.
  b. Check for a femoral pulse.
  c. Take the client's blood pressure on that thigh.
  d. Ask another nurse to try to locate the pulse.

28–5. Which of the following represents expected findings during assessment of the older adult?
  a. facial hair becomes finer and softer
  b. decreased peripheral, color, and night vision
  c. increased sensitivity to odors
  d. respiratory rate and rhythm are irregular at rest

Readings and References

Suggested Readings

Hines, S. E. (2000). Performing a focused physical examination. *Patient Care, 34*(23), 76–78, 87–89, 93–94, 99, 103–104, 106.
    Although this article was aimed at physicians, it is relevant for nurses also. The author expresses concern that physicians do not have adequate physical examination skills, especially to conduct a thorough examination in less than one hour. Thus, she reviews the proper technique for examination of the carotid artery, eye, heart, lungs, skin, abdomen, breast, and musculoskeletal system. The article is well written and easy to follow.

Related Research

Barton, M. B., Harris, R., & Fletcher, S. W. (1999). Does this patient have breast cancer? The screening clinical breast examination: Should it be done? How? *Journal of the American Medical Association, 282,* 1270–1280.
Lillibridge, J., & Wilson, M. (1999). Registered nurses' descriptions of their health assessment practices. *International Journal of Nursing Practice, 5*(1), 29–37.

References

Smith, R. A., Cokkinides, V., von Eschenbach, A. C., Levin, B., Cohen, C, Runowicz, C. D., et al. (2002). American Cancer Society recommendations for early detection of cancer. *CA: A Cancer Journal for Clinicians, 52,* 8–22.

Selected Bibliography

Addison, R. (1999). Practical procedures for nurses. Digital rectal examination. *Nursing Times, 95*(41), insert 2p.

Ayello, E. A. (2000). On the lookout for peripheral vascular disease. *Nursing, 30*(6), 64hh1–hh2, 64hh–hh4.
Faria, S. H. (1999). Assessment of peripheral arterial pulses. *Home Care Provider, 4,* 140–141.
Greenberger, N. J. (1998). Techniques for physical assessment of acute abdominal pain: Getting the most out of the history and physical exam. *Journal of Critical Illness, 13,* 735–742.
Hayko, D. M. (1998). Clinical practice: Peripheral vascular assessment of the lower extremities. *Home Health Focus, 5*(1), 1, 2, 5.
Hayko, D. M. (1999). Clinical practice: Assessing the lungs. *Home Health Focus, 5*(10), 73, 75.
Hood, B. (1999). Physical assessment of the older adult receiving IV therapy at home, CINA conference '99. *Official Journal of the Canadian Intravenous Nurses Association, 15,* 27–30.
Jackson, R., Alghareeb, M., Alaradi, I., & Tomi, Z. (1999). The diagnosis of skin disease. *Dermatology Nursing, 11,* 275, 278–283.
Kacker, A., Gonzales, D. A., & Selesnick, S. H. (1999). The otoscopic examination: What to look for: Where to search. *Consultant 39,* 2397–2402, 2405–2406.
Klingman, L. (1999). Assessing the male genitalia. *American Journal of Nursing, 99*(7), 47–50.
Klingman, L. (1999). Assessing the female reproductive system: A guide through the gynecologic exam. *American Journal of Nursing, 99*(8), 37–43.
Langan, J. C. (1998). Abdominal assessment in the home: From A to ZZZ. *Home Healthcare Nurse, 16,* 51–57.

LoBuono, C. (2001). How to perform an effective clinical breast exam. *Patient Care, 35*(24), 11–17.
O'Hanlon-Nichols, T. (1998). Basic assessment series: A review of the adult musculoskeletal system: A guide to a key aspect of patient care. *American Journal of Nursing, 98*(6), 48–52.
O'Hanlon-Nichols, T. (1998). Basic assessment series: Gastrointestinal system. *American Journal of Nursing, 98*(4), 48–53.
O'Hanlon-Nichols, T. (1998). Basic assessment series: The adult pulmonary system. *American Journal of Nursing, 98*(2) Continuing Care Extra Ed. 39–45.
O'Hanlon-Nichols, T. (1999). Neurologic assessment. *American Journal of Nursing, 99*(6), 44–50.
Owen, A. (1998). Respiratory assessment revisited: Refresh your technique for spotting pulmonary problems. *Nursing, 28*(4), 48–49.
Walton, J. C., Miller, J., & Tordecilla, L. (2001). Elder oral assessment and care. *MEDSURG Nursing, 10*(1), 37–44.
Watson, R. (2000). Assessing cardiovascular functioning in older people. *Nursing Older People, 12*(6), 27–28.
Watson, R. (2001). Assessing the musculoskeletal system in older people. *Nursing Older People, 13*(5), 29–30.
Willis, K. C. (2001). Gaining perspective on peripheral vascular disease. *Nursing, 31*(2), 32hn1–hn4.
Yacone-Morton, L. A. (2002). Perfecting your skills: Cardiac assessment. *RN, 30*(4), 36–39.

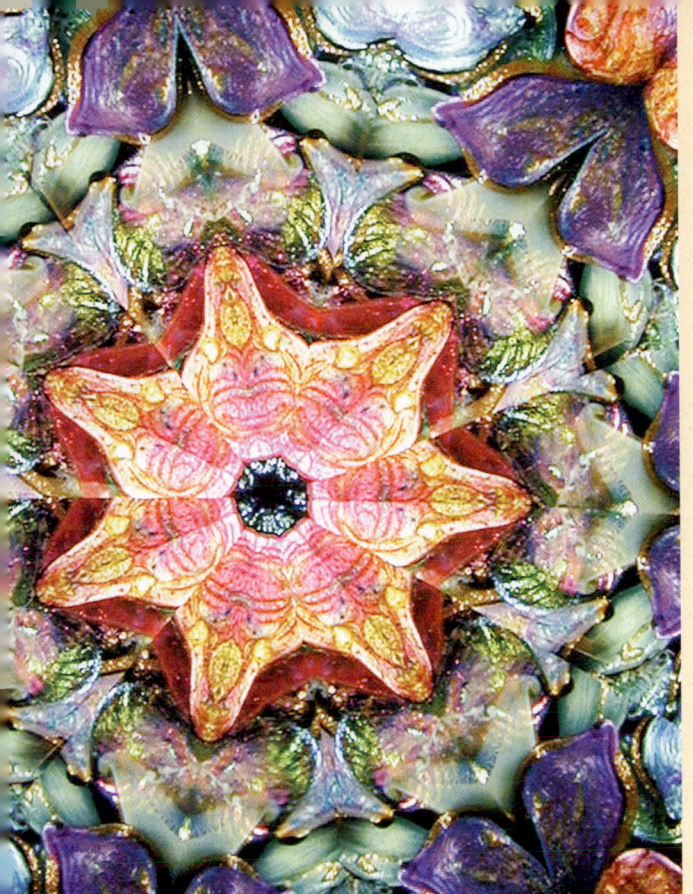

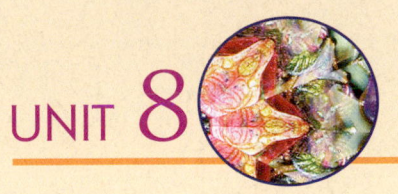

INTEGRAL COMPONENTS OF CLIENT CARE

O*f all the components that are integral to caring for clients, safety is paramount. Concern for safety permeates every element of nursing practice. Nursing activities that promote safety include assessing risk, preventing infection, providing a safe environment, and preventing injury in hospital, outpatient, home, or community-based settings.*

CHAPTER | 29

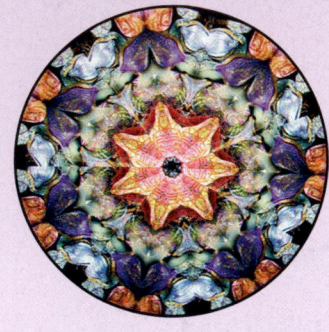

ASEPSIS

LEARNING OUTCOMES

After completing this chapter, you will be able to:

- Explain the concepts of medical and surgical asepsis.

- Identify risks for nosocomial infections.

- Identify signs of localized and systemic infections.

- Identify factors influencing a microorganism's capability to produce an infectious process.

- Identify anatomic and physiologic barriers that defend the body against microorganisms.

- Differentiate active from passive immunity.

- Identify relevant nursing diagnoses and contributing factors for clients at risk for infection and who have an infection.

- Identify interventions to reduce risks for infections.

- Identify measures that break each link in the chain of infection.

- Compare and contrast category-specific, disease-specific, universal, body substance, standard, and transmission-based isolation precaution systems.

- Describe the steps to take in the event of a bloodborne pathogen exposure.

- Correctly implement aseptic practices, including hand washing, donning and removing a facemask, gowning, donning and removing disposable gloves, bagging articles, and managing equipment used for isolation clients.

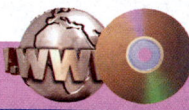

MediaLink

www.prenhall.com/kozier

Additional resources for this chapter can be found on the Student CD-ROM accompanying this textbook, and on the Companion Website at www.prenhall.com/kozier. Click on Chapter 29 to select the activities for this chapter.

CD-ROM
- Audio Glossary
- NCLEX Review

Companion Website
- Additional NCLEX Review
- Case Study: Client with Mycoplasma Pneumonia
- Care Plan Activity: Client on Radiation Therapy and Medication
- MediaLink Application: Go to "Infection Control Today"
- Links to Resources

Nurses are directly involved in providing a biologically safe environment. Microorganisms exist everywhere: in water, in soil, and on body surfaces such as the skin, intestinal tract, and other areas open to the outside (e.g., mouth, upper respiratory tract, vagina, and lower urinary tract). Most microorganisms are harmless, and some are even beneficial in that they perform essential functions in the body. Some microorganisms found in the intestines (e.g., enterobacteria) produce substances called **bacteriocins,** which are lethal to related strains of bacteria. Others produce antibiotic-like substances and toxic metabolites that repress the growth of other microorganisms. Some microorganisms are normal **resident flora** (the collective vegetation in a given area) in one part of the body, yet produce infection in another. For example, *Escherichia coli* is a normal inhabitant of the large intestine but a common cause of infection of the urinary tract. Table 29–1 provides a list of common resident microorganisms.

An **infection** is an invasion of body tissue by microorganisms and their proliferation there. Such a microorganism is called an *infectious agent.* If the microorganism produces no clinical evidence of disease, the infection is called *asymptomatic* or *subclinical.* Some subclinical infections can cause significant damage, for example, cytomegalovirus (CMV) infection in a pregnant woman can lead to significant disease in the unborn child. A detectable alteration in normal tissue function, however, is called **disease.**

Microorganisms vary in their **virulence** (i.e., their ability to produce disease). Microorganisms also vary in the severity of the diseases they produce and their degree of communicability. For example, the common cold virus is more readily transmitted than the bacillus that causes leprosy (*Mycobacterium leprae*). If the infectious agent can be transmitted to an individual by direct or

TABLE 29–1 Examples of Common Resident Microorganisms

Body Area	Microorganisms
Skin	Staphylococcus epidermidis
	Propionibacterium acnes
	Staphylococcus aureus
	Corynebacterium xerosis
	Pityrosporum oxale (yeast)
Nasal passages	Staphylococcus aureus
	Staphylococcus epidermidis
Oropharynx	Streptococcus pneumoniae
Mouth	Streptococcus mutans
	Lactobacillus
	Bacteroides
	Actinomyces
Intestine	Bacteroides
	Fusobacterium
	Eubacterium
	Lactobacillus
	Streptococcus
	Enterobacteriaceae
	Shigella
	Escherichia coli
Urethral orifice	Staphylococcus epidermidis
Urethra (lower)	Proteus
Vagina	Lactobacillus
	Bacteroides
	Clostridium
	Candida albicans

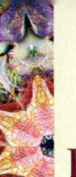

indirect contact, through a vector or vehicle, or as an airborne infection, the resulting condition is called a **communicable disease.**

Pathogenicity is the ability to produce disease; thus a pathogen is a microorganism that causes disease. Many microorganisms that are normally harmless can cause disease under certain circumstances. A "true" pathogen causes disease or infection in a healthy individual. An **opportunistic pathogen** causes disease only in a susceptible individual.

Infectious diseases are the major cause of death worldwide, and a leading cause of illness and death in the United States. The control of the spread of microorganisms and the protection of people from communicable diseases and infections are carried out on the international, national, state, community, and individual level. The World Health Organization is the major regulatory agency at the international level. In the United States, the Centers for Disease Control and Prevention (CDC) is the principal public health agency at the national level concerned with disease prevention and control. At the state level, health departments track epidemics and illnesses as reports are made throughout that area.

Asepsis is the freedom from disease-causing microorganisms. To decrease the possibility of transferring microorganisms from one place to another, asepsis is used. There are two basic types of asepsis: medical and surgical. **Medical asepsis** includes all practices intended to confine a specific microorganism to a specific area, limiting the number, growth, and transmission of microorganisms. In medical asepsis, objects are referred to as **clean,** which means the absence of almost all microorganisms, or **dirty** (soiled, contaminated), which means likely to have microorganisms, some of which may be capable of causing infection.

Surgical asepsis, or **sterile technique,** refers to those practices that keep an area or object free of all microorganisms; it includes practices that destroy all microorganisms and spores. Surgical asepsis is used for all procedures involving the sterile areas of the body.

Sepsis is the state of infection and can take many forms, including septic shock.

TYPES OF MICROORGANISMS CAUSING INFECTIONS

Four major categories of microorganisms cause infection in humans: bacteria, viruses, fungi, and parasites. **Bacteria** are by far the most common infection-causing microorganisms. Several hundred species can cause disease in humans and can live and be transported through air, water, food, soil, body tissues and fluids, and inanimate objects. Most of the microorganisms in Table 29–1 are bacteria. **Viruses** consist primarily of nucleic acid and therefore must enter living cells in order to reproduce. Common virus families include the rhinovirus (causes the common cold), hepatitis, herpes, and human immunodeficiency virus. **Fungi** include yeasts and molds. *Candida albicans* is a yeast considered to be normal flora in the human vagina. **Parasites** live on other living organisms. They include protozoa such as the one that causes malaria, helminths (worms), and arthropods (mites, fleas, ticks).

TYPES OF INFECTIONS

Colonization is the process by which strains of microorganisms become resident flora. In this state, the microorganisms may grow and multiply but do not cause disease. Infection occurs when newly introduced or resident microorganisms succeed in invading a part of the body where the host's defense mechanisms are ineffective and the pathogen causes tissue damage. The infection becomes a disease when the signs and symptoms of the infection are unique and can be differentiated from other conditions.

Infections can be local or systemic. A **local infection** is limited to the specific part of the body where the microorganisms remain. If the microorganisms spread and damage different parts of the body, it is a **systemic infection.** When a culture of the person's blood reveals microorganisms, the condition is called **bacteremia.** When bacteremia results in systemic infection, it is referred to as **septicemia.**

There are also **acute** or **chronic infections.** Acute infections generally appear suddenly or last a short time. A chronic infection may occur slowly, over a very long period, and may last months or years.

NOSOCOMIAL INFECTIONS

Nosocomial infections are classified as infections that are associated with the delivery of health care services in a health care facility. Nosocomial infections can either develop during a client's stay in a facility or manifest after discharge. Nosocomial microorganisms (e.g., tuberculosis and HIV) may also be acquired by health personnel working in the facility and can cause significant illness and time lost from work.

Nosocomial infections have received increasing attention in recent years and are believed to involve about 2 million clients per year. The most common settings where nosocomial infections develop are hospital surgical or medical intensive care units. Reports from the National Nosocomial Infection Surveillance (NNIS) System have revealed that the urinary tract, the respiratory tract, bloodstream, and wounds are the most common nosocomial infection sites (see the NNIS website at http://www.cdc.gov/ncidod/hip/surveill/nnis.htm). The microorganisms that cause nosocomial infections can originate from the clients themselves (an **endogenous** source) or from the hospital environment and hospital personnel (**exogenous** sources). Most nosocomial infections appear to have endogenous sources. *Escherichia coli, Staphylococcus aureus,* and enterococci are the most common infecting microorganisms.

A number of factors contribute to nosocomial infections. **Iatrogenic infections** are the direct result of diagnostic or therapeutic procedures. One example of an iatrogenic infection is bacteremia that results from an intravascular line. Not all nosocomial infections are iatrogenic, nor are all nosocomial infections preventable.

Another factor contributing to the development of nosocomial infections is the compromised host, that is, a client whose normal defenses have been lowered by surgery or illness.

The hands of personnel are a common vehicle for the spread of microorganisms. Insufficient hand washing is thus an important factor contributing to the spread of nosocomial microorganisms.

> **► CLINICAL ALERT**   *A person does not need to have an identified infection in order to pass potentially infective microorganisms to another person. Even normal microorganisms for one person can infect another person.* ■

The cost of nosocomial infections to the client, the facility, and funding sources (e.g., insurance companies and federal, state, or local governments) is great. Nosocomial infections extend hospitalization time, increase clients' time away from work, cause disability and discomfort, and even result in loss of life (see Table 29–2).

CHAIN OF INFECTION

Six links make up the chain of infection (Figure 29–1 ■): the etiologic agent, or microorganism; the place where the organism naturally resides (reservoir); a portal of exit from the reservoir; a method (mode) of transmission; a portal of entry into a host; and the susceptibility of the host.

Etiologic Agent

The extent to which any microorganism is capable of producing an infectious process depends on the number of microorganisms present, the virulence and potency of the microorganisms (pathogenicity), the ability of the microorganisms to enter the body, the susceptibility of the host, and the ability of the microorganisms to live in the host's body.

TABLE 29–2 Nosocomial Infections

Most Common Microorganisms	Causes
Urinary Tract	
Escherichia coli	Improper catheterization technique
Enterococcus species	Contamination of closed drainage system
Pseudomonas aeruginosa	Inadequate hand washing
Surgical Sites	
Staphylococcus aureus	Inadequate hand washing
Enterococcus species	Improper dressing change technique
Pseudomonas aeruginosa	
Bloodstream	
Coagulase-negative staphylococci	Inadequate hand washing
Staphylococcus aureus	Improper intravenous fluid, tubing, and site care technique
Enterococcus species	
Pneumonia	
Staphylococcus aureus	Inadequate hand washing
Pseudomonas aeruginosa	Improper suctioning technique
Enterobacter species	

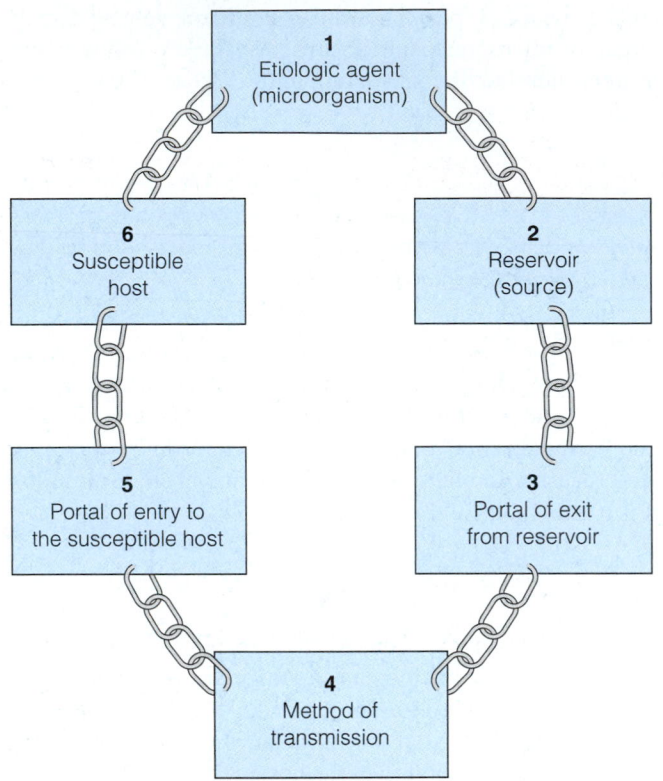

Figure 29–1 ■ The chain of infection.

Some microorganisms, such as the smallpox virus, have the ability to infect almost all susceptible people after exposure. By contrast, microorganisms such as the tuberculosis bacillus infect a relatively small number of the population who are susceptible and exposed, usually people who are poorly nourished, who are living in crowded conditions, or whose immune systems are less competent (such as elders or those with HIV or cancer).

Reservoir

There are many **reservoirs,** or sources of microorganisms. Common sources are other humans, the client's own microorganisms, plants, animals, or the general environment. People are the most common source of infection for others and for themselves (see Table 29–3). For example, the person with an influenza virus frequently spreads it to others. A **carrier** is a person or animal reservoir of a specific infectious agent that usually does not manifest any clinical signs of disease. The *Anopheles* mosquito reservoir carries the malaria parasite but is unaffected by it. The carrier state may also exist in individuals with a clinically recognizable disease such as the dog with rabies. Under either circumstance, the carrier state may be of short duration (temporary or transient carrier) or long duration (chronic carrier). Food, water, and feces also can be reservoirs.

Portal of Exit from Reservoir

Before an infection can establish itself in a host, the microorganisms must leave the reservoir. Common human reservoirs and their associated portals of exit are summarized in Table 29–3.

TABLE 29–3 Human Body Area Reservoirs, Common Infectious Microorganisms, and Portals of Exit

Body Area	Common Infectious Organisms	Portals of Exit
Respiratory tract	Parainfluenza virus	Nose or mouth through sneezing, coughing, breathing, or talking
	Mycobacterium tuberculosis	
	Staphylococcus aureus	
Gastrointestinal tract	Hepatitis A virus	Mouth: saliva, vomitus; anus: feces; ostomies
	Salmonella species	
Urinary tract	*Escherichia coli* enterococci	Urethral meatus and urinary diversion
	Pseudomonas aeruginosa	
Reproductive tract	*Neisseria gonorrhoeae*	Vagina: vaginal discharge; Urinary meatus: semen, urine
	Treponema pallidum	
	Herpes simplex virus type 2	
	Hepatitis B virus (HBV)	
Blood	Hepatitis B virus	Open wound, needle puncture site, any disruption of intact skin or mucous membrane surfaces
	Human immunodeficiency virus (HIV)	
	Staphylococcus aureus	
	Staphylococcus epidermidis	
Tissue	*Staphylococcus aureus*	Drainage from cut or wound
	Escherichia coli	
	Proteus species	
	Streptococcus beta-hemolytic A or B	

Method of Transmission

After a microorganism leaves its source or reservoir, it requires a means of transmission to reach another person or host through a receptive portal of entry. There are three mechanisms:

1. *Direct transmission.* Direct transmission involves immediate and direct transfer of microorganisms from person to person through touching, biting, kissing, or sexual intercourse. Droplet spread is also a form of direct transmission but can occur only if the source and the host are within 3 feet of each other. Sneezing, coughing, spitting, singing, or talking can project droplet spray into the conjunctiva or onto the mucous membranes of the eye, nose, or mouth of another person.

2. *Indirect transmission.* Indirect transmission may be either vehicle-borne or vector-borne.

   a. **Vehicle-borne transmission.** A *vehicle* is any substance that serves as an intermediate means to transport and introduce an infectious agent into a susceptible host through a suitable portal of entry. Fomites (inanimate materials or objects), such as handkerchiefs, toys, soiled clothes, cooking or eating utensils, and surgical instruments or dressings, can act as vehicles. Water, food, blood, serum, and plasma are other vehicles. For example, food or water may become contaminated by a food handler who carries the hepatitis A virus. The food is then ingested by a susceptible host.

   b. **Vector-borne transmission.** A *vector* is an animal or flying or crawling insect that serves as an intermediate means of transporting the infectious agent. Transmission may occur by injecting salivary fluid during biting or by depositing feces or other materials on the skin through the bite wound or a traumatized skin area.

3. *Airborne transmission.* **Airborne transmission** may involve droplets or dust. **Droplet nuclei,** the residue of evaporated droplets emitted by an infected host such as someone with tuberculosis, can remain in the air for long periods. Dust particles containing the infectious agent (e.g., *Clostridium difficile* spores from the soil) can also become airborne. The material is transmitted by air currents to a suitable portal of entry, usually the respiratory tract, of another person.

Portal of Entry to the Susceptible Host

Before a person can become infected, microorganisms must enter the body. The skin is a barrier to infectious agents; however, any break in the skin can readily serve as a portal of entry. Often, microorganisms enter the body of the host by the same route they used to leave the source.

Susceptible Host

A susceptible host is any person who is at risk for infection. A **compromised host** is a person "at increased risk," an individual who for one or more reasons is more likely than others to acquire an infection. Impairment of the body's natural defenses and a number of other factors can affect susceptibility to infec-

tion. Examples include age (the very young or the very old); clients receiving immune suppression treatment for cancer, chronic illness, or following a successful organ transplant; and those with immune deficiency conditions.

BODY DEFENSES AGAINST INFECTION

Individuals normally have defenses that protect the body from infection. These defenses can be categorized as nonspecific and specific. **Nonspecific defenses** protect the person against all microorganisms, regardless of prior exposure. **Specific (immune) defenses,** by contrast, are directed against identifiable bacteria, viruses, fungi, or other infectious agents.

Nonspecific Defenses

Nonspecific body defenses include anatomic and physiologic barriers, and the inflammatory response.

Anatomic and Physiologic Barriers

Intact skin and mucous membranes are the body's first line of defense against microorganisms. Unless the skin and mucosa become cracked and broken, they are an effective barrier against bacteria. Fungi can live on the skin, but they cannot penetrate it. The dryness of the skin also is a deterrent to bacteria. Bacteria are most plentiful in moist areas of the body, such as the perineum and axillae. Resident bacteria of the skin also prevent other bacteria from multiplying. They use up the available nourishment, and the end products of their metabolism inhibit other bacterial growth. Normal secretions make the skin slightly acidic; acidity also inhibits bacterial growth.

The nasal passages have a defensive function. As entering air follows the tortuous route of the passage, it comes in contact with moist mucous membranes and cilia. These trap microorganisms, dust, and foreign materials. The lungs have alveolar **macrophages** (large phagocytes). **Phagocytes** are cells that ingest microorganisms, other cells, and foreign particles.

Each body orifice also has protective mechanisms. The oral cavity regularly sheds mucosal epithelium to rid the mouth of colonizers. The flow of saliva and its partially buffering action help prevent infections. Saliva contains microbial inhibitors, such as lactoferrin, lysozyme, and secretory IgA.

The eye is protected from infection by tears, which continually wash microorganisms away and contain inhibiting lysozyme. The gastrointestinal tract also has defenses against infection. The high acidity of the stomach normally prevents microbial growth. The resident flora of the large intestine help prevent the establishment of disease-producing microorganisms. Peristalsis also tends to move microbes out of the body.

The vagina also has natural defenses against infection. When a girl reaches puberty, lactobacilli ferment sugars in the vaginal secretions, creating a vaginal pH of 3.5 to 4.5. This low pH inhibits the growth of many disease-producing microorganisms. The entrance to the urethra normally harbors many microorganisms. These include *Staphylococcus epidermidis coagulase* (from the skin) and *Escherichia coli* (from feces). It is believed that the urine flow has a flushing and bacteriostatic action that keeps the bacteria from ascending the urethra. An intact mucosal surface also acts as a barrier.

Inflammatory Response

Inflammation is a local and nonspecific defensive response of the tissues to an injurious or infectious agent. It is an adaptive mechanism that destroys or dilutes the injurious agent, prevents further spread of the injury, and promotes the repair of damaged tissue. It is characterized by five signs: (a) pain, (b) swelling, (c) redness, (d) heat, and (e) impaired function of the part, if the injury is severe. Commonly, words with the suffix-*itis* describe an inflammatory process. For example, *appendicitis* means inflammation of the appendix; *gastritis* means inflammation of the stomach.

> **► CLINICAL ALERT** *An easy way to remember the signs of inflammation are the rhyming Latin words:* rubor *(redness),* tumor *(swelling),* color/calor *(heat), and* dolor *(pain).* ■

Injurious agents can be categorized as physical agents, chemical agents, and microorganisms. *Physical agents* include mechanical objects causing trauma to tissues, excessive heat or cold, and radiation. *Chemical agents* include external irritants (e.g., strong acids, alkalis, poisons, and irritating gases) and internal irritants (substances manufactured within the body such as excessive hydrochloric acid in the stomach). *Microorganisms* include the broad groups of bacteria, viruses, fungi, and parasites.

A series of dynamic events is commonly referred to as the three stages of the inflammatory response:

First stage: Vascular and cellular responses
Second stage: Exudate production
Third stage: Reparative phase

VASCULAR AND CELLULAR RESPONSES. At the start of the first stage of inflammation, constriction of the blood vessels occurs at the site of injury, lasting only a few moments. This initial constriction is rapidly followed by dilation of small blood vessels (occurring as a result of histamine released by the injured tissues). Thus more blood flows to the injured area. This marked increase in blood supply is referred to as **hyperemia** and is responsible for the characteristic signs of redness and heat.

Vascular permeability increases at the injured site with the dilation of the vessels in response to cell death, the release of chemical mediators (e.g., bradykinin, serotonin, and prostaglandin), and the release of histamine. The result of this altered permeability is an outpouring of fluid, proteins, and **leukocytes** (white blood cells) into the interstitial spaces, clinically manifested by the characteristic inflammatory signs of swelling (edema) and pain. The pain is caused by the pressure of accumulating fluid on local nerve endings and the chemical mediators, which are thought to irritate the nerve endings. Too much fluid pouring into areas such as the pleural or pericardial cavity can seriously affect organ function. In other areas, such as joints, mobility is impaired.

Blood flow slows in the dilated vessels. This altered rate of flow helps in moving more leukocytes to the injured tissues. Normally, blood cells flow along the center of a blood vessel while plasma without cells streams around them against the walls of the blood vessel. When the blood flow slows, leukocytes aggregate or line up along this inner surface of the blood vessels. This process is known as **margination.** Leukocytes then move through the blood vessel wall into the affected tissue spaces, a process called **emigration.**

The actual passage of blood corpuscles through the blood vessel wall is referred to as **diapedesis.** Leukocytes are attracted to injured cells by **chemotaxis.**

In response to the exit of leukocytes from the blood vessels, the bone marrow produces large numbers of leukocytes and releases them into the bloodstream. This is called **leukocytosis.** The exact mechanism stimulating this increase is unknown, but it is another sign associated with inflammation. A normal leukocyte count of 4,500 to 11,000 per cubic millimeter of blood can rise to 20,000 or more when inflammation occurs.

EXUDATE PRODUCTION. In the second stage of inflammation, the inflammatory **exudate** is produced, consisting of fluid that escaped from the blood vessels, dead phagocytic cells, and dead tissue cells and products that they release. A plasma protein called **fibrinogen** (which is converted to fibrin when it is released into the tissues), thromboplastin (a product released by injured tissue cells), and platelets together form an interlacing network to make a barrier, wall off the area, and prevent spread of the injurious agent. During the second stage, the injurious agent is overcome, and the exudate is cleared away by lymphatic drainage.

The nature and amount of exudate vary according to the tissue involved and the intensity and duration of the inflammation. The major types of exudate are serous, purulent, and hemorrhagic (sanguineous). Descriptions of these exudates are provided in Chapter 34. ∞

REPARATIVE PHASE. The third stage of the inflammatory response involves the repair of injured tissues by regeneration or replacement with fibrous tissue (scar) formation. **Regeneration** is the replacement of destroyed tissue cells by cells that are identical or similar in structure and function. It involves not only replacement of damaged cells one by one but also organization of these cells so that the architectural pattern and function of the tissue are restored. The ability to reproduce cells varies considerably from one type of tissue to another. For example, epithelial tissues of the skin and of the digestive and respiratory tracts have a good regenerative capacity, if their underlying support structures are intact. The same holds true for osseous, lymphoid, and bone marrow tissues. Tissues that have little regenerative capacity include nervous, muscular, and elastic tissues.

When regeneration is not possible, repair occurs by fibrous tissue formation. **Fibrous (scar) tissue** has the capacity to proliferate under the unusual conditions of ischemia and altered pH. The inflammatory exudate with its interlacing network of fibrin provides the framework for this tissue to develop. Damaged tissues are replaced with the connective tissue elements of collagen, blood capillaries, lymphatics, and other tissue-bound substances. In the early stages of this process, the tissue is called **granulation tissue.** It is a fragile, gelatinous tissue, appearing pink or red because of the many newly formed

TABLE 29-4 Types of Immunity

Type	Antigen or Antibody Source	Duration
1. Active	Antibodies are produced by the body in response to an antigen.	Long
a. Natural	Antibodies are formed in the presence of active infection in the body.	Lifelong
b. Artificial	Antigens (vaccines or toxoids) are administered to stimulate antibody production.	Many years; the immunity must be reinforced by booster
2. Passive	Antibodies are produced by another source, animal or human.	Short
a. Natural	Antibodies are transferred naturally from an immune mother to her baby through the placenta or in colostrum.	6 months to 1 year
b. Artificial	Immune serum (antibody) from an animal or another human is injected.	2 to 3 weeks

capillaries. Later in the process, the tissue shrinks (the capillaries are constricted, even obliterated) and the collagen fibers contract, so that a firmer fibrous tissue remains. This is called **cicatrix,** or scar.

Specific Defenses

Specific defenses of the body involve the immune system. An **antigen** is a substance that induces a state of sensitivity or immune responsiveness (**immunity**). If the proteins originate in a person's own body, the antigen is called an **autoantigen.**

The immune response has two components: antibody-mediated defenses and cell-mediated defenses. These two systems provide distinct but overlapping protection.

Antibody-Mediated Defenses

Another name for the *antibody-mediated defenses* is **humoral** (or **circulating**) **immunity** because these defenses reside ultimately in the B lymphocytes and are mediated by antibodies produced by B cells. **Antibodies,** also called **immunoglobulins,** are part of the body's plasma proteins. The antibody-mediated responses defend primarily against the extracellular phases of bacterial and viral infections.

There are two major types of immunity: active and passive (see Table 29–4). In **active immunity,** the host produces antibodies in response to natural antigens (e.g., infectious microorganisms) or artificial antigens (e.g., vaccines). B cells are activated when they recognize the antigen. They then differentiate into plasma cells, which secrete the antibodies and serum proteins that bind specifically to the foreign substance and initiate a variety of elimination responses. The B cell may produce antibody molecules of five classes of immunoglobulins designated by letters and usually written as IgM, IgG, IgA, IgD, and IgE. The presence of IgM in a laboratory analysis shows current infection. Before the antibody response can become effective, the phagocytic cells of the blood bind and ingest foreign substances. The rate of binding and phagocytosis increases if IgG antibodies (which indicate past infection and subsequent immunity) are present. With **passive** (or **acquired**) **immunity,** the host receives natural (e.g., from a nursing mother) or artificial (e.g., from an injection of immune serum) antibodies produced by another source.

Cell-Mediated Defenses

The **cell-mediated defenses,** or **cellular immunity,** occur through the T-cell system. On exposure to an antigen, the lymphoid tissues release large numbers of activated T cells into the lymph system. These T cells pass into the general circulation. There are three main groups of T cells: (a) helper T cells, which help in the functions of the immune system; (b) cytotoxic T cells, which attack and kill microorganisms and sometimes the body's own cells; and (c) suppressor T cells, which can suppress the functions of the helper T cells and the cytotoxic T cells. When cell-mediated immunity is lost, as occurs with human immunodeficiency virus (HIV) infection, an individual is "defenseless" against most viral, bacterial, and fungal infections.

FACTORS INCREASING SUSCEPTIBILITY TO INFECTION

Whether a microorganism causes an infection depends on a number of factors already mentioned. One of the most important factors is host susceptibility, which is affected by age, heredity, level of stress, nutritional status, current medical therapy, and preexisting disease processes.

Age influences the risk of infection. Newborns and older adults have reduced defenses against infection. Infections are a major cause of death of newborns, who have immature immune systems and are protected only for the first 2 or 3 months by immunoglobulins passively received from the mother. Between 1 and 3 months of age, infants begin to synthesize their own immunoglobulins. Immunizations against diphtheria, tetanus, and pertussis are usually started at 2 months, when the infant's immune system can respond (see Table 29–5, page 636).

With advancing age, the immune responses again become weak. Although there is still much to learn about aging, it is known that immunity to infection decreases with advancing age. Because of the prevalence of influenza and its potential for causing death, the CDC recommends annual immunization against influenza for older adults and for persons with chronic cardiac, respiratory, metabolic, and renal disease. Pneumococcal vaccine is recommended for elders last vaccinated more than 5 years previously (see Table 29–5, page 637).

TABLE 29-5 Recommended Childhood and Adolescent Immunization Schedule—United States, 2003

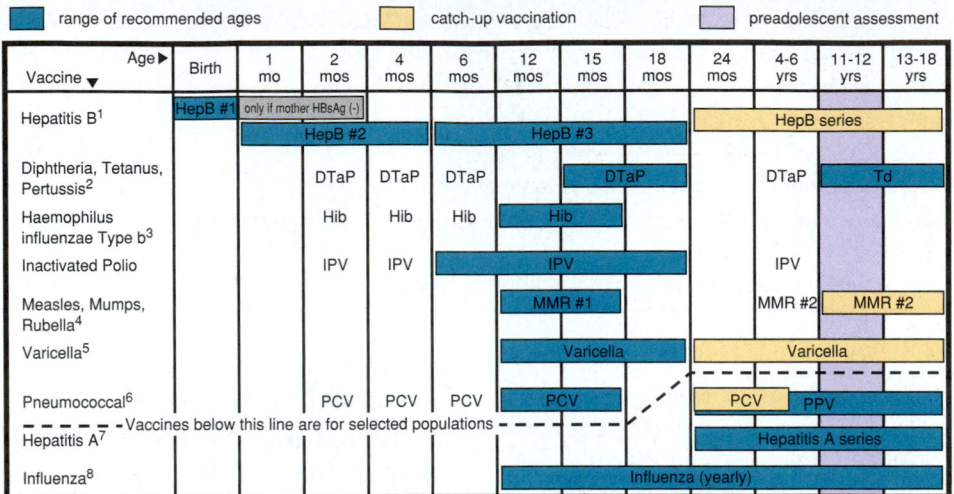

Vaccine ▼ / Age ▶	Birth	1 mo	2 mos	4 mos	6 mos	12 mos	15 mos	18 mos	24 mos	4-6 yrs	11-12 yrs	13-18 yrs
Hepatitis B[1]	HepB #1	only if mother HBsAg (-)	HepB #2			HepB #3				HepB series		
Diphtheria, Tetanus, Pertussis[2]			DTaP	DTaP	DTaP		DTaP			DTaP	Td	
Haemophilus influenzae Type b[3]			Hib	Hib	Hib	Hib						
Inactivated Polio			IPV	IPV		IPV				IPV		
Measles, Mumps, Rubella[4]						MMR #1				MMR #2	MMR #2	
Varicella[5]						Varicella				Varicella		
Pneumococcal[6]			PCV	PCV	PCV	PCV				PCV	PPV	
Hepatitis A[7]										Hepatitis A series		
Influenza[8]						Influenza (yearly)						

Legend: range of recommended ages | catch-up vaccination | preadolescent assessment

Vaccines below this line are for selected populations

This schedule indicates the recommended ages for routine administration of currently licensed childhood vaccines, as of December 1, 2002, for children through age 18 years. Any dose not given at the recommended age should be given at any subsequent visit when indicated and feasible. ☐ Indicates age groups that warrant special effort to administer those vaccines not previously given. Additional vaccines may be licensed and recommended during the year. Licensed combination vaccines may be used whenever any components of the combination are indicated and the vaccine's other components are not contraindicated. Providers should consult the manufacturers' package inserts for detailed recommendations.

1. Hepatitis B vaccine (HepB). All infants should receive the first dose of hepatitis B vaccine soon after birth and before hospital discharge; the first dose may also be given by age 2 months if the infant's mother is HBsAg-negative. Only monovalent HepB can be used for the birth dose. Monovalent or combination vaccine containing HepB may be used to complete the series. Four doses of vaccine may be administered when a birth dose is given. The second dose should be given at least 4 weeks after the first dose, except for combination vaccines which cannot be administered before age 6 weeks. The third dose should be given at least 16 weeks after the first dose and at least 8 weeks after the second dose. The last dose in the vaccination series (third or fourth dose) should not be administered before age 6 months.

Infants born to HBsAg-positive mothers should receive HepB and 0.5 mL Hepatitis B Immune Globulin (HBIG) within 12 hours of birth at separate sites. The second dose is recommended at age 1-2 months. The last dose in the vaccination series should not be administered before age 6 months. These infants should be tested for HBsAg and anti-HBs at 9-15 months of age.

Infants born to mothers whose HBsAg status is unknown should receive the first dose of the HepB series within 12 hours of birth. Maternal blood should be drawn as soon as possible to determine the mother's HBsAg status; if the HBsAg test is positive, the infant should receive HBIG as soon as possible (no later than age 1 week). The second dose is recommended at age 1-2 months. The last dose in the vaccination series should not be administered before age 6 months.

2. Diphtheria and tetanus toxoids and acellular pertussis vaccine (DTaP). The fourth dose of DTaP may be administered as early as age 12 months, provided 6 months have elapsed since the third dose and the child is unlikely to return at age 15-18 months. **Tetanus and diphtheria toxoids (Td)** is recommended at age 11-12 years if at least 5 years have elapsed since the last dose of tetanus and diphtheria toxoid-containing vaccine. Subsequent routine Td boosters are recommended every 10 years.

3. Haemophilus influenzae type b (Hib) conjugate vaccine. Three Hib conjugate vaccines are licensed for infant use. If PRP-OMP (PedvaxHIB® or ComVax®[Merck]) is administered at ages 2 and 4 months, a dose at age 6 months is not required. DTaP/Hib combination products should not be used for primary immunization in infants at ages 2, 4 or 6 months, but can be used as boosters following any Hib vaccine.

4. Measles, mumps, and rubella vaccine (MMR). The second dose of MMR is recommended routinely at age 4-6 years but may be administered during any visit, provided at least 4 weeks have elapsed since the first dose and that both doses are administered beginning at or after age 12 months. Those who have not previously received the second dose should complete the schedule by the 11-12 year old visit.

5. Varicella vaccine. Varicella vaccine is recommended at any visit at or after age 12 months for susceptible children, i.e. those who lack a reliable history of chickenpox. Susceptible persons aged ≥13 years should receive two doses, given at least 4 weeks apart.

6. Pneumococcal vaccine. The heptavalent **pneumococcal conjugate vaccine (PCV)** is recommended for all children age 2-23 months. It is also recommended for certain children age 24-59 months. **Pneumococcal polysaccharide vaccine (PPV)** is recommended in addition to PCV for certain high-risk groups. See *MMWR* 2000;49(RR-9);1-38.

7. Hepatitis A vaccine. Hepatitis A vaccine is recommended for children and adolescents in selected states and regions, and for certain high-risk groups; consult your local public health authority. Children and adolescents in these states, regions, and high risk groups who have not been immunized against hepatitis A can begin the hepatitis A vaccination series during any visit. The two doses in the series should be administered at least 6 months apart. See *MMWR* 1999;48(RR-12);1-37.

8. Influenza vaccine. Influenza vaccine is recommended annually for children age ≥6 months with certain risk factors (including but not limited to asthma, cardiac disease, sickle cell disease, HIV, diabetes, and household members of persons in groups at high risk; see *MMWR* 2002;51(RR-3);1-31), and can be administered to all others wishing to obtain immunity. In addition, healthy children age 6-23 months are encouraged to receive influenza vaccine if feasible because children in this age group are at substantially increased risk for influenza-related hospitalizations. Children aged ≤12 years should receive vaccine in a dosage appropriate for their age (0.25 mL if age 6-35 months or 0.5 mL if aged ≥3 years). Children aged ≤8 years who are receiving influenza vaccine for the first time should receive two doses separated by at least 4 weeks.

For additional information about vaccines, including precautions and contraindications for immunization and vaccine shortages, please visit the National Immunization Program Website at www.cdc.gov/nip or call the National Immunization Information Hotline at 800-232-2522 (English) or 800-232-0233 (Spanish).

Approved by the Advisory Committee on Immunization Practices (www.cdc.gov/nip/acip), the American Academy of Pediatrics (www.aap.org), and the American Academy of Family Physicians (www.aafp.org).

Heredity influences the development of infection in that some people have a genetic susceptibility to certain infections. For example, some may be deficient in serum immunoglobulins, which play a significant role in the internal defense mechanism of the body.

The nature, number, and duration of physical and emotional stressors can influence susceptibility to infection. Stressors elevate blood cortisone. Prolonged elevation of blood cortisone decreases anti-inflammatory responses, depletes energy stores, leads to a state of exhaustion, and decreases resistance to infection. For example, a person recovering from a major operation or injury is more likely to develop an infection than a healthy person.

Resistance to infection depends on adequate nutritional status. Because antibodies are proteins, the ability to synthesize antibodies may be impaired by inadequate nutrition, especially when protein reserves are depleted (e.g., as a result of injury, surgery, or debilitating diseases such as cancer).

Some medical therapies predispose a person to infection. For example, radiation treatments for cancer destroy not only cancerous cells but also some normal cells, thereby rendering them more vulnerable to infection. Some diagnostic procedures may also predispose the client to an infection, especially when the skin is broken or sterile body cavities are penetrated during the procedure.

TABLE 29-5 Recommended Adult Immunization Schedule—United States, 2002–2003

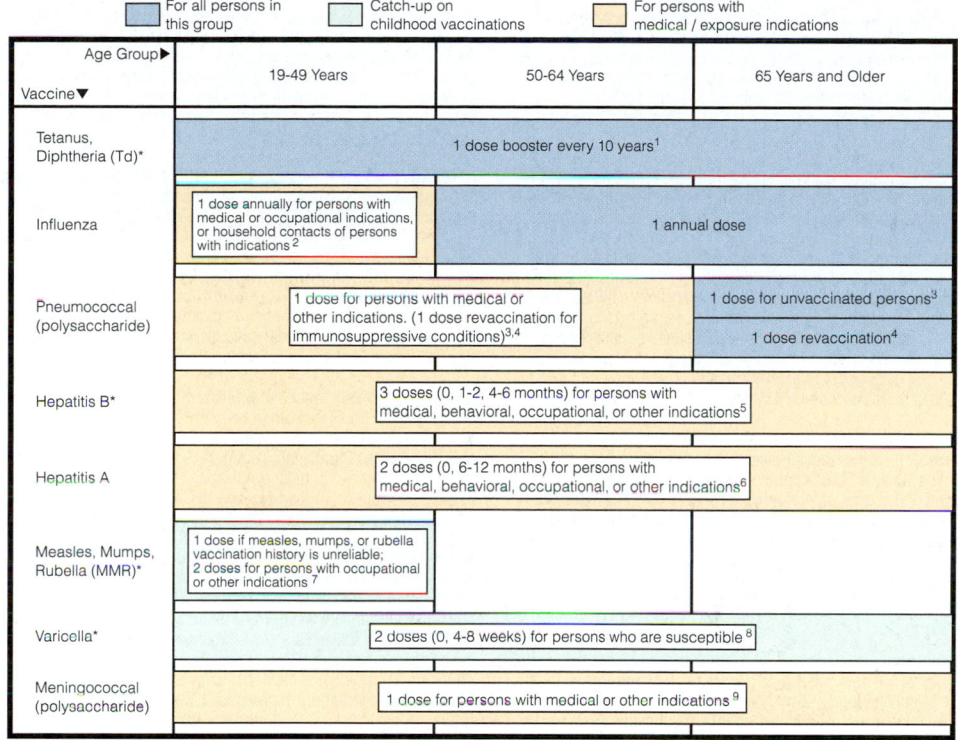

Legend
▨ For all persons in this group
▢ Catch-up on childhood vaccinations
▨ For persons with medical / exposure indications

Vaccine ▼ Age Group ▶	19-49 Years	50-64 Years	65 Years and Older
Tetanus, Diphtheria (Td)*	1 dose booster every 10 years[1]		
Influenza	1 dose annually for persons with medical or occupational indications, or household contacts of persons with indications [2]	1 annual dose	
Pneumococcal (polysaccharide)	1 dose for persons with medical or other indications. (1 dose revaccination for immunosuppressive conditions)[3,4]		1 dose for unvaccinated persons[3] / 1 dose revaccination[4]
Hepatitis B*	3 doses (0, 1-2, 4-6 months) for persons with medical, behavioral, occupational, or other indications[5]		
Hepatitis A	2 doses (0, 6-12 months) for persons with medical, behavioral, occupational, or other indications[6]		
Measles, Mumps, Rubella (MMR)*	1 dose if measles, mumps, or rubella vaccination history is unreliable; 2 doses for persons with occupational or other indications [7]		
Varicella*	2 doses (0, 4-8 weeks) for persons who are susceptible [8]		
Meningococcal (polysaccharide)	1 dose for persons with medical or other indications [9]		

See Footnotes for Recommended Adult Immunization Schedule, United States, 2002-2003 on page 638.

---

*Covered by the Vaccine Injury Compensation Program. For information on how to file a claim call 800-338-2382. Please also visit www.hrsa.gov/osp/vicp To file a claim for vaccine injury write: U.S. Court of Federal Claims, 717 Madison Place, N.W.,Washington D.C. 20005. 202 219-9657.

This schedule indicates the recommended age groups for routine administration of currently licensed vaccines for persons 19 years of age and older. Licensed combination vaccines may be used whenever any components of the combination are indicated and the vaccine's other components are not contraindicated. Providers should consult the manufacturers' package inserts for detailed recommendations.

Report all clinically significant post-vaccination reactions to the Vaccine Adverse Event Reporting System (VAERS). Reporting forms and instructions on filing a VAERS report are available by calling 800-822-7967 or from the VAERS website at www.vaers.org.

For additional information about the vaccines listed above and contraindications for immunization, visit the National Immunization Program Website at www.cdc.gov/nip/ or call the National Immunization Hotline at 800-232-2522 (English) or 800-232-0233 (Spanish).

Approved by the Advisory Committee on Immunization Practices (ACIP), and accepted by the American College of Obstetricians and Gynecologists (ACOG) and the American Academy of Family Physicians (AAFP)

Lifespan Considerations

Elders

Normal aging may predispose elders to increased risk of infection and delayed healing. Organs and biochemical agents that are protective when a person is younger often change in structure and function with increasing age and then provide a decrease in their protective ability. Changes take place in the skin, respiratory tract, gastrointestinal system, kidneys, and immune system. If unchallenged, these systems work well to maintain homeostasis for the individual, but if compromised by stress, illness, infections, treatments, or surgeries, they find it difficult to keep up and therefore are not able to provide adequate protection. Special considerations for elders are:

- Nutrition is often poor in older adults and certain components, especially adequate protein, are necessary to build up and maintain the immune system.
- Diabetes mellitus, which occurs more frequently in elders, increases the risk of infection and delayed healing by causing an alteration in nutrition and impaired peripheral circulation, which decrease the oxygen transport to the tissues.

- The immune system reacts slowly to the introduction of antigens, allowing the antigen to reproduce itself several times before it is recognized by the immune system. T-cell effectiveness is often decreased due to immaturity.
- The normal inflammatory response is delayed. This often causes atypical responses to infections with unusual presentations. Instead of displaying redness, swelling, and fever usually associated with infections, atypical symptoms such as confusion and disorientation, agitation, incontinence, falls, lethargy, and general fatigue are often seen first.

Recognizing these changes in elders is important in early detection and treatment of related potential for infections and delayed healing. Nursing interventions to promote prevention are:

- Provide and teach ways to improve nutritional status.
- Use strict aseptic technique to decrease chance of infections (especially nosocomial infections in health care facilities).
- Encourage elders to have regular immunizations for flu and pneumonia.
- Be alert to subtle atypical signs of infection and act quickly to diagnose and treat.

TABLE 29–5 Footnotes for Recommended Adult Immunization Schedule—United States, 2002–2003

1. Tetanus and diphtheria (Td)—A primary series for adults is 3 doses: the first 2 doses given at least 4 weeks apart and the 3rd dose, 6-12 months after the second. Administer 1 dose if the person had received the primary series and the last vaccination was 10 years ago or longer. *MMWR* 1991; 40 (RR-10): 1-21. The ACP Task Force on Adult Immunization supports a second option: a single Td booster at age 50 years for persons who have completed the full pediatric series, including the teenage/young adult booster. *Guide for Adult Immunization.* 3rd ed.ACP 1994: 20.

2. Influenza vaccination—Medical indications: chronic disorders of the cardiovascular or pulmonary systems including asthma; chronic metabolic diseases including diabetes mellitus, renal dysfunction, hemoglobinopathies, immunosuppression (including immunosuppression caused by medications or by human immunodeficiency virus [HIV]), requiring regular medical follow-up or hospitalization during the preceding year; women who will be in the second or third trimester of pregnancy during the influenza season. Occupational indications: health-care workers. Other indications: residents of nursing homes and other long-term care facilities; persons likely to transmit influenza to persons at high-risk (in-home care givers to persons with medical indications, household contacts and out-of-home caregivers of children birth to 23 months of age, or children with asthma or other indicator conditions for influenza vaccination, household members and care givers of elderly and adults with high-risk conditions); and anyone who wishes to be vaccinated. *MMWR* 2002; 51 (RR-3): 1-31.

3. Pneumococcal polysaccharide vaccination—Medical indications: chronic disorders of the pulmonary system (excluding asthma), cardiovascular diseases, diabetes mellitus, chronic liver diseases including liver disease as a result of alcohol abuse (e.g., cirrhosis), chronic renal failure or nephrotic syndrome, functional or anatomic asplenia (e.g., sickle cell disease or splenectomy), immunosuppressive conditions (e.g., congenital immunodeficiency, HIV infection, leukemia, lymphoma, multiple myeloma, Hodgkins disease, generalized malignancy, organ or bone marrow transplantation), chemotherapy with alkylating agents, anti-metabolites, or long-term systemic corticosteroids. Geographic/other indications: Alaskan Natives and certain American Indian populations. Other indications: residents of nursing homes and other long-term care facilities. *MMWR* 1997; 47 (RR-8): 1-24.

4. Revaccination with pneumococcal polysaccharide vaccine—One time revaccination after 5 years for persons with chronic renal failure or nephrotic syndrome, functional or anatomic asplenia (e.g., sickle cell disease or splenectomy), immunosuppressive conditions (e.g., congenital immunodeficiency, HIV infection, leukemia, lymphoma, multiple myeloma, Hodgkins disease, generalized malignancy, organ or bone marrow transplantation), chemotherapy with alkylating agents, antimetabolites, or long-term systemic corticosteroids. For persons 65 and older, one-time revaccination if they were vaccinated 5 or more years previously and were aged less than 65 years at the time of primary vaccination. *MMWR* 1997; 47 (RR-8): 1-24.

5. Hepatitis B vaccination—Medical indications: hemodialysis patients, patients who receive clotting-factor concentrates. Occupational indications: health-care workers and public-safety workers who have exposure to blood in the workplace, persons in training in schools of medicine, dentistry, nursing, laboratory technology, and other allied health professions. Behavioral indications: injecting drug users, persons with more than one sex partner in the previous 6 months, persons with a recently acquired sexually-transmitted disease (STD), all clients in STD clinics, men who have sex with men. Other indications: household contacts and sex partners of persons with chronic HBV infection, clients and staff of institutions for the developmentally disabled, international travelers who will be in countries with high or intermediate prevalence of chronic HBV infection for more than 6 months, inmates of correctional facilities. *MMWR* 1991; 40 (RR-13): 1-25. (www.cdc.gov/travel/diseases/hbv.htm)

6. Hepatitis A vaccination—For the combined HepA-HepB vaccine use 3 doses at 0, 1, 6 months). Medical indications: persons with clotting-factor disorders or chronic liver disease. Behavioral indications: men who have sex with men, users of injecting and noninjecting illegal drugs. Occupational indications: persons working with HAV-infected primates or with HAV in a research laboratory setting. Other indications: persons traveling to or working in countries that have high or intermediate endemicity of hepatitis A. *MMWR* 1999; 48 (RR-12): 1-37. (www.cdc.gov/travel/diseases/hav.htm)

7. Measles, Mumps, Rubella vaccination (MMR)—Measles component: Adults born before 1957 may be considered immune to measles. Adults born in or after 1957 should receive at least one dose of MMR unless they have a medical contraindication, documentation of at least one dose or other acceptable evidence of immunity. A second dose of MMR is recommended for adults who:
- are recently exposed to measles or in an outbreak setting
- were previously vaccinated with killed measles vaccine
- were vaccinated with an unknown vaccine between 1963 and 1967
- are students in post-secondary educational institutions
- work in health care facilities
- plan to travel internationally

Mumps component: 1 dose of MMR should be adequate for protection. Rubella component: Give 1 dose of MMR to women whose rubella vaccination history is unreliable and counsel women to avoid becoming pregnant for 4 weeks after vaccination. For women of child-bearing age, regardless of birth year, routinely determine rubella immunity and counsel women regarding congenital rubella syndrome. Do not vaccinate pregnant women or those planning to become pregnant in the next 4 weeks. If pregnant and susceptible, vaccinate as early in postpartum period as possible. *MMWR* 1998; 47 (RR-8): 1-57.

8. Varicella vaccination—Recommended for all persons who do not have reliable clinical history of varicella infection, or serological evidence of varicella zoster virus (VZV) infection; health-care workers and family contacts of immunocompromised persons, those who live or work in environments where transmission is likely (e.g., teachers of young children, day care employees, and residents and staff members in institutional settings), persons who live or work in environments where VZV transmission can occur (e.g., college students, inmates and staff members of correctional institutions, and military personnel), adolescents and adults living in households with children, women who are not pregnant but who may become pregnant in the future, international travelers who are not immune to infection. Note: Greater than 90% of U.S. born adults are immune to VZV. Do not vaccinate pregnant women or those planning to become pregnant in the next 4 weeks. If pregnant and susceptible, vaccinate as early in postpartum period as possible. *MMWR* 1996; 45 (RR-11): 1-36, *MMWR* 1999; 48 (RR-6): 1-5.

9. Meningococcal vaccine (quadrivalent polysaccharide for serogroups A, C, Y, and W-135)—Consider vaccination for persons with medical indications: adults with terminal complement component deficiencies, with anatomic or functional asplenia. Other indications: travelers to countries in which disease is hyperendemic or epidemic ("meningitis belt" of sub-Saharan Africa, Mecca, Saudi Arabia for Hajj). Revaccination at 3-5 years may be indicated for persons at high risk for infection (e.g., persons residing in areas in which disease is epidemic). Counsel college freshmen, especially those who live in dormitories, regarding meningococcal disease and the vaccine so that they can make an educated decision about receiving the vaccination. *MMWR* 2000; 49 (RR-7): 1-20.
Note: The AAFP recommends that colleges should take the lead on providing education on meningococcal infection and vaccination and offer it to those who are interested. Physicians need not initiate discussion of the meningococcal quadravalent polysaccharide vaccine as part of routine medical care.

Certain medications also increase susceptibility to infection. Antineoplastic (anticancer) medications may depress bone marrow function, resulting in inadequate production of white blood cells necessary to combat infections. Anti-inflammatory medications, such as adrenal corticosteroids, inhibit the inflammatory response, an essential defense against infection. Even some antibiotics used to treat infections can have adverse effects. Antibiotics may kill resident flora, allowing the proliferation of strains that would not grow and multiply in the body under normal conditions. Certain antibiotics can also induce resistance in some strains of organisms. This resistance has become so wide-spread that the CDC has created a 12-step Campaign to Prevent Antimicrobial Resistance in Healthcare Settings consisting of four strategies: preventing infection, diagnosing and treating infection effectively, using antimicrobials wisely, and preventing transmission.

Any disease that lessens the body's defenses against infection places the client at risk. Examples are chronic pulmonary disease, which impairs ciliary action and weakens the mucous barrier; peripheral vascular disease, which restricts blood flow; burns, which impair skin integrity; chronic or debilitating diseases, which deplete protein reserves; and such immune system diseases as leukemia and aplastic anemia, which alter the production of white blood cells. Diabetes mellitus is a major underlying disease predisposing clients to infection because compromised peripheral vascular status and increased serum glucose levels increase susceptibility.

NURSING MANAGEMENT

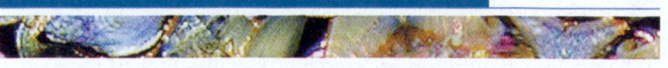

ASSESSING

During the assessing phase of the nursing process, the nurse obtains the client's history, conducts the physical assessment, and gathers laboratory data.

> **► CLINICAL ALERT** *Some common medications such as aspirin and ibuprofen are analgesic (pain relieving), antipyretic (fever reducing), and anti-inflammatory. Acetaminophen, however, is analgesic and antipyretic, but not anti-inflammatory.* ■

Nursing History

During the nursing history, the nurse assesses (a) the degree to which a client is at risk of developing an infection and (b) any client complaints suggesting the presence of an infection. To identify clients at risk, the nurse reviews the client's chart and structures the nursing interview to collect data regarding the factors influencing the development of infection, especially existing disease process, history of recurrent infections, current medications and therapeutic measures, current emotional stressors, nutritional status, and history of immunizations (see the Assessment Interview).

Physical Assessment

Signs and symptoms of an infection vary according to the body area involved. For example, sneezing, watery or mucoid discharge from the nose, and nasal stuffiness commonly occur with an infection of the nose and sinuses; urinary frequency and possible cloudy or discolored urine often occur with a urinary infection. Commonly the skin and mucous membranes are involved in a local infectious process, resulting in

- Localized swelling
- Localized redness
- Pain or tenderness with palpation or movement
- Palpable heat at the infected area
- Loss of function of the body part affected, depending on the site and extent of involvement.

In addition, open wounds may exude drainage of various colors.

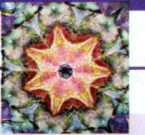

Assessment Interview

CLIENT AT RISK FOR INFECTIONS

- ■ When were you last immunized for diphtheria, tetanus, poliomyelitis, rubella, measles, influenza, hepatitis, and pneumococcal pneumonia?
- ■ When did you last have a tuberculin skin test?
- ■ What infections have you had in the past, and how were these treated?
- ■ Have any of these infections recurred?
- ■ Are you taking any antibiotics, anti-inflammatory medications such as aspirin or ibuprofen, or medications for cancer?
- ■ Have you had any recent diagnostic procedure or therapy that penetrated through your skin or a body cavity?
- ■ What past surgeries have you had?
- ■ How would you describe your eating habits? Do you eat a variety of different types of foods?
- ■ Do you take vitamins?
- ■ On a scale of 1 to 10, how would you rate the stress you have experienced in the last 6 months?
- ■ Have you experienced any loss of energy, loss of appetite, nausea, headache, or other signs associated with specific body systems (e.g., difficulty urinating, urinary frequency, or a sore throat)?

Note: As with all history taking, the nurse must individualize the specific terms used, examples given to the client, and teaching techniques used to validate agreement on the meaning of words according to the client's culture, language spoken, and education or intellectual abilities.

Signs of *systemic infection* include

- Fever
- Increased pulse and respiratory rate, if the fever is high
- Malaise and loss of energy
- Anorexia and, in some situations, nausea and vomiting
- Enlargement and tenderness of lymph nodes that drain the area of infection.

Laboratory Data

Laboratory data that indicate the presence of an infection include the following:

- Elevated leukocyte (white blood cell or WBC) count (4,500 to 11,000/mL is normal).
- Increases in specific types of leukocytes as revealed in the differential WBC count. Specific types of white blood cells are increased or decreased in certain infections. See Chapter 32 ⊙ for normal values for the adult.

- Elevated *erythrocyte sedimentation rate (ESR)*. Red blood cells normally settle slowly, but the rate increases in the presence of an inflammatory process.
- Urine, blood, sputum, or other drainage **cultures** (laboratory cultivations of microorganisms in a special growth medium) that indicate the presence of pathogenic microorganisms.

DIAGNOSING

The NANDA nursing diagnostic label for problems associated with the transmission of microorganisms is *Risk for Infection:* the state in which an individual is at increased risk for being invaded by pathogenic microorganisms.

When using this label, the nurse should identify risk factors:

1. *Inadequate primary defenses* such as broken skin, traumatized tissue, decreased ciliary action, stasis of body fluids, change in pH of secretions, or altered peristalsis
2. *Inadequate secondary defenses* such as leukopenia, immunosuppression, decreased hemoglobin, or suppressed inflammatory response.

Clients who have or are at risk for an existing infection are prime candidates for other physical and psychologic problems. Examples of nursing diagnoses or collaborative problems that may arise from the actual presence of an infection include

- *Potential Complication of Infection: Fever*
- *Impaired Physical Mobility* if the client is fatigued, connected to infusion devices, or in discomfort
- *Imbalanced Nutrition: Less Than Body Requirements* if the client is too ill to eat adequately
- *Acute Pain* if the client is experiencing tissue damage and discomfort
- *Impaired Social Interaction or Social Isolation* if the client is required to be separated from others during a contagious episode
- *Situational Low Self-Esteem* if the client is experiencing negative feelings about self related to the infection process

IDENTIFYING NURSING DIAGNOSES, OUTCOMES, AND INTERVENTIONS

CLIENT AT RISK FOR INFECTION

NURSING DIAGNOSIS/ DEFINITION	SAMPLE DESIRED OUTCOMES [NOC#]/DEFINITION	INDICATORS*	SELECTED INTERVENTIONS [NIC#]/DEFINITION	SAMPLE ACTIVITIES [NIC]
Risk for Infection/At increased risk for being invaded by pathogenic organisms	Knowledge: Infection Control [1807]/*Extent of understanding conveyed about prevention and control of infection*	• Description of mode of transmission • Description of activities to increase resistance to infection	Infection Control [6540]/*Minimizing the acquisition and transmission of infectious agents*	• Instruct patient on proper hand washing techniques • Promote appropriate nutritional intake • Administer antibiotic therapy as indicated

*The measurement scale ranges from None (1) to Extensive (5). See Appendix B.

• *Anxiety* if the client is apprehensive regarding changes in life activities resulting from the infection or its treatment such as absence from work or inability to perform usual functions.

Examples of nursing diagnoses and related outcomes and interventions are shown in Identifying Nursing Diagnoses, Outcomes, and Interventions.

PLANNING

The major goals for clients susceptible to infection are to

• Maintain or restore defenses
• Avoid the spread of infectious organisms
• Reduce or alleviate problems associated with the infection.

Desired outcomes depend on the individual client's condition. Examples of desired outcomes, established in the planning phase, are provided in Identifying Nursing Diagnoses, Outcomes, and Interventions. Nursing strategies to meet the

three broad goals stated above generally include using meticulous medical and surgical aseptic techniques to prevent the spread of potentially infectious microorganisms, implementing measures to support the defenses of a susceptible host, and teaching clients about protective measures to prevent infections and the spread of infectious agents when an infection is present.

Planning for Home Care

Clients being discharged following hospital care for an infection often require continued care to completely eliminate the infection or to adapt to a chronic state. In addition, such clients may be at increased risk for reinfection or development of an opportunistic infection following therapy for existing pathogens.

In preparation for discharge, the nurse needs to know the clients and family's risks, needs, strengths, and resources. The Home Care Assessment box describes the specific assessment data required before establishing a discharge plan. Using the

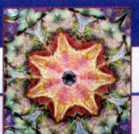

Home Care Assessment

INFECTION

Client and Environment

■ *Self-care abilities for wound care:* Ability to gather and use supplies for clean or aseptic technique to change dressings or care for wounds
■ *Self-care abilities for hygiene and toileting:* Ability to contain potentially infectious material, such as that from coughing or sneezing, and body fluids (urine, stool, drainage); ability to wash hands and implement any required isolation practices
■ *Self-care abilities for medication administration:* Physical dexterity to take pills, administer intravenous antibiotics, store medications safely
■ *Facilities:* Presence of running water, trash containers and disposal, bathroom to facilitate wound care and contain potentially infectious materials.

Family

■ *Caregiver availability, skills, and responses:* Persons able to assist with wound care, medication administration, shopping if client has restricted activity; people able to comprehend infection control activities without excessive personal anxiety
■ *Other susceptible cohabitants:* Presence and immunization status of children, elders, or others who may be at risk of infection from the client.

Community

■ *Resources:* Availability of and familiarity with possible sources of assistance for finances, supplies, home health aid.

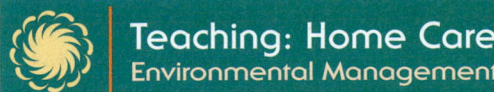

Teaching: Home Care
Environmental Management

- Discuss injury-proofing the home to prevent the possibility of further tissue injury (e.g., use of padding, handrails, removal of hazards).
- Explore ways to control the environmental temperature and airflow (especially if client has an airborne pathogen).
- Determine the advisability of visitors and family members in proximity to the client.
- Describe ways to manipulate the bed, the room, and other household facilities.

Infection Control

- Teach proper hand washing and related hygienic measures to all family members.
- Discuss antimicrobial soaps and effective disinfectants.
- Ensure access to and proper use of gloves and other barriers as indicated by the type of infection or risk.
- Discuss the relationship between hygiene, rest, activity, and nutrition in the chain of infection.
- Instruct about proper administration of medication.
- Instruct about cleaning reusable equipment and supplies.

Infection Protection

- Teach the client and family members the signs and symptoms of infection, and when to contact a health care provider.
- Teach the client and family members how to avoid infections.
- Suggest techniques for safe food preservation and preparation.
- Emphasize the need for proper immunizations of all family members.

Wound Care

- Teach the client and family the signs of wound healing and of wound infection.
- Explain the proper technique for changing the dressing and disposing of the soiled one.
- Delineate the factors that promote wound healing.

Referrals

- Provide appropriate information regarding how to access community resources, home care agencies, sources of supplies, and community or public health departments for immunizations.

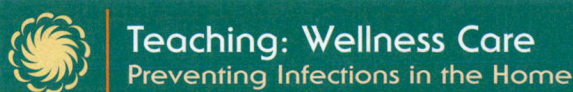

Teaching: Wellness Care
Preventing Infections in the Home

- Wash your hands before handling foods, before eating, after toileting, before and after any required home care treatment, and after touching any body substances (e.g., wound drainage).
- Keep your fingernails short, clean, and well manicured to eliminate rough edges or hangnails, which can harbor microorganisms.
- Do not share personal care items: toothbrush, washcloths, and towels.
- Wash raw fruits and vegetables before eating them.
- Refrigerate all opened and unpackaged foods.
- Clean used equipment (e.g., emesis basin) with soap and water, and disinfect it with a chlorine bleach solution.
- Place contaminated dressings and other disposable items containing body fluids in moisture-proof plastic bags.
- Put used needles in a puncture-resistant container with a screw-top lid. Label so as not to discard in the garbage.
- Clean obviously soiled linen separately from other laundry. Rinse in cold water, wash in hot water if possible, and add a cup of bleach or Lysol to the wash.
- Avoid coughing, sneezing, or breathing directly on others. Cover the mouth and nose to prevent the transmission of airborne microorganisms.
- Be aware of any signs or symptoms of an infection, and report these immediately to your health care contact person.
- Maintain a sufficient fluid intake to promote urine production and output. This helps flush the bladder and urethra of microorganisms.

data gathered about the home situation, the nurse tailors the teaching plan for the client and family (see Teaching: Home Care and Teaching: Wellness Care).

IMPLEMENTING

Whenever possible, the nurse implements strategies to prevent infection. If infection cannot be prevented, the nurse's goal is to prevent the spread of the infection within and between persons, and to treat the existing infection. In the sections that follow, specific nursing activities are described that interfere in the chain of infection to prevent and control transmission of infectious organisms, and that promote care of the infected client. These activities are summarized in Table 29–6.

Preventing Nosocomial Infections

Meticulous use of medical and surgical asepsis is necessary to prevent transport of potentially infectious microorganisms. As discussed previously in this chapter, nosocomial infections are those acquired in relation to health care services. Many nosocomial infections can be prevented using proper hand washing techniques, environmental controls, sterile technique when warranted, and identification and management of clients at risk for infections.

Hand Washing

Hand washing is important in every setting, including hospitals. It is considered one of the most effective infection control measures. Any client may harbor microorganisms that are currently harmless to the client yet potentially harmful to another person or to the same client if they find a portal of entry. It is important that both the nurses' and the clients' hands be washed at the following times to prevent the spread of microorganisms: before eating,

TABLE 29-6 Nursing Interventions that Break the Chain of Infection

Link	Interventions	Rationale
Etiologic agent (microorganism)	Ensure that articles are correctly cleaned and disinfected or sterilized before use.	Correct cleaning, disinfecting, and sterilizing reduce or eliminate microorganisms.
	Educate clients and support persons about appropriate methods to clean, disinfect, and sterilize articles.	Knowledge of ways to reduce or eliminate microorganisms reduces the numbers of microorganisms present and the likelihood of transmission.
Reservoir (source)	Change dressings and bandages when they are soiled or wet.	Moist dressings are ideal environments for microorganisms to grow and multiply.
	Assist clients to carry out appropriate skin and oral hygiene.	Hygienic measures reduce the numbers of resident and transient microorganisms and the likelihood of infection.
	Dispose of damp, soiled linens appropriately.	Damp, soiled linens harbor more microorganisms than dry linens.
	Dispose of feces and urine in appropriate receptacles.	Urine and feces in particular contain many microorganisms.
	Ensure that all fluid containers, such as bedside water jugs and suction and drainage bottles, are covered or capped.	Prolonged exposure increases the risk of contamination and promotes microbial growth.
	Empty suction and drainage bottles at the end of each shift or before they become full, or according to agency policy.	Drainage harbors microorganisms that, if left for long periods, proliferate and can be transmitted to others.
Portal of exit from the reservoir	Avoid talking, coughing, or sneezing over open wounds or sterile fields, and cover the mouth and nose when coughing and sneezing.	These measures limit the number of microorganisms that escape from the respiratory tract.
Method of transmission	Wash hands between client contacts, after touching body substances, and before performing invasive procedures or touching open wounds.	Hand washing is an important means of controlling and preventing the transmission of microorganisms.
	Instruct clients and support persons to wash hands before handling food or eating, after eliminating, and after touching infectious material.	
	Wear gloves when handling secretions and excretions.	Gloves and gowns prevent soiling of the hands and clothing.
	Wear gowns if there is danger of soiling clothing with body substances.	
	Place discarded soiled materials in moisture-proof refuse bags.	Moisture-proof bags prevent the spread of microorganisms to others.
	Hold used bedpans steadily to prevent spillage, and dispose of urine and feces in appropriate receptacles.	Feces in particular contain many microorganisms.
	Initiate and implement aseptic precautions for all clients.	All clients may harbor potentially infectious microorganisms that can be transmitted to others.
	Wear masks and eye protection when in close contact with clients who have infections transmitted by droplets from the respiratory tract.	Masks and eyewear reduce the spread of droplet-transmitted microorganisms.
	Wear masks and eye protection when sprays of body fluid are possible (e.g., during irrigation procedures).	Masks and eye protection provide protection from microorganisms in clients' body substances.
Portal of entry to the susceptible host	Use sterile technique for invasive procedures (e.g., injections, catheterizations).	Invasive procedures penetrate the body's natural protective barriers to microorganisms.
	Use sterile technique when exposing open wounds or handling dressings.	Open wounds are vulnerable to microbial infection.
	Place used disposable needles and syringes in puncture-resistant containers for disposal.	Injuries from needles contaminated by blood or body fluids from an infected client or carrier are a primary cause of HBV and HIV transmission to health care workers.
	Provide all clients with their own personal care items.	People have less resistance to another person's microorganisms than to their own.

TABLE 29–6 Nursing Interventions that Break the Chain of Infection (continued)

Link	Interventions	Rationale
Susceptible host	Maintain the integrity of the client's skin and mucous membranes.	Intact skin and mucous membranes protect against invasion by microorganisms.
	Ensure that the client receives a balanced diet.	A balanced diet supplies proteins and vitamins necessary to build or maintain body tissues.
	Educate the public about the importance of immunizations.	Immunizations protect people against virulent infectious diseases.

Research Note
Will a Soap-and-Water Alternative Increase Compliance with Hand Washing?

Alcohol-based hand gels are available to the general public and to health care institutions as a substitute for soap-and-water hand washing. However, limited research has been conducted on the effectiveness of these gels from the perspectives of their ability to kill microorganisms, affect hand washing frequency, or impact skin condition. In this study by Earl, Jackson, and Rickman (2001), researchers designed three phases to specifically address the question of frequency of hand washing by nurses, physicians, and ancillary personnel (technicians and therapists) in two intensive care units.

In phase I, prior to any intervention, the number of opportunities to wash hands was compared to actual compliance over 4 weeks. In phase II, alcohol gel dispensers were installed inside and outside of patient rooms and both opportunities and occurrences for hand washing with either soap-and-water or gel were counted for 4 weeks. Phase III examined opportunities and occurrences for hand washing between 10 and 14 weeks after installation of the dispensers.

The results were as follows: phase I, 39.6% compliance; phase II, 52.6%; phase III, 57%. The highest rates of compliance were by ancillary personnel, followed by nursing staff, and then physicians. The alcohol gel was used instead of soap about 50% to 60% of the time. Although total amount of required time (including walking to the sinks) was not determined, less actual time was spent in hand antisepsis with gel in phase III (7.5 seconds) than with soap-and-water in phase I (9.4 seconds).

Implications: Although the gel dispensers succeeded in increasing the percent of compliance with hand degerming, the researchers expressed concern that the final rate was still only about 60% of the incidences requiring antisepsis. However, the gel did take less time and was most likely more effective than the inadequate 9-second soap use. The authors recognized weaknesses in the study, including the common Hawthorne effect. This effect states that the participants' behavior may change purely by knowing that a study is being conducted. In this case, the health care providers may have paid more attention to hand antisepsis than they would have had the study not been performed. In addition, it is not possible to extrapolate these results to other institutions and types of care units.

However, this study is an important example of the need to assess, intervene, and reassess effectiveness of procedures designed to increase the safety and health of both providers and clients. The study could easily be replicated in other settings and the results expanded to include other variables such as cost and true time savings.

Note: From "Improved Rates of Compliance with Hand Antisepsis Guidelines: A Three-Phase Observational Study," by M. L. Earl, M. M. Jackson, and L. S. Rickman, 2001, *American Journal of Nursing, 101*(3), pp. 26–33.

after using the bedpan or toilet, and after the hands have come in contact with any body substances, such as sputum or drainage from a wound. In addition, health care workers should wash their hands before and after giving care of any kind.

For routine client care, the CDC recommends antimicrobial foam, hand gel, or vigorous hand washing under a stream of water for at least 10 seconds using granule soap, soap-filled sheets, or antimicrobial liquid soap. Antimicrobial soaps are usually provided in high-risk areas, such as the newborn nursery, and are frequently supplied in dispensers at the sink. Studies have shown that the convenience of antimicrobial foams and gels, which do not require soap and water, may increase health care worker's adherence to hand cleansing (Bischoff, Reynolds, Sessler, Edmond, & Wenzel, 2000). The CDC recommends antimicrobial hand washing agents in the following situations:

- When there are known multiple resistant bacteria
- Before invasive procedures
- In special care units, such as nurseries and ICUs
- Before caring for severely immunocompromised clients.

It is important to recognize that hand washing with either plain soap or antimicrobial soap can damage the skin through the drying effect of the detergents or chemicals (CDC, 2002b). If the nurse develops dermatitis, the client may be at higher risk because hand washing does not decrease bacterial counts on skin with dermatitis. The nurse is also at higher risk because the normal skin barrier has been broken. Although lotions, moisturizers, and emollients have been tried, no research has yet confirmed their effectiveness in decreasing the problem.

Procedure 29–1 describes proper hand washing techniques.

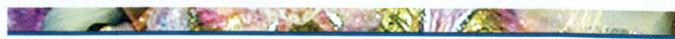

Procedure 29–1 Hand Washing

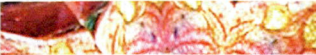

Purposes

- To reduce the number of microorganisms on the hands
- To reduce the risk of transmission of microorganisms to clients
- To reduce the risk of cross-contamination among clients
- To reduce the risk of transmission of infectious organisms to oneself

ASSESSMENT

Determine the client's
- Presence of factors increasing susceptibility to infection
- Use of immunosuppressive medications
- Recent diagnostic procedures or treatments that penetrated the skin or a body cavity
- Current nutritional status

- Signs and symptoms indicating the presence of an infection:
  - Localized signs, such as swelling, redness, pain or tenderness with palpation or movement, palpable heat at site, loss of function of affected body part, presence of exudate
  - Systemic indications, such as fever, increased pulse and respiratory rates, lack of energy, anorexia, enlarged lymph nodes

PLANNING

Determine the location of running water and soap or soap substitutes.

Delegation

The technique of hand washing is identical for all health care providers, including unlicensed assistive personnel. Health care team members are accountable for the implementation of appropriate hand washing procedures by themselves and others.

Equipment
- Soap
- Warm running water
- Disposable or sanitized towels

IMPLEMENTATION

Preparation

Assess the hands.
- Nails should be kept short. *Short, natural nails are less likely to harbor microorganisms, scratch a client, or puncture gloves.* Many agencies do not permit health care workers in direct contact with clients to have any form of artificial nails.
- Remove all jewelry. *Microorganisms can lodge in the settings of jewelry and under rings. Removal facilitates proper cleaning of the hands and arms.*
- Check hands for breaks in the skin, such as hangnails or cuts. *A nurse who has open sores may require a work assignment with decreased risk for transmission of infectious organisms.*

Performance

1. If you are washing your hands where the client can observe you, explain to the client what you are going to do and why it is necessary.
2. Turn on the water, and adjust the flow.
   - There are five common types of faucet controls:
     a. Hand-operated handles.

   b. Knee levers. Move these with the knee to regulate flow and temperature (Figure 29–2 ■).

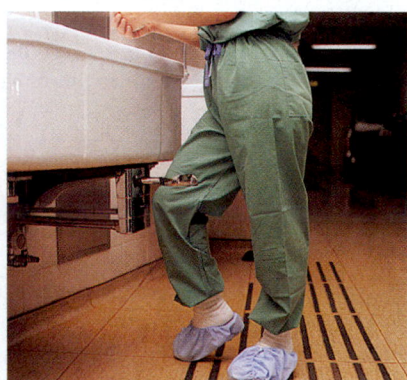

Figure 29–2 ■ A knee-lever faucet control.

   c. Foot pedals. Press these with the foot to regulate flow and temperature (Figure 29–3 ■).

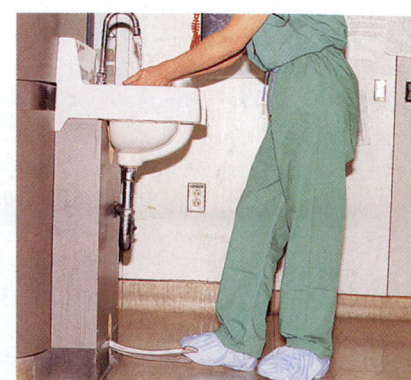

Figure 29–3 ■ A foot-pedal faucet control.

   d. Elbow controls. Move these with the elbows instead of the hands.
   e. Infrared control. Motion in front of the sensor causes water to start and stop flowing automatically.

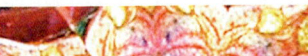

Procedure 29–1 Hand Washing *continued*

IMPLEMENTATION *continued*

- Adjust the flow so that the water is warm. *Warm water removes less of the protective oil of the skin than hot water.*
3. Wet the hands thoroughly by holding them under the running water, and apply soap to the hands.
   - Hold the hands lower than the elbows so that the water flows from the arms to the fingertips. *The water should flow from the least contaminated to the most contaminated area; the hands are generally considered more contaminated than the lower arms.*
   - If the soap is liquid, apply 2 to 4 mL (1 tsp). If it is bar soap, granules, or sheets rub them firmly between the hands.
4. Thoroughly wash and rinse the hands.
   - Use firm, rubbing, and circular movements to wash the palm, back, and wrist of each hand. Interlace the fingers and thumbs, and move the hands back and forth (Figure 29–4 ■). Continue this motion for 10 seconds. *The circular action helps remove microorganisms mechanically. Interlacing*

the fingers and thumbs cleans the interdigital spaces.
   - Rub the fingertips against the palm of the opposite hand. *The nails and fingertips are commonly missed during hand washing.*
   - Rinse the hands.
5. Thoroughly dry the hands and arms.
   - Dry hands and arms thoroughly with a paper towel. *Moist skin becomes chapped readily; chapping produces lesions.*
   - Discard the paper towel in the appropriate container.
6. Turn off the water.
   - Use a new paper towel to grasp a hand-operated control (Figure 29–5 ■). *This prevents the nurse from picking up microorganisms from the faucet handles.*

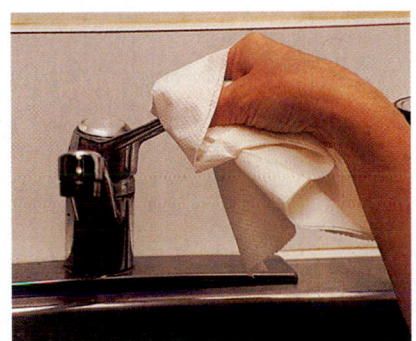

Figure 29–5 ■ Using a paper towel to grasp the handle of a hand-operated faucet.

VARIATION: HAND WASHING BEFORE STERILE TECHNIQUES

- Apply the soap and wash as described in step 4, but hold the hands higher than the elbows during this hand wash. Wet the hands and forearms under the running water, letting it run from the fingertips to the elbows so that the hands become cleaner than the elbows (see Figure 29–6 ■). *In this way, the water runs from the area that now has the fewest microorganisms to areas with a relatively greater number.*

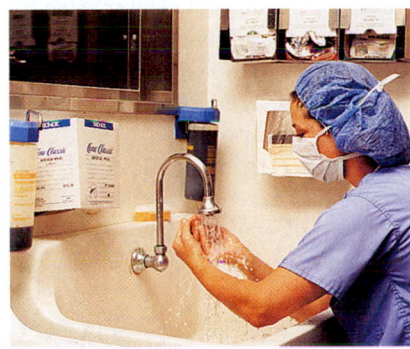

Figure 29–6 ■ The hands are held higher than the elbows during a hand wash before sterile technique.

- Apply the soap and wash as described earlier in step 6, maintaining the hands uppermost.
- After washing and rinsing, use a towel to dry one hand thoroughly in a rotating motion from the fingers to the elbow. Use a new towel to dry the other hand and arm. *A clean towel prevents the transfer of microorganisms from one elbow (least clean area) to the other hand (cleanest area).*

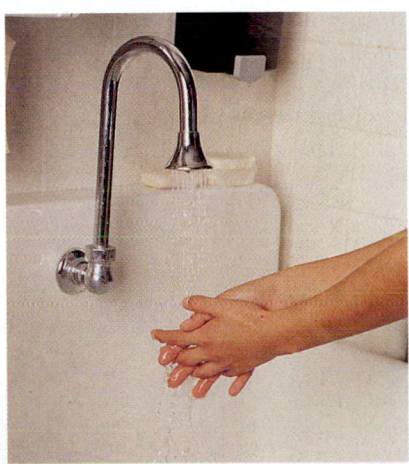

Figure 29–4 ■ Interlacing the fingers during hand washing.

EVALUATION

There is no traditional evaluation of the effectiveness of the individual nurse's hand washing. Institutional quality control departments monitor the occurrence of client infections and investigate those situations in which health care providers are implicated in the transmission of infectious organisms. Research has repeatedly shown the positive impact of careful hand washing on client health associated with prevention of infection (see Readings and References at the end of this chapter).

Supporting Defenses of a Susceptible Host

People are constantly in contact with microorganisms in the environment. Normally a person's natural defenses ward off the development of an infection. *Susceptibility* is the degree to which an individual can be affected, that is, the likelihood of an organism causing an infection in that person. The following measures can reduce a person's susceptibility:

- *Hygiene.* Intact skin and mucous membranes are one barrier against microorganisms entering the body. In addition, good oral care, including flossing the teeth, reduces the likelihood of an oral infection. Regular and thorough bathing and shampooing remove microorganisms and dirt that can result in an infection.
- *Nutrition.* A balanced diet enhances the health of all body tissues, helps keep the skin intact, and promotes the skin's ability to repel microorganisms. Adequate nutrition enables tissues to maintain and rebuild themselves and helps keep the immune system functioning well.
- *Fluid.* Fluid intake permits fluid output that flushes out the bladder and urethra, removing microorganisms that could cause an infection.
- *Rest and sleep.* Adequate rest and sleep are essential to health and to renewing energy. See Chapter 43. 🔗
- *Stress.* Excessive stress predisposes people to infections. Nurses can assist clients to learn stress-reducing techniques. See Chapter 40. 🔗
- *Immunizations.* The use of immunizations has dramatically decreased the incidence of infectious diseases. It is recommended that immunizations begin shortly after birth and be completed in early childhood except for boosters. (See Table 29–5 earlier in this chapter.) Immunizations may be given by injection, inhalation, oral solutions, or nasal sprays. They are frequently given in combination to minimize multiple injection. Because there are frequent changes to immunization schedules, it is advisable to update immunization schedules yearly.

There are immunization programs for high-risk groups such as health care personnel, older adults who are chronically ill, and people traveling to foreign countries. For example, hepatitis B vaccine is recommended for all health care workers.

Cleaning, Disinfecting, and Sterilizing

The first links in the chain of infection, the etiologic agent and the reservoir, are interrupted by the use of **antiseptics** (agents that inhibit the growth of some microorganisms) and **disinfectants** (agents that destroy pathogens other than spores), and by sterilization.

Cleaning

Cleanliness inhibits the growth of microorganisms. When cleaning visibly soiled objects, nurses must always wear gloves to avoid direct contact with infectious microorganisms. Most objects used in the care of clients, whether forceps or drawsheets, can be cleaned by rinsing them in cold water to remove any organic material, washing them with hot soapy water, then rinsing them again to remove the soap. The following steps should be followed when cleaning objects in a hospital.

1. Rinse the article with cold water to remove organic material. *Hot water coagulates the protein of organic material and tends to make it adhere.* Examples of organic material are blood and pus.
2. Wash the article in hot water and soap. *The emulsifying action of soap reduces surface tension and facilitates the removal of substances. Washing dislodges the emulsified substances.*
3. Use an abrasive, such as a stiff-bristled brush, to clean equipment with grooves and corners. *Friction helps dislodge foreign material.*
4. Rinse the article well with warm to hot water.
5. Dry the article; it is now considered clean.
6. Clean the brush and sink. These are considered soiled until they are cleaned appropriately, usually with a disinfectant.

Disinfecting

A disinfectant is a chemical preparation, such as phenol or iodine compounds, used on inanimate objects. Disinfectants are

---

Home Care Considerations

Hand Washing

- Keep fingernails clean, short, and well trimmed.
- Wash hands carefully before and after any hands-on care.
- If there is no running water, use commercially available hand washing agents that require no water.
- You may wish to bring your own bactericidal soap and paper towels for use when washing hands.
- Always turn the water off with a dry paper towel.
- Teach the client and family members hand washing techniques.
- Discuss use of antimicrobial soaps and disinfectants.

- Teach signs and symptoms of infection and when to contact a health care provider.
- Teach how to avoid infections.
  - Do not share personal care items such as toothbrushes.
  - Wash raw fruits and vegetables.
  - Cleanse and disinfect used equipment.
  - Dispose properly contaminated items such as dressings.
  - Dispose properly used sharps such as needles and syringes.
- Emphasize the importance of proper immunizations for all members of the household.

frequently caustic and toxic to tissues. An antiseptic is a chemical preparation used on skin or tissue. Disinfectants and antiseptics often have similar chemical components, but the disinfectant is a more concentrated solution.

Both antiseptics and disinfectants are said to have bactericidal or bacteriostatic properties. A *bactericidal* preparation destroys bacteria, whereas a *bacteriostatic* preparation prevents the growth and reproduction of some bacteria. Although some agents are active against a broad array of bacteria, if a specific microorganism is identified, an agent known to be effective against it should be selected. Spore-forming bacteria such as *Clostridium difficile* (commonly referred to as *C. difficile*), which is a frequent cause of nosocomial diarrhea, and *Bacillus anthracis* (anthrax) may be inhibited by only a few of the agents normally effective against other forms of bacteria. Table 29–7 lists commonly used antiseptics and disinfectants.

When disinfecting articles, nurses need to follow agency protocol and consider the following:

1. The type and number of infectious organisms. Some microorganisms are readily destroyed, whereas others require longer contact with the disinfectant.
2. The recommended concentration of the disinfectant and the duration of contact.
3. The temperature of the environment. Most disinfectants are intended for use at room temperature.
4. The presence of soap. Some disinfectants are ineffective in the presence of soap or detergent.
5. The presence of organic materials. The presence of saliva, blood, pus, or excretions can readily inactivate many disinfectants.
6. The surface areas to be treated. The disinfecting agent must come into contact with all surfaces and areas.

Sterilizing

Sterilization is a process that destroys all microorganisms, including spores and viruses. Four commonly used methods of sterilization are moist heat, gas, boiling water, and radiation.

MOIST HEAT. For sterilizing, moist heat (steam) can be employed in two ways: as steam under pressure or as free steam. Steam under pressure attains temperatures higher than the boiling point. Autoclaves supply steam under pressures of 15 to 17 pounds and temperatures of 121 to 123C (250 to 254F).

Free steam, 100C (212F), is used to sterilize objects that would be destroyed at the higher temperature and pressure of the autoclave. Usually, it is necessary to steam the article for 29 minutes on 3 consecutive days. The intervals are required so that unkilled spores will return to their vegetative state and again become vulnerable to the heat.

GAS. Ethylene oxide gas destroys microorganisms by interfering with their metabolic processes. It is also effective against spores. Its advantages are good penetration and effectiveness for heat-sensitive items. Its major disadvantage is its toxicity to humans.

BOILING WATER. This is the most practical and inexpensive method for sterilizing in the home. The main disadvantage is that spores and some viruses are not killed by this method. The water temperature rises no higher than 100C (212F). Boiling a minimum of 15 minutes is advised for disinfection of articles in the home.

RADIATION. Both ionizing and nonionizing radiation can be used for disinfection and sterilization. Ultraviolet light, a type of nonionizing radiation, can be used for disinfection. Its main drawback is that the ultraviolet rays do not penetrate deeply. Ionizing radiation is used effectively in industry to sterilize foods, drugs, and other items that are sensitive to heat. Its main advantage is that it is effective for items difficult to sterilize; its chief disadvantage is that the equipment is very expensive.

Nurses should be familiar with the cleaning, disinfecting, and sterilizing protocols of the agency in which they practice and should be prepared to teach clients and family members appropriate techniques for home care.

TABLE 29-7 Commonly Used Antiseptics and Disinfectants, Effectiveness, and Use

| Agent | Effective Against | | | | | Use on |
	Bacteria	Tuberculosis	Spores	Fungi	Viruses	
Isopropyl and ethyl alcohol	X	X		X	X	Hands, vial stoppers
Chlorine (bleach)	X	X	X	X	X	Blood spills
Hydrogen peroxide	X	X	X	X	X	Surfaces
Iodophors	X	X	X	X	X	Equipment; intact skin and tissues if diluted
Phenol	X	X		X	X	Surfaces
Chlorhexidine gluconate (Hibiclens)	X				X	Hands
Triclosan (Bacti-Stat)	X					Hands, intact skin

ISOLATION PRECAUTIONS

Isolation refers to measures designed to prevent the spread of infections or potentially infectious microorganisms to health personnel, clients, and visitors. Various infection control measures are used to decrease the risk of transmission of microorganisms in hospitals.

In 1983, the Centers for Disease Control and Prevention established isolation guidelines that allowed health facilities to choose between two systems: category-specific or disease-specific isolation (Garner & Simmons, 1983).

Category-specific isolation precautions were based on seven categories: strict isolation, contact isolation, respiratory isolation, tuberculosis isolation, enteric precautions, drainage/secretions precautions, and blood/body fluid precautions.

Disease-specific isolation precautions provided precautions for specific diseases. These precautions delineated use of private rooms with special ventilation, having the client share a room with other clients infected with the same organism, and gowning to prevent gross soilage of clothes for specific infectious diseases.

In 1987, the CDC presented recommendations (revised in 1988) for **universal precautions (UP),** techniques to be used with all clients to decrease the risk of transmitting unidentified pathogens (CDC, 1987; U.S. Department of Health and Human Services [USDHHS], 1988). Universal precautions interfere with the spread of **bloodborne pathogens,** those microorganisms carried in blood and body fluids that are capable of infecting other persons with serious and difficult to treat viral infections, namely, hepatitis B virus, hepatitis C virus, and HIV. The CDC did not recommend that universal precautions replace disease-specific or category-specific precautions, but that they be used in conjunction with them.

The **body substance isolation (BSI)** system employs generic infection control precautions for all clients except those with the few diseases transmitted through the air. The BSI system (Jackson, 1993), is based on three premises:

1. All people have an increased risk for infection from microorganisms placed on their mucous membranes and non-intact skin.
2. All people are likely to have potentially infectious microorganisms in all of their moist body sites and substances.
3. An unknown portion of clients and health care workers will always be colonized or infected with potentially infectious microorganisms in their blood and other moist body sites and substances.

The term *body substance* includes blood, some body fluids, and urine, feces, wound drainage, oral secretions, and any other body product or tissue.

In addition to other actions and precautions discussed in this chapter, significant emphasis is placed on avoiding injury due to sharp instruments (see Chapter 33 🔗), measures to be taken in case of exposure to bloodborne pathogens, and communication about biohazards to employees. Federal regulations require that in most cases warning labels be affixed to containers of regulated waste and to refrigerators and freezers containing blood or other potentially infectious materials. The la-

Figure 29–7 ■ Biohazard alert. (*Note:* From "Occupational Exposure to Bloodborne Pathogens: Final Rule" (29 CFR Part 1910.1029), by U.S. Department of Labor, Occupational Safety and Health Administration, 1991, *Federal Register, 56*(235), pp. 64175–64182.)

bels required are fluorescent orange or orange-red and feature the biohazard legend shown in Figure 29–7 ■.

CDC (HICPAC) Isolation Precautions (1996)

The Hospital Infection Control Practices Advisory Committee (HICPAC) of the CDC presented new guidelines for isolation precautions in hospitals in 1996 (Garner & HICPAC, 1996). These guidelines designate two tiers of precautions:

> *Tier 1:* Standard Precautions
> *Tier 2:* Transmission-Based Precautions

Standard Precautions

These precautions are used in the care of all hospitalized persons regardless of their diagnosis or possible infection status. They apply to blood, all body fluids, secretions, and excretions except sweat (whether or not blood is present or visible), non-intact skin, and mucous membranes. Thus they combine the major features of UP and BSI. Recommended practices for Standard Precautions are shown in Box 29–1.

Transmission-Based Precautions

These precautions are used in addition to Standard Precautions for clients with known or suspected infections that are spread in one of three ways: by airborne or droplet transmission, or by contact. The three types of Transmission-Based Precautions may be used alone or in combination but always in addition to Standard Precautions. They encompass all of the conditions or diseases previously listed in the category-specific or disease-specific classifications developed by the CDC in 1983. Recommended practices for Transmission-Based Precautions are shown in Box 29–1.

Airborne Precautions are used for clients known to have or suspected of having serious illnesses transmitted by airborne droplet nuclei smaller than 5 microns. Examples of such illnesses include measles (rubeola), varicella (including disseminated zoster), and tuberculosis. (*Note:* The CDC has prepared special guidelines for preventing the transmission of tuberculosis. The

BOX 29–1   ■ Recommended Isolation Precautions in Hospitals

Standard Precautions (Tier One)

- Designed for all clients in hospital.
- These precautions apply to (a) blood; (b) all body fluids, excretions, and secretions except sweat; (c) nonintact (broken) skin; and (d) mucous membranes.
- Designed to reduce risk of transmission of microorganisms from recognized and unrecognized sources.

1. Wash hands after contact with blood, body fluids, secretions, excretions, and contaminated objects whether or not gloves are worn.
   a. Wash hands immediately after removing gloves.
   b. Use a nonantimicrobial soap for routine hand washing.
   c. Use an antimicrobial agent or an antiseptic agent for the control of specific outbreaks of infection.
2. Wear clean gloves when touching blood, body fluids, secretions, excretions, and contaminated items (i.e., soiled gowns).
   a. Clean gloves can be unsterile unless their use is intended to prevent the entrance of microorganisms into the body. See the discussion of sterile gloves in this chapter.
   b. Remove gloves before touching noncontaminated items and surfaces.
   c. Wash hands immediately after removing gloves.
3. Wear a mask, eye protection, or a face shield if splashes or sprays of blood, body fluids, secretions, or excretions can be expected.
4. Wear a clean, nonsterile gown if client care is likely to result in splashes or sprays of blood, body fluids, secretions, or excretions. The gown is intended to protect clothing.
   a. Remove a soiled gown carefully to avoid the transfer of microorganisms to others (i.e., clients or other health care workers).
   b. Wash hands after removing gown.
5. Handle client care equipment that is soiled with blood, body fluids, secretions, or excretions carefully to prevent the transfer of microorganisms to others and to the environment.
   a. Make sure reusable equipment is cleaned and reprocessed correctly.
   b. Dispose of single-use equipment correctly.
6. Handle, transport, and process linen that is soiled with blood, body fluids, secretions, or excretions in a manner to prevent contamination of clothing and the transfer of microorganisms to others and to the environment.
7. Prevent injuries from used scalpels, needles, or other equipment, and place in puncture-resistant containers.

Transmission-Based Precautions (Tier Two)

Airborne Precautions

Use the Tier One precautions as well as the following:

1. Place client in a private room that has negative air pressure, 6 to 12 air changes per hour, and either discharge of air to the outside or a filtration system for the room air.

2. If a private room is not available, place client with another client who is infected with the same microorganism.
3. Wear a respiratory device (N95 respirator) when entering the room of a client who is known or suspected of having primary tuberculosis.
4. Susceptible people should not enter the room of a client who has rubeola (measles) or varicella (chickenpox). If they must enter, they should wear a respirator.
5. Limit movement of client outside the room to essential purposes. Place a surgical mask on the client during transport.

Droplet Precautions

Use the Tier One precautions as well as the following:

1. Place client in private room.
2. If a private room is not available, place client with another client who is infected with the same microorganism.
3. Wear a mask if working within 3 feet of the client.
4. Limit movement of client outside the room to essential purposes. Place a surgical mask on the client during transport.

Contact Precautions

Use the Tier One precautions as well as the following:

1. Place client in private room.
2. If a private room is not available, place client with another client who is infected with the same microorganism.
3. Wear gloves as described in Standard Precautions.
   a. Change gloves after contact with infectious material.
   b. Remove gloves before leaving client's room.
   c. Wash hands immediately after removing gloves. Use an antimicrobial agent.
   d. After hand washing, do not touch possibly contaminated surfaces or items in the room.
4. Wear a gown (see Standard Precautions) when entering a room if there is a possibility of contact with infected surfaces or items, or if the client is incontinent, has diarrhea, a colostomy, or wound drainage not contained by a dressing.
   a. Remove gown in the client's room.
   b. Make sure uniform does not contact possible contaminated surfaces.
5. Limit movement of client outside the room.
6. Dedicate the use of noncritical client care equipment to a single client or to clients with the same infecting microorganisms.

Note: Adapted from "Guidelines for Isolation Precautions in Hospitals," by J. S. Garner and the Hospital Infection Control Practices Advisory Committee (HICPAC), 1996, *Infection Control Hospital Epidemiology, 17,* pp. 53–80, and 1996, *American Journal of Infection Control, 24,* pp. 24–52.

most current information may be found on the CDC Division of Tuberculosis Elimination Web site http:// www.cdc.gov/nchstp/tb).

Droplet Precautions are used for clients known or suspected to have serious illnesses transmitted by particle droplets larger than 5 microns. Examples of such illnesses are diphtheria (pharyngeal); mycoplasma pneumonia; pertussis; mumps; rubella; streptococcal pharyngitis, pneumonia, or scarlet fever in infants and young children; and pneumonic plague.

Contact Precautions are used for clients known or suspected to have serious illnesses easily transmitted by direct client contact or by contact with items in the client's environment. According to the CDC (Garner & HICPAC, 1996), such illnesses include gastrointestinal, respiratory, skin, or wound infections or colonization with multidrug-resistant bacteria; specific enteric infections such as *Clostridium difficile,* and enterohemorrhagic *Escherichia coli 0157:H7, Shigella,* and hepatitis A, for diapered or incontinent clients; respiratory syncytial virus, parainfluenza virus, or enteroviral infections in infants and young children; and highly contagious skin infections such as herpes simplex virus, impetigo, pediculosis, and scabies.

In addition to the preceding conditions, special contact precautions are used for vancomycin-resistant enterococci (VRE) infections. The CDC recommends use of an antimicrobial soap for hand washing and no sharing of equipment among clients with and without VRE. The client should have a private room (or a room with other clients who have VRE), and such isolation should continue until at least three cultures taken 1 week apart are negative (HICPAC, 1995).

Some diseases require a combination of transmission-based precautions. For clients infected with the coronavirus that causes Severe Acute Respiratory Syndrome (SARS) Standard (including eye protection), Contact, and Airborne Precautions are indicated.

Compromised Clients

Compromised clients (those highly susceptible to infection) are often infected by their own microorganisms, by microorganisms on the inadequately washed hands of health care personnel, and by nonsterile items (food, water, air, and client-care equipment). Clients who are severely compromised include those who

- Have diseases, such as leukemia, that depress the client's resistance to infectious organisms
- Have extensive skin impairments, such as severe dermatitis or major burns, which cannot be effectively covered with dressings.

The 1996 (Garner & HICPAC) and 1997 CDC guidelines for severely compromised (immunocompromised) clients include the use of Standard Precautions as described earlier.

ISOLATION PRACTICES

Initiation of practices to prevent the transmission of microorganisms is generally a nursing responsibility and is based on a comprehensive assessment of the client. This assessment takes into account the status of the client's normal defense mechanisms, the client's ability to implement necessary precautions,

and the source and mode of transmission of the infectious agent. The nurse then decides whether to wear gloves, gowns, masks, and protective eyewear. In all client situations, *nurses must wash their hands before and after giving care.*

In addition to the precautions cited within this chapter, the nurse implements aseptic precautions when performing many specific therapies discussed throughout this book. The following are some examples:

- Use strict aseptic technique when performing any invasive procedure (e.g., inserting an intravenous needle or catheter, suctioning an airway, and inserting a urinary catheter) and when changing surgical dressings.
- Handle needles and syringes carefully to avoid needle-stick injuries.
- Change intravenous tubing and solution containers according to hospital policy (e.g., every 48 to 72 hours).
- Check all sterile supplies for expiration date and intact packaging.
- Prevent urinary infections by maintaining a closed urinary drainage system with a downhill flow of urine. Do not irrigate a catheter unless ordered to do so. Provide regular catheter care, and clean the perineal area with soap and water. Keep the drainage bag and spout off the floor.
- Implement measures to prevent impaired skin integrity and to prevent accumulation of secretions in the lungs (for example, encourage the client to move, cough, and breathe deeply at least every 2 hours).

Personal Protective Equipment

All health care providers must apply clean or sterile gloves, gowns, masks, and protective eyewear according to the risk of exposure to potentially infective materials.

Gloves

Gloves are worn for three reasons: First, they protect the hands when the nurse is likely to handle any body substances, for example, blood, urine, feces, sputum, mucous membranes, and nonintact skin. Second, gloves reduce the likelihood of nurses transmitting their own endogenous microorganisms to individuals receiving care. Nurses who have open sores or cuts on the hands must wear gloves for protection. Third, gloves reduce the chance that the nurse's hands will transmit microorganisms from one client or a fomite to another client. In all situations, gloves are changed between client contacts. The hands are washed each time gloves are removed for two primary reasons: (a) The gloves may have imperfections or be damaged during wearing so that they could allow microorganism entry and (b) the hands may become contaminated during glove removal.

Many of the gloves used in infection control are made of latex rubber, as are various other items used in health care (catheters, blood pressure cuffs, rubber sheets, intravenous tubing, stockings and binders, adhesive bandages, and dental dams). Because of the frequent use of gloves, clients with chronic illnesses and health care workers have increasingly reported allergic reactions to latex. Latex gloves lubricated by powder or cornstarch are particularly allergenic because the latex allergen adheres to the powder, which is aerosolized during glove use and inhaled by the user. Latex gloves that are labeled "hypoaller-genic" still contain measurable latex and should not be used by or on persons with known latex sensitivity. Recent studies show some level of latex allergy in 6% to 17% of health care person-nel (Corbin, 2002). The people at greatest risk for developing la-tex allergies are those with other allergic conditions and those who have had frequent or long-term exposure to latex.

Latex allergies can be either local or systemic and may take the form of dermatitis, urticaria (hives), asthma, or anaphylaxis. Clients and health care workers should be assessed for possible allergies through a thorough history taking. Ask clients if they have had any adverse reactions to items such as balloons, con-doms, or dishwashing or utility gloves. Strategies to avoid sensi-tization or exposure to latex include use of nonlatex products, nonlatex barriers between latex products and the skin, and gloves that are unpowdered or washed before use. People with signifi-cant allergies should have no contact with latex products.

Procedure 29–2 describes application and removal of gloves.

Gowns

Clean or disposable impervious (water-resistant) gowns or plastic aprons are worn during procedures when the nurse's uniform is likely to become soiled. *Single-use gown technique* (using a gown only once before it is discarded or laundered) is the usual practice in hospitals. After the gown is worn, the nurse discards it (if it is paper) or places it in a laundry hamper. See Procedure 29–2. Before leaving the client's room, the nurse washes his or her hands.

> ► **CLINICAL ALERT**   *Wearing a patient hospital gown over your uniform does not serve any infection control purpose.*

Sterile gowns may be indicated when the nurse changes the dressings of a client with extensive wounds (e.g., burns).

Face Masks

Masks are worn to reduce the risk for transmission of organ-isms by the droplet contact and airborne routes, and by splat-ters of body substances. The CDC recommends that masks be worn under the following conditions:

1. By those close to the client if the infection (e.g., measles, mumps, or acute respiratory diseases in children) is trans-mitted by large-particle aerosols (droplets). Large-particle aerosols are transmitted by close contact and generally travel short distances (about 1 m, or 3 ft).

2. By all persons entering the room if the infection (e.g., pul-monary tuberculosis and SARS) is transmitted by small-particle aerosols (droplet nuclei). Small-particle aerosols remain suspended in the air and thus travel greater dis-tances by air. Special masks that provide a tighter face seal and better filtration may be used for these infections.

Various types of masks differ in their filtration effective-ness and fit. Single-use disposable surgical masks are effective for use while the nurse provides care to most clients but should be changed if they become wet or soiled. These masks are dis-carded in the waste container after use. Disposable particulate respirators of different types may be effective for droplet transmission, splatters, and airborne microorganisms. Some respirators now available are effective in preventing inhalation of tuberculin organisms. The National Institute for Occupational Safety and Health (NIOSH) tests and certifies such respirators. Currently, the category "N" respirator at 95% efficiency (referred to as an N95 respirator) meets tuberculo-sis and SARS control criteria.

During certain techniques requiring surgical asepsis (sterile technique), masks are worn (a) to prevent droplet contact trans-mission of exhaled microorganisms to the sterile field or to a client's open wound and (b) to protect the nurse from splashes of body substances from the client.

Because the effectiveness of disposable masks and respira-tors against airborne microorganisms is questionable, agencies usually do not assign susceptible caregivers to clients with the specific airborne disease in question. However, caregivers who are immune to specific diseases (e.g., chickenpox, tuberculo-sis, measles, mumps, and rubella) can provide care to clients with these diseases. Guidelines for donning and removing face masks are shown in Procedure 29–2.

Eyewear

Protective eyewear (goggles, glasses, or face shields) and masks may be indicated in situations where body substances may splat-ter the face (see Procedure 29–2). If the nurse wears prescription eyeglasses, goggles may be worn over the glasses. The protec-tive eyewear must extend around the sides of the glasses.

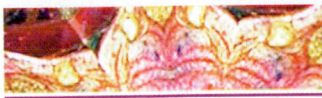

Procedure 29–2 Donning and Removing Personal Protective Equipment (Gloves, Gown, Mask, Eyewear)

Purposes

- To protect health care workers and clients from transmission of potentially infective materials

ASSESSMENT

Consider which activities will be required while the nurse is in the client's room at this time. *This will determine which personal protec-tive equipment is required.*

continued on page 652

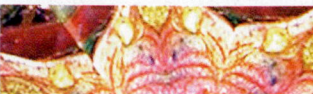

Procedure 29–2 Donning and Removing Personal Protective Equipment (Gloves, Gown, Mask, Eyewear) *continued*

PLANNING

- Application and removal of personal protective equipment can be time consuming. Arrange for the care of your other clients if indicated.
- Determine which supplies are present within the client's room and which must be brought with you.
- Consider if special handling is indicated for removal of any specimens or other materials from the room.

Delegation

Use of personal protective equipment is identical for all health care providers, including unlicensed assistive personnel. Health care team members are accountable for proper implementation of these procedures by themselves and others.

Equipment

As indicated according to which activities will be performed. Ensure that extra supplies are easily available.

- Gown
- Mask
- Eyewear
- Clean gloves

IMPLEMENTATION

Preparation

See Procedure 29–1 for preparation for hand washing. Remove or secure all loose items such as nametags or jewelry.

Performance

1. Explain to the client what you are going to do, why it is necessary, and how he or she can cooperate.
2. Wash your hands.
3. Don a clean gown.
   - Pick up a clean gown, and allow it to unfold in front of you without allowing it to touch any area soiled with body substances.
   - Slide the arms and the hands through the sleeves.
   - Fasten the ties at the neck to keep the gown in place.
   - Overlap the gown at the back as much as possible, and fasten the waist ties or belt (Figure 29–8 ■).

Overlapping securely covers the uniform at the back. Waist ties keep the gown from falling away from the body and prevent inadvertent soiling of the uniform.

4. Don the face mask.
   - Locate the top edge of the mask. The mask usually has a narrow metal strip along the edge.
   - Hold the mask by the top two strings or loops.
   - Place the upper edge of the mask over the bridge of the nose, and tie the upper ties at the back of the head or secure the loops around the ears. If glasses are worn, fit the upper edge of the mask under the glasses. *With the edge of the mask under the glasses, clouding of the glasses is less likely to occur.*
   - Secure the lower edge of the mask under the chin, and tie the lower ties at the nape of the neck (Figure 29–9 ■). *To be effective, a mask must cover both the nose and the mouth, because air moves in and out of both.*

   - If the mask has a metal strip, adjust this firmly over the bridge of the nose. *A secure fit prevents both the escape and the inhalation of microorganisms around the edges of the mask and the fogging of eyeglasses.*
   - Wear the mask only once, and do not wear any mask longer than the manufacturer recommends or once it becomes wet. *A mask should be used only once because it becomes ineffective when moist.*
   - Do not leave a used face mask hanging around the neck.
5. Don protective eyewear if it is not combined with the face mask.
6. Don clean disposable gloves.
   - No special technique is required.
   - If you are wearing a gown, pull the gloves up to cover the cuffs of the gown. If you are not wearing a gown, pull the gloves up to cover the wrists.
7. To remove soiled personal protective equipment, remove the gloves first since they are the most soiled.
   - If wearing a gown that is tied at the waist in front, undo the ties before removing gloves.

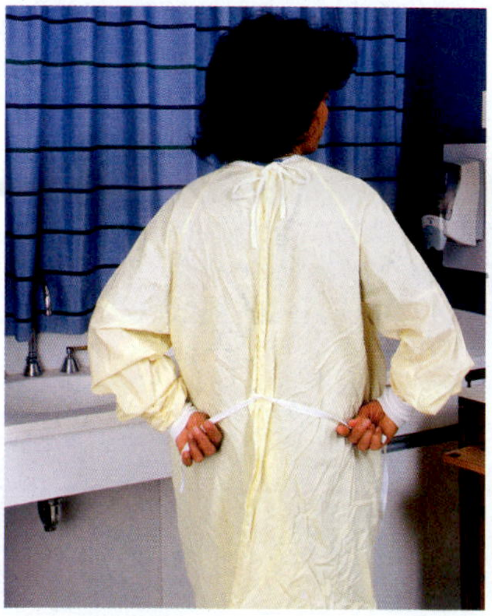

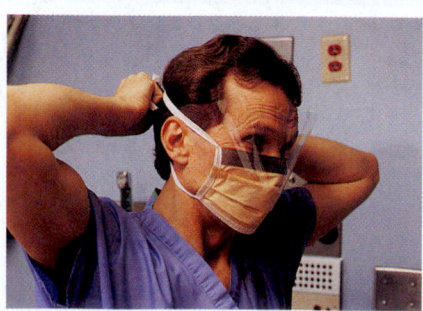

Figure 29–8 ■ Overlapping the gown at the back to cover the nurse's uniform.

Figure 29–9 ■ A facemask and eye protection covering the nose, mouth, and eyes.

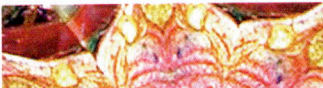

Procedure 29–2 Donning and Removing Personal Protective Equipment (Gloves, Gown, Mask, Eyewear) *continued*

IMPLEMENTATION *continued*

- Remove the first glove by grasping it on its palmar surface just below the cuff, taking care to touch only glove to glove (Figure 29–10 ■). *This keeps the soiled parts of the used gloves from touching the skin of the wrist or hand.*

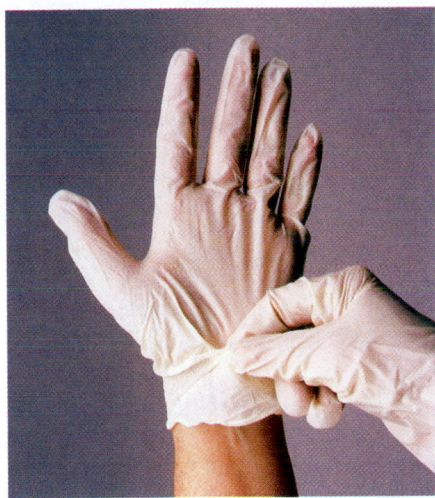

Figure 29–10 ■ Plucking the palmar surface below the cuff of a contaminated glove.

- Pull the first glove completely off by inverting or rolling the glove inside out.
- Continue to hold the inverted removed glove by the fingers of the remaining gloved hand. Place the first two fingers of the bare hand inside the cuff of the second glove (Figure 29–11 ■). *Touching the outside of the second soiled glove with the bare hand is avoided.*

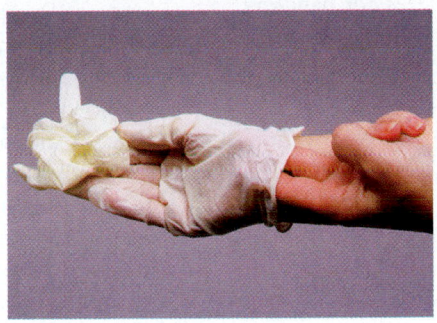

Figure 29–11 ■ Inserting fingers to remove the second contaminated glove.

- Pull the second glove off to the fingers by turning it inside out. This pulls the first glove inside the second glove. *The soiled part of the glove is folded to the inside to reduce the chance of transferring any microorganisms by direct contact.*
- Using the bare hand, continue to remove the gloves, which are now inside out, and dispose of them in the refuse container (Figure 29–12 ■).

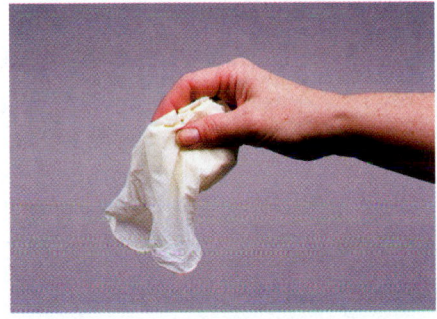

Figure 29–12 ■ Holding contaminated gloves, which are inside out.

8. Wash your hands.
9. Remove the mask.
   - If using a mask with strings, first untie the *lower* strings of the mask. *This prevents the top part of the mask from falling onto the chest.*
   - Untie the top strings and, while holding the ties securely, remove the mask from the face. *This prevents hand contact with the moistened, contaminated portion of the mask.*
     or
     If side loops are present, lift the side loops up and away from the ears and face.
   - Discard a disposable mask in the waste container.
   - Wash the hands again if they have become contaminated by accidentally touching the soiled part of the mask.
10. Remove the gown when preparing to leave the room. Unless a gown is grossly soiled with body substances, no special precautions are needed to remove it. If a gown is grossly soiled:
    - Avoid touching soiled parts on the outside of the gown, if possible. *The top part of the gown may be soiled, for example, if you have been holding an infant with a respiratory infection.*
    - Grasp the gown along the inside of the neck and pull down over the shoulders.
    - Roll up the gown with the soiled part inside, and discard it in the appropriate container.
11. Remove protective eyewear and dispose of properly or place in the appropriate receptacle for cleaning.

EVALUATION

Conduct any follow-up indicated during your care of the client. If there has been any failure of the equipment and exposure to potentially infective materials is suspected, follow the steps in the Practice Guidelines: Steps to Follow after Exposure to Bloodborne Pathogens later in this chapter.

Ensure that an adequate supply of equipment is available for the next health care provider.

Disposal of Soiled Equipment and Supplies

Many pieces of equipment are supplied for single use only and are disposed of after use. Some items, however, are reusable. Agencies have specific policies and procedures for handling soiled equipment (e.g., disposal, cleaning, disinfecting, and sterilizing); the nurse needs to become familiar with these practices in the employing agency. Appropriate handling of soiled equipment and supplies is essential for these reasons:

- To prevent inadvertent exposure of health care workers to articles contaminated with body substances
- To prevent contamination of the environment.

BAGGING. Most articles do not need to be placed in bags unless they are contaminated, or likely to have been contaminated, with infective material such as pus, blood, body fluids, feces, or respiratory secretions. Contaminated articles need to be enclosed in a sturdy bag impervious to microorganisms before they are removed from the room of any client. Some agencies use labels or bags of a particular color that designates them as infective wastes.

CDC guidelines recommend the following methods (USDHHS, 1988):

- A single bag, if it is sturdy and impervious to microorganisms, and if the contaminated articles can be placed in the bag without soiling or contaminating its outside
- Double-bagging if the above conditions are not met

Follow agency protocol, or use the following CDC guidelines to handle and bag soiled items:

- Place garbage and soiled *disposable* equipment, including dressings and tissues, in the plastic bag that lines the waste container. Some agencies separate dry and wet waste material and incinerate dry items, such as paper towels and disposable items. No special precautions are required for disposable equipment that is not contaminated.
- Place *nondisposable* or *reusable* equipment that is visibly soiled in a labeled bag before removing it from the client's room or cubicle, and send it to a central processing area for decontamination. Some agencies may require that glass bottles or jars and metal items be placed in separate bags from rubber and plastic items. Glass and metal can be sterilized in an autoclave, but rubber and plastic are damaged by this process and must be cleaned by other methods, such as gas sterilization.
- Disassemble special procedure trays into component parts. Some components are disposable; others need to be sent to the laundry or central services for cleaning and decontaminating.
- Bag soiled clothing before sending it home or to the agency laundry.

LINENS. Handle soiled linen as little as possible and with the least agitation possible before placing it in the laundry hamper. This prevents gross microbial contamination of the air and persons handling the linen. Close the bag before sending it to the laundry in accordance with agency practice.

LABORATORY SPECIMENS. Laboratory specimens, if placed in a leakproof container with a secure lid with a biohazard label, need no special precautions. Use care when collecting specimens to avoid contaminating the outside of the container. Containers that are visibly contaminated on the outside should be placed inside a sealable plastic bag before sending them to the laboratory. This prevents personnel from having hand contact with potentially infective material.

DISHES. Dishes require no special precautions. Soiling of dishes can largely be prevented by encouraging clients to wash their hands before eating. Some agencies use paper dishes for convenience, which are disposed of in the refuse container.

BLOOD PRESSURE EQUIPMENT. Blood pressure equipment needs no special precautions unless it becomes contaminated with infective material. If it does become contaminated, follow agency practice. Cleaning procedures vary according to whether it is a wall or portable unit.

THERMOMETERS. Nondisposable used thermometers are generally disinfected after use. Check agency practice.

DISPOSABLE NEEDLES, SYRINGES, AND SHARPS. Place needles, syringes, and "sharps" (e.g., lancets, scalpels, and broken glass) into a puncture-resistant container. To avoid puncture wounds, use approved safety or needleless systems and do not detach needles from the syringe or recap the needle before disposal. See Chapter 33 ∞ for how to prevent needlestick injuries.

Transporting Clients with Infections

Transporting clients with infections outside their own rooms is avoided unless absolutely necessary. If a client must be moved, the nurse implements appropriate precautions and measures to prevent soilage of the environment. For example, the nurse ensures that any draining wound is securely covered or places a surgical mask on the client who has an airborne infection. In addition, the nurse notifies personnel at the receiving area of any infection risk so that they can maintain necessary precautions. Follow agency protocol.

Psychosocial Needs of Isolation Clients

Clients requiring isolation precautions can develop several problems as a result of the separation from others and of the special precautions taken in their care. Two of the most common are sensory deprivation and decreased self-esteem related to feelings of inferiority. *Sensory deprivation* occurs when the environment lacks normal stimuli for the client, for example, communication with others. Nurses should therefore be alert to common clinical signs of sensory deprivation: boredom, inactivity, slowness of thought, daydreaming, increased sleeping, thought disorganization, anxiety, hallucinations, and panic.

Chapter 39 ⊙ provides information on the development of self-esteem and self-esteem disturbances. A client's *feeling of inferiority* can be due to the perception of the infection itself or to the required precautions. In North America, many people place a high value on cleanliness, and the idea of being "soiled," "contaminated," or "dirty" can give clients the feeling that they are at fault and substandard. Although this is obviously not true, the infected persons may feel "not as good" as others and blame themselves. An appropriate nursing diagnosis may be *Risk for Situational Low Self-Esteem*.

Nurses need to provide care that prevents these two problems or deals with them positively. Nursing interventions include the following:

1. Assess the individual's need for stimulation.
2. Initiate measures to help meet the need, including regular communication with the client and diversionary activities, such as toys for a child and books, television, or radio for an adult; provide a variety of foods to stimulate the client's sense of taste; stimulate the client's visual sense by providing a view or an activity to watch.
3. Explain the infection and the associated procedures to help clients and their support people understand and accept the situation.
4. Demonstrate warm, accepting behavior. Avoid conveying to the client any sense of annoyance about the precautions or any feelings of revulsion about the infection.

5. Do not use stricter precautions than are indicated by the diagnosis or the client's condition.

STERILE TECHNIQUE

An object is sterile only when it is free of all microorganisms. It is well known that sterile technique is practiced in operating rooms, labor and delivery rooms, and special diagnostic areas. Less known perhaps is that sterile technique is also employed for many procedures in general care areas (such as administering injections, changing wound dressings, performing urinary catheterizations, and administering intravenous therapy). In these situations, all of the principles of surgical asepsis are applied as in the operating or delivery room; however, not all of the sterile techniques that follow are always required. For example, before an operating room procedure, the "scrub" nurse generally puts on a mask and cap, performs a surgical hand scrub, and then dons a sterile gown and gloves. In a general care area, the nurse may only perform a hand wash and don sterile gloves. The basic principles of surgical asepsis, and practices that relate to each principle, appear in Table 29–8.

Sterile Field

A **sterile field** is a microorganism-free area. Nurses often establish a sterile field by using the innermost side of a sterile

TABLE 29–8 Principles and Practices of Surgical Asepsis

Principles	Practices
All objects used in a sterile field must be sterile.	All articles are sterilized appropriately by dry or moist heat, chemicals, or radiation before use.
	Always check a package containing a sterile object for intactness, dryness, and expiration date. Sterile articles can be stored for only a prescribed time; after that, they are considered unsterile. Any package that appears already open, torn, punctured, or wet is considered unsterile.
	Storage areas should be clean, dry, off the floor, and away from sinks.
	Always check chemical indicators of sterilization before using a package. The indicator is often a tape used to fasten the package or contained inside the package. The indicator changes color during sterilization, indicating that the contents have undergone a sterilization procedure. If the color change is not evident, the package is considered unsterile. Commercially prepared sterile packages may not have indicators but are marked with the word sterile.
Sterile objects become unsterile when touched by unsterile objects.	Handle sterile objects that will touch open wounds or enter body cavities only with sterile forceps or sterile gloved hands.
	Discard or resterilize objects that come into contact with unsterile objects.
	Whenever the sterility of an object is questionable, assume the article is unsterile.
Sterile items that are out of vision or below the waist level of the nurse are considered unsterile.	Once left unattended, a sterile field is considered unsterile.
	Sterile objects are always kept in view. Nurses do not turn their backs on a sterile field.
	Only the front part of a sterile gown (from the waist to the shoulder) and 2 inches above the elbows to the cuff of the sleeves are considered sterile.
	Always keep sterile gloved hands in sight and above waist level; touch only objects that are sterile.
	Sterile draped tables in the operating room or elsewhere are considered sterile only at surface level.
	Once a sterile field becomes unsterile, it must be set up again before proceeding.

TABLE 29-8 Principles and Practices of Surgical Asepsis (continued)

Principles	Practices
Sterile objects can become unsterile by prolonged exposure to airborne micro-organisms.	Keep doors closed and traffic to a minimum in areas where a sterile procedure is being performed, because moving air can carry dust and microorganisms.
	Keep areas in which sterile procedures are carried out as clean as possible by frequent damp cleaning with detergent germicides to minimize contaminants in the area.
	Keep hair clean and short or enclose it in a net to prevent hair from falling on sterile objects. Microorganisms on the hair can make a sterile field unsterile.
	Wear surgical caps in operating rooms, delivery rooms, and burn units.
	Refrain from sneezing or coughing over a sterile field. This can make it unsterile because droplets containing microorganisms from the respiratory tract can travel 1 m (3 ft). Some agencies recommend that masks covering the mouth and the nose should be worn by anyone working over a sterile field or an open wound.
	Nurses with mild upper respiratory tract infections refrain from carrying out sterile procedures or wear masks.
	When working over a sterile field, keep talking to a minimum. Avert the head from the field if talking is necessary.
	To prevent microorganisms from falling over a sterile field, refrain from reaching over a sterile field unless sterile gloves are worn and refrain from moving unsterile objects over a sterile field.
Fluids flow in the direction of gravity.	Unless gloves are worn, always hold wet forceps with the tips below the handles. When the tips are held higher than the handles, fluid can flow onto the handle and become contaminated by the hands. When the forceps are again pointed downward, the fluid flows back down and contaminates the tips.
	During a surgical hand wash, hold the hands higher than the elbows to prevent contaminants from the forearms from reaching the hands.
Moisture that passes through a sterile object draws microorganisms from unsterile surfaces above or below to the sterile surface by capillary action.	Sterile moisture-proof barriers are used beneath sterile objects. Liquids (sterile saline or antiseptics) are frequently poured into containers on a sterile field. If they are spilled onto the sterile field, the barrier keeps the liquid from seeping beneath it.
	Keep the sterile covers on sterile equipment dry. Damp surfaces can attract microorganisms in the air.
	Replace sterile drapes that do not have a sterile barrier underneath when they become moist.
The edges of a sterile field are considered unsterile.	A 2.5-cm (1-in.) margin at each edge of an opened drape is considered unsterile because the edges are in contact with unsterile surfaces.
	Place all sterile objects more than 2.5 cm (1 in.) inside the edges of a sterile field.
	Any article that falls outside the edges of a sterile field is considered unsterile.
The skin cannot be sterilized and is unsterile.	Use sterile gloves or sterile forceps to handle sterile items.
	Prior to a surgical aseptic procedure, wash the hands to reduce the number of microorganisms on them.
Conscientiousness, alertness, and honesty are essential qualities in maintaining surgical asepsis.	When a sterile object becomes unsterile, it does not necessarily change in appearance.
	The person who sees a sterile object become contaminated must correct or report the situation.
	Do not set up a sterile field ahead of time for future use.

wrapper or by using a sterile drape. When the field is established, sterile supplies and sterile solutions can be placed on it. Sterile forceps are used in many instances to handle and transfer the sterile supplies.

So that their sterility can be maintained, supplies may be wrapped in a variety of materials. Commercially prepared items are frequently wrapped in plastic, paper, or glass. In the past, it was not unusual for sterile liquids (e.g., sterile water for irrigations) to be supplied in large containers and used many times. This practice is considered undesirable today because once a container has been opened, there can be no assurance that it is sterile. Liquids are preferably packaged in amounts adequate for one use only. Any leftover liquid is discarded.

Procedure 29–3 describes how to establish and maintain a sterile field.

Procedure 29–3 Establishing and Maintaining a Sterile Field

Purposes
- To ensure that sterile items remain sterile

ASSESSMENT

Review the client's record or discuss with the client or other health care team member exactly what procedure will be performed that requires a sterile field. Determine the client's presence or risk for infection and his or her ability to cooperate with the procedure.

PLANNING

Determine, if possible, what supplies and techniques have been used in the past to perform these procedures for this client. Also, attempt to determine if the procedures will be performed again in the future, so that you can conduct appropriate client teaching and have adequate supplies available.

Schedule the procedure at a time consistent with the physician's order, the need for the procedure, and the client's other activities.

Delegation
Sterile procedures are not delegated to unlicensed assistive personnel.

Equipment
- Package containing a sterile drape
- Sterile equipment as needed (e.g., wrapped sterile gauze, wrapped sterile bowl, antiseptic solution, sterile forceps)

IMPLEMENTATION

Preparation
- Ensure that the package is clean and dry; if moisture is noted on the inside of a plastic-wrapped package or the outside of a cloth-wrapped package, it is considered contaminated and must be discarded.
- Check the sterilization expiration dates on the package, and look for any indications that it has been previously opened.
- Follow agency practice about the disposal of possibly contaminated packages.

Performance
1. Explain to the client what you are going to do, why it is necessary, and how he or she can cooperate. Discuss how the results will be used in planning further care or treatments.
2. Observe other appropriate infection control procedures (see Procedures 29–1 and 29–2).
3. Provide for client privacy.
4. Open the package. If the package is inside a plastic cover, remove the cover.

TO OPEN A WRAPPED PACKAGE ON A SURFACE
- Place the package in the center of the work area so that the top flap of the wrapper opens away from you. *This position prevents you from subsequently reaching directly over the exposed sterile contents, which could contaminate them.*

- Reaching around the package (not over it), pinch the first flap on the outside of the wrapper between the thumb and index finger (Figure 29–13 ■). *Touching only the outside of the wrapper maintains the sterility of the inside of the wrapper.*

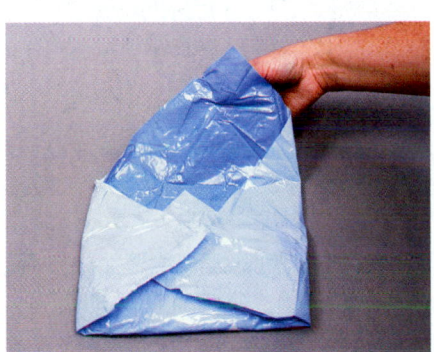

Figure 29–13 ■ Opening the first flap of a sterile wrapped package.

Pull the flap open, laying it flat on the far surface.
- Repeat for the side flaps, opening the top one first. Use the right hand for the right flap, and the left hand for the left flap (Figure 29–14 ■). *By using both hands, you avoid reaching over the sterile contents.*

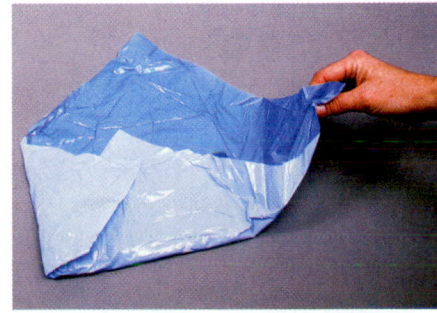

Figure 29–14 ■ Opening the second flap to the side.

- Pull the fourth flap toward you by grasping the corner that is turned down (Figure 29–15 ■). Make sure that the flap does not touch any object. *If the inner surface touches any unsterile article, it is contaminated.*

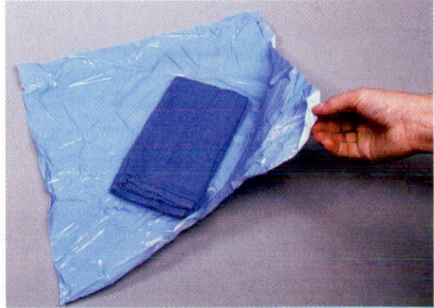

Figure 29–15 ■ Pulling the last flap toward oneself by grasping the corner.

continued on page 658

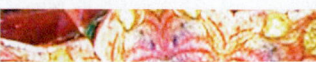

Procedure 29–3 Establishing and Maintaining a Sterile Field *continued*

IMPLEMENTATION *continued*

VARIATION: OPENING A WRAPPED PACKAGE WHILE HOLDING IT

- Hold the package in one hand with the top flap opening away from you.
- Using the other hand, open the package as described above, pulling the corners of the flaps well back (Figure 29–16 ■). *The hands are considered contaminated, and at no time should they touch the contents of the package.*

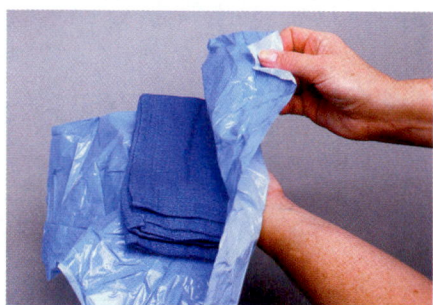

Figure 29–16 ■ Opening a wrapped package while holding it.

VARIATION: OPENING COMMERCIALLY PREPARED PACKAGES

- If the flap of the package has an unsealed corner, hold the container in one hand, and pull back on the flap with the other hand (Figure 29–17 ■).

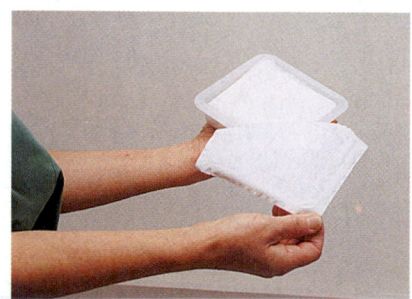

Figure 29–17 ■ Opening a sterile package that has an unsealed corner.

- If the package has a partially sealed edge, grasp both sides of the edge, one with each hand, and pull apart gently (Figure 29–18 ■).

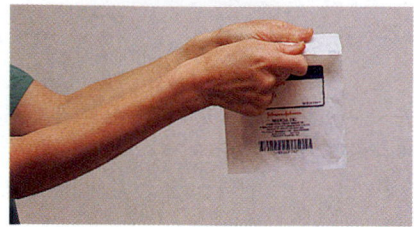

Figure 29–18 ■ Opening a sterile package that has a partially sealed edge.

5. Establish a sterile field by using a drape.
   - Open the package containing the drape as described above.
   - With one hand, pluck the corner of the drape that is folded back on the top.
   - Lift the drape out of the cover, and allow it to open freely without touching any articles (Figure 29–19 ■). *If the drape touches the outside of the package or any unsterile surface, it is considered contaminated.*

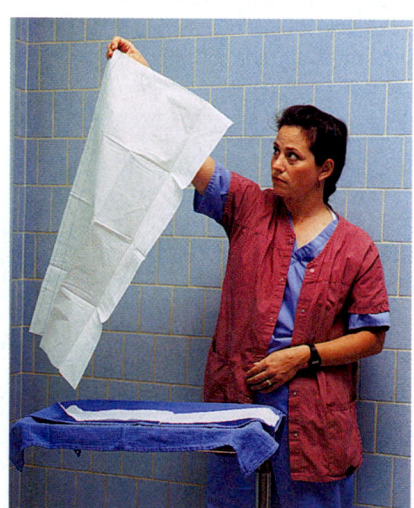

Figure 29–19 ■ Allowing a drape to open freely without touching any objects.

   - Discard the cover.
   - With the other hand, carefully pick up another corner of the drape, holding it well away from you.
   - Lay the drape on a clean and dry surface, placing the bottom (i.e., the freely hanging side) farthest from you (Figure 29–20 ■). *By placing the lowermost side farthest away, you avoid leaning over the sterile field and contaminating it.*
6. Add necessary sterile supplies.

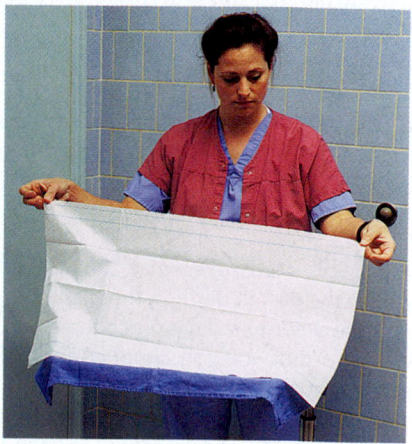

Figure 29–20 ■ Placing a drape on a surface.

TO ADD WRAPPED SUPPLIES TO A STERILE FIELD

- Open each wrapped package as described in the preceding steps.
- With the free hand, grasp the corners of the wrapper, and hold them against the wrist of the other hand (Figure 29–21 ■). *The sterile wrapper now covers the unsterile hand.*

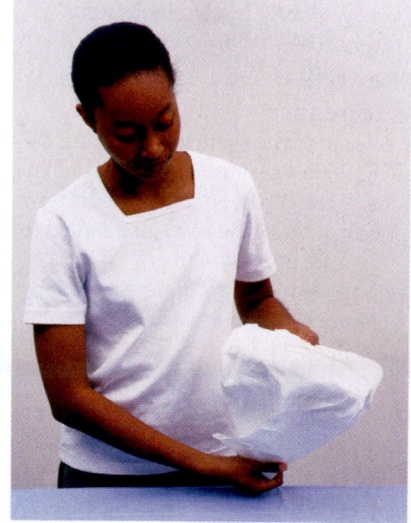

Figure 29–21 ■ Adding wrapped sterile supplies to a sterile field.

- Place the sterile bowl, drape, or other supply on the sterile field by approaching from an angle rather than holding the arm over the field.
- Discard the wrapper.

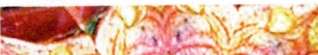

Procedure 29–3 Establishing and Maintaining a Sterile Field *continued*

IMPLEMENTATION *continued*

VARIATION: ADDING COMMERCIALLY PACKAGED SUPPLIES TO A STERILE FIELD

■ Open each package as previously described.
■ Hold the package 15 cm (6 in.) above the field, and allow the contents to drop on the field (Figure 29–22 ■). Keep in mind that 2.5 cm (1 in.) around the edge of the field is considered contaminated. *At a height of 15 cm (6 in.), the outside of the package is not likely to touch and contaminate the sterile field.*

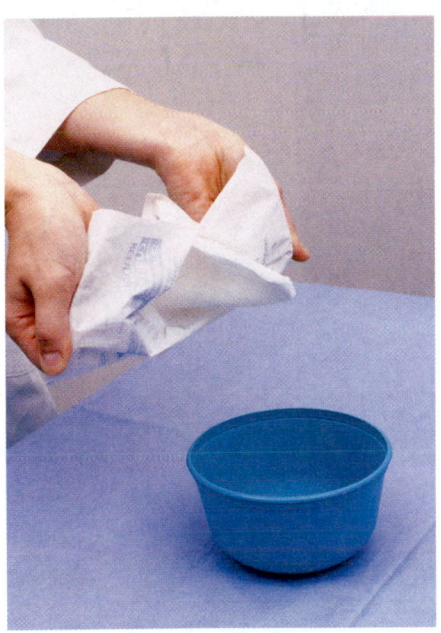

Figure 29–22 ■ Adding commercially packaged gauze to a sterile field.

ADDING SOLUTION TO A STERILE BOWL

Liquids (e.g., normal saline) may need to be poured into containers within a sterile field. Unwrapped bottles or flasks that contain sterile solution are considered sterile on the inside and contaminated on the outside because the bottle may have been handled. Bottles used in an operating room may be sterilized on the outside as well as the inside, however, and these are handled with sterile gloves.

• Before pouring any liquid, read the label three times to make sure you have the correct solution and concentration (strength).

• Obtain the exact amount of solution, if possible. *Once a sterile container has been opened, its sterility cannot be ensured for future use.* Follow agency policy for reuse of open sterile solutions.

• Remove the lid or cap from the bottle and invert the lid before placing it on a surface that is not sterile. *Inverting the lid maintains the sterility of the inside surface because it is not allowed to touch an unsterile surface.*

• Hold the bottle at a slight angle so that the label is uppermost (Figure 29–23 ■). *Any solution that flows down the outside of the bottle during pouring will not damage or obliterate the label.*

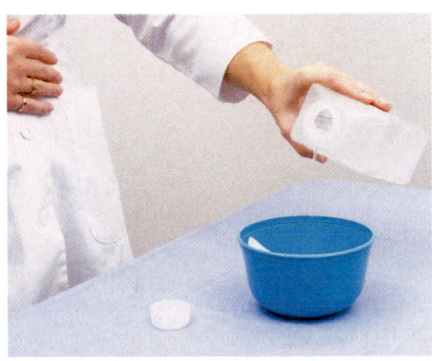

Figure 29–23 ■ Adding a liquid to a sterile bowl.

• Hold the bottle of fluid at a height of 10 to 15 cm (4 to 6 in.) over the bowl and to the side of the sterile field so that as little of the bottle as possible is over the field. *At this height, there is less likelihood of contaminating the sterile field by touching the field or by reaching an arm over it.*

• Pour the solution gently to avoid splashing the liquid. *If a barrier drape (one that has a water-resistant layer) is not used and the drape is on an unsterile surface, moisture will contaminate the field by wicking microorganisms through the drape.*

• If the bottle will be used again, replace the lid securely and write on the label the date and time of opening. *Replacing the lid immediately maintains the sterility of the inner aspect of the lid and the solution.* Depending on agency policy, a sterile container of

solution that is opened may be used only once and then discarded or kept up to 24 hours.

7. Use sterile forceps to handle sterile supplies. Forceps are usually used to move a sterile article from one place to another, for example, transferring sterile gauze from its package to a sterile dressing tray. Forceps may be disposable or resterilized after use. Commonly used forceps include hemostats (Figure 29–24 ■) and tissue forceps (Figure 29–25 ■).

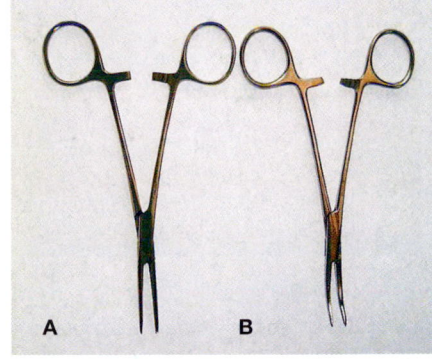

Figure 29–24 ■ Hemostats: *A*, straight; *B*, curved. (Jerry Marshall)

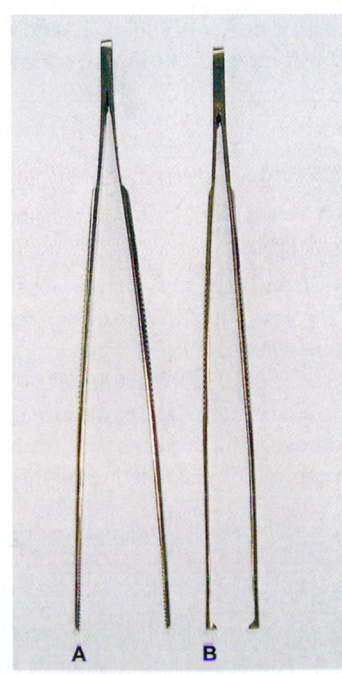

Figure 29–25 ■ Tissue forceps: *A*, plain; *B*, toothed. (Jerry Marshall)

continued on page 660

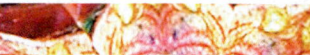

Procedure 29–3 Establishing and Maintaining a Sterile Field *continued*

IMPLEMENTATION *continued*

- Keep the tips of wet forceps lower than the wrist at all times, unless you are wearing sterile gloves (Figure 29–26 ■). *Gravity prevents liquids on the tips of the forceps from flowing to the unsterile handles and later back to the tips.*

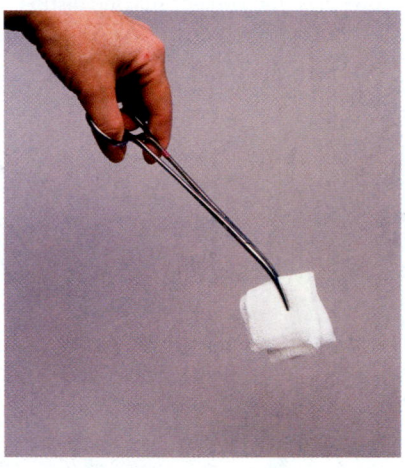

Figure 29–26 ■ Holding forceps with an ungloved hand, keeping the tips lower than the wrist.

- Hold sterile forceps above waist level. *Items held below waist level are considered contaminated.*
- Hold sterile forceps within sight. *While out of sight, forceps may, unknown to the user, become unsterile. Any forceps that go out of sight should be considered unsterile.*
- When using forceps to lift sterile supplies, be sure that the forceps do not touch the edges or outside of the wrapper. *The edges and outside of the sterile field are considered unsterile.*

- When placing forceps whose handles were in contact with the bare hand, position the handles outside the sterile area. *The handles of these forceps harbor microorganisms from the bare hand.*
- Deposit a sterile item on a sterile field without permitting moist forceps to touch the sterile field when the surface under the absorbent sterile field is unsterile and a barrier drape is not used.

8. Document that sterile technique was used in the performance of the procedure.

EVALUATION

Conduct any follow-up indicated during your care of the client. Ensure that adequate numbers and types of sterile supplies are available for the next health care provider.

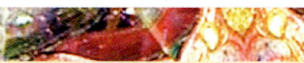

Home Care Considerations

Sterile Field

- Clean and wipe dry a flat surface for the sterile field.
- Keep pets out of the area when setting up for and performing sterile procedures.
- Dispose of all soiled materials in a waterproof bag. Check with the agency as to how to dispose of medical refuse.
- Remove all instruments from the home or other setting where others might accidentally find them. *New or used instruments can be sharp or capable of causing injury. Used instruments may transmit infection.* Check with the agency for instructions on cleansing of reusable supplies and disposal of single-use instruments.
- If appropriate, teach the client and family members the principles of using a sterile field.

Sterile Gloves

Sterile gloves may be donned by the open method or the closed method. The open method is most frequently used outside the operating room because the closed method requires that the nurse wear a sterile gown. Gloves are worn during many procedures to maintain the sterility of equipment and to protect a client's wound.

Sterile gloves are packaged with a cuff of about 5 cm (2 in.) and with the palms facing upward when the package is opened. The package usually indicates the size of the glove (e.g., size 6 or 7½).

Latex, nitrile, and vinyl sterile gloves are available to protect the nurse from contact with blood and body fluids. Latex and nitrile are more flexible than vinyl, mold to the wearer's hands, allow freedom of movement, and have the added feature of re-sealing tiny punctures automatically. Therefore, wear latex or ni-trile gloves when performing tasks (a) that demand flexibility, (b) that place stress on the material (e.g., turning stopcocks, han-dling sharp instruments or tape), and (c) that involve a high risk

of exposure to pathogens. Vinyl gloves should be chosen for tasks unlikely to stress the glove material, requiring minimal pre-cision, and with minimal risk of exposure to pathogens.

Procedure 29–4 describes how to don and remove sterile gloves by the open method.

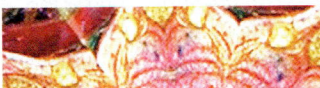

Procedure 29–4 Donning and Removing Sterile Gloves (Open Method)

Purposes

- To enable the nurse to handle or touch sterile objects freely without contaminating them

- To prevent transmission of potentially infective organisms from the nurse's hands to clients at high risk for infection

ASSESSMENT

Review the client's record and orders to determine exactly what procedure will be performed that requires sterile gloves. Check the client record and ask about latex allergies.

PLANNING

Think through the procedure, planning which steps need to be completed before the gloves can be applied. Determine what addi-tional supplies are needed to perform the procedure for this client. Always have an extra pair of sterile gloves available.

Delegation

Sterile procedures are not delegated to unlicensed assistive per-sonnel.

Equipment

- Packages of sterile gloves

IMPLEMENTATION

Preparation

Ensure the sterility of the package of gloves.

Performance

1. Explain to the client what you are go-ing to do, why it is necessary, and how he or she can cooperate. Discuss how the results will be used in planning fur-ther care or treatments.
2. Observe other appropriate infection control procedures (see Procedures 29–1, 29–2, and 29–3).
3. Provide for client privacy.
4. Open the package of sterile gloves.
   - Place the package of gloves on a clean, dry surface. *Any moisture on the surface could contaminate the gloves.*
   - Some gloves are packed in an inner as well as an outer package. Open the outer package without contami-nating the gloves or the inner pack-age. See Procedure 29–3.
   - Remove the inner package from the outer package.
   - Open the inner package as in step 4 of Procedure 29–3 or according to the manufacturer's directions. Some manufacturers provide a numbered sequence for opening the flaps and

folded tabs to grasp for opening the flaps. If no tabs are provided, pluck the flap so that the fingers do not touch the inner surfaces. *The inner surfaces, which are next to the sterile gloves, will remain sterile.*

5. Put the first glove on the dominant hand.
   - If the gloves are packaged so that they lie side by side, grasp the glove for the dominant hand by its folded cuff edge (on the palmar side) with the thumb and first finger of the nondominant hand. Touch only the inside of the cuff (Figure 29–27 ■). *The hands are not sterile. By touching*

only the inside of the glove, the nurse avoids contaminating the outside.
or
   - If the gloves are packaged one on top of the other, grasp the cuff of the top glove as above, using the oppo-site hand.
   - Insert the dominant hand into the glove and pull the glove on. Keep the thumb of the inserted hand against the palm of the hand during inser-tion (Figure 29–28 ■). *If the thumb is kept against the palm, it is less likely to contaminate the outside of the glove.*
   - Leave the cuff turned down.

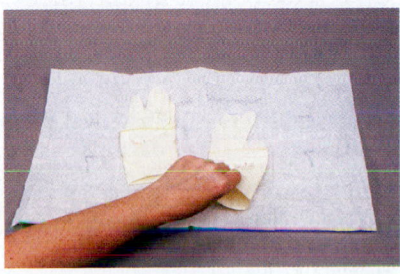

Figure 29–27 ■ Picking up the first sterile glove.

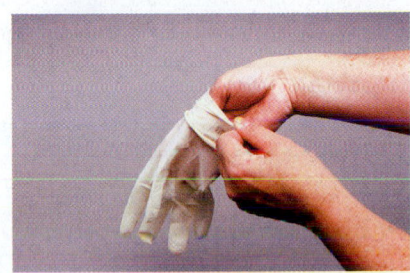

Figure 29–28 ■ Putting on the first sterile glove.

continued on page 662

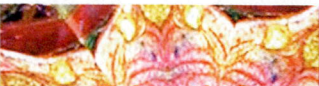

Procedure 29–4 Donning and Removing Sterile Gloves (Open Method) *continued*

IMPLEMENTATION *continued*

6. Put the second glove on the nondominant hand.
   - Pick up the other glove with the sterile gloved hand, inserting the gloved fingers under the cuff and holding the gloved thumb close to the gloved palm (Figure 29–29 ■). *This helps prevent accidental contamination of the glove by the bare hand.*

- Pull on the second glove carefully. Hold the thumb of the gloved first hand as far as possible from the palm (Figure 29–30 ■). *In this position, the thumb is less likely to touch the arm and become contaminated.*

- Adjust each glove so that it fits smoothly, and carefully pull the cuffs up by sliding the fingers under the cuffs.
7. Remove and dispose of used gloves.
   - There is no special technique for removing sterile gloves. If they are soiled with secretions, remove them by turning them inside out. See removal of disposable gloves in Procedure 29–2 on page 652.
8. Document that sterile technique was used in the performance of the procedure.

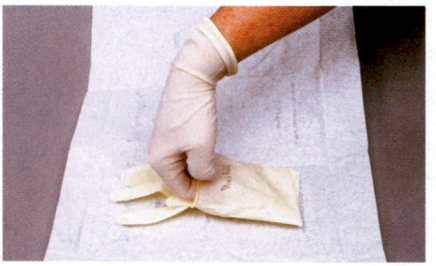

Figure 29–29 ■ Picking up the second sterile glove.

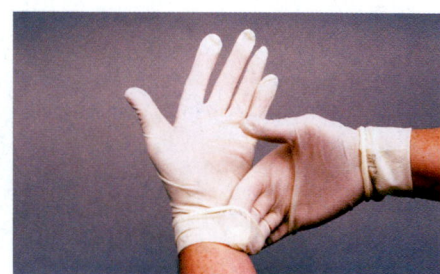

Figure 29–30 ■ Putting on the second sterile glove

EVALUATION

Conduct any follow-up indicated during your care of the client. Ensure that adequate numbers and types of sterile supplies are available for the next health care provider.

Sterile Gowns

Sterile gowning and closed gloving are chiefly carried out in operating or delivery rooms, where surgical asepsis is necessary. The closed method of gloving can be used only when a sterile gown is worn because the gloves are handled through the sleeves of the gown. Before these procedures, the nurse dons a hair cover and a mask, and performs a surgical hand wash.

Procedure 29–5 describes the steps in donning a sterile gown and sterile gloves by the closed method.

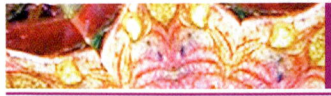

Procedure 29–5 Donning a Sterile Gown and Gloves (Closed Method)

Purposes

- To enable the nurse to work close to a sterile field and handle sterile objects freely

- To protect clients from becoming contaminated with microorganisms on the nurse's hands, arms, and clothing

ASSESSMENT

Review the client's record and orders to determine exactly what procedure will be performed that requires sterile gloves. Check the client record and ask about latex allergies.

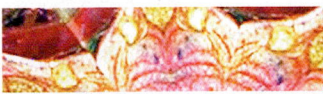

Procedure 29–5 Donning a Sterile Gown and Gloves (Closed Method) *continued*

PLANNING

Think through the procedure, planning which steps need to be completed before the gloves and gown can be applied. Determine what additional supplies are needed to perform the procedure for this client. Always have an extra pair of sterile gloves available.

Delegation

Sterile procedures are not delegated to unlicensed assistive personnel.

Equipment

- Sterile pack containing a sterile gown
- Sterile gloves

IMPLEMENTATION

Preparation

Ensure the sterility of the package of gloves.

Performance

1. Explain to the client what you are going to do, why it is necessary, and how he or she can cooperate. Discuss how the results will be used in planning further care or treatments.
2. Observe other appropriate infection control procedures (see Procedures 29–1, 29–2, and 29–3).
3. Provide for client privacy.

DONNING A STERILE GOWN

4. Open the package of sterile gloves.
   - Remove the outer wrap from the sterile gloves and leave the gloves in their inner sterile wrap on the sterile field. *If the inner wrapper is not touched, it will remain sterile.* See Procedure 29–3, step 4.
5. Unwrap the sterile gown pack.
6. Wash and dry hands carefully. See "Variation" at the end of Procedure 29–1 and review agency practice.
7. Put on the sterile gown.
   - Grasp the sterile gown at the crease near the neck, hold it away from you, and permit it to unfold freely without touching anything, including the uniform. *The gown will be unsterile if its outer surface touches any unsterile objects.*
   - Put the hands inside the shoulders of the gown, and work the arms partway into the sleeves without touching the outside of the gown (Figure 29–31 ■).

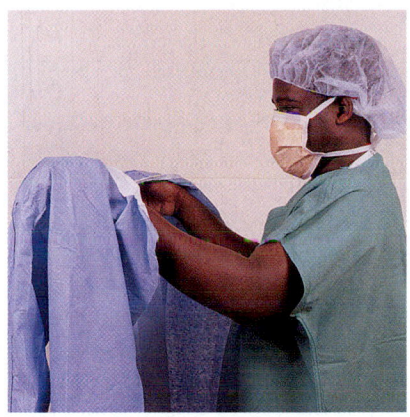

Figure 29–31 ■ Putting on a sterile gown.

   - If donning sterile gloves by using the closed method (see below), work the hands down the sleeves only to the proximal edge of the cuffs.
     or
   - If donning sterile gloves by using the open method, work the hands down the sleeves and through the cuffs.
   - Have a coworker grasp the neck ties without touching the outside of the gown and pull the gown upward to cover the neckline of your uniform in front and back. The coworker ties the neck ties. Gowning continues at step 11.

DONNING STERILE GLOVES (CLOSED METHOD)

8. Open the sterile wrapper containing the sterile gloves.
   - Open the sterile glove wrapper while the hands are still covered by the sleeves (Figure 29–32 ■).

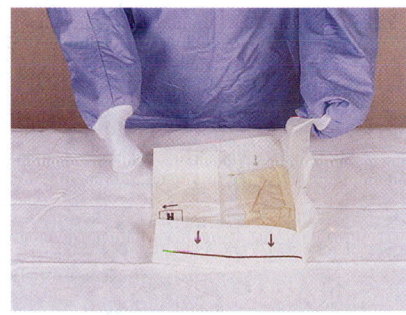

Figure 29–32 ■ Opening the sterile glove wrapper.

9. Put the glove on the nondominant hand. Figures 29–33 ■ through 29–35 ■ show a right-handed person.

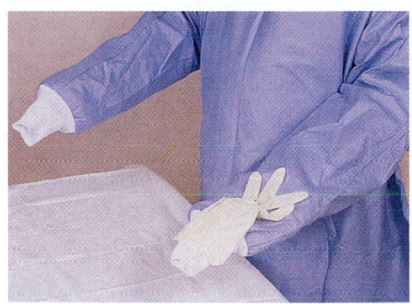

Figure 29–33 ■ Positioning the first sterile glove for the nondominant hand.

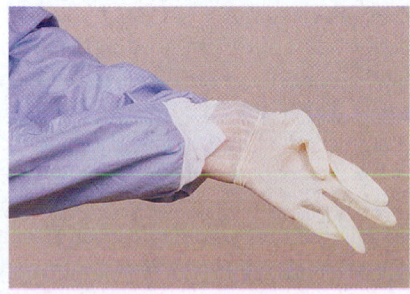

Figure 29–34 ■ Pulling on the first sterile glove.

continued on page 664

Procedure 29–5 Donning a Sterile Gown and Gloves (Closed Method) *continued*

IMPLEMENTATION *continued*

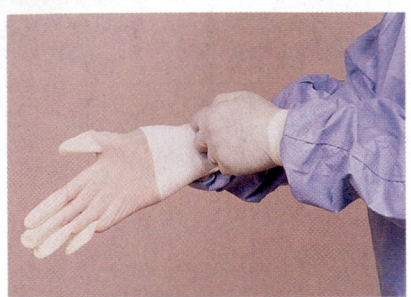

Figure 29–35 ■ Extending the fingers into the second glove of the dominant hand.

- With the dominant hand, pick up the opposite glove with the thumb and index finger, handling it through the sleeve.
- Lay the glove on the opposite gown cuff, thumb side down, with the glove opening pointed toward the fingers (Figure 29–33). Position the dominant hand palm upward inside the sleeve.
- Use the nondominant hand to grasp the cuff of the glove through the gown cuff, and firmly anchor it.

- With the dominant hand working through its sleeve, grasp the upper side of the glove's cuff, and stretch it over the cuff of the gown.
- Pull the sleeve up to draw the cuff over the wrist as you extend the fingers of the nondominant hand into the glove's fingers (Figure 29–34).

10. Put the glove on the dominant hand.
    - Place the fingers of the gloved hand under the cuff of the remaining glove.
    - Place the glove over the cuff of the second sleeve.
    - Extend the fingers into the glove as you pull the glove up over the cuff (Figure 29–35).

COMPLETION OF GOWNING

11. Complete gowning as follows.
    - Have a coworker hold the waist tie of your gown, using sterile gloves or a sterile forceps or drape. *This approach keeps the ties sterile.*
    - Make a three-quarter turn, then take the tie and secure it in front of the gown.

or
- Have a coworker take the two ties at each side of the gown and tie them at the back of the gown, making sure that your uniform is completely covered.
- When worn, sterile gowns should be considered sterile in front from the waist to the shoulder. The sleeves should be considered sterile from 2 inches above the elbow to the cuff, since the arms of a scrubbed person must move across a sterile field. Moisture collection and friction areas such as the neckline, shoulders, underarms, back, and sleeve cuffs should be considered unsterile.

12. Remove and dispose of used gown and gloves.
    - There is no special technique for removing sterile attire. If soiled, remove the attire by turning it inside out. See removal of disposable gowns and gloves in Procedure 29–2.

13. If appropriate, document that sterile technique was used in the performance of the procedure.

EVALUATION

Conduct any follow-up indicated during your care of the client. Ensure that adequate numbers and types of sterile supplies are available for the next health care provider.

INFECTION CONTROL FOR HEALTH CARE WORKERS

NIOSH is part of the CDC and is a research agency of the U.S. Department of Health and Human Services. NIOSH investigates potentially hazardous working conditions and publishes recommendations for preventing workplace illnesses and injuries. For example, NIOSH published a study on preventing needlestick injuries in health care settings in 1999 that found that the majority of needlestick injuries were preventable. This, in part, led to the Needlestick Safety and Prevention Act that went into effect in April 2001.

The Occupational Safety and Health Administration (OSHA), an agency of the U.S. Department of Labor, publishes and enforces regulations to protect health care workers from occupational injuries, including exposure to bloodborne pathogens in the workplace. **Occupational exposure** is defined by OSHA as reasonably anticipated skin, eye, mucous membrane, or parenteral contact with blood or other potentially infectious materials that may result from the performance of an employee's duties (U.S. Department of Labor, OSHA, 1991).

There are three major modes of transmission of infectious materials in the clinical setting:

- Puncture wounds from contaminated needles or other sharps
- Skin contact, which allows infectious fluids to enter through wounds and broken or damaged skin
- Mucous membrane contact, which allows infectious fluids to enter through mucous membranes of the eyes, mouth, and nose.

Using proper precautions with general medical asepsis, appropriately using personal protective equipment (gloves, masks, gowns, goggles, shoe covers, special resuscitative equipment), and avoiding carelessness in the clinical area will place the caregiver at significantly less risk for injury. The chance of a health care worker becoming infected following

Practice Guidelines
Steps to Follow after Exposure to Bloodborne Pathogens

- Report the incident immediately to appropriate personnel within the agency.
- Complete an injury report.
- Seek appropriate evaluation and follow-up. This includes:
  - Identification and documentation of the source individual when feasible and legal
  - Testing of the source for hepatitis B, hepatitis C, and HIV when feasible and consent is given
  - Making results of the test available to the source individual's health care provider
  - Testing of blood of exposed nurse (with consent) for hepatitis B, hepatitis C, and HIV antibodies
  - Postexposure prophylaxis if medically indicated
  - Medical and psychological counseling regarding personal risk of infection or risk of infecting others.
- For a puncture/laceration:
  - encourage bleeding
  - wash/clean the area with soap and water
  - initiate first-aid and seek treatment if indicated.
- For a mucous membrane exposure (eyes, nose, mouth), saline or water flush for 5 to 10 minutes.

Postexposure Protocol (PEP)
HIV:
- For "high-risk" exposure (high blood volume *and* source with a high HIV titer): three-drug treatment is recommended. Must be started within 1 hour.
- For "increased risk" exposure (high blood volume *or* source with a high HIV titer): three-drug treatment is recommended. Must be started within 1 hour.
- For "low-risk" exposure (neither high blood volume nor source with a high HIV titer): two-drug treatment is considered. Must be started within 1 hour.
- Drug prophylaxis continues for 4 weeks.
- Drug regimens vary. Drugs commonly used are zidovudine, lamivudine, didanosine, and indinavir.
- HIV antibody tests done shortly after exposure (baseline), and 6 weeks, 3 months, and 6 months afterward.

Hepatitis B
- Anti-HBs testing 1 to 2 months after last vaccine dose.

Hepatitis C
- Anti-HCV and ALT at baseline and 4 to 6 months after exposure

exposure to pathogens varies widely—estimates range from 30% for hepatitis B (nonimmune workers), to 1.8% for hepatitis C, to 0.3% for HIV (CDC, 2001). Measures to be taken in case of possible exposure to these viruses are delineated by the CDC and outlined in the accompanying Practice Guidelines feature. Hepatitis C, a worldwide epidemic greater than HIV, has become a significant concern to all health care workers since there is currently no vaccine against the virus nor postexposure prophylaxis. Prevention remains the primary goal.

OSHA requires that health care employers make the hepatitis B vaccine and vaccination series available to all employees. Other vaccinations may also be made available (e.g., nurses working in an obstetric area should be vaccinated against rubella to protect pregnant clients and their fetuses).

> **CLINICAL ALERT** *The nurse should consider in advance whether or not he or she would want prophylaxis for HIV exposure since this must be started within 1 hour of exposure.*

ROLE OF THE INFECTION CONTROL NURSE

All health care organizations must have interdisciplinary infection control committees. Representatives from the clinical laboratory, housekeeping, maintenance, dietary, and client care areas are included. An important member of this committee is the infection control nurse. This nurse is specially trained to be knowledgeable about the latest research and practices in preventing, detecting, and treating infections. All infections are reported to the nurse in a manner that allows for recording and analyzing statistics that can assist in improving infection control practices. In addition, the infection control nurse may be involved in employee education and implementation of the bloodborne pathogen exposure control plan mandated by OSHA.

EVALUATING

Using data collected during care—vital signs, lung sounds, skin status, characteristics of urine or other drainage, laboratory blood values, and so on—the nurse judges whether client outcomes have been achieved. Examples of client outcomes and indicators are shown in Identifying Nursing Diagnoses, Outcomes, and Interventions.

If outcomes are not achieved, the nurse may need to consider questions such as the following:

- Were appropriate measures implemented to prevent skin breakdown and lung infection?
- Was strict aseptic technique implemented for invasive procedures?
- Are prescribed medications affecting the immune system?
- Is client placement appropriate to reduce the risk of transmission of microorganisms?
- Did the client and family misunderstand or fail to comply with necessary instructions?

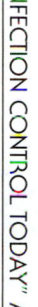

MediaLink GO TO "INFECTION CONTROL TODAY" APPLICATION

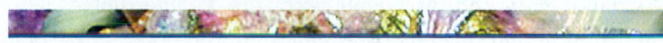

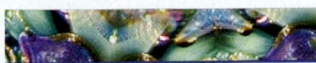

Focus on Critical Thinking

Mrs. Cortez is a 76-year-old woman who is independent, lives alone, and prefers not to rely on others unless absolutely necessary. She was active and healthy until about 6 months ago, at which time she developed a persistent upper respiratory infection. Because she was unable to obtain or prepare foods, she lost weight and became very weak. She finally sought medical attention, but she has not yet fully recovered. Her primary care provider has admitted Mrs. Cortez to the acute care facility for shortness of breath, productive cough, dehydration, and nutritional deficiency.

1. Mrs. Cortez's primary care provider suspects that Mrs. Cortez has pneumonia. What data support Mrs. Cortez's increased risk for such an infection?
2. What other information or assessment data would be helpful to you when planning care for Mrs. Cortez?

3. You recognize that standard precautions are instituted for all hospitalized clients. Explain why the use of such precautions may not prevent the spread of Mrs. Cortez's respiratory infection to other susceptible clients.
4. What can you do to prevent the spread of Mrs. Cortez's infection to other hospitalized clients and at the same time prevent Mrs. Cortez from getting infections from other clients?
5. You see the nursing assistant leaving Mrs. Cortez's room. The assistant stops to wash her hands. She turns on the water handles and soaps and rubs her hands together under running water for about 5 seconds. She then turns off the faucets with her bare hands and proceeds with drying her hands. Should you intervene and, if so, what should you do?

See Critical Thinking Possibilities in Appendix A.

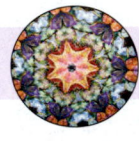 # Chapter Review

EXPLORE MediaLink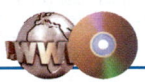

NCLEX review questions, case studies, care plan activities, MediaLink applications, and other interactive resources for this chapter can be found on the Companion Website at www.prenhall.com/kozier. Click on Chapter 29 to select the activities for this chapter.

For more NCLEX review questions, and an audio glossary, access the Student CD-ROM accompanying this textbook.

Chapter Highlights

- Microorganisms are everywhere. Most are harmless and some are beneficial; however, many can cause infection in susceptible persons.
- Effective control of infectious disease is an international, national, community, and individual responsibility.
- Asepsis is the freedom from infection or infectious material.
- Medical aseptic practices limit the number, growth, and transmission of microorganisms.
- Surgical aseptic practices keep an area or objects free of all microorganisms.
- The incidence of nosocomial infections is significant. Major sites for these infections are the respiratory and urinary tracts, the bloodstream, and wounds.
- Factors that contribute to nosocomial infection risks are invasive procedures, medical therapies, the existence of a large number of susceptible persons, inappropriate use of antibiotics, and insufficient hand washing after client contact and after contact with body substances.
- An infection can develop if the links in the chain of infection—infectious agent, reservoir, portal of exit, mode of transmission, portal of entry, and susceptible host—are not interrupted.
- Intact skin and mucous membranes are the body's first line of defense against microorganisms.

- Some normal body flora release bacteriocins and antibiotic-like substances that inhibit microbial growth and destroy foreign bacteria.
- Some body secretions (e.g., saliva and tears) contain enzymes that act as antibacterial agents.
- The inflammatory response limits physical, chemical, and microbial injury and promotes repair of injured tissue.
- Immunity is the specific resistance of the body to infectious agents.
- Acquired immunity is active or passive and in either case may be naturally or artificially induced.
- Especially at risk of acquiring an infection are the very young or old; those with poor nutritional status, a deficiency of serum immunoglobulins, multiple stressors, insufficient immunizations, or an existing disease process; and those receiving certain medical therapies.
- Preventing infections in healthy or ill persons and preventing the transmission of microorganisms from infected clients to others are major nursing functions.
- The nurse must be knowledgeable about sources and modes of transmission of microorganisms.
- Microorganisms are invisible, and nurses have an ethical obligation to ensure that appropriate aseptic measures are taken

to protect clients, support people, and health personnel, including themselves.
- All health care providers must apply clean or sterile gloves, gowns, masks, and protective eyewear according to the risk of exposure to potentially infective materials.

- Should a health care worker be exposed to substances with high risk of transmitting bloodborne pathogens, postexposure practices and consideration of prophylactic treatment must be followed immediately.

Review Questions

29–1. In the situation in which the client is a chronic carrier of infection, in order to prevent the spread of the infection, the most effective action is to
   a. eliminate the reservoir.
   b. block the portal of exit from the reservoir.
   c. block the portal of entry into the host.
   d. decrease the susceptibility of the host.

29–2. Research has shown that the most effective infection control procedure is
   a. hand washing before and after client contact.
   b. wearing gloves and masks for direct client care.
   c. isolation precautions.
   d. broad-spectrum prophylactic antibiotics.

29–3. In caring for a client on contact precautions for a draining infected foot ulcer, correct technique includes
   a. wearing a mask during dressing changes.
   b. providing disposable meal trays and silverware.
   c. following standard precautions in all interactions with the client.

   d. using surgical aseptic technique for all direct contact with the client.

29–4. Which of the following personal protective equipment may be reused by the same nurse during a single shift caring for a single client?
   a. goggles
   b. gown
   c. surgical mask
   d. clean gloves

29–5. While donning sterile gloves (open method), the cuff of the first glove rolls under itself about ¼ inch. The best action for the nurse is to
   a. remove the glove and start over with a new pair.
   b. wait until the second glove is in place and then unroll the cuff with the other sterile hand.
   c. ask a colleague to assist by unrolling the cuff.
   d. leave the cuff rolled under.

Readings and References

Suggested Readings
Bockhold, K. M. (2000). Who's afraid of hepatitis C? *American Journal of Nursing, 100*(5), 26–31. This article focuses on the risks of acquiring the hepatitis C virus from an occupational exposure. Since there is currently no vaccine for hepatitis C, it poses a different risk than hepatitis B. Like B, it can be transmitted through blood and sexual contact. The article reviews techniques for preventing occupational bloodborne pathogen exposure.

Guidelines for preventing opportunistic infections among hematopoietic stem cell transplant recipients (2000). *Morbidity and Mortality Weekly Report, 49*(RR-10), 1–128. Of the 211 guidelines in this CDC report for reducing the chances of infection acquired by patients from health care workers and other exogenous sources, the first and most important is hand washing on entering and leaving the patient's room and prior to any direct contact.

Larson, E. L., & Aiello, A. E. (2001). Hygiene and health: An epidemiologic link? *American Journal of Infection Control, 29*, 232–238. The authors surveyed the literature looking for studies that reported a relationship between personal and household hygiene and the risk of infection. Fifty studies in the past 20 years indicated that reduced incidence of infection was associated with clean water, waste disposal,

and hand washing. In addition, these activities were substantiated in their effectiveness in a variety of settings. The use of special soaps and cleaning techniques was not shown to be particularly effective.

Related Research
Assadian, O., El-Madani, N., Seper, E., Mustafa, S., Aspock, C., Koller, W., et al. (2002). Sensor-operated faucets: A possible source of nosocomial infection? *Infection Control and Hospital Epidemiology, 23*, 44–46.

References
Bischoff, W. E., Reynolds, T. M., Sessler, C. N., Edmond, M. B., & Wenzel, R. P. (2000). Handwashing compliance by health care workers: The impact of introducing an accessible, alcohol-based hand antiseptic. *Archives of Internal Medicine, 160*, 1017–1021.

Centers for Disease Control. (1987). Recommendations for prevention of HIV transmission in health-care settings. *Morbidity and Mortality Weekly Report (suppl.), 36*(2s), 1S–18S.

Centers for Disease Control. (1997). 1997 USPHS/IDSA guidelines for the prevention of opportunistic infections in persons infected with human immunodeficiency virus.

Morbidity and Mortality Weekly Report, 46(RR12), 1–46.

Centers for Disease Control and Prevention. (2001). Updated U. S. Public Health Service guidelines for the management of occupational exposures to HBV, HCV, and HIV and recommendations for post-exposure prophylaxis. *Morbidity and Mortality Weekly Report, 50*(No. RR-11).

Centers for Disease Control and Prevention. (2002). Guideline for hand hygiene in health-care settings: Recommendations of the Healthcare Infection Control Practices Advisory Committee and the HICPAC/SHEA/APIC/IDSA Hand Hygiene Task Force. *Morbidity and Mortality Weekly Report, 51*(No. RR-16).

Centers for Disease Control and Prevention. (2003). *Recommended childhood and adolescent immunization schedule, United States, 2003.* Retrieved March 25, 2003 from http://www.cdc.gov/nip/recs/child-schedule.htm

Corbin, D. E. (2002). Latex allergy & dermatitis. *Occupational Health & Safety, 71*, 36–38, 89.

Earl, M. E., Jackson, M. M., & Rickman, L. S. (2001). Improved rates of compliance with hand antisepsis guidelines: A three-phase observational study. *American Journal of Nursing, 101*(3), 26–33.

Garner, J. S., & Hospital Infection Control Practices Advisory Committee. (1996). Guidelines for isolation precautions in hospitals. *Infection Control Hospital Epidemiology, 17,* 53–80, and *American Journal of Infection Control, 24,* 24–52.

Garner, J. S., & Simmons, B. P. (1983). *CDC guideline for isolation precautions in hospitals* (HHS Publication No. CDC 83-8314). Atlanta, GA: U.S. Department of Health and Human Services, Public Health Service, Centers for Disease Control.

Hospital Infection Control Practices Advisory Committee. (1995). Recommendations for preventing the spread of vancomycin resistance. *American Journal of Infection Control, 23,* 87–94; *Infection Control and Hospital Epidemiology, 16,* 105–113; and *Morbidity and Mortality Weekly Report, 44*(No. RR-12), 1–13.

Jackson, M. M. (1993). Infection precautions: What works and what does not. *CRNA: The Clinical Forum for Nurse Anesthetists, 4* (2), 77–82.

Johnson, M., Maas, M., & Moorhead, S. (Eds.). (2000). *Nursing outcomes classification (NOC)* (2nd ed.). St. Louis, MO: Mosby.

McCloskey, J. C., & Bulechek, G. M. (Eds.). (2000). *Nursing interventions classification (NIC)* (3rd ed.). St. Louis, MO: Mosby.

National Institute for Occupational Safety and Health. (1999). *Preventing needlestick injuries in health care settings.* Cincinnati, OH: U.S. Department of Health and Human Services, Public Health Service, Centers for Disease Control and Prevention, National Institute for Occupational Safety and Health, DHHS Publication No. 2000-108.

NANDA International. (2003). NANDA *nursing diagnoses: Definitions and classification 2003-2004.* Philadelphia: Author.

Notice to readers: Recommended adult immunization schedule—United States, 2002–2003. (2002). *MMWR, 51,* 904–908.

U.S. Department of Health and Human Services, Public Health Service. (1988). Update: Universal precautions for prevention of transmission of human immunodeficiency virus, hepatitis B virus, and other bloodborne pathogens in health care settings. *Morbidity and Mortality Weekly Report, 37*(24), 377–388.

U.S. Department of Labor, Occupational Safety and Health Administration. (1991). Occupational exposure to bloodborne pathogens: Final rule. 29 CFR Part 1910.1029. *Federal Register, 56*(235), 64175–64182.

Selected Bibliography

Bolyard, E. A., Tablan, O. C., Williams, W. W., Pearson, M. L., Shapiro, C. N., & Deitchman, S. D. (1998). Guideline for infection control in healthcare personnel. *Infection Control and Hospital Epidemiology, 19*(6), 407–463.

Centers for Disease Control and Prevention. (2001). Updated U.S. Public Health Service guidelines for the management of occupational exposures to HBV, HCV, and HIV and recommendations for postexposure prophylaxis. *Morbidity and Mortality Weekly Report 50*(RR-11), 1–67.

Friedman, M. M., & Rhinehart, E. (1999). Putting infection control principles into practice in home care. *Nursing Clinics of North America, 34,* 463–482.

Garcia-Martin, M., Lardelli-Claret, P., Jimenez-Moleon, J. J., Bueno-Cavanillas, A., de Dios Luna del Castillo, J., & Galvez-Vargas, R. (2001). Proportion of hospital deaths potentially attributable to nosocomial infection. *Infection Control and Hospital Epidemiology, 22,* 708–714.

Garner, J. S., & Favero, M. S. (1998). Guideline for handwashing and hospital environmental control, 1985, updated. *Morbidity and Mortality Weekly Report, 37*(24). Available from http://www.cdc.gov

Global Consensus Conference. (1999). Final recommendations. *American Journal of Infection Control, 27,* 503–513.

Gritter, M. (1998). The latex threat. *American Journal of Nursing, 98*(9), 26–33.

Hanchett, M. (1998). Implementing standard precautions in home care. *Home Care Manager, 2*(2), 16–20.

Hench, C., & Simpkins, S. (2002, June 17). Hepatitis C: Risk factors, assessment and diagnosis. *NurseWeek,* pp. 19–20.

Hench, C., & Simpkins, S. (2002, July 1). Hepatitis C: Treatment, prevention, and nursing interventions. *NurseWeek,* pp. 22–23.

Jarvis, J. R. (2001). Infection control and changing health-care delivery systems. *Emerging Infectious Diseases, 7,* 170–173.

Kiernan, M. (1999). Handwashing in infection control. *Community Nurse, 5*(7), 19–20.

Kingston, J. (1999). Infection control: Is everybody doing it? *Nursing Times, 95*(44), 60–62.

Lenehan, G. (2002). Latex allergy: Separating fact from fiction. *Nursing, 32*(3), 58–63.

Mayone-Ziomek, J. M. (1998). Handwashing in health care. *Medsurg Nursing, 6,* 364–369.

McConnell, E. A. (1999). Proper hand-washing technique. *Nursing, 29*(4), 26.

Metules, T. J. (2000). Tips for nurses who wash too much. *RN, 63*(3), 34–37.

Metules, T. J. (2001). Protect your eyes. *RN, 64*(10), 69–71.

Occupational Safety and Health Association. (1999). Potential for allergy to natural rubber latex gloves and other natural rubber products. (Technical information bulletin). Retrieved March 23, 2003, from http://www.osha.gov/dts/tib/tib_data/tib19990412.html

Parker, L. J. (1999). Importance of handwashing in the prevention of cross-infection. *British Journal of Nursing, 8,* 716, 718–720.

Perry, C., & Barnett, J. (1998). Principles of universal precautions. *Emergency Nurse, 6*(6), 25–28.

Richards, M. J., Edwards, J. R., Culver, D. H., & Gaynes, R. P. (2000). Nosocomial infections in combined medical-surgical intensive care units in the United States. *Infection Control and Hospital Epidemiology, 21,* 510–515.

Rosenheimer, L. (1999). Establishing an effective infection control and surveillance program in the home care setting. *Home HealthCare Consultant, 6*(12), 38–42.

Schick, R. (1999). Product focus: Hand-washing techniques. *Nursing Homes, 48*(6), 63–67.

Seal, D. V., Hay, R. J., & Middleton, K. R. (2000). *Skin and wound infection: Investigation and treatment in practice.* London: Martin Dunitz.

Shulmeister, L. (1999). I know handwashing is important, but. . . *Clinical Journal of Oncology Nursing, 3,* 139–140.

Stone, S. P. (2001). Hand hygiene: The case for evidence-based education. *Journal of the Royal Society of Medicine, 94,* 278–281.

U.S. Department of Health and Human Services, Centers for Disease Control and Prevention. (1997, September 8). Draft guidelines for infection control in healthcare personnel, 1997. *Federal Register, 62,* 173.

Ward, D. J. (2001). Infection control policies in nursing homes. *Nursing Standard, 15*(46), 40–44.

Wilson, J., & Jenner, E. A. (2001). *Infection control in clinical practice* (2nd ed.). Philadelphia: W. B. Saunders.

Winslow, E. H., & Jacobsen, A. F. (2001). Combatting infection: The case against artificial nails, *Nursing, 31*(10), 30.

Worthington, K. (2001). You've been stuck: What do you do? *American Journal of Nursing, 101*(3), 104.

Xavier, G. (1999). Asepsis. *Nursing Standard, 13*(36), 49–53, 56.

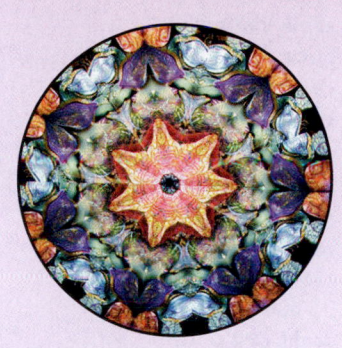

CHAPTER 30

SAFETY

LEARNING OUTCOMES

After completing this chapter, you will be able to:

- Discuss factors that affect people's ability to protect themselves from injury.

- Describe methods to assess clients at risk for injury.

- Identify common potential hazards throughout the life span.

- Give examples of nursing diagnoses, outcomes, and interventions for clients at risk for accidental injury.

- Plan strategies to maintain safety in the health care setting, home, and community, including prevention strategies across the life span for thermal injury, falls, seizures, poisoning, suffocation or choking, excessive noise, electric hazards, firearms, and radiation.

- Explain measures to prevent falls.

- Discuss implementation of seizure precautions.

- Discuss the use and legal implications of restraints.

- Describe alternatives to restraints.

- List desired outcomes to use in evaluating the selected strategies for injury prevention.

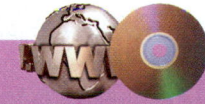

MediaLink

www.prenhall.com/kozier

Additional resources for this chapter can be found on the Student CD-ROM accompanying this textbook, and on the Companion Website at www.prenhall.com/kozier. Click on Chapter 30 to select the activities for this chapter.

CD-ROM
- Audio Glossary
- NCLEX Review
- Animation: Lead Poisoning

Companion Website
- Additional NCLEX Review
- Case Study: Ensuring Client Safety
- Care Plan Activity: Safety at Home
- MediaLink Application: Safety in Nursing Issues
- Links to Resources

A fundamental concern of nurses, which extends from the bedside to the home to the community, is prevention of accidents and injury, as well as assisting the injured. Motor vehicle accidents, falls, drowning, fire and burns, poisoning, inhalation and ingestion of foreign objects, and firearm use are major causes of accidental injury and death.

Nurses need to be aware of what constitutes a safe environment for a particular person or for a group of people in home and community settings. Accidents are often caused by human conduct and can be prevented.

FACTORS AFFECTING SAFETY

The ability of people to protect themselves from injury is affected by such factors as age and development, lifestyle, mobility and health status, sensory-perceptual alterations, cognitive awareness, psychosocial state, ability to communicate, safety awareness, and environmental factors. Nurses need to assess each of these factors when they plan care or teach clients to protect themselves.

Age and Development

Through knowledge and accurate assessment of the environment, people learn to protect themselves from many injuries. Children walking to school learn to stop before crossing the street and wait for oncoming traffic. They also learn not to touch a hot stove. For the very young, learning about the environment is essential. Only through knowledge and experience do children learn what is potentially harmful.

Elders can have difficulty with movement and diminished sensory acuity that contributes to the likelihood of injury. Specific age-related potential hazards and preventive measures are discussed later in this chapter. Box 30–1 summarizes selected hazards for each age group.

Lifestyle

Lifestyle factors that place people at risk include unsafe work environments; residence in neighborhoods with high crime rates; access to guns and ammunition; insufficient income to buy safety equipment or make necessary repairs; and access to illicit drugs, which may also be contaminated by harmful additives. Risk-taking behavior is a factor in some accidents.

Mobility and Health Status

People who have impaired mobility due to paralysis, muscle weakness, and poor balance or coordination are obviously prone to injury. Clients with spinal cord injury and paralysis of both legs may be unable to move even when they perceive discomfort. Hemiplegic clients or clients with

---

BOX 30–1	■ Selected Safety Hazards Throughout the Life Span*

- *Developing fetus:* Exposure to maternal smoking, alcohol consumption, addictive drugs, x-rays (first trimester), certain pesticides
- *Newborns and infants:* Falling, suffocation in crib, choking from aspirated milk or ingested objects, burns from hot water or other spilled hot liquids, automobile accidents, crib or playpen injuries, electric shock, poisoning
- *Toddlers:* Physical trauma from falling, banging into objects, or getting cut by sharp objects; automobile accidents; burns; poisoning; drowning; and electric shock
- *Preschoolers:* Injury from traffic, playground equipment, and other objects; choking, suffocation, and obstruction of airway or ear canal by foreign objects; poisoning; drowning; fire and burns; harm from other people or animals
- *Adolescents:* Vehicular (automobile, bicycle) accidents, recreational accidents, firearms, substance abuse
- *Older adults:* Falling, burns, and pedestrian and automobile accidents

Preventive measures are discussed later in this chapter.

leg casts often have poor balance and fall easily. Clients weakened by illness or surgery are not always fully aware of their condition.

Sensory-Perceptual Alterations

Accurate sensory perception of environmental stimuli is vital to safety. People with impaired touch perception, hearing, taste, smell, and vision are highly susceptible to injury. A person who does not see well may trip over a toy or not see an electric cord. Deaf people do not hear a siren in traffic, and people with impaired olfactory sense may not smell burning food or the sulfur aroma of escaping gas.

Cognitive Awareness

Awareness is the ability to perceive environmental stimuli and body reactions and to respond appropriately through thought and action. Clients with impaired awareness include people lacking sleep; unconscious or semiconscious persons; disoriented people (i.e., those who may not understand where they are or what to do to help themselves); people who perceive stimuli that do not exist; and people whose judgment is altered by disease or medications, such as narcotics, tranquilizers, hypnotics, and sedatives. Mildly confused clients may momentarily forget where they are, wander from their rooms, misplace personal belongings, and so forth.

Emotional State

Extreme emotional states can alter the ability to perceive environmental hazards. Stressful situations can reduce a person's level of concentration, cause errors of judgment, and decrease awareness of external stimuli. People with depression may think and react to environmental stimuli more slowly than usual.

Ability to Communicate

Individuals with diminished ability to receive and convey information are also at risk for injury. Aphasic clients, people with language barriers, and those unable to read are among them. For example, the person unable to interpret the sign "No smoking—oxygen in use" could cause a fire.

Safety Awareness

Information is crucial to safety. Clients in unfamiliar environments frequently need specific safety information. Lack of knowledge about unfamiliar equipment, such as oxygen tanks, intravenous tubing, and hot packs is a potential hazard. Healthy clients need knowledge about water safety, car safety, fire prevention, ways to prevent the ingestion of harmful substances, and many preventive measures related to specific age-related hazards.

Environmental Factors

A safe home requires well-maintained flooring and carpets, a nonskid bathtub or shower surface, functioning smoke alarms that are strategically placed, and knowledge of fire escape routes. Outdoor areas, such as swimming pools, need to be safely secured and maintained. Adequate lighting, both inside and out, will minimize the potential for accidents.

In the workplace, machinery, industrial belts and pulleys, and chemicals may create danger. Worker fatigue, noise and air pollution, or working at great heights or in subterranean areas may also create occupational hazards. The work environment of the nurse may also be unsafe. The health care worker needs to maintain an awareness of potential risk.

Adequate street lighting, safe water and sewage treatment, and regulation of sanitation in food buying and handling all contribute to a healthy, hazard-free community. A safe and secure community strives to be free of excess noise, crime, traffic congestion, dilapidated housing, or unprotected creeks and landfills.

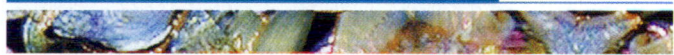

NURSING MANAGEMENT

ASSESSING

Assessing clients at risk for accidents and injury involves (a) noting pertinent indicators in the nursing history and physical examination, (b) using specifically developed risk assessment tools, and (c) evaluating the client's home environment.

Nursing History and Physical Examination

The nursing history and physical examination can reveal considerable data about the client's safety practices and risks for injury. Data include age and developmental level; general health status; mobility status; presence or absence of physiologic or perceptual deficits such as olfactory, visual, tactile, taste, or other sensory impairments; altered thought processes or other impaired cognitive or emotional capabilities; substance abuse; any indications of abuse or neglect; and an accident and injury history. A safety history also needs to include the client's awareness of hazards, knowledge of safety precautions both at home and work, and any perceived threats to safety (Figure 30–1 ■).

Risk Assessment Tools

Risk assessment tools are available to determine clients at risk both for specific kinds of injury, such as falls, or for the general assessment necessary to keep clients safe in their homes and in health care settings. In general, these tools direct the nurse to appraise the factors affecting safety as they have been outlined earlier. The tools summarize specific data contained in the client's nursing history and physical examination. Client risk factors and environmental hazards for falls are discussed later in this chapter (see "Falls").

Home Hazard Appraisal

Hazards in the home are major causes of falls, fire, poisoning, suffocation, and other accidents, such as those caused by improper use of household equipment, tools, and cooking utensils. See Chapter 9 ⊕ for a summary of specific data necessary for a home hazard appraisal.

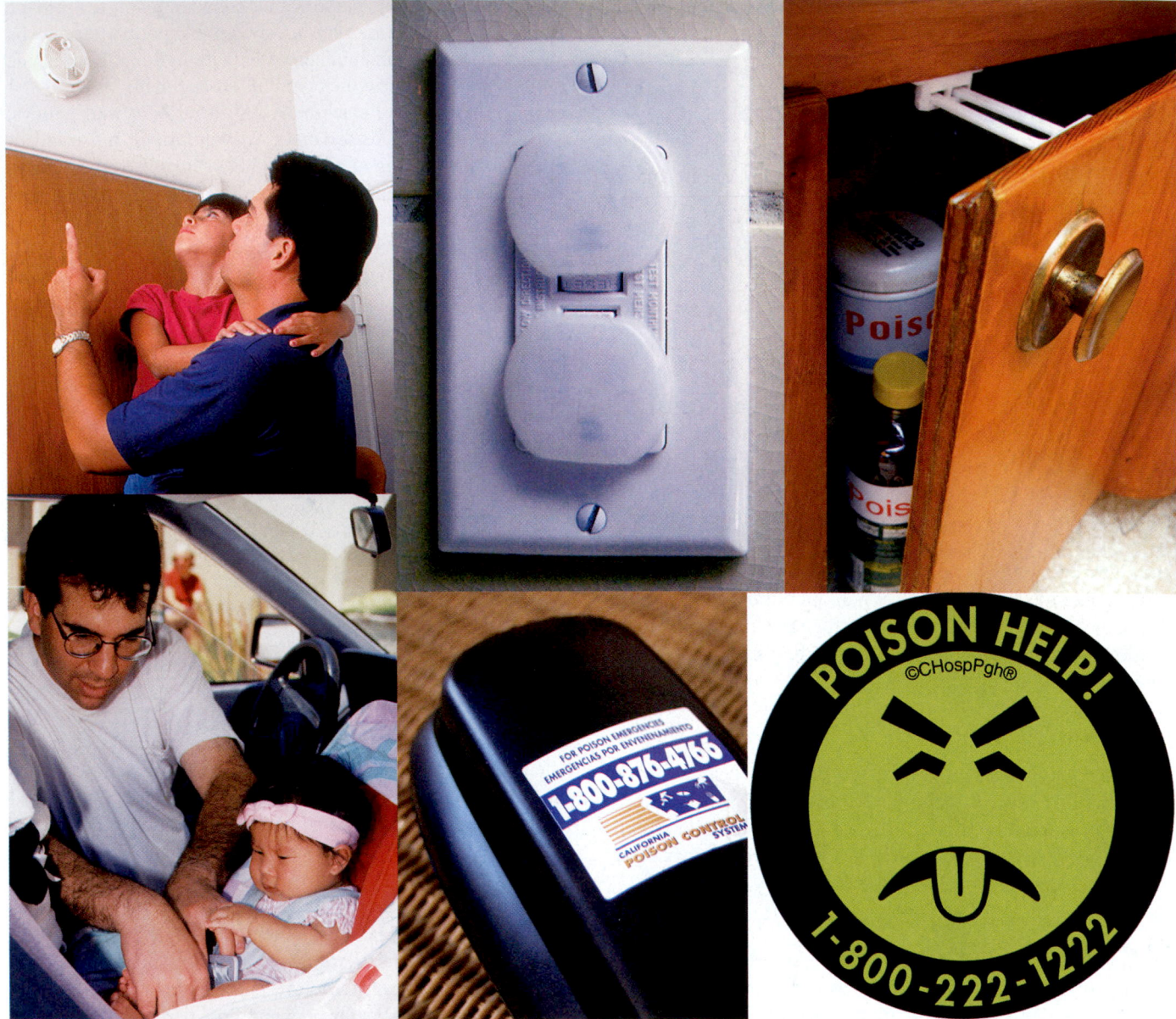

Figure 30–1 ■ Nurses need to teach clients about safety and how to prevent accidents such as by using smoke detectors, safety covers for electrical outlets, childproof locks on drawers and cabinets, Mr. Yuk stickers on toxic substances, and infant car seats, and by placing poison control information near or on the telephone. (Top: Courtesy of Tony Freeman/PhotoEdit; Jerry Marshall; Michael Newman/PhotoEdit; Bottom: Grantpix/Photo Researchers Inc.; Geri Engberg; Children's Hospital Pittsburgh.)

DIAGNOSING

NANDA offers a broad diagnostic label related to safety issues:

- *Risk for Injury:* A state in which the individual is at risk for injury as a result of environmental conditions interacting with the individual's adaptive and defense resources.

This broad label consists of seven subcategories that may be preferred when the nurse wants to describe injury more specifically and or isolate suitable interventions (Wilkinson, 2000):

- *Risk for Poisoning:* Accentuated risk of accidental exposure to, or ingestion of, drugs or dangerous products in doses sufficient to cause poisoning

- *Risk for Suffocation:* Accentuated risk of accidental suffocation (inadequate air available for inhalation)
- *Risk for Trauma:* Accentuated risk of accidental tissue injury (e.g., wound, burn, or fracture)
- *Latex Allergy Response:* An allergic response to natural latex rubber products
- *Risk for Latex Allergy Response:* At risk for allergic response to natural latex rubber products
- *Risk for Aspiration:* At risk for the entry of gastrointestinal secretions, oropharyngeal secretions, solids, or fluids into tracheobronchial passages
- *Risk for Disuse Syndrome:* At risk for deterioration of body systems as the result of prescribed or unavoidable musculoskeletal inactivity.

Another diagnosis the nurse may choose to use is

• *Deficient Knowledge (Accident Prevention):* Inability to state or explain information or demonstrate a required skill related to safety of self and others.

See Identifying Nursing Diagnoses, Outcomes, and Interventions for examples of applying the nursing process for clients at risk for injury.

IDENTIFYING NURSING DIAGNOSES, OUTCOMES, AND INTERVENTIONS

CLIENTS AT RISK FOR SAFETY

DATA CLUSTER	NURSING DIAGNOSIS/ DEFINITION	SAMPLE DESIRED OUTCOMES [NOC#]/DEFINITION	INDICATORS	SELECTED INTERVENTIONS [NIC#]/DEFINITION	SAMPLE NIC ACTIVITIES
Mrs. H. has adopted a toddler. Home assessment reveals many cleaning supplies at floor level, and paint peeling off the walls.	*Risk for Poisoning* related to dangerous products within reach of a child/*Accentuated risk of accidental exposure to, or ingestion of, drugs or dangerous products in doses sufficient to cause poisoning*	Safety Behavior: Home Physical Environment [1910]/*Individual or caregiver actions to minimize environmental factors that might cause physical harm or injury in the home*	Totally adequate • Placement of appropriate hazard warning labels • Storage of hazardous materials to prevent injury • Correction of lead hazard risks • Provision of safe play area	Environmental Management: Safety [6486]/*Monitoring and manipulation of the physical environment to promote safety*	• Identify safety hazards • Remove hazards from the environment, when possible • Initiate and/or conduct screening programs for environmental hazards (e.g., lead) • Educate about environmental hazards • Provide emergency phone numbers (e.g., poison control center)
Mr. P. suffered a stroke resulting in left-sided weakness. As a result, his gait is unsteady. The nurse noticed that his home has several throw rugs and much furniture impeding his mobility. The bathroom does not have grab bars by the toilet or shower.	*Risk for Injury* related to impaired mobility and potential home hazards/*At risk of injury as a result of environmental conditions interacting with the individual's adaptive and defense resources*	Safety Behavior: Home Physical Environment [1910]/*Individual or caregiver actions to minimize environmental factors that might cause physical harm or injury in the home*	Totally adequate • Placement of handrails in bathroom • Arrangement of furniture to reduce risks	Environmental Management: Safety [6486]/*Monitoring and manipulation of the physical environment to promote safety*	• Identify safety needs of client • Identify safety hazards • Modify the environment to minimize hazards and risks • Provide adaptive devices (e.g., handrails) to increase safety of the environment • Monitor the environment for changes in safety status • Educate about environmental hazards

PLANNING

When planning care to prevent accidents and injury, the nurse considers all factors affecting the client's safety, specifies desired outcomes, and selects nursing activities to meet these outcomes. The major goal for clients with safety risks is to prevent accidents and injury. To meet this goal, clients often need to change their health behavior and may need to modify the environment.

Desired outcomes associated with preventing injury depend on the individual client. Examples of desired outcomes, although established in the planning phase, are provided in the "Evaluating" section on page 693.

Nursing interventions to meet desired outcomes are largely directed toward helping the client and family to accomplish the following:

- Identify environmental hazards in home and community.
- Demonstrate safety practices appropriate to the home health care agency, community, and workplace.

- Experience a decrease in the frequency or severity of injury.
- Demonstrate safe childrearing practices or lifestyle practices.

IMPLEMENTING

Hazards to safety occur at all ages and vary according to the age and development level of the individual.

Promoting Safety across the Life Span

Measures to ensure the safety of people of all ages focus on (a) observation or prediction of potentially harmful situations so that harm can be avoided and (b) client education that empowers clients to safeguard themselves and their families from injury. Safety measures covering the life span from infancy to elders are listed in the accompanying Teaching: Wellness Care.

Newborns and Infants.
Accidents are a leading cause of death during infancy, especially during the first year of life. Infants are

---

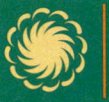

Teaching: Wellness Care
Safety Measures throughout the Life Span

Newborns and Infants
- Use a federally approved car seat at all times (including coming home from hospital). It should be in the back seat, facing backward.
- Never leave the infant unattended on a raised surface.
- Check the temperature of the infant's bath water and formula prior to using.
- Hold the infant upright during feeding. Do not prop the bottle. Cut food in small pieces, and do not feed the infant peanuts or popcorn.
- Investigate the infant's crib for compliance with federal safety regulations: slats no more than 2 3/8 inches apart, lead-free paint, height of crib sides, tight fit of mattress to crib.
- Use a playpen with sides made of small-size netting. Never leave playpen sides down.
- Provide large soft toys with no small detachable or sharp-edged parts.
- Use guard gates on stairs and screens on windows. Supervise the infant in swings and highchairs.
- Cover electric outlets. Coil cords out of reach.
- Place plants, household cleaners, and wastebaskets out of reach. Lock away potential poisons, such as medicines, paint, and gasoline.

Toddlers
- Continue to use federally approved car seats at all times. Place children in back seat when traveling in a car.
- Teach children not to put objects in the mouth, including pills (unless given by parent).
- Keep objects with sharp edges (such as furniture and knives) out of children's reach.
- Place hot pots on back burners with handles turned inward.
- Keep cleaning solutions, insecticides, and medicines in locked cupboards.
- Keep windows and balconies screened.
- Supervise toddlers in the tub.

- Fence in pools, and supervise toddlers, at all times when in or near pools. Do not overfill bathtub. Do not let toddlers play near ditches or wells.
- Teach children not to run or ride a tricycle into the street.
- Obtain a low bed when the child begins to climb.
- Cover outlets with safety covers or plugs.

Preschoolers
- Do not allow children to run with candy or other objects in the mouth.
- Teach children not to put small objects in the mouth, nose, and ears.
- Remove doors from unused equipment such as refrigerators.
- Always supervise preschoolers crossing streets and begin safety teaching about obeying traffic signals and looking both ways.
- Check Halloween treats before allowing children to eat them. Discard loose or open candy.
- Teach children to play in "safe" areas, not on streets and railroad tracks.
- Teach preschoolers the dangers of playing with matches and playing near charcoal, fire, and heating appliances.
- Teach children to avoid strangers and keep parents informed of their whereabouts.
- Teach preschoolers not to walk in front of swings and not to push others off playground equipment.

School-Age Children
- Teach children safety rules for recreational and sports activities: never swim alone, always wear a life jacket when in a boat, and wear a protective helmet and knee and elbow pads when needed.
- Supervise contact sports and activities in which children aim at a target.
- Teach children to obey all traffic and safety rules for bicycling, skateboarding, and roller skating.

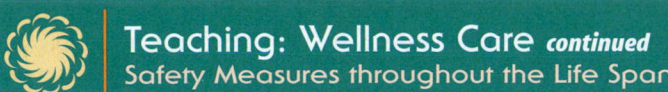

Teaching: Wellness Care *continued*
Safety Measures throughout the Life Span

- Teach children to use light or reflective clothing when walking or cycling at night.
- Teach children safe ways to use the stove, garden tools, and other equipment.
- Supervise children when they use saws, electric appliances, tools, and other potentially dangerous equipment.
- Teach children not to play with fireworks, gunpowder, or firearms. Keep firearms unloaded, locked up, and out of reach.
- Teach children to avoid excavations, quarries, vacant buildings, and playing around heavy machinery.
- Teach children the health hazards of smoking. If you smoke, stop.
- Teach children the effects of drugs and alcohol on judgment and coordination.

Adolescents

- Have adolescents complete a drivers' education course, and take practice drives with them in various kinds of weather.
- Set firm limits on automobile use, namely, never to drive after drinking or using drugs, and never to ride with a driver who has done so. Encourage adolescents to call home for a ride if they have been drinking, assuring them they can do so without a reprimand.
- Restrict number of passengers in car during the first year of driving.
- Teach adolescents to wear a safety helmet when riding motorcycles, scooters, and other sports vehicles. Teach safety rules for water sports.
- Encourage adolescents to use proper equipment when participating in sports. Schedule a physical examination before participation, and be certain there is medical supervision for all athletic activities.
- Encourage adolescents to swim, jog, and go boating in groups so they can obtain help in case of an accident.
- Teach safety measures for use of power tools.
- Teach rules for hunting and the proper care and use of firearms.
- Inform the adolescent of the dangers of drugs, alcohol, and unprotected sex. Include teaching about date rape prevention and defense.
- Teach dangers of sunbathing and tanning beds, as well as use of sun block and protective clothing when doing outdoor activities.
- Be alert to changes in the adolescent's mood and behavior. Listen to and maintain open communication with the adolescent. Open communication is a powerful preventive measure.
- Set a good example of behavior that the adolescent can follow.

Young Adults

- Reinforce motor vehicle safety: Drive defensively, use "designated drivers" if alcohol is consumed, routinely check brakes and tires, and use seat and shoulder belts or car seats for all passengers.
- Remind the young adult to repair potential fire hazards, such as electric wiring.
- Reinforce water safety: Know the depth of a pool or lake before diving; supervise backyard pools and other water activities.
- Discuss evaluating the potential for workplace injuries or death when making decisions about a career or occupation.

- Encourage the young adult to participate actively in programs that reduce occupational hazards.
- Discuss avoiding excessive sun radiation by limiting exposure, using sun-blocking agents, and wearing protective clothing. Explain the skin changes that may indicate a cancerous condition.
- Encourage young adults who are unable to cope with the pressures, responsibilities, and expectations of adulthood to seek counseling.

Middle-Aged Adults

- Reinforce motor vehicle safety: Use seat belts and drive within the speed limit, especially at night. Test visual acuity periodically.
- Make certain stairways are well lighted and uncluttered.
- Equip bathrooms with hand grasps and nonskid bath mats.
- Test smoke detectors and fire alarms regularly.
- Keep all machines and tools in good working condition at work and at home. Follow safety precautions when using machinery.
- Reinforce safety measures taught earlier in life, such as the hazards of excessive sun exposure.

Elders

- Encourage the client to have regular vision and hearing tests.
- Assist the client to have a home hazard appraisal.
- Encourage the client to keep as active as possible.

Preventive measures:

- Ensure eyeglasses are functional.
- Ensure appropriate lighting.
- Mark doorways and edges of steps as needed.
- Keep environment tidy and uncluttered.
- Set safe limits to activities.
- Remove unsafe objects.
- Wear shoes or well-fitted slippers with nonskid soles.
- Use ambulatory devices as necessary (cane, crutches, walker, braces, wheelchair).
- Provide assistance with ambulation as needed.
- Monitor gait and balance.
- Adapt living arrangements to one floor if necessary.
- Encourage exercise and activity as tolerated to maintain muscle strength, joint flexibility, and balance.
- Ensure uncluttered environment with securely fastened rugs.
- Encourage client to request assistance.
- Keep bed in the low position.
- Install grab bars in bathroom.
- Provide raised toilet seat.
- Instruct client to rise slowly from a lying to sitting to standing position, and to stand in place for several seconds before walking.
- Provide a bedside commode as needed.
- Assist with voiding on a frequent and scheduled basis.
- Encourage client to summon help.
- Monitor activity tolerance.
- Attach side rails to the bed.
- Keep rails in place when the bed is in the lowest position.
- Monitor orientation and alertness status.
- Encourage annual or more frequent review of all medications prescribed.

completely dependent on others for care; they are oblivious to such dangers as falling or ingesting harmful substances. Parents may need to learn the amount of observation necessary to maintain infant safety. They also need help to identify and remove common hazards in and around the home, and first-aid information that includes cardiopulmonary resuscitation and interventions for airway obstruction. Common accidents during infancy include burns, suffocation or choking, automobile accidents, falls, and poisoning. Education and support of parents can make them more knowledgeable and better prepared to protect their children from accidents and injuries.

Toddlers. Toddlers are curious and like to feel and taste everything. They are fascinated by potential dangers, such as pools and busy streets, so they need constant supervision and protection (Figure 30–2 ■). Parents can prevent many accidents by

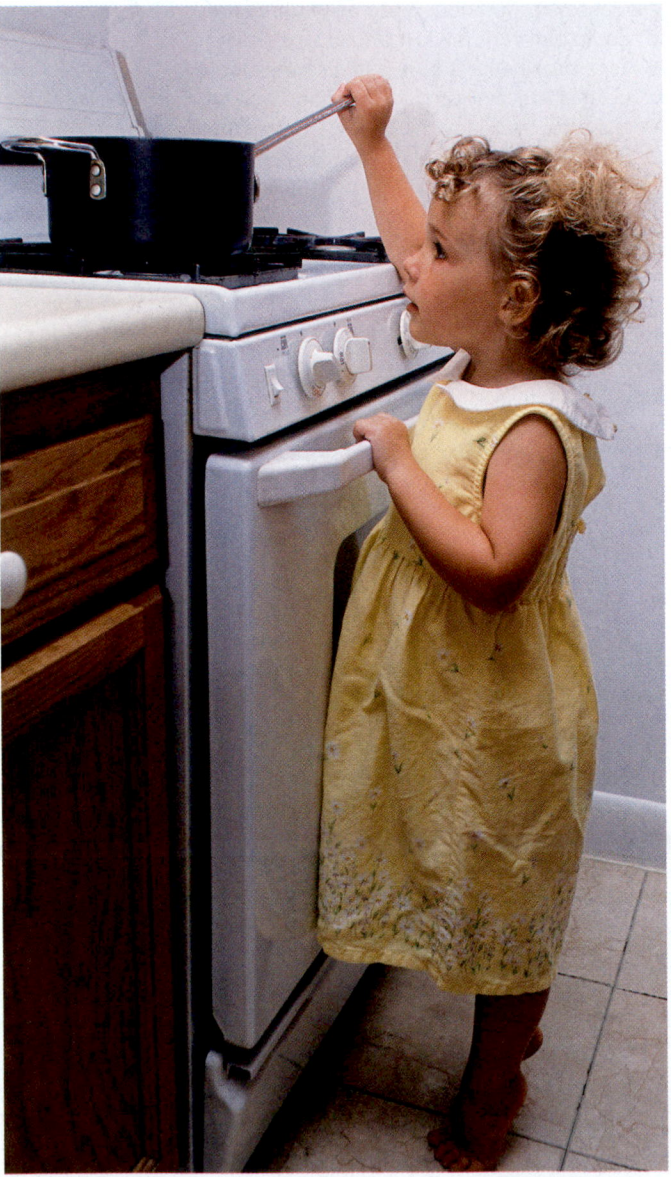

Figure 30–2 ■ Promoting safety (e.g., by placing hot pots on back burners with handles turned inward) is required to keep children from injury.

"toddler-proofing" the home or other setting where the child will be. This practice extends to the use of federally approved car restraints and removing or securing all items that can pose a safety hazard to the child in any setting. It may be necessary to inspect for and remove sources of lead from the environment. Lead poisoning (plumbism) is a risk for children exposed to lead paint chips, fumes from leaded gasoline, or any "leaded" substances. The ingestion of lead-based paint chips is the most common cause of lead poisoning in children.

> ➤ **CLINICAL ALERT** *The remodeling and renovation of older homes (e.g., those built before 1978) accounts for most of the lead poisoning seen today. Nurses need to educate families living in older homes about their children's risk for lead poisoning and provide lead poisoning prevention advice.*

Preschoolers. Children of preschool age are active and often very clumsy, making them susceptible to injury. Control of the environment must continue, keeping hazards such as matches, medicines, and other potential poisons out of reach. Safety education for the child must begin now. Education of the preschooler involves learning how to cross streets, what traffic signals mean, and how to ride bicycles and other wheeled toys safely. Children must be cautioned to avoid hazards, such as busy streets, swimming pools, and other potentially dangerous areas. Parents must maintain careful surveillance; the developmental level of the preschooler does not allow for self-reliance in matters of safety. Parents must also keep in mind that their child's cognitive and motor skills increase quickly; hence, safety measures must keep up with the acquisition of new skills.

School-Age Children. By the time children attend school, they are learning to think before they act. They often prefer adult equipment to toys. They want to be active with other children in such pursuits as bicycling, hiking, swimming, and boating. Although sensitive to peer pressure, the school-age child responds to rules. Children of this age engage in fantasy and magical thinking. They often imitate actions of parents and superheroes with whom they identify.

Accidents are the leading cause of death in school-age children. The most frequent causes of fatalities, in descending order, are motor vehicle accidents, drownings, fires, and firearms. School-age children are also involved in many minor accidents, frequently resulting from outdoor activities and recreational equipment such as swings, bicycles, skateboards, and swimming pools.

Adolescents. Obtaining a driver's license is an important event in the life of an adolescent in North America, but the privilege is not always wisely handled. Teenagers may use driving as an outlet for stress, as a way to assert independence, or as a way to impress peers. When setting limits on automobile use, parents need to assess the teenager's level of responsibility, common sense, and ability to resist peer pressure. The age of the teenager alone does not determine readiness to handle this responsibility.

Adolescents are at risk for sports injuries because their coordination skills are not fully developed. However, sports ac-

MediaLink | LEAD POISONING ANIMATION

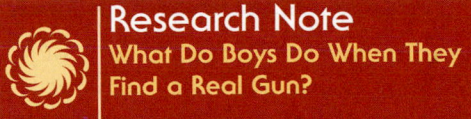

Research Note
What Do Boys Do When They Find a Real Gun?

The researchers conducted a study to compare the beliefs of parents that their son would leave a gun alone or go tell an adult if they found a gun with the child's behavior when they found a gun in a safe environment (Jackman, Farah, Kellerman, & Simon, 2001).

The pilot study consisted of 64 boys, aged 2 to 12 years, in 29 groups of 2 to 3 boys. Each pair or trio of boys was placed in a room with a one-way mirror. Two plastic water pistols were concealed in one drawer within the room and a semiautomatic handgun was placed in a different drawer. The handgun was modified so it could not fire and it also contained a radio transmitter that activated a flashing light to the observers if the trigger was depressed enough to fire the gun. Each group was observed for four behaviors: (a) Did they find the gun? (b) Did they tell an adult? (c) Did they handle the gun? and (d) Did they pull the trigger?

Twenty-one of the groups (72%) discovered the handgun with 16 of the groups (76%) handling it. One or more of the boys in 10 of the groups (48%) pulled the trigger. Almost half of the boys who found the gun thought that it was a toy or were unsure whether it was real. More than 90% of the boys who handled the gun or pulled the trigger stated they had previously received gun safety instruction. The findings of the boy's behaviors contradicted the beliefs of their parents.

Implications: Many 2- to 12-year-old boys will handle a handgun if they find one. This age group is at high risk for unintentional firearm injury. It is important for nurses to emphasize to parents who keep guns the importance of making the guns inaccessible (locked and unloaded) to children or to consider removing guns from the home.

Note: From "Seeing Is Believing: What Do Boys Do When They Find a Real Gun?" by G. A. Jackman, M. M. Farah, A. L. Kellerman, and H. K. Simon, 2001, *Pediatrics, 107*(6), pp. 1247–1250.

tivities are important to the adolescent's self-esteem and overall development. In addition to providing beneficial exercise, sports activities enhance social and personal development. They help the adolescent experience competition, teamwork, and conflict resolution.

Suicide and homicide are two leading causes of death among teenagers. Adolescent males commit suicide at a higher rate than adolescent females, and African Americans commit homicide at a higher rate than European Americans. Suicides by firearms, drugs, and automobile exhaust gases are the most common. Factors influencing the high suicide and homicide rates include economic deprivation, family breakup, and the availability of firearms, which are the most frequently used weapons. Cutting or stabbing tools are the next most frequently used weapons.

Young Adults. Motor vehicle accidents are by far the leading cause of mortality for this group; other causes of accidental death for young adults include drowning, fires, burns, and firearms.

One safety hazard for many young adults is exposure to natural radiation from sunbathing or outdoor activities. Exposure to the sun is directly related to skin cancer. Suicide is another leading cause of death in young adults. Many suicides may actually be mistaken for accidental death (automobile accidents, alcohol intoxication, and drug overdose). In general, suicide results from the young adult's inability to cope with the pressures, responsibilities, and expectations of adulthood.

The nurse's role in the prevention of suicide includes identifying behaviors that may indicate potential problems: depression; a variety of physical complaints including weight loss, sleep disturbances, and digestive disorders; and decreased interest in social and work roles along with an increase in isolation. A young adult identified as at risk for suicide should be referred to a mental health professional or a crisis center. Nurses can also reduce the incidence of suicide by participating in educational programs that provide information about the early signs of suicide.

Middle-Aged Adults. Changing physiologic factors, as well as concern over personal and work-related responsibilities, may contribute to the accident rate of middle-aged persons. Motor vehicle accidents are the most common cause of accidental death in this age group. Decreased reaction times and visual acuity may make the middle-aged adult prone to accidents. Other accidental causes of death for middle-aged adults include falls, fires, burns, poisonings, and drownings. Occupational accidents continue to be a significant safety hazard during the middle years.

Older Adults. Accident prevention is a major concern for older adults. Because vision is limited, reflexes are slowed, and bones are brittle, climbing stairs, driving a car, and even walking require caution. Driving, particularly night driving, requires caution because accommodation of the eye to light is impaired and peripheral vision is diminished. Older persons need to learn to turn the head before changing lanes and should not rely on side vision, for example, when crossing a street. Driving in fog or other hazardous conditions should be avoided.

Fires are a hazard for the elderly person with a failing memory. The older person may forget that the iron or stove has been left on or may not extinguish a cigarette completely. Because of reduced sensitivity to pain and heat, care must be taken to prevent burns when the person bathes or uses heating devices.

Older people at risk for wandering due to organic brain syndromes need to wear identification devices. They can also be registered with the local Alzheimer's Association's Wanderer's Alert Program.

Because older clients who take analgesics or sedatives may become lethargic or confused, they should be monitored regularly and closely. Other measures to induce sleep should be used whenever possible. Nurses can help elderly clients make the home environment safe. Specific hazards can be identified and corrected; for example, handrails can be installed on staircases. The nurse teaches the importance of taking only prescribed medications and contacting a health professional at the first indication of intolerance to them.

> **CLINICAL ALERT**   *Older people have trouble seeing the edges of stairs. Painting white stripes on the edges of the steps will help increase contrast and may prevent falls.*

The incidence of suicide in older adults is increasing and often goes unnoticed when the causes are due to hidden self-destructive behaviors, such as starvation, overdosing with medications, and noncompliance with medical care, treatments, and medications. In older individuals, the suicide attempt is usually more serious, because it is truly intended to end the life, not just to get attention as is often seen in other age groups. Also, the method of suicide is generally more violent in the older person, such as a gunshot wound to the head, or hanging.

Wold (1999) lists important facts regarding suicide of the older adult: (a) White men are the most likely to commit suicide; (b) medical illness is a major contributing factor to suicide; (c) uncontrollable pain, loss of a loved one, and major life changes can be contributing factors, and (d) major depression and social isolation increase the risk of suicide.

Nurses need to be aware of the symptoms and risk factors and see that the person is directed to the appropriate professional or agency for treatment and counseling.

Safety Problems across the Life Span.   Domestic violence is increasing at an alarming rate and involving individuals of all ages, infants to older adults. It includes child abuse, intimate partner abuse, and elder abuse and affects the health and safety of families and the community. Statistics are inaccurate due to the underreporting of incidents. Nurses should be involved in working with all phases of domestic violence: prevention, screening, referrals for treatment, and follow-up care. This usually necessitates collaborative planning with physicians, law enforcement agencies, social services, and other community agencies.

Nurses also have to opportunity to become advocates for community support programs for domestic violence and can become involved in educating other professionals regarding prevention, screening, and treatment.

Domestic violence takes on extra importance because it is known that people who were abused as children often display abusive behavior as an adult. This points to the need for prevention and early intervention to prevent the cycle from continuing. Nurses can be of assistance in restoring dignity, health, and safety to vulnerable individuals.

Preventing Specific Hazards

Implementing measures to prevent specific hazards or accidents such as burns, fire, falls, poisoning, suffocation, electrocution, and so on are critical aspects of nursing care. Teaching clients about safety is another important aspect. Nurses usually have opportunities to teach while providing care.

Scalds and Burns.   A **scald** is a burn from a hot liquid or vapor, such as steam. A **burn** results from excessive exposure to thermal, chemical, electric, or radioactive agents.

Common home hazards causing scalds include the following:

- Pot handles that protrude over the edge of a stove
- Electric appliances used to heat liquids or oils, especially those with dangling cords that are within reach of crawling infants and young children
- Excessively hot bath water.

In health care agencies, the risk of scalds and burns is greater for clients whose skin sensitivity to temperature is impaired. Scalds can occur from overly hot bath water, and burns from therapeutic applications of heat (see Chapter 34). It is important for the nurse to assess how well clients can protect themselves and what special precautions, if any, need to be taken.

Fires.   Fires continue to be a constant risk in both health care settings and homes. Agency fires usually result from malfunctioning electric equipment or combustion of anesthetic gas. Home fires most frequently result from careless disposal of burning cigarettes or matches, from grease, or from faulty electric wiring.

Agency Fires   In health care agencies, fire is particularly hazardous when people are incapacitated and unable to leave the building without assistance. This incapacity makes it extremely important for nurses to be aware of the fire safety regulations and fire prevention practices of the agency in which they work. When a fire occurs the nurse follows four sequential priorities:

1. Protect and evacuate clients who are in immediate danger.
2. Report the fire.
3. Contain the fire.
4. Extinguish the fire.

Extinguishing the fire requires knowledge of three categories of fire, classified according to the type of material that is burning:

> *Class A:* Paper, wood, upholstery, rags, ordinary rubbish
> *Class B:* Flammable liquids and gases
> *Class C:* Electrical

The right type of extinguisher must be used to fight the fire. Extinguishers have picture symbols showing the type of fire for which they are to be used. Directions for use are also attached.

Home Fires   Nursing interventions for home fires focus on teaching fire safety. Preventive measures include the following:

- Keep emergency numbers near the telephone, or stored for speed dialing.
- Be sure the smoke alarms are operable and appropriately located.
- Teach clients to change the batteries in their smoke alarms annually on a special day such as a birthday or January 1.
- Have a family "fire drill" plan. Every member needs to know the plan for the nearest exit from different locations of the home.
- Keep fire extinguishers available and in working order.
- Close windows and doors if possible; cover the mouth and nose with a damp cloth when exiting through a smoke-filled area; and avoid heavy smoke by assuming a bent position with the head as close to the floor as possible.

Falls. People of any age can fall, but infants and older adults are particularly prone to falling and incurring serious injury. Falls are the leading cause of accidents among older adults. They are also a major cause of hospital and nursing home admissions. Most falls occur in the home and are a major threat to the independence of older adults. Fear of falling is common in older adults, even in those who have not experienced a fall. This fear is of particular concern for those who live alone and who anticipate being helpless and unable to summon help after a fall. For these individuals the nurse should encourage daily or more frequent contact with a friend or family member, installation of a personal emergency response system, and measures to maintain a physical environment that prevents falls. Risk factors and associated preventive measures are shown in Table 30–1.

> ➤ CLINICAL ALERT *Falls can break bones and self-confidence, leading to fear of falling causing a decreased activity level and decreased muscle strength. All increase the risk of falling.*

Weak leg muscles, weak knees, poor balance, and loss of flexibility contribute to falls in the elderly. The nurse can use an assessment tool, called the Get Up and Go test, in a hospital, subacute, or home setting. Kimbell (2001) describes the following steps of the test:

1. Observe the client's posture while he sits in a straight-backed chair.
2. Ask the client to stand. Observe if the client stands using only his leg muscles or if he needs to push himself up with his hands.

TABLE 30–1 Risk Factors and Preventive Measures for Falls

Risk Factor	Preventive Measures
Poor vision	Ensure eyeglasses are functional.
	Ensure appropriate lighting.
	Mark doorways and edges of steps as needed.
	Keep the environment tidy.
Cognitive dysfunction (confusion, disorientation, impaired memory, or judgment)	Set safe limits to activities.
	Remove unsafe objects.
Impaired gait or balance and difficulty walking because of lower extremity dysfunction (e.g., arthritis)	Wear shoes or well-fitted slippers with nonskid soles.
	Use ambulatory devices as necessary (cane, crutches, walker, braces, wheelchair).
	Provide assistance with ambulation as needed.
	Monitor gait and balance.
	Adapt living arrangements to one floor if necessary.
	Encourage exercise and activity as tolerated to maintain muscle strength, joint flexibility, and balance.
	Ensure uncluttered environment with securely fastened rugs.
Difficulty getting in and out of chair or in and out of bed	Encourage client to request assistance.
	Keep the bed in the low position.
	Install grab bars in bathroom.
	Provide raised toilet seat.
Orthostatic hypotension	Instruct client to rise slowly from a lying to sitting to standing position, and to stand in place for several seconds before walking.
Urinary frequency or receiving diuretics	Provide a bedside commode.
	Assist with voiding on a frequent and scheduled basis.
Weakness from disease process or therapy	Encourage client to summon help.
	Monitor activity tolerance.
Current medication regimen that includes sedatives, hypnotics, tranquilizers, narcotic analgesics, diuretics	Attach side rails to the bed.
	Keep the rails in place when the bed is in the lowest position.
	Monitor orientation and alertness status.
	Discuss how alcohol contributes to fall-related injuries.
	Encourage client not to mix alcohol and medications and to avoid alcohol when necessary.
	Encourage annual or more frequent review of all medications prescribed.

3. Once the client is comfortable standing, ask him to close his eyes. Does he sway?

4. Ask him to open his eyes, walk 10 feet, turn around and return to the chair. Observe his gait, balance, speed, and stability. How smoothly does he turn?

5. When he gets to the chair, ask him to turn and sit down. Observe how smoothly the client performs this motion.

This quick assessment along with an assessment of the client's environment can help the nurse recommend safety measures to the client and family.

Prevention of falls in health care agencies is an ongoing concern. Health care environments are designed with many safety features to reduce the risk of falls, such as railings along corridors; call bells at each bedside; safety bars in toilet areas; locks on beds, wheelchairs, and stretchers; side rails on beds; night-lights; and so on. In addition, nurses can implement measures to decrease the incidence of falls (see the Practice Guidelines box).

> **CLINICAL ALERT** *When a client falls, the nurse's first duty is to the client. First, assess for injuries. Then, notify the physician.*

Although it may seem that raising the side rails on a bed is an effective method of preventing falls, rails should not be raised routinely for this purpose. Research has shown that persons with memory impairment, altered mobility, nocturia, and other sleep disorders are prone to becoming entrapped in side rails and may, in fact, be more likely to fall trying to get out around or over the raised rails (Capezuti et al., 1999).

Electronic devices are available to detect that clients are attempting to move or get out of bed. A bed or chair **safety monitoring device** has a position-sensitive switch that triggers an audio alarm when the client attempts to get out of the bed or chair. Procedure 30–1 describes how to use these devices.

Practice Guidelines
Preventing Falls in Health Care Agencies

- On admission, orient clients to their surroundings and explain the call system.
- Carefully assess the client's ability to ambulate and transfer. Provide walking aids and assistance as required.
- Closely supervise the clients at risk for falls, especially at night.
- Encourage the client to use the call bell to request assistance. Ensure that the bell is within easy reach.
- Place beside tables and overbed tables near the bed or chair so that clients do not overreach and consequently lose their balance.
- Always keep hospital beds in the low position and wheels locked when not providing care so that clients can move in or out of bed easily.
- Encourage clients to use grab bars mounted in toilet and bathing areas and railings along corridors.
- Make sure nonskid bath mats are available in tubs and showers.
- Encourage the client to wear nonskid footwear.
- Keep the environment tidy; especially keep light cords from underfoot and furniture out of the way.
- Use individualized interventions (e.g., alarm sensitive to client position) rather than side rails for confused clients.

Research Note
Can Psychosocial Group Meetings Empower an Individual to Handle Fear of Falling?

Fear of falling is an important psychological consequence of falling and often leads to decreased function and social interaction. Few studies, however, have identified strategies to reduce fear of falling. The authors of a study on the fear of falling (Gentleman & Malozemoff, 2001) instituted a 10-week research-based clinical intervention with six institutionalized older adults with a history of falls. A weekly "Falls and Feelings" discussion group provided an opportunity for social interaction and a place for the older adults to share their feelings about their falling experiences.

The older adults completed two measurement tools related to self-confidence and sense of life satisfaction before and after the psychosocial discussion group intervention. Over the 10-week intervention, the authors observed increased socialization, concern for others, and cohesiveness among the group members. Three of the six older adults had enhanced scores on the self-confidence and sense of life satisfaction tests.

Implications: The psychosocial aspects of falls are important and the group process nursing intervention described in this study would be easy to implement. Nurses can initiate such a group for institutionalized older adults and encourage them to attend. As the authors indicated, additional research in this area would advance gerontological nursing practice.

Note: From "Falls and Feelings: Description of a Psychosocial Group Nursing Intervention," by B. Gentleman & W. Malozemoff, 2001, Journal of Gerontological Nursing, 27(10), pp. 35–39.

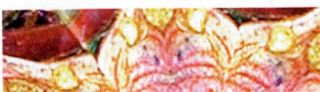

Procedure 30–1 Using a Bed or Chair Exit Safety Monitoring Device

Purposes

- To alert the nurse that the client is attempting to get out of bed
- To help decrease the risk of client falls

ASSESSMENT

Assess

- Mobility status
- Judgment about ability to get out of bed safely
- Proximity of client's room to nurses' station
- Position of side rails
- Functioning status of call light

PLANNING

Determine the appropriate location for the device. If the device will be applied to a thigh, ensure that the location has intact skin.

Delegation

Risk factors for falls may be observed and recorded by persons other than the nurse. The nurse is responsible for assessing the client and confirming that there is a risk of the client falling when getting out of a chair or bed unassisted. The nurse develops a plan of care that includes a variety of interventions that will protect the client. If indicated, use of a safety monitoring device may be delegated to unlicensed assistive personnel (UAP) who have been trained in their application and monitoring.

Equipment

- Alarm and control device
- Sensor
- Connection to nurse call system (optional)

IMPLEMENTATION

Performance

1. Explain to the client what you are going to do, why it is necessary, and how he or she can cooperate. Discuss how the results will be used in planning further care or treatments.
2. Wash hands and observe appropriate infection control procedures.
3. Provide for client privacy.
4. Explain to client and support persons the purpose and procedure of using a safety monitoring device.
   - Explain that the device does not limit mobility in any manner; rather, it alerts the staff when the client is about to get out of bed.
   - Explain that the nurse must be called when the client needs to get out of bed.
5. Test the battery device and alarm sound. *Testing ensures that the device is functioning properly prior to use.*
6. Apply the sensor pad or leg band.
   - Place the leg band according to the manufacturer's recommendation (Figure 30–3 ■). Place the client's leg in a straight horizontal position. *The*

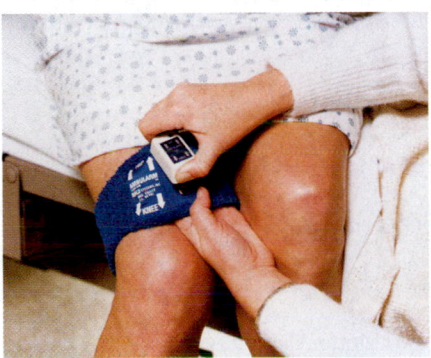

Figure 30–3 ■ Placing the leg band alarm. (Courtesy of Alert Care, Mill Valley, CA.)

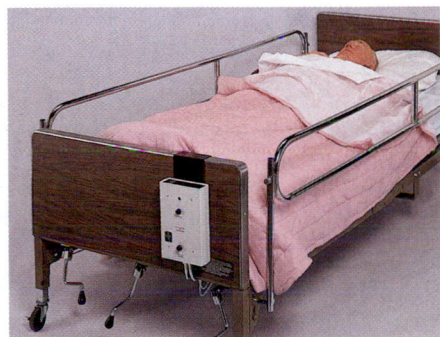

alarm device is position sensitive; that is, when it approaches a near-vertical position (such as in walking, crawling, or kneeling as the client attempts to get out of bed), the audio alarm will be triggered.
   - For the bed or chair device, the sensor is usually placed under the buttocks area (Figure 30–4 ■).

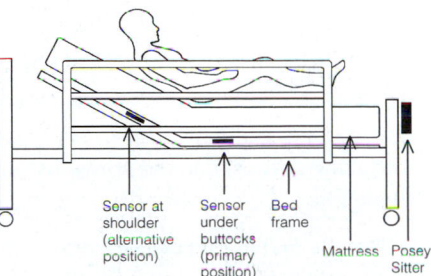

Figure 30–4 ■ Placement of a bed exit monitoring device. (Courtesy of J.T. Posey, Co.)

continued on page 682

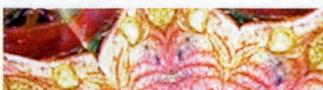

Procedure 30–1 Using a Bed or Chair Exit Safety Monitoring Device *continued*

IMPLEMENTATION *continued*

- For a bed or chair device, set the time delay for determining the client's movement patterns from 1 to 12 seconds.
- Connect the sensor pad to the control unit and the nurse call system.

7. Instruct the client to call the nurse when the client wants or needs to get up, and assist as required.
- When assisting the client up, deactivate the alarm.

- Assist the client back to bed, and reattach the alarm device.

8. Ensure client safety with additional safety precautions.
- Place call light within client reach, lift all side rails, and lower the bed to its lowest position. *The alarm device is not a substitute for other precautionary measures.*

- Place ambulation monitoring stickers on the client's door, chart, and Kardex.

9. Document the type of alarm used, where it was placed, and its effectiveness in the client record using forms or checklists supplemented by narrative notes when appropriate. Record all additional safety precautions and interventions discussed and employed.

EVALUATION

- If the alarm is too sensitive to client movement that is not an attempt to move from bed or chair, reassess and modify accordingly.

- Conduct appropriate follow-up relating to effectiveness of safety precautions.
- Report any difficulties using the device or any falls to the physician.

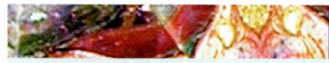

Lifespan Considerations

Preventing Falls

Elders

- Assess for potential personal causes of falls: hypotension, unsteady gait, altered mental responsiveness (such as from medications), poor vision, foot pathology, cognitive changes, and fear.
- In the home or community setting, assess for potential environmental causes of falls:
  - *Lighting:* inadequate amount, inaccessible or inconvenient switches
  - *Floors:* presence of electrical cords, loose rugs, clutter, slippery surfaces

- *Stairs:* absent or unsteady railings, uneven step height or surfaces
- *Furniture:* unsteady base, lack of armrests, cabinets too high or too low
- *Bathroom:* inappropriate toilet height, slippery floors or tub, absence of grab bars
- In the home, consider alternatives to hospital or regular bed if client is extremely prone to fall out of bed:
  - Place the mattress directly onto the floor.
  - Use a water mattress.
  - Place padding on floor next to bed or between client and side rails.

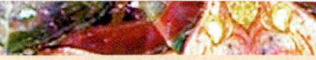

Home Care Considerations

Using a Bed or Chair Exit Safety Monitoring Device

If the device is used in the home, instruct caregivers to do the following:

- Test the monitoring device every 12 to 24 hours to ensure that it is working.
- Check the volume of the alarm to ascertain they can hear it.

Use of the device does not take the place of proper supervision of clients at risk for falling. Assessment of the reasons for falling, especially among elders, can lead to effective prevention.

Seizures. A **seizure** is a sudden onset of a convulsion or other paroxysmal motor or sensory activity. Clients may be prone to seizures due to permanent or temporary medical conditions such as drug reactions, epilepsy, or extreme fever. They are at risk for injury if they experience seizures that involve the entire body such as *grand mal* (tonic-clonic) seizures or any seizure that includes loss of consciousness. **Seizure precautions** are safety measures taken by the nurse to protect clients from injury should they have a seizure. Procedure 30–2 describes how to implement seizure precautions.

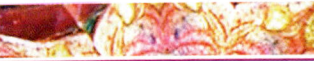

Procedure 30–2 Implementing Seizure Precautions

Purpose

- Protect the client from injury

ASSESSMENT

Assess history of seizures during the admission assessment. If the client has experienced a seizure previously, ask for detailed information, including characteristics of an aura or premonitory symptoms that indicate the seizure is beginning, duration and frequency of the seizures, consequences of the seizures (e.g., incontinence or difficulty breathing), and actions that should be taken to prevent or reduce seizure activity.

PLANNING

Review emergency procedures because the client could have a respiratory arrest or other injury as a result of a seizure.

Delegation

UAP should be familiar with establishing and implementing seizure precautions and methods of obtaining assistance during a client's seizure. Care of the client during a seizure, however, is the responsibility of the nurse due to the importance of careful assessment of respiratory status and potential need for intervention.

Equipment

- Blankets or other linens to pad side rails
- Oral suction equipment
- Oral airway or padded tongue depressor (according to agency policy)
- Oxygen equipment

IMPLEMENTATION

Performance

1. Explain to the client what you are going to do, why it is necessary, and how he or she can cooperate.
2. Wash hands and observe appropriate infection control procedures. If the client is actively seizing, apply clean gloves in preparation for performing respiratory care measures.
3. Provide for client privacy.
4. Pad the bed. Secure blankets or other linens around the head, foot, and side rails of the bed (Figure 30–5 ■).

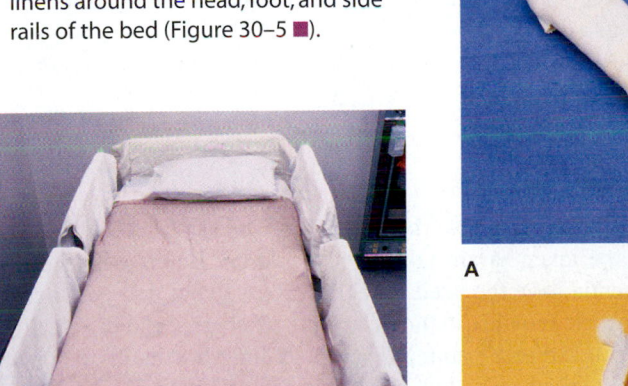

Figure 30–5 ■ Padding a bed for seizure precautions.

5. Put oral suction equipment in place and test to ensure that it is functional.
6. If agency policy prescribes, tape the tongue depressor that has been wrapped with gauze padding or an oral airway within reach of the head of the bed (Figure 30–6 ■).

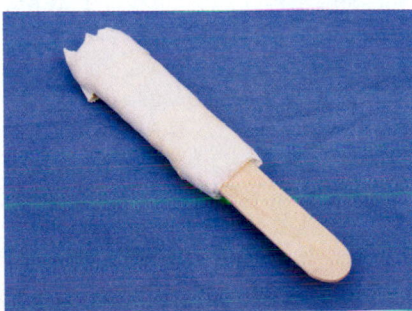

A

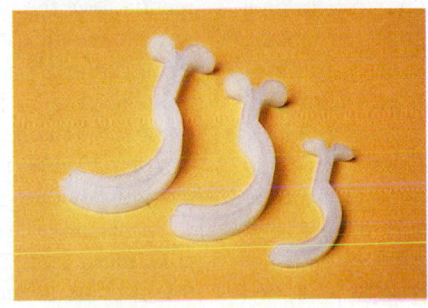

B

Figure 30–6 ■ *A*, Padded tongue blade; *B*, oral airway.

7. If a seizure occurs:
   - Remain with the client and call for assistance if needed.
   - If the client is not in bed, assist client to the floor and protect the head in your lap or on a pillow.
   - According to policy, insert the airway or tongue depressor between the client's upper and lower teeth. *Never force the insertion because forcing can cause damage.* In many agencies, an oral airway is used only for situations in which the client is having continuous seizures **(status epilepticus).** Never place your fingers inside the client's mouth. Loosen any clothing around the neck and chest.
   - Apply oxygen by mask.
   - Turn the client to a lateral position if possible.
   - Time the seizure duration.
   - Move items in the environment to ensure the client does not experience an injury.
   - Observe the progression of the seizure, noting the sequence and type of limb involvement. Observe skin color. When the seizure allows, check pulse and respirations.
   - Administer ordered anticonvulsant medications.
   - Use equipment to suction the oral airway if the client vomits or has excessive oral secretions.

continued on page 684

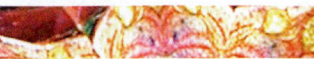

Procedure 30–2 Implementing Seizure Precautions *continued*

IMPLEMENTATION *continued*

- When the seizure has finished, assist client to a comfortable position. Provide hygiene as necessary. Allow the client to verbalize feelings about the seizure.

8. When the seizure has subsided, document it in the client record using forms or checklists supplemented by narrative notes when appropriate

EVALUATION

- Perform a detailed follow-up examination of the client. Administer medications if indicated.

- Report significant deviations from normal to the physician.

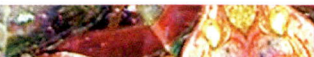

Lifespan Considerations

Implementing Seizure Precautions

Infants

- About 24% of children experience seizures, most during infancy (Ball & Bindler, 2003).

Children

- Febrile seizures occur more commonly than in adults and are usually preventable through antipyretics and tepid baths.

- Determine oxygenation. Apply oxygen if pulse oximetry reading is less than 95% (see Chapter 48).
- Children who have frequent seizures may need to wear helmets for protection.
- Children on anticonvulsant medications should wear a medical identification tag (bracelet or necklace).

Home Care Considerations

Implementing Seizure Precautions

- If clients have frequent or recurrent seizures or take anticonvulsant medications, they should wear a medical identification tag (bracelet or necklace) and carry a card delineating any medications they take.
- When making home visits, inspect anticonvulsant medications and confirm that clients are taking them correctly. Blood level measurements may be required periodically.
- Assist the client in determining which persons in the community should/must be informed of their seizure disorder (e.g.,

employers, health care providers such as dentists, motor vehicle department if driving, companions).
- Discuss safety precautions for inside and out of the home. If seizures are not well controlled, activities that may require restriction or direct supervision by others include tub bathing, swimming, cooking, using electric equipment or machinery, and driving.
- Discuss with the client and family factors that may precipitate a seizure.

Poisoning. The major reasons for poisoning in children are inadequate supervision and improper storage of many household toxic substances. Implementing poison prevention for children is focused on teaching parents to "childproof" the environment, including disposing of unused medications properly by flushing them down a drain. Adolescent and adult poisonings are usually caused by insect or snake bites and drugs used for recreation or in suicide attempts. Implementing poison prevention in these age groups focuses on dissemination of information and counseling. Poisoning in elders usually results from accidental ingestion of a toxic substance (e.g., due to failing eyesight) or an overdose of a prescribed medication (e.g., due to impaired memory). Implementing poison prevention with elders focuses on safeguarding the environment and monitoring the underlying problems.

In elders who have dementia, poisoning is often a safety problem. As cognitive abilities deteriorate, behavior often re-

gresses to resemble that of a child. The same precautions need to be taken as are taken with children. Elders who have dementia have the need to feel everything and will put anything in their mouths, including plants, flowers, candles, small objects, and medications. These and other potentially dangerous items need to be locked up or kept out of reach. A telephone number for the nearest poison control center should be readily available. These precautions are important whether the individual with dementia is being cared for at home or in an institution.

In response to the ever-increasing number of poison hazards, many countries have established poison control centers that provide accurate, up-to-date information about potential hazards and recommend treatment as needed. For certain poisons, specific antidotes or treatments are available; for many, there is no specific therapy.

Nurses intervene in community settings by educating the public about what to do in the event of poisoning: Identify the specific poison by searching for an opened container, empty bottle, or other evidence. Contact the poison control center, indicate the exact quantity of poison the person ingested, and state the person's age and apparent symptoms. Keep the person as quiet as possible and lying on the side or sitting with head placed between the legs to prevent aspiration of vomitus. The Teaching: Client Care feature provides additional guidelines for teaching clients to prevent poisoning.

Carbon Monoxide Poisoning. **Carbon monoxide** (CO) is an odorless, colorless, tasteless gas that is very toxic. Exposure to CO can cause symptoms including headaches, dizziness, weakness, nausea, vomiting, or loss of muscle control. Prolonged exposure to CO can lead to unconsciousness, brain damage, or death. Learning the steps to prevent CO danger is particularly important because all gasoline-powered vehicles, lawn mowers, kerosene stoves, barbecues, and burning wood emit CO. Incomplete or faulty combustion of any fuel, including natural gas used in furnaces, can produce CO. Carbon monoxide detectors are available for the home.

Suffocation or Choking. Suffocation, or **asphyxiation,** is lack of oxygen due to interrupted breathing. Suffocation occurs when the air source is cut off for any reason. One common reason for choking is that food or a foreign object has become lodged in the throat. The universal sign of distress is the victim's grasping the anterior neck and being unable to speak or cough. The emergency response is the **Heimlich maneuver,** or abdominal thrust, which can dislodge the foreign object and reestablish an airway. See Figure 30–7 ■ and Chapter 48. ⚭

Other causes of suffocation are drowning, gas or smoke inhalation, accidental coverage of the nose and mouth by a piece of plastic, accidental strangulation by the shoulder harness of a seat belt, and being trapped in a confined space (e.g., a discarded refrigerator). If a person does not receive immediate relief from suffocation, the interrupted breathing leads to respiratory and cardiac arrest and death. Any obstruction to the air passages must be immediately removed and life support measures instituted when an arrest occurs.

Excessive Noise. Excessive noise is a health hazard that can cause hearing loss, depending on (a) the overall level of noise, (b) the frequency range of the noise, and (c) the duration of exposure and individual susceptibility. Sound levels above 120 decibels (units of loudness) are painful and may cause hearing damage even if a person is exposed for only a short period. Exposure to 85 to 95 decibels for several hours a day can lead to progressive or permanent hearing loss. Noise levels below 85 decibels usually do not affect hearing.

Tolerance of noise is largely individual. The rural dweller may find the city noisy, whereas the city dweller may be oblivious to urban sounds.

When ill or injured, people are frequently sensitive to noises that normally would not disturb them. Loud voices, the clatter of dishes, and even a nearby television can disturb clients, some of whom react angrily. Physiologic effects of noise include (a) increased heart and respiratory rates, (b) increased muscular activity, (c) nausea, and (d) hearing loss, if the noise is sufficiently loud.

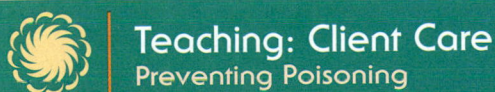

Teaching: Client Care
Preventing Poisoning

- Lock potentially toxic agents, including drugs and cleaning agents, in a cupboard, or attach special plastic hooks to the insides of cabinet doors to keep them securely closed. Unlatching these hooks requires firmer thumb pressure than small children can usually exert.
- Avoid storing toxic liquids or solids in food containers, such as soft drink bottles, peanut butter jars, or milk cartons.
- Do not remove container labels or reuse empty containers to store different substances. Laws mandate that the labels of all poisons specify antidotes.
- Do not rely on cooking to destroy toxic chemicals in plants. Never use anything prepared from nature as a medicine or "tea."
- Teach children never to eat any part of an unknown plant or mushroom and not to put leaves, stems, bark, seeds, nuts, or berries from any plant into their mouths.
- Place poison warning stickers designed for children on containers of bleach, lye, kerosene, solvent, and other toxic substances.
- Do not refer to medicine as candy or pretend false enjoyment when taking medications in front of children; allow them to see the necessity of the medicine without glamorizing it.
- Read and follow label directions on all products before using them.
- Keep syrup of ipecac on hand at all times. Syrup of ipecac is a nonprescription emetic available in single-dose 15-mL vials in all drugstores. Use it only after advice from the local poison control center or the family physician.
- Do not keep poisonous plants in the home, and avoid planting poisonous plants in the yard. The cooperative extension agency in your county can provide a list of poisonous plants.
- Display the phone number of the poison control center near or on all telephones in the home so that it is available to babysitters, family, and friends.

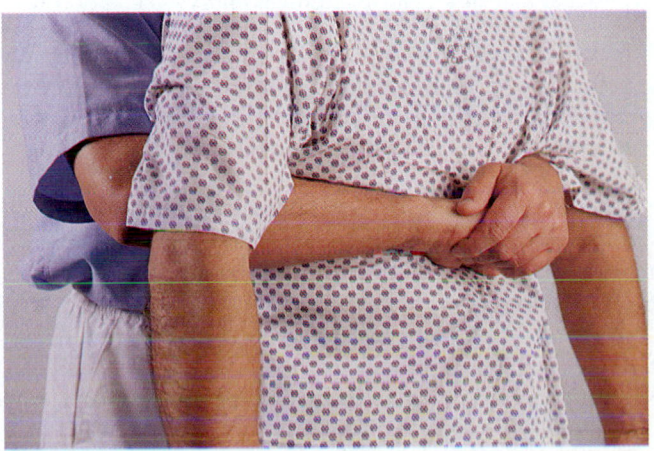

Figure 30–7 ■ Performing the Heimlich maneuver.

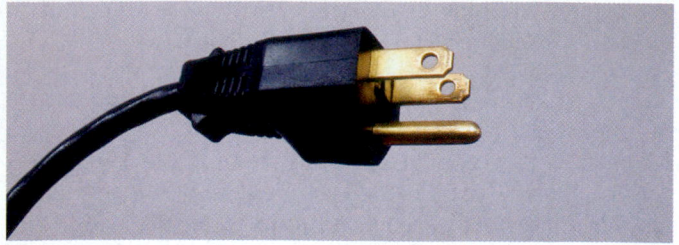

Figure 30–8 ■ Three-pronged grounded plug.

Noise can be minimized in several ways. Acoustic tile on ceilings, walls, and floors as well as drapes and carpeting absorb sound. Background music can mask noise and have a calming effect on some people. It is important for nurses to minimize noise in the hospital setting and to encourage clients to protect their hearing as much as possible.

Electrical Hazards. All electric equipment must be properly grounded. The electric plug of grounded equipment has three prongs. The two short prongs transmit the power to the equipment. The third, longer prong is the grounding device, which carries short circuits or stray electric current to the ground (Figure 30–8 ■). Grounding prongs offer a path of least resistance to stray electric currents.

Faulty equipment (e.g., equipment with a frayed cord) presents a danger of electric shock or may start a fire. For example, an electric spark near certain anesthetic gases or a high concentration of oxygen can cause a serious fire. Actions to reduce electrical hazards are described in Teaching: Client Care.

When major electrical injury (macroshock) does occur, the victim may sustain both superficial and deep burns, muscle contractions, and cardiac and respiratory arrest, necessitating cardiopulmonary resuscitation and life support. **Electric shock** occurs when a current travels through the body to the ground rather than through electric wiring, or from static electricity that builds up on the body. Using machines in good repair, wearing shoes with rubber soles, standing on a nonconductive floor, and using nonconductive gloves can prevent macroshock. However, even with such precautions the rescuer must know that the victim is not to be touched until the electricity is shut off or the victim has been removed from contact with the electric current; otherwise the rescuer may also receive electrical injury.

Firearms. Parents who bring a handgun into the home must accept full responsibility for teaching safety rules to any children who have knowledge of the presence of firearms. The following basic firearm safety rules must be implemented for any gun:

- Store all guns in sturdy locked cabinets without glass and make sure the keys are inaccessible to children.
- Store the bullets in a different location from the guns.
- Tell children never to touch a gun or stay in a friend's house where a gun is accessible.
- Teach children never to point the barrel of a gun at anyone.
- Ensure the firearm is unloaded and the action is open when handing it to someone else.
- Don't handle firearms while affected by alcohol or drugs of any kind, including pharmaceuticals.

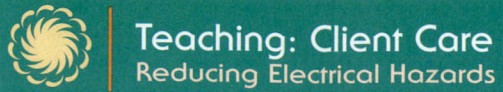

Teaching: Client Care
Reducing Electrical Hazards

- Check cords for fraying or other signs of damage before using an appliance. Do not use if damage is apparent.
- Avoid overloading outlets and fuse boxes with too many appliances.
- Use only grounded outlets and plugs.
- Always pull a plug from the wall outlet by firmly grasping the plug and pulling it straight out. Pulling a plug by its cord can damage the cord and plug unit.
- Never use electric appliances near sinks, bathtubs, showers, or other wet areas, because water readily conducts electricity.
- Keep electric cords and appliances out of the reach of young children.
- Place protective covers over wall outlets to protect young children.
- Have all noninsulated wiring in the home altered to meet safety standards.
- Carefully read instructions before operating electric equipment. Clients who do not understand how to operate the equipment should seek advice.
- Always disconnect appliances before cleaning or repairing them.
- Unplug any appliance that has given a tingling sensation or shock and have an electrician evaluate it for stray current.
- Keep electric cords coiled or taped to the ground away from areas of traffic to prevent others from damaging the cords or tripping over them.

- When cleaning or dry firing a firearm, remove all ammunition to another room, and double-check the firearm when you enter the room you will be using to clean the firearm.
- Have firearms that are regularly used inspected by a qualified gunsmith at least every 2 years.

Radiation. Radiation injury can occur from overexposure to radioactive materials used in diagnostic and therapeutic procedures. Clients being examined using radiography or fluoroscopy generally receive minimal exposure and few precautions are necessary. Nurses need to protect themselves, however, from radiation when some clients are receiving radiation therapy. Exposure to radiation can be minimized by (a) limiting the time near the source, (b) providing as much distance as possible from the source, and (c) using shielding devices such as lead aprons when near the source. Nurses need to become familiar with agency protocols related to radiation therapy.

Procedure- and Equipment-Related Accidents

Risk assessment in the health care setting must include risks related to procedures and equipment. Whether giving a medication or assisting a client out of bed, nurses need to follow safeguards to prevent errors or accidents. Most health care agencies establish protocols that are designed to prevent accidents. When in doubt about a course of action, the nurse should consult the appropriate written guidelines before proceeding.

When an accident or error does occur, most agencies require that the incident be reported. The nurse completes the report immediately after taking whatever action is required to safeguard the client and notifying the charge nurse. For additional information about incident reports, see Chapter 4. ⬭⬭

Restraining Clients

Restraints are protective devices used to limit the physical activity of the client or a part of the body. They can be classified as physical or chemical. **Physical restraints** are any manual method or physical or mechanical device, material, or equipment attached to the client's body; they cannot be removed easily and they restrict the client's movement. **Chemical restraints** are medications such as neuroleptics, anxiolytics, sedatives, and psychotropic agents used to control socially disruptive behavior. The purpose of restraints is to prevent the client from injuring self or others.

Legal Implications of Restraints.

Increasingly, determining the need for safety measures is viewed as an independent nursing function. However, because restraints restrict the individual's freedom, their use has legal implications. Nurses need to know their agency's policies and the state laws about restraining clients. The U.S. Centers for Medicare and Medicaid Services published revised standards for use of restraints in the United States in 2001. These standards apply to all health care organizations and specify two standards for applying restraints: the behavior management standard (client is a danger to self or others) and the acute medical and surgical care standard (temporary immobilization of a client related to a procedure). In the case of the behavior management standard, the nurse may apply restraints but the physician or other licensed independent practitioner must see the client within 1 hour for evaluation. A written restraint order for an adult, following evaluation, is valid for only 4 hours. If the client must be restrained and secluded, there must be continual visual and audio monitoring of the client's status. The medical surgical care standard permits up to 12 hours for obtaining the physician's written order for the restraints. All orders must be renewed daily. See Figure 30–9 ■ for an example of a restraint monitoring and intervention flow sheet.

Standards require that a physician's order for restraints delineate the reason and time period and prohibit the use of a PRN order for restraints. In all cases, restraints should be used *only* after every other possible means of ensuring safety have been tried (and must be documented). See alternatives to the use of restraints in Box 30–2. Restrained clients often become (more) restless and anxious as a result of the loss of self-control. Nurses must document that the need for the restraint was made clear both to the client and to support persons.

Selecting a Restraint.

Before selecting a restraint, nurses need to understand its purpose clearly and measure it against the following five criteria:

1. It restricts the client's movement as little as possible. If a client needs to have one arm restrained, do not restrain the entire body.

2. It does not interfere with the client's treatment or health problem. If a client has poor blood circulation to the hands, apply a restraint that will not aggravate that circulatory problem.

3. It is readily changeable. Restraints need to be changed frequently, especially if they become soiled. Keeping other guidelines in mind, choose a restraint that can be changed with minimal disturbance to the client.

4. It is safe for the particular client. Choose a restraint with which the client cannot self-inflict injury. For example, a physically restrained person could incur injury trying to climb out of bed if one wrist is tied to the bed frame. A jacket restraint would restrain the person more safely.

5. It is the least obvious to others. Both clients and visitors are often embarrassed by a restraint, even though they understand why it is being used. The less obvious the restraint, the more comfortable people feel.

MediaLink | ENSURING CLIENT SAFETY CASE STUDY

BOX 30–2 ■ Alternatives to Restraints

- Assign nurses in pairs to act as "buddies" so that one nurse can observe the client when the other leaves the unit.
- Place unstable clients in an area that is constantly or closely supervised.
- Prepare clients before a move to limit relocation shock and resultant confusion.
- Stay with a client using a bedside commode or bathroom if the client is confused or sedated or has a gait disturbance or a high risk score for falling.
- Monitor all the client's medications and, if possible, attempt to lower or eliminate dosages of sedatives or psychotropics.
- Position beds at their lowest level to facilitate getting in and out of bed.
- Replace full-length side rails with half- or three-quarter-length rails to prevent confused clients from climbing over rails or falling from the end of the bed.
- Use rocking chairs to help confused clients expend some of their energy so that they will be less inclined to wander.

- Wedge pillows or pads against the sides of wheelchairs to keep clients well positioned.
- Place a removable lap tray on a wheelchair to provide support and help keep the client in place.
- To quiet agitated clients, try a warm beverage, soft lights, a back rub, or a walk.
- Use "environmental restraints," such as pieces of furniture or large plants as barriers, to keep clients from wandering beyond appropriate areas.
- Place a picture or other personal item on the door to clients' rooms to help them identify their room.
- Try to determine the causes of the client's sundowner syndrome (nocturnal wandering and disorientation as darkness falls, associated with dementia). Possible causes include poor hearing, poor eyesight, or pain.
- Establish ongoing assessment to monitor changes in physical and cognitive functional abilities and risk factors.

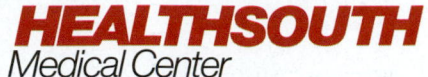
HEALTHSOUTH
Medical Center

ACUTE MEDICAL/SURGICAL CARE
RESTRAINT FLOW SHEET

Restraint Initiated: Date: _____   Time: _____

Order Expires: Date: _____   Time: _____
New verbal order required every 24 hours.

Assessment should be based on individual needs. Patients must be assessed at least every 2 hours.

		0700	0800	0900	1000	1100	1200	1300	1400	1500	1600	1700	1800	1900	2000	2100	2200	2300	2400	0100	0200	0300	0400	0500	0600
Restraints Removed																									
Skin & Circulation Assessed																									
Toileting Offered																									
Food/Fluids Offered																									
Range of Motion & Patient Repositioned																									
Patient Response	R=Restless C=Calm S=Sleeping U=Unaware																								
Effect of Restraint	A=Adequate I=Inadequate (explain)																								
Continued Need	Y=Yes N=No																								
Restraint Reapplied																									
Initials																									

Explain: _____

_____

INIT	SIGNATURE	TITLE

©HRC 2003
HSPI F9440

Figure 30–9 ■ Restraint monitoring and intervention flow sheet. (Courtesy of Health South Medical Center, Birmingham, Alabama.)

Kinds of Restraints. There are several kinds of restraints. Among the most common for adults are jacket restraints, belt restraints, mitt or hand restraints, and limb restraints. Geri chairs and wheelchairs used to confine client activity can also be considered restraints. Restraints for infants and children include mummy restraints, elbow restraints, and crib nets (see Lifespan Considerations later in the chapter). When using restraints, the nurse may find the Practice Guidelines box helpful.

There are several types of vest restraints, but all are essentially sleeveless jackets (vests) with straps (tails) that can be tied to the bed frame under the mattress (Figure 30–10 ■) These body restraints are used to ensure the safety of confused or se-dated clients in beds or wheelchairs. The FDA advises that manufacturers place "front" and "back" labels on vest restraints (USFDA, 1992).

Belt or safety strap body restraints (Figure 30–11 ■) are used to ensure the safety of all clients who are being moved on stretchers or in wheelchairs. Some wheelchairs have a soft, padded safety bar that attaches to side brackets that are installed under the arm rests. To prevent the person from slumping forward, the nurse then attaches a shoulder "Y" strap to the bar and over the client's shoulders to the rear handles. Other safety belt models have a three-loop design. One loop surrounds the person's waist and attaches to the rear handles. If such restraints are

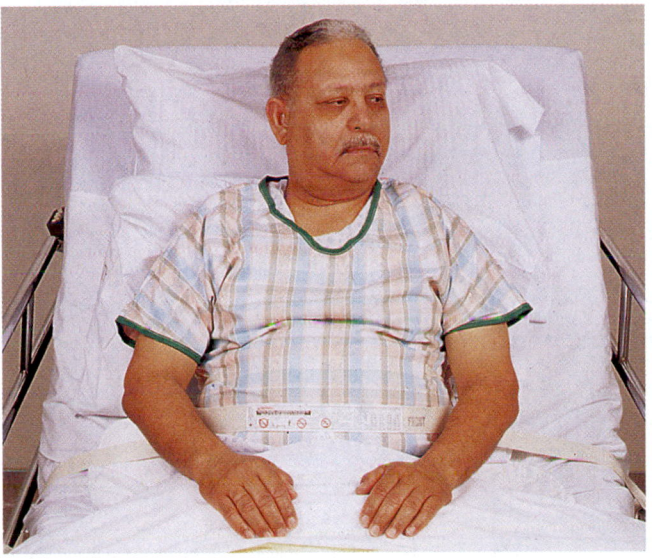

Figure 30–10 ■ A poncho-type vest restraint.

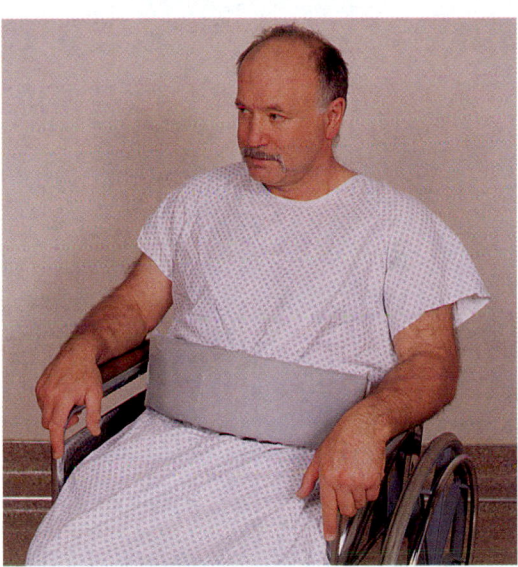

Figure 30–11 ■ A belt restraint.

Practice Guidelines
Applying Restraints

- Obtain consent from the client or guardian.
- Ensure that a physician's order has been provided or, in an emergency, obtain one within 24 hours after applying the restraint.
- Assure the client and the client's support people that the restraint is temporary and protective. A restraint must never be applied as punishment for any behavior or merely for the nurse's convenience.
- Apply the restraint in such a way that the client can move as freely as possible without defeating the purpose of the restraint.
- Ensure that limb restraints are applied securely but not so tightly that they impede blood circulation to any body area or extremity.
- Pad bony prominences (e.g., wrists and ankles) before applying a restraint over them. The movement of a restraint without padding over such prominences can quickly abrade the skin.
- Always tie a limb restraint with a knot (e.g., a clove hitch) that will not tighten when pulled.
- Tie the ends of a body restraint to the part of the bed that moves to elevate the head. Never tie the ends to a side rail or to the fixed frame of the bed if the bed position is to be changed.

- Assess the restraint every 30 minutes. Some facilities have specific forms to be used to record ongoing assessment.
- Release all restraints at least every 2 to 4 hours, and provide range-of-motion (ROM) exercises (see Chapter 42 ⚭) and skin care (see Chapter 34). ⚭
- Reassess the continued need for the restraint at least every 8 hours. Include an assessment of the underlying cause of the behavior necessitating use of the restraints.
- When a restraint is temporarily removed, do not leave the client unattended.
- Immediately report to the nurse in charge and record on the client's chart any persistent reddened or broken skin areas under the restraint.
- At the first indication of cyanosis or pallor, coldness of a skin area, or a client's complaint of a tingling sensation, pain, or numbness, loosen the restraint and exercise the limb.
- Apply a restraint so that it can be released quickly in case of an emergency and with the body part in a normal anatomic position.
- Provide emotional support verbally and through touch.

unavailable, the nurse can place a folded towel or small sheet around the client's waist and fasten it at the back of the wheelchair. Belt restraints may also be used for certain clients confined to bed or to chairs.

A mitt or hand restraint (Figure 30–12 ■) is used to prevent confused clients from using their hands or fingers to scratch and injure themselves. For example, a confused client may need to be prevented from pulling at intravenous tubing or a head bandage following brain surgery. Hand or mitt restraints

allow the client to be ambulatory and/or to move the arm freely rather than be confined to a bed or a chair. Mittens need to be removed on a regular basis to permit the client to wash and exercise the hands. The nurse also needs to take off the mitten to check the circulation to the hand.

Limb restraints (Figure 30–13 ■), which are generally made of cloth, may be used to immobilize a limb, primarily for therapeutic reasons (e.g., to maintain an intravenous infusion). See Procedure 30–3 for applying restraints.

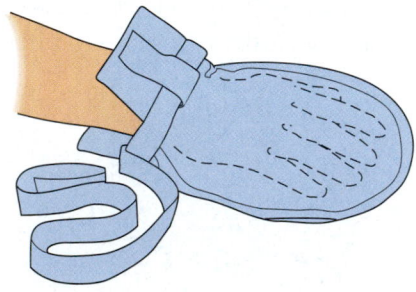

Figure 30–12 ■ A mitt restraint.

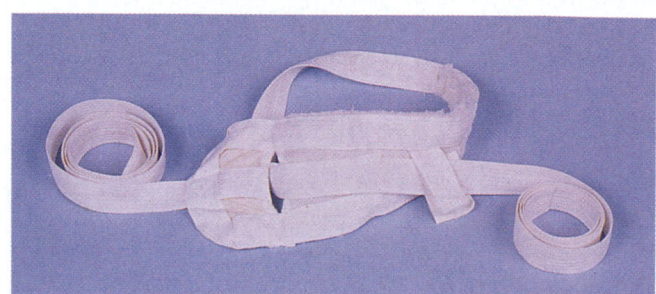

Figure 30–13 ■ A limb restraint.

Procedure 30–3 Applying Restraints

Purposes

- To enable the client to receive treatment
- To allow the treatment to proceed without client interference (e.g., to prevent movements that would disrupt therapy to a limb connected to tubes or appliance)

ASSESSMENT

Assess

- The behavior indicating the possible need for a restraint
- Underlying cause for assessed behavior
- What other protective measures may be implemented before applying a restraint

- Status of skin to which restraint is to be applied
- Circulatory status distal to restraints and of extremities
- Effectiveness of other available safety precautions

PLANNING

Review institutional policy for restraints and seek consultation as appropriate before independently deciding to apply a restraint. All other possible interventions that are less restrictive must have been tried. The physician must be notified prior to using a restraint, unless there is an emergency.

Delegation

The nurse must make the determination that restraints are appropriate in the specific situation, select the proper type of restraints,

evaluate the effectiveness of the restraints, and assess for potential complications from their use. Application of ordered restraints and their temporary removal for skin assessment and care may be delegated to UAP who have been trained in their use.

Equipment

- Appropriate type and size of restraint

IMPLEMENTATION

Performance

1. Explain to the client and family what you are going to do, why it is necessary, and how they can cooperate. Discuss how the results will be used in planning further care or treatments. Allow time for the client to express feelings about being restrained. Provide needed emotional reassurance that the re-

straints will be used only when absolutely necessary and that there will be close contact with the client in case assistance is required.

2. Wash hands and observe appropriate infection control procedures.
3. Provide for client privacy if indicated.
4. Apply the selected restraint.

BELT RESTRAINT (SAFETY BELT)

- Determine that the safety belt is in good order. If a Velcro safety belt is to be used, make sure that both pieces of Velcro are intact.
- If the belt has a long portion and a shorter portion, place the long portion of the belt behind (under) the bedrid-

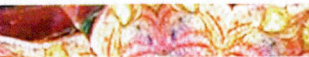

Procedure 30–3 Applying Restraints *continued*

IMPLEMENTATION *continued*

den client and secure it to the movable part of the bed frame. *The long attached portion will then move up when the head of the bed is elevated and will not tighten around the client.* Place the shorter portion of the belt around the client's waist, over the gown. There should be a finger's width between the belt and the client.

or

• Attach the belt around the client's waist, and fasten it at the back of the chair.

or

• If the belt is attached to a stretcher, secure the belt firmly over the client's hips or abdomen. *Belt restraints need to be applied to all clients on stretchers even when the side rails are up.*

JACKET RESTRAINT

• Place vest on client, with opening at the front or the back, depending on the type.
• Pull the tie on the end of the vest flap across the chest, and place it through the slit in the opposite side of the chest.
• Repeat for the other tie.
Use a half-bow knot to secure each tie around the movable bed frame or behind the chair to a chair leg (Figures 30–14 ■ and 30–15 ■). *A half-bow knot does not tighten or slip when the at-*

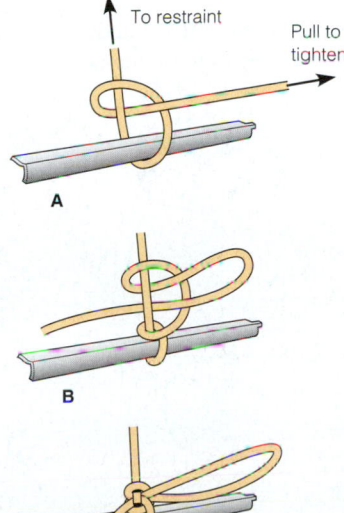

Figure 30–14 ■ To make a half-bow knot (quick-release knot), first place the restraint tie under the side frame of the bed (or around a chair leg). *A,* Bring the free end up, around, under, and over the attached end of the tie and pull it tight. *B,* Again take the free end over and under the attached end of the tie, but this time make a half-bow loop. *C,* Tighten the free end of the tie and the bow until the knot is secure. To untie the knot, pull the end of the tie and then loosen the first cross over the tie.

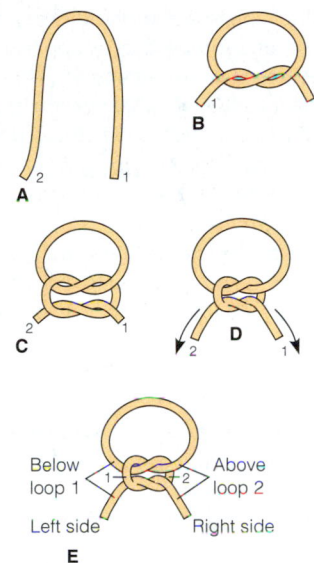

Figure 30–15 ■ Quick-release knot.

tached end is pulled but unties easily when the loose end is pulled.

or

• Fasten the ties together behind the chair using a square (reef) knot (Figure 30–16 ■). *This knot does not tighten with pulling and does not slip when pressure is released.*
• Ensure that the client is positioned appropriately to enable maximum chest expansion for breathing.

MITT RESTRAINT

• Apply the commercial thumbless mitt (Figure 30–12) to the hand to be restrained. Make sure the fingers can be slightly flexed and are not caught under the hand.
• Follow the manufacturer's directions for securing the mitt.
• If a mitt is to be worn for several days, remove it at least every 2 to 4 hours. Wash and exercise the client's hand, then reapply the mitt. Check agency practices about recommended intervals for removal.
• Assess the client's circulation to the hands shortly after the mitt is applied and at regular intervals. *Feelings of numbness or discomfort or inability to move the fingers could indicate impaired circulation to the hand.*

Figure 30–16 ■ To make a square (reef) knot: *A,* Form a "U" loop. *B,* Pass one end (1) over and under the other. *C,* Take the same end (1), and pass it over, under, and over the other. *D,* Pull knot tight. *E,* When the knot is tied correctly, the ties on each side are both either above or below the loop.

WRIST OR ANKLE RESTRAINT

• Pad bony prominences on the wrist or ankle if needed to prevent skin breakdown.
• Apply the padded portion of the restraint around the ankle or wrist.
• Pull the tie of the restraint through the slit in the wrist portion or through the buckle (Figure 30–17 ■).

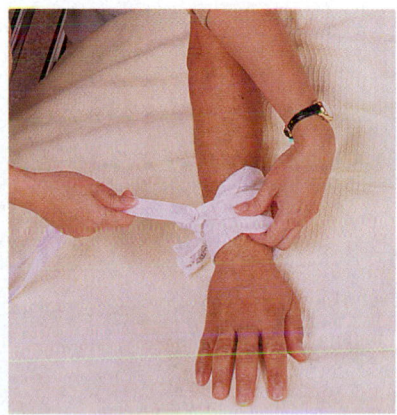

Figure 30–17 ■ Ensure that two fingers can be inserted between the restraint and the wrist or ankle.

continued on page 692

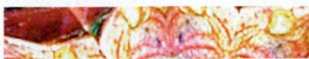

Procedure 30–3 Applying Restraints *continued*

IMPLEMENTATION *continued*

- Using a half-bow knot (quick-release knot) or a square knot as appropriate, attach the other end of the restraint to the movable portion of the bed frame. *If the ties are attached to the movable portion, the wrist or ankle will not be pulled when the bed position is changed.*
5. Record on the client's chart the behavior(s) indicating the need for the restraint, all other interventions imple-

mented in attempt to avoid the use of restraints and their outcomes, and the time the physician was notified of the need for restraint. Also record:
  - The type of restraint applied, the time it was applied, the goal for its application
  - The client's response to the restraint
  - The times that the restraints were removed and skin care given

- Any other assessments and interventions
- Explanations given to the client and significant others.
6. Adjust the plan of care as required, for example, to include releasing the restraint every 2 hours, providing skin care, and providing range-of-motion exercises.

EVALUATION

- Perform a detailed follow-up of the need for the restraints and the client's response. Relate these findings to previous data if available.
- Evaluate circulatory status of restrained limbs.

- Evaluate skin status beneath restraints.
- Remove the restraints as soon as they are no longer needed and document.
- Report significant deviations from normal to the physician.

Lifespan Considerations

Restraints

Infants

Elbow restraints (Figure 30–18 ■) are used to prevent infants or small children from flexing their elbows to touch or scratch a skin lesion or to reach the head when a scalp vein infusion is in place.

This restraint consists of a piece of material with pockets into which plastic or wooden tongue depressors are inserted to provide rigidity.

- Examine the restraint to make sure that the tongue depressors are intact (i.e., all in place and not broken).
- Place the infant's elbow in the center of the restraint. Make sure that the padded material covers the ends of the tongue depressors. This prevents them from irritating the skin.
- Wrap the restraint smoothly around the arm.
- Secure the restraint, using safety pins, ties, or tape. Ensure that it is not so tight that it obstructs blood circulation.
- *Optional:* After the restraint is applied, pin it to the child's shirt. This prevents is from sliding down the arm.

A mummy restraint (Figure 30–19 ■) is a special folding of a blanket or sheet around the infant to prevent movement during a pro-

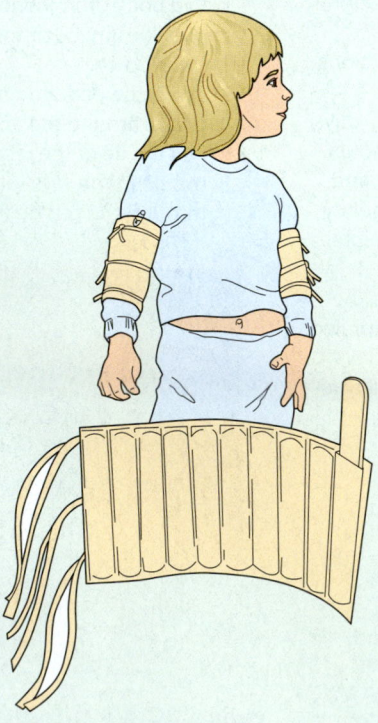

Figure 30–18 ■ An elbow restraint.

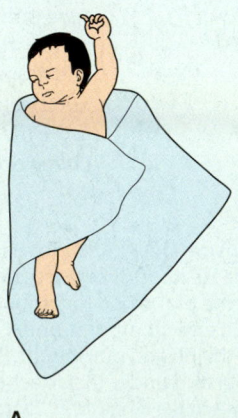

A

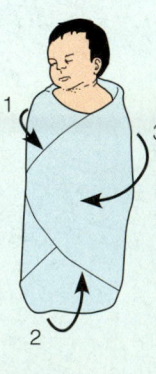

B

Figure 30–19 ■ Making a mummy restraint.

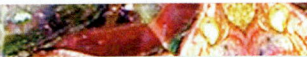
Lifespan Considerations *continued*

cedure such as gastric washing, eye irrigation, or collection of a blood specimen.

- Obtain a blanket or sheet large enough so that the distance between opposite corners is about twice the length of the infant's body. Lay the blanket or sheet on a flat, dry surface.
- Fold down one corner, and place the baby on it in the supine position.
- Fold the right side of the blanket over the infant's body, leaving the left arm free (Figure 30–19, *A*). The right arm is in a natural position at the side.
- Fold the excess blanket at the bottom up under the infant (Figure 30–19, *B*, 2).
- With the left arm in a natural position at the baby's side, fold the left side of the blanket over the infant, including the arm, and tuck the blanket under the body (Figure 30–19, *B*, 3).

- Remain with the infant who is in a mummy restraint until the specific procedure is completed.

Children
A crib net is simply a device placed over the top of a crib to prevent active young children from climbing out of the crib. At the same time, it allows them freedom to move about in the crib. The crib net or dome is not attached to the movable parts of the crib so that the caregiver can have access to the child without removing the dome or net.

- Place the net over the sides and ends of the crib.
- Secure the ties to the springs or frame of the crib. The crib sides can then be freely lowered without removing the net.
- Test with your hand that the net will stretch if the child stands in the crib against it.

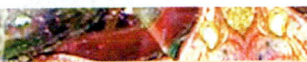
Home Care Considerations

Applying Restraints
Restraints may be necessary for clients in wheelchairs or in the home. Safety guidelines apply in all cases. Assess the knowledge and skill of all caregivers in the use of restraints and educate as indicated.

- Use means other than restraints as much as possible, and stay with the client.

- Pad bony prominences, such as wrists and ankles, if needed before applying a restraint over them.
- Tie restraints with knots that will not tighten when pulled and to parts of the wheelchair that do not move.
- Assess restrained limbs for signs of impaired blood circulation.
- Always stay with a client whose restraint is temporarily removed.

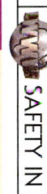

EVALUATING
To prevent client injury, the nurse's role is largely educative and desired outcomes reflect the client's acquisition of knowledge of hazards, behaviors that incorporate safety practices, and skills to perform in the event of certain emergencies. The nurse needs to individualize these for clients. Examples of desired outcomes include the client being able to do the following:

- Describe methods to prevent specific hazards (e.g., falls, suffocation, choking, fires, drowning, electric shock).
- Report use of home safety measures (e.g., fire safety measures, smoke detector maintenance, fall prevention strategies, burn prevention measures, poison prevention measures, safe storage of hazardous materials, firearm safety precautions, electrocution prevention, water safety precautions, bicycle safety, motor vehicle safety).
- Alter home physical environment to reduce the risk of injury.
- Describe emergency procedures for poisoning and fire.
- Describe age-specific risks or work safety risks or community safety risks.
- Demonstrate correct use of child safety seats.
- Demonstrate correct administration of cardiopulmonary resuscitation.

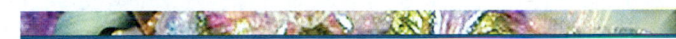

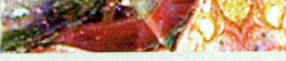
Lifespan Considerations

Elders
Some of the changes due to aging that place the older adult at higher risk for safety concerns are
- Decrease in hearing and sight
- Decrease in response of reflexes
- Fragility of bones and decrease in flexibility of joints and muscles
- Decrease in temperature regulation, increasing the risk of hypothermia and hyperthermia

- Decrease in kidney function, which increases risk of toxicity from medications.

A home environment that was safe when they were younger may need modifications for older adults to decrease the risk of injury. A plan and telephone numbers of those to call should be available for emergency situations.

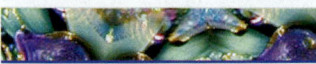

Focus on Critical Thinking

Mr. Moore is a 72-year-old widower who is recovering from a fall in which he fractured his hip and underwent surgical repair 1 week ago. He will be staying with his son for 2 weeks after he is discharged from the hospital, but he is eager to return to his own home. Once he is home, his son will visit nightly after work, he will receive Meals on Wheels once a day, and a home health care attendant will visit weekly to assist him with hygienic care until he is more independent. Mr. Moore's wife died 3 years ago, but he has remained independent and continued his social functions. He lives in a small single-level, house with his dog and cat, and he enjoys gardening. Prior to fracturing his hip he walked his dog daily. You will be his home health care nurse.

1. While hospitalized, Mr. Moore experienced some mild confusion during the night, but his nurses decided not to restrain him. What are the best reasons for avoiding the use of restraints for clients such as Mr. Moore?
2. What are some of the more obvious factors that may affect Mr. Moore's safety as he returns home?
3. What do you need to assess in regard to Mr. Moore's safety and what suggestions can you make for enhancing his safety?
4. What strengths do you note about Mr. Moore that may protect him from injury when he returns home?

See Critical Thinking Possibilities in Appendix A.

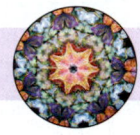 | # Chapter Review

EXPLORE MediaLink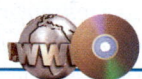

NCLEX review questions, case studies, care plan activities, MediaLink applications, and other interactive resources for this chapter can be found on the Companion Website at www.prenhall.com/kozier. Click on Chapter 30 to select the activities for this chapter.

For animations, more NCLEX review questions, and an audio glossary, access the Student CD-ROM accompanying this textbook.

Chapter Highlights

- Accidents are a major cause of death among individuals of all ages in the United States.
- Nurses need awareness of what constitutes a safe environment for specific individuals and for groups of people in the home, community, and workplace.
- Hazards to safety occur at all ages and vary according to the age and development of the individual.
- Nursing assessment of safety includes assessing factors that can affect safety, for example, age, lifestyle, mobility, sensory alterations, level of awareness, emotional state, and environmental factors.
- Nurses assess clients at risk for injury through methods such as nursing history and physical examintion, risk assessment tools, and home hazard appraisal.
- Major nursing diagnoses for clients at risk for accidental injury can be categorized as *Risk for Injury,* with seven subcategories: *Risk for Poisoning, Risk for Suffocation, Risk for Trauma, Latex Allergy Response, Risk for Latex Allergy Response, Risk for Aspiration,* and *Risk for Disuse Syndrome.*
- When planning to meet safety needs of clients, nurses need to consider physical factors in the environment and the psychologic and physiologic state of the individual. Clients often need to change their health behavior and may need to modify the environment.

- Measures to ensure the safety of people of all ages focus on (a) observation or prediction of situations that are potentially harmful and (b) client education that empowers clients to safeguard themselves and their families from injury. Education is a major health protection strategy in preventing accidents.
- Nurses must be familiar with the fire procedures in the health care agency where they practice. In the event of a fire, the nurse must (a) protect clients from injury, (b) report, (c) contain, and (d) put out the fire.
- Falls are a common cause of injury among older adults.
- Prevention of falls in health care agencies is a continuous concern.
- Side rails do not protect hospitalized clients from falls. It is more likely the client will fall trying to get around or over the side rail.
- Seizure precautions are safety measures taken by the nurse to protect clients from injury should they have a seizure.
- Major reasons for poisoning in children are inadequate supervision and improper storage of household toxic substances.
- Suffocation can occur when foreign objects are swallowed or inhaled, cutting off the person's oxygen supply.
- Prolonged exposure to excessive noise can produce hearing loss.

- Faulty electric equipment and improper grounding pose health hazards in the hospital and the home. Accidents can be prevented by using grounded outlets and plugs, putting protective covers over outlets, keeping appliances in good repair, and making sure that electric wiring and circuits meet safety standards.
- Firearms pose a risk to individuals of all ages. Adults must take full responsibility for following safety procedures when keeping firearms in the home, including storage of ammunition in a separate location.

- In hospitals, radioactive substances are used for both diagnostic and treatment purposes; agency policy should be followed to safeguard clients and staff from unsafe exposure.
- Various alternatives to restraints must be considered before a restraint is applied.
- Because restraints restrict a client's basic freedom to move, careful assessment and accurate, complete documentation are important when restraints are used.

Review Questions

30–1. When a fire occurs in a client's room, the nurse's priority is to
   a. run for help.
   b. protect the client.
   c. put out the fire.
   d. report the fire.

30–2. What is the leading cause of accidents in young and middle-aged adults?
   a. automobile accidents
   b. drowning and firearms
   c. falls
   d. suicide and homicide

30–3. A hospitalized elderly female client who uses a walker is receiving diuretic medication and must use the bathroom several times each night. To promote safety, the nurse should
   a. leave the bathroom light on.
   b. withhold the client's diuretic medication.

   c. provide a bedside commode.
   d. keep the side rails up.

30–4. Which NANDA nursing diagnosis is most applicable for toddlers?
   a. *Risk for Suffocation*
   b. *Risk for Injury*
   c. *Risk for Poisoning*
   d. *Risk for Disuse Syndrome*

30–5. A 75-year-old client is hospitalized with a cerebral vascular accident (stroke). He is unable to ambulate without help, but becomes disoriented at times and tries to get out of bed. What is the most appropriate safety measure for this client?
   a. Restrain the client in bed.
   b. Ask a family member to stay with the client.
   c. Check the client every 15 minutes.
   d. Use a bed exit safety monitoring device.

Readings and References

Suggested Readings

Hall-Long, B. A., Schell, K., & Corrigan, V. (2001). Youth safety education and injury prevention program. *Pediatric Nursing, 27*(2), 141–146. The authors provide an overview of how unintentional injuries are the leading cause of death in U.S. children. They describe a study that was based on the premise that teaching children about safety should start early with developmentally appropriate teaching plans and materials. The article describes a program called Think First for Kids. It is a 6-week injury prevention program for children in first through third grades.

Rogers, P. D., & Bocchino, N. L. (1999). Restraint-free care: Is it possible? Can we make physical restraint a last resort in acute care? *American Journal of Nursing, 99*(10), 26–33. The authors provide helpful suggestions for alternatives to the use of physical restraints.

Talerico, Karen A., & Capezuti, E. (2001). Myths and facts about side rails. *American Journal of Nursing, 101*(7), 43–48. While the use of side rails has been routine practice since the 1970s, nurses now face new

mandates to decrease the use of side rails. The authors review these mandates and frequently held myths about side rails. The facts point out the dangers, including death, of side rails. The safe alternative interventions decision tree is helpful.

Related Research

Dunn, K. S. (2001). The effect of physical restraints on fall rates in older adults who are institutionalized. *Journal of Gerontological Nursing, 27*(10), 41–48.

Grossman, D. C., Cummings, P., Koepsell, T. D., Marshall, J., D'Ambrosio, L., Thompson, R. S., et al. (2000). Firearm safety counseling in primary care pediatrics: A randomized, controlled trial. *Pediatrics, 106*(1), 22–26.

Harrison, B., Booth, D., & Algase, D. (2001). Studying fall risk factors among nursing home residents who fell. *Journal of Gerontological Nursing, 27*(10), 26–34.

Heinzer, M. M. (2002). The walking wounded: The faces of domestic violence in the community. *Holistic Nursing Practice, 16*(3), vi–viii.

Heinzer, M. M., and Krumm, J. R. (2002). Barriers to screening for domestic violence in an emergency department. *Holistic Nursing Practice, 16*(3), 24–33.

Resnick, B. (1999). Falls in a community of older adults: Putting research into practice. *Clinical Nursing Research, 8*(3), 251–266.

References

Ball, J., & Bindler, R. (2003). *Pediatric nursing: Caring for children.* (3rd ed.) Upper Saddle River NJ: Prentice Hall Health.

Capezuti, E., Talerico, K. A., Cochran, I., Becker, H., Strumpf, N., & Evans, L. (1999). Individualized interventions to prevent bed-related falls and reduce siderail use. *Journal of Gerontological Nursing, 25*(11), 26–34.

Gentleman, B., & Malozemoff, W. (2001). Falls and feelings: Description of a psychosocial group nursing intervention. *Journal of Gerontological Nursing, 27*(10), 35–39.

Centers for Medicare & Medicaid Services, Department of Health and Human Services. (2001). *Conditions of participation for hospi-*

tals: Patients' rights (CMS-DHHS Publication No. 42CFR482.13). Retrieved March 31, 2003, from http://www.access.gpo.gov/nara/cfr/waisidx_01/42cfr482_01.html

Jackman, G. A., Farah, M. M., Kellermann, A. L., & Simon, H. K. (2001). Seeing is believing: What do boys do when they find a real gun? *Pediatrics, 107*(6), 1247–1250.

Johnson, M., Maas, M., & Moorhead, S. (Eds.). (2000). *Nursing outcomes classification (NOC)* (2nd ed.). St. Louis, MO: Mosby.

Kimbell, S. (2001). Before the fall. Keeping your patient on his feet. *Nursing, 31*(8), 44–45.

McCloskey, J. C., & Bulechek, G. M. (Eds.). (2000). *Nursing interventions classification (NIC)* (3rd ed.). St. Louis, MO: Mosby.

NANDA International. (2003). *NANDA nursing diagnoses: Definitions and classification 2003-2004.* Philadelphia: Author.

U.S. Food and Drug Administration (1992, July 15). *FDA Safety Alert: Potential hazards with restraint devices.* Rockville, MD: U.S. Department of Health and Human Services.

Wilkinson, J. M. (2000). *Nursing diagnosis handbook with NIC interventions and NOC outcomes* (7th ed.). Upper Saddle River, NJ: Prentice Hall Health.

Wold, G. H. (1999). *Basic geriatric nursing* (2nd ed.). St. Louis, MO: Mosby.

Selected Bibliography

Bernardo, L. M. (2002). Emergency nurses' role in pediatric injury prevention. *Nursing Clinics of North America, 37*(1), 135–143.

Brenner, Z. R. (1999). Toward restraint-free care. *American Journal of Nursing, 98*(12), 16F–16I.

Cohen, S. M. (2001). Lead poisoning: A summary of treatment and prevention. *Pediatric Nursing, 27*(2), 125–130.

Dibartolo, V. (1998). 9 steps to effective restraint use. *RN, 61*(12), 23–24.

Howard, P. K. (2001). Firearm safety and children: Access and attitudes. *Journal of Emergency Nursing, 27*(3), 272–275.

Howard, P. K. (2001). An overview of a few well-known national children's gun safety programs and ENA's newly developed program. *Journal of Emergency Nursing, 27*(5), 485–488.

Jech, A. O. (2001). Of human bondage. Alternatives to restraints help reduce risks to patients. *Nurse Week, 2*(6), 21–22.

Kobs, A. (1998). Questions and answers from the JCAHO. Restraints revisited. *Nursing Management, 29*(1), 17–18.

Melillo, K. D., & Futrell, M. (1998). Wandering and technological devices. Helping caregivers ensure the safety of confused older adults. *Journal of Gerontological Nursing, 24*(8), 32–38.

Morse, J. M. (2001). Preventing falls in the elderly. *Reflections on Nursing Leadership, 27*(1), 26–27.

Patrick, L., & Blodgett, A. (2001). Selecting patients for falls—prevention protocols. An evidence-based approach on a geriatric rehabil-

itation unit. *Journal of Gerontological Nursing, 27*(10), 19–25.

Patrick, L., Leber, M. Scrim, C., Gendron, I., & Eisenrr-Parsche, P. (1999). A standarized assessment and intervention protocol for managing risk for falls on a geriatric rehabilitation unit. *Journal of Gerontological Nursing, 25*(4), 40–47.

Rawsky, E. (1998). Review of literature on falls among the elderly. *Image: Journal of Nursing Scholarship, 30*(1), 47–52.

Rigler, S. K. (1999). Preventing falls in older adults. *Hospital Practice, 34,* 117–120.

Savage, T., & Matheis-Kraft, C. (2001). Fall occurrence in a geriatric psychiatry setting before and after a fall prevention program. *Journal of Gerontological Nursing, 27*(10), 49–53.

Schiff, L. (2002). Market choices: Patient mobility monitors. *RN, 65*(1), 65–66.

Sullivan, G. H. (1999). Legally speaking: Minimizing your risk in patient falls. *RN, 62*(4), 69–72.

Walker, B. L. (1998). Preventing falls. *RN, 61*(5), 40–42

Weiss, C. A. (2001). Fall prevention among the elderly. *Nursing Spectrum Metro Edition, 2*(6), 29–33.

Winslow, E. H., & Jacobson, A. F. (1998). Research for practice: Reducing falls in older patients. *American Journal of Nursing, 98*(10), 22.

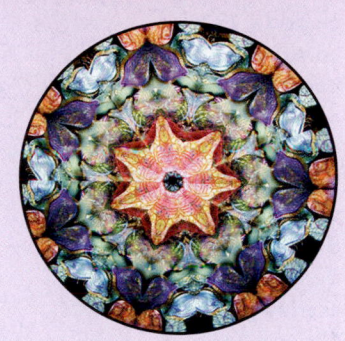

CHAPTER 31

HYGIENE

LEARNING OUTCOMES

After completing this chapter, you will be able to:

- Describe hygienic care that nurses provide to clients.

- Identify factors influencing personal hygiene.

- Identify normal and abnormal assessment findings while providing hygiene care.

- Apply the nursing process to common problems related to hygienic care of the skin, feet, nails, mouth, hair, eyes, ears, and nose.

- Identify the purposes of bathing.

- Describe various types of baths.

- Explain specific ways in which nurses help hospitalized clients with hygiene.

- Describe steps for identified hygienic-care procedures.

- Identify steps in removing contact lenses and inserting and removing artificial eyes.

- Describe steps for removing, cleaning, and inserting hearing aids.

- Identify safety and comfort measures underlying bed-making procedures.

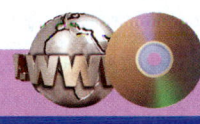

MediaLink

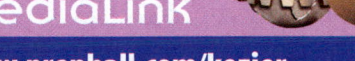

www.prenhall.com/kozier

Additional resources for this chapter can be found on the Student CD-ROM accompanying this textbook, and on the Companion Website at www.prenhall.com/kozier. Click on Chapter 31 to select the activities for this chapter.

CD-ROM
- Audio Glossary
- NCLEX Review

Companion Website
- Additional NCLEX Review
- Case Study: Providing Basic Hygiene Care
- Care Plan Activity: Client on Radiation Therapy
- MediaLink Application: Caring for Dentures
- Links to Resources

Hygiene is the science of health and its maintenance. Personal **hygiene** is the self-care by which people attend to such functions as bathing, toileting, general body hygiene, and grooming. Hygiene is a highly personal matter determined by individual values and practices. It involves care of the skin, hair, nails, teeth, oral and nasal cavities, eyes, ears, and perineal-genital areas.

It is important for nurses to know exactly how much assistance a client needs for hygienic care. Clients may require help after urinating or defecating, after vomiting, and whenever they become soiled, for example, from wound drainage or from profuse perspiration. Table 31–1 lists factors that influence hygiene practices.

HYGIENIC CARE

Nurses commonly use the following terms to describe types of hygienic care. *Early morning care* is provided to clients as they awaken in the morning. This care consists of providing a urinal or bedpan to the client confined to bed, washing the face and hands, and giving oral care. *Morning care* is often provided after clients have breakfast, although it may be provided before breakfast. It usually includes providing for elimination needs, a bath or shower, perineal care, back massages, and oral, nail, and hair care. Making the client's bed is part of morning care. *Afternoon care* often includes providing a bedpan or urinal, washing the hands and face, and assisting with oral care to refresh clients. *Hour of sleep (HS) care* is provided to clients before they retire for the night. It usually involves providing for elimination needs, washing face and hands, giving oral care, and giving a back massage. *As-needed (prn) care* is provided as required by the client. For example, a client who is diaphoretic (sweating profusely) may need more frequent bathing and a change of clothes and linen.

SKIN

The skin is the largest organ of the body. It serves five major functions:

1. It protects underlying tissues from injury by preventing the passage of microorganisms. The skin and mucous membranes are considered the body's first line of defense.
2. It regulates the body temperature. Cooling of the body occurs through the heat loss processes of evaporation of perspiration, and by radiation and conduction of heat from the body when the blood vessels of the skin are vasodilated. Body heat is conserved through lack of perspi-

TABLE 31–1 Factors Influencing Individual Hygienic Practices

Factor	Variables
Culture	North American culture places a high value on cleanliness. Many North Americans bathe or shower once or twice a day, whereas people from some other cultures bathe once a week. Some cultures consider privacy essential for bathing, whereas others practice communal bathing. Body odor is offensive in some cultures and accepted as normal in others.
Religion	Ceremonial washings are practiced by some religions.
Environment	Finances may affect the availability of facilities for bathing. For example, homeless people may not have warm water available; soap, shampoo, shaving lotion, and deodorants may be too expensive for people who have limited resources.
Developmental level	Children learn hygiene in the home. Practices vary according to the individual's age; for example, preschoolers can carry out most tasks independently with encouragement.
Health and energy	Ill people may not have the motivation or energy to attend to hygiene. Some clients who have neuromuscular impairments may be unable to perform hygienic care.
Personal preferences	Some people prefer a shower to a tub bath.

ration and vasoconstriction of the blood vessels. See Chapter 28.

3. It secretes **sebum,** an oily substance that (a) softens and lubricates the hair and skin, (b) prevents the hair from becoming brittle, and (c) decreases water loss from the skin when the external humidity is low. Because fat is a poor conductor of heat, sebum (d) lessens the amount of heat lost from the skin. Sebum also (e) has a **bactericidal** (bacteria-killing) action.

4. It transmits sensations through nerve receptors, which are sensitive to pain, temperature, touch, and pressure.

5. It produces and absorbs vitamin D in conjunction with ultraviolet rays from the sun, which activate a vitamin D precursor present in the skin.

The normal skin of a healthy person has transient and resident microorganisms that are not usually harmful. See Chapter 34.

Sudoriferous (sweat) glands are on all body surfaces except the lips and parts of the genitals. The body has from 2 to 5 million, which are all present at birth. They are most numerous on the palms of the hands and the soles of the feet. Sweat glands are classified as apocrine and eccrine. The **apocrine glands,** located largely in the axillae and anogenital areas, begin to function at puberty under the influence of androgens. Although they produce sweat almost constantly, apocrine glands are of little use in thermoregulation. The secretion of these glands is odorless, but when decomposed or acted on by bacteria on the skin, it takes on a musky, unpleasant odor. The **eccrine glands** are important physiologically. They are more numerous than the apocrine glands and are found chiefly on the palms of the hands, the soles of the feet, and forehead. The sweat they produce cools the body through evaporation. Sweat is made up of water, sodium, potassium, chloride, glucose, urea, and lactate.

Providing Culturally Competent Care

BIOCULTURAL VARIATIONS IN BODY SECRETIONS

- Most Asians and Native North Americans have a mild to absent body odor, whereas Whites and African Americans tend to have strong body odor.
- Eskimos have made an environmental adaptation where they sweat less than Whites on their trunks and extremities but more on their faces. This adaptation allows for temperature regulation without the need to change clothes because of perspiration.
- The amount of chloride excreted by sweat glands varies widely. African Americans have lower salt concentrations in their sweat than Whites.

Note: From Transcultural Concepts in Nursing Care, 4th ed. (pp. 59–60), by M. M. Andrews and J. S. Boyle, 2003, Philadelphia: Lippincott Williams & Wilkins. Adapted with permission.

NURSING MANAGEMENT

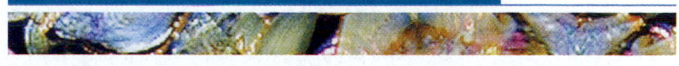

ASSESSING

Assessment of the client's skin and hygienic practices includes (a) a nursing health history to determine the client's skin care practices, self-care abilities, and past or current skin problems; (b) physical assessment of the skin; and (c) identification of clients at risk for developing skin impairments.

Nursing History

Data about the client's skin care practices enable the nurse to incorporate the client's needs and preferences as much as possible in the plan of care. Andrews and Boyle (2003, p. 55) state that people in most cultures in the United States and Canada try to disguise natural body odors by bathing frequently and using deodorant, cologne, or perfumes. Immigrants from other countries where water is scarce may bathe less often than people from countries where water is more accessible.

Assessment of the client's self-care abilities determines the amount of nursing assistance and the type of bath (e.g., bed, tub, or shower) best suited for the client. Important considerations include the client's balance (for tub and shower), ability to sit unsupported (in the tub or bed), activity tolerance, coordination, adequate muscle strength, appropriate joint range of motion, vision, and the client's preferences. Cognition and motivation are also essential. Clients whose cognitive function is impaired or whose illness alters energy levels and motivation will usually need more assistance. It is important for the nurse to determine the client's functional level and to maintain and promote as much client independence as possible. This also enables the nurse to identify the client's potential for growth and rehabilitation. There are several models of functional levels of self-care. One example is shown in Table 31–2.

The presence of past or current skin problems alerts the nurse to specific nursing interventions or referrals the client may require. Many skin care conditions have implications for hygienic care. The client may provide descriptions of these problems during the nursing health history, or the nurse may observe some during the physical examination that follows. Common skin problems and implications for nursing interventions are shown in Table 31–3. Questions to elicit data about the client's skin care practices, self-care abilities, and skin problems are shown in the accompanying Assessment Interview.

Physical Assessment

Physical assessment of the skin, which involves inspection and palpation, is described in Chapter 28. When assisting with bathing and other hygienic care, the nurse often has the opportunity to collect data about skin color, uniformity of color, texture, turgor, temperature, intactness, and lesions.

TABLE 31–2 Definitions and Descriptors for Functional Level

	(0)	(+ 1)	Semidependent (+ 2)	Moderately Dependent (+ 3)	Totally Dependent (+ 4)
	Completely Independent	Requires use of equipment or device	Requires help from another person for assistance, supervision, or teaching	Requires help from another person and equipment or device	Dependent, does not participate in activity
Bathing			Nurse provides all equipment; positions client in bed/bathroom. Client completes bath, except for back and feet.	Nurse supplies all equipment; positions client; washes back, legs, perineum, and all other parts, as needed. Client can assist.	Client needs complete bath; cannot assist at all.
Oral hygiene			Nurse provides equipment; client does task.	Nurse prepares brush, rinses mouth, positions client.	Nurse completes entire procedure.
Dressing/grooming			Nurse gathers items for client; may button, zip, or tie clothing. Client dresses self.	Nurse combs client's hair, assists with dressing, buttons and zips clothing, ties shoes.	Client needs to be dressed and cannot assist the nurse; nurse combs client's hair.
Toileting			Client can walk to bathroom/commode with assistance; nurse helps with clothing.	Nurse provides bedpan, positions client on or off bedpan, places client on commode.	Client is incontinent; nurse places client on bedpan or commode.

Note: From Nursing Diagnosis Handbook with NIC Interventions and NOC Outcomes, 7th ed. (pp. 382, 385, 393), by J. M. Wilkinson, 2000. Upper Saddle River, NJ: Prentice Hall Health. Adapted with permission.

Research Note
Is the Traditional Self-Reporting of ADL Useful?

For more than 30 years the self-reporting of activities of daily living (ADL) has been the sole measure of functional assessment for older adults. Researchers are now challenging this process because the results of a client's self-report of functional ability can vary depending on these reasons: inaccurate perceptions of their abilities due to not recognizing gradual changes, their interpretations of the ADL questions may vary from those of the interviewer, and personal reasons for under- or overreporting functional abilities. Research results show that performance measures may contribute more information than self-reporting. The performance tests of standing balance, walking speed, and chair-rise time are simple tests that can be administered in a short period of time and in a small space with no need for special equipment. Researchers question whether these lower extremity function tests may also be predictive of future functional disability.

Implications: When elderly clients report little or no difficulty with ADL tasks, the nurse can conduct objective lower extremity performance tests to further assess functional ability. Early recognition of potential functional disability may allow for timely intervention and improve an elder's quality of life.

Note: From "Activities of Daily Living: Old-Fashioned or Still Useful?" by J. A. Bennett, 1999, Journal of Gerontological Nursing, 25(5), pp. 22–29.

TABLE 31-3 Common Skin Problems

Problem and Appearance	Nursing Implications
Abrasion Superficial layers of the skin are scraped or rubbed away. Area is reddened and may have localized bleeding or serous weeping.	1. Prone to infection; therefore, wound should be kept clean and dry. 2. Do not wear rings or jewelry when providing care to avoid causing abrasions to clients. 3. Lift, do not pull, a client across a bed.
Excessive Dryness Skin can appear flaky and rough.	1. Prone to infection if the skin cracks; therefore, provide alcohol-free lotions to moisturize the skin and prevent cracking. 2. Bathe client less frequently; use no soap, or use nonirritating soap and limit its use. Rinse skin thoroughly because soap can be irritating and drying. 3. Encourage increased fluid intake if health permits to prevent dehydration.
Ammonia Dermatitis (Diaper Rash) Caused by skin bacteria reacting with urea in the urine. The skin becomes reddened and is sore.	1. Keep skin dry and clean by applying protective ointments containing zinc oxide to areas at risk (e.g., buttocks and perineum). 2. Boil an infant's diapers or wash them with an antibacterial detergent to prevent infection. Rinse diapers well because detergent is irritating to an infant's skin.
Acne Inflammatory condition with papules and pustules.	1. Keep the skin clean to prevent secondary infection. 2. Treatment varies widely.
Erythema Redness associated with a variety of conditions, such as rashes, exposure to sun, elevated body temperature.	1. Wash area carefully to remove excess microorganisms. 2. Apply antiseptic spray or lotion to prevent itching, promote healing, and prevent skin breakdown.
Hirsutism Excessive hair on a person's body and face, particularly in women.	1. Remove unwanted hair by using depilatories, shaving, electrolysis, or tweezing. 2. Enhance client's self-concept.

Assessment Interview

SKIN HYGIENE

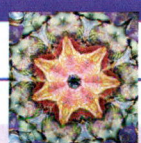

Skin Care Practices

- What are your usual showering or bathing times?
- What hygienic products do you routinely use (e.g., bath oils, powder, facial cleansing creams, body lotions or creams, deodorants, antiperspirants)?
- What facial cosmetic products do you use?
- How and when do you clean makeup applicators and puffs? (Applicators should be kept clean, and products used around the eyes in particular should be discarded after 4 months to prevent bacterial and fungal infections.)
- What hygienic or cosmetic products do you not use because of the skin problems they create (e.g., skin dryness or allergic reactions)?

Self-Care Abilities

- Do you have any problems managing your hygienic practices (e.g., baths and facial care)? If so, what are these?
- How can the nurses best help you?

Skin Problems

- Do you have any tendency toward skin dryness, itchiness, rashes, bruising, excessive perspiration, or lack of perspiration? Have you had skin or scalp lesions in the past?
- Do you have any allergic tendencies? If so, what?

Positive responses to any of these require further exploration in terms of duration (When did it start?); frequency (How often have you had this?); description of lesion or rash; any associated signs, such as fever or nausea; aggravating factors (e.g., season of the year, stress, occupation, medication, recent travel, housing, personal contact); alleviating factors (e.g., medications, lotions, home remedies); and any family history of the problem.

DIAGNOSING

Self-Care Deficit diagnoses are used for clients who have problems performing hygiene care. Three of NANDA's four self-care deficit diagnoses, specified as *Self-Care Deficit: Bathing/ Hygiene, Self-Care Deficit: Dressing/ Grooming,* and *Self-Care Deficit: Toileting* are discussed in this chapter. The fourth diagnosis, *Self-Care Deficit: Feeding,* is discussed in Chapter 45. 🔗

Difficulties encountered by the client in performing bathing activities include the inability to wash the body or body parts, to obtain or get to a water source, and to regulate water temperature or flow. Difficulties in dressing and grooming include inability to obtain, put on, take off, fasten, or replace articles of clothing; and to maintain appearance at a satisfactory level. Toileting problems may involve difficulties getting to the toilet or commode or sitting on and rising from it. In addition, the client may experience problems manipulating clothing for toileting, carrying out proper toilet hygiene, or flushing the toilet or emptying the commode. The reasons (etiologies or related factors) for these problems are varied (see Box 31–1).

Clinical examples of assessment data clusters, related nursing diagnoses, outcomes and interventions are shown in the accompanying Identifying Nursing Diagnoses, Outcomes, and Interventions.

Examples of associated diagnoses include:

- *Deficient Knowledge* related to
  a. Lack of experience with skin condition (acne) and need to prevent secondary infection
  b. New therapeutic regimen to manage skin problems
  c. Lack of experience in providing hygiene care to dependent person
  d. Unfamiliarity with devices available to facilitate sitting on or rising from toilet
- *Situational Low Self-Esteem* related to
  a. Visible skin problem (e.g., acne or alopecia)
  b. Body odor.

The diagnoses *Risk for Impaired Skin Integrity* and *Impaired Skin Integrity* are discussed in Chapter 34. 🔗

BOX 31–1	■ **Etiologies of Self-Care Deficits**

- Decreased or lack of motivation
- Weakness or tiredness
- Pain or discomfort
- Perceptual or cognitive impairment
- Inability to perceive body part or spatial relationship
- Neuromuscular or musculoskeletal impairment
- Medically imposed restriction
- Therapeutic procedure restraining mobility (e.g., intravenous infusion, cast)
- Severe anxiety
- Environmental barriers

PLANNING

In planning care, the nurse and, if appropriate, the client and/or family set outcomes for each nursing diagnosis. The nurse then performs nursing interventions and activities to achieve the client outcomes.

The specific, detailed nursing activities taken by the nurse may include assisting dependent clients with bathing, skin care, and perineal care; providing back massages to promote circulation; instructing clients/families about appropriate hygienic practices and alternative methods for dressing; and demonstrating use of assistive equipment and adaptive activities. Although the nursing interventions discussed in this chapter focus on hygienic measures, the etiology of the nursing diagnoses established may point to other interventions that promote circulation, promote self-esteem, restore nutritional status, correct fluid deficits or excesses, or prevent problems associated with immobility. Nursing strategies to deal with these etiologies are provided in other chapters.

Planning to assist a client with personal hygiene includes consideration of the client's personal preferences, health, and limitations; the best time to give the care; and the equipment, facilities, and personnel available. A client's personal preferences—about when and how to bathe, for example—should be followed as long as they are compatible with the client's health and the equipment available. Nurses need to provide whatever assistance the client requires, either directly or by delegating this task to other nursing personnel.

Planning for Home Care

To provide for continuity of care, it is important that the nurse assess the client's and family's abilities for care and the need for referrals and home health services (see Home Care Assessment on page 704.) In addition, the nurse needs to determine the client's learning needs.

IMPLEMENTING

The nurse applies the general guidelines for skin care while providing one of the various types of baths available to clients. Procedure 31–1 describes how to bathe an adult or pediatric client.

General Guidelines for Skin Care

1. *An intact, healthy skin is the body's first line of defense.* Nurses need to ensure that all skin care measures prevent injury and irritation. Scratching the skin with jewelry or long, sharp fingernails must be avoided. Harsh rubbing or use of rough towels and washcloths can cause tissue damage, particularly when the skin is irritated or when circulation or sensation is diminished. Bottom bedsheets are kept taut and free from wrinkles to reduce friction and abrasion to the skin. Top bed linens are arranged to prevent undue pressure on the toes. When necessary, bed cradles on footboards are used to keep bedclothes off the feet.
2. *The degree to which the skin protects the underlying tissues from injury depends on the general health of the cells, the amount of subcutaneous tissue, and the dryness of the skin.* Skin that is poorly nourished and dry is less easily protected

IDENTIFYING NURSING DIAGNOSES, OUTCOMES, AND INTERVENTIONS

CLIENTS WITH SKIN PROBLEMS

DATA CLUSTER	NURSING DIAGNOSIS/ DEFINITION	SAMPLE DESIRED OUTCOME [NOC #]/DEFINITION	INDICATORS	SELECTED INTERVENTIONS [NIC #]/DEFINITION	SAMPLE NIC ACTIVITIES
Stan Bailey, 75 years old, suffered a "stroke" 2 weeks ago resulting in paralysis of his left side. He states, "I don't want a bath. I can wash myself. I just want to be left alone." He is withdrawn and uncommunicative.	*Self-Care Deficit: Bathing/Hygiene* related to paralyzed left upper and lower limbs and lack of motivation/*Impaired ability to perform or complete bathing/hygiene activities for oneself*	Self-Care: Bathing [0301]/*Ability to cleanse own body*	Requires assistive person • Gets in and out of bathroom • Regulates water temperature • Bathes in shower • Washes body • Dries body	Self-Care Assistance: Bathing/Hygiene [1801]/*Assisting client to perform personal hygiene*	• Place towels, soap, deodorant, shaving equipment, and other needed accessories at bedside/bathroom • Facilitate client's bathing self, as appropriate • Provide assistance until client is fully able to assume self-care
Mark Drake, 15 year old, has facial pustules and papules. Facial skin is inflamed. He states, "I hate going to school or anywhere looking like this. I don't think any girl wants to go out with me. Can you do something to get rid of this?"	*Situational Low Self-Esteem* related to acne/*Development of a negative perception of self-worth in response to a current situation (Specify)*	Self-Esteem [1205]/*Personal judgment of self-worth*	Often positive • Verbalizations of self acceptable • Maintenance of grooming/ hygiene • Description of success in social groups	Self-Esteem Enhancement [5400]/*Assisting a client to increase his/her personal judgment of self-worth*	• Encourage client to identify strengths • Convey confidence in client's ability to handle situation • Assist client to re-examine negative perceptions of self • Assist client to identify the impact of peer group on feelings of self-worth

and more vulnerable to injury. When the skin is dry, lotions or creams with lanolin can be applied, and bathing is limited to once or twice a week because frequent bathing removes the natural oils of the skin and causes dryness.

3. *Moisture in contact with the skin for more than a short time can result in increased bacterial growth and irritation.* After a bath, the client's skin is dried carefully. Particular attention is paid to areas such as the axillae, the groin, beneath the breasts, and between the toes, where the potential for irritation is greatest. A nonirritating dusting powder, such as cornstarch, tends to reduce moisture and can be applied to these areas after they are dried. Clients who are incontinent of urine or feces or who perspire excessively are provided with immediate skin care to prevent skin irritation.

4. *Body odors are caused by resident skin bacteria acting on body secretions.* Cleanliness is the best deodorant. Commercial deodorants and antiperspirants can be applied only after the skin is cleaned. Deodorants diminish odors, whereas antiperspirants reduce the amount of perspiration. Neither is applied immediately after shaving, because of the possibility of skin irritation, nor are they used on skin that is already irritated.

5. *Skin sensitivity to irritation and injury varies among individuals and in accordance with their health.* Generally

Home Care Assessment
HYGIENE

Client and Environment

- *Self-care abilities for hygiene:* Assess the client's ability to bathe, to regulate water faucets, to dress and undress, to groom, and to use the toilet.
- *Self-care aids required:* Determine if there is a need for a tub/shower seat (see Figure 31–1 ■), a hand shower, a nonskid surface or mat in the tub or shower, hand bars on the sides of the tub (see Figure 31–2 ■), or a raised toilet seat.
- *Facilities:* Check for the presence of laundry facilities and running water.
- *Mechanical barriers:* Note furniture obstructing access to the bathroom and toilet, or a doorway too narrow for a wheelchair.

Family

- *Caregiver availability, skills, and responses:* Determine whether individuals are available and able to assist with bathing, dressing, toileting, nail care, hair shampoo, shopping for hygienic or grooming aids, and so on.

- *Education needs:* Assess whether the caregiver needs instruction in how to assist the client in and out of the tub, on and off the toilet, and so on.
- *Family role changes and coping:* Assess effects of client's illness on financial status, parenting, spousal roles, sexuality, and social roles.

Community

- Explore resources that will provide assistance with bathing, laundry, and foot care (e.g., home health aid, podiatrist).
- Consult a social worker as needed to coordinate placement of a client unable to remain in the home or to identify community resources that will help the client stay in the home.
- Consider a consult with (a) a physical therapist to assess, develop, and improve the client's motor function; (b) a home health nurse to provide follow-up for care, teaching, and support; and (c) an occupational therapist to assess and develop abilities to perform activities of daily living.

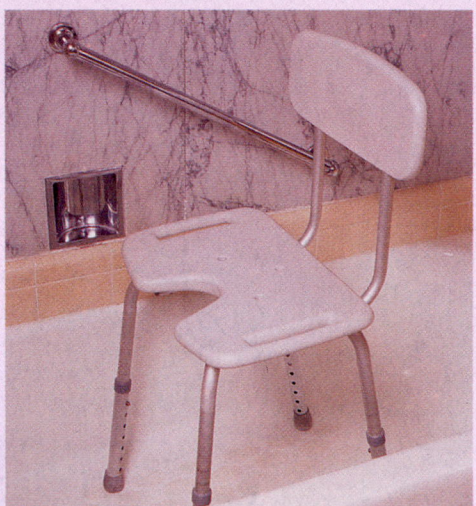

Figure 31–1 ■ Tub/shower seat in the home.

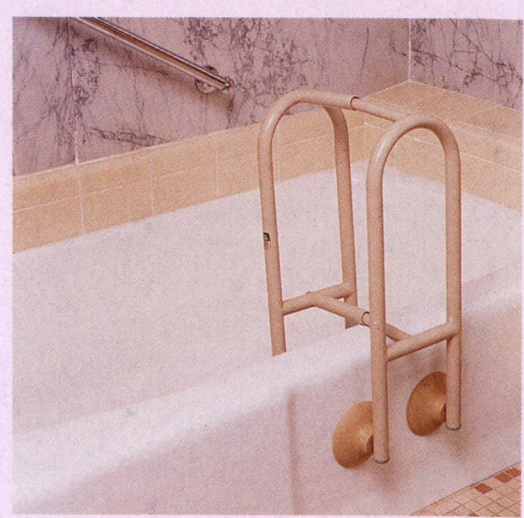

Figure 31–2 ■ Hand bars on the sides of the bathtub.

speaking, skin sensitivity is greater in infants, very young children, and older people. A person's nutritional status also affects sensitivity. Emaciated or obese persons tend to experience more skin irritation and injury. The same tendency is seen in individuals with poor dietary habits and insufficient fluid intake. Even in healthy persons, skin sensitivity is highly variable. Some people's skin is sensitive to chemicals in skin care agents and cosmetics. Hypoallergenic cosmetics and soaps or soap substitutes are now available for these people. The nurse needs to ascertain whether the client has any sensitivities and what agents are appropriate to use.

6. *Agents used for skin care have selective actions and purposes.* Commonly used agents are described in Table 31–4.

Bathing

Bathing removes accumulated oil, perspiration, dead skin cells, and some bacteria. The nurse can appreciate the quantity of oil and dead skin cells produced when observing a person after the removal of a cast that has been on for 6 weeks. The skin is crusty, flaky, and dry underneath the cast. Applications of oil over several days are usually necessary to remove the debris.

Excessive bathing, however, can interfere with the intended lubricating effect of the sebum, causing dryness of the skin. This is an important consideration, especially for older adults, who produce less sebum.

In addition to cleaning the skin, bathing also stimulates circulation. A warm or hot bath dilates superficial arterioles,

TABLE 31–4 Agents Commonly Used on the Skin

Soap	Lowers surface tension and thus helps in cleaning. Some soaps contain antibacterial agents, which can change the natural flora of the skin.
Detergent	Used instead of soap for cleaning. Some people who are allergic to soaps may not be allergic to detergents, and vice versa.
Bath oil	Used in bathwater; provides an oily film on the skin that softens and prevents chapping. Oils can make the tub surface slippery, and clients should be instructed about safety measures (e.g., using nonskid tub surface or mat).
Skin cream, lotion	Provides a film on the skin that prevents evaporation and therefore chapping.
Powder	Can be used to absorb water and prevent friction. For example, powder under the breasts can prevent skin irritation. Some powders are antibacterial.
Deodorant	Masks or diminishes body odors.
Antiperspirant	Reduces the amount of perspiration.

bringing more blood and nourishment to the skin. Vigorous rubbing has the same effect. Rubbing with long smooth strokes from the distal to proximal parts of extremities (from the point farthest from the body to the point closest) is particularly effective in facilitating venous blood flow unless there is some underlying condition (e.g., blood clot) that would preclude this.

Bathing also produces a sense of well-being. It is refreshing and relaxing and frequently improves morale, appearance, and self-respect. Some people take a morning shower for its refreshing, stimulating effect. Others prefer an evening bath because it is relaxing. These effects are more evident when a person is ill. For example, it is not uncommon for clients who have had a restless or sleepless night to feel relaxed, comfortable, and sleepy after a morning bath.

Bathing offers an excellent opportunity for the nurse to assess all clients. The nurse can observe the condition of the client's skin and physical conditions such as sacral edema or rashes. While assisting a client with a bath, the nurse can also assess the client's psychosocial needs, such as orientation to time and ability to cope with the illness. Learning needs, such as a diabetic client's need to learn foot care, can also be assessed.

Categories. Two categories of baths are given to clients: cleaning and therapeutic. **Cleaning baths** are given chiefly for hygiene purposes and include these types:

- *Complete bed bath.* The nurse washes the entire body of a dependent client in bed.
- *Self-help bed bath.* Clients confined to bed are able to bathe themselves with help from the nurse for washing the back and perhaps the feet.
- *Partial bath (abbreviated bath).* Only the parts of the client's body that might cause discomfort or odor, if neglected, are washed: the face, hands, axillae, perineal area, and back. Omitted are the arms, chest, abdomen, legs, and feet. The nurse provides this care for dependent clients and assists self-sufficient clients confined to bed by washing their backs. Some ambulatory clients prefer to take a partial bath at the sink. The nurse can assist them by washing their backs.
- *Towel bath.* The towel bath is an in-bed bath that uses a quick-drying solution containing a disinfectant, a cleaning agent, and a softening agent mixed with water. This commercially prepared solution is used at a temperature of 43.3 to 48.9C (110 to 120F). The solution dries in a few seconds, avoiding the need to dry the client and thereby speeding the bathing process. The following procedure is suggested:
  - Fold a large terry cloth towel in a plastic bag and saturate it with the solution provided.
  - Wring out the towel, then unroll it over the client, at the same time moving the top bed linen off the client.
  - Fold excess towel under the client's chin for subsequent use.
  - Use a gentle massaging motion to clean the body, starting at the feet and working toward the head.
  - Fold the towel upward after the massage and replace with a clean sheet.
  - Use the part of the towel folded under the chin to clean the client's face, neck, and ears.
  - Remove the towel, then roll the client to one side and apply the clean side of the towel to the back of the neck, the back, and the buttocks.
  - Remove the towel.
  - Place clean linen on the bed, dress the client, and position the client appropriately.
- *Bag bath.* The "bag bath" is an adaptation of the towel bath. The equipment needed is a plastic bag, 10 to 12 washcloths, and a nonrinsable cleaner and water mixture. The solution and washcloths are warmed in a microwave. The warming time is about 1 minute, but the nurse needs to determine how long it takes to attain a desirable temperature. Each area of the body is cleaned with a different cloth and then air dried. Because the body is not rubbed dry, the emollient in the solution remains on the skin. Commercially prepared kits are available that provide presoaked disposable cloths in a pack that is heated in a microwave.
- *Tub bath.* Tub baths are often preferred to bed baths because it is easier to wash and rinse in a tub. Tubs are also used for

therapeutic baths. The amount of assistance the nurse offers depends on the abilities of the client. There are specially designed tubs for dependent clients. These tubs greatly reduce the work of the nurse in lifting clients in and out of the tub and offer greater benefits than a sponge bath in bed.

Sponge baths are suggested for the newborn because daily tub baths are not considered necessary. After the bath, the infant should be immediately dried and wrapped to prevent heat loss. Parents need to be advised that the infant's ability to regulate body temperature has not yet fully developed. Infants perspire minimally, and shivering starts at a lower temperature than it does in adults; therefore, infants lose more heat before shivering begins. In addition, because the infant's body surface area is very large in relation to body mass, the body loses heat readily.

- *Shower.* Many ambulatory clients are able to use shower facilities and require only minimal assistance from the nurse. Clients in long-term care settings are often given showers with the aid of a shower chair. The wheels on the shower chair allow clients to be transported from their room to the shower. The shower chair also has a commode seat to facilitate cleansing of the client's perineal area during the shower process (see Figure 31–3 ■).

The water for a bath should feel comfortably warm to the client. People vary in their sensitivity to heat; generally, the temperature should be 43 to 46C (110 to 115F). Most clients will verify a suitable temperature. Clients with decreased circulation or cognitive problems will not be able to verify the temperature. Therefore, the nurse must check the water temperature to avoid burning the client with water that is too hot. The water for a bed bath should be changed when it becomes dirty or cold.

Therapeutic baths are given for physical effects, such as to soothe irritated skin or to treat an area (e.g., the perineum). Medications may be placed in the water. A therapeutic bath is generally taken in a tub one-third or one-half full. The client remains in the bath for a designated time, often 20 to 30 minutes. If the client's back, chest, and arms are to be treated, these ar-

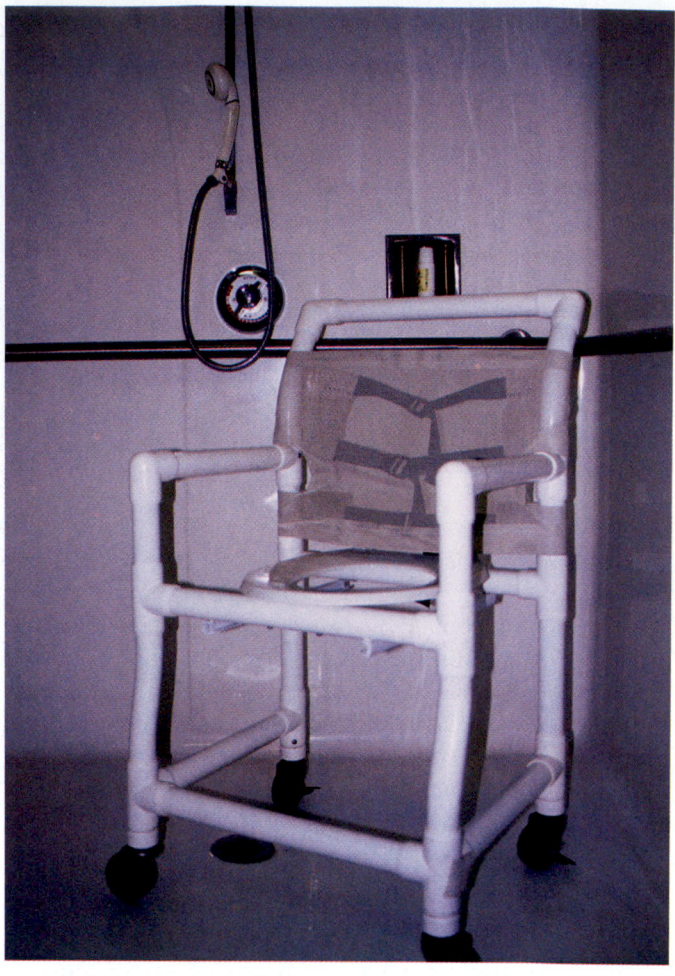

Figure 31–3 ■ A shower chair.

eas need to be immersed in the solution. The bath temperature is generally included in the order; 37.7 to 46C (100 to 115F) may be ordered for adults and 40.5C (105F) is usually ordered for infants. Procedure 31–1 provides guidelines for bathing clients.

Procedure 31–1 Bathing an Adult or Pediatric Client

Purposes

- To remove transient microorganisms, body secretions and excretions, and dead skin cells
- To stimulate circulation to the skin
- To produce a sense of well-being
- To promote relaxation and comfort
- To prevent or eliminate unpleasant body odors

ASSESSMENT

Assess:

- Condition of the skin (color, texture and turgor, presence of pigmented spots, temperature, lesions, excoriations, and abrasions)
- Fatigue
- Presence of pain and need for adjunctive measures (e.g., an analgesic) before the bath
- Range of motion of the joints
- Any other aspect of health that may affect the client's bathing process (e.g., mobility, strength, cognition)
- Need for use of clean gloves during the bath

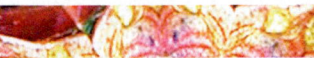
Procedure 31–1 Bathing an Adult or Pediatric Client *continued*

PLANNING

Delegation

The nurse often delegates the skill of bathing to UAP. However, the nurse remains responsible for assessment and client care. The nurse needs to do the following:

- Inform the UAP of the type of bath appropriate for the client and precautions, if any, specific to the needs of the client.
- Remind the UAP to notify the nurse of any concerns or changes (e.g., redness, skin breakdown, rash) so the nurse can assess, intervene if needed, and document.
- Instruct the UAP to encourage the client to perform as much self-care as appropriate in order to promote independence and self-esteem.
- Obtain a complete report about the bathing experience from the UAP.

Equipment

- Basin or sink with warm water (between 43 and 46C or 110 and 115F)
- Soap and soap dish
- Linens: bath blanket, two bath towels, washcloth, clean gown or pajamas or clothes as needed, additional bed linen and towels, if required
- Gloves, if appropriate (e.g., presence of body fluids or open lesions)
- Personal hygiene articles (e.g., deodorant, powder, lotions)
- Shaving equipment for male clients
- Table for bathing equipment
- Laundry hamper

IMPLEMENTATION

Preparation

Before bathing a client, determine (a) the purpose and type of bath the client needs; (b) self-care ability of the client; (c) any movement or positioning precautions specific to the client; (d) other care the client may be receiving, such as physical therapy or x-rays, in order to coordinate all aspects of health care and prevent unnecessary fatigue; (e) client's comfort level with being bathed by someone else; and (f) necessary bath equipment and linens.

Caution is needed when bathing clients who are receiving intravenous therapy. Easy-to-remove gowns that have Velcro or snap fasteners along the sleeves may be used. If a special gown is not available, the nurse needs to pay special attention when changing the client's gown after the bath (or whenever the gown becomes soiled). General guidelines are provided in Box 31–2. These guidelines do not apply if the client has an IV pump or controller. In this situation, either use a special gown or do not put the sleeve of a gown over the client's involved arm.

Performance

1. Explain to the client what you are going to do, why it is necessary, and how he or she can cooperate. Discuss with the client the plan for bathing and explain any unfamiliar procedures to the client.
2. Wash hands and observe other appropriate infection control procedures.
3. Provide for client privacy by drawing the curtains around the bed or closing the door to the room. Some agencies provide signs indicating the need for privacy. *Hygiene is a personal matter.*
4. Prepare the client and the environment.
   - Invite a family member or significant other to participate if desired.
   - Close windows and doors to ensure the room is a comfortable temperature. *Air currents increase loss of heat from the body by convection.*
   - Offer the client a bedpan or urinal or ask whether the client wishes to use the toilet or commode. *Warm water and activity can stimulate the need to void. The client will be more comfortable after voiding, and voiding before cleaning the perineum is advisable.*
   - Encourage the client to perform as much personal self-care as possible. *This promotes independence, exercise, and self-esteem.*
   - During the bath, assess each area of the skin carefully.

FOR A BED BATH

5. Prepare the bed and position the client appropriately.
   - Position the bed at a comfortable working height. Lower the side rail on the side close to you. Keep the other side rail *up.* Assist the client to move near you. *This avoids undue reaching and straining and promotes good body mechanics.*

BOX 31–2 ■ Changing a Hospital Gown for a Client with an Intravenous Infusion

- Slip the gown completely off the arm without the infusion and onto the tubing connected to the arm with the infusion.
- Holding the container above the client's arm, slide the sleeve up over the container to remove the used gown.
- Place the clean gown sleeve for the arm with the infusion over the container as if it were an extension of the client's arm, from the inside of the gown to the sleeve cuff.
- Rehang the container. Slide the gown carefully over the tubing toward the client's hand.
- Guide the client's arm and tubing into the sleeve, taking care not to pull on the tubing.
- Assist the client to put the other arm into the second sleeve of the gown, and fasten as usual.
- Count the rate of flow of the infusion to make sure it is correct before leaving the bedside.

continued on page 708

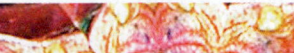

Procedure 31–1 Bathing an Adult or Pediatric Client *continued*

IMPLEMENTATION *continued*

- Place bath blanket over top sheet. Remove the top sheet from under the bath blanket by starting at client's shoulders and moving linen down toward client's feet (Figure 31–4 ■). Ask the client to grasp and hold the top of the bath blanket while pulling linen to the foot of the bed. *The bath blanket provides comfort, warmth, and privacy. Note:* If the bed linen is to be reused, place it over the bedside chair. If it is to be changed, place it in the linen hamper.
- Remove client's gown while keeping the client covered with the bath blanket. Place gown in linen hamper.

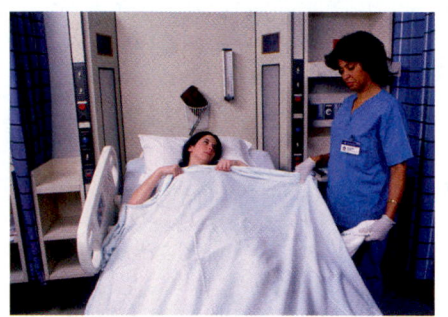

Figure 31–4 ■ Remove top sheet from under the bath blanket.

Figure 31–5 ■ Making a bath mitt, triangular method. (A) Lay your hand on the washcloth; (B) fold the top corner over your hand; (C) fold the side corners over your hand; (D) tuck the second corner under the cloth on the palm side to secure the mitt.

6. Make a bath mitt with the washcloth. *A bath mitt retains water and heat better than a cloth loosely held and prevents ends of washcloth from dragging across the skin.* See Figure 31–5 ■ for the triangular method and Figure 31–6 ■ for the rectangular method.

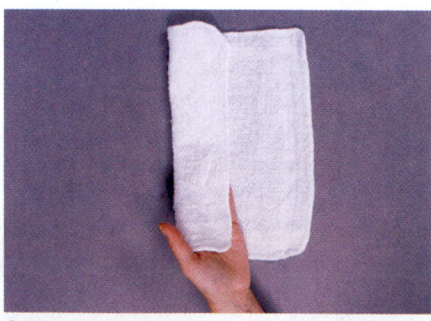

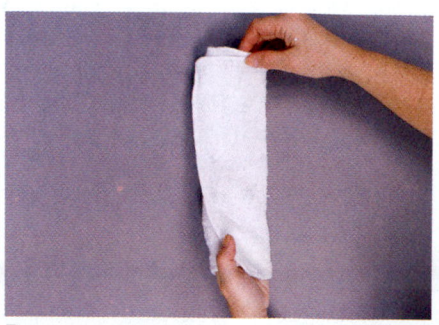

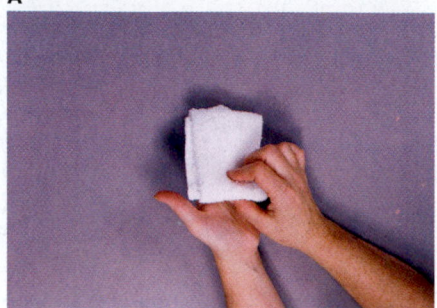

Figure 31–6 ■ Making a bath mitt, rectangular method. (A) Lay your hand on the washcloth and fold one side over your hand; (B) fold the second side over your hand; (C) fold the top of the cloth down and tuck it under the folded side against your palm to secure the mitt.

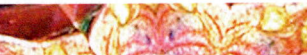

Procedure 31–1 Bathing an Adult or Pediatric Client *continued*

IMPLEMENTATION *continued*

7. Wash the face. *Begin the bath at the cleanest area and work downward toward the feet.*
   - Place towel under client's head.
   - Wash the client's eyes with water only and dry them well. Use a separate corner of the washcloth for each eye. *Using separate corners prevents transmitting microorganisms from one eye to the other.* Wipe from the inner to the outer canthus (Figure 31–7 ■). *This prevents secretions from entering the nasolacrimal ducts.*
   - Ask whether the client wants soap used on the face. *Soap has a drying effect, and the face, which is exposed to the air more than other body parts, tends to be drier.*
   - Wash, rinse, and dry the client's face, ears, and neck.
   - Remove the towel from under the client's head.

8. Wash the arms and hands. (Omit the arms for a partial bath.)
   - Place a towel lengthwise under the arm away from you. *It protects the bed from becoming wet.*
   - Wash, rinse, and dry the arm by elevating the client's arm and supporting the client's wrist and elbow (Figure 31–8 ■). Use long, firm strokes from wrist to shoulder, including the axillary area. *Firm strokes from distal to proximal areas promote circulation by increasing venous blood return.*
   - Apply deodorant or powder if desired.
   - (Optional) Place a towel on the bed and put a washbasin on it. Place the client's hands in the basin. *Many clients enjoy immersing their hands in the basin and washing themselves. Soaking loosens dirt under the nails.* Assist the client as needed to wash, rinse, and dry the hands, paying particular attention to the spaces between the fingers.
   - Repeat for hand and arm nearest you. Exercise caution if an intravenous infusion is present, and check its flow after moving the arm.

9. Wash the chest and abdomen. (Omit the chest and abdomen for a partial bath. However, the areas under a woman's breast may require bathing if this area is irritated or if the client has significant perspiration under the breast.)
   - Place bath towel lengthwise over chest. Fold bath blanket down to the client's pubic area. *Keeps the client warm while preventing unnecessary exposure of the chest.*
   - Lift the bath towel off the chest, and bathe the chest and abdomen with your mitted hand using long, firm strokes (Figure 31–9 ■). Give special attention to the skin under the breasts and any other skin folds particularly if the client is overweight. Rinse and dry well.
   - Replace the bath blanket when the areas have been dried.

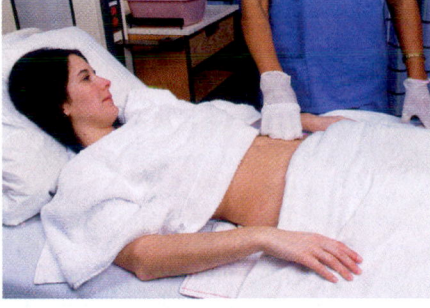

Figure 31–9 ■ Washing the chest and abdomen.

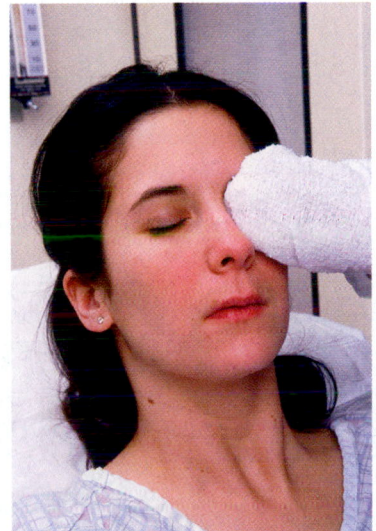

Figure 31–7 ■ Using a separate corner of the washcloth for each eye, wipe from the inner to the outer canthus.

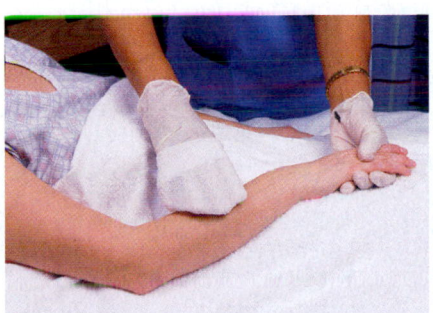

Figure 31–8 ■ Washing the far arm using long, firm strokes from wrist to shoulder area.

continued on page 710

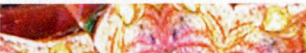

Procedure 31–1   Bathing an Adult or Pediatric Client *continued*

IMPLEMENTATION *continued*

10. Wash the legs and feet. (Omit legs and feet for a partial bath.)
    - Expose the leg farthest from you by folding the bath blanket toward the other leg being careful to keep the perineum covered. *Covering the perineum promotes privacy and maintains the client's dignity.*
    - Lift leg and place the bath towel lengthwise under the leg. Wash, rinse, and dry the leg using long, smooth, firm strokes from the ankle to the knee to the thigh (Figure 31–10 ■). *Washing from the distal to proximal areas promotes circulation by stimulating venous blood flow.*

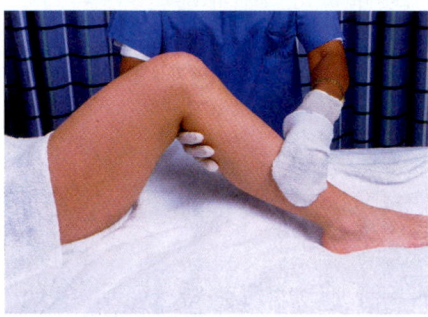

Figure 31–10 ■ Washing far leg.

- Reverse the coverings and repeat for the other leg.
- Wash the feet by placing them in the basin of water (Figure 31–11 ■).
- Dry each foot. Pay particular attention to the spaces between the toes. If you prefer, wash one foot after that leg before washing the other leg.

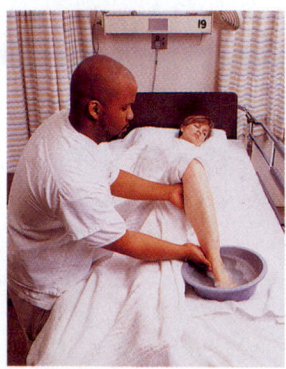

Figure 31–11 ■ Soaking a foot in a basin.

- Obtain fresh, warm bathwater now or when necessary. *Water may become dirty or cold.* Because surface skin cells are removed with washing, the bathwater from dark-skinned clients may be dark, however, this does not mean the client is dirty. Raise side rails when refilling basin. *This ensures the safety of the client.*

11. Wash the back and then the perineum.
    - Assist the client into a prone or side-lying position facing away from you. Place the bath towel lengthwise alongside the back and buttocks while keeping the client covered with the bath blanket as much as possible. *This provides warmth and undue exposure.*
    - Wash and dry the client's back, moving from the shoulders to the buttocks, and upper thighs, paying attention to the gluteal folds (Figure 31–12 ■).

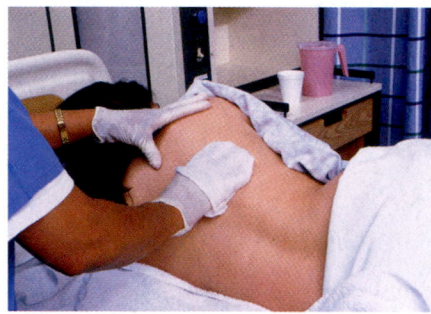

Figure 31–12 ■ Washing the back.

- Perform a back massage now or after completion of bath. (See Procedure 43–1). 🔗
- Assist the client to the supine position and determine whether the client can wash the perineal area independently. If the client cannot do so, drape the client as shown in Procedure 31–2 and wash the area.

12. Assist the client with grooming aids such as powder, lotion, or deodorant.
    - Use powder sparingly. Release as little as possible into the atmosphere. *This will avoid irritation of the respiratory tract by powder inhalation. Excessive powder can cause caking, which leads to skin irritation.*

- Help the client put on a clean gown or pajamas.
- Assist the client to care for hair, mouth, and nails. Some people prefer or need mouth care prior to their bath.

FOR A TUB BATH OR SHOWER

13. Prepare the client and the tub.
    - Fill the tub about one-third to one-half full of water at 43 to 46C (110 to 115F). *Sufficient water is needed to cover the perineal area.*
    - Cover all intravenous catheters or wound dressings with plastic coverings, and instruct the client to prevent wetting these areas if possible.
    - Put a rubber bath mat or towel on the floor of the tub if safety strips are not on the tub floor. *These prevent slippage of the client during the bath or shower.*

14. Assist the client into the shower or tub.
    - Assist the client taking a standing shower with the initial adjustment of the water temperature and water flow pressure, as needed. Some clients need a chair to sit on in the shower because of weakness. Hot water can cause elderly people to feel faint.
    - If the client requires considerable assistance with a tub bath, a hydraulic bathtub chair may be required (see "Variation").
    - Explain how the client can signal for help, leave the client for 2 to 5 minutes, and place an "occupied" sign on the door. For safety reasons, do not leave a client with decreased cognition or clients who may be at risk (e.g., history of seizures, syncope).

15. Assist the client with washing and getting out of the tub.
    - Wash the client's back, lower legs, and feet, if necessary.
    - Assist the client out of the tub. If the client is unsteady, place a bath towel over the client's shoulders and drain the tub of water before the client attempts to get out of it. *Draining the water first lessens the likelihood of a fall. The towel prevents chilling.*

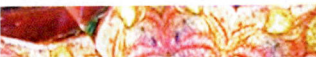

Procedure 31–1 Bathing an Adult or Pediatric Client *continued*

IMPLEMENTATION *continued*

16. Dry the client, and assist with follow-up care.
    - Follow step 12.
    - Assist the client back to his or her room.
    - Clean the tub or shower in accordance with agency practice, discard the used linen in the laundry hamper, and place the "unoccupied" sign on the door.

17. Document
    - Type of bath given (i.e., complete, partial, or self-help). This is usually recorded on a flowsheet.
    - Skin assessment, such as excoriation, erythema, exudates, rashes, drainage, or skin breakdown.
    - Nursing interventions related to skin integrity.
    - Ability of the client to assist or cooperate with bathing.
    - Client response to bathing.
    - Educational needs regarding hygiene.
    - Information or teaching shared with the client or their family.

VARIATION: BATHING USING A HYDRAULIC BATHTUB CHAIR

A hydraulic lift, often used in long-term care or rehabilitation settings, can facilitate the transfer of a client who is unable to ambulate to a tub. The lift also helps eliminate strain on the nurse's back.

- Bring the client to the tub room in a wheelchair or shower chair.
- Fill the tub and check the water temperature with a bath thermometer *to avoid thermal injury to the client.*
- Lower the hydraulic chair lift to its lowest point, outside the tub.
- Transfer the client to the chair lift and secure the seat belt (Figure 31–13 ■).
- Raise the chair lift above the tub.
- Support the client's legs as the chair is moved over the tub *to avoid injury to the legs.*
- Position the client's legs down into the water and slowly lower the chair lift into the tub.
- Assist in bathing the client, if appropriate.

- Reverse the procedure when taking the client out of the tub.
- Dry the client and transport him or her to the room.

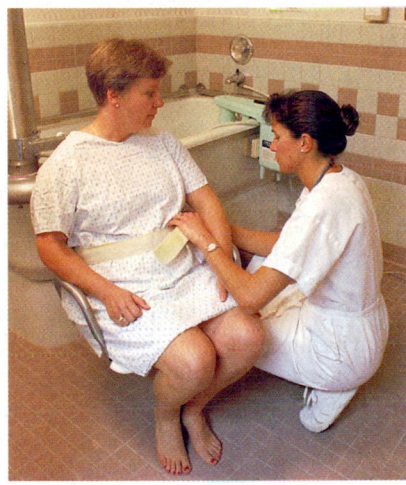

Figure 31–13 ■ Secure the seat belt before moving the client in a hydraulic bathtub chair.

EVALUATION

- Note the client's tolerance of the procedure (e.g., respiratory rate and effort, pulse rate, behaviors, statements regarding comfort).
- Conduct appropriate follow up, such as
  - Condition and integrity of skin (dryness, turgor, redness, lesions, and so on)
  - Client strength
  - Percentage of bath done without assistance.
- Relate to prior assessment data, if available.

Lifespan Considerations

Bathing

Infants
- Sponge baths are suggested for the newborn because daily tub baths are not considered necessary. After the bath, the infant should be immediately dried and wrapped. Parents need to be advised that the infant's ability to regulate body temperature has not yet fully developed and newborns' bodies lose heat readily.

Children
- Encourage a child's participation appropriate for developmental level.
- Closely supervise children in the bathtub. Do not leave them unattended.

Adolescents
- Assist adolescents as needed to choose deodorants and antiperspirants. Secretions from newly active sweat glands react with bacteria on the skin, causing a pungent odor.

Elders
- Changes of aging can decrease the protective function of the skin in elders. These changes include fragile skin, less oil and moisture, and a decrease in elasticity.
- To minimize skin dryness in elders, avoid excessive use of soap. The ideal time to moisturize the skin is immediately after bathing.
- Avoid powder because it causes moisture loss and is a hazardous inhalant. Cornstarch should also be avoided because in the presence of moisture it breaks down into glucose and can facilitate the growth of organisms.
- Protect elders and children from injury related to hot water burns.

Home Care Considerations

Hygiene

Suggest that the client or family do the following:

- Consider purchasing a bath seat that fits in the tub or shower.
- Install a hand shower for use with a bath seat and shampooing.
- Use a nonskid surface on the tub or shower.

- Install hand bars on both sides of the tub or shower to facilitate transfers in and out of the tub or shower.
- Carefully monitor the temperature of the bathwater.
- Apply lotion and oil *after* a bath, not during, because these solutions can make a tub surface slippery.

Long-Term Care Setting. From a historical perspective, the bath has always been a part of nursing care and considered a component of the "art" of nursing. In today's nursing world, however, the bath is seen as "basic" and often delegated to nonprofessionals (Hektor & Touhy, 1997).

In spite of the previously listed therapeutic values associated with bathing, the choice of bathing procedure often depends on the amount of time available to the nurse or unlicensed assistive personnel (UAP) and the client's self-care ability. Nursing authors (Brawley, 2002; Hektor & Touhy, 1997; Rader, Lavelle, Hoeffer, & McKenzie, 1996; Skewes, 1997) challenge nurses to switch from a task-centered approach to an individualized and aesthetic approach to bathing, especially for the older person in a long-term care setting.

The bath routine (e.g., day, time, and number/week) for clients in health care settings is often determined by agency policy, such that the bath becomes routine and depersonalized versus therapeutic, satisfying, and person focused. An individualized approach focusing on therapeutic and comforting outcomes of bathing is especially important for clients with dementia. Miller (1997) found that hygienic care (in the form of showering) of persons with cognitive impairment could cause client distress and precipitate physically aggressive behavior toward staff.

Rader et al. (1996) encourages nurses in the long-term care setting to view the bath from the individual's perspective. For example, what is their usual method of maintaining cleanliness? Are there any past negative experiences related to bathing? Are factors such as pain or fatigue increasing the client's difficulty with the demands and stimuli associated with bathing or showering? A client's resistance to the bathing experience can be a cue to the nurse to consider other methods of maintaining cleanliness. For example, if the shower causes distress, is there another form of bathing (such as the towel bath) that may be more therapeutic and comforting?

Providing personal hygiene to a client with dementia is often an ongoing challenge. Being sensitive to the rhythm of their behavior and looking for cues can often offset problems related to this. Clients with dementia, whether they are at home or in a health care facility, often have certain times of the day when they are more agitated—these are times to avoid doing things that will increase their fear and agitation. It is sometimes helpful to wait awhile (e.g., half an hour or so) and then try giving the bath because they may forget that they were protesting and be willing to participate.

Collaboration between the nurse and UAP is a critical element to implementing the individualized person-focused approach for cognitively impaired clients who exhibit aggressive behavior during bathing. After observing a difficult bathing situation, the nurse and UAP should discuss possible alternative strategies or methods they might implement for the client. Hoeffer, Rader, McKenzie, Lavelle, and Stewart (1997) point out that nursing assistants are concerned that they may be perceived as not doing their job if they vary from the standard routine of the agency. Validation and support by the nurse is critical to the willingness of the UAP to try new approaches.

Perineal-Genital Care

Perineal-genital care is also referred to as *perineal care* or *peri-care.* Perineal care as part of the bed bath is embarrassing for many clients. Nurses also may find it embarrassing initially, particularly with clients of the opposite sex. Most clients who require a bed bath from the nurse are able to clean their own genital areas with minimal assistance. The nurse may need to hand a moistened washcloth and soap to the client, rinse the washcloth, and provide a towel.

Because some clients are unfamiliar with terminology for the genitals and perineum, it may be difficult for nurses to explain what is expected. Most clients, however, understand what is meant if the nurse simply says, "I'll give you a washcloth to finish your bath." Older clients may be familiar with the term *private parts.* Whatever expression the nurse uses, it needs to be one that the client understands and one that is comfortable for the nurse to use.

The nurse needs to provide perineal care efficiently and matter-of-factly. Nurses should wear gloves while providing this care for the comfort of the client and to protect themselves from infection. Procedure 31–2 explains how to provide perineal-genital care.

> **CLINICAL ALERT**   *Always wash or wipe from "clean to dirty." For a female, cleanse perineal area from front to back. For a male, cleanse the urinary meatus by moving in a circular motion from center of urethral opening around the glans.*

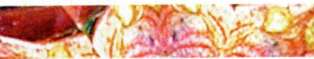

Procedure 31–2 Providing Perineal-Genital Care

Purposes
- To remove normal perineal secretions and odors
- To promote client comfort

ASSESSMENT

Assess for the presence of
- Irritation, excoriation, inflammation, swelling
- Excessive discharge
- Odor; pain or discomfort
- Urinary or fecal incontinence

- Recent rectal or perineal surgery
- Indwelling catheter

Determine
- Perineal-genital hygiene practices
- Self-care abilities

PLANNING

Delegation
Perineal-genital care can be delegated to UAP. If the client has recently had perineal, rectal, or genital surgery, the nurse needs to assess if it is appropriate for the UAP to perform perineal-genital care.

Equipment
Perineal-genital care provided in conjunction with the bed bath
- Bath towel
- Bath blanket
- Clean gloves
- Bath basin with water at 43 to 46C (110 to 115F)
- Soap

- Washcloth

Special perineal-genital care
- Bath towel
- Bath blanket
- Clean gloves
- Cotton balls or swabs
- Solution bottle, pitcher, or container filled with warm water or a prescribed solution
- Bedpan to receive rinse water
- Moisture-resistant bag or receptacle for used cotton swabs
- Perineal pad

IMPLEMENTATION

Preparation
- Determine whether the client is experiencing any discomfort in the perineal-genital area.
- Obtain and prepare the necessary equipment and supplies.

Performance
1. Explain to the client what you are going to do, why it is necessary, and how he or she can cooperate, being particularly sensitive to any embarrassment felt by the client.
2. Wash hands and observe other appropriate infection control procedures (e.g., clean gloves).
3. Provide for client privacy by drawing the curtains around the bed or closing the door to the room. Some agencies provide signs indicating the need for privacy. *Hygiene is a personal matter.*
4. Prepare the client:
   - Fold the top bed linen to the foot of the bed and fold the gown up to expose the genital area.
   - Place a bath towel under the client's hips. *The bath towel prevents the bed from becoming soiled.*
5. Position and drape the client and clean the upper inner thighs.

FOR FEMALES
- Position the female in a back-lying position with the knees flexed and spread well apart.
- Cover her body and legs with the bath blanket. Drape the legs by tucking the bottom corners of the bath blanket under the inner sides of the legs (Figure 31–14 ■). *Minimum exposure lessens embarrassment and helps to provide warmth.* Bring the middle portion of the base of the blanket up over the pubic area.
- Put on gloves, wash and dry the upper inner thighs.

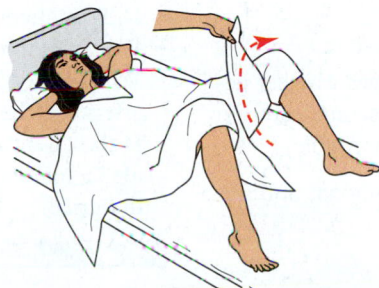

Figure 31–14 ■ Draping the client for perineal-genital care.

FOR MALES
- Position the male client in a supine position with knees slightly flexed and hips slightly externally rotated.
- Put on gloves, wash and dry the upper inner thighs.
6. Inspect the perineal area.
   - Note particular areas of inflammation, excoriation, or swelling, especially between the labia in females and the scrotal folds in males.
   - Also note excessive discharge or secretions from the orifices and the presence of odors.
7. Wash and dry the perineal-genital area.

FOR FEMALES
- Clean the labia majora. Then spread the labia to wash the folds between the labia majora and the labia minora (Figure 31–15 ■). *Secretions that tend to collect around the labia minora facilitate bacterial growth.*
- Use separate quarters of the washcloth for each stroke, and wipe from the pubis to the rectum. For menstruating women and clients with indwelling catheters, use clean

continued on page 714

Procedure 31–2 Providing Perineal-Genital Care *continued*

IMPLEMENTATION *continued*

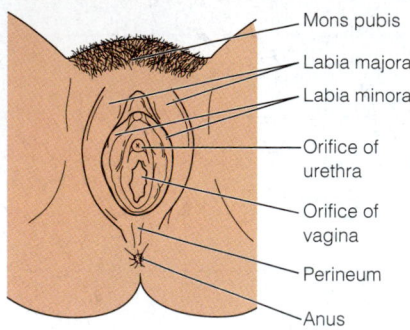

Figure 31–15 ■ Female genitals.

wipes, cotton balls, or gauze. Take a clean ball for each stroke. *Using separate quarters of the washcloth or new cotton balls or gauzes prevents the transmission of microorganisms from one area to the other. Wipe from the area of least contamination (the pubis) to that of greatest (the rectum).*

• Rinse the area well. You may place the client on a bedpan and use a periwash or solution bottle to pour warm water over the area. Dry the perineum thoroughly, paying particular attention to the folds between the labia. *Moisture supports the growth of many microorganisms.*

FOR MALES

• Wash and dry the penis, using firm strokes. *Handling the penis firmly may prevent an erection.*

• If the client is uncircumcised, retract the prepuce (foreskin) to expose the glans penis (the tip of the penis) for cleaning. Replace the foreskin after cleaning the glans penis (Figure 31–16 ■). *Retracting the foreskin is necessary to remove the smegma that collects under the foreskin and facilitates bacterial growth. Replacing the foreskin prevents constriction of the penis, which may cause edema.*

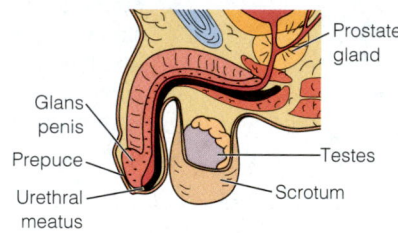

Figure 31–16 ■ Male genitals.

• Wash and dry the scrotum. The posterior folds of the scrotum may need to be cleaned when the but-

tocks are cleaned (see step 9). *The scrotum tends to be more soiled than the penis because of its proximity to the rectum; thus it is usually cleaned after the penis.*

8. Inspect perineal orifices for intactness.
   • Inspect particularly around the urethra in clients with indwelling catheters. *A catheter may cause excoriation around the urethra.*

9. Clean between the buttocks.
   • Assist the client to turn onto the side facing away from you.
   • Pay particular attention to the anal area and posterior folds of the scrotum in males. Clean the anus with toilet tissue before washing it, if necessary.
   • Dry the area well.
   • For postdelivery or menstruating females, apply a perineal pad as needed from front to back. *This prevents contamination of the vagina and urethra from the anal area.*

10. Document any unusual findings such as redness, excoriation, skin breakdown, discharge or drainage and any localized areas of tenderness.

EVALUATION

■ Relate current assessments to previous assessments.
■ Conduct appropriate follow-up such as prescribed ointment for excoriation.

■ Report any deviation from normal to the physician.

Client Teaching Clients often need information about dry skin, skin rashes, and acne.

EVALUATING

Using data collected during care, the nurse judges whether desired outcomes have been achieved. If the outcomes are not achieved, the nurse explores reasons why. For example:

• Did the nurse overestimate the client's functional abilities (physical, mental, emotional) for self-care?
• Were provided instructions not clear?

• Were appropriate assistive devices or supplies not available to the client?
• Did the client's condition change?
• Were required analgesics provided before hygienic care?
• What currently prescribed medications and therapies could affect the client's abilities or tissue integrity?
• Is the client's fluid and food intake adequate or appropriate to maintain skin and mucous membrane moisture and integrity?

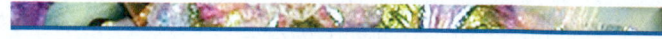

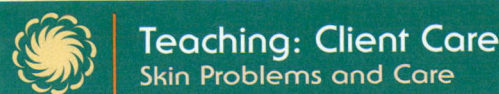

Teaching: Client Care
Skin Problems and Care

Dry Skin

- Use cleansing creams to clean the skin rather than soap or detergent, which cause drying and, in some cases, allergic reactions.
- Use bath oils, but take precautions to prevent falls caused by slippery tub surfaces.
- Thoroughly rinse soap or detergent, if used, from the skin.
- Bathe less frequently when environmental temperature and humidity are low.
- Increase fluid intake.
- Humidify the air with a humidifier or by keeping a tub or sink full of water.
- Use moisturizing or emollient creams that contain lanolin, petroleum jelly, or cocoa butter to retain skin moisture.

Skin Rashes

- Keep the area clean by washing it with a mild soap. Rinse the skin well, and pat it dry.

- To relieve itching, try a tepid bath or soak. Some over-the-counter preparations, such as Caladryl lotion, may help but should be used with full knowledge of the product.
- Avoid scratching the rash to prevent inflammation, infection, and further skin lesions.
- Choose clothing carefully. Too much can cause perspiration and aggravate a rash.

Acne

- Wash the face frequently with soap or detergent and hot water to remove oil and dirt.
- Avoid using oily creams, which aggravate the condition.
- Avoid using cosmetics that block the ducts of the sebaceous glands and the hair follicles.
- Never squeeze or pick at the lesions. This increases the potential for infection and scarring.

FEET

The feet are essential for ambulation and merit attention even when people are confined to bed. Each foot contains 26 bones, 107 ligaments, and 19 muscles. These structures function together for both standing and walking.

Developmental Variations

At birth, a baby's foot is relatively unformed. The arches are supported by fatty pads and do not take their full shape until 5 to 6 years of age. During childhood, the bones and small muscles of the feet are easily damaged by tight, binding stockings and ill-fitting shoes. For normal development, it is important that the arches be supported and that the bony structure and the feet grow with no external restrictions. Feet are not fully grown until about age 20. Healthy feet remain relatively unchanged during life. However, the elderly often require special attention for their feet. For example, reduced blood supply and accompanying arteriosclerosis can make a foot prone to ulcers and infection following trauma.

> ▶ **CLINICAL ALERT** *Clients with diabetes are at high risk for lower extremity amputations (LEA). Routine foot assessment and client education in proper foot care can significantly reduce the risk for LEA.*

NURSING MANAGEMENT

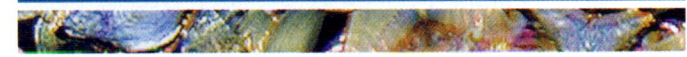

ASSESSING

Assessment of the client's feet includes a nursing health history, physical assessment of the feet, and identifying clients at risk for foot problems.

Nursing Health History

The nurse determines the client's history of (a) normal nail and foot care practices, (b) type of footwear worn, (c) self-care abilities, (d) presence of risk factors for foot problems, (e) any foot discomfort, and (f) any perceived problems with foot mobility. To elicit such data, the nurse asks the client the questions provided in the accompanying Assessment Interview.

Physical Assessment

Each foot and toe is inspected for shape, size, and presence of lesions and is palpated to assess areas of tenderness, edema, and circulatory status. Normally, the toes are straight and flat. Table 31–5 lists physical assessment methods for the feet. Common foot problems include calluses, corns, unpleasant odors, plantar warts, fissures between the toes, and fungal infections such as athlete's foot.

A **callus** is a thickened portion of epidermis, a mass of keratotic material. Most calluses are painless and flat and are

Assessment Interview
FOOT HYGIENE

Foot Care Practices

- How often do you wash your feet and cut your toenails?
- What hygiene products do you usually use on your feet (e.g., soap, foot powder or deodorant, lotion, or cream)?
- What type of shoes and socks do you wear?
- How often do you change your socks or put on clean socks?
- Do you ever go barefoot? If so, when, where, and how often?

Self-Care Abilities

- Do you have any problems managing your foot care? If so, what are these?
- How can the nurses best help you?

Foot Problems and Risk Factors

- Do you have any problems with foot odor?
- Do you have any foot discomfort? If so, where? When does this occur? What do you do to relieve the discomfort? Does this discomfort affect how you walk?
- Have you noticed any problems with foot mobility (e.g., joint stiffness)?
- Do you have diabetes, any circulatory problems with feet (e.g., swelling, changes in skin color, arthritis), or any instances of prolonged exposure to chemicals or water?

found on the bottom or side of the foot over a bony prominence. Calluses are usually caused by pressure from shoes. They can be softened by soaking the foot in warm water with Epsom salts, and abraded with pumice stones or similar abrasives. Creams with lanolin help to keep the skin soft and prevent the formation of calluses.

A **corn** is a keratosis caused by friction and pressure from a shoe. It commonly occurs on the fourth or fifth toe, usually on a bony prominence such as a joint. Corns are usually conical (circular and raised). The base is the surface of the corn and the apex is in deeper tissues, sometimes even attached to bone. Corns are generally removed surgically. They are prevented from reforming by relieving the pressure on the area (i.e., wearing comfortable shoes), and massaging the tissue to promote circulation. The use of oval corn pads should be avoided because they increase pressure and decrease circulation.

Unpleasant odors occur as a result of perspiration and its interaction with microorganisms. Regular and frequent washing of the feet and wearing clean hosiery help to minimize odor. Foot powders and deodorants also help to prevent this problem.

Plantar warts appear on the sole of the foot. These warts are caused by the virus papovavirus hominis. They are moderately contagious. The warts are frequently painful and often make walking difficult. The physician may curettage the warts, freeze them with solid carbon dioxide several times, or apply salicylic acid.

Fissures, or deep grooves, frequently occur between the toes as a result of dryness and cracking of the skin. The treatment of choice is good foot hygiene and application of an antiseptic to prevent infection. Often a small piece of gauze is inserted between the toes in applying the antiseptic and left in place to assist healing by allowing air to reach the area.

> ►**CLINICAL ALERT** *Clients with diabetes often have extremely dry skin. Tell them to use a nonperfumed lotion and to avoid putting lotion between the toes. Advise to not soak their feet in water because it is drying to the skin.*

Athlete's foot, or **tinea pedis** (ringworm of the foot), is caused by a fungus. The symptoms are scaling and cracking of the skin, particularly between the toes. Sometimes small blisters form, containing a thin fluid. In severe cases, the lesions may also appear on other parts of the body, particularly the hands. Treatments usually involve the application of commercial antifungal ointments or powders. Prevention is

TABLE 31–5 Assessment of the Feet

Method	Normal Findings	Deviations from Normal
Inspect all skin surfaces, particularly between the toes, for cleanliness, odor, dryness, inflammation, swelling, abrasions, or other lesions.	Intact skin Absence of swelling or inflammation	Excessive dryness Areas of inflammation or swelling (e.g., corns, calluses) Fissures Scaling and cracking of skin (e.g., athlete's foot) Plantar warts
Palpate anterior and posterior surfaces of ankles and feet for edema.	No swelling	Swelling or pitting edema
Palpate dorsalis pedis pulse on dorsal surface of foot.	Strong, regular pulses in both feet	Weak or absent pulses
Compare skin temperature of both feet.	Warm skin temperature	Cool skin temperature in one or both feet

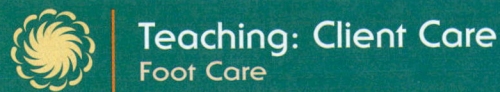

Teaching: Client Care
Foot Care

- Wash the feet daily, and dry them well, especially between the toes.
- When washing, inspect the skin of the feet for breaks or red or swollen areas. Use a mirror if needed to visualize all areas.
- To prevent burns, check the water temperature before immersing the feet.
- Use creams or lotions to moisten the skin, or soak the feet in warm water with Epsom salts to avoid excessive drying of the skin of the feet. Lotion will also soften calluses. A lotion that reduces dryness effectively is a mixture of lanolin and mineral oil.
- To prevent or control an unpleasant odor due to excessive foot perspiration, wash the feet frequently and change socks and shoes at least daily. Special deodorant sprays or absorbent foot powders are also helpful.
- File the toenails rather than cutting them to avoid skin injury. File the nails straight across the ends of the toes. If the nails are too thick or misshapen to file, consult a podiatrist.
- Wear clean stockings or socks daily. Avoid socks with holes or darns that can cause pressure areas.
- Wear correctly fitting shoes that neither restrict the foot nor rub on any area; rubbing can cause corns and calluses. Check worn shoes for rough spots in the lining. Break in new shoes

- gradually by increasing the wearing time 30 to 60 minutes each day.
- Avoid walking barefoot, because injury and infection may result. Wear slippers in public showers and in change areas to avoid contracting athlete's foot or other infections.
- Several times each day exercise the feet to promote circulation. Point the feet upward, point them downward, and move them in circles.
- Avoid wearing constricting garments such as knee-high elastic stockings and avoid sitting with the legs crossed at the knees, which may decrease circulation.
- When the feet are cold, use extra blankets and wear warm socks rather than using heating pads or hot water bottles, which may cause burns. Test bathwater before stepping into it.
- Wash any cut on the foot thoroughly, apply a mild antiseptic, and notify the physician.
- Avoid self-treatment for corns or calluses. Pumice stones and some callus and corn applications are injurious to the skin. Consult a podiatrist or physician first.
- Notify the physician if you notice abnormal sores or drainage, pain, or changes in temperature, color, and sensation of the foot.

---

important. Common preventive measures are keeping the feet well ventilated, drying the feet well after bathing, wearing clean socks or stockings, and not going barefoot in public showers.

An **ingrown toe nail,** the growing inward of the nail into the soft tissues around it, most often results from improper nail trimming. Pressure applied to the area causes localized pain. Treatment involves frequent, hot antiseptic soaks and surgical removal of the portion of nail embedded in the skin. Preventing recurrence involves appropriate instruction and adherence to proper nail-trimming techniques.

Identifying Clients at Risk

Because of reduced peripheral circulation to the feet, clients with diabetes or peripheral vascular disease are particularly prone to infection if skin breakage occurs. Many foot problems can be prevented by teaching the client simple foot care guidelines (see Teaching: Client Care).

DIAGNOSING

A number of nursing diagnoses may apply to clients with foot or foot care problems. The most common diagnostic labels, along with possible related or contributing factors, are as follows:

- *Self-Care Deficit: Hygiene* (foot care) related to
  a. Visual impairment
  b. Impaired hand coordination
  c. Other related or contributing factors (see Box 31–1).

- *Risk for Impaired Skin Integrity* related to
  a. Altered tissue perfusion: peripheral (associated with edema, inadequate arterial circulation)
  b. Poorly fitting shoes.
- *Risk for Infection* related to
  a. Impaired skin integrity (ingrown toenail, corn, trauma)
  b. Deficient nail or foot care.
- *Deficient Knowledge* (diabetic foot care) related to
  a. Lack of teaching/learning activities about diabetic foot care
  b. Newly established medical diagnosis (diabetes) and necessary foot hygiene practices.

Examples of assessment data clusters, related nursing diagnoses, outcomes, and interventions are shown in Identifying Nursing Diagnoses, Outcomes, and Interventions.

PLANNING

Planning involves (a) identifying nursing interventions that will help the client maintain or restore healthy foot care practices and (b) establishing desired outcomes for each client. Interventions may include teaching the client about correct nail and foot care, proper footwear, wearing the correct size, and ways to prevent potential foot problems (e.g., infection, injury, and decreased circulation). For clients with self-care difficulties, the nurse plans a schedule for soaking the client's feet and assisting with regular cleaning and trimming of nails (if not contraindicated). Foot and nail care is often provided during the client's bath but may be provided at any time in the day to accommodate the client's preference or schedule. The frequency

IDENTIFYING NURSING DIAGNOSES, OUTCOMES, AND INTERVENTIONS

CLIENTS WITH FOOT PROBLEMS

DATA CLUSTER	NURSING DIAGNOSIS/ DEFINITION	SAMPLE DESIRED OUTCOME [NOC #]/DEFINITION	INDICATORS	SELECTED INTERVENTIONS [NIC #]/DEFINITION	SAMPLE NIC ACTIVITIES
Sally Brown, an 83-year-old widow, lives alone. Has home-maker services twice a week and Meals on Wheels service daily. Manages to shower once a week with daughter's help. Has pronounced hand tremors and obvious cataracts. States, "I can't see well enough to cut my nails and even if I could see, my hands shake so badly."	Self-Care Deficit: (Foot Care) Hygiene related to impaired hand coordination and visual impairment/Impaired ability to perform or complete bathing/hygiene activities for oneself	Self-Care: Grooming [0304]/Ability to maintain kempt appearance	Dependent, does not participate • Cares for nails	Foot Care [1660]/ Cleansing and inspecting the feet for the purposes of relaxation, cleanliness, and healthy skin	• Inspect skin for irritation, cracking, lesions, corns, calluses, or edema • Instruct family on the importance of foot care • Cut normal-thickness toenails when soft, using a toenail clipper and using the curve of the toe as a guide • Refer to podiatrist for trimming of thickened nails, as appropriate
Kyle Stevens, 14 years old, lives with his mother and eight sisters and brothers in a three-room walk-up. Bathroom down the hall is shared with other tenants in the building. Shoes are ragged and fit poorly. States, "I can't get new ones."	Risk for Impaired Skin Integrity related to poorly fitting shoes and limited access to bathing facilities/At risk for skin being adversely altered	Tissue Integrity: Skin & Mucous Membranes [1101]/Structural intactness and normal physiologic function of skin and mucous membranes	Not compromised • Skin intactness	Skin Surveillance [3590]/Collection and analysis of client data to maintain skin and mucous membrane integrity	• Monitor skin for areas of redness and breakdown • Monitor skin for excessive dryness and moisture • Institute measures to prevent deterioration of skin • Instruct client and family about signs of skin breakdown

of foot care is determined by the nurse and client and is based on objective assessment data and the client's specific problems. For some clients, the feet need to be bathed daily; for those whose feet perspire excessively, bathing more than once a day may be necessary (see Identifying Nursing Diagnoses, Outcomes, and Interventions).

IMPLEMENTING

Procedure 31–3 describes how to provide foot care. See also the discussion of nails. During these procedures, the nurse has the opportunity to teach the client appropriate methods for foot care, that is, methods designed to prevent tissue injury and infection (see earlier Teaching: Client Care feature).

IDENTIFYING NURSING DIAGNOSES, OUTCOMES, AND INTERVENTIONS *continued*

CLIENTS WITH FOOT PROBLEMS *continued*

DATA CLUSTER	NURSING DIAGNOSIS/ DEFINITION	SAMPLE DESIRED OUTCOME [NOC#]/DEFINITION	INDICATORS	SELECTED INTERVENTIONS [NIC#]/DEFINITION	SAMPLE NIC ACTIVITIES
Jim Wakefield, 64 years old, was recently diagnosed with diabetes mellitus. States he has heard of "diabetes" and is worried because a friend of his father's had diabetes and, after cutting his foot, had his leg amputated.	*Deficient Knowledge* (Diabetic Foot Care) related to misinterpretation of information/ *Absence or deficiency of cognitive information related to a specific topic*	Knowledge: Diabetes Management [1820]/*Extent of understanding conveyed about diabetes mellitus and its control*	Substantial knowledge • Description of preventive foot care practices	Teaching: Disease Process [5602]/ *Assisting the client to understand information related to a specific disease process*	• Appraise the client's current level of knowledge related to diabetes • Provide information to the client about diabetes, as appropriate • Discuss lifestyle changes that may be required to prevent future complications or control the disease process • Describe rationale behind foot care management • Instruct the client on which signs and symptoms to report to health care provider, as appropriate

---

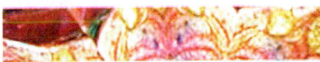

Procedure 31–3 Providing Foot Care

Purposes

- To maintain the skin integrity of the feet
- To prevent foot infections
- To prevent foot odors
- To assess or monitor foot problems

ASSESSMENT

Determine

- History of any problems with foot odor, foot discomfort, foot mobility, circulatory problems (e.g., swelling, changes in skin color and/or temperature, and pain), structural problems (e.g., bunion, hammer toe, or overlapping digits)
- Usual foot care practices (e.g., frequency of washing feet and cutting nails, foot hygiene products used, how often socks are changed, whether the client ever goes barefoot, whether the client see a podiatrist)

Assess

- Skin surfaces for cleanliness, odor, dryness, and intactness
- Each foot and toe for shape, size, presence of lesions (e.g., corn, callus, wart, or rash), and areas of tenderness, ankle edema
- Skin temperatures of the two feet to assess circulatory status and the dorsalis pedis pulses
- Self-care abilities (e.g., any problems managing foot care)

continued on page 720

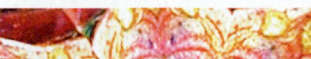 **Procedure 31–3 Providing Foot Care** *continued*

PLANNING

Delegation

Foot care for the *nondiabetic* client can be delegated to UAP. Remind the UAP to notify the nurse of anything that looks out of the ordinary. Review with the UAP the agency policy about cutting or trimming nails.

Equipment

- Washbasin containing warm water
- Pillow
- Moisture-resistant disposable pad
- Towels
- Soap
- Washcloth
- Toenail cleaning and trimming equipment
- Lotion or foot powder

IMPLEMENTATION

Performance

1. Explain to the client what you are going to do, why it is necessary, and how he or she can cooperate.
2. Wash hands and observe other appropriate infection control procedures.
3. Provide for client privacy by drawing the curtains around the bed or closing the door to the room. Some agencies provide signs indicating the need for privacy. *Hygiene is a personal matter.*
4. Prepare the equipment and the client.
   - Fill the washbasin with warm water at about 40 to 43C (105 to 110F). *Warm water promotes circulation, comforts, and refreshes.*
   - Assist the ambulatory client to a sitting position in a chair, or the bed client to a supine or semi-Fowler's position.
   - Place a pillow under the bed client's knees. *This provides support and prevents muscle fatigue.*
   - Place the washbasin on the moisture-resistant pad at the foot of the bed for a bed client or on the floor in front of the chair for an ambulatory client.
   - For a bed client, pad the rim of the washbasin with a towel. *The towel prevents undue pressure on the skin.*
5. Wash the foot and soak it.
   - Place one of the client's feet in the basin and wash it with soap, paying particular attention to the interdigi-

tal areas. Prolonged soaking is generally not recommended for diabetic clients or individuals with peripheral vascular disease. *Prolonged soaking may remove natural skin oils, thus drying the skin and making it more susceptible to cracking and injury.*
   - Rinse the foot well to remove soap. *Soap irritates the skin if not properly removed.*
   - Rub callused areas of the foot with the washcloth. *This helps remove dead skin layers.*
   - If the nails are brittle or thick and require trimming, replace the water and allow the foot to soak for 10 to 20 minutes. *Soaking softens the nails and loosens debris under them.*
   - Clean the nails as required with an orange stick. *This removes excess debris that harbors microorganisms.*
   - Remove the foot from the basin and place it on the towel.
6. Dry the foot thoroughly and apply lotion or foot powder.
   - Blot the foot gently with the towel to dry it thoroughly, particularly between the toes. *Harsh rubbing can damage the skin. Thorough drying reduces the risk of infection.*
   - Apply lotion or lanolin cream. *This lubricates dry skin.*

or
   - Apply a foot powder containing a nonirritating deodorant if the feet tend to perspire excessively. *Foot powders have greater absorbent properties than regular bath powders; some also contain menthol, which makes the feet feel cool.*
7. If agency policy permits, trim the nails of the first foot while the second foot is soaking.
   - See the discussion on nails for the appropriate method to trim nails. Note that in many agencies toenail trimming requires a physician's order or is contraindicated for clients with diabetes mellitus, toe infections, and peripheral vascular disease, unless performed by a podiatrist, general practice physician, or advanced practice provider such as a nurse practitioner.
8. Document any foot problems observed.
   - Foot care is not generally recorded unless problems are noted.
   - Record any signs of inflammation, infection, breaks in the skin, corns, troublesome calluses, bunions, and pressure areas. This is of particular importance for clients with peripheral vascular disease and diabetes.

EVALUATION

- Inspect nails and skin after the soak.
- Compare to prior assessment data.
- Report any abnormalities to the physician.

EVALUATING

Examples of desired outcomes for foot hygiene include the client being able to

- Participate in self-care (foot hygiene) to optimal level of capacity (specify)
- Describe hygienic and other interventions (e.g., proper footwear) to maintain skin integrity, prevent infection, and maintain peripheral tissue perfusion
- Demonstrate optimal foot hygiene, as evidenced by
  a. Intact, pink, smooth, soft, hydrated, and warm skin
  b. Intact cuticles and skin surrounding nails
  c. Correct foot care and nail care practices.

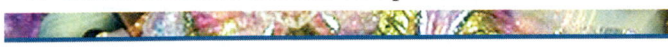

NAILS

Nails are normally present at birth. They continue to grow throughout life and change very little until people are elderly. At that time, the nails tend to be tougher, more brittle, and in some cases thicker. The nails of an older person normally grow less quickly than those of a younger person and may be ridged and grooved.

NURSING MANAGEMENT

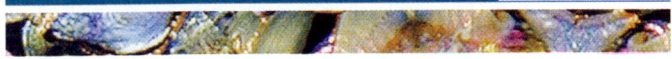

ASSESSING

During the nursing health history, the nurse explores the client's usual nail care practices, self-care abilities, and any problems associated with them (see accompanying Assessment Interview). Physical assessment involves inspection of the nails (e.g., nail shape and texture, nailbed color, and tissues surrounding the nails). See Chapter 28.

DIAGNOSING

Nursing diagnoses related to nail care and nail problems include *Self-Care Deficit* and *Risk for Infection*. Examples of these nursing diagnoses and contributing factors follow:

- *Self-Care Deficit: Grooming* related to
  a. Impaired vision
  b. Impaired hand coordination.

- *Risk for Infection* around the nail bed related to
  a. Impaired skin integrity of cuticles
  b. Altered peripheral circulation.

PLANNING

The nurse identifies measures that will assist the client to develop or maintain healthy nail care practices. A schedule of nail care needs to be established.

IMPLEMENTING

To provide nail care, the nurse needs a nail cutter or sharp scissors, a nail file, an orange stick to push back the cuticle, hand lotion or mineral oil to lubricate any dry tissue around the nails, and a basin of water to soak the nails if they are particularly thick or hard.

One hand or foot is soaked, if needed, and dried; then the nail is cut or filed straight across beyond the end of the finger or toe (see Figure 31–17 ■). Avoid trimming or digging into nails at the lateral corners. This predisposes the client to ingrown toenails. Clients who have diabetes or circulatory problems should have their nails filed rather than cut; inadvertent injury to tissues can occur if scissors are used. After the initial cut or filing, the nail is filed to round the corners, and the nurse cleans under the nail. The nurse then gently pushes back the cuticle, taking care not to injure it. The next finger or toe is cared for in the same manner. Any abnormalities, such as an infected cuticle or inflammation of the tissue around the nail, are recorded and reported.

EVALUATING

Examples of desired outcomes for nail hygiene include the client being able to

- Demonstrate healthy nail care practices, as shown by
  a. Clean, short nails with smooth edges
  b. Intact cuticles and hydrated surrounding skin
- Describe factors contributing to the nail problem
- Describe preventive interventions for the specific nail problem
- Demonstrate nail care as instructed.

In addition, the client should have pink nail beds and quick return of nail bed color after blanch test

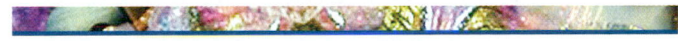

Assessment Interview

NAIL HYGIENE

- What are your usual nail care practices?
- Do you have any problems managing your nail care? If so, what are these?
- Have you had any problems associated with your nails (e.g., inflammation of the tissue surrounding the nail, injury, prolonged exposure to water or chemicals, circulatory problems)?

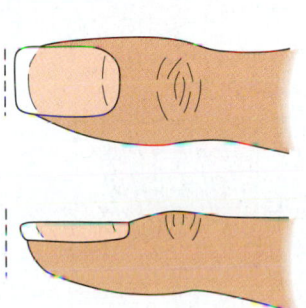

Figure 31–17 ■ Fingernails are trimmed straight across.

MOUTH

Each tooth has three parts: the crown, the root, and the pulp cavity (Figure 31–18 ■). The crown is the exposed part of the tooth, which is outside the gum. It is covered with a hard substance called enamel. The ivory-colored internal part of the crown below the enamel is the dentin. The root of a tooth is embedded in the jaw and covered by a bony tissue called cementum. The pulp cavity in the center of the tooth contains the blood vessels and nerves.

Developmental Variations

Teeth usually appear 5 to 8 months after birth. Baby-bottle syndrome may result in decay of all of the upper teeth and the lower posterior teeth (Pillitteri, 2003, p. 824). This syndrome occurs when an infant is put to bed with a bottle of sugar water, formula, milk, or fruit juice. The carbohydrates in the solutions causes demineralization of the tooth enamel, which leads to tooth decay.

By the time children are 2 years old, they usually have all 20 of their temporary teeth (Figure 31–19 ■). At about age 6 or 7, children start losing their deciduous teeth, and these are gradually replaced by the 31 permanent teeth (Figure 31–20 ■). By age 25, most people have all of their permanent teeth.

The incidence of periodontal disease increases during pregnancy because the rise in female hormones affects gingival tissue and increases its reaction to bacterial plaque. Many pregnant women experience more bleeding from the gingival sulcus during brushing and increased redness and swelling of the **gingiva** (the gum).

Some older adults may have few permanent teeth left, and some have dentures. Loss of teeth occurs mainly because of **periodontal disease** (gum disease) rather than **dental caries** (cavities); however, caries are also common in middle-aged adults.

Some receding of the gums and a brownish pigmentation of the gums occur with age. Because saliva production decreases with age, dryness of the oral mucosa is a common finding in older people.

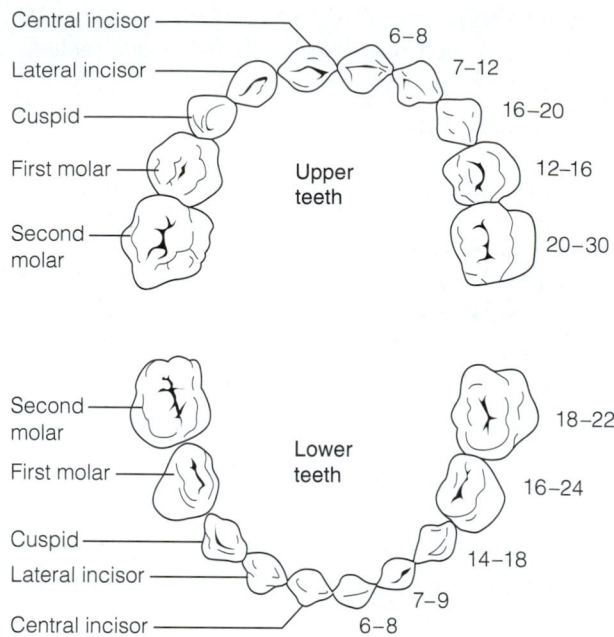

Figure 31–19 ■ Temporary teeth and their times of eruption (stated in months).

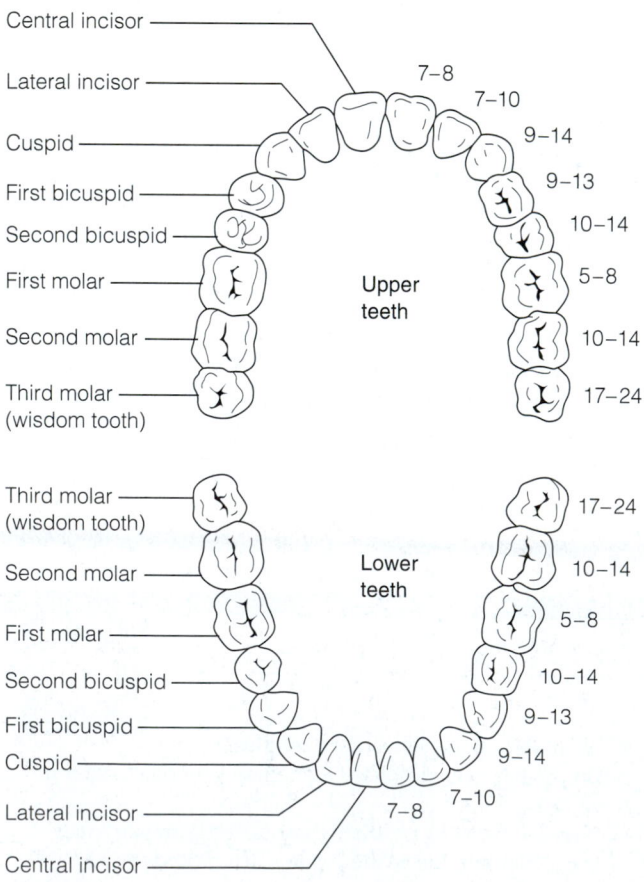

Figure 31–20 ■ Permanent teeth and their times of eruption (stated in years).

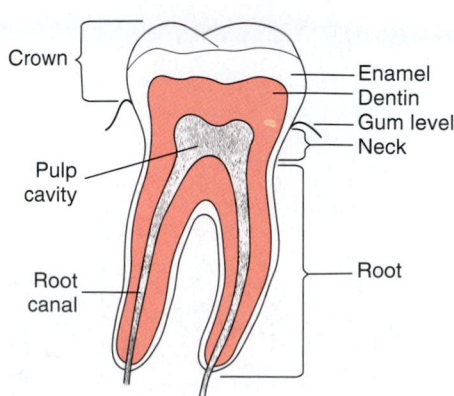

Figure 31–18 ■ The anatomic parts of a tooth.

Providing Culturally Competent Care

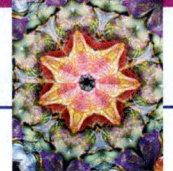

BIOCULTURAL VARIATION IN TEETH

- It is rare for a White baby to be born with teeth; however, the incidence exists among Alaskan Tlingit Indian and Canadian Eskimo infants.
- The size of teeth varies with the teeth of Whites being the smallest, followed by Blacks and then Asians and Native North Americans.
- Whites have more tooth decay than Blacks. Complete tooth loss occurs more often in Whites than in African Americans even though African Americans have a higher incidence of periodontal disease. The difference in tooth decay may be explained by the fact that African Americans have harder and denser tooth enamel.

Note: From *Transcultural Concepts in Nursing Care*, 4th ed. (p. 62), by M. M. Andrews and J. S. Boyle, 2003, Philadelphia: Lippincott Williams & Wilkins. Adapted with permission.

NURSING MANAGEMENT

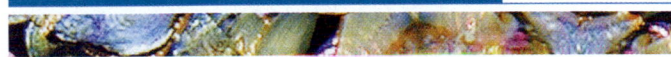

ASSESSING

Assessment of the client's mouth and hygiene practices includes (a) a nursing health history, (b) physical assessment of the mouth, and (c) identification of clients at risk for developing oral problems.

Nursing Health History

During the nursing health history, the nurse obtains data about the client's oral hygiene practices, including dental visits, self-care abilities, and past or current mouth problems. Data about the client's oral hygiene help the nurse determine learning needs and incorporate the client's needs and preferences in the plan of care. Assessment of the client's self-care abilities determines the amount and type of nursing assistance to provide. Clients whose hand coordination is impaired, whose cognitive function is impaired, whose illness alters energy levels and motivation, or whose therapy imposes restrictions on activities will need assistance from the nurse. Information about past or current problems alerts the nurse to specific interventions required or referrals that may be necessary. Questions to elicit this information are shown in the accompanying Assessment Interview.

Physical Assessment

For information about mouth assessment, see Chapter 28. 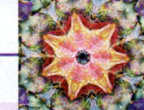 Dental caries (cavities) and periodontal disease are the two problems that most frequently affect the teeth. Both problems are commonly associated with plaque and tartar deposits. **Plaque** is an *invisible* soft film that adheres to the enamel surface of teeth;

Assessment Interview

ORAL HYGIENE

Oral Hygiene Practices

- What are your usual mouth care and/or denture care practices?
- What oral hygiene products do you routinely use (e.g., mouthwash, type of toothpaste, dental floss, denture cleaner)?
- When was your last dental examination, and how often do you see your dentist?

Self-Care Abilities

- Do you have any problems managing your mouth care?

Past or Current Mouth Problems

- Have you had or do you have any problems such as bleeding, swollen or reddened gums, ulcerations, lumps, or tooth pain?

it consists of bacteria, molecules of saliva, and remnants of epithelial cells and leukocytes. When plaque is unchecked, tartar (dental calculus) is formed. **Tartar** is a visible, hard deposit of plaque and dead bacteria that forms at the gum lines. Tartar buildup can alter the fibers that attach the teeth to the gum and eventually disrupt bone tissue. Periodontal disease is characterized by **gingivitis** (red, swollen gingiva), bleeding, receding gum lines, and the formation of pockets between the teeth and gums. In advanced periodontal disease (**pyorrhea**), the teeth are loose and pus is evident when the gums are pressed. Table 31–6 lists additional problems of the mouth.

Identifying Clients at Risk

Certain clients are prone to oral problems because of lack of knowledge or the inability to maintain oral hygiene. Among these are seriously ill, confused, comatose, depressed, and dehydrated clients. In addition, people with nasogastric tubes or receiving oxygen are likely to develop dry oral mucous membranes, especially if they breathe through their mouths. Clients who have had oral or jaw surgery must have meticulous oral hygiene care to prevent the development of infections.

> ➤ **CLINICAL ALERT** *Clients in long-term care settings are at high risk for oral health problems. The nurse must assess the client's oral health and teach the UAP about the importance of and methods to promote oral hygiene.*

Healthy-appearing individuals, too, may be at risk. High-risk variables such as inadequate nutrition, lack of money and/or insurance for dental care, excessive intake of refined sugars, and family history of periodontal disease also need to be identified. Some older people may also be at risk, for example, those who choose salty and enamel-eroding sugary foods because of a decline in their number of taste buds. The decreased

TABLE 31–6 Common Problems of the Mouth

Problem	Description	Nursing Implications
Halitosis	Bad breath	Teach or provide regular oral hygiene.
Glossitis	Inflammation of the tongue	As above
Gingivitis	Inflammation of the gums	As above
Periodontal disease	Gums appear spongy and bleeding	As above
Reddened or excoriated mucosa		Check for ill-fitting dentures.
Excessive dryness of the buccal mucosa		Increase fluid intake as health permits.
Cheilosis	Cracking of lips	Lubricate lips, use antimicrobial ointment to prevent infection.
Dental caries	Teeth have darkened areas, may be painful	Advise client to see a dentist.
Sordes	Accumulation of foul matter (food, micro-organisms, and epithelial elements) in the mouth	Teach or provide regular cleaning.
Stomatitis	Inflammation of the oral mucosa	Teach or provide regular cleaning.
Parotitis	Inflammation of the parotid salivary glands	Teach or provide regular oral hygiene.

saliva production in older adults, which produces a dry mouth and thinning of the oral mucosa, is another factor.

A dry mouth can be aggravated by poor fluid intake, heavy smoking, alcohol use, high salt intake, anxiety, and many medications. Medications that can cause dryness of the mouth include diuretics; laxatives, if used excessively; and tranquilizers, such as chlorpromazine (Thorazine) and diazepam (Valium). Some chemotherapeutic agents used to treat cancer also cause oral dryness and lesions. A common side effect of the anticonvulsant drug phenytoin (Dilantin) is gingival hyperplasia. Optimal oral hygiene (e.g., brushing with a soft toothbrush and flossing) is needed.

Clients who are receiving or have received radiation treatments to the head and neck may have permanent damage to salivary glands. This results in a very dry mouth and can often be treated by providing a thick liquid called *artificial saliva*. Some clients prefer to just sip on liquids to moisten their mouth. Radiation can also cause damage to teeth and jaw structure, with actual damage occurring years after the radiation.

DIAGNOSING

Three nursing diagnoses related to problems with oral hygiene and the oral cavity are *Self-Care Deficit, Impaired Oral Mucous Membrane,* and *Deficient Knowledge.* Note that the North American Nursing Diagnosis Association (NANDA, 2003) includes oral hygiene in the diagnostic label *Self-Care Deficit: Bathing/Hygiene.* In this book the diagnosis *Self-Care Deficit: Oral Hygiene* will be used for clients unable to perform oral care independently. This includes the inability to brush or floss teeth or clean dentures.

The nursing diagnosis *Impaired Oral Mucous Membrane* refers to the state in which an individual experiences disruptions in the tissue layers of the oral cavity. Manifestations in-

clude a coated tongue; dry mouth; dental caries; halitosis; gingivitis; oral plaque, pain, discomfort, erythema, lesions, or ulcers; and lack of or decreased salivation. These may be the result of inadequate oral hygiene, physical injury or drying effect (e.g., mouth breathing, oxygen therapy, decreased salivation, temperature extreme, NPO), mechanical trauma (e.g., surgery, injury from oral tube, broken teeth or ill-fitting dentures), chemical trauma (e.g., side effects of medications), or radiation injury. The diagnosis *Deficient Knowledge* is discussed in Chapter 25.

Clinical examples of assessment data clusters, related nursing diagnoses, outcomes, and interventions are shown in the Identifying Nursing Diagnoses, Outcomes, and Interventions box.

PLANNING

In planning care, the nurse and, if appropriate, the client and/or family set outcomes for each nursing diagnosis. The nurse then performs nursing interventions and activities to achieve the client outcomes.

During the planning phase, the nurse also identifies interventions that will help the client achieve these goals. Specific, detailed nursing activities taken by the nurse may include the following:

- Monitor every shift for dryness of the oral mucosa.
- Monitor for signs and symptoms of glossitis (inflammation of the tongue) and stomatitis (inflammation of the mouth).
- Assist dependent clients with oral care.
- Provide special oral hygiene for clients who are debilitated, unconscious, or have lesions of the mucous membranes or other oral tissues.
- Teach clients about good oral hygiene practices and other measures to prevent tooth decay.
- Reinforce oral hygiene regimen as part of discharge teaching.

IDENTIFYING NURSING DIAGNOSES, OUTCOMES, AND INTERVENTIONS

CLIENTS WITH ORAL CAVITY PROBLEMS

DATA CLUSTER	NURSING DIAGNOSIS/ DEFINITION	SAMPLE DESIRED OUTCOME [NOC #]/DEFINITION	INDICATORS	SELECTED INTERVENTIONS [NIC #]/DEFINITION	SAMPLE NIC ACTIVITIES
Mary Brown, 77 years old, suffered a cerebrovascular accident. Is unconscious and breathing through the mouth via O₂ face mask. 2,500 mL intravenous fluid ordered daily.	*Self-Care Deficit: Oral Hygiene* related to cognitive inability (unconsciousness)/ *Impaired ability to perform or complete bathing/hygiene activities for oneself*	Self-Care: Oral Hygiene [0308]/*Ability to care for own mouth and teeth*	Dependent, does not participate • Clean mouth, gums, and tongue	Oral Health Maintenance [1710]/ *Maintenance and promotion of oral hygiene and dental health for the client at risk for developing oral or dental lesions*	• Establish a mouth care routine • Apply lubricant to moisten lips and oral mucosa, as needed • Monitor for signs and symptoms of glossitis and stomatitis
Joe Kwan, 46 years old, was admitted with a fractured femur. Teeth stained from heavy smoking. One large cavity evident in 2nd lower left molar, tartar buildup along gum margins, and pronounced halitosis. Gums are reddened in some areas and bleed when flossed. States, "I can't remember when I last saw a dentist."	*Impaired Oral Mucous Membrane* related to ineffective oral hygiene/*Disruption of the lips and soft tissue of the oral cavity*	Oral Health [1100]/ *Condition of the mouth, teeth, gums, and tongue*	Not compromised • Cleanliness of teeth • Cleanliness of gums • Breath free of halitosis • Free of bleeding	Oral Health Restoration [1730]/*Promotion of healing for a client who has an oral mucosa or dental lesion*	• Use a soft toothbrush for removal of dental debris • Use toothettes or disposable foam swabs to stimulate gums and clean oral cavity • Encourage flossing between teeth twice daily with unwaxed dental floss, if platelet levels are above 50,000/mm³ • Discourage smoking • Reinforce oral hygiene regimen as part of discharge teaching

IMPLEMENTING

Good oral hygiene includes daily stimulation of the gums, mechanical brushing and flossing of the teeth, and flushing of the mouth. The nurse is often in a position to help people maintain oral hygiene by helping or teaching them to clean the teeth and oral cavity, by inspecting whether clients (especially children) have done so, or by actually providing mouth care to clients who are ill or incapacitated. The nurse can also be instrumental in identifying problems that require the intervention of a dentist or oral surgeon and arranging a referral.

Promoting Oral Health Through the Life Span

A major role of the nurse in promoting oral health is to teach clients about specific oral hygienic measures.

Infants and Toddlers. Most dentists recommend that dental hygiene should begin when the first tooth erupts and be practiced after each feeding. Cleaning can be accomplished by using a wet washcloth or a cotton ball or small gauze moistened with water.

Dental caries occur frequently during the toddler period, often as a result of the excessive intake of sweets or a prolonged use of the bottle during naps and at bedtime. The nurse should give parents the following instructions to promote and maintain dental health:

- Beginning at about 18 months of age, brush the child's teeth with a soft toothbrush. Use only a toothbrush moistened with water at first and introduce toothpaste later. Use one that contains fluoride.
- Give a fluoride supplement daily or as recommended by the physician or dentist, unless the drinking water is fluoridated.
- Schedule an initial dental visit for the child at about 2 or 3 years of age, as soon as all 20 primary teeth have erupted.
- Some dentists recommend an inspection type of visit when the child is about 18 months old to provide an early pleasant introduction to the dental examination.
- Seek professional dental attention for any problems such as discoloring of the teeth, chipping, or signs of infection such as redness and swelling.

Preschoolers and School-Age Children. Because deciduous teeth guide the entrance of permanent teeth, dental care is essential to keep these teeth in good repair. Abnormally placed or lost deciduous teeth can cause misalignment of permanent teeth. Fluoride remains important at this stage to prevent dental caries. Preschoolers need to be taught to brush their teeth after eating and to limit their intake of refined sugars. Parental supervision may be needed to ensure the completion of these self-care activities. Regular dental checkups are required during these years when permanent teeth appear.

Adolescents and Adults. Proper diet and tooth and mouth care should be evaluated and reinforced to adolescents and adults. Specific measures to prevent tooth decay and periodontal disease are listed in Teaching: Wellness Care.

Brushing and Flossing the Teeth

Thorough brushing of the teeth is important in preventing tooth decay. The mechanical action of brushing removes food particles that can harbor and incubate bacteria. It also stimulates circulation in the gums, thus maintaining their healthy firmness. One of the techniques recommended for brushing teeth is called the sulcular technique, which removes plaque and cleans under the gingival margins. Many toothpastes are marketed. Fluoride toothpaste is often recommended because of its antibacterial protection. An effective dentifrice can also be made by combining two parts table salt to one part baking soda.

Caring for Artificial Dentures

Some people have artificial teeth in the form of a plate—a complete set of teeth for one jaw. A person may have a lower plate or an upper plate or both. When only a few artificial teeth are needed, the individual may have a bridge rather than a plate. A bridge may be fixed or removable. Artificial teeth are fitted to the individual and usually will not fit another person. People who wear dentures or other types of oral prostheses should be encouraged to use them. Those who do not wear their prostheses are prone to shrinkage of the gums, which results in further tooth loss.

Like natural teeth, artificial dentures collect microorganisms and food. They need to be cleaned regularly, at least once a day. They can be removed from the mouth, scrubbed with a toothbrush, rinsed, and reinserted. Some people use a dentifrice for cleaning teeth, and others use commercial cleaning compounds for plates.

Assisting Clients with Oral Care

When providing mouth care for partially or totally dependent clients, the nurse should wear gloves to guard against infections. Other required equipment includes a curved basin that fits snugly under the client's chin (e.g., a kidney basin) to receive the rinse water and a towel to protect the client and the bedclothes. See Procedure 31–4.

Foam swabs are often used in health care agencies to clean the mouths of dependent clients (Figure 31–21 ■). These swabs

---

✿ Teaching: Wellness Care
Measures to Prevent Tooth Decay

- Brush the teeth thoroughly after meals and at bedtime. Assist children or inspect their mouths to be sure the teeth are clean. If the teeth cannot be brushed after meals, vigorous rinsing of the mouth with water is recommended.
- Floss the teeth daily.
- Ensure an adequate intake of nutrients, particularly calcium, phosphorus, vitamins A, C, and D, and fluoride.
- Avoid sweet foods and drinks between meals. Take them in moderation at meals.
- Eat coarse, fibrous foods (cleansing foods), such as fresh fruits and raw vegetables.
- Have topical fluoride applications as prescribed by the dentist.
- Have a checkup by a dentist every 6 months.

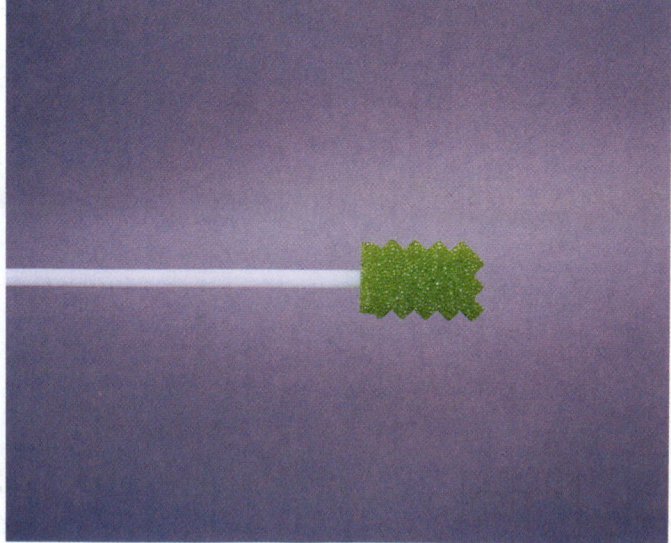

Figure 31–21 ■ Example of foam swab used to clean mouth of a dependent client.

are convenient and effective in removing excess debris from the teeth and mouth but should be used infrequently and for short periods (i.e., less than 3 days) because they do not remove plaque that is at the base of the teeth.

Most people prefer privacy when they take their artificial teeth out to clean them. Many do not like to be seen without their teeth; one of the first requests of many postoperative clients is "May I have my teeth in, please?" The "Variation" section in Procedure 31–4 describes how to clean artificial dentures.

Clients with Special Oral Hygiene Needs

For the client who is debilitated or unconscious or who has excessive dryness, sores, or irritations of the mouth, it may be necessary to clean the oral mucosa and tongue in addition to the teeth. Agency practices differ in regard to special mouth care and the frequency with which it is provided. Depending on the health of the client's mouth, special care may be needed every 2 to 8 hours.

Mouth care for unconscious or debilitated people is important because their mouths tend to become dry and consequently predisposed to infections. Saliva has antiviral, antibacterial, and antifungal effects (Walton, Miller, & Tordecilla, 2001, p. 40). Dryness occurs because the client cannot take fluids by mouth, is often breathing through the mouth, or may be receiving oxygen, which tends to dry the mucous membranes.

The nurse can use commercially prepared applicators or foam swabs to clean the mucous membranes. Normal saline solution is recommended for oral hygiene for the dependent client.

> **➤ CLINICAL ALERT** *Long-term use of lemon-glycerine swabs can lead to further dryness of the mucosa and changes in tooth enamel. Mineral oil is contraindicated because aspiration of it can initiate an infection (lipid pneumonia). Hydrogen peroxide is not recommended for use in oral care because it irritates healthy oral mucosa and may alter the microflora of the mouth.*

Procedure 31–5 focuses on oral care for the unconscious person but may be adapted for conscious persons who are seriously ill or have mouth problems.

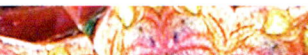

Procedure 31–4 Brushing and Flossing the Teeth

Purposes
- To remove food particles from around and between the teeth
- To remove dental plaque
- To enhance the client's feelings of well-being
- To prevent sores and infection of the oral tissues

ASSESSMENT
- Determine the extent of the client's self-care abilities.
- Assess the client's usual mouth care practices.
- Inspect lips, gums, oral mucosa, and tongue for deviations from normal.
- Identify presence of oral problems such as tooth caries, halitosis, gingivitis, and loose or broken teeth.
- Check if the client has bridgework or wears dentures. If the client has dentures, ask if any tenderness or soreness is present and, if so, the location of the area(s) for ongoing assessment.

PLANNING

Delegation
Oral care, brushing and flossing of teeth, and denture care can be delegated to the UAP. After performing the above assessment, the nurse should instruct the UAP as to the type of oral care and amount of assistance needed by the client. Remind the UAP to report changes in the client's oral mucosa.

Equipment

BRUSHING AND FLOSSING
- Towel
- Disposable gloves
- Curved basin (emesis basin)
- Toothbrush
- Cup of tepid water
- Dentifrice (toothpaste)
- Mouthwash
- Dental floss, at least two pieces 20 cm (8 in.) in length
- Floss holder (optional)

FOR CLEANING ARTIFICIAL DENTURES
- Disposable gloves
- Tissue or piece of gauze
- Denture container
- Clean washcloth
- Toothbrush or stiff-bristled brush
- Dentifrice or denture cleaner
- Tepid water
- Container of mouthwash
- Curved basin (emesis basin)
- Towel

continued on page 728

Procedure 31–4 Brushing and Flossing the Teeth *continued*

IMPLEMENTATION

Preparation

Assemble all the necessary equipment.

Performance

1. Explain to the client what you are going to do, why it is necessary, and how he or she can cooperate.
2. Wash hands and observe other appropriate infection control procedures (e.g., disposable gloves). *Wearing gloves while providing mouth care prevents the nurse from acquiring infections. Gloves also prevent transmission of microorganisms to the client.*
3. Provide for client privacy by drawing the curtains around the bed or closing the door to the room. Some agencies provide signs indicating the need for privacy. *Hygiene is a personal matter.*
4. Prepare the client.
   - Assist the client to a sitting position in bed, if health permits. If not, assist the client to a side-lying position with the head turned *so liquid may be prevented from draining down the client's throat.*
5. Prepare the equipment.
   - Place the towel under the client's chin.
   - Put on disposable gloves.
   - Moisten the bristles of the toothbrush with tepid water and apply the dentrifice to the toothbrush.
   - Use a soft toothbrush (a small one for a child) and the client's choice of dentifrice.
   - For the client who must remain in bed, place or hold the curved basin under the client's chin, fitting the small curve around the chin or neck.
   - Inspect the mouth and teeth.
6. Brush the teeth.
   - Hand the toothbrush to the client, or brush the client's teeth as follows:
     a. Hold the brush against the teeth with the bristles at a 45-degree angle. The tips of the outer bristles should rest against and penetrate under the gingival sulcus (Figure 31–22 ■). The brush will clean under the sulcus of two or three teeth at one time. *This sulcular technique removes plaque and cleans under the gingival margins.*

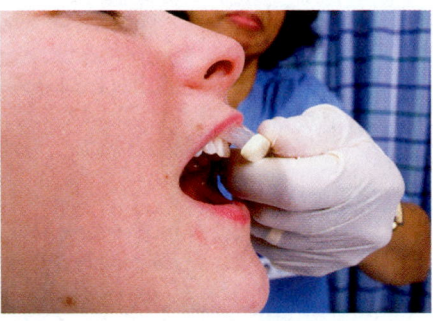

Figure 31–22 ■ The sulcular technique: Place the bristles at a 45-degree angle with the tips of the outer bristles under the gingival margins.

   b. Move the bristles up and down using a vibrating or jiggling motion from the sulcus to the crowns of the teeth (Figure 31–23 ■).

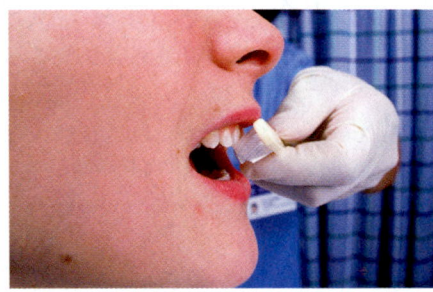

Figure 31–23 ■ Brushing from the sulcus to the crown of the teeth.

   c. Repeat until all outer and inner surfaces of the teeth and sulci of the gums are cleaned.
   d. Clean the biting surfaces by moving the brush back and forth over them in short strokes (Figure 31–24 ■).

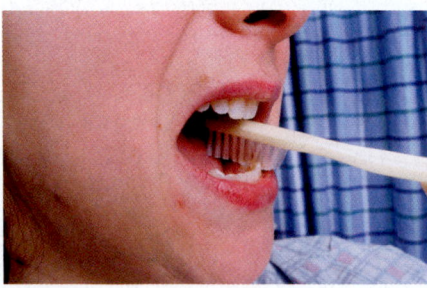

Figure 31–24 ■ Brushing the biting surfaces.

   e. If the tongue is coated, brush it gently with the toothbrush. *Brushing removes accumulated materials and coatings. A coated tongue may be caused by poor oral hygiene and low fluid intake. Brushing gently and carefully helps prevent gagging or vomiting.*
   - Hand the client the water cup or mouthwash to rinse the mouth vigorously. Then ask the client to spit the water and excess dentifrice into the basin. Some agencies supply a standard mouthwash. Alternatively, a mouth rinse of normal saline can be an effective cleaner and moisturizer. *Vigorous rinsing loosens food particles and washes out already loosened particles.*
   - Repeat the preceding steps until the mouth is free of dentifrice and food particles.
   - Remove the curved basin and help the client wipe the mouth.
7. Floss the teeth.
   - Assist the client to floss independently, or floss the teeth as follows. Waxed floss is less likely to fray than unwaxed floss; particles between the teeth attach more readily to unwaxed floss than to waxed floss. Some believe that waxed floss leaves a residue on the teeth and that plaque then adheres to the wax.
     a. Wrap one end of the floss around the third finger of each hand (Figure 31–25 ■).

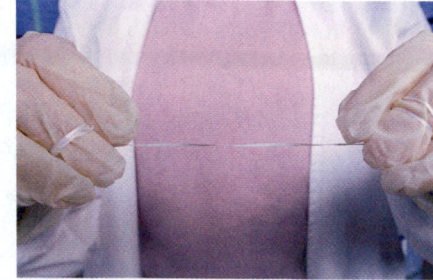

Figure 31–25 ■ Stretching the floss between the third finger of each hand.

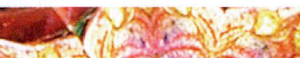

Procedure 31-4 Brushing and Flossing the Teeth *continued*

IMPLEMENTATION *continued*

b. To floss the upper teeth, use your thumb and index finger to stretch the floss. Move the floss up and down between the teeth from the tops of the crowns to the gum and along the gum lines as far as possible. Make a "C" with the floss around the tooth edge being flossed. Start at the back on the right side and work around to the back of the left side, or work from the center teeth to the back of the jaw on either side.

c. To floss the lower teeth, use your index fingers to stretch the floss (Figure 31-26 ■).

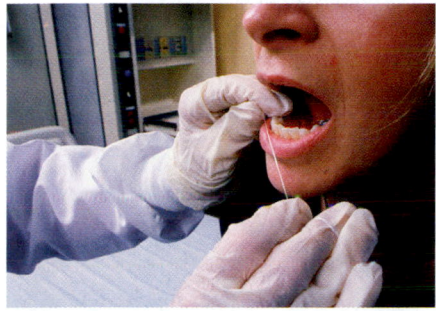

Figure 31-26 ■ Flossing the lower teeth by using the index fingers to stretch the floss.

- Give the client tepid water or mouthwash to rinse the mouth and a curved basin in which to spit the water.
- Assist the client in wiping the mouth.

8. Remove and dispose of equipment appropriately.
   - Remove and clean the curved basin.
   - Remove and discard the gloves.

9. Document assessment of the teeth, tongue, gums, and oral mucosa. Include any problems such as sores or inflammation, bleeding and swelling of the gums. Brushing and flossing teeth are not usually recorded.

VARIATION: ARTIFICIAL DENTURES

1. Remove the dentures.
   - Put on gloves. *Wearing gloves protects the nurse and client from infection.*
   - If the client cannot remove the dentures, take the tissue or gauze, grasp

the upper plate at the front teeth with your thumb and second finger, and move the denture up and down slightly (Figure 31-27 ■). *The slight movement breaks the suction that holds the plate on the roof of the mouth.*

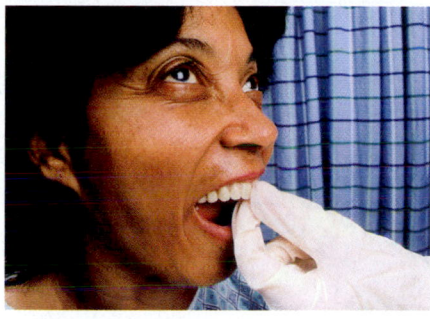

Figure 31-27 ■ Removing the top dentures by first breaking the suction.

- Lower the upper plate, move it out of the mouth, and place it in the denture container.
- Lift the lower plate, turning it so that the left side, for example, is slightly lower than the right, to remove the plate from the mouth without stretching the lips. Place the lower plate in the denture container.
- Remove a partial denture by exerting equal pressure on the border of each side of the denture, not on the clasps, which can bend or break.

2. Clean the dentures.
   - Take the denture container to a sink. Take care not to drop the dentures *as they may break.* Place a washcloth in the bowl of the sink *to prevent damage if the dentures are dropped.*
   - Using a toothbrush or special stiff-bristled brush, scrub the dentures with the cleaning agent and tepid water. Hot water is not used *because heat will change the shape of some dentures.*
   - Rinse the dentures with tepid running water. *Rinsing removes the cleaning agent and food particles.*
     a. If the dentures are stained, soak them in a commercial cleaner. Be sure to follow the manufacturer's directions. To prevent corrosion,

dentures with metal parts should not be soaked overnight.

3. Inspect the dentures and the mouth.
   - Observe the dentures for any rough, sharp, or worn areas that could irritate the tongue or mucous membranes of the mouth, lips, and gums.
   - Inspect the mouth for any redness, irritated areas, or indications of infection.
   - Assess the fit of the dentures. People who have them should see a dentist at least once a year to check the fit and the presence of any irritation to the soft tissues of the mouth. Clients who need repairs to their dentures or new dentures may need a referral for financial assistance.

4. Return the dentures to the mouth.
   - Offer some mouthwash and a curved basin to rinse the mouth. If the client cannot insert the dentures independently, insert the plates one at a time. Hold each plate at a slight angle while inserting it, to avoid injuring the lips (Figure 31-28 ■).

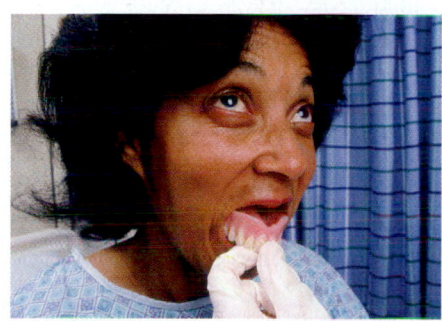

Figure 31-28 ■ Inserting the dentures at a slight angle.

5. Assist the client as needed.
   - Wipe the client's hands and mouth with the towel.
   - If the client does not want to or cannot wear the dentures, store them in a denture container with water. Label the container with the client's name and identification number.

6. Remove and discard gloves.

7. Document all assessments and include any problems such as an irritated area on the mucous membrane.

Procedure 31–5 Providing Special Oral Care

Purposes

- To maintain the intactness and health of the lips, tongue, and mucous membranes of the mouth
- To prevent oral infections
- To clean and moisten the membranes of the mouth and lips

ASSESSMENT

- Inspect lips, gums, oral mucosa, and tongue for deviations from normal.
- Identify presence of oral problems such as tooth caries, halitosis, gingivitis, and loose or broken teeth.
- Assess for gag reflex, when appropriate.

PLANNING

Delegation

Special oral care may be delegated to UAP; however, the nurse needs to assess for the gag reflex. Dependent on this assessment, the nurse needs to inform the UAP of the correct positioning of the client and how to use the oral suction catheter, if needed. Remind the UAP to report changes in the client's oral mucosa.

Equipment

- Towel
- Curved basin (emesis basin)
- Disposable clean gloves
- Bite-block to hold the mouth open and teeth apart (optional)
- Toothbrush
- Cup of tepid water
- Dentifrice or denture cleaner
- Tissue or piece of gauze to remove dentures (optional)
- Denture container as needed
- Mouthwash
- Rubber-tipped bulb syringe
- Suction catheter with suction apparatus (optional)
- Foam swabs and cleaning solution for cleaning the mucous membranes
- Petroleum jelly (Vaseline)

Performance

1. Explain to the client and the family what you are going to do and why it is necessary.
2. Wash hands and observe other appropriate infection control procedures (e.g., disposable gloves).
3. Provide for client privacy by drawing the curtains around the bed or closing the door to the room. Some agencies provide signs indicating the need for privacy. *Hygiene is a personal matter.*
4. Prepare the client.
   - Position the unconscious client in a side-lying position, with the head of the bed lowered. *In this position, the saliva automatically runs out by gravity rather than being aspirated into the lungs.* This position is the one of choice for the unconscious client receiving mouth care. If the client's head cannot be lowered, turn it to one side. *The fluid will readily run out of the mouth or pool in the side of the mouth, where it can be suctioned.*
   - Place the towel under the client's chin.
   - Place the curved basin against the client's chin and lower cheek to receive the fluid from the mouth (Figure 31–29 ■).
   - Put on gloves.

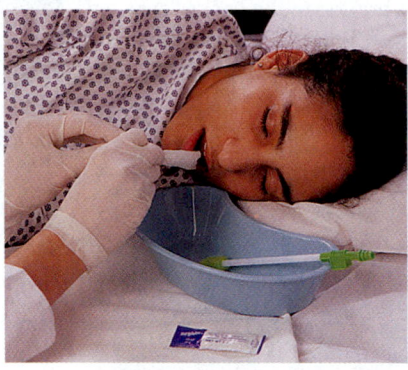

Figure 31–29 ■ Position of client and placement of curved basin when providing special mouth care.

5. Clean the teeth and rinse the mouth.
   - If the person has natural teeth, brush the teeth as described in Procedure 31–4. Brush gently and carefully to avoid injuring the gums. If the client has artificial teeth, clean them as described in the "Variation" component of Procedure 31–4.
   - Rinse the client's mouth by drawing about 10 mL of water or alcohol-free mouthwash into the syringe and injecting it gently into each side of the mouth. *If the solution is injected with force, some of it may flow down the client's throat and be aspirated into the lungs.*
   - Watch carefully to make sure that all the rinsing solution has run out of the mouth into the basin. If not, suction the fluid from the mouth. *Fluid remaining in the mouth may be aspirated into the lungs.*
   - Repeat rinsing until the mouth is free of dentifrice, if used.
6. Inspect and clean the oral tissues.
   - If the tissues appear dry or unclean, clean them with the foam swabs or gauze and cleaning solution following agency policy.
   - Picking up a moistened foam swab, wipe the mucous membrane of one cheek. If no foam swabs are available, wrap a small gauze square around a tongue blade and moisten it. Discard the swab or tongue blade in a waste container; use a fresh one to clean the next area. *Using separate applicators for each area of the mouth prevents the transfer of microorganisms from one area to another.*
   - Clean all mouth tissues in an orderly progression, using separate applicators: the cheeks, roof of the mouth, base of the mouth, and tongue.

Procedure 31–5 Providing Special Oral Care *continued*

PLANNING *continued*

- Observe the tissues closely for inflammation and dryness.
- Rinse the client's mouth as described in step 5.
- Remove and discard gloves.
7. Ensure client comfort.
    - Remove the basin, and dry around the client's mouth with the towel. Replace artificial dentures, if indicated.
    - Lubricate the client's lips with petroleum jelly. *Lubrication prevents cracking and subsequent infection.* If the client is on

oxygen therapy, do *not* use petroleum jelly, because it can cause burns to the skin and mouth. Use another mouth care product that does not have petroleum in it.

8. Document assessment of the teeth, tongue, gums, and oral mucosa. Include any problems such as sores or inflammation and swelling of the gums

EVALUATION

- Consider the client's medical diagnosis and treatment (e.g., chemotherapy, oxygen) and the necessary nursing interventions related to oral hygiene.
- Conduct an ongoing assessment, if appropriate, of the oral mucosa, gums, tongue, and lips.

- Report deviations from normal to the physician.
- Conduct appropriate follow-up such as a referral to a dentist for dental caries.

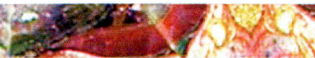

Lifespan Considerations

Oral Hygiene

Infants
- Most dentists recommend that dental hygiene should begin when the first tooth erupts and be practiced after each feeding. Cleaning can be accomplished by using a wet washcloth or a cotton ball or small gauze moistened with water.

Children
- Beginning at about 18 months of age, brush the child's teeth with a soft toothbrush. Use only a toothbrush moistened with water. Introduce toothpaste later and use one that contains fluoride.

Elders
- Oral care is often difficult for certain elders to perform due to problems with dexterity or cognitive problems with dementia.
- Most long-term health care facilities have dentists that come on a regular basis to see clients with special needs.
- Dryness of the oral mucosa is a common finding in elders because saliva production decreases with age.
- Promoting good oral hygiene can have a positive effect on the elders' ability to eat.

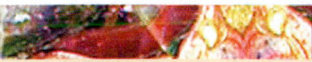

Home Care Considerations

Oral Hygiene
- Assess the oral hygiene practices and attitude toward oral hygiene of family members and the client.

- The client with a nasogastric tube or who is receiving oxygen is likely to develop dry oral mucous membranes, especially if they breathe through their mouths. More frequent oral hygiene will be needed.

EVALUATING

Using data collected during care—status of oral mucosa, lips, tongue, teeth, and so on—the nurse judges whether desired outcomes have been achieved.

If outcomes are not achieved, the nurse and client need to explore the reasons before modifying the care plan. Examples of questions to consider are as follows:

- Did the nurse overestimate the client's functional abilities?
- Is the client's hand coordination or cognitive function impaired?
- Did the client's condition change?
- Has there been a change in the client's energy level and/or motivation?

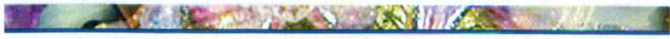

HAIR

The appearance of the hair often reflects a person's feelings of self-concept and sociocultural well-being. Becoming familiar with hair care needs and practices that may be different than our own is an important aspect of providing competent nursing care to all clients. People who feel ill may not groom their hair as before. A dirty scalp and hair are itchy, uncomfortable, and can have an odor. The hair may also reflect state of health (e.g., excessive coarseness and dryness may be associated with endocrine disorders such as hypothyroidism).

Each person has particular ways of caring for hair. Many dark-skinned people need to oil their hair daily because it tends to be dry. Oil prevents the hair from breaking and the scalp from drying. A wide-toothed comb is usually used because finer combs pull and break the hair. Some people brush their hair vigorously before retiring; others comb their hair frequently.

Developmental Variations

Newborns may have **lanugo** (the fine hair on the body of the fetus, also referred to as *down* or *woolly hair*) over their shoulders, back, and sacrum. This generally disappears, and the hair distribution on the eyebrows, head, and eyelashes of young children subsequently becomes noticeable. Some newborns have hair on their scalps; others are free of hair at birth but grow hair over the scalp during the first year of life.

Pubic hair usually appears in early puberty followed in about 6 months by the growth of axillary hair. Boys develop facial hair in later puberty.

In adolescence, the sebaceous glands increase in activity as a result of increased hormone levels. As a result, hair follicle openings enlarge to accommodate the increased amount of sebum, which can make the adolescent's hair more oily.

In older adults, the hair is generally thinner, grows more slowly, and loses its color as a result of aging tissues and diminishing circulation. Men often lose their scalp hair and may become completely bald. This phenomenon may occur even when a man is relatively young. The older person's hair also tends to be drier than normal. With age, axillary and pubic hair becomes finer and scanter, in contrast to the eyebrows, which become bristly and coarse. Many women develop hair on their faces, which may be a concern to them.

NURSING MANAGEMENT

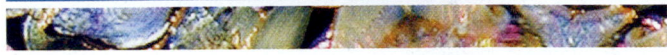

ASSESSING

Assessment of the client's hair, hair care practices, and potential problems includes a nursing health history and physical assessment.

Nursing Health History

During the nursing history the nurse elicits data about usual hair care, self-care abilities, history of hair or scalp problems, and con-

ditions known to affect the hair. Chemotherapeutic agents and radiation of the head may cause **alopecia** (hair loss). Hypothyroidism may cause the hair to be thin, dry, and/or brittle. Use of some hair dyes and curling or straightening preparations can cause the hair to become dry and brittle. Questions to elicit these data are shown in the accompanying Assessment Interview.

Physical Assessment

Physical assessment of the hair is discussed in Chapter 28. Problems include dandruff, hair loss, ticks, pediculosis, scabies, and hirsutism.

Dandruff. Often accompanied by itching, **dandruff** appears as a diffuse scaling of the scalp. In severe cases it involves the auditory canals and the eyebrows. Dandruff can usually be treated effectively with a commercial shampoo. In severe or persistent cases, the client may need the advice of a physician.

Hair Loss. Hair loss and growth are continual processes. Some permanent thinning of hair normally occurs with aging. Baldness, common in men, is thought to be a hereditary problem for which there is no known remedy other than the wearing of a hairpiece or a costly surgical hair transplant, in which hair is taken from the back or the sides of the scalp and surgically moved to the hairless area. Although some medications are being developed, their long-term outcomes are unknown.

Ticks. Small gray-brown parasites that bite into tissue and suck blood, **ticks** transmit several diseases to people, in particular Rocky Mountain spotted fever, Lyme disease, and tularemia. To remove a tick, use a blunt tweezers or gloved fingers and grasp the tick as close to the skin as possible. Gently pull the tick away using perpendicular traction to remove the tick. Be careful to not twist or squeeze the tick's body. If the head breaks off and remains in the skin, use tweezers to remove in a manner similar to that used for removing a splinter. Wash the area with antibacterial soap. Save the tick in a bottle of rubbing alcohol in case the physician wants to identify the type of tick. The following practices to remove a tick are ineffective or dangerous: applying heat with a match and applying substances such as petroleum jelly or gasoline (Gammons & Salam, 2002).

Pediculosis (Lice). Lice are parasitic insects that infest mammals. Infestation with lice is called **pediculosis.** Hundreds of varieties of lice infest humans. Three common kinds are *Pediculus capitis* (the head louse), *Pediculus corporis* (the body louse), and *Pediculus pubis* (the crab louse).

Pediculus capitis is found on the scalp and tends to stay hidden in the hairs; similarly, *Pediculus pubis* stays in pubic hair. *Pediculus corporis* tends to cling to clothing, so that when a client undresses, the lice may not be in evidence on the body; these lice suck blood from the person and lay their eggs on the clothing. The nurse can suspect their presence in the clothing if (a) the person habitually scratches, (b) there are scratches on the skin, and (c) there are hemorrhagic spots on the skin where the lice have sucked blood.

Head and pubic lice lay their eggs on the hairs; the eggs look like oval particles, similar to dandruff, clinging to the hair. Bites and pustular eruptions may also be noticed at the hair lines and behind the ears.

Lice are very small, grayish white, and difficult to see. The crab louse in the pubic area has red legs. Lice may be contracted from infested clothes and direct contact with an infested person.

The treatment often includes topical pediculicides such as pyrethrins (e.g., RID, Pyrinate), permethrin (e.g., Nix), and lindane (e.g., Kwell). The current recommended treatment of choice for head lice is Nix because it is the least toxic (Frankowski & Weiner, 2002). Natural products offered by health food stores are also available; however, clients need to be reminded that natural products are not required to meet the Federal Drug Administration standards. Another treatment, occlusive agents, is used by some. The idea is that an oily substance, such as olive oil, smothers the lice and they die.

Removal of nits (eggs) after applying the treatment is not necessary to prevent spread but most people remove them for aesthetic reasons (Frankowski & Weiner, 2002). Fine-toothed "nit" combs are available. Transmission is from head-to-head contact and it is suggested that the hair care items and bedding of the person who has the lice infestation be washed with hot water.

Scabies. **Scabies** is a contagious skin infestation by the itch mite. The characteristic lesion is the burrow produced by the female mite as it penetrates into the upper layers of the skin. Burrows are short, wavy, brown or black, threadlike lesions most commonly observed between the webs of the fingers and the folds of the wrists and elbows. The mites cause intense itching that is more pronounced at night because the increased warmth of the skin has a stimulating effect on the parasites. Secondary lesions caused by scratching include vesicles, papules, pustules, excoriations, and crusts. Treatment involves thorough cleansing of the body with soap and water to remove scales and debris from crusts, and then an application of a scabicide lotion. All bed linens and clothing should be washed in very hot or boiling water.

Hirsutism. The growth of excessive body hair is called **hirsutism.** The acceptance of body hair in the axillae and on the legs is largely dictated by culture. In North America, the well-groomed woman, as depicted in magazines, has no hair on her legs or under her axillae. In many European cultures, it is not customary for well-groomed women to remove this hair.

Excessive facial hair on a woman is thought unattractive in most Western and Asian cultures. For example, some Japanese brides follow the custom of shaving their faces the day before the wedding.

The cause of excessive body hair is not always known. Older women may have some on their faces, and women in menopause may also experience the growth of facial hair. Excessive body hair may be due to the action of the endocrine system. Heredity is also thought to influence the pattern of hair distribution.

DIAGNOSING

Nursing diagnoses related to hair hygiene and hair and scalp problems include *Self-Care Deficit: Grooming, Impaired Skin Integrity, Risk for Infection,* and *Disturbed Body Image.* Examples of these nursing diagnoses with contributing factors follow:

- *Self-Care Deficit: Grooming* related to
  a. Activity intolerance
  b. Imposed immobility (bed rest)
  c. Pain in upper extremities
  d. Altered level of consciousness
  e. Lack of motivation associated with depression.
- *Impaired Skin Integrity* related to
  a. Scalp laceration
  b. Insect bite.
- *Risk for Infection* related to
  a. Scalp laceration
  b. Insect bite.
- *Disturbed Body Image* related to alopecia.

PLANNING

In planning care, the nurse and, if appropriate, the client and/or family set outcomes for each nursing diagnosis. The nurse then performs nursing interventions and activities to achieve the client outcomes. Identifying Nursing Diagnoses, Outcomes, and Interventions provides suggested outcomes and interventions for hair grooming.

The specific, detailed nursing activities taken by the nurse to assist the client should take into account the client's personal preferences, health, and energy resources as well as the time, equipment, and personnel available. Often, clients like to receive hair care after a bath, before receiving visitors, and before retiring. Nursing interventions may include instructing the client/family in alternative methods for hair care including facilitating the assistance of a barber or beautician, as necessary. At some agencies, shampoos can be given to clients only after a physician's order.

IDENTIFYING NURSING DIAGNOSES, OUTCOMES, AND INTERVENTIONS

HAIR GROOMING

NURSING DIAGNOSIS/ DEFINITION	SAMPLE DESIRED OUTCOME [NOC#]/DEFINITION	INDICATORS*	SELECTED INTERVENTIONS [NIC#]/DEFINITION	SAMPLE NIC ACTIVITIES
Self-Care Deficit: Dressing/Grooming/ Impaired ability to perform or complete dressing and grooming activities for self	Self-Care: Grooming [0304]/*Ability to maintain kempt appearance*	• Shampoos hair • Combs or brushes hair • Maintains neat appearance	Hair Care [1670]/ *Promotion of neat, clean, attractive hair*	• Wash hair, as needed and desired • Dry hair with hair dryer • Brush/comb hair daily or more frequently, as needed • Monitor scalp daily • Braid or otherwise arrange hair as client wishes • Use hair care products of client's preference, as available

*The measurement scale ranges from Dependent, does not participate (1) to Completely independent (5). See Appendix B.

IMPLEMENTING

Hair needs to be brushed or combed daily and washed, as needed, to keep it clean. Nurses may need to provide hair care for clients who cannot meet their own self-care needs.

Brushing and Combing Hair

To be healthy, hair needs to be brushed daily. Brushing has three major functions: It stimulates the circulation of blood in the scalp, it distributes the oil along the hair shaft, and it helps to arrange the hair.

Long hair may present a problem for clients confined to bed because it may become matted. It should be combed and brushed at least once a day to prevent this. A brush with stiff bristles provides the best stimulation to blood circulation in the scalp. The bristles should not be so sharp that they injure the client's scalp, however. A comb with dull, even teeth is advisable. A comb with sharp teeth might injure the scalp; combs that are too fine can pull and break the hair. Some clients are pleased to have their hair tied neatly in the back or braided until other assistance is available or until they feel better and can look after it themselves. Braiding also prevents tangling and matting for clients confined to bed.

Dark-skinned people often have thicker, drier, curlier hair than light-skinned people. Very curly hair may stand out from the scalp. Although the shafts of curly or kinky hair look strong and wiry, they have less strength than straight hair shafts and can break easily. Many African American people have hair that is naturally curly, and it can become matted and tangled in just an 8-hour period of time (Jackson, 1998).

Cultural groups often have their own vocabulary for describing personal activities.

Some African Americans have their hair straightened. Even if straightened, the hair tends to tangle and mat easily, especially at the back and the sides if the client is confined to bed. Other African Americans style their hair in small braids (see Figure 31–30 ■). These braids do not have to be un-

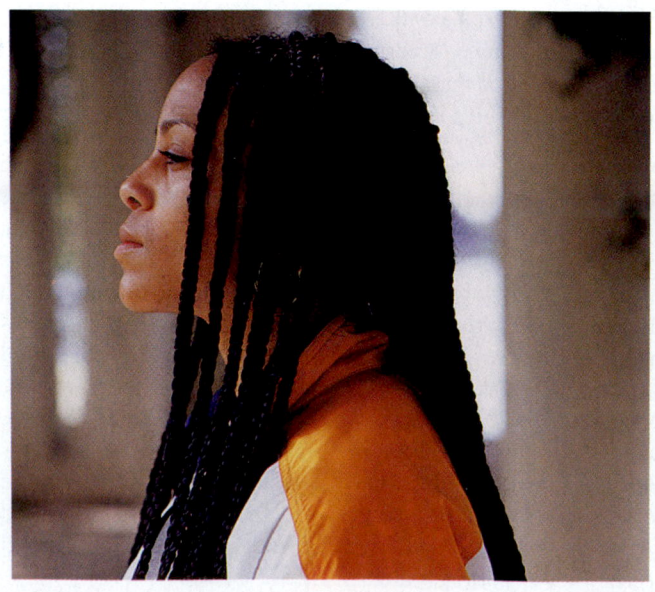

Figure 31–30 ■ An African American's hair styled with braids.

Providing Culturally Competent Care

HAIR CARE

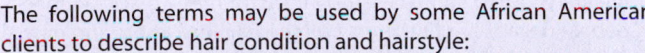

The following terms may be used by some African American clients to describe hair condition and hairstyle:

- *Nappy/kinky.* This means that the hair is very difficult to comb and is very curly, maybe even tangled at the root. The hair "draws" up and appears shorter than it really is because of this extreme curliness. It may have a rough, "steel wool" appearance.
- *Pressed.* The hair is straightened using a hot comb. However, if it gets wet, for example, from sweating, high humidity, shampoo, or "getting caught in the rain," it reverts back to being kinky.
- *Permanent.* This is a chemical means of straightening the hair. The hair will remain straight for 4 to 6 weeks, even if it gets wet. This is the major advantage of the permanent over using the hot comb.
- *Grease.* A client may request some "grease." They are not asking for vegetable shortening. This is a request to apply either lotion to the skin or hair oil to the scalp.
- *Braids/extensions.* Synthetic hair is braided into the person's real hair. The length is variable, usually shoulder length or longer. If the braids are left hanging, the ends are burned with a small lighter to keep them from unraveling and a small rubber band applied. The braids should be left intact, but care of

the scalp is still very important. Products are made especially for those with extensions that can be used to moisturize the hair and scalp. The hair can be shampooed when fixed in this style. Some place a stocking cap over the hair. Others just shampoo the hair gently, use a towel to press excess water from the hair, and keep it covered until the hair and scalp are completely dry. If the synthetic braid extensions need to be removed for some reason, care must be taken not to cut the client's real hair.

- *Dreadlocks.* Made popular by the Rastafarian religion, which reportedly originated in Jamaica. Not everyone who wears dreadlocks is a Rastafarian. Dreadlocks are worn by men, women, and children of all ages. The hair is not combed or picked—ever. Most people keep their locks extremely clean. The locks attract lint. Use tweezers to remove lint that's on top of the hair. With long dreadlocks, removing lint from inside the lock can destroy it. The lint acts as a bonding cement that holds the lock together. Since the hair is shampooed often, this lint is clean. Gently shampoo the hair, taking care not to destroy the locks. Some individuals use a stocking cap, others just gently shampoo the hair. Dreadlocks take a long time to dry when wet. Protect the client from drafts until the hair is dry.

Note: From "The ABC's of Black Hair and Skin Care," by F. Jackson, 1998, *The ABNF Journal, 9*(5), p. 101. Reprinted with permission.

Mediaink PROVIDING BASIC HYGIENE CARE CASE STUDY

braided for shampooing and washing. If, however, unbraiding becomes necessary, the nurse should obtain the client's permission to do so. Some African American clients need to oil their hair daily because it tends to be dry. Oil also prevents the hair strands from breaking and the scalp from becoming too dry. Not all African American individuals have curly or kinky hair. Some have naturally straight hair. Keeping the scalp and hair clean and oiled remains important and necessary. Procedure 31–6 describes how to provide hair care for clients.

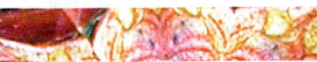

Procedure 31–6 Providing Hair Care for Clients

Purposes

- To stimulate the blood circulation to the scalp
- To distribute hair oils and provide a healthy sheen
- To increase the client's sense of well-being

- To assess or monitor hair or scalp problems (e.g., matted hair or dandruff)

ASSESSMENT

Determine

- History of the following conditions or therapies: recent chemotherapy, hypothyroidism, radiation of the head, unexplained hair loss, and growth of excessive body hair
- Usual hair care practices and routinely used hair care products (e.g., hair spray, shampoo, conditioners, hair oil preparation, hair dye, curling or straightening preparations)
- Whether wetting the hair will make it difficult to comb. Kinky hair is easier to comb when wet, however, it is very difficult to comb when it dries (Jackson, 1998, p. 102).

Assess

- Condition of the hair and scalp. Is the hair straight, curly, kinky? Is the hair matted or tangled? Is the scalp dry?
- Evenness of hair growth over the scalp, in particular, any patchy loss of hair; hair texture, oiliness, thickness, or thinness; presence of lesions, infections, or infestations on the scalp; presence of hirsutism
- Self-care abilities (e.g., any problems managing hair care).

continued on page 736

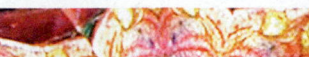

Procedure 31–6 Providing Hair Care for Clients *continued*

PLANNING

Delegation

Brushing and combing hair, shampooing hair, and shaving facial hair can be delegated to UAP unless the client has a condition in which the procedure would be contraindicated (e.g., cervical spinal injury or trauma). The nurse needs to assess the UAP's knowledge and experience of hair care for clients of other cultures, if appropriate.

Equipment

- Clean brush and comb
- A wide-toothed comb is usually used for many black-skinned people because finer combs pull the hair into knots and may also break the hair
- Towel
- Hair oil preparation, if appropriate

IMPLEMENTATION

Performance

1. Explain to the client what you are going to do, why it is necessary, and how he or she can cooperate.
2. Wash hands and observe other appropriate infection control procedures.
3. Provide for client privacy by drawing the curtains around the bed or closing the door to the room. Some agencies provide signs indicating the need for privacy. *Hygiene is a personal matter.*
4. Position and prepare the client appropriately.
   - Assist the client who can sit to move to a chair. *Hair is more easily brushed and combed when the client is in a sitting position.* If health permits, assist a client confined to a bed to a sitting position by raising the head of the bed. Otherwise, assist the client to alternate side-lying positions, and do one side of the head at a time.
   - If the client remains in bed, place a clean towel over the pillow and the client's shoulders. Place it over the sitting client's shoulders. *The towel collects any removed hair, dirt, and scaly material.*
   - Remove any pins or ribbons in the hair.
5. Remove any mats or tangles gradually.
   - Mats can usually be pulled apart with fingers or worked out with repeated brushings.
   - If the hair is very tangled, rub alcohol or an oil, such as mineral oil, on the strands to help loosen the tangles.
   - Comb out tangles in a small section of hair toward the ends. Stabilize the hair with one hand and comb toward the ends of the hair with the other hand. *This avoids scalp trauma.*
6. Brush and comb the hair.
   - For short hair, brush and comb one side at a time. Divide long hair into two sections by parting it down the middle from the front to the back. If the hair is very thick, divide each section into front and back subsections or into several layers.
7. Arrange the hair as neatly and attractively as possible, according to the individual's desires.
   - Braiding long hair helps prevent tangles.
8. Document assessments and special nursing interventions. Daily combing and brushing of the hair are not normally recorded.

VARIATION: HAIR CARE FOR AFRICAN AMERICAN CLIENTS

- Position and prepare the client.
- Untangle the hair first, if appropriate.
   - Use fingers to reduce hair breakage and discomfort. Move fingers in a circular motion starting at the roots and gently moving up to the tip of the hair.

- Comb the hair.
   - Apply hair oil preparation as the client indicates.
   - Using a large and open-toothed comb, grasp a small section of hair and, holding the hair at the tip, start untangling at the tip and work down toward the scalp (Jackson, 1998, p. 102).

OIL SHAMPOO An oil shampoo is composed of one part alcohol and four parts mineral oil. The alcohol is an antiseptic and both the alcohol and mineral oil are cleansing agents (Jackson, 1998, p. 102).

- Warm the mixture.
- Pour it into the hair and gently massage.
- Comb the hair
- Remove excess oil with a towel.

OILING THE HAIR If a water-based shampoo was used it may be necessary to oil and massage the scalp.

- Part the hair in sections.
- Place a small amount of hair oil on the scalp. *The hair is so dense that oiling the top of the hair will not help a dry scalp.*
- Ask the client if he or she would like the hair braided. *Braiding will decrease tangling, however, the choice is the client's.*

> **CLINICAL ALERT**   *Excessively matted or tangled hair may be infested with lice.*

EVALUATION

- Conduct ongoing assessments for problems such as dandruff, alopecia, pediculosis, scalp lesions, or excessive dryness or matting.

- Evaluate effectiveness of medication (e.g., for treating pediculosis), if appropriate.

Shampooing the Hair

Hair should be washed as often as needed to keep it clean. There are several ways to shampoo clients' hair, depending on their health, strength, and age. The client who is well enough to take a shower can shampoo while in the shower. The client who is unable to shower may be given a shampoo while sitting on a chair in front of a sink. The back-lying client who can move to a stretcher can be given a shampoo on a stretcher wheeled to a sink. The client who must remain in bed can be given a shampoo with water brought to the bedside. Volunteer beauticians with portable shampoo chairs may be available to assist with hair care.

Shampoo basins to catch the water and direct it to the washbasin or other receptacle are usually made of plastic or metal. A pail or large washbasin can be used as a receptacle for the shampoo water. If possible, the receptacle should be large enough to hold all shampoo water so that it does not have to be emptied during the shampoo.

Water used for the shampoo should be 40.5C (105F) for an adult or child to be comfortable and not injure the scalp. Usually the client will supply a liquid or cream shampoo. If the shampoo is being given to destroy lice, a medicated shampoo should be used. Dry shampoos are also available. They will remove some of the dirt, odor, and oil. Their main disadvantage is that they dry the hair and scalp.

How often a person needs a shampoo is highly individual, depending largely on the person's activities and the amount of sebum secreted by the scalp. Oily hair tends to look stringy and dirty, and it feels unclean to the person. Procedure 31–7 explains how to provide a shampoo for a client confined to bed.

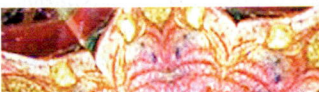

Procedure 31–7 Shampooing the Hair of a Client Confined to Bed

Purposes

- To stimulate the blood circulation to the scalp through massage
- To clean the hair and increase the client's sense of well-being

ASSESSMENT

- Determine routinely used shampoo products
- Assess:
  - Any scalp problems
  - Activity tolerance of the client

PLANNING

Delegation (see Procedure 31–6)

Equipment

- Comb and brush
- Plastic sheet or pad
- Two bath towels
- Shampoo basin
- Washcloth or pad
- Bath blanket
- Receptacle for the shampoo water
- Cotton balls (optional)
- Pitcher of water
- Bath thermometer
- Liquid or cream shampoo
- Hair dryer

IMPLEMENTATION

Preparation

- Determine whether a physician's order is needed before a shampoo can be given. *Some agencies require an order.*
- Determine the type of shampoo to be used (e.g., medicated shampoo).
- Determine the best time of day for the shampoo. Discuss this with the client. A person who must remain in bed may find the shampoo tiring. Choose a time when the client is rested and can rest after the procedure.

Performance

1. Explain to the client what you are going to do, why it is necessary if appropriate, and how he or she can cooperate.
2. Wash hands and observe other appropriate infection control procedures as needed.
3. Provide for client privacy by drawing the curtains around the bed or closing the door to the room. Some agencies provide signs indicating the need for privacy. *Hygiene is a personal matter.*

4. Position and prepare the client appropriately.
   - Assist the client to the side of the bed from which you will work.
   - Remove pins and ribbons from the hair, and brush and comb it to remove any tangles.
5. Arrange the equipment.
   - Put the plastic sheet or pad on the bed under the head. *The plastic keeps the bedding dry.*

continued on page 738

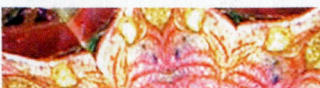

Procedure 31–7 Shampooing the Hair of a Client Confined to Bed *continued*

IMPLEMENTATION *continued*

- Remove the pillow from under the client's head, and place it under the shoulders unless there is some underlying condition (e.g., neck surgery, arthritis of the neck). *This hyperextends the neck.*
- Tuck a bath towel around the client's shoulders. *This keeps the shoulders dry.*
- Place the shampoo basin under the head (Figure 31–31 ■), putting a folded washcloth or pad where the client's neck rests on the edge of the basin. If the client is on a stretcher, the neck can rest on the

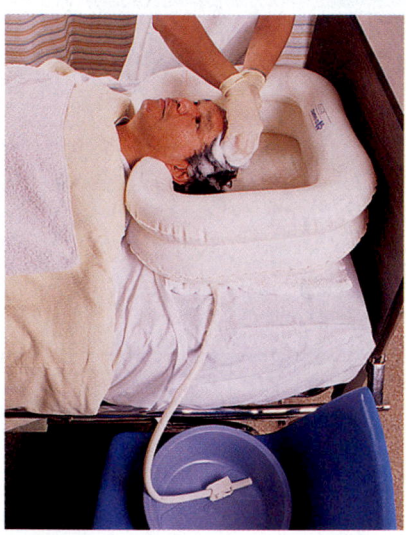

Figure 31–31 ■ Shampooing the hair of a client confined to bed. Note the shampoo basin and the receptacle below.

edge of the sink with the washcloth as padding. *Padding supports the muscles of the neck and prevents undue strain and discomfort.*
- Fanfold the top bedding down to the waist, and cover the upper part of the client with the bath blanket. *The folded bedding will stay dry, and the bath blanket, which can be discarded after the shampoo, will keep the client warm.*
- Place the receiving receptacle on a table or chair at the bedside. Put the spout of the shampoo basin over the receptacle.

6. Protect the client's eyes and ears.
- Place a damp washcloth over the client's eyes. *The washcloth protects the eyes from soapy water. A damp washcloth will not slip.*
- Place cotton balls in the client's ears if indicated. *These keep water from collecting in the ear canals.*

7. Shampoo the hair.
- Wet the hair thoroughly with the water.
- Apply shampoo to the scalp. Make a good lather with the shampoo while massaging the scalp with the pads of your fingertips. Massage all areas of the scalp systematically, for example, starting at the front and working toward the back of the head. *Massaging stimulates the blood circulation in the scalp. The pads of the fingers are used so that the fingernails will not scratch the scalp.*

- Rinse the hair briefly, and apply shampoo again.
- Make a good lather and massage the scalp as before.
- Rinse the hair thoroughly this time to remove all shampoo. *Shampoo remaining in the hair may dry and irritate the hair and scalp.*
- Squeeze as much water as possible out of the hair with your hands.

8. Dry the hair thoroughly.
- Rub the client's hair with a heavy towel.
- Dry the hair with the dryer. Set the temperature at "warm."
- Continually move the dryer to prevent burning the client's scalp.

9. Ensure client comfort.
- Assist the person confined to bed to a comfortable position.
- Arrange the hair using a clean brush and comb.

10. Document the shampoo and any assessments.

EVALUATION

- Conduct ongoing assessments such as any scalp problems or intolerance to the procedure. Report any problems noted to the nurse in charge.

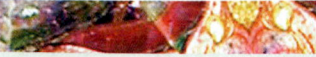

Lifespan Considerations

Hair Care

Infants

- Shampoo an infant's hair daily to prevent seborrhea.

Children

- Monitor school-age children for nits (pediculosis).

Elders

- Ensure adequate warmth for elders when shampooing their hair, because they are susceptible to chilling.

BOX 31–3 ■ Using a Safety Razor to Shave Facial Hair

- Wear gloves in case facial nicks occur and you come in contact with blood.
- Apply shaving cream or soap and water to soften the bristles and make the skin more pliable.
- Hold the skin taut, particularly around creases, to prevent cutting the skin.
- Hold the razor so that the blade is at a 45-degree angle to the skin, and shave in short, firm strokes in the direction of hair growth (Figure 31–32 ■).
- After shaving the entire area, wipe the client's face with a wet washcloth to remove any remaining shaving cream and hair.
- Dry the face well, then apply aftershave lotion or powder as the client prefers.
- To prevent irritating the skin, pat on the lotion with the fingers and avoid rubbing the face.

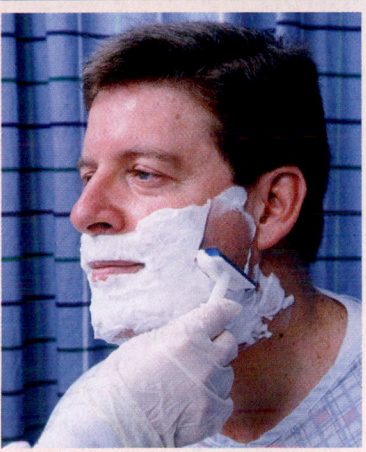

Figure 31–32 ■ Shaving in the direction of hair growth.

Beard and Mustache Care

Beards and mustaches also require daily care. The most important aspect of the care is to keep them clean. Food particles tend to collect in beards and mustaches, and they need washing and combing periodically. Clients may also wish a beard or mustache trim to maintain a well-groomed appearance.

> **CLINICAL ALERT** *A beard or mustache should not be shaved off without the client's consent.*

Male clients often shave or are shaved after a bath. Frequently clients supply their own electric or safety razors. See Box 31–3 for the steps involved in shaving facial hair with a safety razor.

EVALUATING

Using data collected during care, the nurse judges whether desired outcomes have been achieved. Examples of client outcomes that are measureable or observable include the client being able to

- Perform hair grooming with assistance (specify)
- Exhibit clean, well-groomed, resilient hair with a healthy sheen
- Reduce or get rid of scalp lesions or infestations
- Describe factors, interventions, and preventive measures for specific hair problem (e.g., dandruff).

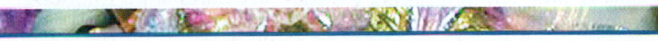

EYES

Normally eyes require no special hygiene, because lacrimal fluid continually washes the eyes, and the eyelids and lashes prevent the entrance of foreign particles. Special interventions are needed, however, for unconscious clients and for clients recovering from eye surgery or having eye injuries, irritations, or infections. In unconscious clients, the blink reflex may be ab-

sent, and excessive drainage may accumulate along eyelid margins. In clients with eye trauma or eye infections, excessive discharge or drainage is common. Excessive secretions on the lashes need to be removed before they dry on the lashes as crusts. Clients who wear eyeglasses, contact lenses, or an artificial eye also may require instruction from and care by the nurse.

NURSING MANAGEMENT

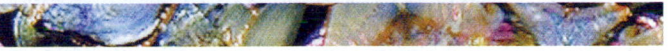

ASSESSING

Assessment of the client's eyes includes a nursing health history and physical assessment.

Nursing Health History

During the nursing history, the nurse obtains data about the client's eyeglasses or contact lenses, recent examination by an ophthalmologist, and any history of eye problems and related treatments. Questions to elicit these data are shown in the accompanying Assessment Interview.

Physical Assessment

In physical assessment, all external eye structures are inspected for signs of inflammation, excessive drainage, encrustations, or other obvious abnormalities. Inspection of the external eye structures is discussed in Chapter 28. ∞

DIAGNOSING

Nursing diagnoses related to eye problems may include *Self-Care Deficit, Risk for Infection,* and *Risk for Injury.* Examples of these diagnoses and possible contributing factors follow:

- *Self-Care Deficit* (contact lens insertion, removal, and cleaning) related to
  a. Deficient knowledge
  b. Impaired vision associated with cataracts.

Assessment Interview

EYES

For Clients Who Wear Eyeglasses

- When do you use your glasses?
- What is your vision like with and without the glasses?

For Clients Who Wear Contact Lenses

- How often do you wear lenses? Daily? On special occasions?
- How long do you wear your lenses in a given day, including sleep time?
- Do you have any problems with the lenses (e.g., cleaning, insertion, removal, damage)?
- Do you carry an emergency identification label to alert others to remove the lenses and ensure appropriate care in an emergency? (If not, advise the client to acquire one.)
- What are your insertion and removal procedures?
- What are your cleaning and storage procedures?
- Have you had any problems with either or both eyes or eyelids, such as excessive tearing, burning, redness, sensitivity to light, swelling, or feelings of dryness? Describe them.
- Are you using any eyedrops or ointments? (These medications can combine chemically with soft lenses and cause lens damage and eye irritation.)

For All Clients

- When did you last have your eyesight tested?
- Are you currently taking any eye medication? If so, provide name, dosage, and frequency.
- Do you have any of the following eye problems: difficulty reading or seeing objects, blurring of vision, tearing, spots or floaters, photophobia (sensitivity to light), burning, itching, pain, double vision, flashing lights, or halos around lights?

- *Risk for Infection* related to
  a. Improper contact lens hygiene
  b. Accumulation of secretions on eyelids.
- *Risk for Injury* related to
  a. Prolonged wearing of contact lenses
  b. Absence of blink reflex associated with unconsciousness.

PLANNING

In planning care, the nurse identifies nursing activities that will assist the client to maintain the integrity of the eye structures or a prosthesis and to prevent eye injury and infection.

IMPLEMENTING

Nursing activities may include teaching clients about how to insert, clean, and remove contact lenses or a prosthesis and ways to protect the eyes from injury and strain.

Eye Care

Dried secretions that have accumulated on the lashes need to be softened and wiped away. Soften dried secretions by placing a sterile cotton ball moistened with sterile water or normal saline over the lid margins. Wipe the loosened secretions from the in-

---

BOX 31–4 ■ Eye Care for the Comatose Client

When a comatose client's corneal reflex is impaired, eye care is essential to keep moist the areas of the cornea that are exposed to air.

- Administer moist compresses to cover the eyes every 2 to 4 hours.
- Clean the eyes with saline solution and cotton balls. Wipe from the inner to outer canthus. This prevents debris from being washed into the nasolacrimal duct.
- Use a new cotton ball for each wipe. This prevents extending infection in one eye to the other eye.
- Instill ophthalmic ointment or artificial tears into the lower lids as ordered. This keeps the eyes moist.
- If the client's corneal reflex is absent, keep the eyes moist with artificial tears and protect the eye with a protective shield. These should be ordered by a physician.
- Monitor the eyes for redness, exudate, or ulceration.

---

ner canthus of the eye to the outer canthus to prevent the particles and fluid from draining into the lacrimal sac and nasolacrimal duct.

If the client is unconscious and lacks a blink reflex or cannot close the eyelids completely, drying and irritation of the cornea must be prevented. Lubricating eye drops may be ordered. Box 31–4 gives suggestions for providing eye care for the comatose client.

Eyeglass Care

It is essential that the nurse exercise caution when cleaning eyeglasses to prevent breaking or scratching the lenses. Glass lenses can be cleaned with warm water and dried with a soft tissue that will not scratch the lenses. Plastic lenses are easily scratched and may require special cleaning solutions and drying tissues. When not being worn, all glasses should be placed in an appropriately labeled case and stored in the client's bedside table drawer.

Contact Lens Care

Contact lenses, thin curved discs of hard or soft plastic, fit on the cornea of the eye directly over the pupil. They float on the tear layer of the eye. For some people, contact lenses offer several advantages over eyeglasses: (a) They cannot be seen and thus have cosmetic value; (b) they are highly effective in correcting some astigmatisms; (c) they are safer than glasses for some physical activities; (d) they do not fog, as eyeglasses do; and (e) they provide better vision in many cases.

Contact lenses may be either hard or soft or a compromise between the two types—gas-permeable lenses. *Hard contact lenses* are made of a rigid, unwettable, airtight plastic that does not absorb water or saline solutions. They usually cannot be worn for more than 12 to 14 hours and are rarely recommended for first-time wearers.

Soft contact lenses cover the entire cornea. Being more pliable and soft, they mold to the eye for a firmer fit. The duration

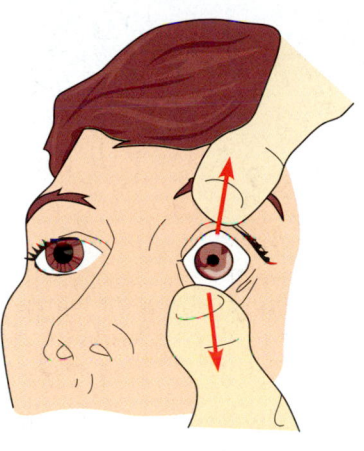
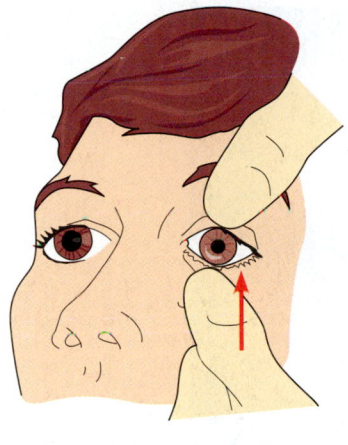
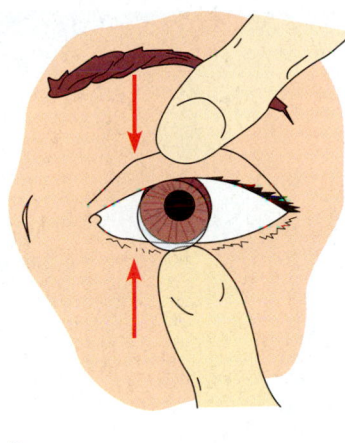

A   B   C

Figure 31–33 ■ Removing hard contact lenses.

of extended wear varies by brand from 1 to 30 days or more. Eye specialists recommend that long-wear brands be removed and cleaned at least once a week. These lenses require scrupulous care and handling.

Gas-permeable lenses are rigid enough to provide clear vision but are more flexible than the traditional hard lens. They permit oxygen to reach the cornea, thus providing greater comfort, and will not cause serious damage to the eye if left in place for several days.

Most clients normally care for their own contact lenses. In general, each lens manufacturer provides detailed cleaning instructions. Depending on the type of lens and cleaning method used, warm tap water, normal saline, or special rinsing or soaking solutions may be used.

All users should have a special container for their lenses. Some contain a solution so that the lenses are stored wet; in others, the lenses are dry. Each lens container has a slot or cup with a label indicating whether it is for the right or left lens. It is essential that the correct lens be stored in the appropriate slot so that it will be placed in the correct eye.

Removing Contact Lenses. Hard contact lenses must be positioned directly over the cornea for proper removal. If the lens is displaced, the nurse asks the client to look straight ahead, and gently exerts pressure on the upper and lower lids to move the lens back onto the cornea. Figure 31–33 ■ shows the steps needed to remove a hard lens. To avoid lens mixups, the nurse places the first lens in its designated cup in the storage base before removing the second lens (Figure 31–34 ■).

Removal of soft lenses varies in two ways. First, have the client look forward. Retract the lower lid with one hand. Using the pad of the index finger of the other hand, move the lens down to the inferior part of the sclera. This reduces the risk of damage to the cornea. Second, remove the lens by gently pinching the lens between the pads of the thumb and index finger. Pinching causes the lens to double up, so that air enters underneath the lens, overcoming the suction and allowing removal. Use the pads of the fingers to prevent scratching the eye

or the lens with the fingernails. Figure 31–35 ■ shows a client removing her own contact lens using the method described. Please note their a nurse would need to wear gloves.

Inserting Contact Lenses. Seriously ill clients whose contact lenses have been removed will not need them reinserted until they become more active in their care and require the lenses to see properly. Contact lenses need to be lubricated in a sterile, nonirritating wetting solution (usually a saline solution) before

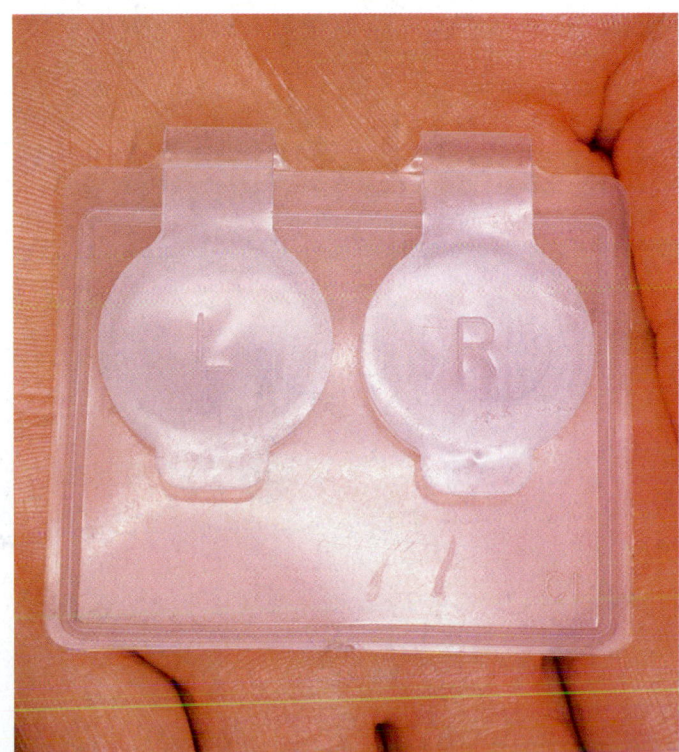

Figure 31–34 ■ Storing lenses. Place the first lens in its designated cup in the storage case before removing the second lens. This avoids mixing up two potentially different lenses. (David Parker/Science Photo Library/Photo Researchers, Inc.)

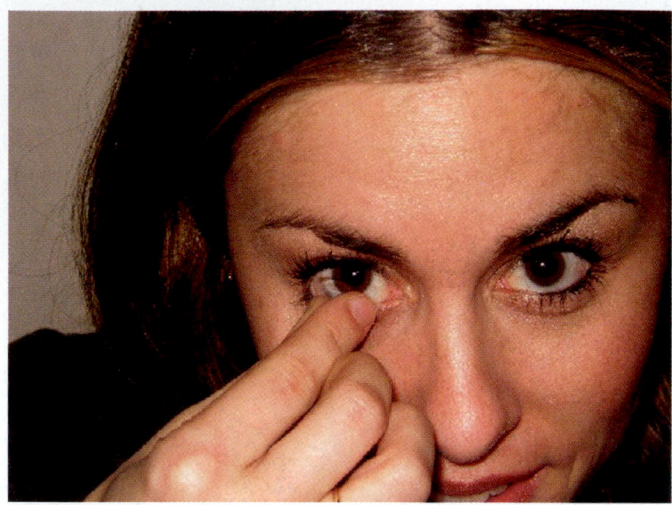

Figure 31–35 ■ Removing a soft lens by pinching it between the pads of the thumb and index finger. (Lester Lefkowitz/Corbis.)

they are inserted. The wetting solution helps the lens glide over the cornea, thus reducing the risk of injury. Most clients, when well, will reinsert the lenses independently.

Artificial Eyes

Artificial eyes are usually made of glass or plastic. Some are permanently implanted; others are removed regularly for cleaning. Most clients who wear a removable artificial eye follow their own care regimen. Even for an unconscious client, daily removal and cleaning are not necessary.

To remove an artificial eye, the nurse puts on clean gloves and retracts the client's lower eyelid down over the infraorbital bone while exerting slight pressure below the eyelid to overcome the suction (Figure 31–36 ■). An alternate method is to compress a small rubber bulb and apply the tip directly to the eye. As the nurse gradually releases the finger pressure on the

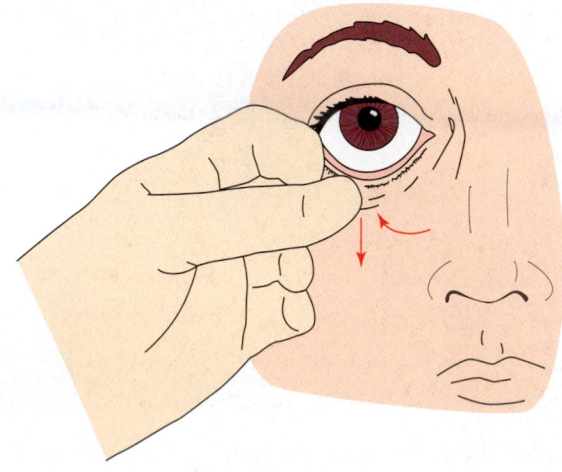

Figure 31–36 ■ Removing an artificial eye by retracting the lower eyelid and exerting slight pressure below the eyelid.

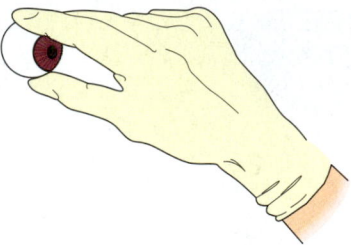

Figure 31–37 ■ Holding an artificial eye between the thumb and index finger for insertion.

bulb, the suction of the bulb counteracts the suction holding the eye in the socket and draws the eye out of the socket.

The eye is cleaned with warm normal saline and placed in a container filled with water or saline solution. The socket and tissues around the eye are usually cleaned with cotton wipes and normal saline. To reinsert the eye, the nurse uses the thumb and index finger of one hand to retract the eyelids, exerting pressure on the supraorbital and infraorbital bones. Holding the eye between the thumb and index finger of the other hand, the nurse slips the eye gently into the socket (Figure 31–37 ■).

General Eye Care

Many clients may need to learn specific information about care of the eyes. Some examples follow:

- Avoid home remedies for eye problems. Eye irritations or injuries at any age should be treated medically and immediately.
- If dirt or dust gets into the eyes, clean them copiously with clean, tepid water as an emergency treatment.
- Take measures to guard against eyestrain and to protect vision, such as maintaining adequate lighting for reading and obtaining shatterproof lenses for glasses.
- Schedule regular eye examinations, particularly after age 40, to detect problems such as cataracts and glaucoma.

EVALUATING

Using data collected during care, the nurse judges whether desired outcomes have been achieved. Examples of desired outcomes to evaluate the effectiveness of nursing interventions follow:

- Conjunctive and sclera free of inflammation
- Eyelids free of secretions
- No tearing
- No eye discomfort
- Demonstrates appropriate methods of caring for contact lenses
- Describes interventions to prevent eye injury and infection

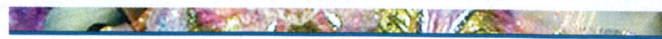

EARS

Normal ears require minimal hygiene. Clients who have excessive **cerumen** (earwax) and dependent clients who have hearing aids may require assistance from the nurse. Hearing aids are usually removed before surgery.

Cleaning the Ears

The auricles of the ear are cleaned during the bed bath. The nurse or client must remove excessive cerumen that is visible or that causes discomfort or hearing difficulty. Visible cerumen may be loosened and removed by retracting the auricle up and back. If this measure is ineffective, irrigation is necessary. Clients need to be advised never to use bobby pins, toothpicks, or cotton-tipped applicators to remove cerumen. Bobby pins and toothpicks can injure the ear canal and rupture the tympanic membrane; cotton-tipped applicators can cause wax to become impacted within the canal.

Care of Hearing Aids

A hearing aid is a battery-powered, sound-amplifying device used by persons with hearing impairments. It consists of a microphone that picks up sound and converts it to electric energy, an amplifier that magnifies the electric energy electronically, a receiver that converts the amplified energy back to sound energy, and an earmold that directs the sound into the ear. There are several types of hearing aids:

- *Behind-the-ear (BTE, or postaural) aid.* This is the most widely used type because it fits snugly behind the ear. The hearing aid case, which holds the microphone, amplifier, and receiver, is attached to the earmold by a plastic tube (Figure 31–38 ■).
- *In-the-ear aid (ITE, or intra-aural).* This one-piece aid has all its components housed in the earmold (Figure 31–39 ■).
- *In-the-canal (ITC) aid.* This is the most compact and least visible aid, fitting completely inside the ear canal. In addition to having cosmetic appeal, the ITC does not interfere with telephone use or the wearing of eyeglasses. However, it is not suitable for clients with progressive hearing loss; it requires adequate ear canal diameter and length for a good fit; and it tends to plug with cerumen more than other aids.
- *Eyeglasses aid.* This is similar to the behind-the-ear aid, but the components are housed in the temple of the eyeglasses. A hearing aid can be in one or both temples of the glasses.

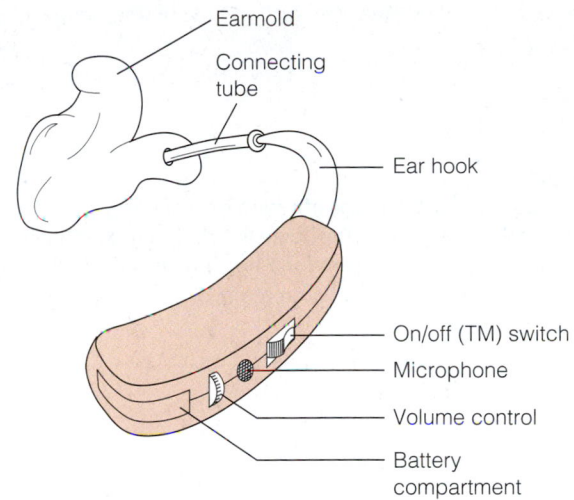
Figure 31–38 ■ A behind-the-ear hearing aid.

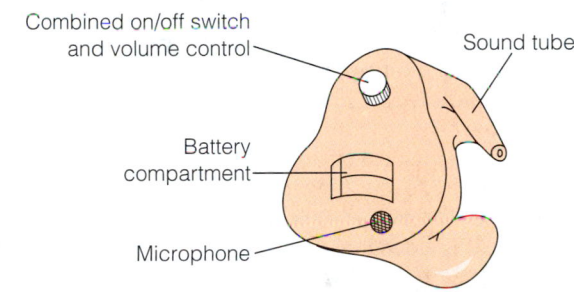
Figure 31–39 ■ An in-the-ear hearing aid.

- *Body hearing aid.* This pocket-sized aid, used for more severe hearing losses, clips onto an undergarment, shirt pocket, or harness carrier supplied by the manufacturer. The case, containing the microphone and amplifier, is connected by a cord to the receiver, which snaps into the earpiece.

For correct functioning, hearing aids require appropriate handling during insertion and removal, regular cleaning of the earmold, and replacement of dead batteries. With proper care, hearing aids generally last 5 to 10 years. Earmolds generally need readjustment every 2 to 3 years. Procedure 31–8 describes how to remove, clean, and insert a hearing aid.

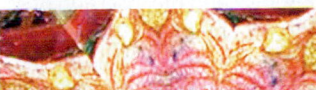
Procedure 31–8 Removing, Cleaning, and Inserting a Hearing Aid

Purpose
- To maintain proper hearing aid function

ASSESSMENT

Determine if the client has experienced any problems with the hearing aid and hearing aid practices. Assess for the presence of inflammation, excessive wax, drainage or discomfort in the external ear.

continued on page 744

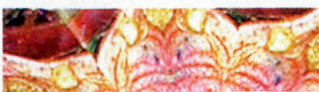

Procedure 31–8 Removing, Cleaning, and Inserting a Hearing Aid *continued*

PLANNING

Delegation

A nurse can delegate the task of caring for a hearing aid to the UAP. It is important, however, for the nurse to first determine that the UAP knows the correct way to care for a hearing aid. Inform the UAP to report the presence of ear inflammation, discomfort, excess wax or drainage to the RN.

Equipment

- Client's hearing aid
- Soap, water, and towels or a damp cloth
- Pipe cleaner or toothpick (optional)
- New battery (if needed)

IMPLEMENTATION

Performance

1. Explain to the client what you are going to do, why it is necessary, and how he or she can cooperate.
2. Wash hands and observe other appropriate infection control procedures.
3. Provide for client privacy by drawing the curtains around the bed or closing the door to the room. Some agencies provide signs indicating the need for privacy. *Hygiene is a personal matter.*
4. Remove the hearing aid.
   - Turn the hearing aid off and lower the volume. The on/off switch may be labeled "O" (off), "M" (microphone), "T" (telephone), or "TM" (telephone/microphone). *The batteries continue to run if the hearing aid is not turned off.*
   - Remove the earmold by rotating it slightly forward and pulling it outward.
   - If the hearing aid is not to be used for several days, remove the battery. *Removal prevents corrosion of the hearing aid from battery leakage.*
   - Store the hearing aid in a safe place and label with client's name. Avoid exposure to heat and moisture. *Proper storage prevents loss or damage.*
5. Clean the earmold.
   - Detach the earmold if possible. Disconnect the earmold from the receiver of a body hearing aid or from the hearing aid case of behind-the-ear and eyeglass hearing aids where the tubing meets the hook of the case. Do not remove the earmold if it is glued or secured by a small metal ring. *Removal facilitates cleaning and prevents inadvertent damage to the other parts.*

   - If the earmold is detachable, soak it in a mild soapy solution. Rinse and dry it well. Do not use isopropyl alcohol. *Alcohol can damage the hearing aid.*
   - If the earmold is not detachable or is for an in-the-ear aid, wipe the earmold with a damp cloth.
   - Check that the earmold opening is patent. Blow any excess moisture through the opening or remove debris (e.g., earwax) with a pipe cleaner or toothpick.
   - Reattach the earmold if it was detached from the rest of the hearing aid.
6. Insert the hearing aid.
   - Determine from the client if the earmold is for the left or the right ear.
   - Check that the battery is inserted in the hearing aid. Turn off the hearing aid, and make sure the volume is turned all the way down. *A volume that is too loud is distressing.*
   - Inspect the earmold to identify the ear canal portion. Some earmolds are fitted for only the ear canal and concha; others are fitted for all the contours of the ear. The canal portion, common to all, can be used as a guide for correct insertion.
   - Line up the parts of the earmold with the corresponding parts of the client's ear.
   - Rotate the earmold slightly forward, and insert the ear canal portion.
   - Gently press the earmold into the ear while rotating it backward.
   - Check that the earmold fits snugly by asking the client if it feels secure and comfortable.

   - Adjust the other components of a behind-the-ear or body hearing aid.
   - Turn the hearing aid on, and adjust the volume according to the client's needs.
7. Correct problems associated with improper functioning.
   - If the sound is weak or there is no sound:
     a. Ensure that the volume is turned high enough.
     b. Ensure that the earmold opening is not clogged.
     c. Check the battery by turning the hearing aid on, turning up the volume, cupping your hand over the earmold, and listening. A constant whistling sound indicates the battery is functioning. If necessary, replace the battery. Be sure that the negative (−) and positive (+) signs on the battery match those where indicated on the hearing aid.
     d. Ensure that the ear canal is not blocked with wax, which can obstruct sound waves.
   - If the client reports a whistling sound or squeal after insertion:
     a. Turn the volume down.
     b. Ensure that the earmold is properly attached to the receiver.
     c. Reinsert the earmold.
8. Document pertinent data.
   - The removal and the insertion of a hearing aid are not normally recorded.
   - Report and record any problems the client has with the hearing aid.

EVALUATION

- Speak to the client in a normal conversational tone and observe client behaviors.
- Compare the client's hearing ability to previous assessments.
- Report to the physician any deviations from normal for the client.

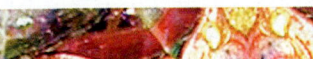

Home Care Considerations

Hearing Aids

- People who need a hearing aid may not wear one because they view the hearing aid as a stigma of old age.
- It is important for the client who just purchased a hearing aid to know that it often takes weeks or even months to adjust to the hearing aid. At first, the sounds will seem shrill as they start hearing high-frequency sounds that had been forgotten. Remind them that it is a hearing aid, not a hearing cure. Encourage them to not give up.

- The client needs to adjust to the hearing aid gradually by increasing the amount of time each day until the aid can be worn for a full day (Anderson, 1998).
- Encourage clients to purchase their hearing aids from a company that has a minimum warranty of a 30-day return policy.
- Emphasize the importance of maintaining the hearing aid, that is, having it cleaned and checked regularly.

NOSE

Nurses usually need not provide special care for the nose, because clients can ordinarily clear nasal secretions by blowing gently into a soft tissue. When the external nares are encrusted with dried secretions, they should be cleaned with a cotton-tipped applicator or moistened with saline or water. The applicator should not be inserted beyond the length of the cotton tip; inserting it further may cause injury to the mucosa.

SUPPORTING A HYGIENIC ENVIRONMENT

Because people are usually confined to bed when ill, often for long periods, the bed becomes an important element in the client's life. A place that is clean, safe, and comfortable contributes to the client's ability to rest and sleep and to a sense of well-being. Basic furniture in a health care facility includes the bed, bedside table, overbed table, one or more chairs, and a storage space for clothing. Most bed units also have a call light, light fixtures, electric outlets, and hygienic equipment in the bedside table. Three types of equipment often installed in an acute care facility are a suction outlet for several kinds of suction, an oxygen outlet for most oxygen equipment, and a sphygmomanometer to measure the client's blood pressure. Some long-term care agencies also permit clients to have personal furniture, such as a television, a chair, and lamps, at the bedside. In the home a client often has personal and medical equipment.

Environment

When providing a comfortable environment it is important to consider the client's age, severity of illness, and level of activity.

Room Temperature

The very young, the very old, and the acutely ill frequently need a room temperature higher than normal. A room temperature between 20 and 23C (68 and 74F) is comfortable for most clients.

Ventilation

Good ventilation is important to remove unpleasant odors and stale air. Odors caused by urine, draining wounds, or vomitus, for example, can be offensive to people. Room deodorizers can help eliminate odors. However, good hygienic practices are the best way to prevent offensive body and breath odors. Hospitals are required to monitor smoking. Hospitals often have a smoking area for clients and prohibit smoking in client rooms.

Noise

Ill persons are usually sensitive to noise such as clanging of metal equipment, loud talking, and laughter. Nurses should try to control noise in health care settings.

Hospital Beds

The frame of a hospital bed is divided into three sections. This permits the head and the foot to be elevated separately. Most hospital beds have electric motors to operate the movable joints. The motor is activated by pressing a button or moving a small lever, located either at the side of the bed or on a small panel separate from the bed but attached to it by a cable, which the client can readily use. Common bed positions are shown in Table 31–7.

Hospital beds are usually 66 cm (26 in.) high and 0.9 m (3 ft) wide, narrower than the usual bed, so that the nurse can reach the client from either side of the bed without undue stretching. The length is usually 1.9 m (6.5 ft). Some beds can be extended in length to accommodate very tall clients. Long-term care facilities for ambulatory clients usually have low beds to facilitate movement in and out of bed. Most hospital beds have "high" and "low" positions that can be adjusted either mechanically or electrically by a button or lever. The high position permits the nurse to reach the client without undue stretching or stooping. The low position allows the client to step easily to the floor.

Mattresses

Mattresses are usually covered with a water-repellent material that resists soiling and can be cleaned easily. Most mattresses have handles on the sides called lugs by which the mattress can be moved.

Many special mattresses are also used in hospitals to relieve pressure on the body's bony prominences, such as the heels. They are particularly helpful for clients confined to bed for a long time. For additional information about mattresses, see Chapter 34.

TABLE 31-7 Commonly Used Bed Positions

Flat Foot of bed Head of bed	Mattress is completely horizontal.	Client sleeping in a variety of bed positions, such as back-lying, side-lying, and prone (face down) To maintain spinal alignment for clients with spinal injuries To assist clients to move and turn in bed Bed-making by nurse
Fowler's position 	Semisitting position in which head of bed is raised to angle of at least 45°. Knees may be flexed or horizontal.	Convenient for eating, reading, visiting, watching TV Relief from lying positions To promote lung expansion for client with respiratory problem To assist a client to a sitting position on the edge of the bed
Semi-Fowler's position 	Head of bed is raised only to 30° angle.	Relief from lying position To promote lung expansion
Trendelenburg's position 	Head of bed is lowered and the foot raised in a straight incline.	To promote venous circulation in certain clients To provide postural drainage of basal lung lobes
Reverse Trendelenburg's position 	Head of bed raised and the foot lowered. Straight tilt in direction opposite to Trendelenburg's position.	To promote stomach emptying and prevent esophageal reflex in client with hiatal hernia

Side Rails

Side rails, or safety sides, are used on both hospital beds and stretchers. They are of various shapes and sizes and are usually made of metal. A bed can have two full-length side rails or four half- or quarter-length side rails (also called split rails). Devices to raise and lower side rails differ. Often one or two knobs are pulled to release the side and permit it to be moved. When side rails are being used, it is important that the nurse never leave the bedside while the rail is lowered. Some side rails have two positions: up and down. Others have three: high, intermediate, and low.

For decades, the use of side rails has been routine practice with the rationale that the side rails serve as a safe and effective means of preventing clients from falling out of bed. Research, however, has not validated this assumption. In fact, several studies have shown that raised side rails do not deter older clients from getting out of bed unassisted and have led to more

serious falls, injuries, and even death (Talerico & Capazuti, 2001). The Health Care Financing Administration now mandates that nurses in both acute care and long-term care decrease the routine use of side rails. Alternatives to side rails do exist and can include low-height bed, mats placed at the side of the bed, motion sensors, and bed alarms (see Chapter 30).

> **CLINICAL ALERT** *Side rail entrapment, injuries, and deaths do occur. When side rails are used, the nurse must assess the client's physical and mental status and closely monitor high-risk (frail, elderly, or confused) clients.*

Footboard or Footboot

These are used to support the immobilized client's foot in a normal right angle to the legs to prevent plantar flexion contractures (see Chapter 42).

Bed Cradles

A bed cradle is a device designed to keep the top bedclothes off the feet, legs, and even abdomen of a client. The bedclothes are arranged over the device and may be pinned in place. There are several types of bed cradles. One of the most common is a curved metal rod that fits over the bed. Part of the cradle fits under the mattress, and small metal brackets press down on each side of the mattress to keep the cradle in place. The frame of some cradles extends over half of the width of the bed, above one leg.

Intravenous Rods

Intravenous rods (poles, stands, standards), usually made of metal, support intravenous (IV) infusion containers while fluid is being administered to a client. These rods were traditionally freestanding on the floor beside the bed. Now, intravenous rods are often attached to the hospital beds. Some hospital units have overhead hanging rods on a track for IVs.

MAKING BEDS

Nurses need to be able to prepare hospital beds in different ways for specific purposes. In most instances, beds are made after the client receives certain care and when beds are unoccupied. At times, however, nurses need to make an occupied bed or prepare a bed for a client who is having surgery (an anesthetic, postoperative, or surgical bed). Regardless of what type of bed equipment is available, whether the bed is occupied or unoccupied, or the purpose for which the bed is being prepared, certain practice guidelines pertain to all bed-making.

Unoccupied Bed

An unoccupied bed can be either closed or open. Generally the top covers of an open bed are folded back (thus the term *open*

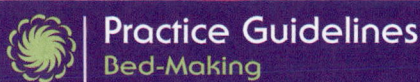

Practice Guidelines
Bed-Making

- Wash hands thoroughly after handling a client's bed linen. Linens and equipment that have been soiled with secretions and excretions harbor microorganisms that can be transmitted to others directly or by the nurse's hands or uniform.
- Hold soiled linen away from uniform.
- Linen for one client is never (even momentarily) placed on another client's bed.
- Place soiled linen directly in a portable linen hamper or tucked into a pillow case at the end of the bed before it is gathered up for disposal.
- Do not shake soiled linen in the air because shaking can disseminate secretions and excretions and the microorganisms they contain.
- When stripping and making a bed, conserve time and energy by stripping and making up one side as much as possible before working on the other side.
- To avoid unnecessary trips to the linen supply area, gather all linen before starting to strip a bed.

bed) to make it easier for a client to get in. Open and closed beds are made the same way, except that the top sheet, blanket, and bedspread of a *closed bed* are drawn up to the top of the bed and under the pillows.

Beds are often changed after bed baths. The linen can be collected before the bath. The linen is not usually changed unless it is soiled. Check the policy at each clinical agency. Unfitted sheets, blankets, and bedspreads are mitered at the corners of the bed. The purpose of mitering is to secure the bedclothes while the bed is occupied. Figure 31–40 ■ shows how to miter the corner of a bed. Procedure 31–9 explains how to change an unoccupied bed.

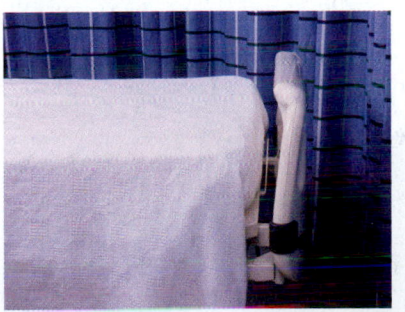

A

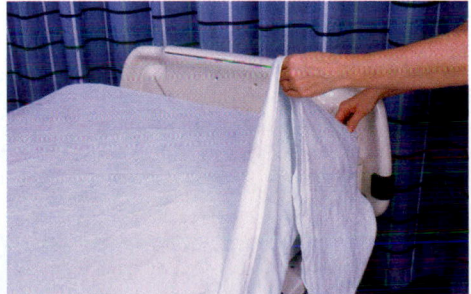

B

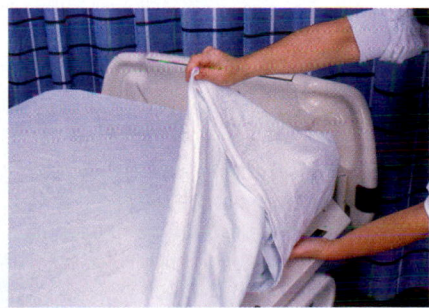

C

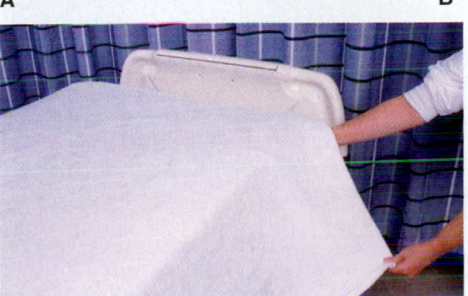

D

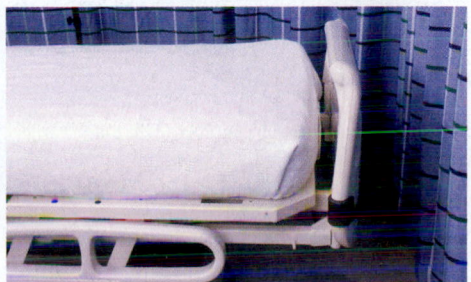

E

Figure 31–40 ■ Mitering the corner of a bed.

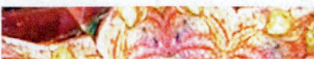

Procedure 31–9 Changing an Unoccupied Bed

Purposes

- To promote the client's comfort
- To provide a clean neat environment for the client
- To provide a smooth, wrinkle-free bed foundation, thus minimizing sources of skin irritation

ASSESSMENT

- Assess the client's health status to determine that the person can safely get out of bed. In some hospitals it is necessary to have a written order if the client has been in bed continuously.
- Assess the client's pulse and respirations if indicated.
- Note all the tubes and equipment connected to the client *because this may influence the need for additional linens or waterproof pads.*

PLANNING

Delegation

Bed-making is usually delegated to UAP. If appropriate, inform the UAP of the proper disposal method of linens that contain drainage. Ask the UAP to inform you immediately if any tubes or dressings become dislodged or removed. Stress the importance of the call light being readily available while the client is out of bed.

Equipment

- Two flat sheets or one fitted and one flat sheet
- Cloth drawsheet (optional)
- One blanket
- One bedspread
- Waterproof drawsheet or waterproof pads (optional)
- Pillowcase(s) for the head pillow(s)
- Plastic laundry bag or portable linen hamper, if available

IMPLEMENTATION

Preparation

Determine what linens the client may already have in the room *to avoid stockpiling of unnecessary extra linens.*

Performance

1. Explain to the client what you are going to do, why it is necessary, and how he or she can cooperate.
2. Wash hands and observe other appropriate infection control procedures.
3. Provide for client privacy.
4. Place the fresh linen on the client's chair or overbed table; do not use another client's bed. *This prevents cross-contamination (the movement of microorganisms from one client to another) via soiled linen.*
5. Assess and assist the client out of bed.
   - Make sure that this is an appropriate and convenient time for the client to be out of bed.
   - Assist the client to a comfortable chair.
6. Raise the bed to a comfortable working height.
7. Strip the bed.
   - Check bed linens for any items belonging to the client, and detach the call bell or any drainage tubes from the bed linen.
   - Loosen all bedding systematically, starting at the head of the bed on the far side and moving around the bed up to the head of the bed on the near side. *Moving around the bed systematically prevents stretching and reaching and possible muscle strain.*
   - Remove the pillowcases, if soiled, and place the pillows on the bedside chair near the foot of the bed.
   - Fold reusable linens, such as the bedspread and top sheet on the bed, into fourths. First, fold the linen in half by bringing the top edge even with the bottom edge, and then grasp it at the center of the middle fold and bottom edges (Figure 31–41 ■). *Folding linens saves time and energy when reapplying the linens on the bed.*
   - Remove the waterproof pad and discard it if soiled.
   - Roll all soiled linen inside the bottom sheet, hold it away from your uniform, and place it directly in the linen hamper (Figure 31–42 ■). *These actions are essential to prevent the transmission of microorganisms to the nurse and others.*
   - Grasp the mattress securely, using the lugs if present, and move the mattress up to the head of the bed.

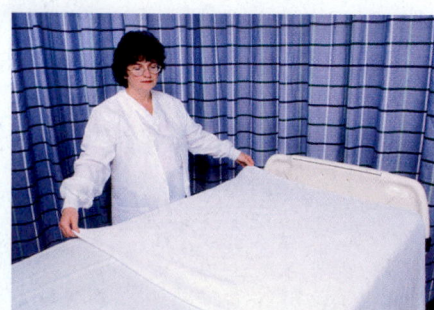

Figure 31–41 ■ Fold reusable linens into fourths when removing them from the bed.

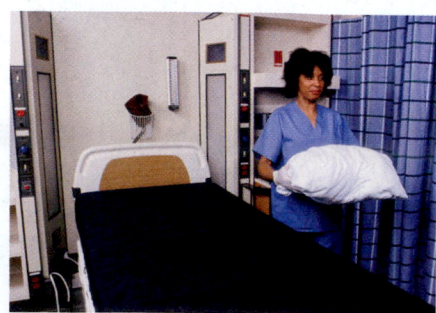

Figure 31–42 ■ Roll soiled linen inside bottom sheet and hold away from body.

IMPLEMENTATION *continued*

7. Apply the bottom sheet and draw-sheet.
   - Place the folded bottom sheet with its center fold on the center of the bed. Make sure the sheet is hem side down for a smooth foundation. Spread the sheet out over the mattress, and allow a sufficient amount of sheet at the top to tuck under the mattress (Figure 31–43 ■). *The top of the sheet needs to be well tucked under to remain securely in place, especially when the head of the bed is elevated.* Place the sheet along the edge of the mattress at the foot of the bed and do not tuck it in (unless it is a contour or fitted sheet).

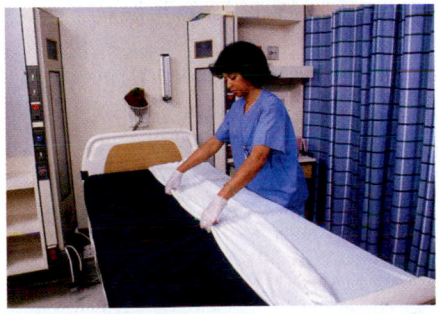

Figure 31–43 ■ Placing bottom sheet on bed.

   - Miter the sheet at the top corner on the near side (Figure 31–41, earlier) and tuck the sheet under the mattress, working from the head of the bed to the foot.
   - If a waterproof drawsheet is used, place it over the bottom sheet so that the centerfold is at the centerline of the bed and the top and bottom edges extend from the middle of the client's back to the area of the midthigh or knee. Fanfold the uppermost half of the folded drawsheet at the center or far edge of the bed and tuck in the near edge (Figure 31–44 ■).
   - Lay the cloth drawsheet over the waterproof sheet in the same manner.
   - *Optional:* Before moving to the other side of the bed, place the top linens on the bed hemside up, unfold them, tuck them in, and miter the bottom corners. *Completing one*

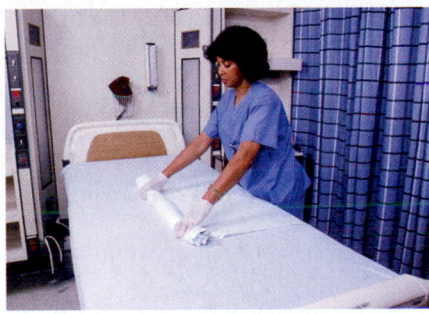

Figure 31–44 ■ Placing drawsheet on bed.

entire side of the bed at a time saves time and energy.

8. Move to the other side and secure the bottom linens.
   - Tuck in the bottom sheet under the head of the mattress, pull the sheet firmly, and miter the corner of the sheet.
   - Pull the remainder of the sheet firmly so that there are no wrinkles. *Wrinkles can cause discomfort for the client.* Tuck the sheet in at the side.
   - Complete this same process for the drawsheet(s).
9. Apply or complete the top sheet, blanket, and spread.
   - Place the top sheet, hemside up, on the bed so that its centerfold is at the center of the bed and the top edge is even with the top edge of the mattress.
   - Unfold the sheet over the bed.
   - *Optional:* Make a vertical or a horizontal toe pleat in the sheet to provide additional room for the client's feet.
     a. *Vertical toe pleat:* Make a fold in the sheet 5 to 10 cm (2 to 4 in.) perpendicular to the foot of the bed (Figure 31–45 ■).

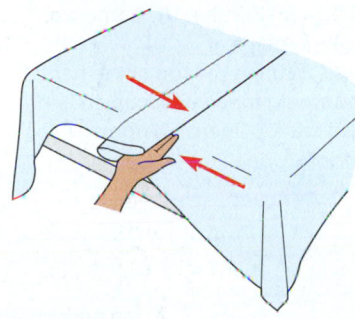

Figure 31–45 ■ A vertical toe pleat.

   b. *Horizontal toe pleat:* Make a fold in the sheet 5 to 10 cm (2 to 4 in.) across the bed near the foot (Figure 31–46 ■).

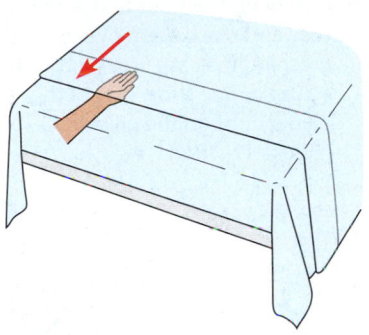

Figure 31–46 ■ A horizontal toe pleat.

Loosening the top covers around the feet after the client is in bed is another way to provide additional space.
   - Follow the same procedure for the blanket and the spread, but place the top edges about 15 cm (6 in.) from the head of the bed to allow a cuff of sheet to be folded over them.
   - Tuck in the sheet, blanket, and spread at the foot of the bed, and miter the corner, using all three layers of linen. Leave the sides of the top sheet, blanket, and spread hanging freely unless toe pleats were provided.
   - Fold the top of the top sheet down over the spread, providing a cuff (Figure 31–47 ■). *The cuff of sheet makes it easier for the client to pull the covers up.*
   - Move to the other side of the bed and secure the top bedding in the same manner.

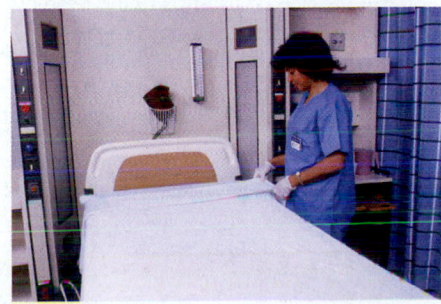

Figure 31–47 ■ Making a cuff of the top linens.

continued on page 750

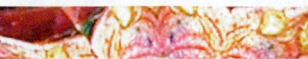

Procedure 31–9 Changing an Unoccupied Bed *continued*

IMPLEMENTATION *continued*

10. Put clean pillowcases on the pillows as required.
    - Grasp the closed end of the pillowcase at the center with one hand.
    - Gather up the sides of the pillowcase and place them over the hand grasping the case. Then grasp the center of one short side of the pillow through the pillowcase (Figure 31–48 ■).

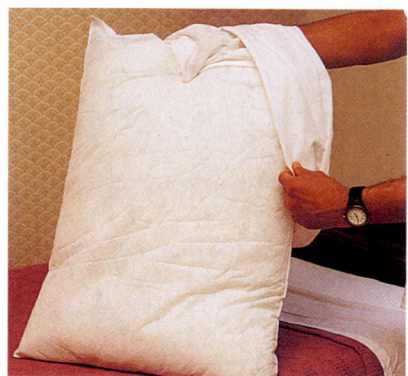

Figure 31–48 ■ Method for putting a clean pillowcase on a pillow.

    - With the free hand, pull the pillowcase over the pillow.
    - Adjust the pillowcase so that the pillow fits into the corners of the case and the seams are straight. *A smoothly fitting pillowcase is more comfortable than a wrinkled one.*
    - Place the pillows appropriately at the head of the bed.

11. Provide for client comfort and safety.
    - Attach the signal cord so that the client can conveniently use it. Some cords have clamps that attach to the sheet or pillowcase. Others are attached by a safety pin.
    - If the bed is currently being used by a client, either fold back the top covers at one side or fanfold them down to the center of the bed. *This makes it easier for the client to get into the bed.*

    - Place the bedside table and the overbed table so that they are available to the client.
    - Leave the bed in the high position if the client is returning by stretcher, or place in the low position if the client is returning to bed after being up.

12. Document and report pertinent data.
    - Bed-making is not normally recorded.
    - Record any nursing assessments, such as the client's physical status and pulse and respiratory rates before and after being out of bed, as indicated.

VARIATION: SURGICAL BED

While the client is in the operating room, the client's bed is prepared for the postoperative phase. In some agencies, the client is brought back to the unit on a stretcher and transferred to the bed in the room. In other agencies, the client's bed is brought to the surgery suite and the client is transferred there. In the latter situation, the bed needs to be made with clean linens as soon as the client goes to surgery so that it can be taken to the operating room when needed.

- Strip the bed.
- Place and leave the pillows on the bedside chair. *Pillows are left on a chair to facilitate transferring the client into the bed.*
- Apply the bottom linens as for an unoccupied bed. Place a bath blanket on the foundation of the bed if this is agency practice. *A flannel bath blanket provides additional warmth.*
- Place the top covers (sheet, blanket, and bedspread) on the bed as you would for an unoccupied bed. Do not tuck them in, miter the corners or make a toe pleat.
- Make a cuff at the top of the bed as you would for an unoccupied bed. Fold the top linens up from the bottom.

- On the side of the bed where the client will be transferred, fold up the two outer corners of the top linens so they meet in the middle of the bed forming a triangle (Figure 31–49 ■).

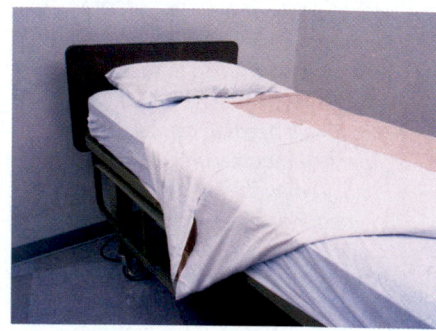

Figure 31–49 ■ Fold up the two outer corners of the top linens forming a triangle.

- Pick up the apex of the triangle and fanfold the top linens lengthwise to the other side of the bed *to facilitate the client's transfer into the bed* (Figure 31–50 ■).

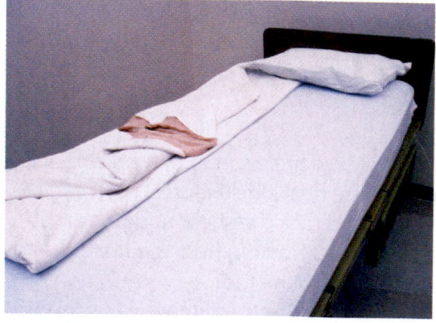

Figure 31–50 ■ Surgical bed. The linens are horizontally fanfolded to the other side of the bed to facilitate transfer of the client into the bed.

- Leave the bed in high position with the side rails down. *The high position facilitates the transfer of the client.*
- Lock the wheels of the bed if the bed is not to be moved. *Locking the wheels keeps the bed from rolling when the client is transferred from the stretcher to the bed.*

EVALUATION

- Make sure the call light is accessible to the client.
- Relate client parameters of activity (e.g., pulse and respirations) to previous assessment data particularly if the client has been

on bedrest for an extended period of time or it is the first time that the client is getting out of bed after surgery.

Changing an Occupied Bed

Some clients may be too weak to get out of bed. Either the nature of their illness may contraindicate their sitting out of bed, or they may be restricted in bed by the presence of traction or other therapies. When changing an occupied bed, the nurse works quickly and disturbs the client as little as possible to conserve the client's energy, using the following guidelines:

- Maintain the client in good body alignment. Never move or position a client in a manner that is contraindicated by the client's health. Obtain help if necessary to ensure safety.
- Move the client gently and smoothly. Rough handling can cause the client discomfort and abrade the skin.
- Explain what you plan to do throughout the procedure before you do it. Use terms that the client can understand.
- Use the bed-making time, like the bed bath time, to assess and meet the client's needs.

Procedure 31–10 Changing an Occupied Bed

Purposes

- To conserve the client's energy and maintain current healthy status
- To promote client comfort

- To provide a clean, neat environment for the client
- To provide a smooth, wrinkle-free bed foundation, thus minimizing sources of skin irritation

ASSESSMENT

- Note specific orders or precautions for moving and positioning the client.
- Determine presence of incontinence or excessive drainage from other sources indicating the need for protective waterproof pads.

- Assess skin condition and need for special mattress (e.g., egg crate), footboard, or heel protectors.

PLANNING

Delegation

Bed-making is usually delegated to UAP. Inform the UAP to what extent the client can assist or if another person will be needed to assist the UAP. Instruct the UAP about the handling of any dressings and/or tubes of the client and also the need for special equipment (e.g., footboard, heel protectors), if appropriate.

Equipment

- Two flat sheets or one fitted and one flat sheet
- Cloth drawsheet (optional)

- One blanket
- One bedspread
- Waterproof drawsheet or waterproof pads (optional)
- Pillowcase(s) for the head pillow(s)
- Plastic laundry bag or portable linen hamper, if available

IMPLEMENTATION

Performance

1. Explain to the client what you are going to do, why it is necessary, and how he or she can cooperate.
2. Wash hands and observe other appropriate infection control procedures. Put on disposable gloves if linen is soiled with body fluids.
3. Provide for client privacy.
4. Remove the top bedding.
   - Remove any equipment attached to the bed linen, such as a signal light.
   - Loosen all the top linen at the foot of the bed, and remove the spread and the blanket.
   - Leave the top sheet over the client (the top sheet can remain over the client if it is being changed and if it will provide sufficient warmth), or

replace it with a bath blanket as follows:
Spread the bath blanket over the top sheet.
   a. Ask the client to hold the top edge of the blanket.
   b. Reaching under the blanket from the side, grasp the top edge of the sheet and draw it down to the foot of the bed, leaving the blanket in place (Figure 31–51 ■).
   c. Remove the sheet from the bed and place it in the soiled linen hamper.
5. Change the bottom sheet and drawsheet.
   - Assist the client to turn on the side facing away from the side where the clean linen is.

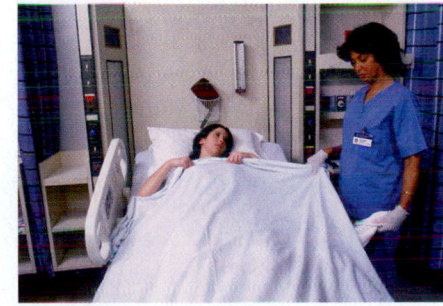

Figure 31–51 ■ Removing top linens under a bath blanket.

- Raise the side rail nearest the client. *This protects the client from falling.* If there is no side rail, have another nurse support the client at the edge of the bed.

continued on page 752

Procedure 31-10 Changing an Occupied Bed *continued*

IMPLEMENTATION *continued*

- Loosen the foundation of the linen on the side of the bed near the linen supply.
- Fanfold the drawsheet and the bottom sheet at the center of the bed (Figure 31–52 ■), as close to the client as possible. *Doing this leaves the near half of the bed free to be changed.*

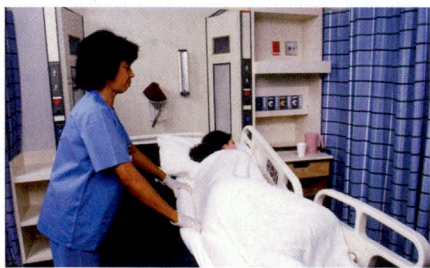

Figure 31–52 ■ Moving soiled linen as close to the client as possible.

- Place the new bottom sheet on the bed, and vertically fanfold the half to be used on the far side of the bed as close to the client as possible (Figure 31–53 ■). Tuck the sheet under the near half of the bed and miter the corner if a contour sheet is not being used.

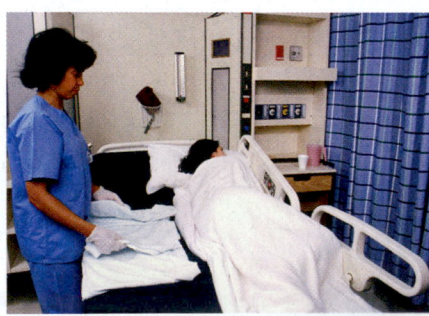

Figure 31–53 ■ Placing new bottom sheet on half of the bed.

- Place the clean drawsheet on the bed with the center fold at the center of the bed. Fanfold the uppermost half vertically at the center of the bed and tuck the near side edge under the side of the mattress (Figure 31–54 ■).

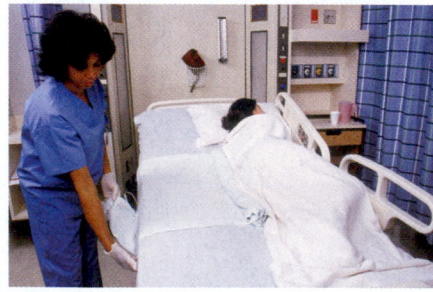

Figure 31–54 ■ Placing clean drawsheet on the bed.

- Assist the client to roll over toward you onto the clean side of the bed. The client rolls over the fanfolded linen at the center of the bed.
- Move the pillows to the clean side for the client's use. Raise the side rail before leaving the side of the bed.
- Move to the other side of the bed and lower the side rail.
- Remove the used linen and place it in the portable hamper.
- Unfold the fanfolded bottom sheet from the center of the bed.
- Facing the side of the bed, use both hands to pull the bottom sheet so that it is smooth and tuck the excess under the side of the mattress.
- Unfold the drawsheet fanfolded at the center of the bed and pull it tightly with both hands. Pull the sheet in three sections: (a) Face the side of the bed to pull the middle section, (b) face the far top corner to pull the bottom section, and (c) face the far bottom corner to pull the top section.
- Tuck the excess drawsheet under the side of the mattress.

6. Reposition the client in the center of the bed.
   - Reposition the pillows at the center of the bed.
   - Assist the client to the center of the bed. Determine what position the client requires or prefers and assist the client to that position.
7. Apply or complete the top bedding.
   - Spread the top sheet over the client and either ask the client to hold the top edge of the sheet or tuck it under the shoulders. The sheet should remain over the client when the bath blanket or used sheet is removed (Figure 31–55 ■).
   - Complete the top of the bed.

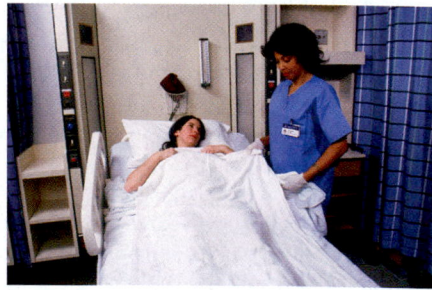

Figure 31–55 ■ Client holds top edge of sheet while nurse removes bath blanket.

8. Ensure continued safety of the client.
   - Raise the side rails. Place the bed in the low position before leaving the bedside.
   - Attach the signal cord to the bed linen within the client's reach.
   - Put items used by the client within easy reach.
9. Bed-making is not normally recorded.

EVALUATION

- Conduct appropriate follow-up, such as determining client's comfort and safety, patency of all drainage tubes, and client's access to call light to summon help when needed.

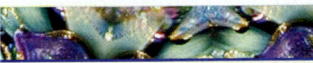

Focus on Critical Thinking

It is the fourth day following a female client's abdominal surgery. She is progressing well, is ambulating several times each day, has been providing for her own hygienic needs, and is planning on going home tomorrow. During your early morning assessment you note that the client's hair is oily and matted and she has an unpleasant body odor. Her dentures in a container at the bedside are in need of cleaning. You check her abdominal incision and verify that there is no drainage, redness, or signs of infection. You inquire about her ability to take care of her own bath and personal needs, and offer to assist her with her bath. She replies that she had a bath yesterday, doesn't feel that she needs another one today, and requests to omit her personal care for the day.

1. You are considering *Self-Care Deficit: Bathing/Hygiene* as an appropriate nursing diagnosis for the client. You review the defining characteristics and related factors and discover what?
2. What else should you ask the client?
3. Why is it important that you obtain the assessments you have already completed along with the above questions you asked?
4. What approaches might you use if you feel that the client does need her hair shampooed and needs to have her personal care attended to?
5. What advantages does performing baths and personal hygiene for clients offer to the nurse?

See Critical Thinking Possibilities in Appendix A.

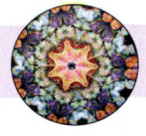

Chapter Review

EXPLORE MediaLink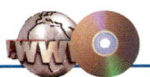

NCLEX review questions, case studies, care plan activities, MediaLink applications, and other interactive resources for this chapter can be found on the Companion Website at www.prenhall.com/kozier. Click on Chapter 31 to select the activities for this chapter.

For more NCLEX review questions, and an audio glossary, access the Student CD-ROM accompanying this textbook.

Chapter Highlights

- Clients' hygienic practices are influenced by numerous factors including culture, religion, environment, developmental level, health and energy, and personal preferences.
- The major functions of the skin are to protect underlying tissues, to help regulate body temperature, to secrete sebum, to transmit sensations through nerve receptors for sensory perception, and to produce and absorb vitamin D in conjunction with ultraviolet rays from the sun.
- When planning hygiene care, the nurse must take the client's preferences into consideration.
- Nurses provide perineal-genital care for clients who are unable to do so for themselves.
- Nurses can often teach clients how to prevent foot problems.
- Oral hygiene should include daily dental flossing and mechanical brushing of the teeth.

- Regular dental checkups and fluoride supplements are recommended to maintain healthy teeth.
- Nurses provide special oral care to clients who are unconscious or debilitated.
- Hair care includes daily combing and brushing and regular shampooing.
- African American clients' hair may require special care.
- Nurses may need to assist dependent clients with their artificial eyes, eyeglasses, and contact lenses.
- Clients with a hearing aid may require nursing assistance with the device.
- Changing bed linens is a part of maintaining hygiene.
- It is important to keep beds clean and comfortable for clients.

Review Questions

31–1. A client can bathe most of her body except for the back, hands, and feet. She also can walk to and from the bathroom and dress herself when given clothing. How would you describe this client's functional level?

a. totally dependent (+4)
b. moderately dependent (+3)
c. semidependent (+2)
d. independent (0)

31–2. The client is unresponsive and requires total care by nursing staff. Prior to providing special oral care, the nurse should assess for
  a. presence of pain.
  b. condition of the skin.
  c. gag reflex.
  d. range of motion.

31–3. A client with diabetes has very dry skin on her feet and lower extremities. To maintain intact skin the nurse should plan to inform the client to
  a. soak her feet frequently.
  b. use a nonperfumed lotion.
  c. apply foot powder.
  d. avoid knee-high elastic stockings.

31–4. The client wears an in-the-ear hearing aid and because of arthritis needs someone to insert the hearing aid. The nurse teaches the UAP to do which of the following actions before inserting the client's hearing aid?
  a. Turn the hearing aid off.
  b. Soak the hearing aid in soapy solution to clean it.
  c. Turn the volume all the way up.
  d. Remove the batteries.

31–5. The client is in surgery and will be returning to his bed via a stretcher. The nurse plans ahead by making which type of bed and placing the bed in which position?
  a. an open bed in low position
  b. an occupied bed in low position
  c. a closed bed in high position
  d. a surgical bed in high position

Readings and References

Suggested Readings

Beuscher, T. L. (1998). Community outreach foot care for the elderly: A winning proposition. *Home Healthcare Nurse, 16*(1), 37–44.
  Beuscher describes one home health agency's development of a foot care program for the elderly. Monthly foot care clinics were begun in six community senior centers and staffed by home health nurses. A modest fee was charged to cover costs. The nurses learned new skills, clients received care they were unable to perform, and senior centers were able to offer a new program to their members.

Brawley, E. C. (2002). Bathing environments: How to improve the bathing experience. *Alzheimer's Care Quarterly, 3*(1), 38–41.
  The author emphasizes that bathing is about more than hygiene. A successful bathing experience should also be a pleasant experience. Accomplishing this for a client with Alzheimer's disease is often challenging for the caregiver. Brawley discusses how the design of the bath environment must consciously create a sense of calm and attempt to reduce risk, noise, glare, and odor.

Hektor, L. M., & Touhy, T. A. (1997). The history of the bath: From art to task? *Journal of Gerontological Nursing, 23*(5), 7–15.
  The authors outline a historical perspective of how the bath has been a major focus of nursing care. The concept of personal cleanliness, started by Nightingale, helped to combat disease (e.g., "germ theory") and change social values and roles. Hektor and Touhy review the many types of therapeutic baths: cold bath, hot bath, acid steam bath, sedative bath, medicated bath, heliotherapy, vapor bath, and sun bath. After pointing out a historical appreciation of the comfort and therapeutic nature of the bath, they compare the current perspective of the bath: a task delegated to unlicensed personnel. They urge the nurse to focus on the person-focused comfort and caring outcomes of bathing.

Related Research

Norwood-Chapman, L., & Burchfield, S. B. (1999). Nursing home personnel knowledge and attitudes about hearing loss and hearing aids. *Gerontology and Geriatrics Education, 20*(2), 37–47.

Pyle, M. A., Massie, M., & Nelson, S. (1998). A pilot study on improving oral care in long-term care settings. *Journal of Gerontological Nursing, 24*(10), 31–38.

References

Anderson, E. G. (1998). Deafness is a scourge (and you can say that again). *Geriatrics, 53*(8), 65–69.

Andrews, M. M., & Boyle, J. S. (2003). *Transcultural Concepts in Nursing Care* (4th ed.) Philadelphia: Lippincott Williams & Wilkins.

Bennett, J. A. (1999). Activities of daily living: Old-fashioned or still useful? *Journal of Gerontological Nursing, 25*(5), 22–29.

Brawley, E. C. (2002). Bathing environments: How to improve the bathing experience. *Alzheimer's Care Quarterly, 3*(1), 38–41.

Frankowski, B. L., & Weiner, L. B. (2002). Head lice. *Pediatrics, 110*(3), 638–643.

Gammons, M., & Salam, G. (2002). Tick removal. *American Family Physician, 66*(4), 643–645.

Hektor, L. M., & Touhy, T. A. (1997). The history of the bath: From art to task? *Journal of Gerontological Nursing, 23*(5), 7–15.

Hoeffer, B., Rader, J., McKenzie, D., Lavelle, M., & Stewart, B. (1997). Reducing aggressive behavior during bathing cognitively impaired nursing home residents. *Journal of Gerontological Nursing, 23*(5), 16–23.

Jackson, F. (1998). The ABC's of black hair and skin care. *The ABNF Journal, 9*(5), 100–104.

Johnson, M., Maas, M., & Moorhead, S. (2000). *Nursing outcomes classification (NOC)* (2nd ed.). St. Louis MD: Mosby.

McCloskey, J. C., & Bulechek, G. M. (2000). *Nursing interventions classification (NIC)* (3rd ed.). St. Louis, MO: Mosby.

Miller, M. F. (1997). Physically aggressive resident behavior during hygienic care. *Journal of Gerontological Nursing, 23*(5), 24–39.

NANDA International. (2003). NANDA *nursing diagnoses: Definitions & classification 2003–2004.* Philadelphia: Author.

Pillitteri, A. (2003). *Maternal and Child Health Nursing: Care of the Childbearing and Childrearing Family* (4th ed.). Philadelphia: Lippincott Williams & Wilkins.

Rader, J., Lavelle, M., Hoeffer, B., & McKenzie, D. (1996). Maintaining cleanliness: An individualized approach. *Journal of Gerontological Nursing, 22*(3), 31–38.

Skewes, S. (1997). Bathing: It's a tough job! *Journal of Gerontological Nursing, 23*(5), 45–49.

Stone, C. M. (1999). Preventing cerumen impaction in nursing facility residents. *Journal of Gerontological Nursing, 25*(5), 43–45.

Talerico, K. A., & Capezuti, E. (2001). Myths and facts about side rails. *American Journal of Nursing, 101*(7), 43–48.

Walton, J. C., Miller, J., & Tordecilla, L. (2001). Elder oral assessment and care. *MEDSURG Nursing, 10*(1), 37–44.

Wilkinson, J. M. (2000). *Nursing diagnosis handbook with NIC interventions and NOC outcomes* (7th ed.). Upper Saddle River, NJ: Prentice Hall Health.

Selected Bibliography

Cavendish, R. (1998). Clinical snapshot: Adult hearing loss. *American Journal of Nursing, 98*(8), 50–51.

Cavendish, R. (1999). Clinical snapshot: Periodontal disease. *American Journal of Nursing, 99*(3), 36–37.

Dempster, J. (1999). The advantages of the bag bath in resident hygiene care. *Canadian Nursing Home, 10*(2), 15–17.

Feldman, C. B. (1998). Caring for feet: Patients and nurse practitioners working together. *Nurse Practitioner Forum, 9*(2), 87–93.

Freeman, E. M. (1997). International perspectives on bathing. *Journal of Gerontological Nursing, 23*(5), 40–44.

Halpin-Landry, J. E., & Goldsmith, S. (1999). Feet first: Diabetes care. *American Journal of Nursing, 99*(2), 26–33.

McConnell, E. A. (1998). Clinical do's & don'ts. Communicating with a hearing-impaired patient. *Nursing, 28*(1), 31.

McConnell, E. A. (1998). Clinical do's & don'ts. Teaching a patient with diabetes how to protect her feet. *Nursing, 28*(12), 31.

McNeill, H. E. (2000). Biting back at poor oral hygiene. *Intensive and Critical Care Nursing, 16*(6), 367–372.

Rakow, P. L. (2000). Perspective on contact lenses. What lens is that new patient wearing? Identifying, inspecting, and verifying the parameters of rigid and soft contact lenses. *Journal of Ophthalmic Nursing and Technology, 19*(6), 304–310.

Ramponi, D. R. (2001). Eye on contact lens removal. *Nursing, 31*(8), 56–57.

Rawlins, C. A., & Trueman, I. W. (2001). Effective mouth care for seriously ill patients. *Professional Nurse, 16*(4), 1025–1028.

Roberts, S. S. (2001). Top ways to prevent dental problems. *Diabetes Forecast, 54*(4), 71–72.

Schwartz, M. (2000). The oral health of the long-term care patient. *Annals of Long Term Care, 8*(12), 41–46.

Sheppard, C. M., & Brenner, P. S. (2000). The effects of bathing and skin care practices on skin quality and satisfaction with an innovative product. *Journal of Gerontological Nursing, 26*(10), 36–45, 55–56.

Sommer, S. K., & Sommer, N. W. (2002). When your patient is hearing impaired. *RN, 65*(12), 28–32.

Whitmyer, C., Terezhalmy, G., Miller, D., & Hujer, M. (1998). Clinical evaluation of the efficacy and safety of an ultrasonic toothbrush system in an elderly patient population. *Geriatric Nursing, 19*(1), 29–33.

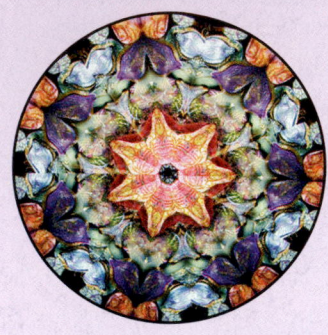

CHAPTER 32

DIAGNOSTIC TESTING

LEARNING OUTCOMES

After completing this chapter, you will be able to:

- Describe the nurse's role for each of the phases involved in diagnostic testing.

- List common blood tests.

- Accurately measure blood glucose from a capillary blood specimen using a blood glucose meter.

- Discuss the nursing responsibilities for specimen collection.

- Explain the rationale for the collection of each type of specimen.

- Collect and test stool specimens.

- Compare and contrast the different types of urine specimens.

- Collect sputum and throat specimens.

- Describe visualization procedures that may be used for the client with gastrointestinal, urinary, and cardiopulmonary alterations.

- Compare and contrast CT, MRI, and nuclear imaging studies.

- Describe the nurse's role in caring for clients undergoing aspiration/biopsy procedures.

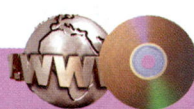

MediaLink

www.prenhall.com/kozier

Additional resources for this chapter can be found on the Student CD-ROM accompanying this textbook, and on the Companion Website at www.prenhall.com/kozier. Click on Chapter 32 to select the activities for this chapter.

CD-ROM
- Audio Glossary
- NCLEX Review
- Animation: PET and SPECT Scans

Companion Website
- Additional NCLEX Review
- Case Study: Checking Lab Results
- Care Plan Activity: Client Waiting for Diagnosis
- MediaLink Application: Diagnostic Tests
- Links to Resources

DIAGNOSTIC TESTING PHASES

Diagnostic and laboratory tests (commonly called lab tests) are tools that provide information about the client. Tests may be used as basic screening as part of a wellness check. Frequently tests are used to help confirm a diagnosis, monitor an illness, and provide valuable information about the client's response to treatment. Nurses need knowledge of the most common lab and diagnostic tests because one primary role of the nurse is to teach the client and family or significant other how to prepare for the test and the care that may be required following the test. Nurses must also know the implications of the test results in order to provide the most appropriate nursing care for the client.

Diagnostic testing occurs in many environments. The traditional sites include hospitals, clinics, and the physician's office. Many test sites, however, are moving to the community. Examples include the home, workplace, shopping malls, and mobile units. The more complex diagnostic tests are performed at diagnostic centers specifically built for those tests.

Diagnostic testing involves three phases: pretest, intratest, and post-test.

Pretest

The major focus of the pretest phase is client preparation. A thorough assessment and data collection (e.g., biologic, psychologic, sociologic, cultural, and spiritual) assist the nurse in determining communication and teaching strategies. Prior to radiologic studies it is important to ask female clients if pregnancy is possible. Special precautions may be necessary or the test may need to be postponed.

The nurse also needs to know what equipment and supplies are needed for the specific test. Common questions include these: What type of sample will be needed and how will it be collected? Does the client need to stop oral intake for a certain number of hours prior to the test? Does the test include administration of dye (contrast media) and, if so, is it injected or swallowed? Are fluids restricted or forced? Are medications given or withheld? How long is the test? Is a consent form required? Answers to these type of questions can help avoid costly mistakes and reduce inconvenience to all involved. Most facilities have information about the tests available to the health care team. The laboratory at the facility can also act as a resource for information.

Intratest

This phase focuses on specimen collection and performing or assisting with certain diagnostic testing. The nurse uses standard precautions and sterile technique as appropriate. During the procedure the nurse provides emotional and physical support while monitoring the client as needed (e.g., vital

---

Teaching: Client Care
Preparing for Diagnostic Testing

- Instruct the client and family about requirements or restrictions (e.g., when and what to eat or drink, how long to fast).
- Provide information about what the client may feel (e.g., a temporary flushing and feeling of warmth when the dye is injected).
- Ask the client if a description of pictures of the involved equipment would help prepare him or her for the test.

- Encourage questions about dialogue about fears and apprehensions. Find out what the client may have heard about the test from others.
- Inform the client of the time period before the results will be available.
- Document teaching. Include the client's response. Record names of audiovisual and reading materials, if used.

Note: From A Manual of Laboratory & Diagnostic Tests, 6th ed., by F. Fischbach, 2000, Philadelphia: Lippincott; and Nurses' Quick Reference to Common Laboratory and Diagnostic Tests, 3rd ed., by F. Fischbach, 2002, Philadelphia: Lippincott. Adapted with permission.

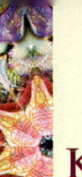

KEY TERMS

abdominal paracentesis, 774
angiography, 773
anoscopy, 773
arterial blood gases, 760
ascites, 774
aspiration, 774
biopsy, 774
blood chemistry, 760
blood urea nitrogen (BUN), 760
cannula, 774
clean-catch, 765
clean voided, 765
colonoscopy, 773
complete blood count (CBC), 758
computed tomography (CT), 773
creatinine, 760
cystoscope, 773
cystoscopy, 773
echocardiogram, 773
electrocardiogram (ECG), 773
electrocardiography, 773
expectorate, 771
guaiac test, 764
hematocrit, 758
hemoglobin, 758
hemoglobin A$_{1c}$, 760
hemoptysis, 771
intravenous pyelography (IVP), 773
kidneys/ureters/bladder (KUB), 773
leukocyte, 758
lumbar puncture, 774
lung scan, 773
magnetic resonance imaging (MRI), 774
manometer, 774
midstream urine specimen, 765
occult blood, 764
peak level, 760
phlebotomist, 758
polycythemia, 758
positron emission tomography (PET), 774
proctoscopy, 773
proctosigmoidoscopy, 773
radiopharmaceutical, 774
reagent, 770
red blood cell (RBC) indices, 758

signs, pulse oximetry, ECG). The nurse ensures correct labeling, storage, and transportation of the specimen to avoid invalid test results.

Post-Test

The focus of this phase is on nursing care of the client and follow-up activities and observations. As appropriate, the nurse compares the previous and current test results and modifies nursing interventions as needed. The nurse also reports the results to appropriate health team members.

Nursing Diagnoses

Nursing diagnoses are based on client data and need. Examples can include

- *Anxiety* or *Fear* related to possible diagnosis of acute or chronic illness pending conclusion of diagnostic testing
- *Impaired Physical Mobility* related to prescribed bedrest and restricted movement of involved extremity
- *Deficient Knowledge* (state diagnostic test) related to misperceptions received from others regarding process for test.

BLOOD TESTS

Blood tests are one of the most commonly used diagnostic tests and can provide valuable information about the hematologic system and many other body systems. A **venipuncture** (puncture of a vein for collection of a blood specimen) can be performed by various members of the health care team. Usually a **phlebotomist,** a person from a laboratory who performs venipuncture, collects the blood specimen for the tests ordered by the physician. In some institutions, nurses may also draw blood samples. The nurse needs to know the guidelines for drawing blood samples for the facility and also the state's nurse practice act.

Complete Blood Count

Specimens of venous blood are taken for a **complete blood count (CBC),** which includes hemoglobin and hematocrit measurements, erythrocyte (RBC) count, leukocyte (WBC) count, red blood cell (RBC) indices, and a differential white cell count. The CBC is a basic screening test and one of the most frequently ordered blood tests (see Table 32–1).

The **hemoglobin** is a measure of the total amount of hemoglobin in the blood. The **hematocrit** measures the percentage of red blood cells in the total blood volume. Normal values for both hemoglobin and hematocrit vary, with males having higher levels than females. Hemoglobin and hematocrit increase with dehydration as the blood becomes more concentrated, and decrease with hypervolemia and resulting hemodilution. Both the hemoglobin and hematocrit are related to the RBC count, the number of RBCs per cubic millimeter of whole blood. It also varies by gender and age. Low RBC counts are indicative of anemia. Clients with chronic hypoxia may develop higher than normal counts, a condition known as **polycythemia. Red blood cell (RBC) indices** may be performed as part of the CBC to evaluate the size, weight, and hemoglobin concentration of RBCs.

The **leukocyte** or **white blood cell (WBC)** count determines the number of circulating WBCs per cubic millimeter of whole blood. High WBC counts are often seen in the presence of a bacterial infection; by contrast, WBC counts may be low if a viral infection is present. In the WBC differential, leukocytes are identified by type, and the percentage of each type is determined. This information is useful in diagnosing certain disorders that have characteristic patterns of distribution.

Serum Electrolytes

Serum electrolytes are often routinely ordered for any client admitted to a hospital as a screening test for electrolyte and acid–base imbalances. Serum electrolytes also are routinely assessed for clients at risk in the community, for example, clients who are being treated with a diuretic for hypertension or heart failure. The most commonly ordered serum tests are for sodium, potassium,

TABLE 32–1 Complete Blood Count with Clinical Implications

Component	Normal Findings (Adult)	Possible Causes of Abnormal Findings	
		Increased	Decreased
Red blood cells count (RBC)	M: $4.7–6.1 \times 10^6$/mL^3 F: $4.2–5.4 \times 10^6$/mL^3	Dehydration Pulmonary fibrosis	Hemorrhage Anemia Pregnancy Dietary deficiency
Hemoglobin (Hgb)	M: 14–18 g/dL or 8.7–11.2 mmol/L F: 12–16 g/dL or 7.4–9.9 mmol/L	Polycythemia Dehydration Severe burns COPD	Hemorrhage Anemia Cancer Kidney disease Sickle cell anemia
Hematocrit (Hct)	M: 42–52% F: 37–47%	Polycythemia Dehydration Burns COPD	Hemorrhage Anemia Hyperthyroidism Dietary deficiency Pregnancy
Red blood cell indices (RBC indices)			
Mean corpuscular volume (MCV)	80–95 µm^3	Liver disease Alcoholism Pernicious anemia	Iron deficiency anemia
Mean corpuscular hemoglobin (MCH)	27–31 pg	Macrocytic anemia	Microcytic anemia Hypochromic anemia
Mean corpuscular hemoglobin concentration (MCHC)	32–36 g/dL	Intravascular hemolysis	Iron deficiency anemia
White blood cell count (WBC)	$5–10 \times 10^3$/mL^3	(Leukocytosis) Infection Inflammation Trauma	(Leukopenia) Autoimmune disease Drug toxicity Bone marrow failure
Differential count:			
Neutrophils	55–70%	Stress Acute infection	Aplastic anemia Dietary deficiency Radiation therapy
Lymphocytes	20–40%	Chronic infection Viral infection Mononucleosis	Leukemia Sepsis Immunodeficiency diseases
Monocytes	2–8%	Chronic inflammatory disorders Tuberculosis Chronic ulcerative colitis	Drug therapy: Prednisone
Eosinophils	1–4%	Parasitic infections Allergic reactions Leukemia	Increased adrenosteroid production
Basophils	0.5–1%	Leukemia	Acute allergic reaction Hyperthyroidism
Platelet count	$150–400 \times 10^3$/mL^3	Malignant disorder Polycythemia Rheumatoid arthritis Iron deficiency anemia	Hemorrhage Leukemia Pernicious anemia Hemolytic anemia Chemotherapy

Note: From *Diagnostic and Laboratory Test Reference*, 5th ed., by K. D. Pagana and T. J. Pagana, 2001, St. Louis, MO: Mosby. Reprinted with permission from Elsevier Science.

BOX 32–1	■ Normal Electrolyte Values for Adults*	
Venous blood		
Sodium	135–145 mEq/L	
Potassium	3.5–5.0 mEq/L	
Chloride	95–105 mEq/L	
Calcium (total)	4.5–5.5 mEq/L or 8.5–10.5 mg/dL	
(ionized)	56% of total calcium (2.5 mEq/L or 4.0–5.0 mg/dL)	
Magnesium	1.5–2.5 mEq/L or 1.6–2.5 mg/dL	
Phosphate (phosphorus)	1.8–2.6 mEq/L	
Serum osmolality	280–300 mOsm/kg water	

Normal laboratory values vary from agency to agency.

chloride, and bicarbonate ions. Normal values of commonly measured electrolytes are shown in Box 32–1.

Blood levels of two metabolically produced substances, urea and creatinine, are routinely used to evaluate renal function. The kidneys, through filtration and tubular secretion, normally eliminate both. Urea, the end product of protein metabolism, is measured as **blood urea nitrogen (BUN). Creatinine** is produced in relatively constant quantities by the muscles and is excreted by the kidneys. Thus, the amount of creatinine in the blood relates to renal excretory function.

Serum Osmolality

Serum osmolality is a measure of the solute concentration of the blood. The particles included are sodium ions, glucose, and urea (BUN). Serum osmolality can be estimated by doubling the serum sodium, because sodium and its associated chloride ions are the major determinants of serum osmolality. Serum osmolality values are used primarily to evaluate fluid balance. Normal values are 280 to 300 mOsm/kg. An increase in serum osmolality indicates a fluid volume deficit; a decrease reflects a fluid volume excess.

Drug Monitoring

Therapeutic drug monitoring is often conducted when a client is taking a medication with a narrow therapeutic range (e.g, digoxin, theophylline, aminoglycosides). This monitoring includes drawing blood samples for peak and trough levels to determine if the blood serum levels of a specific drug are at a therapeutic level and not a subtherapeutic or toxic level. The **peak level** indicates the highest concentration of the drug in the blood serum and the **trough level** represents the lowest concentration. Ideally, a client's peak and trough levels fall within the therapeutic range (Shirrell, Gibbar-Clements, Dooley, & Free, 1999).

Arterial Blood Gases

Measurement of **arterial blood gases** is another important diagnostic procedure (see Chapter 48). ⊕ Specialty nurses or medical technicians normally take specimens of arterial blood from the radial, brachial, or femoral arteries. Because of the relatively great pressure of the blood in these arteries, it is important to prevent hemorrhaging by applying pressure to the puncture side for about 5 to 10 minutes after removing the needle.

Blood Chemistry

A number of other tests may be performed on blood serum (the liquid portion of the blood). These are often are referred to as a **blood chemistry.** In addition to serum electrolytes, common chemistry examinations include determining certain enzymes that may be present (including lactic dehydrogenase [LDH], creatine kinase [CK], aspartate aminotransferase [AST], and alanine aminotransferase [ALT]), serum glucose, hormones such as thyroid hormone, and other substances such as cholesterol and triglycerides. These tests provide valuable diagnostic cues. For example, cardiac markers (e.g., CPK-MB, myoglobin, Troponin T, and Troponin I) are released into the blood during a myocardial infarction (MI, or heart attack). Elevated levels of these markers in the venous blood can help differentiate between an MI and chest pain from a different cause such as angina or pleuritic pain.

A common lab test is the glycosylated hemoglobin or **hemoglobin A_{1C}** (HbA$_{1C}$), which is a measurement of blood glucose that is bound to hemoglobin. Hemoglobin A_{1C} is a reflection of how well blood glucose levels have been controlled during the prior 3 to 4 months. An elevated HbA$_{1C}$ reflects hyperglycemia in diabetics.

Capillary Blood Glucose

A capillary blood specimen is often taken to measure blood glucose when frequent tests are required or when a venipuncture cannot be performed. This technique is less painful than a venipuncture and easily performed. Hence, clients can perform this technique on themselves.

The development of home glucose test kits and reagent strips has simplified the testing of blood glucose and greatly fa-

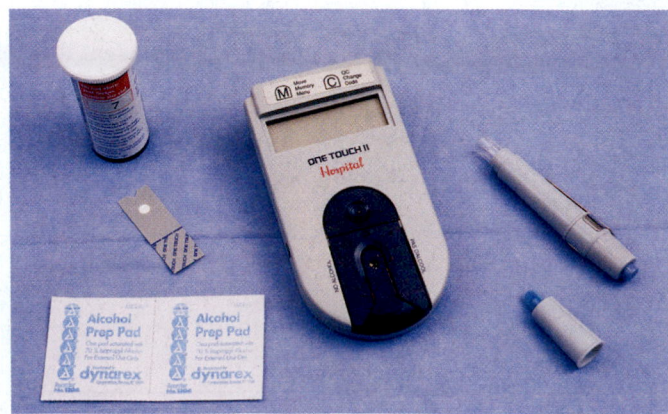

Figure 32–1 ■ Blood glucose monitor, test strips, and lancet injector.

cilitated the management of home care by diabetic clients. A number of manufacturers have developed blood glucose meters (Figure 32–1 ■). Most meters permit measurements between 20 and 600 mg/dL or 100 mL of blood. Meters differ and with the development of new technology, it is imperative that the nurse or client review the manufacturer's operating guidelines. Being familiar with the proper use of the equipment helps ensure accurate readings.

Capillary blood specimens are commonly obtained from the lateral aspect or side of the finger in adults. This site avoids the nerve endings and calloused areas at the fingertip. The earlobe may be used if the client is in shock or the fingers are edematous. Some newer monitors allow for obtaining specimens from areas on the arms and legs.

Procedure 32–1 describes how to obtain a capillary blood specimen and measure blood glucose using a portable meter.

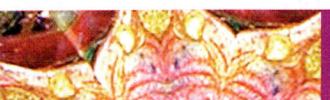

Procedure 32–1   Obtaining a Capillary Blood Specimen and Measuring Blood Glucose

Purposes

- To determine or monitor blood glucose levels of clients at risk for hyperglycemia or hypoglycemia
- To promote blood glucose regulation by the client
- To evaluate the effectiveness of insulin administration

ASSESSMENT

- Before obtaining a capillary blood specimen, determine
  - The frequency and type of testing
  - The client's understanding of the procedure
  - The client's response to previous testing.
- Assess the client's skin at the puncture site to determine if it is intact and the circulation is not compromised.

- Review the client's record for medications that may prolong bleeding such as anticoagulants.
- Assess the client's self-care abilities that may affect accuracy of test results, such as visual impairment and finger dexterity.

PLANNING

Delegation

Check the applicable nurse practice act and the facility policy and procedure manual to determine who can perform this skill. It is usually considered an invasive technique and one that requires problem solving and application of knowledge. It is the responsibility of the nurse to know the results of the test.

Equipment

- Blood glucose meter
- Blood glucose reagent strip compatible with the meter

- Paper towel
- Warm cloth or other warming device (optional)
- Antiseptic swab
- Disposable gloves
- Sterile lancet or #19 or #21-gauge needle
- Lancet injector (optional)
- Cotton ball to wipe the glucose reagent strip (dry wipe method)

IMPLEMENTATION

Preparation

Review the type of meter and manufacturer's instructions. Assemble the equipment at the bedside.

Performance

1. Explain to the client what you are going to do, why it is necessary, and how he or she can cooperate. Discuss how the results will be used in planning further care or treatments.
2. Wash hands and observe other appropriate infection control procedures (e.g., gloves).
3. Provide for client privacy.

4. Prepare the equipment.
   - Obtain a reagent strip from the container and place it on a clean, dry paper towel. *Moisture can change the strip, thereby altering the test results.*
   - Calibrate the meter and run a control sample according to the manufacturer's instructions.
5. Select and prepare the vascular puncture site.
   - Choose a vascular puncture site (e.g., the side of an adult's finger). Avoid sites beside bone. Wrap the finger first in a warm cloth for 30 to 60 seconds (optional), *or* hold a finger in a

dependent position and massage it toward the site. If the earlobe is used, rub it gently with a small piece of gauze. *These actions increase the blood flow to the area, ensure an adequate specimen, and reduce the need for a repeat puncture.*
   - Clean the site with the antiseptic swab and allow it to dry completely *because alcohol can affect accuracy.*
6. Obtain the blood specimen.
   - Put on gloves.
   - Place the injector, if used, against the site, and release the needle, thus permitting it to pierce the skin.

continued on page 762

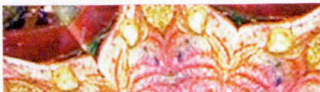

Procedure 32–1 Obtaining a Capillary Blood Specimen and Measuring Blood Glucose *continued*

IMPLEMENTATION *continued*

Make sure the lancet is perpendicular to the site. *The lancet is designed to pierce the skin at a specific depth when it is in a perpendicular position relative to the skin* (Figure 32–2 ■).

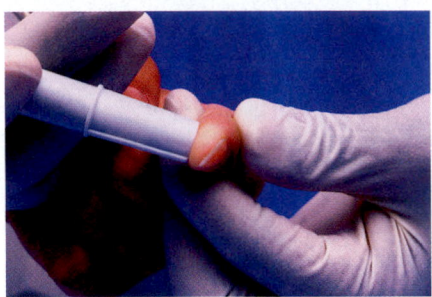

Figure 32–2 ■ Place the injector against the site.

or

- Prick the site with a lancet or needle, using a darting motion.
- Wipe away the first drop of blood with a cotton ball. *The first blood usually contains a greater proportion of serous fluid, which can alter test results.*
- Gently squeeze (but do not touch) the puncture site until a large drop of blood forms.
- Hold the reagent strip under the puncture site until enough blood covers the indicator square. The pad will absorb the blood and a chemical reaction will occur. Do not smear the blood. *This will cause an inaccurate reading* (Figure 32–3 ■).
- Ask the client to apply pressure to the skin puncture site with a cotton ball. *Pressure will assist hemostasis.*

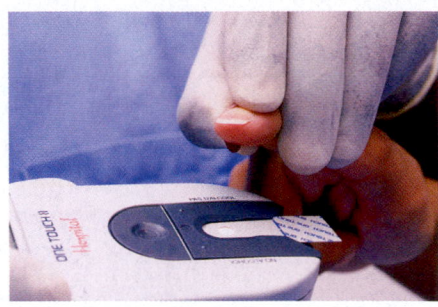

Figure 32–3 ■ Gently squeeze a large drop of blood onto the reagent strip.

7. Expose the blood to the test strip for the period and the manner specified by the manufacturer. As soon as the blood is placed on the test strip:
   - Follow the manufacturer's recommendations on the glucose meter and monitor for the amount of time indicated by the manufacturer (e.g., 60 seconds). *The blood must remain in contact with the test pad for a prescribed time to obtain accurate results.*
   - If indicated, lay the glucose strip on a paper towel or on the side of the timer. *The strip should be kept flat so that blood will not pool on only one part of the pad.*
8. Measure the blood glucose.
   - Place the strip into the meter according to the manufacturer's instructions. Some devices require that the strip be wiped or blotted after a designated period of time before being inserted in the meter. Other strips do not require blotting or wiping. Refer to the specific manufacturer's recommendations for the specific procedure.

- After the designated time most glucose meters will display the glucose reading automatically. Correct timing ensures accurate results (Figure 32–4 ■).
- Turn off the meter and discard the test strip and cotton balls.

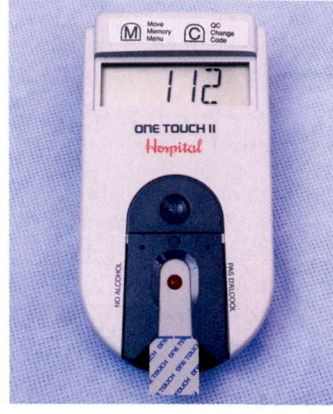

Figure 32–4 ■ The glucose meter will display the glucose reading.

9. Document the method of testing and results on the client's record. If appropriate, record the client's understanding and ability to demonstrate the technique. The client's record may also include a flowsheet on which capillary blood glucose results and the amount, type, route, and time of insulin administration are recorded.
10. Check for orders for sliding scale insulin based on capillary blood glucose results. Administer insulin as indicated.

EVALUATION

- Compare glucose meter reading with normal blood glucose level, status of puncture site, and motivation of the client to perform the test independently.
- Relate blood glucose reading to previous readings and the client's current health status.

- Report abnormal results to the physician.
- Conduct appropriate follow-up such as asking the client to explain the meaning of the results and/or demonstrating the procedure at the next scheduled test.

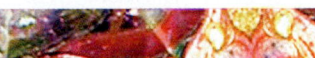

Lifespan Considerations

Capillary Blood Glucose

Infants
- The outer aspect of the heel is the most common site for neonates and infants. Placing a warm cloth on the infant's heel often increases the blood flow to the area.

Children
- Use a fingertip for a young client older than age 2, unless contraindicated.
- Allow the child to choose the puncture site, when possible.

- Praise the young client for cooperating and assure the child that the procedure is not a punishment.

Elders
- Elders may have arthritic joint changes, poor vision, or hand tremors and may need assistance using the glucose meter.
- Elders may have difficulty obtaining diabetic supplies due to financial concerns or homebound status.
- Elders often have poor circulation. Warming the hands by wrapping with a warm washcloth for 10 to 15 minutes may help in obtaining a blood sample.

Home Care Considerations

Capillary Blood Glucose

- Assess the client or caregiver's ability and willingness to perform blood glucose monitoring at home.
- Teach the proper use of the lancet and glucose monitor, and provide written guidelines. Allow time for a return demonstration. The client may need several visits to completely learn the procedure.
- Ensure the client's ability to obtain supplies and purchase reagent strips. The strips are relatively expensive and may not be covered by the client's insurance.

- Instruct the client on how to record the blood glucose levels and when to notify the health care provider.
- Diabetic children who need to perform finger sticks should be taught about safe practices for cleaning blood from surfaces (household bleach is best) and for safe storage of equipment to prevent young children from having access to it. Identify a place in the school where the child can store glucose-monitoring equipment and perform the procedure in private.

SPECIMEN COLLECTION

The nurse contributes to the assessment of a client's health status by collecting specimens of body fluids. All hospitalized clients have at least one laboratory specimen collected during their stay at the health care facility. Laboratory examination of specimens such as urine, blood, stool, sputum and wound drainage provides important adjunct information for diagnosing health care problems and also provides a measure of the responses to therapy.

Nurses often assume the responsibility for specimen collection. Depending on the type of specimen and skill required, the nurse may be able to delegate this task to unlicensed assistive personnel (UAP) under the supervision of the professional nurse.

Nursing responsibilities associated with specimen collection include the following:

- Provide client comfort, privacy, and safety. Clients may experience embarrassment or discomfort when providing a specimen. The nurse should provide the client with as much privacy as possible and handle the specimen discretely. The nurse needs to be nonjudgmental and sensitive to possible sociocultural beliefs that may affect the client's willingness to participate in the specimen collection.

- Explain the purpose of the specimen collection and the procedure for obtaining the specimen. Clients may experience anxiety about the procedure, especially if it is perceived as being intrusive or if they fear an unknown test result. A clear explanation will facilitate the client's cooperation in the collection of the specimen. With proper instruction, many clients are able to collect their own specimen, which promotes independence and reduces or avoids embarrassment.
- Use the correct procedure for obtaining a specimen or ensure that the client or staff follows the correct procedure. Aseptic technique is used in specimen collection to prevent contamination that can cause inaccurate test results. A nursing procedure or laboratory manual is often available if the nurse is unfamiliar with the procedure. If there is any question about the procedure, the nurse calls the laboratory for directions before collecting the specimen.
- Note relevant information on the laboratory requisition slip, for example, medications the client is taking that may affect the results.
- Transport the specimen to the laboratory promptly. Fresh specimens provide more accurate results.
- Report abnormal laboratory findings to the health care provider in a timely manner consistent with the severity of the abnormal results.

Stool Specimens

Analysis of stool specimens can provide information about a client's health condition. Some of the reasons for testing feces include the following:

- To determine the presence of **occult** (hidden) **blood.** Bleeding can occur as a result of ulcers, inflammatory disease, or tumors. The test for occult blood, often referred to as the **guaiac test,** can be readily performed by the nurse in the clinical area or by the client at home. Guaiac paper used in the test is sensitive to fecal blood content.
- To analyze for dietary products and digestive secretions. For example, an excessive amount of fat in the stool (**steatorrhea**) can indicate faulty absorption of fat from the small intestine. A decreased amount of bile can indicate obstruction of bile flow from the liver and gallbladder into the intestine. For these kinds of tests, the nurse needs to collect and send the total quantity of stool expelled at one time instead of a small sample.
- To detect the presence of ova and parasites. When collecting specimens for parasites, it is important that the sample be transported immediately to the lab while it is still warm. Usually three stool specimens are evaluated to confirm the presence of and to identify the organism so that appropriate treatment can be ordered (Kee, 1999).
- To detect the presence of bacteria or viruses. Only a small amount of feces is required because the specimen will be cultured. Collection containers or tubes must be sterile and aseptic technique used during collection. Stools need to be sent immediately to the laboratory. The nurse needs to note on the lab requisition if the client is receiving any antibiotics.

Collecting Stool Specimens

The nurse is responsible for collecting stool specimens ordered for laboratory analysis. Before obtaining a specimen, the nurse needs to determine the reason for collecting the stool specimen and the correct method of obtaining and handling (i.e., how much stool to obtain, whether a preservative needs to be added to the stool, and whether it needs to be sent immediately to the laboratory). It may be necessary to confirm this information by checking with the agency laboratory. In many situations only a single specimen is required; in others, timed specimens are necessary, and every stool passed is collected within a designated time period.

UAP may obtain and collect stool specimen(s). The nurse, however, needs to consider the collection process before delegating this task. For example, a random stool specimen collected in a specimen container may be delegated, but a stool culture requiring a sterile swab in a test tube should be done by the nurse. An incorrect collection technique can cause inaccurate test results.

The task of obtaining and testing a stool specimen for occult blood may be performed by UAP. It is important that the nurse instruct the UAP to tell the nurse if blood is detected and/or whether the test is positive. In addition, the stool specimen should be saved to allow the nurse to repeat the test.

Nurses need to give clients the following instructions:

- Defecate in a clean bedpan or bedside commode.
- Do not contaminate the specimen, if possible, with urine or menstrual discharge. Void before the specimen collection.
- Do not place toilet tissue in the bedpan after defecation. Contents of the paper can affect the laboratory analysis.
- Notify the nurse as soon as possible after defecation, particularly for specimens that need to be sent to the laboratory immediately.

When obtaining stool samples, that is, when handling the client's bedpan, when transferring the stool sample to a specimen container, and when disposing of the bedpan contents, the nurse follows medical aseptic technique meticulously. Wear disposable gloves to prevent hand contamination and take care not to contaminate the outside of the specimen container. Use one or two clean tongue blades to transfer the specimen to the container and then wrap them in a paper towel before disposing of them in the waste container. This practice reduces the chance of contact with other articles and the spread of microorganisms. The amount of stool to be sent depends on the purpose for which the specimen is collected. Usually about 2.5 cm (1 in.) of formed stool or 15 to 30 mL of liquid stool is adequate. For some timed specimens, however, the entire stool passed may need to be sent. Visible pus, mucus, or blood should be included in sample specimens. For a stool culture, the nurse dips a sterile swab into the specimen, preferably where purulent fecal matter is present and, using sterile technique, places the swab in a sterile test tube.

Ensure that the specimen label and the laboratory requisition have the correct information on them and are securely attached to the specimen container. Inappropriate identification of the specimen risks errors of diagnosis or therapy for the client.

Because fresh specimens provide the most accurate results, the nurse sends the specimen to the laboratory immediately. If this is not possible, the nurse follows the directions on the specimen container. In some instances refrigeration is indicated, because bacteriologic changes take place in stool specimens left at room temperature. To prevent contamination, never place a stool specimen in a refrigerator that contains food or medication.

Document all relevant information. Record the collection of the specimen on the client's chart and on the nursing care plan. Include in the recording the date and time of the collection and all nursing assessments (e.g., color, odor, consistency, and amount of feces); presence of abnormal constituents, such as blood or mucus; results of test for occult blood if obtained; discomfort during or after defecation; status of perianal skin; and any bleeding from the anus after defecation.

Testing Feces for Occult Blood

A commonly used test product to measure occult blood is the Hemoccult test, which uses a chemical reagent substance to detect the presence of the enzyme peroxidase in the hemoglobin molecule. To perform the test, the nurse or client uses a tongue blade to place a small amount of stool on a slide or card and then closes the card. The card is turned over and a few drops of

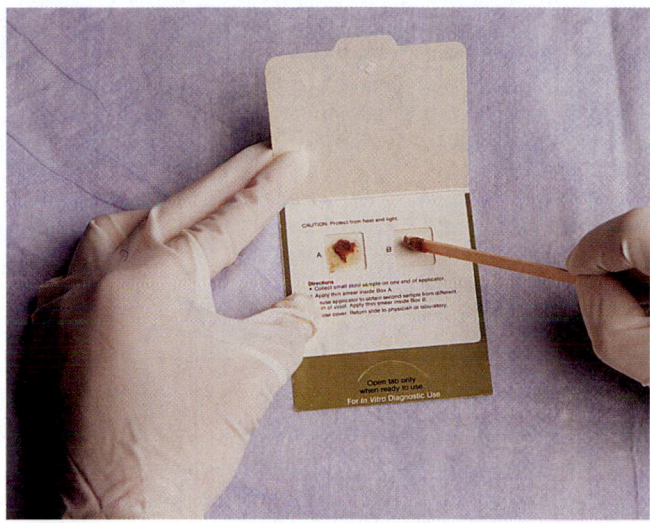

A

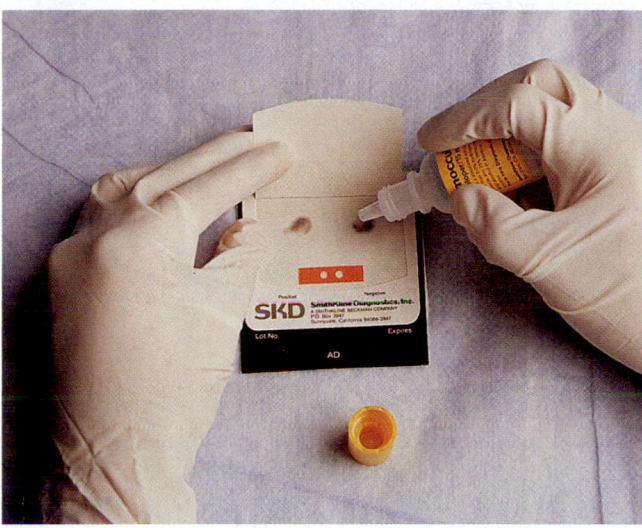

B

Figure 32–5 ■ A, Opening the front cover of a Hemoccult slide and applying a thin smear of feces on the slide. B, Opening the flap on the back of the slide and applying two drops of developing fluid over each smear.

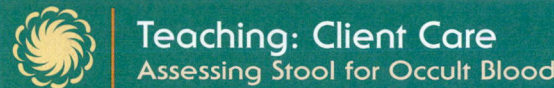

Teaching: Client Care
Assessing Stool for Occult Blood

- Avoid restricted foods, medications, and vitamin C for the period recommended by the manufacturer and during the test. Usually specified foods and vitamin C are restricted for 3 days before the test and specified medications for 7 days before the test.
- Use a ballpoint pen to label the specimens with your name, address, age, and date of specimen. Usually three specimens are collected from consecutive and different bowel movements. Each specimen must be dated accurately.
- Avoid collecting specimens during your menstrual period and for 3 days afterward, and while you have bleeding hemorrhoids or blood in your urine.
- Remove toilet bowl cleaners from the toilet bowl. Flush the toilet twice before proceeding with the test.
- Avoid contaminating the specimen with urine or toilet tissue. Empty your bladder before the test. To facilitate specimen collection, transfer the stool to a clean, dry container. Wear disposable gloves.
- Use the tongue blade provided to transfer the specimen to the test folder or tape. Only a small amount of stool is required. Take the sample from the center of a formed stool to ensure a uniform sample.
- Wrap the tongue blade in a paper towel and dispose of it in the waste receptacle. Do not flush the stick.
- Follow the manufacturer's directions explicitly for the test product being used. Test products vary. For example, for the Hemoccult test, a thin layer of feces is smeared over the boxes inside the envelope, and a drop of developing solution is applied on the opposite side of the specimen paper. For the Hematest, a thin layer of feces is smeared onto guaiac filter paper, a tablet is placed in the middle of the specimen, and two or three drops of water are added to the tablet. If there is space for two specimens in the test folder, take the sample from two different areas of the stool specimen.
- Consult your health care provider if there is any problem understanding the instructions.
- Return completed specimens to your physician or laboratory as instructed.

a reagent are placed onto the smear on the back of the card. The nurse then observes for a color change (Figure 32–5 ■). A blue color indicates a guaiac positive result, that is, the presence of occult blood. No color change or any color other than blue is a negative finding, indicating the absence of blood in the stool.

Certain foods, medications, and vitamin C can produce inaccurate test results. False-positive results can occur if the client has recently ingested (a) red meat (beef, lamb, liver, and processed meats); (b) raw vegetables or fruits, particularly radishes, turnips, horseradish, and melons; or (c) certain medications that irritate the gastric mucosa and cause bleeding, such as aspirin or other nonsteroidal anti-inflammatory drugs, steroids, iron preparations, and anticoagulants. False-negative results can occur if the client has taken more than 250 mg per day of vitamin C from all sources (dietary and supplemental) up to 3 days before the test—even if bleeding is present.

Guidelines for instructing clients to assess their stool for occult blood are listed in the Teaching: Client Care.

Urine Specimens

The nurse is responsible for collecting urine specimens for a number of tests: **clean voided** specimens for routine urinalysis, **clean-catch** or **midstream urine specimens** for urine culture, and timed urine specimens for a variety of tests that depend on the client's specific health problem. Urine specimen collection may require collection via straight catheter insertion. If this is necessary, refer to Chapter 47, Procedure 47–2. ⚭

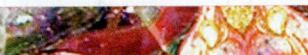

Lifespan Considerations

Stool Specimen

Infants
- To collect a stool specimen for an infant, the stool is scraped from the diaper.

Children
- A child who is toilet trained should be able to provide a fecal specimen, but may prefer being assisted by a parent.

- When explaining the procedure to the child, use words appropriate for the child's age rather than medical terms. Ask the parent what words the family normally uses to describe a bowel movement.

Elders
- Elders may need assistance if serial stool specimens are required.

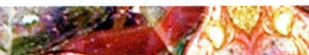

Home Care Considerations

Stool Specimen
- Ask the client or caregiver to call when the stool specimen is obtained. If a laboratory test is needed, the nurse can pick up the specimen or a family member may take it to the laboratory.

- Place the stool specimen inside a plastic biohazard bag. Carry the bag in a sealed container marked "biohazard" and take it to the laboratory promptly. Do not expose the specimen to extreme temperatures in the car.

Clean Voided Urine Specimen

A clean voided specimen is usually adequate for routine examination. Many clients are able to collect a clean voided specimen and provide the specimen independently with minimal instructions. Male clients generally are able to void directly into the specimen container, and female clients usually sit or squat over the toilet, holding the container between their legs during voiding. Routine urine examination is usually done on the first voided specimen in the morning because it tends to have a higher, more uniform concentration and a more acidic pH than specimens later in the day.

At least 10 mL of urine is generally sufficient for a routine urinalysis. Clients who are seriously ill, physically incapacitated, or disoriented may need to use a bedpan or urinal in bed; others may require supervision or assistance in the bathroom. Whatever the situation, clear and specific directions are required:

- The specimen must be free of fecal contamination, so urine must be kept separate from feces.
- Female clients should discard the toilet tissue in the toilet or in a waste bag rather than in the bedpan because tissue in the specimen makes laboratory analysis more difficult.
- Put the lid tightly on the container to prevent spillage of the urine and contamination of other objects.
- If the outside of the container has been contaminated by urine, clean it with a disinfectant.

The nurse must (a) make sure that the specimen label and the laboratory requisition carry the correct information and (b) attach them securely to the specimen. Inappropriate identification of the specimen can lead to errors of diagnosis or therapy for the client.

UAP may be assigned to collect a routine urine specimen. Provide the UAP with clear directions on how to instruct the client to collect his or her own urine specimen or how to cor-rectly collect the specimen for the client who may need to use a bedpan or urinal.

> **▶ CLINICAL ALERT** *Kidney function directly relates to cardiac output. Therefore, any health problem that changes cardiac output may affect urine output.*

Clean-Catch or Midstream Urine Specimen

Clean-catch or midstream voided specimens are collected when a urine culture is ordered to identify microorganisms causing urinary tract infection. Although some contamination by skin bacteria may occur with a clean-catch specimen, the risk of introducing microorganisms into the urinary tract through catheterization is more significant. Care is taken to ensure that the specimen is as free as possible from contamination by microorganisms around the urinary meatus. Clean-catch specimens are collected into a sterile specimen container with a lid. Disposable clean-catch kits are available (Figure 32–6 ■). Procedure 32–2 explains how to collect a clean-catch urine specimen for culture.

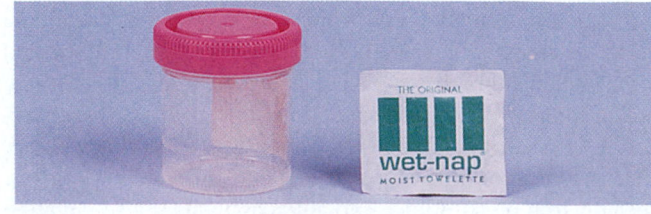

Figure 32–6 ■ Disposable clean-catch specimen equipment.

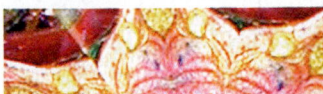

Procedure 32–2 Collecting a Urine Specimen for Culture and Sensitivity by Clean Catch

Purpose

- To determine the presence of microorganisms, the type of organism(s), and the antibiotics to which the organisms are sensitive

ASSESSMENT

- Determine the ability of the client to provide the specimen.
- Assess the color, odor, and consistency of the urine and the presence of clinical signs of urinary tract infection (e.g., frequency, urgency, dysuria, hematuria, flank pain, cloudy urine with foul odor).

PLANNING

Delegation

UAP may perform the collection of a clean-catch or midstream urine specimen. It is important, however, that the nurse inform the unlicensed person about how to instruct the client in the correct process for obtaining the specimen. Proper cleansing of the urethra should be emphasized to avoid contaminating the urine specimen.

Equipment

Equipment used varies from agency to agency. Some agencies use commercially prepared disposable clean-catch kits. Others are agency-prepared sterile trays. Both prepared trays and kits generally contain the following items:

- Clean gloves
- Antiseptic towelette, such as povidone-iodine
- Sterile cotton balls or 2 × 2 gauze pads
- Sterile specimen container
- Specimen identification label

In addition the nurse needs to obtain:

- Completed laboratory requisition form
- Urine receptacle, if the client is not ambulatory
- Basin of warm water, soap, washcloth, and towel for the nonambulatory client

IMPLEMENTATION

Preparation

Gather the necessary equipment needed for the collection of the specimen. Use visual aids, if available, to assist the client to understand the midstream collection technique.

Performance

1. Explain to the client that a urine specimen is required, give the reason, and explain the method to be used to collect it. Discuss how the results will be used in planning further care or treatments.
2. Wash hands and observe other appropriate infection control procedures.
3. Provide for client privacy.
4. For an ambulatory client who is able to follow directions, instruct the client on how to collect the specimen.
   - Direct or assist the client to the bathroom.
   - Ask the client to wash and dry the genitals and perineal area with soap and water. *Washing the perineal area reduces the number of skin and transient bacteria, decreasing the risk of contaminating the urine specimen.*
   - Instruct the client on how to clean the urinary meatus with antiseptic towelettes. *The antiseptic further re-*

duces bacterial contamination of the urinary meatus and the risk of contaminating the specimen.

FOR FEMALE CLIENTS

- Use each towelette only once. Clean the perineal area from front to back and discard the towelette. Use all towelettes provided (usually two or three). *Cleaning from front to back cleans the area of least contamination to the area of greatest contamination* (Figure 32–7 ■).

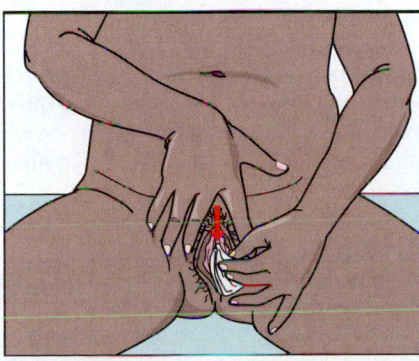

Figure 32–7 ■ Cleansing the female urinary meatus. Spread the labia minora with one hand and with the other hand, cleanse perineal area from front to back.

FOR MALE CLIENTS

- If uncircumcised, retract the foreskin slightly to expose the urinary meatus.
- Using a circular motion, clean the urinary meatus and the distal portion of the penis. Use each towelette only once, then discard. Clean several inches down the shaft of the penis. *This cleans from the area of least contamination to the area of greatest contamination* (Figure 32–8 ■).

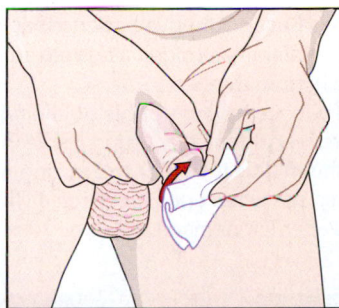

Figure 32–8 ■ Cleansing the male urinary meatus. Retract the foreskin if needed. Using a towelette, cleanse the urinary meatus by moving in a circular motion from the center of the urethral opening around the glans and down the distal portion of the shaft of the penis.

continued on page 768

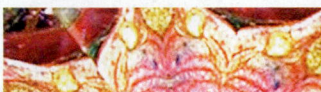

Procedure 32–2 Collecting a Urine Specimen for Culture and Sensitivity by Clean Catch *continued*

IMPLEMENTATION *continued*

5. For a client who requires assistance, prepare the client and equipment.
   - Wash the perineal area with soap and water, rinse, and dry.
   - Assist the client onto a clean commode or bedpan. If using a bedpan or urinal, position the client as upright as allowed or tolerated. *Assuming a normal anatomic position for voiding facilitates urination.*
   - Open the clean-catch kit, taking care not to contaminate the inside of the specimen container or lid. *It is important to maintain sterility of the specimen container to prevent contamination of the specimen.*
   - Put on clean gloves.
   - Clean the urinary meatus and perineal area as described in step 4.
6. Collect the specimen from a nonambulatory client or instruct an ambulatory client on how to collect it.

- Instruct the client to start voiding. *Bacteria in the distal urethra and at the urinary meatus are cleared by the first few milliliters of urine expelled.*
- Place the specimen container into the stream of urine and collect the specimen, taking care not to touch the container to the perineum or penis. *It is important to avoid contaminating the interior of the specimen container and the specimen itself.*
- Collect 30 to 60 mL of urine in the container.
- Cap the container tightly, touching only the outside of the container and the cap. *This prevents contamination or spilling of the specimen.*
- If necessary, clean the outside of the specimen container with disinfectant. *This prevents transfer of microorganisms to others.*
7. Label the specimen and transport it to the laboratory.

- Ensure that the specimen label and the laboratory requisition carry the correct information. Attach them securely to the specimen. *Inaccurate identification or information on the specimen container risks errors in diagnosis or therapy.*
- Arrange for the specimen to be sent to the laboratory immediately. *Bacterial cultures must be started immediately before any contaminating organisms can grow, multiply, and produce false results.*
8. Document pertinent data.
   - Record collection of the specimen, any pertinent observations of the urine such as color, odor, or consistency, and any difficulty in voiding that the client experienced.
   - Indicate on the lab slip if the client is taking any current antibiotic therapy or if the client is menstruating.

EVALUATION

- Report lab results to the physician.
- Discuss findings of the laboratory test with physician and client.
- Conduct appropriate follow-up nursing interventions as needed, such as administering ordered medications and client teaching.

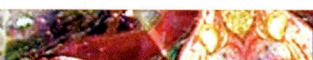

Lifespan Considerations

Urine Specimen

Infants
- The process for cleaning the perineal area and the urethral opening is similar to the process for an adult. A specimen bag, however, is used to collect the urine specimen. The specimen bag has an adhesive backing that attaches to the skin. After the infant has voided a desired amount, gently remove the bag from the skin.
- If you are having trouble obtaining a bagged urine specimen from an infant, try cutting a hole in the diaper (front for a boy and middle for a girl) and pulling part of the bag through. You can see when urine is collected without having to untape the diaper. (Lindemann, 2000).

Children
- When collecting a routine urine specimen, explain the procedure in simple nonmedical terms to the child and ask the child to void using a potty chair or a bedpan placed inside the toilet.
- Give the child a clean specimen container to play with.
- Allow a parent to assist the child, if possible. The child may feel more comfortable with a parent present.

Elders
- For a clean-catch urine specimen, Elders may have difficulty controlling the stream of urine.
- Elder women with arthritis may have difficulty holding the labia apart during the collection of clean-catch urine.

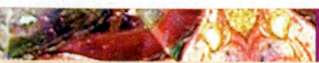

Home Care Considerations

Urine Specimen
- Assess the client's ability and willingness to collect a timed urine specimen. If poor eyesight or hand tremors are a problem, suggest using a clean funnel to pour the urine into the container.
- Always wash hands well with warm, soapy water before and after collecting urine samples.
- Always wear gloves if handling another person's urine.

The home should have a refrigerator or other method for cooling the urine samples. Tell the client to keep the specimen container in a plastic or paper bag in the refrigerator, separate from other refrigerator contents. The client may also use a cooler with ice.

Timed Urine Specimen

Some urine examinations require collection of all urine produced and voided over a specific period of time, ranging from 1 to 2 hours to 24 hours. Timed specimens generally either are refrigerated or contain a preservative to prevent bacterial growth or decomposition of urine components. Each voiding of urine is collected in a small, clean container and then emptied immediately into the large refrigerated bottle or carton.

Some of the tests performed on timed urine specimens include the following purposes:

- To assess the ability of the kidney to concentrate and dilute urine
- To determine disorders of glucose metabolism, for example, diabetes mellitus
- To determine levels of specific constituents, for example, albumin, amylase, creatinine, urobilinogen, certain hormones (e.g., estriol or corticosteroids) in the urine.

To collect a timed urine specimen, follow these steps:

- Obtain a specimen container with preservative (if indicated) from the laboratory. Label the container with identifying information for the client, the test to be performed, time started, and time of completion.
- Provide a clean receptacle to collect urine (bedpan, commode, or toilet collection device).
- Post signs in the client's chart, Kardex, room, and bathroom alerting personnel to save all urine during the specified time.
- At the start of the collection period, have the client void and discard this urine.
- Save all urine produced during the timed collection period in the container, refrigerating or placing the container on ice as indicated. Avoid contaminating the urine with toilet paper or feces.
- At the end of the collection period, instruct the client to completely empty the bladder and save this voiding as part of the specimen. Take the entire amount of urine collected to the laboratory with the completed requisition.
- Record collection of the specimen, time started and completed, and any pertinent observations of the urine on appropriate records.

> **► CLINICAL ALERT** *If the client or staff forgets and discards the client's urine during a timed collection, the procedure must be restarted from the beginning.*

Indwelling Catheter Specimen

Sterile urine specimens can be obtained from closed drainage systems by inserting a sterile needle attached to a syringe through a drainage port in the tubing. Aspiration of urine from catheters can be done only with self-sealing rubber catheters—not plastic, silicone, or Silastic catheters. When self-sealing rubber catheters are used, the needle is inserted just above the location where the catheter is attached to the drainage tubing. The area from which to obtain urine may be marked by a patch on the catheter (see Figure 32–9 ■).

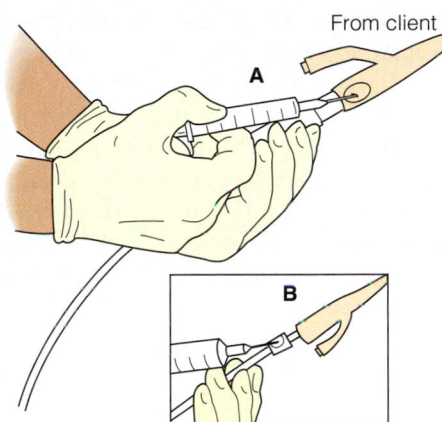

Figure 32–9 ■ Obtaining a urine specimen from a retention catheter. A, From a specific area near the end of the catheter; B, from an access port in the tubing.

To collect a specimen from a Foley (retention) catheter or a drainage tube, follow these steps:

- Put on disposable gloves.
- If there is no urine in the catheter, clamp the drainage tubing for about 30 minutes. This allows fresh urine to collect in the catheter.
- Wipe the area where the needle will be inserted with a disinfectant swab. The site should be distal to the tube leading to the balloon to avoid puncturing this tube. Disinfecting the needle insertion site removes any microorganisms on the surface of the catheter, thereby avoiding contamination of the needle and the entrance of microorganisms into the catheter.
- Insert the needle at a 30- to 45-degree angle (Figure 32–9). This angle of entrance facilitates self-sealing of the rubber.
- Unclamp the catheter.
- Withdraw the required amount of urine, for example, 3 mL for a urine culture or 30 mL for a routine urinalysis.
- Transfer the urine to the specimen container. If a sterile culture tube is used, make sure the needle does not touch the outside of the container.
- Without recapping the needle, discard the syringe and needle in an appropriate sharps container.
- Cap the container.
- Remove gloves and discard appropriately.
- Label the container, and send the urine to the laboratory immediately for analysis or refrigeration.
- Record collection of the specimen and any pertinent observations of the urine on the appropriate records.
- Note that this procedure can be followed if needleless port systems are being used.

Urine Testing

Several simple urine tests are often done by nurses on the nursing units. These include tests for specific gravity, pH, and the presence of abnormal constituents such as glucose, ketones, protein, and occult blood.

Nurses in a health care facility or clients in the home setting can use many commercially prepared kits to test abnormal constituents in the urine. These kits contain the required equipment and an appropriate **reagent** (substance used in a chemical reaction to detect a specific substance). Reagents may be in the form of a tablet, fluid, or paper test strips or dipsticks. When the urine contacts the reagent a chemical reaction occurs, causing a color change that is then compared with a chart to interpret the significance of the color (Figure 32–10 ■). Specific directions for the amount of urine needed, the time required for the chemical reaction, and the meaning of the colors produced vary among manufacturers. Thus it is essential that nurses and clients read and follow directions supplied by each manufacturer. In addition, testing materials need to be checked to ascertain that they are not outdated.

Urine testing may be performed by UAP. It is important that the UAP understands the specific specimen collection procedure and reports the results of the test to the nurse. Inform the UAP to save the urine sample to allow the nurse to repeat the test if necessary.

SPECIFIC GRAVITY. **Specific gravity** is an indicator of urine concentration, or the amount of solutes (metabolic wastes and electrolytes) present in the urine. A *urinometer* or *hydrometer* in a cylinder of urine (Figure 32–11 ■) or a *spectrometer* or *refractometer* is used to measure the specific gravity. The specific gravity of distilled water is 1.00; the specific gravity of urine normally ranges from 1.010 to 1.025. As urine becomes more concentrated, its specific gravity increases. Excess fluid intake or diseases affecting the ability of the kidneys to concentrate urine can result in low specific gravity readings. A high specific gravity may indicate fluid deficit or dehydration, or excess solutes such as glucose in the urine. Steps to measure specific gravity are outlined in the accompanying Practice Guidelines.

URINARY PH. Urinary pH is measured to determine the relative acidity or alkalinity of urine and assess the client's acid–base status. Quantitative measurements of urine pH can be performed in the laboratory, but dipsticks or litmus paper often are used on nursing units or in clinics to obtain less precise pH measurements. Urine normally is slightly acidic, with an aver-

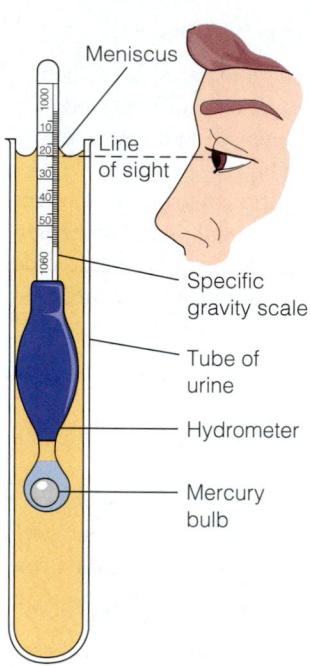

Figure 32–11 ■ A urinometer measurement of the specific gravity of the urine is taken at the base of the meniscus.

Practice Guidelines
Measuring Specific Gravity of Urine

To measure with a urinometer:
- Put on gloves and pour at least 20 mL of a fresh urine sample in the glass cylinder, or fill the cylinder three-quarters full.
- Place the urinometer into the cylinder and give it a gentle spin to prevent it from adhering to the sides of the cylinder.
- Hold the urinometer at eye level and read the measurement at the base of the meniscus at the surface of the urine (Figure 32–11). The concentration of the urine affects the degree to which the urinometer will float. The depth to which it sinks indicates the specific gravity.

To measure with a spectrometer or refractometer:
- Be sure to follow the manufacturer's directions.
- Put on gloves, and place one or two drops of urine on the slide.
- Turn on the instrument light, and look into the instrument. The specific gravity will appear on a scope.
- Write down the number, then turn off the instrument.
- Remove the urine with a damp towel or gauze.

Following the test:
- Discard the urine. Clean the equipment with soap and water. Remove gloves.
- Document the results of the test on the client's record.

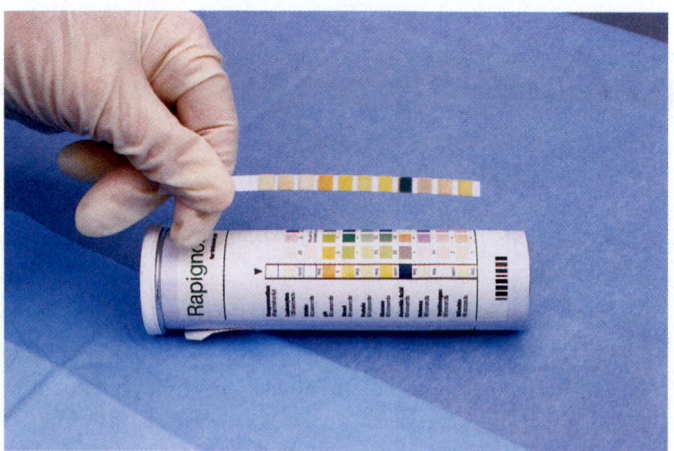

Figure 32–10 ■ After dipping the reagent strip into fresh urine, wait the stated time period and compare the results to the color chart.

age pH of 6 (7 is neutral, less than 7 is acidic, greater than 7 is alkaline). Because the kidneys play a critical role in regulating acid–base balance, assessment of urine pH can be useful in determining whether the kidneys are responding appropriately to acid–base imbalances. In metabolic acidosis, urine pH should decrease as the kidneys excrete hydrogen ions; in metabolic alkalosis, the pH should increase (see Chapter 50).

GLUCOSE. Urine is tested for glucose to screen clients for diabetes mellitus and to assess clients during pregnancy for abnormal glucose tolerance. Normally, the amount of glucose in the urine is negligible, although individuals who have ingested large amounts of sugar may show small amounts of glucose in their urine.

Testing urine for glucose is not a measure of current blood glucose level and is considered an inadequate measurement. The American Diabetes Association (2000, p. 66) states that testing urine for glucose is *only* for people who *cannot or will not* test their blood glucose levels. It is important for clients to understand that urine testing is considered an inadequate measurement of blood glucose.

KETONES. Ketone bodies, a product of the breakdown of fatty acids, normally are not present in the urine. They may, however, be found in the urine of clients with poorly controlled diabetes. Urine testing for ketone level is advised for Type I diabetics who are at home and not feeling well, running a fever, or their blood glucose is consistently over 240 mg/dL (American Diabetes Association, 2000). Urine ketone testing with reagent tablets or a dipstick is also used to evaluate ketoacidosis in clients who are alcoholic, fasting, starving, or consuming high-protein diets.

PROTEIN. Protein molecules normally are too large to escape from glomerular capillaries into the filtrate. If the glomerular membrane has been damaged, however (e.g., because of an inflammatory process such as glomerulonephritis), it can become "leaky," allowing proteins to escape. Urine testing for the presence of protein generally is done with a reagent strip (commonly referred to as a *dipstick*).

OCCULT BLOOD. Normal urine is free from blood. When blood is present, it may be clearly visible or not visible (occult). Commercial reagent strips are used to test for occult blood in the urine.

> **CLINICAL ALERT** *The appearance of blood in the urine is one of the early indications of renal disease. Check again using a freshly collected specimen (Fischbach, 2002, p. 708).*

OSMOLALITY. **Urine osmolality** is a measure of the solute concentration of urine that is a more exact measurement of urine concentration than specific gravity. It is also used to monitor fluid and electrolyte balance. The particles included are nitrogenous wastes, such as creatinine, urea, and uric acid. Normal values are 500 to 800 mOsm/kg. An increased urine osmolality indicates a fluid volume deficit; a decreased urine osmolality reflects a fluid volume excess. This test is sent to the laboratory rather than being tested at the bedside like the previous tests.

Sputum Specimens

Sputum is the mucous secretion from the lungs, bronchi, and trachea. It is important to differentiate it from **saliva,** the clear liquid secreted by the salivary glands in the mouth, sometimes referred to as "spit." Healthy individuals do not produce sputum. Clients need to cough to bring sputum up from the lungs, bronchi, and trachea into the mouth in order to expectorate it into a collecting container.

A UAP can obtain a sputum specimen that is expectorated by a client. It is important to instruct the UAP on when to collect the specimen, how to position the client, and how to correctly collect the specimen. Obtaining a sputum specimen by use of pharyngeal suctioning, however, should be performed by the nurse because it is an invasive, sterile process and requires knowledge application and problem solving. A "sputum trap" is used when the specimen is obtained by suctioning. See Chapter 48, Procedure 48–3. ∞

Sputum specimens are usually collected for one or more of the following reasons:

- For culture and sensitivity to identify a specific microorganism and its drug sensitivities.
- For cytology to identify the origin, structure, function, and pathology of cells. Specimens for cytology often require serial collection of three early-morning specimens and are tested to identify cancer in the lung and its specific cell type.
- For acid-fast bacillus (AFB), which also requires serial collection, often for 3 consecutive days, to identify the presence of tuberculosis (TB). Some agencies use a special glass container when the presence of AFB is suspected.
- To assess the effectiveness of therapy.

Sputum specimens are often collected in the morning. Upon awakening, the client can cough up the secretions that have accumulated during the night. Sometimes specimens are collected during postural drainage, when the client can usually produce sputum. When a client cannot cough, the nurse must sometimes use pharyngeal suctioning to obtain a specimen.

To collect a sputum specimen, the nurse follows these steps:

- Offer mouth care so that the specimen will not be contaminated with microorganisms from the mouth.
- Ask the client to breathe deeply and then cough up 1 to 2 tablespoons, or 15 to 30 mL (4 to 8 fluid drams), of sputum.
- Wear gloves to avoid direct contact with the sputum. Follow special precautions if tuberculosis is suspected, obtaining the specimen in a room equipped with a special airflow system or ultraviolet light, or outdoors. If these options are not available, wear a mask capable of filtering droplet nuclei.
- Ask the client to **expectorate** (spit out) the sputum into the specimen container. Make sure the sputum does not contact the outside of the container (Figure 32–12 ■). If the outside of the container does become contaminated, wash it with a disinfectant.
- Following sputum collection, offer mouthwash to remove any unpleasant taste.
- Label and transport the specimen to the laboratory. Ensure that the specimen label and the laboratory requisition contain the correct information. Arrange for the specimen to be sent to the laboratory immediately or refrigerated. Bacterial cultures must be started immediately before any contaminating organisms can grow, multiply, and produce false results.
- Document the collection of the sputum specimen on the client's chart. Include the amount, color, odor, consistency (thick, tenacious, watery), presence of **hemoptysis** (blood in

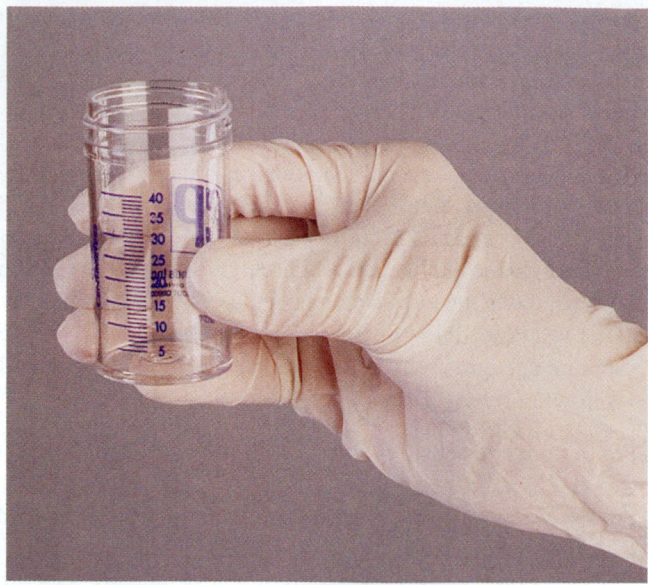

Figure 32–12 ■ Sputum specimen container.

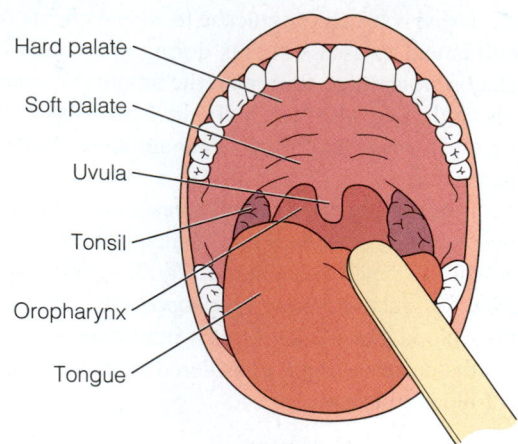

Figure 32–13 ■ Depressing the tongue to view the pharynx.

Labels on Figure 32–13: Hard palate, Soft palate, Uvula, Tonsil, Oropharynx, Tongue

the sputum), odor of the sputum, any measures needed to obtain the specimen (e.g., postural drainage), and any discomfort experienced by the client.

Throat Culture

A throat culture sample is collected from the mucosa of the oropharynx and tonsillar regions using a culture swab. The sample is then cultured and examined for the presence of disease-producing microorganisms. Obtaining a throat culture is an invasive procedure that requires the application of scientific knowledge and potential problem solving to ensure client safety. Thus, it is best for the nurse to perform this procedure.

To obtain a throat culture specimen, the nurse puts on clean gloves, then inserts the swab into the oropharynx and runs the swab along the tonsils and areas on the pharynx that are reddened or contain exudate. The gag reflex, active in some clients, may be decreased by having the client sit upright if health permits, open the mouth, extend the tongue, and say "ah," and by taking the specimen quickly. The sitting position and extension of the tongue help expose the pharynx; saying "ah" relaxes the throat muscles and helps minimize contraction of the constrictor muscle of the pharynx (the gag reflex). If the posterior pharynx cannot be seen, use a light and depress the tongue with a tongue blade (see Figure 32–13 ■).

Lifespan Consideration

Sputum and Throat Specimens

Infants
- Avoid occluding an infant's nose because infants normally breathe only through the nose.

Children
- The young child will need to be restrained gently while the throat specimen is collected. Allow the parents to assist and explain that the procedure will be over quickly.
- Cooperative children can be asked to put their hands under their buttocks, open their mouth, and laugh or pant like a dog (Bindler & Ball, 2003).

- Observe for signs of an ear infection (e.g., rubbing the ears). A child's short respiratory tract allows bacteria to migrate easily to the ears.

Elders
- Elders may need encouragement to cough because a decreased cough reflex occurs with aging.
- Allow time for elders to rest and recover between coughs when obtaining a sputum specimen.

Home Care Considerations

Specimen Collection
- If specimen collection is done on an outpatient basis or in the home, the nurse teaches the client how to obtain the specimens. Provide written instructions and specimen containers to ensure correct and safe performance of the procedure.
- Ensure that the laboratory knows where to send the test results.

VISUALIZATION PROCEDURES

Visualization procedures include *indirect visualization* (noninvasive) and *direct visualization* (invasive) techniques for visualizing body organ and system functions.

Clients with Gastrointestinal Alterations

Direct visualization techniques include **anoscopy,** the viewing of the anal canal; **proctoscopy,** the viewing of the rectum; **proctosigmoidoscopy,** the viewing of the rectum and sigmoid colon; and **colonoscopy,** the viewing of the large intestine. Indirect visualization of the gastrointestinal tract is achieved by roentgenography. X-rays of the gastrointestinal tract can detect strictures, obstructions, tumors, ulcers, inflammatory disease, or other structural changes such as hiatal hernias. Visualization of the tract is enhanced by the introduction of a radiopaque substance such as barium. For examination of the upper gastrointestinal tract or small bowel, the client drinks the barium sulfate. This examination is often referred to as a *barium swallow.* For examination of the lower gastrointestinal tract, the client is given an enema containing the barium. This examination is commonly referred to as a *barium enema.* These x-rays usually include fluoroscopic examination; that is, projection of the x-ray films onto a screen, which permits continuous observation of the flow of barium.

Clients with Urinary Alterations

Visualization procedures also may be used to evaluate urinary function. An x-ray of the **kidneys/ureters/bladder** is commonly referred to as a **KUB. Intravenous pyelography (IVP)** and **retrograde pyelography** also are radiographic studies used to evaluate the urinary tract. In an intravenous pyelogram, contrast medium is injected intravenously; during retrograde pyelography, the contrast medium is instilled directly into the kidney pelvis via the urethra, bladder, and ureters. Following injection or instillation of the contrast medium, x-rays are taken to evaluate urinary tract structures. Renal **ultrasonography** is a noninvasive test that uses reflected sound waves to visualize the kidneys. During a **cystoscopy,** the bladder, ureteral orifices, and urethra can be directly visualized using a **cystoscope,** a lighted instrument inserted through the urethra. Nurses are responsible for preparing clients before these studies and for follow-up care.

Clients with Cardiopulmonary Alterations

A number of visualization procedures can be done to examine the cardiovascular system and respiratory tract.

Electrocardiography provides a graphic recording of the heart's electrical activity. Electrodes placed on the skin transmit the electrical impulses to an oscilloscope or graphic recorder. With the wave forms recorded, the **electrocardiogram** or **ECG,** can then be examined to detect dysrhythmias and alterations in conduction indicative of myocardial damage, enlargement of the heart, or drug effects.

Stress electrocardiography uses ECGs to assess the client's response to an increased cardiac workload during exercise. As the body's demand for oxygen increases with exercising, the cardiac workload increases, as does the oxygen demand of the heart muscle itself. Clients with coronary artery disease may develop chest pain and characteristic ECG changes during exercise.

Angiography is an invasive procedure requiring informed consent of the client. A radiopaque dye is injected into the vessels to be examined. Using fluoroscopy and x-rays, the flow through the vessels is assessed and areas of narrowing or blockage can be observed. Coronary angiography is performed to evaluate the extent of coronary artery disease; pulmonary angiography may be performed to assess the pulmonary vascular system, particularly if pulmonary emboli are suspected. Other vessels that may be studied include the carotid and cerebral arteries, the renal arteries, and the vessels of the lower extremities.

An **echocardiogram** is a noninvasive test that uses ultrasound to visualize structures of the heart and evaluate left ventricular function. Images are produced as ultrasound waves reflect back to a transducer after striking cardiac structures. The nurse should tell the client that this test causes no discomfort, although the conductive gel used may be cold.

X-ray examination of the chest is done both to diagnose disease and to assess the progress of a disease. For an x-ray examination, the nurse needs to inform the client that jewelry and clothing from the waist up must be removed.

A **lung scan,** also known as a V/Q [ventilation/perfusion] scan, records the emissions from radioisotopes that indicate how well gas and blood are traveling through the lungs. The *perfusion scan* (Q scan—P usually stands for "pulmonary", so apparently the next letter in the alphabet was used for "perfusion.") is used to assess blood flow through the pulmonary vascular system. For this, the radioisotope is injected intravenously and measured as it circulates through the lung. The *ventilation scan* (V scan) detects ventilation abnormalities, particularly in clients with emphysema. For this scan, the client inhales a radioactive gas through a mask and then exhales it into room air. The client needs to be informed that no radiation precautions are necessary because as the amount of radioactivity is very small. The scan may take 20 to 40 minutes.

Laryngoscopy and bronchoscopy are sterile procedures that are conducted with a laryngoscope and bronchoscope, respectively. Tissue samples may also be taken for biopsy. A local anesthetic is usually given before the examination. A local anesthetic is sprayed on the client's pharynx to prevent gagging; alternatively, the client gargles with an anesthetic to anesthetize the throat. The bronchoscope is then inserted to visualize the larynx or bronchi. Informed consent is required for these procedures.

Computed Tomography

Computed tomography (CT), also called *CT scanning, computerized tomography,* or *computerized axial tomography (CAT),* is a painless, noninvasive x-ray procedure that has the unique capability of distinguishing minor differences in the density of tissues. The CT produces a three-dimensional image of the organ or structure making it more sensitive than the x-ray machine.

Magnetic Resonance Imaging

Magnetic resonance imaging (MRI) is a noninvasive diagnostic scanning technique in which the client is placed in a magnetic field. Clients with implanted metal devices (e.g., pacemaker, metal hip prosthesis) cannot undergo an MRI because of the strong magnetic field. There is no exposure to radiation. If a contrast media is injected during the procedure, it is not an iodine contrast. Another advantage to the MRI is that it provides a better contrast between normal and abnormal tissue than the CT scan. It is, however, more costly.

The MRI is commonly used for visualization of the brain, spine, limbs and joints, heart, blood vessels, abdomen, and pelvis. The procedure involves the client lying on a platform that moves into either a narrow, closed, high-magnet scanner, or into an open, low-magnet scanner. The client must lie very still. A two-way communication system is used to monitor the client's response and to help relieve feelings of claustrophobia. Earplugs are offered to the client to reduce the discomfort from the loud noises that occur during the test. The procedure lasts between 60 and 90 minutes.

Nuclear Imaging Studies

Fischbach (2000, p. 689) states that nuclear scans study the "physiology or function" of an organ system in contrast to other studies (e.g., CT, MRI, x-ray) which visualize "anatomic" structures. A **radiopharmaceutical,** a pharmaceutical (targeted to a specific organ) labeled with a radioisotope, is administered through various routes for the test. Clients retain the radioisotope for a relatively short time with the most common radiopharmaceutical having a half-life of 6 hours (Fischbach, 2002). A gamma camera is placed over the part of the body under study. The camera, which is networked with a computer, converts the emission of the radioisotope and forms a detailed image. An equal distribution of color is normal, however, darker spots ("hot" spots) indicate hyperfunction and lighter areas ("cold" spots) indicate hypofunction (Kee, 1999). **Positron emission tomography (PET)** is a noninvasive radiologic study that involves the injection or inhalation of a radioisotope. Images are created as the radioisotope is distributed in the body. This allows study of various aspects of organ function and may include evaluation of blood flow and tumor growth, for example.

ASPIRATION/BIOPSY

Aspiration is the withdrawal of fluid that has abnormally collected (e.g., pleural cavity, abdominal cavity) or to obtain a specimen (e.g., cerebral spinal fluid). A **biopsy** is the removal and examination of tissue. Usually the biopsy is performed to determine a diagnosis or to detect malignancy. Both aspiration and biopsy are invasive procedures and require strict sterile technique.

Lumbar Puncture

In a **lumbar puncture** (LP, or spinal tap), cerebrospinal fluid (CSF) is withdrawn through a needle (Figure 32–14 ■) inserted into the subarachnoid space of the spinal canal between the third and fourth lumbar vertebrae or between the fourth and fifth lumbar vertebrae. At this level the needle avoids damaging the spinal cord and major nerve roots (Figure 32–15 ■). The client is positioned laterally with the head bent toward the chest, the knees flexed onto the abdomen, and the back at the edge of the bed or examining table (Figure 32–16 ■). In this position the back is arched, increasing the spaces between the vertebrae so that the spinal needle can be inserted readily. During a lumbar puncture, the physician frequently takes CSF pressure readings using a **manometer,** a glass or plastic tube calibrated in millimeters (Figure 32–17 ■).

Abdominal Paracentesis

Normally the body creates just enough peritoneal fluid for lubrication. The fluid is continuously formed and absorbed into the lymphatic system. However, in some disease processes, a large amount of fluid accumulates in the abdominal cavity; this condition is called **ascites.** Normal ascitic fluid is serous, clear, and light yellow in color. An **abdominal paracentesis** is carried out to obtain a fluid specimen for laboratory study and to relieve pressure on the abdominal organs due to the presence of excess fluid.

A physician performs the procedure with the assistance of a nurse. Strict sterile technique is followed. A common site for abdominal paracentesis is midway between the umbilicus and the symphysis pubis on the midline (Figure 32–18 ■). The physician makes a small incision with a scalpel, inserts the **trocar** (a sharp, pointed instrument) and **cannula** (tube), and then withdraws the trocar, which is inside the cannula (Figure 32–19 ■). Tubing is attached to the cannula and the fluid flows

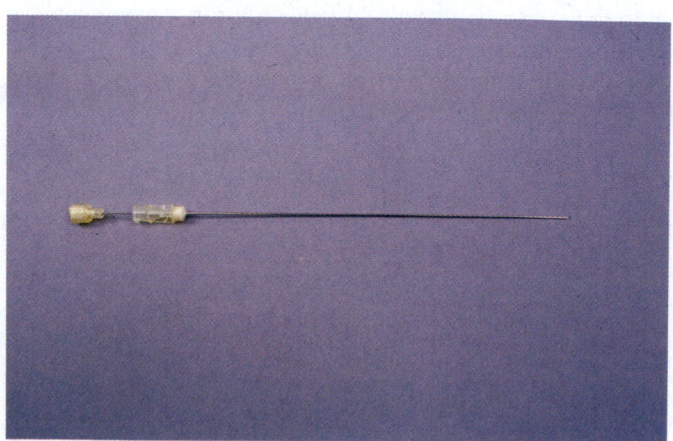

Figure 32–14 ■ A spinal needle with the stylet protruding from the hub.

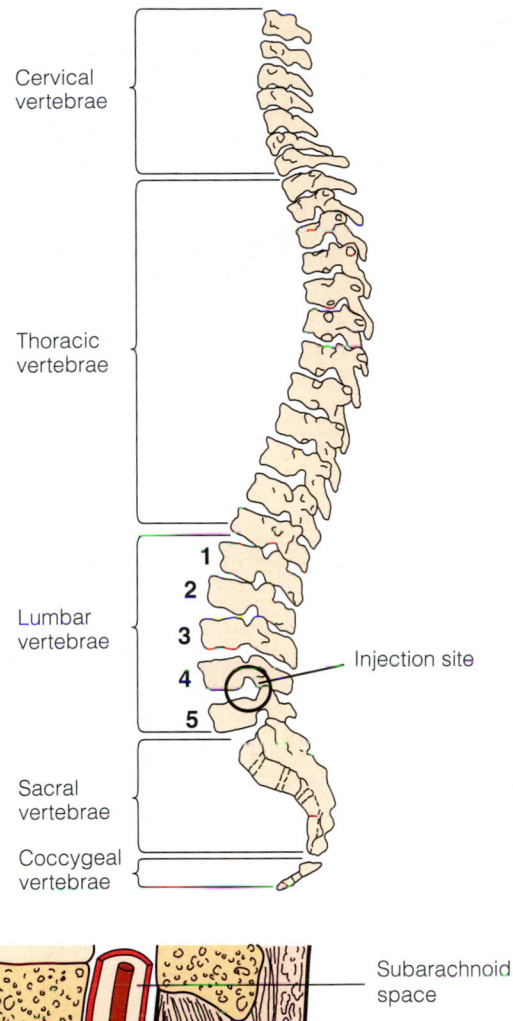

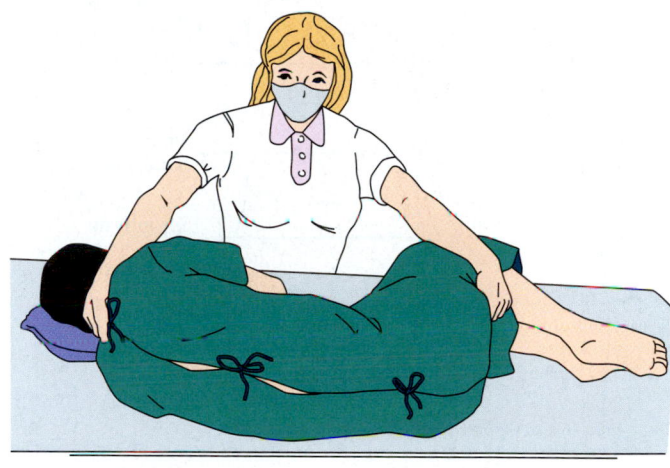

Figure 32–16 ■ Supporting the client for a lumbar puncture.

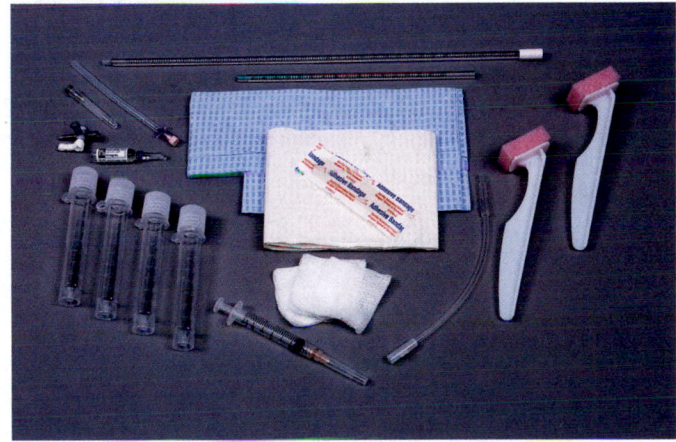

Figure 32–17 ■ A preassembled lumbar puncture set. Note the manometer at the top of the set.

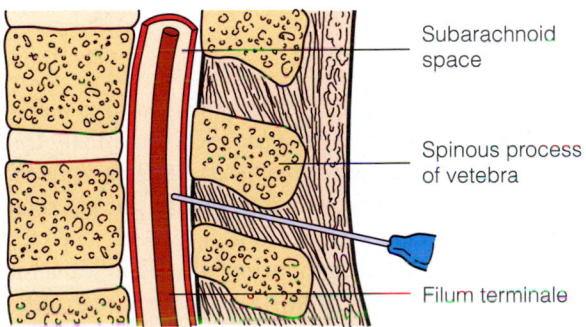

Figure 32–15 ■ A diagram of the vertebral column, indicating a site for insertion of the lumbar puncture needle into the subarachnoid space of the spinal canal.

through the tubing into a receptacle. If the purpose of the paracentesis is to obtain a specimen, the physician may use a long aspirating needle attached to a syringe rather than making an incision and using a trocar and cannula. Normally about 1,500 mL is the maximum amount of fluid drained at one time to avoid hypovolemic shock. The fluid is drained very slowly for the same reason. Some fluid is placed in the specimen container before the cannula is withdrawn. The small incision may or may not be sutured; in either case, it is covered with a small sterile bandage.

Lifespan Considerations

Lumbar Puncture

Children
- Briefly demonstrate the procedure on a doll or stuffed animal. Allow time to answer questions.
- One member of the health care team should maintain eye contact with the young client and provide reassurance during the procedure.

Elders
- Some clients need help maintaining the flexed position due to arthritis, weakness, or tremors.
- Provide an extra blanket to keep the client warm during the procedure. Elders have a decreased metabolism and less subcutaneous fat.
- If the client has a hearing loss, speak slowly and distinctly, especially when unable to make eye contact.

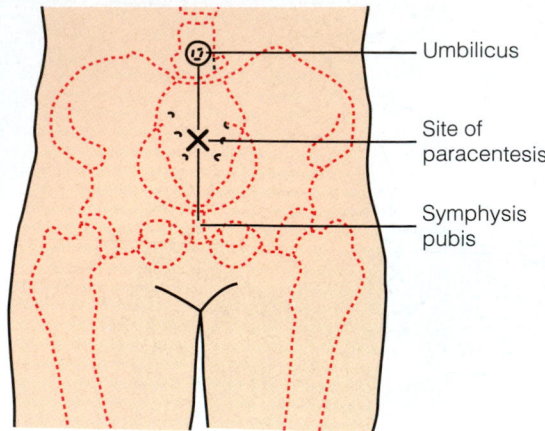

Figure 32–18 ■ A common site for an abdominal paracentesis.

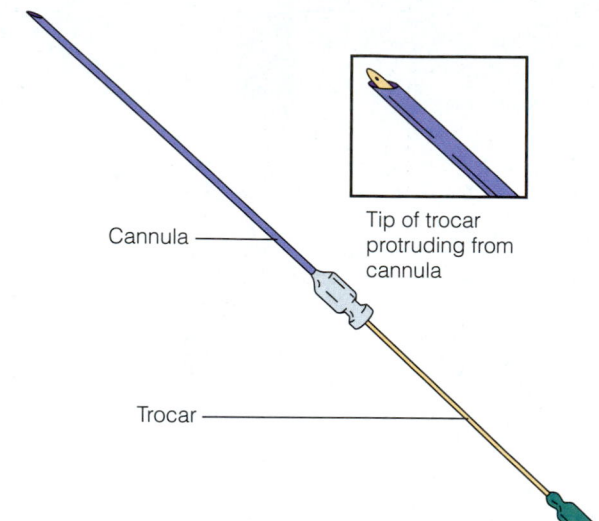

Figure 32–19 ■ A trocar and cannula may be used for an abdominal paracentesis.

Lifespan Considerations

Abdominal Paracentesis

Elders
- Provide pillows and blankets to help elders remain comfortable during the procedure.
- Ask the client to empty the bladder just before the procedure. Elders may need to void more frequently and in smaller amounts.

- Remove ascitic fluid slowly and monitor the client for signs of hypovolemia. Elders have less tolerance for fluid loss and may develop hypovolemia if a large volume of fluid is drained rapidly.

Thoracentesis

Normally, only sufficient fluid to lubricate the pleura is present in the pleural cavity. However, excessive fluid can accumulate as a result of injury, infection, or other pathology. In such a case or in the case of pneumothorax, a physician may perform a **thoracentesis** to remove the excess fluid or air to ease breathing. Thoracentesis is also performed to introduce chemotherapeutic drugs intrapleurally.

The nurse assists the client to assume a position that allows easy access to the intracostal spaces. This is usually a sitting position with the arms above the head, which spreads the ribs and enlarges the intercostal space. Two positions commonly used are one in which the arm is elevated and stretched forward (Figure 32–20 ■, *A*) and one in which the client leans forward over a pillow (Figure 32–20 ■, *B*). To make sure that the needle is inserted below the fluid level when fluid is to be removed

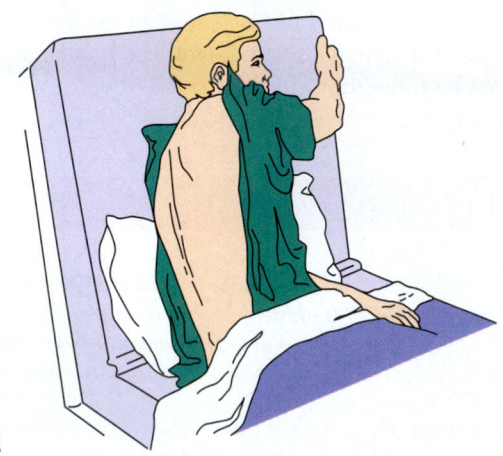

A

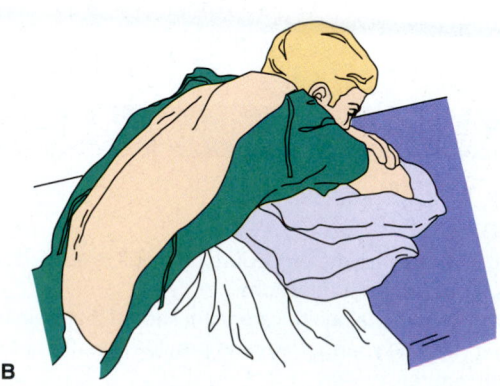

B

Figure 32–20 ■ Two positions commonly used for a thoracentesis. A, Sitting on one side with arm held to the front and up; B, sitting and leaning forward over a pillow.

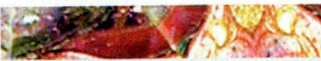

Lifespan Considerations

Thoracentesis

Elders
- Some elders will need help maintaining the proper position due to arthritis, tremors, or weakness.
- Provide support with pillows during the procedure.

- Absence of body fat in elders can help the physician locate the intercostal spaces.
- Provide an extra blanket to keep your client warm during the procedure. Elders have a decreased metabolism and less subcutaneous fat.

(or above any fluid if air is to be removed), the physician will palpate and percuss the chest and select the exact site for insertion of the needle. A site on the lower posterior chest is often used to remove fluid, and a site on the upper anterior chest is used to remove air. A chest x-ray prior to the procedure will help pinpoint the best insertion site.

The physician and the assisting nurse follow strict sterile technique. The physician attaches a syringe and/or stopcock to the aspirating needle. The stopcock must be in the closed position so that no air will enter the pleural space. The physician inserts the needle through the intercostal space to the pleural cavity. In some instances, the physician threads a small plastic tube through the needle and then withdraws the needle. (The tubing is less likely to puncture the pleura.)

If a syringe is used to collect the fluid, the plunger is pulled out to withdraw the pleural fluid as the stopcock is opened. If a large container is used to receive the fluid, the tubing is attached from the stopcock to the adapter on the receiving bottle. When the adapter and stopcock are opened, gravity allows fluid to drain from the pleural cavity into the container, which should be kept below the level of the client's lungs. After the fluid has been withdrawn, the physician removes the needle or plastic tubing.

Bone Marrow Biopsy

Another type of diagnostic study is the *biopsy*. A biopsy is a procedure whereby tissue is obtained for examination. Biopsies are performed on many different types of tissues, for example, bone marrow, liver, breast, lymph nodes, and lung.

A bone marrow biopsy is the removal of a specimen of bone marrow for laboratory study. The biopsy is used to detect specific diseases of the blood, such as pernicious anemia and leukemia. The bones of the body commonly used for a bone marrow biopsy are the sternum, iliac crests, anterior or posterior iliac spines, and proximal tibia in children (Pagana & Pagana, 2001, p. 172). *The posterior superior iliac crest is the preferred site with the client placed prone or on the side* (Figure 32–21 ■).

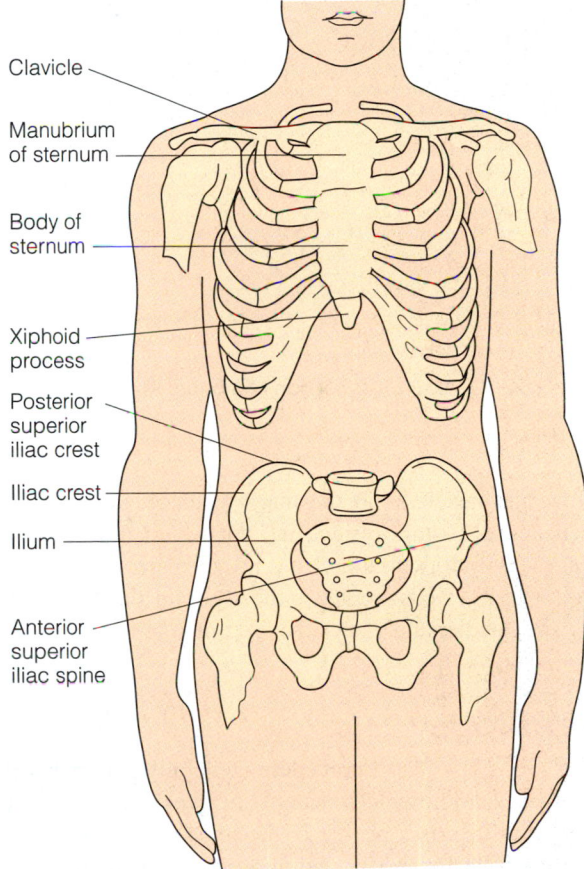

Figure 32–21 ■ The sternum and the iliac crests are common sites for a bone marrow biopsy.

After injecting a local anesthetic, a small incision may be made with a scalpel to avoid tearing the skin or pushing skin into the bone marrow with a needle. The physician then introduces a bone marrow needle with stylet into the red marrow of the spongy bone (Figure 32–22 ■).

Lifespan Considerations

Bone Marrow Biopsy

Children
- Young clients need emotional support due to the pain and pressure associated with this procedure.
- Young clients may require gentle restraint to prevent movement during the procedure.

Elders
- Elders with osteoporosis will experience less needle pressure.
- Ask the client to empty the bladder for comfort before the procedure.
- Provide pillows and blankets to help elders remain comfortable during the procedure.

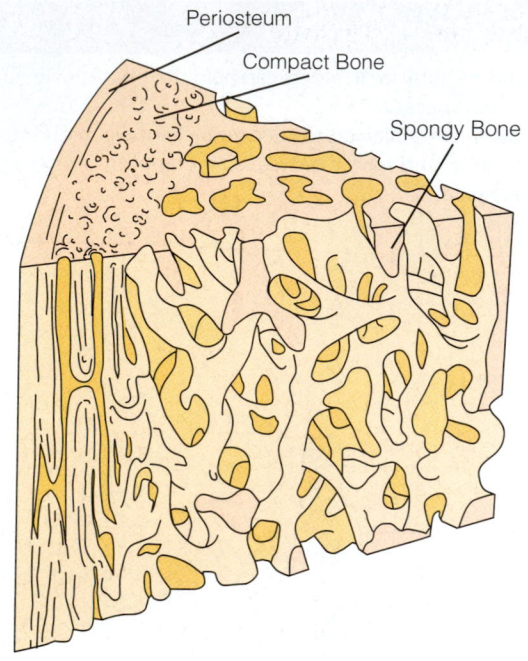

Figure 32–22 ■ A cross section of a bone.

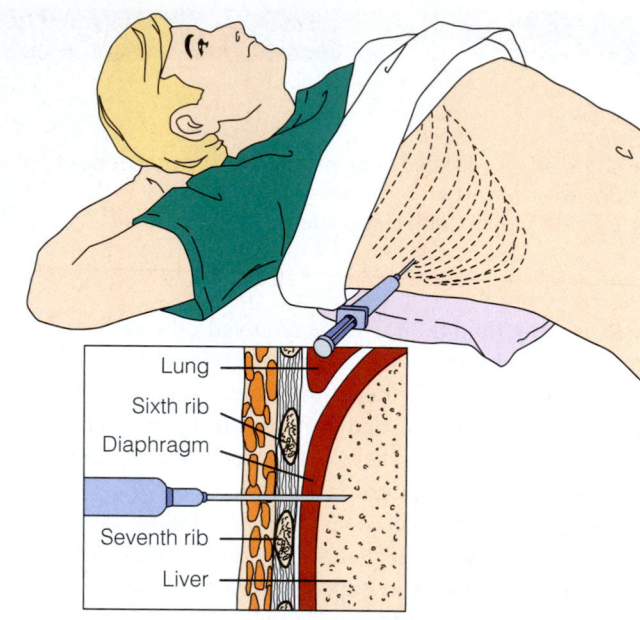

Figure 32–23 ■ A common site for a liver biopsy.

Once the needle is in the marrow space, the stylet is removed and a 10-mL syringe is attached to the needle. The plunger is withdrawn until 1 to 2 mL of marrow has been obtained. The physician replaces the stylet in the needle, withdraws the needle, and places the specimen in test tubes and/or on glass slides.

Liver Biopsy

A liver biopsy is a short procedure, generally performed at the client's bedside, in which a sample of liver tissue is aspirated. A physician inserts a needle in the intercostal space between two of the right lower ribs and into the liver (Figure 32–23 ■) or through the abdomen below the right rib cage (subcostally).

The client exhales and stops breathing while the physician inserts the biopsy needle, injects a small amount of sterile normal saline to clear the needle of blood or particles of tissue picked up during insertion, and aspirates liver tissue by drawing back on the plunger of the syringe. After the needle is withdrawn, the nurse applies pressure to the site to prevent bleeding, often by positioning the client on the biopsy site (Figure 32–24 ■).

Because many clients with liver disease have blood clotting defects and are prone to bleeding, prothrombin time and platelet

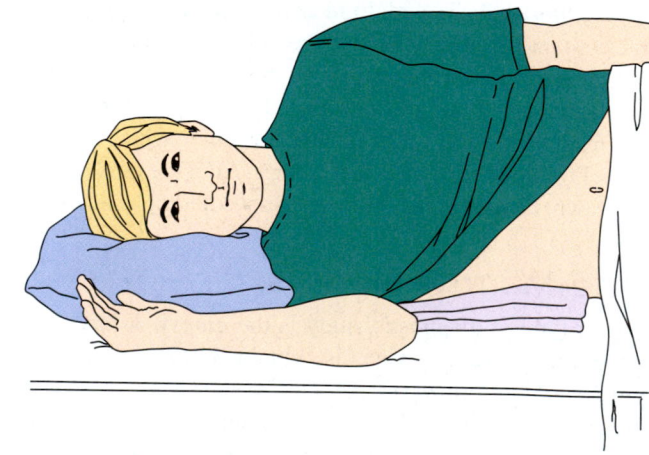

Figure 32–24 ■ The position to provide pressure on a liver biopsy site.

count are normally taken well in advance of the test. If the test results are abnormal, the biopsy may be contraindicated.

Table 32–2 describes how the nurse assists with the above aspiration/biopsy procedures.

Lifespan Considerations

Liver Biopsy

Elders

■ Observe for skin irritation from tape applied to the sterile dressing. Elders often have fragile skin.

■ Ask the client to empty the bladder before the procedure. Elders may need to void more often and in smaller amounts.

TABLE 32-2 Assisting with Aspiration and Biopsy

Procedure	Before the Procedure	During the Procedure	After the Procedure
Lumbar puncture	Prepare the client: • Explain the procedure to the client and support persons. The physician will be taking a small sample of spinal fluid from the lower spine. A local anesthetic will be given to minimize discomfort. Explain when and where the procedure will occur (e.g., the bedside or in a treatment room) and who will be present (e.g., the physician and the nurse) Explain that it will be necessary to lie in a certain position without moving for about 15 minutes. A slight pinprick will be felt when the local anesthetic is injected and a sensation of pressure as the spinal needle is inserted. • Have the client empty the bladder and bowels prior to the procedure to prevent unnecessary discomfort. • Position and drape the client. • Open the lumbar puncture set.	Support and monitor the client throughout: • Stand in front of the client and support the back of the neck and knees if the client needs help remaining still. • Reassure the client throughout the procedure by explaining what is happening. Encourage normal breathing and relaxation. • Observe the client's color, respirations, and pulse during the procedure. Ask the client to report headache or persistent pain at the insertion site. Handle specimen tubes appropriately: • Wear gloves when handling test tubes. • Label the specimen tubes in sequence. • Send the CSF specimens to the lab immediately. Place a small sterile dressing over the puncture site.	Ensure the client's comfort and safety: • Assist the client to a dorsal recumbent position with only one head pillow. The client remains in this position for 1 to 12 hours, depending on the physician's orders. • Determine whether analgesics are ordered and can be given for headaches. • Offer oral fluids frequently, unless contraindicated, to help restore the volume of CSF. Monitor the client: • Observe for swelling or bleeding at the puncture site. • Monitor changes in neurologic status. • Determine whether the client is experiencing any numbness, tingling, or pain radiating down the legs. Document the procedure on the client's chart: • Include date and time performed; the physician's name; the color, character, and amount of CSF; and the number of specimens obtained. Also document CSF pressure and the nurse's assessments and interventions.
Abdominal paracentesis	Prepare the client: • Explain the procedure: obtaining the specimen usually takes about 15 minutes. Emphasize the importance of remaining still during the procedure. Tell the client when and where the procedure will occur and who will be present. • Have the client void just before the paracentesis to reduce the possibility of puncturing the urinary bladder. • Help the client assume a sitting position in bed, in a chair, or on the edge of the bed supported by pillows. • Maintain the client's privacy and provide blankets for warmth.	Assist and monitor the client: • Support the client verbally and describe the steps of the procedure as needed. • Observe the client closely for signs of distress (e.g., abnormal pulse rate, skin color, and blood pressure). • Observe for signs of hypovolemic shock induced by the loss of fluid: pallor, dyspnea, diaphoresis, drop in BP and restlessness, or increased anxiety. • Place a small sterile dressing over the site of the incision after the cannula or aspirating needle is withdrawn.	Monitor the client closely: • Observe for hypovolemic shock. • Observe for scrotal edema with male clients. • Monitor VS, urine output, and drainage from the puncture site every 15 minutes for at least 2 hours and every hour for 4 hours or as the client's condition indicates. • Measure the abdominal girth at the level of the umbilicus. Document all relevant information: • Include date and time performed; the physician's name; abdominal girth before and after; the color, clarity, and amount of drained fluid; and the nurse's assessments and interventions. Transport the correctly labeled specimens to the laboratory.
Thoracentesis	Prepare the client: • Explain the procedure to the client. Normally, the client may experience some discomfort and a feeling of pressure when the needle is inserted. The procedure may bring considerable relief if breathing has been difficult. The procedure takes only a few minutes, depending primarily on the time it takes for the fluid to drain from the pleural	Support and monitor the client throughout: • Support the client verbally and describe the steps of the procedure as needed. • Observe the client for signs of distress, such as dyspnea, pallor and coughing. Collect drainage and laboratory specimens.	Monitor the client • Assess pulse rate and respiratory rate and skin color. • Don't remove more than 1,000 mL of fluid from the pleural cavity within the first 30 minutes. • Observe changes in the client's cough, sputum, respiratory depth, breath sounds, and note complaints of chest pain.

continued on page 780

TABLE 32–2 Assisting with Aspiration and Biopsy (continued)

Procedure	Before the Procedure	During the Procedure	After the Procedure
	cavity. To avoid puncturing the lungs, it is important for the client not to cough while the needle is inserted. Explain when and where the procedure will occur and who will be present. • Help position the client and cover the client as needed with a bath blanket.	Place a small sterile dressing over the site of the puncture.	Position the client appropriately: • Some agency protocols recommend that the client lie on the unaffected side with the head of the bed elevated 30 degrees for at least 30 minutes because this position facilitates expansion of the affected lung and eases respirations. Document all relevant information: • Include date and time performed; the physician's name; the amount, color, and clarity of fluid drained; and nursing assessments and interventions provided. Transport the specimens to the laboratory.
Bone marrow biopsy	Prepare the client: • Explain the procedure. The client may experience pain when the marrow is aspirated and hear a crunching sound as the needle is pushed through the cortex of the bone. The procedure usually takes 15 to 30 minutes. Explain when and where the procedure will occur, who will be present, and which site will be used. • Help the client assume a supine position (with one pillow if desired) for a biopsy of the sternum (sternal puncture) or a prone position for a biopsy of either iliac crest. Fold the bedclothes back or drape the client to expose the area. • Administer a sedative as ordered.	Monitor and support the client throughout: • Describe the steps of the procedure as needed and provide verbal support. • Observe the client for pallor, diaphoresis, and faintness due to bleeding or pain. Place a small dressing over the site of the puncture after the needle is withdrawn: • Some agency protocols recommend direct pressure over the site for 5 to 10 minutes to prevent bleeding. Assist with preparing specimens as needed.	Monitor the client: • Assess for discomfort and bleeding from the site. The client may experience some tenderness in the area. Bleeding and hematoma formation need to be assessed for several days. Report bleeding or pain to the nurse in charge. • Provide an analgesic as needed and ordered. Document all relevant information: • Include date and time of the procedure, the physician's name; and any nursing assessments and interventions. Document any specimens obtained. Transport the specimens to the laboratory.
Liver Biopsy	Prepare the client: • Give preprocedural medications as ordered. Vitamin K may be given for several days before the biopsy to reduce the risk of hemorrhage. • Explain the procedure and tell the client that the physician will take a small sample of liver tissue by putting a needle into the client's side or abdomen. That a sedative and local anesthetic will be given, so the client will feel no pain. Explain when and where the procedure will occur, who will be present, the time required, and what to expect as the procedure is being performed (e.g., the client may experience mild discomfort when the local anesthetic is injected and slight pressure when the biopsy needle is inserted). • Ensure that the client fasts for at least 2 hours before the procedure.	Monitor and support the client throughout: • Support the client in a supine position. • Instruct the client to take a few deep inhalations and exhalations and to hold the breath after the final exhalation for up to 10 seconds as the needle is inserted, the biopsy obtained, and the needle withdrawn. Holding the breath after exhalation immobilizes the chest wall and liver and keeps the diaphragm in its highest position, avoiding injury to the lung and laceration of the liver. • Instruct the client to resume breathing when the needle is withdrawn.	Position the client appropriately: • Assist the client to a right side-lying position with a small pillow or folded towel under the biopsy site. Instruct the client to remain in this position for several hours. Monitor the client. • Assess the client's VS every 15 minutes for the first hour following the test or until the signs are stable. Then monitor vital signs every hour for 24 hours or as needed. • Determine whether the client is experiencing abdominal pain. Severe abdominal pain may indicate bile peritonitis. • Check the biopsy site for localized bleeding. Pressure dressings may be required if bleeding does occur. Document all relevant information. • Include date and time performed; the physician's name; and all nursing assessments and interventions.

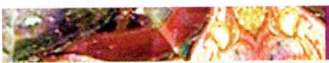

TABLE 32-2 Assisting with Aspiration and Biopsy (continued)

Procedure	Before the Procedure	During the Procedure	After the Procedure
	• Administer the appropriate sedative about 30 minutes beforehand or at the specified time. • Help the client assume a supine position with the upper right quadrant of the abdomen exposed. Cover the client with the bedclothes so that only the abdominal area is exposed.	• Apply pressure to the site of the puncture to help stop any bleeding. Apply a small dressing to the site of the puncture.	Transport the specimens to the laboratory.

Lifespan Considerations

General Considerations

Elders

■ In elders, homeostatic mechanisms are not as efficient as in the younger person. When undergoing diagnostic tests that challenge these functions, care must be taken to accurately monitor functions and note any changes. Examples:

• Dehydration can occur from laxative preps given before bowel diagnostic tests, such as a colonoscopy.

• Fluid restrictions and NPO status for a length of time can lead to hypovolemia and electrolyte imbalances.

• Many dye contrasts used for x-rays and scans can cause renal damage (especially in diabetics).

• Sedation used for certain procedures may require a longer recovery time for older clients.

• Having several tests at a time or for several days compounds these potential problems.

Interventions should focus on ensuring that the client is hydrated during and after these diagnostic tests, monitoring intake and output and vital signs frequently and accurately, and noting any mental status changes that might suggest electrolyte imbalance. Identification of clients at risk (persons with diabetes, kidney disease, or on certain meds) will help initiate measures to prevent injuries or complications from diagnostic tests.

Research Note

Do Non-English-Speaking Clients Have More Diagnostic Tests Ordered Than English-Speaking Clients?

A prospective, comparative, observational study on this topic was conducted at a public hospital emergency department (ED) (Waxman & Levitt, 2000). The population consisted of 172 non-English-speaking clients and 152 English-speaking clients who presented to the ED with complaints of nontraumatic abdominal pain or chest pain. The purpose of the study was to determine provider decision making for these specific clients in the ED setting. The outcome measurements included diagnostic test ordering, admission rate, and length of stay in the ED.

It was hypothesized that there would be more diagnostic tests ordered, a higher admission rate, and a longer ED length of stay in the non-English-speaking clients. The results, however, did not support all of the hypotheses. Significantly more tests were ordered for the non-English-speaking clients with abdominal pain. Of note, three times as many abdominal computed tomographic (CT) scans were ordered. In contrast, there was no increase in test ordering for the non-English-speaking clients with complaints of chest pain. Finally, there were no statistically significant differences in admission rates or length of stay in the ED between the two groups.

Implications: The researchers were surprised, because the results of this study were not consistent with other studies, except for the higher number of diagnostic tests. The greater number of abdominal CT scans ordered may have an impact on health care costs. The authors suggested that a higher use of professional translators instead of lay translators (e.g., family members) may be helpful and a direction for future research.

Note: From "Are Diagnostic Testing and Admission Rates Higher in Non-English-Speaking Versus English-Speaking Patients in the Emergency Department?" by M. A. Waxman and M. A. Levitt, 2000, *Annuals of Emergency Medicine, 36*(5), pp. 456–461.

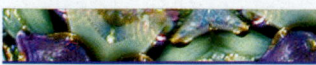

Focus on Critical Thinking

Ms. Angyal, 68, is admitted with fever, nausea, vomiting, and abdominal pain. She informs you that she is a "borderline diabetic" and "only has to watch what she eats." She tells you that she has not eaten for 3 days and has had difficulty "keeping liquids down." While doing the nursing history, she describes her urine as dark and foul smelling. Upon further questions, she states she does have some burning upon urination. She describes her abdominal pain as constant, generalized, and rates it as a 5 or 6 on a scale of 0 to 10. The physician called in the following orders:

CBC and electrolytes STAT
Capillary blood glucose STAT and q 4 hr
VS and TPR q 4 hr
Urine specimen for C & S
CXR
Flat plate abdominal x-ray

1. When measuring Ms. Angyal's capillary blood glucose, you do not obtain enough blood to cover the indicator square on the reagent strip. What could be possible reasons and what should you do?

The lab work returns with the following results: WBC = 17 × 10^3/mL^3 with neutrophils = 80%; Hct = 43.2.

1. Based on the above lab work, what are your nursing interventions?

2. The physician orders IV fluids and an antibiotic with the first dose to be given STAT. You have not obtained the urine specimen yet. Which has priority (e.g., starting the IV, administrating the antibiotic, or obtaining the urine specimen) and why?

3. Three days later, Ms. Angyal has the following lab results: Hct = 39.2 and WBC = 10.8 × 10^3/mL^3. What do those results indicate to you?

4. The abdominal x-ray shows a possible mass. An MRI of the abdomen is ordered. Ms. Angyal is quite anxious because she has heard from her friend that the procedure is claustrophobic for people. How will you respond?

See Critical Thinking Possibilities in Appendix A.

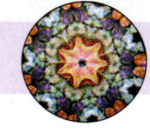 | **Chapter Review**

EXPLORE MediaLink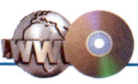

NCLEX review questions, case studies, care plan activities, MediaLink applications, and other interactive resources for this chapter can be found on the Companion Website at www.prenhall.com/kozier. Click on Chapter 32 to select the activities for this chapter.

For animations, more NCLEX review questions, and an audio glossary, access the Student CD-ROM accompanying this textbook.

Chapter Highlights

- Diagnostic testing involves three phases. Client preparation is the focus during the pretest phase. During the intratest phase, the nurse performs or assists with the diagnostic test and collects the specimen. Providing nursing care of the client and follow-up activities and observations are the role of the nurse during the post-test phase.
- Blood tests are one of the most commonly used diagnostic tests. Routinely ordered blood tests can include complete blood count (CBC) and serum electrolytes.
- A capillary blood glucose is a frequent test performed by nurses and clients. This test is used to monitor glucose levels of clients at risk for hyper- and hypoglycemia. It also evaluates the effectiveness of insulin administration.
- Nursing responsibilities associated with specimen collection include (a) providing client comfort, privacy, and safety; (b) explaining the purpose of and procedure for the

- specimen collection; (c) using correct procedure for obtaining the specimen; (d) noting relevant information on the laboratory requisition slip; (e) transporting the specimen promptly; and (f) reporting abnormal findings.
- Clients may need assistance to obtain stool specimens for laboratory analysis. In many agencies, nurses test the stool for occult blood.
- Nurses collect urine specimens for a number of tests. A clean voided specimen is used for routine examination. A clean-catch or midstream voided specimen is collected when a urine culture is ordered to identify microorganisms. Timed urine specimens are collected for a variety of tests depending on the client's health problem. Nurses can complete some simple urine tests (e.g., specific gravity, pH, ketones, protein) at the bedside.
- Sputum and throat culture specimens help determine the presence of disease-producing organisms.

- Visualization procedures include indirect visualization (non-invasive) and direct visualization (invasive) techniques for visualizing body organs and system functions. Examples of invasive procedures include colonoscopy, barium enema, intravenous pyelography, and angiography. Noninvasive procedures include lung scan, echocardiogram, electrocardiography, x-ray, CT, and MRI.

- Examples of aspiration/biopsy tests include lumbar puncture, abdominal paracentesis, thoracentesis, bone marrow biopsy, and liver biopsy. These tests are invasive procedures and require strict sterile technique. After the procedure, the nurse assesses the client for possible complications and provides appropriate nursing interventions as needed.

Review Questions

32–1. The nurse would call the physician immediately for which of the following lab results?
   a. Hgb = 16 g/dL for male client
   b. Hct = 22% for female client
   c. WBC = $9 \times 10^3/mL^3$
   d. platelets = $300 \times 10^3/mL^3$

32–2. Mr. Jones, 78, needs to complete a 24-hour urine specimen. In planning his care, which of the following measures is most important?
   a. At the beginning of the test, instructing him to empty his bladder and save this voiding to start the collection.
   b. Use a sterile receptacle to collect the urine.
   c. Place a sign stating "Save All Urine" in the bathroom.
   d. Keep the urine specimen in the refrigerator.

32–3. The client has a urinary health problem. Which of the following procedures is performed using indirect visualization?
   a. IVP
   b. KUB
   c. retrograde pyelography
   d. cystoscopy

32–4. Which procedure provides information regarding the physiology of an organ?
   a. x-ray
   b. CT
   c. MRI
   d. nuclear scan

32–5. When assisting with a bone marrow biopsy, the nurse should take which of the following actions?
   a. Assist the client to a right side-lying position after the procedure.
   b. Observe for signs of dyspnea, pallor, and coughing.
   c. Assess for bleeding and hematoma formation for several days after the procedure.
   d. Stand in front of the client and support the back of the neck and knees.

Readings and References

Suggested Readings

Cook, L. (1999). The value of lab values. Incorporate lab results into the nursing diagnosis. *American Journal of Nursing, 99*(5), 66–75. This article provides information about common lab tests and how to examine lab values to differentiate between the health conditions of dehydration versus renal failure and protein malnutrition versus renal failure. One scenario also follows the course of an acute infection looking at the WBC differential.

Frizzell, J. (1998). Avoiding lab test pitfalls. *American Journal of Nursing, 98*(2), 34–37. The author focuses on appropriate specimen collection and storage and transportation of specimens. Potential problems with portable diagnostic equipment (e.g., blood glucose monitoring) are reviewed. Also, issues related to interpreting test results are presented.

Hinkle, J. L. (2002). SPECT: A powerful imaging tool. *American Journal of Nursing, 102*(3), 24A–24G. The author reviews how the imaging tool SPECT (single-photon emission computed tomography) is used as part of the diagnostic workup for many neurologic and psychiatric conditions. The advantage to SPECT is that it depicts an organ's function versus the imaging techniques of the CT and MRI, which show only an organ's anatomy.

Related Research

Barton, S. J., & Holmes, S. S. (1998). Practice applications of research. A comparison of reagent strips and the refractometer for measurement of urine specific gravity in hospitalized children. *Pediatric Nursing, 24*(5), 480–482.

Cupples, S. A., Paige-Dobson, B., & Armstrong, D. (1998). Psychophysiological manifestations of anxiety in patients undergoing electrophysiology studies. *Heart & Lung, 27*(6), 374–386.

O'Connor, G., & Cotter, S. (1998). Value of interpersonal encounter endorsed by patients as intervention in magnetic resonance imaging. *The College of Radiographers, 4,* 101–105.

Murphy, F. (2001). Understanding the humanistic interaction with medical imaging technology. *The College of Radiographers, 7,* 193–201.

References

American Diabetes Association. (2000). Resource guide 2000: Urine testing. *Diabetes Forecast Supplement,* January 2000, 66–67.

Bindler, R., & Ball, J. (2003). *Clinical skills for pediatric nursing* (3rd ed.). Upper Saddle River, NJ: Prentice Hall.

Fischbach, F. T. (2000). *A manual of laboratory & diagnostic tests* (6th ed.). Philadelphia: Lippincott.

Fischbach, F. T. (2002). *Nurses' quick reference to common laboratory and diagnostic tests* (3rd ed.). Philadelphia: Lippincott.

Kee, J. L. (1999). *Laboratory and diagnostic tests with nursing implications* (5th ed.). Stamford, CT: Appleton & Lange.

Lindemann, M. (2000). Tips & timesavers. *Nursing, 30*(3), 70.

Pagana, K. D., & Pagana, T. J. (2001). *Diagnostic and laboratory test reference* (5th ed.). St. Louis, MO: Mosby.

Shirrell, D. J., Gibbar-Clements, T., Dooley, R., & Free, C. (1999). Understanding therapeutic drug monitoring. *American Journal of Nursing, 99*(1), 42–44.

Waxman, M. A., & Levitt, M. A. (2000). Are diagnostic testing and admission rates higher in non-English-speaking versus English-speaking patients in the emergency department? *Annals of Emergency Medicine, 36,* 456–461.

Selected Bibliography

American Diabetes Association. (2000). Resource guide 2000: Blood glucose monitors and data management. *Diabetes Forecast Supplement,* January 2000, 42–56.

Ayers, D. M. M. (2002). Eye on diagnostics: EBCT: Beaming in on coronary artery disease. *Nursing, 32*(4), 81.

Ball, J., & Bindler, R. (2003). *Pediatric nursing: Caring for children* (3rd ed.). Upper Saddle River NJ: Prentice Hall Health.

Barker, E. (1998). The xenon CT: A new neuro tool. *RN, 61*(2), 22–25.

Brazier, A. M., & Palmer, M. H. (1995). Collecting clean-catch urine in the nursing home: Obtaining the uncontaminated specimen. *Geriatric Nursing: American Journal of Care for the Aging, 16*(5), 217–224.

Connolly, M. A. (1999). Postdural puncture headache. *American Journal of Nursing, 99*(11), 48–49.

Corbett, J. V. (1998). Laboratory tests and diagnostic procedures in orthopedic nursing practice. *Nursing Clinics of North America, 33,* 685–700.

Dammel, T. (1997). Fecal occult blood testing: Looking for hidden danger. *Nursing, 27*(7), 44–45.

Fann, B. D. (1998). Fluid and electrolyte balance in the pediatric patient. *Journal of Intravenous Nursing, 21*(3), 153–159.

Harvey, M. A. (1999). Point-of-care laboratory testing in critical care. *American Journal of Critical Care, 8*(2), 72–85.

Kumar, D. (1998). Diagnostic tests: PET scanning. Applications for treating epilepsy. *American Journal of Nursing, 98*(7), 16G–17G.

Louie, R. F., Tang, Z., Shelby, D. G., & Kost, G. J. (2000). Point-of-care testing: Millennium technology for critical care. *Laboratory Medicine, 31,* 402–408.

Parini, S. (2000). How to collect specimens. *Nursing, 30*(5), 66–67.

Passanza, C. (2001). Diabetes update: Monitor options. *RN, 64*(6), 36–42.

Ryan, D. (2000). Is it an MI? A lab primer. *RN, 63*(1), 26–30.

Semple, M., & Elley, K. (1998). Practical procedures for nurses. Collecting a sputum specimen. *Nursing Times, 94*(48), 2–8.

Teaching your patient about cardiovascular tests. (2002). *Nursing, 32*(1), 62–64.

Tasota, F. J. (2001). Eye on diagnostics: Digital mammography: Enhanced imaging in real time. *Nursing 31*(4), 70.

Tasota, F. J. (2002). Eye on diagnostics: Full-body scans: Screening for problems. *Nursing, 32*(7), 22.

Tasota, F. J., & Davies, P. (2001). Eye on diagnostics: Diagnosing pulmonary embolism with spiral CT. *Nursing, 31*(5), 75.

Tasota, F. J., & Tate, J. (2001). Eye on diagnostics: Interpreting the highs and lows of platelet counts. *Nursing, 31*(2), 25.

Tasota, F. J., & Tate, J. (2001). Eye on diagnostics: Using PET to detect abnormalities. *Nursing, 31*(11), 24.

Tate, J., & Tasota, F. J. (2001). Eye on diagnostics: Assessing thyroid function with serum tests. *Nursing, 31*(1), 22.

Tate, J., & Tasota, F. J. (2001). Eye on diagnostics: Teaching patients about lipid levels. *Nursing, 31*(3), 68.

Shopping around for the perfect blood glucose meter. (2000). *Nursing, 30*(8), 60–61.

Valentine, V. (2002). Using a laser to make a point. *Nursing, 32*(10), 56–57.

Wilkinson, J. M. (2000). *Nursing diagnosis handbook with NIC interventions and NOC outcomes* (7th Ed.). Upper Saddle River, NJ: Prentice Hall Health.

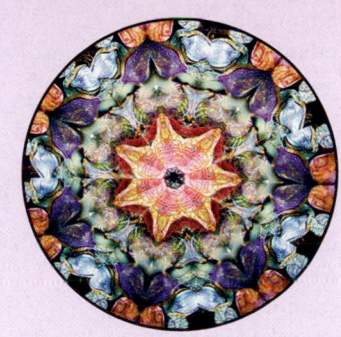

CHAPTER 33

MEDICATIONS

LEARNING OUTCOMES

After completing this chapter, you will be able to:

- Define selected terms related to the administration of medications.
- Describe legal aspects of administering medications.
- Identify physiologic factors and individual variables affecting medication action.
- Describe various routes of medication administration.
- Identify essential parts of a medication order.
- Give examples of various types of medication orders.
- Recognize abbreviations commonly used in medication orders.
- Recognize systems of measurement that are used in the administration of medications.
- List six essential steps to follow when administering medication.
- State the six "rights" to accurate medication administration.
- Describe physiologic changes in older adults that alter medication administration and effectiveness.
- Outline steps required to administer oral medications safely.
- Outline steps required for nasogastric and gastrostomy tube medication administration.
- Identify equipment required for parenteral medications.
- Describe how to mix selected drugs from ampules and vials.
- Identify sites used for intradermal, subcutaneous, and intramuscular injections.
- Describe essential steps for safely administering parenteral medications by intradermal, subcutaneous, intramuscular, and intravenous routes.
- Describe essential steps in safely administering topical medications: dermatologic, ophthalmic, otic, nasal, vaginal, respiratory inhalation, and rectal preparations.

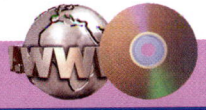

MediaLink

www.prenhall.com/kozier

Additional resources for this chapter can be found on the Student CD-ROM accompanying this textbook, and on the Companion Website at www.prenhall.com/kozier. Click on Chapter 33 to select the activities for this chapter.

CD-ROM
- Audio Glossary
- NCLEX Review
- Animations:
  Agonist/Antagonist Mechanism
  of Action
  Injections
- Videos:
  Metered Dose Inhaler (MDI)
  Small Volume Nebulizer (SVN)
  Treatment

Companion Website
- Additional NCLEX Review
- Case Study: Preparing Medications
- Care Plan Activity: Client on Insulin
- MediaLink Application: Calculating
  Dosages
- Links to Resources

A **medication** is a substance administered for the diagnosis, cure, treatment, or relief of a symptom or for prevention of disease. In the health care context, the words *medication* and *drug* are generally used interchangeably. The term **drug** also has the connotation of an illicitly obtained substance such as heroin, cocaine, or amphetamines. Medications have been known and used since antiquity. Crude drugs, such as opium, castor oil, and vinegar, were used in ancient times. Over the centuries the number of drugs available has increased greatly, and knowledge about these drugs has become correspondingly more accurate and detailed.

In the United States and Canada, medications are usually dispensed on the order of physicians and dentists. In some U.S. states, specially qualified nurse practitioners or other advanced practice nurses and physician's assistants may prescribe drugs. The written direction for the preparation and administration of a drug is called a **prescription.** One drug can have as many as four kinds of names: its generic name, official name, chemical name, and trademark or brand name. The **generic name** is given before a drug becomes official. The **official name** is the name under which it is listed in one of the official publications (e.g., the *United States Pharmacopeia*). The **chemical name** is the name by which a chemist knows it; this name describes the constituents of the drug precisely. The **trademark,** or **brand name,** is the name given by the drug manufacturer. Because one drug may be manufactured by several companies, it can have several trade names; for example, the drug hydrochlorothiazide (official name) is known by the trade names Esidrix and HydroDIURIL. Medications are often available in a variety of forms (see Table 33–1).

Pharmacology is the study of the effect of drugs on living organisms. **Pharmacy** is the art of preparing, compounding, and dispensing drugs. The word also refers to the place where drugs are prepared and dispensed. Drugs are prepared by a **pharmacist,** a person licensed to prepare and dispense drugs and to make up prescriptions. A clinical pharmacist is a specialist who often guides the physician in prescribing drugs. A pharmacy technician is a member of the health team who in some states administers drugs to clients.

DRUG STANDARDS

Drugs may have natural (e.g., plant, mineral, and animal) sources, or they may be synthesized in the laboratory. For example, digitalis and opium are plant derived, iron and sodium chloride are minerals, insulin and vaccines have animal or human sources, and the sulfonamides and propoxyphene hydrochloride (the analgesic Darvon) are the products of laboratory synthesis. Early drugs were derived from the three natural sources only. More and more drugs, however, are being produced synthetically.

Drugs vary in strength and activity. Drugs derived from plants, for example, vary in strength according to the age of the plant, the variety, the place in which it is grown, and the method by which it is preserved. Drugs must be pure and of uniform strength if drug dosages are to be predictable in their effect. Drug standards have therefore been developed to ensure uniform quality. In the United States, official drugs are those so designated by the federal Food, Drug, and Cosmetic Act. These drugs are officially listed in the *United States Pharmacopeia (USP)* and described according to their source, physical and chemical properties, tests for purity and identity, method of storage, assay, category, and normal dosages. In Canada, the *British Pharmacopoeia* is used for the same purpose, although some drugs used in Canada conform to the *USP* because they are obtained from the United States. There is a trend for people to purchase "natural" vitamins and supplements from health food stores or over the counter at pharmacies. An example of this is a thyroid supplement. The natural form varies in strength and is difficult to regulate, while the synthetic thyroid is much more predictable in strength and management of symptoms for clients who need to take a thyroid supplement.

A **pharmacopoeia** (also spelled *pharmacopeia*) is a book containing a list of products used in medicine, with descriptions of the product, chemical tests for determining identity and purity, and formulas and prescriptions. The United States' *National Formulary* lists drugs and their therapeutic value and can include drugs that may still be used but not listed in the *USP.* The *Canadian Formulary* lists drugs used extensively in Canada but not necessarily listed in the *British Pharmacopoeia.*

Pharmacopoeias and formularies are invaluable reference sources for nurses and nursing students. Nurses not only administer thousands of medications but also are responsible for assessing their effectiveness and recognizing unfavorable reactions to drugs. Because it is impossible to commit to memory all pertinent information about a very large number of drugs, nurses must have a reliable reference readily available.

TABLE 33-1 Types of Drug Preparation

Type	Description
Aerosol spray or foam	A liquid, powder, or foam deposited in a thin layer on the skin by air pressure
Aqueous solution	One or more drugs dissolved in water
Aqueous suspension	One or more drugs finely divided in a liquid such as water
Caplet	A solid form, shaped like a capsule, coated and easily swallowed
Capsule	A gelatinous container to hold a drug in powder, liquid, or oil form
Cream	A nongreasy, semisolid preparation used on the skin
Elixir	A sweetened and aromatic solution of alcohol used as a vehicle for medicinal agents
Extract	A concentrated form of a drug made from vegetables or animals
Gel or jelly	A clear or translucent semisolid that liquefies when applied to the skin
Liniment	A medication mixed with alcohol, oil, or soapy emollient and applied to the skin
Lotion	A medication in a liquid suspension applied to the skin
Lozenge (troche)	A flat, round, or oval preparation that dissolves and releases a drug when held in the mouth
Ointment (salve, unction)	A semisolid preparation of one or more drugs used for application to the skin and mucous membrane
Paste	A preparation like an ointment, but thicker and stiff, that penetrates the skin less than an ointment
Pill	One or more drugs mixed with a cohesive material, in oval, round, or flattened shapes
Powder	A finely ground drug or drugs; some are used internally, others externally
Suppository	One or several drugs mixed with a firm base such as gelatin and shaped for insertion into the body (e.g., the rectum); the base dissolves gradually at body temperature, releasing the drug
Syrup	An aqueous solution of sugar often used to disguise unpleasant-tasting drugs
Tablet	A powdered drug compressed into a hard small disc; some are readily broken along a scored line; others are enteric coated to prevent them from dissolving in the stomach
Tincture	An alcoholic or water-and-alcohol solution prepared from drugs derived from plants
Transdermal patch	A semipermeable membrane shaped in the form of a disc or patch that contains a drug to be absorbed through the skin over a long period of time

LEGAL ASPECTS OF DRUG ADMINISTRATION

The administration of drugs in both the United States and Canada is controlled by law. Table 33–2 provides a summary of U.S. drug legislation. Table 33–3 summarizes Canadian drug legislation.

Nurses need to (a) know how nursing practice acts in their areas define and limit their functions and (b) be able to recognize the limits of their own knowledge and skill. To function beyond the limits of nursing practice acts or one's ability is to endanger clients' lives and leave oneself open to malpractice suits. Under the law, nurses are responsible for their own actions regardless of whether there is a written order. If a physician writes an incorrect order (e.g., Demerol 500 mg instead of Demerol 50 mg), *a nurse who administers the written incorrect dosage is responsible for the error as well as the physician.* Therefore, nurses should question any order that appears unreasonable and refuse to give the medication until the order is clarified.

TABLE 33-2 United States Drug Legislation

Legislation	Content
Food, Drug, and Cosmetic Act (1938)	Implemented by Food and Drug Administration (FDA); requires that labels be accurate and that all drugs be tested for harmful effects.
Durkham-Humphrey Amendment (1952)	Clearly differentiates drugs that can be sold only with a prescription, those that can be sold without a prescription, and those that should not be refilled without a new prescription.
Kefauver-Harris Amendment (1962)	Requires proof of safety and efficacy of a drug for approval.
Comprehensive Drug Abuse Prevention and Control Act (1970) (Controlled Substances Act)	Categorizes controlled substances and limits how often a prescription can be filled; established government-funded programs to prevent and treat drug dependence.

TABLE 33-3 Canadian Drug Legislation

Legislation	Content
Proprietary or Patent Medicine Act (1908)	Protects the public against unsafe and ineffective over-the-counter drugs.
Canada Food and Drugs Act (1953)	Prohibits advertising any food, drug, cosmetic, or device as a cure for certain specified diseases. Sets standards for manufacture, distribution, and sale of all drugs, with the exception of narcotics.
Canadian Narcotic Control Act (1961)	Allows only authorized people to possess narcotics. Specifies records about narcotics that must be kept.

Another aspect of nursing practice governed by law is the use of controlled substances. In hospitals, controlled substances are kept in a locked drawer, cupboard, medication cart, or computer-controlled dispensing system. Agencies may have special inventory forms for recording the use of controlled substances. The information required usually includes the name of the client, the date and time of administration, the name of the drug, the dosage, and the signature of the person who prepared and gave the drug. The name of the physician who ordered the drug may also be part of the record. Before removing a controlled substance, the nurse verifies the number actually available with the number indicated on the narcotic or controlled substance inventory record (Figure 33–1 ■). If the number is not the same, the nurse must investigate and correct the discrepancy before proceeding.

Included on the record are the controlled substances wasted during preparation. When a portion or all of a controlled substance dose is discarded, the nurse must ask a second nurse to witness the discarding. Both nurses must sign the control inventory form.

In most agencies, counts of controlled substances are taken at the end of each shift. The count total should tally with the total at the end of the last shift minus the number used. If the totals do not tally and the discrepancy cannot be resolved, it must be reported immediately to the nurse manager, nursing supervisor, and pharmacy according to agency policy. In facilities that use a computerized dispensing system, manual counts are not required, because the dispensing system runs a continuous count; however, discrepancies must be accounted for.

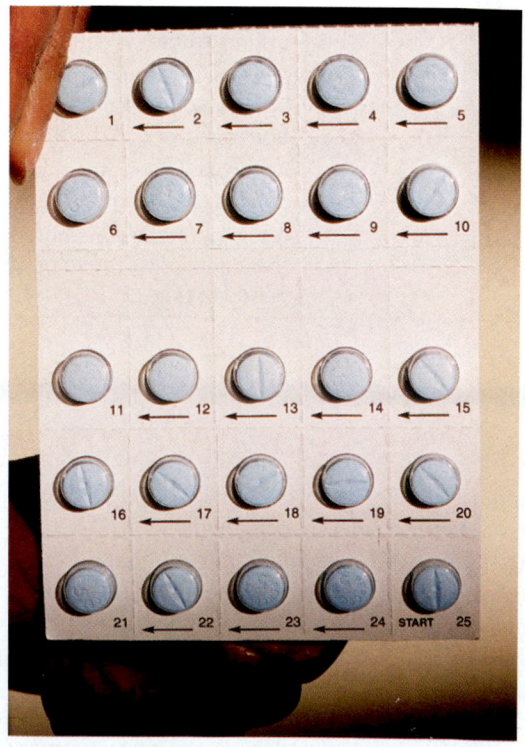

Figure 33-1 ■ Some narcotics are kept in specially designed packages or plastic containers that are sectioned and numbered.

TABLE 33–4 Therapeutic Actions of Drugs

Drug Type	Description	Examples
Palliative	Relieves the symptoms of a disease but does not affect the disease itself.	Morphine sulfate, aspirin for pain
Curative	Cures a disease or condition.	Penicillin for infection
Supportive	Supports body function until other treatments or the body's response can take over.	Norepinephrine bitartrate for low blood pressure; aspirin for high body temperature
Substitutive	Replaces body fluids or substances.	Thyroxine for hypothyroidism, insulin for diabetes mellitus
Chemotherapeutic	Destroys malignant cells.	Busulfan for leukemia
Restorative	Returns the body to health.	Vitamin, mineral supplements

EFFECTS OF DRUGS

The **therapeutic effect** of a drug, also referred to as the **desired effect,** is the primary effect intended, that is, the reason the drug is prescribed. For example, the therapeutic effect of morphine sulfate is analgesia, and the therapeutic effect of diazepam is relief of anxiety. See Table 33–4 for kinds of therapeutic actions.

A **side effect,** or secondary effect, of a drug is one that is unintended. Side effects are usually predictable and may be either harmless or potentially harmful. For example, digitalis increases the strength of myocardial contractions (desired effect), but it can have the side effect of inducing nausea and vomiting. Some side effects are tolerated for the drug's therapeutic effect; more severe side effects, also called **adverse effects,** may justify the discontinuation of a drug.

Drug toxicity (deleterious effects of a drug on an organism or tissue) results from overdosage, ingestion of a drug intended for external use, and buildup of the drug in the blood because of impaired metabolism or excretion (cumulative effect). Some toxic effects are apparent immediately; some are not apparent for weeks or months. Fortunately, most drug toxicity is avoidable if careful attention is paid to dosage and monitoring for toxicity. An example of a toxic effect is respiratory depression due to the cumulative effect of morphine sulfate in the body.

A **drug allergy** is an immunologic reaction to a drug. When a client is first exposed to a foreign substance (antigen), the body may react by producing antibodies. A client can react to a drug as to an antigen and thus develop symptoms of an allergic reaction.

Allergic reactions can be either mild or severe. A mild reaction has a variety of symptoms, from skin rashes to diarrhea (see Table 33–5). An allergic reaction can occur anytime from a few minutes to 2 weeks after the administration of the drug. A severe allergic reaction usually occurs immediately after the administration of the drug and is called an **anaphylactic reaction.** This response can be fatal if the symptoms are not noticed immediately and treatment is not obtained promptly. The earliest symptoms are acute shortness of breath, acute hypotension, and tachycardia.

Drug tolerance exists in a person who has unusually low physiologic response to a drug and who requires increases in the dosage to maintain a given therapeutic effect. Drugs that commonly produce tolerance are opiates, barbiturates, ethyl alcohol, and tobacco. A **cumulative effect** is the increasing response to repeated doses of a drug that occurs when the rate of administration exceeds the rate of metabolism or excretion. As a result, the amount of the drug builds up in the client's body unless the dosage is adjusted. Toxic symptoms may occur. An **idiosyncratic effect** is unexpected and individual. Underresponse and overresponse to

TABLE 33–5 Common Mild Allergic Responses

Symptom	Description/Rationale
Skin rash	Either an intraepidermal vesicle rash or a rash typified by an urticarial wheal or macular eruption; rash is usually generalized over the body
Pruritus	Itching of the skin with or without a rash
Angioedema	Edema due to increased permeability of the blood capillaries
Rhinitis	Excessive watery discharge from the nose
Lacrimal tearing	Excessive tearing
Nausea, vomiting	Stimulation of these centers in the brain
Wheezing and dyspnea	Shortness of breath and wheezing on inhalation and exhalation due to accumulated fluids and swelling of the respiratory tissues
Diarrhea	Irritation of the mucosa of the large intestine

a drug may be idiosyncratic. Also, the drug may have a completely different effect from the normal one or cause unpredictable and unexplainable symptoms in a particular client.

A **drug interaction** occurs when the administration of one drug before, at the same time as, or after another drug alters the effect of one or both drugs. The effect of one or both drugs may be either increased (**potentiating** or **synergistic effect**) or decreased (**inhibiting effect**). Drug interactions may be beneficial or harmful. For example, probenecid, which blocks the excretion of penicillin, can be given with penicillin to increase blood levels of the penicillin for longer periods (potentiating effect). Two analgesics, such as aspirin and codeine, are often given together because together they provide greater pain relief (additive effect). In this example of aspirin and codeine, using a combination of drugs often decreases the total dose of narcotics needed. In addition, certain foods may interact adversely with a medication (see Table 45–1 in Chapter 45). 🔗

Iatrogenic disease (disease caused unintentionally by medical therapy) can be due to drug therapy. Hepatic toxicity resulting in biliary obstruction, renal damage, and malformations of the fetus as a result of specific drugs taken during pregnancy are examples.

DRUG MISUSE

Drug misuse is the improper use of common medications in ways that lead to acute and chronic toxicity. Both over-the-counter drugs and prescription drugs may be misused. Laxatives, antacids, vitamins, headache remedies, and cough and cold medications are often self-prescribed and overused. Most people suffer no harmful effects from these drugs, but some people do. A persistent cough may go undiagnosed until the underlying problem becomes serious and advanced.

Drug abuse is inappropriate intake of a substance, either continually or periodically. By definition, drug use is abusive when society considers it abusive. For example, the intake of alcohol at work may be considered alcohol abuse, but intake at a social gathering may not. Drug abuse has two main facets, drug dependence and habituation. **Drug dependence** is a person's reliance on or need to take a drug or substance. The two types of dependence, physiologic and psychologic, may occur separately or together. **Physiologic dependence** is due to biochemical changes in body tissues, especially the nervous system. These tissues come to require the substance for normal functioning. A dependent person who stops using the drug experiences withdrawal symptoms. **Psychologic dependence** is emotional reliance on a drug to maintain a sense of well-being, accompanied by feelings of need or cravings for that drug. There are varying degrees of psychologic dependence, ranging from mild desire to craving and compulsive use of the drug.

Drug habituation denotes a mild form of psychologic dependence. The individual develops the habit of taking the substance and feels better after taking it. The habituated individual tends to continue the habit even though it may be injurious to health.

Illicit drugs, also called *street drugs,* are those sold illegally. Illicit drugs are of two types: (a) drugs unavailable for purchase under any circumstances, such as heroin (in the United States), and (b) drugs normally available with a prescription that are being obtained through illegal channels. Illicit drugs often are taken because of their mood-altering effect; that is, they make the person feel happy or relaxed.

ACTIONS OF DRUGS ON THE BODY

The action of a drug in the body can be described in terms of its half-life, the time interval required for the body's elimination processes to reduce the concentration of the drug in the body by one-half. For example, if a drug's half-life is 8 hours, then the amount of drug in the body is as follows:

Initially: 100%
After 8 hours: 50%
After 16 hours: 25%
After 24 hours: 12.5%
After 32 hours: 6.25%

Because the purpose of most drug therapy is to maintain a constant drug level in the body, repeated doses are required to maintain that level. When an orally administered drug is absorbed from the gastrointestinal tract into the blood plasma, its concentration in the plasma increases until the elimination rate equals the rate of absorption. This point is known as the *peak plasma level* (Figure 33–2 ■). Unless the client receives another dose of the drug, the concentration steadily decreases. Key terms related to drug actions are as follows:

- **Onset of action:** The time after administration when the body initially responds to the drug
- **Peak plasma level:** The highest plasma level achieved by a single dose when the elimination rate of a drug equals the absorption rate
- **Drug half-life (elimination half-life):** The time required for the elimination process to reduce the concentration of the drug to one-half what it was at initial administration

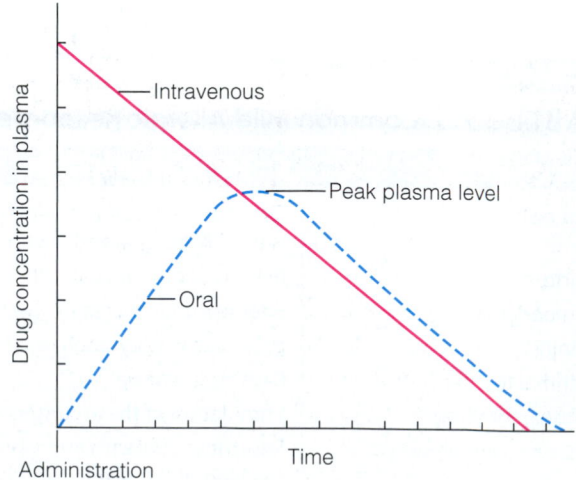

Figure 33–2 ■ A graphic plot of drug concentration in the blood plasma following a single dose.

- **Plateau:** A maintained concentration of a drug in the plasma during a series of scheduled doses

Pharmacodynamics

Pharmacodynamics is the process by which a drug alters cell physiology. One of the mechanisms is the drug interaction with a cellular receptor to produce a response known as an **agonist.** Drugs that have no special pharmacologic action of their own but that inhibit or prevent the action of an agonist are called **specific antagonists.** Drugs may also produce a response by stimulating enzyme activity or hormone production. They have a syngeristic effect.

Pharmacokinetics

Pharmacokinetics is the study of the absorption, distribution, biotransformation, and excretion of drugs.

Absorption

Absorption is the process by which a drug passes into the bloodstream. Unless the drug is administered directly into the bloodstream, absorption is the first step in the movement of the drug through the body. For absorption to occur, the correct form of the drug must be given by the route intended.

The rate of absorption of a drug in the stomach is variable. Food, for example, can delay the dissolution and absorption of some drugs as well as their passage into the small intestine, where most drug absorption occurs. Food can also combine with molecules of certain drugs, thereby changing their molecular structure and subsequently inhibiting or preventing their absorption. Another factor that affects the absorption of some drugs is the acid medium in the stomach. Acidity can vary according to the time of day, foods ingested, and the age of the client. Some drugs do not dissolve or have limited ability to dissolve in the gastrointestinal fluids, decreasing their absorption into the bloodstream. Some drugs are absorbed by tissues before they reach the stomach. For example, nitroglycerin is administered under the tongue, where it is absorbed into the blood vessels that carry it directly to the heart, the intended site of action. If swallowed, this drug will be absorbed into the bloodstream and carried to the liver, where it will be destroyed.

A drug administered directly into the bloodstream, that is, intravenously, is immediately in the vascular system without having to be absorbed. This, then, is the route of choice for rapid action. Because subcutaneous tissue has a poorer blood supply than muscle tissue, absorption from subcutaneous tissue is slower. The rate of absorption of a drug can be accelerated by the application of heat, which increases blood flow to the area; conversely, absorption can be slowed by the application of cold. In addition, the injection of a vasoconstrictor drug such as epinephrine into the tissue can slow absorption of other drugs. Some drugs intended to be absorbed slowly are suspended in a low-solubility medium, such as oil. The absorption of drugs from the rectum into the bloodstream tends to be unpredictable. Therefore, this route is normally used when other routes are unavailable or when the intended action is localized to the rectum or sigmoid colon.

Distribution

Distribution is the transportation of a drug from its site of absorption to its site of action. When a drug enters the bloodstream, it is carried to the most vascular organs—that is, liver, kidneys, and brain. Body areas with lower blood supply—that is, skin and muscles—receive the drug later. The chemical and physical properties of a drug largely determine the area of the body to which the drug will be attracted. For example, fat-soluble drugs will accumulate in fatty tissue, whereas other drugs may bind with plasma proteins.

Biotransformation

Biotransformation, also called **detoxification** or **metabolism,** is a process by which a drug is converted to a less active form. Most biotransformation takes place in the liver, where many drug-metabolizing enzymes in the cells detoxify the drugs. The products of this process are called **metabolites.** There are two types of metabolites: active and inactive. An *active metabolite* has a pharmacologic action itself, whereas an *inactive metabolite* does not.

Biotransformation may be impaired if a person is older or has an unhealthy liver. Nurses must be alert to the accumulation of the active drug in these clients and to subsequent toxicity.

Excretion

Excretion is the process by which metabolites and drugs are eliminated from the body. Most metabolites are eliminated by the kidneys in the urine; however, some are excreted in the feces, the breath, perspiration, saliva, and breast milk. Certain drugs, such as general anesthetic agents, are excreted in an unchanged form via the respiratory tract. The efficiency with which the kidneys excrete drugs and metabolites diminishes with age. Older people may require smaller doses of a drug because the drug and its metabolites may accumulate in the body.

FACTORS AFFECTING MEDICATION ACTION

A number of factors other than the drug itself can affect its action. A person may not respond in the same manner to successive doses of a drug. In addition, the identical drug and dosage may affect different clients differently.

Developmental Factors

During pregnancy women must be very careful about taking medications. Drugs taken during pregnancy pose a risk throughout the pregnancy, but pose the highest risk during the first trimester, due to the formation of vital organs and functions of the fetus during this time. Most drugs are contraindicated because of the possible adverse effects on the fetus.

Infants usually require small dosages because of their body size and the immaturity of their organs, especially the liver and kidneys. They often do not have all of the enzymes required for drug metabolism and therefore may require different medications than adults. In adolescence or adulthood, allergic reactions may occur to drugs formerly tolerated.

MediaLink | AGONIST/ANTAGONIST MECHANISM OF ACTION ANIMATION

Older adults have different responses to medications due to physiologic changes that accompany aging. These changes include decreased liver and kidney function, which can result in the accumulation of the drug in the body. In addition, the older person may be on multiple drugs and incompatibilities may occur.

Older adults often experience decreased gastric mobility and decreased gastric acid production and blood flow, which can impair drug absorption. Increased adipose tissue and decreased total body fluid proportionate to the body mass can increase the possibility of drug toxicity. Older adults may also experience a decreased number of protein-binding sites and changes in the blood–brain barrier. The latter permits fat-soluble drugs to move readily to the brain, often resulting in dizziness and confusion. This is particularly evident with beta blockers.

Gender

Differences in the way men and women respond to drugs are chiefly related to the distribution of body fat and fluid and hormonal differences. Because most drug research is done on men, more research on women is required to reflect the effects of hormonal changes on drug actions in women.

Cultural, Ethnic, and Genetic Factors

A client's response to a drug is influenced by age, gender, size, and body composition. This variation in response is called **drug polymorphism** (Kudzma, 1999). Research studies indicate that ethnicity may contribute to differences in responses to medication. Kudzma (1999) points out that drug metabolism is genetically determined and, as a result, race may effect a drug response. This is called *genetic polymorphism.* The genes that control liver metabolism vary and some clients may have slow metabolism, whereas others are rapid metabolizers. Research has shown that certain medication may work well at usual therapeutic dosages for certain ethnic groups but be toxic for others. Kudzma (1999) provides the example of antipsychotic and antianxiety drugs being effective for African Americans, Caucasians, and Hispanics; however, clients of Asian descent may need a lower dosage because of slower metabolism of that drug classification, which results in them being more prone to an adverse reaction. Cultural factors and practices (e.g., values and beliefs) can also affect a drug's action. For example, an herbal remedy (e.g., the Chinese herb ginseng) may speed up or slow down the metabolism of prescribed medications. The Providing Culturally Competent Care feature provides guidelines for nurses who care for clients from other cultures.

Diet

Nutrients can affect the action of a medication. For example, vitamin K found in green leafy vegetables can counteract the effect of an anticoagulant such as warfarin (Coumadin) (see Table 45–1 in Chapter 45).

Environment

The client's environment can affect the action of drugs, particularly those used to alter behavior and mood. Therefore, nurses assessing the effects of a drug need to consider the drug in the context of the client's personality and milieu.

Environmental temperature may also affect drug activity. When environmental temperature is high the peripheral blood vessels dilate, thus intensifying the action of vasodilators. In contrast, a cold environment and the consequent vasoconstriction inhibit the action of vasodilators but enhance the action of vasoconstrictors. A client who takes a sedative or analgesic in a busy, noisy environment may not benefit as fully as if the environment were quiet and peaceful.

Psychologic Factors

A client's expectations about what a drug can do can affect the response to the medication. For example, a client who believes that codeine is ineffective as an analgesic may experience no relief from pain after it is given.

Illness and Disease

Illness and disease can also affect the action of drugs. For example, aspirin can reduce the body temperature of a feverish client but has no effect on the body temperature of a client without fever. Drug action is altered in clients with circulatory, liver, or kidney dysfunction.

Time of Administration

The time of administration of oral medications affects the relative speed with which they act. Orally administered medications are absorbed more quickly if the stomach is empty.

Providing Culturally Competent Care

MEDICATIONS FOR CLIENTS FROM OTHER CULTURES

Ask about health beliefs and practices.

- Observe for unusual medication responses and adverse drug effects.
- Ask about herbal and folk or home remedies the client may be using.
- Determine the notion of time. What is the sense of time and importance of time frames for the client and family?
- Remember that there is considerable diversity within cultural groups.
- Include culturally sensitive information in health teaching.
- Use printed and visual materials that are in the language of the client.
- Encourage clients to voice their concerns and questions about medications. Be aware of nonverbal behaviors.

Note: From "Culturally Competent Drug Administration," by E. C. Kudzma, 1999, *American Journal of Nursing, 99*(8), pp. 46–51; *Nurse as Educator,* 2nd ed., by S. B. Bastable, 2003, Boston: Jones and Bartlett Publishing. Adapted with permission.

Thus oral medications taken 2 hours before meals act faster than those taken after meals. However, some medications, for example iron preparations, irritate the gastrointestinal tract and need to be given after a meal, when they will be better tolerated. A client's sleep–wake rhythm may affect the action of a drug. Circadian variations in urine output and blood circulation, for example, may affect a client's response to a drug.

ROUTES OF ADMINISTRATION

Pharmaceutical preparations are generally designed for one or two specific routes of administration (see Table 33–6). The route of administration should be indicated when the drug is ordered. When administering a drug, the nurse should ensure that the pharmaceutical preparation is appropriate for the route specified.

TABLE 33–6 Routes of Administration

Route	Advantages	Disadvantages
Oral	Most convenient Usually least expensive Safe, does not break skin barrier Administration usually does not cause stress	Inappropriate for clients with nausea or vomiting. Drug may have unpleasant taste or odor Inappropriate when gastrointestinal tract has reduced motility. Inappropriate if client cannot swallow or is unconscious Cannot be used before certain diagnostic tests or surgical procedures Drug may discolor teeth, harm tooth enamel Drug may irritate gastric mucosa Drug can be aspirated by seriously ill clients
Sublingual	Same as for oral, *plus* Drug can be administered for local effect More potent than oral route because drug directly enters the blood and bypasses the liver	If swallowed, drug may be inactivated by gastric juice Drug must remain under tongue until dissolved and absorbed Drug is rapidly absorbed into the bloodstream
Buccal	Same as for sublingual	Same as for sublingual
Rectal	Can be used when drug has objectionable taste or odor Drug released at slow, steady rate	Dose absorbed is unpredictable
Vaginal	Provides a local therapeutic effect	Limited use
Topical	Provides a local effect Few side effects	May be messy and may soil clothes Drug can enter body through abrasions and cause systemic effects
Transdermal	Prolonged systemic effect Few side effects Avoids gastrointestinal absorption problems	Leaves residue on the skin that may soil clothes
Subcutaneous	Onset of drug action faster than oral	Must involve sterile technique because breaks skin barrier More expensive than oral Can administer only small volume Slower than intramuscular administration Some drugs can irritate tissues and cause pain Can produce anxiety
Intramuscular	Pain from irritating drugs is minimized Can administer larger volume than subcutaneous Drug is rapidly absorbed	Breaks skin barrier Can produce anxiety
Intradermal	Absorption is slow (this is an advantage in testing for allergies)	Amount of drug administered must be small Breaks skin barrier
Intravenous	Rapid effect	Limited to highly soluble drugs Drug distribution inhibited by poor circulation
Inhalation	Introduces drug throughout respiratory tract Rapid localized relief Drug can be administered to unconscious client	Drug intended for localized effect can have systemic effect Of use only for the respiratory system

Oral

Oral administration is the most common, least expensive, and most convenient route for most clients. In oral administration, the drug is swallowed. Because the skin is not broken as it is for an injection, oral administration is also a safe method.

The major disadvantages are possibly unpleasant taste of the drugs, irritation of the gastric mucosa, irregular absorption from the gastrointestinal tract, slow absorption, and, in some cases, harm to the client's teeth. For example, the liquid preparation of ferrous sulfate (iron) can stain the teeth.

Sublingual

In **sublingual** administration a drug is placed under the tongue, where it dissolves (Figure 33–3 ■). In a relatively short time, the drug is largely absorbed into the blood vessels on the underside of the tongue. The medication should not be swallowed. Nitroglycerin is one example of a drug commonly given in this manner.

Buccal

Buccal means "pertaining to the cheek." In buccal administration, a medication (e.g., a tablet) is held in the mouth against the mucous membranes of the cheek until the drug dissolves (Figure 33–4 ■). The drug may act locally on the mucous membranes of the mouth or systemically when it is swallowed in the saliva.

Parenteral

The **parenteral** route is defined as other than through the alimentary or respiratory tract; that is, by needle. The following are some of the more common routes for parenteral administration:

- **Subcutaneous (hypodermic)**—into the subcutaneous tissue, just below the skin
- **Intramuscular**—into a muscle
- **Intradermal**—under the epidermis (into the dermis)
- **Intravenous**—into a vein

Some of the less commonly used routes for parenteral administration are intra-arterial (into an artery), intracardiac (into the

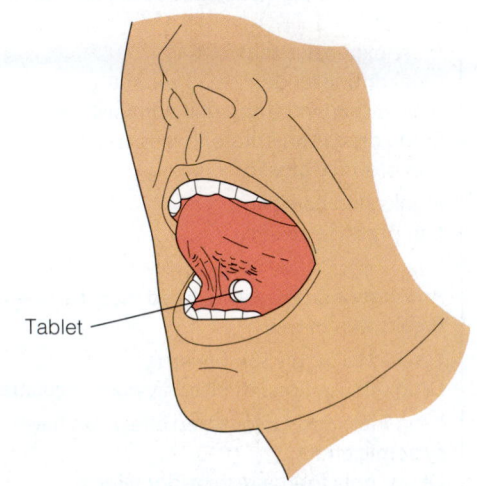

Figure 33–3 ■ Sublingual administration of a tablet.

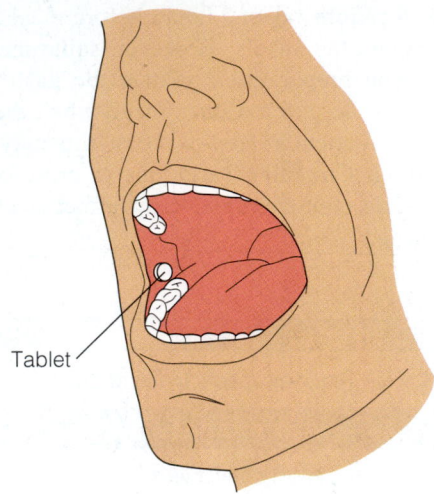

Figure 33–4 ■ Buccal administration of a tablet.

heart muscle), intraosseous (into a bone), **intrathecal** or **intraspinal** (into the spinal canal), intrapleural (into the pleural space), **epidural** (into the epidural space), and intra-articular (into a joint). Sterile equipment and sterile drug solution are essential for all parenteral therapy. The main advantage is fast absorption.

Topical

Topical applications are those applied to a circumscribed surface area of the body. They affect only the area to which they are applied. Topical applications include the following:

- Dermatologic preparations—applied to the skin
- Instillations and irrigations—applied into body cavities or orifices, such as the urinary bladder, eyes, ears, nose, rectum, or vagina
- Inhalations—administered into the respiratory tract by a nebulizer or positive pressure breathing apparatus. Air, oxygen, and vapor are generally used to carry the drug into the lungs.

MEDICATION ORDERS

A physician usually determines the client's medication needs and orders medications, although in some settings nurse practitioners and physician's assistants now order some drugs. Each health agency will have its own policies. Usually the order is written, although telephone and verbal orders are acceptable in a number of agencies. Nursing students need to know the agency policies about medication orders. In some hospitals, for example, only licensed nurses are permitted to accept telephone and verbal orders.

Policies about physicians' orders vary considerably from agency to agency. For example, a client's orders are frequently automatically canceled after surgery or an examination involving an anesthetic agent. New orders must then be written. Most agencies also have lists of abbreviations officially accepted for use in the agency. Both nurses and physicians may need to refer to these lists if they have been working in a different agency. These abbreviations can be used on legal documents, such as clients' charts (see Table 33–7).

TABLE 33–7 Common Abbreviations Used in Medication Orders

Abbreviation	Explanation	Example of Administration Time
ac	before meals	0700, 1100, and 1700 hours
ad lib	freely, as desired	
aq	water	
bid	twice a day	0900 and 2100 hours
c̄	with	
cap	capsule	
dil	dissolve, dilute	
ʒ	dram	
elix	elixir	
g, gm, or Gm	gram	
gr	grain	
gtt	drop	
h	an hour	
hs	at bedtime (hour of sleep)	
ID	intradermal	
IM	intramuscular	
IV	intravenous	
kg or Kg	kilogram	
l or L	liter	
M or m	mix	
mcg or μg	microgram	
mg or mgm	milligram	
OD	right eye	
OS	left eye	
OU	both eyes	
ʒ	ounce	
pc	after meals	0900, 1300, and 1900 hours
po or PO	by mouth	
prn	when needed	
q	every	
qAM	every morning	1000 hours
qh (q1h)	every hour	
q2h	every 2 hours	0800, 1000, 1200 hours, and so on
q3h	every 3 hours	0900, 1200, 1500 hours, and so on
q4h	every 4 hours	1000, 1400, 1800 hours, and so on
q6h	every 6 hours	0600, 1200, 1800, 2400 hours
qid	four times a day	1000, 1400, 1800, 2200 hours
qod	every other day	0900 hours on odd dates
qs	sufficient quantity	
Rx	take	
s̄	without	
sc or Sc or sq	subcutaneous	
ss or s̄s̄	one-half	
stat	at once	
sup or supp	suppostory	
susp	suspension	
tab	tablet	
tid	three times a day	1000, 1400, and 1800 hours
Tr or tinct	tincture	

Types of Medication Orders

Four common medication orders are the stat order, the single order, the standing order, and the prn order.

1. A **stat order** indicates that the medication is to be given immediately and only once (e.g., Demerol 100 mg IM stat).
2. The **single order** or *one-time order* is for medication to be given once at a specified time (e.g., Seconal 100 mg hs before surgery).
3. The **standing order** may or may not have a termination date. A standing order may be carried out indefinitely (e.g., multiple vitamins daily) until an order is written to cancel it, or it may be carried out for a specified number of days (e.g., Demerol 100 mg IM q4h × 5 days). In some agencies, standing orders are automatically canceled after a specified number of days and must be reordered.
4. A **prn order,** or *as needed order,* permits the nurse to give a medication when, in the nurse's judgment, the client requires it (e.g., Amphojel 15 mL prn). The nurse must use good judgment about when the medication is needed and when it can be safely administered.

Essential Parts of a Drug Order

The drug order has seven essential parts, as listed in Box 33–1. In addition, unless it is a standing order it should state the number of doses or the number of days the drug is to be administered.

The *client's full name,* that is, the first and last names and middle initials or names, should always be used to avoid confusion between two clients who have the same last name. In some agencies, the client's identification number and physician's name are put on the order as further identification. Some hospitals imprint the client's name, identification number, and room number on all forms while some agencies use stickers with similar information.

In addition to the *day,* the *month,* and the *year* the order was written, some agencies also require that the time of day be written. Writing the *time of day* on the order can eliminate errors when the nursing shifts change and makes clear when certain orders automatically terminate. For example, in some settings narcotics can be ordered only for 48 hours after surgery. Therefore, a drug that is ordered at 1600 hours November 1,

---

2003, is automatically canceled at 1600 November 3, 2003. Many health agencies use the 24-hour clock, which eliminates confusion between morning and afternoon times. Time with the 24-hour clock starts at midnight, which is 0000 hours (see Chapter 20).

The *name of the drug to be administered* must be clearly written. In some settings only generic names are permitted; however, trade names are widely used in hospitals and health agencies.

The *dosage of the drug* includes the amount, the times or *frequency of administration,* and in many instances the strength; for example, tetracycline 250 mg (amount) four times a day (frequency); potassium chloride 10% (strength) 5 mL (amount) three times a day with meals (time and frequency). Dosages can be written in apothecaries' or metric systems.

Also included in the order is the *route of administration* of the drug. This part of the order, like other parts, is frequently abbreviated. Table 33–7 lists abbreviations of routes of administration. It is not unusual for a drug to have several possible routes of administration; therefore, it is important that the route be included in the order.

The *signature* of the ordering physician or nurse makes the drug order a legal request. *An unsigned order has no validity,* and the ordering physician or nurse needs to be notified if the order is unsigned.

When a physician writes a prescription for a client, the prescription also includes information for the pharmacist. Therefore, a prescription's content differs from that of a medication order in a hospital. Compare the parts of a prescription listed in Box 33–2 with those shown in Figure 33–5 ■.

Communicating a Medication Order

A drug order is written on the client's chart by a physician or by a nurse receiving a telephone or verbal order from a physician. Most acute care agencies have a specified time frame (e.g., 24 or 48 hours) in which the physician issuing the telephone or verbal order must cosign the order written by the nurse. The medication order is then copied by a nurse or clerk to a Kardex or medication administration record (MAR). Increasingly, nurses are being provided with computer printouts of a client's medications instead of copying the physi-

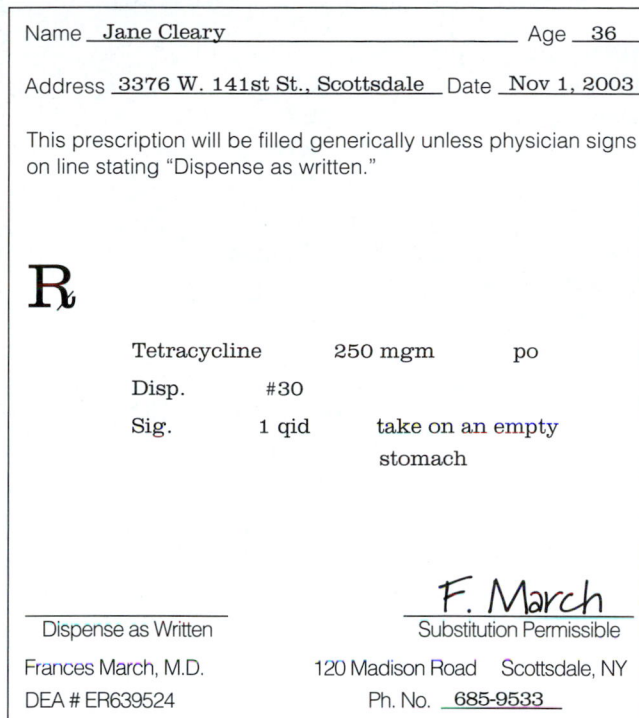

Name	Jane Cleary	Age 36
Address	3376 W. 141st St., Scottsdale	Date Nov 1, 2003

This prescription will be filled generically unless physician signs on line stating "Dispense as written."

R

Tetracycline	250 mgm	po
Disp.	#30	
Sig.	1 qid	take on an empty stomach

F. March

Dispense as Written	Substitution Permissible
Frances March, M.D.	120 Madison Road Scottsdale, NY
DEA # ER639524	Ph. No. 685-9533

Figure 33–5 ■ A prescription filled out by a physician.

cian's order. This method avoids errors of copying and saves nursing time.

> **CLINICAL ALERT**   *If your assigned client receives new medication orders, double check the transcribed information with the physician's order. This ensures client safety.*

Medication administration records (Figure 33–6 ■) vary in form, but all include the client's name, room, and bed number; drug name and dose; and times and method of administration. In some agencies, the date the order was prescribed and the date the order expires are also included.

The nurse should always question the physician about any order that is ambiguous, unusual (e.g., an abnormally high dosage of a medication), or contraindicated by the client's condition. When the nurse judges a physician-ordered medication inappropriate, the following actions are required:

- Contact the physician and discuss the rationale for believing the medication or dosage to be inappropriate.
- Document in notes the following: when the physician was notified, what was conveyed to the physician, and how the physician responded.
- If the physician cannot be reached, document all attempts to contact the physician and the reason for withholding the medication.
- If someone else gives the medication, document data about the client's condition before and after the medication.
- If an incident report (see Chapter 4 ⬭) is indicated, clearly document factual information.

SYSTEMS OF MEASUREMENT

Three systems of measurement are used in North America: the metric system, the apothecaries' system, and the household system, which is similar to the apothecaries' system.

Metric System

The metric system, devised by the French in the latter part of the 18th century, is the system prescribed by law in most European countries and in Canada. The metric system is logically organized into units of 10; it is a decimal system. Basic units can be multiplied or divided by 10 to form secondary units. Multiples are calculated by moving the decimal point to the right, and division is accomplished by moving the decimal point to the left.

Basic units of measurement are the *meter,* the *liter,* and the *gram.* Prefixes derived from Latin designate subdivisions of the basic unit: *deci* (1/10 or 0.1), *centi* (1/100 or 0.01), and *milli* (1/1,000 or 0.001). Multiples of the basic unit are designated by prefixes derived from Greek: *deka* (10), *hecto* (100), and *kilo* (1,000). Only the measurements of volume (the liter) and of weight (the gram) are discussed in this chapter. These are the measures used in medication administration (see Figure 33–7 ■). In nursing practice, the *kilogram* (kg) is the only multiple of the gram used, and the *milligram* (mg) and *microgram* (mcg or µg) are subdivisions. Fractional parts of the liter are usually expressed in *milliliters* (mL), for example, 600 mL; multiples of the liter are usually expressed as *liters* or milliliters, for example, 2.5 liters or 2,500 mL.

Apothecaries' System

The apothecaries' system, older than the metric system, was brought to the United States from England during the colonial period. The basic unit of weight in the apothecaries' system is the *grain* (gr), likened to a grain of wheat, and the basic unit of volume is the **minim,** a volume of water equal in weight to a grain of wheat. The word *minim* means "the least." In ascending order, the other units of weight are the *scruple,* the *dram,* the *ounce,* and the *pound.* Today, the scruple (scr) is seldom used. The units of volume are, in ascending order, the fluid dram, the fluid ounce, the pint, the quart, and the gallon.

Quantities in the apothecaries' system are often expressed by lowercase Roman numerals, particularly when the unit of measure is abbreviated. The Roman numeral follows rather than precedes the unit of measure. For example, two ounces are written as ℥ ii, and 4 ounces are written as ℥ iv. Quantities less than 1 are expressed as a fraction, for example, gr 1/6.

Household System

Household measures may be used when more accurate systems of measure are not required. Included in household measures are drops, teaspoons, tablespoons, cups, and glasses. Although pints and quarts are often found in the home, they are defined as apothecaries' measures.

MEDICATION ADMINISTRATION RECORD

PRN#:
MRN#:   AGE:
ADM: 08-04-03   SEX:
DOB: HT:
DR.   HT:

VERIFIED BY: _____ DATE: _____

DIAGNOSIS: *#ALOC
             *#PNEUMONIA

ALLERGIES: NO KNOWN DRUG ALLERGIES

GENERATED: 08-07-03   07:32am
FOR PERIOD: 08-07-03   08:00
THROUGH: 08-08-03   07:59

START	STOP	MEDICATION/I.V./IVPB/IRRIGATION		0800-1559	1600-2359	0000-0759
08-06 17	09-05 16	FERROUS SULFATE 300MG=5ML TWICE A DAY PO (FES04)	(973539)	09	17	
08-06 17	09-05 16	DOCUSATE SODIUM 100MG=1UDCUP TWICE A DAY PO (COLACE) 100MG/30ML UD HOLD FOR LOOSE STOOL	(973532)	09	17	
08-05 09	09-04 08	ASCORBIC ACID 500MG=1TAB TWICE A DAY PO (VITAMIN C) 500MG TAB	(972096)	09	17	
08-05 09	09-04 08	LEVOTHYROXINE 0.05MG=1TAB DAILY PO (SYNTHROID) 0.05MG TAB	(972095)	09		
08-05 09	09-04 08	ASPIRIN 325MG=1 TAB DAILY PO (ASPIRIN) 325MG TAB *W/FOOD TO AVOID GI UPSET	(972094)	09		
08-04 23	08-14 22	CEFUROXIME ADDV. 1.500GM=1VIAL EVERY 8 HOURS IV (KEFUROX) 1.5GM ADDV *ATTACH TO D5W 50ML ADDV BAG *ACTIVATE BEFORE INFUSION* * INFUSE OVER 30 MINS*	(971776)	14	22	06
		——— PRN ORDERS ———				
08-04 23	09-03 22	ACETAMINOPHEN 650MG=1SUPP EVERY 4 HOURS AS NEEDED PR (TYLENOL) 650MG SUPP	(971779)			

INITIALS	SIGNATURE	SHIFT	INITIALS	SIGNATURE	SHIFT	INITIALS	SIGNATURE	SHIFT

SITE CODES:
A. Right Upper Outer Quadrant Gluteus   C. Right Outer Aspect Arm   E. Right Ventrogluteal   G. Abdomen   I. Left Thigh
B. Left Upper Outer Quadrant Gluteus   D. Left Outer Aspect Arm   F. Left Ventrogluteal   H. Right Thigh

Figure 33–6 ■ Sample medication administration record.

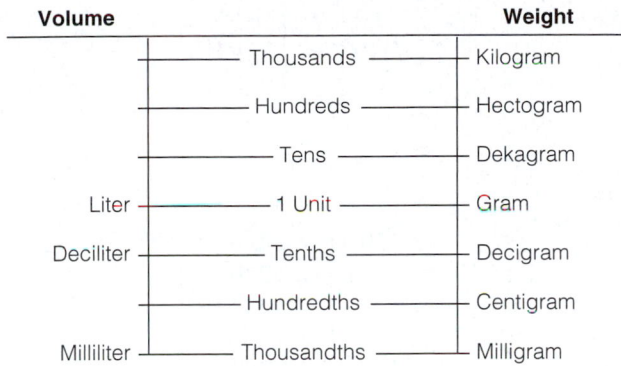

Figure 33–7 ■ Basic metric measurements of volume and weight.

Converting Units of Weight and Measure

Sometimes drugs are dispensed from the pharmacy in grams when the order specifies milligrams, or they are dispensed in milligrams though ordered in grains. For example, a physician orders morphine gr 1/4. The medication is available labeled only in milligrams. The nurse knows that 1 mg = 1/60 gr or 60 mg = 1 grain. To convert the ordered dose to milligrams, the nurse calculates as follows:

If 60 mg = 1 gr
Then x mg = 1/4 gr (0.25 gr)
$$x = \frac{(60 \times 0.25)}{1}$$
$$x = 15 \text{ mg}$$

Converting Weights within the Metric System

It is relatively simple to arrive at equivalent units of weight within the metric system because the system is based on units of 10. Only three metric units of weight are used for drug dosages, the gram (g), milligram (mg), and microgram (mcg or μg): 1,000 mg or 1,000,000 mcg equals 1 g. Equivalents are computed by dividing or multiplying; for example, to change milligrams to grams, the nurse divides the number of milligrams by 1,000. The simplest way to divide by 1,000 is to move the decimal point three places to the left:

500 mg = ? g

Move the decimal point three places to the *left:*

Answer = 0.5 g

Conversely, to convert grams to milligrams, multiply the number of grams by 1,000, or move the decimal point three places to the right:

0.006 g = ? mg

Move the decimal point three places to the *right:*

Answer = 6 mg

Converting Weights and Measures between Systems

When preparing client medications, a nurse may need to convert weights or volumes from one system to another. As an example, the pharmacy may dispense milligrams or grams of chloral hydrate, yet the nurse must administer an order that reads "chloral hydrate gr v̄īīss." To prepare the correct dose, the nurse must convert from the apothecaries' to the metric system. To give clients a useful, realistic measure for home use, the nurse may have to convert from the apothecaries' or metric system to the household system. All conversions are approximate, that is, not totally precise.

Converting Units of Volume

Commonly used approximate equivalents are shown in Table 33–8. By learning these equivalents, the nurse can make many conversions readily. For example, 15 minims = approximately 15 drops (gtt); therefore, 1 minim is approximately 1 drop. Similarly, 1 quart approximates 1,000 mL, and 1 gallon approximates 4,000 mL.

The following are some situations in which nurses need to apply a knowledge of volume conversion:

- Milliliter dosages may need to be fractionalized. The nurse can fractionalize milliliter dosages by remembering that 1 mL contains 15 drops or minims.
- Fluid drams and ounces are commonly used in prescribing liquid medications, such as cough syrups, laxatives, antacids, and antibiotics for children. The fluid ounce is frequently converted to milliliters when measuring a client's fluid intake or output.

TABLE 33–8 Approximate Volume Equivalents: Metric, Apothecaries', and Household Systems

Metric		Apothecaries'		Household
1 mL	=	15 minims (min or m)	=	15 drops (gtt)
15 mL	=	4 fluid drams (3)	=	1 tablespoon (Tbsp)
30 mL	=	1 fluid ounce (3)	=	same
500 mL	=	1 pint (pt)	=	same
1,000 mL	=	1 quart (qt)	=	same
4,000 mL	=	1 gallon (gal)	=	same

- Liters and milliliters are the volumes commonly used in preparing solutions for enemas, irrigating solutions for douches, bladder irrigations, and solutions for cleaning open wounds. In some situations, the nurse needs to convert the volumes of such solutions.

Converting Units of Weight

The units of weight most commonly used in nursing practice are the gram, milligram, and kilogram and the grain and the pound. Household units of weight are generally not applicable.

Table 33–9 shows metric and apothecaries' approximate equivalents. Learning these equivalents helps the nurse make weight conversions readily, as for example in the following situations:

- Converting grams and milligrams to grains and vice versa, for example, when preparing medications
- Converting pounds to kilograms and vice versa, for example, a person's weight.

When converting units of weight from the metric system to the apothecaries' system, the nurse should keep in mind that a milligram is smaller than a grain (1 mg = 1/60 grain and 1 grain = 60 mg). The result of converting a smaller unit (milligram) to a larger unit (grain) is a smaller number. Thus, the nurse must divide (by 60 if converting from milligrams to grains). Conversely, when converting from a larger unit to a smaller unit, the nurse multiplies (by 60 if converting from grains to milligrams), and the product is a larger number. In other words:

$$\text{Small units (mg) to large units (grains)} = \text{a smaller number}$$
$$\text{Large units (grains) to small units (mg)} = \text{a larger number}$$
$$\frac{3{,}000 \text{ mg}}{60} = 50 \text{ grains}$$
$$50 \text{ grains} \times 60 = 3{,}000 \text{ mg}$$

When converting pounds to kilograms, the nurse applies the same rule. The pound is a smaller unit than the kilogram, and the nurse converts by dividing or multiplying by 2.2:

$$2.2 \text{ lb} = 1 \text{ kg}$$
$$110 \text{ lb} = x \text{ kg}$$
$$x = \frac{110 \times 1}{2.2}$$
$$= 50 \text{ kg}$$

or

$$50 \text{ kg} = x \text{ lb}$$
$$1 \text{ kg} = 2.2 \text{ lb}$$
$$x = \frac{2.2 \times 50}{1}$$
$$= 110 \text{ lb}$$

The conversion of milligrams to grams was previously discussed. The decimal point is moved three spaces to the left:

$$3{,}000 \text{ mg} = 3 \text{ g}$$

Calculating Dosages

Several formulas can be used to calculate drug dosages. One formula uses ratios:

$$\frac{\text{Dose on hand}}{\text{Quantity on hand}} = \frac{\text{desired dose}}{\text{quantity desired } (x)}$$

For example, erythromycin 500 mg is ordered. It is supplied in a liquid form containing 250 mg in 5 mL. To calculate the dosage, the nurse uses the formula

$$\frac{\text{Dose on hand (250 mg)}}{\text{Quantity on hand (5 mL)}} = \frac{\text{desired dose (500 mg)}}{\text{quantity desired } (x)}$$

Then the nurse cross-multiplies:

$$250\, x = 5 \text{ mL} \times 500 \text{ mg}$$
$$x = \frac{5 \text{ mL} \times 500 \text{ mg}}{250 \text{ mg}}$$
$$x = 10 \text{ mL}$$

Therefore, the dose ordered is 10 mL. The nurse can also use this formula to calculate dosages:

$$\text{Amount to administer } (x) = \frac{\text{desired dose}}{\text{dose on hand}} \times \text{quantity on hand}$$

For example, heparin is often distributed in vials in prepared dilutions of 10,000 units per milliliter. If the order calls for 5,000 units, the nurse can use the preceding formula to calculate

$$x = \frac{5{,}000}{10{,}000} \times 1$$
$$x = 1/2 \text{ mL}$$

Therefore, the nurse injects 0.5 mL for a 5,000-unit dose.

Dosages for Children

Although dosage is stated in the medication order, nurses must understand something about the safe dosage for children. Unlike adult dosages, children's dosages are not always standard. Body size significantly affects dosage.

TABLE 33–9 Approximate Weight Equivalents: Metric and Apothecaries' Systems

Metric		Apothecaries'
1 mg	=	1/60 grain
60 mg	=	1 grain
1 g	=	15 grains
4 g	=	1 dram
30 g	=	1 ounce
500 g	=	1.1 pound (lb)
1,000 g (1 kg)	=	2.2 lb

Body Surface Area

Body surface area is determined by using a nomogram and the child's height and weight. This is considered to be the most accurate method of calculating a child's dose. Standard nomograms give a child's body surface area according to weight and height (Figure 33–8 ■). The formula is the ratio of the child's body surface area to the surface area of an average adult (1.7 square meters, or 1.7 m^2), multiplied by the normal adult dose of the drug:

$$\text{Child's dose} = \frac{\text{surface area of child (m}^2)}{1.7 \text{ m}^2} \times \text{normal adult dose}$$

For example, a child who weighs 10 kg and is 50 cm tall has a body surface area of 0.4 m^2. Therefore, the child's dose of tetracycline corresponding to an adult dose of 250 mg would be as follows:

$$\text{Child's dose} = \frac{0.4 \text{ m}^2}{1.7 \text{ m}^2} \times 250 \text{ mg}$$

$$= 0.23 \times 250 = 58.82 \text{ mg}$$

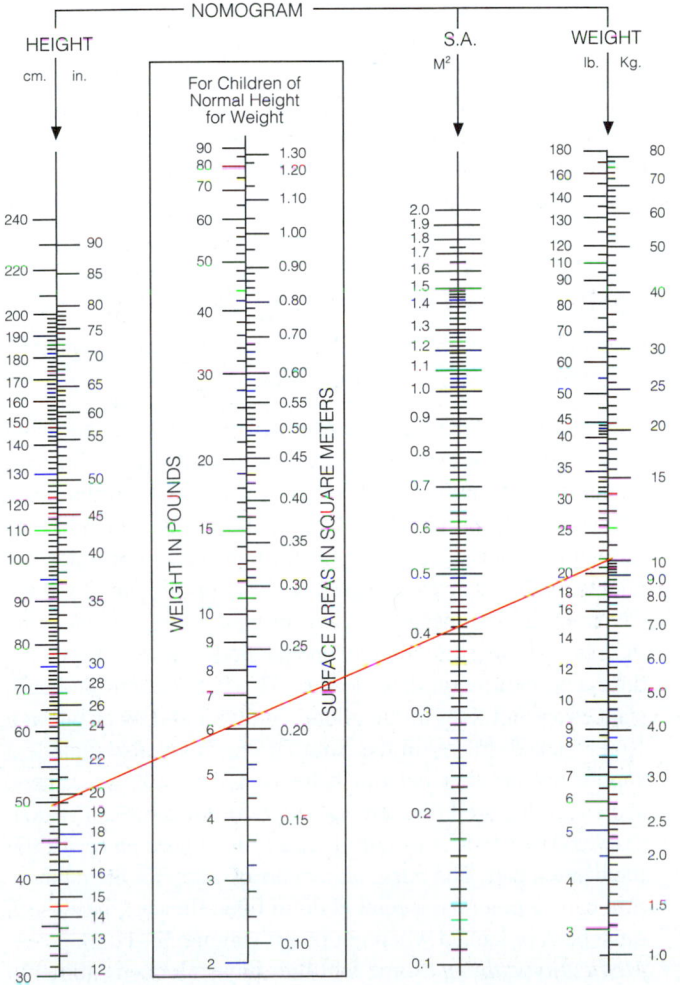

Figure 33–8 ■ Nomogram with estimated body surface area. A straight line is drawn between the child's height (on the left) and the child's weight (on the right). The point at which the line intersects the surface area column is the estimated body surface area.

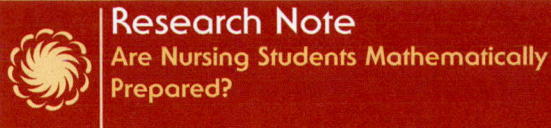

Research Note
Are Nursing Students Mathematically Prepared?

Nurses need to be competent in mathematics to prevent drug administration errors. Brown (2002) reviewed studies, conducted at baccalaureate and associate degree nursing programs, that found a large percentage of nursing students could not pass a basic arithmetic test on entry to the program.

The purpose of this study was to identify the weak links in computational mathematical abilities. The population group consisted of first-semester associate degree nursing students from NLN accredited programs. The students were administered a standard basic mathematic ability test for which each item had four response choices. There was no time limit and no calculators were allowed.

In addition, nursing faculty were asked to review the math test and indicate what percentage of the nursing students should be able to answer all items correctly. The mean student score was 75% and the mean score expected by faculty was 87.9%.

Examination of individual test items provided more information, however, than just the group means. At least 70% could calculate math problems dealing with whole numbers. When the items dealt with fractions, decimals, and percents, however, the correct response rate dropped between 30% and 65%. One of the lowest correct response rate was: 1/400 = (change to a decimal), which is common in medication administration. For example, atropine sulfate 0.4 mg is ordered and available as "gr 1/150."

Implications: Nursing students are mathematically underprepared. The author stressed the importance of the ability to calculate medication dosages correctly and suggested the following strategies: Require students to take a math placement test, provide math remedial courses, and administer a math skills test each semester.

Note: From "Does 1 + 1 Still Equal 2? A Study of the Mathematic Competencies of Associate Degree Nursing Students," by D. L. Brown, 2002, *Nurse Educator, 27*(3), pp. 132–135.

ADMINISTERING MEDICATIONS SAFELY

The nurse should always assess a client's health status and obtain a medication history prior to giving any medication. The extent of the assessment depends on the client's illness or current condition, the intended drug, and the route of administration. For example, if a patient has dyspnea, the nurse assesses respirations carefully before administering any medication that might affect breathing. It is important to determine whether the route of administration is suitable. For example, a client who is nauseated may not be able to keep down a drug taken orally. In general, the nurse assesses the client *prior* to administering any medication to obtain baseline data by which to evaluate the effectiveness of the medication.

The medication history includes information about the drugs the client is taking currently or has taken recently. This

Practice Guidelines
Administering Medications

- Nurses who administer medications are responsible for their own actions. Question any order that is illegible or that you consider incorrect. Call the person who prescribed the medication for clarification.
- Be knowledgeable about the medications you administer. You need to know why the client is receiving the medication. Look up the necessary information if you are not familiar with the medication.
- Federal laws govern the use of narcotics and barbiturates. Keep these medications in a locked place.
- Use only medications that are in a clearly labeled container.
- Do not use liquid medications that are cloudy or have changed color.
- Calculate drug doses accurately. If you are uncertain, ask another nurse to double check your calculations.
- Administer only medications personally prepared.

- Before administering a medication, identify the client correctly using the appropriate means of identification, such as checking the identification bracelet, asking a client to state her name, or both.
- Do not leave medications at the bedside, with certain exceptions (e.g., nitroglycerin, cough syrup). Check agency policy.
- If a client vomits after taking an oral medication, report this to the nurse in charge, or the physician, or both.
- Take special precautions when administering certain medications, for example, have another nurse check the dosages of anticoagulants, insulin, and certain IV preparations.
- Most hospital policies require new orders from the physician for a client's postsurgery care.
- When a medication is omitted for any reason, record the fact together with the reason.
- When a medication error is made, report it immediately to the nurse in charge, the physician, or both.

includes prescription drugs; over-the-counter drugs such as antacids, alcohol, and tobacco; and nonsanctioned drugs such as marijuana. Sometimes an incompatibility with one or more of these drugs affects the choice of a new medication.

Older adults often take vitamins, herbs, food supplements, and/or use folk remedies that they do not list in their medication history. Because many of these have unknown or unpredictable actions and side effects, they need to be noted, with attention paid to possible incompatibilities with other prescribed medications.

An important part of the history is clients' knowledge of their drug allergies. Some clients can tell a nurse, "I am allergic to penicillin, adhesive tape, and curry." Other clients may not be sure about allergic reactions. An illness occurring after a drug was taken may not be identified as an allergy, but the client may associate the drug with an illness or unusual reaction. The client's physician can often give information about allergies. During the history, the nurse tries to elicit information about drug dependencies. How often drugs are taken and the client's perceived need for them are measures of dependence.

Also included in the history are the client's normal eating habits. Sometimes the medication schedule needs to be coordinated with mealtimes or the ingestion of foods. Where a medication must be taken with food on a specified schedule, clients can often adjust their mealtime or have a snack (e.g., with a bedtime medication). In addition, certain foods are incompatible with certain medications, for example, milk is incompatible with tetracycline.

Any problems the client may have in self-administering a medication must also be identified. A client with poor eyesight, for example, may require special labels for the medication container; elderly clients with unsteady hands may not be able to hold a syringe or to inject themselves or another person. Obtaining information as to how and where the client stores his medications is also important. If the client has difficulty opening certain containers, he may change containers, but leave old labels on, which increases the risk of medication errors.

Socioeconomic factors need to be considered for all clients, but especially for elders. Two common problems are lack of transportation to obtain medications and inadequate finances to purchase medications. If the nurse is aware of these problems, proper resources can be obtained for the client.

Medication Dispensing Systems

Medical facilities vary in their medication dispensing systems. The systems can include the following:

- *Medication cart.* The medication cart is on wheels allowing the nurse to move the cart to outside the client's room. The cart contains small numbered drawers that correlate to the room numbers on the nursing unit. The small drawer is labeled with the name of the client currently in that room and holds the clients medications for the shift or 24 hours (Figure 33–9 ■). The medication is usually in unit-dose packaging in which the drug is packaged individually and labeled with the drug name, dose, and expiration date (Figure 33–10 ■). Controlled substances are not kept in the client's individual drawer but in a larger locked drawer in the cart. The cart may also include a supply drawer that contains client-labeled bulk containers, such as Metamucil, that are too large for the small individual drawer. The MAR is usually located in a binder on top of the medication cart. The nurse either carries a key for the medication cart or enters a special code to open the cart, because it must be kept locked when not in use (Figure 33–11 ■).
- *Medication cabinet.* Some facilities have a locked cabinet in the client's room. This cabinet holds the client's unit-dose medications and MAR. Controlled substances are not kept in this cabinet but at another location on the nursing unit. The nurse carries a key for opening the client's medication cabinet, because it must be locked when not in use.

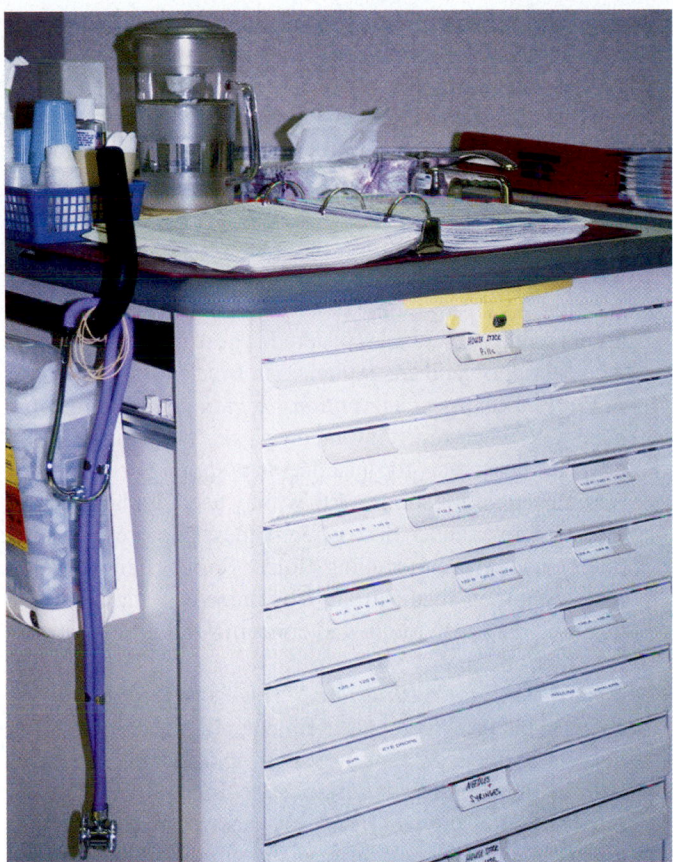

Figure 33–9 ■ Medication cart.

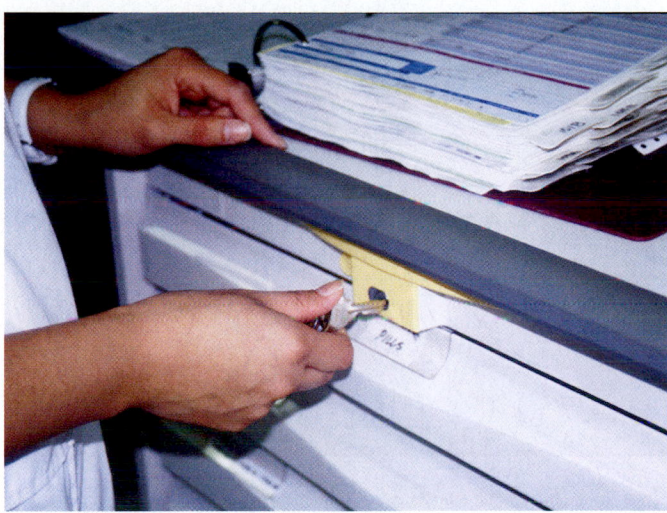

Figure 33–11 ■ The medication cart is kept locked when not in use. The nurse is using a key to access client medications.

- *Medication room.* Depending on the facility, a medication room may be used for a variety of purposes. For example, the medication carts, when not in use, may be placed in this room. The medication room may also be the central location for stock medications, controlled medications, and/or drugs used for emergencies. The medication room is often kept locked. Check agency policy.
- *Computerized medication access system.* This system (Figure 33–12 ■) automates the distribution, management, and control of medications. Similar to automated teller machines, the nurse uses a password to access the system and select the medication (Figure 33–13 ■).

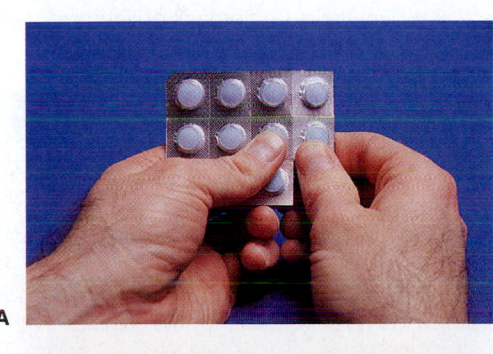

A

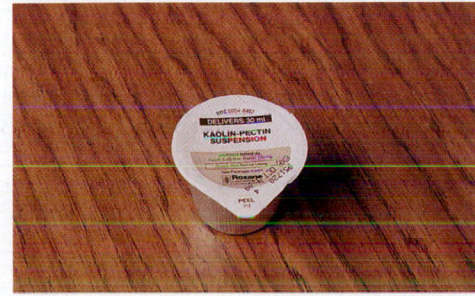

B

Figure 33–10 ■ Unit-dose packages: *A*, tablets; *B*, liquid medications.

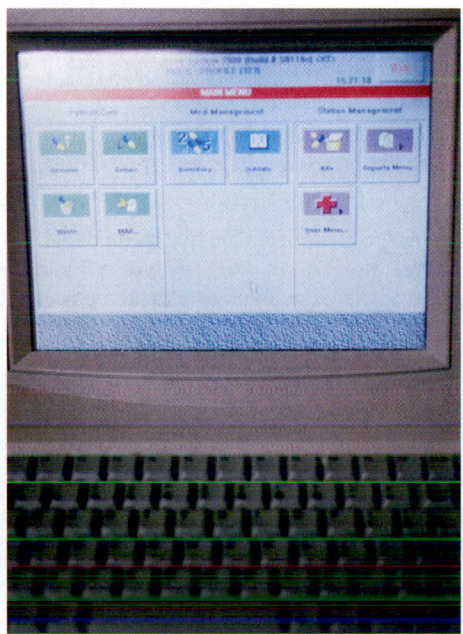

Figure 33–12 ■ Computerized medication access system.

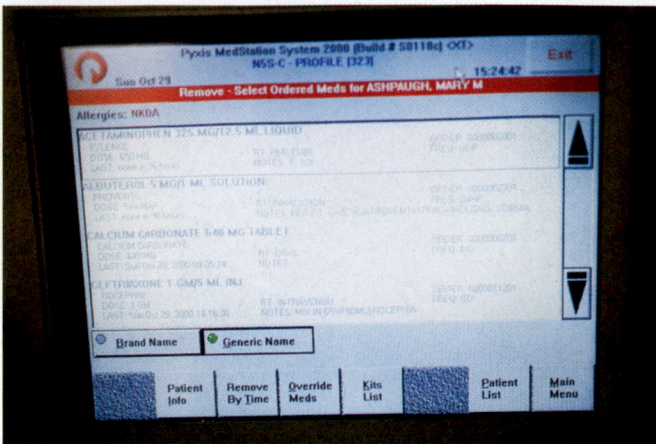

Figure 33–13 ■ Client profile in a computerized medication access system.

Process of Administering Medications

When administering any drug, regardless of the route of administration, the nurse must do the following:

1. *Identify the client.* Errors can and do occur, usually because one client gets a drug intended for another. In hospitals, most clients wear some sort of identification, such as a wristband with name and hospital identification number. Before giving the client any drug, always check the client's identification band. As a double check, the nurse can ask the alert client to state his or her name or can ask another nurse to identify the client before administering any medication.

> ➤ **CLINICAL ALERT**   *Do not ask "Are you John Jones?" because the client may answer "yes" to the wrong name.*

2. *Inform the client.* If the client is unfamiliar with the medication, the nurse should explain the intended action as well as any side effects or adverse effects that might occur.

3. *Administer the drug.* Read medication orders and records carefully and check against the name on the medication envelope or on the drawer in which the client's medications are kept if a medication cart is used. Then administer the medication in the prescribed dosage, by the route ordered, at the correct time. There are six aspects of medication administration which are important for the nurse to check each time a medication is administered. These are referred to as the six "rights" and are explained in Box 33–3.

4. *Provide adjunctive interventions as indicated.* Clients may need help when receiving medications. They may require physical assistance, for instance, in assuming positions for intramuscular injections, or they may need guidance about measures to enhance drug effectiveness and prevent complications, such as drinking fluids. Some clients convey fear about their medications. The nurse can allay fears by listening carefully to clients' concerns and giving correct information.

5. *Record the drug administered.* The facts recorded in the chart, in ink or by computer printout, are name of the drug, dosage, method of administration, specific relevant data such as pulse rate (taken in most settings prior to the administration of digitalis), and any other pertinent information. The record should also include the exact time of administration and the signature of the nurse providing the medication. Many medication records are designed so that the nurse signs once on the page and initials each medication administered. Often, medications that are given regularly are recorded on a special flow record. PRN (as needed) or stat (at once) medications are recorded separately.

6. *Evaluate the client's response to the drug.* The kinds of behavior that reflect the action or lack of action of a drug and

---

BOX 33–3	■ Six "Rights" of Medication Administration

Right Medication
- The medication given was the medication ordered.

Right Dose
- The dose ordered is appropriate for the client.
- Give special attention if the calculation indicates multiple pills/tablets or a large quantity of a liquid medication.
- Double check calculations that appear questionable.
- Know the usual dosage range of the medication.
- Question a dose outside of the usual dosage range.

Right Time
- Give the medication at the right frequency and at the time ordered according to agency policy.
- Medications given within 30 minutes before or after the scheduled time are considered to meet the right time standard.

Right Route
- Give the medication by the ordered route.
- Make certain that the route is safe and appropriate for the client.

Right Client
- Medication is given to the intended client.
- Check the client's identification band with each administration of a medication.
- Know the agency's name alert procedure when clients with the same or similar last names are on the nursing unit.

Right Documentation
- Document medication administration after giving it, not before.
- If time of administration differs from prescribed time, note the time on the MAR and explain reason and follow-through activities (e.g., pharmacy states medication will be available in 2 hours) in nursing notes.
- If a medication is not given, follow the agency's policy for documenting the reason why.

its untoward effects (both minor and major) are as variable as the purposes of the drugs themselves. The anxious client may show the desired effects of a tranquilizer by behavior that reflects a lowered stress level (e.g., slower speech or fewer random movements). The effectiveness of a sedative can often be measured by how well a client slept, and the effectiveness of an antispasmodic by how much pain the client feels. In all nursing activities, nurses need to be aware of the medications that a client is taking and record their effectiveness as assessed by the client and the nurse on the client's chart. The nurse may also report the client's response directly to the nurse manager and physician.

Developmental Considerations

It is important for the nurse to be aware of how growth and development impacts administration of medications for all age groups, particularly the very young and the very old.

Infants and Children

Knowledge of growth and development is essential for the nurse administering medications to children. Oral medications for children are usually prepared in sweetened liquid form to make them more palatable. The parents may provide suggestions about what method is best for their child. Necessary foods such as milk or orange juice should not be used to mask the taste of medications, because the child may develop unpleasant associations and refuse that food in the future.

Children tend to fear any procedure in which a needle is used because they anticipate pain or because the procedure is unfamiliar and threatening. The nurse needs to acknowledge that the child will feel some pain; denying this fact only deepens the child's distrust. After the injection, the nurse (or the parent) can cuddle and speak softly to the infant and give the child a toy to dispel the child's association of the nurse only with pain.

Elders

Elders can have special problems, most of which are related to physiologic changes, to past experiences, and to established attitudes toward medications. The physiologic changes in elders that may affect the administration and effectiveness of medications are listed in Box 33–4.

Many of these changes enhance the possibility of cumulative effects and toxicity. For example, impaired circulation delays the action of medications given intramuscularly or subcutaneously. Digitalis, which is frequently taken by elders, can accumulate to toxic levels and be lethal. It is not uncommon for elders to take several different medications daily. The possibility of error increases with the number of medications taken, whether self-administered at home or administered in a hospital. The greater number of medications also compounds the problem of drug interactions. A general rule to follow is that elders should take as few medications as possible.

Elders usually require smaller dosages of drugs, especially sedatives and other central nervous system depressants. Reactions of elders to medications, particularly sedatives, are unpredictable and often bizarre. It is not uncommon to see irritability, confusion, disorientation, restlessness, and incontinence as a result of sedatives. Nurses therefore need to observe clients carefully for untoward reactions. Physicians often follow the unwritten rule to "start low and go slow" when prescribing medications for elders. The initial prescribed dosage will often be low and then be gradually increased with careful monitoring of actions and side effects of the drug.

Attitudes of elders toward medical care and medications vary. Elders tend to believe in the wisdom of the physician more readily than younger people. Some older people are bewildered by the prescription of several medications and may passively accept their medications from nurses but not swallow them, spitting out tablets or capsules after the nurse leaves the room. For this reason, the nurse is advised to stay with clients until they have swallowed the medications. Others may be suspicious of medications and actively refuse them.

Elders are mature adults capable of reasoning. Therefore, the nurse needs to explain the reasons for and the effects of medications. This education can prevent clients from continuing to take a medication long after there is a need for it or discontinuing a drug too quickly. For example, clients should know that diuretics will cause them to urinate more frequently and may reduce ankle edema. Instructions about medications need to be given to all clients. These instructions should include when to take the drugs, what effects to expect, and when to consult a physician.

BOX 33–4	■ Physiologic Changes Associated with Aging That Influence Medication Administration and Effectiveness

- Altered memory
- Less acute vision
- Decrease in renal function, resulting in slower elimination of drugs and higher drug concentrations in the bloodstream for longer periods
- Less complete and slower absorption from the gastrointestinal tract
- Increased proportion of fat to lean body mass, which facilitates retention of fat-soluble drugs and increases potential for toxicity

- Decreased liver function, which hinders biotransformation of drugs
- Decreased organ sensitivity, which means that the response to the same drug concentration in the vicinity of the target organ is less in older people than in the young
- Altered quality of organ responsiveness, resulting in adverse effects becoming pronounced before therapeutic effects are achieved
- Decrease in manual dexterity due to arthritis and/or decrease in flexibility

Because some clients are required to take several medications daily and because visual acuity and memory may be impaired, the nurse needs to develop simple, realistic plans for clients to follow at home. For example, remembering to take drugs can be difficult for most people, including elders. If medications are scheduled to be taken with meals or at bedtime, clients are not as likely to forget. Some clients may take their medications and then an hour later not remember whether they took them. One solution to forgetfulness is to use a special container or glass strictly for medications. An empty glass or container indicates that the person took the pills. Loss of visual acuity presents problems that can be overcome by writing out the plan in block letters large enough to be read. In some situations the help of a spouse, son, or daughter can be enlisted.

Elders often have a decrease in dexterity due to arthritis or stiffness of their hands and fingers due to aging. This causes difficulty in opening medication containers or in self-administration of other medications such as eye drops, ear drops, insulin injections, and inhalers. Nurses can help clients make the necessary changes or enlist the assistance of another person to help them administer their medications.

ORAL MEDICATIONS

The oral route is the most common route by which medications are given. As long as a client can swallow and retain the drug in the stomach, this is the route of choice (see Procedure 33–1). Oral medications are contraindicated when a client is vomiting, has gastric or intestinal suction, or is unconscious and unable to swallow. Such clients in a hospital are usually on orders for "nothing by mouth" (Latin is *nil per os:* **NPO**).

Research Note
Why Do Medication Administration Errors Occur?

A survey was conducted by Wakefield, Wakefield, Uden-Holman, and Blegen (1998) in which they received 1,384 surveys from nurses in rural and urban acute care hospitals in one state. The following two individual items on the survey had the highest mean values: "interrupted while administering medications" and "doctor's orders not legible."

Five categories of factors were identified and included, in order of frequency: physician (e.g., orders not legible), systems (e.g., interrupted to do other duties), pharmacy (e.g., not all doses delivered), individual (e.g., order not transcribed correctly), and knowledge (e.g., similar names of medications).

Implications: The authors stress that medication administration is a complex process and not a simple psychomotor task. Survey findings such as these provide a basis to begin discussion about improving the system.

Note: From "Nurses' Perceptions of Why Medication Administration Errors Occur," by B. J. Wakefield, D. S. Wakefield, T. Uden-Holman, and M. A. Blegen, 1998, *MEDSURG Nursing, 7*(1), pp. 39–44.

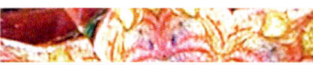
Procedure 33–1 Administering Oral Medications

Purpose
- To provide a medication that has systemic effects or local effects on the gastrointestinal tract or both (see specific drug action).

ASSESSMENT

Assess
- Allergies to medication(s)
- Clients ability to swallow the medication
- Presence of vomiting or diarrhea that would interfere with the ability to absorb the medication
- Specific drug action, side effects, interactions, and adverse reactions

- Client's knowledge of and learning needs about the medication Perform appropriate assessments (e.g., vital signs, laboratory results) specific to the medication.

Determine if the assessment data influence administration of the medication (i.e., is it appropriate to administer the medication or does the medication need to be held and the physician notified?).

PLANNING

Delegation
In acute care settings, the administration of oral/enteral medications is performed by the nurse and is not delegated to unlicensed assistive personnel (UAP). The nurse can inform the UAP of the intended therapeutic effects and/or specific side effects of the medication and request the UAP to report specific client observations to the nurse for follow-up. In some long-term care settings, UAP may be trained to administer certain medications to stable clients. It is important, however, for the nurse to remember that the medication knowledge of the UAP is limited and *assessment and evaluation of the effectiveness of the medication remains the responsibility of the nurse.*

Equipment
- Medication cart
- Disposable medication cups: small paper or plastic cups for tablets and capsules, waxed or plastic calibrated medication cups for liquids

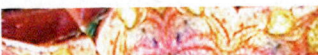

Procedure 33–1 Administering Oral Medications *continued*

PLANNING *continued*

- MAR or computer printout
- Pill crusher

- Straws to administer medications that may discolor the teeth or to facilitate the ingestion of liquid medication for certain clients
- Drinking glass and water or juice

IMPLEMENTATION

Preparation

1. Know the reason why the client is receiving the medication, the drug classification, contraindications, usual dosage range, side effects, and nursing considerations for administering and evaluating the intended outcomes for the medication.
2. Check the MAR
   - Check the MAR for the drug name, dosage, frequency, route of administration, and expiration date for administering the medication, if appropriate. *Certain medications (e.g., narcotics, antibiotics) have a specified time frame at which they expire and need to be reordered.*
   - If the MAR is unclear or pertinent information is missing, compare the MAR with the most recent physician's written order.
   - Report any discrepancies to the charge nurse or the physician, as agency policy dictates.
3. Verify the client's ability to take medication orally.
   - Determine whether the client can swallow, is NPO, is nauseated or vomiting, has gastric suction, or has diminished or absent bowel sounds.
4. Organize the supplies.
   - Place the medication cart outside the client's room.
   - Assemble the MAR(s) for each client together so that medications can be prepared for one client at a time. *Organization of supplies saves time and reduces the chance of error.*

Performance

1. Wash hands and observe other appropriate infection control procedures.
2. Unlock the medication cart.
3. Obtain appropriate medication.
   - Read the MAR and take the appropriate medication from the shelf, drawer, or refrigerator. The medication may be dispensed in a bottle, box, or unit-dose package.

- Compare the label of the medication container or unit-dose package against the order on the MAR (Figure 33–14 ■) or computer printout. *This is a safety check to ensure that the right medication is given.* If these are not identical, recheck the client's chart. If there is still a discrepancy, check with the nurse in charge or the pharmacist.
- Check the expiration date of the medication. Return expired medications to the pharmacy. *Outdated medications are not safe to administer.*
- Use only medications that have clear, legible labels *to ensure accuracy.*

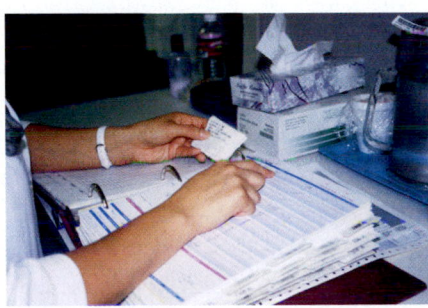

Figure 33–14 ■ Compare the medication label to the MAR.

4. Prepare the medication.
   - Calculate medication dosage accurately.
   - Prepare the correct amount of medication for the required dose, without contaminating the medication. *Aseptic technique maintains drug cleanliness.*
   - While preparing the medication, recheck each prepared drug and container with the MAR again. *This second safety check reduces the chance of error.*

TABLETS OR CAPSULES
   - Place packaged unit-dose capsules or tablets directly into the medicine cup. Do not remove the medication from the wrapper until at the bedside. *The wrapper keeps the medication clean. Not removing the medication from the wrapper facilitates identification of the medication in the event the client refuses the drug or assessment data indicate the drug should be held. Unopened unit-dose packages can usually be returned to the medication cart.*
   - If using a stock container, pour the required number into the bottle cap, and then transfer the medication to the disposable cup without touching the tablets.
   - Keep narcotics and medications that require specific assessments, such as pulse measurements, respiratory rate or depth, or blood pressure, separate from the others. *This reminds the nurse to complete the needed assessment(s) in order to decide whether to give the medication or to withhold the medication if indicated.*
   - Break only scored tablets if necessary to obtain the correct dosage. Use a file or cutting device if needed (Figure 33–15 ■). Check the agency policy as to whether unused portions of a medication can be discarded and, if so, how they are to be discarded.

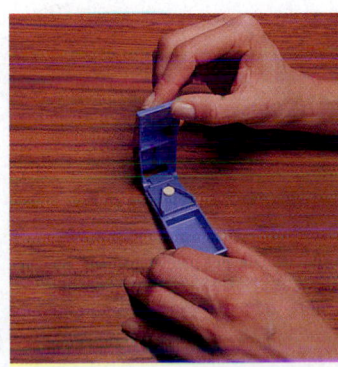

Figure 33–15 ■ A cutting device can be used to divide tablets.

continued on page 808

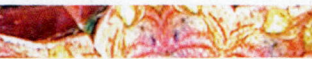

Procedure 33–1 Administering Oral Medications *continued*

IMPLEMENTATION *continued*

- If the client has difficulty swallowing, crush the tablets to a fine powder with a pill crusher or between two medication cups. Then, mix the powder with a small amount of soft food (e.g., custard, applesauce). Some medications should not be crushed. An example of tablets that should not be crushed is oxycontin, a long-acting narcotic, which normally lasts 12 hours after administration. If the tablet is crushed, the client gets a surge of action in the first 2 hours, then may start having severe pain again in 4 to 6 hours, as the effects wear off too soon. The crushing of these tablets causes an uneven effect and the "continuous" pain control is lost.

> ► **CLINICAL ALERT** *Check with the pharmacy before crushing tablets. Sustained-action, enteric-coated, buccal, or sublingual tablets should not be crushed.*

LIQUID MEDICATION

- Thoroughly mix the medication before pouring. Discard any medication that has changed color or turned cloudy.
- Remove the cap and place it upside down on the countertop *to avoid contaminating the inside of the cap.*
- Hold the bottle so the label is next to your palm and pour the medication away from the label (Figure 33–16 ■). *This prevents the label from becoming soiled and illegible as a result of spilled liquids.*

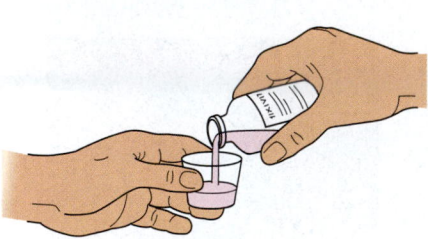

Figure 33–16 ■ Pouring a liquid medication from a bottle.

- Hold the medication cup at eye level and fill it to the desired level, using the bottom of the **meniscus** (crescent-shaped upper surface of a column of liquid) to align with container scale (Figure 33–17 ■). *This method ensures accuracy of measurement.*
- Before capping the bottle, wipe the lip with a paper towel. *This prevents the cap from sticking.*
- When giving small amounts of liquids (e.g., < 5 mL), prepare the medication in a sterile syringe without the needle.
- Keep unit-dose liquids in their package and open them at the bedside.

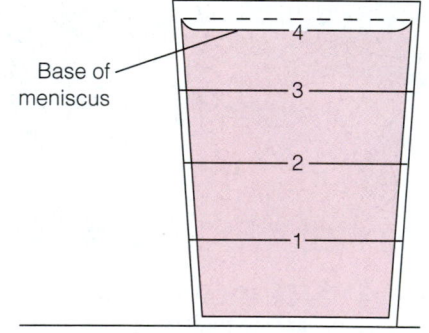

Base of meniscus

Figure 33–17 ■ The *bottom* of the meniscus is the measuring guide.

ORAL NARCOTICS

- If an agency uses a manual recording system for controlled substances, check the narcotic record for the previous drug count and compare it with the supply available. Some medications, including narcotics, are kept in plastic containers that are sectioned and numbered.

- Remove the next available tablet and drop it in the medicine cup.
- After removing a tablet, record the necessary information on the appropriate narcotic control record and sign it.
- *Note:* Computer-controlled dispensing systems allow access only to the selected drug and automatically record its use.

ALL MEDICATIONS

- Place the prepared medication and MAR together on the medication cart.
- Recheck the label on the container before returning the bottle, box, or envelope to its storage place. *This third check further reduces the risk of error.*
- Avoid leaving prepared medications unattended. *This precaution prevents potential mishandling errors.*
- Lock the medication cart before entering the client's room. *This is a safety measure because medication carts are not to be left open when unattended.*
- Check the room number against the MAR if agency policy does not allow the MAR to be removed from the medication cart. *This is another safety measure to ensure that the nurse is entering the correct client room.*
5. Provide for client privacy.
6. Prepare the client.
   - Check the client's identification band. *This ensures that the right client receives the medication.*
   - Assist the client to a sitting position or, if not possible, to a side-lying position. *These positions facilitate swallowing and prevent aspiration.*
   - If not previously assessed, take the required assessment measures, such as pulse and respiratory rates or blood pressure. Take the apical pulse rate before administering digitalis preparations. Take blood pressure before giving antihypertensive

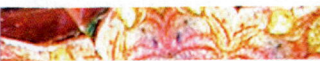

Procedure 33-1 Administering Oral Medications *continued*

IMPLEMENTATION *continued*

drugs. Take the respiratory rate prior to administering narcotics. *Narcotics depress the respiratory center.* If any of the findings are above or below the predetermined parameters, consult the physician before administering the medication.

7. Explain the purpose of the medication and how it will help, using language that the client can understand. Include relevant information about effects; for example, tell the client receiving a diuretic to expect an increase in urine output. *Information facilitates acceptance of and compliance with the therapy.*

8. Administer the medication at the correct time.
   - Take the medication to the client within the time frame of 30 minutes before or after the scheduled time.
   - Give the client sufficient water or preferred juice to swallow the medication. Before using juice, check for any food and medication incompatibilities. *Fluids ease swallowing and facilitate absorption from the gastrointestinal tract.* Liquid medications other than antacids or cough preparations are generally diluted with 15 mL (1/2 oz) of water to facilitate absorption.

   - If the client is unable to hold the pill cup, use the pill cup to introduce the medication into the client's mouth, and give only one tablet or capsule at a time. *Putting the cup to the client's mouth maintains the cleanliness of the nurse's hands. Giving one medication at a time eases swallowing.*
   - If an older child or adult has difficulty swallowing, ask the client to place the medication on the back of the tongue before taking the water. *Stimulation of the back of the tongue produces the swallowing reflex.*
   - If the medication has an objectionable taste, ask the client to suck a few ice chips beforehand, or give the medication with juice, applesauce, or bread if there are no contraindications. *The cold of the ice chips will desensitize the taste buds, and juices or bread can mask the taste of the medication.*
   - If the client says that the medication you are about to give is different from what the client has been receiving, do not give the medication without first checking the original order. *Most clients are familiar with the appearance of medications taken previously. Unfamiliar medications may signal a possible error.*

   - Stay with the client until all medications have been swallowed. *The nurse must see the client swallow the medication before the drug administration can be recorded.* A physician's order or agency policy is required for medications left at the bedside.

9. Document each medication given.
   - Record the medication given, dosage, time, any complaints or assessments of the client, and your signature.
   - If medication was refused or omitted, record this fact on the appropriate record; document the reason, when possible, and the nurse's actions according to agency policy.

10. Dispose of all supplies appropriately.
    - Replenish stock (e.g., medication cups) and return the cart to the appropriate place.
    - Discard used disposable supplies.

11. Evaluate the effects of the medication.
    - Return to the client when the medication is expected to take effect (usually 30 minutes) to evaluate the effects of the medication on the client.

EVALUATION

- Conduct appropriate follow-up.
- Desired effect (e.g., relief of pain or decrease in body temperature)
- Any adverse effects or side effects (e.g., nausea, vomiting, skin rash, change in vital signs)

- Relate to previous findings, if available.
- Report significant deviations from normal to the physician.

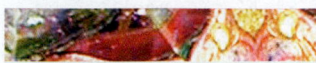

Lifespan Considerations

Administering Oral Medications

Infants

- A syringe or dropper provides the best control for administering medications.
- Place small amounts of liquid along the side of the infant's mouth. To prevent aspiration or spitting out, wait for the infant to swallow before giving more (Bindler & Ball, 2003).
- Another method for giving liquid medications to infants is to have the infant suck the liquid through a nipple. Other methods should be used, however, for unpleasant tasting medicine so that the infant will not associate the unpleasant taste with the nipple. Medication should never be added to the infant's formula for the same reason.
- If using a spoon, retrieve and refeed medication that is thrust outward by the infant's tongue.

Children

- Knowledge of growth and development is essential for the nurse administering medications to children.
- Whenever possible, give children a choice between the use of a spoon, dropper, or syringe.
- Dilute the oral medication, if indicated, with a small amount of water. Many oral medications are readily swallowed if they are diluted with a small amount of water. If large quantities of water are used, the child may refuse to drink the entire amount and receive only a portion of the medication.
- Oral medications for children are usually prepared in sweetened liquid form to make them more palatable. Crush medications that are not supplied in liquid form and mix them with substances available on most pediatric units, such as honey, flavored syrup, jam, or a fruit puree.
- Necessary foods such as milk or orange juice should not be used to mask the taste of medications because the child may develop unpleasant associations and refuse that food in the future.

- Disguise disagreeable-tasting medications with sweet-tasting substances mentioned previously. However, present any altered medication to the child honestly and not as a food or treat.
- Place the young child or toddler on your lap or a parent's lap in a sitting position.
- Administer the medication slowly with a measuring spoon, plastic syringe, or medicine cup.
- To prevent nausea, pour a carbonated beverage over finely crushed ice and give it before or immediately after the medication is administered.
- Follow medication with a drink of water, juice, a soft drink, or a Popsicle or frozen juice bar. This removes any unpleasant aftertaste.
- For children who take sweetened medications on a long-term basis, follow the medication administration with oral hygiene. These children are at high risk for dental caries.

Elders

- The physiologic changes associated with aging influence medication administration and effectiveness. Examples include altered memory, less acute vision, decrease in renal function, less complete and slower absorption from the gastrointestinal tract, and decreased liver function. Many of these changes enhance the possibility of cumulative effects and toxicity.
- Elders usually require smaller dosages of drugs, especially sedatives and other central nervous system depressants.
- Elders are mature adults capable of reasoning. The nurse, therefore, needs to explain the reasons for and the effects of the client's medications.
- Socioeconomic factors such as lack of transportation and decreased finances may influence obtaining medications when needed.
- An increase in marketing and availability of vitamins, herbs, and supplements alerts the nurse to include this information in a medication history.

Home Care Considerations

Administering Medications

Instruct the client to:

- Learn the names of the medications as well as their actions and possible adverse effects.
- Keep all medications out of reach of children and pets.
- If using a syringe to administer the medication to an infant or child, remove and dispose of the plastic cap that fits on the end of the syringe. Infants and small children have been known to choke on these caps.
- Take the medications only as prescribed. Immediately consult the nurse, pharmacist, or physician about any problems with the medication.
- Always check the medication label to make sure the correct medication is being taken.
- Request labels printed with larger type on medication containers if there is difficulty reading the label.

- Check the expiration date and discard outdated medications.
- Ask the pharmacist to substitute childproof caps with ones that are more easily opened, as necessary.
- If a dose or more is missed, do not take two or more doses; ask the pharmacist or physician for directions.
- Do not crush or cut a tablet or capsule without first checking with the physician or pharmacist. Doing so may affect the medication's absorption.
- Never stop taking the medication without the physician's permission.
- Always check with the pharmacist before taking any nonprescription medications. Some over-the-counter medications can interact with the prescribed medication.
- Set up a medication plan may schedule. Weekly pill containers (available at pharmacies) or a written plan may be helpful.

NASOGASTRIC AND GASTROSTOMY MEDICATIONS

For clients who cannot take anything by mouth (NPO) and have **nasogastric tubes** or a **gastrostomy tube** in place, an alternative route for administering medications is through the nasogastric or gastrostomy tube. A nasogastric (NG) tube is inserted by way of the nasopharynx and is placed into the client's stomach for the purpose of feeding the client or to remove gastric secretions. A gastrostomy tube is surgically placed directly into the client's stomach and provides another route for administering medications and nutrition (see Chapter 45). Guidelines for administering medications by nasogastric tubes and gastrostomy tubes are shown in the Practice Guidelines box below.

PARENTERAL MEDICATIONS

Parenteral administration of medications is a common nursing procedure. Nurses give parenteral medications intradermally (ID), subcutaneously (SC or SQ), intramuscularly (IM), or intravenously (IV). Because these medications are absorbed more quickly than oral medications and are irretrievable once injected, the nurse must prepare and administer them carefully and accurately. Administering parenteral drugs requires the same nursing knowledge as for oral and topical drugs; however, because injections are invasive procedures, aseptic technique must be used to minimize the risk of infection.

Equipment

To administer parenteral medications, nurses use syringes and needles to withdraw medication from ampules and vials.

Syringes

Syringes have three parts: the tip, which connects with the needle; the barrel, or outside part, on which the scales are printed; and the plunger, which fits inside the barrel (Figure 33–18 ■). When handling a syringe, the nurse may touch the outside of the

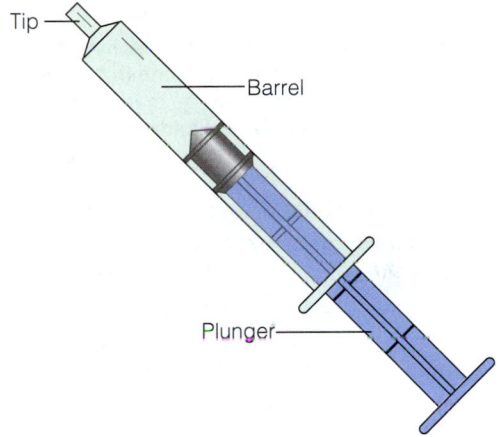

Figure 33–18 ■ The three parts of a syringe.

Practice Guidelines
Administering Medications by Nasogastric or Gastrostomy Tube

- Always check with the pharmacist to see if the client's medications come in a liquid form because these are less likely to cause tube obstruction.
- If medications do not come in liquid form, check to see if they may be crushed. (Note that enteric-coated, sustained action, buccal, and sublingual medications should never be crushed.)
- Crush a tablet into a fine powder and dissolve in at least 30 mL of warm water. Cold liquids may cause client discomfort. Use only water for mixing and flushing.
- Read medication labels carefully before opening a capsule. Open capsules and mix the contents with water only with the pharmacist's advice.
- Do not administer whole or undissolved medications because they will clog the tube.
- Assess tube placement (see Chapter 45 for methods to verify tube placement).
- Before giving the medication, aspirate all the stomach contents and measure the residual volume. Check agency policy if residual volume is greater than 100 mL.
- When administering the medication(s):
  - Remove the plunger from the syringe and connect the syringe to a pinched or kinked tube. Pinching or kinking the tube prevents excess air from entering the stomach and causing distention.
  - Put 15 to 30 mL (5 to 10 mL for children) of water into the syringe barrel to flush the tube before administering the first medication. Raise or lower the barrel of the syringe to adjust the flow as needed. Pinch or clamp the tubing before all the water is instilled to avoid excess air entering the stomach.
  - Pour liquid or dissolved medication into syringe barrel and allow to flow by gravity into the enteral tube.
  - If you are giving several medications, administer each one separately and flush with at least 15 to 30 mL (5 mL for children) of tap water between each medication.
  - When you have finished administering all medications, flush with another 15 to 30 mL (5 to 10 mL for children) of warm water to clear the tube.
- If the tube is connected to suction, disconnect the suction and keep the tube clamped for 20 to 30 minutes after giving the medication to enhance absorption.

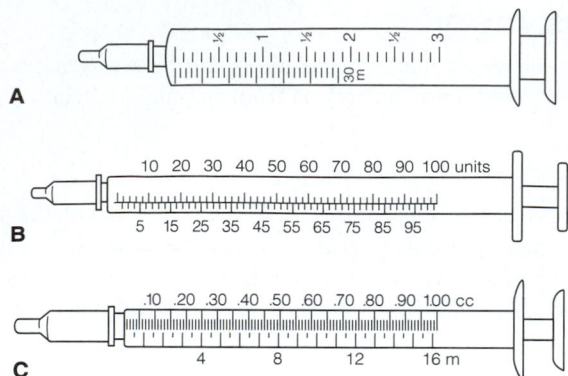

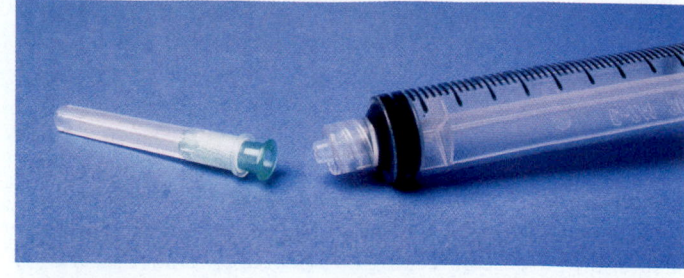

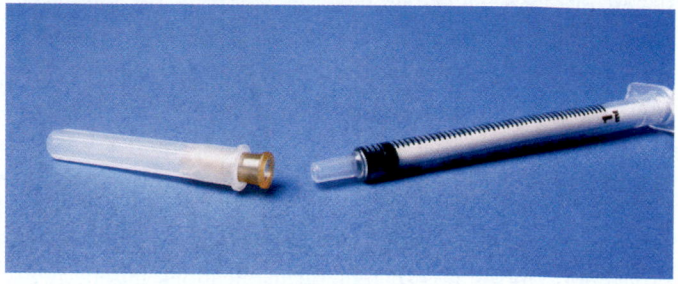

Figure 33–19 ■ Three kinds of syringes: *A,* hypodermic syringe marked in tenths (0.1) of milliliters and in minims; *B,* insulin syringe marked in 100 units; *C,* tuberculin syringe marked in tenths and hundredths (0.01) of cubic millimeters and in minims.

barrel and the handle of the plunger; however, the nurse must *avoid letting any unsterile object contact the tip or inside of the barrel, the shaft of the plunger, or the shaft or tip of the needle.*

There are several kinds of syringes, differing in size, shape, and material. The three most commonly used types are the standard hypodermic syringe, the insulin syringe, and the tuberculin syringe (Figure 33–19 ■). A **hypodermic syringe** comes in 2-, 2.5-, and 3-mL sizes. The syringe usually has two scales marked on it: the minim and the milliliter. The milliliter scale is the one normally used; the minim scale is used for very small dosages.

An **insulin syringe** is similar to a hypodermic syringe, but the scale is specially designed for insulin: a 100-unit calibrated scale intended for use with U-100 insulin. Several low-dose insulin syringes are also available and frequently have a nonremovable needle. All insulin syringes are calibrated on the 100-unit scale in North America. The correct choice of syringe is based on the amount of insulin required.

The **tuberculin syringe** was originally designed to administer tuberculin. It is a narrow syringe, calibrated in tenths and hundredths of a milliliter (up to 1 mL) on one scale and in sixteenths of a minim (up to 1 minim) on the other scale. This type of syringe can also be useful in administering other drugs, particularly when small or precise measurement is indicated (e.g., pediatric dosages).

Syringes are made in other sizes as well (e.g., 5, 10, 20, and 50 mL). These are not generally used to administer drugs directly but can be useful for adding medications to intravenous solutions or for irrigating wounds. The tip of a syringe varies and is classified as either a Luer-Lok or non-Luer-Lok. A Luer-Lok syringe has a tip that requires the needle to be twisted onto it to avoid accidental removal of the needle (see Figure 33–20 ■). The non-Luer-Lok syringe has a smooth graduated tip onto which needles are slipped. The non-Luer-Lok syringe is often used for irrigation purposes (e.g., wounds, tubes).

Most syringes used today are made of plastic, are individually packaged for sterility in a paper wrapper or a rigid plastic container (Figure 33–21 ■), and are disposable. The syringe and needle may be packaged together or separately. Needleless

Figure 33–20 ■ Tips of syringes: *A,* Luer-Lok syringe (note threaded tip); *B,* non-Luer-Lok syringe (note the smooth graduated tip).

systems are also available in which the needle is replaced by a plastic cannula.

Injectable medications are frequently supplied in disposable **prefilled unit-dose systems.** These are available as (a) prefilled syringes ready for use or (b) prefilled sterile cartridges and needles that require the attachment of a reusable holder (injection system) before use (Figure 33–22 ■). Examples of the latter sys-

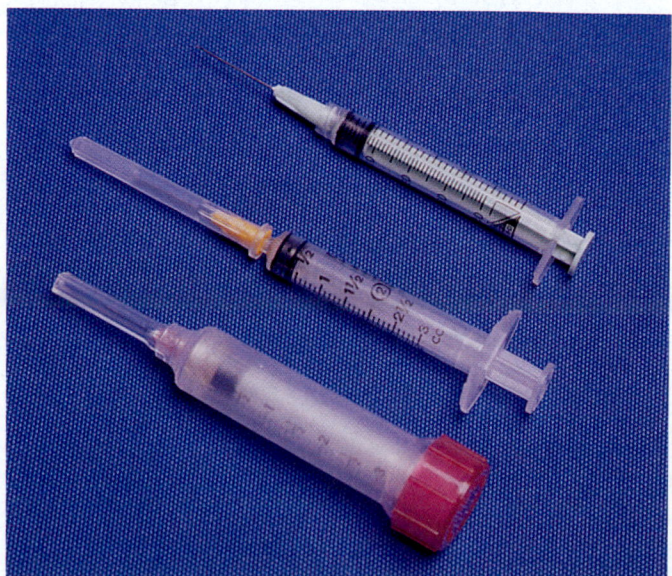

Figure 33–21 ■ Disposable plastic syringes and needles: *Top,* with syringe and needle exposed; *Middle,* with plastic cap over the needle; *Bottom,* with plastic case over the needle and syringe.

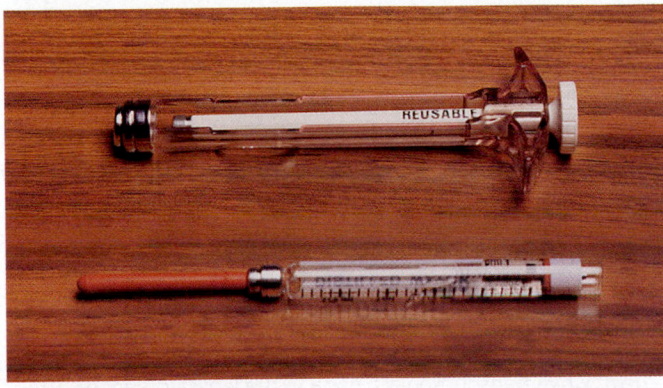

A

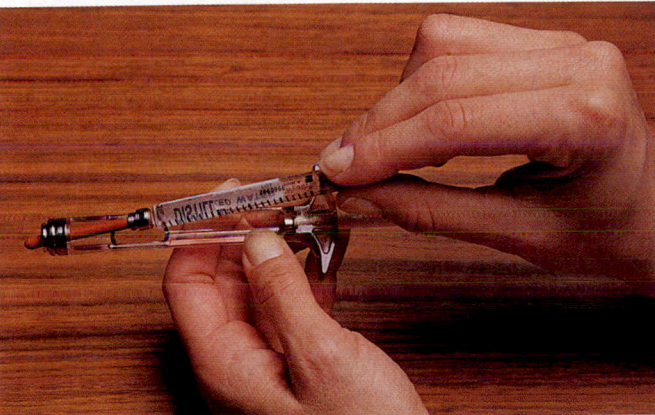

B

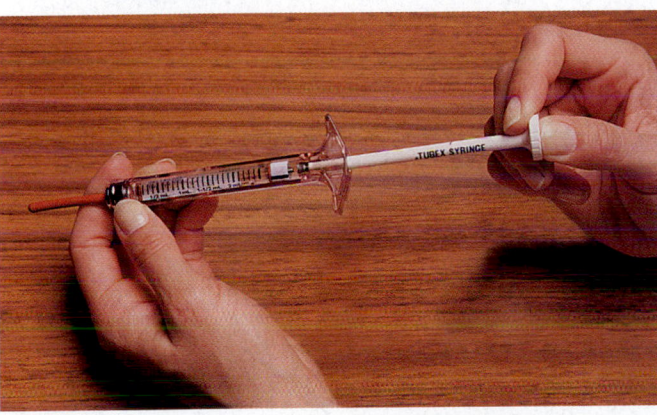

C

Figure 33–22 ■ *A,* Syringe and prefilled sterile cartridge with needle; *B,* assembling the device; *C,* the cartridge slides into the syringe barrel, turns, and locks at the needle end. The plunger then screws into the cartridge end.

tem are the Tubex and Carpuject injection systems. The manufacturers provide specific directions for use. Because most prefilled cartridges are overfilled, excess medication must be ejected before the injection to ensure the right dosage. Because the needle is fused to the syringe, the nurse cannot change the gauge or length of the needle. The nurse, however, can transfer the medication into a regular syringe if the assessment of the client necessitates a different needle gauge or length.

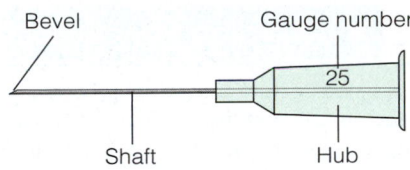

Figure 33–23 ■ The parts of a needle.

Needles

Needles are made of stainless steel, and most are disposable. Reusable needles (e.g., for special procedures) need to be sharpened periodically before resterilization because the points become dull with use and are occasionally damaged or acquire burrs on the tips. A dull or damaged needle should *never* be used.

A needle has three discernible parts: the **hub,** which fits onto the syringe; the **cannula,** or **shaft,** which is attached to the hub; and the **bevel,** which is the slanted part at the tip of the needle (Figure 33–23 ■). A disposable needle has a plastic hub. Needles used for injections have three variable characteristics:

1. *Slant or length of the bevel.* The bevel of the needle may be short or long. Longer bevels provide the sharpest needles and cause less discomfort. They are commonly used for subcutaneous and intramuscular injections. Short bevels are used for intradermal and intravenous injections because a long bevel can become occluded if it rests against the side of a blood vessel.
2. *Length of the shaft.* The shaft length of commonly used needles varies from 1/2 to 2 inches. The appropriate needle length is chosen according to the client's muscle development, the client's weight, and the type of injection.
3. **Gauge** *(or diameter) of the shaft.* The gauge varies from #18 to #28. The larger the gauge number, the smaller the diameter of the shaft. Smaller gauges produce less tissue trauma, but larger gauges are necessary for viscous medications, such as penicillin.

For an adult requiring a subcutaneous injection, it is appropriate to use a needle of #24 to #26 gauge and 3/8 to 5/8 inch long. Obese clients may require a 1-inch needle. For intramuscular injections, a longer needle (e.g., 1 to 1 1/2 inches) with a larger gauge (e.g., #20 to #22 gauge) is used. Slender adults and children usually require a shorter needle. The nurse must assess the client to determine the appropriate needle length.

Preventing Needlestick Injuries

One of the most potentially hazardous procedures that health care personnel face is using and disposing of needles and sharps. Needlestick injuries present a major risk for infection with hepatitis B virus, human immunodeficiency virus (HIV), and many other pathogens. Standards have been set by OSHA to prevent such injuries. Some of these are summarized in Box 33–5. If an accidental needlestick injury occurs, the nurse needs to follow specific steps outlined by the agency.

BOX 33–5 ■ **Avoiding Puncture Injuries**

■ Use appropriate puncture-proof disposal containers to dispose of uncapped needles and sharps. These are provided in all client areas (Figure 33–24 ■). Never throw sharps in wastebaskets. Sharps include any items that can cut or puncture skin such as:
  Needles
  Surgical blades
  Lancets
  Razors
  Broken glass
  Broken capillary pipettes
  Exposed dental wires
  Reusable items (e.g., large-bore needles, hooks, rasps, drill points)
  ANY SHARP INSTRUMENT!
■ Never bend or break needles before disposal.
■ Never recap used needles except under specified circumstances (e.g., when transporting a syringe to the laboratory for an arterial blood gas or blood culture).
■ When recapping a needle:
  • Use a safety mechanical device that firmly grips the needle cap and holds it in place until it is ready to recap.
  • Use a one-handed "scoop" method. This is performed by (a) placing the needle cap and syringe with needle horizontally on a flat surface, (b) inserting the needle into the cap, using one hand (Figure 33–25 ■), and then (c) using your other hand to pick up the cap and tighten it to the needle hub.

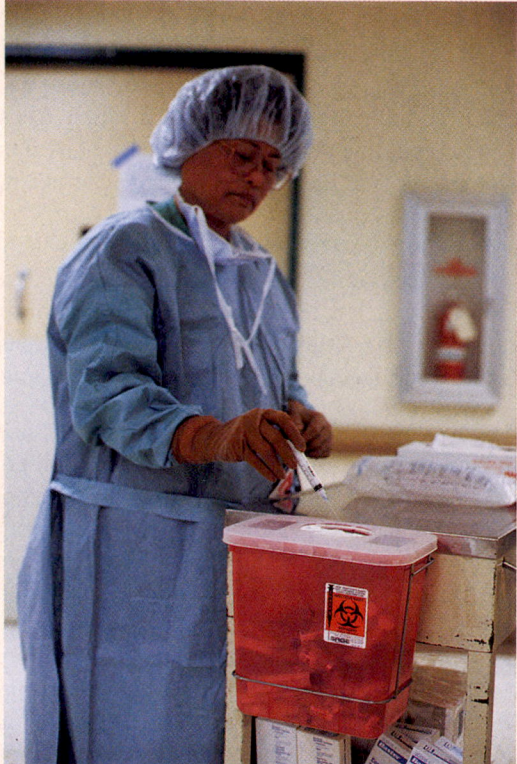

Figure 33–24 ■ A disposal container for contaminated needles and other sharps.

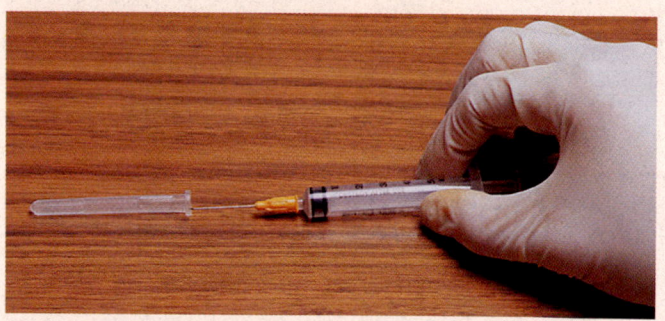

Figure 33–25 ■ Recapping a used needle using the one-handed scoop method.

Safety syringes have been designed in recent years to protect health care workers. Safety devices are categorized as either *passive* or *active*. The nurse does not need to activate the passive safety device. For example, for some syringes, after injection, the needle retracts immediately into the barrel (Figure 33–26 ■).

In contrast, the active safety device requires the nurse to manually activate the safety feature. For example, the nurse activates a mechanism to retract the needle into the syringe barrel or the nurse, after injection, manually pulls a plastic sheath or guard over the needle (Figure 33–27 ■).

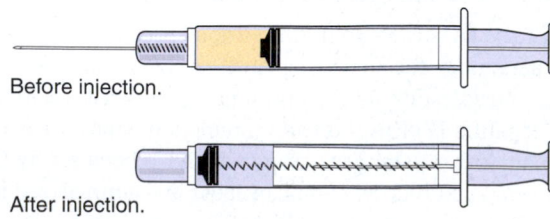

Before injection.

After injection.

Figure 33–26 ■ Passive safety device. The needle retracts immediately into the barrel after injection.

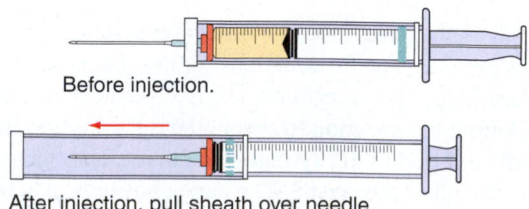

Before injection.

After injection, pull sheath over needle.

Figure 33–27 ■ Active safety device. The nurse manually pulls the sheath or guard over the needle after injection.

Preparing Injectable Medications

Injectable medications can be prepared by withdrawing the medication from an ampule or vial into a sterile syringe, using prefilled syringes, or using needleless injection systems. Figure 33–28 ■ shows an example of a needleless system used to access medication from a vial.

Ampules and Vials

Ampules and vials (Figure 33–29 ■) are frequently used to package sterile parenteral medications. An **ampule** is a glass container usually designed to hold a single dose of a drug. It is made of clear glass and has a distinctive shape with a constricted neck. Ampules vary in size from 1 to 10 mL or more. Most ampule necks have colored marks around them, indicating where they are prescored for easy opening.

To access the medication in an ampule, the ampule must be broken at its constricted neck. Traditionally, files have been used to score the ampule. Today ampule openers are available that prevent injury from broken glass. The device consists of a plastic cap that fits over the top of an ampule and a cutter within the cap that scores the neck of the ampule when rotated. The head of the ampule, when broken, remains inside the cap where it can then be ejected into a sharps container. If an ampule opener is not available, the neck should be filed with a small file, then broken off at that point. Once the ampule is broken, the fluid is aspirated into a syringe using a filter needle. This prevents aspiration of any glass particles.

A **vial** is a small glass bottle with a sealed rubber cap. Vials come in different sizes, from single to multidose vials. They

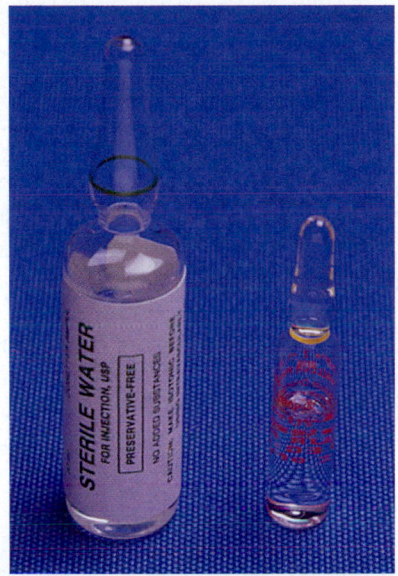

A

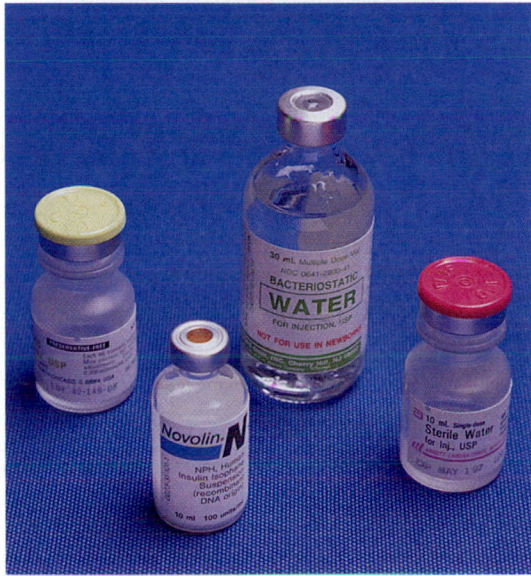

B

Figure 33–29 ■ *A,* Ampules; *B,* Vials.

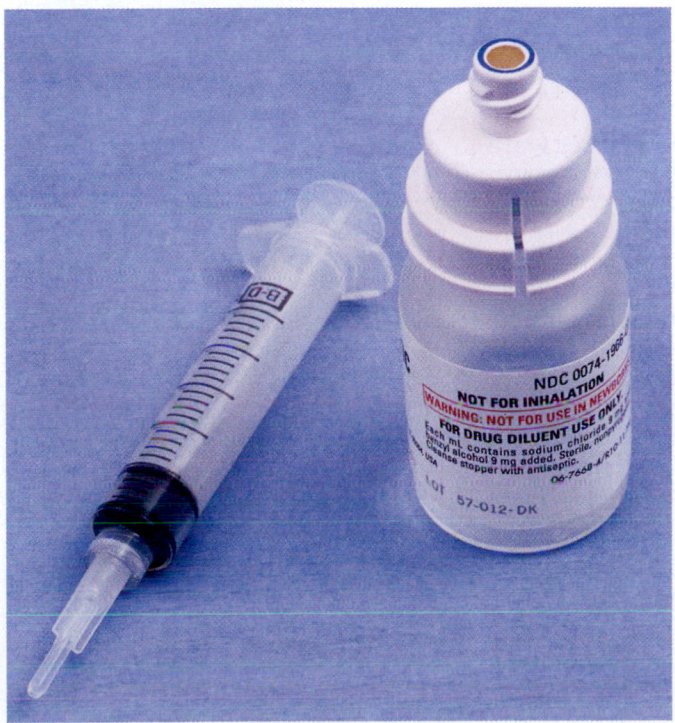

Figure 33–28 ■ A needleless system can extract medication from a vial.

usually have a metal or plastic cap that protects the rubber seal. To access the medication in a vial, the vial must be pierced with a needle. In addition, air must be injected into a vial before the medication can be withdrawn. Failure to inject air before withdrawing the medication leaves a vacuum within the vial that makes withdrawal difficult.

Several drugs (e.g., penicillin) are dispensed as powders in vials. A liquid (solvent or diluent) must be added to a powdered medication before it can be injected. The technique of adding a solvent to a powdered drug to prepare it for administration is called **reconstitution.** Powdered drugs usually have printed instructions (enclosed with each packaged vial) that describe the amount and kind of solvent to be added. Commonly used solvents are sterile water or sterile normal saline. Some preparations are supplied in individual-dose vials; others come in multidose vials. The following are two examples of the preparation of powdered drugs:

1. *Single-dose vial:* Instructions for preparing a single-dose vial direct that 1.5 mL of sterile water be added to the sterile dry powder, thus providing a single dose of 2 mL. The volume of the drug powder was 0.5 mL. Therefore, the 1.5 mL of water plus the 0.5 mL of powder results in 2 mL of solution. In other instances, the addition of a solution does not increase the volume. Therefore, it is important to follow the manufacturer's directions.

2. *Multidose vial:* A dose of 750 mg of a certain drug is ordered for a client. On hand is a 10-g multidose vial. The directions for preparation read: "Add 8.5 mL of sterile water, and each milliliter will contain 1.0 g or 1,000 mg." To determine the amount to inject, the nurse calculates as follows:

$$1 \text{ mL} = 1,000 \text{ mg}$$
$$x \text{ mL} = 750 \text{ mg}$$
(cross multiply)

$$x = \frac{750 \times 1}{1,000}$$
$$x = 0.75$$

The nurse will give 0.75 mL of the medication.

Glass and rubber particulate have been found in medications withdrawn from ampules and vials using a regular needle. As a result, it is strongly recommended that the nurse use a filter needle when withdrawing medications from ampules and vials to prevent withdrawing glass and rubber particles. After drawing the medication into the syringe, the filter needle is replaced with the regular needle for injection. This prevents tracking of the medication through the client's tissues during the insertion of the needle, which minimizes discomfort.

Procedures 33–2 and 33–3 describe how to prepare medications from ampules and vials. Additionally, it is important to remember that when powdered drugs have been reconstituted, the date and time should be written on the label of the vial. Many of these drugs have to be used immediately, so nurses need to know the expiration time after it has been reconstituted.

Procedure 33–2 Preparing Medications from Ampules

PLANNING

Delegation

Preparing medications from ampules and vials involves knowledge and use of aseptic technique. Therefore, these techniques are not delegated to UAP.

Equipment
- MAR or computer printout
- Ampule of sterile medication
- File (if ampule is not scored) and small gauze square
- Antiseptic swabs
- Needle and syringe
- Filter needle

IMPLEMENTATION

Preparation

1. Check the medication administration order.
   - Check the label on the ampule carefully against the MAR to make sure that the correct medication is being prepared.
   - Follow the three checks for administering medications. Read the label on the medication (1) when it is taken from the medication cart, (2) before withdrawing the medication, and (3) after withdrawing the medication.
2. Organize the equipment.

Performance
1. Wash hands and observe other appropriate infection control procedures.
2. Prepare the medication ampule for drug withdrawal.
   - Flick the upper stem of the ampule several times with a fingernail, or, holding the upper stem of the ampule, shake the ampule similar to shaking down a mercury thermometer. *This will bring all medication down to the main portion of the ampule.*
   - Partially file the neck of the ampule, if necessary, to start a clean break.
   - Place a piece of sterile gauze between your thumb and the ampule neck or around the ampule neck, and break off the top by bending it toward you (Figure 33–30 ■). *The sterile gauze protects the fingers from the broken glass and any glass fragments will spray away from the nurse.*
   or
   - Place the antiseptic wipe packet over the top of the ampule before breaking off the top. *This method ensures that all glass fragments fall into the packet and reduces the risk of cuts.*
   - Dispose of the top of the ampule in the sharps container.

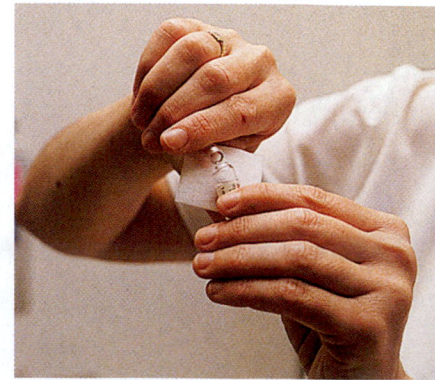

Figure 33–30 ■ Breaking the neck of an ampule.

3. Withdraw the medication.
   - Place the ampule on a flat surface.
   - Using a filter needle to withdraw the medication, disconnect the regular needle, leaving its cap on, and attach the filter needle to the syringe. *The*

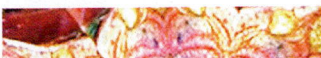

Procedure 33-2 Preparing Medications from Ampules *continued*

IMPLEMENTATION *continued*

filter needle prevents glass particles from being withdrawn with the medication.

- Remove the cap from the filter needle and insert the needle into the center of the ampule. Do not touch the rim of the ampule with the needle tip or shaft. *This will keep the needle sterile.* Withdraw the amount of drug required for the dosage.

- With a single-dose ampule, hold the ampule slightly on its side, if necessary, to obtain all medication (Figure 33–31 ■).
- Replace the filter needle with a regular needle and tighten the cap at the hub of the needle before injecting the client.

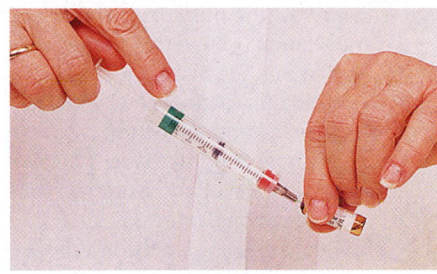

Figure 33–31 ■ Withdrawing a medication from an ampule.

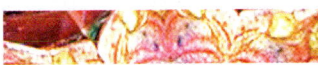

Procedure 33-3 Preparing Medications from Vials

PLANNING

Equipment

- MAR or computer printout
- Vial of sterile medication
- Antiseptic swabs

- Needle and syringe
- Filter needle (check agency policy)
- Sterile water or normal saline, if drug is in powdered form

IMPLEMENTATION

Preparation

- Same preparation as described in Procedure 33–2.

Performance

1. Wash hands and observe other appropriate infection control procedures.
2. Prepare the medication vial for drug withdrawal.
   - Mix the solution, if necessary, by rotating the vial between the palms of the hands, not by shaking. *Some vials contain aqueous suspensions, which settle when they stand. In some instances, shaking is contraindicated because it may cause the mixture to foam.*
   - Remove the protective cap, or clean the rubber cap of a previously opened vial with an antiseptic wipe by rubbing in a circular motion. *The antiseptic cleans the cap of dust or grease and reduces the number of microorganisms.*
3. Withdraw the medication.
   - Attach a filter needle, as agency practice dictates, to draw up premixed liquid medications from multidose vials. *Using the filter needle*

prevents any solid particles from being drawn up through the needle.
- Ensure that the needle is firmly attached to the syringe.
- Remove the cap from the needle, then draw up into the syringe the amount of air equal to the volume of the medication to be withdrawn.
- Carefully insert the needle into the upright vial through the center of the rubber cap, maintaining the sterility of the needle.
- Inject the air into the vial, keeping the bevel of the needle above the surface of the medication (Figure 33–32 ■). *The air will allow the medication to be drawn out easily because negative pressure will not be created inside the vial. The bevel is kept above the medication to avoid creating bubbles in the medication.*

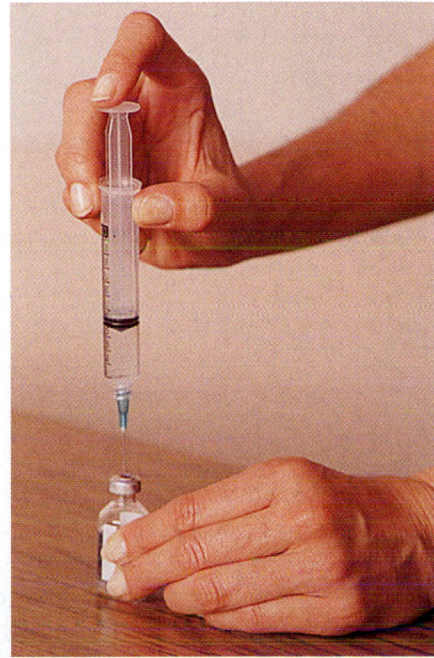

Figure 33–32 ■ Injecting air into a vial.

continued on page 818

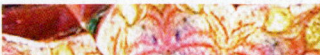

Procedure 33–3 Preparing Medications from Vials *continued*

IMPLEMENTATION *continued*

- Withdraw the prescribed amount of medication using either of the following methods:
  a. Hold the vial down (i.e., with the base lower than the top), move the needle tip so that it is below the fluid level, and withdraw the medication (Figure 33–33 ■). Avoid drawing up the last drops of the vial. *Proponents of this method say that keeping the vial in the upright position while withdrawing the medication allows particulate matter to precipitate out of the solution. Leaving the last few drops reduces the chance of withdrawing foreign particles.*

or
  b. Invert the vial; ensure the needle tip is *below* the fluid level; and gradually withdraw the medication (Figure 33–34 ■). *Keeping the tip of the needle below the fluid level prevents air from being drawn into the syringe.*

- Hold the syringe and vial at eye level to determine that the correct dosage of drug is drawn into the syringe. Eject air remaining at the top of the syringe into the vial.

- When the correct volume of medication is obtained, withdraw the needle from the vial, and replace the cap over the needle using the scoop method, thus maintaining its sterility.
- If necessary, tap the syringe barrel to dislodge any air bubbles present in the syringe. *The tapping motion will cause the air bubbles to rise to the top of the syringe where they can be ejected out of the syringe.*
- Replace the filter needle, if used, with a regular needle and cover of the correct gauge and length before injecting the client.

VARIATION: PREPARING AND USING MULTIDOSE VIALS

- Read the manufacturer's directions.
- Withdraw an equivalent amount of air from the vial before adding the diluent, unless otherwise indicated by the directions.
- Add the amount of sterile water or saline indicated in the directions.
- If a multidose vial is reconstituted, label the vial with the date and time it was prepared, the amount of drug contained in each milliliter of solution, and your initials. *Time is an important factor to consider in the expiration of these medications.*
- Once the medication is reconstituted, store it in a refrigerator or as recommended by the manufacturer.

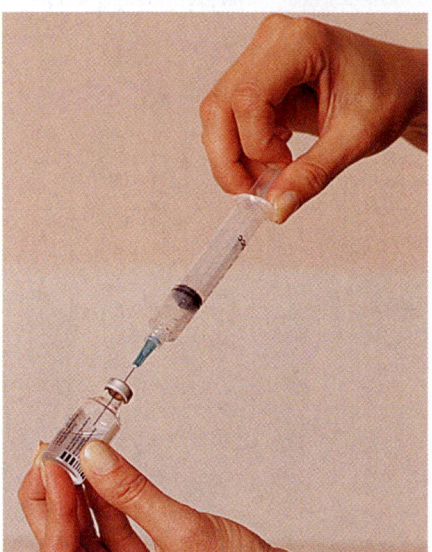

Figure 33–33 ■ Withdrawing a medication from a vial that is held with the base down.

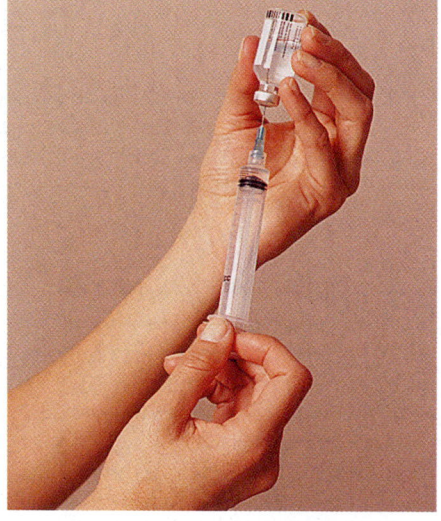

Figure 33–34 ■ Withdrawing a medication from an inverted vial.

Mixing Medications in One Syringe

Frequently, clients need more than one drug injected at the same time. To spare the client the experience of being injected twice, two drugs (if compatible) are often mixed in one syringe and given as one injection. It is common, for instance, to combine two types of insulin in this manner or to combine injectable preoperative medications such as morphine or meperidine (Demerol) with atropine or scopolamine. Drugs can also be mixed in intravenous solutions. When uncertain about drug compatibilities, the nurse should consult a pharmacist or check a compatibility chart before mixing the drugs.

The nurse must also exercise caution when mixing short- and long-acting insulins, because they vary in content. Chemically, insulin is a protein that, when hydrolyzed in the body, yields a number of amino acids. Some insulin preparations contain an additional modifying protein, such as globulin or protamine, that slows absorption. This fact is particularly relevant to mixing two insulin preparations for injection because many insulin syringes have needles that cannot be changed. A vial of insulin that does not have the added protein (i.e., regular insulin) should *never* be contaminated with insulin that does have the added protein (i.e., Lente or NPH insulin). Procedure 33–4 describes how to mix medications in one syringe.

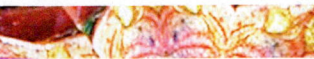

Procedure 33–4 Mixing Medications Using One Syringe

PLANNING

Delegation
Mixing medications in one syringe involves knowledge and use of aseptic technique. Therefore, this procedure is not delegated to UAP.

Equipment
■ MAR or computer printout

■ Two vials of medication; one vial and one ampule; two ampules; or one vial or ampule and one cartridge
■ Antiseptic swabs
■ Sterile hypodermic or insulin syringe and needle (if insulin is being given, use a small-gauge hypodermic needle, e.g., #26 gauge)
■ Additional sterile subcutaneous or intramuscular needle (optional)

IMPLEMENTATION

Preparation
1. Check the MAR.
   - Check the label on the medications carefully against the MAR to make sure that the correct medication is being prepared.
   - Follow the three checks for administering medications. Read the label on the medication (1) when it is taken from the medication cart, (2) before withdrawing the medication, and (3) after withdrawing the medication.
   - Before preparing and combining the medications, ensure that the total volume of the injection is appropriate for the injection site.
2. Organize the equipment.

Performance
1. Wash hands and observe other appropriate infection control procedures.
2. Prepare the medication ampule or vial for drug withdrawal.
   - See Procedure 33–2, step 2, for an ampule.
   - Inspect the appearance of the medication for clarity. Some medications are always cloudy. *Preparations that have changed in appearance should be discarded.*
   - If using insulin, thoroughly mix the solution in each vial prior to administration. Rotate the vials between the palms of the hands and invert the vials. *Mixing ensures an adequate concentration and thus an accurate dose. Shaking insulin vials can make the medication frothy, making precise measurement difficult.*
   - Clean the tops of the vials with antiseptic swabs.
3. Withdraw the medications.

MIXING MEDICATIONS FROM TWO VIALS
■ Take the syringe and draw up a volume of air equal to the volume of medications to be withdrawn from both vials A *and* B.
■ Inject a volume of air equal to the volume of medication to be withdrawn into vial A. Make sure the needle does not touch the solution. *This prevents cross-contamination of the medications.*
■ Withdraw the needle from vial A and inject the remaining air into vial B.
■ Withdraw the required amount of medication from vial B. *The same needle is used to inject air into and withdraw medication from the second vial. It must not be contaminated with the medication in vial A.*
■ Using a newly attached sterile needle, withdraw the required amount of medication from vial A. Avoid pushing the plunger as that will introduce medication B into vial A. If using a syringe with a fused needle, withdraw the medication from vial A. The syringe now contains a mixture of medications from vials A and B. *With this method, neither vial is contaminated by microorganisms or by medication from the other vial.* Be careful to withdraw only the ordered amount and to not create air bubbles. *The syringe now contains two medications and an excess amount cannot be returned to the vial.*

See also the Variation later in this procedure.

MIXING MEDICATIONS FROM ONE VIAL AND ONE AMPULE
■ First prepare and withdraw the medication from the vial. *Ampules do not require the addition of air prior to withdrawal of the drug.*

■ Then withdraw the required amount of medication from the ampule.

MIXING MEDICATIONS FROM ONE CARTRIDGE AND ONE VIAL OR AMPULE
■ First ensure that the correct dose of the medication is in the cartridge. Discard any excess medication and air.
■ Draw up the required medication from a vial or ampule into the cartridge. Note that when withdrawing medication from a vial, an equal amount of air must first be injected into the vial.
■ If the total volume to be injected exceeds the capacity of the cartridge, use a syringe with sufficient capacity to withdraw the desired amount of medication from the vial or ampule, and transfer the required amount from the cartridge to the syringe.

VARIATION: MIXING INSULINS
The following is an example of mixing 10 units of regular insulin and 30 units of neutral protamine Hagedorn (NPH) insulin, which contains protamine.
■ Inject 30 units of air into the NPH vial and withdraw the needle. (There should be no insulin in the needle.) The needle should not touch the insulin (Figure 33–35 ■, step 1).
■ Inject 10 units of air into the regular insulin vial and immediately withdraw 10 units of regular insulin (Figure 33–35, steps 2 and 3). Always withdraw the regular insulin first *to minimize the possibility of contamination.*
■ Reinsert the needle into the NPH insulin vial and withdraw 30 units of NPH insulin (Figure 33–35, step 4). (The air was previously injected into the vial.) Be careful to withdraw only the ordered amount and to not create air bubbles. *The syringe now contains two medications, and an excess amount cannot be returned to the vial.*

continued on page 820

Procedure 33–4 Mixing Medications Using One Syringe *continued*

IMPLEMENTATION *continued*

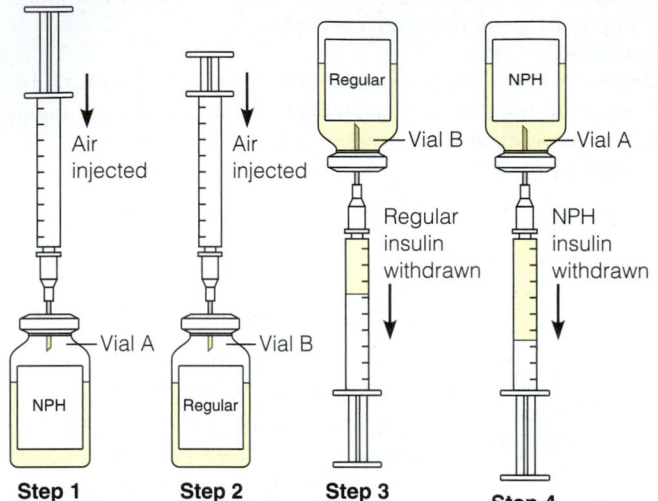

| Step 1 | Step 2 | Step 3 | Step 4 |

Figure 33–35 ■ Mixing two types of insulin.

By using this method, you avoid adding NPH insulin to the regular insulin.

> ➤ **CLINICAL ALERT**   *One way to determine which insulin to withdraw first is to remember the saying "Clear before cloudy."*

Intradermal Injections

An **intradermal (ID) injection** is the administration of a drug into the dermal layer of the skin just beneath the epidermis. Usually only a small amount of liquid is used, for example, 0.1 mL. This method of administration is frequently used for allergy testing and tuberculosis (TB) screening. Common sites for intradermal injections are the inner lower arm, the upper chest, and the back beneath the scapulae (Figure 33–36 ■). The left arm is commonly used for TB screening and the right arm is used for all other tests. The steps for administering an intradermal are described in Procedure 33–5.

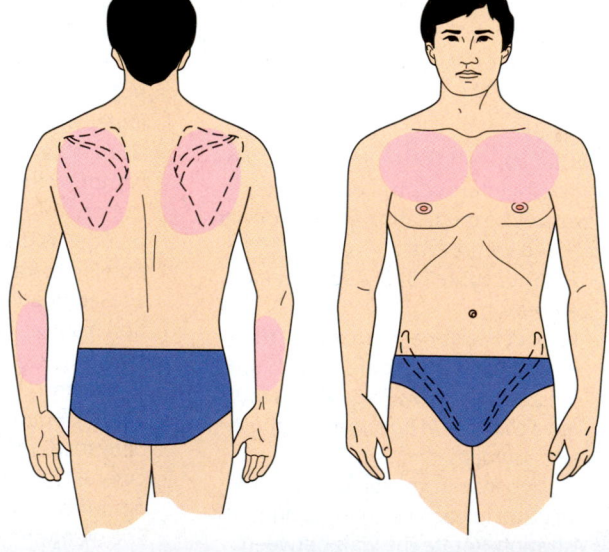

Figure 33–36 ■ Body sites commonly used for intradermal injections.

Procedure 33–5 Administering an Intradermal Injection

Purpose

■ To provide a medication that the client requires for allergy testing and TB screening

ASSESSMENT

Assess

■ Appearance of injection site
■ Specific drug action and expected response

■ Client's knowledge of drug action and response
Check agency protocol about sites to use for skin tests.

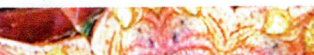

Procedure 33–5 Administering an Intradermal Injection *continued*

PLANNING

Delegation

The administration of intradermal injections is an invasive technique that involves the application of nursing knowledge, problem solving, and sterile technique. This technique is not delegated to UAP. The nurse, however, can inform the UAP about symptoms of allergic reactions and the necessity to report those observations immediately to the nurse.

Equipment

■ Vial or ampule of the correct medication

■ Sterile 1-mL syringe calibrated into hundredths of a milliliter (i.e., tuberculin syringe) and a # 25- to # 27-gauge needle that is 1/4 to 5/8 inch long

■ Alcohol swabs

■ 2-in. × 2-in. sterile gauze square (optional)

■ Clean gloves (according to agency protocol)

■ Bandage (optional)

■ Epinephrine (a bronchodilator and antihistamine) on hand

IMPLEMENTATION

Preparation

1. Check the MAR.
   • Check the label on the medication carefully against the MAR to make sure that the correct medication is being prepared.
   • Follow the three checks for administering medications. Read the label on the medication (1) when it is taken from the medication cart, (2) before withdrawing the medication, and (3) after withdrawing the medication.
2. Organize the equipment.

Performance

1. Wash hands and observe other appropriate infection control procedures (e.g., clean gloves).
2. Prepare the medication from the vial or ampule for drug withdrawal.
   • See Procedures 33–2 and 33–3.
3. Prepare the client
   • Check the client's identification band. *This ensures that the right client receives the medication.*
4. Explain to the client that the medication will produce a small wheal, sometimes called a *bleb*. A *wheal* is a small raised area, like a blister. The client will feel a slight prick as the needle enters the skin. Some medications are absorbed slowly through the capillaries into the general circulation, and the bleb gradually disappears. Other drugs remain in the area and interact with the body tissues to produce redness and induration (hardening), which will need to be interpreted at a particular time (e.g., in 24 or 48 hours). This reaction will also gradually disappear. *Information facilitates acceptance of and compliance with the therapy.*

5. Provide for client privacy.
6. Select and clean the site.
   • Select a site (e.g., the forearm about a hand's width above the wrist and three or four fingerwidths below the antecubital space).
   • Avoid using sites that are tender, inflamed, or swollen and those that have lesions.
   • Put on gloves as indicated by agency policy.
   • Cleanse the skin at the site using a firm circular motion starting at the center and widening the circle outward. Allow the area to dry thoroughly.
7. Prepare the syringe for the injection.
   • Remove the needle cap while waiting for the antiseptic to dry.
   • Expel any air bubbles from the syringe. Small bubbles that adhere to the plunger are of no consequence. *A small amount of air will not harm the tissues.*
   • Grasp the syringe in your dominant hand, holding it between thumb and forefinger. Hold the needle almost parallel to the skin surface, with the bevel of the needle up. *The possibility of the medication entering the subcutaneous tissue increases when using an angle greater than 15 degrees or if the bevel is down.*
8. Inject the fluid.
   • With the nondominant hand, pull the skin at the site until it is taut. For example, if using the ventral forearm, grasp the client's dorsal forearm and gently pull it to tighten the ventral skin. *Taut skin allows for easier entry of the needle and less discomfort for the client.*

• Insert the tip of the needle far enough to place the bevel through the epidermis into the dermis (Figure 33–37 ■, *A*). The outline of the bevel should be visible under the skin surface.

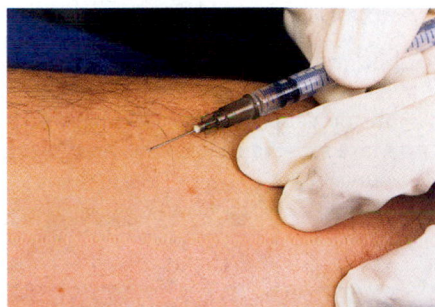

A

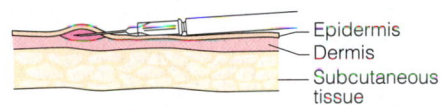

Epidermis
Dermis
Subcutaneous tissue

B

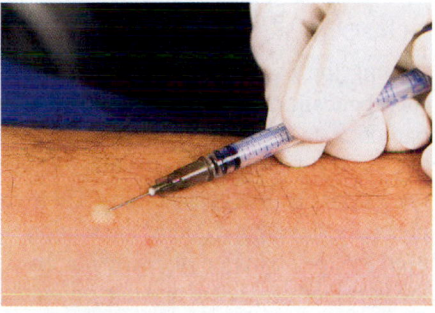

C

Figure 33–37 ■ For an intradermal injection: *A*, the needle enters the skin at a 5- to 15-degree angle; *B, C*, the medication forms a bleb under the epidermis.

continued on page 822

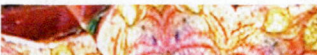

Procedure 33–5 Administering an Intradermal Injection *continued*

IMPLEMENTATION *continued*

- Stabilize the syringe and needle, inject the medication carefully and slowly so that it produces a small wheal on the skin (Figure 33–37, *B, C*). *This verifies that the medication entered the dermis.*
- Withdraw the needle quickly at the same angle at which it was inserted. Apply a bandage if indicated.

- Do not massage the area. *Massage can disperse the medication into the tissue or out through the needle insertion site.*
- Dispose of the syringe and needle safely. *Do not recap the needle in order to prevent needlestick injuries.*

- Remove gloves.
- Circle the injection site with ink to observe for redness or induration (hardening), per agency policy.
9. Document all relevant information.
   - Record the testing material given, the time, dosage, route, site, and nursing assessments.

EVALUATION

- Evaluate the client's response to the testing substance. *Some medications used in testing may cause allergic reactions.* An antidote drug (e.g., epinephrine) may need to be used.

- Evaluate the condition of the site in 24 or 48 hours, depending on the test. Measure the area of redness and induration in millimeters at the largest diameter and document findings.

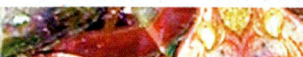

Lifespan Considerations

Administering an Intradermal Injection

Children

- A small child or infant will need to be gently restrained during the procedure. *This prevents injury from sudden movement.*
- Make sure the child understands that the procedure is not a punishment.

- Ask the child not to rub or scratch the injection site. Place a stockinet or gauze dressing over the site if needed. *Rubbing the site can interfere with test results by irritating the underlying tissue.*

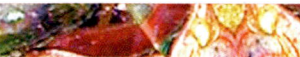

Home Care Considerations

Administering an Intradermal Injection

- Be certain the client understands the need for a follow-up visit to examine the injection site. Set up an appointment for the visit.

- Instruct the client not to wash, rub, or scratch the injection site.

Subcutaneous Injections

Among the many kinds of drugs administered subcutaneously (just beneath the skin) are vaccines, preoperative medications, narcotics, insulin, and heparin. Common sites for subcutaneous (SC or SQ) injections are the outer aspect of the upper arms and the anterior aspect of the thighs. These areas are convenient and normally have good blood circulation. Other areas that can be used are the abdomen, the scapular areas of the upper back, and the upper ventrogluteal and dorsogluteal areas (Figure 33–38 ■). Only small doses (0.5 to 1 mL) of medication are usually injected via the subcutaneous route. Check agency policy.

The type of syringe used for subcutaneous injections depends on the medication to be given. Generally a 2-mL syringe is used for most SC injections. However, if insulin is being administered, an insulin syringe is used; and if heparin is being administered, a tuberculin syringe or prefilled cartridge may be used.

Needle sizes and lengths are selected based on the client's body mass, the intended angle of insertion, and the planned site. Generally a #25-gauge, 5/8-inch needle is used for adults of normal weight and the needle is inserted at a 45-degree angle; a 3/8-inch needle is used at a 90-degree angle. A child may need a 1/2-inch needle inserted at a 45-degree angle.

One method nurses use to determine length of needle is to pinch the tissue at the site and select a needle length that is half the width of the skinfold. To determine the angle of insertion, a general rule to follow relates to the amount of tissue that can be bunched or grasped at the site. A 45-degree angle is used when 1 inch of tissue can be grasped at the site; a 90-degree angle is used when 2 inches of tissue can be grasped.

When administering insulin to adults, the current standard needle gauge is #30 gauge and short needles (5/16 inch) are now available on 30-, 50-, and 100-unit syringes (Fleming,

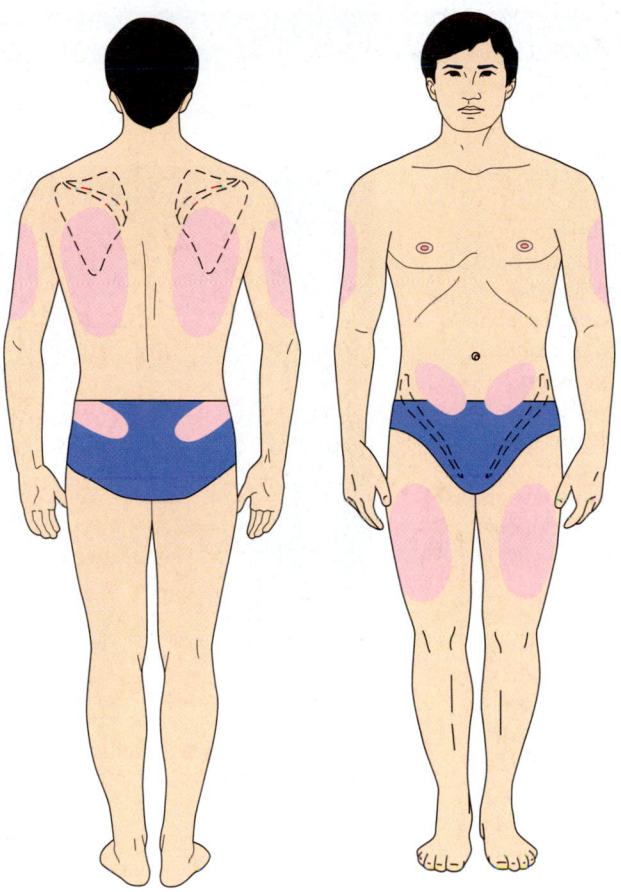

Figure 33–38 ■ Body sites commonly used for subcutaneous injections.

1999). Most clients prefer the shorter and thinner needles because they are less painful. The risk of injecting into the muscle is lessened with the shorter needle.

Subcutaneous injection sites need to be rotated in an orderly fashion to minimize tissue damage, aid absorption, and avoid discomfort. This is especially important for clients who must receive repeated injections, such as diabetics. Because insulin is absorbed at different rates at different parts of the body, the diabetic client's blood glucose levels can vary when various sites are used. Insulin is absorbed most quickly when injected into the abdomen and then into the arms, and most slowly when injected into the thighs and buttocks. Current recommendations include rotating injections within an anatomical area (Fleming, 1999).

Nurses have traditionally been taught to aspirate by pulling back on the plunger after inserting the needle and before injecting the medication. The nurse could then determine whether the needle had entered a blood vessel. Absence of blood was believed to indicate that the needle was in subcutaneous tissue and not in the more vascular muscular tissue. Fleming (1999) challenges the traditional practice of aspiration for insulin subcutaneous injections because it "is cumbersome, rarely yields blood, and isn't a reliable indicator of correct needle placement, and there are no clinical studies confirming or rejecting it" (p. 73). As a result, the practice of aspirating subcutaneous injections varies among nurses.

The steps for administering a subcutaneous injection are described in Procedure 33–6.

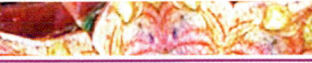

Procedure 33–6 Administering a Subcutaneous Injection

Purposes

- To provide a medication the client requires (see specific drug action)

- To allow slower absorption of a medication compared with either the intramuscular or intravenous route

ASSESSMENT

Assess

- Allergies to medication
- Specific drug action, side effects, and adverse reactions
- Client's knowledge and learning needs about the medication

- Status and appearance of subcutaneous site for lesions, erythema, swelling, ecchymosis, inflammation, and tissue damage from previous injections
- Ability of client to cooperate during the injection
- Previous injection sites used

PLANNING

Delegation

The administration of subcutaneous injections is an invasive technique that involves the application of nursing knowledge, problem solving, and sterile technique. Therefore, this procedure is not delegated to UAP. The nurse, however, can inform the UAP of the intended therapeutic effects and/or specific side effects of the medication and direct the UAP to report specific client observations to the nurse for follow-up.

Equipment

- Clients MAR or computer printout
- Vial or ampule of the correct sterile medication
- Syringe and needle (e.g., 2-mL syringe, #25-gauge needle, 3/8 or 5/8 inch long)
- Antiseptic swabs
- Dry sterile gauze for opening an ampule (optional)
- Clean gloves

continued on page 824

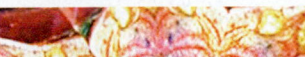

Procedure 33–6 Administering a Subcutaneous Injection *continued*

IMPLEMENTATION

Preparation

1. Check the MAR.
   - Check the label on the medication carefully against the MAR to make sure that the correct medication is being prepared.
   - Follow the three checks for administering medications. Read the label on the medication (1) when it is taken from the medication cart, (2) before withdrawing the medication, and (3) after withdrawing the medication.
2. Organize the equipment.

Performance

1. Wash hands and observe other appropriate infection control procedures (e.g., clean gloves).
2. Prepare the medication from the ampule or vial for drug withdrawal.
   - See Procedure 33–2 (ampule) or 33–3 (vial).
3. Provide for client privacy.
4. Prepare the client
   - Check the client's identification band. *This ensures that the right client receives the medication.*
   - Assist the client to a position in which the arm, leg, or abdomen can be relaxed, depending on the site to be used. *A relaxed position of the site minimizes discomfort.*
   - Obtain assistance in holding an uncooperative client. *This prevents injury due to sudden movement after needle insertion.*
5. Explain the purpose of the medication and how it will help, using language that the client can understand. Include relevant information about effects of the medication. *Information facilitates acceptance of and compliance with the therapy.*
6. Select and clean the site.
   - Select a site free of tenderness, hardness, swelling, scarring, itching, burning, or localized inflammation. Select a site that has not been used frequently. *These conditions could hinder the absorption of the medication and also increase the likelihood of injury and discomfort at the injection site.*
   - Put on clean gloves.

- As agency protocol indicates, clean the site with an antiseptic swab. Start at the center of the site and clean in a widening circle to about 5 cm (2 in.). Allow the area to dry thoroughly. *The mechanical action of swabbing removes skin secretions, which contain microorganisms.*
- Place and hold the swab between the third and fourth fingers of the nondominant hand, or position the swab on the client's skin above the intended site. *Using this technique keeps the swab readily accessible when the needle is withdrawn.*

7. Prepare the syringe for injection.
   - Remove the needle cap while waiting for the antiseptic to dry. Pull the cap straight off to avoid contaminating the needle by the outside edge of the cap. *The needle will become contaminated if it touches anything but the inside of the cap, which is sterile.*
8. Inject the medication.
   - Grasp the syringe in your dominant hand by holding it between your thumb and fingers. With palm facing to the side or upward for a 45-degree angle insertion, or with the palm downward for a 90-degree angle insertion, prepare to inject (Figure 33–39 ■).

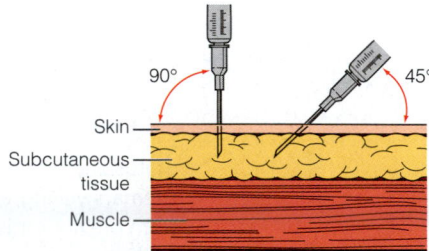

Figure 33–39 ■ Inserting a needle into the subcutaneous tissue using 90- and 45-degree angles.

- Using the nondominant hand, pinch or spread the skin at the site, and insert the needle using the dominant hand and a firm steady push (Figure 33–40 ■).

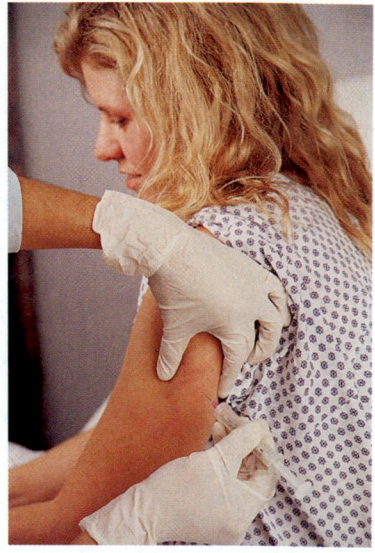

Figure 33–40 ■ Administering a subcutaneous injection into pinched tissue.

Recommendations vary about whether to pinch or spread the skin and at what angle to administer subcutaneous injections. The most important consideration is the depth of the subcutaneous tissue in the area to be injected. If the client has more than 1/2 inch of adipose tissue in the injection site, it would be safe to administer the injection at a 90-degree angle with the skin spread. If the client is thin or lean and lacks adipose tissue, the subcutaneous injection should be given with the skin pinched and at a 45- to 60-degree angle.

- When the needle is inserted, move your nondominant hand to the end of the plunger. Some nurses find it easier to move the nondominant hand to the barrel of the syringe and the dominant hand to the end of the plunger.
- Dependent upon personal choice *and* type of medication, aspirate by pulling back on the plunger. If blood appears in the syringe, withdraw the needle, discard the syringe, and prepare a new injection. If blood does not appear, continue

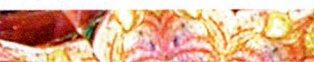

Procedure 33–6 Administering a Subcutaneous Injection *continued*

IMPLEMENTATION *continued*

to administer the medication. *This allows the nurse to determine whether the needle has entered a blood vessel. Subcutaneous medications may be dangerous if placed directly into the bloodstream; they are intended for the subcutaneous tissues, where the absorption time is greater.* See variation for administering a heparin injection.

- Inject the medication by holding the syringe steady and depressing the plunger with a slow, even pressure. *Holding the syringe steady and injecting the medication at an even pressure minimizes discomfort for the client.*

9. Remove the needle.
   - Remove the needle slowly and smoothly, pulling along the line of insertion while depressing the skin with your nondominant hand. *Depressing the skin places countertraction on it and minimizes the client's discomfort when the needle is withdrawn.*
   - If bleeding occurs, apply pressure to the site with dry sterile gauze until it stops. *Bleeding rarely occurs after subcutaneous injection.*

10. Dispose of supplies appropriately.
    - Discard the uncapped needle and attached syringe into designated receptacles. *Proper disposal protects the nurse and others from injury and contamination. The Centers for Disease Control and Prevention (CDC) recommends not capping the needle before disposal to reduce the risk of needlestick injuries.*
    - Remove gloves. Wash hands.

11. Document all relevant information.
    - Document the medication given, dosage, time, route, and any assessments.
    - Many agencies prefer that medication administration be recorded on the medication record. The nurse's notes are used when PRN medications are given or when there is a special problem.

12. Assess the effectiveness of the medication at the time it is expected to act.

VARIATION: ADMINISTERING A HEPARIN INJECTION

The subcutaneous administration of heparin requires special precautions because of the drug's anticoagulant properties.

- Select a site on the abdomen away from the umbilicus and above the level of the iliac crests. Some agencies support the practice of subcutaneous injection of heparin in the thighs or arms as alternate sites to the abdomen.
- Use a 3/8-inch, #25- or #26-gauge needle, and insert it at a 90-degree angle. If a client is very lean or wasted, use a needle longer than 3/8 inch and insert it at a 45-degree angle. The arms or thighs may be used as alternate sites.
- Do *not* aspirate when giving heparin by subcutaneous injection. *Aspiration can possibly damage the surrounding tissue and cause bleeding as well as bruising.*
- Do not massage the site after the injection. *Massaging could cause bleeding and ecchymoses (bruises) and hasten drug absorption.*
- Alternate the sites of subsequent injections.

EVALUATION

- Conduct appropriate follow-up such as desired effect (e.g., relief of pain, sedation, lowered blood sugar, a prothrombin time within preestablished limits), any adverse effects (e.g., nausea, vomiting, skin rash), and clinical signs of side effects.
- Relate to previous findings if available.
- Report deviations from normal to the physician.

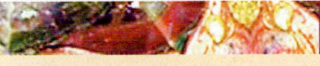

Home Care Considerations

Subcutaneous Injections

- If the client has impaired vision, consider prefilling syringes and storing them in an appropriate environment (e.g., the refrigerator).
- For frequent injections, develop a plan for site rotation with the client.
- For cost-saving measures, teach able clients to safely reuse disposable syringes. Diabetic clients in the home can safely use disposable syringes until the needles become dull, which can vary from 2 to 10 times (Fleming, 1999). Any client reusing syringes should have the ability to safely and correctly recap needles. Clients with poor personal hygiene, acute concurrent illness, open wounds on the hands, or decreased resistance to infection should be discouraged from reusing syringes.
- For insulin-dependent clients, ensure that at least one knowledgeable support person can correctly inject insulin in an emergency situation and recognize and treat hypoglycemia.

Intramuscular Injections

Injections into muscle tissue, or **intramuscular (IM) injections,** are absorbed more quickly than subcutaneous injections because of the greater blood supply to the body muscles. Muscles can also take a larger volume of fluid without discomfort than subcutaneous tissues can, although the amount varies among individuals, chiefly with muscle size and condition and with the site used. An adult with well-developed muscles can usually safely tolerate up to 4 mL of medication in the gluteus medius and gluteus maximus muscles (Figure 33–41 ■). A volume of 1 to 2 mL is usually recommended for adults with less developed muscles. In the deltoid muscle, volumes of 0.5 to 1 mL are recommended.

Usually a 2- to 5-mL syringe is needed. The size of syringe used depends on the amount of medication being administered. The standard prepackaged intramuscular needle is 1½ inches and #21 or #22 gauge. Several factors indicate the size and length of the needle to be used:

- The muscle
- The type of solution
- The amount of adipose tissue covering the muscle
- The age of the client.

For example, a smaller needle such as a #23- to #25-gauge needle 1 inch long is commonly used for the deltoid muscle. More viscous solutions require a larger gauge (e.g., #20 gauge). Very obese clients may require a needle longer than 1½ inches (e.g., 2 inches) and emaciated clients may require a shorter needle (e.g., 1 inch).

A major consideration in the administration of intramuscular injections is the selection of a safe site located away from large blood vessels, nerves, and bone. Several body sites can be used for intramuscular injections. These sites are discussed in detail next. Contraindications for using a specific site include tissue injury and the presence of nodules, lumps, abscesses, tenderness, or other pathology.

Ventrogluteal Site

The ventrogluteal site is in the gluteus medius muscle, which lies over the gluteus minimus (Figure 33–41). The ventrogluteal site is the *preferred* site for intramuscular injections because the area:

- Contains no large nerves or blood vessels
- Provides the greatest thickness of gluteal muscle consisting of both the gluteus medius and gluteus minimus
- Is sealed off by bone
- Contains consistently less fat than the buttock area, thus eliminating the need to determine the depth of subcutaneous fat.

This site is suitable for children over 7 months and adults. The client position for the injection can be a back, prone, or side-lying position. The side-lying position, however, helps locate the ventrogluteal site more easily. Position the client on his or her side with the knee bent and raised slightly toward the chest. The trochanter will protrude, which facilitates locating the ventrogluteal site. To establish the exact site, the nurse places the heel of the hand on the client's greater trochanter, with the fingers pointing toward the client's head. The right hand is used for the left hip, and the left hand for the right hip. With the index finger on the client's anterior superior iliac spine, the nurse stretches the middle finger dorsally (toward the buttocks), palpating the crest of the ilium and then pressing below it. The triangle formed by the index finger, the third finger, and the crest of the ileum is the injection site (Figures 33–42 ■ and 33–43 ■).

Vastus Lateralis Site

The vastus lateralis muscle is usually thick and well developed in both adults and children. It is recommended as the site of choice for intramuscular injections for infants 7 months and younger. Because there are no major blood vessels or nerves in the area, it is desirable for infants whose gluteal muscles are poorly developed. It is situated on the anterior lateral aspect of

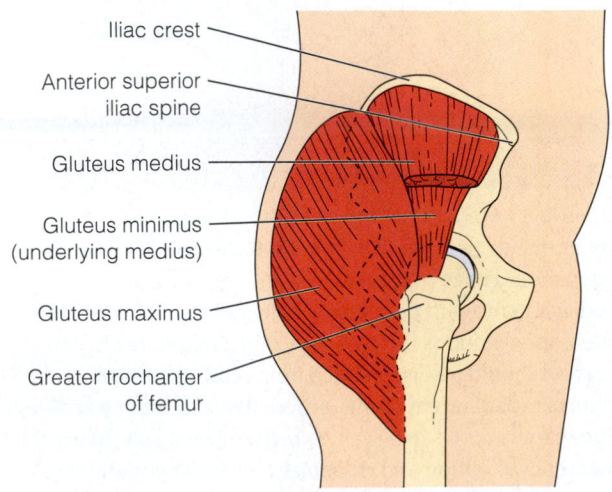

Figure 33–41 ■ Lateral view of the right buttock showing the three gluteal muscles used for intramuscular injections

Iliac crest
Anterior superior iliac spine
Gluteus medius
Gluteus minimus (underlying medius)
Gluteus maximus
Greater trochanter of femur

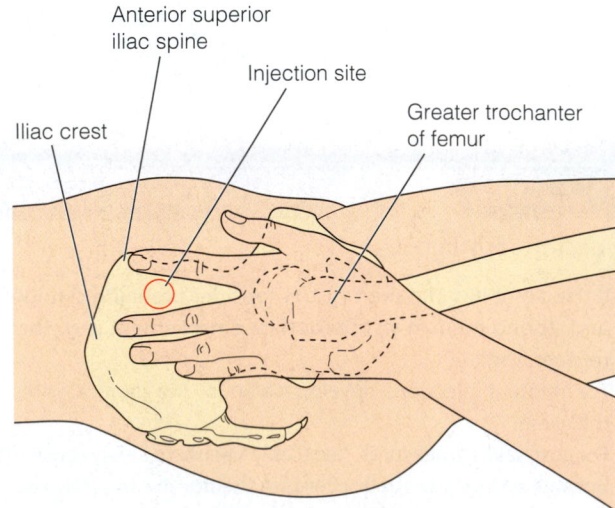

Figure 33–42 ■ Landmarks for the ventrogluteal site for an intramuscular injection.

Anterior superior iliac spine
Injection site
Greater trochanter of femur
Iliac crest

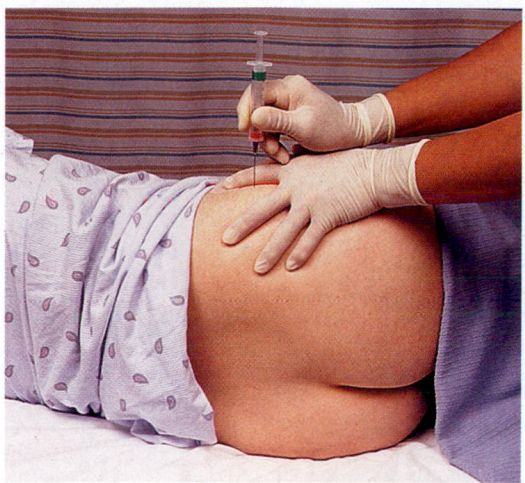

Figure 33–43 ■ Administering an intramuscular injection into the ventrogluteal site.

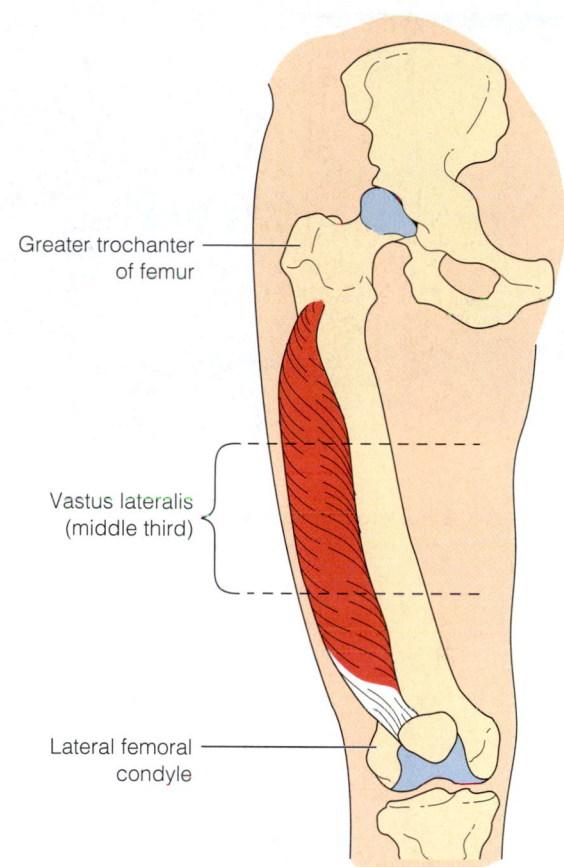

Figure 33–45 ■ Landmarks for the vastus lateralis site of an adult's right thigh, used for an intramuscular injection.

the infant's thigh (Figure 33–44 ■). The middle third of the muscle is suggested as the site. In the adult, the landmark is established by dividing the area between the greater trochanter of the femur and the lateral femoral condyle into thirds and selecting the middle third (Figures 33–45 ■ and 33–46 ■). The client can assume a back-lying or a sitting position for an injection into this site.

Dorsogluteal Site

The dorsogluteal site is composed of the thick gluteal muscles of the buttocks (Figure 33–41). The dorsogluteal site can be used for adults and for children with well-developed gluteal muscles. Because these muscles are developed by walking, this site should not be used for children under 3 years unless the child has been walking for at least 1 year. The nurse must choose the injection site carefully to avoid striking the sciatic nerve, major blood vessels, or bone.

The nurse palpates the posterior superior iliac spine, then draws an imaginary line to the greater trochanter of the femur. This line is lateral to and parallel to the sciatic nerve. The injection site is lateral and superior to this line (Figure 33–47 ■). Palpating the ilium and the trochanter is important; visual calculations alone can result in an injection that is placed too low and injures other structures.

The client needs to assume a prone position with the toes pointed inward or a side-lying position with the upper knee flexed and in front of the lower leg. These positions promote muscle relaxation and therefore minimize discomfort from the injection.

Deltoid Site

The deltoid muscle is found on the lateral aspect of the upper arm. It is not used often for intramuscular injections because it is a relatively small muscle and is very close to the radial nerve and radial artery. It is sometimes considered for use in adults because of rapid absorption from the deltoid area, but no more than 1 mL of solution can be administered. This site is recommended for the administration of hepatitis B vaccine in adults.

The upper landmark for the deltoid site is located by the nurse placing four fingers across the deltoid muscle with the first finger on the acromion process. The top of the axilla is the line that marks the lower border landmark (Figure 33–48 ■). A triangle within

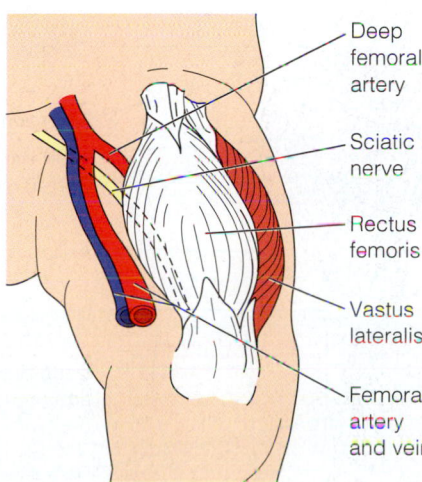

Figure 33–44 ■ The vastus lateralis muscle of an infant's upper thigh, used for intramuscular injections.

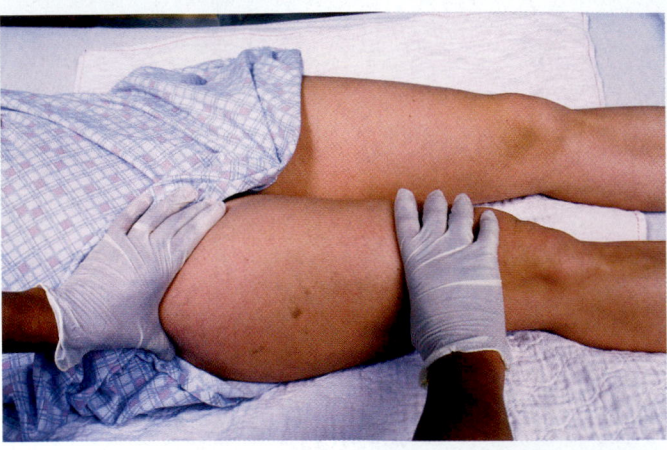

A

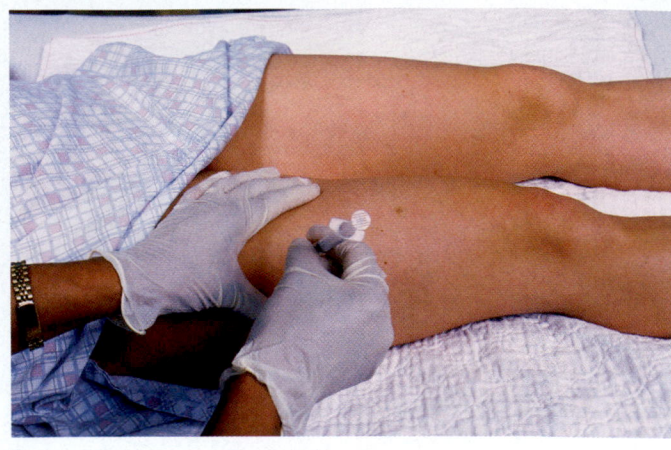

B

Figure 33–46 ■ *A,* Determining landmarks and *B,* Administering an intramuscular injection into the vastus lateralis site.

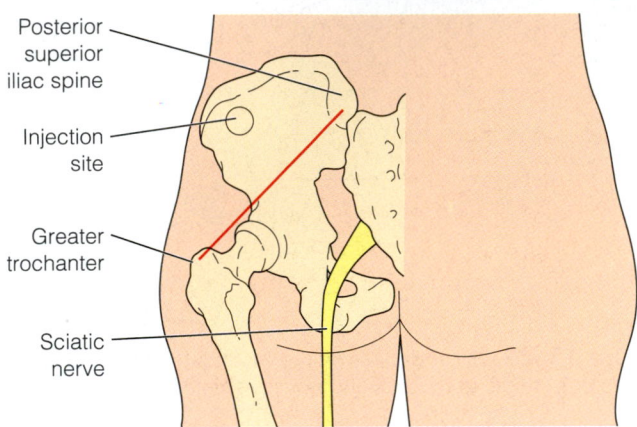

Posterior
superior
iliac spine

Injection
site

Greater
trochanter

Sciatic
nerve

Figure 33–47 ■ Landmarks for the dorsogluteal site for an intramuscular injection.

these boundaries indicates the deltoid muscle about 5 cm (2 in.) below the acromion process (Figures 33–49 ■ and 33–50 ■).

The use of a pinch-grasp technique can reduce the discomfort of an IM injection into the deltoid muscle. This technique involves grasping the muscle, pulling it about 1/2 to 1 inch toward the nurse, and applying a pinching pressure hard enough to cause mild discomfort. The injection is given at a 90-degree angel (McCaffery & Pasero, 1999). It is important for the nurse to inform the client about pinching the skin and explain the purpose.

Rectus Femoris Site

The rectus femoris muscle, which belongs to the quadriceps muscle group, is used only occasionally for intramuscular injections. It is situated on the anterior aspect of the thigh (Figure 33–51 ■).

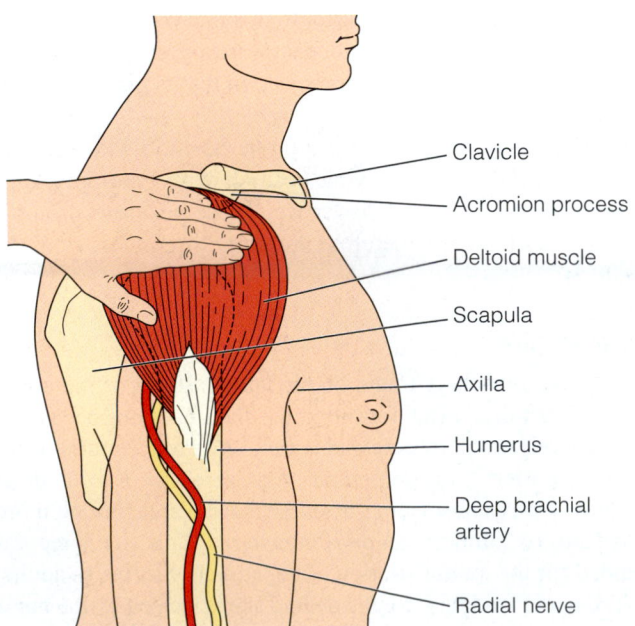

Clavicle

Acromion process

Deltoid muscle

Scapula

Axilla

Humerus

Deep brachial
artery

Radial nerve

Figure 33–48 ■ A method of establishing the deltoid muscle site for an intramuscular injection.

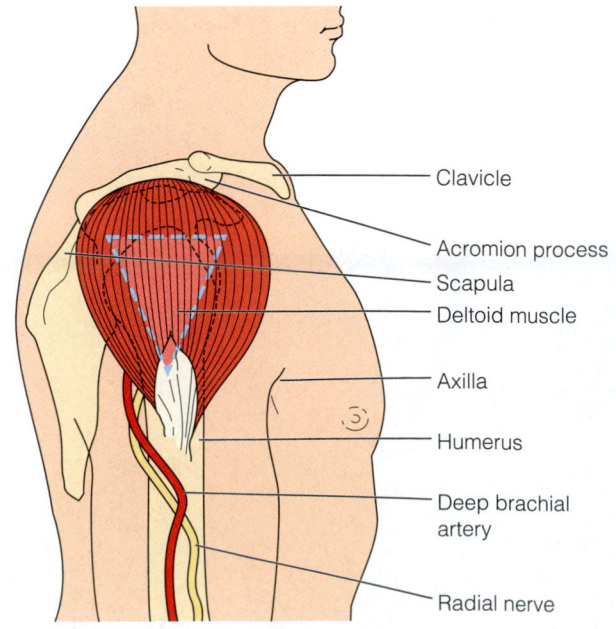

Clavicle

Acromion process

Scapula

Deltoid muscle

Axilla

Humerus

Deep brachial
artery

Radial nerve

Figure 33–49 ■ Landmarks for the deltoid muscle of the upper arm, used for intramuscular injections.

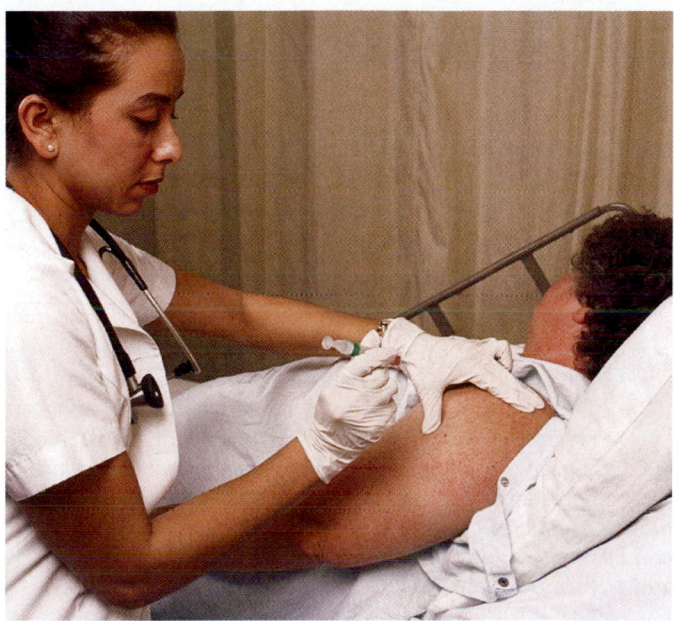

Figure 33–50 ■ Administering an intramuscular injection into the deltoid site.

Its chief advantage is that clients who administer their own injections can reach this site easily. Its main disadvantage is that an injection here may cause considerable discomfort for some people.

IM Injection Technique

Procedure 33–7 describes how to administer an intramuscular injection using the Z-track technique, which is recommended

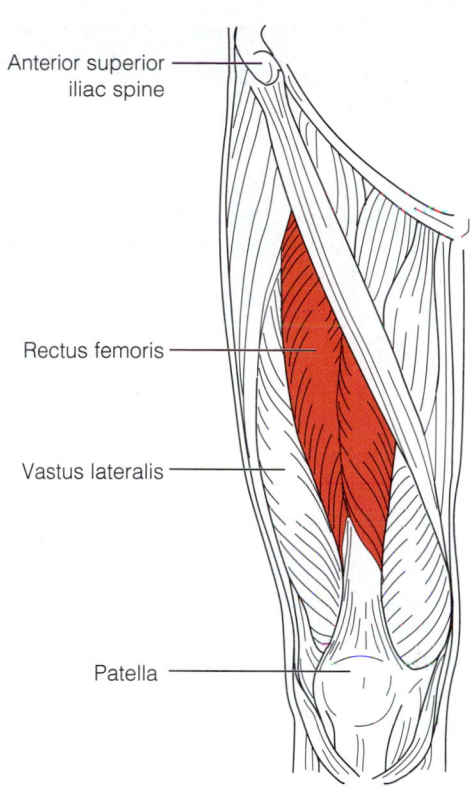

Anterior superior iliac spine

Rectus femoris

Vastus lateralis

Patella

Figure 33–51 ■ Landmarks for the rectus femoris muscle of the upper right thigh, used for intramuscular injections.

for any intramuscular injection. The Z-track method has been found to be less painful than the traditional injection technique (McCaffery & Pasero, 1999).

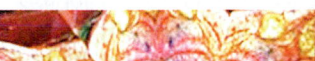 **Procedure 33–7 Administering an Intramuscular Injection**

Purpose

■ To provide a medication the client requires (see specific drug action)

ASSESSMENT

Assess

■ Client allergies to medication(s)
■ Specific drug action, side effects, and adverse reactions
■ Client's knowledge of and learning needs about the medication
■ Tissue integrity of the selected site
■ Client's age and weight to determine site and needle size
■ Client's ability or willingness to cooperate

Determine whether the size of the muscle is appropriate to the amount of medication to be injected. An average adult's deltoid muscle can usually absorb 0.5 mL of medication, although some authorities believe 1 mL can be absorbed by a well-developed deltoid muscle. The gluteus medius muscle can often absorb 1 to 4 mL, although 4 mL may be very painful.

PLANNING

Delegation

The administration of IM injections is an invasive technique that involves the application of nursing knowledge, problem solving, and sterile technique. Delegation to UAP would be inappropriate.

The nurse, however, can inform the UAP of the intended therapeutic effects and/or specific side effects of the medication and direct the UAP to report specific client observations to the nurse for follow-up.

---

continued on page 830

Procedure 33–7 Administering an Intramuscular Injection *continued*

PLANNING *continued*

Equipment
- MAR or computer printout
- Sterile medication (usually provided in an ampule or vial)
- Syringe and needle of a size appropriate for the amount of solution to be administered
- Antiseptic swabs
- Clean gloves

IMPLEMENTATION

Preparation
1. Check the MAR.
   - Check the label on the medication carefully against the MAR to make sure that the correct medication is being prepared.
   - Follow the three checks for administering the medication and dose. Read the label on the medication (1) when it is taken from the medication cart, (2) before withdrawing the medication, and (3) after withdrawing the medication.
   - Confirm that the dose is correct.
2. Organize the equipment.

Performance
1. Wash hands and observe other appropriate infection control procedures (e.g., clean gloves).
2. Prepare the medication from the ampule or vial for drug withdrawal.
   - See Procedure 33–2 (ampule) or 33–3 (vial).
   - Whenever feasible, change the needle on the syringe before the injection. *Because the outside of a new needle is free of medication, it does not irritate subcutaneous tissues as it passes into the muscle.*
   - Invert the syringe needle uppermost and expel all excess air.
3. Provide for client privacy.
4. Prepare the client
   - Check the client's identification band. *This ensures that the right client receives the medication.*
   - Assist the client to a supine, lateral, prone, or sitting position, depending on the chosen site. If the target muscle is the gluteus medius (ventrogluteal site), have the client in the supine position flex the knee(s); in the lateral position, flex the upper leg; and in the prone position, toe in. *Appropriate positioning promotes relaxation of the target muscle.*
   - Obtain assistance in holding an uncooperative client. *This prevents in-*

jury due to sudden movement after needle insertion.

5. Explain the purpose of the medication and how it will help, using language that the client can understand. Include relevant information about effects of the medication. *Information facilitates acceptance of and compliance with the therapy.*
6. Select, locate, and clean the site.
   - Select a site free of skin lesions, tenderness, swelling, hardness, or localized inflammation and one that has not been used frequently.
   - If injections are to be frequent, alternate sites. Avoid using the same site twice in a row. *This is to reduce the discomfort of intramuscular injections.* If necessary, discuss with the prescribing physician an alternative method of providing the medication.
   - Locate the exact site for the injection. See the discussion of sites earlier in this chapter.
   - Put on clean gloves.
   - Clean the site with an antiseptic swab. Using a circular motion, start at the center and move outward about 5 cm (2 in.).

- Transfer and hold the swab between the third and fourth fingers of your nondominant hand in readiness for needle withdrawal, or position the swab on the clients skin above the intended site. Allow skin to dry prior to injecting medication *because this will help reduce the discomfort of the injection.*
7. Prepare the syringe for injection.
   - Remove the needle cover without contaminating the needle.
   - If using a prefilled unit-dose medication, take caution to avoid dripping medication on the needle prior to injection. If this does occur, wipe the medication off the needle with a sterile gauze. *Medication left on the needle can cause pain when it is tracked through the subcutaneous tissue.*
8. Inject the medication using a Z-track technique.
   - Use the ulnar side of the nondominant hand to pull the skin approximately 2.5 cm (1 inch) to the side (Figure 33–52 ■). Under some circumstances, such as for an emaciated client or an infant, the muscle

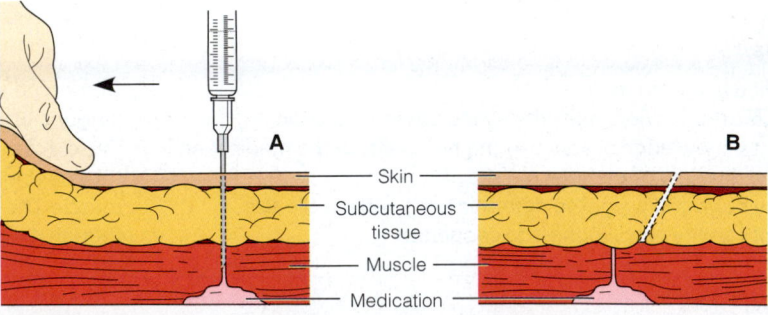

Figure 33–52 ■ Inserting an intramuscular needle at a 90-degree angle using the Z-track method: *A,* skin pulled to the side; *B,* skin released. *Note:* When the skin returns to its normal position after the needle is withdrawn, a seal is formed over the intramuscular site. This prevents seepage of the medication into the subcutaneous tissues and subsequent discomfort.

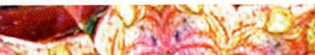

Procedure 33–7 Administering an Intramuscular Injection *continued*

IMPLEMENTATION *continued*

may be pinched. *Pulling the skin and subcutaneous tissue or pinching the muscle makes it firmer and facilitates needle insertion.*

- Holding the syringe between the thumb and forefinger (as if holding a pencil), pierce the skin quickly and smoothly at a 90-degree angle (Figure 33–43), and insert the needle into the muscle. *Using a quick motion lessens the client's discomfort.*
- Hold the barrel of the syringe steady with your nondominant hand and aspirate by pulling back on the plunger with your dominant hand. Aspirate for 5 to 10 seconds. *If the needle is in a small blood vessel, it takes time for the blood to appear.* If blood appears in the syringe, withdraw the needle, discard the syringe,

and prepare a new injection. *This step determines whether the needle has been inserted into a blood vessel.*
- If blood does not appear, inject the medication steadily and slowly (approximately 10 seconds per milliliter) while holding the syringe steady. *Injecting medication slowly promotes comfort and allows time for tissue to expand and begin absorption of the medication. Holding the syringe steady minimizes discomfort.*
- After injection, wait 10 seconds *to permit the medication to disperse into the muscle tissue, thus decreasing the client's discomfort.*

9. Withdraw the needle.
- Withdraw the needle smoothly at the same angle of insertion. *This minimizes tissue injury.*

- Apply gentle pressure at the site with a dry sponge. Do not massage the site. *Massaging the site can increase discomfort of the injection and can result in tissue irritation.*
- If bleeding occurs, apply pressure with a dry sterile gauze until it stops.

10. Discard the uncapped needle and attached syringe into the proper receptacle.
- Remove gloves. Wash hands.

11. Document all relevant information.
- Include the time of administration, drug name, dose, route, and the client's reactions.

12. Assess effectiveness of the medication at the time it is expected to act.

EVALUATION

- Conduct appropriate follow-up, such as
  - Desired effect (e.g., relief of pain or vomiting)
  - Any adverse reactions or side effects
  - Local skin or tissue reactions at injection site (e.g., redness, swelling, pain, or other evidence of tissue damage)

- Relate to previous findings, if available
- Report significant deviation from normal to physician.

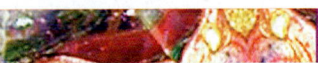

Lifespan Considerations

Intramuscular Injections

Infants

- The ventrogluteal site cannot be used for children under 7 months of age.
- The vastus lateralis site is recommended as the site of choice for intramuscular injections for infants 7 months and younger. Because there are no major blood vessels or nerves in the area, it is desirable for infants whose gluteal muscles are poorly developed. It is situated on the anterior lateral aspect of the thigh (see Figure 33–44).
- Obtain assistance to immobilize an infant or young child. The parent may hold the infant or young child. This prevents accidental injury during the procedure.

Children

- Infants and young children usually require smaller, shorter needles (#22 to #25 gauge, 5/8 to 1 inch long) for intramuscular injection.
- The gluteal muscles are developed by walking. Therefore, the dorsogluteal site should not be used for children under 3 years unless the child has been walking for at least 1 year.

Elders

- Older clients may have a decreased muscle mass or muscle atrophy. A shorter needle may be needed. Assessment of appropriate injection site is critical. Absorption of medication may occur more quickly than expected.

Intravenous Medications

Because intravenous (IV) medications enter the client's bloodstream directly by way of a vein, they are appropriate when a rapid effect is required. This route is also appropriate when medications are too irritating to tissues to be given by other routes. When an intravenous line is already established, this route is desirable because it avoids the discomfort of other par-

enteral routes. Medications are administered intravenously by the following methods:

- Large-volume infusion of intravenous fluid
- Intermittent intravenous infusion (piggyback or tandem setups)
- Volume-controlled infusion (often used for children)
- Intravenous push or bolus
- Intermittent injection ports (device)

In all of these methods, the client has an existing intravenous line or an IV access site such as a saline or heparin lock. Most agencies have procedures and policies about who may administer an IV medication. Chapter 50 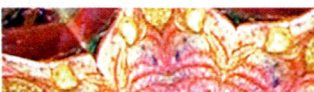 describes the technique for performing a venipuncture and establishing an IV line.

With all IV medication administration it is very important to observe clients closely for signs of adverse reactions. Because the drug enters the bloodstream directly and acts immediately, there is no way it can be withdrawn or its action terminated. Therefore, the nurse must take special care to avoid any errors about the preparation of the drug and the calculation of the dosage. When the drug being administered is particularly potent, an antidote to the drug should be available. In addition, the vital signs are assessed before, during, and after infusion of the drug.

Before adding any medications to an existing intravenous infusion, the nurse must check for the six "rights" and check compatability of the drug and the existing intravenous fluid. Be aware of any incompatabilities of the drug and the fluid that is infusing. For example, the drug dilantin is incompatible with

glucose and will form a precipitate if injected through a port in an intravenous line with glucose infusing.

Large-Volume Infusions

Mixing a medication into a large-volume IV container is the safest and easiest way to administer a drug intravenously. The drugs are diluted in volumes of 1,000 mL or 500 mL of compatible fluids. It may be necessary to consult a pharmacist to confirm compatibility. Fluids such as IV normal saline or Ringer's lactate are frequently used. Commonly added drugs are potassium chloride and vitamins. It may also be necessary to ensure the compatibility of some drugs with the plastic IV bag and tubing. A glass IV bottle and special tubing may be used in special situations. See Procedure 33–8.

The main danger of infusing a large volume of fluid is circulatory overload (hypervolemia) (see Chapter 49).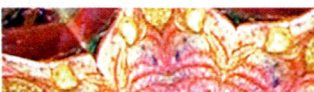

The medication can be added to the fluid container that is running or before it is hung and infusing. In some hospitals the pharmacist adds the medication to the container.

Procedure 33–8 Adding Medications to Intravenous Fluid Containers

Purposes

- To provide and maintain a constant level of a medication in the blood
- To administer well-diluted medications at a continuous and slow rate

ASSESSMENT

- Inspect and palpate the intravenous insertion site for signs of infection, infiltration, or a dislocated catheter.
- Inspect the the surrounding skin for redness, pallor, or swelling.
- Palpate the surrounding tissues for coldness and the presence of edema, which could indicate leakage of the IV fluid into the tissues.

- Take vital signs for baseline data if the medication being administered is particularly potent.
- Determine if the client has allergies to the medication(s).
- Check the compatibility of the medication(s) and IV fluid.

PLANNING

Delegation

Adding medications to IV fluid containers involves the application of nursing knowledge and critical thinking. The nurse does not delegate this procedure to UAP. However, the nurse can inform the UAP of the intended therapeutic effects and/or specific side effects of the medication(s) in the IV and direct the UAP to report specific client observations to the nurse for follow-up.

Equipment
- MAR or computer printout
- Correct sterile medication

- Diluent for medication in powdered form (see manufacturer's instructions)
- Correct solution container, if a new one is to be attached
- Antiseptic or alcohol swabs
- Sterile syringe of appropriate size (e.g., 5 or 10 mL) and a 1- to 1½-inch, #20- or #21-gauge sterile needle or equivalent from needleless system
- IV additive label

IMPLEMENTATION

Preparation
1. Check the MAR.
   - Check the label on the medication carefully against the MAR to make

sure that the correct medication is being prepared.
   - Follow the three checks for administering medications. Read the label on

the medication (1) when it is taken from the medication cart, (2) before withdrawing the medication, and (3) after withdrawing the medication.

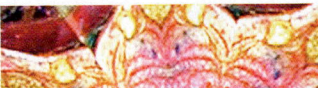

Procedure 33–8 Adding Medications to Intravenous Fluid Containers *continued*

IMPLEMENTATION *continued*

- Confirm that the dosage and route is correct.
- Verify which infusion solution is to be used with the medication.
- Consult a pharmacist, if required, to confirm compatibility of the drugs and solutions being mixed.
2. Organize the equipment.

Performance

1. Wash hands and observe other appropriate infection control procedures.
2. Prepare the medication ampule or vial for drug withdrawal.
   - See Procedure 33–2 (ampule) or 33–3 (vial).
   - Check the agency's practice for using a filter needle or a needleless system to withdraw premixed liquid medications from multidose vials or ampules.
3. Add the medication.

To New IV Container

- Locate the injection port and carefully remove its cover. Clean the port with the antiseptic or alcohol swab. *This reduces the risk of introducing microorganisms into the container when the needle is inserted.*
- Remove the needle cap from the syringe, insert the needle through the center of the injection port, and inject the medication into the bag or bottle (Figure 33–53 ■).

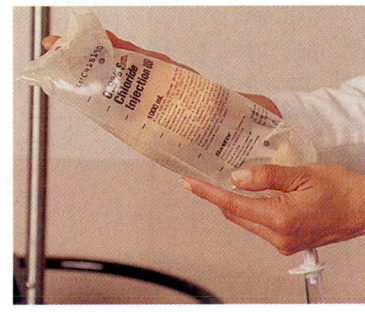

Figure 33–53 ■ Inserting a medication through the injection port of an infusing container.

- Mix the medication and solution by gently rotating the bag or bottle (Figure 33–54 ■). *This should disperse the medication throughout the solution.*

Figure 33–54 ■ Rotating an intravenous bag to distribute a medication.

- Complete the IV additive label with name and dose of medication, date, time, and nurse's initials. Attach it upside down on the bag or bottle (Figure 33–55 ■). *This documents that medication has been added to the solution. When the label is attached upside down, it is easily read when the bag is hanging up.*

MEDICATION ADDED

DRUG

AMOUNT

ADDED BY

DATE   TIME

THIS LABEL MUST BE AFFIXED TO ALL INFUSION
FLUIDS CONTAINING ADDITIONAL MEDICATION

WRAP AROUND IV TUBING	I.V. SET—72 Hours Only
	RN initial
	START—date/hr.
	DISCARD—date/hr.

Figure 33–55 ■ *Top,* label indicating a medication added to an IV infusion; *Bottom,* label indicating time for IV tubing change.

- Clamp the IV tubing. Spike the bag or bottle with IV tubing and hang the IV. *Clamping prevents rapid infusion of the solution.*
- Regulate infusion rate as ordered.

To an Existing Infusion

Determine that the IV solution in the container is sufficient for adding the medication. *Sufficient volume is necessary to dilute the medication adequately.*

- Confirm the desired dilution of the medication, that is, the amount of medication per milliliter of solution.
- Close the infusion clamp. *This prevents the medication from infusing directly into the client as it is injected into the bag or bottle.*
- Wipe the medication port with the alcohol or disinfectant swab. *This reduces the risk of introducing microorganisms into the container when the needle is inserted.*
- Remove the needle cover from the medication syringe.
- While supporting and stabilizing the bag with your thumb and forefinger, carefully insert the syringe needle through the port and inject the medication. *The bag is supported during the injection of the medication to avoid punctures.* If the bag or bottle is too high to reach easily, lower it from the IV pole.
- Remove the bag or bottle from the pole and gently rotate the bottle or bag. *This will mix the medication and solution.*
- Rehang the container and regulate the flow rate. *This establishes the correct flow rate.*
- Complete the medication label and apply to the IV container.
4. Dispose of the equipment and supplies according to agency practice. *This prevents inadvertent injury to others and the spread of microorganisms.*
5. Document the medication(s) on the appropriate form in the client's record.

Intermittent Intravenous Infusions

An intermittent infusion is a method of administering a medication mixed in a small amount of IV solution, such as 50 or 100 mL (Figure 33–56 ■). The drug is administered at regular intervals, such as every 4 hours, with the drug being infused for a short period of time such as 30 to 60 minutes. Two commonly used additive or secondary IV setups are the **tandem** and the **piggyback.**

In a tandem setup, a second container is attached to the line of the first container at the lower, secondary port (Figure 33–57 ■, A). It permits medications to be administered intermittently or simultaneously with the primary solution.

In the piggyback alignment, a second set connects the second container to the tubing of the primary container at the upper port (Figure 33–57 ■, B). This setup is used solely for intermittent drug administration. Various manufacturers describe these sets differently, so the nurse must check the manufacturer's labeling and directions carefully. Traditionally the tubing of the secondary set has been attached to ports of the primary infusion by inserting a needle through the port and taping it in place. Needleless

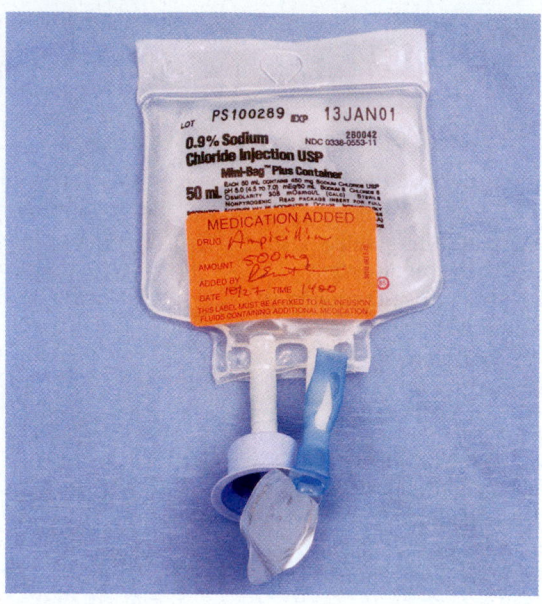

Figure 33–56 ■ Medication in a labeled infusion bag.

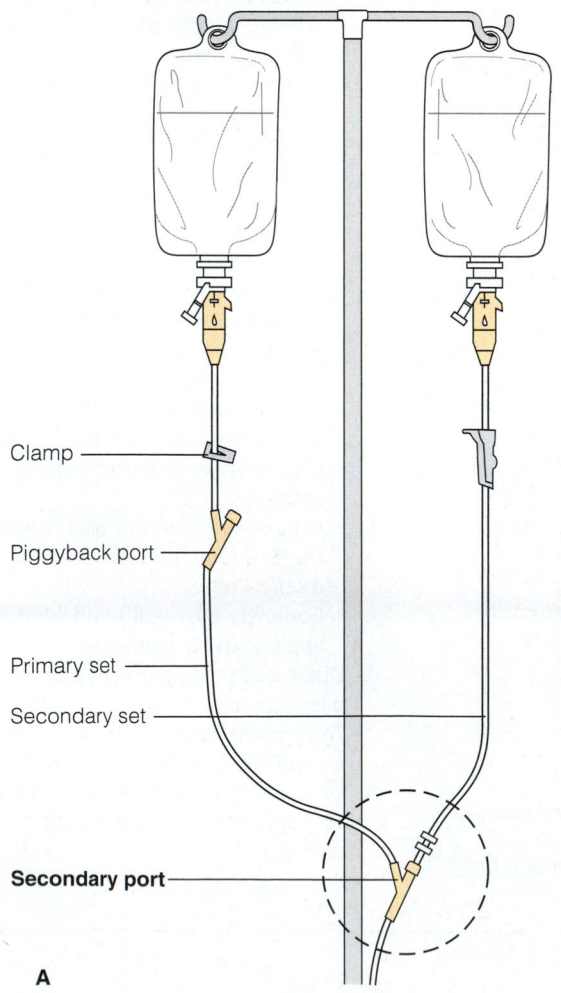

A

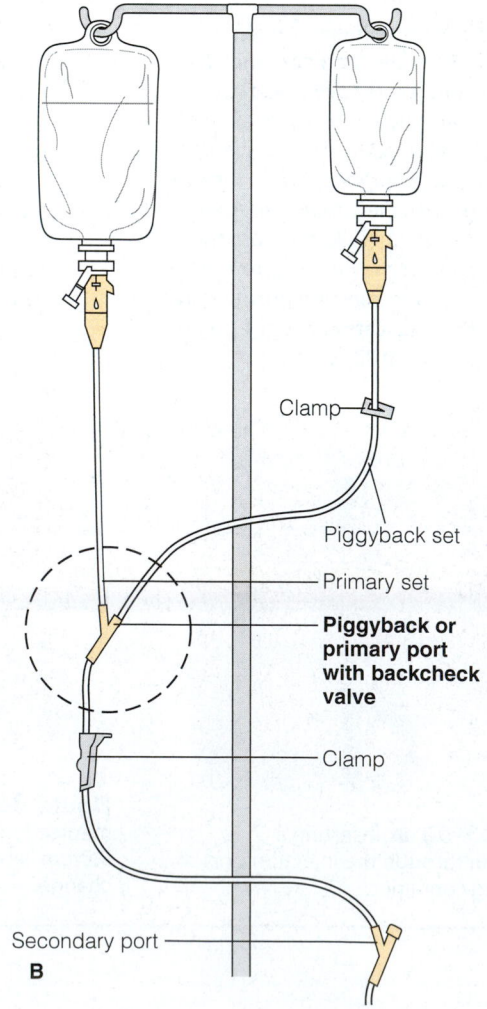

B

Figure 33–57 ■ Secondary intravenous lines: *A,* a tandem intravenous alignment; *B,* an intravenous piggyback (IVPB) alignment.

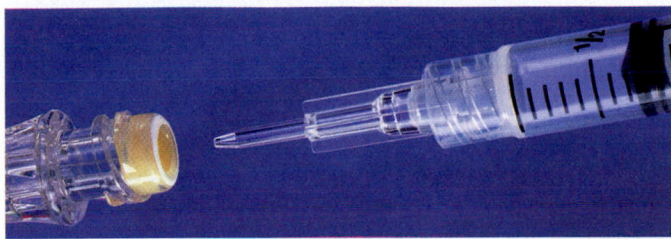

Figure 33–58 ■ A blunt plastic cannula replaces the sharp steel needle. (Photograph reprinted courtesy of (BD) Becton, Dickinson and Company.)

systems are now available (Figure 33–58 ■). These needleless systems can use threaded-lock or lever-lock cannulae to connect the secondary set to the ports of the primary infusion (Figure 33–59 ■). This design prevents needlestick injuries and also prevents touch contamination at the IV connection site.

Another method of intermittently administering an IV medication is by a syringe pump or mini-infuser. The medication is mixed in a syringe that is connected to the primary IV line via a mini-infuser (see Figure 33–60 ■).

Volume-Control Infusions

Intermittent medications may also be administered by a **volume-control infusion set** such as Buretrol, Soluset, Volutrol, and Pediatrol (Figure 33–61 ■). They are small fluid containers (100

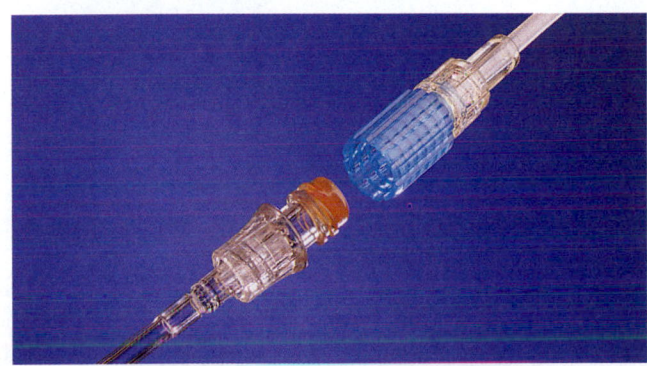

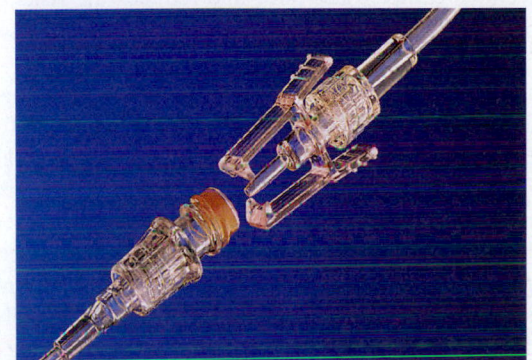

Figure 33–59 ■ Needleless cannulae used to connect the tubing of secondary sets to primary infusions: *A*, threaded-lock cannula; *B*, lever-lock cannula. (photo a) Photograph reprinted courtesy of (BD) Becton, Dickinson and Company and courtesy of Baxter Healthcare Corporation. All rights reserved. (photo b) Photograph reprinted courtesy of (BD) Becton, Dickinson and Company and courtesy of Baxter Healthcare Corporation.

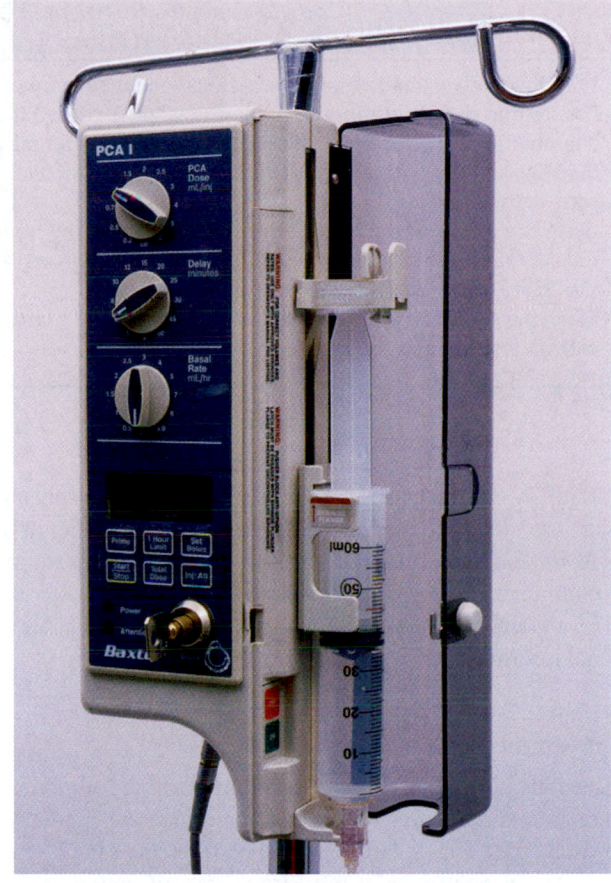

Figure 33–60 ■ Syringe pump or mini-infuser for administration of IV medications.

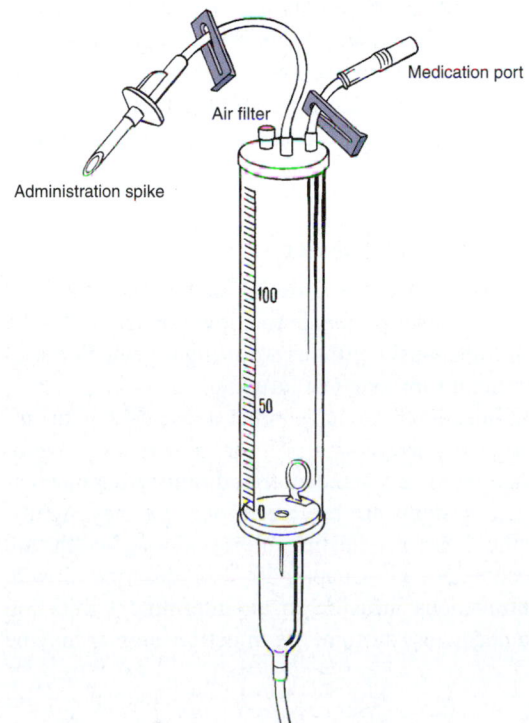

Figure 33–61 ■ A volume-control infusion set.

BOX 33–6 ■ **Adding a Medication to a Volume-Control Infusion Set**

- Withdraw the required dose of the medication into a syringe.
- Ensure that there is sufficient fluid in the volume-control fluid chamber to dilute the medication. Generally, at least 50 mL of fluid is used. Check the directions from the drug manufacturer or consult the pharmacist.
- Close the inflow to the fluid chamber by adjusting the upper roller or slide clamp above the fluid chamber; also ensure that the clamp on the air vent of the chamber is open.
- Clean the medication port on the volume-control fluid chamber with an antiseptic swab.

- Inject the medication into the port of the partially filled volume control set.
- Gently rotate the fluid chamber until the fluid is well mixed.
- Open the line's upper clamp, and regulate the flow by adjusting the lower roller or slide clamp below the fluid chamber.
- Attach a medication label to the volume-control fluid chamber.
- Document relevant data, and monitor the client and the infusion.

---

to 150 mL in size) attached below the primary infusion container so that the medication is administered through the client's IV line. Volume-control sets are frequently used to infuse solutions into children and older clients when the volume administered is critical and must be carefully monitored. Box 33–6 provides additional information.

Intravenous Push

Intravenous push (IVP) (bolus) is the intravenous administration of an undiluted drug directly into the systemic circulation. It is used when a medication cannot be diluted or in an emergency. An IV bolus can be introduced directly into a vein by venipuncture or into an existing IV line through an injection port or through an IV lock.

There are two major disadvantages to this method of drug administration: Any error in administration cannot be corrected after the drug has entered the client, and the drug may be irritating to the lining of the blood vessels. Before administering a bolus, the nurse should look up the maximum concentration recommended for the particular drug and the rate of administration. The administered medication takes effect immediately (see Procedure 33–9).

Intermittent Infusion Devices

Intermittent infusion devices (Figure 33–62 ■) may be affixed to an intravenous catheter or needle to allow medications to be administered intravenously without requiring repeated needlesticks or a continuous intravenous infusion.

Intermittent injection ports have either a resealable latex injection site for needle access or a port that allows a syringe or a needleless adapter to be connected for administering medications. Needleless systems are preferred, because they significantly reduce the risk of needlestick injuries among health care workers. Procedure 50–5 in Chapter 50 🔗 describes how to convert an intravenous infusion to an intermittent injection port. With the needleless system, the injection adapter may be

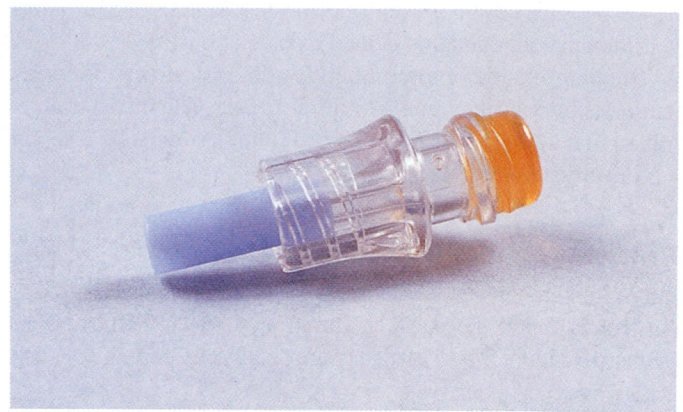

Figure 33–62 ■ Intermittent infusion device with injection port. (Courtesy of Baxter Healthcare Corporation. All rights reserved.)

affixed at the time of intravenous catheter placement, allowing a closed system to be maintained.

Intermittent injection ports may be flushed with sterile saline prior to medication administration, and with saline or heparinized saline afterward. Flushing the port maintains patency of the intravenous catheter and port, and reduces the risks of mixing incompatible medications within the system (see Procedure 33–9).

Clients who require long-term venous access for administering medications (e.g., people receiving chemotherapy for cancer treatment) may have a specialized catheter or port to allow central venous access. The catheter may be tunneled subcutaneously and accessed through an intermittent injection port attached to the distal end of the venous catheter. Other devices have an implantable port or vascular access port surgically inserted under the skin so that no portion of the device exits the body. To administer medications, the port is accessed using a specialized needle through the skin. See Chapter 50 🔗 for more information about central venous lines.

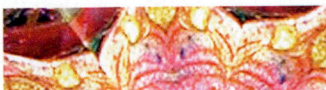

Procedure 33–9 Administering Intravenous Medications Using IV Push

Purpose
- To achieve immediate and maximum effects of a medication

ASSESSMENT

- Inspect and palpate the IV insertion site for signs of infection, infiltration, or a dislocated catheter.
- Inspect the surrounding skin for redness, pallor, or swelling.
- Palpate the surrounding tissues for coldness and the presence of edema, which could indicate leakage of the IV fluid into the tissues.

- Take vital signs for baseline data if the medication being administered is particularly potent.
- Determine if the client has allergies to the medication(s).
- Check the compatibility of the medication(s) and IV fluid.
- Determine specific drug action, side effects, normal dosage, recommended administration time, and peak action time.
- Check patency of IV line by assessing flow rate.

PLANNING

Delegation
The administration of intravenous medication via IV push involves the application of nursing knowledge and critical thinking. This procedure is not delegated to UAP. The nurse, however, can inform the UAP of the intended therapeutic effects and/or specific side effects of the medication and direct the UAP to report specific client observations to the nurse for follow-up.

Equipment

IV PUSH FOR AN EXISTING LINE
- Medication in a vial or ampule
- Sterile syringe (3 to 5 mL) (to prepare the medication)
- Sterile needles #21 to #25 gauge, 2.5 cm (1 in.), or equivalent from a needleless system
- Antiseptic swabs

- Watch with a digital readout or second hand
- Clean gloves

IV PUSH FOR AN IV LOCK
- Medication in a vial or ampule
- Sterile syringe (3 to 5 mL) (to prepare the medication)
- Sterile syringe (3 mL) (for the saline or heparin flush)
- Vial of normal saline to flush the IV catheter or vial of heparin flush solution or both depending on agency practice. *These maintain the patency of the IV lock. Saline is frequently used for peripheral locks.*
- Sterile needles (#21 gauge) or equivalent from a needleless system
- Antiseptic swabs
- Watch with a digital readout or second hand
- Disposable gloves

IMPLEMENTATION

Preparation
1. Check the MAR.
   - Check the label on the medication carefully against the MAR to make sure that the correct medication is being prepared.
   - Follow the three checks for correct medication and dose. Read the label on the medication (1) when it is taken from the medication cart, (2) before withdrawing the medication, and (3) after withdrawing the medication.
   - Calculate medication dosage accurately.
   - Confirm that the route is correct.
2. Organize the equipment.

Performance
1. Wash hands and observe other appropriate infection control procedures.
2. Prepare the medication.

Existing Line
- Prepare the medication according to the manufacturer's direction. *It is important to have the correct dose and the correct dilution.*

IV Lock
a. Flushing with saline
   - Prepare two syringes, each with 1 mL of sterile normal saline.
b. Flushing with heparin and saline
   - Prepare one syringe with 1 mL of heparin flush solution.
   - Prepare two syringes with 1 mL each of sterile, normal saline.
   - Draw up the medication into a syringe.
3. Put a small-gauge needle on the syringe if using a needle system.

4. Wash hands and put on clean gloves. *This reduces the transmission of microorganisms and reduces the likelihood of the nurse's hands contacting the client's blood.*
5. Provide for client privacy.
6. Prepare the client.
   - Check the client's identification band. *This ensures that the right client receives the medication.*
   - If not previously assessed, take the appropriate assessment measures necessary for the medication. If any of the findings are above or below the predetermined parameters, consult the physician before administering the medication.
7. Explain the purpose of the medication and how it will help, using language that the client can understand. Include relevant information about the effects of the medication.
8. Administer the medication by IV push.

continued on page 838

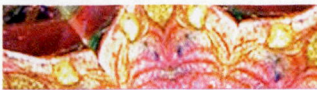

Procedure 33–9 Administering Intravenous Medications Using IV Push *continued*

IMPLEMENTATION *continued*

IV Lock with Needle
- Clean the diaphragm with the antiseptic swab. *This prevents microorganisms from entering the circulatory system during the needle insertion.*
- Insert the needle of the syringe containing normal saline through the center of the diaphragm and aspirate for blood (Figure 33–63 ■). *The presence of blood confirms that the catheter or needle is in the vein. In some situations, blood will not return even though the lock is patent.*

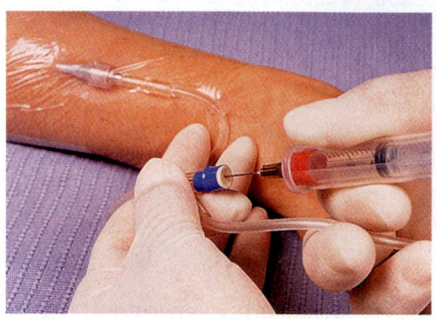

Figure 33–63 ■ Inserting a needle through the diaphragm of an IV lock.

- Flush the lock by injecting 1 mL of saline slowly. *This removes blood and heparin (if present) from the needle and the lock.*
- Remove the needle and syringe.
- Clean the lock's diaphragm with an antiseptic swab. *This prevents the transfer of microorganisms.*
- Insert the needle of the syringe containing the prepared medication through the center of the diaphragm.
- Inject the medication slowly at the recommended rate of infusion. Use a watch or digital readout to time the injection. Observe the client closely for adverse reactions. Remove the needle and syringe when all medication is administered. *Injecting the drug too rapidly can have a serious untoward reaction.*
- Withdraw the needle and syringe.
- Clean the diaphragm of the lock.
- Attach the second saline syringe, and inject 1 mL of saline. *The saline*

injection flushes the medication through the catheter and prepares the lock for heparin if this medication is used. Heparin is incompatible with many medications.
- If heparin is to be used, insert the heparin syringe and inject the heparin slowly into the lock.

IV Lock with Needleless System
- Remove the protective cap from the needleless port.
- Insert syringe containing normal saline into the lock.
- Flush the lock with 1 mL sterile saline. *This clears the lock of blood.*
- Remove the syringe.
- Insert the syringe containing the medication into the valve (Figure 33–64 ■).
- Inject the medication following the precautions described previously.
- Withdraw the syringe.
- Repeat injection of 1 mL of saline.
- Place a new sterile cap over the lock.

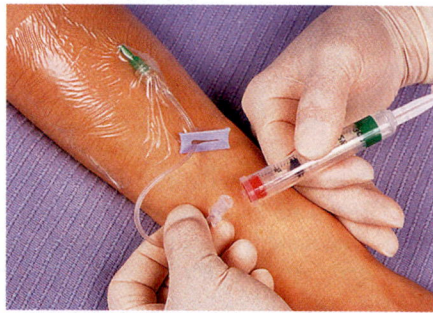

Figure 33–64 ■ Using a needleless system to inject a medication into an IV lock.

Existing Line
- Identify the injection port closest to the client. Some ports have a circle indicating the site for the needle insertion. *An injection port must be used because it is self-sealing. Any puncture to the plastic tubing will leak.*
- Clean the port with an antiseptic swab.
- Stop the IV flow by closing the clamp or pinching the tubing above the injection port.

- Connect the syringe to the IV system.
  a. Needle system
    - Hold the port steady.
    - Insert the needle of the syringe that contains the medication through the center of the port (Figure 33–65 ■). *This prevents damage to the IV line and to the diaphragm of the port.*

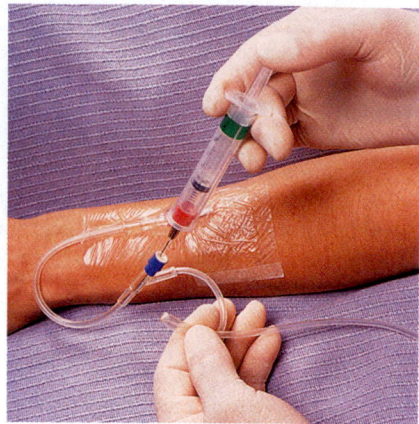

Figure 33–65 ■ Injecting a medication by IV push to an existing IV using a needle system.

  b. Needleless system
    - Remove the cap from the needleless injection port. Connect the tip of the syringe directly to the port (Figure 33–66 ■).

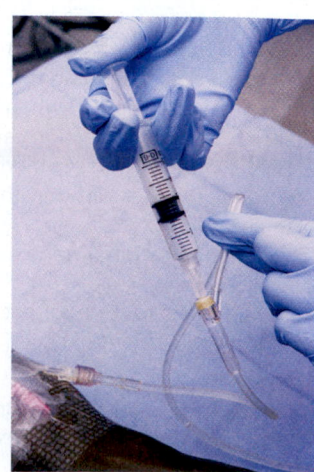

Figure 33–66 ■ Injecting a medication by IV push to an existing IV using a needleless system.

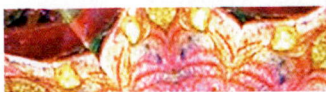

Procedure 33–9 Administering Intravenous Medications Using IV Push *continued*

IMPLEMENTATION *continued*

- Pull back on the plunger of the syringe in order to aspirate a small amount of blood. *This confirms that the port is patent and that the medication will enter the bloodstream.*
- After observing the blood, continue to keep the clamp closed and inject the medication at the ordered rate. Use the watch or digital readout to time the medication administration. *This ensures safe drug administration*

because a too rapid injection could be dangerous.
- Release the clamp or tubing.
- After injecting the medication, withdraw the needle, or for a needleless system, detach the syringe, and attach a new sterile cap to the port.

9. Dispose of equipment according to agency practice. *This reduces needlestick injuries and spread of microorganisms.*
10. Remove and dispose of gloves. Wash hands.

11. Observe the client closely for adverse reactions.
12. Determine agency practice about recommended times for changing the IV lock. Some agencies advocate a change every 48 to 72 hours for peripheral IV devices.
13. Document all relevant information.
    - Record the date, time, drug, dose, and route; client response; and assessments of infusion or heparin lock site if appropriate.

EVALUATION

- Conduct appropriate follow-up such as desired effect of medication, any adverse reactions or side effects, or change in vital signs.
- Reassess status of IV lock site and patency of IV infusion, if running.

- Relate to previous findings, if available.
- Report significant deviations from normal to the physician.

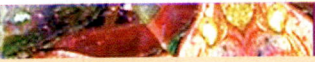

Home Care Considerations

Administering IV Push Antibiotics
Shortened hospital stays and the need to cut costs have led to clients or their caregivers being taught to administer IV push antibiotics at home. The antibiotic is delivered IV push directly into a venous access device with pre- and postadministration flushing (Skokal, 2000).

The nurse must

- Know which antibiotics are unsuitable for IV push administration.
- Know the adverse side effects:
  - Phlebitis (pain and tenderness over the vein, erythema, swelling, and warmth)
  - Speed shock (systemic reaction when a drug is given too rapidly)

  - Venous spasm (cramping and pain above infusion site)
  - Infiltration
- Assess caregiver or client's eyesight and manual dexterity. Both are needed for safe administration of the antibiotic.
- Provide thorough teaching about
  - Venous access device
  - Administration rate (minutes/dose)
  - Schedule for medication administration
  - Flushing technique
  - Adverse reactions
  - Signs that indicate an emergency and the need to call 911
  - Proper storage of medication
- Inspect appearance of medication and check expiration date.

Topical Medications

A topical medication is applied locally to the skin or to mucous membranes in areas such as the eye, external ear canal, nose, vagina, and rectum. Most topical applications used therapeutically are not absorbed well, completely, or predictably when applied to intact skin because the skin's thick outer layer serves as a natural barrier to drug diffusion. This route of absorption through the skin, called **percutaneous,** can be increased if the skin is altered by a laceration, burn, or some other problem. However, if high concentrations or large amounts of a topical medication are applied to the skin, especially if it is done re-

peatedly, sufficient amounts of the drug can enter the bloodstream to cause systemic effects, usually undesirable ones.

A particular type of topical or dermatologic medication delivery system is the **transdermal patch.** This system administers sustained-action medications (e.g., nitroglycerin, estrogen, and nicotine) via multilayered films containing the drug and an adhesive layer. The rate of delivery of the drug is controlled and varies with each product (e.g., from 12 hours to 1 week). Generally, the patch is applied to a hairless, clean area of skin that is not subject to excessive movement or wrinkling (i.e., the trunk or lower abdomen). It may also be applied on the side, lower back, or buttocks. Patches should not be applied to areas with cuts, burns, or abrasions, or on distal parts of extremities (e.g., the forearms). If hair is likely to interfere with patch adhesion or removal, clipping may be necessary before application.

Reddening of the skin with or without mild local itching or burning, as well as allergic contact dermatitis, may occasionally occur. Upon removal of the patch, any slight reddening of the skin usually disappears within a few hours. All applications should be changed regularly to prevent local irritation, and each successive application should be placed on a different site. All clients need to be assessed for allergies to the drug and to materials in the patch before the patch is applied. If a client has a transdermal patch on and develops a fever, the medication may be absorbed and metabolize at a faster rate than normal. The client will need to be monitored for changes in effects of the medication.

When transdermal patches are removed, care needs to be taken as to how and where they are discarded. In the home environment, if they are simply discarded into a trash can, pets or children can be exposed to them, causing effects from any drug remaining on the patch. When removed, they should be folded with the medication side to the inside, and put into a closed container and kept out of reach of children and pets.

> **CLINICAL ALERT**   *The nurse should wear gloves when applying a transdermal patch to avoid getting any of the medication on his or her skin, which can result in the nurse receiving the effect of the medication.*

Skin Applications

Topical skin or dermatologic preparations include ointments, pastes, creams, lotions, powders, sprays, and patches. See Table 33–1 earlier in this chapter. See Practice Guidelines for applying topical medications. Before applying a dermatologic preparation, thoroughly clean the area with soap and water and dry it with a patting motion. Skin encrustations harbor microorganisms and these as well as previously applied applications can prevent the medication from coming in contact with the area to be treated. Nurses should wear gloves when administering skin applications and always use surgical asepsis when an open wound is present.

Ophthalmic Medications

Medications may be administered to the eye using irrigations or instillations. An eye irrigation is administered to wash out the conjunctival sac to remove secretions or foreign bodies or to remove chemicals that may injure the eye. Medications for the eyes, called **ophthalmic** medications, are instilled in the form of liquids or ointments. Eye drops are packaged in monodrip plastic containers that are used to administer the preparation. Ointments are usually supplied in small tubes. All containers must state that the medication is for ophthalmic use. Sterile preparations and sterile technique are indicated. Prescribed liquids are usually dilute, for example, less than 1% strength.

Procedure 33–10 illustrates how to administer ophthalmic instillations.

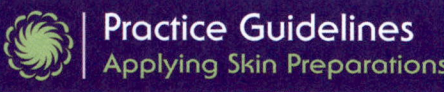

Practice Guidelines
Applying Skin Preparations

Powder

Make sure the skin surface is dry. Spread apart any skin folds, and sprinkle the site until the area is covered with a fine *thin* layer. Cover the site with a dressing if ordered.

Suspension-Based Lotion

Shake the container before use to distribute suspended particles. Put a little lotion on a small gauze dressing or pad, and apply the lotion to the skin by stroking it evenly in the direction of the hair growth.

Creams, Ointments, Pastes, and Oil-Based Lotions

Warm and soften the preparation in gloved hands to make it easier to apply and to prevent chilling (if a large area is to be treated). Smear it evenly over the skin using long strokes that follow the direction of the hair growth. Explain that the skin may feel somewhat greasy after application. Apply a sterile dressing if ordered by the physician.

Aerosol Spray

Shake the container well to mix the contents. Hold the spray container at the recommended distance from the area (usually about 15 to 30 cm [6 to 12 inches] but check the label). Cover the client's face with a towel if the upper chest or neck is to be sprayed. Spray the medication over the specified area.

Transdermal Patches

Select a clean, dry area that is free of hair and matches the manufacturer's recommendations. Remove the patch from its protective covering, holding it without touching the adhesive edges, and apply it by pressing firmly with the palm of the hand for about 10 seconds. Advise the client to avoid using a heating pad over the area to prevent an increase in circulation and the rate of absorption. Remove the patch at the appropriate time, folding the medicated side to the inside so it is covered.

MediaLink | PREPARING MEDICATIONS CASE STUDY

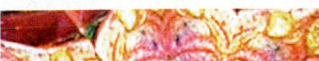

Procedure 33–10 Administering Ophthalmic Instillations

Purpose

- To provide an eye medication the client requires (e.g., an antibiotic) to treat an infection or for other reasons (see specific drug action)

ASSESSMENT

In addition to the assessment performed by the nurse related to the admininstration of any medication, prior to applying ophthalmic medications, assess:

- Appearance of eye and surrounding structures for lesions, exudate, erythema, or swelling
- The location and nature of any discharge, lacrimation, and swelling of the eyelids or of the lacrimal gland

- Client complaints (e.g., itching, burning pain, blurred vision, and photophobia)
- Client behavior (e.g., squinting, blinking excessively, frowning, or rubbing the eyes)

Determine if assessment data influence administration of the medication (i.e., is it appropriate to administer the medication or does the medication need to be held and the physician notified?).

PLANNING

Delegation

Due to the need for assessment, interpretation of client status, and use of sterile technique, ophthalmic medication administration is not delegated to UAP.

Equipment

- Clean gloves
- Sterile absorbent sponges soaked in sterile normal saline
- Medication

- Sterile eye dressing (pad) as needed and paper eye tape to secure it

For irrigation, add:

- Irrigating solution (e.g., normal saline) and irrigating syringe or tubing
- Dry sterile absorbent sponges
- Moisture-resistant towel
- Basin (e.g., emesis basin)

IMPLEMENTATION

Preparation

1. Check the MAR.
   - Check the MAR for the drug name, dose, and strength. Also confirm the prescribed frequency of the instillation and which eye is to be treated. Abbreviations are frequently used to identify the eye: OD (right eye), OS (left eye), OU (both eyes).
   - If the MAR is unclear or pertinent information is missing, compare it with the most recent physician's written order.
   - Report any discrepancies to the charge nurse or physician, as agency policy dictates.
2. Know the reason why the client is receiving the medication, the drug classification, contraindications, usual dose range, side effects, and nursing considerations for administering and evaluating the intended outcomes of the medication.

Performance

1. Compare the label on the medication tube or bottle with the medication record and check the expiration date.
2. If necessary, calculate the medication dosage.

3. Explain to the client what you are going to do, why it is necessary, and how he or she can cooperate. The administration of an ophthalmic medication is not usually painful. Ointments are often soothing to the eye, but some liquid preparations may sting initially. Discuss how the results will be used in planning further care or treatments.
4. Wash hands and observe appropriate infection control procedures.
5. Provide for client privacy.
6. Prepare the client.
   - Check the client's identification band, and ask the client's name. *This ensures that the right client receives the medication.*
   - Assist the client to a comfortable position, either sitting or lying.
7. Clean the eyelid and the eyelashes.
   - Put on clean gloves.
   - Use sterile cotton balls moistened with sterile irrigating solution or sterile normal saline, and wipe from the inner canthus to the outer canthus. *If not removed, material on the eyelid and lashes can be washed into the eye. Cleaning toward the outer*

canthus prevents contamination of the other eye and the lacrimal duct.

8. Administer the eye medication.
   - Check the ophthalmic preparation for the name, strength, and number of drops if a liquid is used. *Checking medication data is essential to prevent a medication error.* Draw the correct number of drops into the shaft of the dropper if a dropper is used. If ointment is used, discard the first bead. *The first bead of ointment from a tube is considered to be contaminated.*
   - Instruct the client to look up to the ceiling. Give the client a dry sterile absorbent sponge. *The person is less likely to blink if looking up. While the client looks up, the cornea is partially protected by the upper eyelid. A sponge is needed to press on the nasolacrimal duct after a liquid instillation or to wipe excess ointment from the eyelashes after an ointment is instilled.*
   - Expose the lower conjunctival sac by placing the thumb or fingers of your nondominant hand on the

continued on page 842

Procedure 33–10 Administering Ophthalmic Instillations *continued*

IMPLEMENTATION *continued*

client's cheekbone just below the eye and gently drawing down the skin on the cheek. If the tissues are edematous, handle the tissues carefully to avoid damaging them. *Placing the fingers on the cheekbone minimizes the possibility of touching the cornea, avoids putting any pressure on the eyeball, and prevents the person from blinking or squinting.*

- Approach the eye from the side and instill the correct number of drops onto the outer third of the lower conjunctival sac. Hold the dropper 1 to 2 cm (0.4 to 0.8 in.) above the sac (Figure 33–67 ■). *The client is less likely to blink if a side approach is used. When instilled into the conjunctival sac, drops will not harm the cornea as they might if dropped directly on it. The dropper must not touch the sac or the cornea.*

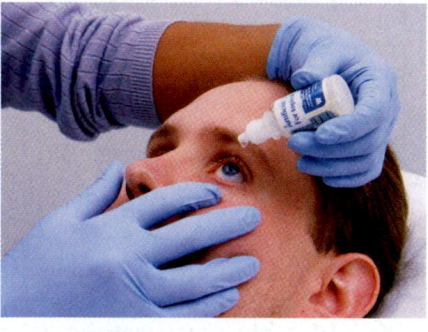

Figure 33–67 ■ Instilling an eyedrop into the lower conjunctival sac.

or
- Holding the tube above the lower conjunctival sac, squeeze 2 cm (0.8 in.) of ointment from the tube into the lower conjunctival sac from the inner canthus outward (Figure 33–68 ■).
- Instruct the client to close the eyelids but not to squeeze them shut. *Closing the eye spreads the medication over the eyeball. Squeezing can injure the eye and push out the medication.*

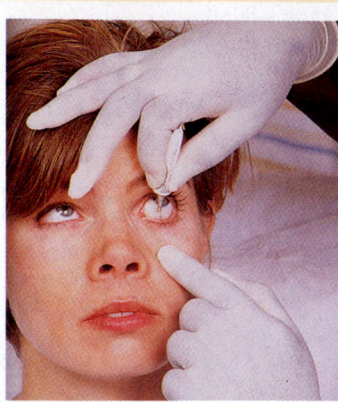

Figure 33–68 ■ Instilling an eye ointment into the lower conjunctival sac.

- For liquid medications, press firmly or have the client press firmly on the nasolacrimal duct for at least 30 seconds (Figure 33–69 ■). *Pressing on the nasolacrimal duct prevents the medication from running out of the eye and down the duct.*

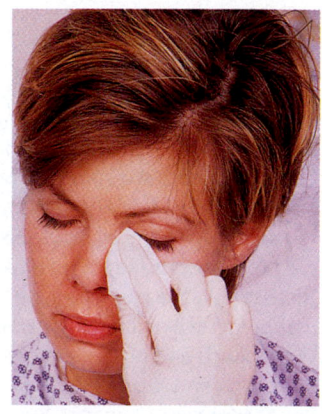

Figure 33–69 ■ Pressing on the nasolacrimal duct.

Variation: Irrigation
- Place absorbent pads under the head, neck, and shoulders. Place an emesis basin next to the eye to catch drainage. Some eye medications cause systemic reactions such as confusion or a decrease in heart rate and blood pressure if the eye

drops go down the nasolacrimal duct and get into the systemic circulation.

- Expose the lower conjunctival sac. Or, to irrigate in stages, first hold the lower lid down, then hold the upper lid up. Exert pressure on the bony prominences of the cheekbone and beneath the eyebrow when holding the eyelids. *Separating the lids prevents reflex blinking. Exerting pressure on the bony prominences minimizes the possibility of pressing the eyeball and causing discomfort.*
- Fill and hold the eye irrigator about 2.5 cm (1 in.) above the eye. *At this height the pressure of the solution will not damage the eye tissue, and the irrigator will not touch the eye.*
- Irrigate the eye, directing the solution onto the lower conjunctival sac and from the inner canthus to the outer canthus. *Directing the solution in this way prevents possible injury to the cornea and prevents fluid and contaminants from flowing down the nasolacrimal duct.*
- Irrigate until the solution leaving the eye is clear (no discharge is present) or until all the solution has been used.
- Instruct the client to close and move the eye periodically. *Eye closure and movement help to move secretions from the upper to the lower conjunctival sac.*

9. Clean and dry the eyelids as needed. Wipe the eyelids gently from the inner to the outer canthus to collect excess medication.
10. Apply an eye pad if needed, and secure it with paper eye tape.
11. Assess the client's response immediately after the instillation or irrigation and again after the medication should have acted.
12. Document all relevant assessments and interventions. Include the name of the drug or irrigating solution, the strength, the number of drops if a liquid medication, the time, and the response of the client.

EVALUATION

- Perform follow-up based on findings of the effectiveness of the administration or outcomes that deviated from expected or normal for the client. Relate findings to previous data if available.
- Report significant deviations from normal to the physician.

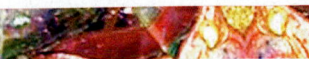

Lifespan Considerations

Administering Ophthalmic Medications

Infants/Children

- Explain the technique to the parents of an infant or child.
- For a young child or infant, obtain assistance to immobilize the arms and head. The parent may hold the infant or young child. *This prevents accidental injury during medication administration.*
- For a young child, use a doll to demonstrate the procedure. *This facilitates cooperation and decreases anxiety.*
- An intravenous (IV) bag and tubing may be used to deliver irrigating fluid to the eye (Figure 33–70 ■).

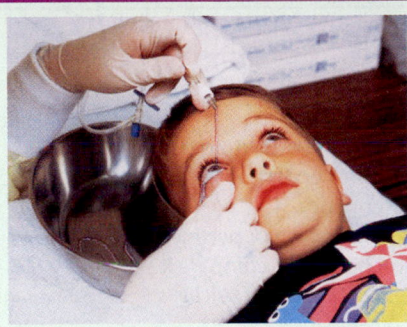

Figure 33–70 ■ Eye irrigation using IV tubing.

Otic Medications

Instillations or irrigations of the external auditory canal are referred to as **otic** and are generally carried out for cleaning purposes. Sometimes applications of heat and antiseptic solutions are prescribed. Irrigations performed in a hospital require aseptic technique so that microorganisms will not be introduced into the ear. Sterile technique is used if the eardrum is perforated. The position of the external auditory canal varies with age. In the child under 3 years of age, it is directed upward. In the adult, the external auditory canal is an S-shaped structure about 2.5 cm (1 inch) long.

Procedure 33–11 explains how to administer otic instillations.

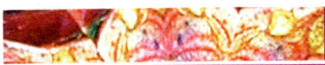

Procedure 33–11   Administering Otic Instillations

Purpose

- To soften earwax so that it can be readily removed at a later time
- To provide local therapy to reduce inflammation, destroy infective organisms in the external ear canal, or both

- To relieve pain

ASSESSMENT

In addition to the assessment performed by the nurse related to the administration of any medications, prior to applying otic medications, assess:

- Appearance of the pinna of the ear and meatus for signs of redness and abrasions
- Type and amount of any discharge

Determine if assessment data influence administration of the medication (i.e., is it appropriate to administer the medication or does the medication need to be held and the physician notifed?)

PLANNING

Delegation

Due to the need for assessment, interpretation of client status, and use of aseptic technique, otic medication administration is not delegated to UAP.

Equipment

- Clean gloves
- Cotton-tipped applicator
- Correct medication bottle with a dropper
- Flexible rubber tip (optional) for the end of the dropper, which prevents injury from sudden motion, for example, by a disoriented client

- Cotton fluff

For irrigation, add:

- Moisture-resistant towel
- Basin (e.g., emesis basin)
- Irrigating solution at the appropriate temperature, about 500 mL (16 oz) or as ordered
- Container for the irrigating solution
- Syringe (rubber bulb or Asepto syringe is frequently used)

continued on page 844

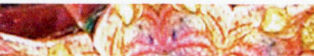

Procedure 33–11 Administering Otic Instillations *continued*

IMPLEMENTATION

Preparation

1. Check the MAR.
   - Check the MAR for the drug name, strength, number of drops, and prescribed frequency.
   - If the MAR is unclear or pertinent information is missing, compare it with the most recent physician's written order.
   - Report any discrepancies to the charge nurse or physician, as agency policy dictates.
2. Know the reason why the client is receiving the medication, the drug classification, contraindications, usual dose range, side effects, and nursing considerations for administering and evaluating the intended outcomes of the medication.

Performance

1. Compare the label on the medication container with the medication record and check the expiration date.
2. If necessary, calculate the medication dosage.
3. Explain to the client what you are going to do, why it is necessary, and how he or she can cooperate. The administration of an otic medication is not usually painful. Discuss how the results will be used in planning further care or treatments.
4. Wash hands and observe appropriate infection control procedures.
5. Provide for client privacy.
6. Prepare the client.
   - Check the client's identification band, and ask the client's name. *This ensures that the right client receives the medication.*
   - Assist the client to a comfortable position for eardrops, lying with the ear being treated uppermost.
7. Clean the pinna of the ear and the meatus of the ear canal.
   - Put on gloves if infection is suspected.
   - Use cotton-tipped applicators and solution to wipe the pinna and auditory meatus. *This removes any discharge present before the instillation so that it won't be washed into the ear canal.*

8. Administer the ear medication.
   - Warm the medication container in your hand, or place it in warm water for a short time. *This promotes client comfort.*
   - Partially fill the ear dropper with medication.
   - Straighten the auditory canal. Pull the pinna upward and backward (Figure 33–71 ■). *The auditory canal is straightened so that the solution can flow the entire length of the canal.*

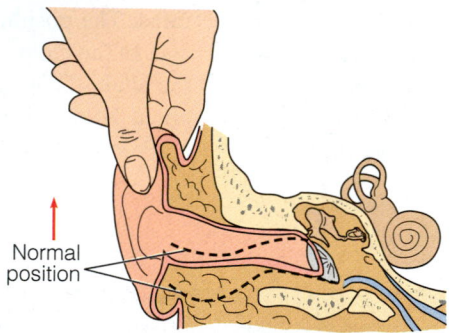

Normal position

Figure 33–71 ■ Straightening the adult ear canal by pulling pinna upward and backward.

- Instill the correct number of drops along the side of the ear canal (Figure 33–72 ■).

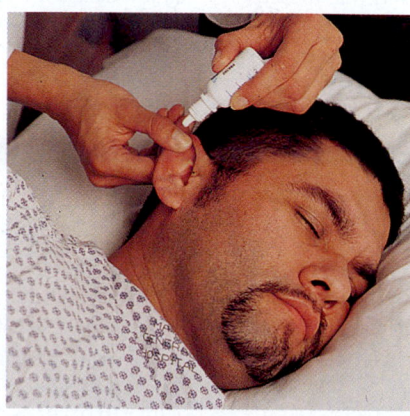

Figure 33–72 ■ Instilling eardrops.

- Press gently but firmly a few times on the tragus of the ear (the cartilaginous projection in front of the exterior meatus of the ear). *Pressing on the tragus assists the flow of medication into the ear canal.*
- Ask the client to remain in the side-lying position for about 5 minutes. *This prevents the drops from escaping and allows the medication to reach all sides of the canal cavity.*
- Insert a small piece of cotton fluff loosely at the meatus of the auditory canal for 15 to 20 minutes. Do not press it into the canal. *The cotton helps retain the medication when the client is up. If pressed tightly into the canal, the cotton would interfere with the action of the drug and the outward movement of normal secretions.*

Variation: Ear Irrigation

- Explain that the client may experience a feeling of fullness, warmth, and, occasionally, discomfort when the fluid comes in contact with the tympanic membrane.
- Assist the client to a sitting or lying position with head turned toward the affected ear. *The solution can then flow from the ear canal to a basin.*
- Place the moisture-resistant towel around the client's shoulder under the ear to be irrigated, and place the basin under the ear to be irrigated.
- Fill the syringe with solution.
or
- Hang up the irrigating container, and run solution through the tubing and the nozzle. *Solution is run through to remove air from the tubing and nozzle.*
- Straighten the ear canal.
- Insert the tip of the syringe into the auditory meatus, and direct the solution gently upward against the top of the canal. *The solution will flow around the entire canal and out at the bottom. The solution is instilled gently because strong pressure from the fluid can cause discomfort and damage the tympanic membrane.*

Procedure 33–11 Administering Otic Instillations *continued*

IMPLEMENTATION *continued*

- Continue instilling the fluid until all the solution is used or until the canal is cleaned, depending on the purpose of the irrigation. Take care not to block the outward flow of the solution with the syringe.
- Assist the client to a side-lying position on the affected side. *Lying with the affected side down helps drain the excess fluid by gravity.*

- Place a cotton fluff in the auditory meatus to absorb the excess fluid.
9. Assess the client's response and the character and amount of discharge, appearance of the canal, discomfort, and so on, immediately after the instillation and again when the medication is expected to act. Inspect the cotton ball for any drainage.

10. Document all nursing assessments and interventions relative to the procedure. Include the name of the drug or irrigating solution, the strength, the number of drops if a liquid medication, the time, and the response of the client.

EVALUATION

- Perform follow-up based on findings of the effectiveness of the administration or outcomes that deviated from expected or normal for the client. Relate findings to previous data if available.

- Report significant deviations from normal to the physician.

Lifespan Considerations

Administering Otic Medications

Infants/Children

- Obtain assistance to immobilize an infant or young child. This prevents accidental injury due to sudden movement during the procedure.
- Because in infants and children under 3 years of age, the ear canal is directed upward, to administer medication, gently pull the pinna down and back (Figures 33–73 ■ and 33–74 ■). For a child *older* than 3 years of age, pull the pinna upward and backward (see Figure 33–71).

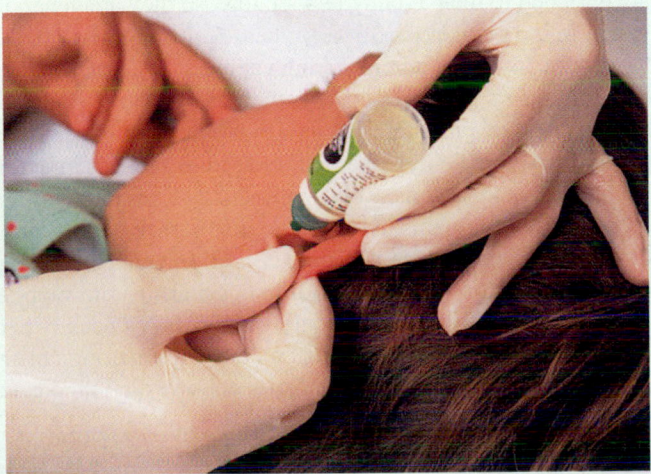

Figure 33–73 ■ Straightening the ear canal of a child by pulling the pinna down and back.

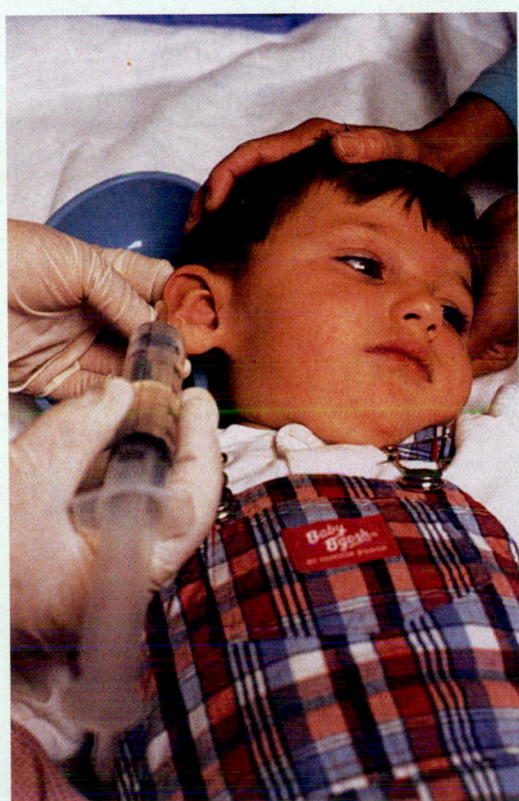

Figure 33–74 ■ Ear irrigation.

Nasal Medications

Nasal instillations (nose drops and sprays) usually are instilled for their astringent effect (to shrink swollen mucous membranes), to loosen secretions and facilitate drainage, or to treat infections of the nasal cavity or sinuses. Nasal decongestants are the most common nasal instillations. Many of these products are available without a prescription. Clients need to be taught to use these agents with caution. Chronic use of nasal decongestants may lead to a rebound effect, that is, an increase in nasal congestion. If excess decongestant solution is swallowed, serious systemic effects may also develop, especially in children. Saline drops are safer as a decongestant for children.

Usually clients self-administer sprays. In the supine position with the head tilted back, the client holds the tip of the container just inside the nares and inhales as the spray enters the nasal passages. For clients who use nasal sprays repeatedly, the nares need to be assessed for irritation. In children, nasal sprays are given with the head in an upright position to prevent excess spray from being swallowed.

Nasal drops are used to treat sinus infections. Clients need to learn ways to position themselves to effectively treat the affected sinus:

- To treat the ethmoid and sphenoid sinuses, instruct the client to lie back with the head over the edge of the bed or a pillow under the shoulders so that the head is tipped backward (Figure 33–75 ■).
- To treat the maxillary and frontal sinuses, instruct the client to assume the same back-lying position, with the head turned toward the side to be treated (Figure 33–76 ■). The client should

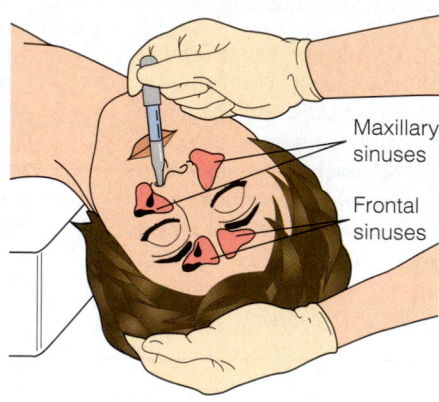

Figure 33–76 ■ Position of the head to instill drops into the maxillary and frontal sinuses.

also be instructed to (a) breathe through the mouth to prevent aspiration of medication into the trachea and bronchi, (b) remain in a back-lying position for at least 1 minute so that the solution will come into contact with all of the nasal surface, and (c) avoid blowing the nose for several minutes.

Vaginal Medications

Vaginal medications, or instillations, are inserted as creams, jellies, foams, or suppositories to treat infection or to relieve vaginal discomfort (e.g., itching or pain). Medical aseptic technique is usually used. Vaginal creams, jellies, and foams are applied by using a tubular applicator with a plunger. Suppositories are inserted with the index finger of a gloved hand. Suppositories are designed to melt at body temperature, so they are generally stored in the refrigerator to keep them firm for insertion. See Procedure 33–12 for administering vaginal instillations.

A vaginal irrigation (douche) is the washing of the vagina by a liquid at a low pressure. Vaginal irrigations are not necessary for ordinary female hygiene but are used to prevent infection by applying an antimicrobial solution that discourages the growth of microorganisms, to remove an offensive or irritating discharge, and to reduce inflammation or prevent hemorrhage by the application of heat or cold. In hospitals, sterile supplies and equipment are used; in a home, sterility is not usually necessary because people are accustomed to the microorganisms in their environments. Sterile technique, however, is indicated if there is an open wound.

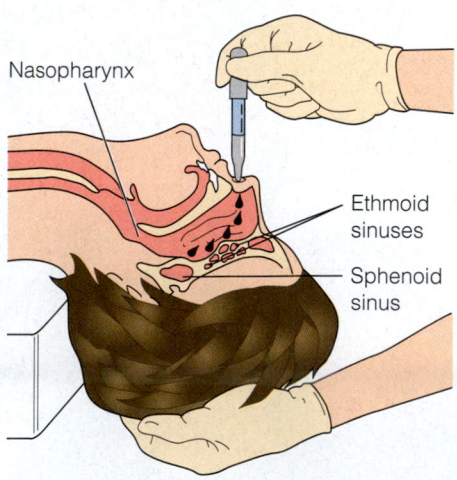

Figure 33–75 ■ Position of the head to instill drops into the ethmoid and sphenoid sinuses.

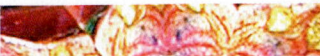

Procedure 33–12 Administering Vaginal Instillations

Purpose

- To treat or prevent infection
- To reduce inflammation
- To relieve vaginal discomfort

ASSESSMENT

In addition to the assessment performed by the nurse related to the administration of any medications, prior to applying vaginal medications, assess:

- The vaginal orifice for inflammation; amount, character, and odor of vaginal discharge

- For complaints of vaginal discomfort (e.g., burning or itching) Determine if assessment data influence administration of the medication (i.e., is it appropriate to administer the medication or does the medication need to be held and the physician notified?).

PLANNING

Delegation

Due to the need for assessments and interpretation of client status, vaginal medication administration is not delegated to UAP.

Equipment

- Drape
- Correct vaginal suppository or cream
- Applicator for vaginal cream
- Clean gloves
- Lubricant for a suppository

- Disposable towel
- Clean perineal pad

For an irrigation, add:

- Moisture-proof pad
- Vaginal irrigation set (these are often disposable) containing a nozzle, tubing and a clamp, and a container for the solution
- IV pole
- Irrigating solution

IMPLEMENTATION

Preparation

1. Check the MAR.
   - Check the MAR for the drug name, strength, and prescribed frequency.
   - If the MAR is unclear or pertinent information is missing, compare it with the most recent physician's written order.
   - Report any discrepancies to the charge nurse or physician, as agency policy dictates.
2. Know the reason why the client is receiving the medication, the drug classification, contraindications, usual dose range, side effects, and nursing considerations for administering and evaluating the intended outcomes of the medication.

Performance

1. Compare the label on the medication container with the medication record and check the expiration date.
2. If necessary, calculate the medication dosage.
3. Explain to the client what you are going to do, why it is necessary, and how she can cooperate. Explain to the client that a vaginal instillation is normally a painless procedure, and in fact may bring relief from itching and burning if an infection is present. Many people feel embarrassed about this procedure, and some may prefer to perform the procedure themselves if instruction is provided. Discuss how the results will be used in planning further care or treatments.
4. Wash hands and observe appropriate infection control procedures.
5. Provide for client privacy.
6. Prepare the client.
   - Check the client's identification band, and ask the client's name. *This ensures that the right client receives the medication.*
   - Ask the client to void. *If the bladder is empty, the client will have less discomfort during the treatment, and the possibility of injuring the vaginal lining is decreased.*
   - Assist the client to a back-lying position with the knees flexed and the hips rotated laterally.
   - Drape the client appropriately so that only the perineal area is exposed.
7. Prepare the equipment.
   - Unwrap the suppository, and put it on the opened wrapper.

   or
   - Fill the applicator with the prescribed cream, jelly, or foam. Directions are provided with the manufacturer's applicator.
8. Assess and clean the perineal area.
   - Put on gloves. *Gloves prevent contamination of the nurse's hands from vaginal and perineal microorganisms.*
   - Inspect the vaginal orifice, note any odor of discharge from the vagina, and ask about any vaginal discomfort.
   - Provide perineal care to remove microorganisms. *This decreases the chance of moving microorganisms into the vagina.*
9. Administer the vaginal suppository, cream, foam, jelly, or irrigation.

   SUPPOSITORY
   - Lubricate the rounded (smooth) end of the suppository, which is inserted first. *Lubrication facilitates insertion.*
   - Lubricate your gloved index finger.
   - Expose the vaginal orifice by separating the labia with your nondominant hand.

continued on page 848

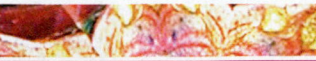

Procedure 33–12 Administering Vaginal Instillations *continued*

IMPLEMENTATION *continued*

- Insert the suppository about 8 to 10 cm (3 to 4 in.) along the posterior wall of the vagina, or as far as it will go (Figure 33–77 ■). *The posterior wall of the vagina is about 2.5 cm (1 in.) longer than the anterior wall because the cervix protrudes into the uppermost portion of the anterior wall.*
- Ask the client to remain lying in the supine position for 5 to 10 minutes following insertion. The hips may also be elevated on a pillow. *This position allows the medication to flow into the posterior fornix after it has melted.*

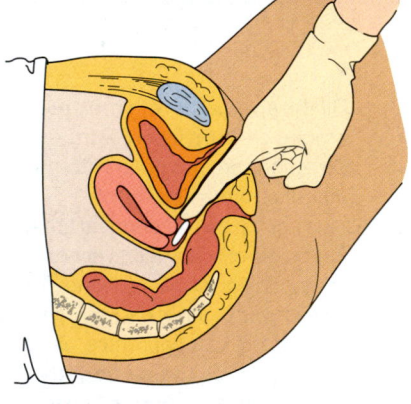

Figure 33–77 ■ Instilling a vaginal suppository.

VAGINAL CREAM, JELLY, OR FOAM

- Gently insert the applicator about 5 cm (2 in.).
- Slowly push the plunger until the applicator is empty (Figure 33–78 ■).

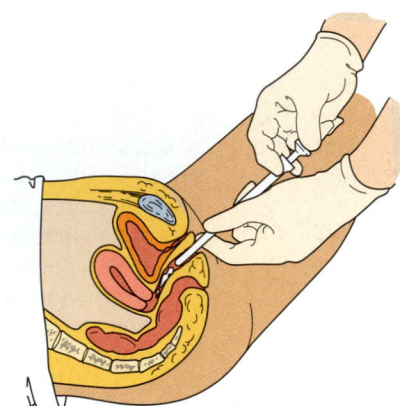

Figure 33–78 ■ Using an applicator to instill a vaginal cream.

- Remove the applicator and place it on the towel. *The applicator is put on the towel to prevent the spread of microorganisms.*
- Discard the applicator if disposable or clean it according to the manufacturer's directions.
- Ask the client to remain lying in the supine position for 5 to 10 minutes following the insertion.

IRRIGATION

- Place the client on a bedpan.
- Clamp the tubing. Hang the irrigating container on the IV pole so that the base is about 30 cm (12 in.) above the vagina. *At this height, the pressure of the solution should not be great enough to injure the vaginal lining.*
- Run fluid through the tubing and nozzle into the bedpan. *Fluid is run through the tubing to remove air and to moisten the nozzle.*
- Insert the nozzle carefully into the vagina. Direct the nozzle toward the sacrum, following the direction of the vagina.
- Insert the nozzle about 7 to 10 cm (3 to 4 in.), start the flow, and rotate the nozzle several times. *Rotating the nozzle irrigates all parts of the vagina.*
- Use all of the irrigating solution, permitting it to flow out freely into the bedpan.
- Remove the nozzle from the vagina.
- Assist the client to a sitting position on the bedpan. *Sitting on the bedpan will help drain the remaining fluid by gravity.*
10. Ensure client comfort.
    - Dry the perineum with tissues as required.
    - Apply a clean perineal pad if there is excessive drainage.
11. Document all nursing assessments and interventions relative to the procedure. Include the name of the drug or irrigating solution, the strength, the time, and the response of the client.

EVALUATION

- Perform follow-up based on findings of the effectiveness of the administration or outcomes that deviated from expected or normal for the client. Relate findings to previous data if available.
- Report significant deviations from normal to the physician.

Rectal Medications

Insertion of medications into the rectum in the form of suppositories is a frequent practice. Rectal administration is a convenient and safe method of giving certain medications. Advantages include the following:

- It avoids irritation of the upper gastrointestinal tract in clients who encounter this problem.
- It is advantageous when the medication has an objectionable taste or odor.

- The drug is released at a slow but steady rate.
- Rectal suppositories are thought to provide higher bloodstream levels (titers) of medication because the venous blood from the lower rectum is not transported through the liver.

To insert a rectal suppository:

- Assist the client to a left lateral position, with the upper leg flexed.
- Fold back the top bedclothes to expose the buttocks.
- Put on a glove on the hand used to insert the suppository.

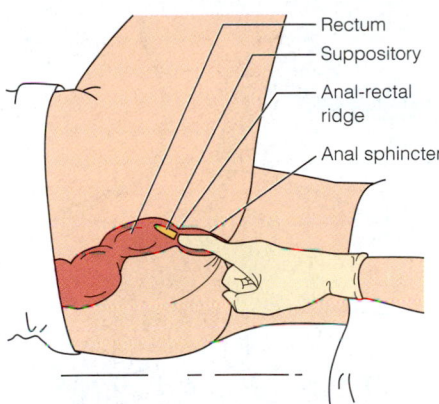

Figure 33–79 ■ Inserting a rectal suppository beyond the internal sphincter and along the rectal wall.

- Unwrap the suppository and lubricate the smooth rounded end, or see manufacturer's instructions. The rounded end is usually inserted first and lubricant reduces irritation of the mucosa.
- Lubricate the gloved index finger.
- Encourage the client to relax by breathing through the mouth. This usually relaxes the external anal sphincter.
- Insert the suppository gently into the anal canal, rounded end first (or according to manufacturer's instructions), along the rectal wall using the gloved index finger. For an adult, insert the suppository beyond the internal sphincter (i.e., 10 cm [4 in.]) (see Figure 33–79 ■).
- Avoid embedding the suppository in feces in order for the suppository to be absorbed effectively.
- Press the client's buttocks together for a few minutes.
- Ask the client to remain in the left lateral or supine position for at least 5 minutes to help retain the suppository. The suppository should be retained for at least 30 to 40 minutes or according to manufacturer's instructions.

RESPIRATORY INHALATION

Nebulizers deliver most medications administered through the inhaled route. A nebulizer is used to deliver a fine spray (fog or mist) of medication or moisture to a client. There are two kinds of nebulization: *atomization* and *aerosolization*. In atomization, a device called an *atomizer* produces rather large droplets for inhalation. In aerosolization, the droplets are suspended in a gas, such as oxygen. The smaller the droplets, the further they can be inhaled into the respiratory tract. When a medication is intended for the nasal mucosa, it is inhaled through the nose;

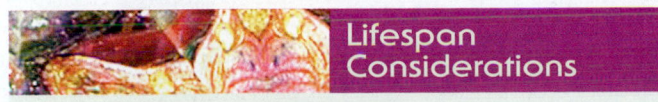

Lifespan Considerations

Administering Rectal Medications

Infants/Children
- Obtain assistance to immobilize an infant or young child. This prevents accidental injury due to sudden movement during the procedure.
- For a child or infant, insert a suppository 5 cm (2 in.) or less.

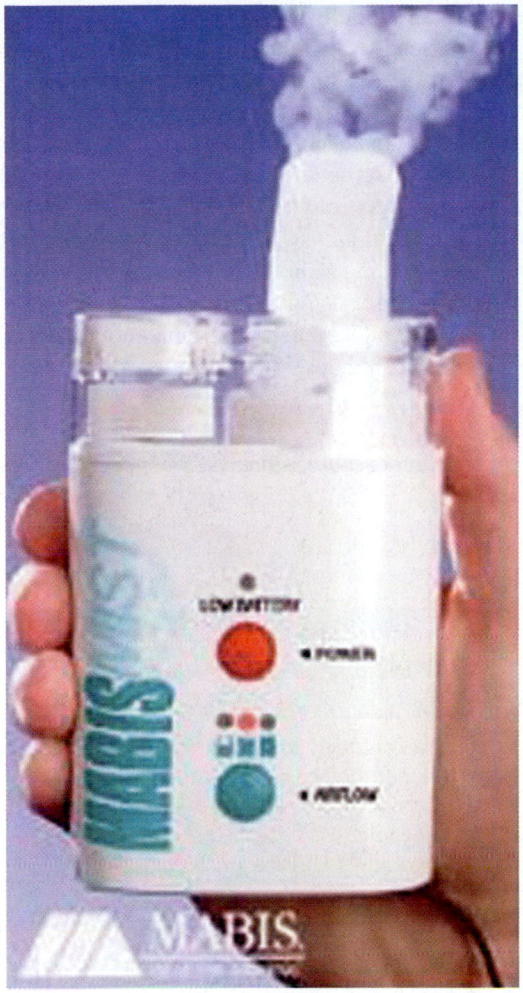

Figure 33–80 ■ Ultrasonic nebulizer. (Courtesy of Mabis Healthcare, Inc.)

MediaLink | METERED DOSE INHALER (MDI) VIDEO

when it is intended for the trachea, bronchi, and/or lungs, it is inhaled through the mouth.

A large-volume nebulizer can provide a heated or cool mist. It is used for long-term therapy, such as that following a tracheostomy. The ultrasonic nebulizer (Figure 33–80 ■) provides 100% humidity and can provide particles small enough to be inhaled deeply into the respiratory tract.

The **metered-dose inhaler (MDI),** a handheld nebulizer, (Figure 33–81 ■), is a pressurized container of medication that can be used by the client to release the medication through a nose-piece or mouthpiece. The force with which the air moves through the nebulizer causes the large particles of medicated solution to break up into finer particles, forming a mist or fine spray.

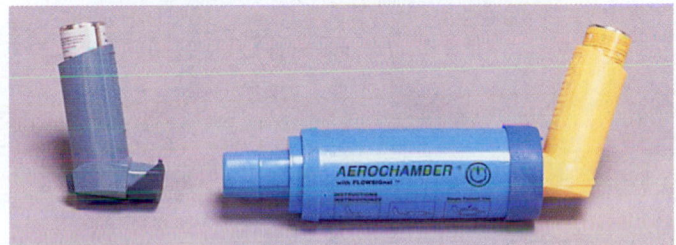

Figure 33–81 ■ Metered-dose inhaler.

To ensure correct delivery of the prescribed medication by MDIs, nurses need to instruct clients to use aerosol inhalers correctly. The client compresses the medication canister by hand to release medication through a mouthpiece. An extender or spacer may be attached to the mouthpiece to facilitate medication absorption for better results (Figure 33–82 ■). Spacers are holding chambers into which the medication is fired and from which the client inhales, so that the dose is not lost by exhalation. The Teaching: Client Care feature provides instructions for clients about using an MDI. Newer breath-activated MDIs are being produced in which inhalation triggers the release of a premeasured dose of medication.

> **CLINICAL ALERT**   *A client's ability to use an MDI correctly decreases over time (Togger & Brenner, 2001). It is important for the nurse to continuously assess if the client is using the MDI correctly.*

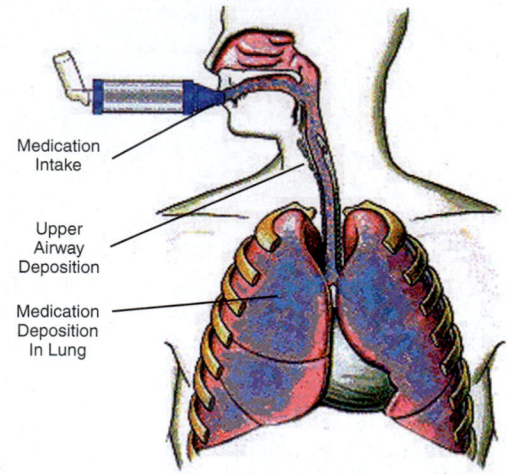

Figure 33–82 ■ Delivery of medication to the lungs using a metered-dose inhaler extender. (Courtesy of Trudell Medical International.)

Medication Intake

Upper Airway Deposition

Medication Deposition In Lung

Teaching: Client Care
Using a Metered-Dose Inhaler

- Make sure the canister is firmly and fully inserted into the inhaler.
- Remove the mouthpiece cap and, holding the inhaler upright, shake the inhaler vigorously for 3 to 5 seconds to mix the medication evenly.
- Exhale comfortably (as in a normal full breath).
- Hold the canister upside down.
  a. Hold the MDI 2 to 4 cm (1 to 2 in.) from the open mouth (Figure 33–83 ■).
  or
  b. Put the mouthpiece far enough into the mouth with its opening toward the throat. Close the lips tightly around the mouthpiece. An MDI with a spacer or extender is always placed in the mouth (Figure 33–84 ■).

Administering the Medication
- Press down *once* on the MDI canister (which releases the dose) and inhale slowly and deeply through the mouth.
- Hold your breath for 10 seconds. *This allows the aerosol to reach deeper airways.*
- Remove the inhaler from or away from the mouth.

- Exhale slowly through *pursed* lips. *Controlled exhalation keeps the small airways open during exhalation.*
- Repeat the inhalation if ordered. Wait 20 to 30 seconds between inhalations of bronchodilator medications *so the first inhalation has a chance to work and the subsequent dose reaches deeper into the lungs.*
- After the inhalation is completed, rinse mouth with tap water to remove any remaining medication and reduce irritation and risk of infection.
- Clean the MDI mouthpiece after each use. Use mild soap and water, rinse it, and let it air dry before replacing it on the device.
- Store the canister at room temperature. Avoid extremes of temperature.
- Report adverse reactions such as restlessness, palpitations, nervousness, or rash to the physician.
- Many MDIs contain steroids for an anti-inflammatory effect. Prolonged use increases the risk of fungal infections in the mouth.

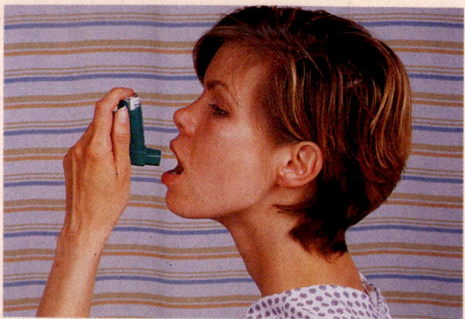

Figure 33–83 ■ Inhaler positioned away from the open mouth.

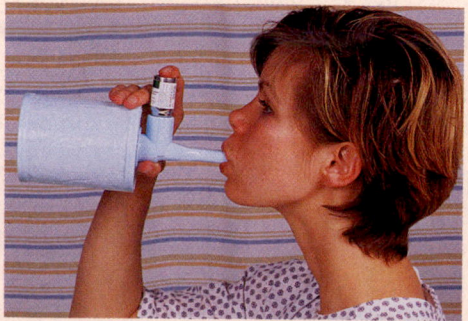

Figure 33–84 ■ An extender spacer attached to a mouthpiece placed in the mouth.

Note: From "Metered Dose Inhalers," by D. A. Togger and P. S. Brenner, 2001, *American Journal of Nursing, 101*(10), pp. 26–32. Reprinted with permission.

SMALL VOLUME NEBULIZER (SVN) TREATMENT VIDEO

MediaLink

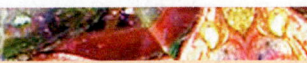

Home Care Considerations

Metered-Dose Inhalers

■ Disinfect the metered-dose inhaler mouthpieces weekly by soaking for 20 minutes in one pint of water with 2 ounces of vinegar added.

■ Teach clients how to determine the amount of medication remaining in a metered-dose inhaler canister:

• Calculate the number of days' doses in a canister. Divide the number of doses (puffs) in the canister (on the label) by the number of puffs taken per day. According to Togger and

Brenner (2001), this is the only accurate method. The previous method of floating the canister in water is not accurate because some of the propellant may remain (even after the medication is gone), which leads the client to incorrectly believe he is receiving medication.

■ Review instructions for using an inhaler spacer or chamber. Research shows that these devices assist in delivering the medication deeply into the lungs rather than only to the oropharynx (see Figure 33–82).

IRRIGATIONS

An **irrigation (lavage)** is the washing out of a body cavity by a stream of water or other fluid that may or may not be medicated. Irrigation is performed for one or more of the following reasons:

• To clean the area, that is, to remove a foreign object or excessive secretions or discharge
• To apply heat or cold
• To apply a medication, such as an antiseptic
• To reduce inflammation
• To relieve discomfort.

Surgical asepsis is required when there is a break in the skin (e.g., in a wound irrigation) or whenever a sterile body cavity (e.g., the bladder) is entered. Some irrigations (e.g., a vaginal, rectal, or gastric irrigation) are often safely conducted using medical asepsis.

Different kinds of syringes are used for irrigations. The most common are the Asepto and the rubber bulb (Figure 33–85 ■). The syringes are often calibrated, permitting the nurse to determine the amount of irrigant being delivered at any given time.

The Asepto syringe is a plastic (or glass) syringe with a rubber bulb. Squeezing the air out of the bulb produces neg-

ative pressure, and fluid can be sucked into the syringe. When the bulb is squeezed again, the fluid is ejected from the syringe. Asepto syringes come in several sizes ranging from 30 mL (1 oz) to 120 mL (4 oz).

The rubber bulb syringe is often used for irrigating the ears. Like the Asepto syringe, the rubber bulb syringe comes in a range of sizes.

Other syringes that can be used are the piston syringe, which has a tip to which a catheter can be attached, and the Pomeroy syringe. Catheters may be used for deep-wound irrigations and for some types of bladder irrigations. The Pomeroy syringe is a metal syringe commonly used for ear irrigations. A shield near the tip prevents the solution from spraying outward. Plastic squeezable bottles are also available for irrigations. These are commonly used for perineal irrigations and some wound irrigations.

The type, amount, temperature, and strength of the solution and the frequency of the irrigation are ordered by the physician. Generally, normal saline at body temperature (37C [98.6F]) is used unless specified otherwise. The amount of solution used varies with the site and purpose of the irrigation. Guidelines for administering eye and ear irrigations are given in Procedures 33–10 (eye) and 33–11 (ear).

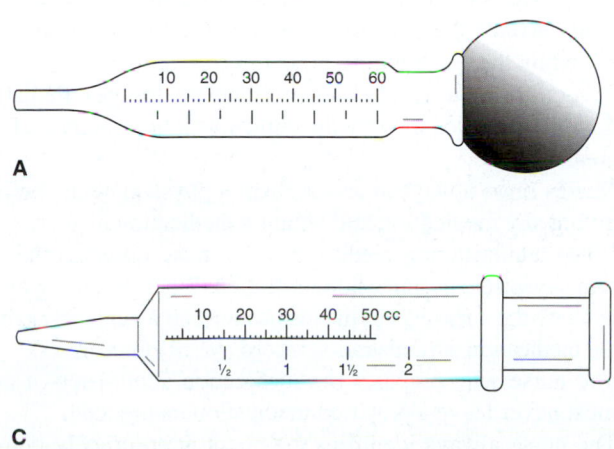

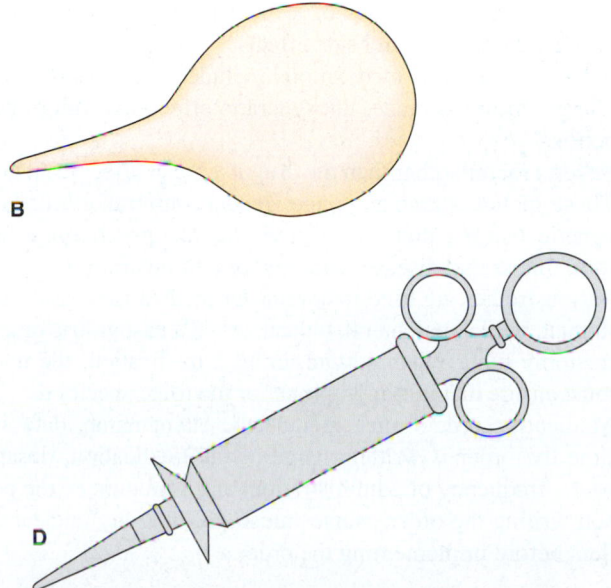

Figure 33–85 ■ Four types of syringes used for irrigations: *A,* Asepto; *B,* rubber bulb; *C,* piston syringe; *D,* Pomeroy.

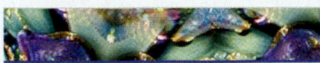

Focus on Critical Thinking

Mr. Ketron is a 20-year-old client who just returned to the nursing unit from surgery after undergoing an emergency appendectomy. He is awake and complaining of mild incisional pain, his dressing is dry and intact, and he has an intravenous infusion of lactated Ringer's solution running at 125 mL/hr. He is to receive Ancef (a cephalosporin antibiotic) 1 g intravenously every 4 hr until he is able to tolerate fluids, at which time he will be placed on oral Suprax (cefixime) 200 mg twice daily until discharged and for 1 week after returning home. He also has an order for morphine sulfate 2.5 mg to be given every 4 hours IVP as necessary for pain.

1. It is always possible that a person receiving antibiotic drugs may experience side effects or an allergic reaction. How does an allergic reaction differ from a drug side effect?

2. Predict the possible consequences of not obtaining a medication history from Mr. Ketron despite the fact that he will be receiving antibiotics and pain medication.
3. Mr. Ketron is complaining of pain and you have prepared his IVP morphine. What assessments will you make before giving the morphine?
4. What precautions should you take, if any, prior to administering Mr. Ketron's intravenous antibiotic medication?
5. Mr. Ketron will be placed on the oral antibiotic when he can tolerate food and oral fluids. What difference, if any, does it make if this drug is given before or after meals?

See Critical Thinking Possibilities in Appendix A.

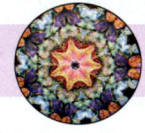 | # Chapter Review

EXPLORE MediaLink

NCLEX review questions, case studies, care plan activities, MediaLink applications, and other interactive resources for this chapter can be found on the Companion Website at www.prenhall.com/kozier. Click on Chapter 33 to select the activities for this chapter.

For animations, more NCLEX review questions, and an audio glossary, access the Student CD-ROM accompanying this textbook.

Chapter Highlights

- Federal drug legislation regulates the production, prescription, distribution, and administration of drugs.
- Nursing practice acts define limits on the nurse's responsibilities regarding medications.
- Medications have several names. Nurses need to know the generic and trade names of a medication and be aware of both its therapeutic and side effects.
- Adverse effects of medications include drug toxicity, drug allergy, drug tolerance, idiosyncratic effect, and drug interactions.
- Several factors other than the drug itself can affect its action. These include pregnancy; age; gender; cultural, ethnic, and genetic factors; diet; client environment; psychologic factors; illness and disease; and time of administration.
- Various routes are used to administer medications: oral, sublingual, buccal, parenteral, topical, or via a nasogastric or gastrostomy tube. When administering a medication, the nurse must ensure that it is appropriate for the route specified.
- Medication orders must include the client name, date and time the order is written, name of the medication, dosage, route, frequency of administration, and signature of the person writing the order. Nurses must question any unclear orders before implementing the order.

- Telephone or verbal orders must be cosigned by the physician within a time specified by agency policy (usually 24 to 48 hours).
- Three systems of measurement are used in North America: the metric system, the apothecaries' system, and the household system. Weights and measures may need to be converted by the nurse within these three systems.
- Several formulas can be used to calculate dosages. Pediatric dosages are calculated by the child's weight or body surface area.
- Nurses must always assess a client's physical status before giving any medication and obtain a medication history.
- When administering medications the nurse observes the six rights to ensure accurate administration. When preparing medications, the nurse checks the medication container label against the medication administration record (MAR) three times.
- The nurse who prepares the medication administers it and must never leave a prepared medication unattended.
- The nurse always identifies the client appropriately before administering a medication and stays with the client until the medication is taken.
- Medications, once given, are documented as soon as possible after administration.

- Medications given parenterally act more quickly than those given orally or topically and must be prepared using sterile technique.
- When preparing two insulins to be mixed in the same syringe, a vial of unmodified insulin should never be contaminated with modified insulin.
- Proper site selection is essential for an intramuscular injection to prevent tissue, bone, and nerve damage. The nurse should always palpate anatomic landmarks when selecting a site.
- The Z-track method for intramuscular injection is recommended to prevent discomfort caused by seepage of the medication into subcutaneous tissues.
- Clients receiving a series of injections should have the injection sites rotated.
- After use, needles should not be recapped but must be placed in puncture-resistant containers.
- Intravenous medications can be administered by various methods: in a large-volume infusion of intravenous fluid, by intermittent intravenous infusion, by volume-controlled infusion, by intravenous push (IVP) or bolus, or by intermittent venous access. In all of these methods the client has an existing intravenous line or an IV access site such as a heparin or saline lock.
- Topical medications are applied to the skin and mucous membranes primarily for their local effects, although some systemic effects may occur.
- A metered-dose inhaler (MDI) is a handheld nebulizer that can be used by clients to self-administer measured doses of an aerosol medication. To ensure correct delivery of the prescribed medication by MDIs, nurses need to instruct clients to use aerosol inhalers correctly.
- Irrigations of body cavities may be performed (a) to remove a foreign object or excessive secretions or discharge, (b) to apply heat or cold, (c) to apply a medication, such as an antiseptic, (d) to reduce inflammation, or (e) to relieve discomfort.
- Surgical asepsis for an irrigation is required when there is a break in the skin (e.g., in a wound irrigation), or whenever a sterile body cavity (e.g., the bladder) is entered.

Review Questions

33–1. Which medication order will be given every other day?
 a. qh
 b. bid
 c. qod
 d. qd

33–2. A client tells the nurse, "This pill is a different color than the one that I usually take at home." Which is the best response by the nurse?
 a. "The doctor ordered a different medication."
 b. "Go ahead and take your medicine."
 c. "I'll leave the pill here while I check with the doctor."
 d. "I will recheck your medication orders."

Digoxin has a half-life of 36 hours. Use this information for Questions 33–3a and 33–3b:

33–3a. What is the amount of drug left in the body after 24 hours?
 a. 12.5%
 b. 25%
 c. 50%
 d. 83%

33–3b. How many days would it take for the digoxin to be eliminated with approximately 3% remaining in the body?
 a. 7.5
 b. 6
 c. 4.5
 d. 3

33–4. Presume that the full name of the client, the date and time that the order was written, and the physician's signature are present on the physician's order sheet. The following medications are listed on the MAR. Which would you question?
 a. Lasix 40 mg, po, STAT
 b. Ampicillin 500 mg, q 6 hr, IVPB
 c. Humulin L (Lente) insulin 36 u, sc, q am, ac
 d. Codeine q 4–6 hr, po, PRN for pain

What size syringe, needle gauge, and needle length would you consider for the following four situations?
 a. A tuberculin syringe, #25–#27 gauge, ¼- to ⅝-inch needle
 b. Two 3-mL syringes, #20–#23 gauge, 1½-inch needle
 c. 2-mL syringe, #25 gauge, ⅝-inch needle
 d. 2-mL syringe, #20–#23 gauge, 1-inch needle

33–5a. The order is for 5 mL of a medication to be given deep IM. The client is a 40-year-old female who weighs 135 pounds and is 5'7" tall.

33–5b. Administer 0.75 mL subcutaneously in the upper arm to a 50-year-old 300-pound client. The nurse can grasp approximately 2 inches of the client's tissue at the upper arm.

33–5c. Administer a tuberculin test to a 22-year-old male who is 6 feet tall and weighs 180 pounds.

33–5d. Administer 0.5 mL of a medication by IM injection to an elderly emaciated client.

Readings and References

Suggested Readings

Clarke, K. (2002). New insulin therapy. No needles needed. *Nursing, 32*(5), 49–51.
 A photo guide in which the author shows how to use the new needleless injector for delivering insulin. The pressure-driven injector requires no needles and is virtually painless.

Smetzer, J. (2001). Take 10 giant steps to medication safety. *Nursing, 31*(11), 49–53.
 A thorough review of 10 key factors to remember to prevent medication errors.

Togger, D. A., & Brenner, P. S. (2001). Metered dose inhalers. *American Journal of Nursing, 101*(10), 26–32.

A previous study completed by one of the authors indicated that many nurses were not able to correctly complete all the steps involved in using an inhaler with and without a spacer. The authors review how to use a MDI effectively to ensure that clients receive all of their inhaled medication.

Related Research

Katsma, D. L., & Katsma, R. (2000). The myth of the 90-angle intramuscular injection. *Nurse Educator, 25*(1), 34–37.

Klingman, L. (2000). Effects of changing needles prior to administering heparin subcutaneously. *Heart & Lung, 29*(1), 70.

References

Bastable, S. B. (2003). *Nurse as educator* (2nd ed.). Boston: Jones and Bartlett Publishing.

Bindler, R. C., & Ball, J. W. (2003). *Clinical skills manual for pediatric nursing: Caring for children* (3rd ed.). Upper Saddle River, NJ: Prentice Hall.

Brown, D. L. (2002). Does 1 + 1 still equal 2? A study of the mathematic competencies of associate degree nursing students. *Nurse Educator, 27*(3), 132–135.

Fleming, D. R. (1999). Challenging traditional insulin injection practices. *American Journal of Nursing, 99*(2), 72–74.

Kudzma, E. C. (1999). Culturally competent drug administration. *American Journal of Nursing, 99*(8), 46–51.

McCaffery, M., & Pasero, C. (1999). *Pain clinical manual* (2nd ed.). St. Louis, MO: Mosby.

Skokal, W. (2000). IV push at home? *RN, 63*(10), 26–29.

Togger, D. A., & Brenner, P. S. (2001). Metered dose inhalers. *American Journal of Nursing, 101*(10), 26–32.

Wakefield, B. J., Wakefield, D. S., Uden-Holman, T., & Blegen, M. A. (1998). Nurses' perceptions of why medication administration errors occur. *MEDSURG Nursing, 7*(1), 39–44.

Selected Bibliography

Avalos-Beck, S. (2001). The hard truth about the PPD skin test. *Nursing, 31*(6), 56–57.

Dayer-Berenson, L. (2001). Polypharmacy in the elderly. *Nursing Spectrum West Region Metro Edition, 2*(4), 29–33.

Fiesta, J. (1998). Legal aspects of medication administration. *Nursing Management, 29*(1), 22–23.

Greenly, M., & Gugerty, B. (2002). How bar coding reduces medication errors. *Nursing, 32*(5), 70.

Ignatavicius, D. D. (2000). Asking the right questions about medication safety. *Nursing, 30*(9), 51–54.

Jagger, J., & Perry, J. (2002). Exposure safety: Realistic expectations for safety devices. *Nursing, 32*(3), 72.

Johnson, C., & Horton, S. (2001). Owning up to errors. Put an end to the blame game. *Nursing, 31*(6), 54–55.

Karch, A. M., & Karch, F. E. (2001). Practice errors: The naked decimal point. *American Journal of Nursing, 101*(12), 22.

Logue, R. M. (2002). Self-medication and the elderly: How technology can help. *American Journal of Nursing, 102*(7), 51–55.

Martin, D. (1998). Needle-free injection. *Nursing, 28*(7), 52–53.

McConnell, E. A. (1998). How to choose and use needle-stick prevention devices. *Nursing, 28*(5), 32hn6–32hn8.

McConnell, E. A. (1999). Clinical do's & don'ts. Administering a Z-track IM injection. *Nursing, 29*(1), 26.

McConnell, E. A. (1999). Clinical do's & don't's: Administering an insulin injection. *Nursing, 29*(12), 18.

McConnell, E. A. (2000). Clinical do's & don't's: Administering an intradermal injection. *Nursing, 30*(3), 17.

McConnell, E. A. (2000). Infusion perfusion: IV pumps for every need. *Nursing Management, 31*(4), 53–55.

McConnell, E. A. (2001). Clinical do's and don'ts. Applying nitroglycerin ointment. *Nursing, 31*(6), 17.

McConnell, E. A. (2001). Clinical do's and don'ts. Instilling eyedrops. *Nursing, 31*(9), 17.

McConnell, E. A. (2002). Clinical do's and don'ts. Teaching your patient to use a metered-dose inhaler. *Nursing, 32*(2), 73.

Miller, D., & Miller, H. (2000). To crush or not to crush. *Nursing, 30*(2), 50–52.

Nagle, B. M. (1998). Low molecular weight heparin. *RN, 61*(4), 40–43.

Pope, B. B. (2002). How to administer subcutaneous and intramuscular injections. *Nursing, 32*(1), 50–51.

Quillen, T. (2000). Tips and timesavers: Crushing advice. *Nursing, 30*(4), 30.

Satarawala, R. (2000). Confronting the legal perils of IV therapy. *Nursing, 30*(8), 44–47.

Service Employees International Union. (1998). *SEIU's Guide to Preventing Needlestick Injuries* (3rd ed.). Washington, DC: Service Employees International Union.

Smetzer, J. L. (1998). Beyond blaming individuals. Lesson from Colorado. *Nursing, 28*(5), 48–51.

Wilburn, S. (2000). Preventing needlesticks in your facility. *American Journal of Nursing, 100*(2), 96.

Wolf, Z. R. (2001). Understanding medication errors. *Nursing Spectrum West Region Metro Edition, 2*(5), 29–33.

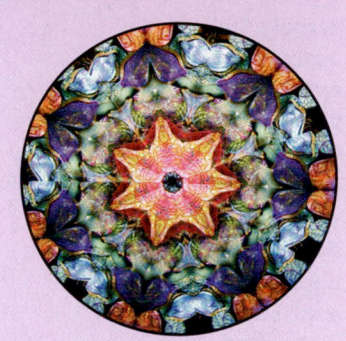

CHAPTER 34

SKIN INTEGRITY AND WOUND CARE

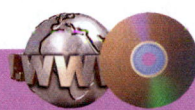

MediaLink

www.prenhall.com/kozier

Additional resources for this chapter can be found on the Student CD-ROM accompanying this textbook, and on the Companion Website at www.prenhall.com/kozier. Click on Chapter 34 to select the activities for this chapter.

CD-ROM
• Audio Glossary
• NCLEX Review
• Animations:
  Pressure Ulcer
  Feature Integument
  Layers of the Skin
  Integumentary Repair

Companion Website
• Additional NCLEX Review
• Case Study: Clients with Chronic Illnesses
• Care Plan Activity: Client with Pressure Ulcer
• MediaLink Application: Enterostomal Therapist
• Links to Resources

LEARNING OUTCOMES

After completing this chapter, you will be able to:

- Describe factors affecting skin integrity.
- Identify clients at risk for pressure ulcer formation.
- Describe the four stages of pressure ulcer development.
- Differentiate primary and secondary wound healing.
- Describe the three phases of wound healing.
- Identify three major types of wound exudate.
- Identify the main complications of and factors that affect wound healing.
- Identify assessment data pertinent to skin integrity, pressure sites, and wounds.
- Identify nursing diagnoses associated with impaired skin integrity.
- Identify essential aspects of planning care to maintain skin integrity and promote wound healing.
- Discuss measures to prevent pressure ulcer formation.
- Describe nursing strategies to treat pressure ulcers, promote wound healing, and prevent complications of wound healing.
- Identify purposes of commonly used wound dressing materials and binders.
- Identify physiologic responses to heat and cold and purposes of heat and cold.
- Describe methods of applying dry and moist heat and cold.
- Identify essential steps of obtaining wound specimens, applying dressings, and irrigating a wound.

The skin is the largest organ in the body and serves a variety of important functions in maintaining health and protecting the individual from injury. Important nursing functions are maintaining skin integrity and promoting wound healing. Impaired skin integrity is not a frequent problem for most healthy people but is a threat to older people; to clients with restricted mobility, chronic illnesses, or trauma; and to those undergoing invasive health care procedures. To protect the skin and manage wounds effectively, the nurse must understand the factors affecting skin integrity, the physiology of wound healing, and specific measures that promote optimal skin conditions.

SKIN INTEGRITY

Intact skin refers to the presence of normal skin and skin layers uninterrupted by wounds. Chapter 28 ⚭ provides details regarding physical examination of the integument. The appearance of the skin and skin integrity are influenced by internal factors such as genetics, age, and the underlying health of the individual as well as external factors such as activity.

Genetics and heredity determine many aspects of a person's skin, including skin color, sensitivity to sunlight, and allergies. Age influences skin integrity in that the skin of both the very young and the very old is more fragile and susceptible to injury than that of most adults. Wounds tend to heal more rapidly in infants and children, however.

Many chronic illnesses and their treatments affect skin integrity. People with impaired peripheral arterial circulation may have skin on the legs that appears shiny, has lost its hair distribution, and damages easily. Some medications, corticosteroids for example, cause thinning of the skin and allow it to be much more readily harmed. Many medications increase sensitivity to sunlight and can predispose one to severe sunburns. Some of the most common ones that cause this damage are certain antibiotics, chemotherapy drugs for cancer, and some psychotherapeutic drugs. Poor nutrition alone can interfere with the appearance and function of normal skin.

TYPES OF WOUNDS

Body wounds are either intentional or unintentional. *Intentional* trauma occur during therapy. Examples are operations or venipunctures. Although removing a tumor, for example, is therapeutic, the surgeon must cut into body tissues, thus traumatizing them. *Unintentional* wounds are accidental; for example, a person may fracture an arm in an automobile collision. If the tissues are traumatized without a break in the skin, the wound is closed. The wound is open when the skin or mucous membrane surface is broken.

Wounds may be described according to how they are acquired (see Table 34–1). They also can be described according to the likelihood and degree of wound contamination.

- *Clean wounds* are uninfected wounds in which minimal inflammation is encountered and the respiratory, alimentary, genital, and urinary tracts are not entered. Clean wounds are primarily closed wounds.
- *Clean-contaminated wounds* are surgical wounds in which the respiratory, alimentary, genital, or urinary tract has been entered. Such wounds show no evidence of infection.
- *Contaminated wounds* include open, fresh, accidental wounds and surgical wounds involving a major break in sterile technique or a large amount of spillage from the gastrointestinal tract. Contaminated wounds show evidence of inflammation.
- *Dirty* or *infected wounds* include wounds containing dead tissue and wounds with evidence of a clinical infection, such as purulent drainage.

Wounds are also classified by depth, that is, the tissue layers involved in the wound (see Box 34–1).

PRESSURE ULCERS

Pressure ulcers were previously called **decubitus ulcers,** *pressure sores,* or *bedsores.* A pressure ulcer is any lesion caused by unrelieved **pressure** (a compressing downward force on a body area) that results in damage to underlying tissue, as defined by the U.S. Public Health Service's Panel for the Prediction and Prevention of Pressure Ulcers in Adults (PPPPUA, 1992b).

TABLE 34–1 Types of Wounds

Type	Cause	Description and Characteristics
Incision	Sharp instrument (e.g., knife or scalpel)	Open wound; deep or shallow
Contusion	Blow from a blunt instrument	Closed wound, skin appears ecchymotic (bruised) because of damaged blood vessels
Abrasion	Surface scrape, either unintentional (e.g., scraped knee from a fall) or intentional (e.g., dermal abrasion to remove pockmarks)	Open wound involving the skin
Puncture	Penetration of the skin and often the underlying tissues by a sharp instrument, either intentional or unintentional	Open wound
Laceration	Tissues torn apart, often from accidents (e.g., with machinery)	Open wound; edges are often jagged
Penetrating wound	Penetration of the skin and the underlying tissues, usually unintentional (e.g., from a bullet or metal fragments)	Open wound

Pressure ulcers are a problem in both acute care settings and long-term care settings, including homes. The best estimate of the incidence of pressure ulcers in hospital settings is 15%; data reported for long-term facilities and homes are less reliable (Cuddigan, Berlowitz, & Ayello, 2001). *Healthy People 2010* has established the objective of reducing the prevalence of pressure ulcers in nursing homes by 50%—from 16/1,000 residents reported in 1997 to 8/1,000.

Etiology of Pressure Ulcers

Pressure ulcers are due to localized **ischemia,** a deficiency in the blood supply to the tissue. The tissue is caught between two hard surfaces, usually the surface of the bed and the bony skeleton. When blood cannot reach the tissue, the cells are deprived of oxygen and nutrients, the waste products of metabolism accumulate in the cells, and the tissue consequently dies. Prolonged, unrelieved pressure also damages the small blood vessels.

After the skin has been compressed, it appears pale, as if the blood had been squeezed out of it. When pressure is relieved, the skin takes on a bright red flush, called **reactive hyperemia,** which is the body's mechanism for preventing pressure ulcers. The flush is due to **vasodilation,** a process in which extra blood floods to the area to compensate for the preceding period of impeded blood flow. Reactive hyperemia usually lasts one-half to three-quarters as long as the duration of impeded blood flow to the area (PPPPUA, 1992a). If the redness disappears in that time, no tissue damage can be anticipated. If, however, the redness does not disappear, then tissue damage has occurred.

Two other factors frequently act in conjunction with pressure to produce pressure ulcers: friction and shearing force.

<table>
<tr><td colspan="2" style="background:#e94e1b;color:white">BOX 34–1   ■ Classifying Wounds by Depth</td></tr>
</table>

Partial thickness: Confined to the skin, that is, the dermis and epidermis; heal by regeneration
Full thickness: Involving the dermis, epidermis, subcutaneous tissue, and possibly muscle and bone; require connective tissue repair

Friction is a force acting parallel to the skin surface. For example, sheets rubbing against skin create friction. Friction can abrade the skin, that is, remove the superficial layers, making it more prone to breakdown.

Shearing force is a combination of friction and pressure. It occurs commonly when a client assumes a Fowler's position in bed. In this position, the body tends to slide downward toward the foot of the bed. This downward movement is transmitted to the sacral bone and the deep tissues. At the same time, the skin over the sacrum tends not to move because of the adherence between the skin and the bedsheets. The skin and superficial tissues are thus relatively unmoving in relation to the bed surface, whereas the deeper tissues are firmly attached to the skeleton and move downward. This causes a shearing force in the area where the deeper tissues and the superficial tissues meet. The force damages the blood vessels and tissues in this area.

Risk Factors

Several factors contribute to the formation of pressure ulcers: immobility and inactivity, inadequate nutrition, fecal and urinary incontinence, decreased mental status, diminished sensation, excessive body heat, advanced age, and the presence of certain chronic conditions.

Immobility

Immobility refers to a reduction in the amount and control of movement a person has. Normally people move when they experience discomfort due to pressure on an area of the body. Healthy people rarely exceed their tolerance to pressure. However, paralysis, extreme weakness, pain, or any cause of decreased activity can hinder a person's ability to change positions independently and relieve the pressure, even if the person can perceive the pressure.

Inadequate Nutrition

Prolonged inadequate nutrition causes weight loss, muscle atrophy, and the loss of subcutaneous tissue. These three reduce the amount of padding between the skin and the bones, thus increasing the risk of pressure ulcer development. More

MediaLink | PRESSURE ULCER ANIMATION

specifically, inadequate intake of protein, carbohydrates, fluids, and vitamin C contribute to pressure ulcer formation.

Hypoproteinemia (abnormally low protein content in the blood), due either to inadequate intake or abnormal loss, predisposes the client to dependent edema. Edema (the presence of excess fluid in the tissues) makes skin more prone to injury by decreasing its elasticity, resilience, and vitality. Edema increases the distance between the capillaries and the cells, thereby slowing the diffusion of oxygen to the tissue cells and of metabolites away from the cells.

Fecal and Urinary Incontinence

Moisture from incontinence promotes skin **maceration** (tissue softened by prolonged wetting or soaking) and makes the epidermis more easily eroded and susceptible to injury. Digestive enzymes in feces also contribute to skin **excoriation** (area of loss of the superficial layers of the skin also known as *denuded* area). Any accumulation of secretions or excretions is irritating to the skin, harbors microorganisms, and makes an individual prone to skin breakdown and infection.

Decreased Mental Status

Individuals with a reduced level of awareness, for example, those who are unconscious or heavily sedated, are at risk for pressure ulcers because they are less able to recognize and respond to pain associated with prolonged pressure.

Diminished Sensation

Paralysis, stroke, or other neurologic disease may cause loss of sensation in a body area. Loss of sensation reduces a person's ability to respond to injurious heat and cold and to feel the tingling ("pins and needles") that signals loss of circulation.

Excessive Body Heat

Body heat is another factor in the development of pressure ulcers. An elevated body temperature increases the metabolic rate, thus increasing the cells' need for oxygen. This increased need is particularly severe in the cells of an area under pressure, which are already oxygen deficient. Severe infections with accompanying elevated body temperatures may affect the body's ability to deal with the effects of tissue compression.

Advanced Age

The aging process brings about several changes in the skin and its supporting structures, making the older person more prone to impaired skin integrity. These changes include the following:

- Loss of lean body mass
- Generalized thinning of the epidermis
- Decreased strength and elasticity of the skin due to changes in the collagen fibers of the dermis
- Increased dryness due to a decrease in the amount of oil produced by the sebaceous glands
- Diminished pain perception due to a reduction in the number of cutaneous end organs responsible for the sensation of pressure and light touch.

Research Note
Does a New Mattress Overlay Decrease Pressure Ulcers in Surgical Clients?

A 1999 study by Schultz, Bien, Dumond, Brown, and Meyers was designed to identify the cause and occurrence of sacral/coccyx, heel, and elbow pressure ulcers in a surgical sample and to test the effectiveness of a new mattress overlay and heel and elbow protectors during surgery. The randomized sample was 413 surgical clients selected to receive standard padding and repositioning (control group) or a new mattress overlay during surgery. Preoperative data obtained included height and weight, history of diabetes, tobacco use, Braden scale scores, age, gender, hemoglobin, hematocrit, WBC, albumin, total protein, and blood pressure. During surgery, nurses recorded any position changes, shifting, or shearing.

The clients were evaluated for skin changes the first 6 days after surgery. The incidence of pressure ulcer formation rate in the overlay group was 26.6% as compared to 16.4% in the control group. Of the total 139 ulcers, 15 were more severe than stage I: nine stage II ulcers (6 of the 9 in the overlay group) and one stage IV ulcer. The clients with pressure ulcers were statistically older, had diabetes, were smaller in body mass, and had lower Braden scale scores on admission. The findings demonstrated client risks for developing pressure ulcers during surgery and that the test overlay mattress was not an effective prevention measure.

Implications: Clients undergoing surgical procedures are often in one position for a long time and also have the risk of friction and shearing while being repositioned or transferred. The standard use of padding and positioning devices proved to be more effective in preventing pressure ulcers than the mattress overlay in this study. Identification of risk factors for clients having surgery should increase awareness of importance of proper padding and positioning to prevent development of ulcers during surgery and postoperatively.

Note: From "Etiology and Incidence of Pressure Ulcers in Surgical Patients," by A. Schultz, M. Bien, K. Dumond, K. Brown and A. Meyers, 1999, *AORN Journal, 70,* pp. 434, 437–440, 443–444, 446–448.

Chronic Medical Conditions

Certain chronic conditions such as diabetes and cardiovascular disease are risk factors for skin breakdown and delayed healing. These conditions compromise oxygen delivery to tissues by poor perfusion and thus cause poor and delayed healing and increase risk of pressure sores.

Other Factors

Other factors contributing to the formation of pressure ulcers are poor lifting techniques, incorrect positioning, repeated injections in the same area, hard support surfaces, and incorrect application of pressure-relieving devices.

Stages of Pressure Ulcer Formation

The four recognized stages of pressure ulcer formation related to observable tissue damage are shown in Figure 34–1 ■.

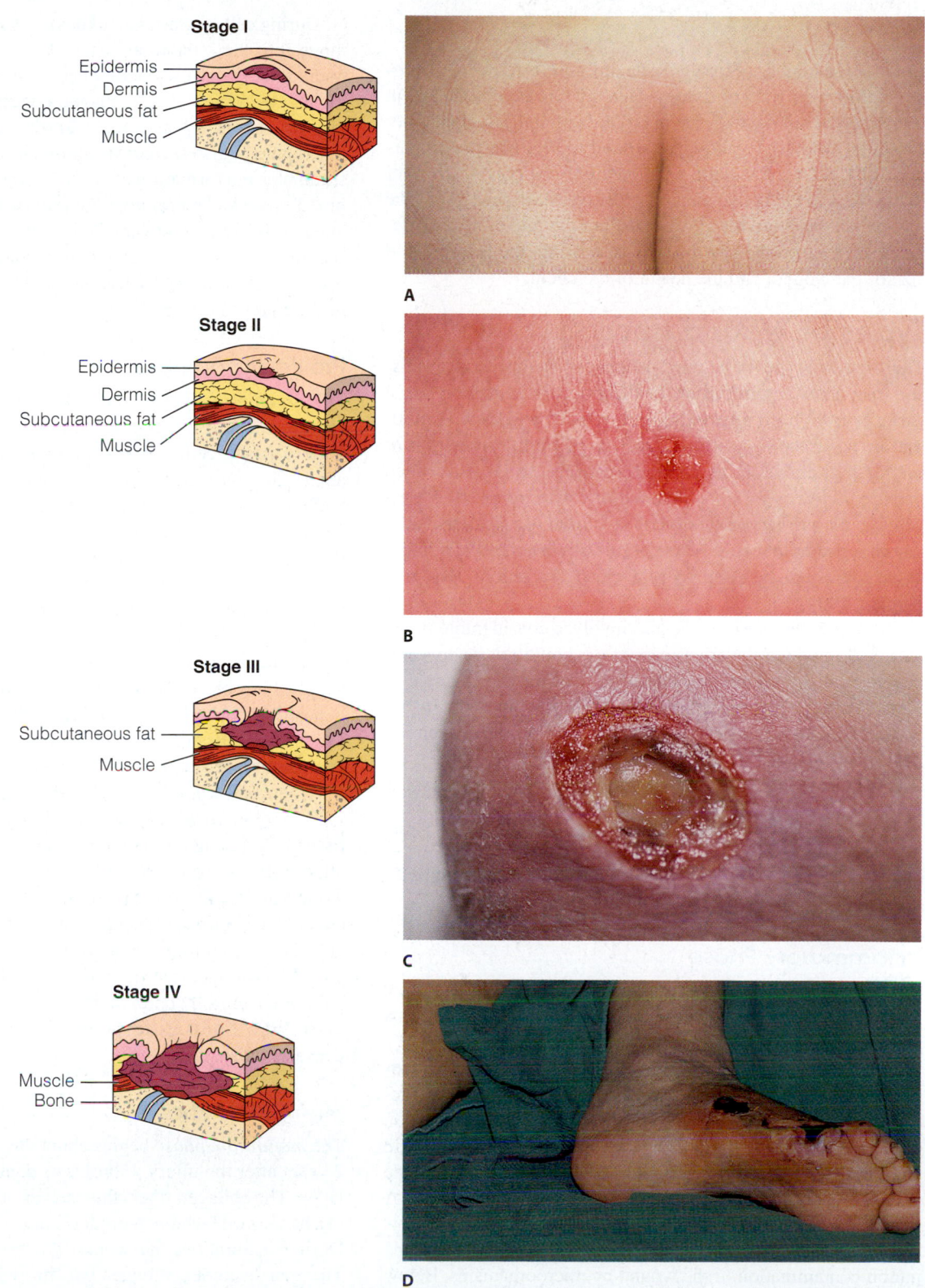

Figure 34–1 ■ Four stages of pressure ulcers. *A,* stage I: nonblanchable erythema signaling potential ulceration; *B,* stage II: partial-thickness skin loss (abrasion, blister, or shallow crater) involving the epidermis and possibly the dermis; *C,* stage III: full-thickness skin loss involving damage or necrosis of subcutaneous tissue that may extend down to, but not through, underlying fascia. The ulcer presents clinically as a deep crater with or without undermining of adjacent tissue. *D,* stage IV: full-thickness skin loss with tissue necrosis or damage to muscle, bone, or supporting structures, such as a tendon or joint capsule. Undermining and sinus tracts may also be present. (Line Art From "Clinical Practice Guideline, Pressure Ulcers in Adults: Prediction and Prevention," by U.S. Department of Health and Human Services, PPPPUA, Pub. no. 92-0047, 1992, Rockville, MD: Public Health Service. Reprinted with permission.)

WOUND HEALING

Healing is a quality of living tissue, it is also referred to as **regeneration** (renewal) of tissues. Healing can be considered in terms of *types of healing,* having to do with the caregiver's decision on whether to allow the wound to seal itself or to purposefully close the wound, and *phases of healing,* which refer to the steps in the body's natural processes of tissue repair. The phases are the same for all wounds, but the rate of healing depends on factors such as the type of healing, the location and size of the wound, and the health of the client.

Types of Wound Healing

There are two types of healing, influenced by the amount of tissue loss. **Primary intention healing** occurs where the tissue surfaces have been **approximated** (closed) and there is minimal or no tissue loss; it is characterized by the formation of minimal granulation tissue and scarring. It is also called *primary union* or *first intention healing.* An example of wound healing by primary intention is a closed surgical incision. Another example would be the use of tissue adhesive, a liquid "glue" that can be used to seal clean lacerations (King & Kinney, 2001).

A wound that is extensive and involves considerable tissue loss, and in which the edges cannot or should not be approximated, heals by **secondary intention healing.** An example of wound healing by secondary intention is a pressure ulcer. Secondary intention healing differs from primary intention healing in three ways: (a) The repair time is longer, (b) the scarring is greater, and (c) the susceptibility to infection is greater.

Phases of Wound Healing

Wound healing can be broken down into three phases: inflammatory, proliferative, and maturation or remodeling.

Inflammatory Phase

The *inflammatory phase* is initiated immediately after injury and lasts 3 to 6 days. Two major processes occur during this phase: hemostasis and phagocytosis.

Hemostasis (the cessation of bleeding) results from vasoconstriction of the larger blood vessels in the affected area, retraction (drawing back) of injured blood vessels, the deposition of **fibrin** (connective tissue), and the formation of blood clots in the area. The blood clots, formed from blood platelets, provide a matrix of fibrin that becomes the framework for cell repair. A scab also forms on the surface of the wound. Consisting of clots and dead and dying tissue, this scab serves to aid hemostasis and inhibit contamination of the wound by microorganisms. Below the scab, epithelial cells migrate into the wound from the edges. The epithelial cells serve as a barrier between the body and the environment, preventing the entry of microorganisms.

The inflammatory phase also involves vascular and cellular responses intended to remove any foreign substances and dead and dying tissues. The blood supply to the wound increases, bringing with it oxygen and nutrients needed in the healing process. The area appears reddened and edematous as a result.

During cell migration, leukocytes (specifically, neutrophils) move into the interstitial space. These are replaced about 24 hours after injury by macrophages, which arise from the blood monocytes. These macrophages engulf microorganisms and cellular debris by a process known as **phagocytosis.** The macrophages also secrete an angiogenesis factor (AGF), which stimulates the formation of epithelial buds at the end of injured blood vessels. The microcirculatory network that results sustains the healing process and the wound during its life. This inflammatory response is essential to healing, and measures that impair inflammation, such as steroid medications, can place the healing process at risk.

Proliferative Phase

The *proliferative phase,* the second phase in healing, extends from day 3 or 4 to about day 21 postinjury. Fibroblasts (connective tissue cells), which migrate into the wound starting about 24 hours after injury, begin to synthesize collagen. **Collagen** is a whitish protein substance that adds tensile strength to the wound. As the amount of collagen increases, so does the strength of the wound, thus the chance that the wound will open progressively decreases. If the wound is sutured, a raised "healing ridge" appears under the intact suture line. In a wound that is not sutured, the new collagen is often visible.

Capillaries grow across the wound, increasing the blood supply. Fibroblasts move from the bloodstream into the wound, depositing fibrin. As the capillary network develops, the tissue becomes a translucent red color. This tissue, called **granulation tissue,** is fragile and bleeds easily.

When the skin edges of a wound are not sutured, the area must be filled in with granulation tissue. When the granulation tissue matures, marginal epithelial cells migrate to it, proliferating over this connective tissue base to fill the wound. If the wound does not close by epithelialization, the area becomes covered with dried plasma proteins and dead cells. This is called **eschar.** Initially, wounds healing by secondary intention seep blood-tinged (serosanguineous) drainage. Later, if they are not covered by epithelial cells, they become covered with thick, gray, fibrinous tissue that is eventually converted into dense scar tissue.

Maturation Phase

The *maturation phase* begins about day 21 and can extend 1 or 2 years after the injury. Fibroblasts continue to synthesize collagen. The collagen fibers themselves, which were initially laid in a haphazard fashion, reorganize into a more orderly structure. During maturation, the wound is remodeled and contracted. The scar becomes stronger but the repaired area is never as strong as the original tissue. In some individuals, particularly dark-skinned persons, an abnormal amount of collagen is laid down. This can result in a hypertrophic scar, or **keloid.**

One method of documenting the progress of healing in pressure ulcers is to use the Pressure Ulcer Scale for Healing (PUSH) tool (National Pressure Ulcer Advisory Panel [NPUAP], 2002). This well-validated tool assigns scores to the ulcer length, width, amount of exudate, and tissue type. The change in the total score over time can be used as an indication of healing.

Kinds of Wound Drainage

Exudate is material, such as fluid and cells, that has escaped from blood vessels during the inflammatory process and is deposited in tissue or on tissue surfaces. The nature and amount of exudate vary according to the tissue involved, the intensity and duration of the inflammation, and the presence of microorganisms.

There are three major types of exudate: serous, purulent, and sanguineous (hemorrhagic). A **serous exudate** consists chiefly of serum (the clear portion of the blood) derived from blood and the serous membranes of the body, such as the peritoneum. It looks watery and has few cells. An example is the fluid in a blister from a burn.

A **purulent exudate** is thicker than serous exudate because of the presence of **pus,** which consists of leukocytes, liquefied dead tissue debris, and dead and living bacteria. The process of pus formation is referred to as **suppuration,** and the bacteria that produce pus are called **pyogenic bacteria.** Not all microorganisms are pyogenic. Purulent exudates vary in color, some acquiring tinges of blue, green, or yellow. The color may depend on the causative organism.

A **sanguineous (hemorrhagic) exudate** consists of large amounts of red blood cells, indicating damage to capillaries that is severe enough to allow the escape of red blood cells from plasma. This type of exudate is frequently seen in open wounds.

> **► CLINICAL ALERT** *A bright sanguineous exudate indicates fresh bleeding, whereas dark sanguineous exudate denotes older bleeding.*

Mixed types of exudates are often observed. A *serosanguineous* (consisting of clear and blood-tinged drainage) exudate is commonly seen in surgical incisions. A *purosanguineous* discharge (consisting of pus and blood) is often seen in a new wound that is infected.

Complications of Wound Healing

Several untoward events can occur to interfere with the healing of a wound. These include excessive bleeding, infection, and dehiscence.

Hemorrhage

Some escape of blood from a wound is normal. **Hemorrhage** (massive bleeding), however, is abnormal. It may be caused by a dislodged clot, a slipped stitch, or erosion of a blood vessel, for example.

Internal hemorrhage may be detected by swelling or distention in the area of the wound and, possibly, by sanguineous drainage from a surgical drain. Some clients will have a **hematoma,** a localized collection of blood underneath the skin that may appear as a reddish blue swelling (bruise). A large hematoma may be dangerous in that it places pressure on blood vessels and can thus obstruct blood flow.

The risk of hemorrhage is greatest during the first 48 hours after surgery. Hemorrhage is an emergency; the nurse should apply pressure dressings to the area and monitor the client's vital signs. In many instances, the client must be taken to the operating room for surgical intervention.

Infection

Contamination of a wound surface with microorganisms (colonization) is an inevitable result. Because the colonizing organisms compete with new cells for oxygen and nutrition, and because their by-products can interfere with a healthy surface condition, the presence of contamination can impair wound healing and lead to infection. When the microorganisms colonizing the wound multiply excessively or invade tissues, infection occurs. Infection suggested by the presence of a change in wound color, pain, or drainage is confirmed by performing a culture of the wound (see Chapter 32). ⊙⊙ Severe infection causes fever and elevated white blood cell count. Clients who are immunosuppressed, such as those with HIV or receiving myelosuppressive treatment for cancer, are especially susceptible to wound infections.

A wound can be infected with microorganisms at the time of injury, during surgery, or postoperatively. Wounds that occur as a result of injury (e.g., bullet and knife wounds) are most likely to be contaminated at the time of injury. Surgery involving the intestines can also result in infection from the microorganisms inside the intestine. Surgical infection is most likely to become apparent 2 to 11 days postoperatively.

Dehiscence with Possible Evisceration

Dehiscence is the partial or total rupturing of a sutured wound. Dehiscence usually involves an abdominal wound in which the layers below the skin also separate. **Evisceration** is the protrusion of the internal viscera through an incision. A number of factors, including obesity, poor nutrition, multiple trauma, failure of suturing, excessive coughing, vomiting, and dehydration, heighten a client's risk of wound dehiscence. Wound dehiscence is more likely to occur 4 to 5 days postoperatively before extensive collagen is deposited in the wound.

Dehiscence may be preceded by sudden straining, such as coughing or sneezing. It is not unusual for a client to feel that "something has given away." When dehiscence or evisceration occurs, the wound should be quickly supported by large sterile dressings soaked in sterile normal saline. Place the client in bed with knees bent to decrease pull on the incision. The surgeon must be notified because immediate surgical repair of the area may be necessary.

Factors Affecting Wound Healing

Characteristics of the individual such as age, nutritional status, lifestyle, and medications influence the speed of wound healing.

Developmental Considerations

Healthy children and adults often heal more quickly than older people, who are more likely to have chronic diseases that hinder healing. For example, reduced liver function can impair the

<table>
<tr><td>BOX 34–2</td><td>■ Factors Inhibiting Wound Healing in Older Adults</td></tr>
</table>

- Vascular changes associated with aging, such as atherosclerosis and atrophy of capillaries in the skin, can impair blood flow to the wound.
- Collagen tissue is less flexible, which increases the risk of damage from pressure, friction, and shearing.
- Scar tissue is less elastic.
- Changes in the immune system may reduce the formation of the antibodies and monocytes necessary for wound healing.
- Nutritional deficiencies may reduce the numbers of red blood cells and leukocytes, thus impeding the delivery of oxygen and the inflammatory response essential for wound healing. Oxygen is needed for the synthesis of collagen and the formation of new epithelial cells.
- Having diabetes or cardiovascular disease increases the risk of delayed healing due to impaired oxygen delivery to these tissues.
- Cell renewal is slower, leading to delayed healing.

synthesis of blood clotting factors. Box 34–2 lists factors inhibiting wound healing in older adults.

Nutrition

Wound healing places additional demands on the body. Clients require a diet rich in protein, carbohydrates, lipids, vitamins A and C, and minerals, such as iron, zinc, and copper. Malnourished clients may require time to improve their nutritional status before surgery, if this is possible. Obese clients are at increased risk of wound infection and slower healing because adipose tissue usually has a minimal blood supply.

Lifestyle

People who exercise regularly tend to have good circulation and because blood brings oxygen and nourishment to the wound, they are more likely to heal quickly. Smoking reduces the amount of functional hemoglobin in the blood, thus limiting the oxygen-carrying capacity of the blood, and constricts arterioles.

Medications

Anti-inflammatory drugs (e.g., steroids and aspirin) and antineoplastic agents interfere with healing. Prolonged use of antibiotics may make a person susceptible to wound infection by resistant organisms.

NURSING MANAGEMENT

ASSESSING

Assessment of Skin Integrity

The nurse conducts an examination of the integument as part of a routine assessment and during regular care.

Nursing History and Physical Assessment. During the review of systems as part of the nursing history, information regarding skin diseases, previous bruising, general skin condition, skin lesions, and usual healing of sores is elicited. Inspection and palpation of the skin focus on determination of skin color distribution, skin turgor, presence of edema, and characteristics of any lesions that are present. Particular attention is paid to skin condition in areas most likely to break down: in skinfolds such as under the breasts, in areas that are frequently moist such as the perineum, and in areas that receive extensive pressure such as the coccyx and trochanters (see Figure 34–2 ■). The accompanying Practice Guidelines describe guidelines for assessing

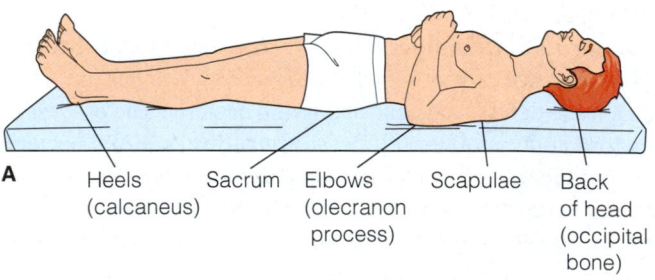

A   Heels (calcaneus)   Sacrum   Elbows (olecranon process)   Scapulae   Back of head (occipital bone)

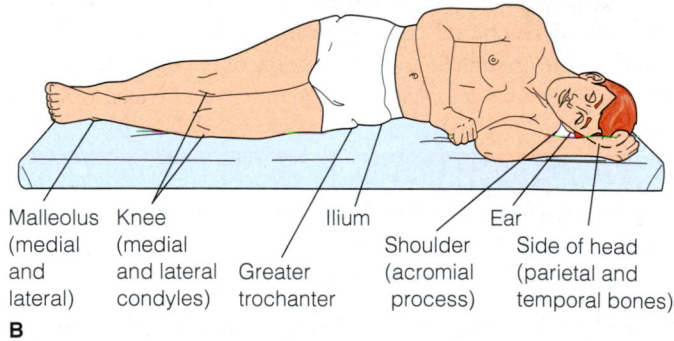

B   Malleolus (medial and lateral)   Knee (medial and lateral condyles)   Greater trochanter   Ilium   Shoulder (acromial process)   Ear   Side of head (parietal and temporal bones)

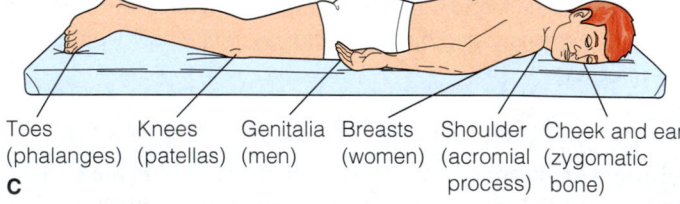

C   Toes (phalanges)   Knees (patellas)   Genitalia (men)   Breasts (women)   Shoulder (acromial process)   Cheek and ear (zygomatic bone)

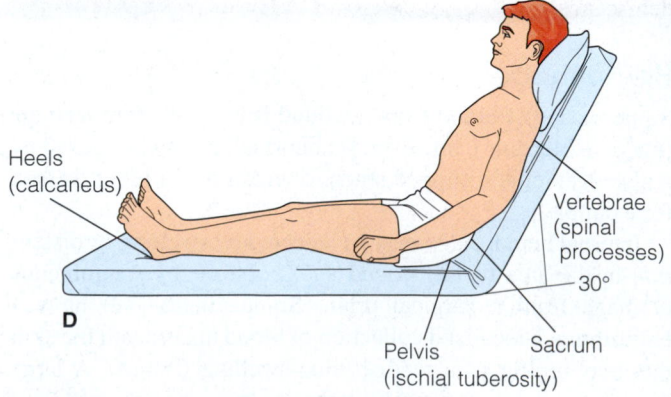

D   Heels (calcaneus)   Vertebrae (spinal processes)   30°   Pelvis (ischial tuberosity)   Sacrum

Figure 34–2 ■ Body pressure areas: in *A*, supine position; *B*, lateral position; *C*, prone position; *D*, Fowler's position.

Practice Guidelines
Assessing Common Pressure Sites

- Be sure the lighting is good, preferably natural or fluorescent, because incandescent lights can create a transilluminating effect.
- Regulate the environment before beginning the assessment so that the room is neither too hot nor too cold. Heat can cause the skin to flush; cold can cause the skin to blanch or become cyanotic.
- Inspect pressure areas (see Figure 34–2) for any whitish or reddened spots; discoloration can be caused by impaired blood circulation to the area. It should disappear in a few minutes when rubbing restores circulation.
- Inspect pressure areas for abrasions and excoriations. An abrasion can occur when skin rubs against a sheet (e.g., when the client is pulled). Excoriations can occur when the skin has prolonged contact with body secretions or excretions or with dampness in skinfolds.
- Palpate the surface temperature of the skin over the pressure areas (warm your hands first). Normally, the temperature is the same as that of the surrounding skin. Increased temperature is abnormal and may be due to inflammation or blood trapped in the area.
- Palpate over bony prominences and dependent body areas for the presence of edema, which feels spongy.

the common pressure sites. Refer to Chapter 28 🔗 for further detail regarding skin assessment.

Risk Assessment Tools. Although clients may be at risk for developing a number of different alterations in skin integrity, the most common and most preventable are pressure ulcers. Several risk assessment tools are available that provide the nurse with systematic means of identifying clients at high risk for pressure ulcer development. The PPPPUA (1992a) recommends that the tool include data collection in the areas of immobility, incontinence, nutrition, and level of consciousness.

In 1987 Bergstrom, Braden, Laguzza, and Holman published the Braden Scale for Predicting Pressure Sore Risk. Their scale consists of six subscales: sensory perception, moisture, activity, mobility, nutrition, and friction and shear (see Figure 34–3 ■). A total of 23 points is possible. An adult who scores 15 to 18 points is considered at risk, scores of 13 to 14 indicate moderate risk, 10 to 12 high risk, and 9 or less very high risk (Ayello & Braden, 2001). For best results, nurses should be trained in proper use of the scale.

Norton's Pressure Area Risk Assessment Form Scale (Table 34–2) includes the categories of general physical condition, mental state, activity, mobility, and incontinence. A category of medications was added in 1987, resulting in a possible score of 24. Scores of 15 or 16 should be viewed as indicators, not predictors, of risk (Anthony, 1987). The Braden and Norton tools should be used when the client first enters the health care agency and whenever the client's condition changes. In some long-term care facilities, a risk assessment scale such as the Braden or Norton scale is done on admission and then on a regular basis,

usually weekly. This increases awareness of specific risk factors and serves as assessment data from which to plan goals and interventions to either maintain or improve skin integrity.

> **CLINICAL ALERT**   *The two validated assessment tools supported by the PPPPUA are the Braden scale and the Norton scale.*

Assessment of Wounds

Nurses commonly assess both untreated and treated wounds. Although a pressure ulcer can be categorized as an untreated or treated wound, the specific assessment of pressure ulcers is discussed separately.

Untreated Wounds. Untreated wounds usually are seen shortly after an injury (e.g., at the scene of an accident or in an emergency center). Assessment for these wounds is shown in the accompanying Practice Guidelines. Guidelines for care follow:

- Control severe bleeding by (a) applying direct pressure over the wound and (b) elevating the involved extremity.
- Prevent infection by (a) cleaning or flushing abrasions or lacerations with water and (b) covering the wound with a clean dressing, if possible (a sterile dressing is preferred). When applying a dressing, wrap the wound tightly enough to apply pressure and approximate the wound edges, if possible. If the first layer of dressing becomes saturated with blood, apply a second layer. Do so without removing the first layer of dressing, because blood clots might be disturbed, resulting in more bleeding.
- Control swelling and pain by applying ice over the wound and surrounding tissues.
- If bleeding is severe or if internal bleeding is suspected, and if emergency equipment is available, assess the client for signs of shock (rapid thready pulse, cold clammy skin, pallor, lowered blood pressure).

Treated Wounds. Treated wounds, or sutured wounds, are usually assessed to determine the progress of healing. These wounds may be inspected during changing of a dressing. If the wound itself cannot be directly inspected, the dressing is inspected and other data regarding the wound (e.g., the presence of pain) are

Practice Guidelines
Assessing Untreated Wounds

- Assess the size and severity of the wound.
- Inspect the wound for bleeding. The amount of bleeding varies according to the type of wound and location. Penetrating wounds may cause internal bleeding.
- Inspect the wound for foreign bodies (soil, broken glass, shreds of cloth, or other foreign substances).
- Assess associated injuries such as fractures, internal bleeding, spinal cord injuries, or head trauma.
- If the wound is contaminated with foreign material, determine when the client last had a tetanus toxoid injection. A tetanus immunization or booster may be necessary.

BRADEN SCALE FOR PREDICTING PRESSURE SORE RISK

Patient's Name _____ Evaluator's Name _____ Date of Assessment _____

SENSORY PERCEPTION
Ability to respond meaningfully to pressure-related discomfort

1. Completely Limited:
Unresponsive (does not moan, flinch, or grasp) to painful stimuli, due to diminished level of consciousness or sedation,
OR
limited ability to feel pain over most of body surface.

2. Very Limited:
Responds only to painful stimuli. Cannot communicate discomfort except by moaning or restlessness,
OR
has a sensory impairment which limits the ability to feel pain or discomfort over 1/2 of body.

3. Slightly Limited:
Responds to verbal commands but cannot always communicate discomfort or need to be turned,
OR
has some sensory impairment which limits ability to feel pain or discomfort in 1 or 2 extremities.

4. No Impairment:
Responds to verbal commands. Has no sensory deficit which would limit ability to feel or voice pain or discomfort.

MOISTURE
Degree to which skin is exposed to moisture

1. Constantly Moist:
Skin is kept moist almost constantly by perspiration, urine, etc. Dampness is detected every time patient is moved or turned.

2. Moist:
Skin is often but not always moist. Linen must be changed at least once a shift.

3. Occasionally Moist:
Skin is occasionally moist, requiring an extra linen change approximately once a day.

4. Rarely Moist:
Skin is usually dry; linen requires changing only at routine intervals.

ACTIVITY
Degree of physical activity

1. Bedfast:
Confined to bed.

2. Chairfast:
Ability to walk severely limited or nonexistent. Cannot bear own weight and/or must be assisted into chair or wheelchair.

3. Walks Occasionally:
Walks occasionally during day but for very short distances, with or without assistance. Spends majority of each shift in bed or chair.

4. Walks Frequently:
Walks outside the room at least twice a day and inside room at least once every 2 hours during waking hours.

MOBILITY
Ability to change and control body position

1. Completely Immobile:
Does not make even slight changes in body or extremity position without assistance.

2. Very Limited:
Makes occasional slight changes in body or extremity position but unable to make frequent or significant changes independently.

3. Slightly Limited:
Makes frequent though slight changes in body or extremity position independently.

4. No Limitations:
Makes major and frequent changes in position without assistance.

NUTRITION
Usual food intake pattern

1. Very Poor:
Never eats a complete meal. Rarely eats more than 1/3 of any food offered. Eats 2 servings or less of protein (meat or dairy products) per day. Takes fluids poorly. Does not take a liquid dietary supplement,
OR
is NPO and/or maintained on clear liquids or IV's for more than 5 days.

2. Probably Inadequate:
Rarely eats a complete meal and generally eats only about 1/2 of any food offered. Protein intake includes only 3 servings of meat or dairy products per day. Occasionally will take a dietary supplement,
OR
receives less than optimum amount of liquid diet or tube feeding.

3. Adequate:
Eats over half of most meals. Eats a total of 4 servings of protein (meat, dairy products) each day. Occasionally will refuse a meal, but will usually take a supplement if offered,
OR
is on a tube feeding or TPN regimen, which probably meets most of nutritional needs.

4. Excellent:
Eats most of every meal. Never refuses a meal. Usually eats a total of 4 or more servings of meat and dairy products. Occasionally eats between meals. Does not require supplementation.

FRICTION AND SHEAR

1. Problem:
Requires moderate to maximum assistance in moving. Complete lifting without sliding against sheets is impossible. Frequently slides down in bed or chair, requiring frequent repositioning with maximum assistance. Spasticity, contractures, or agitation leads to almost constant friction.

2. Potential Problem:
Moves feebly or requires minimum assistance. During a move skin probably slides to some extent against sheets, chair, restraints, or other devices. Maintains relatively good position in chair or bed most of the time but occasionally slides down.

3. No Apparent Problem:
Moves in bed and in chair independently and has sufficient muscle strength to lift up completely during move. Maintains good position in bed or chair at all times.

Total Score _____

Figure 34–3 ■ Braden Scale for Predicting Pressure Sore Risk. (From "Clinical Practice Guideline, Pressure Ulcers in Adults: Prediction and Prevention," by U.S. Department of Health and Human Services, PPPPUA Pub no. 92-0047, pp. 16–17, 1992, Rockville, MD: Public Health Service. Copyright © Barbara Braden and Nancy Bergstrom, 1988. Reprinted with permission.)

TABLE 34–2 Norton's Pressure Area Risk Assessment Form (Scoring System)

A. General Physical Condition		B. Mental State		C. Activity		D. Mobility		E. Incontinence	
Good	4	Alert	4	Ambulatory	4	Full	4	Absent	4
Fair	3	Apathetic	3	Walks with help	3	Slightly limited	3	Occasional	3
Poor	2	Confused	2	Chairbound	2	Very limited	2	Usually urinary	2
Very bad	1	Stuporous	1	Bedfast	1	Immobile	1	Double	1

Note: From *An Investigation of Geriatric Nursing Problems in Hospitals*, by D. Norton, R. McLaren, and A. N. Exton-Smith, 1975, Edinburgh, UK: Churchill Livingstone. Reprinted with permission.

assessed. Many treated wounds are covered with a transparent occlusive dressing that permits observation of the wound without removing the dressing.

Assessment of a treated wound involves observation of its appearance, size, drainage, and the presence of swelling, pain, and status of drains or tubes. In some long-term facilities, home care situations, and outpatient clinics, photographs are taken weekly for a visual record of the progress of pressure sores and wounds. Other assessments are documented and dated along with the photograph. Details about these assessments and signs of healing for a surgical incision are discussed with surgical wounds in Chapter 35. 🔗

Sometimes, the wound reaches under the skin surface (called undermining). The edges of the wound around an open center may be raw or appear healed but the undermining can result in a sinus tract or tunnel that extends the wound many centimeters beyond the main wound surface. To fully assess the size of the wound, the nurse gently explores the undermined area with a thin, flexible probe. Do not use a cotton-tipped swab since it can leave fibers behind in the wound. Once the end of the tract is reached, gently raise the probe so that the bulge created by the end can be seen and its length measured on the skin surface. Sinus tracts are often caused by infection and have significant drainage. They may be treated using antibiotics, irrigation, surgical incision to open and drain the tract, or vacuum therapy for large tracts (Butcher, 2002).

Pressure Ulcers. When a pressure ulcer is present, the nurse notes

- Location of the lesion
- Size of lesion in centimeters (Measure length, width, and depth, beginning with length [head to toe] and then width

[side to side]. To measure depth, insert a sterile gloved finger or applicator stick at the deepest part of the wound, and then measure it against a measuring guide.)
- Presence of undermining or sinus tracts
- Stage of the ulcer (see Figure 34–1)
- Color of the wound bed and location of necrosis or eschar
- Condition of the wound margins
- Integrity of surrounding skin
- Clinical signs of infection, such as redness, warmth, swelling, pain, odor, and exudate (note color of exudate).

Laboratory Data. Laboratory data can often support the nurse's clinical assessment of the wound's progress in healing. A decreased leukocyte count can delay healing and increase the possibility of infection. A hemoglobin level below normal range indicates poor oxygen delivery to the tissues. Blood coagulation studies are also significant. Prolonged coagulation times can result in excessive blood loss and prolonged clot absorption. Hypercoagulability can lead to intravascular clotting. Intra-arterial clotting can result in a deficient blood supply to the wound area. Serum protein analysis provides an indication of the body's nutritional reserves for rebuilding cells. Albumin is an important indicator of nutritional status. A value below 3.5 g/dL indicates poor nutrition and may increase the risk of poor healing and infection. Wound cultures can either confirm or rule out the presence of infection. Sensitivity studies are helpful in the selection of appropriate antibiotic therapy. The nurse obtains a wound culture whenever an infection is suspected.

Procedure 34–1 provides guidelines to obtain a specimen of wound drainage.

Procedure 34-1 Obtaining a Wound Drainage Specimen

Purposes

- To identify the microorganisms potentially causing an infection and the antibiotics to which they are sensitive
- To evaluate the effectiveness of antibiotic therapy

ASSESSMENT

Assess

- Appearance of the wound and surrounding tissue. Check the character and amount of wound drainage. Is the client complaining of pain at the wound site?
- For signs of infection such as fever, chills, or elevated white blood cell count (WBC)

continued on page 866

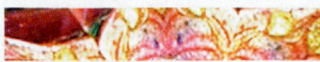

Procedure 34-1   Obtaining a Wound Drainage Specimen *continued*

PLANNING

Before obtaining a specimen of wound drainage determine (a) whether the wound should be cleaned before taking the specimen and (b) whether the site from which to take the specimen has been specified.

Delegation

Obtaining a wound culture is an invasive procedure that requires the application of sterile technique, knowledge of wound healing, and potential problem solving to ensure client safety; therefore, the nurse needs to perform this skill and does not delegate it to unlicensed assistive personnel (UAP).

Equipment
- Clean gloves
- Sterile gloves
- Moisture-proof bag
- Sterile dressing set
- Normal saline and irrigating syringe
- Culture tube with swab and culture medium (aerobic and anaerobic tubes are available) and/or sterile syringe with needle for anaerobic culture
- Completed labels for each container
- Completed requisition to accompany the specimens to the laboratory

IMPLEMENTATION

Preparation

Check the medical orders to determine if the specimen is to be collected for an **aerobic** (growing only in the presence of oxygen) or **anaerobic** (growing only in the absence of oxygen) culture. Aerobic organisms are generally found on the surface of the wound, whereas anaerobic organisms would be found in deep wounds, tunnels, and cavities. Administer an analgesic 30 minutes before the procedure if the client is complaining of pain at the wound site.

Performance

1. Explain to the client what you are going to do, why it is necessary, and how he or she can cooperate. Discuss how the results will be used in planning further care or treatments.
2. Wash hands and observe other appropriate infection control procedures (e.g., gloves).
3. Provide for client privacy.
4. Remove any moist outer dressings that cover the wound.
   - Put on clean gloves.
   - Remove the outer dressing, and observe any drainage on the dressing. Hold the dressing so that the client does not see the drainage because *the appearance of the drainage could upset the client.*
   - Determine the amount of the drainage, for example, "one 2 × 2 gauze saturated with pale yellow drainage."
   - Discard the dressing in the moisture-proof bag. Handle it carefully so that the dressing does not touch the outside of the bag. *Touching the outside of the bag will contaminate it.*

   - Remove your gloves and dispose of them properly.
5. Open the sterile dressing set using sterile technique (see Procedure 29–3).
6. Assess the wound.
   - Put on sterile gloves (see Procedure 29–4).
   - Assess the appearance of the tissues in and around the wound and the drainage. Infection can cause reddened tissues with a thick discharge, which may be foul smelling, whitish, or colored.
7. Clean the wound.
   - Irrigate the wound with normal saline until all visible exudates have been washed away (see Procedure 34–4 later in this chapter).
   - After irrigating, apply a sterile gauze pad to the wound. *This absorbs excess saline.*
   - If a topical antimicrobial ointment or cream is being used to treat the wound, use a swab to remove it. *Residual antiseptic must be removed prior to culture.*
   - Remove and discard sterile gloves.
8. Obtain the aerobic culture.
   - Open a specimen tube and place the cap upside down on a firm, dry surface so that the inside will not become contaminated, or if the swab is attached to the lid, twist the cap to loosen the swab. Hold the tube in one hand and take out the swab in the other (see Figure 34–4 ■).
   - Rotate the swab back and forth over clean areas of granulation tissue from the sides or base of the wound. *Microorganisms most likely*

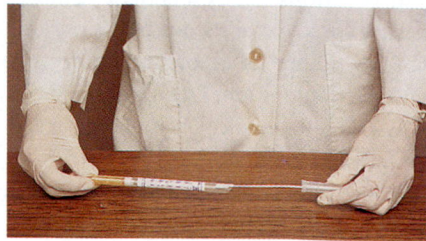

Figure 34–4 ■ A culturette tube for a wound specimen.

to be responsible for a wound infection reside in viable tissue.
   - Do not use pus or pooled exudates to culture. *These secretions contain a mixture of contaminants that are not the same as those causing the infection.*
   - Avoid touching the swab to intact skin at the wound edges. *This prevents the introduction of superficial skin organisms into the culture.*
   - Return the swab to the culture tube, taking care not to touch the top or the outside of the tube. *The outside of the container must remain free of pathogenic microorganisms to prevent their spread to others.*
   - Crush the inner ampule containing the medium for organism growth at the bottom of the tube. *This ensures that the swab with the specimen is surrounded by culture medium.*
   - Twist the cap to secure.
   - If a specimen is required from another site, repeat the steps. Specify the exact site (e.g., inferior drain site or lower aspect of incision) on the

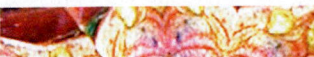

Procedure 34-1 Obtaining a Wound Drainage Specimen *continued*

IMPLEMENTATION *continued*

label of each container. Be sure to put each swab in the appropriately labeled tube.

9. Dress the wound.
   • Apply any ordered medication to the wound.
   • Cover the wound with a sterile moist transparent wound dressing (see Procedure 34–2 later in this chapter).

10. Arrange for the specimen to be transported to the laboratory immediately. Be sure to include the completed requisition.

11. Document all relevant information.
    • Record on the client's chart the taking of the specimen and source.
    • Include the date and time, the appearance of the wound, the color, consistency, amount, and odor of any drainage, the type of culture collected, and any discomfort experienced by the client.

VARIATION: OBTAINING A SPECIMEN FOR ANAEROBIC CULTURE

■ Insert a sterile 10-mL syringe (without needle) into the wound, and aspirate 1 to 5 mL of drainage into the syringe.

■ Attach the needle to the syringe, and expel all air from the syringe and needle.
■ Immediately inject the drainage into the anaerobic culture tube and cap the tube tightly.
   or
■ Use an anaerobic culture swab system in which the swab is immediately placed into a tube filled with an oxygen-free gas or gel environment.
■ Label the tube or syringe appropriately.
■ Send the tube or syringe of drainage to the laboratory immediately. Do not refrigerate the specimen.

EVALUATION

■ Compare findings of wound assessment and drainage to previous assessments to determine any changes.
■ Report the culture results to the physician.

■ Conduct appropriate follow-up such as administering medications as ordered.

DIAGNOSING

The NANDA nursing diagnoses (2003) that relate to clients who have skin wounds or who are at risk for skin breakdown are

• *Risk for Impaired Skin Integrity:* At risk for skin being adversely altered
• *Impaired Skin Integrity:* Altered epidermis and/or dermis
• *Impaired Tissue Integrity:* Damage to mucous membrane, corneal, integumentary, or subcutaneous tissues.

Impaired Skin Integrity commonly applies to pressure ulcers and to wounds extending through the epidermis but not through the dermis. *Impaired Tissue Integrity* applies to pressure ulcers and to wounds extending into subcutaneous tissue, muscle, or bone. Examples of clinical applications of these diagnoses using NANDA, NIC and NOC designations are shown in Identifying Nursing Diagnoses, Outcomes, and Interventions.

Additional nursing diagnoses may be appropriate for clients with existing impaired skin or tissue integrity. Examples of these diagnoses include

• *Risk for Infection* if the skin impairment is severe, the client is immunosuppressed, or the wound is caused by trauma
• *Pain* related to nerve involvement within the tissue impairment or as a consequence of procedures used to treat the wound.

PLANNING

The major goals for clients at *Risk for Impaired Skin Integrity* (pressure ulcer development) are to maintain skin integrity and to avoid potential associated risks. Clients with *Impaired Skin Integrity* need to demonstrate progressive wound healing and regain intact skin (see Identifying Nursing Diagnoses, Outcomes, and Interventions).

Planning for Home Care

Increasingly, wound care is provided in the home rather than in health care facilities. The client and family assume much of the responsibility for assessing and treating existing wounds and for helping to prevent pressure ulcers. The accompanying Home Care Assessment feature outlines appropriate assessment for clients who have wounds or pressure ulcers or are at risk for developing pressure ulcers. In planning for client discharge, nurses are accountable for teaching the client and family wound preventive and care measures. See Teaching: Home Care for a model. A critical pathway can also be useful for planning client care at home (see the example on page 870).

IMPLEMENTING

Nursing interventions for maintaining skin integrity and wound care involve supporting wound healing, preventing pressure ulcers, treating pressure ulcers, dressing and cleaning wounds, applying heat and cold, and supporting and immobilizing wounds.

Supporting Wound Healing

There are three major areas in which nurses can help clients develop optimal conditions for wound healing: obtaining sufficient nutrition and fluids, preventing wound infections, and proper positioning.

Nutrition and Fluids. Clients should be assisted to take in at least 2,500 mL of fluids a day unless conditions contraindicate this amount. Although there is no evidence that excessive doses of vitamins or minerals enhance wound healing, adequate amounts are extremely important. The nurse should ensure that clients receive sufficient protein, vitamins C, A, B_1, and B_5, and zinc.

IDENTIFYING NURSING DIAGNOSES, OUTCOMES, AND INTERVENTIONS

CLIENTS AT RISK FOR OR WITH IMPAIRED SKIN INTEGRITY

DATA CLUSTER	NURSING DIAGNOSIS/ DEFINITION	SAMPLE DESIRED OUTCOMES [NOC#]/DEFINITION	INDICATORS	SELECTED INTERVENTIONS [NIC#]/DEFINITION	SAMPLE NIC ACTIVITIES
Juanita Perez, an 85-year-old, is pale, emaciated, and listless. Weight 90 lb. Is incontinent of urine and stool, and is bedridden.	*Risk for Impaired Skin Integrity* related to incontinence and immobility/*At risk for skin being adversely altered*	Tissue Integrity: Skin and Mucous Membranes [1101]/ *Structural intactness and normal physiological function of skin and mucous membranes*	Mildly compromised • Elasticity in expected range. • Tissue lesion free	Positioning [0840]/ *Deliberative placement of the patient or a body part to promote physiological and/or psychological well-being.* Pressure Ulcer Prevention [3540]/*Prevention of pressure ulcers for a patient at high risk for developing them*	• Explain to the patient that she is going to be turned • Position in proper body alignment • Place on an appropriate therapeutic mattress or bed • Document skin status • Remove moisture from the skin caused by urinary and fecal incontinence • Apply protective barriers such as creams or pads to absorb excess moisture
Matthew Brown, an obese 70-year-old hemiplegic, complains of discomfort in his left heel after attempting to move in bed. Superficial skin abrasion 1.2 cm in diameter present at base of left heel.	*Impaired Skin Integrity* (stage II pressure ulcer) related to friction/*Altered epidermis and/or dermis*	Wound Healing: Secondary Intention [1103]/*The extent to which cells and tissues in an open wound have regenerated*	Substantial • Granulation • Resolution of wound size	Pressure Ulcer Care [3520]/*Facilitation of healing in pressure ulcers*	• Cleanse the skin around the ulcer with mild soap and water • Note characteristics of any drainage • Ensure adequate nutrition • Apply a transparent wound barrier • Use devices on the bed (e.g., sheepskin) that protect the patient

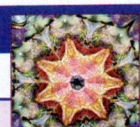

Home Care Assessment
WOUND CARE AND PREVENTION OF PRESSURE ULCERS

Client and Environment

- *Current level of knowledge:* Understanding of the cause of the wound or risk for developing a pressure ulcer; prevention or treatment strategies
- *Self-care abilities for mobility:* Physical ability to change position, ambulate, and transfer including the use of assistive devices
- *Self-care abilities for wound care:* Manual dexterity and visual acuity necessary to perform skin assessments and wound treatments
- *Facilities:* Presence of running water, garbage, bathroom needed to perform wound care and contain potentially infectious materials
- *Current level of nutrition:* Eating habits and preferences, laboratory values indicating need for teaching or other intervention

Family

- *Caregiver availability, skills, and responses:* Willingness to assist with wound care and actions to prevent pressure ulcers
- *Family role changes and coping:* Effect on financial status, parenting and spousal roles, sexuality, social roles
- *Alternate potential primary or respite caregivers:* For example, other family members, volunteers, church members, paid caregivers or housekeeping services; available community respite care (adult day care, senior centers, etc.)

Community

- *Resources:* Availability and familiarity with possible sources of assistance such as equipment and supply companies, organizations that offer medical supplies or financial assistance, home health agencies

---

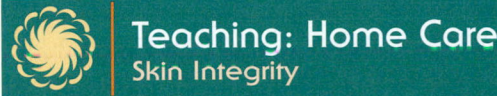

Teaching: Home Care
Skin Integrity

Maintaining Intact Skin

- Discuss relationship between adequate nutrition (especially fluids, protein, vitamins B and C, iron, and calories) and healthy skin.
- Demonstrate appropriate positions for pressure relief.
- Establish a turning or repositioning schedule.
- Demonstrate application of appropriate skin protection agents and devices.
- Instruct to report persistent reddened areas.
- Identify potential sources of skin trauma and means of avoidance.

Promoting Wound Healing

- Discuss importance of adequate nutrition (especially fluids, protein, vitamins B and C, iron, and calories).
- Instruct in wound assessment and provide mechanism for documenting.
- Emphasize principles of asepsis, especially hand washing and proper methods of handling used dressings.
- Provide information about signs of wound infection and other complications to report.
- Reinforce appropriate aspects of pressure ulcer prevention.
- Demonstrate wound care techniques such as wound cleansing and dressing changing.
- Discuss pain control measures, if needed.

Preventing Infection. There are two main aspects to controlling wound infection: preventing microorganisms from entering the wound, and preventing the transmission of bloodborne pathogens to or from the client to others. See Table 34–3, and see Chapter 29 ⊖⊃ for more information about infection control.

Positioning. To promote wound healing, clients must be positioned to keep pressure off the wound. Changes of position and transfers can be accomplished without shear or friction damage. In addition to proper positioning, the client should be assisted to be as mobile as possible because activity enhances circulation. If the client cannot move independently, range-of-motion exercises and a turning schedule are implemented.

Preventing Pressure Ulcers

To reduce the likelihood of pressure ulcer development in all clients, the nurse employs a variety of preventive measures (i.e., skin hygiene) to maintain the skin integrity and instructs the client, support people, and caregivers in how to prevent pressure ulcers.

Providing Nutrition. Because an inadequate intake of calories, protein, vitamins, and iron is believed to be a risk factor for pressure ulcer development, nutritional supplements should be considered for nutritionally compromised clients. The diet should be similar to that which supports wound healing, as discussed earlier. Monitor weight regularly to help assess nutritional status. Pertinent lab work should also be monitored including lymphocyte count, protein (especially albumin), and hemoglobin.

Maintaining Skin Hygiene. Obtain baseline data using the established tool and then reassess the skin at least daily in the hospital and weekly at home. When bathing the client, the nurse should minimize the force and friction applied to the skin, using mild cleansing agents that minimize irritation and dryness and that do not disrupt the skin's "natural barriers." Also, avoid using hot water, which increases skin dryness and irritation. Nurses can minimize dryness by avoiding exposure to cold and low humidity. Dry skin is best treated with moisturizing lotions applied while the skin is moist after bathing. The client's skin should be kept clean and dry and free of irritation and maceration by urine, feces, sweat, incomplete drying after a bath, soap,

CRITICAL PATHWAY FOR WOUND MANAGEMENT

ASSESSMENT DATA

Nursing Assessment for José Alonzo

José Alonzo is a 42-year-old construction worker who was injured at work when a wheelbarrow filled with cement rolled into him and pushed him off a 4-foot ledge. He suffered several bruises and one 9-cm (3.5-in.) laceration on the anterior aspect of the lower left leg. The laceration was covered with a sterile compression dressing at the scene by paramedics. Prior to irrigation and cleansing with normal saline and peroxide, the wound contained particles of cement and dirt. Marcella James, a nurse practitioner, sutured the wound with silk suture and discharged Mr. Alonzo to home care. Mr. Alonzo is to return to the outpatient clinic for suture removal in 10 days. He asks the nurse whether he can use an aloe herbal ointment on the wound and drink a healing herbal tea that his wife makes.

PHYSICAL EXAMINATION

Height: 177.8 cm (5'10")
Weight: 72.7 kg (160 lb)
Temperature: 37C (98.6F)
Pulse rate: 88 bpm
Respirations: 24/min
Blood pressure: 136/90 mm Hg

EXPECTED LENGTH OF TREATMENT: 7 to 10 days

Outcomes	Client verbalizes understanding of teaching, including wound care, signs and symptoms to report, follow-up care.	At time of suture removal • Client is afebrile. • Client has a dry, clean wound with edges well approximated, healing by first intention.
	Date _____ Outpatient setting	**Date** _____ Daily for 10 days (Client activities)
Deficient Knowledge	Provide simple, brief instructions regarding injury and treatment. Encourage client to ask questions and seek assistance. Assess the client's knowledge about wound care. Review written instruction sheet for wound care with client and provide copy.	Follow written discharge teaching regarding wound care and dressing change. Call physician with questions or problems and return to office in 10 days for suture removal.
Diet	Instruct client about foods high in protein and vitamin C and encourage adequate intake.	Diet high in protein and vitamin C. Cultural remedies that will not interfere with healing.
Wound care	Irrigate and clean the wound with normal saline. Surgical consultation for wound closure. Following wound closure, apply dry sterile dressing.	Change dressing daily and prn to keep dressing dry and clean. Inspect wound daily and report any signs and symptoms of infection (redness, pain, warmth, drainage, redness, or fever).
Medications	Tetanus toxoid if indicated.	Only if ordered.

TABLE 34-3 Guidelines for Preventing Infection and the Transmission of Bloodborne Pathogens

Standard Precautions
- Wear gloves when touching blood and body fluids, mucous membranes, or nonintact skin of all clients, and when handling items or surfaces soiled with blood or body fluids.
- Wash hands thoroughly after removing gloves, and if contaminated with blood or body fluids.

Wound Care
- Wash hands before and after caring for wounds.
- Wear gloves, surgical masks, and protective eyewear as appropriate if procedures commonly cause droplets or splashing of blood or body fluids (e.g., wound irrigation).
- Touch an open or fresh surgical wound only when wearing sterile gloves or using a sterile instrument.
- Remove or change dressings over closed wounds when they become wet.

or alcohol. Apply skin protection if indicated. Moisture or skin barriers, also called *skin preps,* are available in liquid, spray, and moist wipe format and are very effective in preventing moisture or drainage from collecting on the skin. In most cases, the nurse can apply these without a physician's order.

In addition, massage over bony prominences should be avoided. Traditionally, nurses have used massage to stimulate blood circulation, with the intention of preventing pressure ulcers. However, scientific evidence does not support this belief, in fact, vigorous massage may lead to deep tissue trauma (NPUAP, 2001; PPPPUA, 1992a).

Avoiding Skin Trauma. Providing the client with a smooth, firm, and wrinkle-free foundation on which to sit or lie helps prevent skin trauma. To prevent injury due to friction and shearing forces, clients must be positioned, transferred, and turned correctly. Friction injuries can be reduced by applying a thin layer of cornstarch to the bedsheet or wheelchair seat cover or by using protective films, such as transparent dressings and skin sealants. For bedridden clients, shearing force can be reduced by elevating the head of the bed to no more than 30 degrees, if this position is not contraindicated by the client's condition. (For example, clients with respiratory disorders may find it easier to breathe in Fowler's position.) When the head of the bed is raised, the skin and superficial fascia stick to the bed linen while the deep fascia and skeleton slide down toward the bottom of the bed. As a result, blood vessels in the sacral area become twisted, and the tissues in the area can become ischemic and necrotic.

Frequent shifts in position, even if only slight, effectively change pressure points. The client should shift weight every 15 to 30 minutes and, whenever possible, exercise or ambulate to stimulate blood circulation.

When lifting a client to change position, nurses should use a lifting device such as a trapeze rather than dragging the client across or up in bed. The friction that results from dragging the skin against a sheet can cause blisters and abrasions, which may contribute to more extensive tissue damage. Therefore, using devices that lift the client's weight off the bed surface is the method of choice.

Any at-risk client confined to bed—even when a special support mattress is used—should be repositioned at least every 2 hours, depending on the client's need, to allow another body surface to bear the weight. Six body positions can usually be used: prone, supine, right and left lateral (side-lying), and right and left Sims' positions. When a lateral position is used, the nurse should avoid positioning the client directly on the trochanter and instead position the client on a 30-degree angle. A written schedule should be established for turning and repositioning.

Providing Supportive Devices. In order for circulation to remain uncompromised, pressure on the bony prominences should remain below capillary pressure for as much time as possible through a combination of turning, positioning, and use of pressure-relieving surfaces. Mean capillary pressure can be estimated at 20 mm Hg although this varies (de Graaff, Ubbink, Lagarde, & Jacobs, 2002). Although some research has been conducted evaluating the effectiveness of pressure-reducing

support surfaces in preventing pressure ulcers in clients at low, intermediate, or high risk, the results are often inconclusive (Cullum, Deeks, Sheldon, Song, & Fletcher, 2001). The nurse should review the manufacturer's product descriptions that report the amount of time that the pressure between the surface and the bony prominence is above or below specified levels and determine if this is adequate to protect a particular client.

For clients confined to bed, three types of support surfaces can be used to relieve pressure. The overlay mattress is applied on top of the standard bed mattress. A replacement mattress is used instead of the standard mattress; most are made of foam and gel combinations. Specialty beds replace hospital beds. They provide pressure relief, eliminate shearing and friction, and decrease moisture. Examples are high-air-loss beds, low-air-loss beds, and beds that provide kinetic therapy. Kinetic beds provide continuous passive motion or oscillation therapy, which is intended to counteract the effects of a client's immobility. Table 34–4 lists selected mechanical devices for reducing pressure on body parts.

When a client is confined to bed or to a chair, pressure-reducing devices, such as pillows made of foam, gel, air, or a combination of these, can be used. When the client is sitting, weight should be distributed over the entire seating surface so that pressure does not center on just one area. To protect a client's heels in bed, supports such as wedges or pillows can be used to raise the heels completely off the bed. Doughnut-type devices should not be used since they limit blood flow and can cause tissue damage to the areas in direct contact with the device.

Treating Pressure Ulcers

Pressure ulcers are a challenge for nurses because of the number of variables involved (e.g., risk factors, types of ulcers, and degrees of impairment) and the numerous treatment measures advocated. Existing and potential infections are the most serious complications of pressure ulcers. In treating pressure ulcers, nurses should follow the agency protocols and the physician's orders, if any. Prompt treatment can prevent further tissue damage and pain and facilitate wound healing. See the accompanying Practice Guidelines feature regarding treating pressure ulcers, and Table 34–5 for dressings for pressure ulcers.

The RYB Color Code. To guide wound care, the nurse can use the RYB color code of wounds. This concept is based on the color of an open wound—red, yellow, or black (RYB)—rather than the depth or size of a wound. On this scheme, the goals of wound care are to protect (cover) red, cleanse yellow, and debride black.

Wounds that are red are usually in the late regeneration phase of tissue repair (i.e., developing granulation tissue). They need to be protected to avoid disturbance to regenerating tissue. The nurse protects red wounds by (a) gentle cleansing (i.e., use of an approved wound cleanser applied without pressure), (b) avoiding the use of dry gauze or wet-to-dry dressings, (c) applying a topical antimicrobial agent, (d) applying an appropriate dressing such as gauze, transparent film, or hydrocolloid dressing, and (e) changing the dressing as infrequently as possible.

Yellow wounds are characterized primarily by liquid to semiliquid "slough" that is often accompanied by purulent drainage.

TABLE 34–4 Mechanical Devices for Reducing Pressure on Body Parts

Device	Description/Comments	
Gel flotation pads	Polyvinyl, silicone, or Silastic pads filled with a gelatinous substance similar to fat.	
Sheepskins (natural and artificial)	Some manufacturers produce mixed natural and synthetic pads; artificial pads are less likely to be damaged by washing but are more likely than natural skins to make the client hot (Figure 34–5 ■).	**Figure 34–5** ■ Sheepskins. (Courtesy of Aussie Slans.)
Pillows and wedges (foam, gel, air, fluid)	Can raise a body part (e.g., heels) off the bed or surface.	
Heel protectors (sheepskin boots, padded splints, foam wedges)	Limit pressure on heels when the client is in bed (Figure 34–6 ■).	**Figure 34–6** ■ Heel protector. (Courtesy of Gaymar Industries, Inc.)
Egg crate mattress	Polyurethane foam mattress resembling an egg crate; some types are flammable (see Figure 34–7 ■).	
Foam mattress	Foam molds to the body.	**Figure 34–7** ■ An egg crate mattress provides comfort and helps to distribute body weight evenly, then helping to reduce pressure on bony prominences.

The nurse cleanses yellow wounds to remove nonviable tissue. Methods used may include applying wet-to-damp dressings, irrigating the wound, using absorbent dressing materials such as impregnated nonadherent, hydrogel dressings, or other exudate absorbers, and consulting with the physician about the need for a topical antimicrobial to minimize bacterial growth.

Black wounds are covered with thick necrotic tissue, or eschar. Black wounds require **debridement** (removal of the necrotic material). Removal of nonviable tissue from a wound must occur before the wound can heal. Debridement may be achieved in four different ways: sharp, mechanical, chemical, and autolytic. In *sharp debridement* a scalpel or scissors is used to separate and remove dead tissue. In many settings, specially trained nurses, physical therapists, and physician's assistants are permitted to perform sharp debridement. *Mechanical debridement* is accomplished through scrubbing force or wet-to-damp

TABLE 34–4 Mechanical Devices for Reducing Pressure on Body Parts (continued)

Device	Description/Comments	
Alternating pressure mattress	Composed of a number of cells in which the pressure alternately increases and decreases; uses a pump (see Figure 34–8 ■).	**Figure 34–8** ■ Alternating pressure mattress (Ease). (Courtesy of EASE.)
Water bed	Special mattress filled with water; controls temperature of water.	
Air-fluidized (AF) bed (static high-air-loss bed)	Forced temperature-controlled air is circulated around millions of tiny silicone-coated beads, producing a fluidlike movement. Provides uniform support to body contours. Decreases skin maceration by its drying effect. Moisture from the client penetrates the bedsheet and soaks the beads. Air flow forces the beads away from the client and rapidly dries the sheet. A major disadvantage is that the head of the bed cannot be elevated (see Figure 34–9 ■).	**Figure 34–9** ■ Air-fluidized bed. (Clinitron). (Courtesy of Hill-Rom Services, Inc. Reprinted with permission. All rights reserved.)
Static low-air-loss (LAL) bed	Consists of many air-filled cushions divided into four or five sections. Separate controls permit each section to be inflated to a different level of firmness; thus pressure can be reduced on bony prominences but increased under other body areas for support (see Figure 34–10 ■).	**Figure 34–10** ■ Low-air-loss bed. (Therapulse® II-Kinetic Concepts Inc.).
Active or second-generation LAL bed	Like the static LAL, but in addition greatly pulsates or rotates from side to side, thus stimulating capillary blood flow and facilitating movement of pulmonary secretions.	

TABLE 34–5 Dressings for Pressure Ulcers

Dressing	Mechanism of Action	Stage			
		I	II	III	IV
Dry gauze	Wicks drainage away from wound surface.			✓	✓
Wet-to-damp gauze	Maintains moist wound environment, wicks drainage away from wound surface.			✓	✓
Transparent barrier	Retains wound moisture, allows gas exchange, does not stick to wound surface.	✓	✓		
Hydrocolloid	Occlusive, repels moisture and dirt, maintains moist wound environment.	✓		✓	
Hydrogel	Maintains moist wound environment.		✓	✓	✓
Alginate	Maintains moist wound environment, absorbs exudate.			✓	✓

Note: Some dressings may be used on other pressure ulcer stages.

Practice Guidelines
Treating Pressure Ulcers

- Minimize direct pressure on the ulcer. Reposition the client at least every 2 hours. Make a schedule, and record position changes on the client's chart.
- Clean the pressure ulcer with every dressing change. The method of cleaning depends on the stage of the ulcer and agency protocol. For example, a whirlpool bath may be indicated for a stage I ulcer and a wound irrigation for a stage IV ulcer. Procedure 34–4 details the steps involved in irrigating a wound.
- Clean and dress the ulcer using surgical asepsis. Refrain from using antiseptics, such as alcohol, that are vasoconstrictors and reduce blood flow to the area.
- If the pressure ulcer is infected, obtain a sample of the drainage for culture and sensitivity to antiseptic agents (see Procedure 34–1).
- If the client cannot keep weight off the pressure ulcer, use pressure-relieving devices.
- Teach the client to move, even if only slightly, to relieve pressure.
- Provide range-of-motion (ROM) exercises as the client's condition permits.

Research Note
Can Radiant Heat Help Heal Pressure Ulcers?

Kloth, Berman, Nett, Papanek, and Dumit-Minkel (2002) reported previous evidence that warming of wounds using noncontact radiant heat at body temperature increased healing. This is referred to as *noncontact normothermic wound therapy* (NNWT). The purpose of this study was to compare the use of NNWT to standard therapy in stage III and IV pressure ulcers randomly assigned to treatment. Standard therapy consisted of use of moisture-retentive dressings, changed daily after irrigating the wound with normal saline. Only hydrofibers, alginates, hydrogels, hydrocolloids, saline-moistened gauze, and saline—impregnated gauze were used; no products containing enzymes, pastes, and other impregnated dressings were allowed. For the wounds in the experimental group, the wound was irrigated daily and a sterile noncontact wound dressing was applied constantly. A radiant heating element in the dressing was activated to give constant heat at 38C for 1 hour, three times a day for 12 weeks or until the wound was healed. The results of the study indicated that the 21 NNWT wounds healed faster than the 22 control wounds, especially when the large wounds in each group were compared.

Implications: Due to the extreme impact of pressure ulcers on clients and the health care system, new and more effective means of healing these wounds should always be explored. The use of heat to enhance blood flow to wound areas has been used for many years but former methods of heat delivery such as "heat lamps" and heating pads have not shown positive results and, sometimes, caused additional injury. NNWT uses normothermic (body temperature) heat and thus avoids the risk of burning or the body's compensatory vasoconstriction that can occur with higher temperatures. Additional research will be needed to determine if these results can be repeated with larger numbers and diverse populations.

Note: From "A Randomized Controlled Clinical Trial to Evaluate the Effects of Noncontact Normothermic Wound Therapy on Chronic Full-Thickness Pressure Ulcers," by W. C. Kloth, J. E. Berman, M. Nett, P. E. Papanek, and S. Dumit-Minkel, 2002, *Advances in Skin & Wound Care,* 15, p. 276.

---

dressings. *Chemical debridement* is more selective than sharp or mechanical techniques. Collagenase enzyme agents such as papain-urea are currently most recommended for this use. In *autolytic debridement,* dressings that contain wound moisture, such as transparent films, trap the wound drainage against the eschar. The body's own enzymes in the drainage break down the necrotic tissue. Although this method takes longer than the other three, it is the most selective and therefore causes the least damage to healthy surrounding and healing issues. When the eschar is removed, the wound is treated as yellow, then red. When more than one color is present, the nurse treats the most serious color first, that is, black, then yellow, then red.

Dressing Wounds

Dressings are applied for the following purposes:

- To protect the wound from mechanical injury
- To protect the wound from microbial contamination
- To provide or maintain high humidity of the wound
- To provide thermal insulation
- To absorb drainage or debride a wound or both
- To prevent hemorrhage (when applied as a pressure dressing or with elastic bandages)
- To splint or immobilize the wound site and thereby facilitate healing and prevent injury.

Types of Dressing. Various dressing materials are available to cover wounds. The type of dressing used depends on (a) the location, size, and type of the wound; (b) the amount of exudate; (c) whether the wound requires debridement or is infected; and (d) such considerations as frequency of dressing change, ease or difficulty of dressing application, and cost. Table 34–6 describes these materials.

Common gauze dressings (Figure 34–11 ■) and other dressing materials are used for specific types and conditions of wounds.

Transparent Wound Barriers. Transparent wound barriers are often applied to wounds including ulcerated or burned skin areas. These dressings offer several advantages:

- They act as temporary skin.
- They are nonporous, self-adhesive dressings that do not require changing as other dressings do. They are often left in place until healing has occurred or as long as they remain intact.
- Because they are transparent, the wound can be assessed through them.

TABLE 34-6 Selected Types of Wound Dressings

Dressing	Description	Purpose	Examples
Transparent adhesive films/ wound barriers	Adhesive plastic, semipermeable, nonabsorbent dressings allow exchange of oxygen between the atmosphere and wound bed. They are impermeable to bacteria and water.	To provide protection against contamination and friction; to maintain a clean moist surface that facilitates cellular migration; to provide insulation by preventing fluid evaporation; and to facilitate wound assessment	Op-Site, Tegaderm, Bioclusive
Impregnated nonadherent dressings	Woven or nonwoven cotton or synthetic materials are impregnated with petrolatum, saline, zinc-saline, antimicrobials, or other agents. Require secondary dressings to secure them in place, retain moisture, and provide wound protection.	To cover, soothe, and protect partial-and full-thickness wounds without exudate	Adaptic, Carrasyn, Xeroform
Hydrocolloids	Waterproof adhesive wafers, pastes, or powders. Wafers, designed to be worn for up to 7 days, consist of two layers. The inner adhesive layer has particles that absorb exudate and form a hydrated gel over the wound; the outer film provides a seal.	To absorb exudate; to produce a moist environment that facilitates healing but does not cause maceration of surrounding skin; to protect the wound from bacterial contamination, foreign debris, and urine or feces; and to prevent shearing	DuoDerm, Comfeel, Tegasorb, Restore, Replicare
Hydrogels	Glycerin or water-based non-adhesive jellylike sheets, granules, or gels are oxygen permeable, unless covered by a plastic film. May require secondary occlusive dressing.	To liquefy necrotic tissue or slough, rehydrate the wound bed, and fill in dead space	Aquasorb, Elasto-Gel, Vigilon
Polyurethane foams	Nonadherent hydrocolloid dressings; these need to have their edges taped down or sealed. Require secondary dressings to obtain an occlusive environment. Surrounding skin must be protected to prevent maceration.	To absorb light to moderate amounts of exudate; to debride wounds	Lyofoam, Allevyn, Vigifoam, Flexzan
Exudate absorbers (alginates)	Nonadherent dressings of powder, beads or granules, ropes, sheets, or paste conform to the wound surface and absorb up to 20 times their weight in exudate; require a secondary dressing.	To provide a moist wound surface by interacting with exudate to form a gelatinous mass; to absorb exudate; to eliminate dead space or pack wounds; and to support debridement	Debrisan, Sorbsan, Kaltostat, Algiderm

- Because they are occlusive, the wound remains moist and retains the serous exudate, which promotes epithelial growth, hastens healing, and reduces the risk of infection.
- Because they are elastic, they can be placed over a joint without disrupting the client's mobility.
- They adhere only to the skin area around the wound and not to the wound itself because they keep the wound moist.

- They allow the client to shower or bathe without removing the dressing.
- They can be removed without damaging wound tissues.

Procedure 34–2 describes how to apply a transparent wound barrier.

Figure 34–11 ■ Some frequently used dressing materials (clockwise from bottom left): surgipad or abdominal pad, 2 × 2 gauze, 2-in. roller gauze, 4 × 4 gauze, 4-in. roller gauze, and nonadherent absorbent dressing.

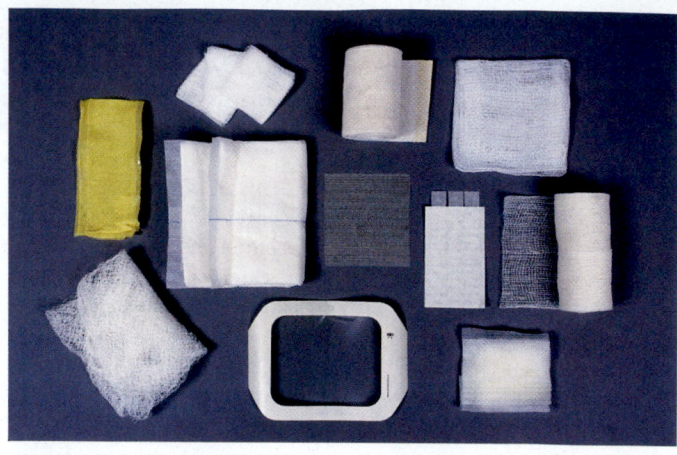

Procedure 34-2 Applying a Transparent Wound Barrier

Purposes

- To provide a moist wound environment and promote wound healing
- To protect the wound from trauma and infectious agents
- To facilitate assessment of wound healing

ASSESSMENT

Assess

- Appearance and size of the wound or at-risk skin area
- Amount and character of exudate
- For complaints of discomfort
- For signs of infection such as fever, chills, or elevated WBC count

PLANNING

If possible, review the client record to note details regarding previous transparent wound dressing changes.

Delegation

Applying a transparent wound dressing requires the use of sterile technique, knowledge of wound healing, and potential problem solving to ensure client safety; therefore, the nurse needs to perform this skill and does not delegate it to UAP.

Equipment
- Clean gloves
- Sterile gloves (optional)
- Hair scissors or clippers
- Alcohol or acetone
- Moisture-proof bag
- Sterile gauze and the wound-cleaning agents specified by the physician or agency (e.g., sterile saline)
- Wound barrier dressing
- Scissors
- Paper tape

IMPLEMENTATION

Preparation

Review the order regarding frequency and type of dressing change, and determine agency protocol about solutions used to clean the wound and whether clean or sterile technique is to be used. Many agencies recommend clean rather than sterile technique for chronic wounds such as a pressure ulcer. If possible, schedule the dressing change at a time convenient for the client. Some dressing changes require only a few minutes and others can take much longer.

Performance

1. Explain to the client what you are going to do, why it is necessary, and how he or she can cooperate. Discuss how the results will be used in planning further care or treatments.
2. Wash hands and observe appropriate infection control procedures.
3. Provide for client privacy. Assist the client to a comfortable position in which the wound can be readily exposed. Expose only the wound area, using a bath blanket to cover the client, if necessary. *Undue exposure is physically and psychologically distressing to most people.*
4. Apply clean gloves and remove the existing dressing, discarding it into the moisture-proof bag.
5. Thoroughly clean the skin area around the wound.
   - Put on clean gloves.
   - Clean the skin well with normal saline or a mild cleansing agent. Always rinse the adjacent skin well before applying a dressing.
   - Clip the hair about 5 cm (2 in.) around the wound area if indicated.
   - Remove gloves and dispose of them in the moisture-proof bag.

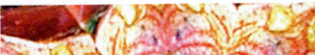

Procedure 34-2 Applying a Transparent Wound Barrier *continued*

IMPLEMENTATION *continued*

6. Clean the wound if indicated.
   - Put on clean or sterile gloves in accordance with agency practice.
   - Clean the wound with the prescribed solution.
   - Dry the surrounding skin with dry gauze.
7. Assess the wound.
8. Apply the wound barrier.
   - Review the instructions on the barrier package. Remove part of the paper backing on the dressing (Figure 34–12 ■).
   - Apply the dressing at one edge of the wound site, allowing at least 2.5-cm (1-in.) coverage of the skin surrounding the wound.
   - Gently lay or press the barrier over the wound. Keep it free of wrinkles, but avoid stretching it too tightly. *A stretched dressing restricts mobility.*
   - Remove and dispose of gloves appropriately.
9. Reinforce the dressing only if absolutely needed.

- Apply paper or other porous tape to "window frame" the edges of the dressing.
10. Assess the wound at least daily.
    - Determine the extent of serous fluid accumulation under the dressing, wound healing, and the need to repair the dressing.

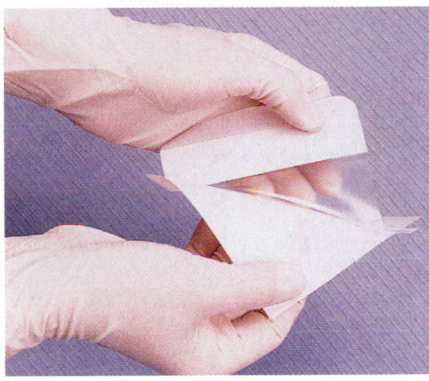

Figure 34–12 ■ A transparent wound dressing.

- If excessive serum has accumulated, consider replacing the transparent wound barrier with a more absorbent type of dressing, such as hydrocolloid.
- If the dressing is leaking, remove it and apply another dressing.
11. Document the dressing change, wound status, and the client's response in the client record using forms or checklists supplemented by narrative notes when appropriate. Many agencies use a designated wound/skin documentation sheet (Figure 34–13 ■).

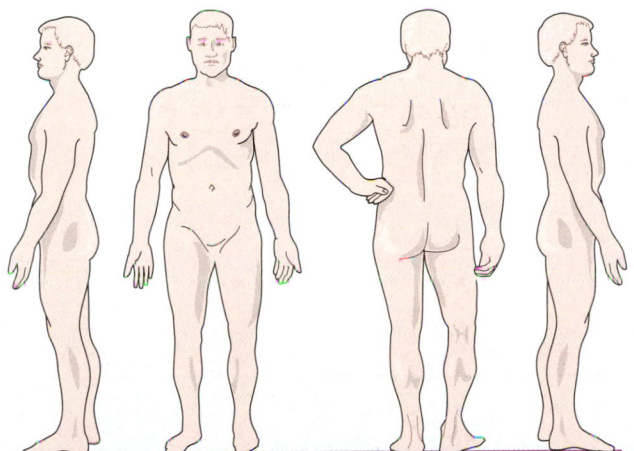

Description of Pressure Ulcers & Classification

Stage I: Characterized by erythema that does not resolve within minutes of pressure relief. Skin remains intact.

Stage II: Partial thickness loss of skin involving the epidermis or dermis – may involve both. The ulcer is superficial and may present as a blister, abrasion, or shallow crater. Free of eschar.

Stage III: Full thickness loss which goes through the dermis to the subcutaneous tissue but does not extend through the underlying fascia. Appears as a crater and may include undermining.

Stage IV: Full thickness skin loss with extensive damage through the subcutaneous tissue to the fascia and may involve muscle layers, joint, and/or bone.

| | | | | |
| 1 cm | 2 cm | 3 cm | 4 cm | 5 cm |

- IDENTIFY LOCATION OF ALL PRESSURE ULCERS ABOVE BY NUMBERING (1, 2, 3): IF MORE THAN 3, USE ADDITIONAL SHEET.

- COMPLETE CHART BELOW FOR SITE #1, USE REVERSE SIDE FOR SITES 2 & 3.

Patient Admitted On: _____

Date Sheet Initiated: _____

Pressure relief methods in use:

❑ Low Airloss Bed

❑ Low Airloss Mattress Overlay

❑ Turning Q2h when pt. supine and Q1h if HOB↑

❑ Pressure Reducing Mattress Overlay

❑ Other _____

Date MD notified of ulcer:

_____

Figure 34–13 ■ Wound/skin documentation sheet.

continued on page 878

Procedure 34-2 Applying a Transparent Wound Barrier *continued*

IMPLEMENTATION *continued*

DOCUMENT WEEKLY AND P.R.N. SIGNIFICANT CHANGE IN ULCER'S APPEARANCE

SITE #1: LOCATION	DESCRIBE TREATMENT:			FREQUENCY:
DATE / TIME				
DIMENSIONS: LENGTH (in. cm.)				
WIDTH				
DEPTH				
ODOR (None or Foul)				
DESCRIBE DRAINAGE (Purulent, Serous, Serosanguinous) & AMOUNT (Scant, Moderate, Copious)				
STAGE (See Above)				
COMMENTARY: ie: Describe tissue surrounding ulcer: is there undermining? % necrotic vs % granular, etc.				
NURSE				

WOUND/SKIN DOCUMENTATION SHEET

Figure 34–13 ■ Wound/skin documentation sheet. *continued*

EVALUATION

■ Perform follow-up based on findings that deviate from expected or normal for the client. Relate findings to previous assessment data if available.

■ Report significant deviations from normal to the physician.

Hydrocolloid Dressings. Hydrocolloid dressings (see Table 34–6) are frequently used over venous stasis leg ulcers and pressure ulcers. These dressings offer several advantages:

• They last a long time.
• They do not need a "cover" dressing and are water resistant, so the client can shower or bathe.

• They can be molded to uneven body surfaces.
• They act as temporary skin and provide an effective bacterial barrier.
• They decrease pain and thus reduce the need for analgesics.
• They absorb some drainage and therefore can be used on draining wounds.
• They contain wound odor.

These dressings have certain limitations, however:

- They are opaque and obscure wound visibility.
- They have a limited absorption capacity.
- They can facilitate anaerobic bacterial growth.
- They can soften and wrinkle at the edges with wear and movement.
- They can be difficult to remove and may leave a residue on the skin.

Because of these limitations, hydrocolloid dressings should not be used for infected wounds or those with deep tracts or *fistulas* (abnormal passage that develops between a hollow organ and the skin or between two hollow organs).

Procedure 34–3 describes how to apply hydrocolloid dressings.

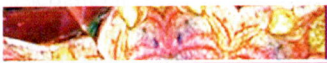

Procedure 34-3 Applying a Hydrocolloid Dressing

Purposes

- To maintain a moist wound surface and promote healing
- To prevent the entrance of microorganisms into the wound
- To minimize wound discomfort
- To promote autolysis of necrotic material by white blood cells
- To decrease the frequency of dressing changes

ASSESSMENT

Assess

- Appearance and size of the wound or at-risk skin area
- Amount and character of exudate
- For complaints of discomfort
- For signs of infection such as fever, chills, or elevated WBC count

PLANNING

If possible, review the client record to note details regarding previous hydrocolloid dressing changes.

Delegation

Applying a hydrocolloid dressing requires the use of sterile technique, knowledge of wound healing, and potential problem solving to ensure client safety; therefore, the nurse needs to perform this skill and does not delegate it to UAP.

Equipment

- Clean gloves
- Sterile gloves (optional)
- Dressing set including scissors and paper tape
- Moisture-proof bag
- Sterile gauze and the wound-cleaning agents specified by the physician or agency (e.g., sterile saline)
- Hydrocolloid dressing at least 3–4 cm (1.5 in.) larger than wound on all four sides
- Skin barrier or skin prep (optional)

IMPLEMENTATION

Preparation

- Review the order regarding frequency and type of dressing change, and determine agency protocol about solutions used to clean the wound and whether clean or sterile technique is to be used. Many agencies recommend clean rather than sterile technique for chronic wounds such as a pressure ulcer.
- Change the dressing if it leaks, is dislodged, or develops an odor. Otherwise, it may remain in place up to 1 week.
- If possible, schedule the dressing change at a time convenient for the client. Some dressing changes require only a few minutes and others can take much longer.

Performance

1. Explain to the client what you are going to do, why it is necessary, and how he or she can cooperate. Discuss how the results will be used in planning further care or treatments.
2. Wash hands and observe appropriate infection control procedures.
3. Provide for client privacy. Assist the client to a comfortable position in which the wound can be readily exposed. Expose only the wound area, using a bath blanket to cover the client, if necessary. *Undue exposure is physically and psychologically distressing to most people.*
4. Apply clean gloves and remove the existing dressing, discarding it into the moisture-proof bag.
5. Thoroughly clean the skin area around the wound.
   - Put on clean gloves.
   - Clean the skin well but gently with normal saline or a mild cleansing agent. Always rinse the adjacent skin well before applying a dressing.
   - Clip the hair about 5 cm (2 in.) around the wound area if indicated.
   - Leave the residue that is difficult to remove on the skin. It will wear off in time. Attempts to remove residue can irritate the surrounding skin.
   - Remove gloves and dispose of them in the moisture-proof bag.

continued on page 880

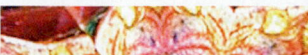

Procedure 34-3 Applying a Hydrocolloid Dressing *continued*

IMPLEMENTATION *continued*

6. Clean the wound if indicated.
   - Put on clean or sterile gloves in accordance with agency practice.
   - Clean the wound with the prescribed solution.
   - Dry the surrounding skin with dry gauze.
7. Assess the wound.
8. Apply the dressing.
   - Follow the manufacturer's instructions. Hold the dressing in place for about 1 minute with your hand. *The warmth helps the dressing conform and adhere.*

- Remove and dispose of the gloves.
- Optional: Apply tape to "window frame" the edges of the dressing or according to agency protocol. *Taping prevents the dressing from sticking to bed linens and the edges from lifting.*
9. Assess and change the dressing as indicated.
   - Inspect the dressing at least daily for leakage, dislodgement, odor, and wrinkling.

- Change the dressing if any of these signs are present.
10. Document the dressing change and the client's response in the client record using forms or checklists supplemented by narrative notes when appropriate. Many agencies use a designated wound/skin documentation sheet (see Figure 34–13).

EVALUATION

■ Perform follow-up based on findings that deviate from expected or normal for the client. Relate findings to previous assessment data if available.

■ Report significant deviations from normal to the physician.

Securing Dressings. The nurse tapes the dressing over the wound, ensuring that the dressing covers the entire wound and does not become dislodged. The correct type of tape must be selected for the purpose. Elastic tape can provide pressure; nonallergenic tape is used when a client is allergic to other tape. The nurse follows these steps:

1. Place the tape so that the dressing cannot be folded back to expose the wound. Place strips at the ends of the dressing, and space tapes evenly in the middle (see Figure 34–14 ■, *A*).
2. Ensure that the tape is long and wide enough to adhere to several inches of skin on each side of the dressing, but not so long or wide that the tape loosens with activity (see Figure 34–14 ■, *B*).
3. Place the tape in the opposite direction from the body action, for example, across a body joint or crease, not lengthwise (see Figure 34–15 ■).

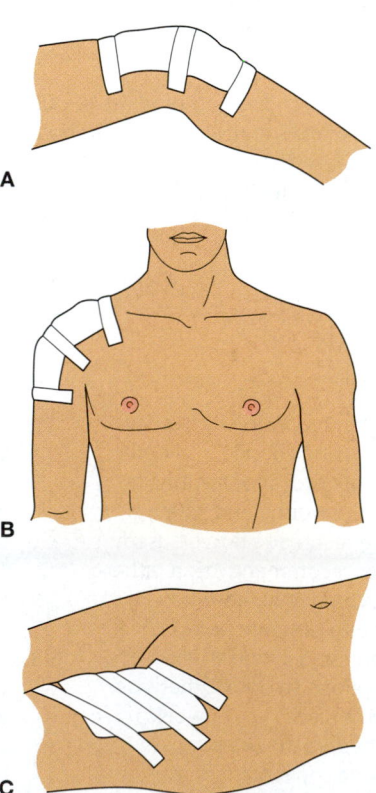

B

C

Figure 34–15 ■ Dressings over moving parts must remain secure in spite of the client's movement. Place the tape over a joint at a right angle to the direction, the joint moves.

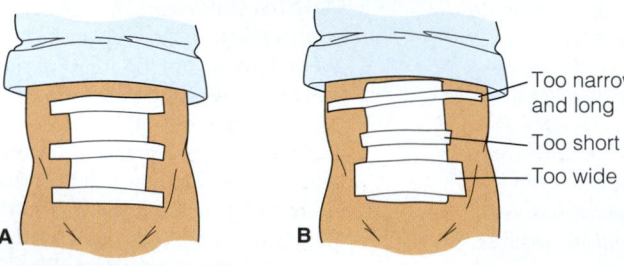

Too narrow and long
Too short
Too wide

A   **B**

Figure 34–14 ■ The strips of tape should be placed at the ends of the dressing and must be sufficiently long and wide to secure the dressing. The tape should adhere to intact skin.

Montgomery straps (tie tapes) are used for wounds requiring frequent dressing changes (see Figure 34–16 ■). These straps prevent skin irritation and discomfort caused by removing the adhesive each time the dressing is changed.

Cleaning Wounds

Wound cleaning involves the removal of debris (i.e., foreign materials, excess slough, necrotic tissue, bacteria, and other microorganisms). The choices of cleaning agent and method depend largely on agency protocol and the physician's preference. Recommended guidelines for cleaning wounds are shown in the accompanying Practice Guidelines.

Commonly used methods to clean a surgical wound and drain site are shown in Chapter 35. ∞

Wound Irrigation and Packing.

An **irrigation (lavage)** is the washing or flushing out of an area. Sterile technique is required for a wound irrigation because there is a break in the skin integrity.

Using piston syringes instead of bulb syringes to irrigate a wound reduces the risk of aspirating drainage and provides safe, effective pressure. For deep wounds with small openings, a sterile straight catheter may also be necessary. Irrigation pressures should range from 4 to 15 pounds per square inch (psi). Below 4 psi, the irrigation may not be effective, and above 15 psi it may damage tissues. A 35-mL syringe with a 19-gauge needle or catheter provides approximately 8 psi (Bergstrom et al., 1994). Some providers advocate the use of a commercial oral water jet for wound cleansing. This can be effective if kept at the lowest setting that provides the desired pressure. Frequently used irrigation solutions are sterile normal saline, lactated Ringer's solution, and antibiotic solutions. Procedure 34–4 details the steps involved in irrigating a wound.

Gauze **packing** using the wet-to-damp technique has been used to pack wounds that require debridement. In this technique, moist 4 × 4 non-cotton-filled gauzes are packed in the

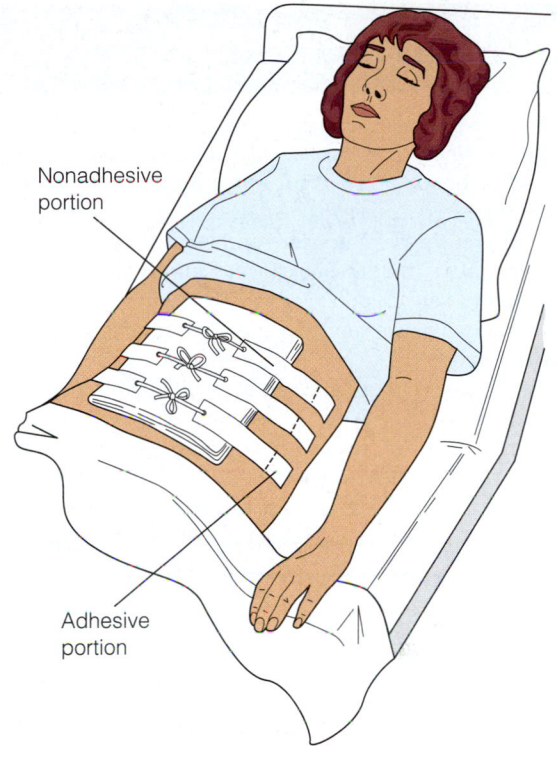

Nonadhesive portion

Adhesive portion

Figure 34–16 ■ Montgomery straps, or tie tapes, are used to secure large dressings that require frequent changing.

MediaLink | www | ENTEROSTOMAL THERAPIST APPLICATION

wound to absorb exudate but they are not allowed to dry before removal. However, research has shown that newer advanced dressing materials have significant advantages over the use of gauze (Ovington, 2001b). See the accompanying Practice Guidelines for issues related to using wet-to-damp dressings.

Practice Guidelines
Cleaning Wounds

- Use solutions such as isotonic saline or tap water to clean or irrigate wounds (Ovington, 2001a). If antimicrobial solutions are used, make sure they are well diluted.
- When possible, warm the solution to body temperature before use. *This prevents lowering the wound temperature, which slows the healing process.*
- If a wound is grossly contaminated by foreign material, bacteria, slough, or necrotic tissue, clean the wound at every dressing change. *Foreign bodies and devitalized tissue act as a focus for infection and can delay healing.*
- If a wound is clean, has little exudate, and reveals healthy granulation tissue, avoid repeated cleaning. *Unnecessary cleaning can delay wound healing by traumatizing newly produced, delicate tissues, reducing the surface temperature of the wound, and removing exudate which itself may have bactericidal properties.*

- Use gauze squares. Avoid using cotton balls and other products that shed fibers onto the wound surface. *The fibers become embedded in granulation tissue and can act as foci for infection. They may also stimulate "foreign body" reactions, prolonging the inflammatory phase of healing and delaying the healing process.*
- Clean superficial noninfected wounds by irrigating them with normal saline. *The hydraulic pressure of an irrigating stream of fluid dislodges contaminating debris and reduces bacterial colonization.*
- *To retain wound moisture,* avoid drying a wound after cleaning it.
- Hold cleaning sponges with forceps or with a sterile gloved hand.
- Clean from the wound in an outward direction to avoid transferring organisms from the surrounding skin into the wound.
- Consider not cleaning the wound at all if it appears to be clean.

Practice Guidelines
Issues Related to the Use of Wet-to-Damp Dressings

- To keep the gauze damp, change or remoisten with saline frequently. *If the gauze is allowed to dry out, removal results in pain and disruption of wound healing through drying of the surface and tissue adherence to the gauze.*
- A wound requires moisture and warmth for optimal healing. Evaporation of the saline causes wound cooling, vasoconstriction, and dehydration.
- Moistened gauze cannot prevent introduction of bacteria into the wound.
- Gauze is easy to use and can be manipulated to fit almost any wound.
- The diversity of advanced dressings may be confusing for clients and health care providers.
- Although gauze is much less expensive than advanced dressings (e.g., polymers, alginates, collagens), the cost per week can

be higher due to the number of dressing changes required. Including the price of the dressing, gloves, saline, and tape, the materials cost for a gauze dressing change twice per day versus an advanced dressing three times per week is very similar. However, at approximately $100 per nurse home visit, the gauze dressing is almost five times as expensive.
- Wounds have been shown to heal twice as quickly with advanced dressings compared to gauze (Ovington, 2001b).

Conclusions: Practitioners should become familiar with the range and uses of advanced dressing materials. The selection of dressing materials must consider time, material cost, client comfort, and speed of wound healing.

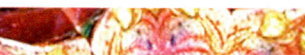

Procedure 34-4 Irrigating a Wound

Purposes

- To clean the area
- To apply heat and hasten the healing process
- To apply an antimicrobial solution

ASSESSMENT

Assess

- The client's record to determine previous appearance and size of the wound
- The character of the exudate
- Presence of pain and the time of the last pain medication
- Clinical signs of systemic infection
- Allergies to the wound irrigation agent or tape

PLANNING

- Before irrigating a wound, determine (a) the type of irrigating solution to be used, (b) the frequency of irrigations, and (c) the temperature of the solution.
- If possible, schedule the irrigation at a time convenient for the client. Some irrigations require only a few minutes and others can take much longer.

Delegation

Due to the need for aseptic technique and assessment skills, wound irrigations are not delegated to UAP. However, UAP may observe the wound and dressing during usual care and must report abnormal findings to the nurse. Abnormal findings must be validated and interpreted by the nurse.

Equipment
- Sterile dressing equipment and dressing materials
- Sterile syringes (e.g., a 30- to 60-mL syringe) with a catheter of an appropriate size (e.g., #18 or #19) or an irrigating (catheter) tip syringe
- Sterile basin for the irrigating solution
- Moisture-proof bag
- Basin to receive the irrigation returns
- Irrigating solution, usually 200 mL (6.5 oz) of solution warmed to body temperature, according to the agency's or physician's choice
- Clean gloves
- Sterile gloves
- Moisture-proof sterile drape

IMPLEMENTATION

Preparation

Check that the irrigating fluid is at the proper temperature.

Performance

1. Explain to the client what you are going to do, why it is necessary, and how

he or she can cooperate. Discuss how the results will be used in planning further care or treatments.
2. Wash hands and observe appropriate infection control procedures.

3. Provide for client privacy.
4. Prepare the client.
   - Assist the client to a position in which the irrigating solution will flow by gravity from the upper end

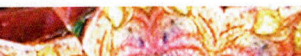

Procedure 34-4 Irrigating a Wound *continued*

IMPLEMENTATION *continued*

of the wound to the lower end and then into the basin.
- Place the waterproof drape over the client and the bed.
- Put on clean gloves and remove and discard the old dressing.
- If indicated, clean the wound from the center of the wound outward, using circular strokes.
- Use a separate swab for each stroke, and discard each swab after use. *This prevents the introduction of microorganisms to other wound areas.*
- Assess the wound and drainage.
- Remove and discard clean gloves.

5. Prepare the equipment.
   - Open the sterile dressing set and supplies.
   - Pour the ordered solution into the solution container.
   - Position the basin below the wound to receive the irrigating fluid.

6. Irrigate the wound.
   - Instill a steady stream of irrigating solution into the wound. Make sure all areas of the wound are irrigated.

- Use either a syringe with a catheter attached or with an irrigating tip to flush the wound (Figure 34–17 ■).

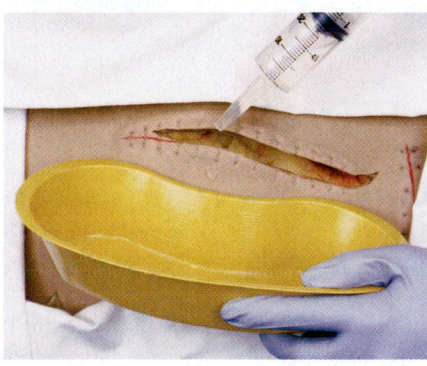

Figure 34–17 ■ Irrigating a wound.

- If you are using a catheter to reach tracks or crevices, insert the catheter into the wound until resistance is met. Do not force the catheter. *Forcing the catheter can cause tissue damage.*

- Continue irrigating until the solution becomes clear (no exudate is present). *The irrigation washes away tissue debris and drainage so that later returns are clearer.*
- Dry the area around the wound. *Moisture left on the skin promotes the growth of microorganisms and can cause skin irritation and breakdown.*

7. Assess and dress the wound.
   - Assess the appearance of the wound again, noting in particular the type and amount of exudate still present and the presence and extent of granulation tissue.
   - Using sterile technique, apply a dressing to the wound based on the amount of drainage expected (see Table 34–6).

8. Document the irrigation and the client's response in the client record using forms or checklists supplemented by narrative notes when appropriate. Many agencies use a designated wound/skin documentation sheet (see Figure 34–13).

EVALUATION

- Perform follow-up based on findings that deviate from expected or normal for the client. Relate findings to previous assessment data if available.

- Report significant deviations from normal to the physician.

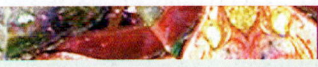

Lifespan Considerations

Pressure Ulcer and Wound Care

Children
- Remind the child not to touch the wound, drains, or dressing. Cover with an appropriate bandage that will remain intact during the child's usual activities. Cover a transparent dressing with opaque material if viewing the site is distressing to the child. Restrain only when all alternatives have been tried and when absolutely necessary.
- Demonstrate wound care on a doll. Reassure that the wound will not be permanent and does not mean anything will fall out of the body.

Elders
- Hold wrinkled skin taut during application of a transparent dressing. Obtain assistance if needed.

- Skin is more fragile and can easily tear with removal of tape (especially adhesive tape). Use paper tape and tape remover as indicated, keeping tape use to the minimum required. Use extreme caution during tape removal.
- Older adults who are in long-term care facilities often have the following factors: immobility, malnutrition, and incontinence—all of which increase the risk for development of skin breakdown.
- Skin breakdown can occur as quickly as within 2 hours, so assessments should be done with each repositioning of the client.
- A thorough assessment of a client's heels should be done every shift. The skin can break down quickly from friction of movement in bed.

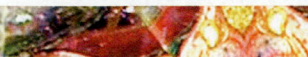

Home Care Considerations

Wound Care

- Perform appropriate client teaching for promoting wound healing and maintenance of healthy skin.
- Instruct the client and family on where to obtain needed supplies. Be sensitive to the cost of dressings (e.g., transparent barriers are costly) and suggest less expensive alternatives if necessary. Be creative in the use of household items for padding pressure areas.

- Instruct the client and family in proper disposal of contaminated dressings. All contaminated items should be double bagged in moisture-proof bags.
- Verify how the client may bathe with the wound (i.e., does the wound need to be covered with a waterproof barrier or should it be cleansed in the shower?).

Many of the techniques described here for dressing wounds may be combined depending on the specific type of wound. In addition, therapies are constantly being designed and evaluated. One example is *vacuum-assisted closure* (VAC), which refers to the use of suction equipment to apply negative pressure to a variety of large or nonhealing wounds. This therapy has been shown to speed tissue generation, reduce swelling around the wound, and enhance wound healing by providing a moist and protected environment (Mendez-Eastman, 2002).

Heat and Cold Applications

Heat and cold are applied to the body for local and systemic effects. Table 34–7 lists the physiologic effects of heat and cold.

Local Effects of Heat. Heat is an old remedy for aches and pains, and people often equate heat with comfort and relief. Heat causes vasodilation and increases blood flow to the affected area, bringing oxygen, nutrients, antibodies, and leukocytes.

Application of heat promotes soft tissue healing and increases suppuration. A possible disadvantage of heat is that it increases capillary permeability, which allows extracellular fluid and substances such as plasma proteins to pass through the capillary walls and may result in edema or an increase in preexisting edema. Heat is often used for clients with musculoskeletal problems such as joint stiffness from arthritis, contractures, and low back pain.

Local Effects of Cold. Generally, the physiologic effects of cold are opposite to the effects of heat. Cold lowers the temperature of the skin and underlying tissues and causes **vasoconstriction.** Vasoconstriction reduces blood flow to the af-

fected area and thus reduces the supply of oxygen and metabolites, decreases the removal of wastes, and produces skin pallor and coolness. Prolonged exposure to cold results in impaired circulation, cell deprivation, and subsequent damage to the tissues from lack of oxygen and nourishment. The signs of tissue damage due to cold are a bluish purple mottled appearance of the skin, numbness, and sometimes blisters and pain. Cold is most often used for sports injuries (e.g., sprains, strains, fractures) to limit postinjury swelling and bleeding.

Systemic Effects of Heat and Cold. Heat applied to a localized body area, particularly a large body area, may cause excessive peripheral vasodilation, which produces a drop in blood pressure. A significant drop in blood pressure can cause fainting. Clients who have heart or pulmonary disease and who have circulatory disturbances such as arteriosclerosis are more prone to this effect than healthy people. With extensive cold applications and vasoconstriction, a client's blood pressure can increase because blood is shunted from the cutaneous circulation to the internal blood vessels. Shivering, a generalized effect of prolonged cold, is a normal response as the body attempts to warm itself.

Thermal Tolerance. Various parts of the body differ in tolerance to heat and cold. The physiologic tolerance of individuals also varies (see Box 34–3). Specific conditions necessitate precautions in the use of hot or cold applications:

- *Neurosensory impairment.* People with sensory impairments are unable to perceive that heat is damaging the tissues and are at risk for burns or are unable to perceive discomfort from cold and prevent tissue injury.
- *Impaired mental status.* People who are confused or have an altered level of consciousness need monitoring during applications to ensure safe therapy.
- *Impaired circulation.* People with peripheral vascular disease, diabetes, or congestive heart failure lack the normal ability to dissipate heat via the blood circulation, which puts them at risk for tissue damage with heat and cold applications.
- *Immediately after injury or surgery.* Heat increases bleeding and swelling.
- *Open wounds.* Cold can decrease blood flow to the wound, thereby inhibiting healing.

Adaptation of Thermal Receptors. Heat and cold receptors adapt to temperature changes. When they are subjected to an

TABLE 34–7 Physiologic Effects of Heat and Cold

Heat	Cold
Vasodilation	Vasoconstriction
Increases capillary permeability	Decreases capillary permeability
Increases cellular metabolism	Decreases cellular metabolism
Increases inflammation	Slows bacterial growth, decreases inflammation
Sedative effect	Local anesthetic effect

■ **Variables Affecting Physiologic Tolerance to Heat and Cold**

Body part. The back of the hand and foot are not very temperature sensitive. In contrast, the inner aspect of the wrist and forearm, the neck, and the perineal area are temperature sensitive.
Size of the exposed body part. The larger the area exposed to heat and cold, the lower the tolerance.
Individual tolerance. The very young and the very old generally have the lowest tolerance. Persons who have neurosensory impairments may have a high tolerance, but the risk of injury is greater.
Length of exposure. People feel hot and cold applications most while the temperature is changing. After a period of time, tolerance increases.
Intactness of skin. Injured skin areas are more sensitive to temperature variations.

abrupt change in temperature, the receptors are strongly stimulated initially. This strong stimulation declines rapidly during the first few seconds and then more slowly during the next half hour or more as the receptors adapt to the new temperature.

Nurses and clients need to understand this adaptive response when applying heat and cold. Clients may be tempted to change the temperature of a thermal application because of the change in thermal sensation following adaptation. Increasing the temperature of a hot application after adaptation can result in serious burns. Decreasing the temperature of a cold application can result in pain and serious impairment of circulation to the body part. Table 34–8 lists temperatures of hot and cold applications.

Rebound Phenomenon.

The rebound phenomenon occurs at the time the maximum therapeutic effect of the hot or cold application is achieved and the opposite effect begins. For example, heat produces maximum vasodilation in 20 to 30 minutes; continuation of the application beyond 30 to 45 minutes brings tissue congestion, and the blood vessels then constrict for reasons unknown. If the heat application is continued, the client is at risk for burns because the constricted blood vessels are unable to dissipate the heat adequately via the blood circulation.

With cold applications, maximum vasoconstriction occurs when the involved skin reaches a temperature of 15C (60F). Below 15C, vasodilation begins. This mechanism is protective: It helps to prevent freezing of body tissues normally exposed to cold, such as the nose and ears. It also explains the ruddiness of the skin of a person who has been walking in cold weather.

An understanding of the rebound phenomenon is essential for the nurse and client. Thermal applications must be halted before the rebound phenomenon begins.

Applying Heat and Cold

Heat can be applied to the body in both dry and moist forms. Dry heat is applied locally by means of a hot water bottle, aquathermia pad, disposable heat pack, or electric pad. Moist heat can be provided by compress, hot pack, soak, or sitz bath. Selected indications for the use of heat and cold are found in Table 34–9.

Dry cold is generally applied locally by means of a cold pack, ice bag, ice glove, or ice collar. Moist cold can be provided by compress or a cooling sponge bath.

For all local applications of heat or cold, the nurse needs to follow these guidelines:

- Determine the client's ability to tolerate the therapy.
- Identify conditions that might contraindicate treatment (e.g., bleeding, circulatory impairment).
- Explain the application to the client.
- Assess the skin area to which the heat or cold will be applied.
- Ask the client to report any discomfort.
- Return to the client 15 minutes after starting the heat or cold, and observe the local skin area for any untoward signs (e.g., redness). Stop the application if any problems occur.
- Remove the equipment at the designated time, and dispose of it appropriately.
- Examine the area to which the heat or cold was applied, and record the client's response.

For contraindications to the use of heat or cold, see Box 34–4.

Hot Water Bag.

A hot water bag or bottle is a common source of dry heat used in the home. It is convenient and relatively inexpensive. However, because of the danger of burning from improper use, many agencies use other means.

TABLE 34–8 Temperatures for Hot and Cold Applications

Description	Temperature	Application
Very cold	Below 15C (59F)	Ice bags
Cold	15–18C (59–65F)	Cold pack
Cool	18–27C (65–80F)	Cold compresses
Tepid	27–37C (80–98F)	Alcohol sponge bath
Warm	37–40C (98–105F)	Warm bath, aquathermia pads
Hot	40–46C (105–115F)	Hot soak, irrigations, hot compresses
Very hot	Above 46C (above 115F)	Hot water bags for adults

TABLE 34–9 Selected Indications of Heat and Cold

Indication	Effect of Heat	Effect of Cold
Muscle spasm	Relaxes muscles and increases their contractility.	Relaxes muscles and decreases muscle contractility.
Inflammation	Increases blood flow, softens exudates.	Vasoconstriction decreases capillary permeability, decreases blood flow, slows cellular metabolism.
Pain	Relieves pain, possibly by promoting muscle relaxation, increasing circulation, and promoting psychologic relaxation and a feeling of comfort; acts as a counterirritant.	Decreases pain by slowing nerve conduction rate and blocking nerve impulses; produces numbness, acts as a counterirritant, increases pain threshold.
Contracture	Reduces contracture and increases joint range of motion by allowing greater distention of muscles and connective tissue.	
Joint stiffness	Reduces joint stiffness by decreasing viscosity of synovial fluid and increasing tissue distensibility.	
Traumatic injury		Decreases bleeding by constricting blood vessels, decreases edema by reducing capillary permeability.

BOX 34–4 ■ Contraindications to the Use of Heat and Cold

Determine the presence of any conditions contraindicating the use of heat:

- *The first 24 hours after traumatic injury.* Heat increases bleeding and swelling.
- *Active hemorrhage.* Heat causes vasodilation and increases bleeding.
- *Noninflammatory edema.* Heat increases capillary permeability and edema.
- *Localized malignant tumor.* Because heat accelerates cell metabolism and cell growth and increases circulation, it may accelerate metastases (secondary tumors).
- *Skin disorder that causes redness or blisters.* Heat can burn or cause further damage to the skin.

Determine the presence of any conditions contraindicating the use of cold:

- *Open wounds.* Cold can increase tissue damage by decreasing blood flow to an open wound.
- *Impaired circulation.* Cold can further impair nourishment of the tissues and cause tissue damage. In clients with Raynaud's disease, cold increases arterial spasm.

- *Allergy or hypersensitivity to cold.* Some clients have an allergy to cold that may be manifested by an inflammatory response, for example, erythema, hives, swelling, joint pain, and occasional muscle spasm. Some react with a sudden increase in blood pressure, which can be hazardous if the person is hypersensitive.

Determine the presence of any conditions indicating the need for special precautions during heat and cold therapy:

- *Neurosensory impairment.* Persons with sensory impairments are unable to perceive that heat is damaging the tissues and are at risk for burns, or they are unable to perceive discomfort from cold and are unable to prevent tissue injury.
- *Impaired mental status.* Persons who are confused or have an altered level of consciousness need monitoring and supervision during applications to ensure safe therapy.
- *Impaired circulation.* Persons with peripheral vascular disease, diabetes, or congestive heart failure lack the normal ability to dissipate heat via the blood circulation, which puts them at risk for tissue damage with heat applications. Cold applications are contraindicated for these people.
- *Open wounds.* Tissues around an open wound are more sensitive to heat and cold.

The following temperatures of the water in the bag are considered safe in most situations and provide the desired effect: normal adult and child over 2 years, 46 to 52C (115 to 125F), debilitated or unconscious adult, or child under 2 years, 40.5 to 46C (105 to 115F).

To apply a hot water bag, the nurse should

- Measure the temperature of the water using a bath thermometer.
- Fill the bag about two-thirds full.
- Expel the remaining air and secure the top. With the air removed, the bag can be molded to the body part.

- Dry the bag and hold it upside down to test for leakage.
- Wrap the bag in a towel or cover and place it on the body site.
- Remove after 30 minutes or in accordance with agency protocol.

Aquathermia Pad. The aquathermia or aquamatic pad (also referred to as a K-pad) is a pad constructed with tubes containing water. The pad is attached by tubing to an electrically powered control unit that has an opening for water and a temperature gauge (Figure 34–18 ■). Some aquathermia pads have an absorbent surface through which moist heat can be applied. The other surface of the pad is waterproof. These pads are disposable.

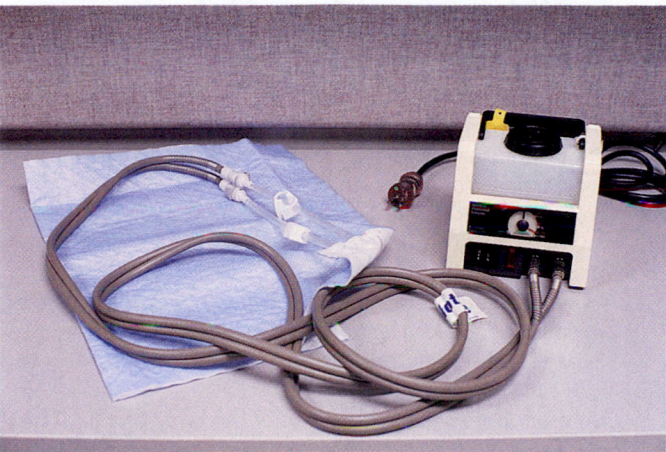

Figure 34–18 ■ An aquathermia heating unit.

To apply an aquathermia pad, the nurse carries out the following steps:

- Fill the reservoir of the unit two-thirds full of distilled water.
- Set the desired temperature. Check the manufacturer's instructions. Most units are set at 40.5C (105F) for adults.
- Cover the pad and plug in the unit. Some manufacturers suggest warming the pad before applying it.
- Apply the pad to the body part. The treatment is usually continued for 30 minutes. Check orders and agency protocol.

Hot and Cold Packs. Commercially prepared hot and cold packs (Figure 34–19 ■) provide heat or cold for a designated time. Directions on the package tell how to initiate the heating or cooling process, for example, by striking, squeezing, or kneading the pack.

Electric Pads. Electric pads provide a constant, even heat, are lightweight, and can be molded to a body part. Electric pads, however, can burn if the setting is too high. Some models have waterproof covers for use when the pad is placed over a moist dressing.

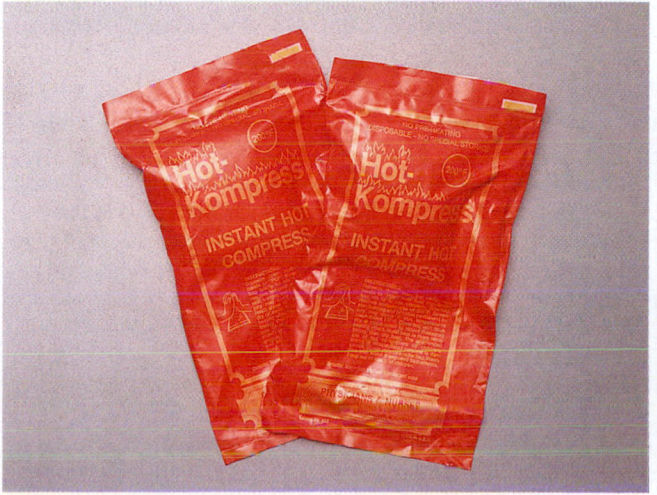

Figure 34–19 ■ Commercially prepared disposable hot packs.

In applying electric pads, the nurse follows these guidelines:

- Do not insert sharp objects (e.g., pins) into the pad. The pin could damage a wire and cause an electric shock.
- Ensure that the body area is dry unless there is a waterproof cover on the pad. Electricity in the presence of water can cause a shock.
- Use pads with a preset heating switch so a client cannot increase the heat.
- Do not place the pad under the client. Heat will not dissipate, and the client may be burned.

Ice Bags, Ice Gloves, and Ice Collars. Ice bags, ice gloves, and ice collars are filled either with ice chips or with an alcohol-based solution. They are applied to the body to provide cold to a localized area (e.g., a collar is often applied to the throat following a tonsillectomy). Always wrap the container in a towel or cover.

Compresses. Compresses can be either warm or cold. A **compress** is a moist gauze dressing applied to a wound. When hot compresses are ordered, the solution is heated to the temperature indicated by the order or according to agency protocol, for example, 40.5C (105F). When there is a break in the skin or when the body part (e.g., an eye) is vulnerable to microbial invasion, sterile technique is necessary; therefore, sterile gloves are needed to apply the compress and all materials must be sterile.

Soak. A soak refers to immersing a body part (e.g., an arm) in a solution or to wrapping a part in gauze dressings and then saturating the dressing with a solution. Sterile technique is generally indicated for open wounds, such as a burn or an unhealed surgical incision. Determine agency protocol regarding the temperature of the solution. Hot soaks are frequently done to soften and remove encrusted secretions and dead tissue.

Sitz Bath. A **sitz bath,** or hip bath, is used to soak a client's pelvic area. The client sits in a special tub or chair and is usually immersed from the midthighs to the iliac crests or umbilicus. Special tubs or chairs are preferred because when the legs are also immersed, as in a regular bathtub, blood circulation to the perineum or pelvic area is decreased. Disposable sitz baths are also available.

The temperature of the water should be from 40 to 43C (105 to 110F), unless the client is unable to tolerate the heat. Determine agency protocol. Some sitz tubs have temperature indicators attached to the water taps. The duration of the bath is generally 15 to 20 minutes, depending on the client's health. To provide a sitz bath

- Assist the client into the tub. Provide support for the client's feet; a footstool can prevent pressure on the backs of the thighs.
- Provide a bath blanket for the client's shoulders, and eliminate drafts to prevent chilling.
- Observe the client closely during the bath for signs of faintness, dizziness, weakness, accelerated pulse rate, and pallor.
- Maintain the water temperature.
- Following the sitz bath, assist the client out of the tub. Help the client to dry.

Cooling Sponge Bath. The purpose of a cooling sponge bath is to reduce a client's fever by promoting heat loss through conduction and vaporization. Cool sponge baths are used with extreme caution, and only for clients with very high temperatures such as over 40C (104F), because rapid skin temperature drop can cause chills that actually increase heat production. The bath is accompanied by antipyretic medication that acts to reset the hypothalamus set point. The temperatures for cooling sponge baths range from 18 to 32C (65 to 93F).

To provide a cooling sponge bath, the nurse should

- Sponge the face, arms, legs, back, and buttocks. The chest and abdomen are not usually sponged. Each area is sponged slowly and gently. Rubbing may increase heat production.
- Leave each area wet and cover with a damp towel.
- Place ice bags and cold packs, if used, or a cool cloth on the forehead for comfort and in each axilla and at the groin. These areas contain large superficial blood vessels that help the transfer of heat.
- Sponge one body part and then another. The sponge bath should take about 30 minutes. A bath given more quickly tends to increase the body's heat production by causing shivering.
- Discontinue the bath if the client becomes pale or cyanotic or shivers, or if the pulse becomes rapid or irregular.
- Reassess the vital signs at 15 minutes and after completing the sponge bath.

Supporting and Immobilizing Wounds

Bandages and binders serve various purposes:

- Supporting a wound (e.g., a fractured bone)
- Immobilizing a wound (e.g., a strained shoulder)
- Applying pressure (e.g., elastic bandages on the lower extremities to improve venous blood flow)
- Securing a dressing (e.g., for an extensive abdominal surgical wound)
- Retaining warmth (e.g., a flannel bandage on a rheumatoid joint)

There are several types of bandages and binders and several ways in which they are applied. When correctly applied, they promote healing, provide comfort, and can prevent injury (see accompanying Practice Guidelines).

Bandages. A **bandage** is a strip of cloth used to wrap some part of the body. Bandages are available in various widths, most commonly 1.5 to 7.5 cm (0.5 to 3 in.) and are usually supplied in rolls for easy application to a body part.

Many types of materials are used for bandages. Gauze is one of the most commonly used, because it is light and porous and readily molds to the body. It is also relatively inexpensive, so it is generally discarded when soiled. Gauze is used to retain dressings on wounds and to bandage the fingers, hands, toes, and feet. It supports dressings and at the same time permits air to circulate; it can be impregnated with petroleum jelly or other medications for application to wounds.

Elasticized bandages are applied to provide pressure to an area. They are commonly used as tensor bandages or as partial

Practice Guidelines
Bandaging

- Whenever possible, bandage the part in its normal position, with the joint slightly flexed *to avoid putting strain on the ligaments and the muscles of the joint.*
- Pad between skin surfaces and over bony prominences *to prevent friction from the bandage and consequent abrasion of the skin.*
- Always bandage body parts by working from the distal to the proximal end *to aid the return flow of venous blood.*
- Bandage with even pressure *to prevent interference with blood circulation.*
- Whenever possible, leave the end of the body part (e.g., the toe) exposed *so that you will be able to determine the adequacy of the blood circulation to the extremity.*
- Cover dressings with bandages at least 5 cm (2 in.) beyond the edges of the dressing *to prevent the dressing and wound from becoming contaminated.*
- Face the client when applying a bandage *to maintain uniform tension and the appropriate direction of the bandage.*

stockings to provide support and improve the venous circulation in the legs.

The width of the bandage used depends on the size of the body part to be bandaged. For example, a 2.5-cm (1-in.) bandage is used for a finger, a 5-cm (2-in.) bandage for an arm, and a 7.5-cm or 10-cm (3-in. or 4-in.) bandage for a leg. Padding (e.g., abdominal pads and gauze squares) is frequently used to cover bony prominences (e.g., the elbow) or to separate skin surfaces (e.g., the fingers).

Before applying a bandage, the nurse needs to know its purpose and to assess the area requiring support (see accompanying Practice Guidelines). When bandages are used to secure dressings, the nurse wears gloves to prevent contact with body fluids.

Practice Guidelines
Assessing before Applying Bandages or Binders

- Inspect and palpate the area for swelling.
- Inspect for the presence of and status of wounds (open wounds will require a dressing before a bandage or binder is applied).
- Note the presence of drainage (amount, color, odor, viscosity).
- Inspect and palpate for adequacy of circulation (skin temperature, color, and sensation). Pale or cyanotic skin, cool temperature, tingling, and numbness can indicate impaired circulation.
- Ask the client about any pain experienced (location, intensity, onset, quality).
- Assess the ability of the client to reapply the bandage or binder when needed.
- Assess the capabilities of the client regarding activities of daily living (e.g., to eat, dress, comb hair, bathe) and assess the assistance required during the convalescence period.

Basic Turns for Roller Bandages. Applying bandages to various parts of the body involves one or more of five basic bandaging turns: circular, spiral, spiral reverse, recurrent, and figure-eight. *Circular* turns are used to anchor bandages and to terminate them. Circular turns usually are not applied directly over a wound because of the discomfort the bandage would cause.

Spiral turns are used to bandage parts of the body that are fairly uniform in circumference, for example, the upper arm or upper leg. *Spiral reverse* turns are used to bandage cylindrical parts of the body that are not uniform in circumference, for example, the lower leg or forearm. *Recurrent* turns are used to cover distal parts of the body, for example, the end of a finger, the skull, or the stump of an amputation. *Figure-eight* turns are used to bandage an elbow, knee, or ankle, because they permit some movement after application.

Circular Turns

- Hold the bandage in your dominant hand, keeping the roll uppermost, and unroll the bandage about 8 cm (3 in.). This length of unrolled bandage allows good control for placement and tension.
- Apply the end of the bandage to the part of the body to be bandaged. Hold the end down with the thumb of the other hand (Figure 34–20 ■).
- Encircle the body part a few times or as often as needed, making sure that each layer overlaps one-half to two-thirds of the previous layer. This provides even support to the area.
- The bandage should be firm, but not too tight. Ask the client if the bandage feels comfortable. A tight bandage can interfere with blood circulation, whereas a loose bandage does not provide adequate protection.
- Secure the end of the bandage with tape or a safety pin over an uninjured area. Pins can cause discomfort when situated over an injured area.

Spiral Turns

- Make two circular turns. Two circular turns anchor the bandage.
- Continue spiral turns at about a 30-degree angle, each turn overlapping the preceding one by two-thirds the width of the bandage (Figure 34–21 ■).

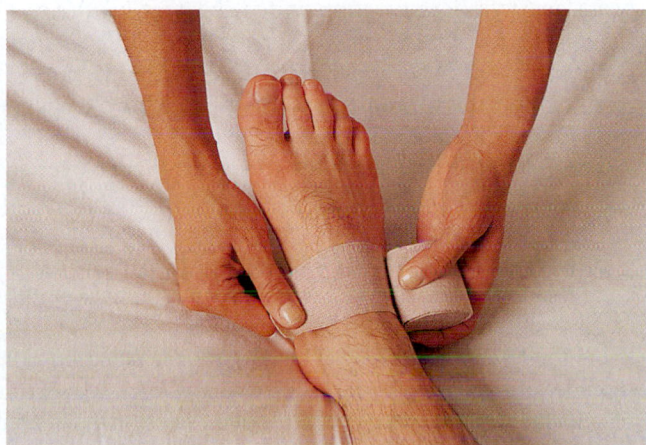

Figure 34–20 ■ Starting a bandage with two circular turns.

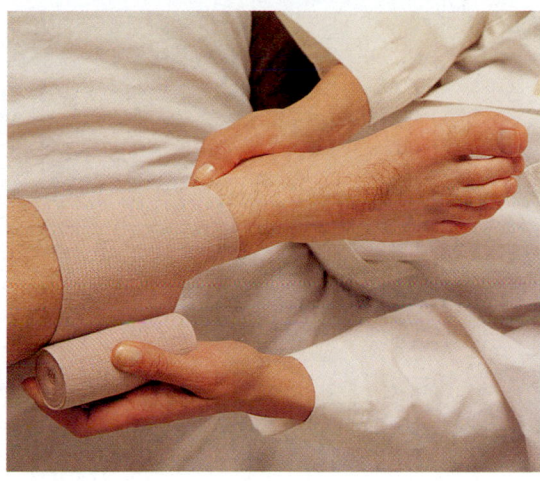

Figure 34–21 ■ Applying spiral turns.

- Terminate the bandage with two circular turns, and secure the end as described for circular turns.

Spiral Reverse Turns

- Anchor the bandage with two circular turns, and bring the bandage upward at about a 30-degree angle.
- Place the thumb of your free hand on the upper edge of the bandage (Figure 34–22 ■, *A*). The thumb will hold the bandage while it is folded on itself.
- Unroll the bandage about 15 cm (6 in.), and then turn your hand so that the bandage falls over itself (Figure 34–22 ■, *B*).
- Continue the bandage around the limb, overlapping each previous turn by two-thirds the width of the bandage. Make each bandage turn at the same position on the limb so that the turns of the bandage will be aligned (Figure 34–22 ■, *C*).
- Terminate the bandage with two circular turns, and secure the end as described for circular turns.

Recurrent Turns

- Anchor the bandage with two circular turns.
- Fold the bandage back on itself, and bring it centrally over the distal end to be bandaged (Figure 34–23 ■).
- Holding it with the other hand, bring the bandage back over the end to the right of the center bandage but overlapping it by two-thirds the width of the bandage.
- Bring the bandage back on the left side, also overlapping the first turn by two-thirds the width of the bandage.
- Continue this pattern of alternating right and left until the area is covered. Overlap the preceding turn by two-thirds the bandage width each time.
- Terminate the bandage with two circular turns (Figure 34–24 ■). Secure the end appropriately.

Figure-Eight Turns

- Anchor the bandage with two circular turns.
- Carry the bandage above the joint, around it, and then below it, making a figure-eight (Figure 34–25 ■).
- Continue above and below the joint, overlapping the previous turn by two-thirds the width of the bandage.

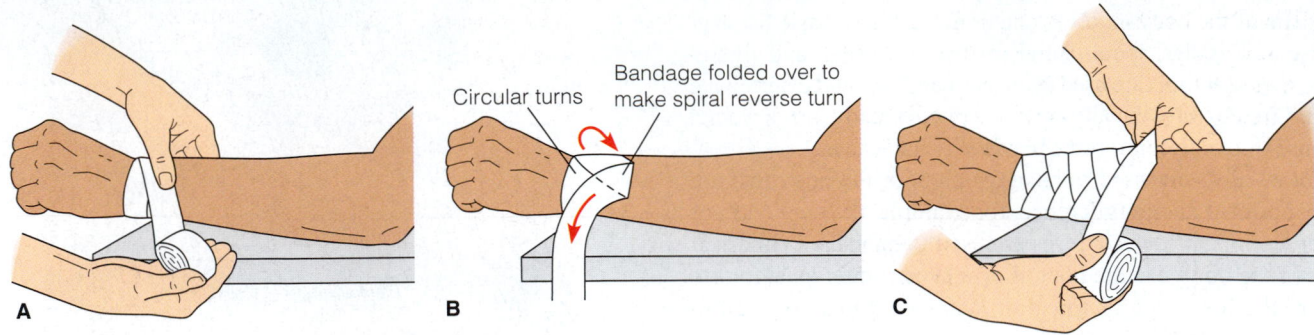

Figure 34–22 ■ Applying spiral reverse turns.

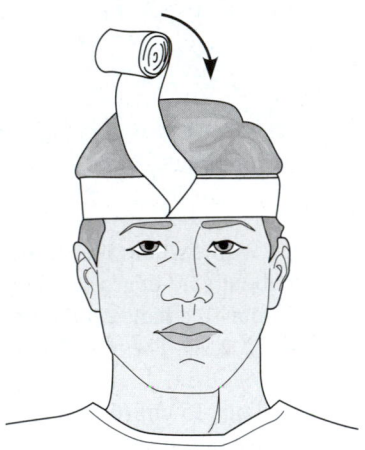

Figure 34–23 ■ Starting a recurrent bandage.

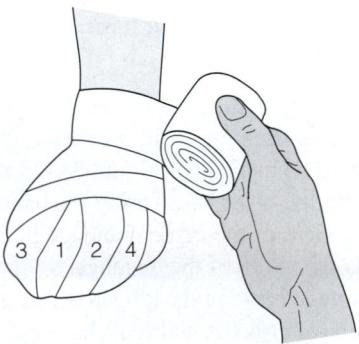

Figure 34–24 ■ Completing a recurrent bandage.

- Terminate the bandage above the joint with two circular turns, and then secure the end appropriately.

Binders. A **binder** is a type of bandage designed for a specific body part, for example, the triangular binder (sling) fits the arm. Binders are used to support large areas of the body, such as the abdomen, arm, or chest.

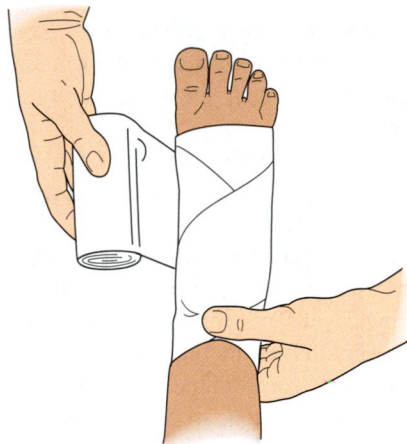

Figure 34–25 ■ Applying a figure-eight bandage.

Triangular Arm Sling

- Ask the client to flex the elbow to an 80-degree angle or less, depending on the purpose. The thumb should be facing upward or inward toward the body. *An 80-degree angle is sufficient to support the forearm, to prevent swelling of the hand, and to relieve pressure on the shoulder joint (e.g., to support the paralyzed arm of a stroke client whose shoulder might otherwise become dislocated).* A more acute angle is preferred if there is swelling of the hand (see how to apply a sling for maximum hand elevation, below).
- Place one end of the unfolded triangular binder over the shoulder of the uninjured side so that the binder falls down the front of the chest of the client with the point of the triangle (apex) under the elbow of the injured side.
- Take the upper corner, and carry it around the neck until it hangs over the shoulder on the injured side.
- Bring the lower corner of the binder up over the arm to the shoulder of the injured side. Using a square knot, secure this corner to the upper corner at the side of the neck on the injured side (Figure 34–26 ■, *A*). *A square knot will not slip. Tying the*

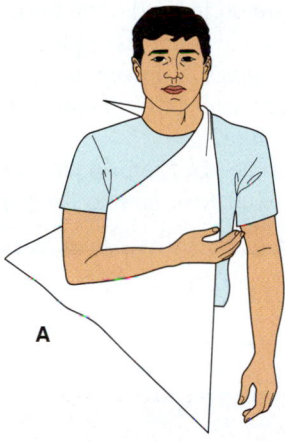

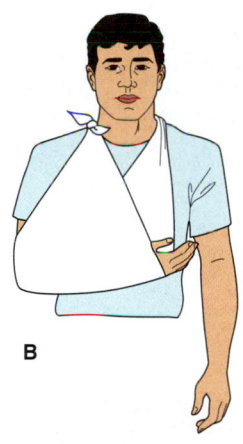

Figure 34–26 ■ Large arm sling.

MediaLink | CLIENTS WITH CHRONIC ILLNESSES CASE STUDY

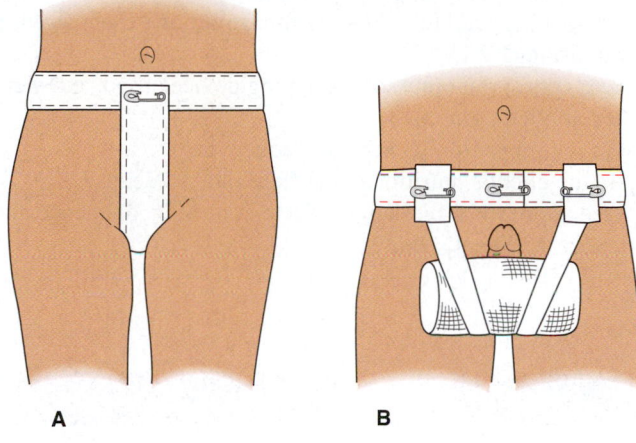

Figure 34–27 ■ T-binders: *A,* single tail; *B,* two tails.

Straight Abdominal Binder

- With the client in a supine position, place the binder smoothly under the body, with the upper border of the binder at the waist and the lower border at the level of the gluteal fold. *A binder placed over the waist interferes with respiration; one placed too low interferes with elimination and walking.*
- Apply padding over the iliac crests if the client is thin.
- Bring the ends around the client, overlap them, and secure them with pins or Velcro (Figure 34–28 ■). Place the top pin horizontally at the waist to allow for comfort when moving.

EVALUATING

The goals established during the planning phase are evaluated according to specific desired outcomes also established in that phase (see Identifying Nursing Diagnoses, Outcomes, and Interventions earlier). To judge whether client outcomes have been achieved, the nurse uses data collected during care, such as skin status over bony prominences and perineal area, nutritional and fluid intake, mental status, signs of healing if an ulcer is present, and so on. If outcomes are not achieved, the nurse should explore the reasons why:

- Has the client's physical condition changed?
- Were risk factors correctly identified?

knot at the side of the neck prevents pressure on the bony prominences of the vertebral column at the back of the neck.
- Make sure the wrist is supported, to maintain alignment.
- Fold the sling neatly at the elbow, and secure it with safety pins or tape. It may be folded and fastened at the front (Figure 34–26 ■, *B*).
- Remove the sling periodically to inspect the skin for indications of irritation, especially around the site of the knot.

T-Binder

- Select the appropriate binder for the client, and place it smoothly under the person with the waistband at waist level.
- Bring the waist tails around the client, overlap them, and secure them with a pin placed horizontally. *The pins placed horizontally allow comfort when bending at the waist and moving.*
- Bring the center tail up between the legs (Figure 34–27 ■, *A*). The two tails of the double T-binder are brought up on either side of the penis (Figure 34–27 ■, *B*). When dressings are in place, take care to touch only the outside of the dressings to prevent contamination of the wound or yourself.
- Fasten the ties at the waist with a safety pin placed horizontally.

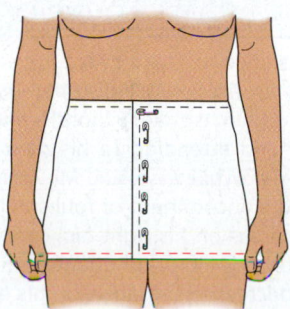

Figure 34–28 ■ A straight abdominal binder.

- Were appropriate devices and techniques used?
- Did the client fail to comply with instructions about moving and turning? Why?
- Were appropriate pressure-relieving devices used, and were they applied correctly?
- Was the repositioning schedule adhered to?
- Are the client's nutritional and fluid intake adequate?
- Were appropriate measures used to control incontinence and protect the client's skin?

- Was the wound supported and immobilized effectively?
- Were stringent aseptic practices implemented when cleaning and changing dressings to prevent infection?
- Was the client receiving anti-inflammatory medications that interfere with healing?
- Was the appropriate dressing applied to keep the wound moist or absorb exudate or both as needed?

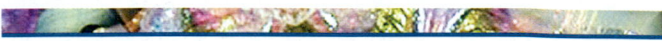

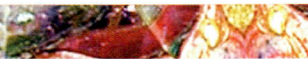

Lifespan Considerations

Applying Bandages and Binders

Children

- Allow the child to help with the procedure by holding supplies, opening boxes, counting turns, and so on.
- If a young client is apprehensive, demonstrate the procedure on a doll or stuffed animal.
- Encourage the child to decorate the bandage.
- Teach the caregivers to apply bandages and binders safely.

Elders

- Older clients may need extra support during the procedure, especially if arthritis, contractures, or tremors are present.
- Avoid constricting the client's circulation with a tight bandage or binder. Observe skin and bony prominences frequently for signs of impaired circulation. The risk for skin breakdown increases with age.

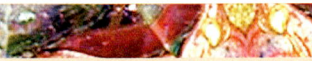

Home Care Considerations

Applying Bandages and Binders

- Assess the client's or caregiver's ability and willingness to perform the bandaging procedure.
- Ensure that the client has the proper supplies and knows how to obtain replacement supplies.
- The client should have two binders so that there is one to wear while the other is being washed. Bandages and binders should be washed inside a mesh laundry bag to keep them from becoming twisted and to prevent Velcro or hooks from catching on other laundry.

- Instruct the client's caregiver to
  a. Wash hands thoroughly before handling dressing supplies and applying the bandage.
  b. Report skin breakdown, redness, pain, or pallor of the affected area.
  c. Check for adequate peripheral circulation after applying the bandage.

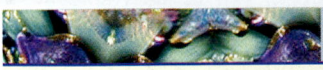

Focus on Critical Thinking

You have been assigned to care for Mr. Johns, a 74-year-old client being treated for a urinary tract disorder. Mr. Johns suffered a cerebrovascular accident (stroke) 6 months ago and has had difficulty ambulating and attending to his own needs because of right-sided weakness. While assessing Mr. Johns you note that he is thin for his height, incontinent of foul-smelling urine, and has deeply reddened areas on his right hip, coccyx, and entire peritoneal area. Mr. Johns is alert and oriented to person, place, and time, but he has decreased sensation on his entire right side. He spends most of his time in bed or sitting at his bedside in a chair due to his difficulty with ambulation.

1. What data suggest that Mr. Johns is particularly vulnerable to pressure ulcer development?
2. What additional information do you need in order to use the Braden scale to determine Mr. Johns' potential for pressure ulcer development?
3. What independent measures can you take to protect Mr. Johns' skin from further breakdown?
4. Considering that Mr. Johns does not have any areas of skin breakdown, why is it important to institute treatment for pressure ulcers at this time?

See Critical Thinking Possibilities in Appendix A.

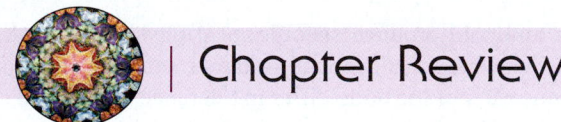 | Chapter Review

EXPLORE MediaLink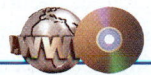

NCLEX review questions, case studies, care plan activities, MediaLink applications, and other interactive resources for this chapter can be found on the Companion Website at www.prenhall.com/kozier. Click on Chapter 34 to select the activities for this chapter.

For animations, more NCLEX review questions, and an audio glossary, access the Student CD-ROM accompanying this textbook.

Chapter Highlights

- Maintaining skin integrity is an important independent function of nursing.
- Wounds are described as intentional or unintentional, closed or open, and clean, clean-contaminated, contaminated, or dirty (infected). Wounds are also classified by depth as partial thickness or full thickness. In addition, wounds are classified according to how they are acquired, as incisions, contusions, abrasions, punctures, lacerations, and penetrating wounds.
- A pressure ulcer is any lesion caused by unrelieved pressure that results in damage to underlying tissues. Pressure ulcers usually occur over bony prominences.
- Two other factors that act in conjunction with pressure to produce a pressure ulcer are friction and shearing forces.
- Several factors increase the risk for the development of pressure ulcers: immobility and inactivity, inadequate nutrition, fecal and urinary incontinence, decreased mental status, diminished sensation, excessive body heat, and advanced age.
- There are four stages of pressure ulcer development, which vary according to the degree of tissue damage.
- There are two types of wound healing, which are distinguished by the amount of tissue loss: primary intention healing and secondary intention healing.
- The wound-healing process has three phases: inflammatory, proliferative, and maturation.
- Major types of wound exudate are serous, purulent, and sanguineous (hemorrhagic). Exudate can be a combination of two or three of these types (e.g., serosanguineous). The process of pus formation is referred to as suppuration.
- The main complications of wound healing are hemorrhage, infection, dehiscence, and evisceration, each of which is identifiable by specific clinical signs and symptoms.
- Factors affecting wound healing include developmental stage, nutritional status, lifestyle, medications, and the presence of infection.
- Several risk assessment tools are available to identify clients at risk for pressure ulcer development. They include scoring systems to evaluate a person's degree of risk.
- Meticulous skin examination of common pressure ulcer sites by the nurse is an important ongoing assessment activity for clients at risk.
- When a pressure ulcer is present, the nurse describes the ulcer in terms of location, size, depth, stage, color, status of wound margins and surrounding skin, and specific signs of infection, if present.
- Wound assessment is an ongoing process to evaluate healing. The nurse assesses wounds by visual inspection, palpation, and the sense of smell. Essential data for assessing wounds include wound appearance, size, drainage, swelling, pain, and the presence of tubes and drains.
- Laboratory data that may be used to assess the progress of wound healing include leukocyte count, hemoglobin, blood coagulation studies, serum protein analysis, and wound cultures. Nurses are usually responsible for obtaining specimens of wound drainage for culture.
- The NANDA nursing diagnoses *Risk for Impaired Skin Integrity, Impaired Skin Integrity,* and *Impaired Tissue Integrity* apply to clients at risk for developing and to those with pressure ulcers.
- Nursing diagnoses related to clients with wounds may include *Risk for Infection* and *Pain.*
- Major goals for clients at risk for developing pressure ulcers are to maintain skin integrity and to avoid potential associated risks.
- Nursing interventions to prevent the formation of pressure ulcers include conducting ongoing assessment of risk factors and skin status, providing skin care to maintain skin integrity, ensuring adequate nutrition, implementing measures to avoid skin trauma, providing supportive devices, and client teaching.
- Treatment for pressure ulcers varies according to the stage of the ulcer and agency protocol.
- Major nursing responsibilities related to wound care include assisting the client in obtaining sufficient nutrition and fluids, preventing wound infections, and proper positioning.
- Wound care may involve cleaning wounds, changing dressings, irrigating, applying heat and cold, and applying bandages and binders.
- Various dressing materials are available to protect wounds, absorb exudate, and keep the wound bed moist, thus facilitating healing.
- Synthetic dressings have been developed for use with specific types of wounds. These include transparent adhesive films, impregnated nonadherent dressings, hydrocolloids, hydrogels, polyurethane foams, and exudate absorbers. The

nurse must be aware of the specific purposes of each and their indications for use.

- The type of dressing used depends on (a) location, size, and type of the wound; (b) amount of exudate; (c) whether or not the wound requires debridement, is infected, or has sinus tracts; and (d) such considerations as frequency of dressing change, ease or difficulty of dressing applications, and cost.
- The RYB color code of wounds can assist nurses to provide appropriate nursing interventions for wounds that heal by secondary intention. In this scheme, the nurse protects red, cleanses yellow, and debrides black.

- Heat and cold produce specific local physiologic and systemic responses that account for their therapeutic effects.
- Various parts of the body differ in tolerance to heat and cold. The physiologic tolerance of individuals also varies. Specific conditions such as neurosensory and circulatory impairments necessitate precautions when applying heat or cold.
- When applying heat and cold, clients and nurses need to be aware of the effects of thermal receptor adaptation and the rebound phenomenon.

Review Questions

34–1. Your client has a Braden scale score of 17. The appropriate nursing action is:
  a. assess the client again in 24 hours; the score is within normal limits.
  b. implement a turning schedule; the client is at increased risk of skin breakdown.
  c. apply a transparent wound barrier to major pressure sites, the client is at moderate risk of skin breakdown.
  d. request an order for a special low-air-loss bed; the client is at very high risk of skin breakdown.

34–2. Proper technique for performing a wound culture includes
  a. cleansing the wound prior to obtaining the specimen.
  b. swabbing for the specimen in the area with the largest collection of drainage.
  c. removing crusts or scabs with sterile forceps and then culturing the site beneath.
  d. waiting 8 hours following a dose of antibiotic to obtain the specimen.

34–3. The client has a pressure ulcer with a shallow, partial skin thickness, eroded area but no necrotic areas. The nurse would treat the area with which of the following dressings?
  a. alginate
  b. dry gauze
  c. hydrocolloid
  d. no dressing is indicated

34–4. When you return to your client to remove the heating pad 30 minutes after application, the client requests that you leave it in place. You explain to the client that
  a. heat application for longer than 30 minutes can actually cause the opposite effect (constriction) of the one desired (dilation).
  b. it will be acceptable to leave the pad in place if the temperature is reduced to between 40.6–46C (105 and 115F).
  c. it will be acceptable to leave the pad in place for another 30 minutes if the site appears satisfactory when assessed.
  d. it will be acceptable to leave the pad in place as long as it is moist heat.

34–5. Which statement, if made by the client or family member, would indicate the need for further teaching?
  a. If a skin area gets red but then the red goes away after turning, I should report it to the nurse.
  b. Putting a sheepskin under the heels or other bony areas can help decrease pressure.
  c. If a person cannot turn himself or herself in bed, someone should help them change position every 4 hours.
  d. The skin should be washed with only warm water (not hot) and lotion put on while it is still a little wet.

Readings And References

Suggested Readings

Hawkins-Bradley, B. (2002). After the fall: The nuts and bolts of wound repair. *Advance for Providers of Post-Acute Care, 5*(1), 48–50. This article reviews the three phases of wound healing and applies them to the example of a client being cared for at home with a large abdominal incision.

Ovington, L. (2001). Wound care products: How to choose. *Home Healthcare Nurse, 19,* 224–232, 240.

This is a very useful article. It describes the "performance-based approach to dressing use" and asks the questions: "What does the wound need? What does the product do? How well does the product perform? What does the patient need? What is available in this setting? What is practical?" It also provides a clear description of various products' abilities to adhere to skin, conform to the wound, absorb exudate, hydrate the wound, debride, and prevent infection.

Related Research

Antle, D., & Leafgreen, P. (2001). Reducing the incidence of pressure ulcer development in the ICU. *American Journal of Nursing, 101*(5), 24EE–24II.

Pieper, B., Sugrue, M., Weiland, M., Sprague, K., & Heiman, C. (1998). Risk factors, prevention methods, and wound care for patients with pressure ulcers. *Clinical Nurse Specialist, 12*(1), 7–14.

References

Anthony, D. (1987). Norton revises risk scores. *Nursing Times, 83*, 6.

Ayello, E. A., & Braden, B. (2001). Why is pressure ulcer risk assessment so important? *Nursing, 31*(11), 74–79.

Bergstrom, N., Allman, R. M., Alvarez, A. M., Bennett, M. A., Carlson, C. E., Frantz, R. A., et al. (1994). *Pressure Ulcer Treatment: Clinical Practice Guideline Number 15. Quick Reference Guide for Clinicians* (Publication No. 95-0653). Rockville, MD: Agency for Health Care Policy and Research, Public Health Service, U.S. Department of Health and Human Services.

Butcher, M. (2002). Wound care: Managing wound sinuses. *Nursing Times, 98*(2), 63–65.

Cuddigan, J., Berlowitz, D. R., & Ayello, E. A. (2001). Pressure ulcers in America: Prevalence, incidence, and implications for the future. *Advances in Skin and Wound Care, 14*, 208–214.

Cullum, N., Deeks, J., Sheldon, T. A., Song, F., & Fletcher, A. W. (2001). Beds, mattresses and cushions for pressure sore prevention and treatment (Cochrane Review). *The Cochrane Library, Issue 4*, Oxford: Update Software.

de Graaff, J. C., Ubbink, D., Lagarde, S. M., & Jacobs, M. J. (2002). The feasibility and reliability of capillary blood pressure measurements in the fingernail fold. *Microvascular Research, 63*, 270–278.

Johnson, M., Maas, M., & Moorhead, S. (Eds.). (2000). *Nursing outcomes classification (NOC)* (2nd ed.). St. Louis, MO: Mosby.

King, M. E., & Kinney, A. Y. (2001). A sticky solution to wound repair. *Nursing, 31*(3), 52–53.

Kloth, W. C., Berman, J. E., Nett, M., Papanek, P. E., & Dumit-Minkel, S. (2002). A randomized controlled clinical trial to evaluate the effects of noncontact normothermic wound therapy on chronic full-thickness pressure ulcers. *Advances in Skin & Wound Care, 15*, 270–276.

McCloskey, J. C., & Bulechek, G. M. (Eds.). (2000). *Nursing interventions classification (NIC)* (3rd ed.). St. Louis, MO: Mosby.

Mendez-Eastman, S. (2002). Negative-pressure wound therapy. *Nursing, 32*(5), 58–63.

National Pressure Ulcer Advisory Panel. (2001). *Pressure ulcer prevention: RN competency-cased curriculum*. Reston, VA: Author

National Pressure Ulcer Advisory Panel. (2002). PUSH Tool. Retrieved May 27, 2003, from http://www.npuap.org/pushins.htm

NANDA International. (2003). *Nursing diagnoses: Definitions and classification 2003-2004*. Philadelphia: Author.

Norton, D., McLaren, R., & Exton-Smith, A. N. (1975). *An investigation of geriatric nursing problems in hospital*. Edinburgh, UK: Churchill Livingstone.

Ovington, L. G. (2001a). Battling bacteria in wound care. *Home Healthcare Nurse, 19*, 622–631.

Ovington, L. G. (2001b). Hanging wet-to-dry dressings out to dry. *Home Healthcare Nurse, 19*, 477–484.

Panel for the Prediction and Prevention of Pressure Ulcers in Adults. (1992a). *Clinical practice guideline, pressure ulcers in adults: Prediction and prevention* (Publication No. 92-0047). Rockville, MD: Agency for Health Care Policy and Research, Public Health Service, U.S. Department of Health and Human Services.

Panel for the Prediction and Prevention of Pressure Ulcers in Adults. (1992b). *Pressure ulcers in adults: Prediction and prevention. quick reference guide for clinicians* (AHCPR Publication No. 92-0050). Rockville, MD: Agency for Health Care Policy and Research, Public Health Service, U.S. Department of Health and Human Services.

Schultz, A., Bien, M., Dumond, K., Brown, K., & Meyers, A. (1999). Etiology and incidence of pressure ulcers in surgical patients. *AORN Journal, 70*, 434, 437–440, 443–444. 446–448.

U.S. Department of Health and Human Services (2000). *Healthy people 2010: Understanding and improving health* (2nd ed.). Washington, DC: U.S. Government Printing Office.

Selected Bibliography

Bergquist, S., & Frantz, R. (1999). Pressure ulcers in community-based older adults receiving home health care: Prevalence, incidence and associated risk factors. *Advances in Wound Care, 12*, 339–351.

Berlowitz, D. R., Bezerra, H. Q., Brandeis, G. H., Kader, B., & Anderson, J. J. (2000). Are we improving the quality of nursing home care? The case of pressure ulcers. *Journal of the American Geriatrics Society, 48*, 59–62.

Berlowitz, D. R., Brandeis, G. H., Anderson, J. J., Ash, A. S., Kader, B., Morris, J. N., et al. (2001). Evaluation of a risk-adjustment model for pressure ulcer development using the minimum data set. *Journal of the American Geriatrics Society, 49*, 872–876.

Berlowitz, D. R., Brandeis, G. H., Morris, J. N., Ash, A. S., Anderson, J. J., Kader, B., et al. (2001). Deriving a risk-adjustment model for pressure ulcer development using the minimum data set. *Journal of the American Geriatrics Society, 49*, 866–871.

Boykin, J. V. (2002). How hyperbaric oxygen therapy helps heal chronic wounds. *Nursing, 32*(6), 24.

Bryant, R. A. (Ed.). (2000). *Acute and chronic wounds: Nursing management* (2nd ed.). St Louis, MO: Mosby.

Dolynchuk, K., Keast, D., Campbell, K., Houghton, P., Orsted, H., Sibbald, G., et al. (2000). Best practices for the prevention and treatment of pressure ulcers. *Ostomy Wound Management, 46*(11), 38–52.

Hess, C. T. (2000). *Nurse's clinical guide to wound care* (3rd ed.). Springhouse, PA: Springhouse.

Inman, K. J., Dymock, K., Fysh, N., Robbins, B., Rutledge, F. S., & Sibbald, W. J. (1999). Pressure ulcer prevention: A randomized controlled trial of 2 risk-directed strategies for patient surface assignment. *Advances in Wound Care, 12*, 72–80.

Jordan, R. (2001). Supporting healing. *Advance for Providers of Post-Acute Care, 4*(5), 74–75, 77.

Krasner, D. (1999). The AHCPR pressure ulcer infection control recommendations revisited. *Ostomy Wound Management, 45*(1A Suppl), 88s–91s.

Krasner, D. L., Rodeheaver, G. T., & Sibbald, R. G. (Eds.). (2001). *Chronic wound care: A clinical source book for healthcare professionals* (3rd ed.). Wayne, PA: HMP Communications.

Maklebust, J., & Sieggreen, M. (2001). *Pressure ulcers: Guidelines for prevention and nursing management* (3rd ed.). Springhouse, PA: Springhouse.

McConnell, E. A. (1998). Clinical do's and don'ts: Applying cold treatment. *Nursing, 28*(6), 26.

Morison, M. J. (Ed.). (2001). *The prevention and treatment of pressure ulcers*. St. Louis, MO: Mosby.

Pieper, B., Templin, T. N., Dobal, M., & Jacox, A. (1999). Wound prevalence, types, and treatments in home care. *Advances in Wound Care, 12*, 117–126.

Rudolph, D. (2002). Why won't this wound heal? *American Journal of Nursing, 102*(2), Critical Care Extra: 24DD–HH.

Singhal, A., Reis, E. D., & Kerstein, M. D. (2001). Options for nonsurgical debridement of necrotic wounds. *Advances in Skin and Wound Care, 14*, 96–103.

Sprigle, S., Linden, M., McKenna, D., Davis, K., & Riordan, B. (2001). Clinical skin temperature measurement to predict incipient pressure ulcers. *Advances in Skin and Wound Care 14*, 133–137.

Stotts, N. A. (1999). Risk of pressure ulcer development in surgical patients: A review of the literature. *Advances in Wound Care, 12*, 127–136.

Sussman, C., & Bates-Jensen, B. M. (2001). *Wound care: A collaborative practice manual for physical therapists and nurses* (2nd ed.). Gaithersburg, MD: Aspen.

Van Rijswijk, L., & Braden, B. J. (1999). Pressure ulcer patient and wound assessment: An AHCPR clinical practice guideline update. *Ostomy Wound Management, 45*(1A suppl), 56–68.

Whittington, K., Patrick, M., & Roberts, J. L. (2000). A national study of pressure ulcer prevalence and incidence in acute care hospitals. *Journal of Wound Ostomy Continence Nursing, 27*, 209–215.

Williams, D. F., Stotts, N. A., & Nelson, K. (2000). Patients with existing pressure ulcers admitted to acute care. *Journal of Wound Ostomy Continence Nursing, 27*, 216–226.

WOCN. (2000). *Wound clinical pathway framework* (Report No. 445–37). Laguna Beach, CA: Wound Ostomy and Continence Nurses Society.

CHAPTER | 35

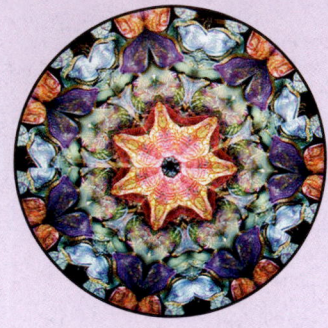

PERIOPERATIVE NURSING

LEARNING OUTCOMES

After completing this chapter, you will be able to:

- Describe the phases of the perioperative period.

- Discuss various types of surgery according to degree of urgency, degree of risk, and purpose.

- Identify essential aspects of preoperative assessment.

- Give examples of pertinent nursing diagnoses for surgical clients.

- Identify nursing responsibilities in planning perioperative nursing care.

- Describe essential preoperative teaching, including pain control, moving, leg exercises, and coughing and deep-breathing exercises.

- Describe essential aspects of preparing a client for surgery, including skin preparation.

- Compare various types of anesthesia.

- Identify essential nursing assessments and interventions during the immediate postanesthetic phase.

- Demonstrate ongoing nursing assessments and interventions for the postoperative client.

- Identify potential postoperative complications and describe nursing interventions to prevent them.

- Identify essential aspects of managing gastrointestinal suction.

- Describe appropriate wound care for a postoperative client.

- Evaluate the effectiveness of perioperative nursing interventions.

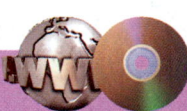

MediaLink

www.prenhall.com/kozier

Additional resources for this chapter can be found on the Student CD-ROM accompanying this textbook, and on the Companion Website at www.prenhall.com/kozier. Click on Chapter 35 to select the activities for this chapter.

CD-ROM
- Audio Glossary
- NCLEX Review

Companion Website
- Additional NCLEX Review
- Case Study: Clients Having Surgical Procedures
- Care Plan Activity: Coronary Artery Bypass Procedure
- MediaLink Application: Developing Operative Care Policies
- Links to Resources

Surgery is a unique experience of a planned physical alteration encompassing three phases: preoperative, intraoperative, and postoperative. These three phases are together referred to as the **perioperative period.**

The **preoperative phase** begins when the decision to have surgery is made and ends when the client is transferred to the operating table. The nursing activities associated with this phase include assessing the client, identifying potential or actual health problems, planning specific care based on the individual's needs, and providing preoperative teaching for the client and support people.

The **intraoperative phase** begins when the client is transferred to the operating table and ends when the client is admitted to the postanesthesia care unit (PACU), also called the postanesthetic room or recovery room. The nursing activities related to this phase include a variety of specialized procedures designed to create and maintain a safe therapeutic environment for the client and the health care personnel.

The **postoperative phase** begins with the admission of the client to the postanesthesia area and ends when healing is complete. During the postoperative phase, nursing activities include assessing the client's response (physiologic and psychologic) to surgery, performing interventions to facilitate healing and prevent complications, teaching and providing support to the client and support people, and planning for home care. The goal is to assist the client to achieve the most optimal health status possible.

Many surgeries are performed in an outpatient setting. Outpatient surgeries are often performed at **ambulatory surgery centers (ASC),** which are facilities where surgeries that do not require hospital admission are performed (Federated Ambulatory Surgery Association, 2002). Ambulatory surgery centers may also be referred to as same-day surgery centers, day surgery centers, or outpatient surgery centers. The client goes to the ASC or to the hospital the day of surgery, has the operation, and leaves the same day. In these instances, the three phases of the perioperative period are shortened and the postoperative phase continues at home. The nurse's role in assessing, teaching, and following up is vital to successful outcomes for the client who undergoes day surgery.

TYPES OF SURGERY

Surgical procedures are commonly grouped according to (a) purpose, (b) degree of urgency, and (c) degree of risk.

Purpose

Surgical procedures may be categorized according to their purpose (see Box 35–1).

Degree of Urgency

Surgery is classified by its urgency and necessity to preserve the client's life, body part, or body function. **Emergency surgery** is performed immediately to preserve function or the life of the client. Surgeries to control internal hemorrhage or repair a fracture are examples of emergency surgeries. **Elective surgery** is performed when surgical intervention is the preferred treatment for a condition that is not imminently life threatening (but may ultimately threaten life or well-being)

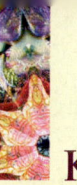

BOX 35–1	■ Purposes of Surgical Procedures
Diagnostic	Confirms or establishes a diagnosis; for example, biopsy of a mass in a breast.
Palliative	Relieves or reduces pain or symptoms of a disease; it does not cure; for example, resection of nerve roots.
Ablative	Removes a diseased body part; for example, removal of a gallbladder (cholecystectomy).
Constructive	Restores function or appearance that has been lost or reduced; for example, breast implant.
Transplant	Replaces malfunctioning structures; for example, hip replacement.

or to improve the client's life. Examples of elective surgeries include cholecystectomy for chronic gallbladder disease, hip replacement surgery, and plastic surgery procedures such as breast reduction surgery.

Degree of Risk

Surgery is also classified as major or minor according to the degree of risk to the client. **Major surgery** involves a high degree of risk, for a variety of reasons: It may be complicated or prolonged, large losses of blood may occur, vital organs may be involved, or postoperative complications may be likely. Examples are organ transplant, open heart surgery, and removal of a kidney. In contrast, **minor surgery** normally involves little risk, produces few complications, and is often performed in a "day surgery." Examples are breast biopsy, removal of tonsils, and knee surgery.

The degree of risk involved in a surgical procedure is affected by the client's age, general health, nutritional status, use of medications, and mental status.

Age

Very young and elder clients are greater surgical risks than children and adults. Age and developmental status affect children's ability to cope with the physiologic and psychologic stresses of surgery. The physiologic response of an infant to surgery is substantially different from an adult's. The blood volume in an infant is small, and its fluid reserves limited. This increases the risk of volume depletion during surgery resulting in inadequate oxygenation of body tissues. Because of the infant's relatively large body surface area and immature temperature regulatory mechanisms, the risk of hypothermia during surgery is significant. Other organ systems, such as the kidneys, liver, and immune system, also have not achieved maturity in infants, affecting their ability to metabolize and eliminate drugs and resist infection.

Toddlers and older children are better able to withstand surgery physiologically, but they often fear separation from their parents, painful events (e.g., "shots"), and either not waking up after surgery or waking up during surgery and feeling what is happening. The child's developmental level, the parent–child relationship, the parents' coping abilities, and preoperative teaching and support will affect how well the child is able to deal with these fears and the level of anxiety the child experiences.

The older adult often has fewer physiologic reserves to meet the extra demands caused by surgery. Because of a lower percentage of body water, decreased kidney function, and a decreased thirst response, elders are at greater risk for fluid and electrolyte imbalances. Many elders demonstrate changes in liver and kidney function, both of which can affect response to anesthesia and other medications that may be administered during the perioperative period. The older adult may be poorly nourished, which can impair healing. Declines in sensory function (hearing in particular) or the presence of dementia make it more difficult to understand directions and teaching. In addition, the elder is more likely to have a chronic disease such as cardiovascular disease, chronic lung disease, or diabetes that affects healing and responses to medication and surgery.

General Health

Surgery is least risky when the client's general health is good. Any infection or pathophysiology increases the risk. Of particular concern are upper respiratory tract infections, which together with a general anesthetic can adversely affect respiratory function. Where there is a high risk of infection, antibiotics may be administered parenterally within 1 hour of surgery and continued for 24 to 72 hours. This practice allows time for drugs to reach therapeutic levels in the tissues but does not permit bacterial resistance to develop. Common health problems that increase surgical risk and may lead to the decision to postpone or cancel surgery are listed in Box 35–2.

Nutritional Status

Adequate nutrition is required for normal tissue repair. Surgery increases the body's need for nutrients for the needed tissue healing and prevention of infection required during the postoperative period. Obesity and malnutrition increase surgical risk.

Obesity contributes to postoperative complications such as pneumonia, wound infections and wound separation. Both the

---

BOX 35–2   ■ Health Problems that Increase Surgical Risk

- Malnutrition can lead to delayed wound healing, infection, and reduced energy. Protein and vitamins are needed for wound healing; vitamin K is essential for blood clotting.
- Obesity leads to hypertension, impaired cardiac function, and impaired respiratory ventilation. Obese clients are also more likely to have delayed wound healing and wound infection because adipose tissue impedes blood circulation and its delivery of nutrients, antibodies, and enzymes required for wound healing.
- Cardiac conditions such as angina pectoris, recent myocardial infarction, hypertension, and heart failure weaken the heart. Well-controlled cardiac problems generally pose minimal operative risk.
- Blood coagulation disorders may lead to severe bleeding, hemorrhage, and subsequent shock.

- Upper respiratory tract infections or chronic obstructive lung diseases such as emphysema adversely affect pulmonary function, especially when exacerbated by the effects of general anesthesia. They also predispose the client to postoperative lung infections.
- Renal disease impairs regulation of the body's fluids and electrolytes and excretion of drugs and other toxins.
- Diabetes mellitus predisposes the client to wound infection and delayed healing.
- Liver disease (e.g., cirrhosis) impairs the liver's abilities to detoxify medications used during surgery, produce the prothrombin necessary for blood clotting, and metabolize nutrients essential for healing.
- Uncontrolled neurologic disease such as epilepsy may result in seizures during surgery or recovery.

obese and underweight client are vulnerble to pressure ulcer formation due to positioning required for surgery. The perioperative nurse provides padding and other measures to protect the client's skin over pressure points during surgery.

A malnurouished client is at risk for delayed wound healing, wound infection and fluid and electrolyte alterations. Malnutrition is evident in approximately 20% of elderly hospitalized clients (Bailes, 2000, p. 192). If a client has serious malnutrition, the surgery may be postponed to improve the nutritional status. If the surgery cannot be delayed, parenteral or enteral nutrition may be initiated.

Medications

The regular use of certain medications can increase surgical risk. Consider these examples:

- *Anticoagulants* increase blood coagulation time.
- *Tranquilizers* may interact with anesthetics, increasing the risk of respiratory depression.
- *Corticosteroids* may interfere with wound healing and increase the risk of infection.
- *Diuretics* may affect fluid and electrolyte balance.

Clients may be unaware of the potential adverse interactions of medications and may fail to report the use of medications for conditions unrelated to the indication for surgery. The astute nurse interviewer should question the client and family about the use of commonly prescribed medications, over-the-counter preparations, and any herbal remedies for specific conditions mentioned during the nursing history.

Mental Status

Disorders that affect cognitive function, such as mental illness, mental retardation, or developmental delay, affect the client's ability to understand and cope with the stresses of surgery. These clients also may require medication such as anticonvulsants or antipsychotic drugs that can interact with anesthetic and analgesic medications used during and after surgery.

Clients with dementia may have difficulty understanding proposed surgical procedures and may respond unpredictably to anesthetics. Manifestations of dementia such as confusion, disorientation, and agitation also may be aggravated by the change of environment in the hospital, interfering with the client's ability to cooperate with pre- and postoperative care.

Extreme anxiety also increases surgical risk and interferes with the client's ability to process information and respond appropriately to instructions. In some instances, professional counseling is indicated prior to surgery. It is also important to determine whether clients have coping skills and support systems to help them.

PREOPERATIVE PHASE

Preoperative Consent

Prior to any surgical procedure, clients must sign a consent form, which is generally supplied by the agency. This requirement protects clients from having any surgical procedure they do not want

or do not understand. It also protects the hospital and the health personnel from a claim by the client or family that permission was not granted. The consent form becomes a part of the client's record and goes to the operating room with the client.

Although the surgeon maintains legal responsibility for ensuring that the client is giving informed consent, the nurse may witness the client's signature on the consent form. In doing so, the nurse should ensure that the client understands the procedure to be performed. If it is not clear that the client understands and consents to the surgery, the nurse should contact the surgeon before surgery proceeds.

Preoperative informed consent should include

- Nature and intention of the surgery
- Name and qualifications of the person performing the surgery
- Risks, including tissue damage, disfigurement, or even death
- Chances of success
- Possible alternative measures
- The right of the client to refuse consent or later withdraw consent.

Informed consent is only possible when the client understands the information being provided, that is, speaks the language and is conscious, mentally competent, and not sedated. It may not be given by a minor. Specific guidelines regarding consent for minors vary among the states in the United States and in the provinces in Canada. Nurses must be aware of their responsibilities regarding consents and of the particular hospital's policies (see Chapter 4).

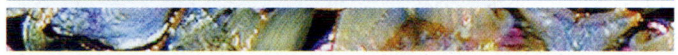

NURSING MANAGEMENT

ASSESSING

Preoperative assessment includes collecting and reviewing specific client data to determine the client's needs both pre- and postoperatively. Physical, psychologic, and social needs are determined during assessment.

Nursing History

The nursing history obtained before surgery provides client data that help the nurse plan preoperative and postoperative care. Although forms vary considerably among agencies, essential preoperative information that should be included is summarized in Box 35–3.

Physical Assessment

Preoperatively, the nurse performs a brief but complete physical assessment, paying particular attention to systems that could affect the client's response to anesthesia or surgery. A brief or "mini" mental status examination provides valuable baseline data for evaluating the client's mental status and alertness after surgery. It is also important to evaluate the client's ability to understand what is happening. Assessment of hearing and vision help guide teaching postoperatively. Respiratory and cardiovascular assessments not only provide baseline data for evaluating the client's postoperative status but also may alert care providers to a problem (e.g., a respiratory infection or irregular pulse rate) that

BOX 35–3   ■ Nursing History

■ *Current health status.* Essential information includes general health status and the presence of any chronic diseases, such as diabetes or asthma, that may affect the client's response to surgery or anesthesia. Note any physical limitations that may affect the client's mobility or ability to communicate after surgery, as well as any prostheses such as hearing aids or contact lenses.

■ *Allergies.* Include allergies to prescription and nonprescription drugs, food allergies, and allergies to tape, latex, soaps, or antiseptic agents. Some food allergies may indicate a potential reaction to drugs or substances used during surgery or diagnostic procedures; for example, an allergy to seafood alerts the nurse to a potential allergy to iodine-based dyes commonly used in radiologic procedures.

■ *Medications.* List all current medications. It may be vital to maintain a blood level of some medications (e.g., anticonvulsants) throughout the surgical experience; others, such as anticoagulants or aspirin, increase the risks of surgery and anesthesia and need to be discontinued several days prior to surgery. It is important to include in the list any herbal remedies the client currently takes.

■ *Previous surgeries.* Previous surgical experiences may influence the client's physical and psychologic responses to surgery or may reveal unexpected responses to anesthesia.

■ *Mental status.* The client's mental status and ability to understand and respond appropriately can affect the entire perioperative experience. Note any developmental disabilities, mental illness, history of dementia, or excessive anxiety related to the procedure.

■ *Understanding of the surgical procedure and anesthesia.* The client should have a good understanding of the planned procedure and what to expect during and after surgery as well as the expected outcome of the procedure.

■ *Smoking.* Smokers may have more difficulty clearing respiratory secretions after surgery, increasing the risk of postoperative complications such as pneumonia and atelectasis.

■ *Alcohol and other mind-altering substances.* Use of substances that affect the central nervous system, liver, or other body systems can affect the client's response to anesthesia and surgery, and postoperative recovery.

■ *Coping.* Clients with a healthy self-concept who have successfully employed appropriate coping mechanisms in the past are better able to deal with the stressors associated with surgery.

■ *Social resources.* Determine the availability of family or other caregivers as well as the client's social support network. These resources are important to the client's recovery, particularly for the client undergoing same-day or short-stay surgery.

■ *Cultural considerations.* Culture influences the client's response to surgery; respecting cultural beliefs and practices can reduce preoperative anxiety and improve recovery.

---

may affect the client's response to surgery and anesthesia. Other systems (gastrointestinal, genitourinary, and musculoskeletal) are examined to provide baseline data (see Chapter 28). ⚮

Screening Tests

The physician orders preoperative diagnostic tests and examinations. Abnormalities may warrant treatment prior to surgery.

The nurse's responsibility is to check the orders carefully, to see that they are carried out, and to ensure that the results are obtained and in the client's record prior to surgery. Table 35–1 lists routine preoperative screening tests. In addition to these routine tests, diagnostic tests directly related to the client's disease are usually appropriate (e.g., gastroscopy to clarify the pathologic condition before gastric surgery).

TABLE 35–1   Routine Preoperative Screening Tests

Test	Rationale
Complete blood count (CBC)	RBCs, hemoglobin (Hgb), and hematocrit (Hct) are important to the oxygen-carrying capacity of the blood; WBCs are an indicator of immune function
Blood grouping and cross-matching	Determined in case blood transfusion is required during or after surgery
Serum electrolytes (Na^+, K^+, Ca^{2+}, Mg^{2+}, Cl^-, HCO_3^-)	To evaluate fluid and electrolyte status
Fasting blood glucose	High levels may indicate undiagnosed diabetes mellitus
Blood urea nitrogen (BUN) and creatinine	To evaluate renal function
ALT, AST, LDH, and bilirubin	To evaluate liver function
Serum albumin and total protein	To evaluate nutritional status
Urinalysis	To determine urine composition and possible abnormal components (e.g., protein or glucose) or infection
Chest x-ray	To evaluate respiratory status and heart size
Electrocardiogram (ECG)	To identify preexisting cardiac problems or disease

DIAGNOSING

Nursing diagnoses that may be appropriate for the preoperative client include

- *Deficient Knowledge* (preoperative routines and postoperative care)
- *Fear* related to
  - Effects of surgery on ability to function in usual roles
  - Outcome of exploratory surgery for malignancy
  - Risk of death
  - Loss of control during anesthesia or waking up during anesthesia
  - Perceived inadequate postoperative analgesia
- *Disturbed Sleep Pattern* related to
  - Hospital routines
  - Psychologic stress
- *Anticipatory Grieving* related to
  - Perceived loss of body part associated with planned surgery
- *Ineffective Coping* related to
  - Conflicting values (e.g., need for blood transfusion versus the religious values for a Jehovah's Witness)
  - Lack of clear outcomes of surgery
  - Unresolved past negative experience with surgery.

Examples of clinical application of some of these diagnoses using NANDA, NIC, and NOC designations are shown in Identifying Nursing Diagnoses, Outcomes, and Interventions.

PLANNING

The overall goal in the preoperative period is to ensure that the client is mentally and physically prepared for surgery. Examples of nursing activities to meet this goal are discussed in the "Implementing" section that follows.

Planning should involve the client and support people. The length of the preoperative period affects preoperative care and planning. When the client is admitted several days before surgery, a nursing care plan and teaching plan can be developed. When the client is admitted the day of surgery, preoperative care planning and teaching may be done on an outpatient basis or by community-based nurses (e.g., nurses in the surgeon's office or same-day surgery unit).

Examples of clinical application of NOC outcomes and NIC interventions are shown in Identifying Nursing Diagnoses, Outcomes, and Interventions.

Planning for Home Care

For the perioperative client, discharge planning begins on or before admission for the planned procedure. Early planning to meet the discharge needs of the client is particularly important

IDENTIFYING NURSING DIAGNOSES, OUTCOMES, AND INTERVENTIONS

THE PREOPERATIVE CLIENT

DATA CLUSTER	NURSING DIAGNOSIS/ DEFINITION	SAMPLE DESIRED OUTCOME [NOC#]/DEFINITION	INDICATORS	SELECTED INTERVENTIONS [NIC#]/DEFINITION	SAMPLE NIC ACTIVITIES
Mr. Taylor, 62 years old, has disabling osteoarthritis and is scheduled for a total knee replacement tomorrow. This is his first surgical experience and he is asking many questions about what to expect before and after surgery. He says, "The more I know, the less anxious I feel."	*Deficient Knowledge (Surgery)/Absence or deficiency of cognitive information related to a specific topic*	*Knowledge: Treatment Procedure(s) [1814]/ Extent of understanding conveyed about procedure(s) required as part of a treatment regimen*	Substantial • Description in steps of procedure (e.g., preoperative process) • Performance of treatment procedure (e.g., deep breathing and coughing, leg exercises)	Teaching: Preoperative [5610]/ *Assisting a patient to understand and mentally prepare for surgery and the postoperative recovery period.*	• Provide time for the patient to ask questions and discuss concerns • Describe the preoperative routines (e.g., anesthesia, diet, tests/lab, voiding, IV therapy, family waiting area) as appropriate • Instruct the patient on the technique of splinting his/her incision, coughing, and deep breathing • Evaluate the patient's ability to return demonstrate leg exercise

for the day-surgery client who is to be discharged soon after recovering from anesthesia.

Discharge planning incorporates an assessment of the client's and support people's abilities and resources for care, their financial resources, and the need for referrals and home health services. However, the extent of discharge planning and home care will vary significantly for clients having different types of surgery.

IMPLEMENTING

The major nursing activity to ensure that the client is prepared for surgery is preoperative teaching.

Preoperative Teaching

Preoperative teaching is a vital part of nursing care. Studies have shown that preoperative teaching reduces clients' anxiety and postoperative complications and increases their satisfaction with the surgical experience. Good preoperative teaching also facilitates the client's return to work and other activities of daily living. Four dimensions of preoperative teaching have been identified as important to clients:

- *Information, including what will happen to the client, when, and what the client will experience, such as expected sensations and discomfort.* The nurse needs to listen carefully and attentively to the client to identify specific concerns and fears. Typical questions are these: What will happen during surgery? How will I feel after the operation? What will the surgeon find? How long will I be in the hospital?

- *Psychosocial support to reduce anxiety.* The nurse provides support by actively listening and providing accurate information. It is important to rectify any misperceptions the client may have.

- *The roles of the client and support people in preoperative preparation, the surgical procedure, and during the postoperative phase.* Understanding his or her role during the perioperative experience increases the client's sense of control and reduces anxiety. This includes what will be expected of the client, desired behaviors, self-care activities, and what the client can do to facilitate recovery.

- *Skills training.* This includes moving, deep breathing, coughing, splinting incisions with the hands or a pillow, and using an incentive spirometer.

If the client is scheduled for same-day surgery, preoperative teaching is often provided before the day of surgery using some combination of videos and verbal and written instructions. The client may have an appointment with day-surgery staff (usually scheduled to coincide with preoperative diagnostic testing) to discuss preoperative concerns, or teaching may be completed by a nurse working with the surgeon. Written instructions are provided, especially when surgery is scheduled several days or weeks hence. Teaching is then reinforced on admission to the surgery unit, and immediate or continuing concerns are addressed. Preoperative instructions are summarized in Box 35–4.

BOX 35–4 ■ Preoperative Instructions

Preoperative Regimen
- Explain the need for preoperative tests (e.g., laboratory, x-ray, ECG).
- Discuss bowel preparation, if required.
- Discuss skin preparation, including operative area and preoperative bath or shower.
- Discuss preoperative medications, if ordered.
- Explain individual therapies ordered by the physician, such as intravenous therapy, the insertion of a urinary catheter or nasogastric tube, use of a spirometer, or antiemboli stockings.
- Discuss the visit by the anesthetist.
- Explain the need to restrict food and oral fluids at least 8 hours before surgery.
- Provide a general timetable for perioperative events, including the time of surgery.
- Discuss the need to remove jewelry, make-up, and all prostheses (e.g., eyeglasses, hearing aids, complete or partial dentures, wig) immediately before surgery.
- Inform client about the preoperative holding area, and give the location of the waiting room for support people.
- Teach deep-breathing and coughing exercises, leg exercises, ways to turn and move (see Procedure 35–1), and splinting techniques.
- Complete the preoperative checklist.

Postoperative Regimen
- Discuss the postanesthesia recovery room's routines and emergency equipment.

- Review type and frequency of assessment activities.
- Discuss pain management.
- Explain usual activity restrictions and precautions related to getting up for the first time postoperatively.
- Describe usual dietary alterations.
- Discuss postoperative dressings and drains.
- Provide an explanation and tour of intensive care unit if client is to be transferred there postoperatively.

Day-Surgery Clients
- Confirm place and time of surgery, including when to arrive (e.g., 1 to 1½ hours before scheduled surgery) and where to register (e.g., reception desk).
- Discuss what to wear (e.g., clients having hand surgery should wear a garment with large sleeve openings to fit over a bulky dressing; all clients need to leave valuables at home).
- Explain the need for a responsible adult to drive or accompany the client home, and arrange a place for them to meet. Include information about discharge criteria and how long the client should expect to stay postoperatively.
- Discuss medications including specific preoperative medications and the client's current medication regimen.
- Review with the client any tests ordered and the need for a urine specimen the morning of surgery.
- Communicate by telephone the evening before surgery to confirm time of surgery and arrival time, and call again the evening after surgery to assess progress.

When the client is a child, addressing the fears and anxieties of both the child and the family is vital. Parents need to know what to expect and to be able to express their concerns. Parents should be considered members of the perioperative team and allowed to participate in providing as much care as possible.

Procedure 35–1 provides guidelines for teaching clients about moving, leg exercises, deep breathing, and coughing.

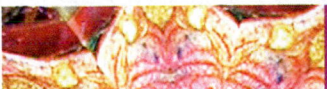

Procedure 35–1 Teaching Moving, Leg Exercises, Deep Breathing, and Coughing

Purposes

MOVING
- To maintain blood circulation
- To stimulate respiratory function
- To decrease stasis of gas in the intestine
- To facilitate early ambulation

LEG EXERCISES
- To stimulate blood circulation, thereby preventing thrombophlebitis and thrombus formation

DEEP BREATHING AND COUGHING
- To facilitate lung aeration, thereby preventing atelectasis and pneumonia

ASSESSMENT

Assess
- Vital signs
- Discomfort
- Temperature and color of feet and legs
- Breath sounds
- Presence of dyspnea or cough
- Learning needs of the client
- Anxiety level of the client
- Client experience with previous surgeries and anesthesia

PLANNING

Before commencing to teach moving, leg exercises, deep-breathing exercises, and coughing, determine (a) the type of surgery, (b) the time of the surgery, (c) the name of the surgeon, (d) the preoperative orders, and (e) the agency's practices for preoperative care. Also, verify that the physician has completed the medical history and physical examination and that the client or the family has signed the consent form.

Delegation
Assessment of the learning needs of the client and his or her support people and determining the teaching content and appropriate strategies for teaching requires application of professional knowledge and critical thinking. Preoperative teaching is conducted by the nurse and is not delegated to unlicensed assistive personnel (UAP). The UAP, however, can reinforce teaching, assist the client with the exercises, and report to the nurse if the client is unable to perform the exercises.

Equipment
- Pillow
- Teaching materials (e.g., videotape, written materials) if available at the agency

IMPLEMENTATION

Preparation
Check that potential distracters (e.g., pain, TV, visitors) to teaching are not present. Include the family in the teaching, if appropriate.

Performance
1. Explain to the client what you are going to do, why it is necessary, and how he or she can cooperate. Discuss how the client's participation in the exercises he or she is going to be taught preoperatively will be helpful during the postoperative recovery.
2. Wash hands and observe appropriate infection control procedures.
3. Provide for client privacy.
4. Show the client ways to turn in bed and to get out of bed.
   - Instruct a client who will have a right abdominal incision or a right-sided chest incision to turn to the left side of the bed and sit up as follows:
     a. Flex the knees.
     b. Splint the wound by holding the left arm and hand or a small pillow against the incision.
     c. Turn to the left while pushing with the right foot and grasping a partial side rail on the left side of the bed with the right hand.
   d. Come to a sitting position on the side of the bed by using the right arm and hand to push down against the mattress and swinging the feet over the edge of the bed.
   - Teach a client with left abdominal or left-sided chest incision to perform the same procedure but splint with the right arm and turn to the right.
   - For clients with orthopedic surgery (e.g., hip surgery), use special aids, such as a trapeze, to assist with movement.

continued on page 904

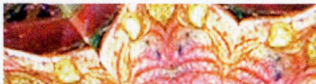

Procedure 35–1 Teaching Moving, Leg Exercises, Deep Breathing, and Coughing *continued*

IMPLEMENTATION

5. Teach the client the following three leg exercises:
   - Alternate dorsiflexion and plantar flexion of the feet. *This exercise is sometimes referred to as calf pumping, because it alternately contracts and relaxes the calf muscles, including the gastrocnemius muscles (see Figure 35–1 ■).*

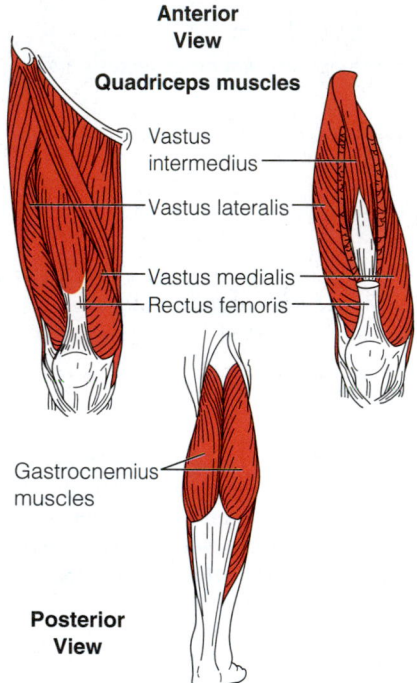

Figure 35–1 ■ Leg muscles: anterior and posterior views.

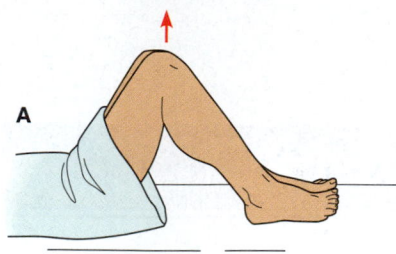

Figure 35–2 ■ Flexing and extending the knees.

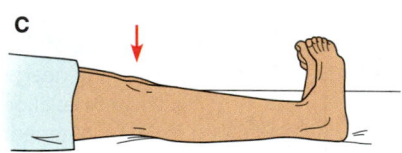

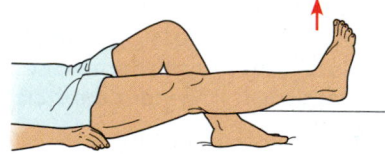

Figure 35–3 ■ Raising and lowering the legs.

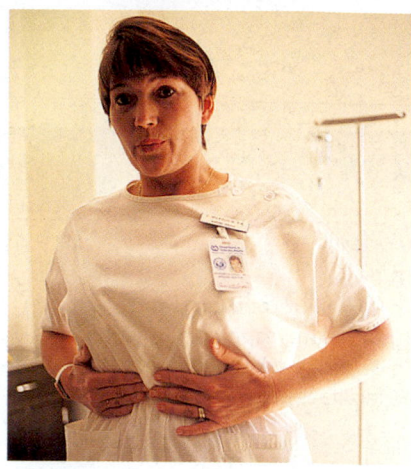

Figure 35–4 ■ Demonstrating deep breathing.

   - Flex and extend the knees, and press the backs of the knees into the bed while dorsiflexing the feet (Figure 35–2 ■). Instruct clients who cannot raise their legs to do isometric exercises that contract and relax the muscles.
   - Raise and lower the legs alternately from the surface of the bed. Flex the knee of the stable leg and extend the knee of the moving leg (Figure 35–3 ■). *This exercise contracts and relaxes the quadriceps muscles.*

6. Demonstrate deep-breathing (diaphragmatic) exercises as follows.
   - Place your hands palms down on the border of your rib cage, and inhale slowly and evenly through the nose until the greatest chest expansion is achieved (Figure 35–4 ■).
   - Hold your breath for 2 to 3 seconds.
   - Then exhale slowly through the mouth.
   - Continue exhalation until maximum chest contraction has been achieved.

7. Help the client perform deep-breathing exercises.
   - Ask the client to assume a sitting position.
   - Place the palms of your hands on the border of the client's rib cage to assess respiratory depth.
   - Ask the client to perform deep breathing, as described in step 6.

8. Instruct the client to cough voluntarily after a few deep inhalations.
   - Ask the client to inhale deeply, hold the breath for a few seconds, and then cough once or twice.
   - Ensure that the client coughs deeply and does not just clear the throat.

9. If the incision will be painful when the client coughs, demonstrate techniques to splint the abdomen.
   - Show the client how to support the incision by placing the palms of the hands on either side of the incision site or directly over the incision site, holding the palm of one hand over the other. *Coughing uses the abdominal and other accessory respiratory muscles. Splinting the incision may reduce pain while coughing if the incision is near any of these muscles.*
   - Show the client how to splint the abdomen with clasped hands and a firmly rolled pillow held against the client's abdomen (Figure 35–5 ■).

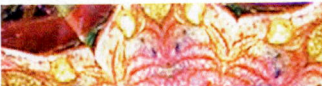

Procedure 35–1 Teaching Moving, Leg Exercises, Deep Breathing, and Coughing *continued*

IMPLEMENTATION *continued*

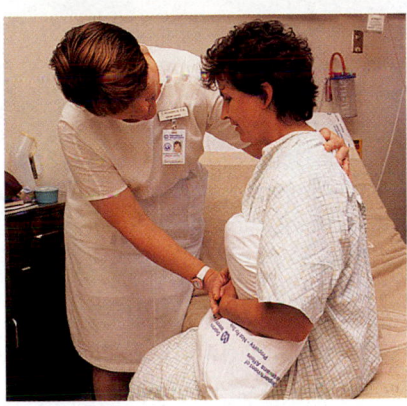

Figure 35–5 ■ Splinting an incision with a pillow while coughing.

10. Inform the client about the expected frequency of these exercises.
   • Instruct the client to start the exercises as soon after surgery as possible.
   • Encourage clients with abdominal or chest surgery to carry out deep breathing and coughing at least every 2 hours, taking a minimum of five breaths at each session. Note, however, that the number of breaths and frequency of deep breathing varies with the client's condition. People who are susceptible to pulmonary problems may need deep-breathing exercises every hour. People with chronic respiratory disease may need special breathing exercises (e.g., pursed-lip breathing, abdominal breathing, exercises using various kinds of incentive spirometers). See Chapter 48. ⊂⊃

11. Document the teaching and all assessments. Some agencies may have a preoperative teaching flow sheet. Check agency policy.

EVALUATION

Conduct appropriate follow-up such as
■ Client's demonstrated ability to perform moving, leg exercises, deep-breathing, and coughing exercises

■ Client's verbalization of key information presented.

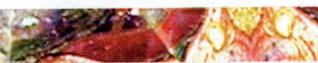

Lifespan Considerations

Preoperative Teaching
Children
■ Parents need to know what to expect and to be able to express their concerns.
■ Separation from parents often is the child's greatest fear; the time of separation should be minimized and parents allowed to interact with the child both immediately preceding and following the surgery.
■ Teaching of the child (both timing and content) should be geared to the child's developmental level and cognitive abilities.
■ Use simple terms to help the child understand (e.g., "You will have a sore tummy").
■ Play is an effective teaching tool with children; the child can put a bandage on an incision on a doll.

Elders
■ Assess hearing ability to ensure the elder client hears the necessary information.
■ Assess short-term memory. Presenting one focused idea at a time and repeating or reinforcing information may be necessary.

■ Elders are at greater risk for postoperative complications, such as pneumonia. Reinforce moving and deep-breathing and coughing exercises.
■ Assess potential postoperative needs at this time. Arrangements can be made preoperatively to obtain necessary items. Examples are medical equipment, such as walkers, raised toilet seats, bed trapezes, Meals on Wheels, and help with transportation.
■ If the elder client will need to be in extended care for a period of time after surgery, this is the time to initiate these plans.
■ Assess the client for risk of pressure ulcer development postoperatively and be extra attentive to use of proper paddings and support devices to prevent injury during positioning and transfers in the operating room. Risks are
   • Older age
   • Poor nutritional status
   • History of diabetes or cardiovascular problems
   • History of taking steroids, which cause increased bruising and skin breakdown.

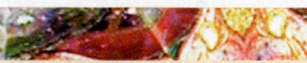

Home Care Considerations

Postoperative Instructions

Adults want information about activities they normally perform while they are recovering at home. This is important information for all surgical clients and particularly clients having the surgery at a same-day surgery center. Discuss the following areas:

- *Food.* Eat small portions at first because anesthesia and pain medications slow gastric emptying.
- *Bowel movements.* Constipation occurs frequently as a result of decreased gastrointestinal mobility due to many causes (e.g., anesthesia, decreased activity, pain medications). Discuss strategies to prevent constipation.
- *Sexual activity.* Intimacy such as gentle hugging and kissing is allowed for clients when they feel like it. Full sexual intercourse takes longer. By the time the wound soreness and tenderness is gone (2 to 4 weeks), the strength of the incision is adequate for sexual intercourse (Fox, 1998).
- *Wound care.* Discuss questions related to wound strength, pain, and infection.

- *Lifting.* Be specific about weight limits, if appropriate. Relate the weight limit to everyday items (e.g., a gallon of milk weighs approximately 8 pounds).
- *Pain.* Provide information about the client's pain medications. Ask the client to describe his or her daily activities and discuss ways to avoid or reduce painful activities.
- *Bathing.* Check with the surgeon because some prefer the wound to be kept dry. There is no evidence that water on a closed wound is harmful or interferes with wound healing. If allowed, inform the client to shower, letting the water wash over the incision for a short time (2 to 3 minutes) and gently pat the incision dry (Fox, 1998).
- *Infection.* Discuss the signs and symptoms of wound infection and when the client should call the physician.
- *Activities.* Advise the client that he or she will tire easily and to plan short activities with frequent rest breaks.

Physical Preparation

Preoperative preparation includes the following areas: nutrition and fluids, elimination, hygiene, medications, rest, care of valuables and prostheses, special orders, and surgical skin preparation. In many agencies a preoperative checklist is used on the day of surgery. The nurse checks the agency's forms and follows appropriate recording procedures. It is essential that (a) all pertinent records (laboratory records, x-ray films, consents)

be assembled and completed so that operating and recovery room personnel can refer to them and (b) all physical preparation is completed to ensure client safety.

Nutrition and Fluids. Adequate hydration and nutrition promote healing. Nurses need to record any signs of malnutrition or fluid imbalance. If the client is on intravenous fluids or on measured fluid intake, nurses must ensure that the fluids are carefully measured.

Research Note
Is "NPO After Midnight" Appropriate Practice?

The practice of NPO after midnight originated in 1946 when reports and animal studies suggested that a higher risk of pulmonary aspiration existed among clients who received general anesthesia and had not fasted. Reevaluation of this tradition began in the 1980s when numerous studies failed to demonstrate that fasting ensured that the stomach would empty. Recent research shows that pulmonary aspiration is a rare complication of modern anesthesia. In addition, prolonged fasting can lead to adverse effects such as irritability, headache, dehydration, hypovolemia, and hypoglycemia. As a result, in 1999, the American Society of Anesthesiology developed guidelines that support more liberal preoperative fasting protocols.

A study by Crenshaw and Winslow (2002) compared the ASA recommendations with the instructions that clients actually received and the period for which they fasted. The results indicated that clients fasted from liquids and solids up to two to three times *longer* than the ASA guidelines. The results also indicated that the majority of clients were not told why they needed to fast, and 32%

received no instructions about whether to take their regular medications on the morning of surgery. A nurse was involved in the preoperative teaching for 63% of the clients.

The authors noted the limitations of the study: It was conducted in only one hospital with a convenience sample of 155 clients. They recommended that similar studies with larger and different samples be conducted to confirm their findings.

Implications: Tradition is difficult to change even with new guidelines based on numerous research studies. Nurses are involved in preoperative teaching and need to provide practice based on evidence rather than tradition. The authors suggest that nurses need to be more assertive in their collaboration with physicians and develop hospital policies consistent with research evidence. It is important to client safety and comfort that accurate, specific information be given about the period of fasting, rationale for fasting, and which medications to take on the day of surgery.

Note: From "Preoperative Fasting: Old Habits Die Hard," by J. T. Crenshaw and E. H. Winslow, 2002, *American Journal of Nursing, 102*(5), pp. 36–44.

The order "NPO after midnight" has been a long-standing tradition because it was believed that anesthestics depress gastrointestinal functioning and there was a danger the client would vomit and aspirate during the administration of a general anesthetic. Reevaluation and research, however, do not support this tradition. As a result, the American Society of Anesthesiology (ASA) revised its practice guidelines for preoperative fasting in healthy clients undergoing elective procedures. According to Crenshaw and Winslow (2002, p. 38), the revised guidelines allow for

- The consumption of clear liquids up to 2 hours before elective surgery requiring general anesthesia, regional anesthesia, or sedation-analgesia
- A light breakfast (e.g., tea and toast) is permitted 6 hours before the procedure
- A heavier meal eight hours before surgery.

> **CLINICAL ALERT** *To help the client cope with thirst during the NPO period, the nurse can teach strategies such as rinsing the mouth, chewing gum, and sucking hard candy.* ■

Elimination. Enemas before surgery are no longer routine, but cleansing enemas may be ordered if bowel surgery is planned. The enemas help prevent postoperative constipation and contamination of the surgical area by feces. After surgery involving the intestines, peristalsis often doesn't return for 24 to 48 hours.

Prior to surgery a retention catheter may be ordered to ensure that the bladder remains empty. This helps prevent inadvertent injury to the bladder, particularly during pelvic surgery. If the client does not have a catheter, it is important to empty the bladder prior to receiving preoperative medications. The bladder must be empty during the operation.

Hygiene. In some settings, clients are asked to bathe or shower the evening or morning of surgery (or both). The purpose of hygienic measures is to reduce the risk of wound infection. The bath includes a shampoo whenever possible.

The client's nails should be trimmed and free of polish and all cosmetics should be removed so that the nail beds, skin, and lips are visible when circulation is assessed during and following surgery.

On the day of surgery, clients in some hospitals may be required to wear a surgical cap. The surgical caps contain the client's hair and any microorganisms on the hair and scalp.

Immediately before surgery, the nurse removes, or asks the client to remove, all hair pins and clips; these may cause pressure or accidental damage to the scalp when the client is unconscious. The client also removes personal clothing and puts on an operating room gown.

Medications. The anesthetist or anesthesiologist may temporarily discontinue routinely taken medications the day of surgery. In some settings preoperative medications are given after the client goes to the operating room; otherwise they are given on the hospital unit. Commonly used preoperative medications include

- *Sedatives* and *tranquilizers* such as secobarbital and diazepam (Valium) to reduce anxiety and ease anesthetic induction
- *Narcotic analgesics* such as morphine and meperidine (Demerol) to provide client sedation and reduce the required amount of anesthetic
- *Anticholinergics* such as atropine, scopolamine, and glycopyrrolate (Robinul) to reduce oral and pulmonary secretions and prevent laryngospasm
- *Histamine-receptor antihistamines* such as cimetidine (Tagamet) and ranitidine (Zantac) to reduce gastric fluid volume and gastric acidity
- *Neuroleptanalgesic* agents such as Innovar to induce general calmness and sleepiness

Preoperative medications must be given at a scheduled time or "on call," that is, when the operating room notifies the nurse to give the medication.

Rest and Sleep. Nurses should do everything to help the client sleep the night before surgery. Often a sedative is ordered. Adequate rest helps the client manage the stress of surgery and helps healing.

Valuables. Valuables such as jewelry and money should be labeled and placed in safekeeping if the client's support people cannot take them home. Removing jewelry also means removing body piercing jewelry as well because there is a risk of injury from burns if an electrosurgical unit is used (AORN Online, 2002). If a client wishes not to remove a wedding band, the nurse can tape it in place. Wedding bands must be removed, however, if there is danger of the fingers swelling after surgery. Situations warranting removal include surgery on or cast application to an arm and a mastectomy that involves removal of the lymph nodes. (Mastectomies may cause edema of the arm and hand.)

Prostheses. All prostheses (artificial body parts, such as partial or complete dentures, contact lenses, artificial eyes, and artificial limbs) and eyeglasses, wigs, and false eyelashes must be removed before surgery. Hearing aids are often left in place and the operating room personnel notified.

In some hospitals, dentures are placed in a locked storage area; in others they are placed in labeled containers and kept at the client's bedside. Partial dentures can become dislodged and obstruct an unconscious client's breathing. The nurse also checks for the presence of chewing gum or loose teeth, a common problem with 5- or 6-year-olds undergoing tonsillectomy. Loose teeth can become dislodged and aspirated during anesthesia.

Special Orders. The nurse checks the surgeon's orders for special requirements (e.g., the insertion of a nasogastric tube prior to surgery, the administration of medications, such as insulin, or the application of antiemboli stockings). For the technique of inserting a nasogastric tube, see Procedure 45–1 in Chapter 45. 🔗

Skin Preparation. In most agencies, skin preparation is carried out during the intraoperative phase.

Vital Signs. Assess and record vital signs for baseline data. Report any abnormal findings, such as elevated blood pressure or elevated temperature.

Antiemboli Stockings. Antiemboli (elastic) stockings are firm elastic hose that compress the veins of the legs and thereby facilitate the return of venous blood to the heart. They also improve arterial circulation to the feet and prevent edema of the legs and feet. These stockings are frequently applied preoperatively as well as postoperatively.

There are several types of stockings. One type extends from the foot to the knee and another from the foot to midthigh. These stockings usually have a partial foot that exposes the heel or toes so that extremity circulation can be assessed. Elastic stockings usually come in small, medium, and large sizes. Procedure 35–2 details the steps required to apply antiemboli stockings.

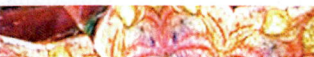

Procedure 35–2 Applying Antiemboli Stockings

Purposes

- To facilitate venous return from the lower extremities
- To prevent venous stasis and venous thrombosis
- To reduce peripheral edema

ASSESSMENT

Assess both lower extremities for
- Rates, volumes, and rhythms of posterior tibial and dorsalis pedis pulses
- Skin color (note pallor, cyanosis, or other pigmentation)
- Skin temperature
- Presence of distended veins or edema
- Skin condition (e.g., thickened, shiny, taut)
- Homans sign (pain in calf with passive dorsiflexion of the foot)

PLANNING

Before applying antiemboli stockings, determine any potential or present circulatory problems and the surgeon's orders involving the lower extremities.

Delegation

UAP frequently remove and apply antiemboli stockings as part of morning and evening hygiene care. The nurse should stress the importance of removing and reapplying the stockings and reporting any changes in the client's skin to the nurse.

Equipment
- Tape measure
- Clean antiemboli stockings of appropriate size and of the type ordered
- Talcum powder or cornstarch (check if the client has an allergy to the powder)

IMPLEMENTATION

Preparation
Take measurements as needed to obtain the appropriate size stockings.
- Measure the length of both legs from the heel to the gluteal fold (for thigh-length stockings) or from the heel to the popliteal space (for knee-length stockings).
- Measure the circumference of each calf and each thigh at the widest point.
- Compare the measurements to the size chart to obtain stockings of correct size. Obtain two sizes if there is a significant difference. *Stockings that are too large for the client do not place adequate pressure on the legs to facilitate venous return, and may bunch, increasing the risk of pressure and skin irritation. Stockings that are too small may impede blood flow to the feet and cause discomfort.*

Performance
1. Explain to the client what you are going to do, why it is necessary, and how he or she can cooperate.

2. Wash hands and observe other appropriate infection control procedures.
3. Provide for client privacy.
4. Select an appropriate time to apply the stockings.
   - Apply stockings in the morning, if possible, before the client arises. *In sitting and standing positions, the veins can become distended so that edema occurs; the stockings should be applied before this happens.*
   - Assist the client who has been ambulating to lie down and elevate the legs for 15 to 30 minutes before applying the stockings. *This facilitates venous return and reduces swelling.*
5. Prepare the client.
   - Assist the client to a lying position in bed.
   - Wash and dry the legs as needed.
   - Dust the ankles with talcum powder or cornstarch. *This eases application.*

6. Apply the stockings.
   - Reach inside the stocking from the top, and grasping the heel, turn the upper portion of the stocking inside out so the foot portion is inside the stocking leg. *Firm elastic stockings are easier to fit over the foot and calf when inverted in this manner rather than bunching up the stocking.*
   - Ask the client to point his or her toes, then position the stocking on the client's foot. With the heel of the stocking down and stretching each side of the stocking, ease the stocking over the toes taking care to place the toe and heel portions of the stocking appropriately (Figure 35–6 ■). *Pointing the toes makes application easier.*

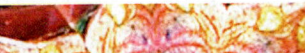

Procedure 35–2 Applying Antiemboli Stockings *continued*

IMPLEMENTATION *continued*

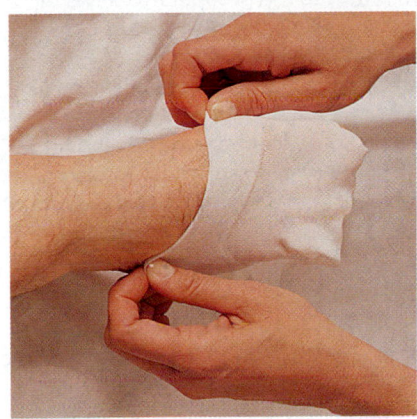

Figure 35–6 ■ Applying the inverted stocking over the toes.

- Grasp the loose portion of the stocking at the ankle and gently pull the stocking over the leg, turning it right side out in the process (Figure 35–7 ■).

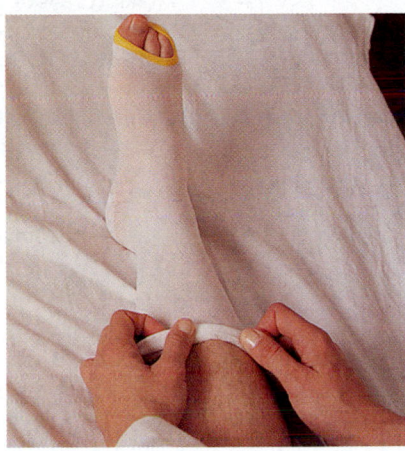

Figure 35–7 ■ Pulling the stocking snugly over the leg.

- Inspect the client's leg and stocking, smoothing any folds or creases. Ensure that the stocking is not rolled down or bunched at the top or ankle. *Folds and creases can cause skin irritation under the stocking; bunching of the stocking can further impair venous return.*
- Remove the stockings for 30 minutes every 8 hours, inspecting the legs and skin while the stockings are off.
- Soiled stockings may be laundered by hand with warm water and mild soap. Hang to dry.
7. Document the procedure. Record the procedure, your assessment data, and when the stockings are removed and reapplied.

EVALUATION

- Conduct appropriate follow-up at least every 4 hours.
- Note the appearance of the legs and skin integrity, any edema, peripheral pulses, skin color and temperature, and compare to previous assessment data, if available.

- If complications occur, remove the stockings and report significant deviations from normal to the physician.

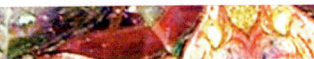

Lifespan Considerations

Antiemboli Stockings

Children
- Antiemboli stockings are infrequently used on children.

Elders
- Because the elastic is quite strong in antiemboli stockings, the elder may need assistance with putting on the stockings. Clients with arthritis may need to have another person put the stockings on for them.

- Many elders have circulation problems and wear antiemboli stockings. It is important to check for wrinkles in the stockings and/or to see if the stocking has rolled down or twisted. If so, correct immediately because the stockings must be evenly distributed over the limb to promote rather than hinder circulation.
- Stockings should be removed once each shift so that a thorough assessment can be made of legs and feet. Redness and skin breakdown on the heels can occur quickly and go undetected if not thoroughly assessed on a regular basis.

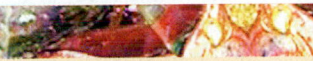

Home Care Considerations

Antiemboli Stockings
- Teach the client or caregiver how to apply the antiemboli stockings.
- Stress the importance of no wrinkles or rolling down of the stockings and the rationale.
- Instruct the client or caregiver to remove the stockings regularly and inspect the skin on the legs.

- Provide instructions about
  - Laundering the stockings
  - The need for two pairs of stockings to allow for one pair to be worn while the other is being laundered
  - Replacing the stockings when they lose their elasticity.

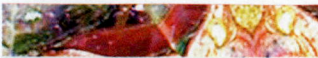

Lifespan Considerations

Postoperative Care
Elders

- Elders have less efficient reserves and may take longer to recover postoperatively. Be attentive to vital signs, intake and output, and mental status and note significant changes.
- Clients with dementia often experience an increase in confusion and agitation from the medications and anesthesia used during surgery. This poses a safety risk during the postoperative period and requires nursing staff to monitor these clients more frequently. It is important to maintain a calm,

reassuring attitude. These changes are often long-lasting, taking days or weeks to return to the preoperative level of cognition.
- Elders may experience more fatigue and weakness after surgery. Encouraging activity is crucial, but needs to be paced to prevent exhaustion.
- When surgery is done on an outpatient basis, nurses should follow up with phone calls that evening and the next day to check on the client's condition and make sure that postoperative instructions were understood.

Sequential Compression Devices. Clients who are undergoing surgery may benefit from a sequential compression device (SCD) to promote venous return from the legs. SCDs inflate and deflate plastic sleeves wrapped around the legs to promote venous flow. SCDs are discussed in Chapter 49 ⟲ (see Procedure 49–1).

EVALUATING

The goals established during the planning phase are evaluated according to specific desired outcomes, also established in that phase. An example of client outcomes and related indicators was shown earlier in Identifying Nursing Diagnoses, Outcomes, and Interventions.

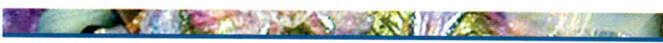

INTRAOPERATIVE PHASE

The intraoperative nurse is a vital member of the surgical team, advocating for the client, maintaining safety, and continually assessing the needs of the client and the team.

Types of Anesthesia

Anesthesia is classified as *general* or *regional.* Anesthetic agents usually are administered by an anesthesiologist or nurse anesthetist. **General anesthesia** is the loss of all sensation and consciousness. Under general anesthesia, protective reflexes such as cough and gag reflexes are lost. A general anesthetic acts by blocking awareness centers in the brain so that amnesia (loss of memory), analgesia (insensibility to pain), hypnosis (artificial sleep), and relaxation (rendering a part of the body less tense) occur. General anesthetics are usually administered by intravenous infusion or by inhalation of gases through a mask or through an endotracheal tube inserted into the trachea.

General anesthesia has certain advantages. Because the client is unconscious rather than awake and anxious, respiration and cardiac function are readily regulated. Also, the anesthesia can be adjusted to the length of the operation and the client's age and physical status. Its chief disadvantage is that it depresses the respiratory and circulatory systems. Some clients become more anxious about a general anesthetic than about the surgery itself. Often this is because they fear losing the capacity to control their own bodies.

Regional anesthesia is the temporary interruption of the transmission of nerve impulses to and from a specific area or region of the body. The client loses sensation in an area of the body but remains conscious. Several techniques are used.

- **Topical (surface) anesthesia** is applied directly to the skin and mucous membranes, open skin surfaces, wounds, and burns. The most commonly used topical agents are lidocaine (Xylocaine) and benzocaine. Topical anesthetics are readily absorbed and act rapidly.
- **Local anesthesia** (infiltration) is injected into a specific area and is used for minor surgical procedures such as suturing a small wound or performing a biopsy. Lidocaine or tetracaine 0.1% may be used.
- A **nerve block** is a technique in which the anesthetic agent is injected into and around a nerve or small nerve group that supplies sensation to a small area of the body. Major blocks involve multiple nerves or a plexus (e.g., the brachial plexus anesthetizes the arm); minor blocks involve a single nerve (e.g., a facial nerve).
- An **intravenous block (Bier block)** is used most often for procedures involving the arm, wrist, and hand. An occlusion tourniquet is applied to the extremity to prevent infiltration and absorption of the injected intravenous agent beyond the involved extremity.
- **Spinal anesthesia** is also referred to as **subarachnoid block (SAB).** It requires a lumbar puncture through one of the interspaces between lumbar disc 2 (L_2) and the sacrum (S_1). An anesthetic agent is injected into the subarachnoid space surrounding the spinal cord. Spinal anesthesia is often categorized as a low, mid, or high spinal. Low spinals (saddle or caudal blocks) are primarily used for surgeries involving the perineal or rectal areas. Mid spinals (below the level of the umbilicus—T_{10}) can be used for hernia repairs or appendectomies, and high spinals (reaching the nipple line—T_4) can be used for surgeries such as cesarean sections.
- **Epidural (peridural) anesthesia** is an injection of an anesthetic agent into the epidural space, the area inside the spinal column but outside the dura mater.

Conscious sedation may be used alone or in conjunction with regional anesthesia for some diagnostic tests and surgical procedures. **Conscious sedation** refers to minimal depression of the level of consciousness in which the client retains the ability to maintain a patent airway and respond appropriately to commands (Kost, 1999). Intravenous narcotics such as morphine or fentanyl (Sublimaze) and antianxiety agents such as diazepam (Valium) or midazolam (Versed) are commonly used to induce and maintain conscious sedation. Conscious sedation increases the client's pain threshold and induces a degree of amnesia but allows for prompt reversal of its effects and a rapid return to normal activities of daily living. Procedures such as endoscopies, incision and drainage of abscesses, and even balloon angioplasty may be performed under conscious sedation.

NURSING MANAGEMENT

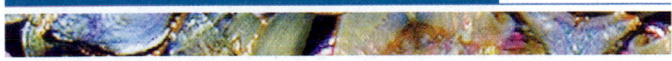

ASSESSING

On the client's admission to the surgical suite or procedure room, the perioperative nurse confirms the client's identity and assesses the client's physical and emotional status. The nurse verifies the information on the preoperative checklist and evaluates the client's knowledge about the surgery and events to follow. The client's response to preoperative medications is assessed, as well as the placement and patency of tubes such as IV lines, nasogastric tubes, and urinary catheters.

Assessment continues throughout surgery, as the nurse and the anesthetist continuously monitor the client's vital signs (including blood pressure, heart rate, respiratory rate, and temperature), ECG, and oxygen saturation. Fluid intake and urinary output are monitored throughout surgery, and blood loss is estimated. In addition, arterial and venous pressures, pulmonary artery pressures, and laboratory values such as blood glucose, hemoglobin, hematocrit, serum electrolytes, and arterial blood gases may be evaluated during surgery. Continual assessment is necessary to rapidly identify adverse responses to surgery or anesthesia and intervene promptly to prevent complications.

DIAGNOSING

NANDA nursing diagnoses that may be appropriate for the intraoperative client include

- *Risk for Aspiration*
- *Ineffective Protection*
- *Impaired Skin Integrity*
- *Risk for Perioperative-Positioning Injury*
- *Risk for Imbalanced Body Temperature*
- *Ineffective Tissue Perfusion*
- *Risk for Deficient Fluid Volume.*

PLANNING

The overall goals of care in the intraoperative period are to maintain the client's safety and to maintain homeostasis. Examples of nursing activities to achieve these goals include the following:

- Position the client appropriately for surgery.
- Perform preoperative skin preparation.

- Assist in preparing and maintaining the sterile field.
- Open and dispense sterile supplies during surgery.
- Provide medications and solutions for the sterile field.
- Monitor and maintain a safe, aseptic environment.
- Manage catheters, tubes, drains, and specimens.
- Perform sponge, sharp, and instrument counts.
- Document nursing care provided and the client's response to interventions.

IMPLEMENTING

During surgery, nurses function as circulating nurses and scrub nurses. **Circulating nurses** assist scrub nurses and the surgeons. They help position the client for the operation and often position any needed equipment. During the surgery, circulating nurses obtain additional supplies as needed, arrange lighting, and so on. **Scrub nurses** assist the surgeons. They wear sterile gowns, gloves, caps, and so on. Their responsibilities include draping the client with sterile drapes and handling sterile instruments and supplies. They also account for used sponges, needles, and instruments. In some surgical settings a surgeon does not close, that is, suture an incision, until the scrub nurse can account for all sponges and instruments. This precaution avoids leaving any supplies inside the client.

Surgical Skin Preparation

Surgical skin preparation involves cleaning the surgical site, removing hair only if necessary, and applying an antimicrobial agent. In most surgery centers skin preparation is done by surgery personnel close to the time of surgery. The purpose of a surgical skin preparation is to reduce the risk of postoperative wound infection. This is done by

- Removing soil and transient microbes from the skin
- Reducing the resident microbial count to subpathogenic amounts in a short time and with the least amount of tissue irritation
- Inhibiting rapid rebound growth of microbes.

The Association of Operating Room Nurses (1996) recommends the following skin preparation practices to reduce the risk of postoperative wound infections:

- Clean the surgical site and surrounding areas. This can be accomplished before the surgical prep by having the client shower and shampoo or wash the surgical site before arriving in the surgical setting, or by washing the surgical site in the surgical setting immediately before applying an antimicrobial agent.
- Assess the surgical site before skin preparation. The nurse assesses the site for moles, warts, rashes, or other skin conditions such as pustules, abrasions, or exudate, and documents their presence before skin preparation.
- Remove hair from the surgical site only when necessary or according to physician's orders or institutional policies and procedures. Personnel skilled in hair removal should remove hair using techniques that preserve skin integrity. Electric clippers or a depilatory cream should be used to reduce the

risk of traumatizing the skin during hair removal. If a depilatory is used, hypersensitivity testing is performed prior to applying it to the surgical site. Skin trauma and abrasions increase the risk of microorganisms colonizing the surgical site. If hair is to be removed, it is done as close to the time of surgery as possible (near the room where the surgical procedure will be performed) to reduce the time for microbial growth.

- Prepare the surgical site and surrounding area with an antimicrobial agent when indicated. A nontoxic antimicrobial agent with a broad range of germicidal action is used to inhibit the growth of microorganisms during and following the surgical procedure. The agent selected depends on the client's history of hypersensitivity reactions, the location of the surgical site, and the skin condition. An area large enough to accommodate extension of the incision and any potential drain sites or additional incisions is prepared.

- Document surgical skin preparation in the client's record. Documentation should include the skin condition, including any growths, abrasions, or rashes; hair removal and the techniques used, if performed; the skin preparation, including cleansing and antimicrobial agent applied; who performed the preoperative skin preparation; and any adverse or hypersensitivity responses noted.

Positioning

Proper positioning of the client during surgery is an important responsibility shared by the nurse, surgeon, and anesthetist. The ideal intraoperative client position provides

- Optimal visualization of and access to the surgical site
- Optimal access for assessing and maintaining anesthesia and vital functions (vital signs, respirations, cardiovascular function)
- Protection of the client from harm.

Positioning is performed after anesthesia is induced and before surgical draping of the client. The client is lifted into position to prevent shearing forces on the skin from sliding or rolling. The exact position for the client depends on the operation, that is, the surgical approach. For example, a lithotomy position is usually used for vaginal surgery.

Positions on the operating table are maintained by straps, and body prominences are frequently padded. The position should consider normal joint range of motion and good body alignment, thereby avoiding strain or injury to muscles, bones, and ligaments.

> **CLINICAL ALERT** *Be especially aware of the intraoperative position required for elders. Because elders are vulnerable to pressure ulcer formation, check the appropriate pressure points of that surgical position on the client.* ■

EVALUATING

The intraoperative nurse uses the goals developed during the planning stage (e.g., maintain client safety) and collects data to evaluate whether the desired outcomes have been achieved.

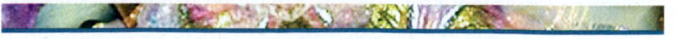

Documentation

Throughout the intraoperative phase the nurse documents client care activities such as IV fluid infusions, positioning, gastric suction, and urinary catheterization.

POSTOPERATIVE PHASE

Nursing during the postoperative phase is especially important for the client's recovery. Anesthesia impairs the ability of clients to respond to environmental stimuli and to help themselves, although the degree of consciousness of clients will vary. Moreover, surgery itself traumatizes the body by disrupting protective mechanisms and homeostasis.

Immediate Postanesthetic Phase

Recovery nurses have specialized skills to care for clients recovering from anesthesia and surgery (Figure 35–8 ■). Once the health status has stabilized, the client is returned to the nursing unit or, in the case of a day-surgery client, to the day-surgery area before discharge. Assessment of the client in the immediate postanesthetic period is summarized in Box 35–5.

During the immediate postanesthetic stage, an unconscious client is positioned on the side, with the face slightly down. A pillow is not placed under the head. In this position, gravity keeps the tongue forward, preventing occlusion of the pharynx and allowing drainage of mucus or vomitus out of the mouth rather than down the respiratory tree.

The nurse ensures maximum chest expansion by elevating the client's upper arm on a pillow. The upper arm is supported because the pressure of an arm against the chest reduces chest expansion potential. An artificial airway is maintained in place, and the client is suctioned as needed until cough and swallowing reflexes return. Generally the client spits out an oropharyngeal airway when coughing returns. Endotracheal tubes are not removed until clients are awake and able to maintain their own airway. The client is then helped to turn, cough, and take deep

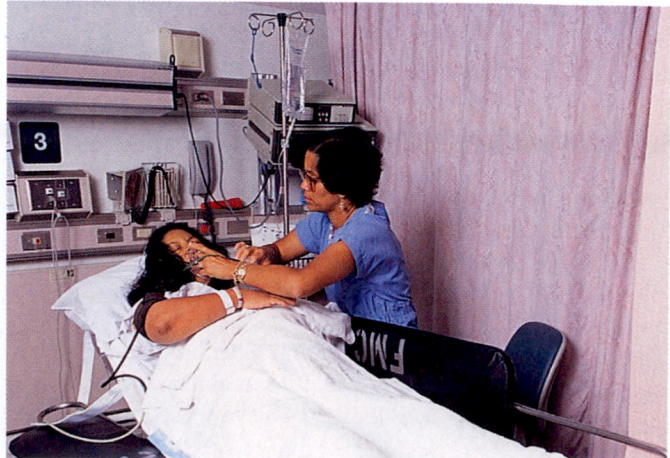

Figure 35–8 ■ Recovery room nurse provides constant assessment and care for clients recovering from anesthesia and surgery.

BOX 35–5 ■ Clinical Assessment

Immediate Postanesthetic Phase

- Adequacy of airway
- Oxygen saturation
- Adequacy of ventilation
  - Respiratory rate, rhythm, and depth
  - Use of accessory muscles
  - Breath sounds
- Cardiovascular status
  - Heart rate and rhythm
  - Peripheral pulse amplitude and equality
  - Blood pressure
  - Capillary filling
- Level of consciousness
  - Not responding
  - Arousable with verbal stimuli
  - Fully awake
  - Oriented to time, person, and place

- Presence of protective reflexes (e.g., gag, cough)
- Activity, ability to move extremities
- Skin color (pink, pale, dusky, blotchy, cyanotic, jaundiced)
- Fluid status
  - Intake and output
  - Status of IV infusions (type of fluid, rate, amount in container, patency of tubing)
  - Signs of dehydration or fluid overload (see Chapter 50)
- Condition of operative site
  - Status of dressing
  - Drainage (amount, type, and color)
- Patency of and character and amount of drainage from catheters, tubes, and drains
- Discomfort (i.e., pain) (type, location, and severity), nausea, vomiting
- Safety (i.e., necessity for side rails, call bell within reach)

---

breaths, provided that vital signs are stable. When spinal anesthesia is used, the client may be required to remain flat for a specified period. See Chapter 48 for information about artificial airways.

The return of the client's reflexes, such as swallowing and gagging, indicates that anesthesia is ending. Time of recovery from anesthesia varies with the kind of anesthetic agent used, its dosage, and the individual's response to it. Nurses should arouse clients by calling them by name, and in a normal tone of voice repeatedly telling them that the surgery is over and that they are in the PACU.

Once the health status has stabilized, the client is returned to the nursing unit or, in the case of a day-surgery client, to the day-surgery area.

Clients are usually discharged from the PACU when

- They are conscious and oriented.
- They are able to maintain a clear airway and deep breathe and cough freely.
- Vital signs have been stable or consistent with preoperative vital signs for at least 30 minutes.
- Protective reflexes (e.g., gag, swallowing) are active.
- They are able to move four extremities.
- Intake and urinary output is adequate (at least 30 mL/hr).
- They are afebrile or a febrile condition has been attended to.
- Dressings are dry and intact; there is no overt drainage.

Preparing for Ongoing Care of the Postoperative Client

While the client is in the operating room, the client's bed and room are prepared for the postoperative phase. In some agencies, the client is brought back to the unit on a stretcher and transferred to the bed in the room. In other agencies, the client's bed is brought to the surgery suite, and the client is transferred there. In the latter situation, the bed needs to be made with clean linens as soon as the client goes to surgery so that it can be taken to the op-

erating room when needed. In addition, the nurse must obtain and set up any special equipment, such as an intravenous pole, suction, oxygen equipment, and orthopedic appliances (e.g., traction). If these are not requested on the client's record, the nurse should consult with the perioperative nurse or surgeon.

NURSING MANAGEMENT

ASSESSING

As soon as the client returns to the nursing unit, the nurse conducts an initial assessment. The sequence of these activities varies with the situation. For example, the nurse may need to check the physician's stat orders before conducting the initial assessment; in such a case, nursing interventions to implement the orders can be carried out at the same time as assessment.

The nurse consults the surgeon's postoperative orders to learn the following:

- Food and fluids permitted by mouth
- Intravenous solutions and intravenous medications
- Position in bed
- Medications ordered (e.g., analgesics, antibiotics)
- Laboratory tests
- Intake and output, which in some agencies are monitored for all postoperative clients
- Activity permitted, including ambulation.

The nurse also checks the PACU record for the following data:

- Operation performed
- Presence and location of any drains
- Anesthetic used
- Postoperative diagnosis
- Estimated blood loss
- Medications administered in the recovery room.

Many hospitals have postoperative protocols for regular assessment of clients. In some agencies, assessments are made every 15 minutes until vital signs stabilize, every hour for the next 4 hours, then every 4 hours for the next 2 days. It is important that the assessments be made as often as the client's condition requires. The nurse assesses the following:

- *Level of consciousness.* Assess orientation to time, place, and person. Most clients are fully conscious but drowsy when returned to their unit. Assess reaction to verbal stimuli and ability to move extremities.
- *Vital signs.* Take the client's vital signs (pulse, respiration, blood pressure, and oxygen saturation level) every 15 minutes until stable or in accordance with agency protocol. Compare initial findings with PACU data. In addition, assess the client's lung sounds and assess for signs of common circulatory problems such as postoperative hypotension, hemorrhage, or shock. Hypovolemia due to fluid losses during surgery is a common cause of postoperative hypotension. Hemorrhage can result from insecure ligation of blood vessels or disruption of sutures. Massive hemorrhage or cardiac insufficiency can lead to shock postoperatively. Common postoperative complications with their manifestations and preventive measures are listed in Table 35–2.
- *Skin color and temperature,* particularly that of the lips and nail beds. The color of the lips and nail beds is an indicator of **tissue perfusion** (passage of blood through the vessels). Pale, cyanotic, cool, and moist skin may be a sign of circulatory problems.

> ➤ **CLINICAL ALERT** *Elders may not show the classic signs of infection (e.g., fever, tachycardia, increased WBC); instead there may be an abrupt change in their mental status.* ■

- *Comfort.* Assess pain with the client's vital signs and as needed between vital sign measurements. Assess the location and intensity of the pain. Do not assume that reported pain is incisional; other causes may include muscle strains, flatus, and angina. Ask the client to rate pain on a scale of 0 to 10, with 0 being no pain and 10 the worst pain imaginable. Evaluate the client for objective indicators of pain: pallor, perspiration, muscle tension, and reluctance to cough, move, or ambulate. Determine when and what analgesics were last administered, and assess the client for any side effects of medication such as nausea and vomiting.
- *Fluid balance.* Assess the type and amount of intravenous fluids, flow rate, and infusion site. Monitor the client's fluid intake and output. In addition to watching for shock, assess the client for signs of circulatory overload, and monitor serum electrolytes. Anesthetics and surgery affect the hormones regulating fluid and electrolyte balance (aldosterone and ADH in particular), placing the client at risk for decreased urine output and fluid and electrolyte imbalances.
- *Dressing and bedclothes.* Inspect the client's dressings and bedclothes underneath the client. Excessive bloody drainage on dressings or on bedclothes, often appearing underneath the client, can indicate hemorrhage. The amount of drainage on dressings is recorded by describing the diameter of the stains or by denoting the number and type of dressings saturated with drainage.
- *Drains and tubes.* Determine color, consistency, and amount of drainage from all tubes and drains. All tubes should be patent, and tubes and suction equipment should be functioning. Drainage bags must be hanging properly.

Document the client's time of arrival and all assessments. Many agencies have progress flow records for this purpose. Alter the frequency, parameters, and priorities to meet the individual needs of the client.

DIAGNOSING

Because surgery can involve many body systems both directly and indirectly and is a complex experience for the client, the nursing diagnoses focus on a wide variety of actual, potential, and collaborative problems.

Actual and potential NANDA diagnoses for the postoperative client include

- *Acute Pain*
- *Risk for Infection*
- *Risk for Injury*
- *Risk for Deficient Fluid Volume*
- *Ineffective Airway Clearance*
- *Ineffective Breathing Pattern*
- *Self-Care Deficit: Bathing/Hygiene, Dressing/Grooming, Toileting*
- *Ineffective Health Maintenance*
- *Disturbed Body Image.*

Collaborative problems that may be experienced by the postoperative client are summarized in Table 35–2. Examples of clinical application of some of these diagnoses using NANDA, NIC, and NOC designations are shown in Identifying Nursing Diagnoses, Outcomes, and Interventions.

PLANNING

Postoperative care planning and discharge planning begin in the preoperative phase when preoperative teaching is implemented. Examples of clinical application of NOC outcomes and NIC interventions are shown in Identifying Nursing Diagnoses, Outcomes, and Interventions.

Planning for Home Care

To provide for continuity of care for the surgical client after discharge, the nurse needs to consider the client's needs for assistance with care in the home setting. Discharge planning for both the day-surgery client and the client who has been hospitalized for several days following surgery incorporates an assessment of the client's and family's abilities for self-care, financial resources, and the need for referrals and home health services. The accompanying Home Care Assessment box outlines a home care assessment for a surgical client; however, it is important to remember that surgical clients have diverse needs, and additional assessment data may be required.

TABLE 35–2 Potential Postoperative Problems

Problem	Description	Cause	Clinical Signs	Preventive Interventions
Respiratory				
Pneumonia	Inflammation of the alveoli	Infection, toxins, or irritants causing inflammatory process	Elevated temperature, cough, expectoration of blood-tinged or purulent sputum, dyspnea, chest pain	Deep-breathing exercises and coughing, moving in bed, early ambulation
Infectious pneumonia	May be limited to one or more lobes (lobar) or occur as scattered patches throughout the lungs (bronchial); also can involve interstitial tissues of lungs	Common organisms include *Streptococcus pneumoniae, Haemophilus influenzae,* and *Staphylococcus aureus*		
Hypostatic pneumonia		Immobility and impaired ventilation result in atelectasis and promote growth of pathogens		
Aspiration pneumonia	Inflammatory process caused by irritation of lung tissue by aspirated material, particularly hydrochloric acid (HCl) from the stomach	Aspiration of gastric contents, food, or other substances; often related to loss of gag reflex		
Atelectasis	A condition in which alveoli collapse and are not ventilated	Mucous plugs blocking bronchial passageways, inadequate lung expansion, analgesics, immobility	Dyspnea, tachypnea, tachycardia; diaphoresis, anxiety; pleural pain, decreased chest wall movement; dull or absent breath sounds; decreased oxygen saturation (SaO_2)	Deep-breathing exercises and coughing, moving in bed, early ambulation
Pulmonary embolism	Blood clot that has moved to the lungs and blocks a pulmonary artery, thus obstructing blood flow to a portion of the lung	Stasis of venous blood from immobility, venous injury from fractures or during surgery, use of oral contraceptives high in estrogen, preexisting coagulation or circulatory disorder	Sudden chest pain, shortness of breath, cyanosis, shock (tachycardia, low blood pressure)	Turning, ambulation, antiemboli stockings, sequential compression devices
Circulatory				
Hypovolemia	Inadequate circulating blood volume	Fluid deficit, hemorrhage	Tachycardia, decreased urine output, decreased blood pressure	Early detection of signs; fluid and/or blood replacement

continued on page 916

TABLE 35–2 Potential Postoperative Problems (continued)

Problem	Description	Cause	Clinical Signs	Preventive Interventions
Hemorrhage	Internal or external bleeding	Disruption of sutures, insecure ligation of blood vessels	Overt bleeding (dressings saturated with bright blood; bright, free-flowing blood in drains or chest tubes), increased pain, increasing abdominal girth, swelling or bruising around incision	Early detection of signs
Hypovolemic shock	Inadequate tissue perfusion resulting from markedly reduced circulating blood volume	Severe hypovolemia from fluid deficit or hemorrhage	Rapid weak pulse, dyspnea, tachypnea; restlessness and anxiety; urine output less than 30 mL/hr; decreased blood pressure; cool, clammy skin, thirst, pallor	Maintain blood volume through adequate fluid replacement, prevent hemorrhage; early detection of signs
Thrombophlebitis	Inflammation of the veins, usually of the legs and associated with a blood clot	Slowed venous blood flow due to immobility or prolonged sitting; trauma to vein, resulting in inflammation and increased blood coagulability	Aching, cramping pain; affected area is swollen, red, and hot to touch; vein feels hard; discomfort in calf when foot is dorsiflexed or when client walks (Homans' sign)	Early ambulation, leg exercises, antiemboli stockings, SCDs, adequate fluid intake
Thrombus	Blood clot attached to wall of vein or artery (most commonly the leg veins)	As for thrombophlebitis for venous thrombi; disruption or inflammation of arterial wall for arterial thrombi	*Venous:* same as thrombophlebitis *Arterial:* pain and pallor of affected extremity; decreased or absent peripheral pulses	*Venous:* same as thrombophlebitis *Arterial:* maintain prescribed position; early detection of signs
Embolus	Foreign body or clot that has moved from its site of formation to another area of the body (e.g., the lungs, heart, or brain).	Venous or arterial thrombus; broken intravenous catheter, fat, or amniotic fluid	In venous system, usually becomes a pulmonary embolus (see pulmonary embolism); signs of arterial emboli may depend on the location	As for thrombophlebitis or thrombus; careful maintenance of IV catheters
Urinary				
Urinary retention	Inability to empty the bladder, with excessive accumulation of urine in the bladder	Depressed bladder muscle tone from narcotics and anesthetics; handling of tissues during surgery on adjacent organs (rectum, vagina)	Fluid intake larger than output; inability to void or frequent voiding of small amounts, bladder distention, suprapubic discomfort, restlessness	Monitoring of fluid intake and output, interventions to facilitate voiding, urinary catheterization as needed
Urinary tract infection	Inflammation of the bladder, ureters, or urethra	Immobilization and limited fluid intake, instrumentation of the urinary tract	Burning sensation when voiding, urgency, cloudy urine, lower abdominal pain	Adequate fluid intake, early ambulation, aseptic straight catheterization only as necessary, good perineal hygiene

TABLE 35–2　Potential Postoperative Problems (continued)

Problem	Description	Cause	Clinical Signs	Preventive Interventions
Gastrointestinal				
Nausea and vomiting		Pain, abdominal distention, ingesting food or fluids before return of peristalsis, certain medications, anxiety	Complaints of feeling sick to the stomach, retching or gagging	IV fluids until peristalsis returns; then clear fluids, full fluids, and regular diet; antiemetic drugs if ordered; analgesics for pain
Constipation	Infrequent or no stool passage for abnormal length of time (e.g., within 48 hours after solid diet started)	Lack of dietary roughage, analgesics (decreased intestinal motility), immobility	Absence of stool elimination, abdominal distention, and discomfort	Adequate fluid intake, high-fiber diet, early ambulation
Tympanites	Retention of gases within the intestines	Slowed motility of the intestines due to handling of the bowel during surgery and the effects of anesthesia	Obvious abdominal distention, abdominal discomfort (gas pains), absence of bowel sounds	Early ambulation; avoid using a straw, provide ice chips or water at room temperature
Postoperative ileus	Intestinal obstruction characterized by lack of peristaltic activity	Handling the bowel during surgery, anesthesia, electrolyte imbalance, wound infection	Abdominal pain and distention; constipation; absent bowel sounds; vomiting	
Wound				
Wound infection	Inflammation and infection of incision or drain site	Poor aseptic technique; laboratory analysis of wound swab identifies causative microorganism	Purulent exudate, redness, tenderness, elevated body temperature, wound odor	Keep wound clean and dry, use surgical aseptic technique when changing dressings
Wound dehiscence	Separation of a suture line before the incision heals,	Malnutrition (emaciation, obesity), poor circulation, excessive strain on suture line	Increased incision drainage, tissues underlying skin become visible along parts of the incision	Adequate nutrition, appropriate incisional support and avoidance of strain
Wound evisceration	Extrusion of internal organs and tissues through the incision	Same as for wound dehiscence	Opening of incision and visible protrusion of organs	Same as for wound dehiscence
Psychologic				
Postoperative depression	Mental disorder characterized by altered mood	Weakness, surprise nature of emergency surgery, news of malignancy, severely altered body image, other personal matter; may be a physiologic response to some surgeries	Anorexia, tearfulness, loss of ambition, withdrawal, rejection of others, feelings of dejection, sleep disturbances (insomnia or excessive sleeping)	Adequate rest, physical activity, opportunity to express anger and other negative feelings

IDENTIFYING NURSING DIAGNOSES, OUTCOMES, AND INTERVENTIONS
THE POSTOPERATIVE CLIENT

DATA CLUSTER	NURSING DIAGNOSIS/ DEFINITION	SAMPLE DESIRED OUTCOME [NOC#]/DEFINITION	INDICATORS	SELECTED INTERVENTIONS [NIC#]/DEFINITION	SAMPLE NIC ACTIVITIES
Mrs. Polk, 65 years old, was scheduled for a right total hip replacement and has returned to her room. Her VS are stable. She is NPO with an IV infusing at 100 cc/hr. Her right hip dressing is dry and intact. A Hemovac drain is an place and draining a small to moderate amount of bloody drainage. Her respirations are 30/min and shallow. Breath sounds are clear but diminished throughout. She is awake and c/o right hip pain which she rates as "8" on a 0–10 scale. She guards her right hip and flinches when someone touches her.	*Acute Pain/Unpleasant sensory and emotional experience arising from actual or potential tissue damage (International Association for the Study of Pain); sudden or slow onset of any intensity from mild to severe with an anticipated or predictable end and a duration of less than 6 months*	Pain Control [1605]/*Personal actions to control pain*	Often demonstrated: • Recognizes causal factors • Recognizes pain onset • Uses analgesics appropriately • Reports symptoms to health care professional • Reports pain controlled	Pain Management [1400]/*Alleviation of pain or a reduction in pain to a level of comfort that is acceptable to the patient*	• Perform a comprehensive assessment of pain to include location, characteristics, onset/duration, intensity or severity of pain and precipitating factors • Assure patient of attentive analgesic care • Consider cultural influences on pain response • Monitor patient satisfaction with pain management at specified intervals
	Ineffective Breathing Pattern/ Inspiration and/or expiration that does not provide adequate ventilation	Respiratory Status: Ventilation [0403]/*Movement of air in and out of the lungs*	Not compromised: • Respiratory rate in expected range • Respiratory rhythm in expected range • Ease of breathing • Adventitious breath sound not present	Respiratory Monitoring [3350]/*Collection and analysis of patient data to ensure airway patency and adequate gas exchange*	• Monitor rate, rhythm, depth, and effort of respirations • Auscultate breath sounds, noting areas of decreased/absent ventilation and presence of adventitious sounds • Monitor patient's ability to cough effectively
	Risk for Infection/At increased risk for being invaded by pathogenic organisms	Wound Healing: Primary Intention [1102]/*The extent to which cells and tissues have regenerated following intentional closure*	Complete: • Skin approximation • Resolution of sanguineous drainage from drain • Resolution of surrounding skin erythema	Infection Control [6540]/*Minimizing the acquisition and transmission of infectious agents*	• Wash hands before and after each patient activity • Institute standard precautions • Ensure appropriate wound care technique

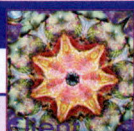

Home Care Assessment
SURGICAL CLIENTS

- **Self-care abilities:**
  Ability to manage hygiene and other self-care, to perform wound care as needed, to manage tubes and stomas, and to manage prescribed medications
- **Supplies required:**
  Wound care supplies such as dressings, hypoallergenic tape, cleansing solutions, binders or slings, elastic wraps, irrigating syringe and solution
- **Assistive devices required:**
  Walker, cane, raised toilet seat, commode, overhead trapeze, grab bars
- **Current level of knowledge:**
  Postoperative pain management, wound care, dressing changes, urinary catheters or other drains, activity restrictions, dietary prescriptions, prescribed exercises (e.g., range-of-motion, postmastectomy exercises), infection control measures such as hand washing

Family

- **Caregiver availability, skills, and responses:**
  Willingness and ability to assume responsibility for care as needed (e.g., wound care, catheter and tube management, meal preparation, assistance with ADLs, shopping, transportation to and from appointments), other available caregivers
- **Family role changes and coping:**
  Effect on parenting and spousal roles, sexuality, social roles, financial status
- **Financial resources:**
  Ability to purchase necessary supplies and equipment; other sources of funding or financial assistance (e.g., Medicare, Medicaid)— see Chapter 6 🔗

Home

- Elicit information from the client and or support person regarding the physical environment of the home and potential issues postoperatively. This may include presence of stairs, access to the home, and accessibility of the kitchen, bathroom, and bedroom

Community

- Available community resources such as equipment and supply companies, support and educational organizations and groups (e.g., ostomy clubs and Reach for Recovery), home health agencies or providers, access to pharmacy services, transportation services for medical care, Meals on Wheels, and other charitable support organizations

IMPLEMENTING

Nursing interventions designed to promote client recovery and prevent complications include (a) pain management, (b) appropriate positioning, (c) incentive spirometry and deep-breathing and coughing exercises, (d) leg exercises, (e) early ambulation, (f) adequate hydration, (g) diet, (h) promoting urinary elimination, (i) suction maintenance, and (j) wound care.

Pain Management

Although pain is a sensory and emotional experience that serves to alert us to harm and initiate responses to avoid or minimize harm, pain in the surgical client has little protective value. It can, in fact, have detrimental effects, leading to stimulation of the sympathetic nervous system, tachycardia, shallow breathing, atelectasis, altered gas exchange, immobility, and immunosuppression (Van Keuren & Eland, 1997). Chapter 44 🔗 provides a more in-depth discussion of pain and pain management.

Pain is usually greatest 12 to 36 hours after surgery, decreasing after the second or third postoperative day. During the initial postoperative period, patient-controlled analgesia (PCA) or continuous analgesic administration through an intravenous or epidural catheter is often prescribed. The nurse monitors the infusion or amount of analgesic administered by PCA, assesses the client's pain relief, and notifies the physician if the client is experiencing unacceptable side effects or inadequate pain relief. "PRN" parenteral or oral analgesics should be administered on a routine basis (every 2 to 6 hours, depending on the drug, route, and dose) for the first 24 to 36 hours. When routine analgesic administration is no longer necessary, the prescribed analgesic is generally given before scheduled activities and rest periods.

An anti-inflammatory agent such as ibuprofen or ketorolac (Toradol) is often administered in conjunction with a narcotic analgesic to enhance pain relief. Clients need to be reminded that analgesics are most effective when taken on a regular basis or before pain becomes severe. Because muscle tension increases pain perception and responses, nurses need to use non-pharmacologic measures in addition to prescribed analgesia. These include ensuring that the client is warm and providing back rubs, position changes, diversional activities, and adjunctive measures such as imagery.

Positioning

Position the client as ordered. Clients who have had spinal anesthetics usually lie flat for 8 to 12 hours. An unconscious or semiconscious client is placed on one side with the head slightly elevated, if possible, or in a position that allows fluids to drain from the mouth. Unless contraindicated, elevation of affected extremities (e.g., following foot surgery) with the distal extremity higher than the heart promotes venous drainage and reduces swelling.

Deep-Breathing and Coughing Exercises

Deep-breathing exercises help remove mucus, which can form and remain in the lungs due to the effects of general anesthetic and analgesics. These drugs depress the action of both the cilia of the mucous membranes lining the respiratory tract and the respiratory center in the brain. By increasing lung expansion and preventing the accumulation of secretions, deep breathing helps prevent pneumonia and **atelectasis** (collapse of the alveoli), which may result from stagnation of fluid in the lungs.

An incentive spirometer is often ordered for the postoperative client to encourage deep breathing. This device measures the flow of air inhaled through a mouthpiece (see Chapter 48). The client is instructed to breathe in through the mouthpiece until a certain level is achieved (usually measured by a ball within an enclosed chamber). Inhalation and ventilation are enhanced using the incentive spirometer.

Deep breathing frequently initiates the coughing reflex. Voluntary coughing in conjunction with deep breathing facilitates the movement and expectoration of respiratory tract secretions.

Encourage the client to do deep-breathing and coughing exercises hourly, or at least every 2 hours, during waking hours for the first few days. Assist the client to a sitting position in bed or on the side of the bed. The client can splint the incision with a pillow when coughing, or the nurse can splint the incision for the client to reduce discomfort.

Leg Exercises

Encourage the client to do leg exercises taught in the preoperative period every 1 to 2 hours during waking hours. Muscle contractions compress the veins, preventing the stasis of blood in the veins, a cause of **thrombus** (stationary clot adhered to the wall of a vessel) formation and subsequent **thrombophlebitis** (inflammation of a vein followed by formation of a blood clot) and **emboli** (a blood clot that has moved). Contractions also promote arterial blood flow.

Moving and Ambulation

Encourage the client to turn from side to side at least every 2 hours. Turning alternates which lung can achieve maximum expansion because it is uppermost. Avoid placing pillows or rolls under the client's knees because pressure on the popliteal blood vessels can interfere with blood circulation to and from the lower extremities. Clients who practice turning before surgery usually find it easier to do after surgery.

The client should ambulate as soon as possible after surgery in accordance with the surgeon's orders. Generally clients begin ambulation the evening of the day of surgery or the first day after surgery, unless contraindicated. Early ambulation prevents respiratory, circulatory, urinary, and gastrointestinal complications. It also prevents general muscle weakness. Schedule ambulation for periods after the client has taken an analgesic or when the client is comfortable. Ambulation should be gradual, starting with the client sitting on the bed and dangling the feet over the side. A client who cannot ambulate is periodically assisted to a sitting position in bed, if allowed, and turned frequently. The sitting position permits the greatest lung expansion.

Hydration

Maintain intravenous infusions as ordered to replace body fluids lost either before or during surgery. When oral intake is permitted, initially offer only small sips of water. Large amounts of water can induce vomiting because anesthetics and narcotic analgesics temporarily inhibit the motility of the stomach. The client who cannot take fluids by mouth may be allowed by the surgeon's orders to suck ice chips. Provide mouth care and place a mouthwash at the client's bedside. Postoperative clients often complain of thirst and a dry, sticky mouth. These discomforts are a result of the preoperative fasting period, preoperative medications (such as atropine), and loss of body fluid.

Measure the client's fluid intake and output for at least 2 days or until fluid balance is stable without an intravenous infusion. Ensuring adequate fluid balance is important. Sufficient fluids keep the respiratory mucous membranes and secretions moist, thus facilitating the expectoration of mucus during coughing. Also, an adequate fluid balance is important to maintain renal and cardiovascular function.

Diet

The surgeon orders the client's postoperative diet. Depending on the extent of surgery and the organs involved, the client may be allowed nothing by mouth for several days or may be able to resume oral intake when nausea is no longer present. When "diet as tolerated" is ordered, offer clear liquids initially. If the client tolerates these with no nausea, the diet can often progress to full liquids and then to a regular diet, provided that gastrointestinal functioning is normal. Assess the return of peristalsis by auscultating the abdomen. Gurgling and rumbling sounds indicate peristalsis. Anesthetic agents, narcotics, handling of the intestines during abdominal surgery, fasting, and inactivity all inhibit peristalsis. Therefore, bowel sounds should be carefully assessed every 4 to 6 hours. Oral fluids and food are usually started after the return of peristalsis. Assist very weak clients to eat.

Observe the client's tolerance of the food and fluids ingested and note and report the passage of flatus or abdominal distention.

Urinary Elimination

Provide measures that promote urinary elimination. For example, help male clients stand at the bedside, or female clients to a bedside commode if allowed, and ensure that fluid intake is adequate. Determine whether the client has any difficulties voiding and assess the client for bladder distention. Report to the surgeon if a client does not void within 8 hours following surgery, unless another time frame is specified.

Anesthetic agents temporarily depress urinary bladder tone, which usually returns within 6 to 8 hours after surgery. Surgery in the pubic area, vagina, or rectum, during which the surgeon may manipulate the bladder, often causes urinary retention. If all measures to promote voiding fail, a urinary catheterization is often ordered (see Chapter 47). Measure the fluid intake and output (I&O) of all new postoperative clients. Generally I&O records are kept for at least 2 days or until the client reestablishes fluid balance without an IV or catheter in place.

Suction

Some clients return from surgery with a gastric or intestinal tube in place and orders to connect the tube to suction. For more information about gastrointestinal tubes, see Chapter 45. The

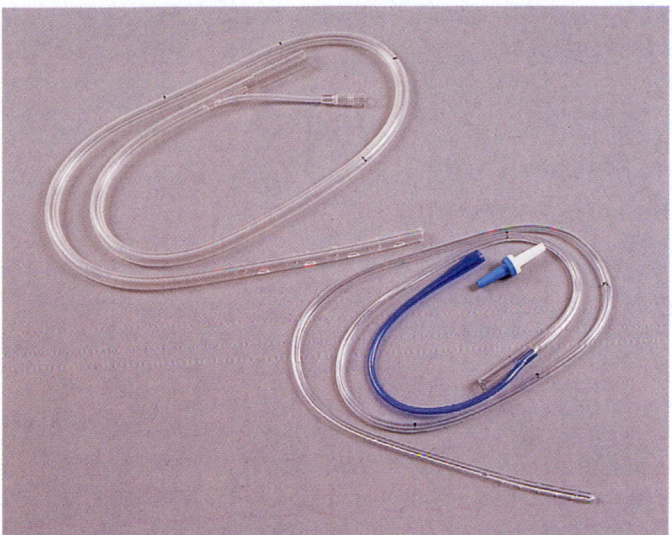

Figure 35–9 ■ Nasogastric tubes used for gastric decompression. *Top left:* Levin (single-lumen) tube; *Lower right:* Salem sump (double-lumen) tube with antireflux valve.

suction ordered can be continuous or intermittent. Intermittent suction is applied when a single-lumen gastric tube is used to reduce the risk of damaging the mucous membrane near the distal port of the tube. Continuous suction may be applied if a double-lumen tube is in place (Figure 35–9 ■). Fluids and electrolytes must be replaced intravenously when gastric suction or continuous drainage is ordered. Nasogastric tubes may be irrigated if the lumen becomes clogged. They are generally irrigated before and after tube feedings or the instillation of medications. Nasogastric irrigation may require a physician's order, particularly following gastrointestinal surgery. Procedure 35–3 describes the management of gastrointestinal suction.

Suction may also be applied to other drainage tubes such as chest tubes or a wound drain. The type and amount of suction is ordered by the physician. Most agencies have wall suction

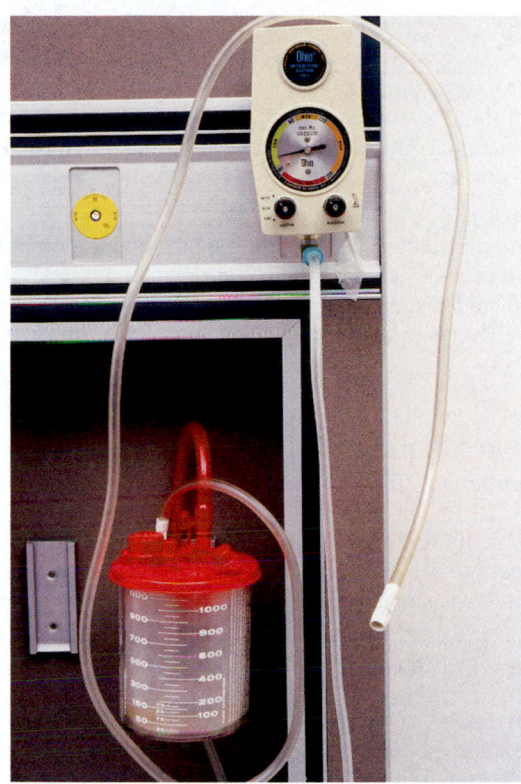

Figure 35–10 ■ Wall suction unit for generating negative pressure for nasogastric suction.

units available (Figure 35–10 ■). A suction regulator with a drainage receptacle connects to a wall outlet that provides negative pressure. Check the receptacle frequently to prevent excess drainage from interfering with the suction apparatus; empty or change the receptacle according to agency policy. Portable electric suction units or pumps (e.g., the Gomco pump) may be used in the home or when wall suction is not available.

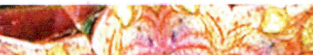
Procedure 35–3 Managing Gastrointestinal Suction

Purposes

- To relieve abdominal distention
- To maintain gastric decompression after surgery
- To remove blood and secretions from the gastrointestinal tract
- To relieve discomfort (i.e., when a client has a bowel obstruction)
- To maintain the patency of the nasogastric tube

ASSESSMENT

Assess

- Presence of abdominal distention on palpation
- Auscultated bowel sounds
- Abdominal discomfort
- Vital signs for baseline data

PLANNING

Before initiating gastric suction, determine (a) whether the suction is continuous or intermittent; (b) the ordered suction pressure (a low suction pressure is between 80 and 100 mm Hg, and a high pressure is between 100 and 120 mm Hg), and (c) whether there is

continued on page 922

Procedure 35–3 Managing Gastrointestinal Suction *continued*

PLANNING *continued*

an order to irrigate the gastrointestinal tube and, if so, the type of solution to use.

Delegation

Managing gastrointestinal suction requires application of knowledge and problem solving and is not delegated to UAP. The UAP, however, can assist with emptying the drainage receptacle and reporting changes in amount and/or color of the drainage to the nurse.

Equipment

INITIATING SUCTION

- Gastrointestinal tube in place in the client
- Basin
- 50-mL syringe with an adapter
- Stethoscope
- Suction device for either continuous or intermittent suction

- Connector and connecting tubing
- Clean gloves

MAINTAINING SUCTION

- Graduated container as required to measure gastric drainage
- Basin of water
- Cotton-tipped applicators
- Ointment or lubricant
- Clean gloves

IRRIGATION

- Clean gloves
- Stethoscope
- Disposable irrigating set containing a sterile 50-mL syringe, moisture-resistant pad, basin, and graduated container
- Sterile normal saline (500 mL) or the ordered solution

IMPLEMENTATION

Performance

1. Explain to the client what you are going to do, why it is necessary, and how he or she can cooperate. Discuss the purpose(s) for the gastrointestinal suction.
2. Wash hands and observe other appropriate infection control procedures (e.g., clean gloves).
3. Provide for client privacy.

Initiating Suction

4. Position the client appropriately.
   - Assist the client to a semi-Fowler's position if it is not contraindicated. *In the semi-Fowler's position, the tube is not as likely to lie against the wall of the stomach and will therefore suction most efficiently. The semi-Fowler's position also prevents reflux of gastric contents, which could lead to aspiration.*
5. Confirm that the tube is in the stomach.
   - Put on clean gloves.
   - Aspirate stomach contents and check the acidity using a pH test strip.
   - Insert air into the tube with the syringe and listen with a stethoscope over the stomach (just below the xiphoid process) for a swish of air.
   - Use other methods in accordance with agency protocol. See Chapter 45, Procedure 45–1. 🔗
6. Set and check the suction.
   - Connect the appropriate suction regulator to the wall suction outlet

and the collection device to the regulator. Intermittent suction regulators generally are used with single-lumen tubes and apply suction for a set interval (15 to 60 seconds), followed by an interval of no suction. Intermittent suction is set at 80 to 100 mm Hg or as ordered by the physician. Check the suction level by occluding the drainage tube and observing the regulator dial during a suction cycle. Continuous suction regulators are used with double-lumen (e.g., Salem sump) nasogastric tubes. Set continuous suction as ordered by the physician, or at 60 to 120 mm Hg.
   - If using a portable suction machine, turn on the machine and regulate the suction as above. The Gomco pump has two settings: low intermittent for single-lumen tubes, and high for double-lumen tubes.
   - Test for proper suctioning by holding the open end of the suction tube to the ear and listening for a sucking noise or by occluding the end of the tube with a thumb.
7. Establish gastric suction.
   - Connect the gastrointestinal tube to the tubing from the suction by using the connector.
   - If a Salem sump tube is in place, connect the larger lumen to the suction equipment. This double-lumen tube has a smaller tube running inside the primary suction

tube. *The smaller tube provides a continuous flow of atmospheric air through the drainage tube at its distal end and prevents excessive suction force on the gastric mucosa at the drainage outlets. Damage to the gastric mucosa is thus avoided.*
   - Always keep the air vent tube of a Salem sump tube open and above the level of the stomach when suction is applied. *Closing the vent would stop the sump action and cause mucosal damage. Keeping the end of the air vent tube higher than the stomach prevents reflux of gastric contents into the air lumen of the tube.*
   - After suction is applied, watch the tubing for a few minutes until the gastric contents appear to be running through the tubing into the receptacle. A Salem sump tube makes a soft, hissing sound when it is functioning correctly.
   - If the suction is not working properly, check that all connections are tight and that the tubing is not kinked.
   - Coil and pin the tubing on the bed so that it does not loop below the suction bottle. *If the tubing falls below the suction bottle, the suction may be obstructed because of the pressure required to push the fluid against gravity.*

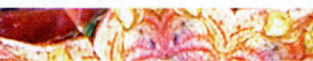

Procedure 35–3 Managing Gastrointestinal Suction *continued*

IMPLEMENTATION *continued*

8. Assess the drainage.
   - Observe the amount, color, odor, and consistency of the drainage. Normal gastric drainage has a mucoid (resembling mucus) consistency and is either colorless or yellow-green because of the presence of bile. A coffee-ground color and consistency may indicate bleeding.
   - Test the gastric drainage for pH and blood (by using Hematest) when indicated. A person who has had gastrointestinal surgery can be expected to have some blood in the drainage.

Maintaining Suction
9. Assess the client and the suction system regularly.
   - Assess the client every 30 minutes until the system is running effectively and then every 2 hours, or as the client's health indicates, to ensure that the suction is functioning properly. If the client complains of fullness, nausea, or epigastric pain or if the flow of gastric secretions is absent in the tubing or in the collection bottle, ineffective suctioning or blockage of the nasogastric tube is likely.
   - Inspect the suction system for patency of the system (e.g., kinks or blockages in the tubing) and tightness of the connections. *Loose connections can permit air to enter and thus decrease the effectiveness of the suction by decreasing the negative pressure.*
10. Relieve blockages if present.
    - Put on clean gloves.
    - Check the suction equipment. To do this, disconnect the nasogastric tube from the suction over a collecting basin (to collect gastric drainage), and then, with the suction on, place the end of the suction tubing in a basin of water. If water is drawn into the drainage bottle, the suction equipment is functioning properly, but the nasogastric tube is either blocked or positioned incorrectly.
    - Reposition the client (e.g., to the other side) if permitted. *This may facilitate drainage.*

- Rotate the nasogastric tube and reposition it. This step is contraindicated for clients with gastric surgery. *Moving the tube may interfere with gastric sutures.*
- Irrigate the nasogastric tube as agency protocol states or on the order of the physician (see steps 14 to 16).
11. Prevent reflux into the vent lumen of a Salem sump tube. *Reflux of gastric contents into the vent lumen may occur when stomach pressure exceeds atmospheric pressure. In this situation, gastric contents follow the path of least resistance and flow out the vent lumen rather than the drainage lumen.* To prevent reflux
    - Place the vent tubing higher than the client's stomach.
    - Keep the drainage collection container below the level of the client's stomach and do not allow it to become too full. A collection device placed above the level of fluid in the stomach or that is too full may interfere with drainage, allowing reflux of gastric contents into the air lumen.
    - Keep the drainage lumen free of particulate matter that may obstruct the lumen (see steps 14 to 16 for irrigating a nasogastric tube).
12. Ensure client comfort.
    - Clean the client's nostrils as needed, using the cotton-tipped applicators and water. Apply a water-soluble lubricant or ointment.
    - Provide mouth care every 2 to 4 hours and as needed. Some postoperative clients are permitted to suck ice chips or a moist cloth to maintain the moisture of the oral mucous membranes.
13. Empty the drainage receptacle according to agency policy or physician's order.
    - Clamp the nasogastric tube and turn off the suction.
    - Put on clean gloves.
    - If the receptacle is graduated, determine the amount of drainage.
    - Disconnect the receptacle.
    - If the receptacle is not graduated, empty the contents into a graduated container and measure.

- Inspect the drainage carefully for color, consistency, and presence of substances (e.g., blood clots).
- Discard and replace a full receptacle or rinse the receptacle with warm water and reattach it to the suction. Check agency policy.
- Turn on the suction and unclamp the nasogastric tube.
- Observe the system for several minutes to make sure function is reestablished.
- Go to step 17.

Irrigating a Gastrointestinal Tube
14. Prepare the client and the equipment.
    - Place the moisture-resistant pad under the end of the gastrointestinal tube.
    - Turn off the suction.
    - Put on clean gloves.
    - Disconnect the gastrointestinal tube from the connector.
    - Determine that the tube is in the stomach. See step 5 above. *This ensures that the irrigating solution enters the client's stomach.*
15. Irrigate the tube.
    - Draw up the ordered volume of irrigating solution in the syringe; 30 mL of solution per instillation is usual, but up to 60 mL may be given per instillation if ordered.
    - Attach the syringe to the nasogastric tube and slowly inject the solution.
    - Gently aspirate the solution. *Forceful withdrawal could damage the gastric mucosa.*
    - If you encounter difficulty in withdrawing the solution, inject 20 mL of air and aspirate again, and/or reposition the client or the nasogastric tube. *Air and repositioning may move the end of the tube away from the stomach wall.* If aspirating difficulty continues, reattach the tube in intermittent low suction, and notify the nurse in charge or physician.
    - Repeat the preceding steps until the ordered amount of solution is used.
    - *Note:* A Salem sump tube can also be irrigated through the vent lumen without interrupting suction. However, only small quantities of irrigant can be injected via this lumen compared to the drainage lumen.

continued on page 924

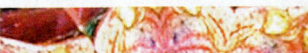

Procedure 35-3 Managing Gastrointestinal Suction *continued*

IMPLEMENTATION *continued*

- After irrigating a Salem sump tube, inject 10 to 20 mL of air into the vent lumen while applying suction to the drainage lumen. *This tests the patency of the vent and ensures sump functioning.*
16. Reestablish suction.
    - Reconnect the nasogastric tube to suction.
    - If a Salem sump tube is used, inject the air vent lumen with 10 mL of air after reconnecting the tube to suction.

- Observe the system for several minutes to make sure it is functioning.
17. Document all relevant information.
    - Record the time suction was started. Also record the pressure established, the color and consistency of the drainage, and nursing assessments.
    - During maintenance, record assessments, supportive nursing measures, and data about the suction system.

- When irrigating the tube, record verification of tube placement; the time of the irrigation; the amount and type of irrigating solution used; the amount, color, and consistency of the returns; the patency of the system following the irrigation; and nursing assessments.

EVALUATION

- Conduct appropriate follow-up such as relief of abdominal distention or discomfort, bowel sounds, character and amount of gastric drainage, integrity of nares, hydration of oral mucous membranes, patency of tube, and system functioning.

- Relate to previous findings if available.
- Report significant deviations from normal to the physician.

Home Care Considerations

GI Suction
Instruct the caregiver to
- Maintain suction as ordered; do *not* increase or decrease the suction without instructions from the nurse or physician.
- Offer mouth care every 2 hours.

- Avoid tension and pulling on the tube by securing it to the gown.
- Check the patency of the tube if nausea or vomiting occurs.
- Report an increasing amount of or bloody drainage.

Wound Care

Most clients return from surgery with a sutured wound covered by a dressing, although in some cases the wound may be left unsutured. Dressings are inspected regularly to ensure that they are clean, dry, and intact. Excessive drainage may indicate hemorrhage, infection, or an open wound.

When dressings are changed, the nurse assesses the wound for appearance, size, drainage, swelling, pain, and the status of a drain or tubes. Details about these assessments are outlined in the accompanying Practice Guidelines.

Because surgical incisions heal by primary intention, the nurse can expect the following sequential signs of healing:

1. *Absence of bleeding and the appearance of a clot binding the wound edges.* The wound edges are well approximated and bound by fibrin in the clot within the first few hours after surgical closure.
2. *Inflammation (redness and swelling) at the wound edges for 1 to 3 days.*
3. *Reduction in inflammation when the clot diminishes,* as granulation tissue starts to bridge the area. The wound is bridged and closed within 7 to 10 days. Increased inflammation associated with fever and drainage is indicative of

wound infection; the wound edges then appear brightly inflamed and swollen.
4. *Scar formation.* Collagen synthesis starts 4 days after injury and continues for 6 months or longer.
5. *Diminished scar size over a period of months or years.* An increase in scar size indicates keloid formation.

See Chapter 34 🔗 for information about wound drainage, cleaning wounds, wound irrigation, hot and cold applications, and supporting and immobilizing wounds.

> ► **CLINICAL ALERT**   *Assess the client immediately if she or he reports a "giving" or "popping" sensation in the incisional area. The client may be experiencing dehiscence or evisceration of the wound.* ■

Surgical Dressings. Not all surgical dressings require changing. Sometimes surgeons in the operating room apply a dressing that remains in place until the sutures are removed, and no further dressings are required. In many situations, however, surgical dressings are changed regularly to prevent the growth of microorganisms.

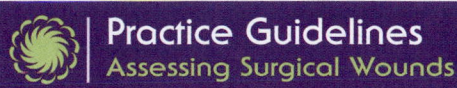

Practice Guidelines
Assessing Surgical Wounds

Appearance
- Inspect color of wound and surrounding area and approximation of wound edges.

Size
- Note size and location of dehiscence, if present.

Drainage
- Observe location, color, consistency, odor, and degree of saturation of dressings. Note number of gauzes saturated or diameter of drainage on gauze.

Swelling
- Observe the amount of swelling; minimal to moderate swelling is normal in early stages of wound healing.

Pain
- Expect severe to moderate postoperative pain for 3 to 5 days; persistent severe pain or sudden onset of severe pain may indicate internal hemorrhaging or infection.

Drains or Tubes
- Inspect drain security and placement, amount and character of drainage, and functioning of collecting apparatus, if present.

In some instances a client may have a Penrose drain inserted (see the next section). In this situation the main surgical incision is considered cleaner than the surgical stab wound made for the drain insertion, because there is usually considerable drainage. The main incision is therefore cleaned first, and under no circumstances are materials that were used to clean the stab wound used subsequently to clean the main incision. In this way, the main incision is kept free of the microorganisms around the stab wound. Cleaning a wound and applying a sterile dressing are detailed in Procedure 35–4.

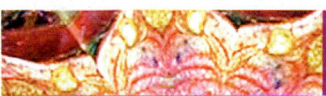

Procedure 35–4 Cleaning a Sutured Wound and Applying a Sterile Dressing

Purposes
- To promote wound healing by primary intention
- To prevent infection
- To assess the healing process
- To protect the wound from mechanical trauma

ASSESSMENT

Assess
- Client allergies to wound cleaning agents
- The appearance and size of the wound
- The amount and character of exudates
- Client complaints of discomfort
- The time of the last pain medication
- Signs of systemic infection (e.g., elevated body temperature, diaphoresis, malaise, leukocytosis)

PLANNING

Before changing a dressing, determine any specific orders about the wound or dressing.

Delegation

Cleaning a newly sutured wound, especially one with a drain, requires application of knowledge, problem solving, and aseptic technique. As a result, this procedure is not delegated to UAP. The nurse can ask the UAP to report soiled dressings that need to be changed or if a dressing has become loose and needs to be reinforced. The nurse is responsible for the assessment and evaluation of the wound.

Equipment
- Bath blanket (if necessary)
- Moisture-proof bag
- Mask (optional)
- Acetone or another solution (if necessary to loosen adhesive)
- Clean gloves
- Sterile gloves
- Sterile dressing set; if none is available, gather the following sterile items:
  - Drape or towel
  - Gauze squares
  - Container for the cleaning solution
  - Cleaning solution (e.g., normal saline)
  - Two pairs of forceps
  - Gauze dressings and surgipads
  - Applicators or tongue blades to apply ointments
- Additional supplies required for the particular dressing (e.g., extra gauze dressings and ointment, if ordered)
- Tape, tie tapes, or binder

continued on page 926

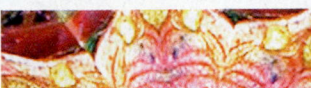

Procedure 35–4   Cleaning a Sutured Wound and Applying a Sterile Dressing   *continued*

IMPLEMENTATION

Preparation

Prepare the client and assemble the equipment.

- Acquire assistance for changing a dressing on a restless or confused adult. *The person might move and contaminate the sterile field or the wound.*
- Assist the client to a comfortable position in which the wound can be readily exposed. Expose only the wound area, using a bath blanket to cover the client, if necessary. *Undue exposure is physically and psychologically distressing to most people.*
- Make a cuff on the moisture-proof bag for disposal of the soiled dressings, and place the bag within reach. It can be taped to the bedclothes or bedside table. *Making a cuff helps keep the outside of the bag free from contamination by the soiled dressings and prevents subsequent contamination of the nurse's hands or of sterile instrument tips when discarding dressing or sponges. Placement of the bag within reach prevents the nurse from reaching across the sterile field and the wound and potentially contaminating these areas.*
- Put on a face mask, if required. *Some agencies require that a mask be worn for surgical dressing changes to prevent contamination of the wound by droplet spray from the nurse's respiratory tract.*

Performance

1. Explain to the client what you are going to do, why it is necessary, and how he or she can cooperate. Discuss how the results will be used in planning further care or treatments.
2. Wash hands and observe other appropriate infection control procedures.
3. Provide for client privacy.
4. Remove binders and tape.
   - Remove binders, if used, and place them aside. Untie tie tapes, if used. Montgomery straps (tie tapes) are commonly used for wounds requiring frequent dressing changes (Figure 35–11 ■). *These straps prevent skin irritation and discomfort caused by removing the adhesive each time the dressing is changed.*

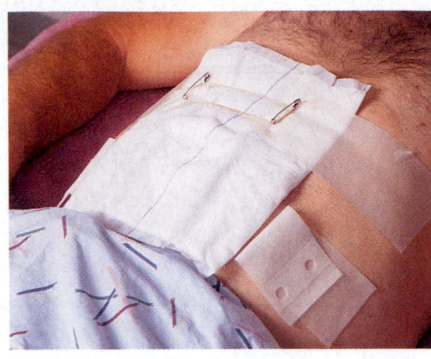

Figure 35–11 ■ Montgomery straps holding dressing.

   - If adhesive tape was used, remove it by holding down the skin and pulling the tape gently but firmly toward the wound. *Pressing down on the skin provides countertraction against the pulling motion. Tape is pulled toward the incision to prevent strain on the sutures or wound.*
   - Use a solvent to loosen tape, if required. *Moistening the tape with acetone or a similar solvent lessens the discomfort of removal, particularly from hairy surfaces.*
5. Remove and dispose of soiled dressings appropriately.
   - Put on clean disposable gloves and remove the outer abdominal dressing or surgipad.
   - Lift the outer dressing so that the underside is *away* from the client's face. *The appearance and odor of the drainage may be upsetting to the client.*
   - Place the soiled dressing in the moisture-proof bag without touching the outside of the bag. *Contamination of the outside of the bag is avoided to prevent the spread of microorganisms to the nurse and subsequently to others.*
   - Remove the under dressings, taking care not to dislodge any drains. If the gauze sticks to the drain, support the drain with one hand and remove the gauze with the other.

- Assess the location, type (color, consistency), and odor of wound drainage, and the number of gauzes saturated or the diameter of drainage collected on the dressings.
- Discard the soiled dressings in the bag as before.
- Remove gloves, dispose of them in the moisture-proof bag, and wash hands.
6. Set up the sterile supplies.
   - Open the sterile dressing set, using surgical aseptic technique.
   - Place the sterile drape beside the wound.
   - Open the sterile cleaning solution and pour it over the gauze sponges in the plastic container.
   - Put on sterile gloves.
7. Clean the wound, if indicated.
   - Clean the wound, using your gloved hands or forceps and gauze swabs moistened with cleaning solution.
   - If using forceps, keep the forceps tips lower than the handles at all times. *This prevents their contamination by fluid traveling up to the handle and nurse's wrist and back to the tips.*
   - Use the cleaning methods illustrated and described in Figure 35–12 ■ or one recommended by agency protocol.
   - Use a separate swab for each stroke and discard each swab after use. *This prevents the introduction of microorganisms to other wound areas.*
   - If a drain is present, clean it next, taking care to avoid reaching across the cleaned incision. Clean the skin around the drain site by swabbing in half or full circles from around the drain site outward, using separate swabs for each wipe (Figure 35–12, C).
   - Support and hold the drain erect while cleaning around it. Clean as many times as necessary to remove the drainage.
   - Dry the surrounding skin with dry gauze swabs as required. Do not dry the incision or wound itself. Moisture facilitates wound healing.

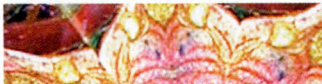

Procedure 35–4 Cleaning a Sutured Wound and Applying a Sterile Dressing *continued*

IMPLEMENTATION *continued*

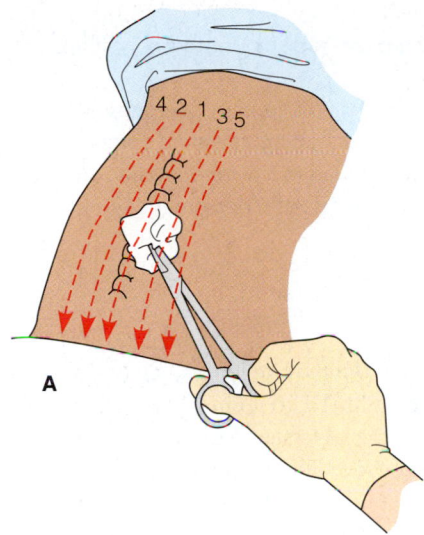

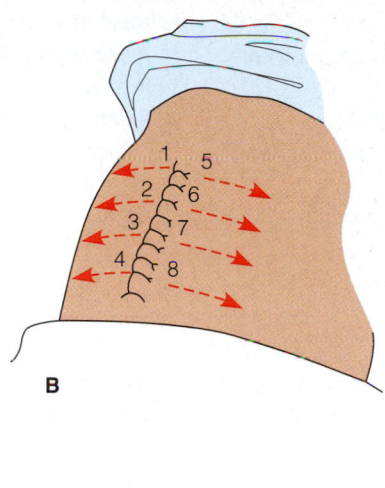

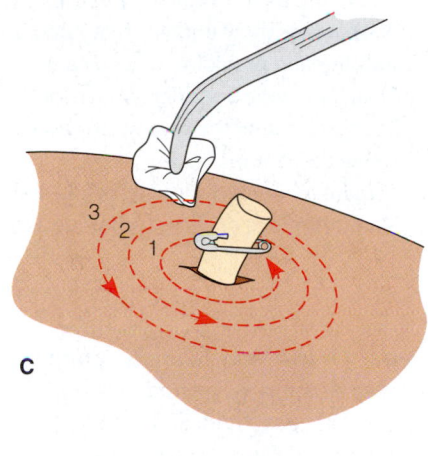

Figure 35–12 ■ Methods of cleaning surgical wounds: *A,* cleaning the wound from top to bottom, starting at the center, *B,* cleaning a wound outward from the incision; *C,* cleaning around a Penrose drain site. For all methods, a clean sterile swab is used for each stroke.

8. Apply dressings to the drain site and the incision.
   • Place a precut 4 in. × 4 in. gauze snugly around the drain (Figure 35–13 ■), or open a 4 in. × 4 in. gauze to 4 in. × 8 in., fold it lengthwise to 2 in. × 8 in., and place the 2 in. × 8 in. gauze around the drain so that the ends overlap. *This dressing absorbs the drainage and helps prevent it from excoriating the skin. Using precut gauze or folding it as described, instead of cutting the gauze, prevents any threads from coming loose and getting into the wound, where they could cause inflammation and provide a site for infection.*

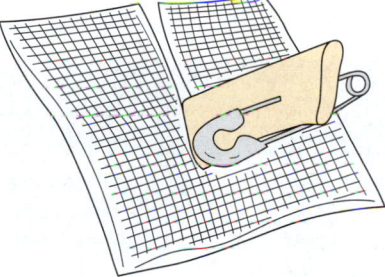

Figure 35–13 ■ Precut gauze in place around a drain.

   • Apply the sterile dressings one at a time over the drain and the incision. Place the bulk of the dressings over the drain area and below the drain, depending on the client's usual position. *Layers of dressings are placed for best absorption of drainage, which flows by gravity.*
   • Apply the final surgipad, remove gloves, and dispose of them. Secure the dressing with tape or ties.
9. Document the procedure and all nursing assessments

EVALUATION

■ Conduct appropriate follow-up, such as amount of granulation tissue or degree of healing; amount of drainage and its color, consistency, and odor; presence of inflammation; and degree of discomfort association with the incision or drain site.

■ Relate to previous findings, if available.
■ Report significant deviations from normal to the physician.

Home Care Considerations

Cleaning a Sutured Wound

Instruct caregivers to

- Provide pain medication approximately 30 minutes before the procedure if the wound care causes pain or discomfort.
- Wash hands thoroughly and dry prior to handling wound care supplies and providing wound care.
- Clean and wipe dry a flat surface for the sterile field.
- Keep pets out of the area when setting up for and performing sterile procedures.
- Acquire all needed supplies before starting a sterile procedure.
- Maintain sterile or clean technique as instructed.

- Handle all sterile supplies from the outside of the wrapper or the edges.
- Do not touch the parts of supplies or equipment that will touch the client.
- Avoid skin injury by using paper tape or Montgomery straps instead of adhesive tape.
- Report any increasing wound drainage, pain, or redness, increasing swelling, or opening or gaping of wound edges.
- Place any soiled dressing materials in a waterproof bag and dispose of it according to public health recommendations.

Wound Drains and Suction. Surgical drains, for example a **Penrose drain,** are inserted to permit the drainage of excessive serosanguineous fluid and purulent material and to promote healing of underlying tissues. These drains may be inserted and sutured through the incision line, but they are most commonly inserted through stab wounds a few centimeters away from the incision line so that the incision itself may be kept dry. Without a drain, some wounds would heal on the surface and trap the discharge inside, and an abscess might form.

Drains vary in length and width. The length can be 25 to 35 cm (10 to 14 in.), and the width 1.2 to 4 cm (0.5 to 1.5 in.). To facilitate drainage and healing of tissues from the inside to the outside, the physician may order that the drain be pulled out or shortened 2 to 5 cm (1 to 2 in.) each day. When a drain is completely removed, the remaining stab wound usually heals within a day or two. Shortening the drain is usually done when the dressing is changed. Steps involved in shortening a drain are given in the accompanying Practice Guidelines.

Practice Guidelines
Shortening a Drain

- Remove dressings, put on sterile gloves, and clean the incision (see Procedure 35–4).
- Clean the drain site appropriately (Figure 35–12,C). Assess the amount and character of drainage, including odor, thickness, and color.
- If the drain has not been shortened before, cut and remove the suture holding it in place. The drain is sutured to the skin during surgery to keep it from slipping into the body cavity.
- Firmly grasp the drain by its full width at the level of the skin, and pull the drain out the required length. Grasping the full width of the drain ensures even traction.

- Insert a sterile safety pin through the base of the drain as close to the skin as possible by holding the drain tightly against the skin edge and inserting the pin above your fingers (Figure 35–14 ■). The pin keeps the drain from falling back into the incision. Holding the drain securely in place at the skin level and inserting the pin above the fingers prevents the nurse from pulling the drain further out or pricking the client during this step.
- With the sterile scissors, cut off the excess drain so that about 2.5 cm (1 in.) remains above the skin (Figure 35–15 ■). Discard the excess in the waste bag.
- Apply dressings to the drain site and the incision.

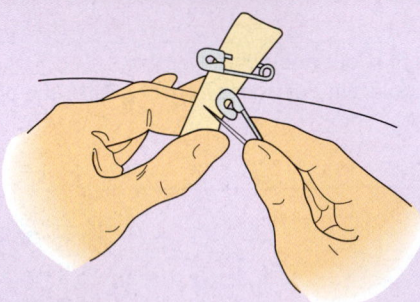

Figure 35–14 ■ Pinning a drain.

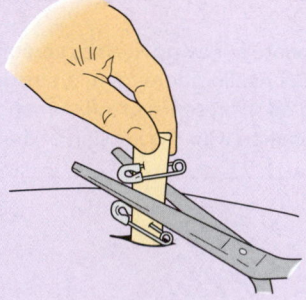

Figure 35–15 ■ Shortening a drain.

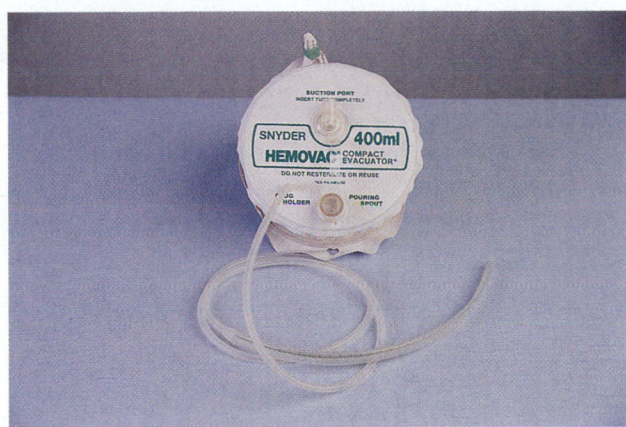

Figure 35–16 ■ Hemovac closed-wound drainage system.

A **closed-wound drainage system** consists of a drain connected to either an electric suction or a portable drainage suction, such as a Hemovac (Figure 35–16 ■) or Jackson-Pratt (Figure 35–17 ■). The closed system reduces the possible entry of microorganisms into the wound through the drain. The drainage tubes are sutured in place and connected to a reservoir. For example, the Jackson-Pratt drainage tube is connected to a reservoir that maintains constant low suction. These portable wound suctions also provide for accurate measurement of the drainage.

The surgeon inserts the wound drainage tube during surgery. Generally the suction is discontinued from 3 to 5 days postoperatively or when the drainage is minimal. Nurses are responsible for maintaining the wound suction, which hastens the healing process by draining excess exudate that might otherwise interfere with the formation of granulation tissue.

Closed-wound drainage systems have directions for use printed on the drainage container. When emptying the container, the nurse should wear gloves and avoid touching the

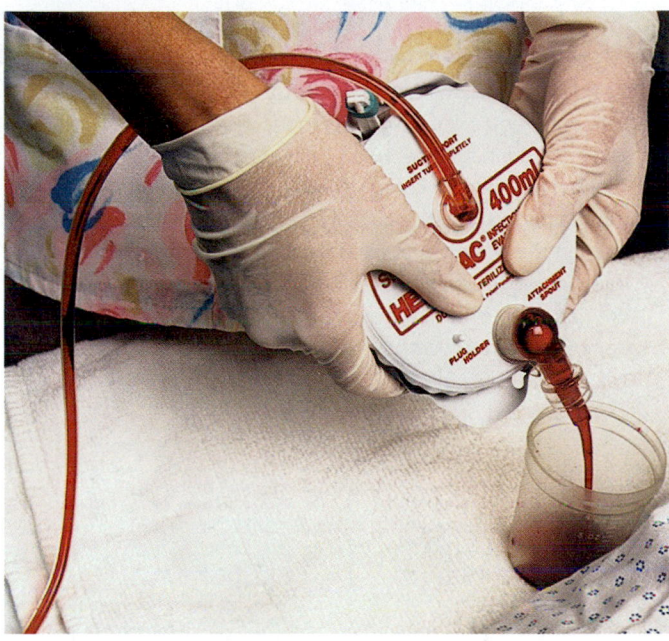

Figure 35–18 ■ Emptying drainage from Hemovac drainage system.

drainage port (Figure 35–18 ■). To reestablish suction, the nurse places the container on a solid, flat surface with the port open. The palm of one hand presses the top and bottom together while the other hand cleanses the opening and plug with an alcohol swab (Figure 35–19 ■). Replace the drainage plug before releasing hand pressure to reestablish the vacuum necessary for the closed drainage system to work.

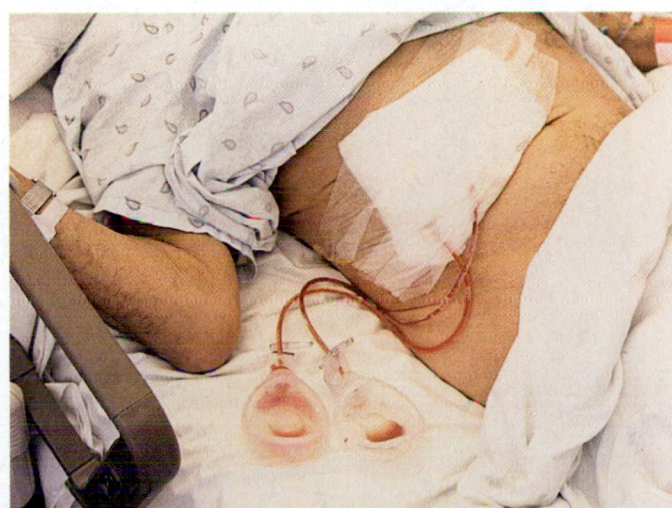

Figure 35–17 ■ Two Jackson-Pratt devices compressed to facilitate collection of exudates.

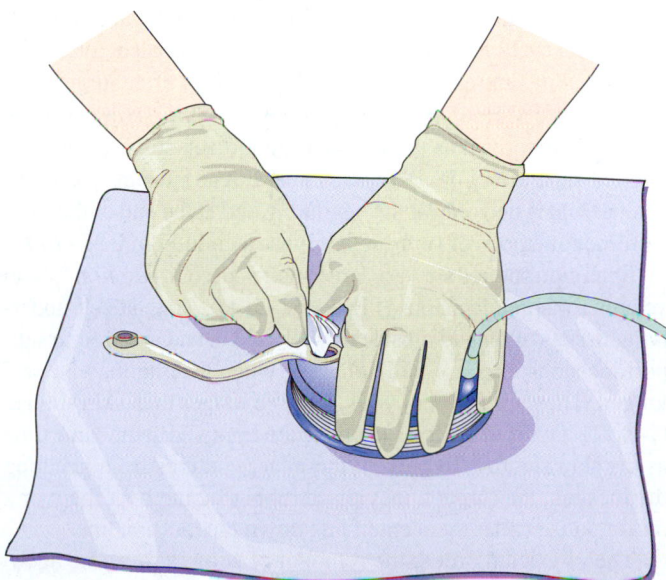

Figure 35–19 ■ With one hand, press the top and bottom together. With the other hand, clean the opening and plug with an alcohol swab. Replace the plug before releasing hand.

Home Care Considerations

Closed-Wound Drainage System

- Schedule regular nursing visits to teach wound care and to observe the drainage site.
- Teach the client or a caregiver to empty, measure, and record the drainage at least once daily.
- Instruct the caregiver to observe the wound daily for signs of infection, such as redness, edema, tenderness, or purulent drainage. The client's temperature should be measured twice daily. *Elevated temperature can indicate infection.*

- Ensure that the client has the proper supplies and knows how to obtain new items as needed.
- Notify the physician of excess drainage, signs of infection, or occlusion of the tube.
- Determine when the physician plans to remove the drain and help the client keep the appointment.

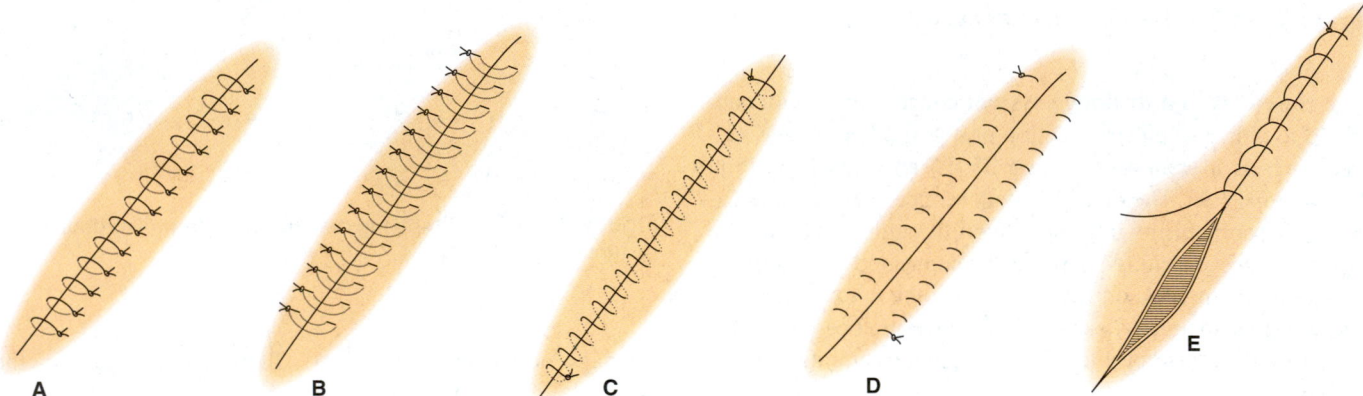

Figure 35–20 ■ Common sutures: *A,* plain interrupted; *B,* mattress interrupted; *C,* plain continuous; *D,* mattress continuous; *E,* blanket continuous.

Sutures. A **suture** is a thread used to sew body tissues together. Sutures used to attach tissues beneath the skin are often made of an absorbable material that disappears in several days. Skin sutures, by contrast, are made of a variety of nonabsorbable materials, such as silk, cotton, linen, wire, nylon, and Dacron (polyester fiber). Silver wire clips or staples are also available. Usually skin sutures are removed 7 to 10 days after surgery.

There are various methods of suturing. Skin sutures can be broadly categorized as either interrupted (each stitch is tied and knotted separately) or continuous (one thread runs in a series of stitches and is tied only at the beginning and at the end of the run). Common methods of suturing are illustrated in Figure 35–20 ■.

Retention sutures are very large sutures used in addition to skin sutures for some incisions (Figure 35–21 ■). They attach underlying tissues of fat and muscle as well as skin and are used to support incisions in obese individuals or when healing may be prolonged. They are frequently left in place longer than skin sutures (14 to 21 days) but in some instances are removed at the same time as the skin sutures. To prevent these large sutures from irritating the incision, the surgeon may place rubber tubing over them or a roll of gauze under them extending down the incision line.

The physician orders the removal of sutures. In some agencies, only physicians remove sutures; in others, registered nurses and nursing students with appropriate supervision may do so. Agency policies about removal of retention sutures vary. The nurse should verify whether they are to be removed and who may remove them.

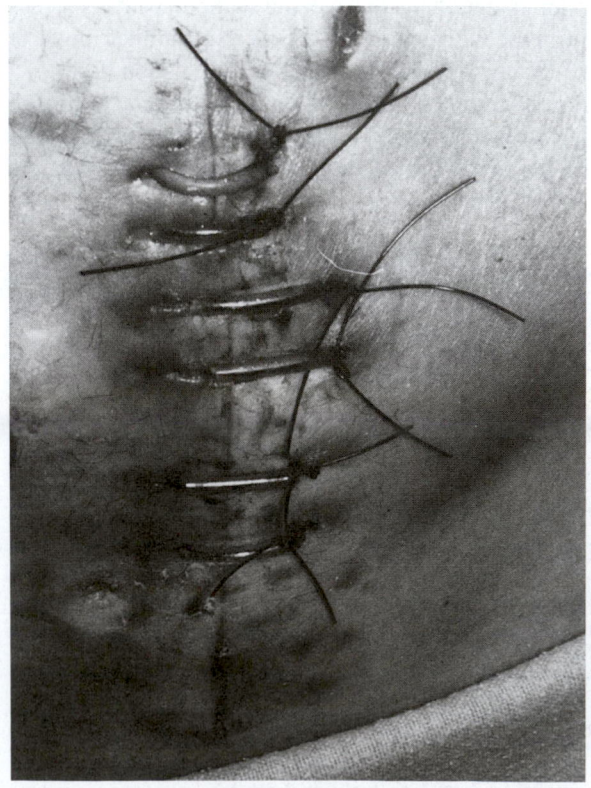

Figure 35–21 ■ A surgical incision with retention sutures.

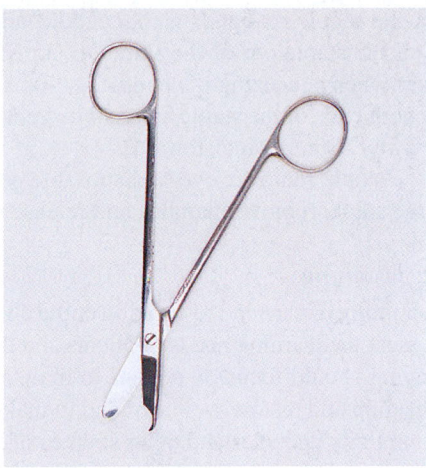

Figure 35–22 ■ Suture scissors.

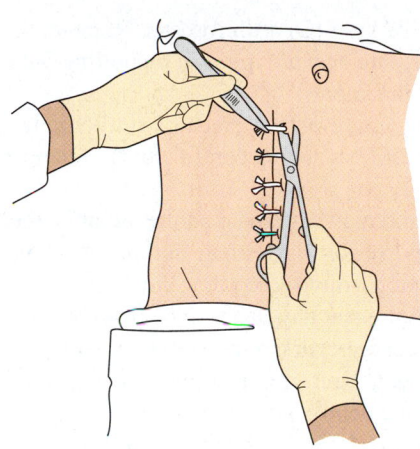

Figure 35–24 ■ Removing a plain interrupted skin suture.

Sterile technique and special suture scissors are used in suture removal. The scissors have a short, curved cutting tip that readily slides under the suture (Figure 35–22 ■). Wire clips or staples are removed with a special instrument that squeezes the center of the clip to remove it from the skin (Figure 35–23 ■). Guidelines for removing sutures and staples follow:

- Before removing skin sutures, verify (a) the orders for suture removal (in many instances, only *alternate* interrupted sutures are removed one day, and the remaining sutures are removed a day or two later) and (b) whether a dressing is to be applied following the suture removal. Some physicians prefer no dressing; others prefer a small, light gauze dressing to prevent friction by clothing.
- Inform the client that suture removal may produce slight discomfort, such as a pulling or stinging sensation, but should not be painful.

- Remove dressings and clean the incision in accordance with agency protocol. Cleaning the suture line with an antimicrobial solution before and after suture removal may help prevent infection.
- Put on sterile gloves.
- Remove plain interrupted sutures as follows:
  a. Grasp the suture at the knot with a pair of forceps.
  b. Place the curved tip of the suture scissors under the suture as close to the skin as possible, either on the side opposite the knot (Figure 35–24 ■) or directly under the knot. Cut the suture. Sutures are cut as close to the skin as possible on one side of the visible part because the suture material that is visible to the eye is in contact with resident bacteria of the skin and must not be pulled beneath the skin during removal. Suture material that is beneath the skin is considered free from bacteria.
  c. With the forceps, pull the suture out in one piece. Inspect the suture carefully to make sure that all suture material is removed. Suture material left beneath the skin acts as a foreign body and causes inflammation.
- Remove mattress interrupted sutures as follows:
  a. When possible, cut the visible part of the suture close to the skin at A and B in Figure 35–25 ■, opposite the knot, and remove this small visible piece. Discard it as described below. In some sutures, the visible part opposite the knot may be so small that it can be cut only once.

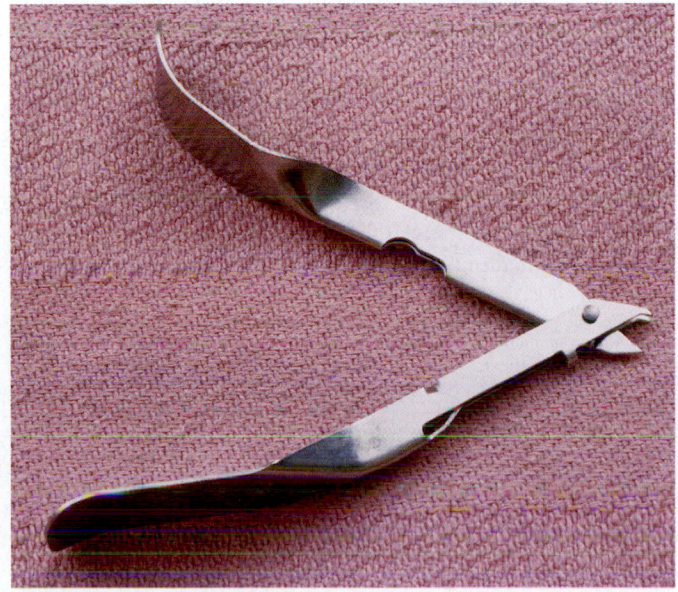

Figure 35–23 ■ Staple remover.

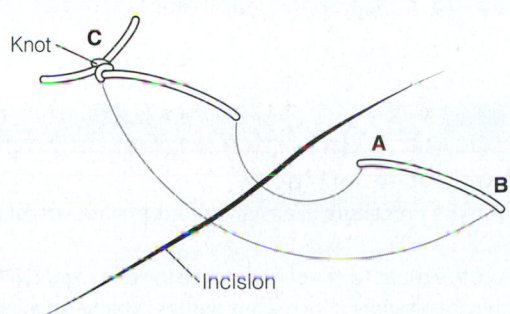

Figure 35–25 ■ Mattress interrupted sutures.

b. Grasp the knot (C) with forceps. Remove the remainder of the suture beneath the skin by pulling out in the direction of the knot.

• Discard the suture onto a piece of sterile gauze or into the moisture-proof bag, being careful not to contaminate the forceps tips.

• Continue to remove alternate sutures, that is, the third, fifth, seventh, and so forth. Alternate sutures are removed first so that remaining sutures keep the skin edges in close approximation and prevent any dehiscence from becoming large.

• If no dehiscence occurs, remove the remaining sutures. If dehiscence does occur, do not remove the remaining sutures, and report the dehiscence to the nurse in charge.

• If Steri-Strips are ordered by the physician, apply them to the wound after removing the sutures or clips. Some physicians order Steri-Strip application to provide additional support to the healing wound.

• Reapply a dressing, if indicated.

• Document the suture removal; number of sutures removed; appearance of the incision; application of a dressing, Steri-Strips, or butterfly tapes (if appropriate); client teaching; and client tolerance of the procedure.

• Remove staples as follows:
  a. Remove dressings and clean the incision in accordance with agency protocol.
  b. Place the lower tips of a sterile staple remover under the staple.
  c. Squeeze the handles together until they are completely closed (Figure 35–26 ■). Pressing the handles together

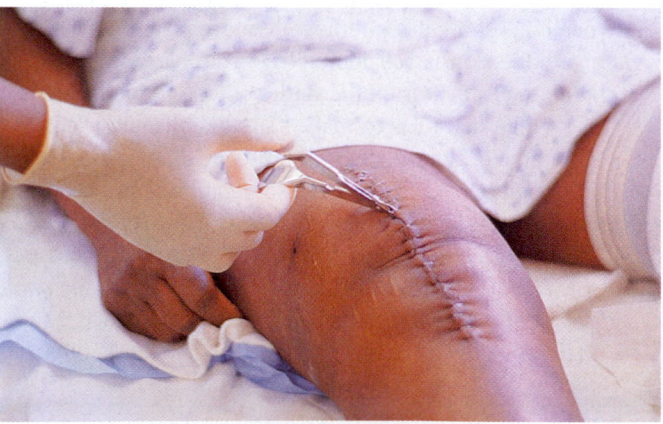

Figure 35–26 ■ Removing surgical clips or staples.

causes the staple to bend in the middle and pulls the edges of the staple out of the skin. Do not lift the staple remover when squeezing the handles.
  d. When both ends of the staple are visible, gently move the staple away from the incision site.
  e. Hold the staple remover over a disposable container, release the staple remover handles and release the staple.

Home Care Teaching

To ensure continuity of care and restoration of the client's health, nurses must meet the learning needs of clients and their support people. Teaching should focus on actions to maintain comfort, to promote healing and restore wellness, and to make use of appropriate community agencies and other sources of help.

Maintaining Comfort

• Instruct the client to use pain medications as ordered, not allowing pain to become severe before taking the prescribed dose.

• If not contraindicated, discuss the use of over-the-counter analgesics such as aspirin or acetaminophen as postoperative pain becomes less severe or if the client is reluctant to use prescription drugs due to side effects.

• Teach the client to avoid using alcohol or other central nervous system depressants while taking narcotic analgesics.

• Discuss the importance of gradually resuming activities, avoiding overexertion.

• Emphasize the importance of paying attention to increasing pain or discomfort. Instruct the client to contact the physician if pain increases after a period of decreasing discomfort.

• Teach the client to use nonpharmacologic measures to help manage pain, such as conscious relaxation, distraction, meditation, or visualization.

Promoting Healing

• If indicated, teach the client how to change wound dressings and perform wound care.

• Emphasize the importance of hygiene and hand washing to prevent infections.

• Instruct the client to report promptly to the physician any increasing redness, swelling, pain, or discharge from the incision or drain sites.

• Discuss any prescribed activity restrictions such as avoiding lifting.

• Discuss the importance of keeping follow-up appointments to monitor healing and recovery after surgery.

Home Care Considerations

Removing Sutures or Staples

■ Perform the procedure in a well-lighted, private area of the home.

■ Instruct the client to observe the incision daily and call the health care provider if increased redness, drainage, or open areas are observed.

■ Provide instructions and supplies for care of the incision, and tell the client when to shower for the first time.

■ Assess the client's ability to keep the incision clean and protected at home.

Restoring Wellness
- Discuss the relationship of increasing activities to restoring wellness and promoting a sense of well-being.
- Teach the client that surgery and stressors can depress immune function and to avoid exposure to illness (e.g., crowded areas and people with upper respiratory illnesses) whenever possible.
- Emphasize the importance of adequate rest for healing and immune function.
- If appropriate, discuss lifestyle changes to promote wellness, such as smoking cessation, increasing activity level, reducing stress, and consuming a healthy diet high in fruits, vegetables, and whole grains with adequate protein to promote healing.

Community Agencies and Other Sources of Help
- Provide information about where durable medical equipment can be purchased, rented, or obtained free of charge; how to access home health and other services; and where to obtain supplies such as dressings or nutritional supplements.
- Suggest additional sources of information, such as the National Rehabilitation Information Center, Reach to Recovery, and United Ostomy Association.

Referrals. The nurse needs to consider appropriate referrals for the client, such as

- Home health agencies for wound care and assessment and for assistance with ADLs if necessary

- Community social services for assistance in obtaining medical and assistive equipment
- Respiratory, physical, or occupational therapy services as indicated

EVALUATING

Using the goals developed during the planning stage, the nurse collects data to evaluate whether the identified goals and desired outcomes have been achieved. Examples of client outcomes and related indicators are shown in the earlier Identifying Nursing Diagnoses, Outcomes, and Interventions boxes.

If the desired outcomes are not achieved, the nurse and client, and support people if helpful, need to explore the reasons before modifying the care plan. For example, if the outcome "Pain control" is not met, questions to be considered include

- What is the client's perception of the problem?
- Does the client understand how to use PCA?
- Is the prescribed analgesic dose adequate for the client?
- Is the client allowing pain to become intense prior to requesting medication or using PCA?
- Where is the client's pain? Could it be due to a problem unrelated to surgery (e.g., chronic arthritis, anginal pain)?
- Is there evidence of a complication that could cause increased pain (an infection, abscess, or hematoma)?

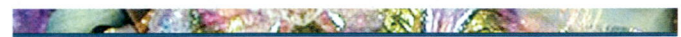

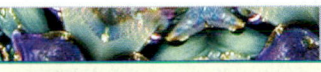 **Focus on Critical Thinking**

Mr. Teng is a 77-year-old client with a history of chronic obstructive pulmonary disease. Currently his respiratory condition is being controlled with medications and he is free of infection. He has just been transferred to the postanesthesia care unit following a hernia repair performed under spinal anesthesia. His blood pressure is 132/88, pulse 84, respirations 28, and tympanic temperature 36.5 C (97.8 F). He is awake and stable.

1. What factors place Mr. Teng at increased risk for the development of complications during and after surgery?
2. Speculate about why Mr. Teng's surgeon and anesthesiologist decided to perform Mr. Teng's surgery under regional anesthesia as opposed to general anesthesia?

3. What preparations were taken during the preoperative period in order to protect Mr. Teng from possible complications during and after his surgery?
4. How will Mr. Teng's postoperative assessments differ from a person who received general anesthesia?
5. What postoperative precautions are especially important to Mr. Teng in view of his chronic lung condition?

See Critical Thinking Possibilities in Appendix A.

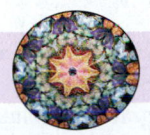 **Chapter Review**

EXPLORE MediaLink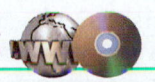

NCLEX review questions, case studies, care plan activities, MediaLink applications, and other interactive resources for this chapter can be found on the Companion Website at www.prenhall.com/kozier. Click on Chapter 35 to select the

activities for this chapter.
For more NCLEX review questions, and an audio glossary, access the Student CD-ROM accompanying this textbook.

Chapter Highlights

- Surgery is a unique experience that creates stress and necessitates physical and psychologic changes.
- The perioperative period includes three phases: preoperative, intraoperative, and postoperative.
- Surgical procedures are categorized by degree of urgency, purpose, and degree of risk.
- Factors such as age, general health, nutritional status, medication use, and mental status affect a client's risk during surgery.
- Clients must agree to surgery and sign an informed consent.
- Nursing history and physical assessment data are important sources for planning preoperative and postoperative care.
- The overall goal of nursing care during the preoperative phase is to prepare the client mentally and physically for surgery.
- Preoperative teaching includes situational information and psychosocial support, the role of the client throughout the perioperative period, expected sensations and discomfort, and training for the postoperative period.
- Preoperative teaching should include moving, leg exercises, and coughing and deep-breathing exercises. Many aspects of preoperative teaching are intended to prevent postoperative complications.
- Physical preparation includes the following areas: nutrition and fluids, elimination, hygiene, rest, medications, care of valuables and prostheses, special orders, and surgical skin preparation.
- Antiemboli stockings or sequential compression devices may be ordered for some clients to facilitate venous return.
- A preoperative checklist provides a guide to and documentation of a client's preparation before surgery.
- Maintaining the client's safety is the overall goal of nursing care during the intraoperative phase.
- Anesthesia may be general or regional. Regional anesthesia includes topical, local, nerve block, intravenous block, spinal anesthesia (subarachnoid block), and epidural.
- A surgical skin preparation should be carried out as close to the time of surgery as possible and is commonly performed during the intraoperative phase.
- Positioning of the client during surgery is important to reduce the risk of tissue and nerve damage.
- Immediate postanesthetic care focuses on assessment and monitoring parameters to prevent complications from anesthesia or surgery.
- Initial and ongoing assessment of the postoperative client includes level of consciousness, vital signs, oxygen saturation, skin color and temperature, comfort, fluid balance, dressings, drains, and tubes.
- The overall goals of nursing care during the postoperative period are to promote comfort and healing, restore the highest possible level of wellness, and prevent associated risks such as infection or respiratory and cardiovascular complications.
- Ongoing postoperative nursing interventions include (a) managing pain, (b) appropriate positioning, (c) encouraging incentive spirometry and deep-breathing and coughing exercises, (d) promoting leg exercises and early ambulation, (e) maintaining adequate hydration and nutritional status, (f) promoting urinary elimination, (g) continuing gastrointestinal suction, and (h) providing wound care.
- Surgical aseptic technique (sterile technique) is used when changing dressings on surgical wounds to promote healing and reduce the risk of infection.
- Penrose drains and Hemovac drainage systems are examples of drains that may be placed in or near surgical wounds to promote drainage of excess serosanguineous or purulent exudate.
- Sutures, wire clips, or staples are used to approximate skin and underlying tissues after surgery. These are generally removed 7 to 10 days after surgery.

Review Questions

35-1. The nurse should check the results of which of the following tests to determine the preoperative status of a client's liver function?
   a. serum electrolytes
   b. BUN, creatinine
   c. ALT, AST, bilirubin
   d. serum albumin

35-2. A client who is having a mastectomy expresses sadness about losing her breast. Based on this information, the nurse would identify that the client is at risk for which nursing diagnosis?
   a. *Body Image Disturbance*
   b. *Anticipatory Grieving*
   c. *Fear*
   d. *Ineffective Coping*

35-3. Which of the following statements by the client would indicate preoperative teaching for gallbladder surgery has been effective?
   a. "I cannot eat or drink anything after midnight."
   b. "I'm not going to cough after surgery because it might open my incision."
   c. "I might have a stroke if I stop taking my anticoagulant."
   d. "The nurse showed me how to contract and relax my calf muscles"

35-4. The nurse assesses a postoperative client who has a rapid, weak pulse; urine output less than 30 mL/hr; and decreased blood pressure. The client's skin is cool and clammy. What complication should the nurse suspect?
   a. thrombophlebitis
   b. hypovolemic shock

c. aspiration pneumonia

d. wound dehiscence

35-5. The nurse can expect that the postoperative client will probably require the most pain medication when?

a. immediately after surgery

b. 4 hours after surgery

c. 12 to 36 hours after surgery

d. 48 to 60 hours after surgery

Readings and References

Suggested Readings

Fox, V. J. (1998). Postoperative education that works. *AORN Journal, 67*(5), 1010, 1012–1017.

Perioperative nurses have acquired greater responsibility for clients' and family members' postoperative education. Recent nursing research indicates that clients may not be getting specific information about dealing with the everyday practical matters they encounter while recovering at home from their surgical procedures. This article addresses some of these issues (e.g., food, sex, driving, bathing, wound care, return to work, limits on activities). The author answers questions most often asked by clients and their family members.

Garbee, D. D., & Beare, P. G. (2001). Creating a positive surgical experience for patients. *AORN Journal, 74*(3), 333–337.

This article presents brief research findings about traditional medical treatments for pain relief and complementary therapies that are available (e.g., music therapy, aromatherapy, hydrotherapy). It concludes with a case study about one hospital that uses all of the therapies to create a positive surgical experience for the client.

Marley, R. A., & Swanson, J. (2001). Patient care after discharge from the ambulatory surgical center. *Journal of PeriAnesthesia Nursing, 16*(6), 339–419.

The authors provide comprehensive information about common postoperative complications described by clients after being discharged home. The information offers helpful interventions and directions that the nurse can teach the client and/or family.

Related Research

Alsop-Shields, L. (2000). Perioperative care of children in a transcultural context. *AORN Journal, 71*(5), 1004–1020.

Greer, S. M., Dalton, J., Carlson, J., & Youngblood, R. (2001). Surgical patients' fear of addiction to pain medication: The effect of an educational program for clinicians. *The Clinical Journal of Pain, 17*(2), 157–164.

Lookinland, S., & Pool, M. (1998). Study on effect of methods of preoperative education in women. *AORN Journal, 67*(1), 203–213.

Mimnaugh, L., Winegar, M., Mabrey, Y., & Davis, J. E. (1999). Sensations experienced during removal of tubes in acute postoperative patients. *Applied Nursing Research, 12*(2), 78–85.

References

AORN Online. (2002). Top ten frequently asked questions. Retrieved April 29, 2003, from http://www.aorn.org/practice/clinical.asp

Association of Operating Room Nurses. (1996). Recommended practices for skin preparation of patients. *AORN Journal, 64*(5), 813–816.

Bailes, B. K. (2000). Perioperative care of the elderly surgical patient. *AORN Journal, 72*(2), 186–207.

Crenshaw, J. T., & Winslow, E. H. (2002). Preoperative fasting: Old habits die hard. *American Journal of Nursing, 102*(5), 36–44.

Federated Ambulatory Surgery Association. Frequently asked questions about ambulatory surgery centers. Retrieved April 29, 2003, from http://www.fasa.org/faqaboutasc.html

Fox, V. J. (1998, May). Postoperative education that works. *AORN Journal, 6*(5), 1010, 1012–1017.

Johnson, M., Maas, M., & Moorhead, S. (2000). *Nursing outcomes classification (NOC)* (2nd ed.). St. Louis, MO: Mosby.

Kost, M. (1999). Conscious sedation. Guarding your patient against complications. *Nursing, 29*(4), 34–39.

McCloskey, J. C., & Bulechek, G. M. (2000). *Nursing interventions classification (NIC)* (3rd ed.). St. Louis, MO: Mosby.

NANDA International. (2003). NANDA *nursing diagnoses: Definitions & classification 2003-2004.* Philadelphia: Author.

Van Keuren, K., & Eland, J. A. (1997). Perioperative pain management in children. *Nursing Clinics of North America, 32*(1), 31–44.

Selected Bibliography

Ben-Hamida, A., & Meyrick-Thomas, J. (1998). How-to guides: Postoperative wound drainage. *Care of the Critically Ill. The Journal for Critical Care Professionals, 14*(2), insert 4p.

Brenner, Z. R. (1999). Preventing postoperative complications: What's old, what's new, what's tried-and-true. *Nursing, 29*(10), 34–39.

Brooks, J. A. (2001). Postoperative nosocomial pneumonia: Nurse-sensitive interventions. *AACN Clinical Issues, 12*(2), 305–323.

Castille, K. (1998). Suturing. *Nursing Standard, 12*(41), 41–46.

Dunn, D. (1998). Preoperative assessment criteria and patient teaching for ambulatory surgery patients. *Journal of PeriAnesthesia Nursing, 13*(5), 274–291.

Eliopoulos, C. (2001). *Gerontological nursing* (5th ed.). Philadelphia: Lippincott.

Ennis, D. (1999). Reducing the risk of surgical site infection. *Nursing, 29*(6), 32hn1–32hn2.

Federated Ambulatory Surgery Association. About FASA. Retrieved April 29, 2003, from http://www.fasa.org/aschistory.html

Frantz, A. K. (2001). Recovery from coronary artery bypass grafting at home: Is your nursing practice current? *Home Healthcare Nurse, 19*, 417–425.

Hrouda, B. S. (2000). How to remove surgical sutures and staples. *Nursing, 30*(2), 54–55.

Hughes, S. (2002). The effects of giving patients pre-operative information. *Nursing Standard, 16*(28), 33–37.

Leinonen, T., Leino-Kilpi, H., Stahlberg, M. R., & Lertola, K. (2001). The quality of perioperative care: Development of a tool for the perceptions of patients. *Methodological Issues in Nursing Research, 35*(2), 294–306.

Malkin, K. F. (2000). Patients' perceptions of a pre-admission clinic. *Journal of Nursing Management, 8*(2), 107–113.

McConnell, E. A. (1998). Managing wound dehiscence and evisceration. *Nursing, 28*(9), 26.

McConnell, E. A. (1999). Using a closed-wound drainage system. *Nursing, 29*(6), 32.

McConnell, E. A. (2001). Emptying a closed-wound drainage device. *Nursing, 31*(2), 17.

McConnell, E. A. (2002). Applying antiembolism stockings. *Nursing, 32*(4), 17.

McConnell, E. A. (2002). Managing a T-tube. *Nursing, 32*(6), 17.

Shaheen, K. W. (1999). Jackson-Pratt drains: Patient discharge instructions. *Plastic Surgical Nursing, 18*(1), 50.

Walton, J. (2001). Helping high-risk surgical patients beat the odds. *Nursing, 31*(3), 54–59.

Ziolkowski, L., & Strzyzewski, N. (2001). Perianesthesia assessment: Foundation of care. *Journal of PeriAnesthesia Nursing, 16*, 359–370.

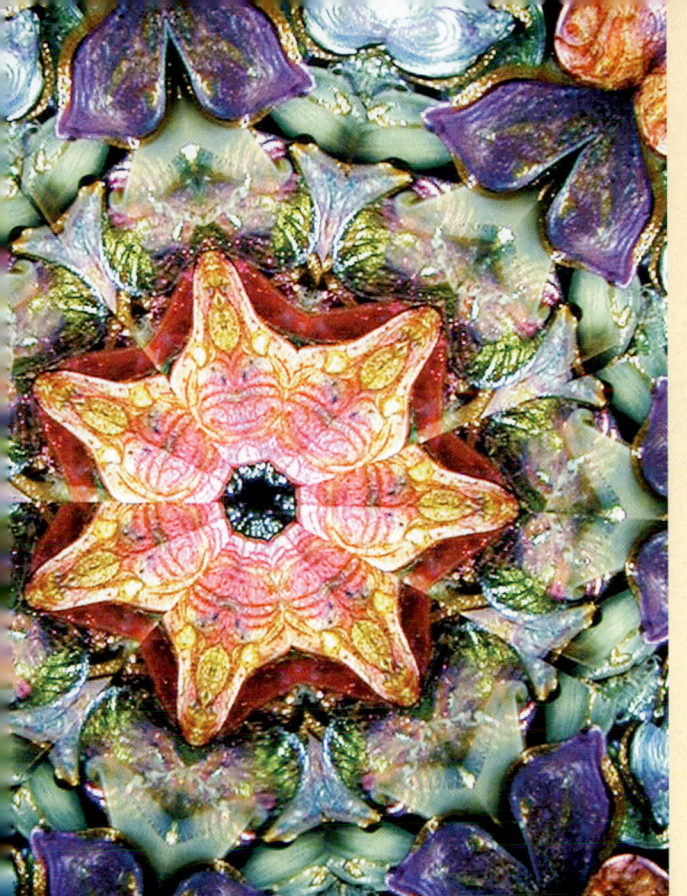

PROMOTING PSYCHOSOCIAL HEALTH

Vital to the art of providing effective and appropriate nursing care is the nurse's ability to convey understanding, sensitivity, and compassion to the client who has a negative self-concept or who confronts a stressful life event. The nurse recognizes the impact of low self-esteem, loss, or other stressors on the individual client as well as on the family and support persons. By providing a supportive environment in which to express feelings, by listening attentively, and by offering comfort, the nurse helps those affected to develop a healthy self-image or cope with stress and to transcend the experience of loss.

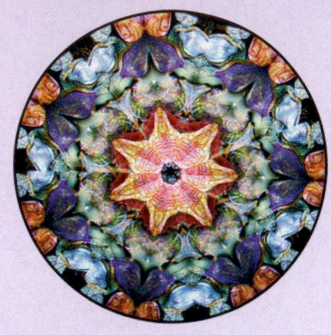

CHAPTER 36

SENSORY PERCEPTION

LEARNING OUTCOMES

After completing this chapter, you will be able to

- Discuss anatomic and physiologic components of the sensory-perception process.

- Describe factors influencing sensory function.

- Discuss factors that place a client at risk for sensory disturbances.

- Describe essential components in assessing a client's sensory-perception function.

- Identify clinical signs and symptoms of sensory overload and deprivation.

- Develop nursing diagnoses and outcome criteria for clients with impaired sensory function.

- Discuss nursing interventions to promote and maintain sensory function.

- Identify strategies to promote and maintain orientation to person, place, time, and situation for the confused client.

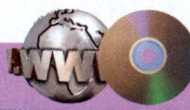

MediaLink

www.prenhall.com/kozier

Additional resources for this chapter can be found on the Student CD-ROM accompanying this textbook, and on the Companion Website at www.prenhall.com/kozier. Click on Chapter 36 to select the activities for this chapter.

CD-ROM
- Audio Glossary
- NCLEX Review
- Animations:
    Brain and Brainstem 3D
    Visceral Effectors A & P Review
    Components of a Reflex Arc
    Meninges of the Brain A & P Review
    Head and Trunk 3D
    The Ear 3D
    The Ear A & P Review
    The Eye 3 D
    The Eye A & P Review
    Lower Limb 3D
    Upper Limb 3D

Companion Website
- Additional NCLEX Review
- Case Study: Clients with Altered Sensory Perception
- Care Plan Activity: The Confused and Agitated Client
- MediaLink Application: Client with Second-Degree Burns
- Links to Resources

An individual's senses are essential for growth, development, and survival. Sensory stimuli give meaning to events in the environment. Any alteration in people's sensory functions can affect their ability to function within the environment. For example, many clients have impaired sensory functions that put them at risk in the health care setting; nurses can help them find ways to function safely in this often confusing environment.

COMPONENTS OF THE SENSORY EXPERIENCE

The sensory process involves two components: reception and perception. **Sensory reception** is the process of receiving stimuli or data. These stimuli are either external or internal to the body. External stimuli are **visual** (sight), **auditory** (hearing), **olfactory** (smell), **tactile** (touch), and **gustatory** (taste). Gustatory stimuli can be internal as well. Other types of internal stimuli are kinesthetic or visceral. **Kinesthetic** refers to awareness of the position and movement of body parts. For example, a person walking is aware of which leg is forward. A related sense is **stereognosis,** the ability to perceive and understand an object through touch by its size, shape, and texture. For example, a person holding a tennis ball is aware of its size, round shape, and soft surface without seeing it. **Visceral** refers to any large organ within the body. Visceral organs may produce stimuli that make a person aware of them (e.g., a full stomach). **Sensory perception** involves the conscious organization and translation of the data or stimuli into meaningful information.

For an individual to be aware of the surroundings, four aspects of the sensory process must be present: a stimulus, a receptor, impulse conduction, and perception.

- *Stimulus.* An agent or act that stimulates a nerve receptor.
- *Receptor.* A nerve cell acts as a receptor by converting the stimulus to a nerve impulse. Most receptors are specific, that is, sensitive to only one type of stimulus, such as visual, auditory, or touch.
- *Impulse conduction.* The impulse travels along nerve pathways to the spinal cord or directly to the brain (see Figure 36–1 ■). For example, auditory impulses travel to the organ of Corti in the inner ear. From there the impulses travel along the eighth cranial nerve to the temporal lobe of the brain.
- *Perception.* Perception, or awareness and interpretation of stimuli, takes place in the brain, where specialized brain cells interpret the nature and the quality of the sensory stimuli. The level of consciousness affects the perception of the stimuli.

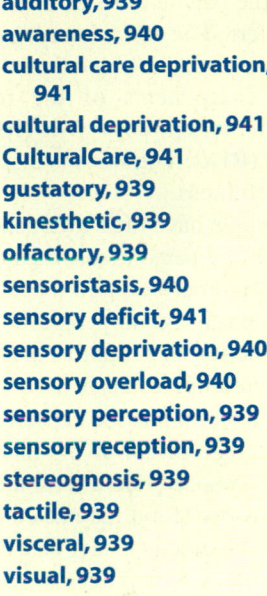

KEY TERMS

auditory, 939
awareness, 940
cultural care deprivation, 941
cultural deprivation, 941
CulturalCare, 941
gustatory, 939
kinesthetic, 939
olfactory, 939
sensoristasis, 940
sensory deficit, 941
sensory deprivation, 940
sensory overload, 940
sensory perception, 939
sensory reception, 939
stereognosis, 939
tactile, 939
visceral, 939
visual, 939

MediaLink | BRAIN AND BRAINSTEM 3D ANIMATION

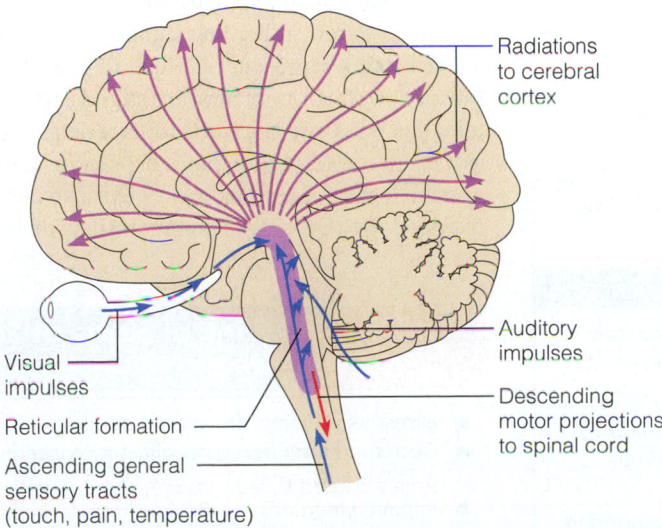

Radiations to cerebral cortex

Auditory impulses

Descending motor projections to spinal cord

Visual impulses

Reticular formation

Ascending general sensory tracts (touch, pain, temperature)

Figure 36–1 ■ The nerve impulses run along the ascending sensory tracts to reach the reticular activating system (RAS); then certain impulses reach the cerebral cortex where they are perceived. (From *Human Anatomy and Physiology,* 4th ed., by Elaine N. Marieb. Copyright © 1998 by Benjamin Cummings Publishing Company. Reprinted with permission.)

Arousal Mechanism

For the person to receive and interpret stimuli, the brain must be alert. The *reticular activating system* (RAS) in the brain stem is thought to mediate the arousal mechanism. There are two components of the reticular activating system, the *reticular excitatory area* (REA) and the *reticular inhibitory area* (RIA). The REA is responsible for stimulus arousal and wakefulness.

People have their own zone of optimum arousal, the level at which the person feels comfortable. **Sensoristasis** is the term used to describe when a person is in optimal arousal. Beyond this comfort zone people must adapt to the increased or decreased sensory stimuli. An absence of stimuli from the RAS to the cerebrum results in the brain's becoming inactive or useless.

The brain has the capacity to adapt to sensory stimuli. For example, a person living in a city may not notice traffic noise that someone from a rural area finds loud and disturbing. Not all sensory stimuli are acted on; some are stored by the memory to be used at a later date. Cognition is cerebral functioning. It involves such processes as conscious thought, reality orientation, problem solving, judgment, and comprehension.

Awareness is the ability to perceive environmental stimuli and body reactions and to respond appropriately through thought and action. The normal, alert person can assimilate many kinds of information at one time. There are several states of awareness (see Table 36–1).

SENSORY ALTERATIONS

People become accustomed to certain sensory stimuli, and when these change markedly the individual may experience discomfort. For example, when clients enter a hospital they usually experience stimuli that differ in quantity and quality from those to which they are accustomed. These changes may cause clients to become confused and disoriented (see Table 36–1).

Nurses are aware of the behaviors that often result from different stimuli. They now pay more attention to color, sound, privacy, and social interaction for clients so that the stimuli more closely resemble those in the home environment. Factors that contribute to alterations in behavior include sensory deprivation, sensory overload, and sensory deficits.

Sensory Deprivation

Sensory deprivation is generally thought of as a decrease in or lack of meaningful stimuli. When a person experiences sensory deprivation, the balance in the reticular activating system is disturbed. The RAS is unable to maintain normal stimulation to the cerebral cortex. Because of this reduced stimulation, a person becomes more acutely aware of the remaining stimuli and often perceives these in a distorted manner. Thus the person often experiences alterations in perception, cognition, and emotion. Box 36–1 lists clinical signs of sensory deprivation.

Sensory Overload

Sensory overload generally occurs when a person is unable to process or manage the amount or intensity of sensory stimuli. Three factors contribute to sensory overload:

- Increased quantity or quality of internal stimuli, such as pain, dyspnea, anxiety
- Increased quantity or quality of external stimuli, such as a noisy health care setting, intrusive diagnostic studies, contacts with many strangers
- Inability to disregard stimuli selectively, perhaps as a result of nervous system disturbances or medications that stimulate the arousal mechanism.

Sensory overload can prevent the brain from ignoring or responding to specific stimuli. Because of the many stimuli, the individual has difficulty perceiving the environment in a way that makes sense. As a result the individual's thoughts race in many directions and restlessness occurs. The person usually feels overwhelmed and does not feel in control. It is important for nurses to remember that sights and sounds that are familiar to them often represent overload to clients. People who have sensory overload may appear fatigued. They often cannot internalize new information and experience cognitive overload as a result of everything that is happening to them. Such factors as pain, lack of sleep, and worry can also contribute to sensory overload. Box 36–2 lists common signs of sensory overload.

TABLE 36–1 States of Awareness

State	Description
Full consciousness	Alert; oriented to time, place, person; understands verbal and written words
Disoriented	Not oriented to time, place, or person
Confused	Reduced awareness, easily bewildered; poor memory, misinterprets stimuli; impaired judgment
Somnolent	Extreme drowsiness but will respond to stimuli
Semicomatose	Can be aroused by extreme or repeated stimuli
Coma*	Will not respond to verbal stimuli

*See Glasgow Coma Scale, Table 28–10 in Chapter 28.

BOX 36–1 ■ Clinical Signs of Sensory Deprivation

- Excessive yawning, drowsiness, sleeping
- Decreased attention span, difficulty concentrating, decreased problem solving
- Impaired memory
- Periodic disorientation, general confusion, or nocturnal confusion
- Preoccupation with somatic complaints, such as palpitations
- Hallucinations or delusions
- Crying, annoyance over small matters, depression
- Apathy, emotional lability

BOX 36–2	■ Clinical Signs of Sensory Overload

- Complaints of fatigue, sleeplessness
- Irritability, anxiety, restlessness
- Periodic or general disorientation
- Reduced problem-solving ability and task performance
- Increased muscle tension
- Scattered attention and racing thoughts

Sensory Deficits

A **sensory deficit** is impaired reception, perception, or both, of one or more of the senses. Blindness and deafness are sensory deficits. When only one sense is affected, other senses may become more acute to compensate for the loss. However, sudden loss of eyesight can result in disorientation.

When the loss of sensory function is gradual, individuals often develop behaviors to compensate for the loss; sometimes these behaviors are unconscious. For example, a person with gradual hearing loss in the right ear may unconsciously turn the left ear toward a speaker. When the loss is sudden, however, compensatory behavior often takes days or weeks to develop.

Some neurologic diseases cause changes in the kinesthetic sense and tactile perceptions. Diseases of the inner ear, for example, can cause loss of kinesthetic sense.

Clients with sensory deficits are at risk of both sensory deprivation and sensory overload. Persons with visual problems may be unable to read, watch television, or recognize nurses by sight. An unfamiliar environment can add to their confusion. Blind people often have highly structured home environments, and the diversity and unfamiliarity of the hospital environment can create sensory overload. At the same time, impaired vision often results in an inability to move around readily or socialize with others.

FACTORS AFFECTING SENSORY FUNCTION

A number of factors affect the amount and quality of sensory stimulation, including a person's developmental stage, culture, level of stress, medications and illness, and lifestyle.

Developmental Stage

Perception of sensation is critical to the intellectual, social, and physical development of infants and children. Infants learn to recognize the face of the mother or caregiver and establish bonding essential to later emotional development. Young children respond to music by singing and dancing as they begin to interact with their peers in groups. As children grow, they learn to interpret visual and auditory signals when preparing to cross the street. Adults have many learned responses to sensory cues. The sudden loss or impairment of any sense, therefore, has a profound effect on both the child and adult. Normal physiologic changes in older adults put them at higher risk for altered sensory function. The diminishing of sensory perception that may come with chronic disease or aging is generally gradual.

Culture

An individual's culture often determines the amount of stimulation that a person considers usual or "normal." For example, a child reared in a big-city Latino neighborhood where extended families share responsibilities for all the children may be accustomed to more stimulation than a child reared in a European American suburb of scattered single-family homes. In addition, the normal amount of stimulation associated with ethnic origin, religious affiliation, and income level, for example, also affects the amount of stimulation an individual desires and believes to be meaningful. A sudden change in cultural surroundings experienced by immigrants or visitors to a new country, especially where there are differences in language, dress, and cultural behaviors, may also result in sensory overload or cultural shock.

Cultural deprivation, or **cultural care deprivation,** is a lack of culturally assistive, supportive, or facilitative acts. Spector (2000) coined the term "**CulturalCare**—professional health care that is culturally sensitive, culturally appropriate, and culturally competent" (p. 281) and points out that CulturalCare is essential for the new millennium (see Chapter 13). It is important that nurses be sensitive to what stimulation is culturally acceptable to a client. For example, in some cultures touching is comforting, whereas in others it is offensive. Some clients find the presence of cultural or religious symbols reassuring and their absence a source of anxiety. Nurses should encourage clients who want to have culturally related symbols present and to follow practices with which they are comfortable, provided that these practices do not endanger health.

Stress

During times of increased stress, people may find their senses already overloaded and thus seek to decrease sensory stimulation. For example, a client dealing with physical illness, pain, hospitalization, and diagnostic tests may wish to have only close support people visit. In addition, the client may need the nurse's help to decrease unnecessary stimuli (e.g., noise) as much as possible. On the other hand, clients may seek sensory stimulation during times of low stress in order to maintain cortical arousal.

Medications and Illness

Certain medications can alter an individual's awareness of environmental stimuli. Narcotics and sedatives, for example, can decrease awareness of stimuli. Some antidepressants can alter perceptions of stimuli. Anyone taking several medications concurrently may show alterations in sensory function; elders are especially at risk and need to be monitored carefully. Certain medications, if taken over a long period of time, become ototoxic, injuring the auditory nerve and causing hearing loss that may be irreversible. Some of these medications are aspirin, furosemide (Lasix), the aminoglycosides, and certain drugs given for cancer chemotherapy.

Certain diseases, such as atherosclerosis, restrict blood flow to the receptor organs and the brain, thereby decreasing awareness and slowing responses. Uncontrolled diabetes mellitus can impair vision and is a leading cause of blindness in the

United States. Some central nervous system diseases cause varying degrees of paralysis and sensory loss.

Lifestyle and Personality

Lifestyle influences the quality and quantity of stimulation to which an individual is accustomed. A client who is employed in a large company may be accustomed to many diverse stimuli, whereas a client who is self-employed and works in the home is exposed to fewer, less diverse stimuli. People's personalities also differ in terms of the quantity and quality of stimuli with which they are comfortable. Some people delight in constantly changing stimuli and excitement, whereas others prefer a more structured life with few changes.

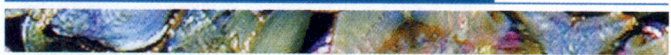

NURSING MANAGEMENT

ASSESSING

Nursing assessment of sensory-perceptual functioning includes six components: (a) nursing history, (b) mental status examination, (c) physical examination, (d) identification of clients at risk, (e) the client's environment, and (f) social support network.

Nursing History

During the nursing history the nurse assesses present sensory perceptions, usual functioning, sensory deficits, and potential problems. In some instances, significant others can provide data the client cannot. For example, support people may reveal signs of recent changes in the client's hearing ability, such as inattention to others, recent mood swings, difficulty following clear instructions, frequent requests to have something repeated, and unusually loud radio or television volumes. Examples of interview questions to elicit data about the client's sensory-perceptual functioning are shown in the accompanying Assessment Interview.

Mental Status

Mental status is critical to any evaluation of the sensory-perceptual process. Usually data on mental status including level of consciousness, orientation, memory, and attention span can be obtained during the nursing history (see Chapter 28).

Physical Examination

Physical assessment determines whether the senses are impaired. During the physical examination the nurse assesses vision and hearing, and the olfactory, gustatory, tactile, and kinesthetic senses. The examination should reveal the client's specific visual and hearing abilities; perception of heat, cold, light touch, and pain in the limbs; and awareness of the position of the body parts. Specific sensory tests include

- Visual acuity, using a Snellen chart or other reading material such as a newspaper, and visual fields
- Hearing acuity, by observing the client's conversation with others and by performing the whisper test and the Weber and Rinne tuning fork tests

Assessment Interview

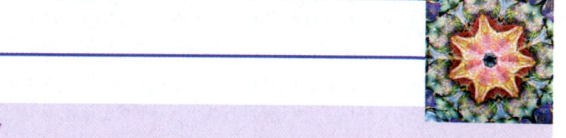

SENSORY-PERCEPTUAL FUNCTIONING

Visual
- How would you rate your vision (excellent, good, fair, or poor)?
- Do you wear eyeglasses or contact lenses?
- Describe any recent changes in your vision.
- Do you have any difficulty seeing near or far objects?
- Do you have any difficulty seeing at night? Have you ever experienced blurred vision, double vision, spots moving in front of your eyes, blind spots, light sensitivity, flashing lights, or halos around objects?
- When did you last visit an eye doctor?

Auditory
- How would you rate your hearing (excellent, good, fair, or poor)?
- Do you wear a hearing aid?
- Describe any recent changes in your hearing.
- Can you locate the direction of sounds and distinguish various voices?
- Do you experience any dizziness or vertigo? Do you experience any ringing, buzzing, humming, crackling noises, or fullness in the ears?

Gustatory
- Have you experienced any changes in taste (e.g., difficulty in differentiating sweet, sour, salty, and bitter tastes)?
- Do you enjoy the taste of foods as you did previously?

Olfactory
- Have you experienced any changes in smell?
- Do things (foods, flowers, perfumes, and so on) smell the same as previously?
- Can you distinguish foods by their odors and tell when something is burning?
- Have you experienced any changes in appetite? (Changes in appetite may be related to an impaired sense of smell.)

Tactile
- Are you experiencing any pain or discomfort?
- Have you experienced any decrease in your ability to perceive heat, cold, or pain in your limbs?
- Do you have any numbness or tingling in your extremities?

Kinesthetic
- Have you noticed any difficulty in perceiving the position of parts of your body?

- Olfactory sense, by identifying specific aromas
- Gustatory sense, by identifying three tastes such as lemon, salt, and sugar
- Tactile sense, by testing light touch, sharp and dull sensation, two-point discrimination, hot and cold sensation, vibration sense, position sense, and stereognosis.

These tests are described in detail in Chapter 28. 🔗 The nurse should also determine whether sensory adaptive devices that the client uses, such as eyeglasses or hearing aids, function properly.

Clients at Risk for Sensory Deprivation or Overload

Clients at risk for sensory-perceptual alterations need to be identified to ensure that preventive measures can be initiated. Box 36–3 describes clients at risk.

Client Environment

The nurse assesses the client's environment for quantity, quality, and type of stimuli. The client's environment may produce insufficient stimuli, placing the client at risk for sensory deprivation, or excessive stimuli, placing the client at risk for sensory overload. Nonstimulating environments include those that (a) severely restrict physical activity and (b) limit social contact with family and friends. Because appropriate or meaningful stimuli decrease the incidence of sensory deprivation, the nurse must consider the client's health care environment for the presence of the following stimuli:

- Radio or other auditory device (e.g., cassette player), television
- Clock or calendar
- Reading material (or toys for children)
- Number and compatibility of roommates
- Number of visitors.

In the client's home, the nurse may also note the presence of a videocassette recorder, pets, bright colors, adequate lighting, and so on.

To assess a health care environment that produces excessive stimuli, the nurse considers, for example, bright lights, noise, therapeutic measures, frequency of assessments and procedures.

> ► **CLINICAL ALERT** *Are you aware of the noise level around you or the noise level you create while providing nursing care? The standard of 45 decibels (dB) for rest and sleep is often not met. For example, studies have shown that sounds in critical care units range from 60 to 83 dB, thereby suggesting sensory overload.* ■

Social Support Network

The degree of isolation a person feels is significantly influenced by the quality and quantity of support from family members and friends. The nurse assesses (a) whether the client lives alone, (b) who visits and when, and (c) any signs indicating social deprivation, such as withdrawal from contact with others to avoid embarrassment or dependence on others, negative self-image, reports of lack of meaningful communication with others, and absence of opportunities to discuss fears or concerns that facilitate coping mechanisms.

DIAGNOSING
Disturbed Sensory Perception as the Diagnostic Label

The North American Nursing Diagnosis Association (NANDA International, 2003) includes the following diagnostic labels for sensory perception alterations:

- *Disturbed Sensory Perception* (Specify: *Visual, Auditory, Kinesthetic, Gustatory, Tactile, Olfactory*): Change in the

---

BOX 36–3 ■ Clients at Risk for Sensory Deprivation and Overload

Sensory Deprivation: Clients who
- are confined in a nonstimulating or monotonous environment in the home or health care agency
- have impaired vision or hearing
- have mobility restrictions such as quadriplegia or paraplegia with bed rest, traction apparatus
- are unable to process stimuli (e.g., clients who have brain damage or who are taking medications that affect the central nervous system)
- have emotional disorders (e.g., depression) and withdraw within themselves
- have limited social contact with family and friends (e.g., clients from a different culture).

Sensory Overload: Clients who
- have pain or discomfort
- are acutely ill and have been admitted to an acute care facility
- are being closely monitored in an intensive care unit (ICU) (Figure 36–2 ■) and have intrusive tubes such as IVs, catheters, or nasogastric or endotracheal tubes
- have decreased cognitive ability (e.g., head injury).

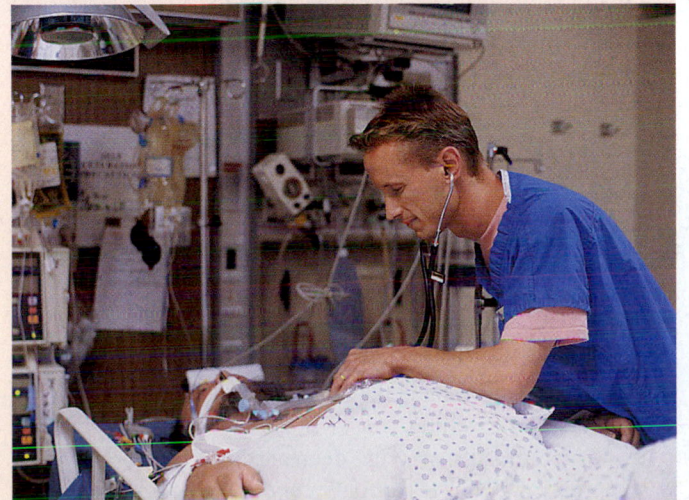

Figure 36–2 ■ A client in an ICU may experience sensory overload.

amount or patterning of incoming stimuli accompanied by a diminished, exaggerated, distorted, or impaired response to such stimuli (NANDA International 2003, p. 163). This diagnostic label is used to describe clients whose perception has been altered by physiologic factors (e.g., pain, sleep deprivation) or disease states such as a stroke (Wilkinson, 2000).

Other diagnostic labels that can relate to sensory perception alterations include

- *Acute Confusion:* The abrupt onset of a cluster of global, transient changes and disturbances in attention, cognition, psychomotor activity level of consciousness, and/or sleep/wake cycle (NANDA International 2003, p. 38).
- *Chronic Confusion:* An irreversible, long-standing, and/or progressive deterioration of intellect and personality characterized by decreased ability to interpret environmental stimuli; and decreased capacity for intellectual thought processes; and manifested by disturbances of memory, orientation, and behavior (NANDA International 2003, p. 39).
- *Impaired Memory:* Inability to remember or recall bits of information or behavior skills. Impaired memory may be attributed to pathophysiological or situational causes that are either temporary or permanent (NANDA International 2003, p. 112).

> ▶ **CLINICAL ALERT**   *It is easy to confuse the two nursing diagnoses* Disturbed Sensory Perception *and* Altered Thought Processes. *You may find it helpful to remember that the diagnosis* Disturbed Sensory Perception *refers to sensory input—the person's ability to accurately interpret stimuli. In contrast, when a person's* cognitive *abilities (because of mental disorders, i.e., dementia) interfere with the ability to interpret stimuli accurately, the diagnosis is more likely* Altered Thought Processes. *Double check your assessment data to see if the primary problem is one of sensory input or cognitive ability.* ■

Examples of clinical application of some of these diagnoses using NANDA, Nursing Interventions Classification (NIC), and Nursing Outcomes Classification (NOC) designations are shown in Identifying Nursing Diagnoses, Outcomes, and Interventions.

Sensory-Perception Problem as the Etiology

Depending on the data obtained, alterations in sensory-perception function may affect other areas of human functioning and indicate other diagnoses. In these instances the sensory-perception problem becomes the etiology.

Examples of nursing diagnoses for which sensory-perception disturbances are the etiology include

- *Risk for Injury* related to sensory-perception disturbance (specify). For example,
  a. Visual impairment (e.g., decreased depth perception)
  b. Reduced tactile sensation secondary to neurologic or circulatory alterations
  c. Decreased sense of smell
  d. Hearing impairment
  e. Decreased kinesthetic sense

- *Impaired Home Maintenance* related to sensory-perception disturbance (declining visual abilities)
- *Risk for Impaired Skin Integrity* related to sensory-perception disturbance (altered tactile sensation)
- *Impaired Verbal Communication* related to sensory-perception disturbance (specify). For example,
  a. Altered level of consciousness
  b. Hearing impairment
  c. Sensory overload
  d. Sensory deprivation
- *Self Care Deficit: Bathing/Hygiene* related to sensory-perception disturbance (specify). For example,
  a. Visual impairment
  b. Diminished kinesthetic sense
  c. Inability to perceive body part or spatial relationship
- *Social Isolation* related to sensory-perception disturbance (specify). For example,
  a. Impaired vision
  b. Impaired hearing.

PLANNING

Planning includes goals associated with the care of clients independent of setting and those specific to the home environment.

Planning Independent of Setting

The overall outcome criteria for clients with sensory-perception alterations are to

- Maintain the function of existing senses
- Develop an effective communication mechanism
- Prevent injury
- Prevent sensory overload or deprivation
- Reduce social isolation
- Perform activities of daily living independently and safely.

The NIC developed by the Iowa Intervention Project can be a guide when planning care (McCloskey & Bulechek, 2000). Appropriate nursing activities may be selected from the following nursing interventions:

- Communication Enhancement: Hearing Deficit
- Communication Enhancement: Visual Deficit
- Nutrition Management
- Environmental Management
- Fall Prevention
- Body Mechanics Promotion
- Peripheral Sensation Management
- Emotional Support
- Surveillance: Safety.

Examples of clinical application of NOC outcomes and NIC interventions are shown in Identifying Nursing Diagnoses, Outcomes, and Interventions.

Planning for Home Care

To provide for continuity of care, the nurse must consider the client's needs for assistance with care in the home or residential treatment setting. Some clients with severe alterations in sensory-perception functioning may be discharged to an assisted living

IDENTIFYING NURSING DIAGNOSES, OUTCOMES, AND INTERVENTIONS

CLIENTS WITH SENSORY PERCEPTION DISTURBANCES

DATA CLUSTER	NURSING DIAGNOSIS/ DEFINITION	SAMPLE DESIRED OUTCOMES [NOC#]/DEFINITION	INDICATORS	SELECTED INTERVENTIONS [NIC#/DEFINITION	SAMPLE NIC ACTIVITIES
Anthony Broom, a 52-year-old lawyer, has multiple sclerosis. Muscle strength and tactile sensation have declined during the past 2 years. He uses a motorized wheelchair to move about. He reports loss of sensation in his lower limbs and fingers and inability to discern temperature differences. His wife assists with bathing and grooming.	Risk for Injury/At risk of injury as a result of environmental conditions interacting with the individual's adaptive and defensive resources	Risk Control [1902]/Actions to eliminate or reduce actual, personal, and modifiable health threats	Often demonstrated: • Acknowledges risk • Monitors environmental risk factors • Develops effective risk control strategies as needed	Risk Identification [6610]/Analysis of potential risk factors, determination of health risks, and prioritization of risk reduction strategies for an individual or group	• Institute routine risk assessment, using reliable and valid instruments • Determine past and current level of functioning • Identify individual's usual coping strategies • Determine presence/absence of basic living needs
Emma Robertson, an 84-year-old widow, lives alone in her apartment. She can hear words spoken clearly and close to the left ear but cannot hear any sounds with the right ear. She says she spends her time listening to the television and radio (at loud volume). She tends to speak loudly and shout when talking with others, and nods and smiles when others speak. Her daughter, who visits, says she refuses to wear a hearing aid. (Ms. Robertson says it doesn't help and is uncomfortable.) Her daughter has recently noted that her mother has become withdrawn, appears absorbed in her own thoughts, and talks and laughs to herself.	Disturbed Sensory Perception (Auditory)/Change in the amount or patterning of incoming stimuli accompanied by a diminished, exaggerated, distorted, or impaired response to such stimuli	Hearing Compensation Behavior [1610]/Actions to identify, monitor and compensate for hearing loss	Often demonstrated: • Positions self to advantage hearing • Reminds others to use techniques that advantage hearing • Uses hearing assistive devices (e.g., light on telephone, fire alarm, door bell)	Communication Enhancement: Hearing Deficit [4974]/Assistance in accepting and learning alternate methods for living with diminished hearing	• Facilitate appointment for hearing examination, as appropriate • Teach that sounds will be experienced differently with the use of a hearing aid • Move closer to less affected ear • Obtain attention through touch
	Impaired Verbal Communication/Decreased, delayed or absent ability to receive, process, transmit, and use a system of symbols	Communication: Receptive Ability [0904]/Ability to receive and interpret verbal and/or nonverbal messages	Mildly compromised: • Interpretation of spoken language • Acknowledgment of messages received	As above	As above plus: • Keep hearing aid clean • Face the client directly, speak slowly, clearly and concisely • Use simple words and short sentences • Use paper, pencil or computer communication when necessary

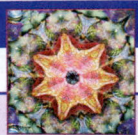

Home Care Assessment
SENSORY PERCEPTION DISTURBANCES

Client and Environment

- *Self-care abilities:* Ability to care for self while adapting to sensory impairment
- *Safety:* Physical safety of client's environment including lighting, noise, access, lack of clutter or obstructions, use of stairs, assistive devices with respect to sensory impairment, such as flashing fire alarms or telephones for hearing impaired

- *Level of knowledge:* Assistive devices available; ways to maximize use of other senses; local, regional, or national organizations that may provide education, training, support, or other assistance, such as the National Braille Association, Guide Dogs for the Blind, the National Association of the Deaf.

---

facility that provides the specific support the client requires. Discharge planning incorporates a reassessment of the client's abilities for self-care, the availability and skills of support people, financial resources, and the need for referrals and home health services. See the accompanying Home Care Assessment for sensory-perception alterations and confusion. A major aspect of discharge planning involves the instructional needs of the client and family. See methods to support visual and auditory function and maintain a safe environment in the next section.

IMPLEMENTING

Nurses can assist clients with sensory alterations by promoting healthy sensory function, by adjusting environmental stimuli, and by helping clients to manage acute sensory deficits.

Promoting Healthy Sensory Function

Detecting sensory problems early is one step toward preventing serious problems. The arousal mechanism for sensation is normally present at birth; however, it is undifferentiated. The special senses are also present at birth, although some changes in function occur during the growth process.

Early screening to detect problems in the visual and hearing functions is essential. All infants should be screened for hearing loss by 1 month of age, preferably before hospital discharge; infants identified with a hearing loss should be enrolled in an intervention program by 6 months of age (Centers for Disease Control and Prevention, 2003). In addition, children with chronic ear infections and people who live or work in an environment where there is a high noise level should receive routine auditory testing. Women who are considering pregnancy should be advised of the importance of testing for syphilis and rubella, which can cause hearing impairments in newborns. Periodic vision screening of all newborns and children is recommended to detect congenital blindness, strabismus, and refractive errors.

Healthy sensory function can be promoted with environmental stimuli that provide appropriate sensory input. This input should vary and be neither excessive nor too limited. As many senses as possible should be stimulated. Various colors, sounds, textures, smells, and body positions can provide various sensations. Nurses can teach parents to stimulate infants and children, and teach family members to stimulate an elderly person. Social activities often help stimulate the mind and the senses.

Nurses should also teach clients at risk of sensory loss how to prevent the loss and should teach general health measures, such as getting regular eye examinations and controlling chronic diseases such as diabetes (see Teaching: Wellness Care).

Teaching: Wellness Care
Preventing Sensory Disturbances

- Have regular health examinations.
- Have regular eye examinations as recommended by the physician or pediatrician to screen for eye problems. For clients ages 40 and over, a medical eye examination is generally recommended every 3 to 5 years, or every 1 to 2 years if there is a family history of glaucoma.
- Seek early medical attention (a) if signs suggesting visual impairment arise, for example, failure to react to light, or reduced eye contact from an infant; (b) if the child complains of an earache or has an ear infection; and (c) for persistent eye redness, discharge or increased tearing, growths on or near the eye, pupil asymmetry or other irregularity, or any pain or discomfort.
- Obtain regular immunizations of children against diseases capable of causing hearing loss (e.g., rubella, mumps, and measles).

- Avoid giving infants and toddlers toys with long pointed handles and keep pointed instruments (e.g., scissors and screwdrivers) out of reach. Supervise preschoolers when they use scissors.
- Make sure that toddlers do not walk or run with a pointed object in hand; teach preschoolers to walk carefully when carrying such objects as sticks or toy weapons.
- Teach school-age children and adolescents the proper use of sports equipment (e.g., hockey sticks) and power tools.
- Wear protective eye goggles when using power tools, riding motorcycles, spraying chemicals, and so on.
- Wear ear protectors when working in an environment with high noise levels or brief loud impulse noises (e.g., blasting).
- Wear dark glasses to avoid damage from ultraviolet rays and never look directly into the sun.

BOX 36–4	■ Preventing Sensory Overload

- Minimize unnecessary light, noise, and distraction. Provide dark glasses and earplugs as needed.
- Control pain as indicated.
- Introduce yourself by name, and address the client by name.
- Provide orienting cues, such as clocks, calendars, equipment, and furniture in the room.
- Provide a private room.
- Limit visitors.
- Plan care to allow for uninterrupted periods for rest or sleep.
- Schedule a routine of care so the client knows when and what to expect (post the schedule for the client wherever possible).

- Speak in a low tone of voice and in an unhurried manner.
- Provide new information gradually to enable the client to process the meaning. When providing information, ask the client to repeat it so that there are no misunderstandings.
- Describe any tests and procedures to the client beforehand.
- Reduce noxious odors. Empty a commode or bedpan immediately after use, keep wounds clean and covered, use a room deodorizer when indicated, and provide good ventilation.
- Take time to discuss the client's problems and to correct misinterpretations.
- Assist the client with stress-reducing techniques.

Adjusting Environmental Stimuli

The client functions best when the environment is somewhat similar to that of the individual's ordinary daily life. Sometimes nurses need to take steps to adjust the client's environment to prevent either sensory overload or sensory deprivation.

Preventing Sensory Overload. For clients who are at risk of overstimulation, nurses should reduce the number and type of environmental stimuli. The nurse can counteract sensory overload by blocking stimuli and by helping the client organize the stimuli and alter responses to the stimuli.

Dark glasses can partially block light rays, and a window shade or drape can reduce visual stimulation. Earplugs reduce auditory stimuli, as do soft background music and earphones. The odor from a draining wound can be minimized by keeping the dressing dry and clean and applying a liquid deodorant on a gauze near the wound.

Another method of blocking stimuli is to reduce novelty and surprise and provide rest intervals free of interruptions. Sometimes the number of visitors and the length of visits must be restricted. Also, if the nurse carries out several nursing measures together, the client can have a scheduled quiet period before the next activity.

By explaining sounds in the environment, the nurse can help the client organize them mentally: A bell signals a change of shift; a buzzer, a change of IV. When clients understand their meaning,

stimuli are frequently less confusing and more easily ignored. People can also learn to alter their responses to the stimuli. Clients can employ relaxation techniques to reduce anxiety and stress despite continual sensory stimulation (see Chapter 40). Box 36–4 provides nursing measures for clients with sensory overload.

Preventing Sensory Deprivation. For clients who are at risk for sensory deprivation, nurses can increase environmental stimuli in a number of ways. For example, newspapers, books, and television can stimulate the visual and auditory senses. Providing objects that are pleasant to touch, such as a pet to stroke, can provide tactile and interactive stimulation. Clocks that differentiate night from day by color can help orient a client to time. The olfactory sense can be stimulated by the presence of fresh flowers or plants.

Arrangements should also be made for people to visit and talk with the client regularly. Many church and community groups provide visitors to "shut-ins," that is, people who are confined to their homes or who reside in nursing homes. Box 36-5 provides measures to prevent sensory deprivation.

Managing Acute Sensory Deficits

When assisting clients who have a sensory deficit, the nurse needs to (a) encourage the use of sensory aids to support residual sensory function, (b) promote the use of other senses, (c) communicate effectively, and (d) ensure client safety.

BOX 36–5	■ Preventing Sensory Deprivation

- Encourage the client to use eyeglasses and hearing aids.
- Address the client by name and touch the client while speaking if this is not culturally offensive.
- Communicate frequently with the client and maintain meaningful interactions (e.g., discuss current events).
- Provide a telephone, radio and/or TV, clock, and calendar.
- Provide murals, pictures, sculptures, and wall hangings. Many libraries and museums will lend artwork free of charge, or a local school may provide art projects developed by their students.
- Have family and friends bring freshly cut flowers and plants.
- Consider having a resident pet such as fish, a cat, or a bird or make arrangements for pets to visit on a regular basis.

- Include different textured objects to feel such as a sheepskin pillow, silk scarf, soft blanket, or other inanimate object.
- Increase tactile stimulation through physical care measures such as back massages, hair care, and foot soaks.
- Encourage social interaction through activity groups or visits by family and friends.
- Encourage the use of crossword puzzles or games to stimulate mental function.
- Encourage environment changes such as a walk through a mall, or for an immobilized client, sitting near a window or at a place on the nursing unit where the client can watch local traffic.
- Encourage the use of self-stimulation techniques such as singing, humming, whistling, or reciting.

MediaLink | UPPER LIMB 3D ANIMATION

MediaLink | LOWER LIMB 3D ANIMATION

BOX 36–6 ■ Sensory Aids for Visual and Hearing Deficits

Visual
- Eyeglasses of the correct prescription, clean and in good repair
- Adequate room lighting, including night-lights
- Sunglasses or shades on windows to reduce glare
- Bright contrasting colors in the environment
- Magnifying glass
- Phone dialer with large numbers
- Clock and wristwatch with large numbers
- Color code or texture code on stoves, washer, medicine containers, and so on
- Colored or raised rims on dishes
- Reading material with large print
- Braille or recorded books
- Seeing-eye dog

Hearing
- Hearing aid in good order
- Lip reading
- Sign language
- Amplified telephones
- Telecommunication device for the deaf (TDD)
- Amplified telephone ringers and doorbells
- Flashing alarm clocks
- Flashing smoke detectors

Sensory Aids. Many sensory aids are available for clients who have visual and hearing deficits. Examples are listed in Box 36–6. Sensory aids can be used in the health care setting as well as in the home. In all situations, the assistance of support people needs to be enlisted whenever possible to help the client deal with the deficit.

Promoting the Use of Other Senses. When one sense is lost, the nurse can teach the client to use other senses to supplement the loss. This stimulation is similar to that provided to prevent sensory deprivation, discussed earlier. However, the type of stimulation needs to be adapted in accordance with the client's specific deficit. For example, for the visually impaired client, stimulation of hearing, taste, smell, and touch can be encouraged. A radio, audiotapes of music or books, clocks that chime, music boxes, and wind chimes can be used for auditory stimulation. Diets that include a variety of flavors, temperatures, and textures can be planned to stimulate the taste buds. Taking sips of water between foods and eating foods separately can emphasize the taste sensation. Fresh flowers, scented candles (safely used), room fragrances, brewing coffee, and baking can stimulate the sense of smell. Clients can also be encouraged to remember pleasant or familiar odors such as the perfume of sweet peas. Measures such as providing a hug, massage, hair brushing, grooming, different textures in clothing and upholstery fabrics, and pets can be used to stimulate touch receptors.

Communicating Effectively. Communication with clients who have sensory deficits should convey respect, enhance the person's self-esteem, and ensure the exchange of correct information. A person with a hearing impairment has to concentrate more than other people and therefore tires more readily. Fatigue compounded by an illness can further reduce the person's ability to hear. A person with a visual impairment is unable to observe most nonverbal cues during communication and relies largely on the spoken word and tone of voice. Guidelines for communicating with people who are visually or hearing impaired are shown in Box 36–7.

Ensuring Client Safety. Nurses must implement safety precautions in health care settings for clients with sensory deficits and teach them special precautions to ensure their safety at home.

Impaired Vision. For clients with visual impairments, nurses need to do the following in a health care setting:

- Orient the client to the arrangement of room furnishings and maintain an uncluttered environment.
- Keep pathways clear and do not rearrange furniture without orienting the client. Ensure that housekeeping personnel are informed about this.
- Organize self-care articles within the client's reach and orient the client to his or her location.
- Keep the call light within easy reach and place the bed in the low position.
- Assist with ambulation by standing at the client's side, walking about 1 foot ahead, and allowing the person to grasp your arm. Confirm whether the client prefers grasping your arm with the dominant or nondominant hand.

Impaired Hearing. Clients with hearing impairments who are unable to hear the alarms of IV pumps and cardiac monitors need to be assessed frequently. They can be taught to use their visual sense to identify kinks in the IV tubing or a loose ECG lead, and so on. For home safety, clients with impaired hearing need to obtain devices that either amplify sounds or respond with flashing lights to sounds such as a doorbell or smoke detector, a baby crying, or a burglar alarm. The sounds of doorbells and alarm clocks may be amplified or changed to a lower frequency or buzzerlike sound. These devices can be obtained from hearing aid dealers, telephone companies, and appliance stores.

Impaired Olfactory Sense. Clients with an impaired sense of smell need to be taught about the dangers of cleaning with chemicals such as ammonia. Because a gas leak can go undetected, clients need to keep gas stoves and heaters in good working order. Strong chemicals such as ammonia used in confined spaces such as a bathroom may affect the client before they are smelled. Food poisoning is a concern with clients who have difficulty detecting spoiled meat or dairy products. These clients need to carefully inspect food for freshness (check its color and texture) and check expiration dates on food packages.

Impaired Tactile Sense. Clients with an impaired sense of touch may not be aware of hot temperatures, which can cause burns, or pressure on bony prominences, which can produce

MediaLink   CLIENT WITH SECOND DEGREE BURNS APPLICATION

BOX 36–7 ■ Communicating with Clients Who Have a Visual or Hearing Deficit

Visual Deficit

- Always announce your presence when entering the client's room and identify yourself by name.
- Stay in the client's field of vision if the client has a partial vision loss.
- Speak in a warm and pleasant tone of voice. Some people tend to speak louder than necessary when talking to a blind person.
- Always explain what you are about to do before touching the person.
- Explain the sounds in the environment.
- Indicate when the conversation has ended and when you are leaving the room.

Hearing Deficit

- Before initiating conversation, convey your presence by moving to a position where you can be seen or by gently touching the person.
- Decrease background noises (e.g., radio) before speaking.
- Talk at a moderate rate and in a normal tone of voice. Shouting does not make your voice more distinct and in some instances makes understanding more difficult.
- Address the person directly. Do not turn away in the middle of a remark or story. Make sure the person can see your face easily and that it is well lighted.
- Avoid talking when you have something in your mouth, such as chewing gum. Avoid covering your mouth with your hand.
- Keep your voice at about the same volume throughout each sentence, without dropping the voice at the end of each sentence.
- Always speak as clearly and accurately as possible. Articulate consonants with particular care.
- Do not "overarticulate"; mouthing or overdoing articulation is just as troublesome as mumbling. Pantomime or write ideas, or use sign language or finger spelling as appropriate.
- Use longer phrases, which tend to be easier to understand than short ones. For example, "Would you like a drink of water?" presents much less difficulty than "Would you like a drink?" Word choice is important: "Fifteen cents" and "fifty cents" may be confused, but "half a dollar" is clear.
- Pronounce every name with care. Make a reference to the name for easier understanding, for example, "Joan, the girl from the office" or "Sears, the big downtown store."
- Change to a new subject at a slower rate, making sure that the person follows the change to the new subject. A key word or two at the beginning of a new topic is a good indicator.

---

pressure ulcers. Clients with decreased sensation to temperature should have the temperature adjusted on their hot water heater and test water temperature with a thermometer before bathing. Clients with decreased sensation to pressure must change their position frequently.

The Confused Client

Confusion can occur in clients of all ages, but it is most commonly seen in older people. Confusion often presents with subtle symptoms, but an attempt should be made to differentiate between acute confusion (*delirium*) and chronic confusion (*dementia*). Delirium is often called acute confusion, has an abrupt onset, and a cause which, when treated, reverses the confusion. Dementia is often called chronic confusion with symptoms that are gradual and irreversible. It is often difficult to differentiate between the two conditions, but it is important to treat causes, if possible, in order to be able to reverse the condition. The most common causes of confusion are

- *Drug effects,* such as potentiating effects of multiple drug use and drug intoxication
- *Physiologic disturbances,* such as hypoxia, dehydration, metabolic or fluid imbalances, neurologic disorders, infectious processes, and nutritional deficiencies
- *Abrupt loss* of a significant person or persons
- *Multiple losses* in a short time span
- *A move* to a radically different environment.

Clients who are confused often know something is wrong and want help. Box 36–8 lists nursing interventions to help ori-

ent the confused person to time, place, person, and situation (see Figure 36–3 ■).

The Unconscious Client

The person who is unconscious and unable to respond to the spoken word nevertheless can often hear what is spoken. It is therefore important that nurses talk to the client as though they

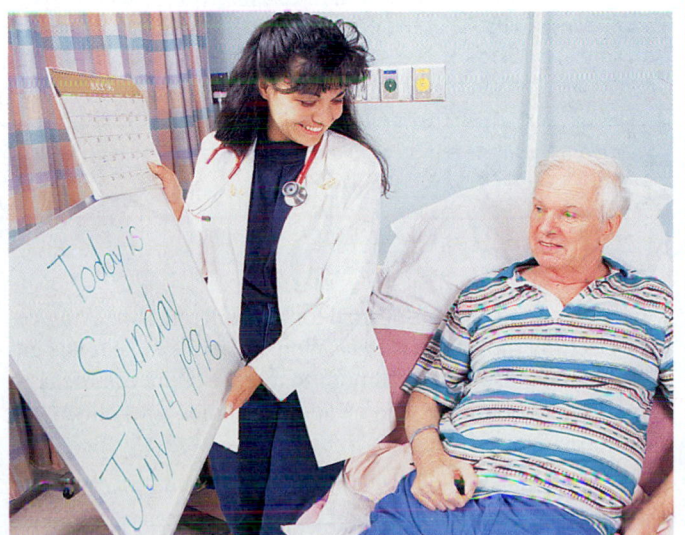

Figure 36–3 ■ Promoting orientation to time and date is essential for clients who are confused or have a memory loss.

BOX 36–8 ■ Promoting Orientation to Time, Place, Person, and Situation

- Wear a readable name tag.
- Address the person by name and introduce yourself frequently: "Good morning, Mr. Richards. I am Betty Brown. I will be your nurse today."
- Identify time and place as indicated: "Today is December 5, and it is 8:00 in the morning."
- Ask the client, "Where are you?" and orient the client to place (e.g., nursing home) if indicated.
- Place a calendar and clock in the client's room. Mark holidays with ribbons, pins, or other means.
- Speak clearly and calmly to the client, allowing time for your words to be processed and for the client to give a response.
- Provide frequent face-to-face contact.
- Provide clear, concise explanations of each treatment procedure or task.

- Reinforce reality by interpreting unfamiliar sounds, sights, and smells; correct any misconceptions of events or situations.
- Schedule activities (e.g., meals, bath, activity and rest periods, treatments) at the same time each day to provide a sense of security. If possible, assign the same caregivers.
- Keep familiar items in the client's environment (e.g., photographs), and keep the environment uncluttered. A disorganized, cluttered environment increases confusion.
- Encourage the client to wear familiar or personal clothing and to arrange personal hygiene articles in order of use as needed.
- Encourage participation in familiar activities or hobbies to emphasize the client's strengths rather than problems.
- Tell the client when you are leaving and when you will return.

Research Note
Are There Predictors of Agitation for Clients with Dementia in an Acute Care Setting?

A client admitted to a hospital experiences changes in patterns of rest, sleep, and activity that may result in periods of sensory overload and sensory deprivation. A client with dementia is even less able to adapt to these changes, which may delay or prevent recovery. To study this phenomenon, Kovach and Wells (2002) used the Model of Imbalances in Sensoristasis, which postulates that some of the agitated behaviors and functional decline of older adults with dementia can be attributed to imbalances in the pacing of sensory stimulating and sensory calming activity. The pacing of activity of persons with dementia in acute care has not been studied.

The research questions asked if agitation scores were associated with type of activity, unpleasantness of the activity, and length of the activity, and also looked into the contribution of sustained (e.g., 90 minutes) versus unsustained activity. Six clients were chosen from two medical units that have a large population of older adult admissions. All of the clients had the diagnosis of dementia on admission. The average age was 82.5. This descriptive study collected data between 7:30 AM and 10 PM over 5 days.

The results showed sustained active activity occurred most often during the day and afternoon hours. Most of the unpleasant activity also occurred in the morning and afternoon hours. The highest agitation scores were recorded in the afternoon and the lowest in the evening. Agitation scores were considerably higher during sustained activity and unpleasant activity. Diagnostic and treatment needs often necessitated sustained unpleasant activity.

Implications: The small number of clients in the study limits generalizability. The authors point out that there are no parameters for guiding the optimal pacing for clients with dementia in acute care. The results, however, suggest that when activity is sustained for 90 minutes, agitation is higher. Possible nursing interventions include balancing active and calming activities—for example, scheduling rest periods during the busy activities involved in being a client on an acute care unit.

Note: From "Pacing of Activity as a Predictor of Agitation for Persons with Dementia in Acute Care," by C. R. Kovach and T. Wells, 2002, *Journal of Gerontological Nursing, 22*(1), pp. 28–35.

were understood, using a normal tone of voice and speaking before touching the client. Nurses should also try to keep the environmental noises at a minimum so that the client can focus on words. The following are some additional measures nurses can take in caring for the unconscious client:

- Orient the unconscious client to self, time, and place.
- Listen carefully to the support person's concerns. Often they simply want to express them.
- Maintain the same schedule each day. Routine gives the client a sense of security.

- Touch and stroke the unconscious client.
- To the support persons, explain what is happening, and encourage them to talk to and touch the client as though the client were conscious. This auditory and tactile stimulation supports the client and may restore some degree of consciousness.
- Always address the client by name, and explain beforehand the care to be provided. Unconscious clients require bathing, skin care, turning, feeding, and assistance with elimination needs.

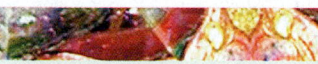

Lifespan Considerations

Elders

Normal changes of aging often result in varying degrees of impairments in sensory perception of the senses—hearing, vision, smell, taste, and touch. Diseases and conditions that are more common in elders and which also alter sensory perception, are strokes and other neurologic disorders such as Parkinson's disease. Nursing interventions need to be very specific and individualized and may be directed to either increase or decrease sensory stimuli.

The goals of nursing care should be focused on maintaining safety and communication with clients who have these impairments. Clients with dementia may have problems that fit more appropriately under "altered thought processes," but the goals should be similar—to maximize their potential, maintain their quality of life and dignity, and at the same time, be aware of safety and communication issues.

EVALUATING

Using the measurable desired outcomes developed during the planning stage as a guide, the nurse collects data needed to judge whether client goals and outcomes have been achieved. Examples of client outcomes and related indicators are shown in the earlier Identifying Nursing Diagnoses, Outcomes, and Interventions and in the Nursing Care Plan. If outcomes are not achieved, the nurse and client, and support people if appropriate, need to explore the reasons before modifying the care plan.

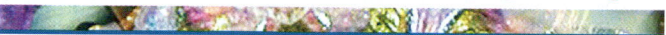

NURSING CARE PLAN FOR SENSORY-PERCEPTION DISTURBANCE

ASSESSMENT DATA		NURSING DIAGNOSIS	OUTCOMES [NOC#]/INDICATORS*
Nursing Assessment Julia Hagstrom is an 80-year-old widow who has recently become a resident of an extended care facility. Just prior to her admission she underwent surgery for the removal of cataracts and also experienced more difficulty with hearing. Her children were concerned about her physical safety and lack of socialization and urged her to enter a nursing home. Mrs. Hagstrom had cared for herself independently for 15 years in her own home. Three days after admission the nurse finds the client somewhat confused and disoriented to person, place, and time. She appears restless, withdrawn, and her syntax is sometimes inappropriate. She states, "I'm afraid of all of these strange creatures in this orphanage."	**Physical Examination** Height: 160 cm (5'3") Weight: 55.3 kg (122 lb) Temperature: 37C (98.6F) Pulse: 72 BPM Respirations: 18/minute Blood Pressure: 128/74 mm Hg Rinne test: negative **Diagnostic Data** Chest x-ray, CBC, and urinalysis all negative	*Sensory Perception Disturbance (Sensory Overload)* related to change in environment, and hearing loss (as evidenced by disorientation to time, place, person; restlessness; and altered behavior)	Cognitive Orientation [0901] as evidenced by consistently demonstrates: • Identifies self • Identifies significant other(s) • Identifies current place • Identifies correct season Hearing Compensation Behavior [1610] as evidenced by often demonstrates: • Positions self to advantage hearing • Reminds others to use techniques that advantage hearing • Eliminates background noise • Using hearing assistive devices

continued on page 952

NURSING CARE PLAN FOR SENSORY-PERCEPTION DISTURBANCE *continued*

NURSING INTERVENTIONS [NIC#] AND SELECTED ACTIVITIES*	RATIONALE
Reality Orientation [4820]	
• Provide a consistent physical environment and a daily routine.	Routine eliminates the element of surprise, overstimulation, and further confusion.
• Provide access to familiar objects, when possible.	Familiarity helps reduce confusion.
• Provide a low-stimulation environment for Mrs. Hagstrom because disorientation may be increased by overstimulation.	A disruption in the quality or quantity of incoming stimuli can affect a person's cognitive status. Sensory overload blocks out meaningful stimuli.
• Provide for adequate rest, sleep, and daytime naps.	Reduces overstimulation and fatigue, which may be contributing factors to confusion.
• Use a calm and unhurried approach when interacting with Mrs. Hagstrom.	Promotes communication that enhances the person's sense of dignity.
• Speak to the client in a slow, distinct manner with appropriate volume.	The client who has difficulty hearing will be better able to lip read and comprehend speech.
• Engage Mrs. Hagstrom in concrete "here and now" activities (that is, ADLs) that focus on something outside the self that is concrete and reality oriented.	Assists the individual to differentiate between own thoughts and reality.
Communication Enhancement: Hearing Deficit [4974]	
• Facilitate use of hearing aids, as appropriate.	Hearing can be enhanced if the volume is appropriate and the hearing aid is consistently used.
• Listen attentively.	Effective listening is essential in a nurse–client relationship. Poor listening skills can undermine trust and block therapeutic communication.
• Use simple words and short sentences, as appropriate.	Using simple terms and short sentences facilitates understanding and minimizes anxiety.
• Obtain Mrs. Hagstrom's attention through touch.	Gaining the attention of a client with a hearing impairment is an essential first step toward effective communication. However, the client's personal space should be respected and permission to touch should be obtained.

EVALUATION

Outcomes met. Mrs. Hagstrom identifies her primary nurse by sight and name on the third day. She is aware that Christmas is 3 weeks away and is anxious to go shopping with the group. She bathes herself each morning and makes her own bed. Her daughter has brought new batteries for her hearing aid, which she wears during the day.

*Outcomes, interventions, and activities selected are only a sample of those suggested by NOC and NIC and should be further individualized for each client.

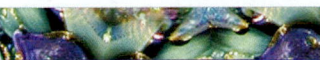

Focus on Critical Thinking

Mrs. Dodd is a 51-year-old client who is being cared for in the critical care unit following an automobile accident in which she suffered extensive traumatic injuries. Mrs. Dodd is connected to several monitoring devices, has an intubation tube and ventilator to assist her with respirations, and is receiving various pain and other medications.

1. Identify factors that place Mrs. Dodd at risk for the development of sensory deprivation or overload.

2. What assessment findings would alert you to Mrs. Dodd's experiencing sensory overload as opposed to sensory deprivation?
3. How can you intervene to help Mrs. Dodd during this stressful event?
4. How might the care of a client in the home setting differ from the care of a client such as Mrs. Dodd who is receiving care in a critical care unit?

See Critical Thinking Possibilities in Appendix A.

CONCEPT MAP   Sensory-Perception Disturbance

JH
80 y.o. ♀
widow

- Lived independently in own home for 15 years
- Recent removal of cataracts
- Experiencing more difficulty hearing
- Children concerned about her safety and lack of socialization and urged her to enter a nursing home
- Became a resident of ECF 3 days ago
- Confused

- Disoriented to person, place, & time
- Restless
- Withdrawn
- Syntax inappropriate at times
- Stated "I'm afraid of all these strange creatures in this orphanage"
- VS: WNL
- CXR, CBC, U/A negative

Sensory-Perception Disturbance
(sensory overload) r/t change
in environment, and hearing loss

Cognitive Orientation aeb constantly demonstrates
- identifies self, others, current place, correct season

Hearing Compensation Behavior aeb often demonstrates
- positions self to advantage hearing
- reminds others to use techniques that advantage hearing
- eliminates background noise
- uses hearing aid

Reality Orientation

Speak slowly
and distinctly

**Communications Enhancement:
Hearing Deficit**

Provide
consistent
physical
environment
and daily
routine

Use calm
unhurried
approach

Provide a low-
stimulation
environment

Facilitate use of
hearing aid

Obtain attention
through touch

Provide access
to families objects

Engage in concrete
"here and now"
activities

Listen
attentively

Use simple words,
short sentences

Provide for
adequate rest
and sleep

Outcomes met
- able to identify her nurse by name
- aware that Christmas is 3 weeks away
- anxious to go shopping with the group
- bathes self and makes own bed
- wears hearing aid during the day

Legend: Assessment ☐ Nursing Diagnosis ☐ Outcomes ☐ Nursing Interventions ▆ Activities ☐ Evaluation/Reassessment ☐

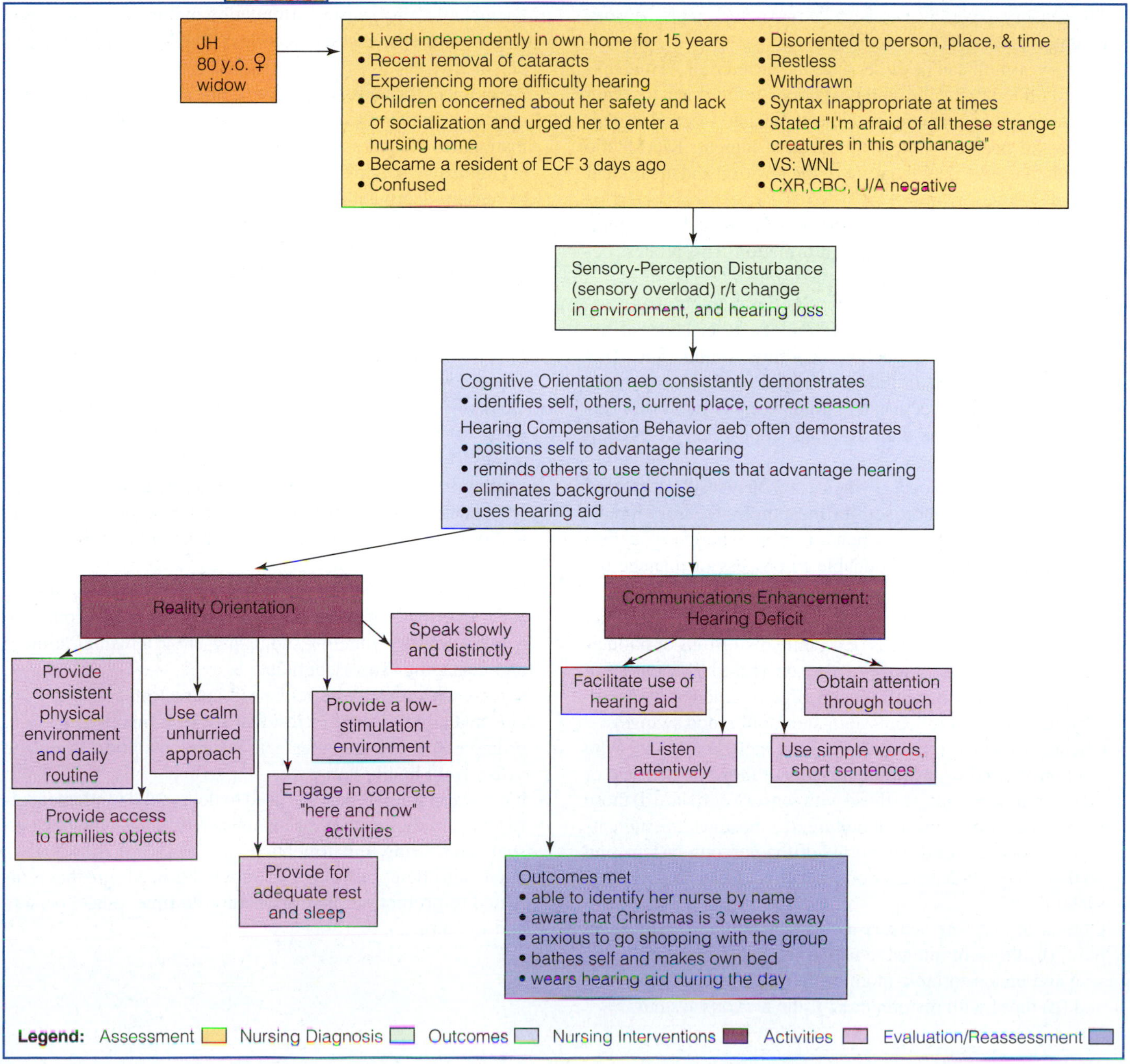

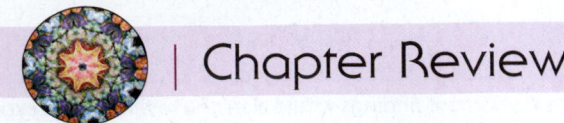

Chapter Review

EXPLORE MediaLink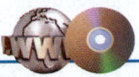

NCLEX review questions, case studies, care plan activities, MediaLink applications, and other interactive resources for this chapter can be found on the Companion Website at www.prenhall.com/kozier. Click on Chapter 36 to select the activities for this chapter.

For animations, more NCLEX review questions, and an audio glossary, access the Student CD-ROM accompanying this textbook.

Chapter Highlights

- The sensory experience consists of two components: sensory reception and sensory perception.
- Sensory stimuli can be either external or internal. Visual, auditory, olfactory, tactile, and gustatory stimuli orient a person to the external environment. Kinesthetic and visceral stimuli orient the person to the internal environment. Kinesthetic stimuli make the person aware of the position and movement of body parts.
- Sensory perception involves the awareness and interpretation of stimuli into meaningful information. This process occurs in the cerebral cortex.
- The reticular activating system (RAS), with its many ascending and descending connections to other areas of the brain, monitors and regulates incoming stimuli. The RAS maintains, enhances, or inhibits cortical arousal.
- The normal, alert person can assimilate many kinds of information at one time and respond appropriately through thought and action.
- Sensory deprivation occurs when a person receives decreased sensory input or monotonous or meaningless sensory input.
- Sensory overload occurs when a person experiences excessive sensory input and is unable to process or manage the stimuli. The person feels overwhelmed and not in control.
- Responses to both sensory deprivation and sensory overload include perceptual changes (e.g., mild distortions or hallucinations), cognitive changes (e.g., decreased concentration and problem-solving ability), and affective changes (e.g., apathy, anxiety, anger, depression, and rapid mood swings).
- Clients at risk for sensory deprivation include (a) those who are homebound or institutionalized, (b) those on bed rest or isolation precautions, (c) those with sensory deficits, (d) those who come from a different culture, (e) those with certain affective disorders or disturbances of the nervous system, and (f) those on certain medications that affect the central nervous system.
- Clients at risk for sensory overload include (a) those in pain, (b) those in intensive care units, (c) those with intrusive and uncomfortable monitoring or treatment equipment, and (d) those with disturbances of the nervous system.

- Factors affecting sensory stimulation include developmental stage, culture, stress, medications, illness, and lifestyle and personality.
- Assessment for sensory-perception disturbances includes (a) a nursing history to identify sensory deficits, (b) physical examination, (c) mental status, (d) identification of clients at risk, (e) immediate environment, and (f) presence of clinical signs of sensory deprivation or overload.
- NANDA nursing diagnoses related to a client's sensory-perception impairments are *Sensory Perception Disturbances: Visual, Auditory, Gustatory, Olfactory, Tactile, Kinesthetic; Acute Confusion; Chronic Confusion; Impaired Memory; Social Isolation; Impaired Verbal Communication; Risk for Impaired Skin Integrity; Self-Care Deficit: Bathing/Hygiene; Impaired Home Maintenance;* and *Risk for Injury.*
- Goals for persons with sensory-perception disturbances include (a) maintaining or promoting the function of existing senses, (b) maintaining or improving communication, (c) preventing injury, (d) avoiding sensory deprivation or overload, (e) reducing social isolation, and (f) maintaining or restoring ability to function safely in the environment and to perform self-care.
- Interventions to prevent or modify sensory deprivation, sensory overload, and sensory deficits include promoting healthy sensory function, adjusting environmental stimuli, and managing sensory deficits.
- Clients with sensory deficits need instruction about sensory aids available to support residual sensory function, ways to promote the use of other senses, and methods to ensure safety from bodily harm.
- Nurses and support persons need to devise and implement effective communication mechanisms for clients who have visual and hearing impairments.
- Confused clients and unconscious clients need care that is directed to promoting their orientation to time, place, person, and situation.

Review Questions

36–1. Which client is at greatest risk for experiencing sensory overload?
  a. a 40-year-old client who has no family and is in isolation
  b. a 28-year-old quadriplegic client in a private room
  c. a 16-year-old listening to loud music
  d. an 80-year-old client admitted for emergency surgery

36–2. An alert 80-year-old client is transferred to a long-term care facility. On the second night he becomes confused and agitated. What is the most appropriate nursing diagnosis?
  a. *Chronic Confusion*
  b. *Impaired Memory*
  c. *Disturbed Sensory Perception*
  d. *Altered Thought Processes*

36–3. The nursing diagnosis *Risk for Impaired Skin Integrity* related to sensory-perception disturbance would best fit a client who
  a. cut foot by stepping on broken glass.
  b. uses a wheelchair due to paraplegia.
  c. has poor vision and wears glasses.
  d. is legally blind and smokes in bed.

36–4. Which statement by a client with decreased hearing indicates a need for a sensory aid in the home?
  a. "I tripped over that throw rug again."
  b. "I can't hear the doorbell."
  c. "My eyesight is good if I wear my glasses."
  d. "I can hear the TV if I turn it up high."

36–5. A hospitalized client is disoriented and believes she is in a train station. Which response by the nurse is most helpful?
  a. "You wouldn't be getting a bath at the train station."
  b. "Let's finish your bath before the train arrives."
  c. "Don't you know where you are?"
  d. "It may seem like a train station sometimes, but this is Valley Hospital."

Readings and References

Suggested Readings

Chitsey, A. M., Haight, B. K., & Jones, M. M. (2002). Snoezelen®. A multisensory environmental intervention. *Journal of Gerontological Nursing, 28*(3), 41–49.
This article describes *Snoezelen*®, a term used to describe an environmental intervention designed to stimulate the primary senses of touch, hearing, sight, smell, and taste. The authors provide a review of the literature for multisensory stimulation studies. In many of these studies, the subjects included "senile" older adults, confused, mentally unstable clients, and older adults with dementia. It was noted that many of these clients suffered from sensory deprivation because of their health condition. Providing sensory stimulation sessions or setting aside a special room equipped with devices to enhance a sensory stimulation session often resulted in positive outcomes. For example, clients became more relaxed, more talkative and sociable, and staff noted a decrease in disruptive behavior. Snoezelen® has been a popular intervention in Great Britain and is just beginning to appear in the United States.

Demers, K. (2001). Try this: Best practices in nursing care to older adults. Hearing screening. *Journal of Gerontological Nursing, 27*(11), 8–9.
The author provides the screening version of the Hearing Handicap Inventory for the Elderly (HHIE-S), which is a 5-minute, 10-item questionnaire developed to assess how the individual perceives the social and emotional effects of hearing loss.

Related Research

Farr, L., Todero, C., & Boen, L. (2001). Reducing disruption of circadian temperature rhythm following surgery. *Biological Research for Nursing, 2*(4), 257–266.

References

Centers for Disease Control and Prevention, National Center on Birth Defects and Developmental Disabilities. (2003). Hearing Loss. Retrieved May 5, 2003, from http://www.cdc.gov/ncbddd/dd/ddhi.htm

Johnson, M., Maas, M., & Moorhead (Eds.). (2000). *Nursing outcomes classification (NOC)* (2nd ed.). St. Louis, MO: Mosby.

Kovach, C. R., & Wells, T. (2002). Pacing of activity as a predictor of agitation for persons with dementia in acute care. *Journal of Gerontological Nursing, 22*(1), 28–35.

McCloskey, J. C., & Bulechek, G. M. (Eds.). (2000). *Nursing interventions classification (NIC)* (3rd ed.) St. Louis, MO: Mosby.

NANDA International. (2003). *NANDA nursing diagnoses: Definitions and classification 2003-2004.* Philadelphia: Author.

Spector, R. E. (2000). *Cultural diversity in health & illness* (5th ed.). Upper Saddle River, NJ: Prentice Hall Health.

Wilkinson, J. M. (2000). *Nursing diagnosis handbook with NIC interventions and NOC outcomes* (7th ed.). Upper Saddle River, NJ: Prentice Hall Health.

Selected Bibliography

Ebersole, P., & Hess, P. (1998). *Toward healthy aging: Human needs and nursing response.* St. Louis, MO: Mosby.

Eliopoulos, C. (2001). *Gerontological nursing* (5th ed.). Philadelphia: Lippincott.

Gammon, J. (1999). The psychological consequences of source isolation: A review of the literature. *Journal of Clinical Nursing, 8*(1), 13–21.

McGregor, D. (2002). Driving over 65: Proceed with caution. *Journal of Gerontological Nursing, 28*(8), 22–26.

Rapp, C. G. (2001). Acute confusion/delirium protocol. *Journal of Gerontological Nursing, 27*(4), 21–33.

Topf, M. (2000). Hospital noise pollution: An environmental stress model to guide research and clinical interventions. *Journal of Advanced Nursing, 31*, 520–528.

Wold, G. H. (1999). *Basic geriatric nursing* (2nd ed.). St Louis, MO: Mosby.

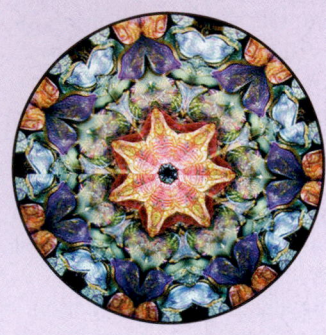

CHAPTER | 37

SELF-CONCEPT

LEARNING OUTCOMES

After completing this chapter, you will be able to:

- Identify four personal and social dimensions of self-concept.
- Give Erikson's explanation of the effects of psychosocial tasks on self-concept and self-esteem.
- Describe the four components of self-concept.
- Identify common stressors affecting self-concept and coping strategies.
- Describe the essential aspects of assessing role relationships.
- Identify nursing diagnoses related to altered self-concept.
- Describe nursing interventions designed to achieve identified outcomes for clients with altered self-concept.
- Describe ways to enhance client self-esteem.

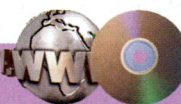

MediaLink

www.prenhall.com/kozier

Additional resources for this chapter can be found on the Student CD-ROM accompanying this textbook, and on the Companion Website at www.prenhall.com/kozier. Click on Chapter 37 to select the activities for this chapter.

CD-ROM
• Audio Glossary
• NCLEX Review

Companion Website
• Additional NCLEX Review
• Case Study: Refusal to Accept a Medical Diagnosis
• Care Plan Activity: Client Who Lost His Job
• MediaLink Application: A Change in Attitude
• Links to Resources

Self-concept is one's mental image of oneself. A positive self-concept is essential to a person's mental and physical health. Individuals with a positive self-concept are better able to develop and maintain interpersonal relationships and resist psychologic and physical illness. An individual possessing a strong self-concept should be better able to accept or adapt to changes that may occur over the life span. How one views oneself affects one's interaction with others.

Nurses have a responsibility not only to identify people with a negative self-concept, but also to identify the possible causes in order to help people develop a more positive view of themselves. Individuals who have a poor self-concept may express feelings of worthlessness, self-dislike, or even self-hatred, which may be projected to others. Individuals with a poor self-concept may feel sad or hopeless and may state they lack energy to perform even the simplest of tasks.

SELF-CONCEPT

Self-concept involves all of the self-perceptions, that is, appearance, values, and beliefs, that influence behavior and that are referred to when using the words *I* or *me*. Self-concept is a complex idea that influences

- How one thinks, talks, and acts
- How one sees and treats another person
- Choices one makes
- Ability to give and receive love
- Ability to take action and to change things.

Four dimensions of self-concept are

- *Self-knowledge:* the knowledge that one has about oneself, including insights into one's abilities, nature, and limitations
- *Self-expectation:* what one expects of oneself; may be a realistic or unrealistic expectation
- *Social self:* how a person is perceived by others and society
- *Social evaluation:* the appraisal of oneself in relationship to others, events, or situations.

People who value "how I perceive me" above "how others perceive me" can be termed *me-centered.* They try hard to live up to their own expectations and compete only with themselves, not others. In contrast, strongly *other-centered* people have a high need for approval from others and try hard to live up to the expectations of others, comparing, competing, and evaluating themselves in relation to others. They tend not to deal with their personal shortcomings, are unable to assert themselves, and fear disapproval. The positive self-concept, therefore, is me-centered and is formed with minimal reference to others' opinions.

Assessing and promoting a positive self-concept is not limited to the nurse acting on the client. A nurse's own self-concept is also important. Nurses who understand the different dimensions of themselves are better able to understand the needs, desires, feelings, and conflicts of their clients. Nurses who feel positive about themselves are more likely to help clients meet their needs.

Self-awareness refers to the relationship between one's perception of himself or herself and others' perceptions of him or her. Thus, a nurse who is very self-aware has perceptions that are very congruent. Becoming more self-aware is a process that requires time and energy and is never complete. One important component of the process is introspection, which involves the nurse considering his or her own beliefs, attitudes, motivations, strengths, and limitations (Eckroth-Bucher, 2001). In addition to using individual reflective exercises, the nurse gains insight into the self through working with other nurses who serve as mentors and by taking seriously and acting on the feedback obtained during regular performance reviews (Rowe, 1999).

Once the nurse has developed a clear understanding and awareness of self, the nurse can respect and avoid projecting his or her own beliefs onto others. While in the caregiver role, the self-aware nurse is able to suspend judgment and focus on the needs of the client, even if they differ from those of the nurse. When conflicts arise, the nurse can analyze his or her reactions through introspection and by asking

- "What is there in me that produces this kind of reaction in the client?
- "Why do I react this way (fear, anger, anxiety, annoyance, anger, worry)?"
- Can I change the way I respond to this situation to impact the client's reaction in a helpful way?" (Eckroth-Bucher, 2001, p. 38).

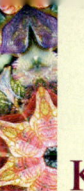

KEY TERMS

body image, 959
core self-concept, 959
global self, 958
global self-esteem, 960
ideal self, 959
role, 960
role ambiguity, 960
role conflicts, 960
role development, 960
role mastery, 960
role performance, 960
role strain, 960
self-concept, 957
self-esteem, 960
specific self-esteem, 960

FORMATION OF SELF-CONCEPT

A person is not born with a self-concept; rather, it develops as a result of social interactions with others. Chapter 21 ⊂⊃ discusses the development of self-concept, including Erikson's stages of development, Piaget's cognitive developmental stages, and Havighurst's developmental tasks.

According to Erikson (1963), throughout life people face developmental tasks associated with eight psychosocial stages that provide a theoretical framework. The success with which a person copes with these developmental tasks largely determines the development of self-concept. Inability to cope results in self-concept problems at the time and, often, later in life. Table 37–1 lists examples of behaviors indicating successful and unsuccessful resolution of these developmental tasks.

There are three broad steps in the development of one's self-concept:

- The infant learns that the physical self is separate and different from the environment.
- The child internalizes others' attitudes toward self.
- The child and adult internalize the standards of society.

The term **global self** refers to the collective beliefs and images one holds about oneself. It is the most complete description that individuals can give of themselves at any one time. It is also a person's frame of reference for experiencing and viewing the world. Some of these beliefs and images represent statements of fact, for example, "I am a woman"; "I am a mother"; "I am short." Others refer to less tangible aspects of self, for instance, "I am competent"; "I am shy."

TABLE 37–1 Examples of Behaviors Associated with Erikson's Stages of Psychosocial Development

Stage: Developmental Tasks	Behaviors Indicating Positive Resolution	Behaviors Indicating Negative Resolution
Infancy: trust vs. mistrust	Requesting assistance and expecting to receive it Expressing belief of another person Being unable to accept assistance Sharing time, opinions, and experiences	Restricting conversation to superficialities Refusing to provide a person with information
Toddlerhood: autonomy vs. shame and doubt	Accepting the rules of a group but also expressing disagreement when it is felt Expressing one's own opinion Easily accepting deferment of a wish fulfillment	Failing to express needs Not expressing one's own opinion when opposed Overconcern about being clean
Early childhood: initiative vs. guilt	Starting projects eagerly Expressing curiosity about many things Demonstrating original thought	Imitating others rather than developing independent ideas Apologizing and being very embarrassed over small mistakes Verbalizing fear about starting a new project
Early school years: industry vs. inferiority	Completing a task once it has been started Working well with others Using time effectively	Not completing tasks started Not assisting with the work of others Not organizing work
Adolescence: identity vs. role confusion	Asserting independence Planning realistically for future roles Establishing close interpersonal relationships	Failing to assume responsibility for directing one's own behavior Accepting the values of others without question Failing to set goals in life
Early adulthood: intimacy vs. isolation	Establishing a close, intense relationship with another person Accepting sexual behavior as desirable Making a commitment to that relationship, even in times of stress and sacrifice	Remaining alone Avoiding close interpersonal relationships
Middle-aged adults: generativity vs. stagnation	Being willing to share with another person Guiding others Establishing a priority of needs, recognizing both self and others	Talking about oneself instead of listening to others Showing concern for oneself in spite of the needs of others Being unable to accept interdependence
Older adults: integrity vs. despair	Using past experience to assist others Maintaining productivity in some areas Accepting limitations	Crying and being apathetic Not accepting changes Demanding unnecessary assistance and attention from others

Each separate image and belief one holds about oneself has a bearing on self-concept. However, self-concept is not simply a sum of its parts, because the various images and beliefs people hold about themselves are not given equal weight and prominence. Each person's self-concept is like a piece of art. At the center of the art are the beliefs and images that are most vital to the person's identity. They constitute **core self-concept.** For example: "I am very smart/of average intelligence"; "I am male/female." Images and beliefs that are less important to the person are on the periphery. For example: "I am left-/right-handed"; "I am athletic/unathletic."

People are thought to base their self-concept on how they perceive and evaluate themselves in these areas:

- Vocational performance
- Intellectual functioning
- Personal appearance and physical attractiveness
- Sexual attractiveness and performance
- Being liked by others
- Ability to cope with and resolve problems
- Independence
- Particular talents.

Maintaining and evaluating one's self-concept is an ongoing process. Events or situations may change the level of self-concept over time. By the time people reach maturity their basic self-concept is relatively well established. Having a basic self-concept includes how we see ourselves and how we are seen by others. There is also the **ideal self,** which is how we should be or would prefer to be. The ideal self is the individual's perception of how one should behave based on certain personal standards, aspirations, goals, and values. Sometimes this ideal self is realistic; sometimes it is not. When perceived self is close to ideal self, people do not wish to be much different from what they believe they already are. A discrepancy between ideal self and perceived self can be an incentive to self-improvement. However, when the discrepancy is great, low self-esteem can result.

Nurses, like other adults, view themselves based on both internal and external inputs acquired over many years. The ability to appraise one's own strengths, the desire to follow in the steps of role models, and the feedback received from colleagues and clients are some of the influences on the nurse's self-concept.

COMPONENTS OF SELF-CONCEPT

There are four components of self-concept: personal identity, body image, role performance, and self-esteem.

Personal Identity

A person's personal identity is the conscious sense of individuality and uniqueness that is continually evolving throughout life. People often view their identity in terms of name, sex, age, race, ethnic origin or culture, occupation or roles, talents, and other situational characteristics (e.g., marital status and education).

Personal identity also includes beliefs and values, personality, and character. For instance, is the person outgoing, friendly, reserved, generous, selfish? Personal identity thus encompasses both the tangible and factual, such as name and sex, and the intangible, such as values and beliefs. Identity is what distinguishes self from others.

A person with a strong sense of identity has integrated body image, role performance, and self-esteem into a complete self-concept. This sense of identity provides a person with a sense of continuity and a unity of personality. Furthermore, the individual sees himself or herself as a unique person.

Body Image

The image of physical self, or **body image,** is how a person perceives the size, appearance, and functioning of the body and its parts. Body image has both cognitive and affective aspects. The cognitive is the knowledge of the material body and its attachments; the affective includes the sensations of the body, such as pain, pleasure, fatigue, and physical movement. Body image is the sum of these attitudes, conscious and unconscious, that a person has toward his or her body.

Body image encompasses the functioning of the body and its parts. It includes clothing, makeup, hairstyle, jewelry, and other things intimately connected to the person (Figure 37–1 ■). It also includes body prostheses, such as artificial limbs, dentures, and

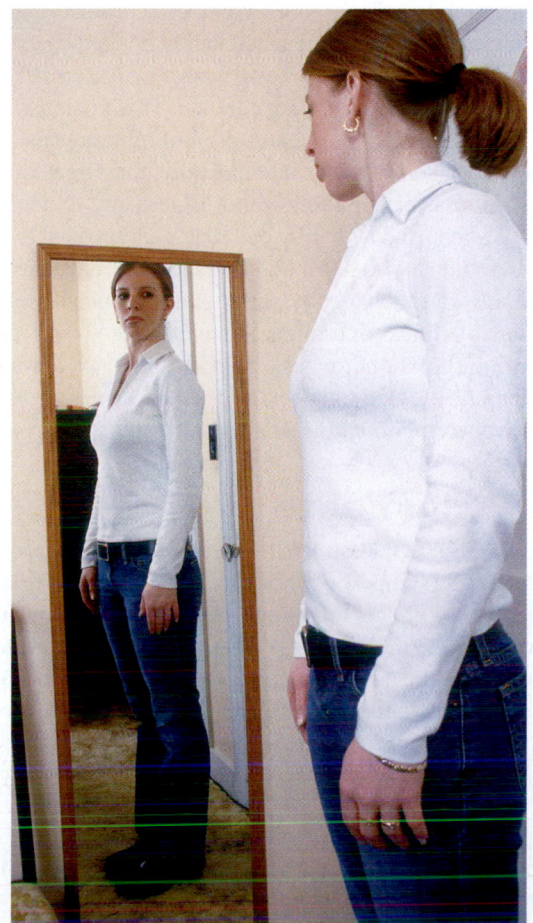

Figure 37–1 ■ Body image is the sum of a person's conscious and unconscious attitudes about his or her body.

hairpieces, as well as devices required for functioning, such as wheelchairs, canes, and eyeglasses. Past as well as present perceptions and how the body has evolved over time are part of one's body image.

A person's body image develops partly from others' attitudes and responses to that person's body and partly from the individual's own exploration of the body. For example, body image develops in infancy as the parents or caregivers respond to the child with smiles, holding, and touching, and as the child explores its own body sensations during breast-feeding, thumb sucking, and the bath. Cultural and societal values also influence a person's body image.

The various information and entertainment media have played a part over the years in how individuals view themselves and others. During adolescence, concerns related to body image are of paramount concern. The "ideal" person portrayed by the media is really an unrealistic goal for many.

If a person's body image closely resembles one's body ideal, the individual is more likely to think positively about the physical and nonphysical components of the self. The body ideal is greatly influenced by cultural standards. For example, currently in North America the fit, well-toned body is admired.

Another aspect of body image is the understanding that different parts of the body have different values for different people. For example, large breasts may be highly important to one woman and unimportant to another, or the occurrence of gray hair may be traumatic to one person and barely noticed by another.

A person with a healthy body image will normally show concern for both health and appearance. This person will seek help if ill and will include health-promoting practices in daily activities. A person who has an unhealthy body image is likely to be overly concerned about minor illness and to neglect activities like sleep and a healthy diet that are important to health.

The individual who has a body image disturbance may hide or not look at or touch a body part that is significantly changed in structure by illness or trauma. Some individuals may also express feelings of helplessness, hopelessness, powerlessness, and vulnerability, and may exhibit self-destructive behavior such as over- or undereating or suicide attempts.

Role Performance

Throughout life people undergo numerous role changes. A **role** is a set of expectations about how the person occupying one position behaves. **Role performance** relates what a person in a particular role does to the behaviors expected of that role. **Role mastery** means that the person's behaviors meet social expectations. Expectations, or standards of behavior of a role, are set by society, a cultural group, or a smaller group to which a person belongs. Each person usually has several roles, such as husband, parent, brother, son, employee, friend, church member. Some roles are assumed for only limited periods, such as client, student, and ill person. **Role development** involves socialization into a particular role. For example, nursing students are socialized into nursing through exposure to their instructors, clinical experience, classes, laboratory simulations, and seminars.

To act appropriately, people need to know who they are in relation to others and what society expects for the positions they hold. **Role ambiguity** occurs when expectations are unclear, and people do not know what to do or how to do it and are unable to predict the reactions of others to their behavior. Failure to master a role creates frustration and feelings of inadequacy, often with consequent lowered self-esteem.

Self-concept is also affected by role strain and role conflicts. People undergoing **role strain** are frustrated because they feel or are made to feel inadequate or unsuited to a role. Role strain is often associated with sex role stereotypes. For example, women in occupations traditionally held by men might be assumed to have less knowledge and competence than men in the same roles.

Role conflicts arise from opposing or incompatible expectations. In an interpersonal conflict, people have different expectations about a particular role. For example, a grandparent may have different expectations than the mother about how she should care for her children. In an interrole conflict, one person's or group's role expectations differ from the expectations of another person or group. For example, a woman who has little flexibility in her full-time job schedule has a role conflict if her husband expects her to handle all child care problems. In a person-role conflict, role expectations violate the beliefs or values of the role occupant. Role conflict can lead to tension, decrease in self-esteem, and embarrassment if needs for achievement, independence, and recognition are unmet.

Self-Esteem

Self-esteem is one's judgment of one's own worth, that is, how that person's standards and performances compare to others and to one's ideal self. If a person's self-esteem does not match with the ideal self, then low self-concept results.

There are two types of self-esteem: global and specific. **Global self-esteem** is how much one likes one's self as a whole. **Specific self-esteem** is how much one approves of a certain part of oneself. Global self-esteem is influenced by specific self-esteem. For example, if a man values his looks, then how he looks will strongly affect his global self-esteem. By contrast, if a man places little value on his cooking skills, then how well or badly he cooks will have little influence on his global self-esteem.

Self-esteem is derived from self and others. In infancy, self-esteem is related to the caregiver's evaluations and acceptances. Later the child's self-esteem is affected by competition with others. As an adult, a person who has high self-esteem has feelings of significance, of competence, of the ability to cope with life, and of control over one's destiny.

> **► CLINICAL ALERT** *If Maslow's level of love and belonging needs are met, the needs for self-esteem are next higher on the hierarchy. When the need for self-esteem is satisfied, the individual strives for self-actualization.* ■

The foundation for self-esteem is established during early life experiences, usually within the family structure. However, an adult's functional level of overall self-esteem may change markedly from day to day and moment to moment. Functional self-esteem is a result of the person's ongoing evaluation of interactions with people and objects. Functional self-esteem can exceed basic self-esteem, or it can regress to a level below that of basic self-esteem. Severe stress—for example, stress related to prolonged illness or unemployment—can substantially lower a person's self-esteem. People frequently focus on their negative aspects and spend less time on their positive aspects. It is important that both strengths and weaknesses be identified.

FACTORS THAT AFFECT SELF-CONCEPT

Many factors affect a person's self-concept. Major factors are development, family and culture, stressors, resources, history of success and failure, and illness.

Development

As an individual develops, the factors that affect the self-concept change. For example, an infant requires a supportive, caring environment, while a child requires freedom to explore and learn.

Family and Culture

A young child's values are largely influenced by the family and culture. Later on, peers influence the child and thereby affect the sense of self. When the child is confronted by differing expectations from family, culture, and peers, the child's sense of self is often confused (Figure 37–2 ■). For example, a child may realize that his parents expect he will not drink alcohol and that he will attend religious services each Saturday evening. At the same time, his peers drink beer and encourage him to spend Saturday evenings with them.

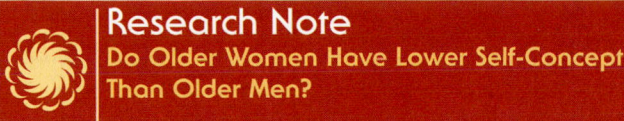

Research Note
Do Older Women Have Lower Self-Concept Than Older Men?

In a meta-analysis, the findings from multiple research studies are examined to see if they are similar enough in definition of terms and concepts to be combined to increase the strength of the results. Pinquart and Sorensen (2001) examined 300 studies that investigated the similarities and differences between older men and women in the areas of subjective well-being (happiness, loneliness, subjective health) and self-concept. They found that there were minimal differences between older men and women in subjective well-being and self-concept when widowhood, health, and socioeconomic status were controlled. There were larger differences (women had lower self-concept) in the upper segments of the age groups.

Implications: One should not make assumptions regarding the differences in the ways older women and men view their health, well-being, and self. A variety of factors influence one's perspective of how healthy, happy, or positive life is to an older person. More research needs to be conducted to establish if there are significantly different variables between men's and women's views or if other factors can be identified. The authors also recommend research into possible differences in the ways men and women react to negative changes in their health and functioning.

Note: From "Gender Differences in Self-Concept and Psychological Well-Being in Old Age: A Meta-Analysis," by M. Pinquart, and S. Sorensen, 2001, *Journals of Gerontology Series B: Psychological Sciences and Social Sciences, 56B*(4), pp. 195–213.

Stressors

Stressors can strengthen the self-concept as an individual copes successfully with problems. On the other hand, overwhelming stressors can cause maladaptive responses including substance abuse, withdrawal, and anxiety. The ability of a person to handle stressors will largely depend on personal resources.

Resources

An individual's resources are internal and external. Examples of internal resources include confidence and values, whereas external resources include support network, sufficient finances, and organizations. Generally the greater the number of resources a person has and uses, the more positive the effect on the self-concept.

History of Success and Failure

People who have a history of failures come to see themselves as failures, whereas people with a history of successes will have a more positive self-concept, making more successes likely.

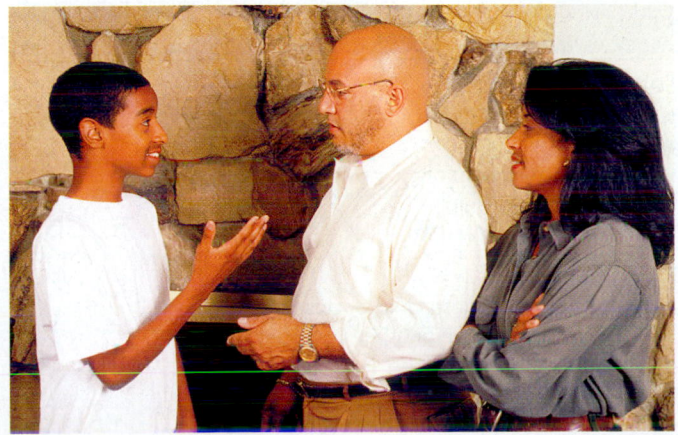

Figure 37–2 ■ A child is often pulled in opposite directions by family and peer expectations. (Jonathan Nourak/PhotoEdit.)

Illness

Illness and trauma can also affect the self-concept. A woman who has a mastectomy may see herself as less attractive, and the loss may affect how she acts and values herself. People respond to stressors such as illness and alterations in function related to aging in a variety of ways: acceptance, denial, withdrawal, and depression are common reactions.

NURSING MANAGEMENT

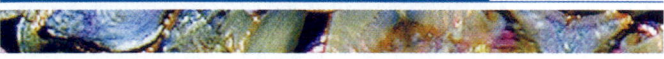

ASSESSING

A thorough assessment includes a psychosocial assessment of the client and the family or support person, because this provides clues to actual or potential problems. The nurse assessing self-concept focuses on the four components: (a) personal identity, (b) body image, (c) role performance, and (d) self-esteem.

Before conducting a psychosocial assessment, the nurse must establish trust and a working relationship with the client. Guidelines for conducting a psychosocial assessment include the following:

- Create a quiet, private environment.
- Minimize interruptions if possible.
- Maintain appropriate eye contact.
- Sit at eye level with the client.
- Demonstrate an interest in the client's concerns.
- Indicate acceptance of the client by not criticizing, frowning, or demonstrating shock.
- Ask open-ended questions to encourage the client to talk rather than close-ended questions that tend to block free sharing.
- Avoid asking more personal questions than are actually needed.
- Minimize writing detailed notes during the interview because this can create client concern that confidential material

Providing Culturally Competent Care

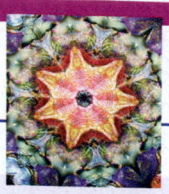

ASSESSING SELF-CONCEPT

It is the nurse's responsibility to use therapeutic communication and to remain sensitive to the effect that cultural influences will have on the client's behaviors and needs. Cultural background is not only assessed directly but is also considered as a factor in the areas of self-perception, role relationships, major stressors, and coping strategies. In the area of behaviors that may suggest low self-esteem, nurses need to ask themselves the following question: Is this really a behavior that would suggest a low self-esteem or is it part of the cultural behavior(s) of the client? In addition, might the client be experiencing cultural dissonance, a situation in which there are conflicting beliefs and attitudes between the client's culture and the one in which the client is living.

is being "recorded" as well as interfere with your ability to focus on what the client is saying.

- Determine whether the family can provide additional information.
- Maintain confidentiality.
- Be aware of your own biases and discomforts that could influence the assessment.
- Consider how the client's behavior is influenced by culture.

It is also important that the nurse identify any stressors that may affect aspects of the self-concept. See Box 37–1 for examples of stressors that may place a client at risk for problems with self-concept.

➤ **CLINICAL ALERT** *The degree to which a stressor is perceived to affect self-concept varies from person to person. For example, whereas some people may respond to repeated failures by trying harder, others may give up.* ■

BOX 37–1 ■ Stressors Affecting Self-Concept

Identity Stressors
- Change in physical appearance (e.g., facial wrinkles)
- Declining physical, mental, or sensory abilities
- Inability to achieve goals
- Relationship concerns
- Sexuality concerns
- Unrealistic ideal self

Body Image Stressors
- Loss of body parts (e.g., amputation, mastectomy, hysterectomy)
- Loss of body functions (e.g., from stroke, spinal cord injury, neuromuscular disease, arthritis, declining mental or sensory abilities)
- Disfigurement (e.g., through pregnancy, severe burns, facial blemishes, colostomy, tracheostomy)
- Unrealistic body ideal (e.g., a muscular configuration that cannot be achieved)

Self-Esteem Stressors
- Lack of positive feedback from significant others
- Repeated failures
- Unrealistic expectations
- Abusive relationship
- Loss of financial security

Role Stressors
- Loss of parent, spouse, child, or close friend
- Change or loss of job or other significant role
- Divorce
- Illness
- Ambiguous or conflicting role expectations
- Inability to meet role expectations

Assessment Interview
PERSONAL IDENTITY

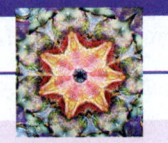

- How would you describe your personal characteristics? *or,* How do you see yourself as a person?
- How do others describe you as a person?
- What do you like about yourself?
- What do you do well?
- What are your personal strengths, talents, and abilities?
- What would you change about yourself if you could?
- Does it bother you a great deal if you think someone doesn't like you?

When stressors are identified, the nurse needs to determine how the client perceives the stressor. A positive, growth-oriented perception of stressful events reinforces self-worth; a negative, hopeless, defeatist perception leads to decreased self-esteem. The nurse should also identify the client's coping style and determine whether this style is effective by asking the client such questions as these:

- When you have a problem or face a stressful situation, how do you usually deal with it?
- Do these methods work?

Personal Identity

When assessing self-concept, the information the nurse first needs is about the client's personal identity. This involves who the client believes he or she is. See the accompanying Assessment Interview for examples of questions to ask.

Body Image

If there are indications of a body image disturbance, the nurse should assess the client carefully for possible functional or physical problems. The disturbance may be a result of a present deformity or malfunction or an anticipated one. In addition to the stated responses about the problem, it is important to assess related behavior. See the accompanying Assessment Interview for examples of questions to ask about body image.

Assessment Interview
BODY IMAGE

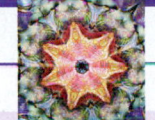

- Is there any part of your body you would like to change?
- Are you comfortable discussing your surgery?
- Do you feel different or inferior to others?
- How do you feel about your appearance?
- What changes in your body do you expect following your surgery?
- How have significant others in your life reacted to changes in your body?

Role Performance

The nurse assesses the client's satisfactions and dissatisfactions associated with role responsibilities and relationships: family roles, work roles, student roles, and social roles. Family roles are especially important to people because family relationships are particularly close. Relationships can be supportive and growth producing or, at the opposite extreme, highly stressful if there is violence or abuse. Assessment of family role relationships may begin with structural aspects such as the number in the family group, ages, and residence location. To obtain data related to the client's family relationships and satisfaction or dissatisfaction with work roles and social roles, the nurse might ask some of the questions shown in the accompanying Assessment Interview, keeping in mind, however, that questions need to be tailored to the individuals and their age and situation.

Self-Esteem

A nurse can ask the following questions to determine a client's self-esteem:

- Are you satisfied with your life?
- How do you feel about yourself?
- Are you accomplishing what you want?
- What goals in life are important to you?

It is important for the nurse to determine the client's cultural background first in order to not misinterpret specific behaviors.

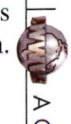

MediaLink | A CHANGE IN ATTITUDE APPLICATION

Assessment Interview
ROLE PERFORMANCE

Family Relationships
- Tell me about your family.
- What is home like?
- How is your relationship with your spouse/partner/significant other (if appropriate)?
- What are your relationships like with your other relatives?
- How are important decisions made in your family?
- What are your responsibilities in the family?
- How well do you feel you accomplish what is expected of you?
- What about your role or responsibilities would you like changed?
- Are you proud of your family members?
- Do you feel your family members are proud of you?

Work Roles and Social Roles
- Do you like your work?
- How do you get along at work?
- What about your work would you like to change if you could?
- How do you spend your free time?
- Are you involved in any community groups?
- Are you most comfortable alone, with one other person, or in a group?
- Who is most important to you?
- Whom do you seek out for help?

The following behaviors might reflect low self-esteem and/or may be misinterpreted due to the client's cultural background:

- Avoids eye contact.
- Stoops in posture and moves slowly.
- Is poorly groomed and has an unkempt appearance.
- Is hesitant or halting in speech.
- Is overly critical of self (e.g., "I'm no good," "I'm ugly," or "People don't like me.").
- May be overly critical of others.
- Is unable to accept positive remarks about self.
- Apologizes frequently.
- Verbalizes feelings of hopelessness, helplessness, and powerlessness, such as "I really don't care what happens," "I'll do whatever anyone wants," "Whatever is destined will happen."

DIAGNOSING

The NANDA nursing diagnostic labels relating specifically to self-concept include the following:

- *Disturbed Body Image*
- *Ineffective Role Performance*
- *Chronic Low Self-Esteem.*

Examples of clinical applications of these diagnoses using NANDA, NIC, and NOC designations are shown in Identifying Nursing Diagnosis, Outcomes, and Interventions.

Additional nursing diagnoses that may apply to clients with problems of self-concept include

- *Disturbed Personal Identity*
- *Anxiety* related to changed physical appearance (e.g., amputation, mastectomy)
- *Impaired Adjustment* to changed physical functioning or appearance
- *Ineffective Coping* with role change related to death of spouse
- *Anticipatory Grieving* or *Dysfunctional Grieving* related to change in physical appearance
- *Hopelessness*
- *Powerlessness*
- *Parental Role Conflict*
- *Rape-Trauma Syndrome*
- *Disturbed Sleep Pattern*
- *Social Isolation*
- *Spiritual Distress*
- *Disturbed Thought Processes.*

PLANNING

The nurse develops plans in collaboration with the client and support people when possible, according to the client's state of health, level of anxiety, resources, coping mechanisms, and sociocultural and religious affiliation. The nurse who has little experience in intervening with clients with altered self-concept

IDENTIFYING NURSING DIAGNOSES, OUTCOMES, AND INTERVENTION
CLIENTS WITH SELF-CONCEPT AND ROLE PROBLEMS

DATA CLUSTER	NURSING DIAGNOSIS/ DEFINITION	SAMPLE DESIRED OUTCOMES [NOC#]/DEFINITION	INDICATORS	SELECTED INTERVENTIONS [NIC#]/DEFINITION	SAMPLE NIC ACTIVITIES
Frank Sawyers had a permanent colostomy 7 days ago for cancer of the sigmoid colon. When the nurse was changing the colostomy appliance, Frank said, "I am really repulsed by this." He avoided looking at the stoma and put his arm over his eyes.	*Disturbed Body Image/Confusion in mental picture of one's physical self*	Body Image [1200]/*Positive perception of own appearance and body functions*	Often positive • Willingness to touch affected body part • Adjustment to changes in body function	Body Image Enhancement [522]/*Improving a patient's conscious and unconscious perceptions and attitudes toward his/her body* Self-Care Assistance [1800]/*Assisting another to perform activities of daily living*	• Assist patient to discuss changes caused by illness/surgery • Assist patient in identifying parts of his body that have positive perceptions associated with them • Facilitate contact with individuals with similar changes in body image • Encourage independence but intervene when patient is unable to perform

continued on page 965

IDENTIFYING NURSING DIAGNOSES, OUTCOMES, AND INTERVENTION

CLIENTS WITH SELF-CONCEPT AND ROLE PROBLEMS continued

DATA CLUSTER	NURSING DIAGNOSIS/ DEFINITION	SAMPLE DESIRED OUTCOMES [NOC#]/DEFINITION	INDICATORS	SELECTED INTERVENTIONS [NIC#]/DEFINITION	SAMPLE NIC ACTIVITIES
Sofie Ferraro, a 73-year-old with right-sided (dominant) hemiplegia, says, "Although the Rehabilitation Center taught me so much about how to manage in my home, my poor husband has to do a lot to help me with cooking meals and cleaning the house."	*Ineffective Role Performance/ Patterns of behavior and self-expression that do not match the environmental context, norms, and expectations*	Caregiver–Patient Relationship [2204]/ *Positive interactions and connections between the caregiver and the care recipient*	Not compromised • Effective communication • Companionship • Collaborative problem solving	Role Enhancement [5370]/*Assisting a patient, significant other, and/or family to improve relationships by clarifying and supplementing specific role relationships*	• Assist patient to identify positive strategies for managing role changes • Facilitate discussion of expectations between patient and significant other in reciprocal role
George Kawazi, a first-year college student, is studying liberal arts and the sciences. George states that even though he attends all his classes and studies every day and on weekends, his grades do not please his father, who expects straight A's. "I've always had trouble measuring up to Father's expectations. He never thought I was as good as my older brother."	*Chronic Low Self-Esteem/ Long-standing negative self-evaluation/feelings about self or self-capabilities*	Self-Esteem [1205]/*Personal judgment of self-worth*	Often positive • Acceptance of self-limitations • Willingness to confront others • Description of success in school	Self-Esteem Enhancement [5400]/*Assisting a patient to increase his/her personal judgment of self-worth*	• Determine patient's confidence in own judgment • Reinforce strengths the patient identifies • Assist in setting realistic goals • Explore previous experiences of success

may wish to consult with a more experienced nurse to develop effective plans. The nurse and client set goals to enhance the client's self-concept.

The goals established will vary according to the diagnoses and defining characteristics related to each individual. Examples of desired outcomes, interventions, and activities are shown in Identifying Nursing Diagnosis, Outcomes, and Interventions. Specific nursing orders associated with each of these activities can be selected to meet the individual needs of the client.

A critical pathway may also be used as a plan of care. See the Critical Pathway for an example of a plan of care for a client undergoing a total mastectomy.

IMPLEMENTING

Nursing interventions to promote a positive self-concept include helping a client to identify areas of strength. In addition, for clients who have an altered self-concept, nurses should establish a therapeutic relationship and assist clients to evaluate themselves and make behavioral changes.

CRITICAL PATHWAY FOR CLIENT FOLLOWING TOTAL MASTECTOMY

	Date _____ First 24 hours postoperative	Date _____ 48 hours postoperative	Date _____ 3 days postoperative
Daily Outcomes	Client will • Be afebrile. • Have clean, dry dressing. • Recover from anesthesia as evidenced by vital signs returning to baseline; being awake, alert, and oriented. • Verbalize understanding and demonstrate cooperation with turning, coughing, deep breathing, and splinting. • Tolerate ordered diet without nausea and vomiting. • Verbalize control of incisional pain. • Verbalize ability to cope.	Client will • Be afebrile. • Have clean, dry wound with edges well approximated, healing by first intention. • Demonstrate cooperation with turning, coughing, deep breathing, and splinting. • Tolerate ordered diet without nausea and vomiting. • Ambulate 4 times per day in hallway. • Verbalize control of incisional pain. • Verbalize beginning ability to cope with changes in body image. • Verbalize ability to cope. • Verbalize beginning understanding of home care instructions.	Client will • Be afebrile. • Have clean, dry wound with edges well approximated, healing by first intention. • Manage pain with oral medications and/or nonpharmacologic measures. • Be independent in self-care. • Be fully ambulatory. • Have resumed preadmission urine and bowel elimination pattern. • Verbalize home care instructions. • Tolerate usual diet. • Verbalize ability to cope with changes in body image and ongoing stressors. • Demonstrate progressive upper extremity exercises that include external rotation and abduction of the affected shoulder when the stitches are removed 7 to 10 days after surgery.
Tests and Treatments	Vital signs and O₂ saturation, neurovascular assessment, dressing and wound drainage assessment q15min × 4; q30min × 4; q1h × 4 and then q4h if stable. NO BLOOD PRESSURES OR VENIPUNCTURE ON AFFECTED ARM. Assess respiratory status q4h and prn. Incentive spirometer q2h. Intake and output q shift. Assess voiding—if unable to void, try suggestive voiding techniques or catheterize q8h or prn.	Vital signs and dressing and wound drainage assessment q4h. NO BLOOD PRESSURES OR VENIPUNCTURE ON AFFECTED ARM. Assess respiratory status q4h. Incentive spirometer q2h until fully ambulatory. Intake and output q shift.	Vital signs and dressing and wound drainage assessment q4h–8h. NO BLOOD PRESSURES OR VENIPUNCTURE ON AFFECTED ARM. Assess respiratory status q4h–8h. Assess wound and apply dry sterile dressing q day and prn.
Knowledge	Orient to room and surroundings. Provide simple, brief instructions. Review preoperative preparation, including hospital and specific postoperative care: turning, coughing, deep breathing, incentive spirometer, mobilization, intravenous infusions, pain management.	Review plan of care and importance of early mobilization. Begin discharge teaching regarding wound care/dressing change, diet, and activity. Review written discharge instructions with client and support person.	Complete discharge teaching to include wound care, diet, follow-up care, signs and symptoms to report, activity, and medication (frequency, dose, route, and side effects). Provide client with written discharge instructions including upper arm and shoulder exercises for affected arm.

continued on page 967

CRITICAL PATHWAY FOR CLIENT FOLLOWING TOTAL MASTECTOMY continued

	Date _____ First 24 hours postoperative	Date _____ 48 hours postoperative	Date _____ 3 days postoperative
Activity	Provide safety precautions. Ambulate 4 times in room. Encourage finger, wrist, and elbow movement and use of affected arm for ADLs and personal hygiene.	Fully ambulatory in room. Walk in hall 4 to 6 times per day. Encourage finger, wrist, and elbow movement and use of affected arm for ADLs and personal hygiene. Instruct client in progressive upper arm exercises.	Fully ambulatory. Encourage finger, wrist, and elbow movement and use of affected arm for ADLs and personal hygiene. Reinforce instructions regarding progressive exercises.
Medications	IV/PCA analgesics. IV antibiotics. IV fluids.	PO or IV/PCA analgesics. IV antibiotics. Intermittent IV device.	PO analgesics. Discontinue IV device.
Body Image	Establish a trusting relationship with client. Encourage client and significant others to verbalize their feelings about the mastectomy. Listen to client and significant others and show interest. Allow the client to respond to loss of body part and changed body image with grieving behaviors. Support the client's strengths and assist her to look at herself in totality.	Maintain trusting relationship with client. Encourage client and significant others to verbalize their feelings about the mastectomy. Listen to client and significant others and show interest and concern. Allow the client to respond to loss of body part and changed body image with grieving behaviors. Support the client's strengths and assist her to look at herself in totality.	Provide opportunities to verbalize ongoing concerns regarding changes in body image and self-concept. Encourage and provide opportunities for self-care of wound and dressing. Provide opportunity for client to meet with volunteer from Reach to Recovery. Assist client to obtain temporary breast prosthesis. Answer questions and provide information on breast reconstruction.
Psychosocial	Assess coping status. Use active listening. Provide a nonthreatening environment. Determine support people and resources available to the client. Assess responses of support people. Allow for client's input regarding sequence of care. Be supportive of client's effective coping behaviors.	Assess coping status. Use active listening. Provide a nonthreatening environment. Determine support people and resources available to the client. Assess responses of support people. Allow for client's input regarding sequence of care. Be supportive of client's effective coping behaviors.	Assess coping status. Use active listening. Provide a nonthreatening environment. Determine support people and resources available to the client. Assess responses of support people. Allow for client's input regarding sequence of care. Be supportive of client's effective coping behaviors.
Transfer/ Discharge Plans	Determine discharge needs with client and support people. Begin home care instructions.	Review progress toward discharge goals. Finalize discharge plans.	Complete discharge instructions.

BOX 37–2 ■ Framework for Identifying Personality Strengths

Note past, present, and anticipated future participation in

- Hobbies and crafts
- Expressive arts such as writing, painting, sketching, or music appreciation
- Sports and outdoor activities, including spectator sports
- Education, training, and related areas (including self-education)
- Work, vocation, job, or position.

In addition, determine

- Sense of humor and the ability to laugh at oneself and take kidding
- Health status including healthy aspects of body function and good health maintenance practices

- Special aptitudes such as sales or mechanical ability; a "green thumb"; ability to recognize and enjoy beauty; ability to solve problems; a liking for adventure or pioneering; having perseverance and the drive needed to get things done
- Relationship strengths including the ability to make people feel comfortable, the capacity to enjoy being with people, being aware of people's needs and feelings, being able to listen
- Emotional strengths including the capacity to give and receive warmth, affection, and love; the ability to "take" anger and to feel and express a wide range of emotions; the capacity for empathy
- Spiritual strengths such as religious faith or love of God, membership and participation in church and related activities.

Identifying Areas of Strength

Healthy people often perceive their problems and weaknesses more easily than their assets and strengths. People with low self-esteem tend to focus even more on their limitations and to be aware of fewer strengths and many more problems. When a client has difficulty identifying personality strengths and assets, the nurse provides the client with a set of guidelines or a framework for identifying personality strengths (Box 37–2).

Nurses can employ the following specific strategies to reinforce strengths:

- Stress positive thinking rather than self-negation.
- Notice and verbally reinforce client strengths.
- Encourage the setting of attainable goals.
- Acknowledge goals that have been attained.
- Provide honest, positive feedback.

Enhancing Self-Esteem

Nurses assisting clients who have an altered self-concept must establish a therapeutic relationship. To do this the nurse must have self-awareness and effective communication skills. The following nursing techniques may help clients analyze the problem and enhance the self-concept:

- Encourage clients to appraise the situation and express their feelings.
- Encourage clients to ask questions.
- Provide accurate information.
- Become aware of distortions, inappropriate or unrealistic standards, and faulty labels in clients' speech.
- Explore clients' positive qualities and strengths.
- Encourage clients to express positive self-evaluation more than negative self-evaluation.
- Avoid criticism.
- Teach clients to substitute negative self-talk ("I can't walk to the store anymore") with positive self-talk ("I can walk half a block each morning"). Negative self-talk reinforces a negative self-concept.

Certain strategies vary depending on the age of the client (see Lifespan Considerations).

Lifespan Considerations

Enhancing Self-Esteem
Children

- Children build strong self-esteem if they develop five basic attitudes: (a) security and trust, (b) identity, (c) belonging, (d) purpose, and (e) personal competence.
- Key ingredients for helping children develop high self-esteem are love, acceptance, firmness, consistency, and the establishment of expectations. Love and acceptance indicate to the child that parents, teachers, and caregivers care and want the best for the child. Adults can demonstrate love and acceptance by taking time to be with the child, to listen, to read, to play, or just to be there. Physical contact—such as a hug—usually conveys warmth and caring.
- Firmness and consistency provide the rules and the consequences for breaking them. Such limits provide a safe and predictable world in which to live. Establishing high but reasonable expectations for the child indicates confidence in the child's abil-

ities. As the child succeeds in meeting those expectations, self-confidence increases. Rules or standards need to be reasonable and broad enough to serve as general guidelines in new situations, such as in a neighbor's house, a friend's yard, or school classroom. Standards needs to be established for the treatment of others, respect for the property of others, the value of honesty, and routines such as getting ready for school in the morning, doing homework, completing chores, and going to bed at night.
- Children need positive feedback from the people of greatest significance to them: parents, grandparents, older siblings, teachers, and close friends. The kind of feedback given can be more significant than the child's actual level of performance. Positive feedback enhances a child's sense of identity and self-concept.
- A sense of purpose provides direction for children and a basis for success, fulfillment, and, therefore, a positive self-concept. Adults can help a child develop a sense of purpose by setting reasonable expectations, by helping the child set realistic

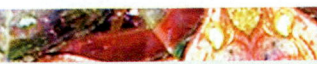

goals, by conveying faith and confidence in the child's ability to achieve the goals, and by helping the child expand interests, talents, and abilities.

- Individuals who grow up in families whose members value each other are likely to feel good about themselves. If adults help children to accomplish goals that are important to them, children are more likely to develop a sense of personal competence and independence.

Adolescents

- Provide increasing levels of responsibility. Adolescents need to experience successes and failures and the consequences of their own behavior.
- Encourage discussion about issues including problems and mistakes.
- Show appreciation for effort and contributions. Emphasize the process, not just the result.
- Ask for their opinions and suggestions.
- Encourage participation in decision making in areas that affect the adolescent. Show confidence in the teen's judgments.
- Avoid comparison with or ridicule or punishment in front of others.
- Assist in the creation of realistic goals and standards.

Adults

- Explore the meaning of self-esteem and how his or her self-esteem has influenced past behaviors and actions (and can influence present and future plans and decisions).
- Assist the client in assessing the internal and external forces contributing to or retarding his or her self-esteem.
- Act in ways that demonstrate belief that the person can cope with the realities and demands of life and is worthy of experiencing joy and happiness.
- Avoid comparisons with other people.
- Discourage statements about the self that are negative.
- Encourage the use of affirmations to enhance your self-esteem: statements such as "I like myself" or "I am a valuable person."
- Encourage associations with positive, supportive people.
- Make positive statements about the person's past successes (major or minor).
- Assist the person to make a list of his or her positive qualities and to review this list often.
- Suggest the person do things for others, making a positive contribution because this enhances positive feelings of self-worth.

Elders

Elders who become increasingly dependent can develop low self-esteem. Old age is frequently accompanied by changes such as reduced income, decline in physical health, loss of friends and family, and retirement. In addition to those actions listed above for use with adults, nurses can use the following techniques to help elders enhance their self-esteem:

- Encourage clients to participate in planning their own care.
- Listen carefully to their concerns.
- Assist clients to identify and use their own strengths.
- Encourage them to participate in activities in which they can be successful.
- Communicate that the client is valued. Use the client's name and ask for advice.
- Encourage elders to stay connected with their memories. Reminiscing by writing or recording an autobiography or storytelling are excellent ways to do this.
- For elders who are in hospitals or nursing homes, make sure that they are always shown respect and dignity and are provided privacy.
- Encourage creativity activities to tap their resources. Examples are music, art, storytelling, quilting, and photography.
- Work with clients to establish goals in small steps that are achievable—this, in itself, can bolster self-esteem.

Weaving the Tapestry of Life

The mainstays of the tapestry of life are the powers in one's life—self-esteem, love of life and humanity, and closeness to and recognition of the Godlife in oneself and others.

The weavings that form the patterns in one's life are experiences, knowledge and dreams. Beauty can be seen throughout, but strength of the fabric increases with age as the tapestry displays interweavings and integration of these special qualities.

As time goes on, aging is often accompanied by a fragileness of the physical body and an increased number of inevitable losses—emotional and social, as well as physical. This is when the integration of those special fibers—strengthening qualities—become so crucial to the overall quality of life of the individual.

When these strengths are displayed in the tapestry of life, the individual is not only given a feeling of self-worth and self-love, but the tapestry is a beautiful gift for all who behold it and are somehow touched by it.

Grace Miller

EVALUATING

To determine whether client outcomes have been achieved, the nurse uses data collected during interactions with the client and significant others (see earlier Identifying Nursing Diagnosis, Outcomes, and Interventions). If outcomes are not achieved, the nurse should explore the reasons, considering questions such as the following:

- Have old situations recurred, triggering feelings or behaviors associated with low self-esteem?

- Have new stressful situations occurred with which the client feels unable to cope, resulting in continuing or recurrent low self-esteem?
- Are new or additional roles causing increased stress in adapting?
- Are significant others supporting the client adequately in attempts to improve self-esteem?
- Did the client follow through on referrals to appropriate agencies? Did the agencies provide the expected services?
- Were the client's expectations too high in relation to the time needed for successful resolution of self-esteem problems?

The nurse, client, and significant others need to understand that to change beliefs, feelings, and behaviors affecting self-esteem requires time and ongoing effort. Unlike many physical problems (e.g., wounds) where healing can be quickly observed, improving one's self-concept can be a continuing concern and is not so easily evaluated. New crises can cause clients to doubt themselves and revert to former feelings of inadequacy. People can learn from each new situation and gain new strategies for feeling satisfied with themselves.

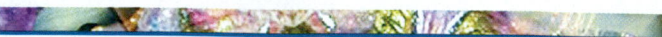

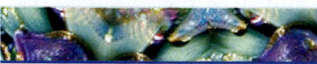

Focus on Critical Thinking

Craig is a 20-year-old male college student who was involved in an automobile accident 3 days ago, suffering a traumatic amputation of his left lower leg. Craig's mother has remained with him since the accident and is very supportive. His father is grief stricken and having difficulty dealing with Craig's condition because Craig was captain of his college basketball team and had aspirations of becoming a professional basketball player. Craig's condition is stable and he is being placed into a rehabilitation program immediately. Soon, he will be fitted for a leg prosthesis. Usually an outgoing individual, Craig is somber and nontalkative. He does not look at his leg when dressings are being changed and he refuses to discuss his rehabilitation program.

1. Given Craig's age, speculate about whether Craig's self-concept is at risk for being adversely affected by his disability.

2. What data suggest that Craig's self-esteem is, or is at risk for being, negatively impacted by his amputation?
3. What factors are likely to affect Craig's adaptation to his amputation and rehabilitation?
4. How would your interventions differ for a client who was 70 years old?
5. What other groups of clients, in addition to those with amputations, are at risk for the development of altered self-esteem or body image?

See Critical Thinking Possibilities in Appendix A.

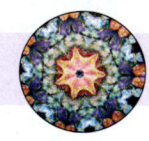 ## Chapter Review

EXPLORE MediaLink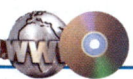

NCLEX review questions, case studies, care plan activities, MediaLink applications, and other interactive resources for this chapter can be found on the Companion Website at www.prenhall.com/kozier. Click on Chapter 37 to select the activities for this chapter.

For more NCLEX review questions and an audio glossary, access the Student CD-ROM accompanying this textbook.

Chapter Highlights

- A positive self-concept is essential to a person's physical and psychologic well-being.
- A person's self-perception can differ from the person's perception of how others see them and from the ideal self, that is, how the person would like to be.
- Interactions with significant others create the conditions that influence self-concept throughout life.
- When individuals are able to conceptualize the self, they begin a lifelong process of deciding whether and to what extent they are valuable and worthy.
- Individuals who grow up in families whose members value each other are likely to feel good about themselves.
- Factors affecting self-concept include development, family and culture, stressors, resources, history of success and failure, and illness.

- The nurse assesses four areas of self-concept: personal identity, body image, self-esteem, and role performance and relationships.
- Because a positive self-concept is basic to health, one of the nurse's major responsibilities is to assist clients whose self-concept is disturbed to develop a more positive and realistic image of themselves.
- A trusting client–nurse relationship is essential for the effective assessment of a client's self-concept, for providing help and support, and for motivating client behavior change.

Review Questions

37–1. In spite of weighing 105 lb, Sally, who is 5′7″ complains of being fat. This may represent a flaw in her
    a. body image.
    b. personal identity.
    c. self-expectation.
    d. core self-concept.

37–2. Students juggling the responsibilities of work, school, and family may be experiencing
    a. role ambiguity.
    b. role strain.
    c. role conflict.
    d. role enhancement.

37–3. An appropriate desired outcome for clients with situational low self-esteem might be
    a. restored self-esteem.
    b. consistently verbalizes self-acceptance.
    c. teaches adaptive skills.
    d. describes preoccupation with altered self.

37–4. An 89-year-old client states "I'm a lost cause. I can't even stand long enough to cook my own meals anymore." An appropriate response from the nurse would be
    a. "That must be difficult. What things are you still able to do?"
    b. "Well, that is to be expected at your age."
    c. "Do you have someone else who can cook for you?"
    d. "Are you a good cook?"

37–5. An adult who has failed to satisfactorily resolve the developmental task of adolescence—identity versus confusion—may show which behavior?
    a. asserts independence
    b. is unable to express personal desires
    c. has difficulty working as a member of a team
    d. goes along with the crowd in all activities

Readings and References

Suggested Readings

Cook, N. F. (1999). Self-concept and cancer: Understanding the nursing role. *British Journal of Nursing, 8,* 318–324.
    It is part of the nurse's role to assist clients with challenges to their self-concept. In cancer, these challenges arise at various points in the disease process, from diagnosis, through treatment, to rehabilitation or death. This article examines adaptation using Roy's Adaptation Model and guides the nurse in using a structured approach to using communication and support strategies.

Related Research

Cowin, L. (2001). Measuring nurses' self-concept. *Western Journal of Nursing Research, 23,* 313–325.
van Baarsen, B. (2002). Theories on coping with loss: The impact of social support and self-esteem on adjustment to emotional and social loneliness following a partner's death in later life. *The Journals of Gerontology, 57B*(1), S33–S42.

References

Eckroth-Bucher, M. (2001). Philosophical basis and practice of self-awareness in psychiatric nursing. *Journal of Psychosocial Nursing & Mental Health Services, 39*(2), 32–39.
Erikson, E. H. (1963). *Childhood and society* (2nd ed.). New York: Norton.
Johnson, M., Maas, M., & Moorhead, S. (Eds.). (2000). *Nursing outcomes classification (NOC)* (2nd ed.). St. Louis, MO: Mosby.
McCloskey, J. C., & Bulechek, G. M. (Eds.). (2000). *Nursing interventions classification (NIC)* (3rd ed.). St. Louis, MO: Mosby.
NANDA International. (2003). *NANDA nursing diagnoses: Definitions and classification 2003-2004.* Philadelphia: Author.
Pinquart, M., & Sorensen, S. (2001). Gender differences in self-concept and psychological well-being in old age: A meta-analysis. *Journals of Gerontology Series B: Psychological Sciences and Social Sciences, 56B*(4), 195–213.

Rowe, J. (1999). Self-awareness: Improving nurse-client interactions. *Nursing Standard, 14*(8), 37–40.

Selected Bibliography

Anderson, J. A. (1999). Adolescent self-esteem: A foundation disposition. *Nursing Science Quarterly, 12,* 62–67.
Castle, D. J., & Phillips, K. A. (Eds.). (2001). *Disorders of body image.* Petersfield, UK: Wrightson Biomedical.
Cox, S. (2002). Emotional competence—the rest of the story. *Nursing Management, 33*(10), 64–66.
Mruk, C. J. (1999). *Self-esteem: Research, theory, and practice* (2nd ed.). New York: Springer.
Norris, J., & Spelic, S. S. (2002). Supporting adaption to body image disruption. *Rehabilitation Nursing, 27*(1), 8–12, 38.
Wilkinson, J. M. (2000). *Nursing diagnosis handbook with NIC interventions and NOC outcomes* (7th ed.). Upper Saddle River, NJ: Prentice Hall Health.

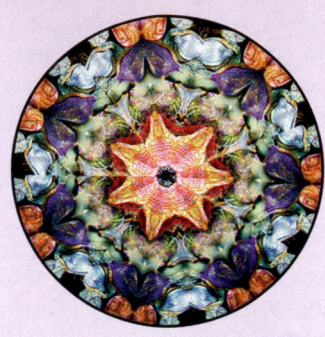

CHAPTER | 38

SEXUALITY

LEARNING OUTCOMES

- After completing this chapter, you will be able to:
- Define sexual health.
- Describe the components of psychologic sexual health.
- Describe sexual development and concerns across the life span.
- Identify factors influencing sexuality.
- Identify common illnesses affecting sexuality.
- Discuss essential aspects of sexual stimulation, intercourse, and the sexual response cycle.
- Describe physiologic changes in males and females during the sexual response cycle.
- Identify the forms of male and female sexual dysfunction.
- Gain the ability to conduct a sexual history.
- Recognize health promotion teaching related to reproductive structures.
- Identify nursing diagnoses and interventions for the client experiencing sexuality problems.

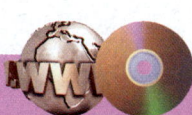

MediaLink

www.prenhall.com/kozier

Additional resources for this chapter can be found on the Student CD-ROM accompanying this textbook, and on the Companion Website at www.prenhall.com/kozier. Click on Chapter 38 to select the activities for this chapter.

CD-ROM
- Audio Glossary
- NCLEX Review
- Animations:
    Female Pelvis 3D
    Male Pelvis 3D
    Spermatogenesis
    Oogenesis and Spermatogenesis Compared
    Oogenesis and Spermatogenesis A & P Review
    Oogenesis and Spermatogenesis Terms and Definitions
    Female Reproductive System A & P Review
    Female Reproductive System Terms & Definitions
    Male Reproductive System A & P Review
    Male Reproductive System Terms & Definitions
    Ovulation A & P Review

Companion Website
- Additional NCLEX Review
- Case Study: Client in an Automobile Accident
- Care Plan Activity: Client with a Mastectomy
- MediaLink Application: Society for Human Sexuality
- Links to Resources

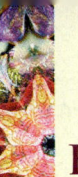

desire phase, 980

dysmenorrhea, 975

erectile dysfunction, 983

excitement/plateau phase, 981

gender, 973

gender identity, 974

hypoactive sexual desire disorder, 983

impotence, 983

menopause, 975

menstruation, 975

orgasmic disorder, 983

orgasmic phase, 982

rapid ejaculation, 983

resolution phase, 982

retarded ejaculation, 983

sex, 973

sexual arousal disorder, 983

sexual health, 973

sexual orientation, 974

sexual pain disorders, 983

sexual self-concept, 974

sexuality, 973

Sexuality is a crucial part of a person's identity. Sex is central to who we are, to our emotional well-being, and to the quality of our lives. All people have the potential to positively experience and pleasurably express their sexuality. One does not have to be in a relationship to be sexual. The idea that you need another person to feel sexual is both disempowering and untrue. Clients do not leave their sexuality behind when they enter the health care system—their sexuality is always a part of them. Professional nurses, as health care providers focusing on the holistic nature of care, have a responsibility to provide effective sexual health care for their clients.

In a holistic approach to client health care, all aspects of being interact. Thus sexuality influences and is influenced by the biologic, psychologic, sociologic, cultural, and spiritual aspects of being. The need to acknowledge and deal with issues of sexuality in health care practice cannot be overlooked.

Sex is the term most commonly used to identify biologic male or female status. The more appropriate and descriptive term, however, is **gender.** The term *sex* is also used to describe sexual behavior in general such as "When is the last time you had sex?" or more specific expressions such as "What are your favorite sex activities?" **Sexuality** includes how you feel about your body, interest in sexual activity, your need for touch, the ability to communicate your sexual needs to a partner, and the ability to engage in satisfying sexual activity. When you create and experience erotic pleasure you are having sex, but you are also experiencing your sexuality (Ellison, 2000).

Sexuality is subject to lifelong dynamic change. Normal developmental alterations and health status may necessitate adaptations in sexual expressions, but individuals continue to express sexuality in a variety of ways throughout their lives.

SEXUAL HEALTH

Like "health," sexual health is difficult to define. For most people sexual health is a phenomenon that is not considered until its absence or an impairment is noticed. The World Health Organization defined **sexual health** in 1975 as "the integration of the somatic, emotional, intellectual, and social aspects of sexual being, in ways that are positively enriching and that enhance personality, communication, and love" (p. 6). This definition recognizes the biologic, psychologic, and sociocultural dimensions of sexuality. Characteristics of sexual health are listed in Box 38–1.

Because sexuality and sexual functioning are aspects of health and well-being, they are a part of nursing care and need to be assessed. When doing so, nurses should make the assessment nonjudgmentally, encouraging clients to discuss their concerns and offer suggestions to assist the return of intimacy and sexual function.

Clients are often hesitant to introduce the topic of sex with their primary health care providers. They may be too embarrassed or they may think that they should not have sexual problems in our liberated times. When health care professionals do not introduce the topic, these individuals are unrecognized and unserved.

BOX 38–1 ■ Characteristics of Sexual Health

- Knowledge about sexuality and sexual behavior
- Ability to express one's full sexual potential, excluding all forms of sexual coercion, exploitation, and abuse
- Ability to make autonomous decisions about one's sexual life within a context of personal and social ethics
- Experience of sexual pleasure as a source of physical, psychologic, cognitive, and spiritual well-being
- Capability to express sexuality through communication, touch, emotional expression, and love
- Right to make free and responsible reproductive choices.
- Ability to access sexual health care for the prevention and treatment of all sexual concerns, problems, and disorders.

Note: From Declaration of Sexual Rights, by the World Association of Sexology, 1999, Adopted at the 14th World Congress of Sexology, Hong Kong and People's Republic of China. Reprinted with permission. See http://www.worldsexology.org

FEMALE PELVIS 3D ANIMATION | MediaLink

> **CLINICAL ALERT** *As a result of culture, age, gender, and personal characteristics, not every nurse will be comfortable discussing sex with every client. However, it is the nurse's responsibility to ensure that someone introduces the topic with the client.* ■

Nurses require six basic skills to help clients in the area of sexuality:

- Self-knowledge and comfort with their own sexuality
- Acceptance of sexuality as an important area for nursing intervention and a willingness to work with clients expressing their sexuality in a variety of ways
- Knowledge of sexual growth and development throughout the life cycle
- Knowledge of basic sexuality, including how certain health problems and treatments may affect sexuality and sexual function and which interventions facilitate sexual expression and functioning
- Therapeutic communication skills
- Ability to recognize the need of the client and family members to have the topic of sexuality introduced not only in written or audiovisual materials but also in a verbal discussion

For purposes of assessing a few of your personal values, complete the statements in Box 38–2.

Components of Sexual Health

Four critical components of sexual health are sexual self-concept, body image, gender identity, and sexual orientation. One's **sexual self-concept** (how one values oneself as a sexual being) determines with whom one will have sex, the gender and kinds of people a person is attracted to, and the values about when, where, with whom, and how one expresses sexuality. A positive sexual self-concept enables people to form intimate relationships throughout life. A negative sexual self-concept may impede the formation of relationships.

Body image, a central part of the sense of self, is constantly changing. Pregnancy, aging, trauma, disease, and therapies can alter an individual's appearance and function, which can affect body image. How a person feels about her or his body is related to one's sexuality. People who feel good about their bodies are likely to be comfortable with and enjoy sexual activity. People who have a poor body image may respond negatively to sexual arousal. A major influence on body image for women is the media focus on physical attractiveness and large breasts.

MALE PELVIS 3D ANIMATION | MediaLink

BOX 38–2	■ **Assessing Personal Sexual Values**

- I believe sexual satisfaction is . . .
- When I think of my parents having sex, I . . .
- If I were to care for a transgendered client I would . . .
- When I think about lesbians, gays, and bisexuals, I . . .
- Masturbation is . . .
- My beliefs about oral sex are . . .

Likewise, many men worry about penis size. The myth that "larger is better," particularly if it is erect and has staying power, is pervasive in North America. A man's body image can suffer when he is unable to achieve an erection.

Gender identity is one's self-image as a female or male. More than just the biologic component, it also includes social and cultural norms. Gender identity is the result of a long series of developmental events that may or may not conform to one's apparent biologic sex. Once gender identity is established, it cannot be easily changed.

Transgender is an umbrella term for people whose gender identity or gender expression differs from their anatomical sex. The term includes the following people:

- *Cross-dressers:* people who routinely wear clothes associated with the other sex. Cross-dressing is a form of gender expression and is not necessarily tied to sexual orientation. Many cross-dressers are heterosexual.
- *Intersexed:* People whose sexual organs are ambiguous at birth. The older term is *hermaphrodite.*
- *Preoperative transsexuals:* people who identify as one gender at all times—a gender that conflicts with their anatomy. Many undergo hormonal treatment and may undergo gender reassignment surgery.
- *Postoperative transsexuals:* people who have had full or partial surgery to change their gender.

Gender-role behavior is the outward expression of a person's sense of maleness or femaleness as well as the expression of what is perceived as gender-appropriate behavior. Each society defines its roles for males and females; boys are given reinforcement for behaving in a "masculine" way, and girls receive reinforcement for exhibiting "feminine" behaviors.

Physical structure, variations in the internal sense of what is male or female, family values, and cultural values all influence gender-role behavior. In North America, expected adult male roles include breadwinner, heterosexual lover, father, and athlete. Expected male behaviors include wearing trousers, demonstrating physical strength, and expressing feelings in a controlled fashion. Women are expected to express their emotions more freely and to be gentler in their physical responses; they also have a broader choice of clothing than men do.

In actuality, however, many people are challenging these stereotypes. Men sport long hair, earrings, and cosmetics. Women wear construction boots, jeans, and men's suits. Men make loving and sensitive single fathers. Women are capably functioning as competitive and assertive executives and world leaders.

One's attraction to people of the same sex, other sex, or both sexes is referred to as **sexual orientation.** Sexual orientation lies along a continuum with a wide range between the two extremes of exclusively heterosexual attraction and exclusively homosexual attraction. Individuals who are attracted to people of both genders are referred to as *bisexuals.*

The origins of sexual orientation are still not well understood. Some biologic theories describe sexual orientation in terms of the genetic composition of the individual. Psychologic theories stress the role of early learning experiences and cognitive processes. Other theories acknowledge the confluence of genetics and the environment in the development of sexual orientation.

Estimates of the percentage of the population with a homosexual orientation vary, although the usual figure is 5% to 10% of men and 2% to 4% of women (Rodgers, 2001). Because these individuals grow up acutely aware of the discrimination they face in North America, many do not disclose their sexual orientation; thus actual figures are not available.

Health care professionals need to develop and convey a nonjudgmental attitude when caring for clients with sexual orientations that differ from their own.

DEVELOPMENT OF SEXUALITY

The development of sexuality begins with conception and continues throughout the life span. Every society develops expectations about acceptable forms of sexual expression. Table 38–1 outlines characteristics of sexual development through the life span, with nursing interventions and teaching guidelines for each developmental stage.

Birth to 12 Years

From birth, infants are assigned the gender of male or female and by 3 years of age begin to develop a gender identity. Preschoolers become increasingly aware of their own and others' body parts. During the school-age years, gender-role behavior is learned.

Adolescence

During early adolescence (12 to 13 years), primary and secondary sex characteristics develop, necessitating information about body changes. For boys, the testes and scrotum increase in size, the skin over the scrotum becomes darker, pubic hair grows, and axillary sweating begins. Development of the genitals to adult size takes about 5 to 6 years. For girls, the pelvis and hips broaden, the breast tissue develops (see "Stages" in Chapter 28), pubic hair grows, axillary sweating begins, vaginal secretions become milky and change from an alkaline to an acid pH.

Girls need to be taught about **menstruation** (monthly uterine bleeding) and related self-care. Teenagers have irregular menstruation initially, which may lead to embarrassment because of stained clothing. They can be taught to be aware of subtle signs of impending menstruation, such as tender breasts, water retention or bloating, or the appearance of skin eruptions or pimples. Girls should also be counseled regarding the variety of feminine hygiene products available (e.g., sanitary pads and tampons) so that they can make intelligent choices. Parents and nurses should advise teenage girls to wash their hands thoroughly before inserting a tampon, to change tampons frequently, to alternate them with sanitary pads, and to use pads at night. These measures will help to decrease infection. Thorough cleaning of the genital area and wiping from front to back will also decrease infection and prevent odors.

Dysmenorrhea (painful menstruation) is prevalent among adolescent females. Cramping, lower abdominal pain radiating to the back and upper thighs, nausea, vomiting, diarrhea, and headaches may occur for a few hours up to 3 days. Dysmenorrhea results from powerful uterine contractions, which cause ischemia and, in turn, cramping pain. The symptoms of dysmenorrhea are treated with bed rest, administration of simple analgesics such as aspirin, application of heat to the abdomen, certain exercises, biofeedback (see Chapter 14), and nonsteroidal anti-inflammatory medications, such as ibuprofen (Motrin or Advil).

All adolescents want to know about sexual behaviors but are often uneasy about discussing these concerns with their parents. Nurses, the schools, and the family need to provide accurate information. During the nursing assessment, teenagers should be asked directly what they know about sex, contraception, and reproduction. Sometimes a lot of the teenager's information is based on popular myths and little, if any, on fact. The nurse should discuss factual information about sex, sexual actions and their consequences, the individual's right to make a decision regarding ways to express oneself sexually, and the responsibilities of each person with respect to sexual activity.

Sexually transmitted diseases (STDs) are the most common bacterial infections among adolescents. Teens need education about these diseases, preventive measures, and early treatment. Table 38–2 lists the common types and symptoms of STDs for which teenagers should seek medical care. The nurse should also inform the teenager about the various methods of birth control: abstinence, pills, diaphragms, intrauterine devices, the rhythm method, and condoms to prevent an unplanned pregnancy. These are discussed later in this chapter.

Young and Middle Adulthood

In young adulthood, many people begin to form intimate relationships with long-term implications. These relationships may take the form of dating, cohabitation, or marriage. Note, however, that some people do not form intimate relationships until late adulthood and that some never form these types of relationships.

Young adult men and women are often concerned about normal sexual response, for both themselves and their partners. In heterosexual relationships, problems may arise because of basic differences in male and female expectations and responses. Gay and lesbian couples often fare better in this respect. Couples need to communicate their needs to one another early in their courtship so that a successful intimate relationship can develop and grow. Young adults should also be aware that because sexual needs and responses may change, each partner should listen and respond to the needs of the other.

During middle adulthood both men and women experience decreased hormone production, causing the climacteric, usually called **menopause** in women. These events often affect the individual's sexual self-concept, body image, and sexual identity.

Women throughout the perimenopausal period experience hot flashes, vasomotor instability, sleep disturbances, vaginal dryness, genital tract atrophy, mood changes, and skin, hair, and nail changes. The incidence of osteoporosis and cardiovascular lipid changes also increases. A tendency to gain weight

MediaLink | SPERMATOGENESIS ANIMATION

TABLE 38-1 Sexual Development throughout Life

Stage	Characteristics	Nursing Interventions and Teaching Guidelines
Infancy Birth to 18 months	Given gender assignment of male or female. Differentiates self from others gradually. External genitals are sensitive to touch. Male infants have penile erections; females, vaginal lubrication.	Self-manipulation of the genitals is normal. Caregivers need to recognize these behaviors as common in children.
Toddler 1–3 years	Continues to develop gender identity. Able to identify own gender.	Body exploration and genital fondling is normal. Use names for body parts. Children from single-parent homes should have contact with adults of both sexes.
Preschooler 4–5 years	Becomes increasingly aware of self. Explores own and playmates' body parts. Learns correct names for body parts. Learns to control feelings and behavior. Focuses love on parent of the other sex.	Answer questions about "where babies come from" honestly and simply. Parental overreaction to exploration of genitals and masturbation can lead to feelings that sex is "bad."
School Age 6–12 years	Has strong identification with parent of same gender. Tends to have friends of the same gender. Has increasing awareness of self. Increased modesty, desire for privacy. Continues self-stimulating behavior. Learns the role and concepts of own gender as part of the total self-concept. At about 8 or 9 years becomes concerned about specific sex behaviors and often approaches parents with explicit concerns about sexuality and reproduction.	Provide parents and children with opportunities to express their concerns and ask questions regarding sex. Answer all questions with factual data and perhaps follow up with appropriate books and other material. Advise parents to discuss basic information about sexual intercourse, menstruation, and reproduction with children at about 10 years of age. Give children reading material and then discuss it with them.
Adolescence 12–18 years	Primary and secondary sex characteristics develop. Menarche usually takes place. Develops relationships with interested partners. Masturbation is common. May participate in sexual activity.	Adolescents require information about body changes. Peer groups have great importance at this time and assist in forming gender roles. Dating helps adolescents prepare for adult roles. Parents influence values and beliefs regarding behavior. Teenagers require information about contraceptive measures and precautions to take in regard to STDs.
Young Adulthood 18–40 years	Sexual activity is common. Establishes own lifestyle and values. Many couples share financial obligations and household tasks.	Young adults often require information about measures to prevent unwanted pregnancies (i.e., abstinence or contraceptive devices). Require information to prevent STDs. Regular communication is required to understand partner's sexual needs and to work through problems and stresses.
Middle Adulthood 40–65 years	Men and women experience decreased hormone production. The menopause occurs in women, usually anywhere between 40 and 55 years. The climacteric occurs gradually in men. Quality rather than the number of sexual experiences becomes important. Individuals establish independent moral and ethical standards.	Women and men may need help adjusting to new roles. People may require counseling to help them reevaluate and direct their energies. Encourage couples to look at the positive aspects of this time of life.

TABLE 38–1 Sexual Development throughout Life (continued)

Stage	Characteristics	Nursing Interventions and Teaching Guidelines
Late Adulthood 65 years and over	Interest in sexual activity often continues. Sexual activity may be less frequent. Women's vaginal secretions diminish, and breasts atrophy. Men produce fewer sperm and need more time to achieve an erection and to ejaculate.	Elders often continue to be sexually active. Couples may require counseling about adapting their affection and sexual needs to physical limitations.

might be a complaint during this time. Up until very recently exogenous hormonal replacement therapy (HRT) was widely used to eliminate the symptoms of menopause. Given evidence for an increased risk for heart disease and breast cancer, many women are choosing not to use HRT and are instead relying on natural products such as soy to manage the uncomfortable symptoms. Like estrogen, testosterone is produced by the ovaries and adrenal glands and declines gradually throughout a woman's life. Research has shown that testosterone improves sexual desire and response in many women (Berman & Berman, 2001).

The climacteric in the male is not as dramatic as in the female; changes are more gradual. Most experts say there is not a true climacteric in the male, but that the decline in male sexual desire is related to the decline in physical strength and aging of all body tissues. Although testosterone levels decline with age, the ability for men to remain fertile may extend into old age.

TABLE 38–2 Clinical Signs of Sexually Transmitted Diseases

Disease	Male	Female
Gonorrhea	Painful urination; urethritis with watery white discharge, which may become purulent.	May be asymptomatic; or vaginal discharge, pain, and urinary frequency may be present.
Syphilis	Chancre, usually on glans penis, which is painless and heals in 4–6 weeks; secondary symptoms—skin eruptions, low-grade fever, inflammation of lymph glands—in 6 weeks to 6 months after chancre heals.	Chancre on cervix or other genital areas, which heals in 4–6 weeks; symptoms same as for male.
Genital warts (condyloma acuminatum)	The infection is caused by the human papilloma virus (HPV). Single lesions or clusters of lesions growing beneath or on the foreskin, at external meatus, or on the glans penis. On dry skin areas, lesions are hard and yellow-gray. On moist areas, lesions are pink or red and soft with a cauliflower-like appearance.	Certain strains of HPV have been linked to cervical cancer. Lesions appear at the bottom part of the vaginal opening, on the perineum, the vaginal lips, inner walls of the vagina, and the cervix.
Chlamydial urethritis	Urinary frequency; watery, mucoid urethral discharge.	Commonly a carrier; vaginal discharge, dysuria, urinary frequency.
Trichomoniasis	Slight itching; moisture on top of penis; slight, early morning urethral discharge. Many males are asymptomatic.	Itching and redness of vulva and skin inside thighs; copious watery, frothy vaginal discharge.
Candidiasis	Itching, irritation, discharge, plaque of cheesy material under foreskin.	Red and excoriated vulva; intense itching of vaginal and vulvar tissues; thick, white, cheesy or curd-like discharge.
Acquired immune deficiency syndrome (AIDS)	Symptoms can appear anytime from several months to several years after acquiring the virus. The person has reduced immunity to other diseases. Symptoms include any of the following for which there is no other explanation: persistent heavy night sweats; extreme fatigue; severe weight loss; enlarged lymph glands in neck, axillae, or groin; persistent diarrhea; skin rashes; blurred vision or chronic headache; harsh, dry cough; thick gray-white coating on tongue or throat.	
Herpes genitalis (herpes simplex of the genitals)	Primary herpes involves the presence of painful sores or large, discrete vesicles that last for weeks; vesicles rupture. Recurrent herpes is itchy rather than painful; it lasts for a few hours to 10 days.	

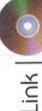

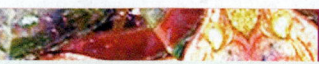

Lifespan Considerations

Elders

It's nice when grown people whisper to each other under the covers. Their ecstasy is more leaf-sigh than bray and the body is the vehicle, not the point. They reach, grown people, for something beyond, way beyond and way, way down underneath tissue. . . . They are inward toward each other.

This quote is from the book *Jazz* by Toni Morrison, 1993 winner of the Nobel Prize in Literature. It is an excellent portrayal of sexuality of most elders. Their sexuality does not change as they get older, but their expression of it does. When they are comfortable with themselves, they can still relate to each other in a meaningful way. Sex-related changes of aging are outlined elsewhere in this chapter, as well as a discussion of other contributing factors for problems related to sexual functioning. Nurses who are sensitive to these changes and challenges to elders can be of great help in developing interventions that can help decrease the problem, and at the same time, help elders maintain their dignity and positive self-worth.

Note: From Jazz *(p. 228), by T. Morrison, 1992, New York: Alfred A. Knopf, Inc. Reprinted with permission from International Creative Management, Inc. Copyright © 1992 by Toni Morrison.*

Older Adulthood

Elders may define sexuality far more broadly and include in their definition such things as touching, hugging, romantic gestures (e.g., giving or receiving roses), comfort, warmth, dressing up, joy, spirituality, and beauty. Interest in sexual activity is not lost as people age. For men, however, more time is needed to achieve an erection and to ejaculate; more direct genital stimulation is required to achieve an erection; the volume of ejaculated fluid decreases; and the intensity of contractions with orgasm may decrease. The refractory period after orgasm is longer.

Older women remain capable of multiple orgasms and may, in fact, experience an increase in sexual desire after menopause; vaginal lubrication and elasticity decrease with menopause and decreased estrogen, and phases of the sexual response cycle may take longer to occur. There is a possibility of pain during sexual activity and intercourse (dyspareunia) related to vaginal dryness or chronic health conditions (e.g., diabetes or arthritis). Lack of privacy may be a concern for older adults who live with family or in a rehabilitation or nursing home facility.

FACTORS INFLUENCING SEXUALITY

Many factors influence a person's sexuality: developmental level (discussed above), culture, religious values, personal ethics, disease processes, and medications.

Culture

Sexuality is regulated by the individual's culture. For example, culture influences the sexual nature of dress, rules about marriage, expectations of role behavior and social responsibilities, and specific sex practices. Societal attitudes vary widely. Attitudes about childhood sexual play with self or children of the same gender or other gender may be restrictive or permissive. Premarital and extramarital coitus and homosexuality may be unacceptable or tolerated. Polygamy (several marriage partners) or monogamy (one marriage partner) may be the norm. Male and female roles also vary. For example, in traditional Iranian culture women are not allowed to work outside the home.

Specific sex practices include puberty rites, body beautification, and female circumcision and genital mutilation. Puberty rites of adolescent males in native African and Australian cultures include circumcision (removal of the foreskin of the penis). Female body beautification carried out in some cultures (e.g., Belgian Congo) to make the body more decorative involves the formation of keloids (scars) at 4 to 5 years of age from above the chest to the groin. Female circumcision or female genital mutilation (FGM), practiced in Africa today, involves either excision of the clitoris, the labia minora, and the labia majora, or closure of the vagina (infibulation). The reasons for sexual mutilation vary. Infibulation may be done to guarantee the bride's virginity. Excision of the clitoris reduces sexual desire and vulnerability to temptation. In 1980, the World Health Organization and the United Nations Children's Fund (UNICEF) unanimously recommended that all forms of female circumcision be abolished. In 1996, the U.S. Congress passed legislation making practicing FGM on girls under 18 a federal criminal offense (Brady, 1998).

Because clients (and colleagues) may differ in their approaches to sexuality, nurses must be aware of and consider cultural factors when approaching sexual issues in health care. See Chapter 13 ∞ for additional information about culture.

Religious Values

Religion influences sexual expression. It provides guidelines for sexual behavior and acceptable circumstances for the behavior, as well as prohibited sexual behavior and the consequences of breaking the sexual rules. The guidelines or rules may be detailed and rigid or broad and flexible. For example, some religions view forms of sexual expression other than male–female intercourse as unnatural and hold virginity before marriage to be the rule.

Many religious values conflict with the more flexible values of society that have developed during the last few decades (often labeled the "sexual revolution"), such as the acceptance of premarital sex, unwed motherhood, homosexuality, and abortion. These conflicts create marked anxiety and potential sexual dysfunctions in some individuals. See Chapter 39 ∞ for additional information about religious values.

MediaLink   OOGENESIS AND SPERMATOGENESIS COMPARED ANIMATION

MediaLink   OOGENESIS AND SPERMATOGENESIS A & P REVIEW ANIMATION

Personal Ethics

Although ethics is integral to religion, ethical thought and ethical approaches to sexuality can be viewed separately from religion. Many individuals and groups have developed written or unwritten codes of conduct based on ethical principles. What one person views as bizarre, perverted, or wrong may be completely natural and right to another. Examples include masturbation, oral or anal intercourse, and cross-dressing. Many people accept sexual expression of various forms if it is performed by consenting adults, is practiced in private, and is not harmful. Couples need to explore and communicate about various types of sexual expression to prevent domination of sexual decision making by one member of the couple.

Health Status

Healthy minds, bodies, and emotions are necessary for sexual well-being. Many health factors can interfere with a person's expression of sexuality. The following are examples of common disorders that may alter sexual expression.

Heart Disease

Heart disease frequently influences sexual expression. Clients experiencing or at risk for myocardial infarction are often anxious about sexual activity. Concerns about the effect of sexual activity on the heart may cause people to restrict or avoid sexual activity. Education by health professionals can alleviate client fears following heart surgery or hospitalization for alterations in heart function. Suggestions as to when to resume activity based on reactions to exercise, avoiding sexual intercourse after large meals or consumption of alcoholic beverages, positions to assume, and signs of distress can provide the couple with information that will help them to make sexual activity decisions (Bedell, Duperval, & Goldberg, 2002).

Prostate Cancer

Millions of American men experience prostate cancer. Gay or straight, men who have prostate cancer can feel victimized twice if the disease or treatment interferes with their earlier sexual abilities. If they lose their erectile ability, they often feel ineffectual and powerless and the impact on intimate relationships can be devastating. Because of anatomic changes in the posterior urethra following surgery, retrograde ejaculation sometimes results; during ejaculation the seminal fluid follows the path of least resistance and goes into the bladder. This affects fertility but does not lessen the sensations of orgasm. Individuals and couples initially respond to the threat of death from prostate cancer and focus on doing everything they can to prevent it. Later they then find themselves dealing with the complex issues of sexuality (Rudberg, Carlsson, Nilsson, & Wikblad, 2002).

Hysterectomy

Hysterectomy, the removal of a woman's uterus, is the second most common pelvic operation in women, after cesarean section. Some women who experienced preoperative pain and bleeding report a general sense of improved health and increased sexual responsiveness. If there is injury to the nerves during the surgery, hysterectomy may have an adverse effect on sexual arousal and orgasm (Berman & Berman, 2001).

Diabetes Mellitus

Many men with long-term diabetes mellitus develop erectile dysfunction related to neurologic changes associated with the disease process. Women who have diabetes may experience orgasmic dysfunction (loss of ability for orgasm), difficulty experiencing arousal, loss of vaginal lubrication, and painful intercourse related to a yeast (*Monilia*) infection of the vagina. The latter commonly occurs with diabetes.

Spinal Cord Injury

Because the level of the injury to the spinal cord determines the effect on sexual functioning, individuals may be capable of erection and ejaculation and be fertile, may have psychogenic or reflexogenic genital arousal, or may have no physiologic genital responses.

Surgical Procedures

Any surgical procedure has the potential to alter a person's body image, especially when the surgery involves mutilating, removing, or altering parts of the body. Examples include amputation of a leg, radical neck surgery, excision of large portions of the lower jaw, and ostomies. The impact is even greater when the surgery alters or removes body parts linked directly with sexual functioning (e.g., mastectomy, hysterectomy, and vaginal excision in women; orchiectomy [removal of the testicles] and penectomy in men). Feelings of ugliness and loss of masculinity or femininity are common after these surgeries.

Many people also have concerns about their reactions to a partner's surgical procedure. Having discussions with both individuals will provide facts in place of potentially erroneous beliefs about surgical procedures altering sexual behaviors.

Joint Disease

Joint disease may indirectly affect sexual function because of pain, stiffness, loss of joint motion, and fatigue. Such symptoms influence sexual motivation as well as sexual positioning and methods.

Chronic Pain

Chronic pain that accompanies many chronic illnesses often decreases sexual motivation. Altered positions for genital sex may be necessary, and alternative ways to achieve sexual stimulation and warmth may need to be emphasized.

Sexually Transmitted Disease

There are numerous STDs, many of which are listed in Table 38–2. The presence of an STD in one partner induces fear of transmission in the other, often resulting in abstinence of sexual contact. In some situations, the presence of an STD is unknown and transmission occurs.

MediaLink OOGENESIS AND SPERMATOGENESIS TERMS & DEFINITION ANIMATION

Mental Disorders

Because the mind and thought processes are involved in sexual functioning, any impairment of the brain may affect sexual expression. In depression, it is relatively common to see decreased interest in sex. In the manic phase of bipolar disorder, people often exhibit increased sexual behavior that is frequently impulsive. In addition, emotional intimacy is problematic when they are argumentative, arrogant, and hostile. Those suffering from schizophrenia may be sexually preoccupied and exhibit socially inappropriate behavior. They may also experience delusions regarding gender identity, sexual orientation, or erotomanic delusions—believing that famous people are in love with them. Individuals who have paranoid characteristics tend to blame any problems on the sexual partner and may be consumed by pathologic jealousy.

Medications

Many prescription medications have side effects that affect sexual functioning. Most frequently, the impact is negative, but sometimes there is a positive impact. Table 38–3 provides an overview of the effects of medications on sexual function. For example, antidepressants may slow ejaculation. This may be a problem for the man who finds himself suddenly feeling unable to ejaculate. If the man is suffering from premature ejaculation, however, the antidepressant may "cure" this problem. Some street drugs such as marijuana, amphetamines, and cocaine enhance sexual functioning. Others, such as opioids and anabolic steroids, interfere with sexual functioning.

SEXUAL RESPONSE AND LOVE PLAY

Sexual response and love play involve people's emotional, psychologic, physical, and spiritual makeup, which plays a significant role in sexual satisfaction. It is within the role of the nurse to support and facilitate healthy sexual expression and accurate knowledge of the sexual response cycle is important to this role.

Sexual Response Cycle

Commonly occurring phases of the human sexual response follow a similar sequence in both females and males regardless of sexual orientation. It does not matter, either, if the motive for being sexually active is true love or passionate lust. Table 38–4 provides a summary of the physiologic changes associated with each of the phases of the cycle.

The response cycle starts in the brain, with conscious sexual desires called the **desire phase.** Sexually arousing stimuli, often called erotic stimuli, may be real or symbolic. Sight, hearing, smell, touch, and imagination (sexual fantasy) can all invoke sexual arousal. Sexual desire fluctuates within each person and varies from person to person. If people suppress or

TABLE 38–3 Effects of Medications on Sexual Function

Medication	Possible Effects*
Alcohol	Moderate amounts: increased sexual functioning; chronic use: decreased sexual desire, orgasmic dysfunction, and impotence
Alpha-blockers	Inability to ejaculate
Amphetamines	Increased sex drive, delayed orgasm
Amyl nitrate	Reported enhanced orgasm; vasodilation, fainting
Anabolic steroids	Decreased sex drive, shrinking of testicles and infertility in men
Antianxiety agents	Decreased sexual desire; orgasmic dysfunction in women; delayed ejaculation
Anticonvulsants	Decreased sexual desire; reduced sexual response
Antidepressants	Decreased sexual desire; orgasmic delay or dysfunction in women; delayed or failed ejaculation; painful erection
Antihistamines	Decreased vaginal lubrication; decreased desire
Antihypertensives	Decreased sexual desire; erectile failure; ejaculation dysfunction
Antipsychotics	Decreased sexual desire; orgasmic dysfunction in women; delayed ejaculation; ejaculatory failure
Barbiturates	In low doses, increased sexual pleasure; in large doses, decreased sexual desire, orgasmic dysfunction, and impotence
Beta-blockers	Decreased sexual desire
Cardiotonics	Decreased sexual desire
Cocaine	Increased intensity of sexual experience; with chronic use, decreased sexual desire and sexual dysfunction
Diuretics	Decreased vaginal lubrication; decreased sexual desire; erectile dysfunction
Marijuana	As above for cocaine, but prolonged use reduces testosterone levels and reduces sperm production
Narcotics	Inhibited sexual desire and response; erectile and ejaculatory dysfunctions

*Nurses and clients must familiarize themselves with the specific medication prescribed or used, because effects vary in each category of drug.

block out conscious sexual desires, they may not experience any physiologic response. Although psychologic causes are the more common cause of a lack of sexual desire, medications, drugs, and hormone imbalances can also block sexual desire.

The **excitement/plateau phase** involves two primary physiologic changes (see Figure 38-1 ■). *Vasocongestion* is an increase in the blood flow to various body parts resulting in erection of the penis and clitoris and swelling of the labia, testes, and breasts. Vasocongestion stimulates sensory receptors within these body parts that in turn transmit messages to the conscious brain where they are usually interpreted as pleasurable sensations. When stimulation is continued, vasocongestion increases

TABLE 38-4 Physiologic Changes Associated with the Sexual Response Cycle

Phase of the Sexual Response Cycle	Signs Present in Both Sexes	Signs Present in Males Only	Signs Present in Females Only
Excitement/Plateau	Muscle tension increases as excitement increases. Sex flush, usually on chest. Nipple erection.	Penile erection; glans size increases as excitement increases. Appearance of a few drops of lubricant, which may contain sperm.	Erection of the clitoris. Vaginal lubrication. Labia may increase 2 to 3 times in size. Breasts enlarge. Inner two-thirds of vagina widens and lengthens; outer third swells and narrows. Uterus elevates.
Orgasmic	Respirations may increase to 40 breaths per minute. Involuntary spasms of muscle groups throughout the body. Diminished sensory awareness. Involuntary contractions of the anal sphincter. Peak heart rate (110–180 BPM), respiratory rate (40/min or greater), and blood pressure (systolic 30–80 mm Hg and diastolic 20–50 mm Hg above normal).	Rhythmic, expulsive contractions of the penis at 0.8-sec intervals. Emission of seminal fluid into the prostatic urethra from contraction of the vas deferens and accessory organs (stage 1 of the expulsive process). Closing of the internal bladder sphincter just before ejaculation to prevent retrograde ejaculation into bladder. Orgasm may occur without ejaculation. Ejaculation of semen through the penile urethra and expulsion from the urethral meatus. The force of ejaculation varies from man to man and at different times but diminishes after the first two to three contractions (stage 2 of the expulsive process).	Approximately 5–12 contractions in the orgasmic platform at 0.8-sec intervals. Contraction of the muscles of the pelvic floor and the uterine muscles. Varied pattern of orgasms, including minor surges and contractions, multiple orgasms, or a simple intense orgasm similar to that of the male.
Resolution	Reversal of vasocongestion in 10–30 min; disappearance of all signs of myotonia within 5 min. Genitals and breasts return to their preexcitement states. Sex flush disappears in reverse order of appearance. Heart rate, respiratory rate, and blood pressure return to normal. Other reactions include sleepiness, relaxation, and emotional outbursts such as crying or laughing.	A refractory period during which the body will not respond to sexual stimulation; varies, depending on age and other factors, from a few moments to hours or days.	

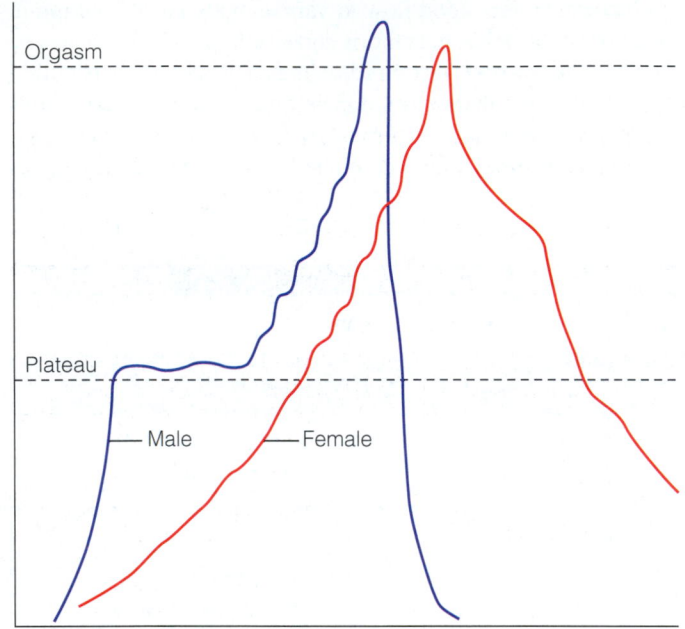

Figure 38–1 ■ Phases of the sexual response cycle.

until it either is released by orgasm or fades away. Likewise, *myotonia,* an increase of tension in muscles, may increase until released by orgasm, or it may also simply fade away.

The **orgasmic phase** is the involuntary climax of sexual tension, accompanied by physiologic and psychologic release. This phase is considered the measurable peak of the sexual experience. Although the entire body is involved, the major focus of the orgasm is felt in the pelvic region. Male orgasms usually last 10 to 30 seconds while female orgasms last 10 to 50 seconds. Men usually have an *ejaculation* and expel semen as part of their orgasm. Before puberty and in later years, males experience orgasms without ejaculation.

The **resolution phase,** the period of return to the unaroused state, may last 10 to 15 minutes after orgasm, or longer if there is no orgasm. This phase in females is quite varied as some women experience multiple successive orgasms followed by a longer period of resolution.

Love Play

Mention love play and many people think of sexual intercourse—of two people caught up in hot passion. Much of our sexual activity, however, does not fit this description.

Over a lifetime, sexual fantasies and solo sex are the most common sexual outlets for women and men, single and coupled persons, and heterosexual, gay/lesbian, and bisexual persons. *Masturbation* is the ongoing love affair that each of us has with ourselves throughout our lifetime. It is the way we discover our erotic feelings and learn about our sexual response. Mutual masturbation can provide sexual pleasuring and intimacy without hurrying to genital interaction before both partners are ready. Masturbation shared with a partner is a safe alternative to unprotected genital sex (Dodson, 2002).

Male-to-female or female-to-female oral–genital sex is known technically as *cunnilingus.* This involves kissing, licking, or sucking of the female genitals including the mons pubis, vulva, clitoris, labia, and vagina. *Fellatio* is oral stimulation of the penis by licking and sucking. *Sixty-nine* is simultaneous oral–genital stimulation by two persons. Preconceptions and myths are a major deterrent for those who have not tried oral sex.

Anal stimulation can be a source of sexual pleasure because the anus has a rich nerve supply. Stimulation may be applied with fingers, mouth, or sex toys such as vibrators. The anus is surrounded by strong muscles and the rectum contains no natural lubrication. Thus inserting a finger or penis in the rectum requires relaxation and water-soluble lubricant.

For older individuals, physical factors such as energy levels, pain, and immobility may have an effect. Libido generally diminishes with general ill health, chronic diseases that cause disability or pain, and depression. Many prescription medications can also diminish sexual desire (see Table 38–3).

A common form of sexual activity for heterosexual couples is *genital intercourse.* Penile–vaginal intercourse can be both physically and emotionally satisfying. There are varieties of positions for this kind of intercourse; the most common is lying face to face (with female or male on top). Side-lying, standing, sitting, and rear-entry positions are also used. Side-lying, female-on-top, and rear-entry positions facilitate clitoral stimulation, either by penile or manual contact. The choice of intercourse positions and activities depends on physical comfort and beliefs, values, and attitudes about different practices.

During intercourse, the man moves the penis back and forth along the vaginal walls by rhythmic thrusting movements of his hips. At the same time the woman may move her own body to match the partner's hip movements. Movements continue until orgasm is achieved by one or both partners. Simultaneous orgasm is difficult to achieve. After coitus, caressing, hugging, and kissing can increase the shared intimacy and should be encouraged.

The other form of genital intercourse is *anal intercourse,* during which the penis is inserted into the anus and rectum of the partner. Anal intercourse is most commonly practiced by gay men, but a number of heterosexual couples engage in it as well. Positions for anal intercourse are similar to those for penile–vaginal intercourse, with minor differences due to the position of the anus.

Current practice dictates the use of a condom in both forms of intercourse to prevent the transmission of disease. Because anorectal tissue is not self-lubricating, a lubricant must be used on the condom. Also, since normal bacterial flora from the bowel can produce infection in other parts of the body, the used condom should be removed and another applied before inserting the penis into other body orifices.

ALTERED SEXUAL FUNCTION

The ability to engage in sexual behavior is of great importance to most people. Many people experience transient problems with their ability to respond to sexual stimulation or to maintain the response. A smaller percentage of people experience long-standing problems.

Male Dysfunction

Three male dysfunctions are erectile dysfunction, rapid ejaculation, and retarded ejaculation. **Erectile dysfunction,** also commonly referred to as **impotence,** is the inability to achieve or maintain an erection sufficient for sexual satisfaction for oneself or one's partner. Erectile dysfunction can be caused by physiologic or psychologic factors. Physiologic factors include (a) neurologic disorders created by spinal cord injuries, injury to the genitals or perineal nerves, extensive surgery such as abdominal-perineal bowel resections, radical perineal prostatectomy, diabetes mellitus, multiple sclerosis, and Parkinson's disease; and (b) prolonged use of drugs, such as alcohol, sedatives, heroin, antidepressants, antipsychotics (phenothiazines), and antihypertensives.

Psychologic factors are often signaled by a sudden rather than a gradual onset. They may include the following: (a) doubts about one's ability to perform or about one's masculinity; (b) fatigue, anger, or stress; (c) traumatic sexual experiences (e.g., rejection); and (d) boredom associated with the specific partner (Rosen, 2000).

Rapid ejaculation occurs when a man is unable to delay ejaculation long enough to satisfy his partner. This usually means that ejaculation occurs after only very limited stimulation of the penis. Often the ejaculation occurs either during penetration (of the vagina, mouth, or anus) or immediately following. The condition may develop when the need for rapid orgasm or performance demands continue over time.

Retarded ejaculation is either the inability to ejaculate into the vagina or a delayed ejaculation. Often, the male has difficulty reaching any kind of orgasm with a partner. Like erectile dysfunction, retarded ejaculation may have physical or psychologic origins.

Female Dysfunction

Four female dysfunctions are hypoactive sexual desire disorder, sexual arousal disorder, orgasmic disorder, and sexual pain disorders. **Hypoactive sexual desire disorder** involves a persistent or recurring absence of sexual thoughts or disinterest in sexual activity. Sexual desire may be changed by various conditions and circumstances. Pregnancy can affect sexual desire if it is associated with physical discomfort, fear of injury to the fetus, or perceived loss of attractiveness. Postpartum hormonal changes, fatigue, and anxiety of new parenthood may contribute to decreased sexual desire. Nursing mothers produce unusually high levels of prolactin, which severely reduces sex drive. Other factors that may influence sexual desire include medications, depression, and menopause (Berman & Berman, 2001).

Sexual arousal disorder is diagnosed when a woman is unable to attain or maintain adequate vaginal lubrication and/or has decreased clitoral and labial sensations. Factors include a decreased vaginal or clitoral blood flow, damage to the genital nerves, or a clinical depression.

Orgasmic disorder is defined as a difficulty or inability to achieve orgasm in spite of stimulation and arousal. If it has always been a problem for a woman, it is referred to as *primary orgasmic disorder.* If it is secondary to surgery, trauma, or lack of hormones, it is referred to as *secondary orgasmic disorder* (Berman & Berman, 2001).

Sexual pain disorders include dyspareunia, vaginismus, and genital pain. *Dyspareunia* describes pain experienced by a woman during intercourse because of inadequate lubrication, scarring, vaginal infection, or hormonal imbalance. *Vaginismus* is diagnosed when involuntary muscle spasms of the lower third of the vagina make insertion of the penis very painful or impossible. It is most frequently a conditioned response. *Genital pain* is diagnosed when the woman experiences pain with any type of sexual stimulation other than intercourse. Causes include vaginal infections, prior genital mutilation, or vestibulitis, an inflammation around the opening of the vagina (Berman & Berman, 2001).

Effects of Medications on Sexual Function

Many prescription medications and social drugs can affect sexual desire and response. These include central nervous system depressants such as narcotics; antianxiety agents such as barbiturates and benzodiazepines; anticholinergic agents such as atropine; cardiovascular agents such as antiarrhythmics, antihypertensives, diuretics, and beta-blocking agents; antidepressants and antipsychotics; and social drugs such as alcohol and marijuana. Clients should be educated about possible alterations in sexual functions. Table 38–3 outlines possible effects of various medications on sexual function.

NURSING MANAGEMENT

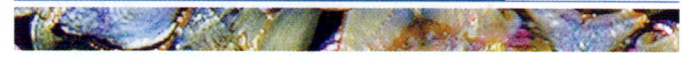

ASSESSING

Information about a client's sexual health status should always be an integral part of a nursing assessment. The amount and kind of data collected depend on the context of the assessment, that is, the client's reason for seeking health care and how the client's sexuality interacts with other problems. The nurse's professional preparation also influences the level of sexual health assessment.

Generally, the nurse conducts a sexual history on the following categories of clients:

- Those receiving care for pregnancy, infertility, contraception, or an STD
- Those whose illness or therapy will affect sexual functioning (e.g., clients with diabetes, gynecologic problem, heart disease)
- Those currently experiencing a sexual problem.

Nursing History

Including a sexual history as part of the general nursing history is important for some clients and not important for other clients. It is critical, however, at least to introduce the topic of sexuality to give permission for clients to bring up any concerns or problems. All nursing histories should at least include

MediaLink | FEMALE REPRODUCTIVE SYSTEM TERMS & DEFINITIONS ANIMATION a question such as "Have there been any changes in your sexual functioning that might be related to your illness or the medications you take?" Nurses might also facilitate communication by saying, "As a nurse, I'm concerned about all aspects of your health. People often have questions about sexual matters, both when they are well and when they are ill. When I take your history, sexual concerns are included to help plan a comprehensive treatment approach."

It is critical that nurses not make assumptions about clients because assumptions interfere with accurate history taking. If you assume that all people do all things, you will be more open to clients than if you make assumptions about who is and who is not sexually active, how many partners they have, or if they do or do not masturbate. Imposing personal values on others is detrimental to the nurse–client relationship.

The accompanying Assessment Interview: Sexual Health History, provides questions that nurses may ask as part of the health history. These questions typically occur later in the assessment process after a rapport has been established.

Physical Examination

Physical examination of the female genitals and reproductive tract and the male genitals is part of a routine physical examination in some agencies. Check agency protocol. See Chapter 28 for details of the examination. If the client has not been examined within 1 year or if data from the recent nursing history indicate a need, the nurse performs a physical examination. Nursing history data indicating the need for a physical examination include the following:

- Suspicion of infertility, pregnancy, or an STD
- Reports of discharge, presence of a lump, or change in color, size, and shape of a genital organ
- Changes in urinary function
- Need for Papanicolaou test
- Request for birth control.

Assessment Interview

SEXUAL HEALTH HISTORY

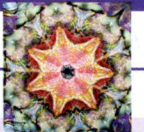

- Are you currently sexually active? With men, women, or both?
- With one or more than one partner?
- Describe the positive and negative aspects of your sexual functioning.
- Do you have difficulty with sexual desire? Arousal? Orgasm? Satisfaction?
- Do you experience any pain with sexual interaction?
- If there are problems, how have they influenced how you feel about yourself? How have they affected your partner? How have they affected the relationship?
- Do you expect your sexual functioning to be altered because of your illness?
- What are your partner's concerns about your future sexual functioning?
- Do you have any other sexual questions or concerns that I have not addressed?

Identifying Clients at Risk

Clients at risk for altered sexual patterns include those experiencing

- Altered body structure or function due to trauma, pregnancy, recent childbirth, anatomic abnormalities of the genitals, or disease (see "Health Status" section earlier in this chapter for common diseases affecting sexuality)
- Physical, psychosocial, emotional, or sexual abuse; sexual assault
- Disfiguring conditions, such as burns, skin conditions, birthmarks, scars (e.g., mastectomy), and ostomies
- Specific medication therapy that causes sexual problems (see Table 38–3)
- Temporary or long-term impaired physical ability to perform grooming and maintain sexual attractiveness
- Value conflicts between personal beliefs and religious doctrine
- Loss of a partner
- Lack of knowledge or misinformation about sexual functioning and expression.

DIAGNOSING

The NANDA nursing diagnoses relating specifically to sexuality include the following:

- *Ineffective Sexuality Pattern*
- *Sexual Dysfunction.*

Examples of clinical applications of these diagnoses using NANDA, NIC and NOC designations are shown in Identifying Nursing Diagnoses, Outcomes, and Interventions.

Sexual problems can also be the etiology of other diagnoses, including the following:

- *Deficient Knowledge* (e.g., about conception, STDs, contraception, or normal sexual changes over the life span) related to misinformation and sexual myths
- *Pain* related to inadequate vaginal lubrication or effects of genital surgery
- *Anxiety* related to loss of sexual desire or functioning
- *Fear* related to history of sexual abuse or dyspareunia
- *Disturbed Body Image* (e.g., mastectomy) related to perceived sexual rejection by spouse.

PLANNING

Overall goals to meet clients' sexual needs include the following:

- Maintain, restore, or improve sexual health.
- Increase knowledge of sexuality and sexual health.
- Prevent the occurrence or spread of STDs.
- Prevent unwanted pregnancy.
- Increase satisfaction with the level of sexual functioning.
- Improve sexual self-concept.

Examples of specific desired outcomes related to some of these goals are provided in Identifying Nursing Diagnoses, Outcomes, and Interventions. Nursing interventions to promote sexual health and function focus largely on the nurse's teaching role. For example, clients need to be taught about normal sexual function, the effects of medications on sexual

IDENTIFYING NURSING DIAGNOSES, OUTCOMES, AND INTERVENTIONS

CLIENTS WITH SEXUALITY PROBLEMS

DATA CLUSTER	NURSING DIAGNOSIS/ DEFINITION	SAMPLE DESIRED OUTCOMES [NOC#]/DEFINITION	INDICATORS	SELECTED INTERVENTIONS [NIC#]/DEFINITION	SAMPLE NIC ACTIVITIES
Marsha Ogilvy, 55 years old, reports vaginal burning and pain whenever she and her husband make love. Her last menses was 14 months ago. She says her husband is concerned about the lack of her usual response to love-making.	*Sexual Dysfunction/Change in sexual function that is viewed as unsatisfying, unrewarding, inadequate*	Physical Aging Status [0113]/*Physical changes that commonly occur with aging*	No deviation from expected range • Sexual functioning	Health Education [5510]/*Developing and providing instruction and learning experiences to facilitate voluntary adaptation of behavior conducive to health in individuals, families, groups, or communities*	• Determine current health knowledge and lifestyle behaviors of individual and family • Incorporate strategies to enhance the client's self-esteem • Teach strategies that can be used to minimize client's discomfort
Larry Stogryn, 52 years old, has a history of hypertension for which he has been taking an anti-hypertensive (reserpine [Serpasil]). He says he has lost interest in sex in the past few months, and when he does have sex, he has trouble keeping an erection.	*Ineffective Sexuality Patterns/Expressions of concern regarding his or her sexuality*	Sexual Functioning [0119]/*Integration of physical, socioemotional, and intellectual aspects of sexual expression*	Often demonstrated • Sustained penile erection • Performs sexually with assistive device as needed • Adapts sexual technique as needed	Sexual Counseling [5248]/*Use of an interactive helping process focusing on the need to make adjustments in sexual practice or enhance coping with a sexual event/disorder*	• Discuss the effect of medication on sexuality • Discuss any alternative forms of sexual expression that might be acceptable to the client • Provide referral to other members of the health care team as appropriate (e.g., primary care provider to explore alternative blood pressure medications or use of medications used for erectile dysfunction such as sildenafil citrate (Viagra); urologist for consideration of prosthesis, penile injections, and other interventions

function, preventing sexually transmitted diseases, and performing breast and testicular self-examinations. In addition to teaching, nurses can do the following to help clients maintain a healthy sexual self-concept:

- Provide privacy during intimate body care.
- Involve the client's partner in physical care.
- Give attention to the client's appearance and dress.
- Give clients privacy to meet their sexual needs alone or with a partner within physically safe limits.

IMPLEMENTING

The interventions the nurse selects are based on the data obtained from the client and the identified nursing diagnoses. Many interventions are directed at preventing problems the client is at risk for and providing information about changes and how to adapt to those changes.

Providing Sexual Health Teaching

Providing education for sexual health is an important component of nursing implementation. Many sexual problems exist because of sexual ignorance; many others can be prevented with effective sexual health teaching. Examples of important areas of teaching are sex education (including self-examination) and responsible sexual behavior.

Sex Education. Nurses can assist clients to understand their anatomies and how their bodies function. For example, understanding the anatomy of the genitals may help women learn how their bodies respond to sexual stimulation. Both men and women need to learn the kind of stimulation that is pleasing and causes arousal. The importance of open communication between partners should also be encouraged. Women may also benefit from learning Kegel exercises. These exercises involve contraction and relaxation of the pubococcygeal muscle, the muscle that contracts when a person prevents urine flow. The benefits of Kegel exercises include increased pelvic floor mus-

cle tone; increased vaginal lubrication during sexual arousal; increased sensation during intercourse; increased genital sensitivity; stronger gripping of the base of the penis; earlier postpartum recovery of the pelvic floor muscle; and increased flexibility of episiotomy scars (Berman & Berman, 2001). The steps to perform Kegel exercises are discussed in Chapter 47 because these exercises are also used in bladder retraining.

Details about physiologic changes that occur during major developmental crises should be provided as part of general health care. For example, the nurse needs to discuss the effects of puberty, pregnancy, menopause, and the male climacteric on sexual function. When clients experience illness or surgery that alters sexual function, the nurse needs to discuss effects of treatment (e.g., medications) and any changes that need to be undertaken to ensure safe sex (e.g., position changes or a safe time to resume sexual intercourse after a heart attack).

Parents often need assistance to learn ways to answer questions and what information to provide for their children starting in the preschool years. Parents need to be the primary educators of children at an early age; however, peers, teachers, media, and toys also teach about sexual issues.

Although there is an increasing awareness today of sexuality and sexual functioning, some people still hold certain myths and misconceptions about sexuality. Many of these are handed down in families and are part of the beliefs in a particular culture. It is highly important that nurses learn about the beliefs clients hold and provide up-to-date information. Table 38–5 lists some common sexual myths and misconceptions.

Teaching Self-Examination. Monthly breast self-examination (BSE) for women and monthly testicular self-examination (TSE) for men can play an important role in early detection of disease resulting in a greater chance of cure and less complex treatment. Clients need to be assured that most lumps discovered are not cancerous, but that it is essential that all lumps or other detected abnormalities be checked by the client's primary care provider

TABLE 38–5 Common Sexual Misconceptions

Misconception	Fact
Nearly all men over 70 years old have erectile dysfunction.	Sexual ability is not lost due to age. Changes may be due to disease or medication.
Masturbation causes certain mental instabilities.	Masturbation is a common and healthy behavior.
Sexual activity weakens a person.	There is no evidence that sexual activity weakens a person.
Women who have experienced orgasm are more likely to become pregnant.	Conceiving is not related to experiencing orgasm.
Nice girls shouldn't feel entitled to their own sexual satisfaction.	As women become more comfortable with their own sexuality, they advocate for their own sexual fulfillment.
A large penis provides greater sexual satisfaction to women than a small penis.	There is no evidence that a large penis provides greater satisfaction.
Alcohol is a sexual stimulant.	Alcohol is a relaxant and central nervous system depressant. Chronic alcoholism is associated with erectile dysfunction.
Intercourse during menstruation is dangerous, (i.e., it will cause vaginal tissue damage).	There is no physiologic basis for abstinence during menses.
The face-to-face coital position is the moral or proper one.	The position that offers the most pleasure and is acceptable to both partners is the correct one.

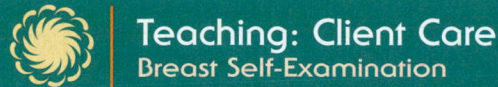

Teaching: Client Care
Breast Self-Examination

Inspection before a Mirror

Look for any change in size or shape; lumps or thickenings; any rashes or other skin irritations; dimpled or puckered skin; any discharge or change in the nipples (e.g., position or asymmetry). Inspect the breasts in all of the following positions:

- Stand and face the mirror with your arm relaxed at your sides or hands resting on the hips; then turn to the right and the left for a side view (look for any flattening in the side view).
- Bend forward from the waist with arms raised over the head.
- Stand straight with the arms raised over the head and move the arms slowly up and down at the sides. (Look for free movement of the breasts over the chest wall.)
- Press your hands firmly together at chin level while the elbows are raised to shoulder level.

Palpation: Lying Position

- Place a pillow under your right shoulder and place the right hand behind your head. This position distributes breast tissue more evenly on the chest.
- Use the finger pads (tips) of the three middle fingers (held together) on your left hand to feel for lumps.

- Press the breast tissue against the chest wall firmly enough to know how your breast feels. A ridge of firm tissue in the lower curve of each breast is normal.
- Use small circular motions systematically all the way around the breast as many times as necessary until the entire breast is covered. (Review Figures 28–70 through 28–72 in Chapter 28 ⊂⊃ for patterns that the client may use.)
- Bring your arm down to your side and feel under your armpit, where breast tissue is also located.
- Repeat the exam on your left breast, using the finger pads of your right hand.

Palpation: Standing or Sitting

- Repeat the examination of both breasts while upright with one arm behind your head. This position makes it easier to check the area where a large percentage of breast cancers are found, the upper outer part of the breast and toward the armpit.
- *Optional:* Do the upright BSE in the shower. Soapy hands glide more easily over wet skin.

Report any changes to your health care provider promptly.

---

for accurate diagnosis. All nursing history assessments of clients need to include the client's understanding and practice of BSE or TSE. Self-examination involves both inspection and palpation procedures and should be conducted once a month.

Although 95% of the more than 200,000 new breast cancers in the United States each year occur in women (Jemal et al., 2003), men with an increased risk of breast cancer due to high estrogen levels or strong family history of breast cancer should also learn BSE. For BSE a regular time is best—such as 1 week following menstruation, when breast tenderness and fullness caused by fluid retention have subsided, or on the same day of the month for men or postmenopausal women. People who examine themselves regularly become familiar with the shape and texture of their breasts. The steps of BSE are very similar to those used when the nurse performs breast examination (see Box 28–28 ⊂⊃ in the Health Assessment chapter). For specific techniques of breast self-examination, see the Teaching: Client Care feature.

Testicular cancer occurs in more than 7,500 American men each year (Jemal et al., 2003). For men, starting at age 15, monthly self-exams of the testicles are an effective way of getting to know this area of their body and thus detecting testicular cancer at an early and very curable stage. The best time for TSE is after a warm bath or shower when the scrotal sac is relaxed. For specific techniques of self-examination, see the Teaching: Client Care feature on page 988.

> **CLINICAL ALERT** *It may be wise for both male and female nurses to request permission from a parent or guardian before teaching testicular self-examination to teenage boys.* ■

Responsible Sexual Behavior. Responsible sexual behavior involves the prevention of sexually transmitted diseases and the prevention of unwanted pregnancy and the avoidance of sexual harassment or abuse.

STD Prevention. The prevention of STDs is an essential part of sexual health teaching (Figure 38–3 ■). Note that *Trichomonas* and *Candida* infections can also be acquired nonsexually. Increases in these diseases are due to two factors: (a) changing sexual morality that has permitted increased sexual activity and (b) an increase in the number of sexual partners. Because the term *sexually transmitted disease* elicits feelings of guilt, shame, and fear, people frequently do not seek medical help as early as they should. Clients need education about these diseases, preventive measures, and early treatment. Many STDs can be treated quickly and effectively. Others may have serious consequences. For example, women may develop pelvic inflammatory disease (PID) resulting in damage to the reproductive structures and possible infertility. AIDS has no cure. The anxiety about AIDS transmission has caused many individuals to alter their sexual behavior, such as using a condom during intercourse.

Table 38–2, earlier in this chapter, lists common signs of STDs for which people should seek medical care. Methods for decreasing exposure to STDs are described in the Teaching: Client care feature on page 988.

Prevention of Unwanted Pregnancies. Prevention of unwanted pregnancies must be addressed not only with adolescents but also with couples who are planning the time of their first birth and want to space children and limit family size. Nurses need to be familiar with various contraceptive methods

MediaLink | SOCIETY FOR HUMAN SEXUALITY APPLICATION

Teaching: Client Care
Testicular Self-Examination

- Choose one day of each month (e.g., the first or last day of each month) to examine yourself.
- Examine yourself when you are taking a warm shower or bath.
- Support the testicle underneath with one hand. Place the fingers of the other hand under the testicle and the thumb on top (this may be easier to do if the leg on that side is raised).
- Roll each testicle between the thumb and fingers of your hand, feeling for lumps, thickening, or a hardening in consistency (Figure 38–2 ■). The testes should feel smooth.
- Palpate the epididymis, a cordlike structure on the top and back of the testicle. The epididymis feels soft and not as smooth as a testicle.
- Locate the spermatic cord, or vas deferens, which extends upward from the scrotum toward the base of the penis. It should feel firm and smooth.

- Using a mirror, inspect your testicles for swelling, any enlargement, or lumps in the skin of the testicle.
- Report any lumps or other changes to your health care provider promptly.

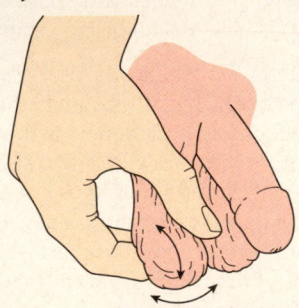

Figure 38–2 ■ Rolling the testicle between the thumb and fingers.

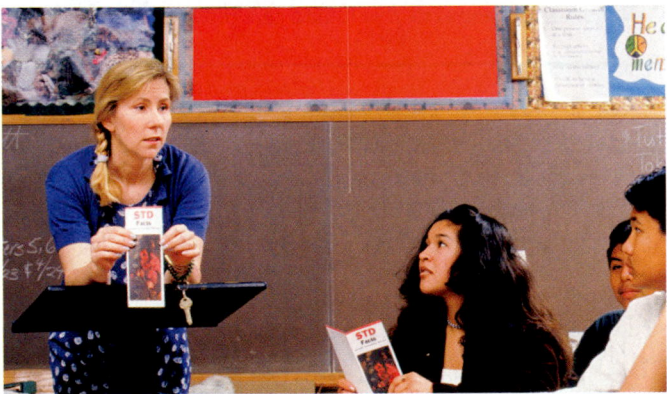

Figure 38–3 ■ Adolescents require age-appropriate teaching about sexuality and STDs. (Will Hart/PhotoEdit.)

and their advantages, disadvantages, contraindications, effectiveness, safety, and cost (Figure 38–4 ■). It is beyond the scope of this text to discuss contraceptives in detail. The various methods are outlined in Box 38–3.

Counseling for Altered Sexual Function

One technique nurses can use to help clients with altered sexual function is the PLISSIT model, developed by Annon (1974) for this purpose. The model involves four progressive levels represented by the acronym PLISSIT:

P	Permission giving
LI	Limited information
SS	Specific suggestions
IT	Intensive therapy

At each level, the nurse provides additional guidance and information to the client and therefore requires more specialized and specific knowledge and skill. All professional nurses should be able to function at the first three levels.

Teaching: Client Care
Preventing Transmission of STDs and HIV

- Limit the number of sexual partners.
- Use condoms in nonmonogamous and homosexual relationships or other relationships that have the potential for STD transmission.
- Talk openly with sexual partners about how to have "safer sex" and be honest about any history of an STD.
- Abstain from high-risk sexual activity with a partner known to have or suspected of having an STD.
- Report to a health care facility for examination whenever in doubt about possible exposure or when signs of an STD are evident.
- When an STD is diagnosed, notify all partners and encourage them to seek treatment.
- Avoid unnecessary transfusions of blood or blood products. Use autologous transfusions (donation of own blood before surgery) for elective surgery whenever possible.

Permission Giving. Clients may feel that they need permission to be sexual beings, to ask questions, to show affection, and to express themselves sexually. Giving permission means that the nurse by attitude or word lets the client know that sexual thoughts, fantasies, and behaviors between informed consenting adults are allowed. Giving permission begins when the nurse acknowledges the client's spoken and unspoken sexual concerns and conveys the attitude that sexual concerns and needs are important to health and recovery.

For example, the nurse might ask a client recuperating from a heart attack the following questions:

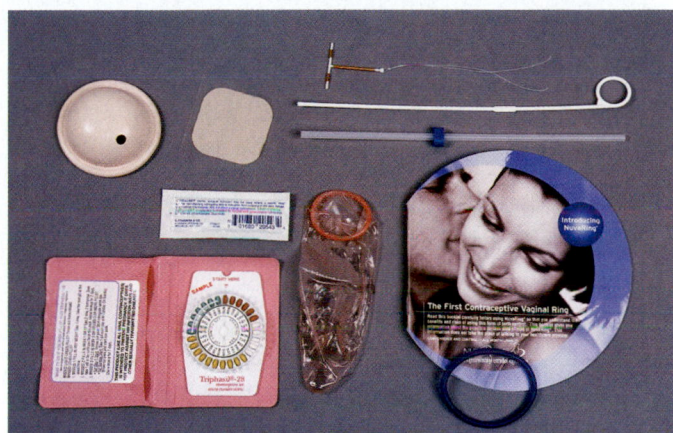

Figure 38–4 ■ Methods of contraception.

"Now that you're recuperating and you've had some time to sort out your feelings, have you thought about how your heart attack might alter your sex life?"

"Have you and your partner discussed how you both feel about it?"

Limited Information. Clients need accurate but concise information. The nurse might explain what is normal; how some medical conditions, treatments, injuries, or surgeries may affect sexuality and sexual functioning; or how aging may affect sexuality and functioning.

Continuing with the preceding example, the nurse shares information and informs the client about how the heart attack might affect the client's sex life, including the following:

"Your heart attack will not alter your capacity for sexual response. Most people can resume intercourse in 4 to 6 weeks, but this should be confirmed by your doctor."

"Many postcoronary clients fear sexual intercourse because of increased heart and respiratory rates associated with it. However, your prescribed program of progressive physical activity will also increase your tolerance for sexual activity."

Many clients recuperating from childbirth, for example, or specific illness or disease (e.g., heart attack) need instruction

---

Research Note
What Are College Students' Perceptions and Practices of Sexual Activities in Sexual Encounters?

An exploratory study of 84 college students examined the understanding college students have of safer sexual encounters that include ideas about what constitutes "safe" sex, expectations for sexual activities, and planning for sexual encounters (von Sadovszky, Keller, & McKinney, 2002). Analysis of three open- and closed-ended questions about sexual activities revealed no significant difference between expectations regarding sexual activities among participants who had risky and safer encounters. Planning of an encounter was not related to safer sexual activities, and what constitutes safer sexual activities was generally misunderstood. Participants believed risky encounters to be safer because of the use of a condom only during vaginal sex, the use of hormone-based birth control pills, or because of the belief that no sex had occurred during oral sex.

Implications: Nurses need to assess the clients' knowledge and beliefs about sexual activities related to STDs and unwanted pregnancy.

Note: From "College Students' Perceptions and Practices of Sexual Activities in Sexual Encounters," by V. von Sadovszky, M. Keller, and K. McKinney, 2002, *Journal of Nursing Scholarship, 34*, pp. 133–138.

---

about safe sexual activities and the effects that therapy may have on sexual functioning. The following topics need to be considered:

- When sexual activity is safe
- Specific sexual activities that are unsafe, and why
- Adaptations needed for resuming a satisfactory sexual life
- The side effects of prescribed medications on sexual functioning, and the need to notify the physician for possible dose or medication adjustment should problems develop.

Specific Suggestions. At this level, the nurse requires specialized knowledge and skill about how sexuality and functioning may be affected by a disease process or therapy and what interventions might be effective. The nurse offers suggestions to help the client adapt sexual activity to promote optimal functioning, such as what measures might be used to alleviate vaginal dryness, safe positions for intercourse following a total hip replacement, safe and unsafe sexual practices following a heart attack, and ways to handle ostomy appliances, Foley catheters, casts, or other devices (e.g., prostheses) during sexual activity. Similarly, nurses on a cardiac unit need specialized knowledge about sexual readjustment during cardiac rehabilitation, and nurses working with clients with spinal cord injuries need information about the sexual consequences of spinal injuries at various levels.

Using the example of the client recuperating from a heart attack, the nurse may offer the following suggestion:

"Many people express concern about the stress of certain positions for intercourse, but you may use whatever position is comfortable for you and your partner, or try side-lying or partner-on-top positions."

BOX 38–3 ■ Methods of Contraception

- Abstinence
- Withdrawal of the penis before ejaculation (coitus interruptus)
- Fertility awareness (identification of the days of the month when conception could take place and abstaining during that time)
- Mechanical barriers: vaginal diaphragm, cervical cap, condom
- Chemical barriers: insertion of spermicidal foams, creams, jellies, or suppositories into the vagina before intercourse
- Intrauterine devices (IUDs)
- Hormonal: oral contraceptives (birth control pills), subdermal implants of synthetic progestin
- Surgical sterilization: tubal ligation and vasectomy
- Abortion

MediaLink | OVULATION A & P REVIEW ANIMATION

Intensive Therapy. Intensive therapy, provided by a clinical nurse specialist or sex therapist, is used when the first three levels of counseling are ineffective. It may involve such issues as sexual motivation, marriage, or self-concept.

Dealing with Inappropriate Sexual Behavior

Nurses may encounter a variety of sexually inappropriate behaviors for a number of reasons. The behavior may be either aggressive or nonaggressive. Clients may act out sexually by

- Exposing themselves
- Asking the nurse to provide intimate physical care, such as bathing genital areas, when they are capable of doing this themselves
- Touching or grabbing the nurse's genitals or buttocks
- Making blatant sexual statements to the nurse
- Offering the nurse sex
- Whistling; making comments about the nurse's attractiveness or desirability
- Making sexual comments to another client in the same room or to visitors about the "sexy" nurse or what they would like to do sexually with the nurse.

Possible reasons for this inappropriate behavior are

- Fear or anxiety over future ability to function sexually
- Unmet need for intimacy and sexual closeness because of hospitalization, injury, illness, treatment, lack of a partner, lack of privacy
- Misinterpretation of the nurse's behavior as sexual or provocative
- Need for reassurance that they are still sexual beings and still sexually attractive
- Need for attention

- Confusion: Neurologic impairment or trauma can lead clients to use profane sexual language, engage in masturbation, expose themselves, or inappropriately touch or grab at the nurse
- Need to control: clients may be experiencing loss of control over their lives because of hospitalization, injury, or illness
- Need for power
- Belief that flirtatious behavior is expected due to media portrayal of nurses as sexy, available, and experienced.

Before implementing any nursing interventions, the nurse should first ensure that the behavior is inappropriate and not an attempt to communicate a physical need. For example, clients may expose themselves if they are febrile, pull at the penis if a catheter is uncomfortable or irritating, or reach for the nurse if unable to communicate verbally. Nursing strategies to deal with inappropriate sexual behavior are listed in Box 38–4.

EVALUATING

The goals established during the planning phase are evaluated according to specific desired outcomes also established during that phase. If any outcomes have not been achieved, the nurse should explore the reasons with questions such as the following:

- Were risk factors correctly identified?
- Did the client convey all significant fears and concerns about sexuality?
- Was the client more comfortable following discussions about sexual matters?
- Did the client understand the nurse's teaching?
- Was the health teaching compatible with the client's culture and religious values?
- Was the client ready to deal with sexuality problems?

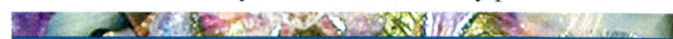

BOX 38–4 ■ Nursing Strategies for Inappropriate Sexual Behavior

- Communicate that the behavior is not acceptable by saying, for example, "I really do not like the things you are saying," or "I see you are not dressed. I will be back in 10 minutes and will help you with breakfast when you get your clothes on."
- Tell the client how the behavior makes you feel: "When you act like that toward me, I am very uncomfortable. It embarrasses me and makes it hard for me to give you the kind of nursing care you need."
- Identify the behavior you expect: "Please call me by my name, not 'honey,'" or "I expect you to keep yourself covered when I am in the room. If you are feeling hot or something is uncomfortable, let me know, and I will try to make you more comfortable."
- Set firm limits: Take the client's hand and move it away, use direct eye contact, and say, "Don't do that!"

- Try to refocus clients from the inappropriate behavior to their real concerns and fears; offer to discuss sexuality concerns: "All morning you have been making very personal sexual comments about yourself. Sometimes people talk like that when they are concerned about the sexual part of their life and how their illness will affect them. Are there things that you have questions about or would like to talk about?"
- Report the incident to your nursing instructor, charge nurse, or clinical nurse specialist. Discuss the incident, your feelings, and possible interventions.
- Assign a nurse who will confront the behavior and relate to the client in a consistent manner.
- Clarify the consequences of continued inappropriate behavior (avoidance, withdrawal of services, no chance to help resolve underlying concerns of client).

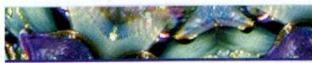

Focus on Critical Thinking

Mr. Curry is a 50-year-old African American male with diabetes who suffered a heart attack 3 weeks ago. He is doing well and is in a cardiac rehabilitation program. His diabetes is controlled with diet and his only medications consist of a daily aspirin and an antihypertensive medication. During a routine checkup you inquire how he is feeling and whether he is doing well on his medications. Reluctantly, he admits that he is having some sexual problems. You encourage further discussion of the matter by displaying interest and explaining that it is okay for him to share his concerns with you. Mr. Curry states that he is having some difficulty achieving erections, but is more concerned that he will have another heart attack if he engages in sexual activities.

1. Speculate about Mr. Curry's reluctance to discuss his sexual concerns.
2. What factors influence nurses' abilities to discuss sexual concerns with their clients?
3. What is the relationship between health and sexual function?
4. How can you best intervene to help Mr. Curry?

See Critical Thinking Possibilities in Appendix A.

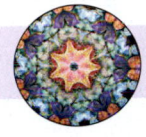 | Chapter Review

EXPLORE MediaLink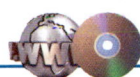

NCLEX review questions, case studies, care plan activities, MediaLink applications, and other interactive resources for this chapter can be found on the Companion Website at www.prenhall.com/kozier. Click on Chapter 38 to select the activities for this chapter.

For animations, more NCLEX review questions, and an audio glossary, access the Student CD-ROM accompanying this textbook.

Chapter Highlights

- Sexuality is important in developing self-identity, interpersonal relationships, intimacy, and love.
- In its broad sense, sexuality involves all aspects of being and behaving.
- The components that contribute to the development of sexuality are numerous; both biologic and psychologic components exist at all ages.
- Factors that affect sexuality include developmental level, culture, religious values, personal ethics, disease processes, and medications.
- Assessing risk for or actual sexual problems is part of the initial nursing assessment. Assessment should also be carried out when clients or support people present cues that problems exist or when clients have an illness that could cause sexual problems.
- Nurses assess attitudes toward sexuality, including factors that affect attitudes and behaviors.
- An understanding of sexual stimuli and response patterns can help individuals have satisfying sexual relationships.
- Before assisting clients with sexual problems, nurses must acquire accurate information about sexuality, identify and accept their own sexual values and behaviors as well as those of others, and be comfortable acquiring and disseminating information about sexuality.
- Sexual problems of adults include erectile dysfunction, rapid ejaculation, retarded ejaculation, sexual arousal disorders, orgasmic disorder, vaginismus, dyspareunia, and vaginal pain.
- Nursing diagnoses for clients with sexual problems are related to many contributing factors, including altered body structure or function, lack of knowledge or misinformation about sexual matters, physical or psychologic abuse, value conflicts, and loss or lack of a partner.
- Nursing interventions focus largely on teaching clients about sexual function and sexuality, responsible sexual behavior that includes the prevention of STDs and unwanted pregnancies, and self-examination of the breasts and testicles.
- Counseling clients with altered sexual functions can be facilitated by using the PLISSIT model: permission giving (P), limited information (LI), and specific suggestions (SS). Intensive therapy (IT) requires intervention by clinical nurse specialists or sex therapists.

Review Questions

38–1. Which is a common reason clients do not introduce the topic of sex with health care providers?
  a. They assume that health care providers know little about sexual functioning.
  b. Most clients have few, if any, questions or problems.
  c. Female clients prefer to discuss problems with female health care providers.
  d. They are too embarrassed to introduce the topic of sex.

38–2. A male client who had a heart attack 3 days ago, grabs the female nurse's breasts and buttocks. What is her best response?
  a. "You may not touch me in this way. I'm guessing that you may have some sexual concerns since your heart attack"
  b. "Take your hands off of me and act your age. This is no way for an adult man to behave."
  c. "If you don't stop touching me like this, I will be forced to have you assigned to a male nurse."
  d. Say nothing. Leave the room and ask the charge nurse to reassign you to another patient.

38–3. Which is a typical gender role behavior in the United States?
  a. Men are given permission to wear a wide variety of clothing.
  b. Men are expected to be nuturing as well as aggressive.
  c. Women are most responsible for child-rearing activities.
  d. Women should express their feelings in a controlled manner.

38–4. Your male client is beginning an antidepressant medication. What should you include in your teaching?
  a. "Your partner will be really happy because your sexual functioning is going to improve."
  b. "You may find that your desire for sex will decrease while on this medication."
  c. "Retrograde ejaculation is a common problem when taking antidepressants."
  d. "Your skin will probably become supersensitive to touch, so be careful."

38–5. Your client, who had a hysterectomy 3 days ago, says to you, "I no longer feel like a real woman." What is your best response?
  a. "Don't worry about that. The feeling will probably go away."
  b. "You should talk to your doctor about how you feel."
  c. "I don't blame you. I would feel like half a woman also."
  d. "I hear your concern. Tell me more about your feelings."

Readings and References

Suggested Readings

Doyle, D., Bisson, D., Janes, N., Lynch, H., & Martin, C. (1999). Human sexuality in long-term care. *Canadian Nurse, 95*(1), 26–29. These authors define sexuality broadly and describe a three-part process they developed at a 577-bed chronic care hospital to acknowledge and support appropriate sexual expression of the residents. The process involves (a) a team meeting of staff members who are guided to answer six questions about the nature of the relationship, (b) a family meeting, and (c) ongoing assessment.

Related Research

Augustus, C. E. (2002). Beliefs and perceptions of African American women who have had hysterectomy. *Journal of Transcultural Nursing, 13,* 296–302.

Forste, R., & Haas, D. W. (2002). The transition of adolescent males to first sexual intercourse: Anticipated or delayed? *Perspectives on Sexual and Reproductive Health, 34,* 184–190.

Rew, L., Fouladi, R. T., & Yockey, R. D. (2002). Sexual health practices of homeless youth. *Journal of Nursing Scholarship, 34,* 139–145.

References

Annon, J. (1974). *The behavioral treatment of sexual problems. Vol. 1. Brief therapy.* New York: Harper & Row.

Bedell, S. E., Duperval, M., & Goldberg, R. (2002). Cardiologists' discussions about sexuality with patients with chronic coronary artery disease. *American Heart Journal, 144,* 239–242.

Berman, J., & Berman, L. (2001). *For women only.* New York: Henry Holt and Company.

Brady, J. M. (1998). Female genital mutilation. *Nursing, 28*(9), 50–51.

Dodson, B. (2002). *Orgasms for two: The joy of partner sex.* New York: Harmony Books.

Ellison, C. R. (2000). *Women's sexualities.* Oakland, CA: New Harbinger.

Jemal, A., Murray, T., Samuels, A., Ghafoor, A., Ward, E., & Thun, M. J. (2003). Cancer statistics, 2003. *CA: A Cancer Journal for Clinicians, 53,* 5–26.

Johnson, M., Maas, M., & Moorhead, S. (Eds.). (2000). *Nursing outcomes classification (NOC)* (2nd ed.). St. Louis, MO: Mosby.

McCloskey, J. C., & Bulechek, G. M. (Eds.). (2000). *Nursing interventions classification (NIC)* (3rd ed.). St. Louis, MO: Mosby.

Morrison, T. (1992). *Jazz.* New York: Alfred A. Knopf, Inc.

NANDA International. (2003). NANDA *nursing diagnoses: Definitions and classification 2003-2004.* Philadelphia: Author.

Rodgers, J. E. (2001). *Sex: A natural history.* New York: Times Books.

Rosen, R. C. (2000). Medical and psychological interventions for erectile dysfunction. In S. R. Leiblum & R. C. Rosen. *Principles and practice of sex therapy* (3rd ed., pp. 276–304). New York: Guilford Press.

Rudberg, L., Carlsson, M., Nilsson, S., & Wikblad, K. (2002). Self-perceived physical, psychologic, and general symptoms in survivors of testicular cancer 3 to 13 years after treatment. *Cancer Nursing, 25,* 187–195.

Von Sadovszky, V., Keller, M., & McKinney, K. (2002). College students' perceptions and practices of sexual activities in sexual encounters. *Journal of Nursing Scholarship, 34,* 133–138.

World Association of Sexology. (1999). *Declaration of sexual rights.* Adopted at the 14th World Congress of Sexology, Hong Kong and People's Republic of China.

World Health Organization. (1975). *Education and treatment in human sexuality: The training of health professionals.* Geneva: Author.

Suggested Bibliography

Alexander, C. J. (Ed.). (1999). *Working with gay men and lesbians in private psychotherapy practice.* Binghamton, NY: Harrington Park Press.

Armishaw, J., & Davis, K. (2002). Women, hepatitis C, and sexuality: A critical feminist exploration. *Contemporary Nurse, 12,* 194–203.

Estes, J. P. (2002). Beyond basic ADLS: Sexual expression is an important but often overlooked activity of daily living. *Rehab Management: The Interdisciplinary Journal of Rehabilitation, 15*(3), 36–37.

Fishman, J. R., & Mamo, L. (2001). What's in a disorder: A cultural analysis of medical and pharmaceutical constructions of male and female sexual dysfunction. *Women and Therapy, 24,* 179–193.

Gross, Z. (2000). *Seasons of the heart: Men and women talk about love, sex, and romance after 60.* Novato, CA: New World Library.

Hock, R. A. (2002). *Insights in human sexuality.* Upper Saddle River, NJ: Prentice Hall Health.

Joannides, P. N. (1999). *The guide to getting it on* (2nd ed.). West Hollywood, CA: Goofy Foot Press.

Jenkins, R. R., & Raine, T. (2000). Helping adolescents prevent unintended pregnancy. *Contemporary Pediatrics, 17*(5), 75–76, 79–80, 82.

Jollery, S. (2002). Taking a sexual history: The role of the nurse. *Nursing Times, 98*(18), 39–41.

Katz, A. (2002). Sexuality after hysterectomy. *Journal of Obstetrics, Gynecologic, and Neonatal Nursing, 31,* 256–262.

King, B. M. (2002). *Human sexuality today* (4th ed.). Upper Saddle River, NJ: Prentice Hall Health.

Klein, E., & Kroll, K. (1999). *Enabling romance: A guide to love, sex, and relationships for the disabled.* New York: Harmony Press.

Maticka-Tyndale, E. (2001). Sexual health and Canadian youth: How do we measure up? *Canadian Journal of Human Sexuality, 10,* 1–16.

Miracle, T., Miracle, A., & Baumeister, R. (2003). *Human sexuality: Meeting your basic needs.* Upper Saddle River, NJ: Prentice Hall Health.

Stipetich, R. L., Abel, L. J., Blatt, H. J., Galbreath, R. W., Lief, J. H., Butler, W. M., et al. (2002). Nursing assessment of sexual function following permanent prostate brachytherapy for patients with early-stage prostate cancer. *Clinical Journal of Oncology Nursing, 6,* 271–274, 280–282.

Tiefer, L. (2001). Arriving at a "new view" of women's sexual problems: Background, theory, and activism. *Women and Therapy, 24,* 63–98.

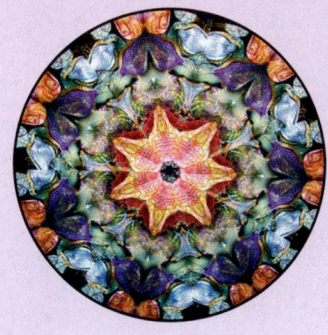

CHAPTER 39

SPIRITUALITY

LEARNING OUTCOMES

After completing this chapter, you will be able to

- Define the concepts of spirituality and religion as they relate to nursing and health care.

- Identify characteristics of spiritual well-being.

- Identify factors associated with spiritual distress and manifestations of it.

- Describe the spiritual development of the individual across the life span.

- Describe the influence of spiritual and religious beliefs about diet, dress, prayer and meditation, and birth and death on health care.

- Assess the spiritual needs of clients and plan nursing care to assist clients with spiritual needs.

- Describe nursing interventions to support clients' spiritual beliefs and religious practices.

- Identify desired outcomes for evaluating the client's spiritual well-being.

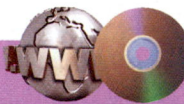

MediaLink

www.prenhall.com/kozier

Additional resources for this chapter can be found on the Student CD-ROM accompanying this textbook, and on the Companion Website at www.prenhall.com/kozier. Click on Chapter 39 to select the activities for this chapter.

CD-ROM
- Audio Glossary
- NCLEX Review

Companion Website
- Additional NCLEX Review
- Case Study: Supporting a Client's Religious Practices
- Care Plan Activity: Treating a Client who is Paralyzed
- MediaLink Application: Researching Atheism as a Client's Religious Preference
- Links to Resources

In holistic nursing, the nurse provides care not only for the physical body and mind but also for the client's spirit. Meeting the client's spiritual needs can decrease suffering and aid in physical and mental healing. To implement spiritual care, nurses need to be skilled in establishing trusting nurse–client relationships. Because involvement in the meeting of spiritual needs is personal for both the nurse and the client, nurses need to communicate with sensitivity and empathy and to have a good understanding of their own values. It is important for nurses to develop a broad concept of spirituality. Nurses cannot rely solely on their own spiritual practices; they need to be aware of the array of religious traditions and spiritual expressions to which their clients may subscribe. Sensitivity in providing care is essential to meet the various levels and depths of clients' spiritual expressions and needs. A client's experience with what is seen as Divine is complex and individual. Thus each client needs to be approached in light of unique needs. Many clients have spiritual strengths that the nurse can nurture to help them attain or maintain a feeling of spiritual well-being, to recover from illness, and to face a peaceful death.

SPIRITUALITY DESCRIBED

Spirituality, faith, and religion are separate entities, yet the words are often used interchangeably. The word *spiritual* derives from the Latin word *spiritus,* which means "to blow" or "to breathe," and has come to connote that which gives life or essence to being human. **Spirituality** refers to that part of being human that seeks meaningfulness through intra-, inter-, and transpersonal connection (Reed, 1991). Spirituality generally involves a belief in a relationship with some higher power, creative force, divine being, or infinite source of energy. For example, a person may believe in "God," "Allah," the "Great Spirit," or a "Higher Power." Spirituality includes the following aspects (Martsolf & Mickley, 1998):

- Meaning (having purpose, making sense of life)
- Value (having cherished beliefs and standards)
- Transcendence (appreciating a dimension that is beyond the self)
- Connecting (relating to others, nature, Ultimate Other)
- Becoming (which involves reflection, allowing life to unfold, and knowing who one is).

Words or concepts reflective of spirituality, such as faith, courage, cheer, and hope, may be used in ordinary speech when discussing spirituality.

Spiritual Needs

Just as everybody has a spiritual dimension, all clients have needs that reflect their spirituality. These needs are often brought forward by an illness or other health crisis. Clients who have well-defined spiritual beliefs may find that their beliefs are challenged by their health situation; clients who have no defined beliefs may suddenly come face to face with challenging questions related to the meaning and purpose of life. Nurses need to be sensitive to indications of the client's spiritual needs and respond appropriately, as discussed later. Meeting clients' spiritual needs can also enhance coping behaviors and expand valuable resources available to the client. Aspects and illustrations of spiritual need are listed in Box 39–1.

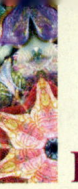

KEY TERMS

agnostic, 997
atheist, 997
faith, 997
holy day, 997
hope, 997
kosher, 999
meditation, 999
monotheism, 997
polytheism, 997
prayer, 999
presencing, 1002
religion, 996
spiritual health, 996
spiritual distress, 996
spiritual well-being, 996
spirituality, 995
transcendence, 997

BOX 39–1 ■ Examples of Spiritual Needs	
■ Need for love	■ Need for meaning to the fullness of life
■ Need for hope	■ Need for values
■ Need for trust	■ Need for creativity
■ Need for forgiveness	■ Need to connect with a God or Higher Power, or a Being greater than oneself
■ Need to be respected and valued	■ Need to belong to a community
■ Need for dignity	

Spiritual Well-Being

Spiritual health, or **spiritual well-being,** is manifested by a feeling of being "generally alive, purposeful, and fulfilled" (Ellison, 1983, p. 332). According to Pilch (1988), spiritual wellness is "a way of living, a lifestyle that views and lives life as purposeful and pleasurable, that seeks out life-sustaining and life-enriching options to be chosen freely at every opportunity, and that sinks its roots deeply into spiritual values and/or specific religious beliefs" (p. 31). Characteristics of spiritual well-being are shown in Box 39–2.

People nurture or enhance their spirituality in many ways. Some focus on development of the inner self or world; others focus on the expression of their spiritual energy with others or the outer world. Relating to one's inner self or soul may be achieved by conducting an inner dialogue with a higher power or with oneself through prayer or meditation, by analyzing dreams, by communing with nature, or by experiencing the inspiration of art (e.g., drama, music, dance). The expression of a person's spiritual energy to others is manifested in loving relationships with and service to others, joy and laughter, participation in religious services and associated fellowship gatherings and activities, and by expression of compassion, empathy, forgiveness, and hope. Nurses who attend to their own spirituality are better able to work with clients who have spiritual needs; it is important to be comfortable with one's own spirituality.

Spiritual Distress

Spiritual distress refers to a challenge to the spiritual well-being or to the belief system that provides strength, hope, and meaning to life. Some factors that may be associated with or contribute to a person's spiritual distress include physiologic problems, treatment-related concerns, and situational concerns. Physiologic problems include having a medical diagnosis of a terminal or debilitating disease, experiencing pain, experiencing the loss of a body part or function, or experiencing a miscarriage or stillbirth. Treatment-related factors include recommendation for blood transfusions, abortion, surgery, dietary restrictions, amputation of a body part, or isolation.

Situational factors include the death or illness of a significant other, inability to practice one's spiritual rituals, or feelings of embarrassment when practicing them (Carpenito, 2002).

NANDA International (2003) offers the following as defining characteristics of spiritual distress:

- Expresses lack of hope, meaning and purpose in life, forgiveness of self
- Expresses being abandoned by or having anger toward God
- Refuses interaction with friends, family
- Sudden changes in spiritual practices
- Requests to see a religious leader
- No interest in nature, reading spiritual literature

No list could be complete, however, considering the complexity and variability of people and their spiritual dimensions.

RELATED CONCEPTS

Because spirituality is a reflection of an inner experience that is expressed individually, it includes as many representations as there are human beings. Concepts related to spirituality include religion, faith, hope, transcendence, and forgiveness.

Religion

Religion is an organized system of beliefs and practices. It offers a way of spiritual expression that provides guidance for believers in responding to life's questions and challenges. According to Vardey (1995, p. xv), the organized religions offer (a) a sense of community bound by common beliefs; (b) the collective study of scripture (the Torah, Bible, Koran, or others); (c) the performance of ritual; (d) the use of disciplines and practices, commandments, and sacraments; and (e) ways of taking care of the person's spirit (such as fasting, prayer, and meditation). Many traditional religious practices and rituals are related to such life events as birth, transition from childhood to adulthood, marriage, illness, and death (Figure 39–1 ■). Religious rules of conduct,

---

BOX 39–2 ■ Characteristics Indicative of Spiritual Well-Being

- Sense of inner peace
- Compassion for others
- Reverence for life
- Gratitude
- Appreciation of both unity and diversity
- Humor
- Wisdom
- Generosity
- Ability to transcend the self
- Capacity for unconditional love

Note: From Spiritual Dimensions of Nursing Practice, by V. B. Carson, 1989, Philadelphia: Saunders. Reprinted with permission from Elsevier.

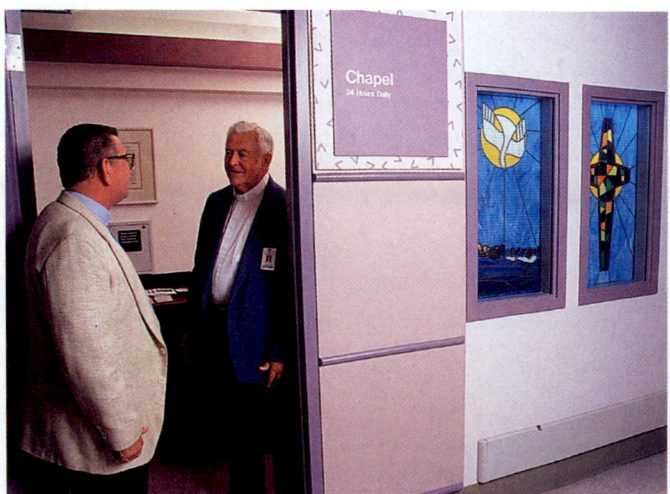

Figure 39–1 ■ Hospital chaplains minister to clients and their families.

typically influenced concurrently by culture, may also apply to matters of daily life such as dress, food, social interaction, menstruation, and sexual relationships.

Religious development of an individual refers to the acceptance of specific beliefs, values, rules of conduct, and rituals. Religious development may or may not parallel spiritual development. For example, a person may follow certain religious practices and yet not internalize the symbolic meaning behind the practices. Yet often religious development undergirds and enhances spirituality by providing a system of belief that can suggest areas of growth to the believer. For example, the daily prayers of the Muslims bring the believers into direct relationship with the profound questions of life several times per day. An **agnostic** is a person who doubts the existence of God or a supreme being or believes the existence of God has not been proved. An **atheist** is one without belief in a God. **Monotheism** is the belief in the existence of one God, while **polytheism** is the belief in more than one god. The moral and ethical codes of agnostics and atheists are not derived from theistic beliefs.

Faith

Faith is to believe in or be committed to something or someone. Fowler (1981) describes faith as being present in both religious and nonreligious people. Faith gives life meaning, providing the individual with strength in times of difficulty. For the client who is ill, faith—whether in a higher authority (e.g., God, Allah, Jehovah), in oneself, in the health care team, or in a combination of all—provides strength and hope.

Hope

Hope is a concept that incorporates spirituality. Stephenson (1991) suggested this definition: "a process of anticipation that involves the interaction of thinking, acting, feeling, and relating, and is directed toward a future fulfillment that is personally meaningful" (p. 1459). In the absence of hope, the client gives up, losing spirit, and illness is likely to progress more rapidly.

Transcendence

The term **transcendence** is often used interchangeably with self-transcendence, which Coward (1990) defined as: "the capacity to reach out beyond oneself, to extend oneself beyond personal concerns and to take on broader life perspectives, activities, and purposes" (p. 162). Transcendence is also thought to involve a person's recognition that there is something other or greater than the self and a seeking and valuing of that greater other, whether it is an ultimate being, force, or value.

Forgiveness

The concept of forgiveness is receiving increased attention among health care professionals. For many clients, illness or disability bring a sense of shame or guilt. The health problem is interpreted as a punishment for past sins (e.g., "Having sex before I got married is why I have breast cancer"). Clients facing imminent death may seek forgiveness from others as well

as from God. Mickley and Cowles' (2001) research suggests that nurses can play a pivotal role in assisting clients to understand the process of forgiveness and to persevere through it.

SPIRITUAL DEVELOPMENT

Just as individuals develop physically, cognitively, and morally, they also develop spiritually. Several theologians have identified specific linear stages through which individuals may progress while maturing spiritually. Westerhoff (1976), for example, described faith as a way of behaving that evolves from a faith guided by parents and others during infancy and childhood to an owned faith that is internalized in adulthood and serves as a directive for action. Table 39–1 describes some of the aspects of spiritual development and healthful religious behaviors during different life stages.

SPIRITUAL PRACTICES AFFECTING NURSING CARE

Clients frequently identify religious practices such as prayer as important strategies for coping with illness (Pargament, 1997). The most common practices affecting the nursing care of clients include holy days, sacred writings, sacred symbols, prayer, meditation, and those associated with diet, nutrition, healing, dress, birth, and death.

> ► **CLINICAL ALERT** *Because expressions of spirituality and religious beliefs are personal, it is possible for a nurse unknowingly to impose religious beliefs or practices on a client. The nurse's ethical behavior depends on thorough self-knowledge as well as sensitivity to the client's statements and responses.* ■

Holy Days

A **holy day** is a day set aside for special religious observance, and all the world religions observe certain holy days. For example, Christians observe Easter and Christmas, Jews observe Yom Kippur and Passover, Buddhists observe the birthday of the Buddha, Muslims observe the month-long holy period of Ramadan, and Hindus observe Mahashivarathri, a celebration of Lord Shiva. Many religions require fasting, extended prayer, and reflection or ritual observances on sacred (or high holy) days; however, believers who are seriously ill are often exempted from such requirements.

The concept of the Sabbath is common to both Christians and Jews, in response to the biblical commandment "Remember the Sabbath day to keep it holy." Most Christians observe the Sabbath on Sunday, whereas Jews and sabbatarian Christians (e.g., Seventh-Day Adventists) observe Saturday as their Sabbath. Clients who are devout in their religious practices may want to avoid any special treatments or other intrusions on their day of rest and reflection.

MediaLink | RESEARCHING ATHEISM AS A CLIENT'S RELIGIOUS PREFERENCE APPLICATION

TABLE 39–1 Stages of Spiritual Development

Developmental Stage	Characteristics
0–3 years	Neonates and toddlers are acquiring fundamental spiritual qualities of trust, mutuality, courage, hope, and love. Transition to next stage of faith begins when child's language and thought begin to allow use of symbolism.
3–7 years	Fantasy-filled, imitative phase when child can be influenced by examples, moods, actions. Child relates intuitively to ultimate conditions of existence through stories and images, the fusion of facts and feelings. Make-believe is experienced as reality (Santa Claus, God as grandfather in the sky).
7–12 years, even into adulthood	Child attempting to sort fantasy from fact by demanding proofs or demonstrations of reality. Stories are important for finding meaning and organizing experience. Child accepts stories and beliefs literally. Ability to learn the beliefs and practices of the culture, religion.
Adolescence	Experience of the world now beyond the family unit and spiritual beliefs can aid understanding of extended environment. Generally conform to the beliefs of those around them; have not yet examined beliefs objectively.
Young adulthood	Development of a self-identity and worldview differentiated from those of others. The individual forms independent commitments, lifestyle, beliefs, and attitudes. Begins to develop personal meaning for symbols of religion and faith.
Mid-adulthood	Newfound appreciation for the past; increased respect for inner voice; more awareness of myths, prejudices, and images that exist because of social background. Attempts to reconcile contradictions in mind and experience and to remain open to others' truths.
Mid- to late adulthood	Able to believe in, and live with a sense of participation in, a nonexclusive community. May work to resolve social, political, economic, or ideological problems in society. Able to embrace life, yet hold it loosely. (Martin Luther King, Jr., Mahatma Gandhi, and Mother Teresa illustrate this stage.)

Note: From *Stages of Faith Development: The Psychology of Human Development and the Quest for Meaning,* by J. W. Fowler, 1981, San Francisco: HarperCollins Publishers, Inc. Adapted with permission from HarperCollins Publishers, Inc.

Muslims follow the practice of prayer fives times a day and the Muslim client may need assistance to maintain this commitment. In addition, Muslims traditionally gather on Friday at noon to worship and learn about their faith. Both Hindus and Buddhists practice meditation, and the nurse may create a quiet time for them to meditate.

Solemn religious observances throughout the year may be referred to as *high holy days* and may include fasting, reflection, and prayer. Examples of such holy days are Rosh Hashanah and Yom Kippur (Jewish), Good Friday (Christian), and Ramadan (Islam). Many hospitals and health organizations facilitate ritual observances for clients and staff on holy days. Because many religions follow calendars other than the Gregorian calendar, a multifaith calendar can be used to identify the holy days of the various religious groups (Griffith, 1996).

Sacred Writings

Each religion has sacred and authoritative scriptures that provide guidance for its adherents' beliefs and behaviors; in addition, sacred writings frequently tell instructive stories of the religion's leaders, kings, and heroes. In most religions, these scriptures are thought to be the word of the Supreme Being as written down by prophets or other human representatives. Christians rely on the Bible, Jews on the Torah and Talmud, and Muslims on the Koran; Hindus have several holy texts, or Vedas, and Buddhists value the teachings of the Tripitakas. Scriptures generally set forth religious law in the form of admonitions and rules for living (e.g., the Ten Commandments).

This religious law may be interpreted in various ways by subgroups of a religion's adherents and may affect a client's willingness to accept treatment suggestions; for example, blood transfusions are in conflict with the religious admonitions of Jehovah's Witnesses.

People often gain strength and hope from reading religious writings when they are ill or in crisis. Examples of scriptural stories that may give comfort to clients are Job's suffering, in both the Jewish and Christian scriptures, and Jesus's healing of people who were physically or mentally ill, in the New Testament.

Sacred Symbols

Sacred symbols include jewelry, medals, amulets, icons, totems, or body ornamentation (e.g., tattoos) that carry religious or spiritual significance. They may be worn to pronounce one's faith, to remind the practitioner of the faith, to provide spiritual protection, or to be a source of comfort or strength. People may wear religious medals at all times, and they may wish to wear them when they are undergoing diagnostic studies, medical treatment, or surgery. People who are Roman Catholic may carry a rosary for prayer; a person who is Muslim may carry a mala, or string of prayer beads (Figure 39–2 ■).

People may have religious icons or statues in their home, car, or place of work as a personal reminder of their faith or as part of a personal place of worship or meditation. Hospitalized clients or long-term care residents may wish to have their spiritual icons or statues with them as a source of comfort.

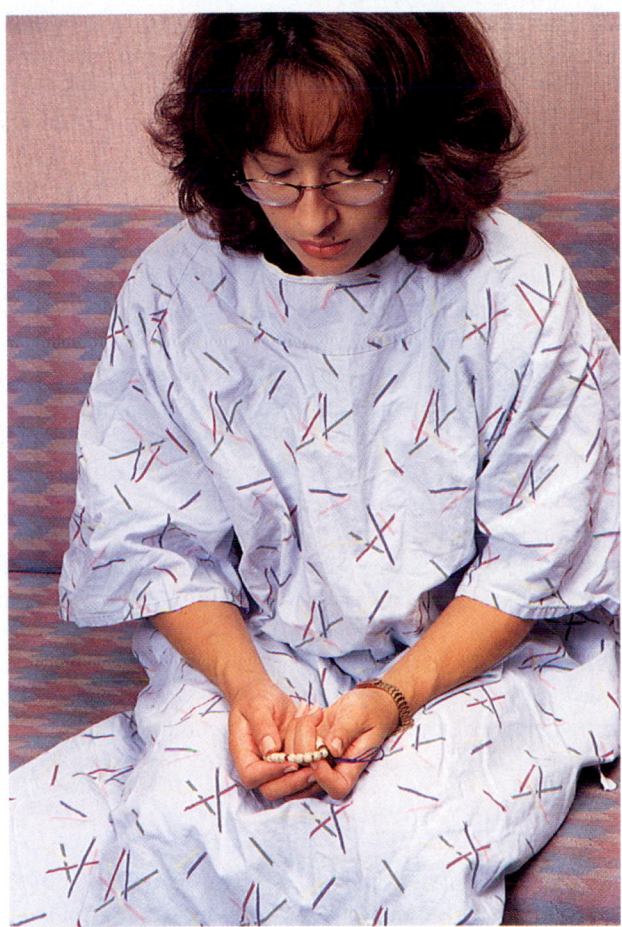

Figure 39–2 ■ Clients may bring objects to the hospital to use in prayer or other religious rituals. Caregivers should respect such objects, because they usually have great significance for clients.

Prayer and Meditation

Prayer is a spiritual practice; for many, it is also a religious practice. An encyclopedia of religion defines **prayer** simply as "human communication with divine and spiritual entities" (Gill, 1987, p. 489). Some argue that because prayer requires a belief in a divine or spiritual entity not all people pray, while others consider prayer a universal phenomenon that does not require such belief. Ulanov and Ulanov (1983), for example, proposed that everyone prays: "People pray whether or not they call it prayer. We pray every time we ask for help, understanding, or strength, in or out of religion . . . who and what we are speak out of us. . . . To pray is to listen to and hear this self who is speaking" (p. 1). Prayer is intention plus love, often communicated with "the Absolute," according to Dossey (1999); that is, prayer is a loving wish or thought for oneself or another, and not an invocation of positive or negative forms of magic.

There are different types of prayer experience. Poloma and Gallup (1991) categorized prayer experiences as follows:

- Ritual (e.g., Hail Mary, memorized prayers that can be repeated)
- Petitionary (e.g., "God, cure me!" or intercessory prayers when one is requesting something of the divine)

- Colloquial (i.e., conversational prayers)
- Meditational (e.g., moments of silence focused on nothing, a meaningful phrase, or on a certain aspect of the divine).

While meditational and colloquial prayer experiences have been found to be associated with spiritual well-being and quality of life in healthy adults, ritual and petitionary prayer experiences may be most comforting and appropriate for those who are ill.

Some religions have prescribed prayers that are printed in a prayer book, such as the Anglican/Episcopal *Book of Common Prayer* or the Catholic *Missal*. Some religious prayers are attributed to the source of faith; for example, the Lord's Prayer for Christians is attributed to Jesus, and the first sutra for Muslims is attributed to Mohammed.

Some religions require daily prayers or dictate specific times for prayer and worship: the five daily prayers, or Salat, of the Muslims (performed while facing east toward Mecca at dawn, noon, midafternoon, sunset, and evening), the daily Kaddish of the Jews, or the seven canonical prayers of the Roman Catholics. People who are ill may want to continue or increase their prayer practices (Moschella et al., 1997). They may need uninterrupted quiet time during which they have their prayer books, rosaries, malas, or other icons available to them.

Meditation is the act of focusing one's thoughts or engaging in self-reflection or contemplation. Some people believe that, through deep meditation, one can influence or control physical and psychologic functioning and the course of illness.

Beliefs Affecting Diet and Nutrition

Many religions have proscriptions regarding diet. There may be rules about which foods and beverages are allowed and which are prohibited. For example, Orthodox Jews are not to eat shellfish or pork, and Muslims are not to drink alcoholic beverages or eat pork. Members of the Church of Jesus Christ of Latter-Day Saints (Mormons) are not to drink caffeinated or alcoholic beverages. Older Catholics may choose not to eat meat on Fridays because it was proscribed in years past. Buddhists and Hindus are generally vegetarian, not wanting to take life to support life. Religious law may also dictate how food is prepared; for example, many Jewish people require **kosher** food, which is food prepared according to Jewish law.

Some solemn religious observances are marked by fasting, which is the abstinence from food for a specified period of time. Some religions also restrict beverages; others allow drinking of water or other sustaining beverages on fast days. Examples of religions that observe fasting include Islam, Judaism, and Catholicism. During the month of Ramadan, devout Muslims eat no food and avoid beverages during daylight hours; the fast is broken after sunset. Members of Jewish synagogues fast on Yom Kippur and devout Catholics may fast on Good Friday. Most religions lift the fasting requirements for seriously ill believers for whom fasting may be a detriment to health (e.g., diabetic clients). Some religions may exempt nursing mothers or menstruating women from fasting requirements.

It is important that health care providers prescribe diet plans with an awareness of the client's dietary and fasting beliefs.

Beliefs Related to Healing

Clients may have religious beliefs that attribute illness to a spiritual disruption. Healing for such clients may appear to be unrelated to current treatment practices. The nurse needs to assess the client's beliefs and, if possible, include in planning some aspects of healing that are part of the client's belief system.

Beliefs Related to Dress

Many religions have laws or traditions that dictate dress. For example, Orthodox and Conservative Jewish men believe that it is important to have their heads covered at all times and therefore wear yarmulkes. Orthodox Jewish women cover their hair with a wig or scarf as a sign of respect to God. Many Muslim women also cover their hair in accordance with their particular ethnic or national background. Mormons may wear temple undergarments in compliance with religious law.

Some religions require that women dress in a conservative manner, which may include wearing sleeves and modestly cut tops, and skirts that cover the knees. Some religions, for example, Islam, may require that the body (torso, arms, and legs) be covered. Hindu women accustomed to wearing saris prefer to cover all of the body except arms and feet (Figure 39–3 ■). Hospital gowns may make women wishing to comply with religious dress codes uneasy and uncomfortable. Clients may be especially disconcerted when undergoing diagnostic tests or treatments, such as mammography, that require body parts to be bared.

Beliefs Related to Birth

For all religions the birth of a child is an important event giving cause for celebration. Many religions have specific ritual

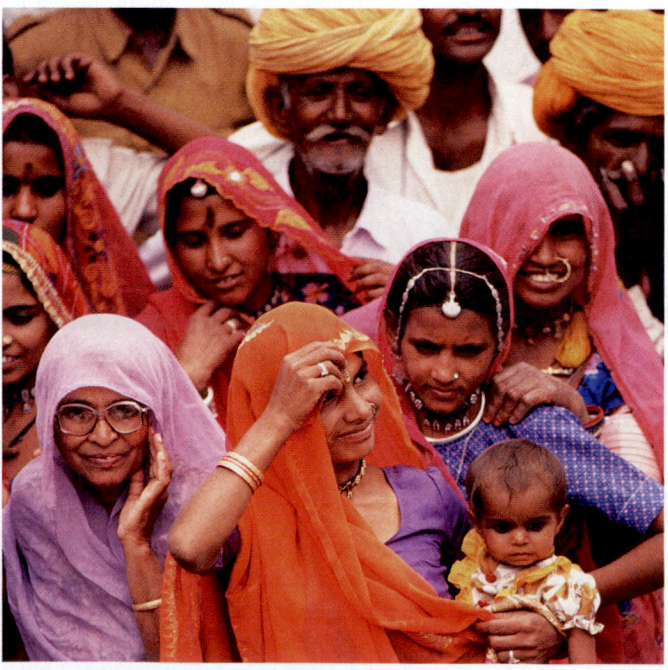

Figure 39–3 ■ Hindu women dressed in saris. (Charlie Westerman/Getty Images.)

ceremonies that consecrate the new child to God. When a Muslim child is born, "someone recites the call to prayer in the infant's ear." On the seventh day after birth, the child is named, and a tuft of hair is shaved from the head (Denny, 1993, p. 682).

In the Christian faith, baptism and christening ceremonies may take place after the birth of a child to confirm that the "infant [was] born into a Christian family as part of the organism of the church" (Frankiel, 1993, p. 556). Christian parents of seriously ill infants may want baptism performed at birth by the nurse or physician, if a chaplain or clergy person is not present.

In the Jewish religion, the ritual circumcision conducted on male children on the eighth day after birth is an expression of the religious bond between the prophet Abraham, his descendants, and their God. Following the ritual circumcision by the trained person, called a *mohel,* the child is named. Girls are named in the synagogue on the Sabbath after the birth (Fishbane, 1993).

When nurses are aware of the religious needs of families and their infants, they can assist families in fulfilling their religious obligations. This is especially important when the newborn infant is seriously ill or in danger of dying because some people believe that if religious obligations are not fulfilled the infant will not be accepted into the community of the faithful after death.

Beliefs Related to Death

Spiritual and religious beliefs play a significant role in the believer's approach to death just as they do in other major life events. Many believe that the person who dies transcends this life for a better place or state of being.

Some religions have special rituals surrounding dying and death that must be observed by the faithful. Observance of these rituals provides comfort to the dying person and their loved ones. Some rituals are carried out while the person is still alive, and can include special prayers, singing or chants, and reading of sacred scriptures. Roman Catholic priests perform the Sacrament of the Sick (previously referred to as the Last Rites) when clients are very ill or near death. Muslims who are dying want their body or head turned toward Mecca (Denny, 1993).

Jews have a tradition of burial within 24 hours following death, except on the Sabbath, and they "sit Shiva" (gather to pay respects), draping any mirrors in black to ensure that guests are focused on memory of the deceased rather than on themselves. Tibetan Buddhists read the *Tibetan Book of the Dead* within 7 days of the death to release the soul of the deceased from the Bardos, or nether worlds. Hindus cremate the body within 24 hours to release the soul from any earthly attachment.

Griffith (1996) suggests that during a terminal illness the client and family should be queried about observances or rituals that follow death. Some religions require that the body of the deceased be touched only by members of that faith. In both the Muslim (Denny, 1993) and the Jewish (Fishbane, 1993) religions, believers may require that a ritual bath be done after death by a family member or by a ritual burial society. Religious symbols or objects should be treated with respect and kept with the body (Griffith, 1996). The nurse can support the family of the deceased by providing an environment conducive to the performance of their traditional death rituals.

> **►CLINICAL ALERT** *Before sharing personal beliefs or practices, a nurse must consider questions such as the following:*
>
> - *For what purpose am I sharing my beliefs or practices? By doing so, am I meeting my needs or my client's?*
> - *Is my spiritual care reflecting a spiritual assessment?*
> - *Am I preying on a vulnerable client?*
> - *Am I offering my beliefs or practices in a manner that allows my client comfortably to refuse?*
> - *Does my spiritual care hurt or contribute to a therapeutic relationship with the client?* ■

SPIRITUAL HEALTH AND THE NURSING PROCESS

The nursing process, which includes assessing, diagnosing, planning, implementing, and evaluating, can be applied to the area of spiritual health.

NURSING MANAGEMENT

ASSESSING

Data about a client's spiritual beliefs are obtained from the client's general history (religious preferences or orientation); through a nursing history; and by clinical observations of the client's behavior, verbalizations, mood, and so on. Nurses should never assume that a client follows all the practices of the client's stated religion.

Nursing History

The Joint Commission on Accreditation for Healthcare Organizations (2000) now mandates that each client admitted to an institution's care must be assessed for spiritual beliefs and practices. Taylor (2002) recommends a two-tiered approach to spiritual assessment. All clients can be asked a general question or two (e.g., "What spiritual beliefs or practices are important to you now while you live with illness?" "How would you like your health care team to support you spiritually?"). Only those who manifest some type of unhealthful spiritual need or are at risk for spiritual distress need be subjected to a more thorough spiritual assessment. Even this assessment can be streamlined to hone in on the particular spiritual concern present.

Although the nurse will continually be assessing, the initial spiritual assessment is best taken at the end of the assessment process, or following the psychosocial assessment, after the nurse has developed a relationship with the client and/or support person. A nurse who has demonstrated sensitivity and personal warmth, earning some rapport, will be more successful during a spiritual assessment.

Assessment Interview
SPIRITUALITY

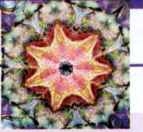

- Are any particular religious practices important to you? If so, could you please tell me about them?
- How will being here interfere with your religious practices?
- How is your faith helpful to you? In what ways is it important to you right now?
- In what ways can I support your spirit? For example, would you like me to read your prayer book to you?
- Would you like a visit from your spiritual counselor or the hospital chaplain? What are your hopes and your sources of strength right now? What comforts you during hard times?

The questions provided in the accompanying Assessment Interview may be suitable. Stoll (1989) suggests nurses obtain data about the client's concept of deity, sources of hope and strength, religious practices and rituals, and any relationship perceived between spiritual beliefs and health.

Clinical Assessment

Cues to spiritual and religious preferences, strengths, concerns, or distress may be revealed by one or more of the following (Shelley & Fish, 1988; Sumner, 1998):

1. *Environment.* Does the client have a Bible, Torah, Koran, other prayer book, devotional literature, religious medals, a rosary, cross, Star of David, or religious get-well cards in the room? Does a church send altar flowers or Sunday bulletins?
2. *Behavior.* Does the client appear to pray before meals or at other times or read religious literature? Does the client have nightmares and sleep disturbances or express anger at religious representatives or at a deity?
3. *Verbalization.* Does the client mention God or a higher power, prayer, faith, the church, synagogue, temple, a spiritual or religious leader, or religious topics? Does the client ask about a visit from the clergy? Does the client express fear of death, concern with the meaning of life, inner conflict about religious beliefs, concern about a relationship with the deity, questions about the meaning of existence or the meaning of suffering, or about the moral or ethical implications of therapy?
4. *Affect and attitude.* Does the client appear lonely, depressed, angry, anxious, agitated, apathetic, or preoccupied?
5. *Interpersonal relationships.* Who visits? How does the client respond to visitors? Does a minister come? How does the client relate to other clients and nursing personnel?

See also specific manifestations of spiritual well-being and spiritual distress on page 996.

DIAGNOSING

In diagnosing spiritual health, the nurse may find that spiritual problems provide the diagnostic label, or that spiritual distress is the etiology of the problem.

Spiritual Problems as the Diagnostic Label

The North American Nursing Diagnosis Association (NANDA International, 2003) recognizes three diagnoses related to spirituality: *Spiritual Distress, Readiness for Enhanced Spiritual Well-Being,* and *Risk for Spiritual Distress.*

- *Spiritual Distress* is "impaired ability to experience and integrate meaning and purpose in life through a person's connectedness with self, others, art, music, literature, nature, or a power greater than oneself" (p. 177). See Identifying Nursing Diagnoses, Outcomes, and Interventions for a clinical illustration of this diagnosis.
- *Readiness for Enhanced Spiritual Well-Being* recognizes that spiritual well-being is the "ability to experience and integrate meaning and purpose in life through a person's connectedness with self, others, art, music, literature, nature, or a power greater than oneself" (p. 180). This wellness diagnosis describing spiritual health acknowledges that some people respond to adversity with an increased sensitivity to spirituality or spiritual maturation.
- *Risk for Spiritual Distress* is defined by NANDA (2003) as being "at risk for an altered sense of harmonious connectedness with all of life and the universe in which dimensions that transcend and empower the self may be disrupted" (p. 179). This diagnosis may be appropriate for a client who presently shows no indication of this disruption of spirit yet may if a nurse fails to intervene.

Spiritual Distress as the Etiology

Spiritual distress may affect other areas of functioning and indicate other diagnoses. In these instances, spiritual distress becomes the etiology. Examples include

- *Fear* related to apprehension about soul's future after death and unpreparedness for death
- *Chronic* or *Situational Low Self-Esteem* related to failure to live within the precepts of one's faith
- *Disturbed Sleep Pattern* related to spiritual distress
- *Ineffective Coping* related to feelings of abandonment by God and loss of religious faith
- *Decisional Conflict* related to conflict between treatment plan and religious beliefs.

PLANNING

In the planning phase, the nurse identifies interventions to help the client achieve the overall goal of maintaining or restoring spiritual well-being so that spiritual strength, serenity, and satisfaction are realized (see Identifying Nursing Diagnoses, Outcomes, and Interventions).

Planning in relation to spiritual needs should be designed to do one or more of the following:

- Help the client fulfill religious obligations.
- Help the client draw on and use inner resources more effectively to meet the present situation.
- Help the client maintain or establish a dynamic, personal relationship with a supreme being in the face of unpleasant circumstances.
- Help the client find meaning in existence and the present situation.

- Promote a sense of hope.
- Provide spiritual resources otherwise unavailable.

IMPLEMENTING

Nursing actions to help clients meet their spiritual needs include (a) providing presence, (b) supporting religious practices, (c) assisting clients with prayer, and (d) referring clients for spiritual counseling.

Providing Presence

Presencing, which is defined as being present, being there, or just being with a client, is a term that identifies one of the competencies incorporated by expert nurses (Zerwekh, 1997). Pettigrew (1990) identified four distinguishing features of presencing:

- Giving of self in the present moment
- Being available with all of the self
- Listening, with full awareness of the privilege of doing so
- Being there in a way that is meaningful to another person.

Fredriksson (1999) noted that presencing is a "gift of self" given by the nurse who maintains an attitude of attentiveness toward the client. Thus, nurses who listen attentively to clients yet fail to give of self (i.e., inwardly "make room") diminish their effectiveness.

There are multiple levels of presencing. Osterman and Schwartz-Barcott (1996) identified four ways of being present for clients:

- Presence (when a nurse is physically present but not focused on the client)
- Partial presence (when a nurse is physically present and attending to some task on the client's behalf but not relating to the client on any but the most superficial level)
- Full presence (when a nurse is mentally, emotionally, and physically present; intentionally focusing on the client)
- Transcendent presence (when a nurse is physically, mentally, emotionally, and spiritually present for a client; involves a transpersonal and transforming experience).

Presencing is often the best and sometimes the only intervention to support a client who suffers under circumstances that medical interventions cannot address. When a client is helpless, powerless, and vulnerable, a nurse's presencing can be most beneficial. Rather than worrying about saying or doing "the right thing," nurses should focus on being fully present (Taylor, 2002).

Supporting Religious Practices

During the assessment of the client, the nurse will have obtained specific information about the client's religious preference and practices. Nurses need to consider specific religious practices that will affect nursing care, such as the client's beliefs about birth, death, dress, diet, prayer, sacred symbols, sacred writings, and holy days as discussed earlier in this chapter. The Practice Guidelines on page 1004 outlines ways the nurse can help clients to continue their usual spiritual practices. Box 39–3 provides health-related information about specific religions.

IDENTIFYING NURSING DIAGNOSES, OUTCOMES, AND INTERVENTIONS

CLIENTS WITH SPIRITUAL DISTRESS

DATA CLUSTER	NURSING DIAGNOSIS/ DEFINITION	SAMPLE DESIRED OUTCOME [NOC#]/DEFINITION	INDICATORS	SELECTED INTERVENTIONS [NIC#]/DEFINITION	SAMPLE NIC ACTIVITIES
Marilyn Eckhardt, 72 years old, is crying, fingering her rosary, and voicing concern that she has not seen her priest for confession since being admitted to the hospital. She states that she is afraid to die without confessing her sins. She also states that she does not want to see the hospital chaplain, but rather her own priest, whose parish is about 30 miles away. The hospital record indicates that Ms. Eckhardt is Roman Catholic.	*Spiritual Distress* related to inability to practice spiritual ritual (confession with parish priest)/ *Impaired ability to experience and integrate meaning and purpose in life through a person's connectedness with self, others, art, music, literature, nature, or a power greater than oneself*	Spiritual Well-Being [2001]/*Personal expressions of connectedness with self, others, higher power, all life, nature, and the universe that transcend and empower the self*	Mildly Compromised • Interaction with spiritual leaders • Participation in spiritual rites and passages • Prayer	Spiritual Support [5420]/*Assisting the client to feel balance and connection with a greater power*	• Refer to spiritual advisor of client's choice • Encourage chapel service attendance, if desired • Encourage the use of spiritual resources, if desired • Provide desired spiritual articles, according to client preferences
John Ames, 42 years old, is in a terminal state with an AIDS-related condition. He has become withdrawn but states to the nurse, "What have I done that God has punished me so?" The nurse observes religious literature on his bedside cabinet.	*Spiritual Distress* related to crisis of illness and impending death/ *Impaired ability to experience and integrate meaning and purpose in life through a person's connectedness with self, others, art, music, literature, nature, or a power greater than oneself*	Dignified Dying [1303]/ *Maintaining personal control and comfort with the approaching end of life*	To a Great Extent • Discusses spiritual experiences • Discusses spiritual concerns • Shares feelings about dying	Spiritual Support [5420]/ *Assisting the client to feel balance and connection with a greater power*	• Be available to listen to client's feelings • Be open to client's feelings about illness and death • Use values clarification techniques to help client clarify beliefs and values, as appropriate • Encourage the use of spiritual resources, if desired

BOX 39-3 ■ Health-related Information about Specific Religions: A Sampler

Amish, Mennonite—Likely will not have insurance coverage; rely on religious community for support.

Anglicans, Episcopalians, Roman Catholics—Appreciate receiving Eucharist (Holy Communion), a ritual of ingesting bread and wine (or grape juice) led by clergy or lay leaders to commemorate death of Jesus. Forehead may be marked by priest with ashes on Ash Wednesday (40 days before Easter); no need to wash off. Lenten season (Ash Wednesday to Easter) may involve some degree of abstention from food.

Buddhist—May be vegetarian. Facilitate meditation (may desire incense, visual focal point, use breathing or chanting, etc.).

Christian Scientist—Typically oppose Western medical interventions, relying instead on lay and professional Christian Science practitioners.

Hindu—Most eat no beef; many are vegetarian. Cleanliness highly valued. Many food preferences (e.g., foods fresh or cooked in oil).

Jehovah's Witnesses—Abstain from most blood products; need to discuss alternative treatments such as blood conservation strategies, autologous techniques, hematopoietic agents, nonblood volume expanders, and so on; contact local Jehovah's Witness hospital liaison committee.

Jews—Some observe kosher diet to varying degrees (e.g., avoid pork and shellfish, do not mix dairy and meat). Sabbath observance varies (e.g., Orthodox Jews avoid traveling in vehicles, writing, turning on electric appliances and lights, etc.).

Latter-Day Saints (LDS or Mormons)—Avoid alcohol, caffeine, smoking. Prefer to wear temple undergarments. Arrange for priestly blessing if requested.

Muslim—Respect modesty, avoid nakedness. Provide same-gender nurse if possible. Support prayers five times daily (may need to assist with ritual washing and positioning beforehand). Allow for family and imam (religious leader) to follow Islamic guidelines for burial when client dies. Eat no pork. Children, pregnant, elderly, and sick exempt from daytime fast during month of Ramadan.

Roman Catholics—Sacrament of the Sick (previously known as Last Rites) appropriate for the ill. Be aware that some may think rite means they are dying.

Seventh-Day Adventists—Avoid unnecessary treatments on Saturday (Sabbath). Sabbath begins Friday sundown, ends Saturday sundown. Adventists prefer restful, spirit-nurturing, family activities on Sabbaths. Likely to be vegetarian and abstain from caffeinated beverages. Do not smoke or drink alcohol.

Assisting Clients with Prayer

Prayer involves a sense of love and connection, as well as a reaching out. It has many health benefits and healing properties (Dossey, 1996). It offers a means for someone to talk to, a mechanism for expressing care, and a sense of serenity and connection with something greater.

Clients may choose to participate in private prayer or want group prayer with family, friends, or clergy. In such situations the nurse's major responsibility is to ensure a quiet environment and privacy. Nursing care may need to be adjusted to accommodate periods for prayer.

Illness can interfere with some clients' ability to pray. Feelings such as anxiety, fear, guilt, grief, despair, and isola-

tion can produce barriers to relationships in general and to the relationship the person has with the Divine. In these instances the client may ask the nurse to pray with them. Prayers with clients should only be done when there is mutual agreement between the clients and those praying with them. Nurses who are unaccustomed to praying aloud or in public may find it helpful to have a formal prayer or a scriptural passage readily available. Because prayer can evoke deep feelings, the nurse needs to spend time with the client following a prayer to enable the client to express these feelings. The accompanying Practice Guidelines provide clinical suggestions for praying with clients.

Practice Guidelines
Supporting Religious Practices

- Create a trusting relationship with the client so that any religious concerns or practices can be openly discussed and addressed.
- If unsure of client religious needs, ask how nurses can assist in having these needs met. Avoid relying on personal assumptions when caring for clients.
- Do not discuss personal spiritual beliefs with a client unless the client requests it. Be sure to assess whether such self-disclosure contributes to a therapeutic nurse–client relationship.
- Inform clients and family caregivers about spiritual support available at your institution (e.g., chapel or meditation room, chaplain services).
- Allow time and privacy for, and provide comfort measures prior to, private worship, prayer, meditation, reading, or other spiritual activities.
- Respect and ensure safety of client's religious articles (e.g., icons, amulets, clothing, jewelry).
- If desired by client, facilitate clergy or spiritual care specialist visitation. Collaborate with chaplain (if available).
- Prepare client's environment for spiritual rituals or clergy visitations as needed (e.g., have chair near bedside for clergy, create private space).
- Make arrangements with dietician so that dietary needs can be met. If institution cannot accommodate client's needs, ask family to bring food. (Most religions have some recommendations about diet, such as espousing vegetarianism, rejecting alcohol.)
- Acquaint yourself with the religions, spiritual practices, and cultures of the area in which you are working.
- Remember the difference between facilitating/supporting a client's religious practice and participating in it yourself.
- Ask another nurse to assist you if a particular religious practice makes you uncomfortable.
- All spiritual interventions must be done within agency guidelines.

Research Note
Spiritual Conflicts Associated with Praying about Cancer

A qualitative study of 30 persons living with cancer was conducted to determine the how, when, what, and outcomes of prayer during life-threatening illness. Because the informants unexpectedly and covertly referred to spiritual conflicts associated with praying, the researchers conducted a secondary analysis of the data. These data, which were collected using in-depth interviews and then content analyzed, revealed several spiritual concerns that occur for some individuals who pray about their illness. Themes included:

- Wondering about "unanswered" prayers
- Hesitancy to pray in a petitionary way
- Inner struggle about releasing control to God
- Questioning the nature of God (e.g., "Is God able or willing to cure me?")

- Wondering why and how a loving, powerful God could allow suffering
- Bargaining with God for something (e.g., to live to see a grandchild born)
- Doubting if prayer works
- Wondering if they are personally worthy, or spiritually good enough
- Wondering if they were praying the "right" way.

These findings extend previous research that reports how clients frequently find prayer a helpful coping strategy. While clients can believe in and use prayer, they may also concurrently have doubts or questions about prayer. Nurses can be sensitive to these spiritual conflicts and provide support.

Note: From "Spiritual Conflicts Associated with Praying about Cancer," by E. J. Taylor, F. H. Outlaw, T. Bernardo, and A. Roy, 1999, *Psycho-Oncology, 8,* pp. 386–394.

Practice Guidelines
Praying with Clients

- Clients' preferences for prayer reflect their personalities. That is, introverts may prefer being alone to pray, and their prayers will reflect their capacity for introspection. In contrast, extroverts' prayers may revolve around their relationships with others and be expressed in creative, verbal ways. Similarly, a prayer of a feeling type of client may be emotion filled, whereas the prayer of a thinking-type client may be based on ideas and logic. Structure prayer interventions accordingly.
- When assessing whether a client would like you to pray, ask to pray in a way that allows both of you to feel comfortable if the answer is no. ("Some people tell me prayer helps them to cope with rough times like this. Would you feel comfortable if I prayed with you?")
- Assess how the client approaches the addressee of prayer. For example, a Baptist may pray to Jesus, whereas a Jew would pray directly to God, or Yahweh. This assessment can usually be made while listening to a client talk about religious beliefs.
- Before praying, assess what they would like for you to pray. Listen carefully. The answer may provide greater insight into their fears and concerns.
- Personalize the prayer. Present your client's name and personal concerns to the Divine.
- Prayer can be used to summarize a conversation. This lets the client know you have heard what was said. It may also help the client to view circumstances more objectively.
- Prayer may be the springboard to further discussion or catharsis. Stay with the client after a prayer until there has been time for conversation.
- Follow a prayer with nonverbal communication (e.g., eye contact or touch) to convey "See, I am me, a person, and you are you, and we have returned from our brief journey inward."

- Remember some clients would like to pray aloud with you, just as you may with them. This can be a beautiful experience that nurtures both the client and nurse. It allows the client to reciprocate caring.
- Be mindful of one difference between magic and prayer. Magic invokes a greater power for personal gain. Prayer allows the greater power to do the greater good ("Thy will be done").
- Praying with a client may not involve verbalization. You may feel it will be more comfortable or appropriate if you remain quiet and fully present, praying silently.
- Facilitate the clients' prayer practices. Schedule time for them when they will be undisturbed, palliate distressing symptoms that interfere with praying, help with articles that accompany prayers (e.g., rosaries, prayer garments, books of prayers), and so on.
- In times of distress, a client or loved one may not be able to construct a prayer spontaneously. You may want to teach a centering prayer that is very brief (e.g., "Lord, have mercy/healing"). Nurses can discuss with care recipients what prayer would benefit them most and encourage them to use it while alone. These prayers may be more beneficial when they are framed in a positive sense. To illustrate, "Jesus loves me" or "The Lord has mercy."
- Encourage clients to think (privately or with you) about what prayer means to them. Offer questions like these: Why do you pray? What do you expect from your praying? Are these expectations appropriate? How content are you with your prayer experiences? Is there a yearning for something more in your prayer experience?

Note: From "Caring for the Spirit," by E. J. Taylor. In *Psychosocial Dimensions of Oncology Nursing Care,* by C. C. Burke (Ed.), 1998, pp. 55–75. Pittsburgh, PA: Oncology Nursing Press. Adapted with permission.

Practice Guidelines
When Nurse–Client Spiritual Values Conflict: Steps to Resolution

- Assess spiritual or religious assumptions or beliefs that determine client's approach to explaining illness and responding to it. For example, What do you think has caused your illness [or distressed your spirit]? What do you think your sickness does to you [spiritually]? How does it work? What do you think are the best things to do for your illness [or spiritual health]? What [spiritual] concerns has your illness caused you? What do you do about them?
- Explain simply to the client your beliefs about the cause (or meaning) and how best to respond to (or cope with) this illness.
- Openly compare with the client how these beliefs differ.

- Objectively discuss how your different religious and cultural backgrounds contribute to these contrasting beliefs.
- Encourage the client to ask questions about your model.
- Support client beliefs and practices that are healthful (from your perspective).
- Accommodate for client beliefs and practices that are neither helpful nor harmful.
- Change and provide alternatives for client beliefs and practices that are harmful without trying to change the underlying belief system, if possible. Engage family member(s) or client's clergy as therapeutic allies.

Note: From "Spirituality, Culture, and Cancer Care," by E. J. Taylor, 2001, *Seminars in Oncology Nursing, 17,* pp. 197–205. Adapted with permission.

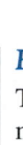
MediaLink | TREATING A PARALYZED CLIENT CARE PLAN ACTIVITY

Referring Clients for Spiritual Counseling

There are times when spiritual care is best referred to other members of the health care team. Referrals can be made for hospitalized clients and their families through the hospital chaplain's office if one is available. Nurses in home and community health settings can identify spiritual resources by checking directories of community service agencies, telephone directories, or religious directories that describe available spiritual counselors and the services provided through the religious community. Many religious counselors will provide assistance to members of their faith who are not members of their specific religious community. For example, a priest may attend a client in the hospital or at home even though the person is not a member of the priest's parish.

Referrals may be necessary when the nurse makes a diagnosis of spiritual distress. In this situation the nurse and religious counselor can work together to meet the client's needs. One situation the nurse may encounter is client refusal of necessary medical intervention because of religious tenets. In this case the nurse encourages the client, physician, and spiritual adviser to discuss the conflict and consider alternative methods of therapy. The nurse's major role is to provide information the client needs to make an informed decision, and to support the client's decision. See the accompanying Practice Guidelines.

EVALUATING

Using the measurable desired outcomes developed during the planning stage, the nurse collects data needed to judge whether client goals and outcomes have been achieved. See the accompanying Nursing Care Plan.

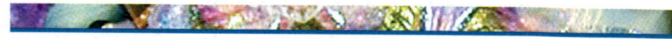

Lifespan Considerations

Elders

```
                    SPIRIT TITER
DIS-SPIRITED _____ INSPIRED
(low)                                        (high)
```

Spirituality can be compared to developmental stages in that individuals are often at different places as a result of life experiences, coping skills, social supports, and, most important, their individual belief systems. Older adults experience multiple changes and losses over their life span and if their spirit titer is low they may become dis-spirited, or depressed. If they have a high spirit titer, they will lean toward being inspired and becoming an inspiration to others in spite of hardships they may have experienced.

Nurses need to direct their goals and planning to assist the client in attaining and maintaining a high spirit titer. This can be done by

- Being a presence with that person, showing acceptance and listening authentically.

- Recognizing and validating inner resources of an individual, such as coping methods, humor, motivation, self-determination, positive attitude, and optimism.
- Assisting the client to leave a legacy by storytelling and/or recording life stories for family and friends.
- Encouraging creative expression, as in art, music, and writing. This keeps the imagination alive and serves to regenerate the body, mind, and spirit.
- Developing ways to keep in touch with nature and maintain a sense of wonder. Recognizing the seasons, the emergence of flowers in spring, the phases of the moon, the migrations of birds, and the unchanging stars provides examples of orderliness in the universe, even in the midst of chaos and loss.

An inspired person will find hope, meaning, purpose, and value in existence.

Note: From *The Transparent Self,* by S. Jourard, 1971, New York: D. Van Nostrand. Adapted with permission.

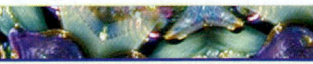

Focus on Critical Thinking

Terry is a 32-year-old male who received several pints of blood following an automobile accident 10 years ago. Five years ago he was diagnosed with acquired immune deficiency syndrome (AIDS) and is now in the hospital with pneumonia and severe diarrhea. He is very ill and very discouraged. While you are caring for Terry, he comments, "I might as well die right now because I'm not going to get well. My folks were Methodist, but I guess I'm being punished because I'm not very religious."

1. Terry stated that he was "not very religious." Does that mean that he is not spiritual? Explain.
2. What data suggest that Terry may be experiencing spiritual distress?
3. How might illness affect one's spiritual beliefs? Religious beliefs?
4. How might a spiritual assessment be of benefit to both you and Terry?

See Critical Thinking Possibilities in Appendix A.

NURSING CARE PLAN FOR SPIRITUAL DISTRESS

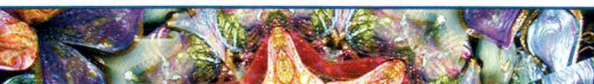

ASSESSMENT DATA		NURSING DIAGNOSIS	DESIRED OUTCOMES [NOC #]/INDICATORS*
Nursing Assessment Mrs. Sally Horton is a 60-year-old hospitalized homemaker who is recovering from a right radical mastectomy. Her physician told her yesterday that due to metastases of the cancer, her prognosis is poor. This morning her nurse finds her tearful, stating she slept poorly and has no appetite. She asks the nurse, "Why has God done this to me? Perhaps it's because I have sinned in my life. I've not gone to church or spoken to a minister in several years. Is there a chapel in the hospital where I could go and pray? I'm terribly afraid of dying and what awaits me."	**Physical Examination** Height: 165.1 cm (5′ 5″) Weight: 54.0 kg (199 lb) Temperature: 36.6C (98F) Pulse: 88 BPM Respirations: 22/minute Blood Pressure: 146/86 mm Hg Large surgical dressing right chest wall and axillary region, dry and intact. Slight edema right hand and arm. **Diagnostic Data** RBC: 3.5×10^6/mL Hgb: 10.5 g/L Hct: 35%	*Spiritual Distress* related to feelings of guilt and alienation from God as evidenced by questioning why "God has done this"; inquiries about praying in a chapel; insomnia; no appetite	Spiritual Well-Being [2001] as evidenced by not compromised • Interacts with spiritual leader of her religion • Uses a type of prayer experience that provides her comfort • Connectedness with others to share thoughts, feelings, and beliefs

NURSING INTERVENTIONS [NIC #] / SELECTED ACTIVITIES*	RATIONALE
Spiritual Support [5420]/ • Be open to Mrs. Horton's feelings about illness and death.	*Encourages expression of inner fears and concerns and teaches the client the value of confronting issues.*
• Assist her to properly express and relieve anger in appropriate ways.	*Anger can be a source of energy and its release a source of freedom when expressed in a constructive manner.*
• Use values clarification techniques to help Mrs. Horton clarify beliefs and values.	*Value conflicts often lead to confusion and indecision. Clarification of beliefs and values will help clients base decisions on their most important values, including those that are spiritual in nature.*
• Observe and listen empathetically to her communication.	*The nature of spiritual care may directly affect the speed and quality of recovery and/or redefining hope and finding meaning in death.*
• Facilitate Mrs. Horton's use of meditation, prayer, and other religious traditions and rituals.	*Spiritual needs may sometimes be overlooked or ignored. Recognizing and respecting the individual's spiritual needs is an important advocacy role for nurses.*
• Provide full or transcendant presencing.	*The nurse's therapeutic presence provides comfort and alleviates a client's sense of aloneness or abandonment—a frequent fear among those who are dying.*

continued on page 1008

NURSING INTERVENTIONS [NIC #] / SELECTED ACTIVITIES*	RATIONALE

Values Clarification [5480]

- Create an accepting, nonjudgmental atmosphere.

- Use appropriate questions to assist Mrs. Horton in reflecting on the situation and what is important personally.

- Encourage her to list values that guide behavior in times of tragedy.

- Help Mrs. Horton to evaluate how her values are in agreement or conflict with those of family members or significant others.

Establishes rapport and the therapeutic relationship, which promotes communication and open expression.

Helps the client explore the whys of how she is feeling and identify personal values that may have an impact on the current situation and future decisions.

Helps the client clarify values and beliefs by reflecting on past behaviors. Experience is a major source for values development.

Decisions and actions may be contradictory to the client's own values if the need to please others is greater than the need to please themselves.

EVALUATION

Outcome met. Mrs. Horton has been visited on several occasions by her minister. She reads scripture each day and has found consolation in reading the Book of Psalms. She states "God is merciful and will help me bear my suffering."

*Outcomes, interventions and activities selected are only a sample of those suggested by NOC and NIC and should be further individualized for each client.

CONCEPT MAP   Spiritual Distress

S.H.
63 y.o. female ♀
Metastatic breast cancer
(R) radical mastectomy
poor prognosis

- Drsg dry/intact
- Sl. edema (R) hand & arm
- Tearful
- States slept poorly
- No appetite

- Height: 165.1 (5'5")
- Weight: 54 kg (147 lb)
- T36.6 C
- P 88/min
- R 22 min
- BP 146/86
- Large surgical drsng (R) chest wall and axillary region
- RBC 3.5×10^6/mL
- Hgb:10.5g/dL
- Hct 35%

- "Why has God done this to me? Perhaps because I have sinned."
- "I haven't gone to church in several years."
- "I'm afraid of dying."
- Asks if there is a chapel in hospital.

Spiritual Distress r/t feelings of guilt and alienation from God

Spiritual Well-Being aeb not compromised
- interacts with spiritual leader of her religion
- uses a type of prayer experience that provides her comfort
- connects with others to share thoughts, feelings, and beliefs

Spiritual Support

- Be open to her feelings about illness and death.
- Facilitate use of meditation, prayer, and other traditions and rituals.
- Observe and listen empathetically.
- Assist her to properly express and relieve anger.
- Provide full or transcendant presencing.

Values Clarification

- Create an accepting, nonjudgmental atmosphere.
- Encourage her to list values that guide behavior in times of tragedy.
- Use appropriate questions to assist her to reflect on the situation and what is important personally.
- Help evaluate how her values agree or are in conflict with family members/ significant others.

Outcome met
- has been visited on several occasions by her minister.
- she reads scripture each day.
- finds consolation in reading the Book of Psalms.
- states "God is merciful and will help me bear my suffering."

Legend: Assessment ☐ Nursing Diagnosis ☐ Outcomes ☐ Nursing Interventions ☐ Activities ☐ Evaluation/Reassessment ☐

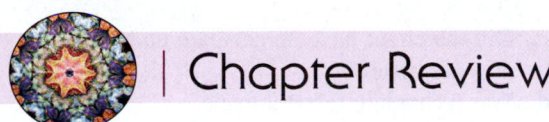

Chapter Review

EXPLORE MediaLink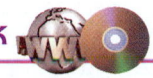

NCLEX review questions, case studies, care plan activities, MediaLink applications, and other interactive resources for this chapter can be found on the Companion Website at www.prenhall.com/kozier. Click on Chapter 39 to select the activities for this chapter.

For more NCLEX review questions, and an audio glossary, access the Student CD-ROM accompanying this textbook.

Chapter Highlights

- To implement spiritual care, nurses need to be skilled in establishing a trusting nurse–client relationship.
- Clients have a right to receive care that respects their individual spiritual and religious values.
- Because spiritual beliefs and practices are highly personal, nurses must respect the rights of people to hold their own spiritual beliefs and to communicate or not communicate these to others.
- Nurses need to be aware of their own spiritual beliefs in order to be comfortable assisting others.
- The spiritual needs of clients and support persons often come into focus at a time of illness. Spiritual beliefs can help people accept illness and plan for what lies ahead.
- Spiritual distress refers to a disturbance in or a challenge to a person's belief or value system that provides strength, hope, and meaning to life. Possible factors in spiritual distress include physiologic problems, treatment-related concerns, and situational concerns. Spiritual distress may be reflected in a number of behaviors, including depression, anxiety, verbalizations of unworthiness, and fear of death.

- Nurses can support clients' religious practices if they understand needs related to holy days, sacred writings, sacred symbols, prayer and meditation, dietary practices, dress requirements or prohibitions, healing, birth rituals, and death rituals.
- A spiritual assessment is best obtained after the nurse has developed a relationship with the client. Information may be elicited about the client's concept of the deity or creative force, the client's source of hope and strength, the significance of religious practices and rituals, and the relationship the client perceives between health and spiritual beliefs.
- Nursing interventions that promote spiritual well-being include offering one's presence, supporting the client's religious practices, praying with a client, and referring the client to a religious counselor.

Review Questions

39–1. When planning care for an elder residing in your skilled nursing facility who is searching to make life meaningful, which nursing action would be most beneficial?
  a. Assess for depression.
  b. Diagnose and document that the client has "spiritual distress."
  c. Keep the client busy with social activities.
  d. Explore with the client the kind of legacy desired to leave.

39–2. Your client's wife asks you to pray for her. What would be the best initial response for a nurse who personally believes in prayer?
  a. "May I call the chaplain to come and pray with you?"
  b. "I know your faith is important to you. It is to me, too."
  c. "For what would you like me to pray?"
  d. "Isn't it wonderful that we have a God with whom we can share our concerns?"

39–3. Your client is experiencing severe pain that cannot be controlled by analgesics. An appropriate intervention is full presencing, which involves:
  a. physical presence.
  b. physical presence with mental awareness of the client.
  c. physical, mental, and emotional presence.
  d. physical, mental, emotional, and spiritual presence.

39–4. Your client reports, "Cancer was the best thing that happened to me! It is making me appreciate life so much more." This statement supports which NANDA diagnosis?
  a. *Spiritual Distress*
  b. *Risk for Spiritual Distress*
  c. *Readiness for Enhanced Spiritual Well-Being*
  d. *Cognitive Denial*

39–5. A dying client states, "Part of what makes dying hard is that I don't know for sure where I'm going. Nurse, what do you believe happens in the hereafter?" In evaluating

spiritual care given to this client, the nurse should consider which of the following?
a. Was the client satisfied with answers provided?
b. Was the therapeutic effectiveness of the nurse–client relationship compromised?

c. Did the client have an accurate understanding of all afterlife beliefs?
d. Was a chaplain referral made?

Readings and References

Suggested Readings

Andrews, M. M., & Hanson, P. A. (2003). Religion, culture, and nursing. In M. M. Andrews & J. S. Boyle (Eds.), *Transcultural concepts in nursing care* (4th ed., pp. 432–502). Philadelphia: Lippincott.
The authors discuss religious practices, holy days, sacraments, beliefs related to healing, and beliefs of major world religions about diet, medications, medical treatment, and surgical procedures. Andrews and Hanson also discuss health issues that may be controversial within the religious group, the religious support system for ill believers, and religion-specific issues related to death and dying.

Burkhardt, M. A., & Nagai-Jacobson, M. G. (2002). *Spirituality: Living our connectedness.* Albany, NY: Delmar.
These nurse authors write thoroughly about ways health care professionals can heal themselves through nurturing their own spirituality. They discuss numerous approaches to spiritual self-care.

O'Brien, M. E. (1999). *Spirituality in nursing: Standing on holy ground.* Sudbury, MA: Jones & Bartlett.
Written by a Roman Catholic nurse academician, this is a text about the relationship between spirituality and health. O'Brien discusses spiritual needs of clients with acute and chronic illness, as well as those of children, families, older adults, and dying persons.

Sumner, H. (1998). Recognizing and responding to spiritual distress. *American Journal of Nursing, 98* (1), 26–31.
This continuing education article includes the scope of spiritual distress, a spiritual needs assessment guide, barriers to spiritual care, and points to consider in providing care that respects the individual spiritual values of clients.

Taylor, E. J. (2002). *Spiritual care: Nursing theory, research, and practice.* Upper Saddle River, NJ: Prentice Hall.
This nurse author describes in practical terms how nurses can nurture spiritual health in their clients. Based on theory and research, she discusses conducting spiritual assessments; documentation and diagnosis of spiritual concerns; how to assist clients in transforming tragedy; how to support spiritual rituals like prayer; and how to nurture spirituality with journal writing, art, dream analysis, empathic listening, and more.

Related Research

Halstead, M. T., & Hull, M. (2001). Struggling with paradoxes: The process of spiritual development in women with cancer. *Oncology Nursing Forum, 28,* 1534–1544.

Moadel, A., Morgan, C., Fatone, A., Grennan, J., Carter, J., Laruffa, et al. (1999). Seeking meaning and hope: Self-reported spiritual and existential needs among an ethnically diverse cancer patient population. *Psycho-Oncology 8,* 378–385.

Taylor, E. J., & Outlaw, F. H. (2002). Use of prayer among persons with cancer. *Holistic Nursing Practice, 16*(3), 46–60.

References

Carpenito, L. J. (2002). *Nursing diagnosis: Application to clinical practice* (9th ed.). Philadelphia: Lippincott.

Carson, V. B. (1989). *Spiritual dimensions of nursing practice.* Philadelphia: Saunders.

Coward, D. D. (1990). The lived experience of self-transcendence in women with advanced breast cancer. *Nursing Science Quarterly, 3*(4), 162–169.

Denny, F. M. (1993). Islam and the Muslim community. In H. Byron Earhart (Ed.), *Religious traditions of the world* (pp. 603–713). New York: HarperSanFrancisco.

Dossey, L. (1996). *Prayer is good medicine. How to reap the benefits of prayer.* New York: HarperCollins.

Dossey, L. (1999). Healing and the nonlocal mind: Interview by Bonnie Horrigan. *Alternative Therapies in Health and Medicine, 5*(6), 85–93.

Ellison, C. W. (1983, April). Spiritual well-being: Conceptualization and measurement. *Journal of Psychology and Theology, 11,* 330–340.

Fishbane, M. (1993). Judaism: Revelation and traditions. In H. Byron Earhart (Ed.), *Religious traditions of the world* (pp. 373–484). New York: HarperSanFrancisco.

Fowler, J. W. (1981). *Stages of faith development: The psychology of human development and the quest for meaning.* San Francisco: Harper & Row.

Frankiel, S. S. (1993). Christianity: A way of salvation. In H. Byron Earhart (Ed.), *Religious traditions of the world* (pp. 484–601). New York: HarperSanFrancisco.

Fredriksson, L. (1999). Modes of relating in a caring conversation: A research synthesis on presence, touch, and listening. *Journal of Advanced Nursing, 30,* 1167–1176.

Gill, S. D. (1987). Prayer. In M. Eliade (Ed.), *The encyclopedia of religion* (pp. 489–492). New York: Macmillan.

Griffith, J. K. (1996). *The religious aspects of nursing care.* Vancouver, BC: Author.

Johnson, M., Maas, M., & Moorhead, S. (2000). *Nursing outcomes classification (NOC)* (2nd ed.). St. Louis, MO: Mosby.

Joint Commission on Accreditation of Healthcare Organizations. (2000). *Hospital accreditation standards.* Oakbrook, IL: Author.

Jourard, S. (1971). *The transparent self.* London: D. Van Nostrand.

Martsolf, D. S., & Mickley, J. R. (1998). The concept of spirituality in nursing theories: Differing world-views and extent of focus. *Journal of Advanced Nursing, 27,* 294–303.

McCloskey, J. C., & Bulechek, G. M. (2000). *Nursing interventions classification (NIC)* (3rd ed.). St. Louis, MO: Mosby.

Mickley, J. R., & Cowles, K. (2001). Ameliorating the tension: Use of forgiveness for healing. *Oncology Nursing Forum, 28,* 31–38.

Moschella, V. D., Pressman, K. R., Pressman, P., & Weissman, D. E. (1997, Spring). The problem of theodicy and religious response to cancer. *Journal of Religion & Health, 36*(1), 17–20.

NANDA International. (2003). *NANDA nursing diagnoses: Definitions and classification 2003-2004.* Philadelphia: Author.

Osterman, P., & Schwartz-Barcott, D. (1996). Presence: Four ways of being there. *Nursing Forum, 31*(2), 23–30.

Pargament, K. I. (1997). *The psychology of religion and coping.* New York: Guilford.

Pettigrew, J. (1990). Intensive nursing care: The ministry of presence. *Critical Care Nursing Clinics of North America, 2,* 503–508.

Pilch, J. J. (1988, May/June). Wellness spirituality. *Health Values, 12,* 28–31.

Poloma, M. M., & Gallup G. H., Jr. (1991). *Varieties of prayer: A survey report.* Philadelphia: Trinity Press International.

Reed, S. (1991). *Spirituality.* Paramus, NJ: Salesiana Publishers.

Shelley, J. A., & Fish, S. (1988). *Spiritual care: The nurse's role* (3rd ed.). Downers Grove, IL: Inter Varsity Press.

Stephenson, C. (1991). The concept of hope revisited for nursing. *Journal of Advances in Nursing, 16,* 1456–1461.

Stoll, R. T. (1989). The essence of spirituality. In Carson, V. B. (Ed.), *Spiritual dimensions of nursing practice.* Philadelphia: Saunders.

Sumner, H. (1998, January). Recognizing and responding to spiritual distress. *American Journal of Nursing, 98,* 26–31.

Taylor, E. J. (1998). Caring for the spirit. In C. C. Burke (Ed.), *Psychosocial dimensions of oncology nursing care.* Pittsburgh: Oncology Nursing Press.

Taylor, E. J. (2001). Spirituality, culture, and cancer care. *Seminars in Oncology Nursing, 17*(3), 197–205.

Taylor, E. J. (2002). *Spiritual care: Nursing theory, research, and practice.* Upper Saddle River, NJ: Prentice Hall.

Taylor, E. J., Outlaw, F. H., Bernardo, T., & Roy, A. (1999). Spiritual conflicts associated with praying about cancer. *Psycho-Oncology, 8,* 386–394.

Ulanov, A., & Ulanov, B. (1983). *Primary speech: A psychology of prayer.* Atlanta, GA: John Knox Press. (Classic.)

Vardey, L. (1996). *God in all worlds.* Toronto: Vintage Canada.

Westerhoff, J. (1976). *Will our children have faith?* New York: Seabury Press.

Wilkinson, J. M. (2000). *Nursing diagnosis handbook with NIC interventions and NOC outcomes* (7th ed). Upper Saddle River, NJ: Prentice Hall Health.

Zerwekh, J. V. (1997). The practice of presencing. *Seminars in Oncology Nursing, 13,* 260–262.

Selected Bibliography

Murray, C. K. (1998). Say a little prayer. *Nursing, 28*(6), 55.

Plotnikoff, G. A. (2000). Should medicine reach out to the spirit? Understanding a patient's spiritual foundation can guide appropriate care. *Postgraduate Medicine, 108*(6), 19–21.

Sherwood, G. D. (2000). The power of nurse-client encounters: Interpreting spiritual themes. *Journal of Holistic Nursing, 18*(2), 159–175.

Sulmasy, D. P. (2001). Addressing the religious and spiritual needs of dying patients. *Western Journal of Medicine, 175*(4), 251–254.

Van Dover, L. J., & Bacon, J. M. (2001). Spiritual care in nursing practice: A close-up view. *Nursing Forum, 36*(3), 18–28.

CHAPTER | 40

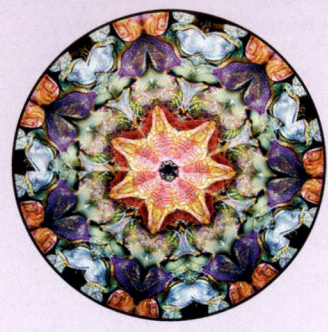

STRESS AND COPING

LEARNING OUTCOMES

After completing this chapter, you will be able to:

- Differentiate the concepts of stress as a stimulus, as a response, and as a transaction.

- Describe the three stages of Selye's general adaptation syndrome.

- Identify physiologic, psychologic, and cognitive indicators of stress.

- Differentiate four levels of anxiety.

- Identify behaviors related to specific ego defense mechanisms.

- Discuss types of coping and coping strategies.

- Identify essential aspects of assessing a client's stress and coping patterns.

- Identify nursing diagnoses related to stress.

- Describe interventions to help clients minimize and manage stress.

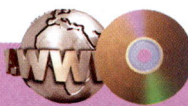

MediaLink

www.prenhall.com/kozier

Additional resources for this chapter can be found on the Student CD-ROM accompanying this textbook, and on the Companion Website at www.prenhall.com/kozier. Click on Chapter 40 to select the activities for this chapter.

CD-ROM
- Audio Glossary
- NCLEX Review

Companion Website
- Additional NCLEX Review
- Case Study: Becoming Parents
- Care Plan Activity: Client Going Through a Divorce
- MediaLink Application: Resources for Helping a Client to Manage Stress
- Links to Resources

Stress is a universal phenomenon. All people experience it. Parents refer to the stress of raising children, working people talk of the stress of their jobs, and students at all levels talk of the stress of school. Stress can result from both positive and negative experiences. For example, a bride preparing for her wedding, a graduate preparing to start a new job, and a husband concerned about caring for his wife and family following a diagnosis of cancer all experience stress reactions.

The concept of stress is important because it provides a way of understanding the person as a being who responds in totality (mind, body, and spirit) to a variety of changes that take place in daily life.

CONCEPT OF STRESS

Stress is a condition in which the person responds to changes in the normal balanced state. A **stressor** is any event or stimulus that causes an individual to experience stress. When a person faces stressors, responses are referred to as *coping strategies, coping responses,* or *coping mechanisms.*

Sources of Stress

There are many sources of stress. They can be broadly classified as internal or external stressors, or developmental or situational stressors. *Internal stressors* originate within a person, for example, cancer or feelings of depression. *External stressors* originate outside the individual, for example, a move to another city, a death in the family, or pressure from peers. *Developmental stressors* occur at predictable times throughout an individual's life. Within each developmental stage, certain tasks must be achieved to prevent or reduce stress. Examples of these tasks are shown in Table 40–1. *Situational stressors* are unpredictable and may occur at

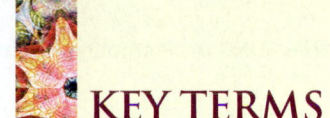

KEY TERMS

alarm reaction, 1015
anger, 1017
anxiety, 1016
burnout, 1026
caregiver burden, 1020
coping, 1020
coping mechanism, 1020
coping strategy, 1020
countershock phase, 1015
crisis counseling, 1025
crisis intervention, 1025
depression, 1017
ego defense mechanisms, 1018
fear, 1017
general adaptation syndrome (GAS), 1015
local adaptation syndrome (LAS), 1015
shock phase, 1015
stage of exhaustion, 1015
stage of resistance, 1015
stimulus-based stress model, 1014
stress, 1013
stressor, 1013
transactional stress theory, 1016

TABLE 40–1 Selected Stressors Associated with Developmental Stages

Developmental Stage	Stressors
Child	Beginning school
	Establishing peer relationships and adjustments
	Coping with peer competition
Adolescent	Accepting changing physique
	Developing relationships involving sexual attraction
	Achieving independence
	Choosing a career
Young adult	Getting married
	Leaving home
	Managing a home
	Getting started in an occupation
	Continuing one's education
	Rearing children
Middle adult	Accepting physical changes of aging
	Maintaining social status and standard of living
	Helping teenage children to become independent
	Adjusting to aging parents
Older adult	Accepting decreasing physical abilities and health
	Accepting changes in residence
	Adjusting to retirement and reduced income
	Adjusting to death of spouse and friends

Figure 40–1 ■ Some disorders that can be caused or aggravated by stress. *(From Health and Wellness: A Holistic Approach, 7th ed. (p. 44), by G. Edlin, E. Golanty, and K. M. Brown, 2002, Boston: Jones & Barlett. Adapted with permission.)*

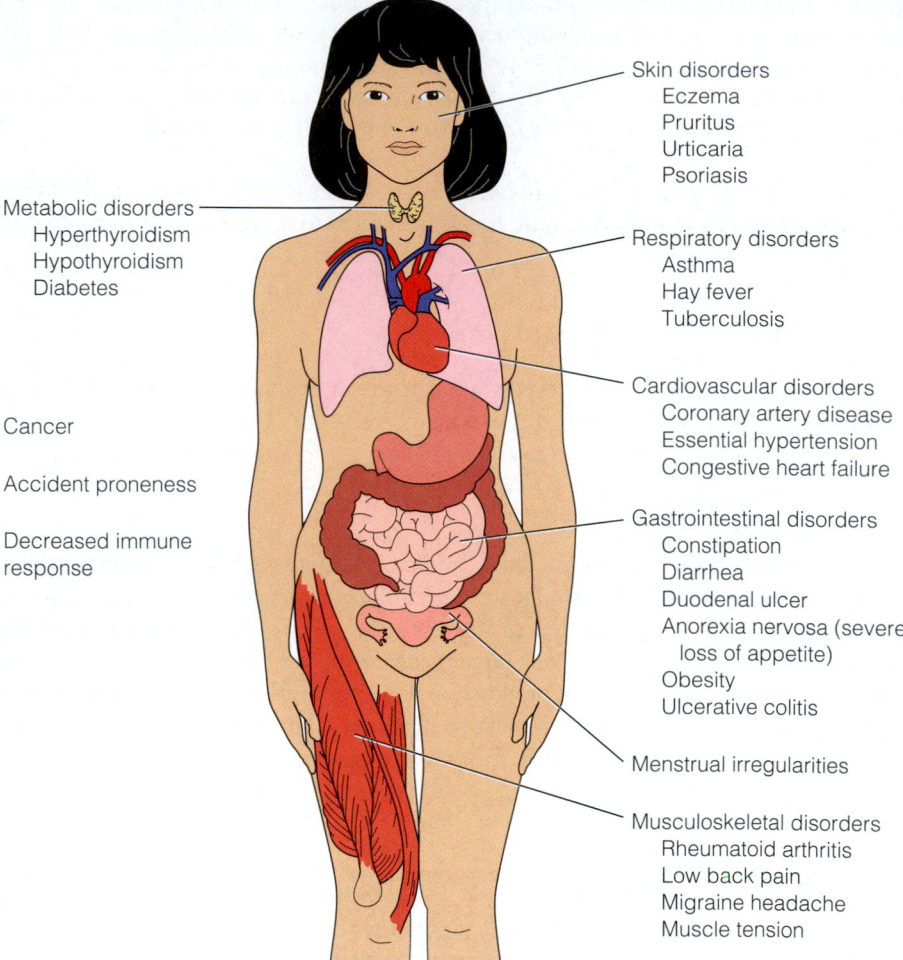

Metabolic disorders
  Hyperthyroidism
  Hypothyroidism
  Diabetes

Cancer

Accident proneness

Decreased immune response

Skin disorders
  Eczema
  Pruritus
  Urticaria
  Psoriasis

Respiratory disorders
  Asthma
  Hay fever
  Tuberculosis

Cardiovascular disorders
  Coronary artery disease
  Essential hypertension
  Congestive heart failure

Gastrointestinal disorders
  Constipation
  Diarrhea
  Duodenal ulcer
  Anorexia nervosa (severe loss of appetite)
  Obesity
  Ulcerative colitis

Menstrual irregularities

Musculoskeletal disorders
  Rheumatoid arthritis
  Low back pain
  Migraine headache
  Muscle tension

any time during life. Situational stress may be positive or negative. Examples of this type of stress include

- Death of a family member
- Marriage or divorce
- Birth of a child
- New job
- Illness.

The degree to which any of these events has positive or negative effects can depend to some extent on an individual's developmental stage. For example, the death of a parent may be more stressful for a 12-year-old than for a 40-year-old.

Effects of Stress

Stress can have physical, emotional, intellectual, social, and spiritual consequences. Usually the effects are mixed, because stress affects the whole person. Physically, stress can threaten a person's physiologic homeostasis. Emotionally, stress can produce negative or nonconstructive feelings about the self. Intellectually, stress can influence a person's perceptual and problem-solving abilities. Socially, stress can alter a person's relationships with others. Spiritually, stress can challenge one's beliefs and values. Many illnesses have been linked to stress (Figure 40–1 ■).

MODELS OF STRESS

Models of stress assist nurses to identify the stressor in a particular situation and to predict the individual's responses. Nurses can use the knowledge of these models to assist clients in strengthening healthy coping responses and in adjusting unhealthy, unproductive responses. Three main models of stress are stimulus based, response based, and transaction based.

Stimulus-Based Models

In **stimulus-based stress models,** stress is defined as a stimulus, a life event, or a set of circumstances that arouses physiologic and/or psychologic reactions that may increase the individual's vulnerability to illness. In their classic work, Holmes and Rahe (1967) assigned a numerical value to 43 life changes or events. The scale of stressful life events is used to document a person's relatively recent experiences, such as divorce, pregnancy, and retirement. In this view, both positive and negative events are considered stressful.

Similar scales have since been developed, but all scales should be used with caution because the degree of stress an event presents is highly individual. For example, a divorce may be highly traumatic to one person and cause relatively little anxiety to another. In addition, many scales have not been tested for age, socioeconomic status, or cultural sensitivity.

Response-Based Models

Stress may also be considered as a response. This definition was developed and described by Selye (1956, 1976) as "the nonspecific response of the body to any kind of demand made upon it" (1976, p. 1). Schafer (2000) defined stress as the "arousal of mind and body in response to demands made upon them" (p. 9).

Selye's stress response is characterized by a chain or pattern of physiologic events called the **general adaptation syndrome (GAS)** or *stress syndrome.* To differentiate the cause of stress from the response to stress, Selye (1976) created the term *stressor* to denote any factor that produces stress and disturbs the body's equilibrium. Because stress is a state of the body, it can be observed only by the changes it produces in the body. This response of the body, the stress syndrome or GAS, occurs with the release of certain adaptive hormones and subsequent changes in the structure and chemical composition of the body. Body organs affected by stress are the gastrointestinal tract, the adrenal glands, and the lymphatic structures. With prolonged stress, the adrenal glands enlarge considerably; the lymphatic structures, such as the thymus, spleen, and lymph nodes, atrophy (shrink); and deep ulcers appear in the lining of the stomach.

In addition to adapting globally, the body can also react locally; that is, one organ or a part of the body reacts alone. This is referred to as the **local adaptation syndrome (LAS).** One example of the LAS is inflammation. Selye (1976) proposed that both the GAS and the LAS have three stages: alarm reaction, resistance, and exhaustion (see Figure 40–2 ■).

Alarm Reaction

The initial reaction of the body is the **alarm reaction,** which alerts the body's defenses. Selye (1976) divided this stage into two parts: the shock phase and the countershock phase.

During the **shock phase,** the stressor may be perceived consciously or unconsciously by the person. In any case, the autonomic nervous system reacts, and large amounts of epinephrine (adrenaline) and cortisone are released into the body. The person is then ready for "fight or flight." This primary response is short lived, lasting from 1 minute to 24 hours.

The second part of the alarm reaction is called the **countershock phase.** During this time, the changes produced in the body during the shock phase are reversed. Thus, a person is best mobilized to react during the shock phase of the alarm reaction.

Stage of Resistance

The second stage in the GAS and LAS syndromes, the **stage of resistance,** is when the body's adaptation takes place. In other words, the body attempts to cope with the stressor and to limit the stressor to the smallest area of the body that can deal with it.

Stage of Exhaustion

During the third stage, the **stage of exhaustion,** the adaptation that the body made during the second stage cannot be main-

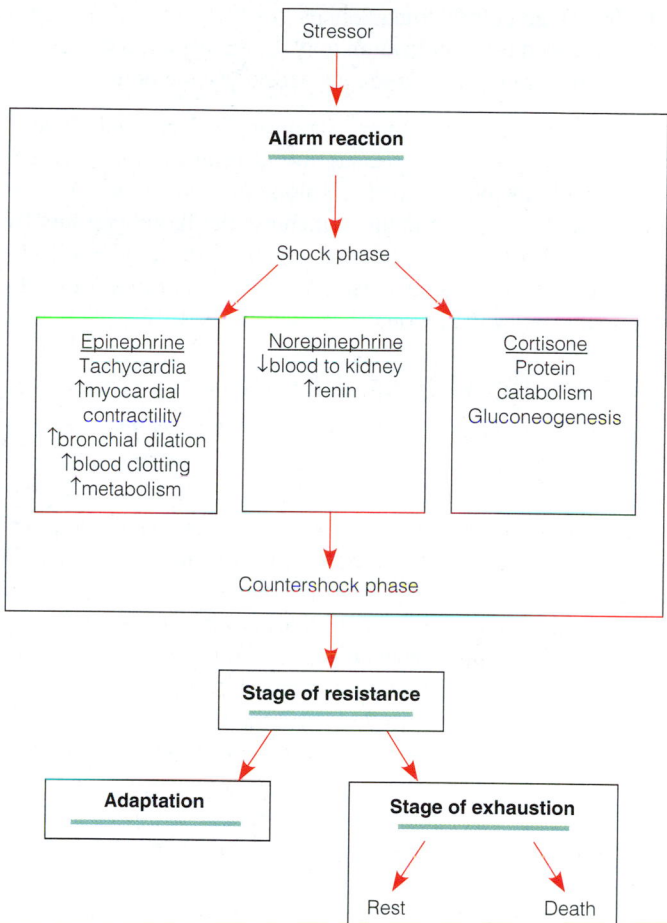

Figure 40–2 ■ The three stages of adaptation to stress: the alarm reaction, the stage of resistance, and the stage of exhaustion.

tained. This means that the ways used to cope with the stressor have been exhausted. If adaptation has not overcome the stressor, the stress effects may spread to the entire body. At the end of this stage, the body may either rest and return to normal, or death may be the ultimate consequence. The end of this stage depends largely on the adaptive energy resources of the individual, the severity of the stressor, and the external adaptive resources that are provided, such as oxygen.

Selye's (1976) general adaptation syndrome encompasses a range of physiologic responses to stressors in the body as a whole (see Figure 40–2). Stressors stimulate the sympathetic nervous system, which in turn stimulates the hypothalamus. The hypothalamus releases corticotropin releasing hormone (CRH), which stimulates the anterior pituitary gland to release adrenocorticotropin (ACTH). During times of stress, the adrenal medulla secretes epinephrine and norepinephrine in response to sympathetic stimulation. Significant body responses to epinephrine include the following:

1. Increased myocardial contractility, which increases cardiac output and blood flow to active muscles
2. Bronchial dilation, which allows increased oxygen intake
3. Increased blood clotting

4. Increased cellular metabolism
5. Increased fat mobilization to make energy available and to synthesize other compounds needed by the body.

The principal effect of norepinephrine is decreased blood to the kidneys and increased secretion of renin. Renin is an enzyme that hydrolyzes one of the blood proteins to produce angiotensin. Angiotensin tends to increase the blood pressure by constricting arterioles. The sum of all of these adrenal hormonal effects permits the person to perform far more strenuous physical activity than would otherwise be possible.

Transaction-Based Models

Transactional theories of stress are based on the work of Lazarus (1966), who states that the stimulus theory and the response theory do not consider individual differences. Neither theory explains which factors lead some people and not others to respond effectively nor interprets why some people are able to adapt for longer periods than are others.

Although Lazarus recognizes that certain environmental demands and pressures produce stress in substantial numbers of people, he emphasizes that people and groups differ in their sensitivity and vulnerability to certain types of events, as well as in their interpretations and reactions. For example, in terms of illness, one person may respond with denial, another with anxiety, and still another with depression. To explain variations among individuals under comparable conditions, the Lazarus model takes into account cognitive processes that intervene between the encounter and the reaction, and the factors that affect the nature of this process. In contrast to Selye, who focuses on physiologic responses, Lazarus includes mental and psychologic components or responses as part of his concept of stress.

The Lazarus **transactional stress theory** encompasses a set of cognitive, affective, and adaptive (coping) responses that arise out of person–environment transactions. The person and the environment are inseparable; each affects and is affected by the other. Stress "refers to any event in which environmental demands, internal demands, or both tax or exceed the adaptive resources of an individual, social system, or tissue system" (Monat & Lazarus, 1991, p. 3). The individual responds to perceived environmental changes by adaptive or coping responses.

INDICATORS OF STRESS

Indicators of an individual's stress may be physiologic, psychologic, or cognitive.

Physiologic Indicators

Responses to stress vary depending on the individual's perception of events. The physiologic signs and symptoms of stress result from activation of the sympathetic and neuroendocrine systems of the body. Box 40–1 lists physiologic indicators of stress.

Psychologic Indicators

Psychologic manifestations of stress include anxiety, fear, anger, depression, and unconscious ego defense mechanisms.

BOX 40–1 ■ Physiologic Indicators of Stress

- Pupils dilate to increase visual perception when serious threats to the body arise.
- Sweat production (diaphoresis) increases to control elevated body heat due to increased metabolism.
- The heart rate and cardiac output increase to transport nutrients and by-products of metabolism more efficiently.
- Skin is pallid because of constriction of peripheral blood vessels, an effect of norepinephrine.
- Sodium and water retention increase due to release of mineralocorticoids, which results in increased blood volume.
- The rate and depth of respirations increase because of dilation of the bronchioles, promoting hyperventilation.
- Urinary output decreases.
- The mouth may be dry.
- Peristalsis of the intestines decreases, resulting in possible constipation and flatus.
- For serious threats, mental alertness improves.
- Muscle tension increases to prepare for rapid motor activity or defense.
- Blood sugar increases because of release of glucocorticoids and gluconeogenesis.

Some of these coping patterns are helpful; others are a hindrance, depending on the situation and the length of time they are used or experienced.

Anxiety

A common reaction to stress is **anxiety,** a state of mental uneasiness, apprehension, dread, or foreboding or a feeling of helplessness related to an impending or anticipated unidentified threat to self or significant relationships. Anxiety can be experienced at the conscious, subconscious, or unconscious level. It differs from fear in four ways:

- The source of anxiety may not be identifiable; the source of fear is identifiable.
- Anxiety is related to the future, that is, to an anticipated event. Fear is related to the present.
- Anxiety is vague, whereas fear is definite.
- Anxiety is the result of psychologic or emotional conflict; fear is the result of a discrete physical or psychologic entity.

► CLINICAL ALERT *Mild or moderate anxiety motivates goal-directed behavior. In this sense, anxiety is an effective coping strategy. For example, mild anxiety motivates students to study. Excessive anxiety, however, often has destructive effects.* ■

Anxiety may be manifested on four levels:

1. Mild anxiety produces a slight arousal state that enhances perception, learning, and productive abilities. Most healthy people experience mild anxiety, perhaps as a feeling of mild restlessness that prompts a person to seek information and ask questions.

2. Moderate anxiety increases the arousal state to a point where the person expresses feelings of tension, nervousness, or concern. Perceptual abilities are narrowed. Attention is focused more on a particular aspect of a situation than on peripheral activities.

3. Severe anxiety consumes most of the person's energies and requires intervention. Perception is further decreased. The person, unable to focus on what is really happening, focuses on only one specific detail of the situation generating the anxiety.

4. Panic is an overpowering, frightening level of anxiety causing the person to lose control. It is less frequently experienced than other levels of anxiety. The perception of a panicked person can be affected to the degree that the person distorts events.

Table 40–2 lists indicators of these levels.

Fear

Fear is an emotion or feeling of apprehension aroused by impending or seeming danger, pain, or other perceived threat. The fear may be in response to something that has already occurred, in response to an immediate or current threat, or in response to something the person believes will happen. The object of fear may or may not be based in reality. For example, the beginning nursing student may be fearful in anticipation of the first experience in a client care setting. The student may fear that the client will not want to be cared for by the student or that the student might inadvertently harm the client.

Anger

Anger is an emotional state consisting of a subjective feeling of animosity or strong displeasure. People may feel guilty when they feel anger because they have been taught that to feel angry is wrong. However, anger can be expressed in a non-alienating verbal manner; it is then considered a positive emotion and a sign of emotional maturity because growth and beneficial interactions result from it.

A verbal expression of anger can be considered a signal to others of one's internal psychologic discomfort and a call for assistance to deal with perceived stress. In contrast, hostility is usually marked by overt antagonism and harmful or destructive behavior; aggression is an unprovoked attack or a hostile, injurious, or destructive action or outlook; and violence is the exertion of physical force to injure or abuse. Verbally expressed anger differs from hostility, aggression, and violence, but it can lead to destructiveness and violence if the anger persists unabated.

A clearly expressed verbal communication of anger, when the angry person tells the other person about the anger and carefully identifies the source, is constructive. This clarity of communication gets the anger out into the open so that the other person can deal with it and help to alleviate it. The angry person "gets it off the chest" and prevents an emotional buildup.

Depression

Depression is a common reaction to events that seem overwhelming or negative. **Depression,** an extreme feeling of sadness, despair, dejection, lack of worth, or emptiness, affects millions of

TABLE 40–2 Indicators of Levels of Anxiety

Category	Level of Anxiety			
	Mild	**Moderate**	**Severe**	**Panic**
Verbalization changes	Increased questioning	Voice tremors and pitch changes	Communication difficult to understand	Communication may not be understandable
Motor activity changes	Mild restlessness	Tremors, facial twitches, and shakiness	Increased motor activity, inability to relax	Increased motor activity, agitation
	Sleeplessness	Increased muscle tension	Fearful facial expression	Unpredictable responses
Perception and attention changes	Feelings of increased arousal and alertness	Narrowed focus of attention	Inability to focus or concentrate	Trembling, poor motor coordination
		Able to focus but selectively inattentive	Easily distracted	Perception distorted or exaggerated
	Uses learning to adapt	Learning slightly impaired	Learning severely impaired	Unable to learn or function
Respiratory and circulatory changes	None	Slightly increased respiratory and heart rates	Tachycardia, hyperventilation	Dyspnea, palpitations, choking, chest pain, or pressure
Other changes	None	Mild gastric symptoms (e.g., "butterflies in the stomach")	Headache, dizziness, nausea	Feeling of impending doom
				Paresthesia, sweating

Note: From *Nursing Diagnosis: Application to Clinical Practice,* 9th ed., by L. J. Carpenito, 2001, Philadelphia: Lippincott; *Mental Health Nursing,* 5th ed. (p. 273), by K. L. Fontaine, and J. S. Fletcher, 2003, Upper Saddle River, NJ: Pearson Education, Inc. Adapted with permission.

Americans a year. The signs and symptoms of depression and the severity of the problem vary with the client and the significance of the precipitating event. Emotional symptoms can include feelings of tiredness, sadness, emptiness, or numbness. Behavioral signs of depression include irritability, inability to concentrate, difficulty making decisions, loss of sexual desire, crying, sleep disturbance, and social withdrawal. Physical signs of depression may include loss of appetite, weight loss, constipation, headache, and dizziness. Many people experience short periods of depression in response to overwhelming stressful events, such as the death of a loved one or loss of a job; prolonged depression, however, is a cause for concern and may require treatment.

Unconscious Ego Defense Mechanisms

Unconscious **ego defense mechanisms** are psychologic adaptive mechanisms or, in the words of Sigmund Freud (1946), mental mechanisms that develop as the personality attempts to defend itself, establish compromises among conflicting impulses, and allay inner tensions. Defense mechanisms are the unconscious mind working to protect the person from anxiety. They can be considered precursors to conscious cognitive coping mechanisms that will ultimately solve the problem. Like some verbal and motor responses, defense mechanisms release tension. Table 40–3 describes these mechanisms and lists examples of their adaptive and maladaptive use.

Cognitive Indicators

Cognitive indicators of stress are thinking responses that include problem solving, structuring, self-control or self-discipline, suppression, and fantasy. *Problem solving* involves thinking through the threatening situation, using specific steps to arrive at a solution. The person assesses the situation or problem, analyzes or defines it, chooses alternatives, carries out the selected alternative, and evaluates whether the solution was successful.

Structuring is the arrangement or manipulation of a situation so that threatening events do not occur. For example, a nurse can structure or control an interview with a client by asking only direct, closed questions. Structuring can be productive in certain situations. A person who schedules a dental examination semiannually to prevent severe dental disease is using productive structuring.

Self-control (*discipline*) is assuming a manner and facial expression that convey a sense of being in control or in charge. When self-control prevents panic and harmful or nonproductive actions in a threatening situation, it is a helpful response that conveys strength. Self-control carried to an extreme, however, can delay problem solving and prevent a person from receiving the support of others, who may perceive the person as handling the situation well, as cold, or as unconcerned.

Suppression is consciously and willfully putting a thought or feeling out of mind: "I won't deal with that today. I'll do it tomorrow." This response relieves stress temporarily but does not solve the problem. A man who keeps ignoring a toothache, pushing it out of his mind because he fears the pain of having a filling, will not obtain relief of his symptoms.

Fantasy or *daydreaming* is likened to make-believe. Unfulfilled wishes and desires are imagined as fulfilled, or a threatening experience is reworked or replayed so that it ends differently from reality. Experiences can be relived, everyday

TABLE 40–3 Defense Mechanisms

Defense Mechanism	Example(s)	Use/Purpose
Compensation Covering up weaknesses by emphasizing a more desirable trait or by overachievement in a more comfortable area.	A high school student too small to play football becomes the star long-distance runner for the track team.	Allows a person to overcome weakness and achieve success.
Denial An attempt to screen or ignore unacceptable realities by refusing to acknowledge them.	A woman, though told her father has metastatic cancer, continues to plan a family reunion 18 months in advance.	Temporarily isolates a person from the full impact of a traumatic situation.
Displacement The transferring or discharging of emotional reactions from one object or person to another object or person.	A husband and wife are fighting, and the husband becomes so angry he hits a door instead of his wife.	Allows for feelings to be expressed through or to less dangerous objects or people.
Identification An attempt to manage anxiety by imitating the behavior of someone feared or respected.	A new graduate suddenly left in charge emulates her faculty role model.	Helps a person avoid self-devaluation.
Intellectualization A mechanism by which an emotional response that normally would accompany an uncomfortable or painful incident is evaded by the use of rational explanations that remove from the incident any personal significance and feelings.	The pain over a parent's sudden death is reduced by saying, "He wouldn't have wanted to live with a disability."	Protects a person from pain and traumatic events.

TABLE 40–3 Defense Mechanisms (continued)

Defense Mechanism	Example(s)	Use/Purpose
Introjection A form of identification that allows for the acceptance of others' norms and values into oneself, even when contrary to one's previous assumptions.	A 7-year-old tells his little sister, "Don't talk to strangers." He has introjected this value from the instructions of parents and teachers.	Helps a person avoid social retaliation and punishment; particularly important for the child's development of superego.
Minimization Not acknowledging the significance of one's behavior.	A person says, "Don't believe everything my wife tells you. I wasn't so drunk I couldn't drive."	Allows a person to decrease responsibility for own behavior.
Projection A process in which blame is attached to others or the environment for unacceptable desires, thoughts, shortcomings, and mistakes.	A mother is told her child must repeat a grade in school, and she blames this on the teacher's poor instruction. A husband forgets to pay a bill and blames his wife for not giving it to him earlier.	Allows a person to deny the existence of shortcomings and mistakes; protects self-image.
Rationalization Justification of certain behaviors by faulty logic and ascribing motives that are socially acceptable but did not in fact inspire the behavior.	A mother spanks her toddler too hard and says it was all right because he couldn't feel it through the diapers anyway.	Helps a person cope with the inability to meet goals or certain standards.
Reaction formation A mechanism that causes people to act exactly opposite to the way they feel.	An executive resents his bosses for calling in a consulting firm to make recommendations for change in his department but verbalizes complete support of the idea and is exceedingly polite and cooperative.	Aids in reinforcing repression by allowing feelings to be acted out in a more acceptable way.
Regression Resorting to an earlier, more comfortable level of functioning that is characteristically less demanding and responsible.	An adult throws a temper tantrum when he does not get his own way. A critically ill client allows the nurse to bathe and feed him.	Allows a person to return to a point in development when nurturing and dependency were needed and accepted with comfort.
Repression An unconscious mechanism by which threatening thoughts, feelings, and desires are kept from becoming conscious; the repressed material is denied entry into consciousness.	A teenager, seeing his best friend killed in a car accident, becomes amnesic about the circumstances surrounding the accident.	Protects a person from a traumatic experience until he or she has the resources to cope.
Sublimation Displacement of energy associated with more primitive sexual or aggressive drives into socially acceptable activities.	A person with excessive sexual drives invests psychic energy into a well-defined religious value system.	Protects a person from behaving in irrational, impulsive ways.
Substitution The replacement of a highly valued, unacceptable, or unavailable object by a less valuable, acceptable, or available object.	A woman wants to marry a man exactly like her dead father and settles for someone who looks a little bit like him.	Helps a person achieve goals and minimizes frustration and disappointment.
Undoing An action or words designed to cancel some disapproved thoughts, impulses, or acts in which the person relieves guilt by making reparation.	A father spanks his child and the next evening brings home a present for him. A teacher writes an exam that is far too easy, then constructs a grading curve that makes it difficult to earn a high grade.	Allows a person to appease guilty feelings and atone for mistakes.

Note: From *Mental Health Nursing,* 5th ed. (pp. 11–12), by K. L. Fontaine and J. S. Fletcher, 2003, Upper Saddle River, NJ: Pearson Education, Inc. Reprinted with permission.

problems solved, and plans for the future made. The outcome of current problems may also be fantasized. For example, a client who is awaiting the results of a breast biopsy may fantasize the surgeon as saying, "You do not have cancer." Fantasy responses can be helpful if they lead to problem solving. For example, the client awaiting breast biopsy results might say to herself, "Even if the doctor says, 'You have cancer,' as long as he also says it can be treated, I can accept that." Fantasies can be destructive and nonproductive if a person uses them to excess and retreats from reality.

COPING

Coping may be described as dealing with problems and situations, or contending with them successfully. A **coping strategy (coping mechanism)** is an innate or acquired way of responding to a changing environment or specific problem or situation. According to Folkman and Lazarus (1991), coping is "the cognitive and behavioral effort to manage specific external and/or internal demands that are appraised as taxing or exceeding the resources of the person" (p. 210).

Two types of coping strategies have been described: problem-focused and emotion-focused coping. *Problem-focused coping* refers to efforts to improve a situation by making changes or taking some action. *Emotion-focused coping* includes thoughts and actions that relieve emotional distress. Emotion-focused coping does not improve the situation, but the person often feels better.

Coping strategies are also viewed as long term or short term. *Long-term coping strategies* can be constructive and realistic. For example, in certain situations talking with others about the problem and trying to find out more about the situation are long-term strategies.

Other long-term strategies include those that involve a change in lifestyle patterns such as eating a healthy diet, exercising regularly, balancing leisure time with working, or using problem solving in decision making instead of anger or other nonconstructive responses.

Short-term coping strategies can reduce stress to a tolerable limit temporarily but are in the end ineffective ways to deal with reality. They may even have a destructive or detrimental effect on the person. Examples of short-term strategies are using alcoholic beverages or drugs, daydreaming and fantasizing, relying on the belief that everything will work out, and giving in to others to avoid anger.

Coping strategies vary among individuals and are often related to the individual's perception of the stressful event. Three approaches to coping with stress are to alter the stressor, adapt to the stressor, or avoid the stressor. A person's coping strategies often change with a reappraisal of a situation. There is never only one way to cope. Some people choose avoidance; others confront a situation as a means of coping. Still others seek information or rely on religious beliefs as a means of coping.

Coping can be adaptive or maladaptive. *Adaptive coping* helps the person to deal effectively with stressful events and minimizes distress associated with them. *Maladaptive coping* can result in unnecessary distress for the person and others associated with the person or stressful event. In nursing literature,

TABLE 40–4 Examples of the Effects of Stress on Basic Human Needs

Needs	Example
Physiologic	Altered elimination pattern
	Change in appetite
	Altered sleep pattern
Safety and security	Expresses nervousness and feelings of being threatened
	Focuses on stressors, inattention to safety measures
Love and belonging	Isolated and withdrawn
	Becomes overly dependent
	Blames others for own problems
Self-esteem	Fails to socialize with others
	Becomes a workaholic
	Draws attention to self
Self-actualization	Preoccupied with own problems
	Shows lack of control
	Unable to accept reality

effective and ineffective coping are often differentiated. *Effective coping* results in adaptation; *ineffective coping* results in maladaptation. Although the coping behavior may not always seem appropriate, the nurse needs to remember that coping is always purposeful.

The effectiveness of an individual's coping is influenced by a number of factors, including

- The number, duration, and intensity of the stressors
- Past experiences of the individual
- Support systems available to the individual
- Personal qualities of the person.

If the duration of the stressors is extended beyond the coping powers of the individual, that person becomes exhausted and may develop increased susceptibility to health problems. Reaction to long-term stress is seen in family members who undertake the care of a person in the home for a long period. This stress is called **caregiver burden** and produces responses such as chronic fatigue, sleeping difficulties, and high blood pressure. Prolonged stress can also result in mental illness. As coping strategies or defense mechanisms (see Table 40–3) become ineffective, the individual may have interpersonal problems, work difficulties, and a significant decrease in abilities to meet basic human needs (see Table 40–4).

NURSING MANAGEMENT

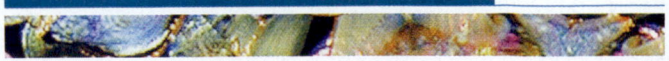

ASSESSING

Nursing assessment of a client's stress and coping patterns includes (a) nursing history and (b) physical examination of the client for indicators of stress (e.g., nail biting, nervousness, weight changes) or stress-related health problems (e.g., hypertension, dyspnea). When obtaining the nursing history, the nurse poses questions about client-perceived stressors or stressful incidents, manifestations of stress, and past and present coping strategies. During the physical examination, the nurse observes for verbal, motor, cognitive, or other physical manifestations of stress. Remember, however, that clinical signs and symptoms may not occur when cognitive coping is effective.

In addition, the nurse should be aware of expected developmental transitions (predictable tasks that must be accomplished if the person is to grow psychologically as well as physically; see Chapters 21 to 23). Persons go through different developmental stages from infancy to old age when certain tasks are expected to be completed or resolved. When these tasks are carried over and not resolved, stress increases as they become older. For example, if an infant does not learn to trust those around him during infancy, this mistrust may accompany him through life, influencing his relationships and possibly being the root of dysfunction, stress, and ineffective coping. This knowledge helps the nurse identify additional stressors that are present and the client's response to them (see Table 40–1). Questions to elicit data about the client's stress and coping patterns are shown in the accompanying Assessment Interview.

Assessment Interview

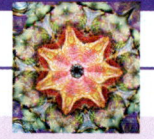

STRESS AND COPING PATTERNS

- On a scale of 1 to 10, where 1 is "very minor" and 10 is "extreme," how would you rate the stress you are experiencing in the following areas?
  a. Home
  b. Work or school
  c. Finance
  d. Recent illness or loss of loved one
  e. Your health
  f. Family responsibilities
  g. Relationships with friends
  h. Relationship with parents or children
  i. Relationship with partner
  j. Recent hospitalization
  k. Other (specify)
- How long have you been dealing with these stressors?
- How do you usually handle stressful situations? If the client does not adequately describe, prompt with the following:
  a. Cry
  b. Get angry
  c. Talk to someone (Who?)
  d. Withdraw from the situation
  e. Control others or situation
  f. Go for a walk or physical exercise
  g. Try to arrive at a solution
  h. Pray
  i. Laugh, joke, or use some other expression of humor
  j. Meditate or use some other relaxation technique such as yoga or guided imagery
- How well does your usual coping strategy work?

DIAGNOSING

NANDA diagnostic labels related to stress, adaptation, and coping include (in alphabetical order)

- *Anxiety:* Vague, uneasy feeling of discomfort or dread accompanied by an autonomic response (the source often nonspecific or unknown to the individual); a feeling of apprehension caused by the anticipation of danger. It is an alerting signal that warns of impending danger and enables the individual to take measures to deal with a threat.
- *Caregiver Role Strain:* Difficulty in performing the caregiver role
- *Compromised Family Coping:* Usually supportive primary person (family member or close friend) provides insufficient, ineffective, or compromised support, comfort, assistance, or encouragement that may be needed by the client to manage or master adaptive tasks related to his or her health challenge
- *Decisional Conflict (Specify):* Uncertainty about course of action to be taken when the choice among competing actions involves risk, loss, or challenge to personal life values
- *Defensive Coping:* Repeated projection of falsely positive self-evaluation based on a self-protective pattern that defends against underlying perceived threats to positive self-regard
- *Disabled Family Coping:* Behavior of significant person (family member or other primary person) that disables his/her capacities and the client's capacities to effectively address tasks essential to either person's adaption to the health challenge
- *Fear:* Response to perceived threat that is consciously recognized as a danger
- *Impaired Adjustment:* Inability to modify lifestyle/behavior in a manner consistent with a change in health status
- *Ineffective Coping:* Inability to form a valid appraisal of the stressors, inadequate choices of practiced responses, and/or inability to use resources
- *Ineffective Denial:* Conscious or unconscious attempt to disavow the knowledge or meaning of an event to reduce anxiety/fear, but leading to the detriment of health
- *Post-Trauma Syndrome:* Sustained maladaptive response to a traumatic, overwhelming event
- *Relocation Stress Syndrome:* Physiologic and/or psychosocial disturbance following transfer from one environment to another.

Examples of clinical applications of these diagnoses using NANDA, NIC, and NOC designations are shown in Identifying Nursing Diagnosis, Outcomes, and Interventions.

PLANNING

The nurse develops plans in collaboration with the client and significant support people when possible, according to the client's state of health (e.g., ability to return to work), level of anxiety, support resources, coping mechanisms, and sociocultural and religious affiliation. The nurse with little experience intervening with clients undergoing stress may wish to consult with a more experienced nurse to develop effective plans. The nurse and client set goals to change the existing client responses to the stressor or stressors.

IDENTIFYING NURSING DIAGNOSES, OUTCOMES, AND INTERVENTIONS
CLIENTS WITH STRESS AND COPING CHALLENGES

DATA CLUSTER	NURSING DIAGNOSIS/ DEFINITION	SAMPLE DESIRED OUTCOMES [NOC#]/DEFINITION	INDICATORS	SELECTED INTERVENTIONS [NIC#]/DEFINITION	SAMPLE NIC ACTIVITIES
Darryl Johnson, a 67-year-old accountant, was diagnosed with a heart attack. He says, "I'm scared about this. My dad died of a heart attack when he was 68 years old. But, I don't think I can give up smoking, take up exercising, and change my diet."	*Impaired Adjustment/Inability to modify lifestyle/behavior in a manner consistent with a change in health status*	Acceptance: Health Status [1300]/ *Reconciliation to health status*	Substantial • Recognition of reality of current health situation • Demonstration of positive self-regard • Clarification of values	Counseling [5240]/*Use of an interactive helping process focusing on the needs, problems, or feelings of the patient and significant others to enhance or support coping, problem-solving, and interpersonal relationships*	• Demonstrate empathy, warmth, and genuineness • Provide factual information as appropriate • Use techniques of reflection and clarification to facilitate expression of feelings
Sonia Park, a 33-year-old mother of three, returned to work after 8 years at home. She says, "I'm so tired since I started work. I'm not keeping up with housekeeping the way I should, and I'm not spending as much time with the kids. I'm too tired to shop and go to my son's baseball game. Everyone is helping out and not complaining, but I just keep thinking they wish I still baked cookies and played more with them. I'm sure not sleeping well, and I'm having awful headaches."	*Decisional Conflict (Work Versus Home Responsibilities Causing Emotional and Physical Stress)/ Uncertainty about a course of action to be taken when the choice among competing actions involves risk, loss, or challenge to personal life values*	Decision Making [0906]/*Ability to choose between two or more options*	Often demonstrated • Identifies alternatives • Identifies resources necessary to support each alternative • Chooses among alternatives	Decision-Making Support [5250]/ *Providing information and support for a patient who is making a decision regarding health care*	• Inform patient of alternative views or solutions • Help patient identify advantages and disadvantages to each alternative • Facilitate patient's articulation of goals

The overall client goals for persons experiencing stress-related responses are to

- Decrease or resolve anxiety
- Increase ability to manage or cope with stressful events or circumstances
- Improve role performance.

Examples of clinical applications of NOC outcomes and NIC interventions are shown in Identifying Nursing Diagnoses, Outcomes, and Interventions. A sample nursing care plan and concept map using NIC interventions and selected activities are shown on pages 1027–1029.

Planning for Home Care

Clients who are experiencing stress may require ongoing nursing support or referral to community agencies that can provide support to meet client needs and enhance client coping. The determination of how much and what type of planning and home care follow-up is needed is based in great part on the nurse's knowledge of how the client and family have coped with previous stressors and the nature of the present stressor. The Home

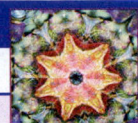

Home Care Assessment
STRESS AND COPING

Client

- **Knowledge:** Client's understanding of the nature of the stressors
- **Current coping strategies:** Effectiveness of current coping strategies and willingness to learn new stress management techniques
- **Self-care abilities:** Physical, emotional, social, and financial ability to minimize associated stressors
- **Role expectations:** Client's perception of the need to return to prior roles and possible stressors associated with these roles

Family

- **Knowledge:** Family members' and significant others' understanding of the nature of the client's stressors and their own relationship with client stressors

- **Family coping strategies:** Effectiveness of family members' and significant others' coping strategies and willingness to learn new stress management techniques
- **Role expectations:** Family members' and significant others' perception of the need for the client to return to family and work roles
- **Support people's availability and skills:** Family members' and significant others' sensitivity to the client's emotional and physical needs and ability to provide a supportive environment

Community

- **Resources:** Availability of and familiarity with possible sources of assistance for stress management such as massage therapists, religious or spiritual centers, physical care providers, support groups, and so on

---

Care Assessment feature describes data to be gathered for home care or follow-up assessment.

IMPLEMENTING

Although stress is part of daily life, it is also highly individual; a situation that to one person is a major stressor may not affect another. Some methods to help reduce stress will be effective for one person; other methods will be appropriate for a different person. A nurse who is sensitive to clients' needs and reactions can choose those methods of intervention that will be most effective for each individual.

Encouraging Health Promotion Strategies

Several health promotion strategies are often appropriate as interventions for clients with stress-related nursing diagnoses. Among these are physical exercise, optimal nutrition, adequate rest and sleep, and time management.

> ➤ **CLINICAL ALERT** *Many persons have "comfort foods"— things they like to eat that actually make them feel better emotionally.* ■

Exercise. Regular exercise promotes both physical and emotional health. Physiologic benefits include improved muscle tone, increased cardiopulmonary function, and weight control. Psychologic benefits include relief of tension, a feeling of well-being, and relaxation. In general, health guidelines recommend exercise at least three times a week for 30 to 45 minutes.

Nutrition. Optimal nutrition is essential for health and in increasing the body's resistance to stress. To minimize the negative effects of stress (e.g., irritability, hyperactivity, anxiety), people need to avoid excesses of caffeine, salt, sugar, and fat, and deficiencies in vitamins and minerals. Guidelines for a well-balanced, healthy diet are detailed in Chapter 45. ∞

Rest and Sleep. Rest and sleep restore the body's energy levels and are an essential aspect of stress management. To ensure adequate rest and sleep, clients may need help to attain comfort (such as pain management) and to learn techniques that promote peace of mind and relaxation. (See "Using Relaxation Techniques" on page 1024.)

Time Management. People who manage their time effectively usually experience less stress because they feel more in control of their circumstances. Clients who feel overwhelmed often need help to prioritize tasks and to consider whether modifications can be made to decrease role demands. Working mothers, for example, may need to consider delegating tasks to family members or hiring part-time help. Controlling the demands of others is also an important aspect of effective time management because requests made by others cannot always be met. Clients may need to learn to develop an awareness of which requests they can meet without undue stress, which ones can be negotiated, and which ones need to be declined. Feelings of control can be enhanced when clients schedule a daily or weekly period of time to deal with specific tasks. Time management must address both what is important to the client and what can realistically be achieved. For example, clients need to consider whether a clean house and time spent with the children can both be accomplished satisfactorily and, if not, which is more important. Clients who are feeling overwhelmed need to reexamine the "should do," "ought to do," and "must do" situations in their lives and develop realistic self-expectations.

Minimizing Anxiety

Nurses carry out measures to minimize clients' anxiety and stress. For example, nurses encourage clients to take deep breaths before an injection, explain procedures before they are implemented including sensations likely to be experienced during the procedure, administer a massage to help the client relax, and offer support to clients and families during times of

BOX 40–2 ■ Minimizing Stress and Anxiety

- Listen attentively; try to understand the client's perspective on the situation.
- Provide an atmosphere of warmth and trust; convey a sense of caring and empathy.
- Determine if it is appropriate to encourage clients' participation in the plan of care; give them choices about some aspects of care but do not overwhelm them with choices.
- Stay with clients as needed to promote safety and feelings of security and to reduce fear.
- Control the environment to minimize additional stressors such as reducing noise, limiting the number of persons in the room, and providing care by the same nurse as much as possible.
- Implement suicide precautions if indicated.
- Communicate in short, clear sentences.
- Help clients to
  a. Determine situations that precipitate anxiety and identify signs of anxiety.
  b. Verbalize feelings, perceptions, and fears as appropriate. Some cultures discourage the expression of feelings.
  c. Identify personal strengths.
  d. Recognize usual coping patterns and differentiate positive from negative coping mechanisms.
  e. Identify new strategies for managing stress (e.g., exercise, massage, progressive relaxation).
  f. Identify available support systems.
- Teach clients about
  a. The importance of adequate exercise, a balanced diet, and rest and sleep to energize the body and enhance coping abilities.
  b. Support groups available such as Alcoholics Anonymous, Weight Watchers or Overeaters Anonymous, and parenting and child abuse support groups.
  c. Educational programs available such as time management, assertiveness training, and meditation groups.

illness. The nurse recognizes that quick action may be necessary to avoid the contagious nature of anxiety. That is, the anxious feeling of one person tends to make others around him or her also anxious. This can include family members, other clients nearby, or health care providers. General guidelines for helping clients who are stressed and feeling anxious are outlined in Box 40–2.

Mediating Anger

Often nurses find clients' anger difficult to handle. Caring for the client who is angry is difficult for two reasons:

- Clients seldom state, "I feel angry or frustrated," or indicate the reason for their anger. Instead, they may refuse treatment, become verbally abusive or demanding, threaten violence, or become overly critical. Their complaints rarely reflect the cause of their anger.
- Anger from clients can elicit fear and anger in the nurse, who may respond in a manner that intensifies the client's anger, even to the point of violence. Nurses tend to respond in a way that reduces their own stress rather than the client's stress.

Fontaine and Fletcher (1999) recommend the following strategies for dealing with clients' anger:

- Know and understand your own response to the feelings and expressions of anger.
- Accept the client's right to be angry; feelings are real and cannot be discounted or ignored.
- Try to understand the meaning of the client's anger.
- Ask the client what contributed to the anger.
- Help the client "own" the anger—do not assume responsibility for her or his feelings.
- Let clients talk about their anger.
- Listen to the client, and act as calmly as possible.
- After the interaction is completed, take time to process your feelings and your responses to the client with your colleagues.

Always ensure the safety of the client and others. Know the agency procedures to call for assistance from other staff or security personnel if you believe someone (including yourself) is in danger.

> ►**CLINICAL ALERT** *A nurse who is concerned for his or her own safety while working with an angry client should withdraw from the situation or obtain support from another individual.* ■

Using Relaxation Techniques

Several relaxation techniques can be used to quiet the mind, release tension, and counteract the fight or flight responses of GAS discussed earlier in this chapter. Nurses can teach these techniques to clients. Nurses should also encourage clients to use these techniques when they encounter stressful health situations. Examples of these situations are (a) during childbirth, (b) postoperatively to cope with pain, and (c) before and during a painful procedure. Many agencies now have relaxation tapes available that the client can borrow or purchase. Some clients make their own recordings. Specific relaxation techniques are discussed in Chapter 14 ⊙⊙ and include

- Breathing exercises
- Massage
- Progressive relaxation
- Imagery
- Biofeedback
- Yoga
- Meditation
- Therapeutic touch
- Music therapy
- Humor and laughter.

Crisis Intervention

A *crisis* is an acute, time-limited state of disequilibrium resulting from situational, developmental, or societal sources of

Research Note
How Do Clients and Nurses Choose to Reduce Client Preoperative Anxiety?

Many studies have examined the use of stress reduction strategies in preoperative clients and some have shown improved recovery rates posited to follow from the reduced level of stress. In addition, the literature has commonly suggested that persons use the same coping strategies that have been successful with previous experiences of stress. One study, performed by a nursing student (Grieve, 2002), involved querying 150 clients in a same-day surgery setting about their feelings before surgery and observing the nursing staff's use of stress reduction techniques. As expected, most clients expressed anxiety, particularly about losing control when under anesthesia. Although some clients expressed that they usually used active coping strategies (e.g., gaining information), the researcher noted that, as the level of anxiety increased, most clients used avoidance coping strategies (e.g., distraction). The two most commonly used nursing strategies to reduce anxiety were distraction, accomplished by conversation or music, and provision of information.

Implications: The researcher concluded that a satisfactory correlation was seen between clients' usual coping strategies and those provided by the nursing staff. He felt, however, that there was inadequate awareness by nurses that a client's coping style could change based on severity of anxiety. He expressed concern that nurses may not have enough time to assess client style and might continue to provide information rather than distraction.

Note: From "Day Surgery Preoperative Anxiety Reduction and Coping Strategies," by R. J. Grieve, 2002, *British Journal of Nursing, 11,* pp. 670–673, 676–678.

BOX 40–3 ■ Common Characteristics of Crises

- All crises are experienced as sudden. The person is usually not aware of a warning signal, even if others could "see it coming." The individual or family may feel that they had little or no preparation for the event or trauma.
- The crisis is often experienced as ultimately life threatening, whether this perception is realistic or not.
- Communication with significant others is often decreased or cut off.
- There may be perceived or real displacement from familiar surroundings or loved ones.

All crises have an aspect of loss, whether actual or perceived. The losses can include an object, a person, a hope, a dream, or any significant factor for that individual.

The traditional steps of the nursing process correspond closely to the steps of crisis intervention. In assessment, the nurse or helper must focus on the person and the problem, collecting data about the client, the client's coping style, the precipitating event, the situational supports, the client's perception of the crisis, and the client's ability to handle the problem. This information is the basis for later decisions about how and when to intervene and whom to call. An individual's perception of the event and personal response will determine the nursing diagnoses. The most common nursing diagnoses for people in crisis are similar to those cited earlier in this chapter. In addition, diagnoses such as *Risk for Self Directed Violence, Risk for Other Directed Violence, Rape Trauma Syndrome,* and *Hopelessness* may be appropriate.

Effective planning for crisis intervention must be based on careful assessment and developed in active collaboration with the person in crisis and the significant people in that person's life.

Implementation involves crisis counseling and home crisis visits. **Crisis counseling** focuses on solving immediate problems and it involves individuals, groups, or families. Crisis intervention centers rely heavily on telephone counseling by volunteers who have professional consultation available to them. Also known as hotlines and often available around the clock, they allow callers to remain anonymous and test what it feels like to ask for assistance. The volunteers usually work within a protocol that indicates what information they need from the client to assess the crisis. Their goal is to plan steps to provide immediate relief and then long-term follow-up if necessary.

Crisis Home visits are made when telephone counseling does not suffice or when the crisis workers need to obtain additional information by direct observation or to reach a client who is unobtainable by telephone. Home visits are appropriate when crisis workers need to initiate contacts rather than waiting for clients to come to them; for example, when a telephone caller is assessed to be highly suicidal or when a concerned neighbor, physician, or clergy member informs the agency of clients in potential crisis.

Stress Management for Nurses

Nurses, like clients, are susceptible to experiencing anxiety and stress. Nursing practice involves many stressors related to both clients and the work environment—understaffing,

stress. A person in crisis is temporarily unable to cope with or adapt to the stressor by using previous methods of problem solving. People in crisis generally have a distorted perception of the event and do not have adequate situational support or coping mechanisms. Common characteristics of crises are shown in Box 40–3.

Crisis intervention is a short-term helping process of assisting clients to (a) work through a crisis to its resolution and (b) restore their precrisis level of functioning. It is a process that includes not only the client in crisis but also various members of the client's support network. Crisis intervention is not the specialty of any one professional group. People who intervene in crises come from the fields of nursing, medicine, psychology, social work, and theology. Police officers, teachers, school guidance counselors, and rescue workers, among others, are often on the spot in moments of crisis.

Because a state of disequilibrium is so uncomfortable, a crisis is self-limiting. However, a person experiencing a crisis alone is more vulnerable to unsuccessful negotiation than is a person working through a crisis with help. Working with another person increases the likelihood that the person in crisis will resolve it in a positive way. Often a state of crisis offers the individual or family great potential for growth and change.

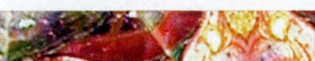

Lifespan Considerations

Middle-Aged Adults

■ Middle-aged adults are often called the "sandwich generation." They find themselves caring for children and grandchildren and often caring for aging parents at the same time. When these activities become time and energy consuming, there is often not enough time left for attention to self. Nurses need to be aware of this and assist in suggesting resources and effective planning to ease the strain.

Elders

■ Elders experience many losses and changes in their lives. They may be incremental and, over time, become stressful and possibly overwhelming. Changes in health, decreased functional ability and independence, need for relocation, loss of family and friends, and becoming a caregiver for a spouse or friend

are a few of the stresses often experienced by elders. Many of them have survived significant challenges in their earlier lives and have learned effective coping skills. Nurses can help them plan, evaluate their strategies, and learn new strategies, if needed. Informal and formal social supports are very important in learning to successfully live with these changes and stress.

■ Some effective coping methods for elders are exercise, learning different relaxation techniques, participation in activities, adequate nutrition and rest, and engaging in expressive creative activities, such as art, music, and journaling. Referral to community resources and supports should be done when appropriate. It is most important to see elders as unique individuals, with unique past experiences and very specific needs as they get older.

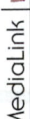

MediaLink | CLIENT GOING THROUGH A DIVORCE CARE PLAN ACTIVITY

increasing severity of client illnesses, adjusting to various work shifts, being expected to assume responsibilities for which one is not prepared, inadequate support from supervisors and peers, visiting homes that are depressing, caring for dying clients, and so on. Although most nurses cope effectively with the physical and emotional demands of nursing, in some situations nurses become overwhelmed and develop **burnout,** a complex syndrome of behaviors that can be likened to the exhaustion stage of the general adaptation syndrome. The nurse with burnout manifests physical and emotional depletion, a negative attitude and self-concept, and feelings of helplessness and hopelessness.

Nurses can prevent burnout by using the techniques to manage stress discussed for clients. Nurses must first recognize their stress and become attuned to such responses as feelings of being overwhelmed, fatigue, angry outbursts, physical illness, and increases in coffee drinking, smoking, or substance abuse. Once attuned to stress and personal reactions, it is necessary to identify which situations produce the most pronounced reactions so that steps may be taken to reduce the stress. Suggestions include:

- Plan a daily relaxation program with meaningful quiet times to reduce tension (e.g., read, listen to music, soak in a tub, or meditate).
- Establish a regular exercise program to direct energy outward.
- Study assertiveness techniques to overcome feelings of powerlessness in relationships with others. Learn to say no.
- Learn to accept failures—your own and others—and make it a constructive learning experience. Recognize that most people do the best they can. Learn to ask for help, to show your feelings with colleagues, and to support your colleagues in times of need.
- Accept what cannot be changed. There are certain limitations in every situation. Get involved in constructive

change efforts if organizational policies and procedures cause stress.
- Develop collegial support groups to deal with feelings and anxieties generated in the work setting.
- Participate in professional organizations to address workplace issues.
- Seek counseling if indicated to help clarify concerns.

EVALUATING

Using the desired outcomes developed during the planning stage as a guide, the nurse collects data needed to determine whether client goals and outcomes have been achieved. Examples of client goals and related outcomes are shown in Identifying Nursing Diagnoses, Outcomes, and Interventions earlier and in the accompanying Nursing Care Plan.

If outcomes are not achieved, the nurse, client, and support people, if appropriate, need to explore the reasons before modifying the care plan. Questions such as the following need to be considered:

- How does the client perceive the problem?
- Is there an underlying problem that has not been identified?
- Have new stressors occurred that interfere with successful coping?
- Were existing coping strategies sufficient to meet intended outcomes?
- How does the client perceive the effectiveness of new coping strategies?
- Did the client implement new coping strategies properly?
- Did the client access and use available resources?
- Have family members and significant others provided effective support?

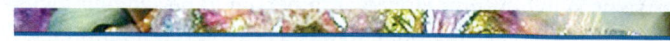

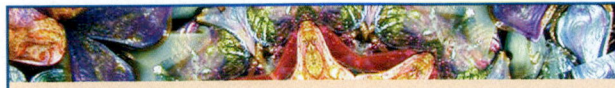

NURSING CARE PLAN FOR INEFFECTIVE COPING

ASSESSMENT DATA		*NURSING DIAGNOSIS*	DESIRED OUTCOMES [NOC#]/INDICATORS*
Nursing Assessment Ruby Smithson is a 55-year-old mother of four children who is hospitalized with breast cancer. She is scheduled for a modified radical mastectomy. Ruby was relatively healthy until she found a lump in her right breast 1 week ago. She and her husband are extremely anxious about the surgery. Ruby confides to the admitting nurse that "I can't stand the idea of having one of my breasts cut off; I don't know how I'm going to be able to even look at myself." Mr. Smithson informs the nurse that Ruby has been abusing alcohol since her diagnosis and neglecting her responsibilities as a mother. She is tearful and doesn't see how she will be able to continue her work as a dress designer.	**Physical Examination** Height: 164 cm (5'5") Weight: 58 kg (158 lb) Temperature: 37C (98.6F) Pulse rate: 88 BPM Respirations: 16/minute Blood pressure: 142/88 mm Hg **Diagnostic Data** Chest x-ray negative, CBC, and urinalysis within normal limits	*Ineffective Coping* related to personal vulnerability secondary to mastectomy (as evidenced by verbalization of inability to cope, substance abuse, inability to meet role expectations)	Coping [1302], as evidenced by often demonstrating ability to • Identify effective and ineffective coping patterns • Verbalize sense of control • Report decrease in negative feelings • Modify lifestyle as needed Social Support [1504], as evidenced by substantial reports of • Willingness to call on others for help • Emotional assistance provided by others

NURSING INTERVENTIONS [NIC#]/SELECTED ACTIVITIES*	*RATIONALE*
Coping Enhancement [5230]/ • Provide an atmosphere of acceptance	*Establishing rapport is essential to a therapeutic relationship and supports the client in self-reflection. Recognizing problems and sharing feelings is best brought about in an atmosphere of warmth and trust.*
• Provide factual information concerning the diagnosis, treatment, and prognosis.	*Factual information serves as a foundation for the individual to explore feelings and alternative coping strategies. Stressed clients often misunderstand facts and require frequent clarification so that appropriate conclusions can be drawn. Having valid information helps relieve stress.*
• Appraise Ruby's adjustment to changes in body image.	*Alteration in body image may be a major issue for Ruby and should be explored to facilitate therapeutic intervention. Coping strategies often change with a reappraisal of the situation.*
• Seek to understand Ruby's perspective of the stressful situation.	*Expressing emotions can decrease the perceived intensity of the stressor and serves as a basis for therapeutic interaction between the client and caregiver.*
• Arrange situations that encourage her autonomy.	*Enhances a sense of control, personal achievement, and self-esteem.*
• Explore with her previous methods of dealing with life problems.	*Present and past coping status assists both the client and caregiver in capitalizing on successful methods, identifying ineffective strategies, and developing new skills more appropriate to the present situation. Also determines risk for inflicting self-harm.*
• Encourage verbalization of feelings, perceptions, and fears.	*Open, nonthreatening discussions facilitate the identification of causative and contributing factors.*
• Encourage Ruby to identify her own strengths and abilities.	*Assists the client to develop appropriate strategies for coping based on personal strengths and previous experiences. Improves self-concept and sense of ability to manage stress.*

continued on page 1028

NURSING CARE PLAN FOR INEFFECTIVE COPING *continued*

NURSING INTERVENTIONS [NIC #] / SELECTED ACTIVITIES*	RATIONALE
• Encourage Ruby to realistically describe changes in her role.	*Individuals experiencing stress may have unrealistic perceptions or reality distortions. Helping Ruby clearly describe her role would be beneficial in developing realistic goals for role achievement.*
• Foster constructive outlets for anger and hostility.	*Assists the individual in channeling potentially harmful emotions and physical energy into constructive behavior.*
• Support the use of appropriate defense mechanisms.	*Denial can be temporarily therapeutic in helping the individual cope and relieve tension. After a time, however, denial and other defense mechanisms are counterproductive.*
Support System Enhancement [5440]	
• Identify the degree of family support.	*Assessing family interaction serves as a basis for identifying Ruby's support systems or lack thereof.*
• Determine barriers to using support systems.	*Although adequate support systems may be available, Ruby may not be using them or may be using them ineffectively.*
• Involve husband, family, and friends in the care and planning.	*Supporting Ruby in acknowledging changes in her appearance conveys acceptance and provides a foundation for her to begin to adjust.*
• Discuss with concerned others how they can help.	*Family and friends are often willing but unsure how to help. Identifying specific strategies such as praise and encouragement during rehabilitation and healing will promote acceptance of change.*
• Refer Ruby to a community-based breast cancer support group.	*Community support is beneficial in helping to meet unresolved needs, decreasing feelings of social isolation, and facilitating a positive self-image.*

EVALUATION

The coping outcome was not met. Following surgery, Ruby was withdrawn. During bathing, she would not assist and turned her head away when the dressing was removed. She refused to learn how to manage the wound drain or to discuss her feelings or plans for the future. Because clients having a mastectomy are often only hospitalized for a few days, it may be that she requires more time to reach the desired outcome. Continue to offer information and demonstrate availability for when she is ready to verbalize feelings. Social support outcome partly met. Ruby allows her husband to provide direct care and emotional support for her. A social worker was consulted and discharge was delayed for 24 hours. Ruby has agreed that the social worker can contact a breast cancer support group and ask the group to call her.

*Outcomes, interventions, and activities selected are only a sample of those suggested by NOC and NIC and should be further individualized for each client.

Applying Critical Thinking

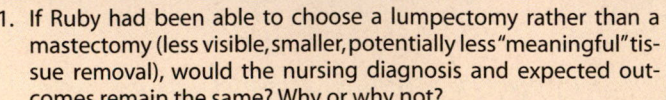

1. If Ruby had been able to choose a lumpectomy rather than a mastectomy (less visible, smaller, potentially less "meaningful" tissue removal), would the nursing diagnosis and expected outcomes remain the same? Why or why not?
2. Does Ruby's situation reflect more of a stimulus-based model or a response-based model? Why?
3. While working with Ruby, she becomes very angry and says to you "You don't understand. You've never had to go through this." How would you respond?

4. Based on the evaluation above, do you believe that Ruby is in crisis? What factors led to your decision? How does your view change the modifications indicated in her care plan?
5. Give one example of how Ruby might use the defense mechanisms described on pages 1018–1019. Explain whether this is adaptive or maladaptive.

See Critical Thinking Possibilities in Appendix A.

CONCEPT MAP For Ineffective Coping

| R.S. 55 y.o. ♀ Medical Dx: Breast cancer | • Lump detected 1 week ago. Very anxious, tearful
• Husband reports alcohol abuse and ineffective mothering since Dx | • Height: 164 cm (5'5")
• Weight: 58 kg (158 lb)
• T37C (98.6F), P:88, R:16, BP142/88
• Chest x-ray negative, CBC, and urinalysis with normal limits |

Ineffective Coping r/t personal vulnerability secondary to mastectomy (as evidenced by verbalization of inability to cope, substance abuse, inability to meet role expectations)

Social Support aeb substantial reports of
• willingness to call on others for help
• emotional assistance provided by others

Coping aeb often demonstrating ability to
• identify effective and ineffective coping patterns
• verbalize sense of control
• report decrease in negative feelings
• modify lifestyle as needed

Support System Enhancement

Identify the degree of family support

Determine barriers to using support systems

Involve husband, family, and friends in the care and planning

Discuss with concerned others how they can help

Refer to a community-based breast cancer support group

Coping Enhancement

Provide factual information concerning the diagnosis, treatment, and prognosis

Arrange situations that encourage her autonomy

Provide an atmosphere of acceptance

Explore with her previous methods of dealing with life problems

Appraise adjustment to changes in body image

Seek to understand perspective of the stressful situation

Support the use of appropriate defense mechanisms

Encourage verbalization of feelings, perceptions, and fears

Encourage to identify her own strengths and abilities

Encourage to realistically describe changes in her role

Foster constructive outlets for anger and hostility

Outcome partly met
• allows her husband to provide direct care and emotional support for her
• a social worker was consulted; discharge delayed 24 hours

Outcome not met
• following surgery, was withdrawn. Did not assist with bathing, turned her head away with dressing removed
• refused to learn to manage wound drain or discuss feelings or plans for the future

Legend: Assessment ▢ Nursing Diagnosis ▢ Outcomes ▢ Nursing Interventions ▢ Activities ▢ Evaluation/Reassessment ▢

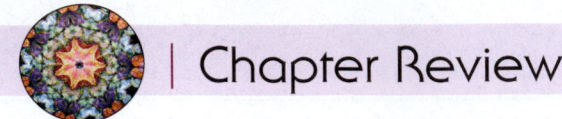

Chapter Review

EXPLORE MediaLink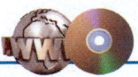

NCLEX review questions, case studies, care plan activities, MediaLink applications, and other interactive resources for this chapter can be found on the Companion Website at www.prenhall.com/kozier. Click on Chapter 40 to select the activities for this chapter.

For more NCLEX review questions, and an audio glossary, access the Student CD-ROM accompanying this textbook.

Chapter Highlights

- Stress is a state of physiologic and psychologic tension that affects the whole person—physically, emotionally, intellectually, socially, and spiritually.
- Models view stress as a stimulus, stress as a response, and stress as a transaction.
- General adaptation syndrome (GAS) is a multisystem response to stress and involves three steps: alarm reaction, stage of resistance, and stage of exhaustion.
- Local adaptation syndrome (LAS) is a localized physiologic response that also expresses the three stages of GAS. An example of LAS is the inflammatory response.
- There are physiologic, psychologic, and cognitive indicators of stress. Physiologic indicators are the result of increased activity of the sympathetic and neuroendocrine systems.
- Common psychologic indicators are anxiety, fear, anger, and depression. Anxiety, the most common response, has four levels: mild, moderate, severe, and panic. Ego defense mechanisms such as denial, rationalization, compensation, and sublimation protect individuals from anxiety.
- Cognitive indicators or thinking responses to stress include problem solving, structuring, self-control (discipline), suppression, and fantasy.

- Coping strategies to deal with stress vary significantly among individuals. Strategies may be problem focused or emotion focused, long term or short term, and effective or ineffective.
- The effectiveness of individual coping depends on the number, duration, and intensity of the stressors; past experience; support systems available; and the personal qualities of the person.
- Prolonged stress and ineffective coping interfere with the meeting of basic needs and can affect physical and mental health.
- Nursing assessment of a client experiencing stress involves a nursing history to identify perceptions of and duration of stressors and coping strategies and also a physical examination for physical indicators of stress.
- Nursing interventions for clients who are stressed are aimed at encouraging health promotion strategies (exercise, healthy diet, adequate rest, and time management), minimizing anxiety, mediating anger, teaching about specific relaxation techniques, and implementing crisis interventions as needed.
- Because nursing practice involves many stressors related to both clients and the work environment, nurses are susceptible to anxiety and burnout. Like clients, they need to implement stress reduction measures.

Review Questions

40–1. At work, several long-term clients have recently died. Which of the following actions is most likely to represent ineffective coping?
  a. The nurse talks at length to her partner about the deaths.
  b. The nurse keeps busy with other actions and doesn't think about the deaths for several days.
  c. The nurse offers to work extra shifts for several weeks.
  d. Several nurses schedule a group session with the agency clergy to discuss the deaths.

40–2. The nurse wishes to help a 50-year-old client identify previously successful coping strategies that may be useful in the current situation of needing to begin taking insulin for diabetes. Which of the following most likely represents a stressor of a similar style to the current one?
  a. interviewing for a new job

  b. death of a pet while the person was a teenager
  c. the person's partner filing for a divorce
  d. starting to wear eyeglasses at age 30

40–3. Two people have been in a car accident and have similar injuries. According to the transaction-based model, their degree of stress from the accident would be
  a. completely individual based on previous experience and personal characteristics.
  b. extremely similar since they had the same stimulus.
  c. the identical physiologic alarm reaction.
  d. different depending on their external resources and support levels.

40–4. Although clients may exhibit calm behavior, physical evidence of stress may still be manifested by
  a. constricted pupils.
  b. dilated peripheral blood vessels (flush).

c. hyperventilation.
d. decreased heart rate.

40–5. The parents of a hospitalized young child have just been informed that the child has leukemia. The father responds by continuing his usual work schedule, rarely visiting, and asking when the child can return to school.

Of the following, which is the least likely to be an appropriate nursing diagnosis at this tine?

a. *Ineffective Denial*
b. *Caregiver Role Strain*
c. *Fear*
d. *Compromised Family Coping*

Readings and References

Suggested Readings

Garbee, D. D., & Gentry, J. A. (2001). Coping with the stress of surgery. *Association of Operating Room Nurses Journal, 73,* 946–951.
This article reviews the viewpoints of problem-focused versus emotion-focused coping with stress. It includes a case study of a client being prepared preoperatively for surgery for cancer of the colon who then develops post-operative complications.

Zook, R. (1998). Learning to use positive defense mechanisms. *American Journal of Nursing, 98*(3), 16B, F, H.
The author describes how people use defense mechanisms. These mechanisms are described as existing on a continuum from healthy adaptive approaches to stress, to minimal, moderate, and high levels of distortion. Zook states that the best known defense mechanism is denial. Included with the article is a glossary of defense mechanisms categorized from highly adaptive to maladaptive (high distortion). Also included is information about recognizing maladaptive behaviors and suggestions on how nurses can help clients drop negative defense mechanisms.

Related Research

Reynaud, S. N., & Meeker, B. J. (2002). Coping styles of older adults with ostomies. *Journal of Gerontological Nursing, 28*(5), 30–36.

References

Carpenito, L. J. (2001). *Nursing diagnosis: Application to clinical practice* (9th ed.). Philadelphia: Lippincott.

Edlin, G., Golanty, E., & Brown, K. M. (2002). *Health and wellness: A holistic approach* (7th ed.). Boston: Jones & Bartlett.

Folkman, S., & Lazarus, R. S. (1991). Coping and emotion. In A. Monat & R. S. Lazarus (Eds.), *Stress and coping* (3rd ed.). New York: Columbia University Press.

Fontaine, K. L., & Fletcher, J. S. (2003). *Mental health nursing* (5th ed.). Upper Saddle River, NJ: Pearson Education, Inc.

Freud, S. (1946). *The ego and the mechanisms of defense.* New York: International Universities Press.

Grieve, R. J. (2002). Day surgery preoperative anxiety reduction and coping strategies. *British Journal of Nursing, 11,* 670–673, 676–678.

Holmes, T. H., & Rahe, R. H. (1967). The social readjustment rating scale. *Journal of Psychosomatic Research, 11,* 213–218.

Johnson, M., Maas, M., & Moorhead, S. (Eds.). (2000). *Nursing outcomes classification (NOC)* (2nd ed.). St. Louis, MO: Mosby.

Lazarus, R. S. (1966). *Psychological stress and the coping process.* New York: McGraw Hill.

McCloskey, J. C., & Bulechek, G. M. (Eds.). (2000). *Nursing interventions classification (NIC)* (3rd ed.). St. Louis, MO: Mosby.

Monat, A., & Lazarus, R. S. (Eds.). (1991). *Stress and coping* (3rd ed.). New York: Columbia University Press.

NANDA International. (2003). *NANDA nursing diagnoses: Definitions and classification 2003-2004.* Philadelphia: Author.

Schafer, W. (2000). *Stress management for wellness* (4th ed.). Stamford, CT: International Thomson Publishing.

Selye, H. (1956). *The stress of life.* New York: McGraw-Hill.

Selye, H. (1976). *The stress of life* (revised ed.). New York: McGraw-Hill.

Selected Bibliography

Gates, D. M. (2001). Stress and coping: A model for the workplace. *AAOHN Journal, 49,* 390–398.

Gold, J., & Thornton, L. (2001). Simple strategies for managing stress. *RN, 64*(12), 65–68.

Grandinetti, D. A. (2002). Two ways to beat stress. *RN, 65*(3), 4–7.

Lynch, S. M., & George, L. K. (2002). Interlocking trajectories of loss related events and depressive symptoms among elders. *The Journals of Gerontology, 57B,* S117–125.

Martin, P., Long, M. V., & Poon, L. W. (2002). Age changes and differences in personality traits and states of the old and very old. *The Journals of Gerontology, 57B,* 144–152.

McGowan, B. (2001). Self reported stress and its effects on nurses. *Nursing Standard, 15*(42), 33–38.

Review anxiety and mood disorders. (2002). *Nursing, 32*(6), 76–77.

Richardson, C., & Poole, H. (2001). Chronic pain and coping: A proposed role for nurses and nursing models. *Journal of Advanced Nursing, 34,* 659–667.

Walters, K. L., & Simoni, J. M. (2002). Reconceptualizing Native women's health: An "indigenist" stress coping model. *Journal of Public Health, 92,* 520–524.

Wu, C., Lee, Y. Y., Baig, K., & Wichaikhum, O. (2001). Coping behaviors of individuals with chronic obstructive pulmonary disease. *Medsurg Nursing, 10,* 315–320.

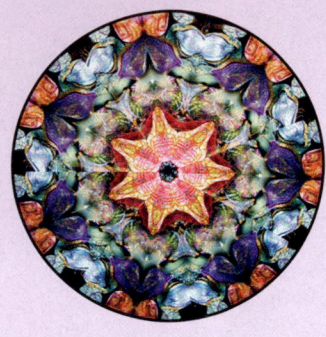

CHAPTER 41

LOSS, GRIEVING, AND DEATH

LEARNING OUTCOMES

After completing this chapter, you will be able to:

- Describe types and sources of losses.
- Discuss selected frameworks for identifying stages of grieving.
- Identify clinical symptoms of grief.
- Discuss factors affecting a grief response.
- Identify measures that facilitate the grieving process.
- List clinical signs of impending and actual death.
- Describe essential aspects of the Patient Self-Determination Act.
- Identify the nurse's legal responsibilities regarding client death and issues such as advance health care directives, autopsy, certification of death, do-not-resuscitate orders, euthanasia, inquests, and organ donation.
- Describe helping clients die with dignity.
- Describe nursing measures for care of the body after death.
- Describe the role of the nurse in working with families or caregivers of dying clients.

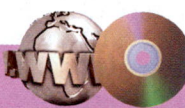

MediaLink

www.prenhall.com/kozier

Additional resources for this chapter can be found on the Student CD-ROM accompanying this textbook, and on the Companion Website at www.prenhall.com/kozier. Click on Chapter 41 to select the activities for this chapter.

CD-ROM
- Audio Glossary
- NCLEX Review

Companion Website
- Additional NCLEX Review
- Case Study: Helping a Family Accept a Terminal Illness
- Care Plan Activity: Client Who Suffered an Arm Amputation
- MediaLink Application: Resource for Client Dealing with a Pet Loss
- Links to Resources

Loss, grieving, and death are experienced by everyone at some time during their life. People may suffer the loss of valued relationships through life changes, such as moving from one city to another, separation, divorce, or the death of a parent, spouse, or friend. People may grieve changing life roles as they watch grown children leave home or they retire from their lifelong work. The loss of valued material objects through theft or natural disaster can evoke feelings of grief and loss. When people's lives are affected by civil or national strife, they may grieve the loss of valued ideals such as safety, freedom, or democracy.

In the clinical setting, the nurse encounters clients who may be experiencing grief related to declining health, loss of a body part, terminal illness, or the impending death of self or a significant other. The nurse may also work with clients in community settings who are grieving losses related to personal crisis (e.g., divorce, separation) or disaster (war, earthquakes, floods, or hurricanes). Therefore, it is important for the nurse to understand the significance of loss and develop the ability to assist clients as they work through the grieving process.

Nurses may interact with dying clients and their families or caregivers in a variety of settings, from a fetal demise (death of an unborn child), to the adolescent victim of an accident, to the elderly client who finally succumbs to a chronic illness. Nurses must recognize the various influences on the dying process—legal, ethical, religious and spiritual, biologic, personal—and be prepared to provide sensitive, skilled, and supportive care to all those affected.

LOSS AND GRIEF

Loss is an actual or potential situation in which something that is valued is changed, no longer available, or gone. People can experience the loss of body image, a significant other, a sense of well-being, a job, personal possessions, beliefs, or a sense of self. Illness and hospitalization often produce losses.

Death is a fundamental loss, both for the dying person and for those who survive. Although death is inevitable, it can stimulate people to grow in their understanding of themselves and others. Death can be viewed as the dying person's final opportunity to experience life in ways that bring significance and fulfillment. People experiencing loss often search for the meaning of the event and it is generally accepted that finding meaning is needed in order for healing to occur. Note, however, that persons can be well adjusted without searching for meaning and that even those who find meaning do not see it as an end point, but rather an ongoing process (Davis, Wortman, Lehman, & Silver, 2000).

Types and Sources of Loss

There are two general types of loss, actual and perceived. Both losses can be anticipatory. An **actual loss** can be recognized by others. A **perceived loss** is experienced by one person but cannot be verified by others. Psychologic losses are often perceived losses in that they are not directly verifiable. For example, a woman who leaves her employment to care for her children at home may perceive a loss of independence and freedom. An **anticipatory loss** is experienced before the loss actually occurs. For example, a woman whose husband is dying may experience actual loss in anticipation of his death.

Loss can be viewed as situational or developmental. The loss of one's job, the death of a child, or the loss of functional ability because of acute illness or injury are *situational losses*. Losses that occur in the process of normal development—such as the departure of grown children from the home, retirement from a career, and the death of aged parents—are *developmental losses* that can to some extent be anticipated and prepared for.

There are many sources of loss: (a) loss of an aspect of oneself—a body part, a physiologic function, or a psychologic attribute; (b) loss of an object external to oneself; (c) separation from an accustomed environment; and (d) loss of a loved or valued person.

Aspect of Self

The loss of an aspect of self changes a person's body image, even though the loss may not be obvious. A face scarred from a burn is generally obvious to people; loss of part of the stomach or loss of ability to feel emotion may not be as obvious. The degree to which these losses affect a person largely depends on the integrity of the person's body image.

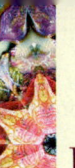

During old age, changes occur in physical and mental capabilities. Again the self-image is vulnerable. Old age is the stage in life when people may experience many losses: of employment, of usual activities, of independence, of health, of friends, and of family.

External Objects

Loss of external objects includes (a) loss of inanimate objects that have importance to the person, such as the loss of money or the burning down of a family's house; and (b) loss of animate (live) objects such as pets that provide love and companionship.

Familiar Environment

Separation from an environment and people who provide security can result in a sense of loss. The 6-year-old is likely to feel loss when first leaving the usual environment to attend school. The university student who moves away from home for the first time also experiences a sense of loss.

Loved Ones

The loss of a loved one or valued person through illness, divorce, separation, or death can be very disturbing. In some illnesses, a person may undergo personality changes that make friends and family feel they have lost that person.

The death of a loved one is a permanent and complete loss. In contemporary American society, death is often denied. People may be uncomfortable talking about death and being around people who are dying. There is a tendency to consider extraordinary measures that prolong and preserve life.

Grief, Bereavement, and Mourning

Grief is the total response to the emotional experience related to loss. Grief is manifested in thoughts, feelings, and behaviors associated with overwhelming distress or sorrow. **Bereavement** is the subjective response experienced by the surviving loved ones after the death of a person with whom they have shared a significant relationship. **Mourning** is the behavioral process through which grief is eventually resolved or altered; it is often influenced by culture, spiritual beliefs, and custom. Grief and mourning are experienced not only by the person who faces the death of a loved one but also by the person who suffers other kinds of loses. Grieving is essential for good mental and physical health. It permits the individual to cope with the loss gradually and to accept it as part of reality. Grief is a social process; it is best shared and carried out with the assistance of others.

Working through one's grief is important because bereavement may have potentially devastating effects on health. Among the symptoms that can accompany grief are anxiety, depression, weight loss, difficulties in swallowing, vomiting, fatigue, headaches, dizziness, fainting, blurred vision, skin rashes, excessive sweating, menstrual disturbances, palpitations, chest pain, and dyspnea. The bereaved may also experience alterations in libido, concentration, and patterns of eating, sleeping, activity, and communication.

Although bereavement can threaten health, a positive resolution of the grieving process can enrich the individual with new insights, values, challenges, openness, and sensitivity. For some, the pain of loss, though diminished, recurs for the rest of their lives.

Types of Grief Responses

A normal grief reaction may be abbreviated or anticipatory. *Abbreviated grief* is brief but genuinely felt. The lost object may not have been sufficiently important to the grieving person or may have been replaced immediately by another, equally esteemed object. **Anticipatory grief** is experienced in advance of the event. The wife who grieves before her ailing husband dies is anticipating the loss. A young girl may grieve in advance of an operation that will leave a scar on her body. Because many of the normal symptoms of grief will have already been expressed in anticipation, the reaction when the loss actually occurs may be quite abbreviated.

Disenfranchised grief occurs when a person is unable to acknowledge the loss to other persons. Situations in which this may occur often relate to a socially unacceptable loss that cannot be spoken about, such as suicide, abortion, or giving a child up for adoption. Other examples include losses of relationships that are socially unsanctioned and may not be known to other people.

Unhealthy grief—that is, pathologic or **dysfunctional grief**—may be unresolved or inhibited. Many factors can contribute to dysfunctional grief, including a prior traumatic loss and the circumstances of the present loss. Other influences include family or cultural barriers to the emotional expression of grief.

Unresolved grief is extended in length and severity. The same signs are expressed as with normal grief, but the bereaved may also have difficulty expressing the grief, may deny the loss, or may grieve beyond the expected time. With *inhibited grief*, many of the normal symptoms of grief are suppressed, and other effects, including somatic, are experienced instead.

Dysfunctional grief after a death may be inferred from the following data or observations:

- The client fails to grieve; for example, a husband does not cry at, or absents himself from, his wife's funeral.
- The client avoids visiting the grave and refuses to participate in memorial services, even though these practices are a part of the client's culture.
- The client becomes recurrently symptomatic on the anniversary of a loss or during holidays.
- The client develops persistent guilt and lowered self-esteem.
- Even after a prolonged period, the client continues to search for the lost person. Some may consider suicide to effect reunion.
- A relatively minor event triggers symptoms of grief.
- Even after a period of time, the client is unable to discuss the deceased with composure; for example, the client's voice cracks and quivers, eyes become moist.
- After the normal period of grief, the client experiences physical symptoms similar to those of the person who died.
- The client's relationships with friends and relatives worsen following the death.

Many factors contribute to unresolved grief after a death:

- Ambivalence (intense feelings, both positive and negative) toward the lost person

TABLE 41-1 Client Responses and Nursing Implications in Kübler-Ross's Stages of Grieving

Stage	Behavioral Responses	Nursing Implications
Denial	Refuses to believe that loss is happening. Is unready to deal with practical problems, such as prosthesis after loss of leg. May assume artificial cheerfulness to prolong denial.	Verbally support client but do not reinforce denial. Examine your own behavior to ensure that you do not share in client's denial.
Anger	Client or family may direct anger at nurse or staff about matters that normally would not bother them.	Help client understand that anger is a normal response to feelings of loss and powerlessness. Avoid withdrawal or retaliation; do not take anger personally. Deal with needs underlying any angry reaction. Provide structure and continuity to promote feelings of security. Allow clients as much control as possible over their lives.
Bargaining	Seeks to bargain to avoid loss. May express feelings of guilt or fear of punishment for past sins, real or imagined.	Listen attentively, and encourage client to talk to relieve guilt and irrational fear. If appropriate, offer spiritual support.
Depression	Grieves over what has happened and what cannot be. May talk freely (e.g., reviewing past losses such as money or job), or may withdraw.	Allow client to express sadness. Communicate nonverbally by sitting quietly without expecting conversation. Convey caring by touch.
Acceptance	Comes to terms with loss. May have decreased interest in surroundings and support people. May wish to begin making plans (e.g., will, prosthesis, altered living arrangements).	Help family and friends understand client's decreased need to socialize. Encourage client to participate as much as possible in the treatment program.

- A perceived need to be brave and in control; fear of losing control in front of others
- Endurance of multiple losses, such as the loss of an entire family, which the bereaved finds too overwhelming to contemplate
- Extremely high emotional value invested in the dead person; failure to grieve in this instance helps the bereaved avoid the reality of the loss
- Uncertainty about the loss—for example, when a loved one is "missing in action"
- Lack of support systems.

Stages of Grieving

Many authors have described stages or phases of grieving, perhaps the most well known of them being Kübler-Ross (1969), who has described five stages: denial, anger, bargaining, depression, and acceptance (Table 41-1). Engel (1964) has identified six stages of grieving: shock and disbelief, developing awareness, restitution, resolving the loss, idealization, and outcome (Table 41-2). Sanders (1998) described five phases of bereavement: shock, awareness, conservation/withdrawal, healing, and renewal (Table 41-3).

Martocchio (1985) discusses five clusters of grief—shock and disbelief; yearning and protest; anguish, disorganization, and despair; identification in bereavement; and reorganization and restitution—and maintains that there is no single cor-

rect way, nor a correct timetable, by which a person progresses through the grief process. Whether a person can succeed in integrating the loss and how this is accomplished are related to that person's individual development and personal makeup. In addition, individuals responding to the very same loss cannot be expected to follow the same pattern or schedule in resolving their grief, even while they support each other.

Rando (1984, 1986, 1991, 1993, 2000) has written extensively on the subject of grief, describing three categories of responses: avoidance, confrontation, and accommodation. Avoidance is similar to Kübler-Ross's phases of denial, anger, and bargaining and Engel's phase of shock and disbelief. Confrontation is the most upsetting phase for the grieving person facing the loss. Accommodation is the phase in which the person begins to resume more usual activities, feels better, and places the loss in perspective.

Manifestations of Grief

The nurse assesses the grieving client or family members following a loss to determine the phase or stage of grieving. Physiologically, the body responds to a current or anticipated loss with a stress reaction. The nurse can assess the clinical signs of this response.

Manifestations of grief that would be considered normal include verbalization of the loss, crying, sleep disturbance, loss

TABLE 41–2 Engel's Stages of Grieving

Stage	Behavioral Responses
Shock and disbelief	Refuses to accept loss.
	Has stunned feelings.
	Accepts the situation intellectually, but denies it emotionally.
Developing awareness	Reality of loss begins to penetrate consciousness.
	Anger may be directed at agency, nurses, or others.
Restitution	Conducts rituals of mourning (e.g., funeral).
Resolving the loss	Attempts to deal with painful void.
	Still unable to accept new love object to replace lost person or object.
	May accept more dependent relationship with support person.
	Thinks over and talks about memories of the lost object.
Idealization	Produces image of lost object that is almost devoid of undesirable features.
	Represses all negative and hostile feelings toward lost object.
	May feel guilty and remorseful about past inconsiderate or unkind acts to lost person.
	Unconsciously internalizes admired qualities of lost object.
	Reminders of lost object evoke fewer feelings of sadness.
	Reinvests feelings in others.
Outcome	Behavior influenced by several factors: importance of lost object as source of support, degree of dependence on relationship, degree of ambivalence toward lost object, number and nature of other relationships, and number and nature of previous grief experiences (which tend to be cumulative).

Note: From "Grief and Grieving," by G. L. Engel, 1964, *American Journal of Nursing, 64*(9), pp. 93–98. Adapted with permission.

of appetite, and difficulty concentrating. Dysfunctional grieving may be characterized by extended time of denial, depression, severe physiologic symptoms, or suicidal thoughts.

Factors Influencing the Loss and Grief Responses

A number of factors affect a person's response to a loss or death. These factors include age, significance of the loss, culture, spiritual beliefs, gender, socioeconomic status, support systems, and the cause of the loss or death. Nurses can learn general concepts about the influence of these factors of the grieving experience, but the constellation of these factors and their significance will vary from individual to individual.

Age

Age affects a person's understanding of and reaction to loss. With familiarity, people usually increase their understanding and acceptance of life, loss, and death.

People do not usually experience the loss of loved ones at regular intervals. As a result, preparation for these experiences is difficult. Coping with other of life's losses, such as the loss of a pet, the loss of a friend, and the loss of youth or a job, can help people anticipate the more severe loss of death of loved ones by teaching them successful coping strategies.

CHILDHOOD. Children differ from adults not only in their understanding of loss and death but also in how they are affected by the loss of others. The loss of a parent or other significant person can threaten the child's ability to develop, and regression sometimes results. Assisting the child with the grief experience includes helping the child regain the normal continuity and pace of emotional development.

Some adults may assume that children do not have the same need as an adult to grieve the loss of others. In situations of crisis and loss, children are sometimes pushed aside or protected from the pain. They can feel afraid, abandoned, and lonely. Careful work with bereaved children is especially necessary because experiencing a loss in childhood can have serious effects later in life.

EARLY AND MIDDLE ADULTHOOD. As people grow, they come to experience loss as part of normal development. By middle age, for example, the loss of a parent through death seems a more normal occurrence compared to the death of a younger person. Coping with the death of an aged parent has even been viewed as a necessary developmental task of the middle-aged adult.

The middle-aged adult can experience losses other than death. For example, losses resulting from impaired health or body function and losses of various role functions can be difficult for the middle-aged adult. How the middle-aged adult responds to such losses is influenced by previous experiences with loss, the person's sense of self-esteem, and the strength and availability of support.

LATE ADULTHOOD. Losses experienced by older adults include loss of health, mobility, independence, and work role. Limited income and the need to change one's living accommodations can also lead to feelings of loss and grieving.

TABLE 41–3 Sander's Phases of Bereavement

Phase	Description	Behavioral Responses
Shock	Survivors are left with feelings of confusion, unreality, and disbelief that the loss has occurred. They are often unable to process the normal thought sequences. Phase may last from a few minutes to many days.	Disbelief Confusion Restlessness Feelings of unreality Regression and helplessness State of alarm Physical symptoms: dryness of mouth and throat, sighing, weeping, loss of muscular control, uncontrolled trembling, sleep disturbance, and loss of appetite Psychologic symptoms: preoccupation with thoughts of the deceased and psychologic distancing
Awareness of loss	Friends and family resume normal activities. The bereaved experience the full significance of their loss.	Separation anxiety Conflicts Acting out emotional expectations Prolonged stress Physical symptoms: crying and sleep disturbance Psychologic symptoms: anger, guilt, frustration, shame, oversensitivity, disbelief and denial, dreaming, sense of presence of the deceased, and fear of death
Conservation/ withdrawal	During this phase, survivors feel a need to be alone to conserve and replenish both physical and emotional energy. The social support available to the bereaved has decreased, and they may experience despair and helplessness.	Physical symptoms: weakness, fatigue, need for more sleep, and a weakened immune system Psychologic symptoms: withdrawal, obsessional review, grief work, and ultimately a renewal of hope
Healing: the turning point	During this phase, the bereaved move from distress about living without their loved one to learning to live more independently.	Assuming control Identity restructuring Relinquishing roles, such as spouse, child, or parent Physical symptoms: increased energy, sleep restoration, immune system restoration, and physical healing Psychologic symptoms: forgiving, forgetting, searching for meaning, and hope
Renewal	In this phase, survivors move on to a new self-awareness, an acceptance of responsibility for self, and learning to live without the loved one.	Functional stability Revitalization Assumption of responsibility for self-care needs Psychologic symptoms: loneliness, anniversary reactions, and a reaching out to others

Note: From Grief: The Mourning After: Dealing with Adult Bereavement, 2nd ed., by C. M. Sanders, 1998, New York: John Wiley & Sons. Adapted with permission.

For older adults, the loss through death of a longtime mate is profound. Although individuals differ in their ability to deal with such a loss, research suggests that health problems for widows and widowers increase following the death of the spouse (Shahar, Schultz, Shahar, & Wing, 2001). Because the majority of deaths occur among elderly people, and because the number of elderly people is increasing in North America, nurses will need to be especially alert to the potential problems of older grieving adults.

Significance of the Loss

The significance of a loss depends on the perceptions of the individual experiencing the loss. One person may experience a great sense of loss over a divorce; another may find it only mildly disrupting. A number of factors affect the significance of the loss:

- Importance of the lost person, object, or function
- Degree of change required because of the loss
- The person's beliefs and values.

For older people who have already encountered many losses, an anticipated loss such as their own death may not be viewed as highly negative, and they may be apathetic about it instead of reactive. More than fearing death, some may fear loss of control or becoming a burden.

Culture

Culture influences an individual's reaction to loss. How grief is expressed is often determined by the customs of the culture. Unless an extended family structure exists, grief is handled by the nuclear family. The death of a family member in a typical nuclear family leaves a great void because the same few individuals fill most of the roles. In cultures where several generations and extended family members either reside in the same household or are physically close, the impact of a family member's death may be softened because the roles of the deceased are quickly filled by other relatives.

Some persons have adopted the belief that grief is a private matter to be endured internally. Therefore, feelings tend to be repressed and may remain unidentified. People who have been socialized to "be strong" and "make the best of the situation" may not express deep feelings or personal concerns when they experience a serious loss.

Some cultural groups value social support and the expression of loss. In some groups, the expression of grief through wailing, crying, physical prostration, and other outward demonstrations are acceptable and encouraged. Other groups may frown on this demonstration as a loss of control, favoring a more quiet and stoic expression of grief. In cultural groups where strong kinship ties are maintained, physical and emotional support and assistance are provided by family members.

Spiritual Beliefs

Spiritual beliefs and practices greatly influence both a person's reaction to loss and subsequent behavior. Most religious groups have practices related to dying, and these are often important to the client and support people. To provide support at a time of death, nurses need to understand the client's particular beliefs and practices.

Gender

The gender roles into which many people are socialized in the United States and Canada affect their reactions at times of loss. Men are frequently expected to "be strong" and show very little emotion during grief, whereas it is acceptable for women to show grief by crying. Often when a wife dies, the husband, who is the chief mourner, is expected to repress his own emotions and to comfort sons and daughters in their grieving.

Gender roles also affect the significance of body image changes to clients. A man might consider his facial scar to be "macho," but a woman might consider hers ugly. Thus the woman, but not the man, would see the change as a loss.

Socioeconomic Status

The socioeconomic status of an individual often affects the support system available at the time of a loss. A pension plan or insurance, for example, can offer a widowed or disabled person a choice of ways to deal with a loss; a person who is confronted with both severe loss and economic hardship may not be able to cope with either.

Support System

The people closest to the grieving individual are often the first to recognize and provide needed emotional, physical, and functional assistance. However, because many people are uncomfortable or inexperienced in dealing with losses, the usual support people may instead withdraw from the grieving individual. In addition, support may be available when the loss is first recognized, but as the support people return to their usual activities, the need for ongoing support may be unmet. Sometimes, the grieving individual is unable or unready to accept support when it is offered.

Cause of Loss or Death

Individual and societal views on the cause of a loss or death may significantly influence the grief response. Some diseases are considered "clean," such as cardiovascular disorders, and engender compassion, whereas others may be viewed as repulsive and less unfortunate. A loss or death that is beyond the control of those involved may be more acceptable than one that is preventable, such as a drunk driving accident. Injuries or deaths occurring during respected activities, such as "in the line of duty," are considered honorable, whereas those occurring during illicit activities may be considered the individual's just rewards.

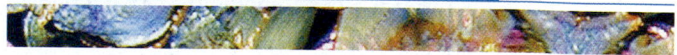

NURSING MANAGEMENT

ASSESSING

Nursing assessment of the client experiencing a loss includes three major components: (a) nursing history, (b) assessment of personal coping resources, and (c) physical assessment. During the routine health assessment of every client, the nurse poses questions regarding previous and current losses. The nature of the loss and the significance of such losses to the client must be explored.

If there is a current or recent loss, greater detail is needed in the assessment. Because clients do not always associate physical ailments with emotional responses such as grief, the nurse may need to probe to identify possible loss-related stresses. If the client reports significant losses, it is important to examine how the client usually copes with loss and what resources are available to assist the client in coping. Data regarding general health status; other personal stressors; cultural and spiritual traditions, rituals, and beliefs related to loss and grieving; and the person's support network will be needed in order to determine a plan of care (see the Assessment Interview). In assessing the client's response to a current loss, the nurse may identify dysfunctional grief best treated by a health care professional who is expert in assisting such clients. If the nursing assessment reveals severe physical or psychologic signs and symptoms, the client should be referred to an appropriate care provider.

DIAGNOSING

Nursing diagnoses (NANDA International, 2003) relating specifically to grieving include the following:

Assessment Interview

LOSS AND GRIEVING

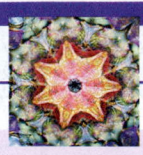

Previous Losses

- Have you ever lost someone or something very important to you?
- Have you or your family ever moved your home?
- What was it like for you when you first started school? Moved away from home? Got a job? Retired?
- Are you physically able to do all the things you used to do?
- Has anyone important or close to you died?
- Do you think there will be any losses in your life in the near future?

If there has been previous grieving:

- Tell me about (the loss). What was losing _____ like for you?
- Did you have trouble sleeping? Eating? Concentrating?
- What kinds of things did you do to make yourself feel better when something like that happened?
- Did you observe any spiritual or cultural practices when you had a loss like that?
- Whom did you turn to if you were very upset about (the loss)?
- How long did it take you to feel more like yourself again and go back to your usual activities?

If there is a current loss:

- What have you been told about (the loss)? Is there anything else you would like to know or don't understand?
- What changes do you think this (illness, surgery, problem) will cause in your life? What do you think it will be like without (the lost object)?
- Have you ever experienced a loss like this before?
- Can you think of anything good that might come out of this?
- What kind of help do you think you will need? Who is going to be helping you with this loss?
- Are there any people or organizations in your community that might be able to help?

Current Grieving

- Are you having trouble sleeping? Eating? Concentrating? Breathing?
- Do you have any pain or other new physical problems?
- What are you doing to help you deal with this loss?
- Are you taking any drugs or medications to help you cope with this loss?

- *Anticipatory Grieving:* Intellectual and emotional responses and behaviors by which individuals, families, communities work through the process of modifying self-concept based on the perception of potential loss
- *Dysfunctional Grieving:* Extended, unsuccessful use of intellectual and emotional responses and behaviors by which individuals, families, communities attempt to work through the process of modifying self-concept based on the perception of loss.

Other nursing diagnoses may include

- *Interrupted Family Processes* if the loss has such impact on the individual and family that usual effective roles and interactions are negatively affected
- *Impaired Adjustment* if the client has great difficulty placing the loss in appropriate perspective to his or her other life activities
- *Risk for Loneliness* related to the loss of relationships with others.

Examples of clinical applications of some of these diagnoses using NANDA, NIC, and NOC designations are shown in Identifying Nursing Diagnoses, Outcomes, and Interventions.

PLANNING

The overall goals for clients who are grieving the loss of body function or a body part are to adjust to the changed ability and to redirect both physical and emotional energy into rehabilitation. The goals for clients who are grieving the loss of a loved one are to remember that person without feeling intense pain

and to redirect emotional energy into one's own life and adjust to the actual or impending loss.

Examples of clinical applications of NOC outcomes and NIC interventions are shown in Identifying Nursing Diagnoses, Outcomes, and Interventions.

Planning for Home Care

Clients who have sustained or anticipate a loss may require ongoing nursing care to assist them in adapting to the loss. The determination of how much and what type of home care follow-up is needed is based in great part on the nurse's knowledge of how the client and family have coped with previous losses. In preparation for home care, the nurse reassesses the client's abilities and needs. The Home Care Assessment on page 1041 describes data to gather for home care or follow-up assessment.

IMPLEMENTING

The skills most relevant to situations of loss and grief are attentive listening, silence, open and closed questioning, paraphrasing, clarifying and reflecting feelings, and summarizing. Less helpful to clients are responses that give advice and evaluation, those that interpret and analyze, and those that give unwarranted reassurance. To ensure effective communication, the nurse must make an accurate assessment of what is appropriate for the client.

Communication with grieving clients needs to be relevant to their stage of grief. Whether the client is angry or depressed affects how the client hears messages and how the nurse interprets the client's statements.

IDENTIFYING NURSING DIAGNOSES, OUTCOMES, AND INTERVENTIONS

CLIENTS WHO ARE GRIEVING

DATA CLUSTER	NURSING DIAGNOSIS/ DEFINITION	SAMPLE DESIRED OUTCOMES [NOC#]/DEFINITION	INDICATORS	SELECTED INTERVENTIONS [NIC#]/DEFINITION	SAMPLE NIC ACTIVITIES
Teresa Jimenez's son Ramon, age 15, has cystic fibrosis of the lungs. Mother and son are waiting for an appropriate donor for a heart-lung transplant. She says, "We've been called to the transplant unit twice, but things didn't work out. Ramon gets his hopes all geared up, and then he's deflated. I can't eat or sleep worrying. I don't know what I'll do if he doesn't get that transplant. He's all I've got since my husband left us six years ago."	*Anticipatory Grieving/Intellectual and emotional responses and behaviors by which individuals, families, communities work through the process of modifying self-concept based on the perception of potential loss*	Grief Resolution [1304]/*Adjustment to actual or impending loss*	To a moderate extent: • Maintains living environment • Seeks social support • Progresses through stages of grief	Grief Work Facilitation [5290]/*Assistance with the resolution of a significant loss*	• Encourage discussion of previous loss experiences • Communicate acceptance of discussing loss • Identify sources of community support • Reinforce progress made in the grieving process
Tom Bauer's wife died 14 months ago of a ruptured aortic aneurysm at age 59. He lives alone, has no children, and refuses to see friends. He reports frequent headaches, inability to concentrate at work, little interest in food, and early morning insomnia. These symptoms increase at the time of his wife's birthday and their anniversary. He says, "I still can't find it in myself to visit her grave. There are times when I'd just like to die and be with her."	*Dysfunctional Grieving/ Extended, unsuccessful use of intellectual and emotional responses and behaviors by which individuals, families, communities attempt to work through the process of modifying self-concept based on the perception of potential loss*	Concentration [0905]/*Ability to focus on a specific stimulus*	Often demonstrated ability: Maintains attention • Maintains focus without being distracted	Mood Management [5330]/*Providing for safety, stabilization, recovery, and maintenance of a patient who is experiencing dysfunctionally depressed or elevated mood*	• Determine whether patient presents safety risk to self or others • Assist patient to maintain a normal cycle of sleep/wakefulness • Provide opportunity for physical activity • Teach decision-making skills • Provide or refer for psychotherapy when appropriate • Assist patient to consciously monitor mood

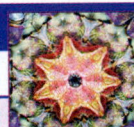

Home Care Assessment
GRIEVING

Client

- **Knowledge:** Client's understanding of the implications of the loss
- **Self-care abilities:** Skill in caring for self based on any physical abilities that may have been altered by the loss
- **Current coping:** Stage in the grieving or bereavement process
- **Current manifestations of the grief response:** Adaptive or maladaptive signs and symptoms; cultural or spiritually based behaviors
- **Role expectations:** Client's perception of the need to return to work or family roles

Family

- **Knowledge:** Various family members' perception of the loss
- **Support people's availability and skills:** Sensitivity to the client's emotional and physical needs; ability to provide an accepting environment
- **Role expectations:** Family perception of client's need to return to work or family roles

Community

- **Resources:** Availability and familiarity with possible sources of assistance such as grief support groups, religious or spiritual centers, counseling services, physical care providers

In addition to using effective communication skills, the nurse implements a plan to provide client and family teaching and to help the client work through the stages of grief.

Facilitating Grief Work

- Explore and respect the client's and family's ethnic, cultural, religious, and personal values in their expressions of grief.
- Teach the client or family what to expect in the grief process, such as that certain thoughts and feelings are normal (acceptable) and that labile emotions, feelings of sadness, guilt, anger, fear, and loneliness will stabilize or lessen over time. Knowing what to expect may lessen the intensity of some reactions.
- Encourage the client to express and share grief with support people. Sharing feelings reinforces relationships and facilitates the grief process.
- Teach family members to encourage the client's expression of grief, not to push the client to move on or enforce his or her own expectations of appropriate reactions. If the client is a child, encourage family members to be truthful and to allow the child to participate in the grieving activities of others.
- Encourage the client to resume normal activities on a schedule that promotes physical and psychologic health. Some clients may try to return to normal activities too quickly. However, a prolonged delay in return may indicate dysfunctional grieving.

Providing Emotional Support

- Use silence and personal presence along with techniques of therapeutic communication. These techniques enhance exploration of feelings and let clients know that the nurse acknowledges their feelings.
- Acknowledge the grief of the client's family and significant others. Family support persons are part of the grieving client's world.
- Offer choices that promote client autonomy. Clients need to have a sense of some control over their own lives at a time when much control may not be possible.
- Provide appropriate information regarding how to access community resources: clergy, support groups, counseling services.

- Suggest additional sources of information and help such as
  a. Grief Recovery Institute
  b. Partnership of Caring: America's Voice for the Dying
  c. American Association of Retired Persons.

Examples of nursing actions appropriate for clients in various stages of the grief process are shown in the Concept Map at the end of the chapter.

EVALUATING

Evaluating the effectiveness of nursing care of the grieving client is difficult because of the long-term nature of the life transition. Criteria for evaluation must be based on goals set by the client and family.

Client goals and related desired outcomes for a grieving client will depend on the characteristics of the loss and the client. Examples of client goals and related outcomes are shown in the accompanying Identifying Nursing Diagnoses, Outcomes, and Interventions.

If outcomes are not achieved, the nurse needs to explore why the plan was unsuccessful. Such exploration begins with reassessing the client in case the nursing diagnoses were inappropriate. Examples of questions guiding the exploration include

- Do the client's grieving behaviors indicate dysfunctional grieving or another nursing diagnosis?
- Is the expected outcome unrealistic for the given time frame?
- Does the client have additional stressors previously not considered that are affecting grief resolution?
- Have nursing orders been implemented consistently, compassionately, and genuinely?

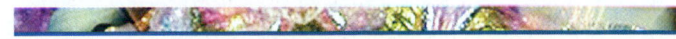

DYING AND DEATH

The concept of death is developed over time, as the person grows, experiences various losses, and thinks about concrete and abstract concepts. In general, humans move from a childhood belief in death as a temporary state, to adulthood in which death is accepted as very real but also very frightening, to older

Medialink | CLIENT WHO SUFFERED AN ARM AMPUTATION CARE PLAN ACTIVITY adulthood in which death may be viewed as more desirable than living with a poor quality of life. Table 41–4 describes some of the specific beliefs common to different age groups. The nurse's knowledge of these developmental stages helps in understanding some of the client's responses to a life-threatening situation.

Responses to Dying and Death

The reaction of any person to another person's impending or real death, or to the potential reality of their own death, depends on all the factors regarding loss and the development of the concept of death. In spite of the individual variations in a person's views about the cause of death, spiritual beliefs, availability of support systems, or any other factor, responses tend to cluster in the phases described by theorists (see Tables 41–1 to 41–3).

Both the client who is dying and the family members grieve as they recognize the loss. Defining characteristics for the nursing diagnosis of *Anticipatory Grieving* include denial, guilt, anger, despair, feelings of worthlessness, crying, and inability to concentrate. They may extend to thoughts of suicide, delusions, and hallucinations. *Fear,* the feeling of disruption that is related to an identifiable source (in this case someone's death),

may also be present. Many of the characteristics seen in a fearful person are similar to those of grieving and include crying, immobility, increased pulse and respirations, dry mouth, anorexia, difficulty sleeping, and nightmares. *Hopelessness* occurs when the person perceives no solutions to a problem—when the death becomes inevitable and the person is unable to see how to move beyond the death. The nurse may observe apathy, pessimism, and inability to make decisions. A person who does perceive a solution to the problem but does not believe that it is possible to implement the solution may be said to experience *Powerlessness.* This loss of control may be manifested by anger, violence, acting out, or depression and passive behavior.

> ➤**CLINICAL ALERT** *Persons who have experienced the deaths of multiple significant others, such as members of the AIDS community, do not necessarily feel the loss or grieve any more or less than those who have experienced fewer deaths.* ■

Caregivers, both professionals and support people, also respond to the impending death. The NANDA diagnosis *Risk for Caregiver Role Strain* may be applied to this group. The ongo-

TABLE 41–4 Development of the Concept of Death

Age	Beliefs/Attitudes
Infancy to 5 years	Does not understand concept of death.
	Infant's sense of separation forms basis for later understanding of loss and death.
	Believes death is reversible, a temporary departure, or sleep.
	Emphasizes immobility and inactivity as attributes of death.
5 to 9 years	Understands that death is final.
	Believes own death can be avoided.
	Associates death with aggression or violence.
	Believes wishes or unrelated actions can be responsible for death.
9 to 12 years	Understands death as the inevitable end of life.
	Begins to understand own mortality, expressed as interest in afterlife or as fear of death.
12 to 18 years	Fears a lingering death.
	May fantasize that death can be defied, acting out defiance through reckless behaviors (e.g., dangerous driving, substance abuse).
	Seldom thinks about death, but views it in religious and philosophic terms.
	May seem to reach "adult" perception of death but be emotionally unable to accept it.
	May still hold concepts from previous developmental stages.
18 to 45 years	Has attitude toward death influenced by religious and cultural beliefs.
45 to 65 years	Accepts own mortality.
	Encounters death of parents and some peers.
	Experiences peaks of death anxiety.
	Death anxiety diminishes with emotional well-being.
65+ years	Fears prolonged illness.
	Encounters death of family members and peers.
	Sees death as having multiple meanings, (e.g., freedom from pain, reunion with already deceased family members).

ing responsibilities for providing physical, economic, psychologic, and social support to a dying person can create extreme stress for the provider. Often, the length of time between a terminal diagnosis and when death will occur is unknown and the people supporting the dying person become fatigued, depressed, and feel empty. There may be anger due to loss of time and resources for personal activities or attention to other people. Within a family that usually functions effectively, death of a member may result in *Impaired Family Processes.* In this situation, the family may be unable to meet the physical, emotional, or spiritual needs of the members and may have difficulty communicating and problem solving.

Professional caregivers, including nurses, may experience role strain due to repeated interactions with dying clients and their families. Although most nurses who work in oncology, hospice, intensive care, emergency, or other areas where client deaths are common have chosen such assignments, there can still be a sense of failure when clients die. Just as there must be support systems for grieving clients, there must also be support systems for grieving health care professionals.

People may think of death as the worst occurrence in life and do their best to avoid thinking or talking about death—especially their own. Nurses are not immune to such attitudes. They need to take time to analyze their own feelings about death before they can effectively help others with a terminal illness. Nurses who are uncomfortable with dying clients tend to impede the clients' attempts to discuss dying and death in these ways:

- Change the subject (e.g., "Let's think of something more cheerful" or "You shouldn't say things like that").
- Offer false reassurance (e.g., "You are doing very well").
- Deny what is happening (e.g., "You don't really mean that," or "You're going to live until you're a hundred").
- Be fatalistic (e.g., "Everyone dies sooner or later," or "God will take you when He wants you").
- Block discussion (e.g., "I don't think things are really that bad") and convey an attitude that stops further discussion of the subject.
- Be aloof and distant or avoid the client.
- "Manage" the client's care and make the client feel increasingly dependent and powerless.

Caring for the dying and the bereaved is one of the nurse's most complex and challenging responsibilities, bringing into play all the skills needed for holistic physiologic and psychosocial care. To be effective, nurses must come to grips with their own attitudes toward loss, death, and dying, because these attitudes will directly affect their ability to provide care.

Definitions and Signs of Death

The traditional clinical signs of death were cessation of the apical pulse, respirations, and blood pressure, also referred to as **heart-lung death.** However, since the advent of artificial means to maintain respirations and blood circulation, identifying death is more difficult. In 1968, the World Medical Assembly adopted the following guidelines for physicians as indications of death:

- Total lack of response to external stimuli
- No muscular movement, especially breathing
- No reflexes
- Flat encephalogram (brain waves).

In instances of artificial support, absence of brain waves for at least 24 hours is an indication of death. Only then can a physician pronounce death, and only after this pronouncement can life-support systems be shut off.

Another definition of death is **cerebral death** or **higher brain death,** which occurs when the higher brain center, the cerebral cortex, is irreversibly destroyed. In this case, there is "presence of cardiac activity, the permanent loss of cerebral function, manifested clinically by the absence of purposive responsiveness to external stimuli; absence of cephalic reflexes, apnea, and an isoelectric electroencephalogram for at least 30 minutes in the absence of hypothermia and poisoning by central nervous system depressants" (Stedman, 2000). People who support this definition of death believe the cerebral cortex, which holds the capacity for thought, voluntary action, and movement, is the individual.

Legalities Related to Death

The nurse's role in legal issues related to death is prescribed by the laws of the region and the policies of the health care institution. For example, in some states, a feeding tube cannot be removed from a person in a persistent vegetative state without a prior directive from the client, but in other states the removal is allowed at the family's request or a physician's order. Some facilities permit do-not-resuscitate orders or protocols that specify the extent of invasive life-sustaining measures. Caring for dying clients who have agreed to organ donation can also be complex in terms of determining which medications, treatments, or equipment must be continued until the time for harvesting the organs has arrived. Many of these legal issues stimulate strong ethical concerns. It is important that the nurse have support from other team members in understanding and providing appropriate care to clients facing death.

Advance Health Care Directives

Advance health care directives include a variety of legal and lay documents that allow persons to specify aspects of care they wish to receive should they become unable to make or communicate their preferences. The Patient Self-Determination Act implemented in 1991 requires all health care facilities receiving Medicare and Medicaid reimbursement to (a) recognize advance directives, (b) ask clients whether they have advance directives, and (c) provide educational materials advising clients of their rights to declare their personal wishes regarding treatment decisions, including the right to refuse medical treatment. Clients and families often have difficulty making advance treatment decisions for end-of-life matters. They need to be reassured that even if they make a decision and have an advance directive, they will always have the option to change their decision. For example, clients may have decided not to have ventilator support if they were terminally ill, but if and when the actual situation occurred, they have the right to change their mind or take more time to make the decision.

Nurses need to assess if clients and families have an accurate understanding of life-sustaining measures. They may misunderstand what actually sustains life and base their decisions on that. Nurses need to incorporate teaching in this area and continue to be supportive of clients' decisions.

There are two types of advance health care directives: the living will and the health care proxy or surrogate. The **living will** provides specific instructions about what medical treatment the client chooses to omit or refuse (e.g., ventilatory support) in the event that the client is unable to make those decisions. For example, the client may later enter a persistent vegetative state or have a terminal illness and need resuscitation to avoid immediate death.

The **health care proxy,** also referred to as a *durable power of attorney for health care,* is a notarized or witnessed statement appointing someone else (e.g., a relative or trusted friend) to manage health care treatment decisions when the client is unable to do so. Figure 41–1 ■ shows an example of an advance health care directive that combines a living will declaration and the durable power of attorney for health care.

Nurses should learn the law regarding patient self-determination for the state in which they practice, as well as the policy and procedures for implementation in the institution where they work. The legally binding nature and specific requirements of advance medical directives are determined by individual state legislation. In most states, advance directives must be witnessed by two people but do not require review by an attorney. Some states do not permit relatives, heirs, or physicians to witness advance directives. As a client advocate, it is important for the nurse to facilitate family discussion about end-of-life concerns and decisions.

Autopsy

An **autopsy** or **postmortem examination** is an examination of the body after death. It is performed only in certain cases. The law describes under what circumstances an autopsy must be performed, for example, when death is sudden or occurs within 48 hours of admission to a hospital. The organs and tissues of the body are examined to establish the exact cause of death, to learn more about a disease, and to assist in the accumulation of statistical data.

It is the responsibility of the physician or, in some instances, of a designated person in the hospital to obtain consent for an autopsy. Consent must be given by the decedent (before death) or by the next of kin. Laws in many states and provinces prioritize the family members who can provide consent as follows: surviving spouse, adult children, parents, and siblings. After an autopsy, hospitals cannot retain any tissues or organs without the permission of the person who consented to the autopsy.

Certification of Death

The formal determination of death, or pronouncement, must be performed by a physician, a coroner, or a nurse. The granting of the authority to nurses to pronounce death is regulated by the state or province. It may be limited to nurses in long-term care, home health, and hospice agencies or to advanced practice nurses. By law, a death certificate must be made out when a person dies. It is usually signed by the attending physician and filed with a local health or other government office. The family is usually given a copy to use for legal matters, such as insurance claims.

Do-Not-Resuscitate Orders

Physicians may order "no code" or **"do-not-resuscitate"** (**DNR**) for clients who are in a stage of terminal, irreversible illness or expected death. A DNR order is generally written when the client or proxy has expressed the wish for no resuscitation in the event of a respiratory or cardiac arrest. Many physicians are reluctant to write such an order if there is any conflict between the client and family members or among family members. A DNR order is written to indicate that the goal of treatment is a comfortable, dignified death and that further life-sustaining measures are not indicated.

The American Nurses Association (ANA) makes the following recommendations related to DNR orders:

- The competent client's values and choices should always be given highest priority, even when these wishes conflict with those of the family or health care providers.
- When the client is incompetent, an advance directive or the proxy decision makers acting for the client should make health care treatment decisions.
- A DNR decision should always be the subject of explicit discussion between the client, family, any designated decision maker acting on the client's behalf, and the health care team.
- DNR orders must be clearly documented, reviewed, and updated periodically to reflect changes in the client's condition. Such documentation is required to meet standards of the Joint Commission on Accreditation of Healthcare Organizations.
- A DNR order is separate from other aspects of a client's care and does not imply that other types of care should be withdrawn, for example, nursing care to ensure comfort or medical treatment for chronic but non-life-threatening illnesses.
- If it is contrary to the nurse's personal beliefs to carry out a DNR order, the nurse should consult the nurse manager for a change in assignment.

The ANA also recommends that each health care organization put into place mechanisms to resolve conflicts between clients, their families, and health care professionals, or between different health care professionals. Institutional ethics committees usually deal with such conflicts. It is important that nurses be represented on these institutional ethics committees so that nursing perspectives can be heard and nurses can be involved in developing DNR policies.

Many states (but not all) permit clients living at home to arrange special orders so that emergency technicians called to the home in the event of a cardiopulmonary arrest will respect the client's wish not to be resuscitated. Some emergency medical services have written policies specifying that staff may withhold CPR if the client has a signed order or approved form or wears a MedicAlert DNR medallion. Nurses should be familiar with the

POWER OF ATTORNEY FOR HEALTH CARE

(1) DESIGNATION OF AGENT: I designate the following individual as my agent to make health care decisions for me: _____

_____
(Name of individual you choose as agent)

_____
(address) (city) (state) (zip code)

_____
(home phone) (work phone)

OPTIONAL: If I revoke my agent's authority or if my agent is not willing, able, or reasonably available to make a health-care decision for me, I designate as my first alternate agent:

_____
(Name of individual you choose as first alternate agent)

_____
(address) (city) (state) (zip code)

_____
(home phone) (work phone)

OPTIONAL: If I revoke the authority of my agent and first alternate agent or if neither is willing, able, or reasonably available to make a health care decision for me, I designate as my second alternate agent:

_____
(Name of individual you choose as second alternate agent)

_____
(address) (city) (state) (zip code)

_____
(home phone) (work phone)

(2) AGENT'S AUTHORITY: My agent is authorized to make all health care decisions for me, including decisions to provide, withhold, or withdraw artificial nutrition and hydration, and all other forms of health care to keep me alive, **except** as I state here:

(3) WHEN AGENT'S AUTHORITY BECOMES EFFECTIVE: My agent's authority becomes effective when my primary physician determines that I am unable to make my own health care decisions unless I mark the following box. If I mark this box [ ], my agent's authority to make health care decisions for me takes effect immediately.

(4) AGENT'S OBLIGATION: My agent shall make health care decisions for me in accordance with this power of attorney for health care, any instructions I give below, and my other wishes to the extent known to my agent. To the extent my wishes are unknown, my agent shall make health care decisions for me in accordance with what my agent determines to be in my best interest. In determining my best interest, my agent shall consider my personal values to the extent known to my agent.

(5) AGENT'S POSTDEATH AUTHORITY: My agent is authorized to make anatomical gifts, authorize an autopsy, and direct disposition of my remains, except as I state here or elsewhere in this form:

INSTRUCTIONS FOR HEALTH CARE
Strike any wording you do not want.

(6) END-OF-LIFE DECISIONS: I direct that my health care providers and others involved in my care provide, withhold, or withdraw treatment in accordance with the choice I have marked below: **(Initial only one box)**
[ ] (a) **Choice NOT To Prolong Life**
I do not want my life to be prolonged if (1) I have an incurable and irreversible condition that will result in my death within a relatively short time, (2) I become unconscious and, to a reasonable degree of medical certainty, I will not regain consciousness, or (3) the likely risks and burdens of treatment would outweigh the expected benefits, **OR**
[ ] (b) **Choice To Prolong Life**
I want my life to be prolonged as long as possible within the limits of generally accepted health care standards.

(7) RELIEF FROM PAIN: Except as I state in the following space, I direct that treatment for alleviation of pain or discomfort should be provided at all times even if it hastens my death:

DONATION OF ORGANS AT DEATH
(8) Upon my death: (mark applicable box)
[ ] (a) I give any needed organs, tissues, or parts,
OR
[ ] (b) I give the following organs, tissues, or parts only: _____
[ ] (c) My gift is for the following purposes:
(strike any of the following you do not want)
(1) Transplant
(2) Therapy
(3) Research
(4) Education

(9) EFFECT OF COPY: A copy of this form has the same effect as the original.

(10) SIGNATURE: Sign and date the form here:

_____ _____
(date)   (sign your name)

_____ _____
(address)   (print your name)

_____ _____
(city)   (state)

(11) WITNESSES: This advance health care directive will not be valid for making health care decisions unless it is either: (1) signed by two (2) qualified adult witnesses who are personally known to you and who are present when you sign or acknowledge your signature; or (2) acknowledged before a notary public.

Figure 41–1 ■ Sample advance health care directive.

federal and state or provincial laws and the policies of their agency concerning withholding life-sustaining measures.

Euthanasia

Euthanasia is the act of painlessly putting to death persons suffering from incurable or distressing disease. It is sometimes referred to as "mercy killing." Regardless of compassion and good intentions or moral convictions, euthanasia is legally wrong in both Canada and the United States and can lead to criminal charges of homicide or to a civil lawsuit for withholding treatment or providing an unacceptable standard of care. Because advanced technology has enabled the medical profession to sustain life almost indefinitely, people are increasingly considering the meaning of quality of life. For some people, the withholding of artificial life-support measures or even the withdrawal of life support is a desired and acceptable practice for clients who are terminally ill or who are incurably disabled and believed unable to live their lives with some happiness and meaning.

Voluntary euthanasia refers to situations in which the dying individual desires some control over the time and manner of death. All forms of euthanasia are illegal except in states where right-to-die statutes and living wills exist. In 1994, the state of Oregon approved the first U.S. physician-assisted suicide law, the Death with Dignity Act, which permits physicians to prescribe lethal doses of medications. The law took effect in November 1997 and, from 1998 through 2002, a total of 129 persons died from the prescriptions they obtained under the act. Since Oregon's action, a number of states have proposed right-to-die laws. Right-to-die statutes legally recognize the client's right to refuse treatment.

Inquest

An inquest is a legal inquiry into the cause or manner of a death. When a death is the result of an accident, for example, an inquest is held into the circumstances of the accident to determine any blame. The inquest is conducted under the jurisdiction of a coroner or medical examiner. A **coroner** is a public official, not necessarily a physician, appointed or elected to inquire into the causes of death, when appropriate. A **medical examiner** is a physician and usually has advanced education in pathology or forensic medicine. Agency policy dictates who is responsible for reporting deaths to the coroner or medical examiner.

Organ Donation

Under the Uniform Anatomical Gift Act and the National Organ Transplant Act in the United States or the Human Tissue Act in Canada, people 18 years or older and of sound mind may make a gift of all or any part of their own bodies for the following purposes: for medical or dental education, research, advancement of medical or dental science, therapy, or transplantation. The donation can be made by a provision in a will or by signing a card-like form. This card is usually carried at all times by the person who signed it. In most states and provinces, the person can revoke the gift, either by destroying the card or by revoking the gift orally in the presence of two witnesses. Nurses may serve as witnesses for people consenting to donate organs.

In almost every case, there is a greater need for transplantation than there are available organs. Thus, in many states, if there is no valid donor document, health care workers are required to discuss with survivors of a potential organ donor the option to make an anatomical gift. Survivors are obliged to grant or withhold donation in accordance with their knowledge of the donor's views on anatomical gifts. The details regarding this process of requesting donation from family members and other legal aspects of organ donation vary by state or province. The nurse needs to be familiar with the appropriate legislation.

Death-Related Religious and Cultural Practices

Various cultural and religious traditions and practices associated with death, dying, and the grieving process help people cope with these experiences. Nurses are often present through the dying process and at the moment of death. Knowledge of the client's religious and cultural heritage helps nurses provide individualized care to clients and their families, even though they may not participate in the rituals associated with death.

In many cultures, people prefer a peaceful death at home rather than in the hospital. Members of some ethnic groups may request that health professionals not reveal the prognosis to dying clients. They believe the person's last days should be free of worry. People in other cultures prefer that a family member (preferably a male in some cultures) be told the diagnosis so that the client can be tactfully informed by a family member in gradual stages or not be told at all. Nurses also need to determine whom to call, and when, as the impending death draws near.

Beliefs and attitudes about death, its cause, and the soul also vary among cultures. Unnatural deaths, or "bad deaths," are sometimes distinguished from "good deaths." In addition, the death of a person who has behaved well in life may be considered less threatening based on the belief that the person will be reincarnated into a good life.

Beliefs about preparation of the body, autopsy, organ donation, cremation, and prolonging life are closely allied to the person's religion. Autopsy, for example, may be prohibited, opposed, or discouraged by Eastern Orthodox religions, Muslims, Jehovah's Witnesses, and Orthodox Jews. Some religions prohibit the removal of body parts and dictate that all body parts be given appropriate burial. Organ donation is prohibited by Jehovah's Witnesses and Muslims, whereas Buddhists in America consider it an act of mercy and encourage it. Cremation is discouraged, opposed, or prohibited by the Mormon, Eastern Orthodox, Islamic, Roman Catholic, and Jewish faiths. Hindus, in contrast, prefer cremation and cast the ashes in a holy river. Prolongation of life is generally encouraged; however, some religions, such as Christian Science, are unlikely to use medical means to prolong life, and the Jewish faith generally opposes prolonging life after irreversible brain damage. In hopeless illness, Buddhists may permit euthanasia.

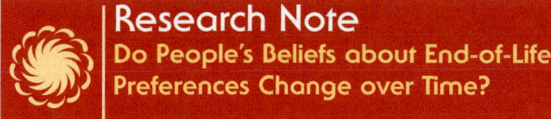

Research Note
Do People's Beliefs about End-of-Life Preferences Change over Time?

In a study by Lockhort, Ditto, Danks, Coppola, and Smucker (2001), 50 elders were queried regarding their views of quality of life in several simulated scenarios. They were also asked whether they would prefer to live or die in situations of coma, chronic severe pain, blindness, deafness, being bedridden, and other situations. The elders completed the questionnaire twice, between 5 and 16 months apart. Surprisingly, 25% to 30% of the elders changed their rating of quality of life and revised their judgment of "worse than death" to "better than death" on the majority of the most severe of the scenarios. The longer the time between the ratings, the more likely it was that their responses would change.

Implications: Two important conclusions can be drawn from this study, even though it used a small sample and needs to be replicated with a much broader group of respondents. First, nurses should not assume that views expressed by elders at any particular point in time about their quality of life and desire to continue living will not change. Ongoing assessment of views and preferences is needed. Second, the relationship between these views and the use of advance directives or DNR orders is integral and reinforces the need to confirm and revise these documents as time passes or conditions change.

Note: From "The Stability of Older Adults' Judgments of Fates Better and Worse than Death," by L. K. Lockhart, P. H. Ditto, P. H. Danks, C. M. Coppola, and W. D. Smucker, 2001, *Death Studies, 25,* pp. 299–317.

Assessment Interview
THE DYING CLIENT

Ask the spouse, partner, or significant others:

- Have you ever been close to someone who was dying before?
- What have you been told about what may happen when death occurs?
- Do you have questions about what may happen at the time of death?
- How do you think you would like to say goodbye?
- How are you taking care of yourself during these times?
- Who can you turn to for help at this time?
- Is there anyone you would like us to contact now or when the death occurs?

Nurses also need to be knowledgeable about the client's death-related rituals, such as last rites, chanting at the bedside, and other rituals, such as special procedures for washing, dressing, positioning, and shrouding the dead. For example, certain cultures retain their native customs, in which family members of the same sex wash and prepare the body for burial and cremation. Muslims also customarily turn the body toward Mecca. Nurses need to ask family members about their preference and verify who will carry out these activities. Burial clothes and other cultural or religious items are often important symbols for the funeral. For example, Mormons are often dressed in their "temple clothes." Some Native Americans may be dressed in elaborate apparel and jewelry and wrapped in new blankets with money. The nurse must ensure that any ritual items present in the health care agency be returned to the family or to the funeral home.

NURSING MANAGEMENT

ASSESSING

To gather a complete database that allows accurate analysis and identification of appropriate nursing diagnoses for dying clients and their families, the nurse first needs to recognize the states of awareness manifested by the client and family members.

In cases of terminal illness, the state of awareness shared by the dying person and the family affects the nurse's ability to communicate freely with clients and other health care team members and to assist in the grieving process. Three types of awareness that have been described are closed awareness, mutual pretense, and open awareness.

In **closed awareness,** the client is unaware of impending death. The family may not completely understand why the client is ill, and they believe the client will recover. The physician may believe it is best not to communicate a diagnosis or prognosis to the client. Nursing personnel are confronted with an ethical problem in this situation. See Chapter 5 🔗 for further information on ethical dilemmas.

With **mutual pretense,** the client, family, and health personnel know that the prognosis is terminal but do not talk about it and make an effort not to raise the subject. Sometimes the client refrains from discussing death to protect the family from distress. The client may also sense discomfort on the part of health personnel and therefore not bring up the subject. Mutual pretense permits the client a degree of privacy and dignity, but it places a heavy burden on the dying person, who then has no one in whom to confide.

With **open awareness,** the client and people around know about the impending death and feel comfortable discussing it, even though it is difficult. This awareness provides the client an opportunity to finalize affairs and even participate in planning funeral arrangements.

Not all people can handle open awareness. Some believe that terminal clients acquire knowledge of their condition even if they are not directly informed. Others believe that clients remain unaware of their condition until the end. It is difficult, however, to distinguish what clients know from what they are willing to accept or acknowledge.

Nursing care and support for the dying client and family include making an accurate assessment of the physiologic signs of approaching death. In addition to signs related to the client's specific disease, certain other physical signs are indicative of impending death. The four main characteristic changes are loss of muscle tone, slowing of the circulation, changes in respirations,

BOX 41-1 ■ Signs of Impending Clinical Death

Loss of Muscle Tone
- Relaxation of the facial muscles (e.g., the jaw may sag)
- Difficulty speaking
- Difficulty swallowing and gradual loss of the gag reflex
- Decreased activity of the gastrointestinal tract, with subsequent nausea, accumulation of flatus, abdominal distention, and retention of feces, especially if narcotics or tranquilizers are being administered
- Possible urinary and rectal incontinence due to decreased sphincter control
- Diminished body movement

Slowing of the Circulation
- Diminished sensation
- Mottling and cyanosis of the extremities

- Cold skin, first in the feet and later in the hands, ears, and nose (the client, however, may feel warm if there is an elevated body temperature)
- Slower and weaker pulse
- Decreased blood pressure

Changes in Respirations
- Rapid, shallow, irregular, or abnormally slow respirations; noisy breathing, referred to as the death rattle, due to collecting of mucus in the throat; mouth breathing, dry oral mucous membranes

Sensory Impairment
- Blurred vision
- Impaired senses of taste and smell

---

and sensory impairment. Box 41–1 lists indications of impending clinical death.

Various consciousness levels may exist just before death. Some clients are alert, whereas others are drowsy, stuporous, or comatose. Hearing is thought to be the last sense lost.

As death approaches, the nurse assists the family and other significant people to prepare. Depending in part on knowledge of the person's state of awareness, the nurse asks questions that help identify ways to provide support during the period before and after death. In particular, the nurse needs to know what the family expects to happen when the person dies so accurate information can be given at the appropriate depth. See the Assessment Interview for sample interview questions. When the family members know what to expect they may be better able to support the dying person and others who are grieving. In addition, they may be able to make certain decisions about events surrounding the death such as whether they will want to view the body after death.

DIAGNOSING

A range of nursing diagnoses, addressing both physiologic and psychosocial needs, can be applied to the dying client, depending on the assessment data. Diagnoses that may be particularly appropriate for the dying client are *Fear, Hopelessness,* and *Powerlessness.* In addition, *Risk for Caregiver Role Strain* and *Impaired Family Processes* are not uncommon diagnoses for caregivers and family members.

Examples of clinical applications of some of these diagnoses using NANDA, NIC, and NOC designations are shown in Identifying Nursing Diagnoses, Outcomes, and Interventions.

PLANNING

Major goals for dying clients are (a) maintaining physiologic and psychologic comfort and (b) achieving a dignified and peaceful death, which includes maintaining personal control and accepting declining health status. When planning care with these clients, the Dying Person's Bill of Rights (Box 41–2) can be a useful guide.

Examples of clinical applications of NOC outcomes and NIC interventions are shown in Identifying Nursing Diagnoses, Outcomes, and Interventions.

Planning for Home Care

People facing death may need help accepting that they have to depend on others. Some dying clients require only minimal care; others need continuous attention and services. People need help, well in advance of death, in planning for the period of dependence. They need to consider what will happen and how and where they would like to die.

BOX 41-2 ■ The Dying Person's Bill of Rights

I have the right to be treated as a living human being until I die.

I have the right to maintain a sense of hopefulness however changing its focus may be.

I have the right to express my feelings and emotions about my approaching death in my own way.

I have the right to participate in decisions concerning my care.

I have the right to expect continuing medical and nursing attention even though cure goals must be changed to comfort goals.

I have the right not to die alone.

I have the right to be free from pain.

I have the right to have my questions answered honestly.

I have the right not to be deceived.

I have the right to have help from and for my family in accepting my death.

I have the right to die in peace and with dignity.

I have the right to retain my individuality and not be judged for my decisions which may be contrary to the beliefs of others.

I have the right to be cared for by caring, sensitive, knowledgeable people who will attempt to understand my needs and will be able to gain some satisfaction in helping me face my death.

Note: From "The Dying Person's Bill of Rights," by A. J. Barbus, 1975, created at the workshop *The Terminally Ill Patient and the Helping Person,* Lansing, MI: South Western Michigan Inservice Education Council.

IDENTIFYING NURSING DIAGNOSES, OUTCOMES, AND INTERVENTIONS

CLIENTS WHO ARE DYING

DATA CLUSTER	NURSING DIAGNOSIS/ DEFINITION	SAMPLE DESIRED OUTCOMES [NOC#]/DEFINITION	INDICATORS	SELECTED INTERVENTIONS [NIC#]/DEFINITION	SAMPLE NIC ACTIVITIES
Keisha Washington, who has multiple sclerosis and is paralyzed from the neck down, has appealed for someone to help her commit suicide. Her mind and speaking ability appear unimpaired. She states, "I dread the same fate as my sister, who also had multiple sclerosis and before death had pain and became blind and mute."	*Hopelessness/ Subjective state in which an individual sees limited or no alternatives or personal choices available and is unable to mobilize energy on own behalf*	Quality of Life [2000]/*An individual's expressed satisfaction with current life circumstances*	Moderate: • Satisfaction with close relationships • Satisfaction with coping ability • Satisfaction with pervasive mood	Hope Instillation [5310]/*Facilitation of the development of a positive outlook in a given situation*	• Assist patient to identify areas of hope in life • Expand the patient's repertoire of coping mechanisms • Facilitate the patient reliving and savoring past achievements and experiences • Provide patient opportunity to be involved with support groups
John Yee, age 63, has metastatic carcinoma of the bowel. He has noticed a rapid deterioration in energy in the past week and feels bloated and nauseated. He has become increasingly jaundiced and says, "I know I haven't long to live. Why can't they just give me a big dose of morphine and get it over with?"	*Powerlessness/ Perception that one's own action will not significantly affect an outcome; a perceived lack of control over a current situation or immediate happening*	Participation: Health Care Decisions [1606]/*Personal involvement in selecting and evaluating health care options*	Sometimes demonstrated: • Seeks information • Defines available options • Identifies available support for achieving desired outcomes	Teaching: Individual [5606]/*Planning, implementation, and evaluation of a teaching program designed to address a patient's particular needs*	• Determine the patient's motivation to learn specific information • Set mutual, realistic learning goals with the patient • Select appropriate learning materials • Select teaching methods/ new methods if previous ones were ineffective • Document the content presented, materials provided, and patient's understanding of the information

A major factor in determining whether a person will die in a health care facility or at home is the availability of willing and able caregivers. If the dying person wishes to be at home, and family or others can provide care to maintain symptom control, the nurse should facilitate a referral to hospice services. Hospice staff and nurses will then conduct a full assessment of the home and care providers' skills.

IMPLEMENTING

The major nursing responsibility for clients who are dying is to assist the client to a peaceful death. More specific responsibilities are the following:

- To provide relief from loneliness, fear, and depression
- To maintain the client's sense of security, self-confidence, dignity, and self-worth
- To help the client accept losses
- To provide physical comfort.

Helping Clients Die with Dignity

Nurses need to ensure that the client is treated with dignity, that is, with honor and respect. Dying clients often feel they have lost control over their lives and over life itself. Helping clients die with dignity involves maintaining their humanity, consistent with their values, beliefs, and culture. By introducing options available to the client and significant others, nurses can restore and support feelings of control. Some choices that clients can make are the location of care (e.g., hospital, home, or hospice), times of appointments with health professionals, activity schedule, use of health resources, and times of visits from relatives and friends.

Clients want to be able to manage the events preceding death so they can die peacefully. Nurses can help clients to determine their own physical, psychologic, and social priorities. Dying people often strive for self-fulfillment more than for self-preservation, and may need to find meaning in continuing to live while suffering. Part of the nurse's challenge, then, is to support the client's will and hope.

Although it is natural for people to be uncomfortable discussing death, steps can be taken to make such discussions easier for both the nurse and the client. Strategies include the following:

- Identify personal feelings about death and how they may influence interactions with clients. Acknowledge personal fears about death, and discuss them with a friend or colleague.
- Focus on the client's needs. The client's fears and beliefs may be different from the nurse's. It is important that the nurse avoid imposing personal fears and beliefs on the client or family.
- Talk to the client or the family about how the client usually copes with stress. Clients will use their usual coping strategies for dealing with impending death. For example, if they are usually quiet and reflective, they will become more quiet and withdrawn when facing terminal illness.
- Establish a communication relationship that shows concern for and commitment to the client. Communication strategies that let the client know you are available to talk about death include the following:

  a. Describe what you see, for example, "You seem sad. Would you like to talk about what's happening to you?"
  b. Clarify your concern, for example, "I'd like to know better how you feel and how I may help you."
  c. Acknowledge the client's struggle, for example, "It must be difficult to feel so uncomfortable. I would like to help you be more comfortable."
  d. Provide a caring touch. Holding the client's hand or offering a comforting massage can encourage the client to verbalize feelings.
- Determine what the client knows about the illness and prognosis.
- Respond with honesty and directness to the client's questions about death.
- Make time to be available to the client to provide support, listen, and respond.

Hospice and Palliative Care

The hospice movement was founded by the physician Cecily Saunders in London, England, in 1967 and was later extended to the United States by Sylvia Lack, also a medical doctor. **Hospice** care focuses on support and care of the dying person and family, with the goal of facilitating a peaceful and dignified death. Hospice care is based on holistic concepts, emphasizes care to improve quality of life rather than cure, supports the client and family through the dying process, and supports the family through bereavement. Assessing the needs of the client's family is just as important as caring for the client who is receiving hospice care. The condition of the client usually deteriorates and attention needs to be focused on the caregivers to ensure that they are receiving support and resources as these changes occur. If the hospice team meets regularly, these needs can be discussed and interventions initiated. Physical needs are usually apparent, but emotional and behavioral signs are often more subtle. A good assessment and ongoing evaluation can help indicate when modifications or changes are needed.

The principles of hospice care can be carried out in a variety of settings, the most common being home and the hospital (or nursing home)-based unit. Services focus on symptom control and pain management. Commonly, clients are eligible for hospice care or hospice insurance benefits when certified by a physician to be likely to die within 6 months. Hospice care is always provided by a team of both health professionals and nonprofessionals to ensure a full range of care services.

Palliative care, as described by the World Health Organization and the Institute of Medicine, focuses on symptom care of clients for whom disease no longer responds to cure-focused treatment. This care may differ from hospice in that the client is not necessarily believed to be imminently dying. Both hospice and palliative care can include **end-of-life care,** that is, the care provided in the final weeks before death.

Meeting the Physiologic Needs of the Dying Client

The physiologic needs of people who are dying are related to a slowing of body processes and to homeostatic imbalances. Interventions include providing personal hygiene measures;

TABLE 41–5 Physiologic Needs of Dying Persons

Problem	Nursing Care
Airway clearance	Fowler's position: conscious clients
	Throat suctioning: conscious clients
	Lateral position: unconscious clients
	Nasal oxygen for hypoxic clients
Bathing/hygiene	Frequent baths and linen changes if diaphoretic
	Mouth care as needed for dry mouth
	Liberal use of moisturizing creams and lotions for dry skin
	Moisture-barrier skin preparations for incontinent clients
Physical mobility	Assist client out of bed periodically, if client is able
	Regularly change bedridden client's position
	Support client's position with pillows, blanket rolls, or towels as needed
	Elevate client's legs when sitting up
	Implement pressure ulcer prevention program and use pressure-relieving surfaces as indicated
Nutrition	Antiemetics or a small amount of an alcoholic beverage to stimulate appetite
	Encourage liquid foods as tolerated
Constipation	Dietary fiber as tolerated
	Stool softeners or laxatives as needed
Urinary elimination	Skin care in response to incontinence of urine or feces
	Bedpan, urinal, or commode chair within easy reach
	Call light within reach for assistance onto bedpan or commode
	Absorbent pads placed under incontinent client; linen changed as often as needed
	Catheterization, if necessary
	Keep room as clean and odor free as possible
Sensory/perceptual changes	Check preference for a light room
	Hearing is not diminished; speak clearly and do not whisper
	Touch is diminished, but client will feel pressure of touch
	Implement pain management protocol if indicated

controlling pain; relieving respiratory difficulties; assisting with movement, nutrition, hydration, and elimination; and providing measures related to sensory changes (also see Table 41–5).

Pain control is essential to enable clients to maintain some quality in their life and their daily activities, including eating, moving, and sleeping. Many drugs have been used to control the pain associated with terminal illness: morphine, heroin, methadone, and alcohol. Usually the physician determines the dosage, but the client's opinion should be considered; the client is the one ultimately aware of personal pain tolerance and fluctuations of internal states. Because physicians usually prescribe dosage ranges for pain medication, nurses use their own judgment as to the amount and frequency of pain medication in providing client relief. Because of decreased blood circulation, analgesics are administered by intravenous infusion, sublingually, rectally, or transdermally rather than subcutaneously or intramuscularly. Clients on narcotic pain medications also require implementation of a protocol to treat opioid-induced constipation.

Providing Spiritual Support

Spiritual support is of great importance in dealing with death. Although not all clients identify with a specific religious faith or belief, most have a need for meaning in their lives, particularly as they experience a terminal illness.

The nurse has a responsibility to ensure that the client's spiritual needs are attended to, either through direct intervention or by arranging access to individuals who can provide spiritual care. Nurses need to be aware of their own comfort with spiritual issues and be clear about their own ability to interact supportively with the client. Nurses have a responsibility to not impose their own religious or spiritual beliefs on a client but to respond to the client in relation to the client's own background and needs. Communication skills are most important in helping the client articulate needs and in developing a sense of caring and trust.

Specific interventions may include facilitating expressions of feeling, prayer, meditation, reading, and discussion with appropriate clergy or a spiritual adviser. It is important for nurses to establish an effective interdisciplinary relationship with spiritual support specialists. For a further discussion of spiritual issues, see Chapter 39. ⊘

Supporting the Family

The most important aspects of providing support to the family members of a dying client involve using therapeutic communication to facilitate their expression of feelings. When nothing can reverse the inevitable dying process, the nurse can provide an empathetic and caring presence. The nurse also serves as a teacher, explaining what is happening and what the family can expect. Due to the effects of the stress of moving through the grieving process, family members may not absorb what they are told and need to have information provided repeatedly. The nurse must have a calm and patient demeanor.

> **► CLINICAL ALERT** *People may use a variety of terms instead of the word* died. *Serious examples include* passed away, gone to a better place, lost, *or* free from suffering. *Humorous examples include* bought the farm, kicked the bucket, *or* croaked. ■

Family members should be encouraged to participate in the physical care of the dying person as much as they wish to and are able. The nurse can suggest they assist with bathing, speak or read to the client, and hold hands. The nurse must not, however, have specific expectations for family members' participation. Those who feel unable to be with the dying person also require support from the nurse and from other family members. They should be shown an appropriate waiting area if they wish to remain nearby.

After the client dies, the family should be encouraged to view the body, because this has been shown to facilitate the grieving process. They may wish to clip a lock of hair as a remembrance. Children should be included in the events surrounding the death if they wish to.

Postmortem Care

Rigor mortis is the stiffening of the body that occurs about 2 to 4 hours after death. It results from a lack of adenosine triphosphate (ATP), which causes the muscles to contract, which in turn immobilizes the joints. Rigor mortis starts in the involuntary muscles (heart, bladder, and so on), then progresses to the head, neck, and trunk, and finally reaches the extremities.

Because the deceased person's family often wants to view the body, and because it is important that the deceased appear natural and comfortable, nurses need to position the body, place dentures in the mouth, and close the eyes and mouth before rigor mortis sets in. Rigor mortis usually leaves the body about 96 hours after death.

Algor mortis is the gradual decrease of the body's temperature after death. When blood circulation terminates and the hypothalamus ceases to function, body temperature falls about 1C (1.8F) per hour until it reaches room temperature.

Simultaneously, the skin loses its elasticity and can easily be broken when removing dressings and adhesive tape.

After blood circulation has ceased, the red blood cells break down, releasing hemoglobin, which discolors the surrounding tissues. This discoloration, referred to as **livor mortis,** appears in the lowermost or dependent areas of the body.

Tissues after death become soft and eventually liquefied by bacterial fermentation. The hotter the temperature, the more rapid the change. Therefore, bodies are often stored in cool places to delay this process. Embalming prevents the process through injection of chemicals into the body to destroy the bacteria.

Nursing personnel may be responsible for care of a body after death. Postmortem care should be carried out according to the policy of the hospital or agency. Because care of the body may be influenced by religious law, the nurse should check the client's religion and make every attempt to comply. If the deceased's family or friends wish to view the body, it is important to make the environment as clean and pleasant as possible and to make the body appear natural and comfortable. All equipment, soiled linen, and supplies should be removed from the bedside. Some agencies require that all tubes in the body remain in place; in other agencies, tubes may be cut to within 2.5 cm (1 in.) of the skin and taped in place; in others, all tubes may be removed.

Normally the body is placed in a supine position with the arms either at the sides, palms down, or across the abdomen. One pillow is placed under the head and shoulders to prevent blood from discoloring the face by settling in it. The eyelids are closed and held in place for a few seconds so they remain closed. Dentures are usually inserted to help give the face a natural appearance. The mouth is then closed.

Soiled areas of the body are washed; however, a complete bath is not necessary, because the body will be washed by the **mortician** (also referred to as an **undertaker**), a person trained in care of the dead. Absorbent pads are placed under the buttocks to take up any feces and urine released because of relaxation of the sphincter muscles. A clean gown is placed on the client, and the hair is brushed and combed. All jewelry is removed, except a wedding band in some instances, which is taped to the finger. The top bed linens are adjusted neatly to cover the client to the shoulders. Soft lighting and chairs are provided for the family.

In the hospital, after the body has been viewed by the family, the deceased's wrist identification tag is left on and additional identification tags are applied. The body is wrapped in a **shroud,** a large piece of plastic or cotton material used to enclose a body after death. Identification is then applied to the outside of the shroud. The body is taken to the morgue if arrangements have not been make to have a mortician pick it up from the client's room. Nurses have a duty to handle the deceased with dignity and to label the corpse appropriately. Mishandling can cause emotional distress to survivors. Mislabeling can create legal problems if the body is inappropriately identified and prepared incorrectly for burial or a funeral.

EVALUATING

To evaluate the achievement of client goals, the nurse collects data in accordance with the desired outcomes established in the planning phase. Evaluation activities may include the following:

- Listening to the client's reports of feeling in control of the environment surrounding death, such as control over pain relief, visitation of family and support people, or treatment plans
- Observing the client's relationship with significant others

- Listening to the client's thoughts and feelings related to hopelessness or powerlessness.

Examples of desired outcomes for dying clients are shown in Identifying Nursing Diagnoses, Outcomes, and Interventions on page 1049. Some of the special needs of elders and their families during death and dying are found in Lifespan Considerations.

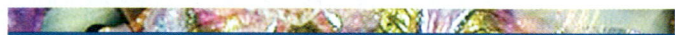

Lifespan Considerations

Elders

Elders who are dying often have a need to know that their lives had meaning. An excellent way to assure them of this is to make audiotapes or videotapes of them telling stories of their lives. This gives the client a sense of value and worth and also lets him or her know that family members and friends will also benefit from it. Doing this with children and grandchildren often eases communication and support during this difficult time.

Caregivers of a dying person need ongoing support and ongoing teaching as the client's condition changes. Some of these needs are

- teaching ways to feed the client when swallowing becomes difficult
- teaching way to transfer and reposition client safely
- teaching ways to communicate if verbalization becomes more difficult
- teaching nonpharmacological methods of pain control
- teaching comfort measures, such as frequent oral care and frequent repositioning.

Focus on Critical Thinking

Mrs. Govinda was a 75-year-old female who was admitted to the hospital after repeated episodes of pneumonia. Despite aggressive antibiotic therapy, Mrs. Govinda's condition rapidly deteriorated and she died unexpectedly 1 week after being admitted to the hospital. Mrs. Govinda's oldest son, who lived nearby and frequently cared for his mother, arranged for the funeral and visited with relatives. He misses his mother and cries occasionally but managed to return to work the following week. The youngest son had difficulty attending the funeral, has been unable to sleep or eat, cannot concentrate at work, and cannot believe that his mother is dead. The middle son did not weep at the funeral and had little to say to his brothers or other relatives. He returned home to another state but has remained distant. He is back to work but feels very fatigued and apathetic.

1. From the data provided, describe the phase of bereavement being experienced by each of the three surviving sons.
2. What factors may have affected how each of the brothers reacted to the death of their mother?
3. What cues, other than physical signs, might have indicated that Mrs. Govinda was dying, even though her death was unexpected?
4. What is the primary factor to consider when trying to make the decision to administer or withhold pain medication from a dying client?
5. How might your own feelings about death affect the care you provide to the dying client?

See Critical Thinking Possibilities in Appendix A.

CONCEPT MAP   The Grieving Client

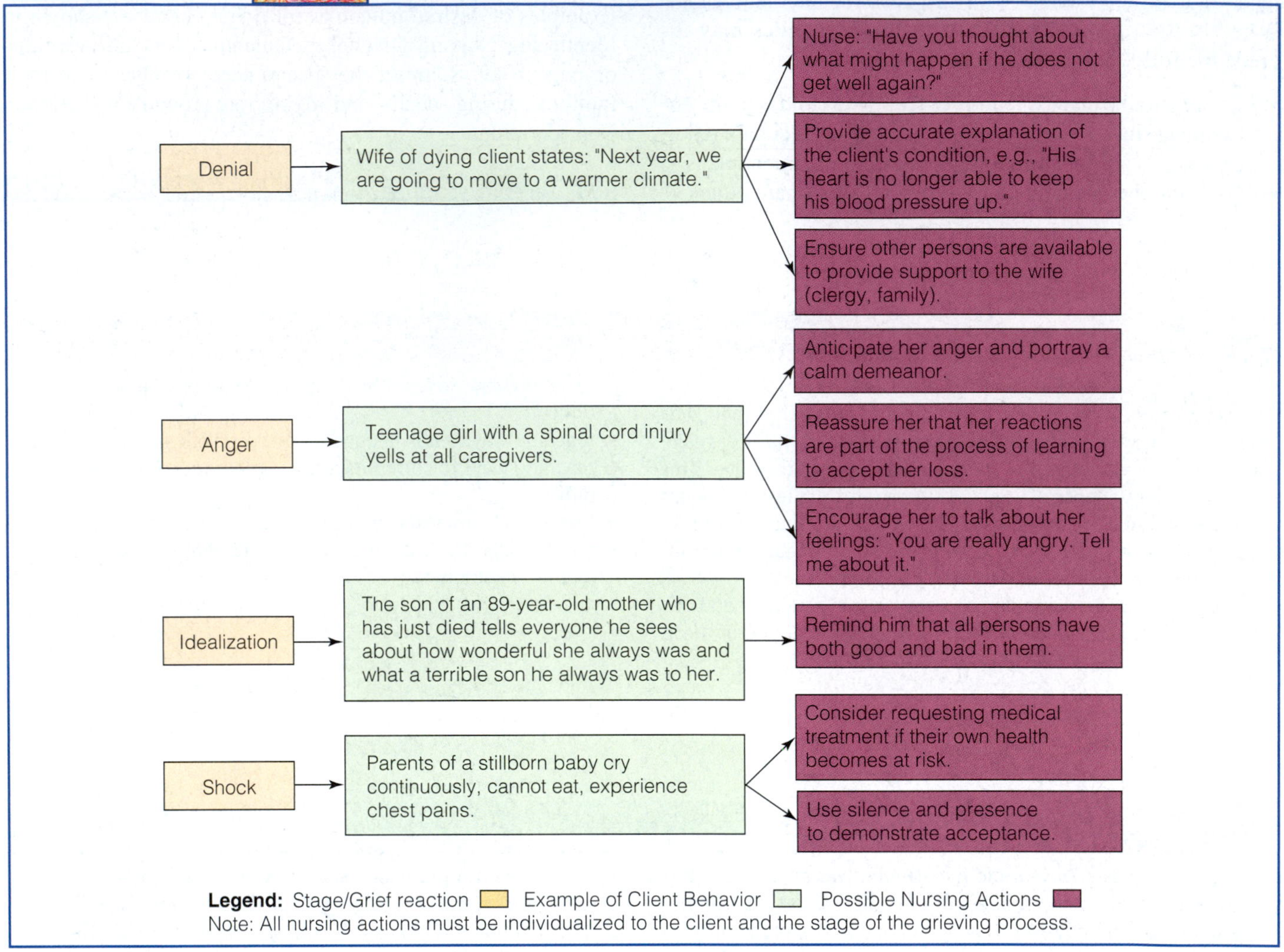

Denial	→	Wife of dying client states: "Next year, we are going to move to a warmer climate."	→	Nurse: "Have you thought about what might happen if he does not get well again?"
				Provide accurate explanation of the client's condition, e.g., "His heart is no longer able to keep his blood pressure up."
				Ensure other persons are available to provide support to the wife (clergy, family).

Anger	→	Teenage girl with a spinal cord injury yells at all caregivers.	→	Anticipate her anger and portray a calm demeanor.
				Reassure her that her reactions are part of the process of learning to accept her loss.
				Encourage her to talk about her feelings: "You are really angry. Tell me about it."

| Idealization | → | The son of an 89-year-old mother who has just died tells everyone he sees about how wonderful she always was and what a terrible son he always was to her. | → | Remind him that all persons have both good and bad in them. |

| Shock | → | Parents of a stillborn baby cry continuously, cannot eat, experience chest pains. | → | Consider requesting medical treatment if their own health becomes at risk. |
| | | | | Use silence and presence to demonstrate acceptance. |

Legend: Stage/Grief reaction ▢   Example of Client Behavior ▢   Possible Nursing Actions ▣
Note: All nursing actions must be individualized to the client and the stage of the grieving process.

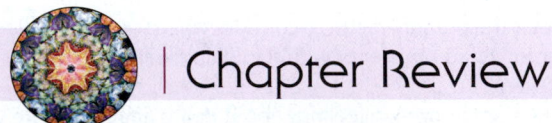

Chapter Review

EXPLORE MediaLink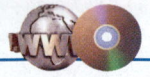

NCLEX review questions, case studies, care plan activities, MediaLink applications, and other interactive resources for this chapter can be found on the Companion Website at www.prenhall.com/kozier. Click on Chapter 41 to select the activities for this chapter.

For more NCLEX review questions, and an audio glossary, access the Student CD-ROM accompanying this textbook.

Chapter Highlights

- Nurses help clients deal with all kinds of losses, including loss of body image, loss of a loved one, loss of a sense of well-being, and loss of a job.

- Loss, especially loss of a loved one or a valued body part, can be viewed as either a situational or a developmental loss and as either an actual or a perceived loss (both of which can be anticipatory).

- Grieving is a normal, subjective emotional response to loss; it is essential for mental and physical health. Grieving allows the bereaved person to cope with loss gradually and to accept it as part of reality.
- Knowledge of different stages or phases of grieving and factors that influence the loss reaction can help the nurse understand the responses and needs of clients.
- How an individual deals with loss is closely related to the individual's stage of development, personal resources, and social support system.
- Caring for the dying and the bereaved is one of the nurse's most complex and challenging responsibilities.

- Nurses' attitudes about death and dying directly affect their ability to provide care.
- Nurses must consider the entire family as requiring care in situations involving loss, especially death.
- Nurses must be knowledgeable about their responsibilities about legal issues surrounding death: advance directives, autopsies, certification of death, DNR orders, euthanasia, inquests, and organ donation.
- Dying clients require open communication, physical help, and emotional and spiritual support to ensure a peaceful and dignified death. They need to maintain a sense of control in managing the events preceding death.

Review Questions

41–1. All of the following may be considered normal or "healthy" types of grief EXCEPT
  a. abbreviated grief.
  b. anticipatory grief.
  c. disenfranchised grief.
  d. dysfunctional grief.

41–2. A patient's family tells you that, in their culture, a dead person may not be left alone before burial. Your hospital policy states that after 6:00 PM when mortuaries are closed, bodies are to be stored in the hospital morgue refrigerator until the next day. How would the nurse best manage this situation?
  a. Gently explain the policy to the family and then implement it.
  b. Inquire of the nursing supervisor how an exception to the policy could be made.
  c. Call the patient's physician for advice.
  d. Move the deceased to an empty room and assign an aide to stay with the body.

41–3. While waiting for the grown children of a deceased patient to arrive, the shift has changed. The oncoming nurse has never met the patient or family. It would be most appropriate for the nurse to greet the family by saying

  a. "I'm very sorry for your loss."
  b. "I'll take you in to view the body."
  c. "I didn't know your father but I am sure he was a wonderful person."
  d. "How long will you want to stay with your father?"

41–4. Which of the following is true regarding a patient with a DNR order?
  a. The patient may no longer make decisions regarding his or her own health care.
  b. The patient and family recognize that the patient will most likely die within the next 48 hours.
  c. Nurses will continue to implement all treatments focused on comfort and symptom management.
  d. A DNR order in place from a previous admission is valid for this and subsequent admissions.

41–5. At which age does a child begin to accept that he or she will someday die?
  a. Less than 5 years old
  b. 5–9 years old
  c. 9–12 years old
  d. 12–18 years old

Readings and References

Suggested Readings

American Journal of Nursing (AJN) bimonthly articles on palliative nursing care and end-of-life issues.
  The goal of this series is to advance the specialty of palliative nursing through the application of current knowledge to clinical care. Beginning May 2002, a special article is published every other month on a specific topic. These are available at http://www.ajnonline.com and http://www.nursingcenter.com. Follow the links to the AJN issues published in odd-numbered months.
American Nurses Association position statements on topics of critical importance to nurses.
  The ANA authors a wide variety of statements on topics of critical importance to nurses.

Several in the area of Ethics and Human Rights are listed below and may be found on the ANA website at these locations:
Assisted Suicide:
  http://nursingworld.org/readroom/position/ethics/etsuic.htm
Promotion of Comfort and Relief of Pain in Dying Patients:
  http://nursingworld.org/readroom/position/ethics/etpain.htm
Nursing Care and Do Not Resuscitate Decisions:
  http://nursingworld.org/readroom/position/ethics/etdnr.htm
Active Euthanasia:
  http://nursingworld.org/readroom/position/ethics/eteuth.htm

Nursing and the Patient Self-Determination Acts:
  http://nursingworld.org/readroom/position/ethics/etsdet.htm
Farella, C. (2001). Assisted suicide: What role for nurses? *Nursing Spectrum, 2*(6), 12–13.
  This article reviews certain aspects of the Oregon Death with Dignity Act and addresses the nurse's role in physician-assisted suicide through several statements from nurses and a case study.
Haynor, P. M. (1998). Meeting the challenge of advance directives. *American Journal of Nursing, 98*(3), 26–33.
  Haynor discusses the requirements specified in the Patient Self-Determination Act and its implications for health care agencies and health

care personnel. Advance directive resources are listed for clients. Haynor uses clinical examples to emphasize the two situations that create the biggest challenges: no advance directive and family opposition. Also included are such topics as how youth complicates the process, how race and culture influence advance directive decisions, educating the public, and questions to pursue.

Related Research

Bonura, D., Fender, M., Roesler, M., & Pacquiao, D. F. (2001). Culturally congruent end-of-life care for Jewish patients and their families. *Journal of Transcultural Nursing, 12,* 211–220.

Freeborne, N., Lynn, J., & Desbiens, N. A. (2000). Insights about dying from the SUPPORT Project: The Study to Understand Prognoses and Preferences for Outcomes and Risks of Treatment. *Journal of the American Geriatric Society, 48,* S199–S205.

Norton, S. A., & Bowers, B. J. (2001). Working toward consensus: Providers' strategies to shift patients from curative to palliative treatment choices. *Research in Nursing and Health, 24,* 258–269.

Steinhauser, K. E., Christakis, N. A., Clipp, E. C., McNeilly, M., Grambow, S., Parker, J., et al. (2001). Preparing for the end of life: Preferences of patients, families, physicians, and other care providers. *Journal of Pain and Symptom Management, 22,* 727–737.

van Baarsen, B. (2002). Theories on coping with loss: The impact of social support and self-esteem on adjustment to emotional and social loneliness following a partner's death in later life. *Journal of Gerontology, 57B,* S33–S42.

References

Barbus, A. J. (1975). *The dying person's bill of rights.* Created at the workshop *The terminally ill patient and the helping person,* Lansing, MI, South Western Michigan Inservice Education Council.

Davis, C., Wortman, C. B., Lehman, D. R., & Silver, R. C. (2000). Searching for meaning in loss: Are clinical assumptions correct? *Death Studies, 24,* 497–540.

Engel, G. L. (1964). Grief and grieving. *American Journal of Nursing, 64,* 93–98.

Johnson, M., Maas, M., & Moorhead, S. (Eds.). (2000). *Nursing outcomes classification (NOC)* (2nd ed.). St. Louis, MO: Mosby.

Kübler-Ross, E. (1969). *On death and dying.* New York: Macmillan.

Lockhart, L. K., Ditto, P. H., Danks, P. H., Coppola, C. M., & Smucker, W. D. (2001). The stability of older adults' judgments of fates better and worse than death. *Death Studies, 25,* 299–317.

Martocchio, B. C. (1985). Grief and bereavement: Healing through hurt. *Nursing Clinics of North America, 20,* 327–341.

McCloskey, J. C., & Bulechek, G. M. (Eds.). (2000). *Nursing interventions classification (NIC)* (3rd ed.). St. Louis, MO: Mosby.

NANDA International. (2003). NANDA *nursing diagnoses: Definitions and classification 2003-2004.* Philadelphia: Author.

Rando, T. A. (1984). *Grief, dying, and death.* Champaign, IL: Research Press.

Rando, T. A. (1986). *Loss and anticipatory grief.* Lexington, MA: Lexington.

Rando, T. A. (1991). *How to go on living when someone you love dies.* New York: Bantam.

Rando, T. A. (1993). *Treatment of complicated mourning.* Champaign, IL: Research Press.

Rando, T. A. (2000). *Clinical dimensions of anticipatory mourning: Theory and practice in working with the dying, their loved ones, and their caregivers.* Champaign, IL: Research Press.

Sanders, C. M. (1998). *Grief: The mourning after: Dealing with adult bereavement* (2nd ed.). New York: John Wiley & Sons.

Shahar, D., R., Schultz, R., Shahar, A., & Wing, R. R. (2001). The effect of widowhood on weight change, dietary intake, and eating behavior in the elderly population. *Journal of Aging and Health, 13,* 186–199.

Stedman, T. L. (2000). *Stedman's medical dictionary* (27th ed.). Philadelphia: Lippincott Williams & Wilkins.

Selected Bibliography

Cox, R., & Parkman, C. A. (2002). The end-of-life movement. *Continuing Care, 21*(2), 20–23, 30.

Ferrell, B. R., & Coyle, N. (Eds.). (2001). *Textbook of palliative care nursing.* Oxford: Oxford University Press.

Ferrell, B. R., & Coyle, N. (2002). An overview of palliative care nursing. *American Journal of Nursing, 102*(5), 26–32.

Fontana, J. S. (2002). Rational suicide in the terminally ill. *Journal of Nursing Scholarship, 34,* 147–151.

Furman, J. (2002). What you should know about chronic grief: Learn to deal with your own lingering emotions when a patient dies. *Nursing, 32*(2), 56.

Hellwig, K. (2000). A family lesson in dying. *RN, 63*(12), 32–33.

Kirk, K. (1998). How Oregon's Death with Dignity Act affects practice. *American Journal of Nursing, 98*(8), 54–55.

Kübler-Ross, E. (1974). *Questions and answers on death and dying.* New York: Macmillan.

Kübler-Ross, E. (1975). *Death: The final stage of growth.* Englewood Cliffs, NJ: Prentice Hall.

Kübler-Ross, E. (1978). *To live until we say goodbye.* Englewood Cliffs, NJ: Prentice Hall.

Matzo, M., & Sherman, D. W. (Eds.). (2001). *Palliative care nursing: Quality care to the end of life.* New York: Springer.

Melvin, C. S., & Heater, B. S. (2001). Organ donation: Moral imperative or outrage? *Nursing Forum, 36*(4), 5–14.

Paice, J. A. (2002). Managing psychological conditions in palliative care. *American Journal of Nursing, 102*(11), 36–42.

Panke, J. T. (2002). Difficulties in managing pain at the end of life. *American Journal of Nursing, 102*(7), 26–33.

Poor, B., & Poirrier, G. P. (2001). *End of life nursing care.* Boston: Jones & Bartlett and the National League for Nursing.

Stroebe, M., & Schut, H. (1999). The dual process model of coping with bereavement: Rationale and description. *Death Studies, 23,* 197–224.

Sulmasy, D. (2001). Addressing the religious and spiritual needs of dying patients. *Western Journal of Medicine, 175,* 251–254.

Tilden, V. P. (2000). Advance directives: Meaningful existence and appropriate care at the end of life. *American Journal of Nursing, 100*(12), 49, 51.

Tuten, M. (2001). A death with dignity in Oregon. *Oncology Nursing Forum, 28,* 58–65.

Valente, S. M. (2001). End-of-life issues. *Geriatric Nursing, 22,* 294–298.

Zilberfein, F. (1999). Coping with death: Anticipatory grief and bereavement. *Generations, 23*(1), 69–74.

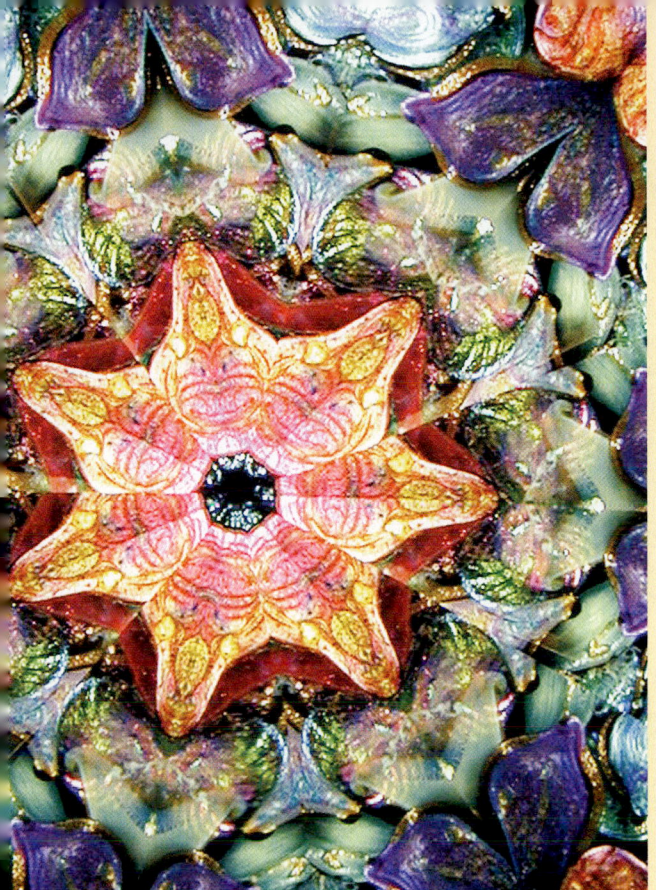

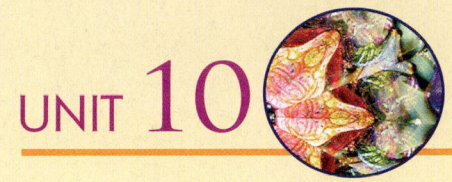

PROMOTING PHYSIOLOGIC HEALTH

The human body consists of a complex network of intricate and interacting systems. Drawing on a comprehensive knowledge base, nurses are cognizant of a host of factors that influence physical health as they provide care to support optimal physiologic function. Efforts to restore, maintain, or improve function include measures that address a client's need for nourishment, comfort, and activity.

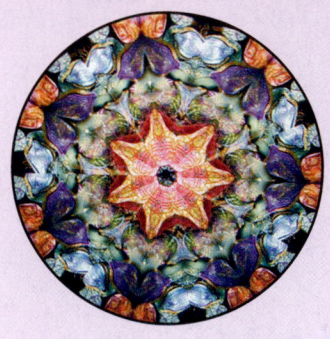

CHAPTER 42

ACTIVITY AND EXERCISE

LEARNING OUTCOMES

After completing this chapter, you will be able to:

- Describe four basic elements of normal movement.

- Differentiate isotonic, isometric, isokinetic, aerobic, and anaerobic exercise.

- Compare the effects of exercise and immobility on body systems.

- Identify factors influencing a person's body alignment and activity.

- Assess activity-exercise pattern, alignment, mobility capabilities and limitations, activity tolerance, and potential problems related to immobility.

- Develop nursing diagnoses, outcomes, and interventions related to activity, exercise, and mobility problems.

- Use proper body mechanics when positioning, moving, lifting, and ambulating clients.

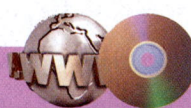

MediaLink

www.prenhall.com/kozier

Additional resources for this chapter can be found on the Student CD-ROM accompanying this textbook, and on the Companion Website at www.prenhall.com/kozier. Click on Chapter 42 to select the activities for this chapter.

CD-ROM
- Audio Glossary
- NCLEX Review
- Animations:
    3D Anatomical
    Joint and Muscle
    Anatomical Movements
    A & P Review

Companion Website
- Additional NCLEX Review
- Case Study: Treating a Client with Mobility Problems
- Care Plan Activity: Activity and Exercise
- MediaLink Application: Promoting Exercise for Seniors
- Links to Resources

An **activity-exercise pattern** refers to a person's routine of exercise, activity, leisure, and recreation. It includes (a) activities of daily living (ADLs) that require energy expenditure such as hygiene, cooking, shopping, eating, working, and home maintenance, and (b) the type, quality, and quantity of exercise, including sports (Gordon, 2002).

Mobility, the ability to move freely, easily, rhythmically, and purposefully in the environment, is an essential part of living. People must move to protect themselves from trauma and to meet their basic needs. Mobility is vital to independence; a fully immobilized person is as vulnerable and dependent as an infant.

People often define their health and physical fitness by their activity because mental well-being and the effectiveness of body functioning depend largely on their mobility status. For example, when a person is upright, the lungs expand more easily, intestinal activity (peristalsis) is more effective, and the kidneys are able to empty completely. In addition, motion is essential for proper functioning of bones and muscles.

The ability to move also influences self-esteem and body image. For most people, self-esteem depends on a sense of independence and a feeling of usefulness or being needed. People with mobility impairments may feel helpless and burdensome to others. Body image can be altered by paralysis, amputations, or any motor impairment. The reaction of others to impaired mobility can also alter self-esteem and body image significantly.

NORMAL MOVEMENT

Normal movement and stability are the result of an intact musculoskeletal system, an intact nervous system, and intact inner ear structures responsible for equilibrium.

Body movement requires coordinated muscle activity and neurologic integration. It involves four basic elements: body alignment (posture), joint mobility, balance, and coordinated movement.

Alignment and Posture

Proper body alignment and posture bring body parts into position in a manner that promotes optimal balance and maximal body function whether the client is standing, sitting, or lying down. A person maintains balance as long as the **line of gravity** (an imaginary vertical line drawn through the body's center of gravity) passes through the **center of gravity** (the point at which all of the body's mass is centered) and the **base of support** (the foundation on which the body rests). In humans, the usual line of gravity begins at the top of the head and falls between the shoulders, through the trunk, slightly anterior to the sacrum, and between the weight-bearing joints and base of support (Figure 42–1 ■). For a person in the upright position, the center of gravity is located in the center of the pelvis approximately midway between the umbilicus and the symphysis pubis. For greatest balance and stability, a standing adult must center body weight symmetrically along the line of gravity. Greater stability and balance are provided in a sitting or lying position than in a standing position. The feet of the chair or bed form a considerably wider base of support, the center of gravity is lower, and the line of gravity is less mobile.

When the body is well aligned, strain on the joints, muscles, tendons, or ligaments is minimized and internal structures and organs are supported. People are usually unaware of the functions of the skeletal muscles that maintain body posture. These muscles function almost continuously, making tiny adjustments that enable an erect or seated posture despite the endless downward pull of gravity. The extensor muscles, often referred to as the *antigravity muscles,* carry the major load.

Proper body alignment enhances lung expansion and promotes efficient circulatory, renal, and gastrointestinal functions. A person's posture is one criterion for assessing general health, physical fitness, and attractiveness. Posture reflects the mood, self-esteem, and personality of an individual.

Joint Mobility

Joints are the functional units of the musculoskeletal system. The bones of the skeleton articulate at the joints and most of the skeletal muscles attach to the two bones at the joint. These muscles are categorized according to the type of joint movement they produce on contraction. Muscles are therefore called flexors, extensors, internal rotators, and the like. The flexor muscles are stronger than the

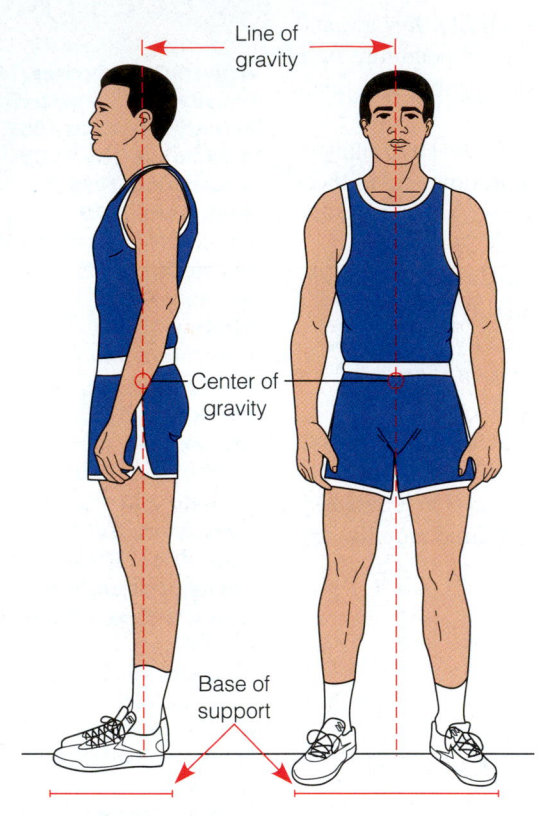

Figure 42–1 ■ The center of gravity and the line of gravity influence standing alignment.

TABLE 42–1 Types of Joint Movements

Movement	Action
Flexion	Decreasing the angle of the joint (e.g., bending the elbow)
Extension	Increasing the angle of the joint (e.g., straightening the arm at the elbow)
Hyperextension	Further extension or straightening of a joint (e.g., bending the head backward)
Abduction	Movement of the bone away from the midline of the body
Adduction	Movement of the bone toward the midline of the body
Rotation	Movement of the bone around its central axis
Circumduction	Movement of the distal part of the bone in a circle while the proximal end remains fixed
Eversion	Turning the sole of the foot outward by moving the ankle joint
Inversion	Turning the sole of the foot inward by moving the ankle joint
Pronation	Moving the bones of the forearm so that the palm of the hand faces downward when held in front of the body
Supination	Moving the bones of the forearm so that the palm of the hand faces upward when held in front of the body

extensor muscles. Thus, when a person is inactive, the joints are pulled into a flexed (bent) position. If this tendency is not counteracted with exercise and position changes, the muscles permanently shorten, and the joint becomes fixed in a flexed position. Types of joint movement are shown in Table 42–1.

The **range of motion (ROM)** of a joint is the maximum movement that is possible for that joint. Joint range of motion varies from individual to individual and is determined by genetic makeup, developmental patterns, the presence or absence of disease, and the amount of physical activity in which the person normally engages. Table 42–2 shows the various joint movements and the usual ranges of motion.

Balance

The mechanisms involved in maintaining balance and posture are complex. Mechanisms of equilibrium (sense of balance) respond, frequently without our awareness, to various head movements. The equilibrium sense depends on informational inputs from the labyrinth (inner ear), vision (vestibulo-ocular input), and from stretch receptors of muscles and tendons (vestibulospinal input). The labyrinth consists of the cochlea, vestibule, and semicircular canals. The cochlea is concerned with hearing and the vestibule and semicircular canals with equilibrium. Under normal conditions the equilibrium receptors in the semicircular canals and vestibule, collectively called the vestibular apparatus, send signals to the brain that initiate

reflexes needed to make required changes in position. The receptors, hairlike cells, respond to displacement of the head in any direction. When the head moves, the fluid flow within the vestibule and semicircular canals stimulates sensory hair cells. Information from these balance receptors goes directly to reflex centers in the brain stem rather than to the cerebral cortex as with other special senses. This enables fast reflexive responses to body imbalance.

Coordinated Movement

Balanced, smooth, purposeful movement is the result of proper functioning of the cerebral cortex, cerebellum, and basal ganglia. The cerebral cortex initiates voluntary motor activity, the cerebellum coordinates the motor activities of movement, and the basal ganglia maintain posture. The cerebral cortex operates movements, not muscles. The cortex, for example, may direct the arm to pick up a cup of coffee. The cerebellum, which operates below the level of consciousness, blends and coordinates the muscles involved in voluntary movement. It does not direct the movement but translates the "instructions" from the cerebral cortex into detailed actions by the many different muscles in the hand, arm, and shoulder. When a client's cerebellum is injured, movements become clumsy, unsure, and uncoordinated.

TABLE 42-2 Selected Joint Movements

Body Part—Type of Joint/Movement	Normal Range	Illustration
Neck—Pivot Joint		
Flexion. Move the head from the upright midline position forward, so that the chin rests on the chest (Figure 42–2 ■).	45° from midline	**Figure 42–2**
Extension. Move the head from the flexed position to the upright position (Figure 42–2).	45° from midline	
Hyperextension. Move the head from the upright position back as far as possible (Figure 42–2).	45° from midline	
Lateral flexion. Move the head laterally to the right and left shoulders (Figure 42–3 ■).	40° from midline	**Figure 42–3**
Rotation. Turn the face as far as possible to the right and left (Figure 42–4 ■).	70° from midline	**Figure 42–4**
Shoulder—Ball-and-Socket Joint		
Flexion. Raise each arm from a position by the side forward and upward to a position beside the head (Figure 42–5 ■).	180° from the side	**Figure 42–5**
Extension. Move each arm from a vertical position beside the head forward and down to a resting position at the side of the body (Figure 42–5).	180° from vertical position beside the head	
Hyperextension. Move each arm from a resting side position to behind the body (Figure 42–5).	50° from side position	
Abduction. Move each arm laterally from a resting position at the sides to a side position above the head, palm of the hand away from the head (Figure 42–6 ■).	180°	**Figure 42–6**
Adduction (anterior). Move each arm from a position at the sides across the front of the body as far as possible (Figure 42–6). The elbow may be straight or bent.	50°	
Circumduction. Move each arm forward, up, back, and down in a full circle (Figure 42–7 ■).	360°	**Figure 42–7**
External rotation. With each arm held out to the side at shoulder level and the elbow bent to a right angle, fingers pointing down, move the arm upward so that the fingers point up (Figure 42–8 ■).	90°	**Figure 42–8**
Internal rotation. With each arm held out to the side at shoulder level and the elbow bent to a right angle, fingers pointing up, bring the arm forward and down so that the fingers point down (Figure 42–8).	90°	

continued on page 1062

TABLE 42–2 Selected Joint Movements (continued)

Body Part—Type of Joint/Movement	Normal Range	Illustration
Elbow—Hinge Joint		
Flexion. Bring each lower arm forward and upward so that the hand is at the shoulder (Figure 42–9 ■).	150°	**Figure 42–9**
Extension. Bring each lower arm forward and downward, straightening the arm (Figure 42–9).	150°	
Rotation for supination. Turn each hand and forearm so that the palm is facing upward (Figure 42–10 ■).	70° to 90°	**Figure 42–10**
Rotation for pronation. Turn each hand and forearm so that the palm is facing downward (Figure 42–10).	70° to 90°	
Wrist—Condyloid Joint		
Flexion. Bring the fingers of each hand toward the inner aspect of the forearm (Figure 42–11 ■).	80° to 90°	**Figure 42–11**
Extension. Straighten each hand to the same plane as the arm (Figure 42–11).	80° to 90°	
Hyperextension. Bend the fingers of each hand back as far as possible (Figure 42–12 ■).	70° to 90°	**Figure 42–12**
Radial flexion (abduction). Bend each wrist laterally toward the thumb side with hand supinated (Figure 42–13 ■).	0° to 20°	**Figure 42–13**
Ulnar flexion (adduction). Bend each wrist laterally toward the fifth finger with the hand supinated (Figure 42–13).	30° to 50°	
Hand and Fingers: Metacarpophalangeal Joints—Condyloid; Interphalangeal Joints—Hinge		
Flexion. Make a fist with each hand (Figure 42–14 ■).	90°	**Figure 42–14**
Extension. Straighten the fingers of each hand (Figure 42–14).	90°	
Hyperextension. Bend the fingers of each hand back as far as possible (Figure 42–14).	30°	
Abduction. Spread the fingers of each hand apart (Figure 42–15 ■).	20°	**Figure 42–15**
Adduction. Bring the fingers of each hand together (Figure 42–15).	20°	
Thumb—Saddle Joint		
Flexion. Move each thumb across the palmar surface of the hand toward the fifth finger (Figure 42–16 ■).	90°	**Figure 42–16**
Extension. Move each thumb away from the hand (Figure 42–16).	90°	
Abduction. Extend each thumb laterally (Figure 42–17 ■).	30°	**Figure 42–17**
Adduction. Move each thumb back to the hand (Figure 42–17).	30°	

TABLE 42–2 Selected Joint Movements (continued)

Body Part—Type of Joint/Movement	Normal Range	Illustration
Opposition. Touch each thumb to the top of each finger of the same hand. The thumb joint movements involved are abduction, rotation, and flexion (Figure 42–18 ■).		**Figure 42–18**
Hip—Ball-and-Socket Joint **Flexion.** Move each leg forward and upward. The knee may be extended or flexed (Figure 42–19 ■).	Knee extended, 90°; knee flexed, 120°	**Figure 42–19**
Extension. Move each leg back beside the other (Figure 42–20 ■). **Hyperextension.** Move each leg back behind the body (Figure 42–20).	90° to 120° 30° to 50°	**Figure 42–20**
Abduction. Move each leg out to the side (Figure 42–21 ■). **Adduction.** Move each leg back to the other leg and beyond in front of it (Figure 42–21).	45° to 50° 20° to 30° beyond other leg	**Figure 42–21**
Circumduction. Move each leg backward, up, to the side, and down in a circle (Figure 42–22 ■).	360°	**Figure 42–22**
Internal rotation. Turn each foot and leg inward so that the toes point as far as possible toward the other leg (Figure 42–23 ■). **External rotation.** Turn each foot and leg outward so that the toes point as far as possible away from the other leg (Figure 42–23).	90° 90°	**Figure 42–23**

continued on page 1064

TABLE 42–2 Selected Joint Movements (continued)

Body Part—Type of Joint/Movement	Normal Range	Illustration
Knee—Hinge Joint **Flexion.** Bend each leg, bringing the heel toward the back of the thigh (Figure 42–24 ■). **Extension.** Straighten each leg, returning the foot to its position beside the other foot (Figure 42–24).	120° to 130° 120° to 130°	**Figure 42–24**
Ankle—Hinge Joint **Extension (plantar flexion).** Point the toes of each foot downward (Figure 42–25 ■). **Flexion (dorsiflexion).** Point the toes of each foot upward (Figure 42–25).	45° to 50° 20°	**Figure 42–25**
Foot—Gliding **Eversion.** Turn the sole of each foot laterally (Figure 42–26 ■). **Inversion.** Turn the sole of each foot medially (Figure 42–26).	5° 5°	**Figure 42–26**
Toes: Interphalangeal Joints—Hinge; Metatarsophalangeal Joints—Hinge; Intertarsal Joints—Gliding **Flexion.** Curl the toe joints of each foot downward (Figure 42–27 ■). **Extension.** Straighten the toes of each foot (Figure 42–27).	35° to 60° 35° to 60°	**Figure 42–27**
Trunk—Gliding Joint **Flexion.** Bend the trunk toward the toes (Figure 42–28 ■). **Extension.** Straighten the trunk from a flexed position (Figure 42–28). **Hyperextension.** Bend the trunk backward (Figure 42–28).	70° to 90° 20° to 30°	**Figure 42–28**
Lateral flexion. Bend the trunk to the right and to the left (Figure 42–29 ■).	35° on each side	**Figure 42–29** 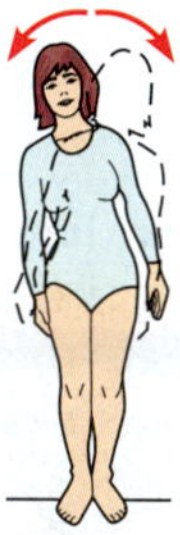
Rotation. Turn the upper part of the body from side to side (Figure 42–30 ■).	30° to 45°	**Figure 42–30** 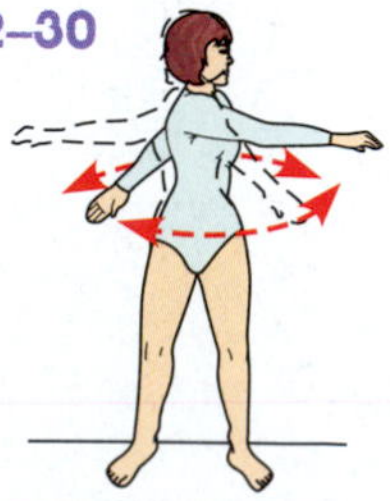

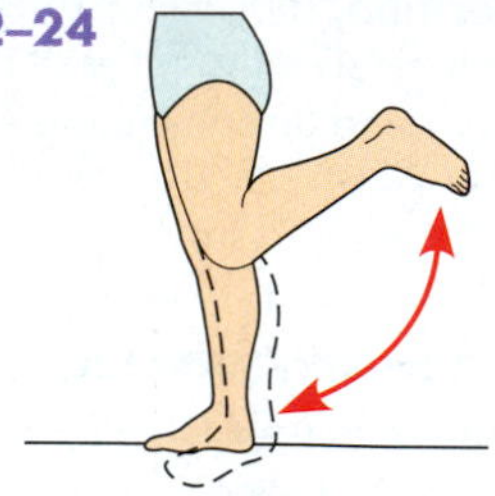

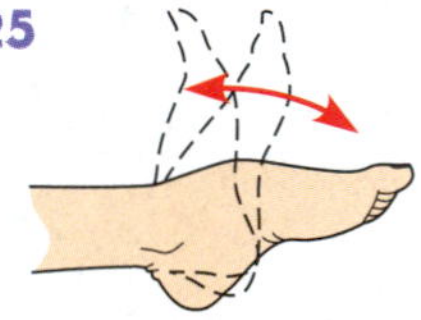

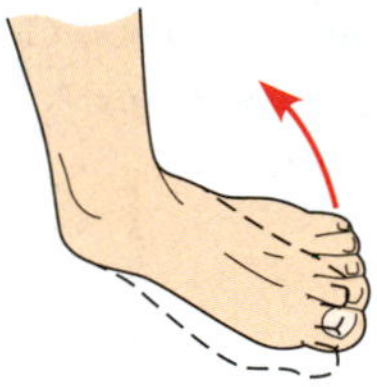

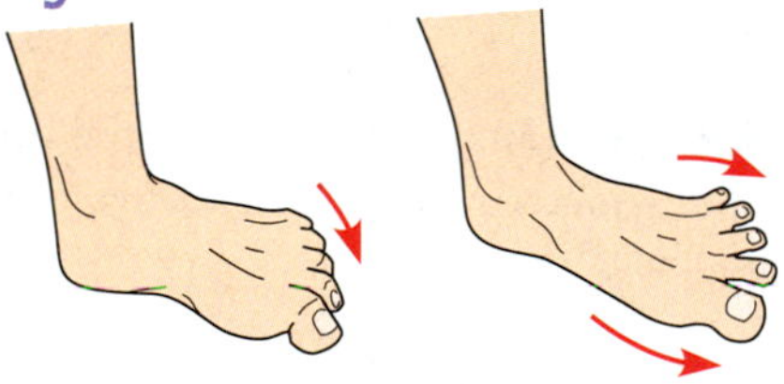

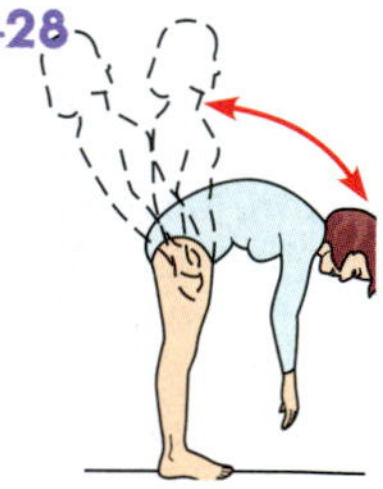

EXERCISE

The National Institutes of Health (NIH) defines exercise and physical activity as follows (1995, p. 3):

- **Physical activity** is "bodily movement produced by skeletal muscles that requires energy expenditure and produces progressive health benefits."
- **Exercise** is "a type of physical activity defined as a planned, structured, and repetitive bodily movement done to improve or maintain one or more components of physical fitness."

People participate in exercise programs to decrease risk factors for cardiovascular disease and to increase their health and well-being. **Activity tolerance** is the type and amount of exercise or daily living activities an individual is able to perform without experiencing adverse effects.

Types of Exercise

Exercise involves the active contraction and relaxation of muscles. Exercises can be classified according to the type of muscle contraction (isotonic, isometric, or isokinetic) and according to the source of energy (aerobic or anaerobic).

Isotonic (dynamic) exercises are those in which the muscle shortens to produce muscle contraction and active movement. Most physical conditioning exercises—running, walking, swimming, cycling, and other such activities—are isotonic, as are ADLs and active ROM exercises (those initiated by the client). Examples of isotonic bed exercises are pushing or pulling against a stationary object, using a trapeze to lift the body off the bed, lifting the buttocks off the bed by pushing with the hands against the mattress, and pushing the body to a sitting position.

Isotonic exercises increase muscle tone, mass, and strength and maintain joint flexibility and circulation. During isotonic exercise, both heart rate and cardiac output quicken to increase blood flow to all parts of the body. Little or no change in blood pressure occurs.

Isometric (static or setting) exercises are those in which there is a change in muscle tension but there is no change in muscle length and no muscle or joint movement. These exercises involve exerting pressure against a solid object and are useful for strengthening abdominal, gluteal, and quadriceps muscles used in ambulation; for maintaining strength in immobilized muscles in casts or traction; and for endurance training. Examples of isometric bed exercise would be extending the leg in a supine position, tensing the thigh muscles, and pressing the knee against the bed, holding it for several seconds. These are often called quadriceps (or quad) sets.

Isometric exercises produce a moderate increase in heart rate and cardiac output, but no appreciable increase in blood flow to other parts of the body.

Isokinetic (resistive) exercises involve muscle contraction or tension against resistance; thus, they can be either isotonic or isometric. During isokinetic exercises, the person moves (isotonic) or tenses (isometric) against resistance. Special ma-

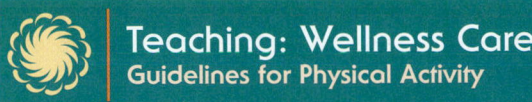

Teaching: Wellness Care
Guidelines for Physical Activity

Frequency	Three times per week
Duration	Cumulative 30 minutes daily (can be divided throughout the day)
Intensity	"Moderate" intensity as measured by the talk test and perceived exertion scale
Type of exercise	Walking, biking, and swimming are recommended for beginners and older adults. Activities that are more strenuous include jogging, running, and jumping rope.
Safety	Outside of the home, use appropriate safety measures such as checking equipment for proper function, wearing a helmet and other protective gear, using reflective devices at night, carrying identification and emergency information.

MediaLink | A & P REVIEW ANIMATION

chines or devices provide the resistance to the movement. These exercises are used in physical conditioning and are often done to build up certain muscle groups; for example, the pectorals (chest muscles) may be increased in size and strength by lifting weights.

Aerobic exercise is activity during which the amount of oxygen taken in the body is greater than that used to perform the activity. Aerobic exercises use large muscle groups, are performed continuously, and are rhythmic in nature. Examples are walking, jogging, running, bicycling, dancing, cross-country skiing, jumping rope, rowing, swimming, and skating. Aerobic exercises improve cardiovascular conditioning and physical fitness. Assessment of physical fitness is discussed in Chapter 8. The accompanying Teaching: Wellness Care feature describes frequency, duration, and intensity of exercise recommended for healthy adults.

Intensity of exercise can be measured in three ways:

1. *Target heart rate.* With this system, the goal is to work up to and sustain a target heart rate during exercise, based on the person's age. To determine the target heart rate, first calculate the person's maximum heart rate by subtracting her or his current age in years from 220. Then obtain the target heart rate by taking 60% to 85% of the maximum. At least 60% of maximum heart rate is the recommended intensity. Because heart rates are so variable among individuals, the tests that follow are replacing this measure.
2. *Talk test.* This test is easier to implement and keeps most people at 60% of maximum heart rate or more. When exercising, the person should be able to carry on a conversation even with some labored breathing. However, exercise intensity should be increased if the person can carry on with unlimited unlabored discussion.
3. *Borg scale of perceived exertion (Borg, 1998).* This scale measures "how difficult" the exercise feels to the person

in terms of heart and lung exertion. The scale progresses as follows:

6	14
7 Very, very light	15 Hard
8	16
9 Very light	17 Very hard
10	18
11 Fairly light	19 Very, very hard
12	20
13 Somewhat hard	

"Very, very hard" corresponds closely to 100% of maximum heart rate. "Very light" is close to 40%. Most people need to strive for the "Somewhat hard" level, which corresponds to 75% of maximum heart rate.

Anaerobic exercise involves activity in which the muscles cannot draw out enough oxygen from the bloodstream, and anaerobic pathways are used to provide additional energy for a short time. This type of exercise is used in endurance training for athletes.

Benefits of Exercise

Regular exercise is essential for healthy functioning of major body systems. The benefits of exercise on these systems follow.

Musculoskeletal System

The size, shape, tone, and strength of muscles (including the heart muscle) are maintained with mild exercise and increased with strenuous exercise. With strenuous exercise, muscles **hypertrophy** (enlarge), and the efficiency of muscular contraction increases. Hypertrophy is commonly seen in the arm muscles of a tennis player, the leg muscles of a skater, and the arm and hand muscles of a carpenter.

Exercise increases joint flexibility and range of motion. Bone density is maintained through weight-bearing. The stress of weight-bearing maintains a balance between osteoblasts (bone-building cells) and osteoclasts (bone-resorption and breakdown cells).

Cardiovascular System

Adequate exercise increases the heart rate, the strength of heart muscle contraction, and the blood supply to the heart and muscles. Cardiac output (the amount of blood pumped by the heart) increases as much as 30 L/min. Normal cardiac output is 5 L/min.

Respiratory System

Ventilation (air circulating into and out of the lungs) increases. In strenuous exercise, the intake of oxygen increases to as much as 20 times normal intake. Normal ventilation is about 5 or 6 L/min. Adequate exercise also prevents pooling of secretions in the bronchi and bronchioles, decreases breathing effort, and improves diaphragmatic excursion.

Gastrointestinal System

Exercise improves the appetite and increases gastrointestinal tract tone, facilitating peristalsis.

Metabolic System

Exercise elevates the metabolic rate, thus increasing the production of body heat and waste products and calorie use. During strenuous exercise, the metabolic rate can increase to as much as 20 times the normal rate. Exercise increases the use of triglycerides and fatty acids, resulting in a reduced level of serum triglycerides and cholesterol. Exercise also enhances the effectiveness of insulin, lowering blood sugar. In diabetics, exercise can reduce their need for injecting supplemental insulin.

Urinary System

As adequate exercise promotes efficient blood flow, the body excretes wastes more effectively. In addition, stasis (stagnation) of urine in the bladder is usually prevented.

Psychoneurologic System

Exercise produces a sense of well-being and improves tolerance to stress. It may also improve self-concept by reducing depression and improving one's body image. Energy level increases and quality of sleep is enhanced.

FACTORS AFFECTING BODY ALIGNMENT AND ACTIVITY

A number of factors affect an individual's body alignment, mobility, and daily activity level. These include growth and development, physical health, mental health, nutrition, personal values and attitudes, and certain external factors.

Growth and Development

A person's age and musculoskeletal and nervous system development affect posture, body proportions, body mass, body movements, and reflexes. Newborn movements are reflexive and random. All extremities are generally flexed but can be passively moved through a full range of motion. The feet are usually inverted but can be passively everted. As the neurologic system matures, control over movement progresses during the first year. Gross motor development precedes fine motor skills. Gross motor development occurs in a head-to-toe fashion, that is, progression from head control, to crawling, to pulling up to a standing position, to standing, and to walking, usually after the first birthday. Initially, walking involves a wide stance and unsteady gait, thus the term toddler. From ages 1 to 5 years, both gross and fine motor skills are refined. For example, preschoolers master riding a tricycle, dancing, running, jumping, using crayons to draw, fastening or using zippers, and brushing their teeth.

From 6 to 12 years, refinement of motor skills continues and exercise patterns for later life are generally determined. Many schools provide physical education and competitive sports programs to enhance physical activity. Posture in school-age children is excellent, often the best during one's lifetime. In adolescence, growth spurts may result in awkwardness that can be manifested in posture. Postural habits formed during adolescence often persist into adulthood.

Adults between 20 and 40 years of age generally have few physical changes affecting mobility with the exception of pregnant women. Pregnancy alters center of gravity, affects balance, and reduces exercise tolerance. As age advances, muscle tone and bone density decrease, joints lose flexibility, reaction time slows, and bone mass decreases, particularly in women who have osteoporosis. **Osteoporosis** is a condition in which the bones become brittle and fragile due to calcium depletion. Osteoporosis is common in older women and primarily affects the weight-bearing joints of the lower extremities and the back, causing compression fractures of the vertebrae and hip fractures. All of these changes affect older adults' posture, gait, and balance. Posture becomes forward leaning and stooped, which shifts the center of gravity forward. To compensate for this shift, the knees flex slightly for support and the base of support is widened. Gait becomes wide based, short stepped, and shuffling.

Physical Health

Mobility and activity tolerance are affected by any disorder that impairs the ability of the nervous system, musculoskeletal system, cardiovascular system, respiratory system, and vestibular apparatus. Congenital problems such as hip dysplasia, spina bifida, cerebral palsy, and the muscular dystrophies affect motor functioning. Disorders of the nervous system such as Parkinson's disease, multiple sclerosis, central nervous system tumors, cerebrovascular accidents (strokes), infectious processes (e.g., meningitis), and head and spinal cord injuries can leave muscle groups weakened, paralyzed, **spastic** (with too much muscle tone), or **flaccid** (without muscle tone). Musculoskeletal disorders affecting mobility include strains, sprains, fractures, joint dislocations, amputations, and joint replacements. Inner ear infections and dizziness can impair balance.

Many other acute and chronic illnesses that limit the supply of oxygen and nutrients needed for muscle contraction and movement can seriously affect activity tolerance. Examples include chronic obstructive lung disease, anemia, congestive heart failure, and angina.

Mental Health

Mental or affective disorders such as depression or chronic stress may affect a person's desire to move. The depressed person may lack enthusiasm for taking part in any activity and may even lack energy for usual hygiene practices. Lack of visible energy is seen in a slumped posture with head bowed. By contrast, happy, confident people usually stand erect. Chronic stress can deplete the body's energy reserves to the point that fatigue discourages the desire to exercise, even though exercise can energize the person and facilitate coping.

Nutrition

Both undernutrition and overnutrition can influence body alignment and mobility. Poorly nourished people may have muscle weakness and fatigue. Vitamin D deficiency causes bone deformity during growth. Inadequate calcium intake increases the risk of osteoporosis. Obesity can distort movement and can adversely affect posture and balance.

Personal Values and Attitudes

Whether people value regular exercise is often the result of family influences. In families that incorporate regular exercise in their daily routine or spend time together in activities, children learn to value physical activity. Sedentary families, on the other hand, participate in sports only as spectators, and this lifestyle is often transmitted to their children. Values about physical appearance also influence some people's participation in regular exercise. People who value a muscular build or physical attractiveness may participate in regular exercise programs to produce the appearance they desire. Choice of physical activity or type of exercise is also influenced by values. Choices may be influenced by geographic location and cultural role expectations.

External Factors

Many external factors affect a person's mobility. Excessively high temperature and high humidity discourage activity, whereas comfortable temperature and humidity are conducive to activity. The availability of recreational facilities also influences activity; for example, lack of money may prohibit a client from joining an exercise club or gymnasium. Neighborhood safety promotes outdoor activity, whereas an unsafe environment discourages people from going outdoors. Adolescents, in particular, may spend many hours sitting at computers, watching television, or playing video games rather than going outside to visit friends or exercise.

> ► **CLINICAL ALERT** *In America, there are increasing numbers of adolescents who are overweight and adolescents who have Type 2 diabetes. Twenty-five percent of children in America watch TV 4 hours or more daily, and only 27% of students in grades 9 through 12 engage in moderate physical activity at least 30 minutes a day on 5 or more days of the week. The Centers for Disease Control and Prevention has instituted the VERB: It's What You Do program—a TV, radio, and Internet media campaign to encourage 9- to 13-year-olds to become more physically active (USDHHS, 2002).* ■

Prescribed Limitations

Limitations to movement may be medically prescribed for some health problems. To promote healing, devices such as casts, braces, splints, and traction are often used to immobilize body parts. Clients who are short of breath may be advised not to walk up stairs. Bed rest may be the therapeutic choice for certain clients, for example, to relieve edema, to reduce metabolic and oxygen needs, to promote tissue repair, or to decrease pain.

The term **bed rest** varies in meaning to some extent. In some agencies bed rest means strict confinement to bed or complete bed rest. Others may allow the client to use a bedside commode or have bathroom privileges. Nurses need to familiarize themselves with the meaning of bed rest in their practice setting.

EFFECTS OF IMMOBILITY

Individuals who have inactive lifestyles or who are faced with inactivity because of illness or injury are at risk for many problems that can affect major body systems. Whether immobility causes any problems often depends on the duration of the inactivity, the client's health status, and the client's sensory awareness. The most obvious signs of prolonged immobility are often manifested in the musculoskeletal system. Clients experience a significant decrease in muscular strength and agility whenever they do not maintain a moderate amount of physical activity. In addition, immobility adversely affects the cardiovascular, respiratory, metabolic, urinary, and psychoneurologic systems. Nurses need to understand these effects and encourage client movement as much as possible. Early ambulation after illness or surgery is an essential measure to prevent complications. Potential effects of immobility on body systems follow.

Musculoskeletal System

- *Disuse osteoporosis.* Without the stress of weight-bearing activity, the bones demineralize. They are depleted chiefly of calcium, which gives the bones strength and density. Regardless of the amount of calcium in a person's diet, the demineralization process, known as *osteoporosis,* continues with immobility. The bones become spongy and may gradually deform and fracture easily.
- *Disuse atrophy.* Unused muscles **atrophy** (decrease in size), losing most of their strength and normal function.
- *Contractures.* When the muscle fibers are not able to shorten and lengthen, eventually a **contracture** (permanent shortening of the muscle) forms, limiting joint mobility. This process eventually involves the tendons, ligaments, and joint capsules; it is irreversible except by surgical intervention. Joint deformities such as foot drop (Figure 42–31 ■) and external hip rotation occur when a stronger muscle dominates the opposite muscle.
- *Stiffness and pain in the joints.* Without movement, the collagen (connective) tissues at the joint become **ankylosed** (permanently immobile). In addition, as the bones demineralize, excess calcium may deposit in the joints, contributing to stiffness and pain.

Cardiovascular System

- *Diminished cardiac reserve.* Decreased mobility creates an imbalance in the autonomic nervous system, resulting in a preponderance of sympathetic activity over cholinergic activity that increases heart rate. Rapid heart rate reduces dias-

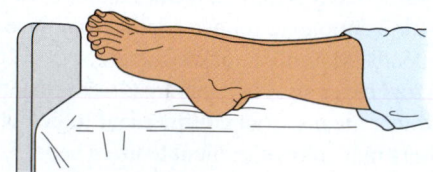

Figure 42–31 ■ Plantar flexion contracture (foot drop).

tolic pressure, coronary blood flow, and the capacity of the heart to respond to any metabolic demands above the basal levels. Because of this diminished cardiac reserve, the immobilized person may experience tachycardia with even minimal exertion.
- *Increased use of the Valsalva maneuver.* The **Valsalva maneuver** refers to holding the breath and straining against a closed glottis. For example, clients tend to hold their breath when attempting to move up in a bed or sit on a bedpan. This builds up sufficient pressure on the large veins in the thorax to interfere with the return blood flow to the heart and coronary arteries. When the client exhales and the glottis again opens, pressure is suddenly released, and a surge of blood flows to the heart. Tachycardia and cardiac arrhythmias can result if the client has cardiac disease.
- *Orthostatic (postural) hypotension.* Orthostatic hypotension is a common result of immobilization. Under normal conditions, sympathetic nervous system activity causes automatic vasoconstriction in the blood vessels in the lower half of the body when a mobile person changes from a horizontal to a vertical posture. Vasoconstriction prevents pooling of the blood in the legs and effectively maintains central blood pressure to ensure adequate perfusion of the heart and brain. During any prolonged immobility, this reflex becomes dormant. When the immobile person attempts to sit or stand, this reconstricting mechanism fails to function properly in spite of increased adrenalin output. The blood pools in the lower extremities, and central blood pressure drops. Cerebral perfusion is seriously compromised, and the person feels dizzy or lightheaded and may even faint. This sequence is usually accompanied by a sudden and marked increase in heart rate, the body's effort to protect the brain from an inadequate blood supply.
- *Venous vasodilation and stasis.* The skeletal muscles of an active person contract with each movement, compressing the blood vessels in those muscles and helping to pump the blood back to the heart against gravity. The tiny valves in the leg veins aid in venous return to the heart by preventing backward flow of blood and pooling. In an immobile person, the skeletal muscles do not contract sufficiently, and the muscles atrophy. The skeletal muscles can no longer assist in pumping blood back to the heart against gravity. Blood pools in the leg veins, causing vasodilation and engorgement. The valves in the veins can no longer work effectively to prevent backward flow of blood and pooling (Figure 42–32 ■). This phenomenon is known as incompetent valves. As the blood continues to pool in the veins, its greater volume increases venous blood pressure, which can become much higher than that exerted by the tissues surrounding the vessel.
- *Dependent edema.* When the venous pressure is sufficiently great, some of the serous part of the blood is forced out of the blood vessel into the interstitial spaces surrounding the blood vessel, causing edema. Edema is most common in parts of the body positioned below the heart. Dependent edema is most likely to occur around the sacrum or heels of a client who sits up in bed or in the feet and lower legs of a client who sits in a chair. Edema further impedes venous return of blood to the

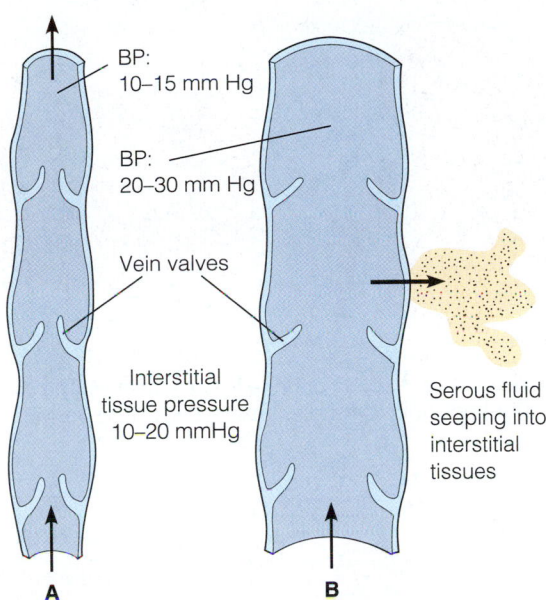

Figure 42–32 ■ Leg veins: *A*, in a mobile person; *B*, in an immobile person.

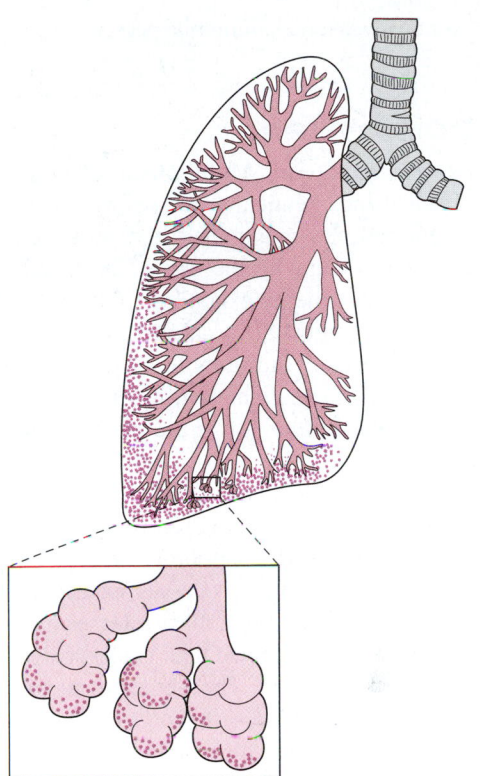

Figure 42–33 ■ Pooling of secretions in the lungs of an immobile person.

heart, causing more pooling and more edema. Edematous tissue is uncomfortable and more susceptible to injury than normal tissue.

- *Thrombus formation.* Three factors collectively predispose a client to the formation of a **thrombophlebitis** (a clot that is loosely attached to an inflamed vein wall): impaired venous return to the heart, hypercoagulability of the blood, and injury to a vessel wall.

  A **thrombus** (clot) is particularly dangerous if it breaks loose from the vein wall to enter the general circulation as an **embolus** (an object that has moved from its place of origin, causing obstruction to circulation elsewhere). Large emboli that enter the pulmonary circulation may occlude the vessels that nourish the lungs to cause an infarcted (dead) area of the lung. If the infarcted area is large, pulmonary function may be seriously compromised, or death may ensue. Emboli traveling to the coronary vessels or brain can produce a similarly dangerous outcome.

Respiratory System

- *Decreased respiratory movement.* In a recumbent, immobile client, ventilation of the lungs is passively altered. The body presses against the rigid bed and curtails chest movement. The abdominal organs push against the diaphragm, restricting lung movement and making it difficult to expand the lungs fully. An immobile recumbent person rarely sighs, partly because overall muscle atrophy also affects the respiratory muscles and partly because there is no stimulus of activity. Without these periodic stretching movements, the cartilaginous intercostal joints may become fixed in an expiratory phase of respiration, further limiting the potential for maximal ventilation. These changes produce shallow respirations and reduce **vital capac-**

ity (the maximum amount of air that can be exhaled after a maximum inhalation).

- *Pooling of respiratory secretions.* Secretions of the respiratory tract are normally expelled by changing positions or posture and by coughing. Inactivity allows secretions to pool by gravity (Figure 42–33 ■), interfering with the normal diffusion of oxygen and carbon dioxide in the alveoli. The ability to cough up secretions may also be hindered by loss of respiratory muscle tone, dehydration (which thickens secretions), or sedatives that depress the cough reflex. Poor oxygenation and retention of carbon dioxide in the blood can, if allowed to continue, predispose the person to respiratory acidosis, a potentially lethal disorder.

- *Atelectasis.* When ventilation is decreased, pooled secretions may accumulate in a dependent area of a bronchiole and effectively block it. Because of changes in regional blood flow, bed rest decreases the amount of surfactant produced. (Surfactant enables the alveoli to remain open.) The combination of decreased surfactant and blockage of a bronchiole with mucus can cause atelectasis (the collapse of a lobe or of an entire lung) distal to the mucous blockage. Immobile elderly, postoperative clients are at greatest risk of atelectasis.

- *Hypostatic pneumonia.* Pooled secretions provide excellent media for bacterial growth. Under these conditions, a minor upper respiratory infection can evolve rapidly into a severe infection of the lower respiratory tract. Pneumonia caused by static respiratory secretions can severely impair oxygen–carbon dioxide exchange in the alveoli and is a fairly common cause of death among weakened, immobile persons, especially heavy smokers.

Metabolic System

- *Decreased metabolic rate.* **Metabolism** refers to the sum of all the physical and chemical processes by which living substance is formed and maintained and by which energy is made available for use by the body. The **basal metabolic rate** is the minimal energy expended for the maintenance of these processes, expressed in calories per hour per square meter of body surface. In immobile clients, the basal metabolic rate and gastrointestinal motility and secretions of various digestive glands decrease as the energy requirements of the body decrease.

- *Negative nitrogen balance.* In an active person, a balance exists between protein synthesis (**anabolism**) and protein breakdown (**catabolism**). Immobility creates a marked imbalance, and the catabolic processes exceed the anabolic processes. Catabolized muscle mass releases nitrogen. Over time, more nitrogen is excreted than is ingested, producing a negative nitrogen balance. The negative nitrogen balance represents a depletion of protein stores that are essential for building muscle tissue and for wound healing.

- *Anorexia.* Loss of appetite (**anorexia**) occurs because of the decreased metabolic rate and the increased catabolism that accompany immobility. Reduced caloric intake is usually a response to the decreased energy requirements of the inactive person. If protein intake is reduced, the nitrogen imbalance may become more pronounced, sometimes so severely that malnutrition ensues.

- *Negative calcium balance.* A negative calcium balance occurs as a direct result of immobility. Greater amounts of calcium are extracted from bone than can be replaced. The absence of weight-bearing and of stress on the musculoskeletal structures is the direct cause of the calcium loss from bones. Weight-bearing and stress are also required for calcium to be replaced in bone.

Urinary System

- *Urinary stasis.* In a mobile person, gravity plays an important role in the emptying of the kidneys and the bladder. The shape and position of the kidneys and active kidney contractions are important in completely emptying the urine from the calyces, renal pelvis, and ureters (Figure 42–34 ■, *A*). The shape and position of the urinary bladder (the detrusor muscle) and active bladder contractions are also important in achieving complete emptying (Figure 42–35 ■, *A*).

  When the person remains in a horizontal position, gravity impedes the emptying of urine from the kidneys and the urinary bladder. To urinate, the person who is supine (in a back-lying position) must push upward, against gravity (Figures 42–34 ■, *B*, and 42–35 ■, *B*). The renal pelvis may fill with urine before it is pushed into the ureters. Emptying is not as complete, and **urinary stasis** (stoppage or slowdown of flow) occurs after a few days of bed rest. Because of the overall decrease in muscle tone during immobilization, in-

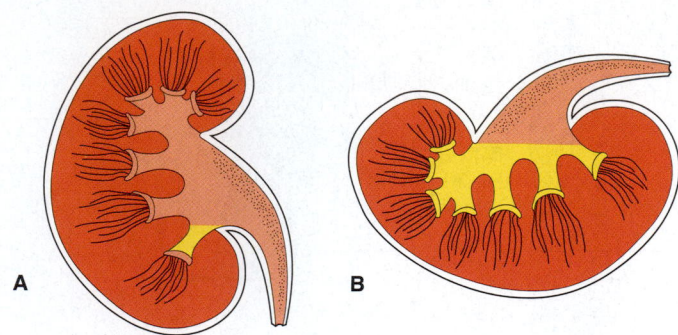

Figure 42–34 ■ Pooling of urine in the kidney: *A*, The client is in an upright position; *B*, the client is in a back-lying position.

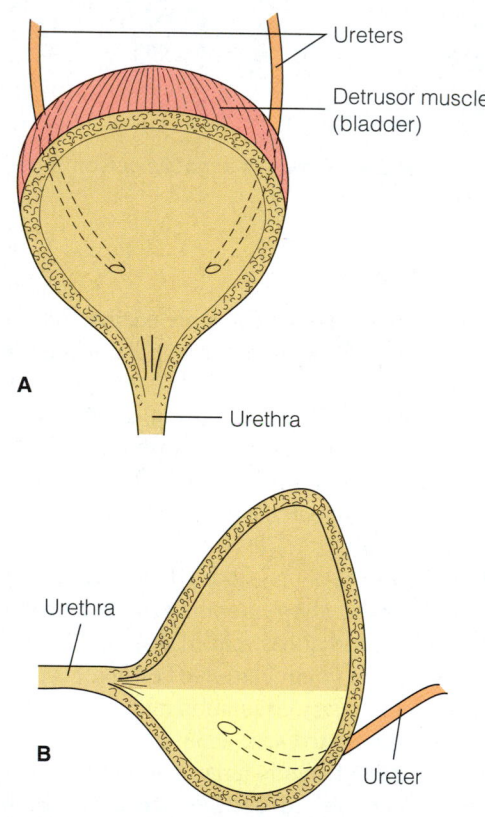

Figure 42–35 ■ Pooling of urine in the urinary bladder: *A*, The client is in an upright position; *B*, the client is in a back-lying position.

cluding the tone of the detrusor muscle, bladder emptying is further compromised.

- *Renal calculi.* In a mobile person, calcium in the urine remains dissolved because calcium and citric acid are balanced in an appropriately acid urine. With immobility and the resulting excessive amounts of calcium in the urine, this balance is no longer maintained. The urine becomes more alkaline, and the calcium salts precipitate out as crystals to form renal **calculi** (stones). In an immobile person in a horizontal position, the renal pelvis filled with stagnant, alkaline urine is an ideal location for calculi to form. The stones usually develop in the renal pelvis and pass through the ureters into the bladder. As the stones pass along the long, narrow ureters, they cause extreme pain and bleeding and can sometimes obstruct the urinary tract.

- *Urinary retention.* The immobile person may suffer from **urinary retention** (accumulation of urine in the bladder), bladder distention, and occasionally **urinary incontinence** (involuntary urination). The decreased muscle tone of the urinary bladder inhibits its ability to empty completely, and the immobilized person is unable to relax the perineal muscles sufficiently to urinate. The discomfort of using a bedpan or urinal, the embarrassment and lack of privacy associated with this function, and the unnatural position for urination combine to make it difficult for the client to relax the perineal muscles sufficiently to urinate while lying in bed.

   When urination is not possible, the bladder gradually becomes distended with urine. The bladder may stretch excessively, eventually inhibiting the urge to void. When bladder distention is considerable, some involuntary urinary "dribbling" may occur (retention with overflow). This does not relieve the urinary distention, because most of the stagnant urine remains in the bladder.

- *Urinary infection.* Static urine provides an excellent medium for bacterial growth. The flushing action of normal, frequent urination is absent, and urinary distention often causes minute tears in the bladder mucosa, allowing infectious organisms to enter. The increased alkalinity of the urine caused by the hypercalcuria supports bacterial growth. The organism most commonly causing urinary tract infections is *Escherichia coli,* which normally resides in the colon. The normally sterile urinary tract may be contaminated by improper perineal care, the use of an indwelling urinary catheter, or occasionally **urinary reflux** (backward flow). During reflux, contaminated urine from an overly distended bladder backs up into the renal pelvis to contaminate the kidney pelvis as well.

Gastrointestinal System

Constipation is a frequent problem for immobilized people because of decreased peristalsis and colon motility. The overall skeletal muscle weakness affects the abdominal and perineal muscles used in defecation. When the stool becomes very hard, more strength is required to expel it. The immobile person may lack this strength.

The bedfast person's unnatural and uncomfortable position on the bedpan does not facilitate elimination. The backward-leaning posture does not promote effective use of the muscles used in defecation. Some people are reluctant to use the bedpan in the presence of others. The embarrassment, lack of privacy, dependence on others to assist with the bedpan, and disruption of normal bowel habits may cause the individual to postpone or ignore the urge for elimination. Repeated postponement eventually suppresses the urge and weakens the defecation reflex.

Some persons may make excessive use of the Valsalva maneuver by straining at stool in an attempt to expel the hard stool. This effort dangerously increases intra-abdominal and intrathoracic pressures and places undue stress on the heart and circulatory system.

Integumentary System

- *Reduced skin turgor.* The skin can atrophy as a result of prolonged immobility. Shifts in body fluids between the fluid compartments can affect the consistency and health of the dermis and subcutaneous tissues in dependent parts of the body, eventually causing a gradual loss in skin elasticity.
- *Skin breakdown.* Normal blood circulation relies on muscle activity. Immobility impedes circulation and diminishes the supply of nutrients to specific areas. As a result, skin breakdown and formation of pressure ulcers can occur.

Psychoneurologic System

People who are unable to carry out the usual activities related to their roles (e.g., as breadwinner, husband, mother, or athlete) become aware of an increased dependence on others. These factors lower the person's self-esteem. Frustration and the decrease in self-esteem may in turn provoke exaggerated emotional reactions. Emotional reactions vary considerably. Some individuals become apathetic and withdrawn, some regress, and some become angry and aggressive.

Because the immobilized person's participation in life becomes much narrower and the variety of stimuli decreases, the person's perception of time intervals deteriorates. Problem-solving and decision-making abilities may deteriorate as a result of lack of intellectual stimulation and the stress of the illness and immobility. In addition, the loss of control over events can cause anxiety.

Immobility can impair the social and motor development of young children.

NURSING MANAGEMENT

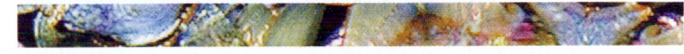

ASSESSING

Assessment relative to a client's activity and exercise includes a nursing history and a physical examination of body alignment, gait, appearance and movement of joints, capabilities and limitations for movement, muscle mass and strength, activity tolerance, problems related to immobility, and physical fitness.

The nurse collects information from the client, from other nurses, and from the client's records. The examination and history are important sources of information about disabilities affecting the client's mobility and activity status, such as contractures, edema, pain in the extremities, or generalized fatigue.

Nursing History

An activity and exercise history is usually part of the comprehensive nursing history form and includes daily activity level, activity tolerance, type and frequency of exercise, factors affecting mobility, and effects of immobility. If the client indicates a recent pattern change or difficulties with mobility, a

Assessment Interview

ACTIVITY AND EXERCISE

Daily Activity Level

- What activities do you carry out during a routine day?
- Are you able to carry out the following tasks independently?
  - a. Eating
  - b. Dressing/grooming
  - c. Bathing
  - d. Toileting
  - e. Ambulating
  - f. Using a wheelchair
  - g. Transferring in and out of bed, bath, and car
  - h. Cooking
  - i. House cleaning
  - j. Shopping
- Where problems exist in your ability to carry out such tasks:
  - a. Would you rate yourself as partially or totally dependent?
  - b. How is the task achieved (by family, friend, agency, or use of specialized equipment)?

Activity Tolerance

- How much and what types of activities make you tired?

- Do you ever experience dizziness, shortness of breath, marked increase in respiratory rate, or other problems following mild or moderate activity?

Exercise

- What type of exercise do you carry out to enhance your physical fitness?
- What is the frequency and length of this exercise session?
- Do you believe exercise is beneficial to your health? Explain.

Factors Affecting Mobility

- Environmental factors. Do stairs, lack of railings or other assistive devices, or an unsafe neighborhood impede your mobility or exercise regimen?
- Health problems. Do any of the following health problems affect your muscle strength or endurance: heart disease, lung disease, stroke, cancer, neuromuscular problems, musculoskeletal problems, visual or mental impairments, trauma, or pain?
- Financial factors. Are your finances adequate to obtain equipment or other aids that you require to enhance your mobility?

more detailed history is required. This detailed history should include the specific nature of the problem, when it first began and its frequency, its causes if known, how the problem affects daily living, what the client is doing to cope with the problem, and whether these methods have been effective. Examples of interview questions to elicit this data are shown in the accompanying Assessment Interview.

Physical Examination

Conduct of the physical examination focusing on activity and exercise emphasizes body alignment, gait, appearance and movement of joints, capabilities and limitations for movement, muscle mass and strength, and activity tolerance.

Body Alignment Assessment of body alignment includes an inspection of the client while the client stands. The purpose of body alignment assessment is to identify

- Normal developmental variations in posture
- Posture and learning needs to maintain good posture
- Factors contributing to poor posture, such as fatigue or low self-esteem
- Muscle weakness or other motor impairments.

To assess alignment, the nurse inspects the client from lateral (Figure 42–36 ■, A), anterior, and posterior perspectives. From the anterior and posterior views, the nurse should observe whether

- The shoulders and hips are level.
- The toes point forward.
- The spine is straight, not curved to either side.

The "slumped" posture (Figure 42–36 ■, B) is the most common problem that occurs when people stand. The neck is

flexed far forward, the abdomen protrudes, the pelvis is thrust forward to create **lordosis** (an exaggerated inward curvature of the lumbar spine), and the knees are hyperextended. Low back pain and fatigue occur quickly in people with poor posture.

Gait The characteristic pattern of a person's **gait** (walk) is assessed to determine the client's mobility and risk for injury due

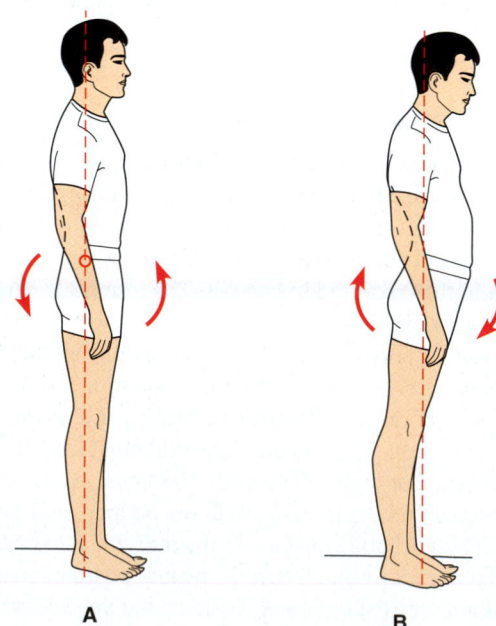

A　　　　　**B**

Figure 42–36 ■ A standing person with A, good trunk alignment; B, poor trunk alignment. The arrows indicate the direction in which the pelvis is tilted.

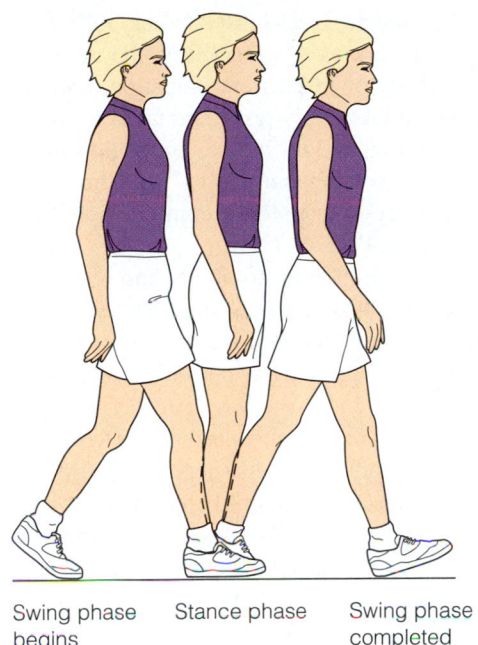

Swing phase   Stance phase   Swing phase
begins   completed

Figure 42–37 ■ The stance and swing phases of a normal gait.

to falling. Two phases of normal gait are stance and swing (Figure 42–37 ■). When one leg is in the swing phase, the other is in the stance phase. In the *stance phase,* (a) the heel of one foot strikes the ground, and (b) body weight is spread over the ball of that foot while the other heel pushes off and leaves the ground. In the *swing phase,* the leg from behind moves in front of the body.

The nurse assesses gait as the client walks into the room or asks the client to walk a distance of 10 feet down a hallway and observes for the following:

- Head is erect, gaze is straight ahead, and vertebral column is upright.
- Heel strikes the ground before the toe.
- Feet are dorsiflexed in the swing phase.
- Arm opposite the swing-through foot moves forward at the same time.
- Gait is smooth, coordinated, and rhythmic, with even weight borne on each foot; it produces minimal body swing from side to side and directs movement straight ahead; and it starts and stops with ease.

The nurse may also assess **pace** (the number of steps taken per minute). A normal walking pace is 70 to 100 steps per minute. The pace of an older person may slow to about 40 steps per minute.

The nurse should also note the client's need for a prosthesis or assistive device, such as a cane or walker. For a client who uses assistive aids, the nurse assesses gait without the device and compares the assisted and unassisted gaits.

Appearance and Movement of Joints. Physical examination of the joints involves inspection, palpation, assessment of range of active motion, and if active motion is not possible, assessment of range of passive motion. The nurse should assess the following:

- Any joint swelling or redness, which could indicate the presence of an injury or an inflammation.
- Any deformity, such as a bony enlargement or contracture, and symmetry of involvement.
- The muscle development associated with each joint and the relative size and symmetry of the muscles on each side of the body
- Any reported or palpable tenderness.
- **Crepitation** (palpable or audible crackling or grating sensation produced by joint motion).
- Increased temperature over the joint. Palpate the joint using the backs of the fingers and compare the temperature with that of the symmetric joint.
- The degree of joint movement. Ask the client to move selected body parts as shown in Table 42–2. If indicated, measure the extent of movement with a goniometer, a device that measures the angle of the joint in degrees. See Figure 28–85, page 601.

Assessment of range of motion should not be unduly fatiguing, and the joint movements need to be performed smoothly, slowly, and rhythmically. No joint should be forced. Uneven, jerky movement and forcing can injure the joint and its surrounding muscles and ligaments.

Capabilities and Limitations for Movement. The nurse needs to obtain data that may indicate hindrances or restrictions to the client's movement and the need for assistance, including the following:

- How the client's illness influences the ability to move and whether the client's health contraindicates any exertion, position, or movement.
- Encumbrances to movement, such as an intravenous line in place or a heavy cast.
- Mental alertness and ability to follow directions. Check whether the client is receiving medications that hinder the ability to walk safely. Narcotics, sedatives, tranquilizers, and some antihistamines cause drowsiness, dizziness, weakness, and orthostatic hypotension.
- Balance and coordination.
- Presence of orthostatic hypotension before transfers. Specifically, assess for any increase in pulse rate, marked fall in blood pressure, dizziness, lightheadedness, and dimming of vision when the client moves from a supine to a vertical posture.
- Degree of comfort. People who have pain may not want to move and can require an analgesic before they are moved.
- Vision. Is it adequate to prevent falls?

The nurse also assesses the amount of assistance the client requires for the following:

- Moving in the bed. In particular, observe for the amount of assistance the client requires for turning
  a. From a supine position to a lateral position
  b. From a lateral position on one side to a lateral position on the other
  c. From a supine position to a sitting position in bed.
- Rising from a lying position to a sitting position on the edge of the bed. Healthy people can normally rise without support from the arms.

- Rising from a chair to a standing position. Normally this can be done without pushing with the arms.
- Coordination and balance. Determine the client's abilities to hold the body erect, to bear weight and keep balance in a standing position on both legs or only one, to take steps, and to push off from a chair or bed.

Muscle Mass and Strength. Before the client undertakes a change in position or attempts to ambulate, it is essential that the nurse assess the client's strength and ability to move. Providing appropriate assistance lowers the risk of muscle strain and body injury to both the client and nurse. Assessment of upper extremity strength is especially important for clients who use ambulation aids, such as walkers and crutches. For information on how to determine muscle mass and strength in lower and upper extremities, see Chapter 28. 🔗

Activity Tolerance. By determining an appropriate activity level for a client, the nurse can predict whether the client has the strength and endurance to participate in activities that require similar expenditures of energy. This assessment is useful in encouraging increasing independence in people who (a) have a cardiovascular or respiratory disability, (b) have been completely immobilized for a prolonged period, (c) have decreased muscle mass or a musculoskeletal disorder, (d) have experienced inadequate sleep, (e) have experienced pain, or (f) are depressed, anxious, or unmotivated.

The most useful measures in predicting activity tolerance are heart rate, strength, and rhythm; respiratory rate, depth, and rhythm; and blood pressure. These data are obtained at the following times:

- Before the activity starts (baseline data), while the client is at rest
- During the activity
- Immediately after the activity stops
- Three minutes after the activity has stopped and the client has rested.

The activity should be stopped immediately in the event of any physiologic change indicating the activity is too strenuous or prolonged for the client. These changes include the following:

- Sudden facial pallor
- Feelings of dizziness or weakness
- Change in level of consciousness
- Heart rate or respiratory rate that significantly exceeds baseline or preestablished levels
- Change in heart or respiratory rhythm from regular to irregular
- Weakening of the pulse
- Dyspnea, shortness of breath, or chest pain
- Diastolic blood pressure change of 10 mm Hg or more

If, however, the client tolerates the activity well, and if the client's heart rate returns to baseline levels within 5 minutes after the activity ceases, the activity is considered safe. This activity, then, can serve as a standard for predicting the client's tolerance for similar activities.

Problems Related to Immobility. When collecting data pertaining to the problems of immobility, the nurse uses the assessment methods of inspection, palpation, and auscultation; checks results of laboratory tests; and takes measurements, including body weight, fluid intake, and fluid output. Specific techniques for assessing immobility problems and abnormal assessment findings related to the complications of immobility are listed in Table 42–3.

It is extremely important to obtain and record baseline assessment data soon after the client first becomes immobile. These baseline data serve as the standard against which all data collected throughout the period of immobilization are compared.

Because a major nursing responsibility is to prevent the complications of immobility, the nurse needs to identify clients at risk of developing such complications before problems arise. Clients at risk include those who (a) are poorly nourished; (b) have decreased sensitivity to pain, temperature, or pressure; (c) have existing cardiovascular, pulmonary, or neuromuscular problems; and (d) have altered level of consciousness.

DIAGNOSING

Mobility problems may be appropriate as the diagnostic label or as the etiology for other nursing diagnoses.

NANDA includes the following nursing diagnostic labels for activity and exercise problems:

- *Activity Intolerance:* Insufficient physiological or psychological energy to endure or complete required or desired daily activities. Four levels that can be used after the diagnostic label include:
  Level I: Walk, regular pace, on level ground indefinitely; climb one flight of stairs or more but more short of breath than normally
  Level II: Walk one city block 500 feet on level ground; climb one flight slowly without stopping
  Level III: Walk no more than 50 feet on level ground without stopping; unable to climb one flight of stairs without stopping
  Level IV: Dyspnea and fatigue at rest
- *Risk for Activity Intolerance:* At risk for experiencing insufficient physiological or psychological energy to endure or complete required or desired daily activities
- *Impaired Physical Mobility:* Limitation in independent, purposeful physical movement of the body or of one or more extremities.
  More specific versions of this diagnosis are
  Impaired Bed Mobility
  Impaired Walking
  Impaired Wheelchair Mobility
  Impaired Transfer Ability.
- *Risk for Disuse Syndrome:* At risk for deterioration of body systems as the result of prescribed or unavoidable musculoskeletal inactivity

A clinical example of this nursing diagnosis is shown in the Nursing Care Plan and the Concept Map on pages 1108–1110.

Depending on the data obtained, problems with mobility often affect other areas of human functioning and indicate other

TABLE 42–3 Assessing Problems of Immobility

Assessment	Problem
Musculoskeletal System	
Measure arm and leg circumferences	Decreased circumference due to decreased muscle mass
Palpate and observe body joints	Stiffness or pain in joints
Take goniometric measurements of joint ROM	Decreased joint ROM, joint contractures
Cardiovascular System	
Auscultate the heart	Increased heart rate
Measure blood pressure	Orthostatic hypotension
Palpate and observe sacrum, legs, and feet	Peripheral dependent edema, increased peripheral vein engorgement
Palpate peripheral	Weak peripheral pulses
Measure calf muscle circumferences	Edema
Observe calf muscle for redness, tenderness, and swelling	Thrombophlebitis
Respiratory System	
Observe chest movements	Asymmetric chest movements, dyspnea
Auscultate chest	Diminished breath sounds, crackles, wheezes, and increased respiratory rate
Metabolic System	
Measure height and weight	Weight loss due to muscle atrophy and loss of subcutaneous fat
Palpate skin	Generalized edema due to low blood protein levels
Urinary System	
Measure fluid intake and output	Dehydration
Inspect urine	Cloudy, dark urine; high specific gravity
Palpate urinary bladder	Distended urinary bladder due to urinary retention
Gastrointestinal System	
Observe stool	Hard, dry, small stool
Auscultate bowel sounds	Decreased bowel sounds due to decreased intestinal motility
Integumentary System	
Inspect skin	Break in skin integrity

diagnoses. In these instances, the mobility problem becomes the etiology. Examples in which *Impaired Physical Mobility* is the etiology follow. The etiology needs to be described more explicitly in terms such as reduced ROM, neuromuscular impairment or musculoskeletal impairment of upper and lower extremities, or joint pain.

- *Fear* (of falling)
- *Ineffective Coping*
- *Low Self-Esteem*
- *Powerlessness*
- *Risk for Injury* (falls)
- *Self-Care Deficit.*

When problems associated with prolonged immobility arise, many other diagnoses may be necessary. Examples include, but are not limited to, the following:

- *Ineffective Airway Clearance* if there is stasis of pulmonary secretions
- *Risk for Infection* if there is stasis of urinary or pulmonary secretions
- *Risk for Injury* if orthostatic hypotension is present.

PLANNING

Positioning, transferring, and ambulating clients are almost always independent nursing functions. The physician usually orders specific body positions only after surgery, anesthesia, or trauma involving the nervous and musculoskeletal systems. All clients should have an activity order written by their physician when they are admitted to the agency for care.

As part of planning, the nurse is responsible for identifying those clients who need assistance with body alignment and determining the degree of assistance they need. The nurse must

MediaLink | TREATING A CLIENT WITH MOBILITY PROBLEMS CASE STUDY

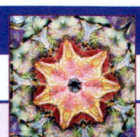

be sensitive to the client's need to function as independently as possible yet provide assistance when the client needs it.

Most clients require some nursing guidance and assistance to learn about, achieve, and maintain proper body mechanics. The nurse should also plan to teach clients applicable skills. For example, a client with a back injury needs to learn how to get out of bed safely and comfortably, a client with an injured leg needs to learn how to transfer from bed to wheelchair safely, and a client with a newly acquired walker needs to learn how to use it safely. Nurses often teach family members or caregivers safe moving, lifting, and transfer techniques in the home setting.

The goals established for clients will vary according to the diagnosis and defining characteristics related to each individual. Examples of overall goals for clients with actual or potential problems related to mobility or activity follow.

The client will have

- Increased tolerance for physical activity.
- Restored or improved capability to ambulate and/or participate in ADLs.
- Absence of injury from falling or improper use of body mechanics.
- Enhanced physical fitness.
- Absence of any complications associated with immobility.
- Improved social, emotional, and intellectual well-being.

Examples of desired outcomes, interventions, and activities are provided in the Nursing Care Plan and Concept Map on pages 1108–1110.

Planning for Home Care

Clients who have been hospitalized for activity or mobility problems often need continued care in the home. In preparation for discharge, the nurse needs to determine the client's actual and potential health problems, strengths, and resources. The

accompanying Home Care Assessment describes the specific assessment data required before establishing a discharge plan for clients with mobility or activity problems. A major aspect of discharge planning involves instructional needs of the client and family. See Teaching: Home Care and other Teaching features throughout this chapter.

IMPLEMENTING

Nursing strategies to maintain or promote body alignment and mobility involve positioning clients appropriately, moving and turning clients in bed, transferring clients, providing ROM exercises, ambulating clients with or without mechanical aids, and strategies to prevent the complications of immobility. Whenever positioning, moving, lifting, and ambulating clients, nurses must use proper body mechanics to avoid musculoskeletal strain and injury.

Using Body Mechanics

Body mechanics is the term used to describe the efficient, coordinated, and safe use of the body to move objects and carry out the activities of daily living. The major purpose of body mechanics is to facilitate the safe and efficient use of appropriate muscle groups to maintain balance, reduce the energy required, reduce fatigue, and decrease the risk of injury. Good body mechanics is essential to both clients and nurses. This section focuses on body mechanics used by nurses when moving and turning clients in bed and transferring clients between beds, wheelchairs, and stretchers.

When the person moves, the center of gravity shifts continuously in the direction of the moving body parts. Balance depends on the interrelationship of the center of gravity, the line of gravity, and the base of support. The closer the line of gravity is to the center of the base of support, the greater the person's stability (Figure 42–38 ■, *A*). Conversely, the closer the line of gravity is to the edge of the base of support, the

---

Home Care Assessment:
MOBILITY AND ACTIVITY PROBLEMS

Client and Environment
- Capabilities or tolerance for required and desired activities: Self-care (feeding, bathing, toileting, dressing, grooming, home maintenance, shopping, cooking); recreational activities
- Mobility aids required: Cane, walker, crutches, wheelchair, transfer boards
- Equipment required if immobilized: Special bed, side rails, pressure-reducing mattress
- Current level of knowledge: Body mechanics for use of mobility aids; specific exercises prescribed
- Home mobility hazard appraisal: Adequacy of lighting; presence of handrails; safety of pathways and stairs; congested areas; unanchored rugs, mats, or electrical cords, and any other obstacles to safe movement; structural adjustments needed for wheelchair access

Family or Caregiver
- Caregiver availability, skills, and willingness: Primary people able to assist client with self-care, movement, shopping, and so on; physical and emotional status to assist with care; learning needs
- Family role changes and coping: Effect on financial status, parenting and spousal roles, social roles
- Availability of caregiver support: Other support people available for occasional duties such as shopping, transportation, housekeeping, cooking, budgeting, respite care

Community
- Resources: Availability and familiarity with sources of medical equipment, financial assistance, homemaker services, hygienic care; Meals on Wheels; spiritual counselors and visitors; sources of respite for caregiver

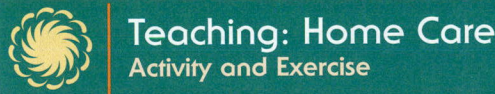

Teaching: Home Care
Activity and Exercise

Maintaining Musculoskeletal Function

- Teach the systematic performance of passive or assistive ROM exercises to maintain joint mobility.
- As appropriate, demonstrate the proper way to perform isotonic, isometric, or isokinetic exercises to maintain muscle mass and tone (collaborate with the physical therapist about these). Incorporate ADLs into exercise program if appropriate.
- Provide a written schedule for the type, frequency, and duration of exercises; encourage the use of a progress graph or chart to facilitate adherence with the therapy.
- Offer an ambulation schedule.
- Instruct in the availability of assistive ambulatory devices and correct use of them.
- Discuss pain control measures required before exercise.

Preventing Injury

- Teach safe transfer and ambulation techniques.
- Discuss safety measures to avoid falls (e.g., locking wheelchairs, wearing appropriate footwear, using rubber tips on crutches, keeping the environment safe, and using mechanical aids such as raised toilet seat, grab bars, urinal, and bedpan or commode to facilitate toileting).

- Teach the use of proper body mechanics.
- Teach ways to prevent postural hypotension.

Managing Energy to Prevent Fatigue

- Discuss activity and rest patterns and develop a plan as indicated; intersperse rest periods with activity periods.
- Discuss ways to minimize fatigue such as performing activities more slowly and for shorter periods, resting more often, and using more assistance as required.
- Provide information about available resources to help with ADLs and home maintenance management.
- Teach ways to increase energy (e.g., increasing intake of high-energy foods, ensuring adequate rest and sleep, controlling pain).
- Teach techniques to monitor activity tolerance as appropriate.

Referrals

- Provide appropriate information about accessing community resources: home care agencies, sources of equipment, and so on.

---

more precarious the balance (Figure 42–38 ■, *B*). If the line of gravity falls outside the base of support, the person falls (Figure 42–38 ■, *C*).

The broader the base of support and the lower the center of gravity, the greater the stability and balance. Body balance, therefore, can be greatly enhanced by (a) widening the base of support and (b) lowering the center of gravity, bringing it closer to the base of support. The base of support is easily widened by spreading the feet farther apart. The center of gravity is readily lowered by flexing the hips and knees until a squatting position is achieved. The importance of these alterations cannot be overemphasized for nurses.

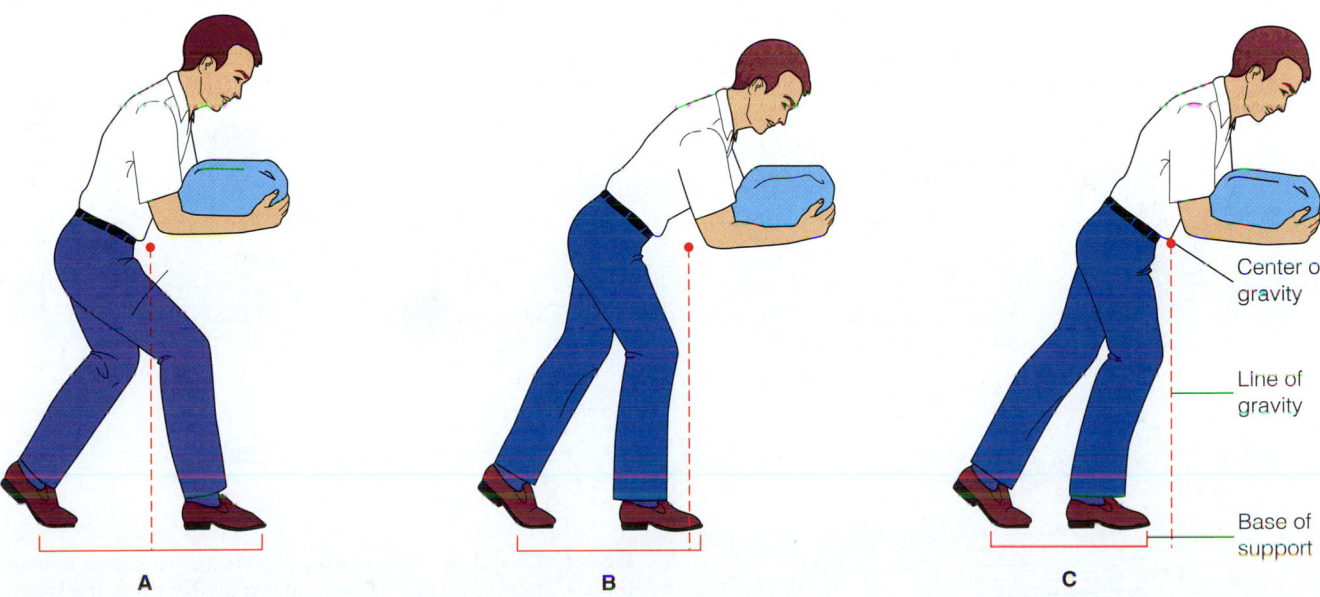

Figure 42–38 ■ *A,* Balance is maintained when the line of gravity falls close to the base of support. *B,* Balance is precarious when the line of gravity falls at the edge of the base of support. *C,* Balance cannot be maintained when the line of gravity falls outside the base of support.

Two movements to avoid because of their potential for causing back injury are twisting (rotation) of the thoracolumbar spine and acute flexion of the back with hips and knees straight (stooping). Undesirable twisting of the back can be prevented by squarely facing the direction of movement, whether pushing, pulling, or sliding, and moving the object directly toward or away from one's center of gravity.

Lifting

When a person lifts or carries an object, for example, a suitcase, the weight of the object becomes part of the person's body weight. This weight affects the location of the person's center of gravity, which is displaced in the direction of the added weight. To counteract this potential imbalance, body parts (e.g., arm and trunk) move in a direction away from the weight. In this way, the center of gravity is maintained over the base of support. By holding the lifted object as close as possible to the body's center of gravity, the lifter avoids undue displacement of the center of gravity and achieves greater stability.

People can lift more weight when they use a lever than when they do not. In the body, the bones of the skeleton act as levers, a joint is a fulcrum (fixed point about which a lever moves), and the muscles exert the force (Figure 42–39 ■). Use of the arms as levers is often applied in clinical practice when the nurse needs to raise a client's head off the bed, for example, or give back care to a client in traction.

Because lifting involves movement against gravity, the nurse must use the major muscle groups of the thighs, knees, upper and lower arms, abdomen, and pelvis to prevent back strain. The nurse can increase overall muscle strength by synchronized use of as many muscle groups as possible during an activity. For instance, when the arms are used in an activity, dividing the work between the arms and legs helps prevent back strain.

Another technique based on the principle of leverage can be used when lifting objects from the floor to waist level. In this technique, the back and knees are flexed until the load is at thigh level, at which point the knees remain flexed to provide thrust as the back begins to straighten (Figure 42–40 ■). This technique provides for balance, leverage, and synchronized use of muscles, which help avoid back pain and injury. When one lifts an object to knee level, the shoulder and arm muscles pull, the abdominal and lumbar muscles contract for leverage and pull, and the thigh and leg muscles exert the upward thrust to bring the object off the floor. When one lifts an object from midthigh to waist level, force is provided essentially by the leg and thigh muscle groups, but the back and lumbar muscles remain contracted.

In all positions, it is important to maintain a distance of at least 30 cm (12 in.) between the feet and to keep the load close to the body, especially when it is at knee level. Before attempting the lift, the nurse must ensure that there are no hazards on the floor, that there is a clear path for moving the object, and that the nurse's base of support is secure.

Pulling and Pushing. When pulling or pushing an object, a person maintains balance with least effort when the base of support is enlarged in the direction in which the movement is to be produced or opposed. For example, when pushing an object, a person can enlarge the base of support by moving the front foot forward. When pulling an object, a person can enlarge the base of support by (a) moving the rear leg back if the person is facing the object or (b) moving the front foot forward if the person is facing away from the object. It is easier and safer to pull an object toward one's own center of gravity than to push it away, because a person can exert more control of the object's movement when pulling it.

Pivoting

Pivoting is a technique in which the body is turned in a way that avoids twisting of the spine. To pivot, place one foot ahead of the other, raise the heels very slightly, and put the body weight on the balls of the feet. When the weight is off the heels, the

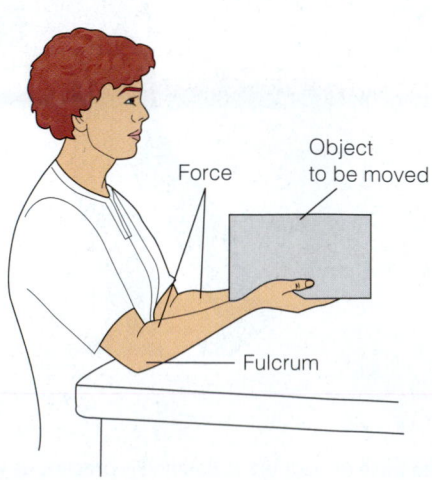

Figure 42–39 ■ Using the arm as a lever.

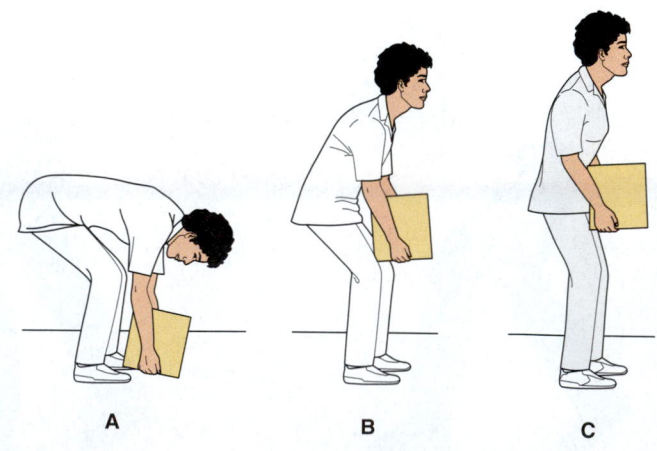

Figure 42–40 ■ Lifting heavy objects from the floor to waist level. *A,* Stand close to the load and flex the back and the knees, lowering the body to grasp the load. *B,* Begin lifting with the back flexed, and gradually straighten the knees so that the leg muscles bear most of the burden. *C,* To hold or walk with the object, maintain a less flexed but not a completely straight position.

frictional surface is decreased and the knees are not twisted when turning. Keeping the body aligned, turn (pivot) about 90 degrees in the desired direction. The foot that was forward will now be behind.

A summary of guidelines and rationale related to body mechanics is shown in Table 42–4.

Preventing Back Injury

Many factors increase the potential for lower back injuries. A major contributor is habitually poor standing and sitting posture, which produces lordosis. Overweight individuals who carry their extra weight over their abdomen, pregnant women, and women who consistently wear high-heeled shoes are at risk

TABLE 42–4 Summary of Guidelines and Principles Related to Body Mechanics

Guidelines	Rationale
Plan the move or transfer carefully. Free the surrounding area of obstacles and move required equipment near the head or foot of the bed.	Appropriate preparation prevents potential falls and injury and safeguards the client and equipment.
Obtain the assistance of other people or use mechanical devices to move objects that are too heavy. Encourage clients to assist as much as possible by pushing or pulling themselves to reduce your muscular effort. Use arms as levers whenever possible to increase lifting power.	The heavier an object, the greater the force needed to move the object.
Adjust the working area to waist level, and keep the body close to the area. Elevate adjustable beds and overbed tables or lower the side rails of beds to prevent stretching and reaching.	Objects that are close to the center of gravity are moved with the least effort.
Provide a firm, smooth, dry bed foundation before moving a client in bed or use a pull sheet.	Less friction between the object moved and the surface on which it is moved requires less energy.
Always face the direction of the movement.	Ineffective use of major muscle groups occurs when the spine is rotated or twisted.
Start any body movement with proper alignment. Stand as close as possible to the object to be moved. Avoid stretching, reaching, and twisting, which may place the line of gravity outside the base of support.	Balance is maintained and muscle strain is avoided as long as the line of gravity passes through the base of support.
Before moving an object, increase your stability by widening your stance and flexing your knees, hips, and ankles.	The wider the base of support and the lower the center of gravity, the greater the stability.
Before moving an object, contract your gluteal, abdominal, leg, and arm muscles to prepare them for action.	The greater the preparatory isometric tensing, or contraction of muscles, before moving an object, the less the energy required to move it, and the less the likelihood of musculoskeletal strain and injury.
Avoid working against gravity. Pull, push, roll, or turn objects instead of lifting them. Lower the head of the client's bed before moving the client up in bed.	Moving an object along a level surface requires less energy than moving an object up an inclined surface or lifting it against the force of gravity.
Use your gluteal and leg muscles rather than the sacrospinal muscles of your back to exert an upward thrust when lifting. Distribute the workload between both arms and legs to prevent back strain.	Pulling creates less friction than pushing.
When pushing an object, enlarge the base of support by moving the front foot forward.	The synchronized use of as many large muscle groups as possible during an activity increases overall strength and prevents muscle fatigue and injury.
When pulling an object, enlarge the base of support by either moving the rear leg back if facing the object or moving the front foot forward if facing away from the object.	Balance is maintained with minimal effort when the base of support is enlarged in the direction in which the movement will occur.
When moving or carrying objects, hold them as close as possible to your center of gravity.	The closer the line of gravity to the center of the base of support, the greater the stability.
Use the weight of the body as a force for pulling or pushing, by rocking on the feet or leaning forward or backward.	Body weight adds force to counteract the weight of the object and reduces the amount of strain on the arms and back.
Alternate rest periods with periods of muscle use to help prevent fatigue.	Continuous muscle exertion can result in muscle strain and injury.

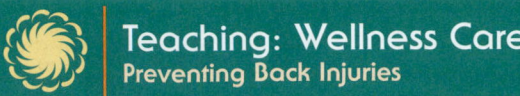

Teaching: Wellness Care
Preventing Back Injuries

- Become consciously aware of your posture and body mechanics.
- When standing for a period of time, periodically flex one hip and knee and rest your foot on an object if possible.
- When sitting, keep your knees slightly higher than your hips.
- Use a firm mattress that provides good body support at natural body curvatures.
- Exercise regularly to maintain overall physical condition; include exercises that strengthen the pelvic, abdominal, and lumbar muscles.
- Avoid exercises that cause pain or require spinal flexion with straight legs (e.g., toe-touching and sit-ups) or spinal rotation (twisting).
- When moving an object, spread your feet apart to provide a wide base of support.
- When lifting an object, distribute the weight between large muscles of the legs and arms. Although there are complex formulas for calculating the maximum weight a person can safely lift using variables such as the starting, carrying, and ending locations of the object, a general guideline is a limit of 15 to 25 pounds held at elbow height.
- Wear a support belt when lifting heavy objects and obtain assistance if indicated (especially if items weigh more than 25 pounds).
- Wear clothing that allows you to use good body mechanics and comfortable low-heeled shoes that provide good foot support and will not cause you to slip, stumble, or turn your ankle.

---

because of the exaggerated lumbar curvature these situations produce. Sedentary persons are at greater risk because of weak back and abdominal muscles.

Low back injuries are preventable. Some guidelines for preventing back injuries are presented in Teaching: Wellness Care.

Positioning Clients

Positioning a client in good body alignment and changing the position regularly and systematically are essential aspects of nursing practice. Clients who can move easily automatically reposition themselves for comfort. Such people generally require minimal positioning assistance from nurses, other than guidance about ways to maintain body alignment and to exercise their joints. However, people who are weak, frail, in pain, paralyzed, or unconscious rely on nurses to provide or assist with position changes. For all clients, it is important to assess the skin and provide skin care before and after a position change.

Any position, correct or incorrect, can be detrimental if maintained for a prolonged period. Frequent change of position helps to prevent muscle discomfort, undue pressure resulting in pressure ulcers, damage to superficial nerves and blood vessels, and contractures. Position changes also maintain muscle tone and stimulate postural reflexes.

When the client is not able to move independently or assist with moving, the preferred method is to have two or more peo-

ple move or turn the client. Appropriate assistance reduces the risk of muscle strain and body injury to both the client and nurse.

When positioning clients in bed, the nurse can do a number of things to ensure proper alignment and promote client comfort and safety:

- Make sure the mattress is firm and level yet has enough give to fill in and support natural body curvatures. A sagging mattress, a mattress that is too soft, or an underfilled waterbed used over a prolonged period can contribute to the development of hip flexion contractures and low back strain and pain. Bed boards made of plywood and placed beneath a sagging mattress are increasingly recommended for clients who have back problems or are prone to them. Some bed boards are hinged across the middle so that they will bend as the head of the bed is raised. It is particularly important in the home setting to inspect the mattress for support.
- Ensure that the bed is clean and dry. Wrinkled or damp sheets increase the risk of pressure ulcer formation. Make sure extremities can move freely whenever possible. For example, the top bedclothes need to be loose enough for the client to move the feet.
- Place support devices in specified areas according to the client's position. Box 42–1 lists commonly used support devices. Use only those support devices needed to maintain alignment and to prevent stress on the client's muscles and joints. If the person is capable of movement, too many devices limit mobility and increase the potential for muscle weakness and atrophy. Common alignment problems that can be corrected with support devices include the following:
  a. Flexion of the neck
  b. Internal rotation of the shoulder
  c. Adduction of the shoulder
  d. Flexion of the wrist
  e. Anterior convexity of the lumbar spine

BOX 42–1   ■ Support Devices

- **Pillows.** Different sizes are available. Used for support or elevation of a body part (e.g., an arm). Specially designed dense pillows can be used to elevate the upper body.
- **Mattresses.** There are two types of mattresses: ones that fit on the bed frame (e.g., standard bed mattress) and mattresses that fit on the standard bed mattress (e.g., egg crate mattress). Mattresses should be evenly supportive.
- **Bed boards.** The boards are usually made of wood and are placed under the mattress to provide support.
- **Chair beds.** These beds can be placed into the position of a chair for clients who cannot move from the bed but require a sitting position.
- **Foot boot.** These are made of a variety of substances. They usually have a firm exterior and padding of foam to protect the skin. They provide support to the feet in a natural position and keep the weight of covers off the toes. Clients who are able to sit may benefit from high-top shoes to maintain foot alignment.
- **Footboard.** A flat panel often made of plastic or wood. It keeps the feet in dorsiflexion to prevent plantar flexion.

f. External rotation of the hips
g. Hyperextension of the knees
h. Plantar flexion of the ankle.

- Avoid placing one body part, particularly one with bony prominences, directly on top of another body part. Excessive pressure can damage veins and predispose the client to thrombus formation. Pressure against the popliteal space may damage nerves and blood vessels in this area.
- Plan a systematic 24-hour schedule for position changes.
- Sometimes a person who appears well aligned may be experiencing real discomfort. Both appearance, in relation to alignment criteria, and comfort are important in achieving effective alignment.

Fowler's Position. **Fowler's position,** or a semisitting position, is a bed position in which the head and trunk are raised 45 to 90 degrees. In **low-Fowler's** or **semi-Fowler's position** (Figure 42–41 ■), the head and trunk are raised 15 to 45 degrees; in **high-Fowler's position,** the head and trunk are raised 90 degrees (see Table 42–5). In this position, the knees may or may not be flexed.

Fowler's position is the position of choice for people who have difficulty breathing and for some people with heart problems. When the client is in this position, gravity pulls the diaphragm downward, allowing greater chest expansion and lung ventilation.

A common error nurses make when aligning clients in Fowler's position is placing an overly large pillow or more than one pillow behind the client's head. This promotes the development of neck flexion contractures. If a client desires several head pillows, the nurse should encourage the client to rest without a pillow for several hours each day to extend the neck fully and counteract the effects of poor neck alignment.

Orthopneic Position. In the **orthopneic position,** the client sits either in bed or on the side of the bed with an overbed table across the lap (Figure 42–42 ■). This position facilitates respiration by allowing maximum chest expansion. It is particularly helpful to clients who have problems exhaling, because they can press the lower part of the chest against the edge of the overbed table.

Dorsal Recumbent Position. In the **dorsal recumbent** (back-lying) **position** (Figure 42–43 ■), the client's head and shoulders are slightly elevated on a small pillow. In some agencies,

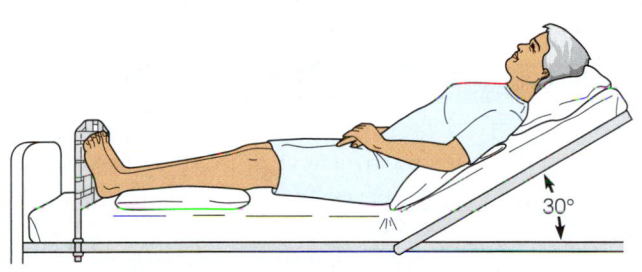

Figure 42–41 ■ Low-Fowler's (semi-Fowler's) position (supported). Note that arm support is omitted in this instance. The amount of support depends on the needs of the individual client.

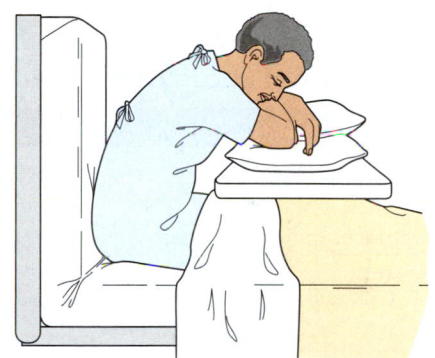

Figure 42–42 ■ Orthopneic position.

TABLE 42–5 Fowler's Position

Unsupported Position	Problem to Be Prevented	Corrective Measure*
Bed-sitting position with upper part of body elevated 30–90° commencing at hips	Posterior flexion of lumbar curvature	Pillow at lower back (lumbar region) to support lumbar region
Head rests on bed surface	Hyperextension of neck	Pillows to support head, neck, and upper back
Arms fall at sides	Shoulder muscle strain, possible dislocation of shoulders, edema of hands and arms with flaccid paralysis, flexion contracture of the wrist	Pillow under forearms to eliminate pull on shoulder and assist venous blood flow from hands and lower arms
Legs lie flat and straight on lower bed surface	Hyperextension of knees	Small pillow under thighs to flex knees
Heels rest on bed surface	Pressure on heels	Pillow under lower legs
Feet are in plantar flexion	Plantar flexion of feet (foot drop)	Footboard to provide support for dorsal flexion

*The amount of correction depends on the needs of the individual client.

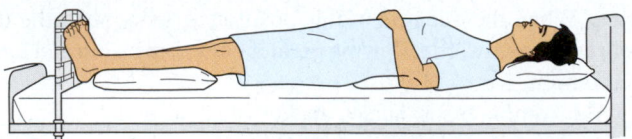

Figure 42–43 ■ Dorsal recumbent position (supported).

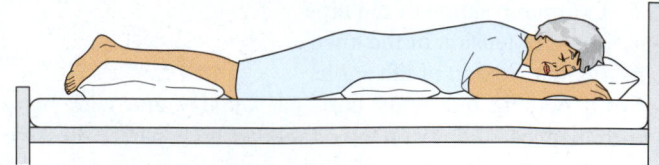

Figure 42–44 ■ Prone position (supported).

the terms *dorsal recumbent* and *supine* are used interchangeably; strictly speaking, however, in the **supine** or **dorsal position** the head and shoulders are not elevated. In both positions, the client's forearms may be elevated on pillows or placed at the client's sides. Supports are similar in both positions, except for the head pillow (see Table 42–6). The dorsal recumbent position is used to provide comfort and to facilitate healing following certain surgeries or anesthetics (e.g., spinal).

Prone Position. In the **prone position,** the client lies on the abdomen with the head turned to one side (Figure 42–44 ■). The hips are not flexed. Both children and adults often sleep in this position, sometimes with one or both arms flexed over their heads. This position has several advantages. It is the only

bed position that allows full extension of the hip and knee joints. When used periodically, the prone position helps to prevent flexion contractures of the hips and knees, thereby counteracting a problem caused by all other bed positions. The prone position also promotes drainage from the mouth and is especially useful for unconscious clients or those clients recovering from surgery of the mouth or throat (see Table 42–7).

The prone position poses some distinct disadvantages. The pull of gravity on the trunk produces a marked lordosis in most people, and the neck is rotated laterally to a significant degree. For this reason, the prone position may not be recommended for people with problems of the cervical or lumbar spine. This position also causes plantar flexion. Some clients with cardiac

TABLE 42–6 Dorsal Recumbent Position

Unsupported Position	Problem to Be Prevented	Corrective Measure*
Head is flat on bed surface	Hyperextension of neck in thick-chested person	Pillow of suitable thickness under head and shoulders if necessary for alignment
Lumbar curvature of spine is apparent	Posterior flexion of lumbar curvature	Roll or small pillow under lumbar curvature
Legs may be externally rotated	External rotation of legs	Roll or sandbag placed laterally to trochanter of femur (optional)
Legs are extended	Hyperextension of knees	Small pillow under thigh to flex knee slightly
Feet assume plantar flexion position	Plantar flexion (foot drop)	Footboard or rolled pillow to support feet in dorsal flexion
Heels on bed surface	Pressure on heels	Pillow under lower legs

*The amount of correction depends on the needs of the individual client.

TABLE 42–7 Prone Position

Unsupported Position	Problem to Be Prevented	Corrective Measure*
Head is turned to side and neck is slightly flexed	Flexion or hyperextension of neck	Small pillow under head unless contraindicated because of promotion of mucous drainage from mouth
Body lies flat on abdomen accentuating lumbar curvature	Hyperextension of lumbar curvature; difficulty breathing; pressure on breasts (women); pressure on genitals (men)	Small pillow or roll under abdomen just below diaphragm
Toes rest on bed surface; feet are in plantar flexion	Plantar flexion of feet (foot drop)	Allow feet to fall naturally over end of mattress, or support lower legs on a pillow so that toes do not touch the bed

* The amount of correction depends on the needs of the individual client.

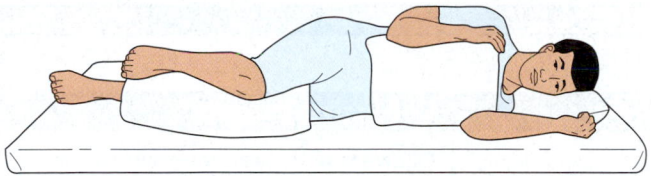

Figure 42–45 ■ Lateral position (supported).

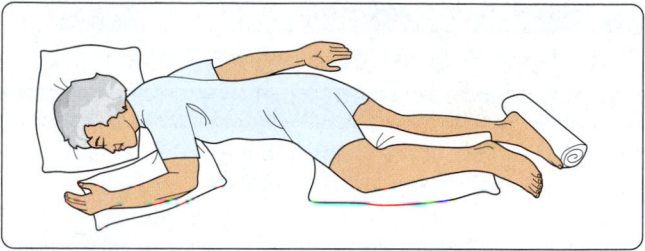

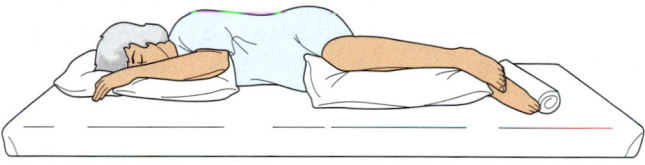

Figure 42–46 ■ Sims' position (supported).

or respiratory problems find the prone position confining and suffocating because chest expansion is inhibited during respirations. The prone position should be used only when the client's back is correctly aligned, only for short periods, and only for people with no evidence of spinal abnormalities.

Lateral Position. In the **lateral** (side-lying) **position** (Figure 42–45 ■), the person lies on one side of the body. Flexing the top hip and knee and placing this leg in front of the body creates a wider, triangular base of support and achieves greater stability. The greater the flexion of the top hip and knee, the greater the stability and balance in this position. This flexion reduces lordosis and promotes good back alignment. For this reason, the lateral position is good for resting and sleeping clients. The lateral position helps to relieve pressure on the sacrum and heels in people who sit for much of the day or who are confined to bed and rest in Fowler's or dorsal recumbent positions much of the time. In the lateral position, most of the body's weight is borne by the lateral aspect of the lower scapula, the lateral aspect of the ilium, and the greater trochanter of the femur. People who have sensory or motor deficits on one side of the body usually find that lying on the uninvolved side is more comfortable (see Table 42–8).

Sims' Position. In **Sims'** (semiprone) **position** (Figure 42–46 ■), the client assumes a posture halfway between the lateral and the prone positions. The lower arm is positioned behind the client, and the upper arm is flexed at the shoulder and the elbow. Both legs are flexed in front of the client. The upper leg is more acutely flexed at both the hip and the knee than is the lower one.

Sims' position may be used for unconscious clients because it facilitates drainage from the mouth and prevents aspiration of fluids. It is also used for paralyzed clients because it reduces pressure over the sacrum and greater trochanter of the hip. It is often used for clients receiving enemas and occasionally for clients undergoing examinations or treatments of the perineal area. Many people, especially pregnant women, find Sims' position comfortable for sleeping. People with sensory or motor deficits on one side of the body usually find that lying on the uninvolved side is more comfortable (see Table 42–9).

Moving and Turning Clients in Bed

Although healthy people usually take for granted that they can change body position and go from one place to another with little effort, ill people may have difficulty moving, even in bed. How much assistance clients require depends on their own ability to move and their health status. Nurses should be sensitive to both the need of people to function independently and their need for assistance to move.

When a nurse assists a person to move, correct body mechanics need to be employed so that the nurse is not injured. Correct body alignment for the client must also be maintained so that undue stress is not placed on the musculoskeletal system.

TABLE 42–8 Lateral Position

Unsupported Position	Problem to Be Prevented	Corrective Measure*
Body is turned to side, both arms in front of body, weight resting primarily on lateral aspects of scapula and ilium	Lateral flexion and fatigue of sternocleidomastoid muscles	Pillow under head and neck to provide good alignment
Upper arm and shoulder are rotated internally and adducted	Internal rotation and adduction of shoulder and subsequent limited function; impaired chest expansion	Pillow under upper arm to place it in good alignment; lower arm should be flexed comfortably
Upper thigh and leg are rotated internally and adducted	Internal rotation and adduction of femur; twisting of the spine	Pillow under leg and thigh to place them in good alignment; shoulders and hips should be aligned

*The amount of correction depends on the needs of the individual client.

TABLE 42–9 Sims' (Semiprone) Position

Unsupported Position	Problem to Be Prevented	Corrective Measure*
Head rests on bed surface; weight is borne by lateral aspects of cranial and facial bones	Lateral flexion of neck	Pillow supports head, maintaining it in good alignment unless drainage from the mouth is required
Upper shoulder and arm are internally rotated	Internal rotation of shoulder and arm; pressure on chest, restricting expansion during breathing	Pillow under upper arm to prevent internal rotation
Upper leg and thigh are adducted and internally rotated	Internal rotation and adduction of hip and leg	Pillow under upper leg to support it in alignment
Feet assume plantar flexion	Foot drop	Sandbags to support feet in dorsal flexion

*The amount of correction depends on the needs of the individual client.

Actions and rationales applicable to moving and lifting clients include these:

- Before moving a client, assess the degree of exertion permitted, the client's physical abilities (e.g., muscle strength, presence of paralysis), ability to understand instructions, degree of comfort or discomfort when moving, client's weight, presence of orthostatic hypotension (particularly important when client will be standing), and your own strength and ability to move the client.
- If indicated, use pain relief modalities or medication prior to moving the client.
- Prepare supportive equipment, e.g., pillows, trochanter roll.
- Obtain required assistance.
- Explain the procedure to the client and listen to any suggestions the client or support people have.
- Provide privacy.
- Wash hands.
- Raise the height of the bed *to bring the client close to your center of gravity.*
- Lock the wheels on the bed, and raise the rail on the side of the bed opposite you *to ensure client safety.*
- Face in the direction of the movement *to prevent spinal twisting.*

- Assume a broad stance *to increase stability and provide balance.*
- Lean your trunk forward, and flex your hips, knees, and ankles *to lower your center of gravity, increase stability, and ensure use of large muscle groups during movements.*
- Tighten your gluteal, abdominal, leg, and arm muscles *to prepare them for action and prevent injury.*
- Rock from the front leg to the back leg when pulling or from the back leg to the front leg when pushing *to overcome inertia, counteract the client's weight, and help attain a balanced, smooth motion.*
- After moving the client, determine the client's comfort, body alignment, tolerance of the activity (e.g., check pulse rate, blood pressure), and safety precautions required (e.g., side rails).

See Procedures 42–1 through 42–4 on moving and turning clients in bed and helping them sit up on the edge of the bed. *Note:* The Assessment, Planning, Delegation, and Equipment sections as listed in Procedure 42–1 are the same for each of these four procedures and are not repeated. The Evaluation section at the end of Procedure 42–4 is also the same for all four procedures and, hence, is not repeated.

Procedure 42–1 Moving a Client Up in Bed

ASSESSMENT

Before moving a client, assess the following:

- The client's physical abilities (e.g., muscle strength, presence of paralysis)
- Ability to understand instructions

- Degree of comfort or discomfort when moving. If needed, administer analgesics or perform other pain-relief measures (see Chapter 44). 🔗
- Client's weight
- Your own strength and ability to move the client

PLANNING

Review the client record to determine if previous nurses have recorded information about the client's ability to move.

Delegation

The skills of moving and turning clients in bed can be delegated to unlicensed assistive personnel (UAP). The nurse may wish to review

proper body mechanics with the UAP to protect the UAP from injury. Emphasize the need for the UAP to report changes in the client's condition that require assessment and intervention by the nurse.

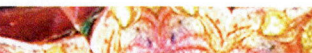 **Procedure 42–1 Moving a Client Up in Bed** *continued*

PLANNING *continued*

Equipment
- Assistive devices such as overhead trapeze, pull and/or turn sheet, and transfer or sliding bar.

Purposes
- Clients who have slid down in bed from the Fowler's position or been pulled down by traction often need assistance to move up in bed.

IMPLEMENTATION:

Preparation
Determine:
- Assistive devices that will be required
- Encumbrances to movement such as an IV or a heavy cast on one leg
- Medications the client is receiving, because certain medications may hamper movement or alertness of the client
- Assistance required from other health care personnel.

Performance
1. Explain to the client what you are going to do, why it is necessary, and how he or she can cooperate. Listen to any suggestions made by the client or support people. Discuss how the results will be used in planning further care or treatments.
2. Wash hands and observe other appropriate infection control procedures.
3. Provide for client privacy.
4. Adjust the bed and the client's position.
   - Adjust the head of the bed to a flat position or as low as the client can tolerate. *Moving the client upward against gravity requires more force and can cause back strain.*
   - Raise the bed to the height of your center of gravity.
   - Lock the wheels on the bed and raise the rail on the side of the bed opposite you.
   - Remove all pillows, then place one against the head of the bed. *This pillow protects the client's head from inadvertent injury against the top of the bed during the upward move.*
5. Elicit the client's help in lessening your workload.
   - Ask the client to flex the hips and knees and position the feet so that they can be used effectively for pushing. *Flexing the hips and knees keeps the entire lower leg off the bed surface preventing friction during movement, and ensures use of the large muscle groups in the client's legs when pushing, thus increasing the force of movement.*

- Ask the client to
   a. Grasp the head of the bed with both hands and pull during the move
   or
   b. Raise the upper part of the body on the elbows and push with the hands and forearms during the move
   or
   c. Grasp the overhead trapeze with both hands and lift and pull during the move. *Client assistance provides additional power to overcome inertia and friction during the move. These actions also keep the client's arms partially off the bed surface, reducing friction during movement, and make use of the large muscle groups of the client's arms to increase the force during movement.*
6. Position yourself appropriately, and move the client.
   - Face the direction of the movement, and then assume a broad stance with the foot nearest the bed behind the forward foot and weight on the forward foot. Lean your trunk forward from the hips. Flex hips, knees, and ankles.
   - Place your near arm under the client's thighs (Figure 42–47 ■).

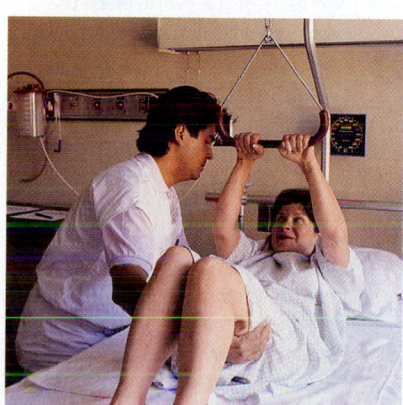

Figure 42–47 ■ Moving a client up in bed.

This supports the heaviest part of the body (the buttocks). Push down on the mattress with the far arm. The far arm acts as a lever during the move.
   - Tighten your gluteal, abdominal, leg, and arm muscles and rock from the back leg to the front leg and back again. Then, shift your weight to the front leg as the client pushes with the heels and pulls with the arms so that the client moves toward the head of the bed.
7. Ensure client comfort.
   - Elevate the head of the bed and provide appropriate support devices for the client's new position.
   - See the sections on positioning clients earlier in this chapter.

VARIATION: A CLIENT WHO HAS LIMITED STRENGTH OF THE UPPER EXTREMITIES
- Assist the client to flex the hips and knees as in step 5 previously. Place the client's arms across the chest. *This keeps them off the bed surface and minimizes friction during movement.* Ask the client to flex the neck during the move and keep the head off the bed surface.
- Position yourself as in step 6 and place one arm under the client's back and shoulders and the other arm under the client's thighs. *This placement of the arms distributes the client's weight and supports the heaviest part of the body (the buttocks).* Shift your weight as in step 6.

VARIATION: TWO NURSES USING A HAND–FOREARM INTERLOCK
Two people are required to move clients who are unable to assist because of their condition or weight. Using the technique described in step 6, with the second staff member on the opposite side of the bed, both of you interlock your forearms (Figure 42–48 ■) under the client's thighs and shoulders and lift the client up in bed.

continued on page 1086

Procedure 42–1 Moving a Client Up in Bed *continued*

IMPLEMENTATION *continued*

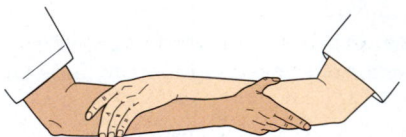

Figure 42–48 ■ Two nurses using a hand–forearm interlock.

VARIATION: TWO NURSES USING A TURN SHEET

Two nurses can use a turn sheet to move a client up in bed. *A turn sheet distributes the client's weight more evenly, decreases fric-tion, and exerts a more even force on the client during the move. In addition, it prevents injury of the client's skin, because the friction created between two sheets when one is moved is less than that created by the client's body moving over the sheet.*

- Place a drawsheet or a full sheet folded in half under the client, extending from the shoulders to the thighs. Each person rolls up or fanfolds the turn sheet close to the client's body on either side.
- Both individuals grasp the sheet close to the shoulders and buttocks of the client. *This draws the weight closer to the nurse's center of gravity and increases the* nurse's balance and stability, permitting a smoother movement. Follow the method of moving clients with limited upper extremity strength as described earlier.

8. Document all relevant information. Record:
   - Time and change of position moved from and position moved to
   - Any signs of pressure areas
   - Use of support devices
   - Ability of client to assist in moving and turning
   - Response of client to moving and turning (e.g., anxiety, discomfort, dizziness).

Procedure 42–2 Turning a Client to the Lateral or Prone Position in Bed

Purposes

- Movement to the lateral (side-lying) position may be necessary when placing a bedpan beneath the client, when changing the client's bed linen, or when repositioning the client.

IMPLEMENTATION

Preparation

Determine:
- Assistive devices that will be required
- Encumbrances to movement such as an IV or a heavy cast on one leg
- Medications the client is receiving, because certain medications may hamper movement or alertness of the client
- Assistance required from other health care personnel.

Performance

1. Explain to the client what you are going to do, why it is necessary, and how he or she can cooperate. Discuss how the results will be used in planning further care or treatments.
2. Wash hands and observe other appropriate infection control procedures.
3. Provide for client privacy.
4. Position yourself and the client appropriately before performing the move.
   - Move the client closer to the side of the bed opposite the side the client will face when turned. *This ensures that the client will be positioned safely in the center of the bed after turning.* Use a pull sheet beneath the client's trunk and thighs to pull the client to the side of the bed. Roll up the sheet as close as possible to the client's body and pull the client to the side of the bed. Adjust the client's head and reposition the legs appropriately.
   - While standing on the side of the bed nearest the client, place the client's near arm across the chest. Abduct the client's far shoulder slightly from the side of the body and externally rotate the shoulder (Figure 42–8 on page 1061). *Pulling the one arm forward facilitates the turning motion. Pulling the other arm away from the body and externally rotating the shoulder prevents that arm from being caught beneath the client's body during the roll.*
   - Place the client's near ankle and foot across the far ankle and foot. *This facilitates the turning motion. Making these preparations on the* side of the bed closest to the client helps prevent unnecessary reaching.
   - Raise the side rail next to the client before going to the other side of the bed. *This ensures that the client, who is close to the edge of the mattress, will not fall.*
   - Position yourself on the side of the bed toward which the client will turn, directly in line with the client's waistline and as close to the bed as possible.
   - Lean your trunk forward from the hips. Flex your hips, knees, and ankles. Assume a broad stance with one foot forward and the weight placed on this forward foot.
5. Pull or roll the client toward you to the lateral position.
   - Place one hand on the client's far hip and the other hand on the client's far shoulder (Figure 42–49, ■ A). *This position of the hands supports the client at the two heaviest parts of the body, providing greater control in movement during the roll.*

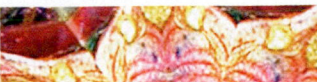

Procedure 42–2 Turning a Client to the Lateral or Prone Position in Bed *continued*

IMPLEMENTATION *continued*

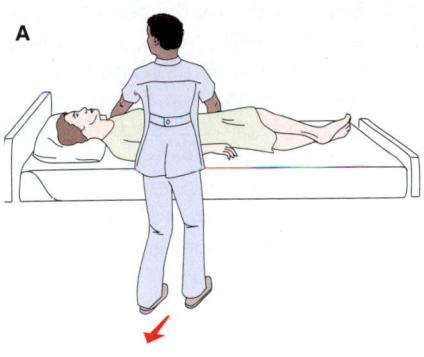

A

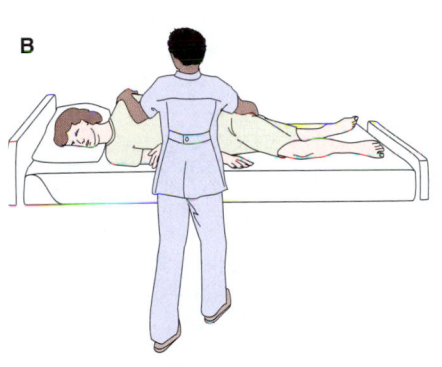

B

Figure 42–49 ■ Moving a client to a lateral position.

- Tighten your gluteal, abdominal, leg, and arm muscles; rock backward, shifting your weight from the forward to the backward foot, and roll the client onto the side of the body to face you (Figure 42–49 ■, *B*). *Turning the client toward you promotes the client's sense of security.*
- Position the client on his or her side with arms and legs positioned and supported properly (see Table 42–8).

VARIATION: TURNING THE CLIENT TO A PRONE POSITION

To turn a client to the prone position, follow the preceding steps, with two exceptions:

- Instead of abducting the far arm, keep the client's arm alongside the body for the client to roll over. *Keeping the arm alongside the body prevents it from being pinned under the client when the client is rolled.*

- Roll the client completely onto the abdomen. *It is essential to move the client as close as possible to the edge of the bed before the turn so that the client will be lying on the center of the bed after rolling.* Never pull a client across the bed while the client is in the prone position. *Doing so can injure a woman's breasts or a man's genitals.*

6. Document all relevant information. Record:
   - Time and change of position moved from and position moved to
   - Any signs of pressure areas
   - Use of support devices
   - Ability of client to assist in moving and turning
   - Response of client to moving and turning (e.g., anxiety, discomfort, dizziness).

Procedure 42–3 Logrolling a Client

Purposes

- **Logrolling** is a technique used to turn a client whose body must at all times be kept in straight alignment (like a log). An example is the client with a spinal injury. Considerable care must be taken to prevent additional injury. This technique requires two nurses or, if the client is large, three nurses. For the client who has a cervical injury, one nurse must maintain the client's head and neck alignment.

IMPLEMENTATION

Preparation

Determine:
- Assistive devices that will be required
- Encumbrances to movement such as an IV or a heavy cast on one leg
- Medications the client is receiving, because certain medications may hamper movement or alertness of the client
- Assistance required from other health care personnel.

Performance

1. Explain to the client what you are going to do, why it is necessary, and how he or she can cooperate. Discuss how the results will be used in planning further care or treatments.
2. Wash hands and observe other appropriate infection control procedures.
3. Provide for client privacy.
4. Position yourselves and the client appropriately before the move.
   - Stand on the same side of the bed, and assume a broad stance with one foot ahead of the other.
   - Place the client's arms across the chest. *Doing so ensures that they will not be injured or become trapped under the body when the body is turned.*
   - Lean your trunk, and flex your hips, knees, and ankles.
   - Place your arms under the client as shown in Figure 42–50 ■ or Figure 42–51 ■, depending on the client's size. *Each staff member then has a major weight area of the client centered between the arms.*
   - Tighten your gluteal, abdominal, leg, and arm muscles.

continued on page 1088

Procedure 42–3 Logrolling a Client *continued*

IMPLEMENTATION *continued*

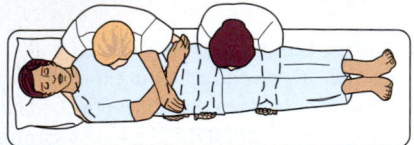

Figure 42–50 ■ Correct arm placement for moving a client to the side of the bed: two nurses.

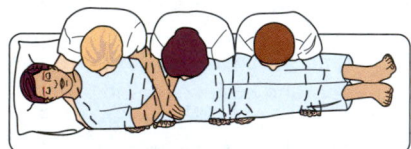

Figure 42–51 ■ Correct arm placement for moving a client to the side of the bed: three nurses.

5. Pull the client to the side of the bed.
   - One nurse counts: One, two, three, go. Then, at the same time, all staff members pull the client to the side of the bed by shifting their weight to the back foot. *Moving the client in unison maintains the client's body alignment.*
   - Elevate the side rail on this side of the bed. *This prevents the client from falling while lying so close to the edge of the bed.*
6. Move to the other side of the bed, and place supportive devices for the client when turned.
   - Place a pillow where it will support the client's head after the turn. *The pillow prevents lateral flexion of the neck and ensures alignment of the cervical spine.*
   - Place one or two pillows between the client's legs to support the upper leg when the client is turned. *This pillow prevents adduction of the upper leg and keeps the legs parallel and aligned.*
7. Roll and position the client in proper alignment.
   - All nurses flex their hips, knees, and ankles and assume a broad stance with one foot forward.
   - All nurses reach over the client and place hands as shown in Figure 42–52 ■. *Doing so centers a major weight area of the client between each nurse's arms.*

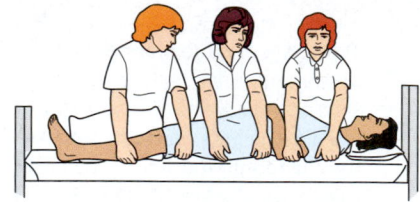

Figure 42–52 ■ Correct hand placement for logrolling a client.

- One nurse counts: One, two, three, go. Then, at the same time, all nurses roll the client to a lateral position.
- Support the client's head, back, and upper and lower extremities with pillows.
- Raise the side rails and place the call bell within the client's reach.

VARIATION: USING A TURN OR LIFT SHEET
- Use a turn sheet to facilitate logrolling. First, stand with another nurse on the same side of the bed. Assume a broad stance with one foot forward, and grasp half of the fanfolded or rolled edge of the turn sheet. On a signal, pull the client toward both of you (Figure 42–53 ■).

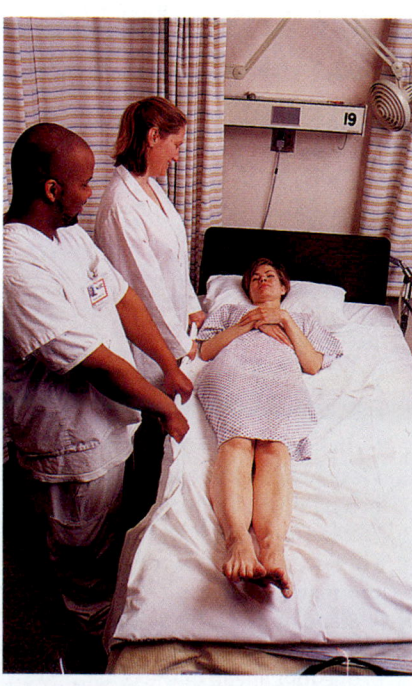

Figure 42–53 ■ Using a turn sheet, the nurses pull the sheet with the client on it to the edge of the bed.

- Before turning the client, place pillow supports for the head and legs, as described in step 6. This helps maintain the client's alignment when turning. Then, go to the other side of the bed (farthest from the client), and assume a stable stance. Reaching over the client, grasp the far edges of the turn sheet, and roll the client toward you (Figure 42–54 ■). The second nurse (behind the client) helps turn the client and provides pillow supports to ensure good alignment in the lateral position.

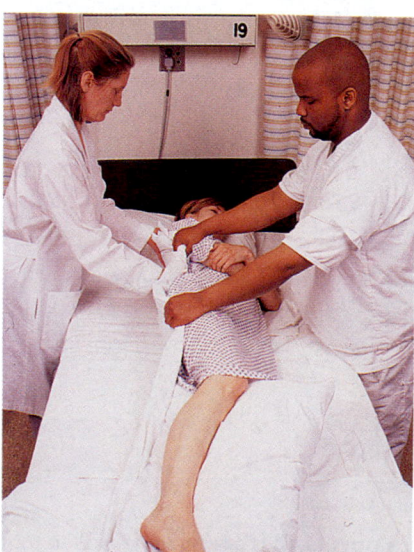

Figure 42–54 ■ The nurse on the right uses the far edge of the sheet to roll the client toward him; the nurse on the left remains behind the client and assists with turning.

8. Document all relevant information. Record:
   - Time and change of position moved from and position moved to
   - Any signs of pressure areas
   - Use of support devices
   - Ability of client to assist in moving and turning
   - Response of client to moving and turning (e.g., anxiety, discomfort, dizziness).

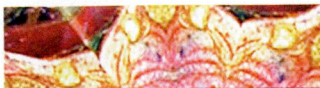

Procedure 42–4 Assisting the Client to Sit on the Side of the Bed (Dangling)

Purposes

■ The client assumes a sitting position on the edge of the bed before walking, moving to a chair or wheelchair, eating, or performing other activities.

IMPLEMENTATION

Preparation

Determine:

■ Assistive devices that will be required
■ Encumbrances to movement such as an IV or a heavy cast on one leg
■ Medications the client is receiving, because certain medications may hamper movement or alertness of the client
■ Assistance required from other health care personnel.

Performance

1. Explain to the client what you are going to do, why it is necessary, and how he or she can cooperate. Discuss how the results will be used in planning further care or treatments.
2. Wash hands and observe other appropriate infection control procedures.
3. Provide for client privacy.
4. Position yourself and the client appropriately before performing the move.
   • Assist the client to a lateral position facing you.
   • Raise the head of the bed slowly to its highest position. *This decreases the distance that the client needs to move to sit up on the side of the bed.*
   • Position the client's feet and lower legs at the edge of the bed. *This enables the client's feet to move easily off the bed during the movement, and the client is aided by gravity into a sitting position.*
   • Stand beside the client's hips and face the far corner of the bottom of the bed (the angle in which movement will occur). Assume a broad stance, placing the foot nearest the client forward. Lean your trunk forward from the hips. Flex your hips, knees, and ankles (Figure 42–55, ■ A).
5. Move the client to a sitting position.
   • Place one arm around the client's shoulders and the other arm beneath both of the client's thighs near the knees (Figure 42–55, A). *Supporting the client's shoulders prevents the client from falling backward*

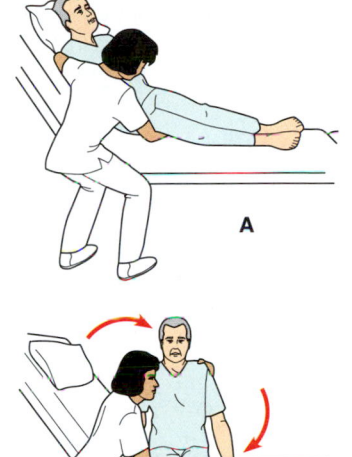

Figure 42–55 ■ Assisting a client to a sitting position on the edge of the bed.

during the movement. Supporting the client's thighs reduces friction of the thighs against the bed surface during the move and increases the force of the movement.
   • Tighten your gluteal, abdominal, leg, and arm muscles.
   • Lift the client's thighs slightly. *This reduces the friction of the client's thighs and the nurse's arm against the bed surface.*
   • Pivot on the balls of your feet in the desired direction facing the foot of the bed while pulling the client's feet and legs off the bed (Figure 42–55 ■, B). *Pivoting prevents twisting of the nurse's spine. The weight of the client's legs swinging downward increases downward movement of the lower body and helps make the client's upper body vertical.*
   • Keep supporting the client until the client is well balanced and comfort-

able. *This movement may cause some clients to faint.*
   • Assess vital signs (e.g., pulse, respirations, and blood pressure) as indicated by the client's health status.

VARIATION: TEACHING A CLIENT HOW TO SIT ON THE SIDE OF THE BED INDEPENDENTLY

A client who has had recent abdominal surgery or who is weak may have too much abdominal pain or too little strength to sit straight up in bed. This person can be taught to assume a dangle position without assistance. Instruct the client to:
   • Roll to the side and lift the far leg over the near leg (Figure 42–56, ■ A).
   • Grasp the mattress edge with the lower arm and push the fist of the upper arm into the mattress (Figure 42–56 ■, B).
   • Push up with the arms as the heels and legs slide over the mattress edge.
   • Maintain the sitting position by pushing both fists into the mattress behind and to the sides of the buttocks.

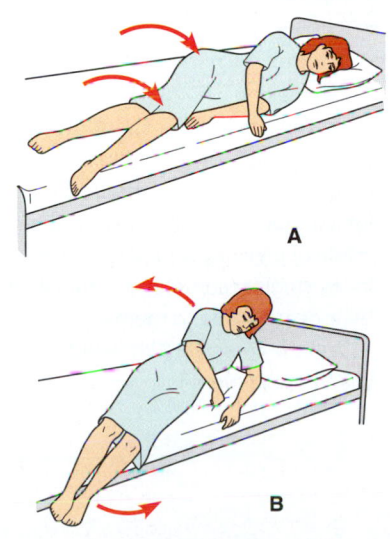

Figure 42–56 ■ Moving to a sitting position independently.

continued on page 1090

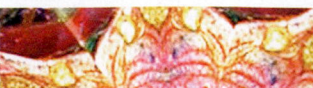

Procedure 42–4 Assisting the Client to Sit on the Side of the Bed (Dangling) *continued*

IMPLEMENTATION *continued*

6. Document all relevant information. Record:
   • Time and change of position moved from and position moved to

   • Any signs of pressure areas
   • Use of support devices
   • Ability of client to assist in moving and turning

   • Response of client to moving and turning (e.g., anxiety, discomfort, dizziness).

EVALUATION

■ Check the skin integrity of the pressure areas from the previous position. Relate findings to previous assessment data if available. Conduct follow-up assessment for previous and/or new skin breakdown areas.

■ Check for proper alignment after the position change. Do a visual check and ask the client for a comfort assessment.

■ Determine that all required safety precautions (e.g., side rails) are in place.

■ Determine client's tolerance of the activity (e.g., vital signs before and after dangling) particularly the first time the client changes position.

■ Report-significant changes to the physician.

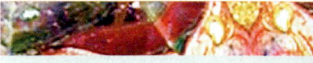

Lifespan Considerations

Positioning, Moving, and Turning Clients
Infants
• Position infants on their side for sleep, particularly after feeding.

Children
• Carefully inspect the dependent skin surfaces of all infants and children confined to bed at least three times in each 24-hour period.

Elders
• Decreased subcutaneous fat and thinning of the skin place elders at risk for skin breakdown. Repositioning at least every 2

hours helps reduce pressure on bony prominences and avoid skin trauma.

• In clients who have had cerebrovascular accidents (strokes), there is a risk of shoulder displacement on the paralyzed side from improper moving or repositioning techniques. Use care when moving, positioning in bed, and transferring. Pillows or foam devices are helpful to support the affected arm and shoulder and prevent injury.

Home Care Considerations

Positioning, Moving, and Turning Clients
• When making a home visit, it is particularly important to inspect the mattress for support. A sagging mattress, a mattress that is too soft, or an underfilled waterbed used over a prolonged period can contribute to the development of hip flexion contractures and low back strain and pain. Bed boards made of plywood and placed beneath a sagging mattress are increasingly recommended for clients who have back problems or are prone to them.
• Assess the caregivers' knowledge and application of body mechanics to prevent injury.

• Demonstrate how to turn and position the client in bed. Observe the caregiver performing a return demonstration.
• Teach caregivers the basic principles of body alignment and how to check for proper alignment after the client has been changed to a new position.
• Teach the caregiver to check the client's skin for redness and integrity after repositioning the client. Stress the importance of informing the nurse about the length of time skin redness remains over pressure areas after the person has been repositioned. Emphasize that reddened areas should not be massaged as it may lead to tissue trauma.

Transferring Clients

Many clients require some assistance in transferring between bed and chair or wheelchair, between wheelchair and toilet, and between bed and stretcher. Before transferring any client, however, the nurse must determine the client's physical and mental

capabilities to participate in the transfer technique. In addition, the nurse must analyze and organize the activity. General guidelines for transfer techniques include these:

• Plan what to do and how to do it. Determine the space in which the transfer is maneuvered (bathrooms, for instance,

Practice Guidelines
Wheelchair Safety

- Always lock the brakes on both wheels of the wheelchair when the client transfers in or out of it.
- Raise the footplates before transferring the client into the wheelchair.
- Lower the footplates after the transfer, and place the client's feet on them.
- Ensure the client is positioned well back in the seat of the wheelchair.
- Use seat belts that fasten behind the wheelchair to protect confused clients from falls. *Note:* Seat belts are a form of restraint and must be used in accordance with policies and procedures that apply to the use of restraints (see Chapter 30).
- Back the wheelchair into or out of an elevator, rear large wheels first.
- Place your body between the wheelchair and the bottom of an incline.

Practice Guidelines
Safe Use of Stretchers

- Lock the wheels of the bed and stretcher before the client transfers in or out of them.
- Fasten safety straps across the client on a stretcher, and raise the side rails.
- Never leave a client unattended on a stretcher unless the wheels are locked and the side rails are raised on both sides and/or the safety straps are securely fastened across the client.
- Always push a stretcher from the end where the client's head is positioned. This position protects the client's head in the event of a collision.
- If the stretcher has two swivel wheels and two stationary wheels:
  a. Always position the client's head at the end with the stationary wheels and
  b. Push the stretcher from the end with the stationary wheels. The stretcher is maneuvered more easily when pushed from this end.
- Maneuver the stretcher when entering the elevator so that the client's head goes in first.

are usually cramped); the number of assistants (one or two) needed to accomplish the transfer safely; the skill and strength of the nurse(s); and the client's capabilities.

- Obtain essential equipment before starting (e.g., transfer belt, wheelchair), and check its function.
- Remove obstacles from the area used for the transfer.
- Explain the transfer to the client, including what the client should do.
- Explain the transfer to the nursing personnel who are helping; specify who will give directions (one person needs to be in charge).
- Always support or hold the client rather than the equipment.
- During the transfer, explain step by step what the client should do, for example, "Move your right foot forward."
- Make a written plan of the transfer, including the client's tolerance (e.g., pulse and respiratory rates).

Because wheelchairs and stretchers are unstable, they can predispose the client to falls and injury. Guidelines for the safe use of wheelchairs and stretchers are shown in the accompanying Practice Guidelines.

Transfer (walking) belts provide the greatest safety. The nurse grasps the belt to control movement of the client during the transfer. An increasing number of hospitals and nursing homes are requiring that personnel use the transfer belt to ambulate or move clients. See Procedure 42–5 for transferring a client between a bed and a chair and Procedure 42–6 for transferring a client between a bed and a stretcher. The Evaluation section at the end of Procedure 42–6 also applies to Procedure 42–5.

Procedure 42–5 Transferring between Bed and Chair

Purposes

- A client may need to be transferred between the bed and a wheelchair or chair, the bed and the commode, or a wheelchair and the toilet. There are numerous variations in the technique.

Which variation the nurse selects depends on factors related to the client, the environment, and the health care provider that are assessed prior to beginning the transfer.

ASSESSMENT

Before transferring a client, assess the following:
- The client's body size
- Ability to follow instructions
- Activity tolerance
- Muscle strength
- Joint mobility
- Presence of paralysis
- Level of comfort

- Presence of orthostatic hypotension
- The technique with which the client is familiar
- The space in which the transfer will need to be maneuvered (bathrooms, for example, are usually cramped)
- The number of assistants (one or two) needed to accomplish the transfer safely
- The skill and strength of the nurse(s).

continued on page 1092

Procedure 42–5   Transferring between Bed and Chair *continued*

PLANNING

Review the client record to determine if previous nurses have recorded information about the client's ability to transfer. Implement pain-relief measures so that they are effective when the transfer begins.

Delegation

The skill of transferring a client can be delegated to UAP who have demonstrated good body mechanics and safe transfer technique for the involved client. It is important for the nurse to assess the client's capabilities and communicate specific information about what the UAP should report back to the nurse.

Equipment
- Robe or appropriate clothing
- Slippers or shoes with nonskid soles
- Transfer (walking) belt
- Chair, commode, wheelchair, or stretcher as appropriate to client need
- Sliding board

IMPLEMENTATION

Preparation
- Plan what to do and how to do it.
- Obtain essential equipment before starting (e.g., transfer belt, wheelchair), and check that it is functioning correctly.
- Remove obstacles from the area used for the transfer.

Performance
1. Explain the transfer process to the client. During the transfer, explain step by step what the client should do, for example, "Move your right foot forward."
2. Wash hands and observe other appropriate infection control procedures.
3. Provide for client privacy.
4. Position the equipment appropriately.
   - Lower the bed to its lowest position so that the client's feet will rest flat on the floor. Lock the wheels of the bed.
   - Place the wheelchair parallel to the bed as close to the bed as possible (Figure 42–57 ■). Put the wheelchair

on the side of the bed that allows the client to move toward his or her stronger side. Lock the wheels of the wheelchair and raise the footplate.
5. Prepare and assess the client.
   - Assist the client to a sitting position on the side of the bed (see Procedure 42–4).
   - Assess the client for orthostatic hypotension before moving the client from the bed.
   - Assist the client in putting on a bathrobe and nonskid slippers or shoes.
   - Place a transfer belt snugly around the client's waist. Check to be certain that the belt is securely fastened.
6. Give explicit instructions to the client. Ask the client to:
   - Move forward and sit on the edge of the bed. *This brings the client's center of gravity closer to the nurse's.*
   - Lean forward slightly from the hips. *This brings the client's center of gravity more directly over the base of support and positions the head and trunk in the direction of the movement.*
   - Place the foot of the stronger leg beneath the edge of the bed and put the other foot forward. *In this way, the client can use the stronger leg muscles to stand and power the movement. A broader base of support makes the client more stable during the transfer.*
   - Place the client's hands on the bed surface or on your shoulders so that the client can push while standing. *This provides additional force for the movement and reduces the potential for strain on the nurse's back.* The client should not grasp your neck for support. *Doing so can injure the nurse.*

7. Position yourself correctly.
   - Stand directly in front of the client. Lean the trunk forward from the hips. Flex the hips, knees, and ankles. Assume a broad stance, placing one foot forward and one back. Mirror the placement of the client's feet, if possible. *This helps prevent loss of balance during the transfer.*
   - Encircle the client's waist with your arms, and grasp the transfer belt at the client's back (Figure 42–58 ■) with thumbs pointing downward. *The belt provides a secure handle for holding on to the client and controlling the movement. Downward placement of the thumbs prevents potential wrist injury as the nurse lifts. By*

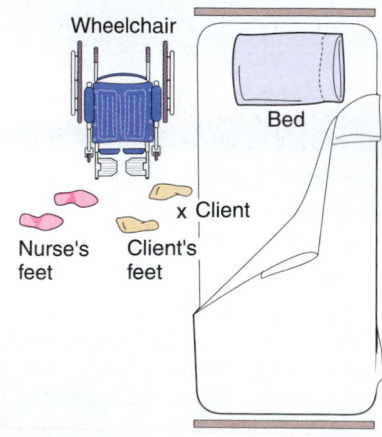

Figure 42–57 ■ The wheelchair is placed parallel to the bed as close to the bed as possible. Note that placement of the nurse's feet mirrors that of the client's feet.

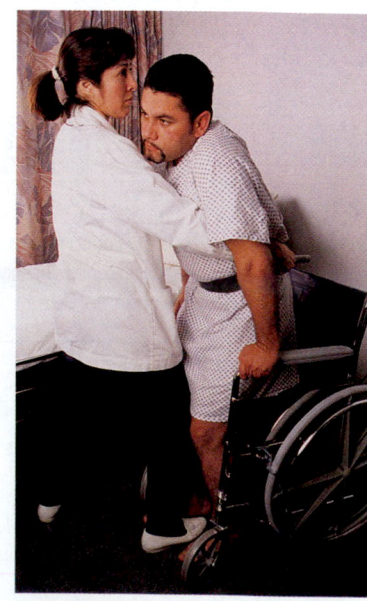

Figure 42–58 ■ Using a transfer (walking) belt.

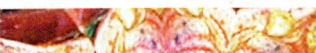

Procedure 42–5 Transferring between Bed and Chair *continued*

IMPLEMENTATION *continued*

supporting the client in this manner, you keep the client from tilting backward during the transfer.
- Tighten your gluteal, abdominal, leg, and arm muscles.

8. Assist the client to stand, and then move together toward the wheelchair.
- On the count of three, ask the client to push with the back foot, rock to the forward foot, and extend (straighten) the joints of the lower extremities. Push or pull up with the hands, while pushing with the forward foot, rock to the back foot, extend the joints of the lower extremities, and pull the client (directly toward your center of gravity) into a standing position.
- Support the client in an upright standing position for a few moments. *This allows the nurse and the client to extend the joints and provides the nurse with an opportunity to ensure that the client is stable before moving away from the bed.*
- Together, pivot or take a few steps toward the wheelchair.

9. Assist the client to sit.
- Ask the client to:
  a. Back up to the wheelchair and place the legs against the seat. *Having the client place the legs against the wheelchair seat minimizes the risk of the client falling when sitting down.*
  b. Place the foot of the stronger leg slightly behind the other. *This supports body weight during the movement.*
  c. Keep the other foot forward. *This provides a broad base of support.*
  d. Place both hands on the wheelchair arms or on your shoulders. *This increases stability and lessens the strain on the nurse.*
- Stand directly in front of the client. Place one foot forward and one back.
- Tighten your grasp on the transfer belt, and tighten your gluteal, abdominal, leg, and arm muscles.
- On the count of three, have the client shift the body weight by rocking to the back foot, lower the body onto the edge of the wheelchair seat by flexing the joints of the legs and arms. Place some body weight

on the arms, while shifting your body weight by stepping back with the forward foot and pivoting toward the chair while lowering the client onto the wheelchair seat.

10. Ensure client safety.
- Ask the client to push back into the wheelchair seat. *Sitting well back on the seat provides a broader base of support and greater stability and minimizes the risk of falling from the wheelchair. A wheelchair can topple forward when the client sits on the edge of the seat and leans far forward.*
- Lower the footplates, and place the client's feet on them.
- Apply a seat belt as required.

VARIATION: ANGLING THE WHEELCHAIR
For clients who have difficulty walking, place the wheelchair at a 45-degree angle to the bed. *This enables the client to pivot into the chair and lessens the amount of body rotation required.*

VARIATION: TRANSFERRING WITHOUT A BELT
- For clients who need minimal assistance, place the hands against the sides of the client's chest (not at the axillae) during the transfer (Figure 42–59 ■). For clients who require more assistance, reach through the client's axillae and place the hands on the client's scapulae during the transfer. Avoid placing hands or pressure on the axillae, especially for clients who have upper extremity paralysis or paresis.

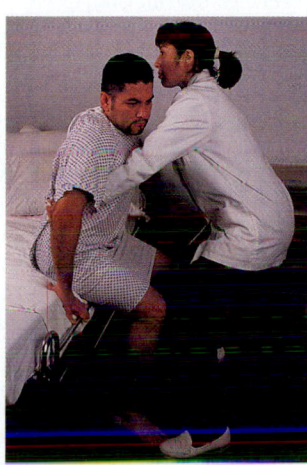
Figure 42–59 ■ Transferring without a belt.

- Follow the steps described previously.

VARIATION: TRANSFERRING WITH A BELT AND TWO NURSES
- When the client is able to stand, position yourselves on both sides of the client, facing the same direction as the client. Flex your hips, knees, and ankle. Grasp the client's transfer belt with the hand closest to the client and with the other hand support the client's elbows.
- Coordinating your efforts, all three of you stand simultaneously, pivot, and move to the wheelchair. Reverse the process to lower the client onto the wheelchair seat.

VARIATION: TRANSFERRING A CLIENT WITH AN INJURED LOWER EXTREMITY
When the client has an injured lower extremity, movement should always occur toward the client's unaffected (strong) side. For example, if the client's right leg is injured and the client is sitting on the edge of the bed preparing to transfer to a wheelchair, position the wheelchair on the client's left side. In this way, the client can use the unaffected leg most effectively and safely.

VARIATION: USING A SLIDING BOARD
- For clients who cannot stand, use a sliding board to help them move without nursing assistance. This method not only promotes clients' sense of independence but also preserves your energy (Figure 42–60 ■).

11. Document relevant information:
- Client's ability to bear weight and pivot
- Number of staff needed for transfer
- Length of time up in chair
- Client response to transfer and being up in chair or wheelchair.

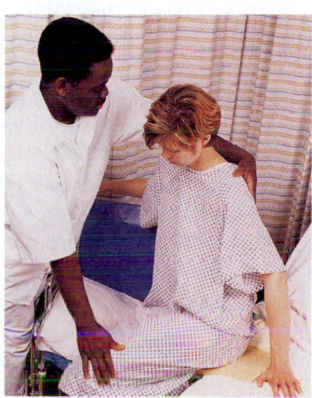
Figure 42–60 ■ Using a sliding board.

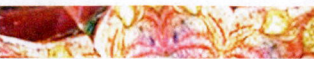

Procedure 42–6 Transferring between Bed and Stretcher

Purposes

- The stretcher, or gurney, is used to transfer supine clients from one location to another. Whenever the client is capable of accomplishing the transfer from bed to stretcher independently, either by lifting onto it or by rolling onto it, the client should be encouraged to do so. If the client cannot move onto the stretcher independently, at least two nurses are needed to assist with the transfer; more are needed if the client is totally helpless or is heavy.

ASSESSMENT

Before transferring a client, assess the following:
- The client's body size
- Ability to follow instructions
- Activity tolerance
- Level of comfort
- The space in which the transfer is maneuvered
- The number of assistants (one or two others) needed to accomplish the transfer safely
- The skill and strength of the nurses

PLANNING

Review the client record to determine if previous nurses have recorded information about how the client tolerated similar transfers. If indicated, implement pain-relief measures so that they are effective when the transfer begins.

Delegation

The skill of transferring a client can be delegated to UAPs who have demonstrated good body mechanics and safe transfer technique for the involved client. It is important for the nurse to assess the client's capabilities and communicate specific information about what the UAPs should report to the nurse.

Equipment
- Stretcher
- Optional: sliding board

IMPLEMENTATION

Preparation

Obtain the necessary equipment and nursing personnel to assist in the transfer.

Performance

1. Explain to the client what you are going to do, why it is necessary, and how he or she can cooperate. Explain the transfer to the nursing personnel who are helping and specify who will give directions (one person needs to be in charge).
2. Wash hands and observe other appropriate infection control procedures.
3. Provide for client privacy.
4. Adjust the client's bed in preparation for the transfer.
   - Lower the head of the bed until it is flat or as low as the client can tolerate.
   - Raise the bed so that it is slightly higher than the surface of the stretcher. *It is easier for the client to move down a slant.*
   - Ensure that the wheels on the bed are locked.
   - Pull the drawsheet out from both sides of the bed.
5. Move the client to the edge of the bed and position the stretcher.
   - Roll the drawsheet as close to the client's side as possible.
   - Pull the client to the edge of the bed and cover the client with a sheet or bath blanket to maintain comfort.
   - Place the stretcher parallel to the bed next to the client and lock the stretcher wheels.
   - Fill the gap that exists between the bed and the stretcher loosely with the bath blankets (optional).
6. Transfer the client securely to the stretcher.
   - In unison with the other staff members, press your body tightly against the stretcher. *This prevents the stretcher from moving.*
   - Roll the pull sheet tightly against the client. *This achieves better control over client movement.*
   - Flex your hips and pull the client on the pull sheet in unison directly toward you and onto the stretcher. *Pulling downward requires less force than pulling along a flat surface.*
   - Ask the client to flex the neck during the move, if possible, and place the arms across the chest. *This prevents injury to these body parts.*
7. Ensure client comfort and safety.
   - Make the client comfortable, unlock the stretcher wheels, and move the stretcher away from the bed.
   - Immediately raise the stretcher side rails and/or fasten the safety straps across the client. *Because the stretcher is high and narrow, the client is in danger of falling unless these safety precautions are taken.*

VARIATION: USING A TRANSFER BOARD

The transfer board is a lacquered or smooth polyethylene board measuring 45 to 55 cm (18 to 22 in.) by 182 cm (72 in.) with handholds along its edges. This device may be used by one nurse alone or up to four nurses together. Turn the client to a lateral position away from you, position the board close to the client's back, and roll the client onto the board. Pull the client and board across the bed to the stretcher. Safety belts may be placed over the chest, abdomen, and legs.

VARIATION: USING A THREE-PERSON CARRY (USE CAUTION)

- Three people of about equal height stand side by side facing the client. Recommendations vary as to which staff member lifts a specific area of the client. Often, the strongest person supports the heaviest part of the client or the tallest person with the longest reach supports the head and shoulders. The stretcher or bed to which the client will be moved is placed at a right angle at the foot of the bed. The wheels of the

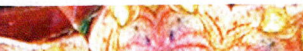

Procedure 42–6 Transferring between Bed and Stretcher *continued*

IMPLEMENTATION *continued*

bed and stretcher are locked. Each person flexes the knees and places the foot nearest to the stretcher slightly forward.

■ The arms of the lifters are put under the client at the head and shoulders, hips and thighs, and upper and lower legs. On the count of 3, the lifters roll the client onto their chests and step back in unison (Figure 42–61 ■). They then pivot around to the stretcher and lower the client by flexing their knees and hips until their elbows are on the surface of the stretcher. The client is then released on the stretcher surface and is aligned and covered and the stretcher side rails are raised.

8. Document relevant information:
   • Equipment used

   • Number of people needed for transfer

   • Destination if reason for transfer is transport from one location to another.

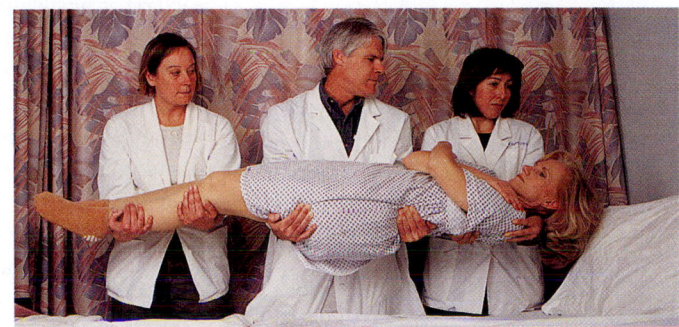

Figure 42–61 ■ The three-person carry.

EVALUATION

■ Compare client capabilities such as weight-bearing, pivoting ability, and strength and control to previous transfers.

■ Report any significant deviations from normal to the physician.

■ Note use of appropriate safety measures (e.g., transfer belt, locking wheels of bed and wheelchair) by UAP during transfer process.

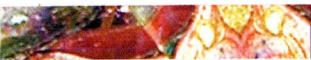

Lifespan Considerations

Transferring Clients
Infants

■ The infant who is lying down, on the side or supine, can be placed in either a bassinet or crib for transport. If the bassinet has a bottom shelf, it can be used for carrying the IV pump or monitor.

Children

■ The toddler should be transported in a high-top crib with the side rails up and the protective top in place. Stretchers should not be used because the mobile toddler may roll or fall off.

Elders

■ Use special caution with older clients to prevent skin tears or bruising during a transfer or when using a hydraulic lift.

■ Since conditions of elders can change from day to day, always assess the situation to ensure that you have the right equipment and enough people to assist when transferring a client.

■ Write the method used to transfer each client—equipment used, best position, number of people needed to assist in transfer—this can be part of the care plan and also be available in the client's room as a guide to all personnel caring for the client.

■ Avoid sudden position changes. They can cause orthostatic hypotension and increase the risk of fainting and falls.

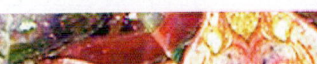

Home Care Considerations

Transferring from Bed to a Chair

■ The caregiver and client should practice transfer technique(s) in the hospital or long-term care setting before being discharged.

■ Assess furniture in the home. Does the client's favorite chair have arms for ease of using and sitting? Examine the fabric—is

it rough? Will it cause skin abrasions? If the client will be using a wheelchair, is there enough space in the bedroom and bathroom for a safe transfer?

Using a Hydraulic Lift

Hydraulic lifts, such as the Hoyer lift, are used primarily for clients who cannot help themselves or who are too heavy for others to lift safely. The lift can be used in transferring the client between the bed and a wheelchair, the bed and the bathtub, and the bed and a stretcher. The Hoyer lift consists of a base on casters, a hydraulic mechanical pump, a mast boom, and a sling (Figure 42–62 ■). The sling may consist of a one-piece or two-piece canvas seat. The one-piece seat stretches from the client's head to the knees. The two-piece seat has one canvas strap to support the client's buttocks and thighs and a second strap extending up to the axillae to support the back. It is important to be familiar with the model used and the practices that accompany use. Before using the lift, the nurse ensures that it is in working order and that the hooks, chains, straps, and canvas seat are in good repair. Most agencies recommend that two nurses operate a lift. Check agency policy.

Providing ROM Exercises

When people are ill, they may need to perform ROM exercises until they can regain their normal activity levels. **Active ROM exercises** are isotonic exercises in which the client moves each joint in the body through its complete range of movement, maximally stretching all muscle groups within each plane over the joint. These exercises maintain or increase muscle strength and endurance and help to maintain cardiorespiratory function in an immobilized client. They also prevent deterioration of joint capsules, ankylosis, and contractures.

Full ROM does not occur spontaneously in the immobilized individual who independently achieves ADLs, moves about in bed, transfers between bed and wheelchair or chair, or ambulates a short distance, because only a few muscle groups are maximally stretched during these activities. Although the client may successfully achieve some active ROM movements of the upper extremities while combing the hair, bathing, and dressing, the immobilized client is very unlikely to achieve any active ROM movements of the lower extremities when these are not used in the normal functions of standing and walking about. For this reason, most wheelchair and many ambulatory clients need active ROM exercises until they regain their normal activity levels.

At first, the nurse may need to teach the client to perform the needed ROM exercises; eventually, the client may be able to accomplish these independently. Instructions for the client performing active ROM exercises are shown in the accompanying Teaching: Client Care feature.

During **passive ROM exercises,** another person moves each of the client's joints through its complete range of movement, maximally stretching all muscle groups within each plane over each joint. Because the client does not contract the muscles, passive ROM exercises are of no value in maintaining muscle strength but are useful in maintaining joint flexibility. For this reason, passive ROM exercises should be performed only when the client is unable to accomplish the movements actively.

Passive ROM exercises should be accomplished for each movement of the arms, legs, and neck that the client is unable to achieve actively. As with active ROM exercises, passive ROM exercises should be accomplished to the point of slight resistance, but not beyond, and never to the point of discomfort. The movements should be systematic, and the same sequence should be followed during each exercise session. Each exercise should consist of three repetitions, and the series of exercises should be done twice daily. Performing one series of exercises along with the bath is helpful. Passive ROM exercises are accomplished most effectively when the client lies supine in bed. General guidelines for providing passive exercises are shown in the accompanying Practice Guidelines.

During active-assistive ROM exercises, the client uses a stronger, opposite arm or leg to move each of the joints of a limb incapable of active motion. The client learns to support and move the weak arm or leg with the strong arm or leg as far as

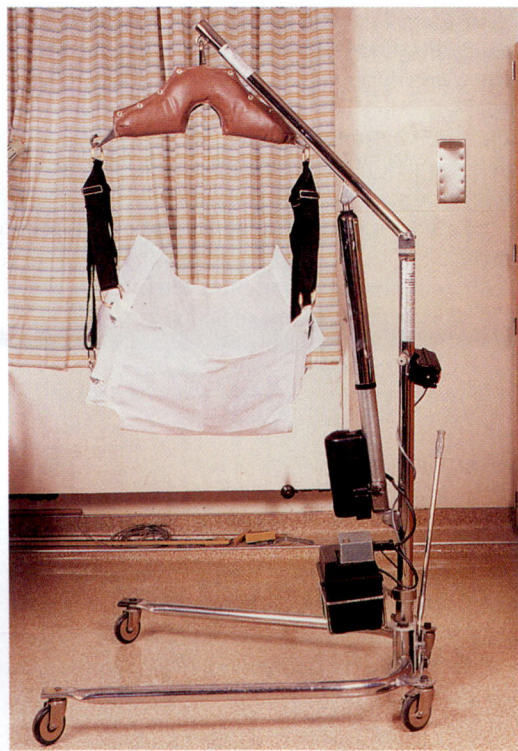

Figure 42–62 ■ A one-piece seat hydraulic lift.

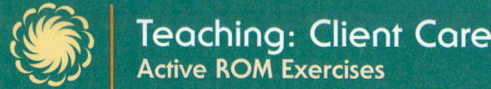

Teaching: Client Care
Active ROM Exercises

- Perform each ROM exercise as taught to the point of slight resistance, but not beyond, and never to the point of discomfort.
- Perform the movements systematically, using the same sequence during each session.
- Perform each exercise three times.
- Perform each series of exercises twice daily.

Elders

- For elders, it is not essential to achieve full range of motion in all joints. Instead, emphasize achieving a sufficient range of motion to carry out ADLs, such as walking, dressing, combing hair, showering, and preparing a meal.

Practice Guidelines
Providing Passive ROM Exercises

- Ensure that the client understands the reason for doing ROM exercises.
- If there is a possibility of hand swelling, make sure rings are removed.
- Clothe the client in a loose gown, and cover the body with a bath blanket.
- Use correct body mechanics when providing ROM exercise to avoid muscle strain or injury to both yourself and the client.
- Position the bed at an appropriate height.
- Expose only the limb being exercised to avoid embarrassing the client.
- Support the client's limbs above and below the joint as needed to prevent muscle strain or injury (Figure 42–63 ■). This may also be done by cupping joints in the palm of your hand or cradling limbs along your forearm (Figure 42–64 ■). If a joint is painful (e.g., arthritic), support the limb in the muscular areas above and below the joint.
- Use a firm, comfortable grip when handling the limb.
- Move the body parts smoothly, slowly, and rhythmically. Jerky movements cause discomfort and, possibly, injury. Fast movements can cause spasticity (sudden, prolonged involuntary muscle contraction) or rigidity (stiffness or inflexibility).
- Avoid moving or forcing a body part beyond the existing range of motion. Muscle strain, pain, and injury can result. This is particularly important for people with flaccid (limp) paralysis, whose muscles can be stretched and joints dislocated without their awareness.
- If muscle spasticity occurs during movement, stop the movement temporarily, but continue to apply slow, gentle pressure on the part until the muscle relaxes; then proceed with the motion.

- If a contracture is present, apply slow firm pressure, without causing pain, to stretch the muscle fibers.
- If rigidity occurs, apply pressure against the rigidity, and continue the exercise slowly.
- Teach client's caregiver the purposes and technique of performing passive ROM at home if appropriate.
- Avoid hypertension of joints in elders if joints are arthritic.
- Use the exercises as an opportunity to also assess skin condition.

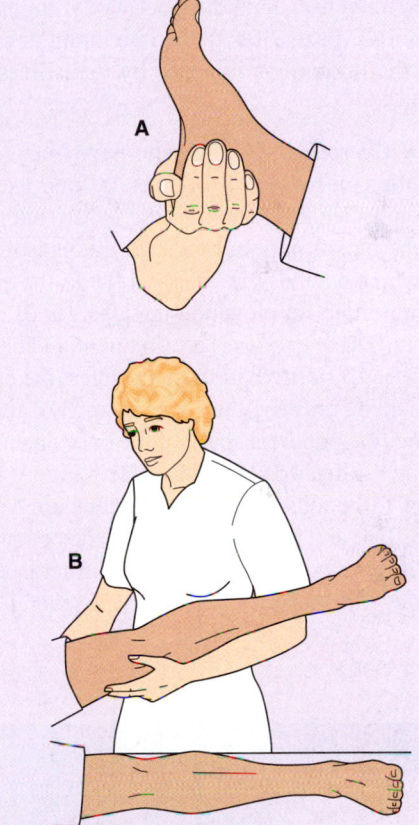

Figure 42–64 ■ Holding limbs for support during passive exercise: *A*, cupping; *B*, cradling.

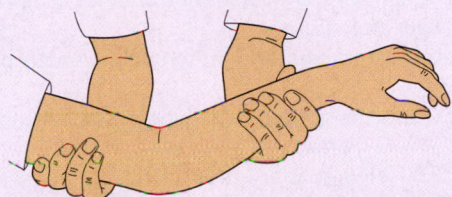

Figure 42–63 ■ Supporting a limb above and below the joint for passive exercise.

possible. Then the nurse continues the movement passively to its maximal degree. This activity increases active movement on the strong side of the client's body and maintains joint flexibility on the weak side. Such exercise is especially useful for stroke victims who are hemiplegic (paralyzed on one-half of the body).

Functional joint flexibility is also maintained in the performance of ADLs. The following are examples:

- Eating, shaving, grooming, and bathing exercise the elbow (flexion and extension) and shoulder (abduction).
- Activities requiring fine motor skills, such as writing and eating, exercise the fingers (flexion, extension, adduction, abduction) and the thumb (opposition).

- Walking exercises the shoulders (flexion, extension), hip (flexion, extension, hyperextension), knee (flexion, extension), and ankle (plantar flexion and dorsiflexion).
- Reaching for articles exercises the shoulders (flexion, extension, and perhaps slight abduction or adduction).
- Dressing involves many joint movements.

> **➤ CLINICAL ALERT**   *Clients who require passive ROM exercises after a disability should have a goal of progressing to active-assistive ROM exercises and, finally, to active ROM exercises.* ■

Ambulating Clients

Ambulation (the act of walking) is a function that most people take for granted. However, when people are ill they are often confined to bed and are thus nonambulatory. The longer clients are in bed, the more difficulty they have walking.

Even 1 or 2 days of bed rest can make a person feel weak, unsteady, and shaky when first getting out of bed. A client who has had surgery, is elderly, or has been immobilized for a longer time will feel more pronounced weakness. The potential problems of immobility are far less likely to occur when clients become ambulatory as soon as possible. The nurse can assist clients to prepare for ambulation by helping them become as independent as possible while in bed. Nurses should encourage clients to perform ADLs, maintain good body alignment, and carry out active ROM exercises to the maximum degree possible yet within the limitations imposed by their illness and recovery program.

Preambulatory Exercises. Clients who have been in bed for long periods often need a plan of muscle tone exercises to strengthen the muscles used for walking before attempting to walk. One of the most important muscle groups is the quadriceps femoris, which extends the knee and flexes the thigh. This group is also important for elevating the legs, for example, for walking upstairs. These exercises are frequently called quadriceps drills or sets. To strengthen these muscles, the client consciously tenses them, drawing the kneecap upward and inward. The client pushes the popliteal space of the knee against the bed surface, relaxing the heels on the bed surface (Figure 42–65 ■). On the count of 1, the muscles are tensed; they are held during the counts of 2, 3, 4; and they are relaxed at the count of 5. The exercise should be done within the client's tolerance, that is, without fatiguing the muscles. Carried out several times an hour during waking hours, this simple exercise significantly strengthens the muscles used for walking.

Assisting Clients to Ambulate. Clients who have been immobilized for even a few days may require assistance with ambulation. The amount of assistance will depend on the client's condition, including age, health status, and length of inactivity. Assistance may mean walking alongside the client while providing physical support (see Procedure 42–7) or providing instruction to the client about the use of assistive devices such as a cane, walker, or crutches.

Some clients experience postural (orthostatic) hypotension on assuming a vertical position from a lying position and may need information about ways to control this problem (see Teaching: Client Care). The client may exhibit some or all of the following symptoms: pallor, diaphoresis, nausea, tachycardia, and dizziness. If any of these are present, the client should be assisted to a supine position in bed and closely assessed.

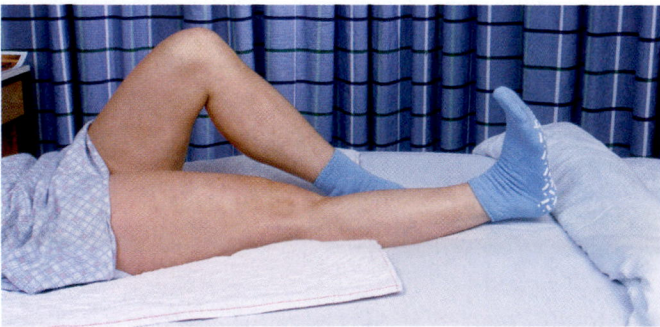

Figure 42–65 ■ Tensing the quadriceps femoris muscles before ambulation.

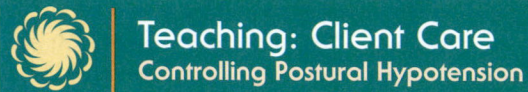

Teaching: Client Care
Controlling Postural Hypotension

- Rest with the head of the bed elevated 8 to 12 inches. This position makes the position change on rising less severe.
- Avoid sudden changes in position. Arise from bed in three stages:
  a. Sit up in bed for 1 minute.
  b. Sit on the side of the bed with legs dangling for 1 minute.
  c. Stand with care, holding onto the edge of the bed or another nonmovable object for 1 minute.
- Never bend down all the way to the floor or stand up too quickly after stooping.
- Postpone activities such as shaving and hair grooming for at least 1 hour after rising.
- Wear elastic stockings at night to inhibit venous pooling in the legs.
- Be aware that the symptoms of hypotension are most severe at the following times:
  a. 30 to 60 minutes after a heavy meal
  b. 1 to 2 hours after taking an antihypertension medication.
- Get out of a hot bath very slowly, because high temperatures can lead to venous pooling.
- Use a rocking chair to improve circulation in the lower extremities. Even mild leg conditioning can strengthen muscle tone and enhance circulation.
- Refrain from any strenuous activity that results in holding the breath and bearing down. This Valsalva maneuver slows the heart rate, leading to subsequent lowering of blood pressure.

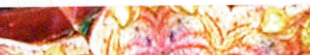

Procedure 42–7 Assisting the Client to Ambulate

Purposes

- To provide a safe condition for the client to walk with whatever support is needed.

ASSESSMENT

Assess

- Length of time in bed and time up previously
- Baseline vital signs
- Range of motion of joints needed for ambulating (e.g., hips, knees, ankles)
- Muscle strength of lower extremities
- Need for ambulation aids (e.g., cane, walker, crutches)
- Client's intake of medications (e.g., narcotics, sedatives, tranquilizers, and antihistamines) that may cause drowsiness, dizziness,

weakness, and orthostatic hypotension and seriously hinder the client's ability to walk safely
- Presence of joint inflammation, fractures, muscle weakness, or other conditions that impair physical mobility
- Ability to understand directions
- Level of comfort

PLANNING

Implement pain-relief measures so that they are effective when the transfer begins.

The amount of assistance needed while ambulating will depend on the client's condition, for example, age, health status, length of inactivity, and emotional readiness. Review any previous experiences with ambulation and the success of such efforts. Plan the length of the walk with the client, in light of the nursing or physician's orders. Be prepared to shorten the walk according to the person's activity tolerance.

Delegation

Ambulation of clients is frequently delegated to UAP. However, the nurse should conduct an initial assessment of the client's abilities in order to direct other personnel in providing appropriate assistance. Any unusual events that arise from assisting the client in ambulation must be validated and interpreted by the nurse.

Equipment

- Transfer belt if the client is known to be unsteady
- Wheelchair for following client or chairs along the route if the client needs to rest

---

IMPLEMENTATION

Preparation

Be certain that others are available to assist you if needed. Also, plan the route of ambulation that has the fewest hazards.

Performance

1. Explain to the client how you are going to assist, why ambulation is necessary, and how he or she can cooperate. Discuss how this activity relates to the overall plan of care.
2. Wash hands and observe appropriate infection control procedures.
3. Ensure that the client is appropriately dressed to walk and has shoes or slippers with nonskid soles.
4. Prepare the client for ambulation.
   - Apply elastic (antiemboli) stockings as required.
   - Assist the client to sit on the edge of the bed.
   - Assess the client carefully for signs and symptoms of orthostatic hypotension (dizziness, lightheadedness, or a sudden increase in heart rate) prior to leaving the bedside.

- Assist the client to stand by the side of the bed until he or she feels secure.
5. Ensure client safety while assisting the client to ambulate.
   - Encourage the client to ambulate independently if he or she is able, but walk beside the client.
   - Remain physically close to the client in case assistance is needed at any point.
   - Use a transfer or walking belt if the client is slightly weak and unstable. Make sure the belt is pulled snugly around the client's waist and fastened securely. Grasp the belt at the client's back, and walk behind and slightly to one side of the client (Figure 42–66 ■).
   - If it is the client's first time out of bed following surgery, injury, or an extended period of immobility, or if the client is quite weak or unstable, have an assistant follow you and the client with a wheelchair in the event that it is needed quickly.

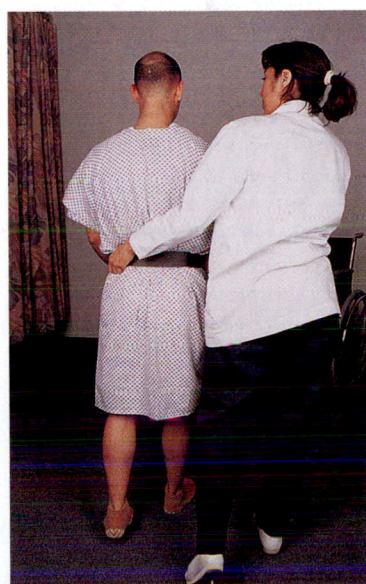

Figure 42–66 ■ Using a transfer (walking) belt to support the client.

continued on page 1100

IMPLEMENTATION *continued*

- If the client is moderately weak and unstable, walk on the client's weaker side and interlock your forearm with the client's closest forearm. Encourage the client to press the forearm against your hip or waist for stability if desired. In addition, have the client wear a transfer or walking belt *so that you can quickly grab the belt and prevent a fall if the client feels faint.*
- If the client is very weak and unstable, place your near arm around the client's waist, and with your other arm support the client's near arm at the elbow. Walk on the client's stronger side. Again, have the client wear a transfer or walking belt in case of an emergency. Encourage the client to assume a normal walking stance and gait as much as possible.

6. Protect the client who begins to fall while ambulating.
   - If a client begins to experience the signs and symptoms of orthostatic hypotension or extreme weakness, quickly assist the client into a nearby wheelchair or other chair, and help the client to lower the head between the knees.
   - Stay with the client. *A client who faints while in this position could fall head first out of the chair.*
   - When the weakness subsides, assist the client back to bed.
   - If a chair is not close by, assist the client to a horizontal position on the floor before fainting occurs (Figure 42–67 ■).
     a. Assume a broad stance with one foot in front of the other. *A broad stance widens your base of support. Placing one foot behind the other allows you to rock backward and use the femoral muscles when supporting the client's weight and lowering the center of gravity (see the next step), thus preventing back strain.*
     b. Bring the client backward so that your body supports the person. *Clients who faint or start to fall usually pitch slightly forward because of the momentum of ambulating. Bringing the client's weight backward against your body al-*

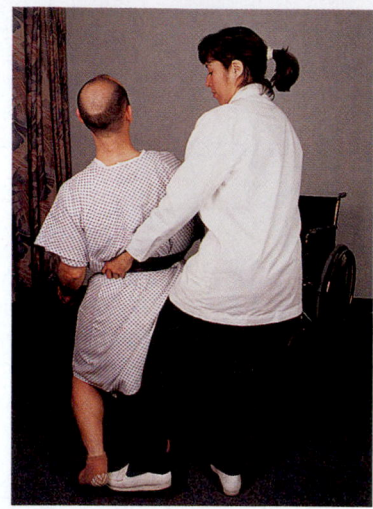

Figure 42–67 ■ Lowering a fainting client to the floor.

lows gradual movement to the floor without injury to the client.
     c. Allow the client to slide down your leg, and lower the person gently to the floor, making sure the client's head does not hit any objects.

VARIATION: TWO NURSES
- After the client stands, assume a position with one nurse at either side. Grasp the inferior aspect of the client's upper arm with your nearest hand and the client's lower arm or hand with your other hand (Figure 42–68 ■). *This provides a secure grip for each nurse.*

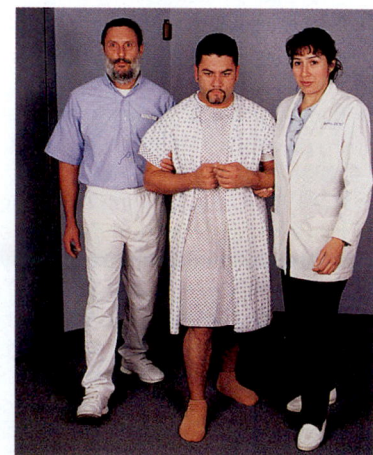

Figure 42–68 ■ Two nurses supporting an ambulatory client.

- *Optional:* Place a walking belt around the client's waist. Each nurse grasps the side handle with the near hand and the lower aspect of the client's upper arm with the other hand.
- Walk in unison with the client, using a smooth, even gait, at the same speed and with steps the same size as the client's. *This gives the client a greater feeling of security.*
- If the client starts to fall and cannot regain strength or balance, slip your arms under the client's axillae, grasp the client's hands, and lower the person gently to the floor or to a nearby chair (Figure 42–69 ■). *Placing the nurse's arms under the client's axillae evenly balances the client's weight between the two nurses, preventing injury to both the nurses and the client.*

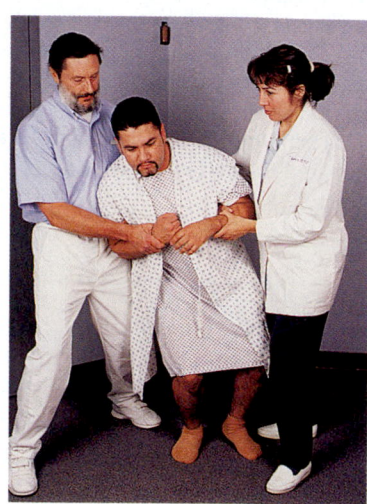

Figure 42–69 ■ Two nurses lowering a fainting client to the floor.

7. Document distance and duration of ambulation in the client record using forms or checklists supplemented by narrative notes when appropriate. Include description of the client's gait (including body alignment) when walking; pace; activity tolerance when walking (e.g., pulse rate, facial color, any shortness of breath, feelings of dizziness, or weakness); degree of support required; and respiratory rate and blood pressure after initial ambulation to compare with baseline data.

EVALUATION

- Establish a plan for continued ambulation based on expected or normal ability for the client.

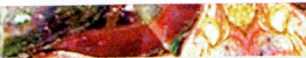

Lifespan Considerations

Assisting the Client to Ambulate
Elders
- Inquire how the client has ambulated previously and modify assistance accordingly.
- Take into account a decrease in speed, strength, resistance to fatigue, reaction time, and coordination due to a decrease in nerve conduction.
- Be cautious when using a transfer belt with a client with osteoporosis. Too much pressure from the belt can increase the risk of vertebral compression fractures.
- If assistive devices, such as a walker or cane are used, make sure clients are supervised in the beginning to learn the proper method of using them. Crutches may be much more difficult for elders due to decreased upper body strength.

- Be alert to signs of activity intolerance, especially in elders with cardiac and lung problems.
- Set small goals and increase slowly to build endurance, strength, and flexibility.
- Be aware of any fall risks the elder may have, such as
  - Effects of medications
  - Neurological disorders
  - Environmental hazards
  - Orthostatic hypotension.
- In elders, the body's responses return to normal more slowly. For instance, an increase in heart rate from exercise may stay elevated for hours before returning to normal.

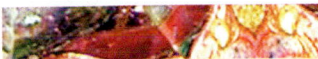

Home Care Considerations

Assisting the Client to Ambulate
- When making a home visit, assess carefully for safety issues for ambulation. Counsel the client and family about unfastened rugs, slippery floors, and loose objects on the floors.

- Check the surroundings for adequate supports such as railings and grab bars.
- Recommend that nonskid strips be placed on outside steps and inside stairs that are not carpeted.

Using Mechanical Aids for Walking

Mechanical aids for ambulation include canes, walkers, and crutches.

Canes. Two types of canes are used today: the standard straight-legged cane and the quad cane, which has four feet and provides the most support (Figure 42–70 ■). Cane tips should have rubber caps to improve traction and prevent slipping. The standard cane is 91 cm (36 in.) long; some aluminum canes can be adjusted from 56 to 97 cm (22 to 38 in.). The length should permit the elbow to be slightly flexed. Clients may use either one or two canes, depending on how much support they require.

Walkers. Walkers are mechanical devices for ambulatory clients who need more support than a cane provides. Walkers come in many different shapes and sizes, with devices suited to individual needs. The standard type is made of polished aluminum. It has four legs with rubber tips and plastic hand grips (Figure 42–73 ■). Many walkers have adjustable legs.

The standard walker needs to be picked up to be used. The client therefore requires partial strength in both hands and wrists, strong elbow extensors, and strong shoulder depressors. The client also needs the ability to bear at least partial weight on both legs.

Four-wheeled and two-wheeled models of walkers (roller walkers) do not need to be picked up to be moved, but they are less stable than the standard walker is. They are used by clients who are too weak or unstable to pick up and move the walker with each step. Some roller walkers have a seat at the back so the client can sit down to rest when desired. An adaptation of the standard and four-wheeled walker is one that has two tips and two wheels. This type provides more stability than the four-wheeled model yet still permits the client to keep the walker in contact with the ground all the time. The client tilts the walker toward the body, lifting the tips while the wheels remain on the ground, and then pushes the walker forward.

The nurse may need to adjust the height of a client's walker so that the hand bar is just below the client's waist and the client's elbows are slightly flexed. This position helps the client assume a more normal stance. A walker that is too low causes

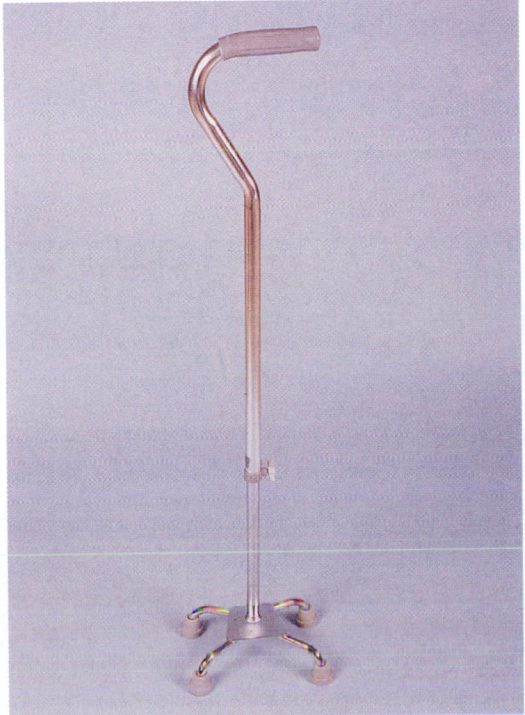

Figure 42–70 ■ A quad cane.

Teaching: Client Care
Using Canes

- Hold the cane with the hand on the stronger side of the body to provide maximum support and appropriate body alignment when walking.
- Position the tip of a standard cane (and the nearest tip of other canes) about 15 cm (6 in.) to the side and 15 cm (6 in.) in front of the near foot, so that the elbow is slightly flexed.

When Maximum Support Is Required

- Move the cane forward about 30 cm (1 ft), or a distance that is comfortable while the body weight is borne by both legs (Figure 42–71 ■, A).
- Then move the affected (weak) leg forward to the cane while the weight is borne by the cane and stronger leg (Figure 42–71 ■, B).

- Next, move the unaffected (stronger) leg forward ahead of the cane and weak leg while the weight is borne by the cane and weak leg.
- Repeat the steps. This pattern of moving provides at least two points of support on the floor at all times.

As You Become Stronger and Require Less Support

- Move the cane and weak leg forward at the same time, while the weight is borne by the stronger leg (Figure 42–72 ■, A).
- Move the stronger leg forward, while the weight is borne by the cane and the weak leg (Figure 42–72 ■, B).

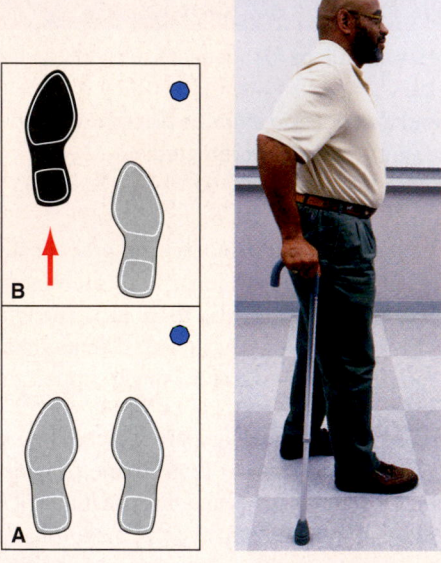

Figure 42–71 ■ Steps involved in using a cane to provide maximum support.

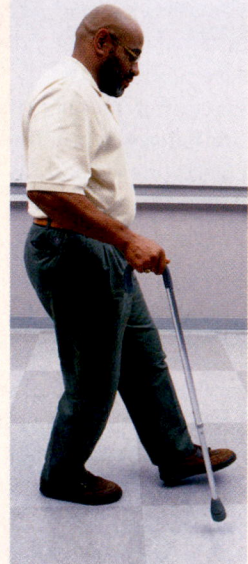

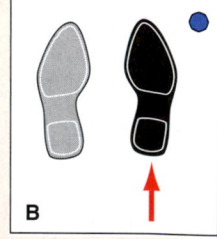

Figure 42–72 ■ Steps involved in using a cane when less than maximum support is required.

the client to stoop; one that is too high makes the client stretch and reach.

Crutches. Crutches may be a temporary need for some people and a permanent one for others. Sometimes clients are discouraged when they attempt crutch walking. Clients confined to bed are often unaware of weakness that becomes apparent when they try to stand or walk. Clients realize that they can no longer take balance for granted when they must cope with the weight of a heavy cast or a paralyzed limb. Frequently, progress may be slower than the client anticipated. Encouragement from the nurse and the setting of realistic goals are especially important.

There are several kinds of crutches. The most frequently used are the underarm crutch, or axillary crutch with hand bars, and the Lofstrand crutch, which extends only to the forearm (Figure 42–74 ■). On the Lofstrand crutch, the metal cuff around the forearm and the metal bar stabilize the wrists and

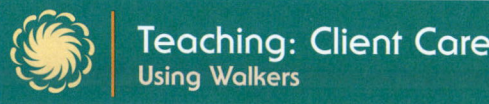

Teaching: Client Care
Using Walkers

When Maximum Support Is Required

- Move the walker ahead about 15 cm (6 in.) while your body weight is borne by both legs.
- Then move the right foot up to the walker while your body weight is borne by the left leg and both arms.
- Next, move the left foot up to the right foot while your body weight is borne by the right leg and both arms.

If One Leg Is Weaker Than the Other

- Move the walker and the weak leg ahead together about 15 cm (6 in.) while your weight is borne by the stronger leg.
- Then move the stronger leg ahead while your weight is borne by the affected leg and both arms.

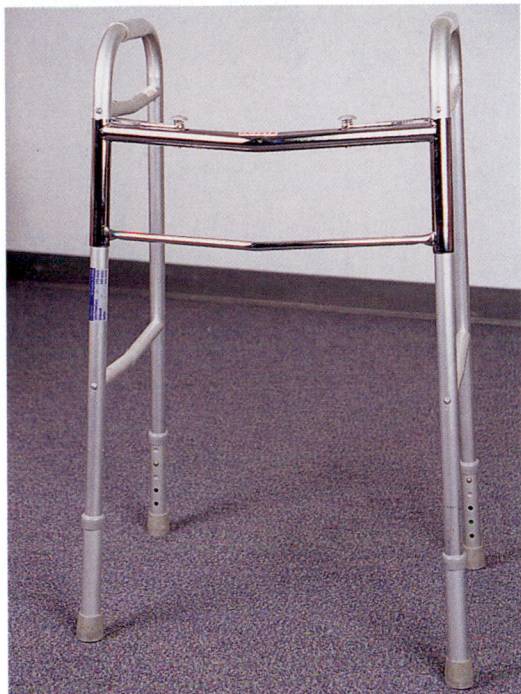

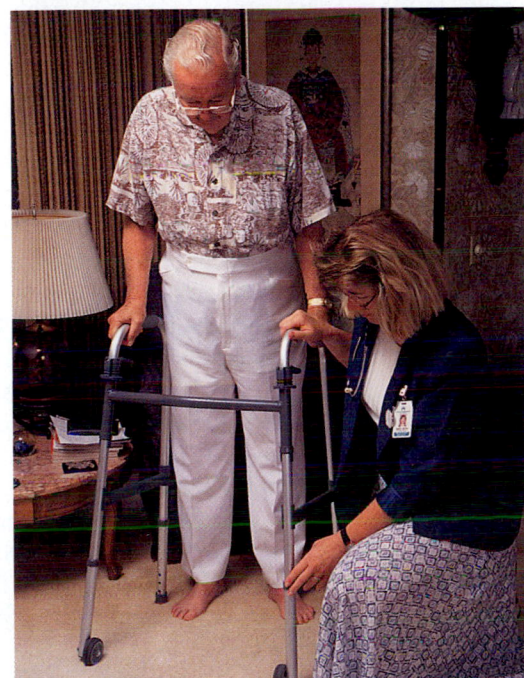

Figure 42–73 ■ *A,* standard walker; *B,* two-wheeled walker.

Research Note
Does Use of a Cane or Walker at Home Herald Level of Function after Hospitalization?

Research was performed on a subset of data gathered for the very large Hospital Outcomes Project for the Elderly (HOPE). Three groups of clients hospitalized for a medical illness were studied: those who used no assistive device before entering the hospital (64%), and those who used either a cane (21%) or a walker (13%). The 1,212 participants completed interviews within 2 days of hospital admission, at discharge, and 3 months after discharge. Results indicated that those who used a walker before admission were more likely to decline in their ability to perform ADLs both in the hospital and at the 3-month follow-up. Those who used a cane also demonstrated lower levels of ADLs at 3 months but values were not as strongly predictive as the walker data. The authors noted that the change in independence was not limited to ability to ambulate. Those who used a cane or walker were at increased risk of developing greater dependence in ADLs overall, including those activities not related to walking. This indicates that the use of the assistive device was a marker of overall functional status.

Implications: The most obvious use of these research findings is to highlight the need for the nurse to diligently institute measures to promote independence and prevent dependence in those who use assistive devices prior to hospital admission. If one can predict those clients who are at increased risk for the complications that may follow illness and hospitalization, there is an increased chance of implementing an effective prevention plan of care.

Note: From "Use of an Ambulation Assistive Device Predicts Functional Decline Associated with Hospitalization," by J. E. Mahoney, M. A. Sager, and M. Jalaluddin, 1999, *American Journal of Gerontology, 54A,* pp. M83–M88.

thus make walking safer and easier. The platform, or elbow extensor, crutch also has a cuff for the upper arm (Figure 42–74). All crutches require suction tips, usually made of rubber, which help to prevent slipping on a floor surface.

In crutch walking, the client's weight is borne by the muscles of the shoulder girdle and the upper extremities. Before beginning crutch walking, exercises that strengthen the upper arms and hands are recommended.

Measuring Clients for Crutches. When nurses measure clients for axillary crutches, it is most important to obtain the

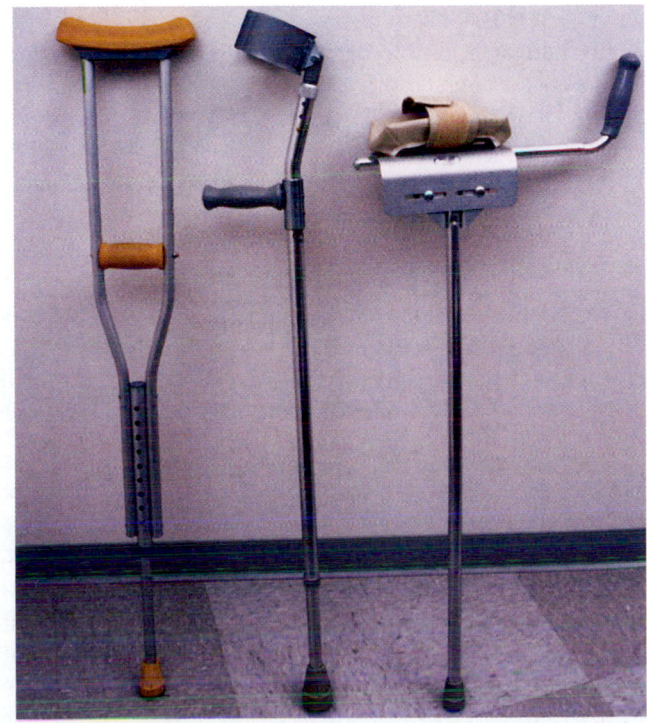

Figure 42–74 ■ Types of crutches: axillary, Lofstrand, and platform.

Teaching: Client Care
Using Crutches

- Follow the plan of exercises developed for you to strengthen your arm muscles before beginning crutch walking.
- Have a health care professional establish the correct length for your crutches and the correct placement of the hand-pieces. Crutches that are too long force your shoulders upward and make it difficult for you to push your body off the ground. Crutches that are too short will make you hunch over and develop an improper body stance.
- The weight of your body should be borne by the arms rather than the axillae (armpits). Continual pressure on the axillae can injure the radial nerve and eventually cause crutch palsy, a weakness of the muscles of the forearm, wrist, and hand.
- Maintain an erect posture as much as possible to prevent strain on muscles and joints and to maintain balance.
- Each step taken with crutches should be a comfortable distance for you. It is wise to start with a small rather than large step.
- Inspect the crutch tips regularly, and replace them if worn.
- Keep the crutch tips dry and clean to maintain their surface friction. If the tips become wet, dry them well before use.
- Wear a shoe with a low heel that grips the floor. Rubber soles decrease the chances of slipping. Adjust shoelaces so they cannot come untied or reach the floor where they might catch on the crutches. Consider shoes with alternate forms of closure (e.g., Velcro), especially if you cannot easily bend to tie laces. Slip-on shoes are acceptable only if they are snug and the heel does not come loose when the foot is bent.

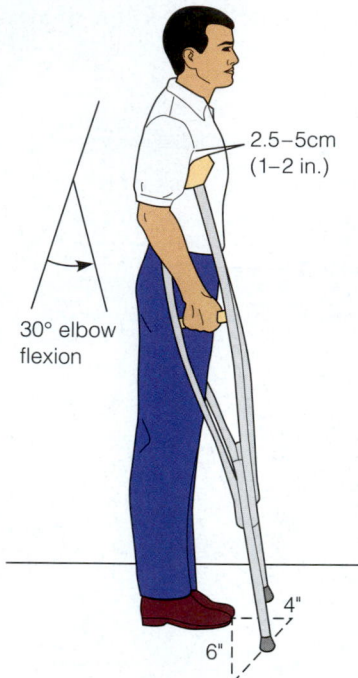

Figure 42–75 ■ The standing position for measuring the correct length for crutches.

correct length for the crutches and the correct placement of the hand piece. There are two methods of measuring crutch length:

1. The client lies in a supine position and the nurse measures from the anterior fold of the axilla to the heel of the foot and adds 2.5 cm (1 in.).
2. The client stands erect and positions the crutch as shown in Figure 42–75 ■. The nurse makes sure the shoulder rest of the crutch is at least three finger widths, that is, 2.5 to 5 cm (1 to 2 in.), below the axilla.

To determine the correct placement of the hand bar:

1. The client stands upright and supports the body weight by the hand grips of the crutches.
2. The nurse measures the angle of elbow flexion. It should be about 30 degrees. A goniometer (Figure 28–85) may be used to verify the correct angle.

Crutch Gaits. The crutch gait is the gait a person assumes on crutches by alternating body weight on one or both legs and the crutches. Five standard crutch gaits are the four-point gait, three-point gait, two-point gait, swing-to gait, and swing-through gait. The gait used depends on the following individual factors: (a) the ability to take steps, (b) the ability to bear weight and keep balance in a standing position on both legs or only one, and (c) the ability to hold the body erect.

Clients also need instruction about how to get into and out of chairs and go up and down stairs safely. All of these crutch

skills are best taught before the client is discharged and preferably before the client has surgery.

Crutch Stance (Tripod Position). Before crutch walking is attempted, the client needs to learn facts about posture and balance. The proper standing position with crutches is called the **tripod (triangle) position** (Figure 42–76 ■). The crutches are placed about 15 cm (6 in.) in front of the feet and out laterally about 15 cm (6 in.), creating a wide base of support. The feet are slightly apart. A tall person requires a wider base than a short person does. Hips and knees are extended, the back is straight, and the head is held straight and high. There should be no hunch to the shoulders and thus no weight borne by the axillae. The elbows are extended sufficiently to allow weight-bearing on the hands. If the client is unsteady, the nurse places a walking belt around the client's waist and grasps the belt from above, not from below. A fall can be prevented more effectively if the belt is held from above.

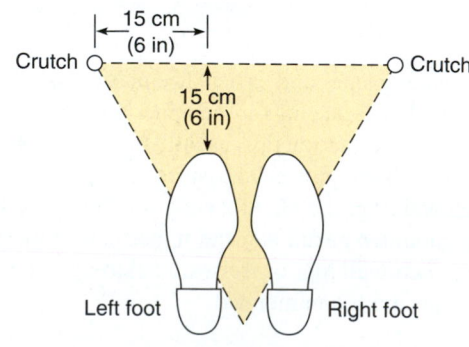

Figure 42–76 ■ The tripod position.

Four-Point Alternate Gait. This is the most elementary and safest gait, providing at least three points of support at all times, but it requires coordination. Clients can use it when walking in crowds because it does not require much space. To use this gait, the client needs to be able to bear weight on both legs (Figure 42–77 ■, reading from bottom to top). The nurse asks the client to

1. Move the right crutch ahead a suitable distance, such as 10 to 15 cm (4 to 6 in.).
2. Move the left front foot forward, preferably to the level of the left crutch.
3. Move the left crutch forward.
4. Move the right foot forward.

Three-Point Gait. To use this gait, the client must be able to bear the entire body weight on the unaffected leg. The two crutches and the unaffected leg bear weight alternately (Figure 42–78 ■, reading from bottom to top). The nurse asks the client to

1. Move both crutches and the weaker leg forward.
2. Move the stronger leg forward.

Two-Point Alternate Gait. This gait is faster than the four-point gait. It requires more balance because only two points support the body at one time; it also requires at least partial weight-bearing on each foot. In this gait, arm movements with the crutches are similar to the arm movements during normal walking (Figure 42–79 ■, reading from bottom to top). The nurse asks the client to

1. Move the left crutch and the right foot forward together.
2. Move the right crutch and the left foot ahead together.

Swing-To Gait. The swing gaits are used by clients with paralysis of the legs and hips. Prolonged use of these gaits results in

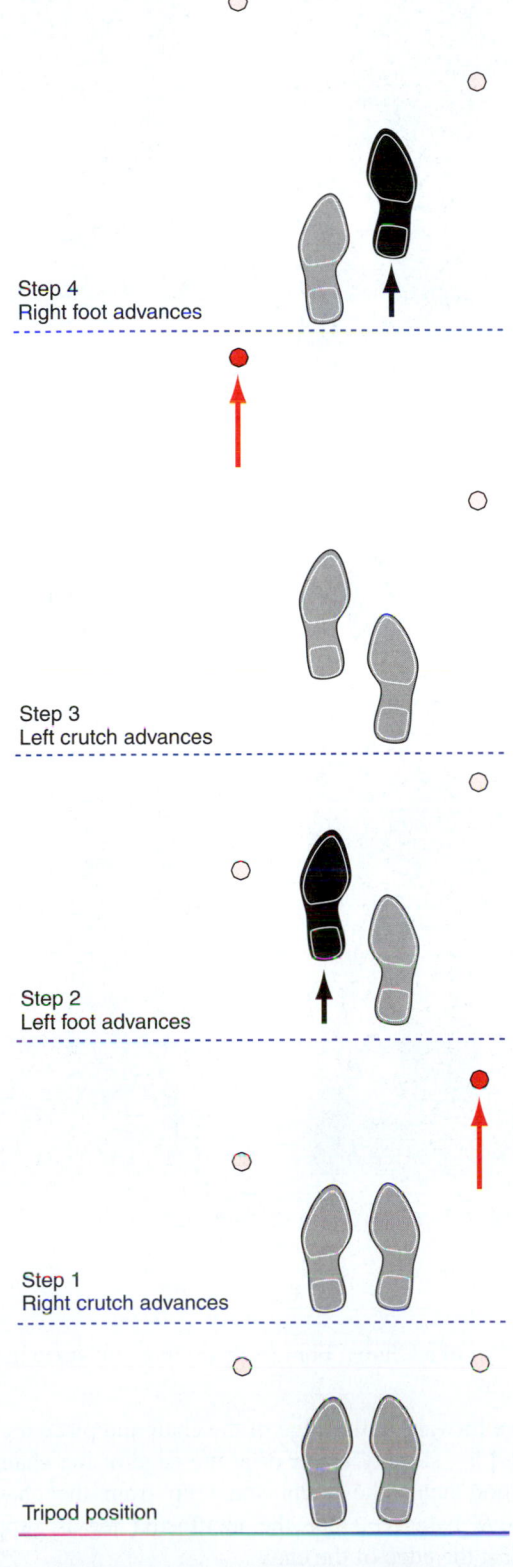

Figure 42–77 ■ The four-point alternate crutch gait.

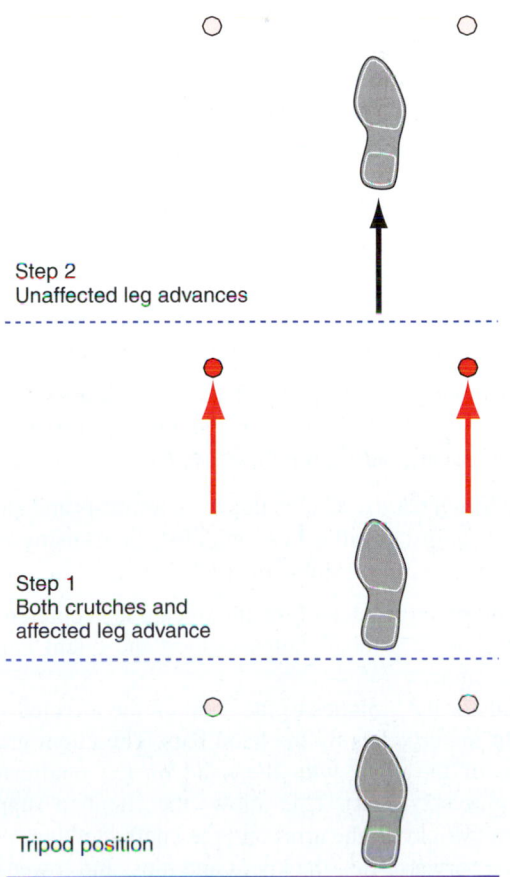

Figure 42–78 ■ The three-point crutch gait.

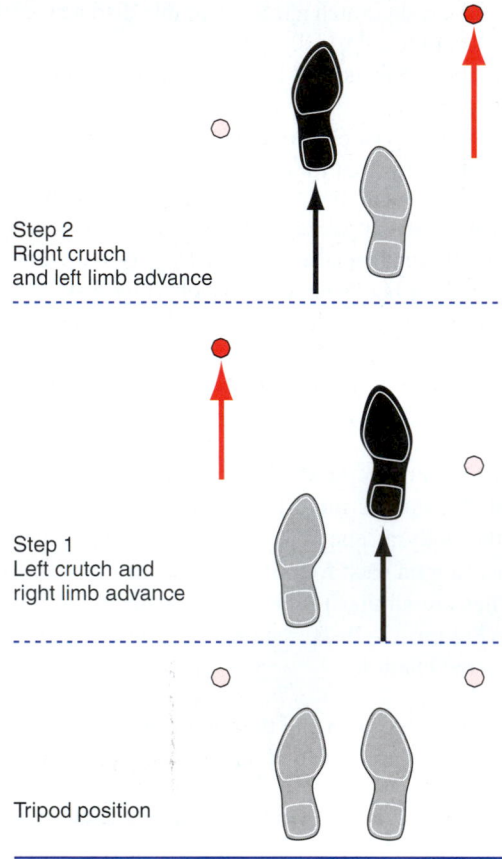

Step 2
Right crutch
and left limb advance

Step 1
Left crutch and
right limb advance

Tripod position

Figure 42–79 ■ The two-point alternate crutch gait.

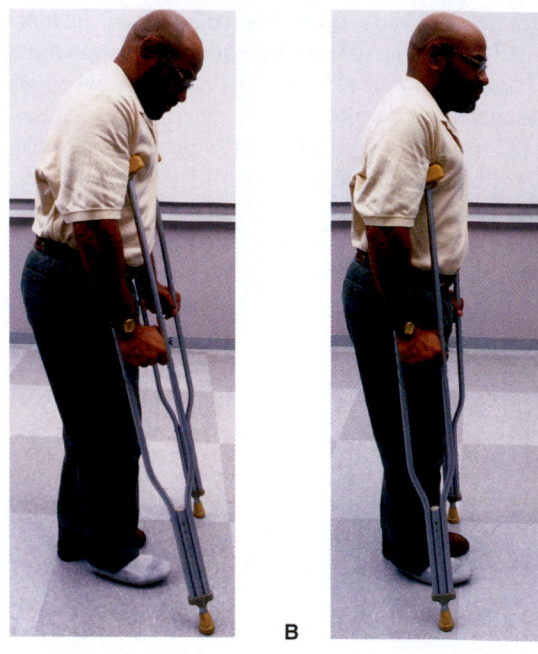

A   B

Figure 42–80 ■ The swing-to crutch gait.

atrophy of the unused muscles. The swing-to gait is the easier of these two gaits. The nurse asks the client to

1. Move both crutches ahead together (Figure 42–80 ■, *A*).
2. Lift body weight by the arms and swing to the crutches (Figure 42–80 ■, *B*).

Swing-Through Gait. This gait requires considerable skill, strength, and coordination. The nurse asks the client to

1. Move both crutches forward together (Figure 42–81 ■, *A*).
2. Lift body weight by the arms and swing through and beyond the crutch (Figure 42–81 ■, *B*).

Getting into a Chair. Chairs that have armrests and are secure or braced against a wall are essential for clients using crutches. For this procedure, the nurse instructs the client to

1. Stand with the back of the unaffected leg centered against the chair. The chair helps support the client during the next steps.
2. Transfer the crutches to the hand on the affected side and hold the crutches by the hand bars. The client grasps the arm of the chair with the hand on the unaffected side (Figure 42–82 ■). This allows the client to support the body weight on the arms and the unaffected leg.
3. Lean forward, flex the knees and hips, and lower into the chair.

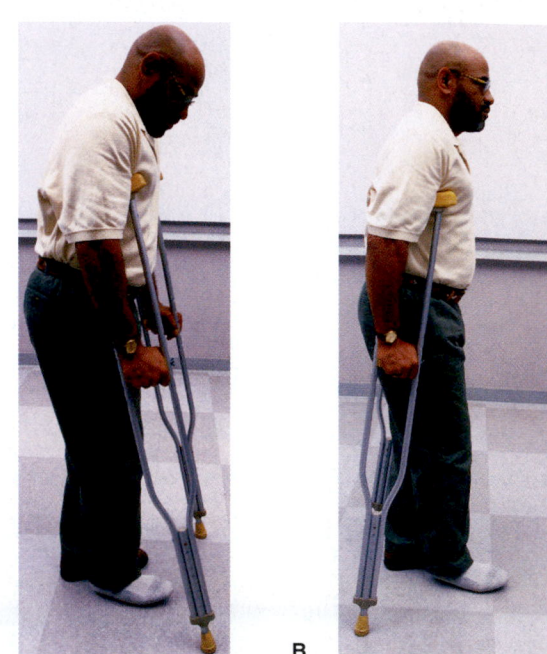

A   B

Figure 42–81 ■ The swing-through crutch gait.

Getting Out of a Chair. For this procedure, the nurse instructs the client to

1. Move forward to the edge of the chair and place the unaffected leg slightly under or at the edge of the chair. This position helps the client stand up from the chair and achieve balance, since the unaffected leg is supported against the edge of the chair.

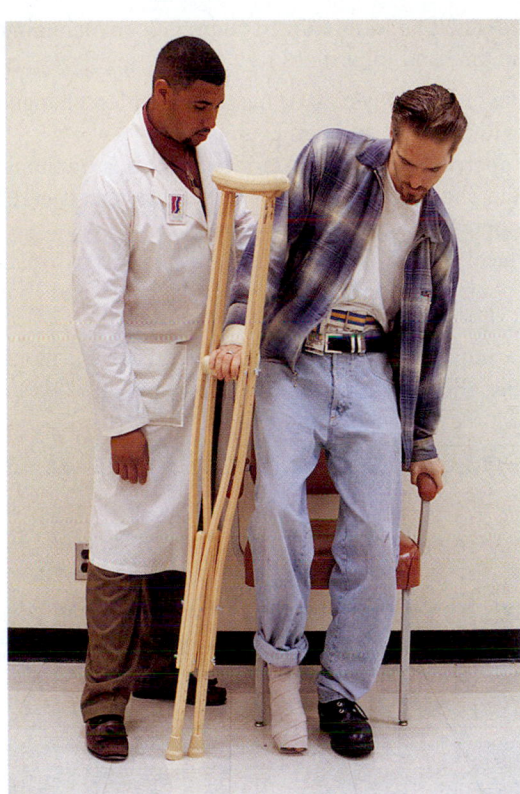

Figure 42–82 ■ A client using crutches getting into a chair.

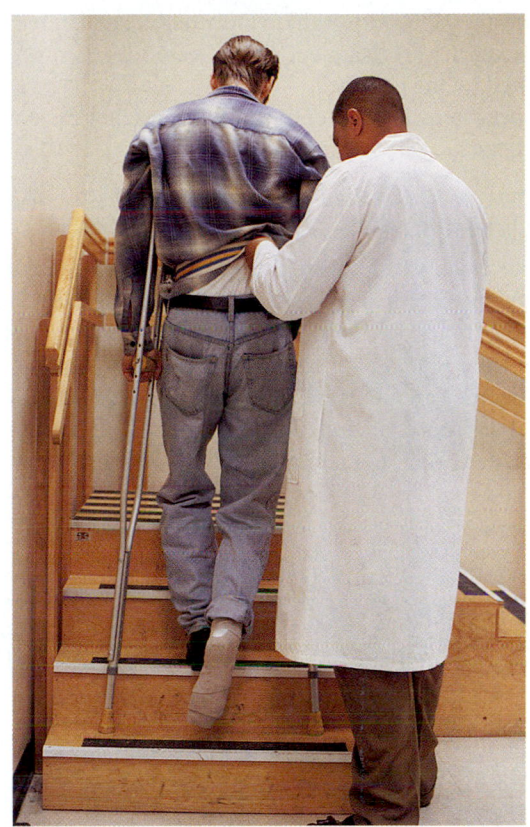

Figure 42–83 ■ Climbing stairs: placing weight on the crutches while first moving the unaffected leg onto a step.

2. Grasp the crutches by the hand bars in the hand on the affected side, and grasp the arm of the chair by the hand on the unaffected side. The body weight is placed on the crutches and the hand on the armrest to support the unaffected leg when the client rises to stand.
3. Push down on the crutches and the chair armrest while elevating the body out of the chair.
4. Assume the tripod position before moving.

Going up Stairs. For this procedure, the nurse stands behind the client and slightly to the affected side if needed. The nurse instructs the client to

1. Assume the tripod position at the bottom of the stairs.
2. Transfer the body weight to the crutches and move the unaffected leg onto the step (Figure 42–83 ■).
3. Transfer the body weight to the unaffected leg on the step and move the crutches and affected leg up to the step. The affected leg is always supported by the crutches.
4. Repeat steps 2 and 3 until the client reaches the top of the stairs.

Going down Stairs. For this procedure, the nurse stands one step below the client on the affected side if needed. The nurse instructs the client to

1. Assume the tripod position at the top of the stairs.
2. Shift the body weight to the unaffected leg, and move the crutches and affected leg down onto the next step (Figure 42–84 ■).

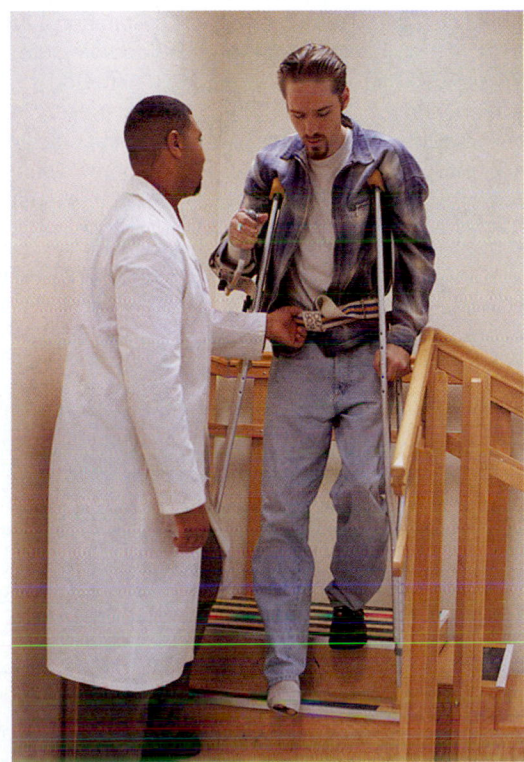

Figure 42–84 ■ Descending stairs: moving the crutches and affected leg to the next step.

3. Transfer the body weight to the crutches, and move the unaffected leg to that step. The affected leg is always supported by the crutches.
4. Repeat steps 2 and 3 until the client reaches the bottom of the stairs.

EVALUATING

The goals established during the planning phase are evaluated according to specific desired outcomes, also established in that phase. Examples of these are shown in the accompanying Nursing Care Plan.

If outcomes are not achieved, the nurse, client, and support person if appropriate need to explore the reasons before modifying the care plan. For example, the following questions may be considered if an immobilized client fails to maintain muscle mass and tone and joint mobility:

- Has the client's physical or mental condition changed motivation to perform required exercise?
- Were appropriate range-of-motion exercises implemented?
- Was the client encouraged to participate in self-care activities as much as possible?
- Was the client encouraged to make as many decisions as possible when developing a daily activity plan and to express concerns?
- Did the nurse provide appropriate supervision and monitoring?
- Was the client's diet adequate to provide appropriate nourishment for energy requirements?

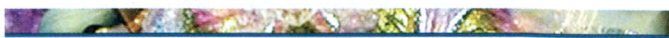

NURSING CARE PLAN FOR RISK FOR DISUSE SYNDROME

ASSESSMENT DATA		NURSING DIAGNOSIS	DESIRED OUTCOMES [NOC #]/INDICATORS*
Nursing Assessment Peter Chan, a 69-year-old, unmarried accountant being treated for congestive heart failure, states he has dyspnea with mild activity. ("I cannot climb a flight of stairs without stopping and resting and become breathless even when walking on level ground.") Prefers the orthopneic position. He works at home and sits at a table for most of the day.	**Physical Examination** Height: 178 cm (5'10") Weight: 102 kg (225 lb) Temperature: 37.8C (100.4F) Pulse rate: 94 BPM Respirations: 20/minute Blood pressure: 174/92 mm Hg Rales present in both lungs. Respirations slightly labored. Color pale. 3+ (5 mm) edema both feet and ankles **Diagnostic Data** CBC, and urinalysis within normal limits. CXR reveals an enlarged heart.	*Risk for Disuse Syndrome* related to decreased activity resulting from inadequate balance between oxygen supply and demand associated with decreased cardiac output and obesity.	Immobility Consequences: Physiological [0204], as evidenced by slight • Pressure ulcers • Decreased muscle strength Immobility Consequences: Psycho-cognitive [0205], as evidenced by slight • Decreased interest and motivation • Sleep disturbances • Decreased self-esteem Muscle Function [0209], as evidenced by mildly compromised • Muscle tone • Steadiness of movement • Strength of muscle contraction

NURSING CARE PLAN FOR RISK FOR DISUSE SYNDROME *continued*

NURSING INTERVENTIONS [NIC #] / SELECTED ACTIVITIES*	RATIONALE
Positioning [0840] • Position to alleviate dyspnea, e.g., high Fowler's.	Clients with increased pulmonary secretions are able to breathe better when upright because abdominal organs are lower and there is greater room for lung and diaphragmatic excursion.
• Provide support to edematous areas, e.g., elevate feet on foot stool when sitting.	Elevating the dependent area assists with decreasing tissue pressure and promoting fluid return to the venous system and the heart.
• Encourage active range of motion exercises.	Active ROM helps keep muscles in current strength and promotes circulation. Mild activity also helps burn unneeded calories.
Self-Awareness Enhancement [5390] • Encourage patient to recognize and discuss thoughts and feelings	In order for the patient to begin to work on enhancing ability to cope with the current situation, he must be aware of his thoughts and feelings and be able to share some of them with the nurse.
• Assist patient to identify the impact of illness on self-concept.	Patients may not be aware of the relationship between their physical illness and their feelings.
Exercise Therapy: Muscle Control [0226] • Collaborate with physical, occupational, and recreational therapists in developing and executing exercise program.	This patient will need a multidisciplinary approach to his care. Each member contributes from his or her area of expertise.
• Explain rationale for type of exercise and protocol to patient.	If the patient understands what the reasons are for activity, he can cooperate better.
• Provide step-by-step cuing for each motor activity during exercise or ADLs.	As-needed reminders help the patient recall what to do next.
• Use visual aids to facilitate learning how to perform exercises.	Some people have better visual memory than auditory memory.

Note: Immobility Managment is a Level 2 class (C) under the NIC Level 1 Basic Physiological Domain: Interventions to manage restricted body movement and the sequelae. See Table 18–7 on page 308.

EVALUATION

Outcomes met. Mr. Chan did not develop any skin breakdown or other evidence of the complications of immobility to date. However, since the risk factors remain, the care plan will be ongoing.

*Outcomes, interventions, and activities selected are only a sample of those suggested by NOC and NIC and should be further individualized for each client.

Applying Critical Thinking

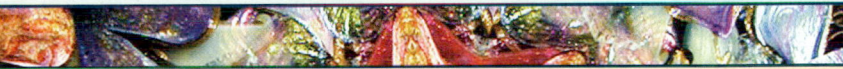

1. What assessment findings alert you that Mr. Chan is developing problems associated with his current state of decreased mobility?
2. Mr. Chan may benefit from using a walker to assist with ambulation at home. What teaching should be done in regard to use of a walker?
3. The care plan does not address one of Mr. Chan's risk factors—obesity. Would you add this to the plan?
4. What assumptions has the nurse made in assigning the desired outcome of "Immobility Consequences: Psycho-Cognitive"?
5. How are the choices of outcomes influenced by the cause of his nursing diagnosis (a chronic illness)?

See Critical Thinking Possibilities in Appendix A. 🔗

CONCEPT MAP   Client at Risk for Disuse Syndrome

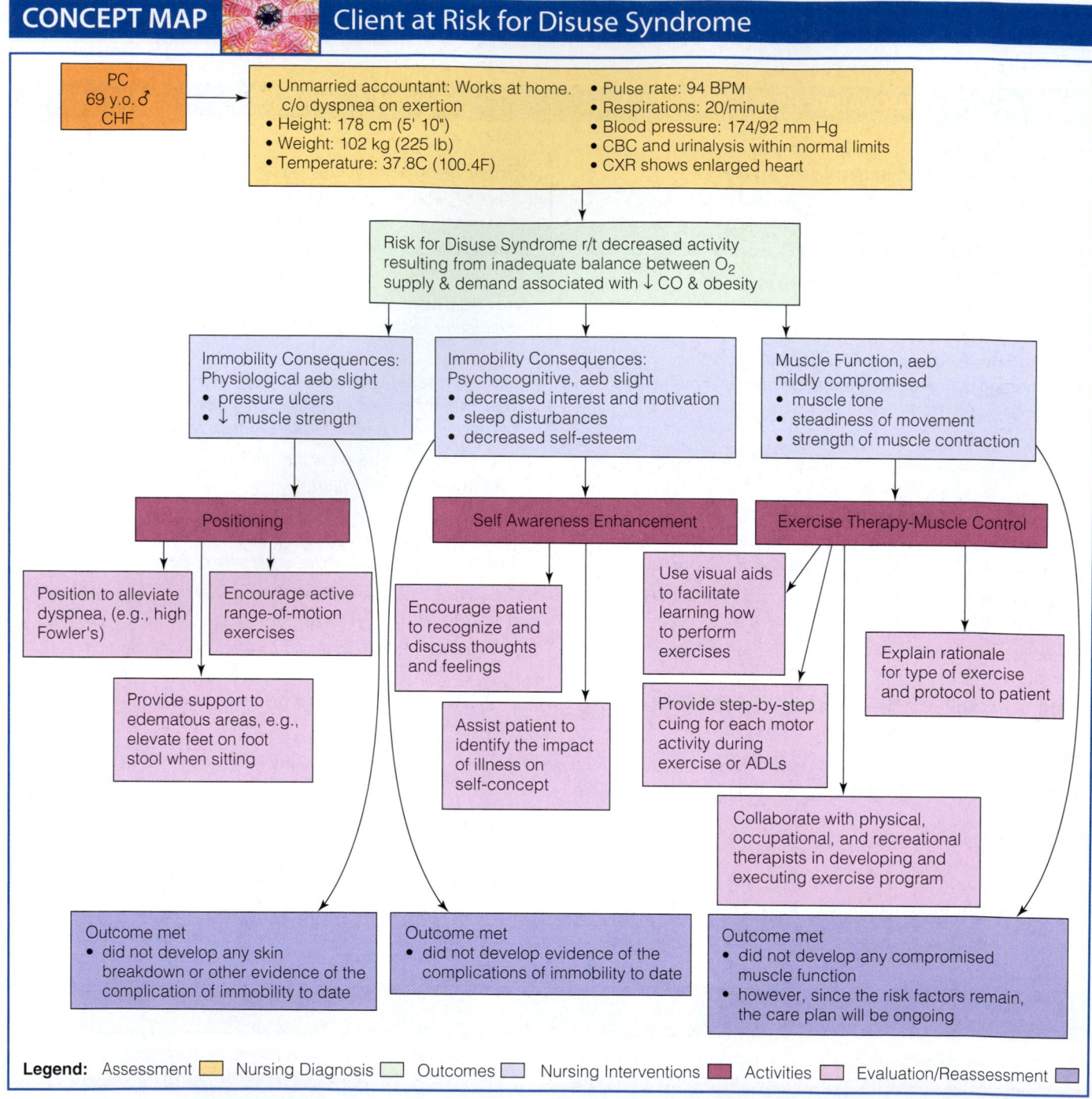

PC
69 y.o. ♂
CHF

- Unmarried accountant: Works at home. c/o dyspnea on exertion
- Height: 178 cm (5' 10")
- Weight: 102 kg (225 lb)
- Temperature: 37.8C (100.4F)
- Pulse rate: 94 BPM
- Respirations: 20/minute
- Blood pressure: 174/92 mm Hg
- CBC and urinalysis within normal limits
- CXR shows enlarged heart

Risk for Disuse Syndrome r/t decreased activity resulting from inadequate balance between O_2 supply & demand associated with ↓ CO & obesity

Immobility Consequences: Physiological aeb slight
- pressure ulcers
- ↓ muscle strength

Immobility Consequences: Psychocognitive, aeb slight
- decreased interest and motivation
- sleep disturbances
- decreased self-esteem

Muscle Function, aeb mildly compromised
- muscle tone
- steadiness of movement
- strength of muscle contraction

Positioning

Self Awareness Enhancement

Exercise Therapy-Muscle Control

Position to alleviate dyspnea, (e.g., high Fowler's)

Encourage active range-of-motion exercises

Encourage patient to recognize and discuss thoughts and feelings

Use visual aids to facilitate learning how to perform exercises

Explain rationale for type of exercise and protocol to patient

Provide support to edematous areas, e.g., elevate feet on foot stool when sitting

Assist patient to identify the impact of illness on self-concept

Provide step-by-step cuing for each motor activity during exercise or ADLs

Collaborate with physical, occupational, and recreational therapists in developing and executing exercise program

Outcome met
- did not develop any skin breakdown or other evidence of the complication of immobility to date

Outcome met
- did not develop evidence of the complications of immobility to date

Outcome met
- did not develop any compromised muscle function
- however, since the risk factors remain, the care plan will be ongoing

Legend: Assessment ☐ Nursing Diagnosis ☐ Outcomes ☐ Nursing Interventions ☐ Activities ☐ Evaluation/Reassessment ☐

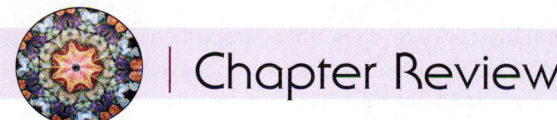

Chapter Review

EXPLORE MediaLink

NCLEX review questions, case studies, care plan activities, MediaLink applications, and other interactive resources for this chapter can be found on the Companion Website at www.prenhall.com/kozier. Click on Chapter 42 to select the activities for this chapter.

For animations more NCLEX review questions, and an audio glossary, access the Student CD-ROM accompanying this textbook.

Chapter Highlights

- The ability to move freely, easily, and purposefully in the environment is essential for people to meet their basic needs.
- Purposeful coordinated movement of the body relies on the integrated functioning of the musculoskeletal system, the nervous system, and the vestibular apparatus of the inner ear.
- Body movement involves four basic elements: body alignment, joint mobility, balance, and coordinated movement.
- People maintain alignment and balance when the line of gravity passes through the center of gravity and the base of support.
- The broader the base of support and the lower the center of gravity, the greater the stability and balance achieved.
- Exercise is physical activity performed to maintain muscle tone and joint mobility, to enhance physiologic functioning of body systems, and to improve physical fitness. Activity tolerance is the type and amount of exercise or daily living activities an individual is able to perform without experiencing adverse effects.
- Exercise is classified as either isotonic, isometric, or isokinetic and as either aerobic or anaerobic.
- Many factors influence body alignment and activity. These include growth and development, physical health, mental health, personal values and attitudes, and prescribed limitations to movement.
- Immobility affects almost every body organ and system adversely; complications also include psychosocial problems. Exercise, by contrast, provides many benefits to the same body organs and systems.
- Problems of immobility include disuse osteoporosis and atrophy; contractures; diminished cardiac reserve; orthostatic hypotension; venous stasis, edema, and thrombus formation; decreased respiratory movement and pooling of secretions; decreased metabolic rate and negative nitrogen balance; urinary stasis, retention, and infection; constipation; and varying emotional reactions.
- The nurse has responsibilities (a) to prevent the complications of immobility and reduce the severity of any problems resulting from immobility and (b) to design exercise programs for clients that promote wellness.
- Assessment relative to a client's activity and exercise includes a nursing history and physical examination of body alignment, gait, joint appearance and movement, capabilities and limitations for movement, muscle mass and strength, activity tolerance, and problems related to immobility.
- An activity and exercise history includes daily activity level, activity tolerance, type and frequency of exercise, and factors affecting mobility.
- NANDA nursing diagnoses that relate to activity and mobility problems include *Activity Intolerance, Risk for Activity Intolerance, Impaired Physical Mobility,* and *Risk for Disuse Syndrome.* Other relevant diagnoses are *Self-Care Deficit, Risk for Injury, Fear* (of falling), *Powerlessness, Low Self-Esteem, Ineffective Coping,* and, if the client is immobilized, many other potential problems such as *Ineffective Airway Clearance* and *Risk for Infection.*
- Body mechanics is the efficient, coordinated, and safe use of the body to move objects and carry out the activities of daily living.
- Nurses must use good body mechanics in their daily work and especially when moving and turning clients in bed and assisting clients to make transfers. Falls and back injuries are the most common and serious consequences of improper body mechanics.
- Positioning a client in good body alignment and changing the position regularly and systematically are essential aspects of nursing practice.
- Before positioning dependent clients, the nurse should plan a systematic 24-hour schedule for position changes, including positions that provide for full extension of the neck, hips, and knees. The nurse also uses appropriate supportive devices to maintain alignment and prevent strain on the client's muscles and joints.
- Before moving, turning, or transferring a client, the nurse must consider the client's health status and degree of exertion permitted, physical ability to assist, ability to comprehend instruction, degree of discomfort, client's weight, and the nurse's own strength and ability.
- Assistance from others or the use of mechanical lifting aids is essential for clients who are too heavy for the nurse to move or lift safely.
- Safety measures must always be employed when the nurse uses a wheelchair or stretcher to move and transfer clients.

- Ambulating techniques that facilitate normal walking gait yet provide needed support are most effective. The nurse can assist clients to prepare for ambulation by helping them become as independent as possible while in bed.

- Preambulatory exercises that strengthen the muscles for walking are essential for clients who have been immobilized for a prolonged period.
- Clients need specific instructions about appropriate use of canes, walkers, and crutches.

Review Questions

42–1. To increase stability during patient transfer, the nurse increases the base of support by
    a. leaning slightly backward.
    b. spacing the feet further apart.
    c. tensing the abdominal muscles.
    d. bending the knees.

42–2. Isotonic exercises such as walking are intended to
    a. increase muscle tone.
    b. increase endurance.
    c. increase muscle size.
    d. deplete muscle oxygen.

42–3. Five minutes after the patient's first postoperative exercise, the patient's vital signs have not yet returned to baseline. An appropriate nursing diagnosis might be
    a. *Activity Intolerance.*
    b. *Risk for Activity Intolerance.*
    c. *Impaired Physical Mobility.*
    d. *Risk for Disuse Syndrome.*

42–4. Which of the following demonstrates proper transfer technique in moving a client from sitting on the side of the bed to a chair?
    a. Have the client grasp the nurse around the neck for stability while standing.
    b. The nurse rocks from the rear foot to the front foot while standing the client.
    c. Place the chair perpendicular (right angled) to the bed.
    d. Have the client sit first on the edge of the chair and then push back fully.

42–5. Which of the following statements from a client with one weak leg regarding use of crutches when using stairs indicates a need for increased teaching?
    a. "Going up, the strong leg goes first, then the weaker leg with both crutches."
    b. "Going down, the weaker leg goes first with both crutches, then the strong leg."
    c. "The weaker leg always goes first with both crutches."
    d. "A cane or single crutch may be used instead of both crutches if held on the weaker side."

Readings and References

Suggested Readings

Metules, T. J. (2001). Watch your back. *RN, 64*(6), 65–66.
    The author points out that conditions for nurses in providing direct patient care that require lifting can cause back injuries, even in nurses who are strong and use proper techniques. The need for ergonomics, "the science of adapting the work environment to the worker" (p. 65), is what is needed. Useful hints are provided.

Related Research

Mathieson, K. M., Kronenfeld, J. J., & Keith, V. M. (2002). Maintaining functional independence in elderly adults: The role of health status and financial resources in predicting home modifications and use of mobility equipment. *The Gerontologist, 42,* 24–31.

References

Borg, G. (1998). *Borg's perceived exertion and pain scales.* Champaign, IL: Human Kinetics.
Centers for Disease Control and Prevention. (n.d.). *Introducing the Youth Media Compaign.* Retrieved May 16, 2003, from http://www.cdc.gov/youthcompaign/index.htm

Gordon, M. (2002). *Manual of nursing diagnosis* (10th ed.). St. Louis, MO: Mosby.
Johnson, M., Maas, M., & Moorhead, S. (Eds.). (2000). *Nursing outcomes classification (NOC)* (2nd ed.). St. Louis, MO: Mosby.
Mahoney, J. E., Sager, M. A., & Jalaluddin, M. (1999). Use of an ambulation assistive device predicts functional decline associated with hospitalization. *American Journal of Gerontology, 54A,* M83–M88.
McCloskey, J. C., & Bulechek, G. M. (Eds.). (2000). *Nursing interventions classification (NIC)* (3rd ed.). St. Louis, MO: Mosby.
National Institutes of Health Consensus Development Conference Statement [Electronic version]. (1995, December 18–20). *Physical Activity and Cardiovascular Health, 13*(3), 1–33. Retrieved May 16, 2003, from http://consensus.nih.gov/cons/101/101_statement.pdf
NANDA International. (2003). *NANDA nursing diagnoses: Definitions and classification 2003-2004.* Philadelphia: Author.

Selected Bibliography

California Department of Occupational Health. (1997). *A back injury prevention guide for*

health care providers. Retrieved May 16, 2003, from www.dir.ca.gov/dosh/dosh_publications/backinj.pdf
Haigh, C., & Peacok, L. (1998, February). Dilemmas in moving and handling patients. *Community Nurse, 4*(1), 26–28.
Jitramentree, N. (2001). Evidence-based protocol: Exercise promotion—encouraging older adults to walk. *Journal of Gerontological Nursing, 29*(10), 7–18.
Konradi, D. B., & Anglin, L. T. (2001). Moderate-intensity exercise: For our patients, for ourselves. *Orthopedic Nursing, 20,* 47–56.
McConnell, E. A. (2001). Applying a hip abduction pillow. *Nursing, 31*(12), 14.
McConnell, E. A. (2002). Using proper body mechanics. *Nursing, 32*(5), 17.
Schiff, L. (2001). Lift and transfer devices. *RN, 64*(8), 61–62.
Wilkinson, J. M. (2000). *Nursing diagnosis handbook with NIC interventions and NOC outcomes* (7th ed.). Upper Saddle River, NJ: Prentice Hall Health.
Wilkinson, J. M. (2001). *Nursing process and critical thinking* (3rd ed.). Upper Saddle River, NJ: Prentice Hall Health.

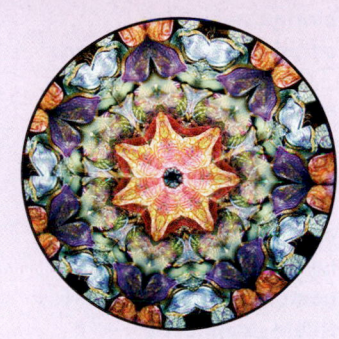

CHAPTER 43

REST AND SLEEP |

LEARNING OUTCOMES

After completing this chapter, you will be able to:

- Explain the functions and the physiology of sleep.

- Identify the characteristics of NREM and REM sleep.

- Identify the four stages of NREM sleep.

- Describe variations in sleep patterns throughout the life span.

- Identify factors that affect normal sleep.

- Describe common sleep disorders.

- Identify the components of a sleep pattern assessment.

- Develop nursing diagnoses, outcomes, and nursing interventions related to sleep problems.

- Describe interventions that promote normal sleep.

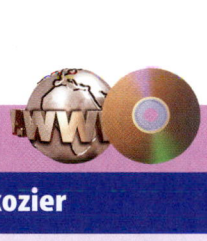

MediaLink

www.prenhall.com/kozier

Additional resources for this chapter can be found on the Student CD-ROM accompanying this textbook, and on the Companion Website at www.prenhall.com/kozier. Click on Chapter 43 to select the activities for this chapter.

CD-ROM
- Audio Glossary
- NCLEX Review

Companion Website
- Additional NCLEX Review
- Case Study: Client Who Has Difficulty Falling Asleep
- Care Plan Activity: Client with Sleep Disorder
- MediaLink Application: Diagnosing Sleep Apnea
- Links to Resources

Rest and sleep are essential for health. People who are ill frequently require more rest and sleep than usual. Often, debilitated people expend excessive amounts of energy to regain health or perform the activities of daily living. As a result, such people experience increased and frequent fatigue and need extra rest and sleep. Rest restores a person's energy, allowing the individual to resume optimal functioning. When people are deprived of rest, they are often irritable, depressed, and tired, and they may have poor control over their emotions. Providing a restful environment for clients is an important function of nurses.

The meaning of rest and the need for rest vary among individuals. **Rest** implies calmness, relaxation without emotional stress, and freedom from anxiety. Therefore, rest does not always imply inactivity; in fact, some people find certain activities such as walking in fresh air restful. When rest is prescribed for a client, both nurse and client must know whether the client is to be inactive and whether that inactivity involves the whole body or a body part (e.g., an arm).

Sleep is a basic human need; it is a universal biological process common to all people. Historically, sleep was considered a state of unconsciousness. More recently, **sleep** has come to be considered an altered state of consciousness in which the individual's perception of and reaction to the environment are decreased. Sleep is characterized by minimal physical activity, variable levels of consciousness, changes in the body's physiologic processes, and decreased responsiveness to external stimuli. Some environmental stimuli, such as a smoke detector alarm, will usually awaken a sleeper, whereas other noises will not. It appears that individuals respond to meaningful stimuli while sleeping and selectively disregard unmeaningful stimuli.

PHYSIOLOGY OF SLEEP

The cyclic nature of sleep is thought to be controlled by centers located in the lower part of the brain. These centers actively inhibit wakefulness, thus causing sleep.

Circadian Rhythms

Biorhythms (rhythmic biologic clocks) exist in plants, animals, and humans. In humans, these are controlled from within the body and synchronized with environmental factors, such as light and darkness, gravity, and electromagnetic stimuli. The most familiar biorhythm is the circadian rhythm. The term circadian is from the Latin *circa dies,* meaning "about a day."

Sleep is a complex biologic rhythm. When a person's biologic clock coincides with sleepwake patterns, the person is said to be in **circadian synchronization;** that is, the person is awake when the physiologic and psychologic rhythms are most active and is asleep when the physiologic and psychologic rhythms are most inactive.

Circadian regularity begins by the third week of life and may be inherited. Babies are awake most often in the early morning and the late afternoon. After 4 months of age, infants enter a 24-hour cycle in which they sleep mostly during the night. By the end of the fifth or sixth month, infants' sleep wake patterns are almost like those of adults.

Stages of Sleep

The **electroencephalogram (EEG)** provides a good picture of what occurs during sleep. Electrodes are placed on various parts of the sleeper's scalp. The electrodes transmit electric energy from the cerebral cortex to pens that record the brain waves on graph paper.

Two types of sleep have been identified: **NREM** (non-REM) **sleep** and **REM** (rapid eye movement) **sleep.**

NREM Sleep

NREM sleep is also referred to as slow-wave sleep because the brain waves of a sleeper are slower than the alpha and beta waves of a person who is awake or alert. Most sleep during a night is NREM sleep. It is a deep, restful sleep and brings a decrease in some physiologic functions. Basically, all metabolic process including vital signs, metabolism, and muscle action slow. Even swallowing and saliva production are reduced (Orr, 2000). See Box 43–1.

NREM sleep is divided into four stages. *Stage I* is the stage of very light sleep. During this stage, the person feels drowsy and relaxed, the eyes roll from side to side, and the heart and res-

- Arterial blood pressure falls.
- Pulse rate decreases.
- Peripheral blood vessels dilate.
- Cardiac output decreases
- Skeletal muscles relax.
- Basal metabolic rate decreases 10% to 30%.
- Growth hormone levels peak.
- Intracranial pressure decreases.

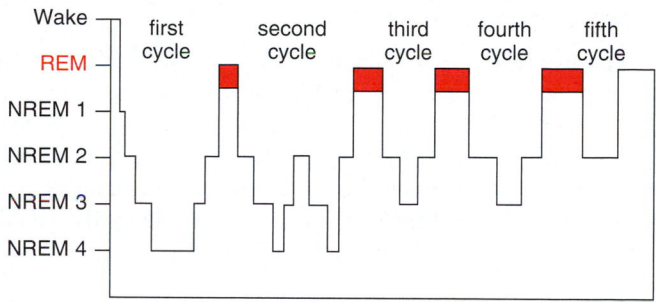

Figure 43–1 ■ Time spent in REM and non-REM stages of sleep cycles.

piratory rates drop slightly. The sleeper can be readily awakened and this stage lasts only a few minutes.

Stage II is the stage of light sleep during which body processes continue to slow down. The eyes are generally still, the heart and respiratory rates decrease slightly, and body temperature falls. Stage II lasts only about 10 to 15 minutes but constitutes 40% to 45% of total sleep.

During *Stage III,* the heart and respiratory rates, as well as other body processes, slow further because of the domination of the parasympathetic nervous system. The sleeper becomes more difficult to arouse. The person is not disturbed by sensory stimuli, the skeletal muscles are very relaxed, reflexes are diminished, and snoring may occur.

Stage IV signals deep sleep, called delta sleep. The sleeper's heart and respiratory rates drop 20% to 30% below those exhibited during waking hours. The sleeper is very relaxed, rarely moves, and is difficult to arouse. Stage IV is thought to restore the body physically. During this stage, the eyes usually roll, and some dreaming occurs.

REM Sleep

REM sleep usually recurs about every 90 minutes and lasts 5 to 30 minutes. REM sleep is not as restful as NREM sleep, and most dreams take place during REM sleep. Furthermore, these dreams are usually remembered; that is, they are consolidated in the memory.

During REM sleep, the brain is highly active, and brain metabolism may increase as much as 20%. This type of sleep is also called paradoxical sleep because it seems a paradox that sleep can take place simultaneously with this type of brain activity. In this phase, the sleeper may be difficult to arouse or may wake spontaneously, muscle tone is depressed, gastric secretions increase, and heart and respiratory rates often are irregular.

Sleep Cycles

During a sleep cycle, people pass through NREM and REM sleep, the complete cycle usually lasting about 1.5 hours in adults. In the first sleep cycle, a sleeper passes through all of the first three NREM stages in a total of about 20 to 30 minutes. Then, stage IV may last about 30 minutes. After stage IV NREM, the sleep passes back through stages III and II over about 20 minutes. Thereafter, the first REM stage occurs, last-

ing about 10 minutes, completing the first sleep cycle. The usual sleeper experiences four to six cycles of sleep during 7 to 8 hours (see Figure 43–1 ■). The sleeper who is awakened during any stage must begin anew at Stage I NREM sleep and proceed through all the stages to REM sleep.

The duration of NREM stages and REM sleep varies throughout the sleep period. As the night progresses, the sleeper becomes less tired and spends less time in Stages III and IV of NREM sleep. REM sleep increases and dreams tend to lengthen. If the sleeper is very tired, REM cycles are often short—for example, 5 minutes instead of 20—during the early portion of sleep. Before sleep ends, periods of near wakefulness occur, and Stages I and II NREM sleep and REM sleep predominate.

FUNCTIONS OF SLEEP

The effects of sleep on the body are not completely understood. Sleep exerts physiologic effects on both the nervous system and other body structures. Sleep in some way restores normal levels of activity and normal balance among parts of the nervous system. Sleep is also necessary for protein synthesis, which allows repair processes to occur.

The role of sleep in psychological well-being is best noticed by the deterioration in mental functioning related to sleep loss. Persons with inadequate amounts of sleep tend to become emotionally irritable, have poor concentration, and experience difficulty making decisions.

NORMAL SLEEP PATTERNS AND REQUIREMENTS

It has been suggested that maintaining a regular sleep wake rhythm is more important than the number of hours actually slept. Some people, for example, can function well on as little as 5 hours of sleep each night. Reestablishing the sleep wake rhythm (e.g., after the disruption of surgery) is an important aspect of nursing.

> ► **CLINICAL ALERT**   *"Health is the first muse, and sleep is the condition to produce it."*
> *Ralph Waldo Emerson, Uncollected Lectures, "Resources" (1932)* ■

Newborns

Newborns sleep 16 to 18 hours a day, usually divided into about seven sleep periods. NREM sleep is characterized by regular respirations, closed eyes, and the absence of body and eye movements. REM sleep has rapid eye movements that are observable through closed lids, body movement, and irregular respirations. Most of the sleep time is spent in Stages III and IV of NREM sleep. Nearly 50% of sleep is REM.

Infants

Some infants sleep as long as 22 hours a day, others 12 to 14 hours a day. About 20% to 30% of sleep is REM sleep. At first, infants awaken every 3 or 4 hours, eat, and then go back to sleep. Periods of wakefulness gradually increase during the first months. By 4 months, most infants sleep through the night and establish a pattern of daytime naps that varies among individuals. They generally awaken early in the morning, however. At the end of the first year, an infant usually takes one or two naps per day and sleeps about 14 of every 24 hours.

About half of the infant's sleep time is spent in light sleep. During light sleep, the infant exhibits a great deal of activity, such as movement, gurgles, and coughing. Parents need to ascertain that infants are truly awake before picking them up for feeding and changing. Many infants begin waking up again in the middle of the night between 5 and 9 months of age. For parents who find this behavior a problem, the nurse needs to assess the infant's total sleep pattern and compare it with the parents' sleep schedule. Parents need reassurance that there is no one correct way to handle this situation. The best solution is one that provides a continuous healthy environment for both the infant and the parents.

Toddlers

The sleep requirements of toddlers decrease to 10 to 12 hours per day. About 20% to 30% is REM sleep. Most still need an afternoon nap, but the need for midmorning naps gradually decreases. The toddler's normal sleep wake cycle is usually established by age 2 or 3 years. The toddler may exhibit a great deal of resistance to going to bed. Parents need assurance that if the child has had adequate attention from them during the day, maintaining a consistent approach with respect to bedtime will promote good sleep habits for the entire family. The child who awakens at night may be afraid of the dark or have experienced night terrors or nightmares.

Preschoolers

The preschool child usually requires 11 to 12 hours of sleep per night, particularly if the child is in preschool. Sleep needs fluctuate in relation to activity and growth spurts. Many children of this age dislike bedtime and resist by requesting another story, game, or television program. The 4- to 5-year-old may become restless and irritable if sleep requirements are not met. A nap or quiet time during the day may be needed to restore energy levels.

Children in this age group still require bedtime rituals. Parents can help children who resist bedtime by warning them that bedtime is approaching and by continuing to use the same firm and consistent approach suggested for the toddler. Preschool children wake up frequently at night. REM sleep is still 20% to 30% higher than for adults; however, Stage I sleep is less.

School-Age Children

The school-age child sleeps between 8 and 12 hours a night without daytime naps. The 8-year-old requires at least 10 hours of sleep each night. As the child approaches 11 or 12 years of age, less sleep is required and bedtime may be as late as 10 PM. The REM sleep of children at this age is reduced to about 20%. Although some children still experience night awakenings due to nightmares, this problem continues to decrease with age.

Adolescents

Most adolescents require 8 to 10 hours of sleep each night to prevent undue fatigue and susceptibility to infections. A change in sleep pattern is common in adolescence. Children who once were early risers begin to sleep late in the mornings and occasionally take afternoon naps. The reason for daytime sleeping is not fully understood, but it is possibly a result of physical maturity and reduced nocturnal sleep. Sleep at this age is about 20% REM.

During adolescence, boys begin to experience **nocturnal emissions** (orgasm and emission of semen during sleep), known as "wet dreams," several times each month. Boys need to be informed about this normal development to prevent embarrassment and fear.

Young Adults

The sleep wake cycle is very important to young adults. They usually have an active lifestyle, and are thought to require 7 to 8 hours of sleep each night but may do well on less.

Middle-Aged Adults

Middle-aged adults generally maintain the sleep pattern established at a younger age. They usually sleep 6 to 8 hours per night. About 20% is REM sleep. The numbers of arousals from sleep increases and the amount of Stage IV sleep begins to decrease.

Elders

The older adult sleeps about 6 hours a night. About 20% to 25% is REM sleep. Stage IV sleep is markedly decreased and in some instances absent. The first REM period is longer. Many elders awaken more often during the night and it often takes them longer to go back to sleep. Because of the change in Stage IV sleep, older people have less restorative sleep (see Lifespan Considerations).

Some elders may be said to have *Sundowner's syndrome.* Although not a sleep disorder directly, it refers to a confusional state that tends to appear at dusk (thus the name) and may happen because of a change in circadian rhythms (changes in the sleep wake cycle), decreased sensory stimulation at the end of the day, a mental condition such as Alzheimer's disease.

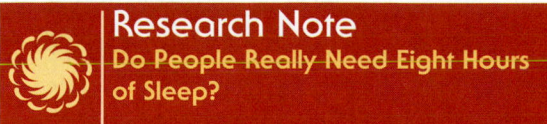

Research Note
Do People Really Need Eight Hours of Sleep?

Often, health care providers attempt to intervene with clients who report receiving less than 8 hours of sleep each night on the unproved assumption that 8 hours is the optimal amount.

Researchers examined this assumption by investigating the relationship between survival and length of sleep (Kripke, Gorfinkel, Wingard, Klauber, & Marler, 2002). After controlling for various other variables, data from more than 1 million adult Americans (collected for other purposes) showed that the best survival was in those who slept 7 hours per night. The worst survival was among those who slept for more than 8.5 hours or less than 3.5 or 4.5 hours each night. No relationship was found between reports of insomnia and mortality.

Implications: This very large study reassures both providers and clients that few if any health dangers are associated with sleeping between 6 and 8 hours per night. The nurse should focus on the client's subjective feelings of being rested and any other aspects of disturbed sleep that may exist rather than the exact length. Eight is not the magic number.

Note: From "Mortality Associated with Sleep Duration and Insomnia," by D. F. Kripke, L. Garfinkel, D. L. Wingard, M. R. Klauber, and M. R. Marler, 2002, *Archives of General Psychiatry, 59*(2), pp. 131–136.

FACTORS AFFECTING SLEEP

Both the quality and the quantity of sleep are affected by a number of factors. *Quality of sleep* refers to the individual's ability to stay asleep and to get appropriate amounts of REM and NREM sleep. *Quantity of sleep* is the total time the individual sleeps.

Illness

Illness that causes pain or physical distress can result in sleep problems. People who are ill require more sleep than normal, and the normal rhythm of sleep and wakefulness is often disturbed. People deprived of REM sleep subsequently spend more sleep time than normal in this stage.

Respiratory conditions can disturb an individual's sleep. Shortness of breath often makes sleep difficult, and people who have nasal congestion or sinus drainage may have trouble breathing and hence may find it difficult to sleep.

People who have gastric or duodenal ulcers may find their sleep disturbed because of pain, often a result of the increased gastric secretions that occur during REM sleep.

Certain endocrine disturbances can also affect sleep. Hyperthyroidism lengthens presleep time, making it difficult for a client to fall asleep. Hypothyroidism, conversely, decreases Stage IV sleep. Women with low levels of estrogen often report excessive fatigue. In addition, they may experience sleep disruptions due, in part, to the discomfort associated with hot flashes or night sweats that can occur with reduced estrogen levels.

Elevated body temperatures can cause some reduction in Stages III and IV NREM sleep and REM sleep.

The need to urinate during the night also disrupts sleep, and people who awaken at night to urinate sometimes have difficulty getting back to sleep.

Environment

Environment can promote or hinder sleep. Any change—for example, noise in the environment—can inhibit sleep. The absence of usual stimuli or the presence of unfamiliar stimuli can prevent people from sleeping. Stage I sleep is the lightest and Stages III and IV the deepest; as a result, louder noises are needed to awaken a person in Stages III and IV. However, over

Lifespan Considerations

Elders

The quality of sleep is often diminished in elders. Some of the leading factors that often are influential in sleep disturbances are

- Side effects of medications
- Gastric reflux disease
- Respiratory and circulatory disorders, which may cause breathing problems or discomfort
- Pain from arthritis, increased stiffness, or impaired immobility
- Nocturia
- Depression
- Loss of life partner and/or close friends
- Disruptions of bedtime rituals/routines when a person is hospitalized or institutionalized
- Confusion related to delirium or dementia.

Interventions to promote sleep and rest can help enhance the rejuvenation and renewal that sleep provides. Rituals and routines that become the rhythm of one's life and have been performed for years are often disrupted by being hospitalized or in-

stitutionalized. The following interventions can help promote sleep and rest is follows:

- Maintain usual bedtime ritual, or develop a new one with the client that will encourage relaxation or sleep, such as music, relaxation techniques, back massage, and warm drinks.
- Be sure their environment is warm and safe, especially if they get out of bed during the night.
- Provide comfort measures, such as analgesics if indicated, and proper positioning.
- Enhance the sense of safety and security by checking on clients frequently and making sure that the call light is within reach.
- If lack of sleep is caused by medications or certain health conditions, work on specific interventions related to these problems.
- Evaluate the situation and find out what the rest and sleep disturbances mean to the client. They may not perceive sleeplessness to be a serious problem, but will just do other activities and sleep when tired.

time people can be habituated to a noise so that the level has less effect.

Discomfort from environmental temperature and lack of ventilation can affect sleep. Light levels can be another factor. A person accustomed to darkness while sleeping may find it difficult to sleep in the light.

Fatigue

It is thought that a person who is moderately fatigued usually has a restful sleep. Fatigue also affects a person's sleep pattern. The more tired the person is, the shorter the first period of paradoxical (REM) sleep. As the person rests, the REM periods become longer.

Lifestyle

A person who does shift work and changes shifts frequently must arrange activities to be ready to sleep at the right time. Moderate exercise usually is conducive to sleep, but excessive exercise can delay sleep. The person's ability to relax before retiring is an important factor affecting the ability to fall asleep.

Emotional Stress

Anxiety and depression frequently disturb sleep. A person preoccupied with personal problems may be unable to relax sufficiently to get to sleep. Anxiety increases the norepinephrine blood levels through stimulation of the sympathetic nervous system. This chemical change results in less Stage IV NREM and REM sleep and more stage changes and awakenings.

Stimulants and Alcohol

Caffeine-containing beverages act as stimulants of the central nervous system, thus interfering with sleep. People who drink an excessive amount of alcohol often find their sleep disturbed. Excessive alcohol disrupts REM sleep, although it may hasten the onset of sleep. While making up for lost REM sleep after some of the effects of the alcohol have worn off, people often experience nightmares. The alcohol-tolerant person may be unable to sleep well and become irritable as a result.

Diet

Weight loss has been associated with reduced total sleep time as well as broken sleep and earlier awakening. Weight gain, on the other hand, seems to be associated with an increase in total sleep time, less broken sleep, and later waking. Dietary L-tryptophan—found, for example, in cheese and milk—may induce sleep, a fact that might explain why warm milk helps some people get to sleep.

Smoking

Nicotine has a stimulating effect on the body, and smokers often have more difficulty falling asleep than nonsmokers do. Smokers are usually easily aroused and often describe themselves as light sleepers. By refraining from smoking after the evening meal, the person usually sleeps better; moreover, many former smokers report that their sleeping patterns improved once they stopped smoking.

BOX 43–2 ■ Drugs that Disrupt Sleep

These drugs may disrupt REM sleep, delay onset of sleep, decrease sleep time, cause nightmares, or increase daytime drowsiness:

- Alcohol
- Amphetamines
- Antidepressants
- Beta-blockers
- Bronchodilators
- Caffeine
- Decongestants
- Narcotics
- Steroids

Motivation

The desire to stay awake can often overcome a person's fatigue. For example, a tired person can probably stay alert while attending an interesting concert. When a person is bored and is not motivated to stay awake, by contrast, sleep often readily ensues.

Medications

Some medications affect the quality of sleep. Hypnotics can interfere with Stages III and IV NREM sleep and suppress REM sleep. Beta-blockers have been known to cause insomnia and nightmares. Narcotics, such as meperidine hydrochloride (Demerol) and morphine, are known to suppress REM sleep and to cause frequent awakenings and drowsiness. Tranquilizers interfere with REM sleep. Amphetamines and antidepressants decrease REM sleep abnormally. A client withdrawing from any of these drugs gets much more REM sleep than usual and as a result may experience upsetting nightmares. Box 43–2 lists drugs that can disrupt sleep.

COMMON SLEEP DISORDERS

A knowledge of common sleep disorders helps nurses obtain and recognize pertinent data. Sleep disorders may be categorized as parasomnias, primary disorders, and secondary disorders.

Parasomnias

A **parasomnia** is behavior that may interfere with sleep or that occurs during sleep. The *International Classification of Sleep Disorders* (American Sleep Disorders Association, 1997) subdivides parasomnias into arousal disorders (e.g., sleepwalking, sleep terrors), sleep wake transition disorders (e.g., sleep talking), parasomnias associated with REM sleep (e.g., nightmares), and others (e.g., bruxism). Box 43–3 describes examples of parasomnias.

Primary Sleep Disorders

Primary sleep disorders are those in which the person's sleep problem is the main disorder. These disorders include insomnia, hypersomnia, narcolepsy, sleep apnea, and sleep deprivation.

BOX 43–3	■ Parasomnias

- *Bruxism.* Usually occurring during Stage II NREM sleep, this clenching and grinding of the teeth can eventually erode dental crowns and cause teeth to come loose.
- *Nocturnal enuresis.* Bed-wetting during sleep can occur in children over 3 years old. More males than females are affected. It often occurs 1 to 2 hours after falling asleep, when rousing from NREM Stages III to IV.
- *Nocturnal erections.* Nocturnal erections and emissions occur during REM sleep. They begin during adolescence and do not present a sleep problem.
- *Periodic limb movements disorder (PLMD).* In this condition, the legs jerk twice or three times per minute during sleep and is most common among elders. This kicking motion can wake

the client and result in poor sleep. The condition may be treated with medications such as those otherwise used for Parkinson's disease. PLMD differs from restless leg syndrome (RLS), which occurs whenever the person is at rest, not just at night when sleeping. RLS may occur during pregnancy or be due to other medical problems that can be treated.
- *Sleeptalking.* Talking during sleep occurs during NREM sleep before REM sleep. It rarely presents a problem to the person unless it becomes troublesome to others.
- *Somnambulism.* Somnambulism (sleepwalking) occurs during Stages III and IV of NREM sleep. It is episodic and usually occurs 1 to 2 hours after falling asleep. Sleepwalkers tend not to notice dangers (e.g., stairs) and often need to be protected from injury.

Insomnia

Insomnia, the most common sleep disorder, is the inability to obtain an adequate amount or quality of sleep. People suffering from insomnia do not feel refreshed on arising. There are three types of insomnia:

1. Difficulty in falling asleep (initial insomnia)
2. Difficulty in staying asleep because of frequent or prolonged waking (intermittent or maintenance insomnia)
3. Early morning or premature waking (terminal insomnia).

Insomnia can result from physical discomfort but more often is a result of mental overstimulation due to anxiety. People who become habituated to drugs or who drink large quantities of alcohol are likely to have insomnia.

Treatment for insomnia frequently requires the client to develop new behavior patterns that induce sleep. The usefulness of sleeping medications is questionable. Such medications do not deal with the cause of the problem, and their prolonged use can create drug dependencies.

Hypersomnia

Hypersomnia, the opposite of insomnia, is excessive sleep, particularly in the daytime. The afflicted person often sleeps until noon and takes many naps during the day. Hypersomnia can be caused by medical conditions, for example, central nervous system damage and certain kidney, liver, or metabolic disorders, such as diabetic acidosis and hypothyroidism. In some instances, a person uses hypersomnia as a coping mechanism to avoid facing the responsibilities of the day.

Narcolepsy

Narcolepsy—from the Greek *narco,* meaning "numbness," and *lepsis,* meaning "seizure"— is a sudden wave of overwhelming sleepiness that occurs during the day; thus, it is referred to as a "sleep attack." Its cause is unknown, although it is believed to be a lack of the chemical hypocretin in the central nervous system that regulates sleep. Onset of symptoms tends to occur between ages 15 and 30. In narcoleptic attacks,

sleep starts with the REM phase. Even though people who have narcolepsy sleep well at night, they nod off several times a day even when conversing with someone or driving a car. Narcolepsy historically has been controlled by central nervous system stimulants and antidepressants but a drug approved by the U. S. Food and Drug Administration in 1999, modafinil, improves alertness without stimulating other body systems or interfering with nighttime sleep.

Sleep Apnea

Sleep apnea is the periodic cessation of breathing during sleep. This disorder needs to be assessed by a sleep expert, but it is often suspected when the person has loud snoring, frequent nocturnal awakenings, excessive daytime sleepiness, insomnia, morning headaches, intellectual deterioration, irritability or other personality changes, and physiologic changes such as hypertension and cardiac arrhythmias. It is most frequent in men over 50 and in postmenopausal women.

The periods of apnea, which last from 10 seconds to 2 minutes, occur during REM or NREM sleep. Frequency of episodes ranges from 50 to 600 per night. These apneic episodes drain the person of energy and lead to excessive daytime sleepiness.

Three common types of sleep apnea are obstructive apnea, central apnea, and mixed apnea. Obstructive apnea occurs when the structures of the pharynx or oral cavity block the flow of air. The person continues to try to breathe; that is, the chest and abdominal muscles move. The movements of the diaphragm become stronger and stronger until the obstruction is removed. Enlarged tonsils, a deviated nasal septum, nasal polyps, and obesity predispose the client to obstructive apnea.

Central apnea is thought to involve a defect in the respiratory center of the brain. All actions involved in breathing, such as chest movement and airflow, cease. Clients who have brain stem injuries and muscular dystrophy, for example, often have central sleep apnea. At this time, there is no available treatment. Mixed apnea is a combination of central apnea and obstructive apnea.

An episode of sleep apnea usually begins with snoring; thereafter, breathing ceases, followed by marked snorting as breathing resumes. Toward the end of each apneic episode, increased carbon dioxide levels in the blood cause the client to wake.

Treatment for sleep apnea can be directed at the cause of the apnea. For example, enlarged tonsils may be removed. Other surgical procedures, including laser removal of excess tissue in the pharynx, reduce or eliminate snoring and may be effective in relieving the apnea. In other cases, the use of a nasal continuous positive airway pressure (CPAP) device at night is effective in maintaining an open airway.

Sleep apnea profoundly affects a person's work or school performance. In addition, prolonged sleep apnea can cause a sharp rise in blood pressure and may lead to cardiac arrest. Over time, apneic episodes can cause cardiac arrhythmias, pulmonary hypertension, and subsequent left-sided heart failure.

> ➤ **CLINICAL ALERT** *Partners of clients with sleep apnea may become aware of the problem because they hear snoring that stops during the apnea period and then restarts. Surgical removal of tonsils or other tissue in the pharynx, if not the cause of the sleep apnea, can actually worsen the situation by removing the snoring and, thus, the warning that apnea is occurring.* ■

Sleep Deprivation

A prolonged disturbance in amount, quality, and consistency of sleep can lead to a syndrome referred to as **sleep deprivation.** This is not a sleep disorder in itself but a result of sleep disturbances. It produces a variety of physiologic and behavioral symptoms, the severity of which depends on the degree of the deprivation. Two major types of sleep deprivation are REM deprivation and NREM deprivation. A combination of the two increases the severity of symptoms. Table 43–1 shows the causes and clinical signs of sleep deprivation.

Secondary Sleep Disorders

Secondary sleep disorders are sleep disturbances caused by other clinical conditions. They may be associated with mental, neurologic, or other conditions. Examples of conditions causing secondary sleep disorders include depression, alcoholism, dementia, Parkinsonism, thyroid dysfunction, chronic obstructive pulmonary disease, and peptic ulcer disease (American Sleep Disorders Association, 1997).

NURSING MANAGEMENT

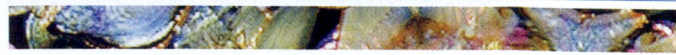

ASSESSING

Assessment relative to a client's sleep includes a sleep history, a sleep diary, a physical examination, and a review of diagnostic studies.

Sleep History

A brief general sleep history, which is usually part of the comprehensive nursing history, is obtained for all clients entering a health care facility. This enables the nurse to incorporate the client's needs and preferences in the plan of care. A general sleep history includes the following:

• Usual sleeping pattern, specifically sleeping and waking times; hours of undisturbed sleep; quality of or satisfaction with sleep (e.g., effect on energy level for daily functioning); and time and duration of naps.

TABLE 43–1 Types, Causes, and Signs of Sleep Deprivation

Type	Causes	Clinical signs
REM deprivation	Alcohol, barbiturates, shift work, jet lag, extended ICU hospitalization, morphine, meperidine hydrochloride (Demerol)	Excitability, restlessness, irritability, and increased sensitivity to pain Confusion and suspiciousness Emotional lability
NREM deprivation	All the above plus diazepam (Valium), flurazepam hydrochloride (Dalmane), hypothyroidism, depression, respiratory distress disorders, sleep apnea, and age (common in the elderly)	Withdrawal, apathy, hyporesponsiveness Feeling physically uncomfortable Lack of facial expression Speech deterioration Excessive sleepiness
Both REM and NREM deprivation	As above	Decreased reasoning ability (judgment) and ability to concentrate Inattentiveness Marked fatigue: blurred vision, itchy eyes, nausea, headache Difficulty performing activities of daily living Lack of memory, mental confusion, visual or auditory hallucinations, illusions

- Bedtime rituals performed to help the person fall asleep (e.g., a glass of hot fluid, reading or other method of relaxing, and special equipment or positioning aids).
- Use of sleep medication and other drugs. Sleep can be disturbed by a variety of drugs, such as stimulants or steroids, if they are taken close to bedtime. Hypnotics and sedating antidepressants may cause excessive daytime sleepiness.
- Sleep environment (e.g., dark room, cool or warm temperature, noise level, night-light).
- Recent changes in sleep patterns or difficulties in sleeping.

If the client indicates a recent pattern change or difficulties in sleeping, a more detailed history is required. This detailed history should explore the exact nature of the problem and its cause, when it first began and its frequency, how it affects daily living, what the client is doing to cope with the problem, and whether these methods have been effective. Questions the nurse might ask the client with a sleeping disturbance are shown in the accompanying Assessment Interview.

Sleep Diary

Sometimes clients with a sleeping problem can provide more precise information if they keep a written record of their sleep pattern and the habits associated with it. Such a sleep diary or log can be kept by clients who are sleeping at home and should be maintained for at least 1 week. A sleep diary may include all or selected aspects of the following information that pertain to the client's specific problem:

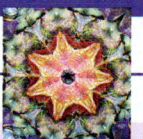

Assessment Interview

SLEEP DISTURBANCES

- How would you describe your sleeping problem? What changes have occurred in your sleeping pattern? How often does this happen?
- Do you have difficulty falling asleep?
- Do you wake up often during the night? If so, how often?
- Do you wake up earlier in the morning than you would like and have difficulty falling back to sleep?
- How do you feel when you wake up in the morning?
- Do you sleep more than usual? If so, how often do you sleep?
- Do you have periods of overwhelming tiredness? If so, when does this happen?
- Have you ever suddenly fallen asleep in the middle of a daytime activity? If so, has any muscle weakness or paralysis occurred?
- Has anyone ever told you that you snore, walk in your sleep, talk in your sleep, or stop breathing for a while when sleeping?
- What have you been doing to deal with this sleeping problem? Does it help?
- What do you think might be causing this problem? Do you have any medical condition that might be causing you to sleep more (or less)? Are you receiving medications for an illness that might alter your sleeping pattern? Are you experiencing any stressful or upsetting events or conflicts that may be affecting your sleep?
- How is your sleeping problem affecting you?

- Total number of sleep hours per day
- Activities performed 2 to 3 hours before bedtime (type, duration, and time)
- Bedtime rituals (e.g., ingestion of food, fluid, or medication) before going to bed
- Time of (a) going to bed, (b) trying to fall asleep, (c) falling asleep (approximate), (d) any instances of waking up and duration of these periods, and (e) waking up in the morning
- Any worries that the client believes may affect sleep
- Factors that the client believes have a positive or negative effect on sleep.

Keeping such a diary may become stressful for some clients and further affect their sleep. The nurse needs to advise the client to obtain the assistance of a bed partner in keeping the diary or to discontinue the diary if it presents a problem. When a diary is completed, the nurse and client can develop flowcharts or graphs that will assist in organizing the data and identifying the specific problem.

Physical Examination

Examination of the client includes observation of the client's facial appearance, behavior, and energy level. Darkened areas around the eyes, puffy eyelids, reddened conjunctiva, glazed or dull-appearing eyes, and limited facial expression are indicative of sleep insufficiency. Behaviors such as irritability, restlessness, inattentiveness, slowed speech, slumped posture, hand tremor, yawning, rubbing the eyes, withdrawal, confusion, and incoordination are also suggestive of sleep problems. Lack of energy may be noted by observing whether the client appears physically weak, lethargic, or fatigued.

In addition, the nurse assesses whether the client has a deviated nasal septum, enlarged neck, or is obese. These findings may be associated with obstructive sleep apnea or snoring.

Diagnostic Studies

Sleep is measured objectively in a sleep disorder laboratory by **polysomnography:** an electroencephalogram (EEG), electromyogram (EMG), and electro-oculogram (EOG) are recorded simultaneously. Electrodes are placed on the center of the scalp to record brain waves (EEG), on the outer canthus of each eye to record eye movement (EOG), and on the chin muscles to record the structural electromyogram (EMG). The following may also be monitored, depending on findings of the initial interview: respiratory effort and airflow, ECG, leg movements, and oxygen saturation. Oxygen saturation is determined by monitoring with a pulse oximeter, a light-sensitive electric cell that attaches to the ear or a finger. Oxygen saturation and ECG assessments are of particular importance if sleep apnea is suspected. Through polysomnography, the client's activity (movements, struggling, noisy respirations) during sleep can be assessed. Such activity of which the client is unaware may be the cause of arousal during sleep.

DIAGNOSING

Disturbed Sleep Pattern, the NANDA (2003) diagnosis given to clients with sleep problems, is usually made more explicit

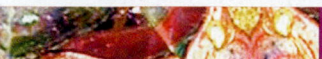

Home Care Consideration

When in the home care setting, remember to assess for the possibility of sleep disruption and deprivation in the caregiver. A sleep-deprived family member may be caring for a well-rested client. Respite care, where someone relieves the caregiver and cares for the client for some time, may be needed.

with descriptions such as "difficulty falling asleep" or "difficulty staying asleep."

Various factors or etiologies may be involved and must be specified for the individual. These include physical discomfort or pain; anxiety about actual or anticipated loss of a loved one, loss of a job, loss of life due to serious disease process, or worry about a family member's behavior or illness; frequent changes in sleep time due to shift work or overtime; and changes in sleep environment or bedtime rituals (e.g., noise or overstimulation of hospital environment, alcohol or other drug dependency, drug withdrawal, misuse of sedatives prescribed for insomnia, and effects of medications such as steroids or stimulants). Examples of clinical applications of this diagnosis using NANDA, NIC, and NOC designations are shown in Identifying Nursing Diagnoses, Outcomes, and Interventions.

Sleep pattern disturbances may also be stated as the etiology of another diagnosis, in which case the nursing interventions are directed toward the sleep disturbance itself. Examples include the following:

- *Risk for Injury* related to somnambulism
- *Ineffective Coping* related to insufficient quality and quantity of sleep
- *Fatigue* related to insomnia
- *Risk for Impaired Gas Exchange* related to sleep apnea
- *Deficient Knowledge* (Nonprescription remedies for insomnia) related to misinformation
- *Disturbed Thought Process* related to chronic insomnia
- *Anxiety* related to sleep apnea and threat of death
- *Activity Intolerance* related to sleep deprivation.

PLANNING

The major goal for clients with sleep disturbances is to maintain (or develop) a sleeping pattern that provides sufficient energy for daily activities. Other goals may relate to enhancing the client's feeling of well-being or improving the quality (as opposed to the quantity) of the client's sleep. The nurse plans specific nursing interventions to reach the goal based on the etiology of each nursing diagnosis. These interventions may include reducing environmental distractions, promoting bedtime rituals, providing comfort measures, scheduling nursing care to provide for uninterrupted sleep periods, and teaching stress reduction, relaxation techniques, or ways to develop good sleep habits.

Examples of NOC outcomes and NIC interventions to assist clients with sleep disturbances are shown in Identifying Nursing Diagnoses, Outcomes, and Interventions. Specific nursing activities associated with each of these interventions can be selected to meet the individual needs of the client. See the Nursing Care Plan and Concept Map for Rest and Sleep at the end of the chapter.

IMPLEMENTING

Nursing interventions to enhance the quantity and quality of clients' sleep involve largely nonpharmacologic measures. These involve health teaching about sleep habits, support of bedtime rituals, the provision of a restful environment, specific measures to promote comfort and relaxation, and essential considerations about the use of sleep medications.

For hospitalized clients, sleep problems are often related to the hospital environment or their illness. Assisting the client to sleep in such instances can be challenging to a nurse, often involving scheduling activities, administering analgesics, and providing a supportive environment. Explanations and a supportive relationship are essential for the fearful or anxious client.

Client Teaching

Healthy individuals need to learn the importance of rest and sleep in maintaining active and productive lifestyles. They need to learn (a) the conditions that promote sleep and those that interfere with sleep, (b) safe use of sleep medications, (c) effects of other prescribed medications on sleep, and (d) effects of their disease states on sleep. Client teaching for promoting sleep is shown in Teaching: Wellness Care on page 1124.

Supporting Bedtime Rituals

Most people are accustomed to bedtime rituals or presleep routines that are conducive to comfort and relaxation. Altering or eliminating such routines can affect a client's sleep. Common prebedtime activities of adults include an evening stroll, listening to music, watching television, taking a soothing bath, and praying. Children, too, are socialized into presleep routines such as a bedtime story, holding onto a favorite toy or blanket, and kissing everyone goodnight. Sleep is also usually preceded by hygienic routines, such as washing the face and hands (or bathing), brushing the teeth, and voiding.

In institutional settings, nurses can provide similar bedtime rituals—assisting with a hand and face wash, providing a massage or hot drink, plumping of pillows, and providing extra blankets as needed. Conversing about accomplishments of the day or enjoyable events such as visits from friends can also help to relax clients and bring peace of mind.

Creating a Restful Environment

All people need a sleeping environment with minimal noise, a comfortable room temperature, appropriate ventilation, and appropriate lighting. Although most people prefer a darkened environment, a low light source may provide comfort for children

IDENTIFYING NURSING DIAGNOSES, OUTCOMES, AND INTERVENTIONS

CLIENTS WITH SLEEP PROBLEMS

DATA CLUSTER	NURSING DIAGNOSIS/ DEFINITION	SAMPLE DESIRED OUTCOMES [NOC#]/DEFINITION	INDICATORS	SELECTED INTERVENTIONS [NIC#]/DEFINITION	SAMPLE NIC ACTIVITIES
Gillian Marks, 51, states she has had a problem falling asleep since her mastectomy 2 months ago. Says fears of prognosis become prominent when she is not active and busy. Has tried reading or watching TV but neither make her sleepy or relaxed. Appears agitated and restless.	Disturbed Sleep Pattern/ Time limited disruption of sleep (natural, periodic suspension of consciousness) amount and quality	Well-Being [2002]/An individual's expressed satisfaction with health status	Not compromised • Satisfaction with ability to relax • Satisfaction with ability to express emotions	Coping Enhancement [5230]/ Assisting a patient to adapt to perceived stressors, changes, or threats that interfere with meeting life demands and roles	• Appraise adjustment to changes in body image • Explore previous methods of dealing with life problems • Encourage verbalization of feelings, perceptions, and fears • Instruct on the use of relaxation techniques
Thomas Strep states that a recent shortage of paramedics has resulted in extensive overtime and frequent "double shifts" and rotations from his usual two weekly 7–3 and 3–7 shifts. States, "All I want to do is go to sleep when I get home, but I can't. I guess I'm too riled up."	Sleep Deprivation/ Prolonged periods of time without sleep (sustained natural, periodic suspension of relative consciousness)	Rest [0003]/Extent and pattern of diminished activity for mental and physical rejuvenation	Not compromised • Amount of rest • Rest pattern • Mentally rested	Progressive Muscle Relaxation [1460]/ Facilitating the tensing and releasing of successive muscle groups while attending to the resulting differences in sensation	• Choose quiet, comfortable setting • Have the patient tense, for 5 to 10 seconds, each of 8 to 16 major muscle groups • Instruct patient to focus on the sensations in the muscles when tensed and when relaxed
				Simple Guided Imagery [6000]/ Purposeful use of imagination to achieve relaxation and/or direct attention away from undesirable sensations	• Discuss an image the patient has experienced that is pleasurable and relaxing, such as lying on a beach, watching a snowfall, floating on a raft • Choose a scene that involves as many of the senses as possible • Have the patient travel mentally to the scene and report how it smells, looks, feels, etc. • Assist the patient to develop a method of ending the imagery such as counting while breathing deeply

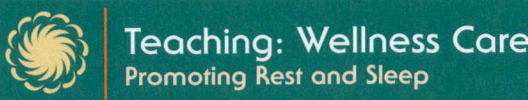

Teaching: Wellness Care
Promoting Rest and Sleep

Sleep Pattern

- Establish a regular bedtime and wake-up time for all days of the week to prevent disruptions in your biologic rhythm. Eliminate lengthy naps, or if a daytime nap is necessary, take it at the same time each day and limit the time to 30 minutes, preferably once a day.
- Get adequate exercise during the day to reduce stress, but avoid excessive physical exertion 2 hours before bedtime.
- Avoid dealing with office work or family problems before bedtime.
- Establish a regular routine before sleep such as reading, listening to soft music, taking a warm bath, or doing some other quiet activity you enjoy.
- When you are unable to sleep, pursue some relaxing activity until you feel drowsy.
- If you have trouble falling asleep, get up and pursue non-strenuous activity until you feel sleepy.
- Use the bed mainly for sleep, so that you associate it with sleep.

Environment

- Ensure appropriate lighting, temperature, and ventilation.
- Keep noise to a minimum; block out extraneous noise as necessary with soft music.

Diet

- Avoid heavy meals 3 hours before bedtime.
- Avoid alcohol and caffeine-containing foods and beverages (coffee, tea, chocolate) at least 4 hours before bedtime. Caffeine can interfere with sleep and both caffeine and alcohol act as diuretics, creating the need to void during sleep time.
- Decrease fluid intake 2 to 4 hours before sleep if necessary to avoid the need to use the bathroom during sleeping hours.
- If a bedtime snack is necessary, consume only light carbohydrates or a milk drink. Heavy or spicy foods can cause gastrointestinal upsets that disturb sleep.

Medications

- Use sleeping medications only as a last resort. Use over-the-counter medications sparingly because many contain antihistamines that cause daytime drowsiness.
- Take analgesics before bedtime to relieve aches and pains.
- Consult with your health care provider about adjusting other medications that may cause insomnia.

---

or those in a strange environment. Infants and children need a quiet room usually separate from the parents' room, a light or warm blanket as appropriate, and a location away from open windows or drafts.

Environmental distractions such as environmental noises and staff communication noise are particularly troublesome for hospitalized clients. Environmental noises include the sound of paging systems, telephones, and call lights; doors closing; elevator chimes; furniture squeaking; and linen carts being wheeled through corridors. Staff communication is a major factor creating noise, particularly at staff change of shift.

To create a restful environment, the nurse needs to reduce environmental distractions, reduce sleep interruptions, ensure a safe environment, and provide a room temperature that is satisfactory to the client. Some interventions to reduce environmental distractions, especially noise, are listed in Box 43–4.

The environment must also be safe so that the client can relax. People who are unaccustomed to narrow hospital beds may feel more secure with side rails.

Additional safety measures include

- Placing beds in low positions
- Using night-lights
- Placing call bells within easy reach.

Promoting Comfort and Relaxation

Comfort measures are essential to help the client fall asleep and stay asleep, especially if the effects of the person's illness interfere with sleep. A concerned, caring attitude, along with the

| BOX 43–4 | ■ Reducing Environmental Distractions in Hospitals |

- Close window curtains if street lights shine through.
- Close curtains between clients in semiprivate and larger rooms.
- Reduce or eliminate overhead lighting; provide a night-light at the bedside or in the bathroom.
- Close the door of the client's room.
- Adhere to agency policy about times to turn off communal televisions or radios.
- Lower the ring tone of nearby telephones.
- Discontinue use of the paging system after a certain hour (e.g., 2100 hours) or reduce its volume.
- Keep required staff conversations at low levels; conduct nursing reports or other discussions in a separate area away from client rooms.
- Wear rubber-soled shoes.
- Ensure that all cart wheels are well oiled.
- Perform only essential noisy activities during sleeping hours.

following interventions, can significantly promote client comfort and sleep:

- Provide loose-fitting nightwear.
- Assist clients with hygienic routines.
- Make sure the bed linen is smooth, clean, and dry.
- Assist or encourage the client to void before bedtime.
- Offer to provide a back massage before sleep (see Procedure 43–1).

- Position dependent clients appropriately to aid muscle relaxation, and provide supportive devices to protect pressure areas.
- Schedule medications, especially diuretics, to prevent nocturnal awakenings.
- For clients who have pain, administer analgesics 30 minutes before sleep.
- Listen to the client's concerns and deal with problems as they arise.

People of any age, but especially elders, are unable to sleep well if they feel cold. Changes in circulation, metabolism, and body tissue density reduce the older person's ability to generate and conserve heat. To compound this problem, hospital gowns have short sleeves and are made of thin polyester. Bed sheets also are often made of polyester rather than a warm fabric, such as cotton flannel. The following interventions can be used to keep elders warm during sleep:

- Before the client goes to bed, warm the bed with prewarmed bath blankets.
- Use 100% cotton flannel sheets or apply thermal blankets between the sheet and bedspread.
- Encourage the client to wear own clothing, such as flannel nightgown or pajamas, socks, leg warmers, long underwear, sleeping cap (if scalp hair is sparse), or sweater, or use extra blankets.

Emotional stress obviously interferes with a person's ability to relax, rest, and sleep, and inability to sleep further aggravates feelings of tension. Sleep rarely occurs until a person is relaxed. Relaxation techniques can be encouraged as part of the nightly routine. Slow, deep breathing for a few minutes followed by slow, rhythmic contraction and relaxation of muscles can alleviate tension and induce calm. Imagery, meditation, and yoga can also be taught. These techniques are discussed in Chapter 14.

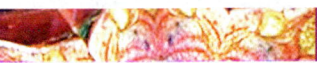

Procedure 43–1 Providing a Back Massage

Effleurage is a type of massage consisting of long, slow, gliding strokes. Research demonstrates that back massage has the ability to elicit a relaxation response (Gauthier, 1999). A simple 3-minute back rub can enhance client comfort and relaxation and have a positive effect on cardiovascular parameters such as blood pressure, heart rate, and respiratory rate. Rowe and Alfred (1999) found that slow-stroke massage could diffuse agitated behaviors in individuals with Alzheimer's disease.

Purposes
- To relieve muscle tension
- To promote physical and mental relaxation
- To relieve insomnia.

ASSESSMENT

Assess

- Behaviors indicating potential need for a back massage, such as a complaint of stiffness, muscle tension in the back or shoulders, or difficulty sleeping related to tenseness or anxiety
- Whether the client is willing to have a massage, because some individuals may not enjoy a massage
- Contraindications for back massage (e.g., impaired skin integrity, back surgery, vertebral, rib fracture).

PLANNING

Ensure that you have the full amount of time available for the massage. Although the actual technique may require only about 5 minutes, the entire process should be conducted in a calm and unhurried manner.

Delegation

The nurse can delegate this skill to UAP; however, the nurse should first assess for any contraindications and client willingness.

Equipment
- Lotion
- Towel for excess lotion

IMPLEMENTATION

Preparation

Determine (a) previous assessments of the skin, (b) special lotions to be used, and (c) positions contraindicated for the client. Arrange for a quiet environment with no interruptions to promote maximum effect of the back massage.

Performance

1. Explain to the client what you are going to do, why it is necessary, and how he or she can cooperate. Encourage the client to give you feedback as to the amount of pressure you are using during the back rub.
2. Wash hands and observe other appropriate infection control procedures.
3. Provide for client privacy.

continued on page 1126

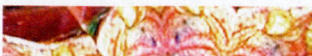

Procedure 43–1 Providing a Back Massage *continued*

IMPLEMENTATION *continued*

4. Prepare the client.
   - Assist the client to move to the near side of the bed within your reach and adjust the bed to a comfortable working height *to prevent back strain.*
   - Establish which position the client prefers. The prone position is recommended for a back rub. The side-lying position can be used if a client cannot assume the prone position.
   - Expose the back from the shoulders to the inferior sacral area. Cover the remainder of the body *to prevent chilling and minimize exposure.*
5. Massage the back.
   - Pour a small amount of lotion onto the palms of your hands and hold it for a minute. The lotion bottle can also be placed in a bath basin filled with warm water. *Back rub preparations tend to feel uncomfortably cold to people. Warming the solution facilitates client comfort.*

- Using your palm, begin in the sacral area using smooth, circular strokes.
- Move your hands up the center of the back and then over both scapulae.
- Massage in a circular motion over the scapulae.
- Move your hands down the sides of the back.
- Massage the areas over the right and left iliac crests (Figure 43–2 ■).
- Apply firm, continuous pressure without breaking contact with the client's skin.
- Repeat above for 3 to 5 minutes obtaining more lotion as necessary.
- While massaging the back, assess for skin redness and areas of decreased circulation.
- Pat dry any excess lotion with a towel.
6. Document that a back rub was performed and the client's response. Record any unusual findings.

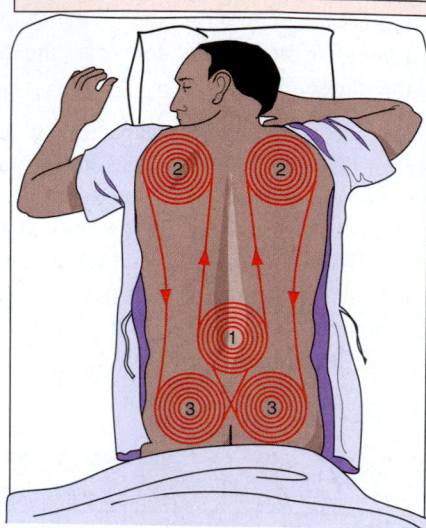

Figure 43–2 ■ One suggested pattern for a back massage.

EVALUATION

Compare the client's current response to his or her previous response. Is there a positive client outcome such as increased relaxation and decrease in pain and anxiety because of the back massage?

Enhancing Sleep with Medications

Sleep medications often prescribed on a prn (as-needed) basis for clients include the sedative-hypnotics, which induce sleep, and antianxiety drugs or tranquilizers, which decrease anxiety and tension. When prn sleep medications are ordered in institutional settings, the nurse is responsible for making decisions with the client about when to administer them. These medications should be administered only with complete knowledge of their actions and effects and only when indicated. Whenever possible, nonpharmacologic interventions to induce and maintain sleep, discussed earlier, are the preferred interventions.

Both nurses and clients need to be aware of the actions, effects, and risks of the specific medication prescribed. Although medications vary in their activity and effects, considerations include the following:

- Sedative-hypnotic medications produce a general central nervous system (CNS) depression and an unnatural sleep; REM or NREM sleep is altered to some extent and daytime drowsiness and a morning hangover effect may occur.
- Antianxiety medications decrease levels of arousal by facilitating the action of neurons in the CNS that suppress responsiveness to stimulation. These medications are contraindicated in pregnant women because of their associated

risk of congenital anomalies, and in nursing mothers because the medication is excreted in breast milk.
- Sleep medications vary in their onset and duration of action and will impair waking function as long as they are chemically active. Some medication effects can last many hours beyond the time that the client's perception of daytime drowsiness and impaired psychomotor skills have disappeared. Clients need to be cautioned about such effects and about driving or handling machinery while the drug is in their system.
- Sleep medications affect REM sleep more than NREM sleep. Clients need to be informed that one or two nights of increased dreaming (REM rebound) are usual after the drug is discontinued.
- Initial doses of medications should be low and increases added gradually, depending on the client's response. Elders, in particular, are susceptible to side effects because of their metabolic changes; they need to be closely monitored for changes in mental alertness and coordination. Clients need to be instructed to take the smallest effective dose and then only for a few nights or intermittently as required.
- Regular use of any sleep medication can lead to tolerance over time (e.g., 4 weeks) and rebound insomnia. In some instances, this may lead clients to increase the dosage. Clients must be cautioned about developing a pattern of drug dependency.

TABLE 43–2 Selected Sedative-Hypnotic Medications Used for Insomnia

Medication	Half-Life
Chloral hydrate (Noctec)	7–10 hours
Ethchlorvynol (Placidyl)	10–20 hours
Flurazepam (Dalmane)	47–100 hours
Glutethimide (Doriden)	1–12 hours
Lorazepam (Ativan)	10–20 hours
Melatonin	1 hour
Temazepam (Restoril)	9–15 hours
Triazolam (Halcion)	1.5–5.5 hours
Zaleplon (Sonata)	1 hour
Zolpidem (Ambien)	2.6 hours

- Abrupt cessation of barbiturate sedative-hypnotics can create withdrawal symptoms such as restlessness, tremors, weakness, insomnia, increased heart rate, seizures, convulsions, and even death. Long-term users need to taper withdrawal by about 25% to 30% weekly.

About half of the clients who seek medical intervention for sleep problems are treated with sedative-hypnotics (Vitiello, 1999). Table 43–2 presents some of the common medications used for enhancing sleep and the half-life of these medications. The half-life represents how long it takes for half of the medication to be metabolized and eliminated by the body; hence, those with shorter half-lives are less likely to cause residual drowsiness after administration.

EVALUATING

Using data collected during care and the desired outcomes developed during the planning stage as a guide, the nurse judges whether client goals and outcomes have been achieved. Data collection may include (a) observations of the duration of the client's sleep and the presence of signs of REM and NREM sleep and (b) questions about how the client feels on awakening, or about the effectiveness of specific interventions such as the use of relaxation techniques, adherence to a consistent sleep wake cycle, or the ingestion of milk products before bedtime. Examples of client goals and related outcomes are shown in Identifying Nursing Diagnoses, Outcomes, and Interventions box earlier in this chapter.

If the desired outcomes are not achieved, the nurse, client, and support people if appropriate should explore the reasons, which may include answers to the following questions:

- Were etiologic factors correctly identified?
- Has the client's physical condition or medication therapy changed?
- Did the client comply with instructions about establishing a regular sleep wake pattern?
- Did the client avoid ingesting caffeine?
- Did the client participate in stimulating daytime activities to avoid excessive daytime naps?
- Were all possible measures taken to provide a restful environment for the client?
- Were bedtime rituals supported?
- Were the comfort and relaxation measures effective?

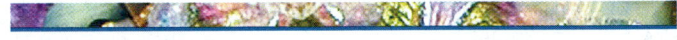

Medialink | CLIENT WHO HAS DIFFICULTY FALLING ASLEEP CASE STUDY

NURSING CARE PLAN FOR REST AND SLEEP

ASSESSMENT DATA		NURSING DIAGNOSIS	DESIRED OUTCOMES [NOC #]/INDICATORS*
Nursing Assessment Jack Harrison is a 36-year-old police officer assigned to a high-crime police precinct. One week ago he received a surface bullet wound to his arm. Today he arrives at the outpatient clinic to have the wound redressed. While speaking with the nurse, Mr. Harrison mentions that he has recently been promoted to the rank of detective and has assumed new responsibilities. He states that since his promotion, he has experienced increasing difficulty falling asleep and sometimes staying asleep. He expresses concern over the danger of his occupation and his desire to do well in his new position. He complains of waking up feeling tired and irritable.	**Physical Examination** Height: 185.4 cm (6'2") Weight: 85.7 kg (189 lb) Temperature: 37.0C (98.6F) Pulse: 80 BPM Respirations: 18/minute Blood pressure: 144/88 mm Hg Pale, drawn, with dark circles under eyes. **Diagnostic Data** CBC within normal range, x-ray left arm: evidence of superficial soft tissue injury	*Sleep Pattern Disturbance* related to anxiety (as evidenced by difficulty falling and remaining asleep, fatigue, irritability, drawn facial appearance, dark circles under eyes)	Sleep [0004] as evidenced by • Describes one or two factors that cause insomnia • Identifies two or three measures that induce sleep • Verbalizes decreased irritability and a greater sense of well-being by day 21 • Recognizes his coping patterns by day 7 • Identifies effective new and old coping strategies by day 10

continued on page 1128

NURSING CARE PLAN FOR REST AND SLEEP *continued*

NURSING INTERVENTIONS [NIC #] / SELECTED ACTIVITIES*	RATIONALE
Sleep Enhancement [1850]	
• Determine the client's sleep and activity pattern	*The amount of sleep an individual needs varies with lifestyle, health, and age.*
• Encourage Mr. Harrison to establish a bedtime routine to facilitate transition from wakefulness to sleep	*Rituals and routines induce comfort, relaxation, and sleep.*
• Encourage him to eliminate stressful situations before bedtime	*Stress interferes with a person's ability to relax, rest, and sleep.*
• Instruct Mr. Harrison and significant others about factors (e.g., physiologic, psychologic, lifestyle, frequent work shift changes, excessively long work hours, and other environmental factors) that contribute to sleep pattern disturbances.	*Knowledge of causative factors can enable the client to begin to control factors that inhibit sleep.*
• Discuss with Mr. Harrison and his family comfort measures, sleep-promoting techniques, and lifestyle changes that can contribute to optimal sleep	*Knowledge of factors that affect sleep enables the client to implement changes in lifestyle and pre-bedtime activities.*
• Monitor bedtime food and beverage intake for items that facilitate or interfere with sleep	*Milk and protein foods contain tryptophan, a precursor of serotonin, which is thought to induce and maintain sleep. Stimulants should be avoided because they inhibit sleep.*
Security Enhancement [5380]	
• Discuss specific situations or individuals that threaten Mr. Harrison or his family	*Fear is reduced when the reality of a situation is confronted in a safe environment. Awareness of factors that cause intensification of fears enhances control.*
• Help Mr. Harrison and his family identify what factors increase their sense of security	*Stress and anxiety can increase a person's risk of stress-related illness. If unable to remove the stressor, the individual can be taught to change ways of responding.*
• Assist him to use coping responses that have been successful in the past	*Feelings of safety and security increase when an individual identifies previously successful ways of dealing with anxiety-provoking or fearful situations.*
Anxiety Reduction [5820]	
• Create an atmosphere that facilitates trust	*Trust is an essential first step in the therapeutic relationship.*
• Seek to understand Mr. Harrison's perspective of a stressful situation	*Anxiety is a feeling aroused by a vague, nonspecific threat. Identifying the client's perspective will facilitate planning for the best approach to anxiety reduction.*
• Encourage verbalization of feelings, perceptions, and fears	*Open expression of feelings facilitates identification of specific emotions such as anger or helplessness, distorted perceptions, and unrealistic fears.*
• Help Mr. Harrison identify situations that precipitate anxiety	*Describing what the person experienced immediately prior to feeling anxious, and identifying associated events, will enable the client to prevent or recognize his anxiety in order to initiate problem solving.*
• Determine the client's decision-making ability	*Maladaptive coping mechanisms are characterized by an inability to make decisions and choices.*

EVALUATION

Outcome met. Mr. Harrison acknowledges his insomnia is a somatic expression of his anxiety regarding job promotion and fear of failing. He states that talking with the police department counselor has been helpful. He is practicing relaxation techniques each night and sleeps an average of 7 hours a night. Mr. Harrison expresses a greater sense of well-being.

---

* Outcomes, interventions, and activities selected are only a sample of those suggested by NOC and NIC and should be further individualized for each client.

Applying Critical Thinking

1. Explain why keeping a sleep diary might be beneficial for Mr. Harrison.
2. What further information would be helpful to obtain from him about his sleep problem?
3. What suggestions can you make that may help him develop better sleep habits?

4. What evidence suggests that Mr. Harrison is experiencing a primary as opposed to a secondary sleep disorder?
5. What are the most common problems that interfere with clients' ability to sleep?

See Critical Thinking Possibilities in Appendix A.

CONCEPT MAP 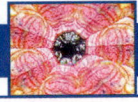 Rest and Sleep

JH
36 y.o. ♂

- Police officer high-crime precinct. Bullet wound to arm 1 week ago. Recently promoted to detective. C/O increasing difficulty falling asleep and sometimes staying asleep. Concern over danger of his occupation and desire to do well in new position. C/O waking up feeling tired and irritable.

- Height: 185.4 cm (6' 2")
- Weight: 85.7 kg (189 lb)
- Temperature: 37.0C (98.6F)
- Pulse rate: 80 BPM
- Respirations: 18/minute
- Blood pressure: 144/88 mm Hg
- Pale, drawn, with dark circles under eyes

- CBC within normal range, x-ray left arm: evidence of superficial soft tissue injury

Sleep Pattern Disturbance r/t anxiety (aeb difficulty falling and remaining asleep, fatigue, irritability, drawn facial appearance, dark circles under eyes)

Sleep aeb
- describes one or two factors that cause insomnia
- identifies two or three measures that induce sleep
- verbalizes decreased irritability and a greater sense of well-being by day 21
- recognizes his coping patterns by day 7
- identifies effective new and old coping strategies by day 10

Anxiety Reduction

Create an atmosphere that facilitates trust

Help him identify situations that precipitate anxiety

Seek to understand his perspective of a stressful situation

Determine his decision-making ability

Encourage verbalization of feelings, perceptions, and fears

Sleep Enhancement

Determine the client's sleep and activity pattern

Monitor bedtime food and beverage intake for items that facilitate or interfere with sleep

Encourage to establish a bedtime routine to facilitate transition from wakefulness to sleep

Discuss with the client and his family comfort measures, sleep-promoting techniques, and lifestyle changes that can contribute to optimal sleep

Encourage to eliminate stressful situations before bedtime

Instruct the client and significant others about factors (e.g., physiologic, psychologic, lifestyle, frequent work shift changes, excessively long work hours, and other environmental factors) that contribute to sleep pattern disturbances

Outcome met
- acknowledges his insomnia is a somatic expression of his anxiety regarding job promotion and fear of failing
- states that talking with the police department counselor has been helpful
- practicing relaxation techniques each night and sleeps an average of 7 hours a night
- expresses a greater sense of well-being

Legend: Assessment ☐ Nursing Diagnosis ☐ Outcomes ☐ Nursing Interventions ☐ Activities ☐ Evaluation/Reassessment ☐

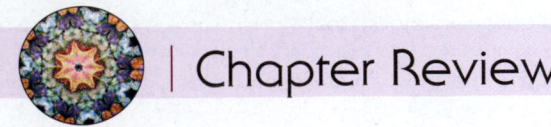

Chapter Review

EXPLORE MediaLink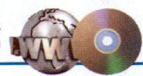

NCLEX review questions, case studies, care plan activities, MediaLink applications, and other interactive resources for this chapter can be found on the Companion Website at www.prenhall.com/kozier. Click on Chapter 43 to select the activities for this chapter.

For more NCLEX review questions, and an audio glossary, access the Student CD-ROM accompanying this textbook.

Chapter Highlights

- Sleep is a naturally occurring altered state of consciousness in which a person's perception and reaction to the environment are decreased.
- Rest and sleep are restorative, protective, and energy conserving.
- The sleep cycle is controlled by specialized areas in the brain stem and is affected by the individual's circadian rhythm.
- During a normal night's sleep, an adult has four to six sleep cycles, each with NREM (quiet sleep) and REM (rapid eye movement) sleep.
- NREM (slow-wave) sleep consists of four stages, progressing from Stage I, very light sleep, to Stage IV, deep sleep. NREM sleep constitutes most of a sleep cycle.
- REM sleep recurs about every 90 minutes, is less restful than NREM sleep, and is often associated with dreaming.
- The ratio of NREM to REM sleep varies with age.

- Many factors can affect sleep, including illness, environment, fatigue, lifestyle, emotional stress, stimulants and alcohol, diet, smoking, motivation, and medications.
- Common sleep disorders include parasomnias (such as bruxism, nocturnal enuresis, sleeptalking, and somnambulism), insomnia, hypersomnia, narcolepsy, sleep apnea, and sleep deprivation.
- Assessment of a client's sleep includes obtaining a sleep history, reviewing a sleep diary, and conducting a physical examination to detect signs of sleep deprivation.
- Nursing responsibilities to help clients sleep include (a) teaching clients ways to enhance sleep and rest, (b) supporting bedtime rituals, (c) creating a restful environment, (d) promoting comfort and relaxation, and (e) using prescribed sleep medications.
- Nonpharmacologic interventions to induce and maintain sleep are always the preferred interventions.

Review Questions

43–1. A client in whom REM sleep predominates over non-REM sleep will most likely
  a. be very relaxed.
  b. have a lowered blood pressure.
  c. feel poorly rested.
  d. be easily awakened.

43–2. The nurse is caring for a client with a history of sleep apnea. It would be common for assessment to also indicate
  a. cardiac irregularities.
  b. nasal obstruction.
  c. chest pain.
  d. insomnia.

43–3. An elderly client complains of difficulty sleeping due to worry over finances. Which of the following would be an appropriate goal for the nursing care plan? "By day 5,
  a. the client will sleep 8 to 10 hours per day."
  b. the client will express feeling adequately rested."
  c. the client will have a plan to pay all the bills."
  d. the client will keep busy until bedtime to decrease thinking about financial problems."

43–4. While performing back massage, the nurse demonstrates proper technique when
  a. Pouring the lotion directly onto the client's skin.
  b. Using the fingertips to perform the stroking motions.
  c. Using firm, continuous pressure.
  d. Continuing the massage for at least 15 minutes.

43–5. A client reports to the nurse taking barbiturate sleeping pills every night for several months and now wishes to stop taking them. The nurse advises the client to
  a. take the last pill on a Friday night so disrupted sleep can be compensated on the weekend.
  b. continue to take the pills since sleeping without them after such a long time will not be possible.
  c. discontinue taking the pills completely all at one time.
  d. begin by skipping the pills every third night then tapering to every other night before completely stopping.

Readings and References

Suggested Readings

Beck-Little, R., & Weinrich, S. P. (1998). Assessment and management of sleep disorders in the elderly. *Journal of Gerontological Nursing, 24*(4), 21–29.
The authors explain that sleep disorders are rarely diagnosed in the elderly. They can affect falling asleep or maintaining sleep or cause excessive sleepiness in the daytime. The authors explain three types of disorders: dyssomnias, parasomnias, and medical-psychiatric sleep disorders. Assessment and interventions are also included.

Redeker, N. S. (2000). Sleep in acute care settings: An integrative review. *Journal of Nursing Scholarship, 32,* 31–38.
The author reviewed the literature on the sleep of hospitalized adults from 1971 to 1999. The findings are organized by correlates of sleep: patient characteristics (symptoms, age, gender, primary sleep disorders) and environmental factors (noise, light, and disruptions), outcomes of sleep, and challenges to studying sleep in this population.

Related Research

Richards, K. C., Sullivan, S. C., Phillips, R. L., Beck, C. K., & Overton-McCoy, A. L. (2001). The effect of individualized activities on sleep. *Journal of Gerontological Nursing, 27*(9), 30–37.

References

American Sleep Disorders Association. (1997). *The international classification of sleep disorders: Diagnostic and coding manual.* Lawrence, KS: Allen Press.

Emerson, R. W. (1932). *Uncollected lectures.* New York: W. E. Rudge.

Gauthier, D. M. (1999). The healing potential of back massage. *Online Journal of Knowledge Synthesis for Nursing, 6*(5). Retrieved May 16, 2003 from http://www.stti.inpui.edu/library/ojksn/abstracts/060005.htm

Johnson, M., Maas, M., & Moorhead, S. (Eds.). (2000). *Nursing outcomes classification (NOC)* (2nd ed.). St. Louis, MO: Mosby.

Kripke, D. F., Garfinkel, L., Wingard, D. L., Klauber, M. R., & Marler, M. R. (2002). Mortality associated with sleep duration and insomnia. *Archives of General Psychiatry, 59*(2), 131–136.

McCloskey, J. C., & Bulechek, G. M. (Eds.). (2000). *Nursing interventions classification (NIC)* (3rd ed.). St. Louis, MO: Mosby.

NANDA International. (2003). *NANDA nursing diagnoses: Definitions and classification 2003-2004.* Philadelphia: Author.

Orr, W. C. (2000). Editorial: Sleep and functional bowel disorders: Can bad bowels cause bad dreams? *American Journal of Gastroenterology, 95,* 1118–1121.

Rowe, M., & Alfred, D. (1999). The effectiveness of slow-stroke massage in diffusing agitated behaviors in individuals with Alzheimer's disease. *Journal of Gerontological Nursing, 25,* 2234.

Vitiello, M. V. (1999). Effective treatments for age-related sleep disturbances. *Geriatrics, 54,* 47–52.

Selected Bibliography

Anonymous. (2001). Nontraditional choices: Trying therapeutic massage. *Nursing, 31*(6), 26.

Aaronson, L. S., Teel, C. S., Cassmeyer, V., Neuberger, G. B., Pallikkathayil, L., Pierce, J., et al. (1999). Defining and measuring fatigue. *Image: Journal of Nursing Scholarship, 31,* 45–50.

Barroso, J. (2002). HIV-related fatigue. *American Journal of Nursing, 102*(5), 83–86.

Davis, K. (2002). Symptomatic treatment of restless legs syndrome. *Patient Care, 36*(8), 10.

Dines-Kalinowski, C. M. (2002). Dream weaver. *Nursing Management, 33*(4), 48–49.

Farella, C. (2002). Quiet riot: Newborn ICUs pump up the care and turn down the volume. *Nursing Spectrum, 3*(6), 16W–17W.

Giron, M. S. T., Forsell, Y., Bernsten, C., Thorslund, M., Winblad, B., & Fastbom, J. (2002). Sleep problems in a very old population: Drug use and clinical correlates. *Journal of Gerontology Series A: Biological Sciences and Medical Sciences, 57,* M236–240.

Hoffart, M. B., & Keene, E. P. (1998). The benefits of visualization. *American Journal of Nursing, 98*(12), 44–47.

Kreiger, A. C., & Redeker, N. S. (2002). Obstructive sleep apnea syndrome: Its relationship with hypertension. *The Journal of Cardiovascular Nursing, 17,* 1–11.

Montgomery, L., Haynes, L. C., & Garner, A. F. (2002). An unusual sleep disorder. *RN, 65*(4), 41–43.

Morin, C. M., Mimeault, V., & Gagné, A. (1999). Nonpharmacological treatment of late-life insomnia. *Journal of Psychosomatic Research, 46,* 103–116.

Stansberry, T. T. (2001). Narcolepsy: Unveiling a mystery. *American Journal of Nursing, 101*(8), 50–53.

Yantis, M. A. (2002). Obstructive sleep apnea. *American Journal of Nursing, 102*(6), 83, 85.

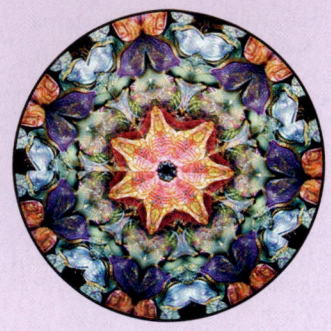

CHAPTER 44

PAIN MANAGEMENT

LEARNING OUTCOMES

After completing this chapter, you will be able to:

- Identify types and categories of pain according to location, etiology, and duration.

- Differentiate pain threshold from pain tolerance.

- Describe the four processes involved in nociception and how pain interventions can work during each process.

- Describe the gate control theory and its application to nursing care.

- Identify subjective and objective data to collect and analyze when assessing pain.

- Identify examples of nursing diagnoses for clients with pain.

- State outcome criteria by which to evaluate a client's response to interventions for pain.

- Identify barriers to effective pain management.

- Describe pharmacologic interventions for pain.

- Define tolerance, dependence, and addiction.

- Describe the World Health Organization's ladder step approach to cancer pain.

- Identify rationales for using various analgesic delivery routes.

- Describe nonpharmacologic pain control interventions.

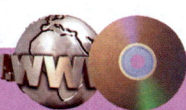

MediaLink

www.prenhall.com/kozier

Additional resources for this chapter can be found on the Student CD-ROM accompanying this textbook, and on the Companion Website at www.prenhall.com/kozier. Click on Chapter 44 to select the activities for this chapter.

CD-ROM
- Audio Glossary
- NCLEX Review

Companion Website
- Additional NCLEX Review
- Case Study: Treating a Client with Stomach Cancer
- Care Plan Activity: Treating Chronic Back Pain
- MediaLink Application: The Mayday Pain Project
- Links to Resources

Pain is a highly unpleasant and very personal sensation that cannot be shared with others. It can occupy all of a person's thinking, direct all activities, and change a person's life. Yet pain is a difficult concept for a client to communicate. A nurse can neither feel nor see a client's pain.

No two people experience pain in exactly the same way. In addition, the differences in individual pain perception and reaction, as well as the many causes of pain, present the nurse with a complex situation when developing a plan to relieve pain and provide comfort. Effective pain management is an important aspect of nursing care.

Pain is more than a symptom of a problem; it is a high-priority problem in itself. Pain presents both physiologic and psychologic dangers to health and recovery. Severe pain is viewed as an emergency situation deserving attention and prompt treatment.

THE NATURE OF PAIN

Although pain is a universal experience, its exact nature remains a mystery. It is known that pain is highly subjective and individual and that it is one of the body's defense mechanisms that indicate a problem. Unrelieved pain presents both physiologic and psychologic dangers to health and recovery. McCaffery defines **pain** as "whatever the experiencing person says it is, existing whenever he (or she) says it does" (McCaffery & Pasero, 1999, p. 5). Basic to this definition is the care provider's willingness to believe that the client is experiencing pain and that the client is the real authority on that pain.

Types of Pain

Pain may be described in terms of duration, location, or etiology. When pain lasts only through the expected recovery period, it is described as **acute pain,** whether it has a sudden or slow onset and regardless of the intensity. **Chronic pain,** on the other hand, is prolonged, usually recurring or persisting over 6 months or longer, and interferes with functioning. Chronic pain can be further classified as chronic malignant pain, when associated with cancer or other life-threatening conditions, or as chronic nonmalignant pain when the etiology is a nonprogressive disorder. Acute and chronic pain result in different physiologic and behavioral responses, as shown in Table 44–1.

Pain can be categorized according to its origin as cutaneous, deep somatic, or visceral. **Cutaneous pain** originates in the skin or subcutaneous tissue. A paper cut causing a sharp pain with some burning is an example of cutaneous pain. **Deep somatic pain** arises from ligaments, tendons, bones, blood vessels, and nerves. It is diffuse and tends to last longer than cutaneous pain. An ankle sprain is an example of deep somatic pain. **Visceral pain** results from stimulation

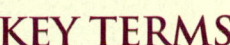

TABLE 44–1 Comparison of Acute and Chronic Pain

Acute Pain	Chronic Pain
Mild to severe	Mild to severe
Sympathetic nervous system responses:	Parasympathetic nervous system responses:
Increased pulse rate	Vital signs normal
Increased respiratory rate	
Elevated blood pressure	
Diaphoresis	Dry, warm skin
Dilated pupils	Pupils normal or dilated
Related to tissue injury; resolves with healing	Continues beyond healing
Client appears restless and anxious	Client appears depressed and withdrawn
Client reports pain	Client often does not mention pain unless asked
Client exhibits behavior indicative of pain: crying, rubbing area, holding area	Pain behavior often absent

of pain receptors in the abdominal cavity, cranium, and thorax. Visceral pain tends to appear diffuse and often feels like deep somatic pain, that is, burning, aching, or a feeling of pressure. Visceral pain is frequently caused by stretching of the tissues, ischemia, or muscle spasms. For example, an obstructed bowel will result in visceral pain.

Pain may also be described according to where it is experienced in the body. **Radiating pain** is perceived at the source of the pain and extends to nearby tissues. For example, cardiac pain may be felt not only in the chest but also along the left shoulder and down the arm. **Referred pain** is pain felt in a part of the body that is considerably removed from the tissues causing the pain. For example, pain from one part of the abdominal viscera may be perceived in an area of the skin remote from the organ causing the pain (Figure 44–1 ■).

Intractable pain is pain that is highly resistant to relief. One example is the pain from an advanced malignancy. When caring for a client experiencing intractable pain, nurses are challenged to use a number of methods, pharmacologic and nonpharmacologic, to provide the client with pain relief.

Neuropathic pain is the result of current or past damage to the peripheral or central nervous system and may not have a stimulus, such as tissue or nerve damage, for the pain. Neuropathic pain is long lasting, unpleasant, and can be described as burning, dull, and aching; episodes of sharp, shooting pain can also be experienced (Hawthorn & Redmond, 1998).

Phantom pain, which is a painful sensation perceived in a body part that is missing (e.g., an amputated leg) or paralyzed by a spinal cord injury, is an example of neuropathic pain. This can be distinguished from *phantom sensation,* that is, the feeling that the missing body part is still present. The incidence of phantom pain can be reduced when analgesics are administered via epidural catheter prior to the amputation.

Certain major pain syndromes have been identified to describe conditions associated with prolonged or severe pain. Common pain syndromes include peripheral pain syndromes, central pain syndromes, and pain with underlying pathology syndromes (see Box 44–1).

Concepts Associated with Pain

When an individual perceives pain from injured tissue, the pain threshold is reached. An individual's **pain threshold** is the amount of pain stimulation a person requires in order to feel pain. People's pain threshold is generally fairly uniform; however, it can change. For example, the same stimuli that once produced mild pain can at another time produce intense pain. Excessive sensitivity to pain is called **hyperalgesia.**

Two additional terms used in the context of pain are pain sensation and pain reaction. **Pain sensation** can be considered the same as pain threshold; **pain reaction** includes the autonomic nervous system and behavioral responses to pain. The autonomic nervous system response is the automatic reaction of the body that often protects the individual from further harm, for example, the automatic withdrawal of the hand from a hot stove. The behavioral response is a learned response used as a method of coping with the pain.

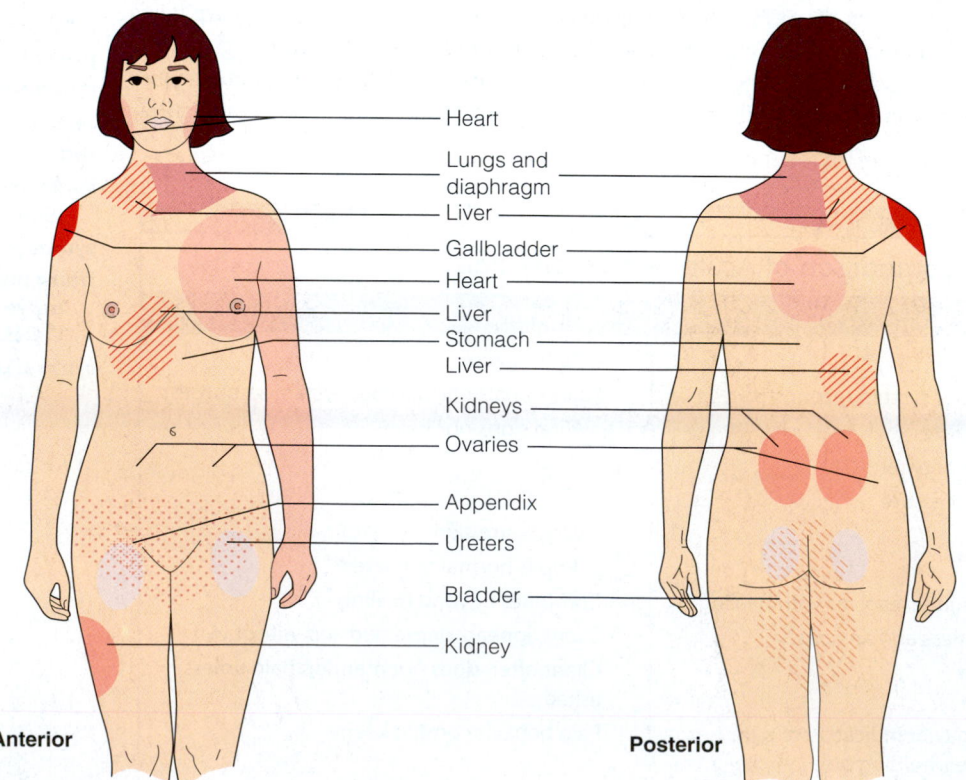

Heart
Lungs and diaphragm
Liver
Gallbladder
Heart
Liver
Stomach
Liver
Kidneys
Ovaries
Appendix
Ureters
Bladder
Kidney

Anterior

Posterior

Figure 44–1 ■ Common sites of referred pain from various body organs.

BOX 44–1   ■ Common Pain Syndromes

Peripheral Pain Syndromes

- Postherpetic neuralgia. An episode of herpes has two phases: a vesicular eruption and neuralgic pain that often encircles the body. The pain ranges from mild to severe. In the postherpetic syndrome, severe pain persists for months or years with lightning-like pain in the area of the original eruption.
- Phantom limb pain. Can occur in anyone who has had a body part amputated. The pain may be severe and is often described as a burning, crushing, or cramping sensation.

Central Pain Syndromes

- Trigeminal neuralgia. This is an intense stablike pain that is distributed by one or more branches of the trigeminal nerve (5th cranial). The pain is usually experienced on parts of the face and head; for example, gums, eye, cheek, and surface of the head.

Pain with Underlying Pathology Syndromes

- Headache. This common somatic pain can be caused by either intracranial or extracranial problems. To establish a plan to prevent or treat headache, the nurse needs to assess the quality, location, onset, duration, and frequency of the pain, as well as any signs and symptoms that precede the headache.
- Cancer pain syndrome. These syndromes can result from the progression of the disease or from efforts to cure or control the disease.
- Myofascial pain syndrome. This pain occurs in the muscles and fascia. It is characterized by muscle spasm, tenderness, stiffness, limitation of movement, and weakness. The pain is often described as dull or aching, and the intensity varies from severe and disabling to mild.

Pain tolerance is the maximum amount and duration of pain that an individual is willing to endure. Some clients are unable to tolerate even the slightest pain, whereas others are willing to endure severe pain rather than be treated for it. Thus pain tolerance varies greatly among people and is widely influenced by psychologic and sociocultural factors.

PHYSIOLOGY OF PAIN

How pain is transmitted and perceived is still incompletely understood. Whether pain is perceived and to what degree depend on the interaction between the body's analgesia system and the nervous system's transmission and interpretation of stimuli.

Nociception

The peripheral nervous system includes primary sensory neurons specialized to detect tissue damage and to evoke the sensation of touch, heat, cold, pain, and pressure. The receptors that transmit pain sensation are called **nociceptors.** These pain receptors or nociceptors can be excited by mechanical, thermal, or chemical stimuli (see Table 44–2). The physiologic processes related to pain perception are described as **nociception.** Four processes are involved in nociception: transduction, transmission, perception, and modulation (Paice, 2002).

Transduction

During the transduction phase, noxious stimuli (tissue injury) trigger the release of biochemical mediators (e.g., prostagladins, bradykinin, serotonin, histamine, substance P) that sensitize nociceptors. Noxious or painful stimulation also causes movement of ions across cell membranes, which excites nociceptors. Pain medications can work during this phase by blocking the production of prostaglandin (e.g., ibuprofen) or by decreasing the movement of ions across the cell membrane (e.g., local anesthetic).

Transmission

The second process of nociception, transmission of pain, includes three segments (McCaffery & Pasero, 1999). During the

---

TABLE 44–2 Types of Pain Stimuli

Stimulus Type	Physiologic Basis of Pain
Mechanical	
1. Trauma to body tissues (e.g., surgery)	Tissue damage; direct irritation of the pain receptors; inflammation
2. Alterations in body tissues (e.g., edema)	Pressure on pain receptors
3. Blockage of a body duct	Distention of the lumen of the duct
4. Tumor	Pressure on pain receptors; irritation of nerve endings
5. Muscle spasm	Stimulation of pain receptors (also see chemical stimuli)
Thermal	
Extreme heat or cold (e.g., burns)	Tissue destruction; stimulation of thermosensitive pain receptors
Chemical	
1. Tissue ischemia (e.g., blocked coronary artery)	Stimulation of pain receptors because of accumulated lactic acid (and other chemicals, such as bradykinin and enzymes) in tissues
2. Muscle spasm	Tissue ischemia secondary to mechanical stimulation (see above)

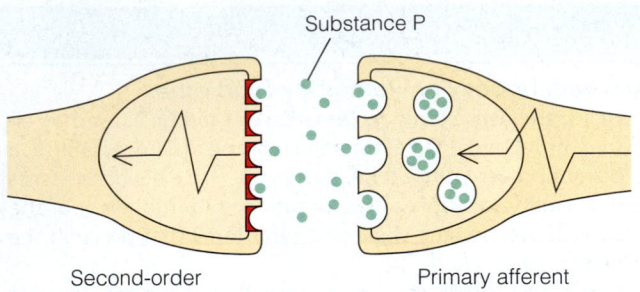

Substance P

Second-order   Primary afferent

Figure 44–2 ■ Substance P assists the transmission of impulses across the synapse from the primary afferent neuron to a second-order neuron in the spinothalamic tract.

first segment, the pain impulse travels from the peripheral nerve fibers to the spinal cord. Substance P serves as a neurotransmitter, enhancing the movement of impulses across the nerve synapse from the primary afferent neuron to the second-order neuron in the dorsal horn of the spinal cord (Figure 44–2 ■). Two types of nociceptor fibers cause this transmission to the dorsal horn of the spinal cord: C fibers, which transmit dull, aching pain, and A-delta fibers, which transmit sharp, localized pain. The second segment is transmission from the spinal cord, and ascension, via spinothalamic tracts, to the brain stem and thalamus (Figure 44–3 ■). The third segment involves trans-

mission of signals between the thalamus to the somatic sensory cortex where pain perception occurs.

Pain control can take place during this second process of transmission. For example, opioids (narcotics) block the release of neurotransmitters, particularly substance P, which stops the pain at the spinal level.

Perception

The third process, perception, is when the client becomes conscious of the pain. It is believed that pain perception occurs in the cortical structures, which allows for different cognitive-behavioral strategies to be applied to reduce the sensory and affective components of pain (McCaffery & Pasero, 1999, p. 22). For example, nonpharmacologic interventions such as distraction, guided imagery, and music can help direct the client's attention away from the pain.

Modulation

Often described as the "descending system," this fourth process occurs when neurons in the brain stem send signals back down to the dorsal horn of the spinal cord (Paice, 2002, p. 75). These descending fibers release substances such as endogenous opioids, serotonin, and norepinephrine, which can inhibit the ascending noxious (painful) impulses in the dorsal horn. These neurotransmitters, however, are taken back by the

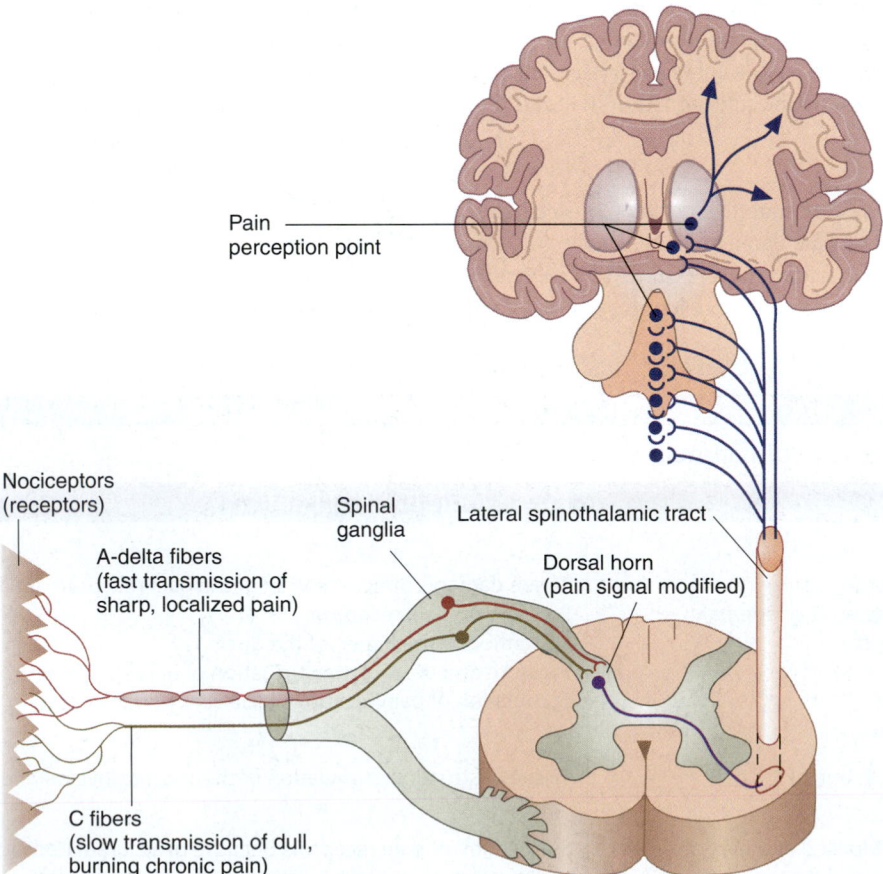

Pain perception point

Nociceptors (receptors)

A-delta fibers (fast transmission of sharp, localized pain)

Spinal ganglia

Lateral spinothalamic tract

Dorsal horn (pain signal modified)

C fibers (slow transmission of dull, burning chronic pain)

Figure 44–3 ■ Physiology of pain perception.

body, which limits their analgesic usefulness (McCaffery & Pasero, 1999). Clients with chronic pain may be prescribed tricyclic antidepressants, which inhibit the reuptake of norepinephrine and serotonin. This action increases the modulation phase that helps inhibit painful ascending stimuli.

Gate Control Theory

According to Melzack and Wall's gate control theory (1965), peripheral nerve fibers carrying pain to the spinal cord can have their input modified at the spinal cord level before transmission to the brain. Synapses in the dorsal horns act as gates that close to keep impulses from reaching the brain or open to permit impulses to ascend to the brain.

Small-diameter nerve fibers carry pain stimuli through a gate, but large-diameter nerve fibers going through the same gate can inhibit the transmission of those pain impulses—that is, close the gate (Figure 44–4 ■). The gate mechanism is thought to be situated in the substantia gelatinosa cells in the dorsal horn of the spinal cord. Because a limited amount of sensory information can reach the brain at any given time, certain cells can interrupt the pain impulses. The brain also appears to influence whether the gate is open or closed. For example, previous experiences with pain are known to affect the way an individual responds to pain. The involvement of the brain helps explain why painful stimuli are interpreted differently by people. Although the gate control theory is not unanimously accepted, it does help explain why electrical and mechanical interventions as well as heat and pressure can relieve pain. For example, a back massage may stimulate impulses in large nerves, which in turn close the gate to back pain.

Responses to Pain

The body's response to pain is a complex process rather than a specific action. It has both physiologic and psychosocial aspects. Initially the sympathetic nervous system responds, resulting in the fight-or-flight response. As pain continues, the body adapts as the parasympathetic nervous system takes over, reversing many of the initial physiologic responses. This adaptation to the pain occurs after several hours or days of pain. The actual pain receptors adapt very little and continue to transmit the pain message. The person may learn to cope with the pain through cognitive and behavioral activities, such as diversions, imagery, and excessive sleeping. The individual may respond to pain by seeking out physical interventions to manage the pain, such as analgesics, massage, and exercise.

A proprioceptive reflex also occurs with the stimulation of pain receptors. Impulses travel along sensory pain fibers to the spinal cord. There they synapse with motor neurons, and the impulses travel back via motor fibers to a muscle near the site of the pain (Figure 44–5 ■). The muscle then contracts in a protective action. For example, when a person touches a hot stove the hand reflexively draws back from the heat even before the person is aware of the pain.

Factors Affecting the Pain Experience

Numerous factors can affect a person's perception of and reaction to pain. These include the person's ethnic and cultural

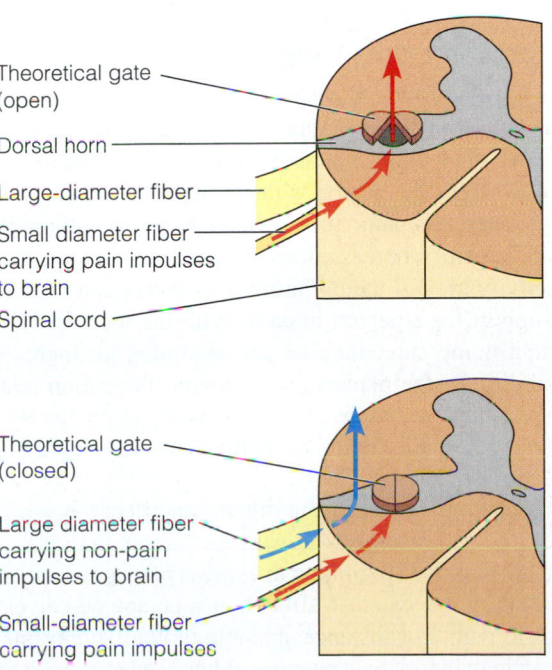

Theoretical gate (open)

Dorsal horn

Large-diameter fiber

Small diameter fiber carrying pain impulses to brain

Spinal cord

Theoretical gate (closed)

Large diameter fiber carrying non-pain impulses to brain

Small-diameter fiber carrying pain impulses

Figure 44–4 ■ A schematic illustration of the gate control theory.

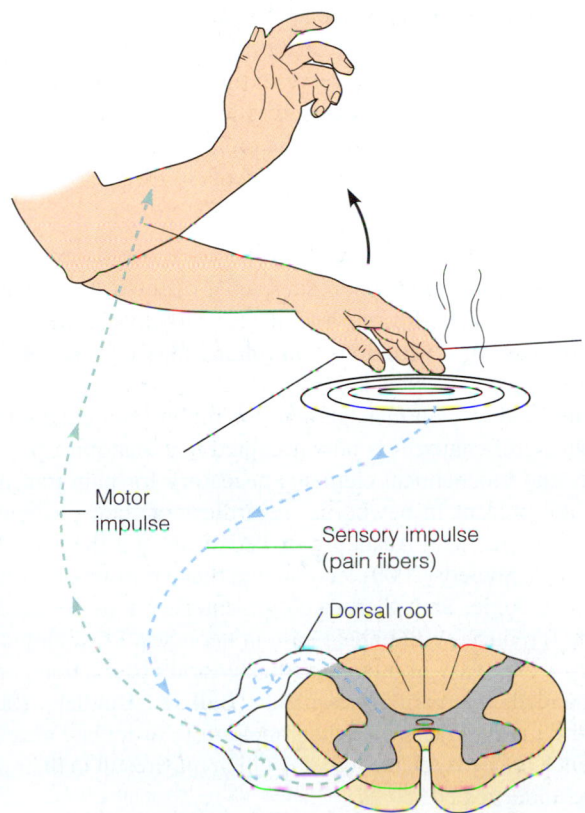

Motor impulse

Sensory impulse (pain fibers)

Dorsal root

Figure 44–5 ■ Proprioceptive reflex to a pain stimulus.

values, developmental stage, environment and support people, previous pain experiences, and the meaning of the current pain, as well as anxiety and stress.

Ethnic and Cultural Values

Ethnic background and cultural heritage have long been recognized as factors that influence both a person's reaction to pain and the expression of that pain. Behavior related to pain is a part of the socialization process. For example, individuals in one culture may have learned to be expressive about pain, whereas individuals from another culture may have learned to keep those feelings to themselves and not bother others.

Although there appears to be little variation in pain threshold, cultural background can affect the level of pain that an individual is willing to tolerate. In some Middle Eastern and African cultures, self-infliction of pain is a sign of mourning or grief. In other groups, pain may be anticipated as part of the ritualistic practices, and therefore tolerance of pain signifies strength and endurance. Additionally, there are significant variations in the expression of pain. Studies have shown that individuals of northern European descent tend to be more stoic and less expressive of their pain than individuals from southern European backgrounds.

Nurses must realize they have their own attitudes and expectations about pain. Andrews and Boyle (2003) point out that health care has been dominated by white Anglo-Saxon Protestants and most nurses have been influenced by these values and beliefs. For example, nurses may place a higher value on silent suffering or self-control in response to pain. Nurses expect people to be objective about pain and to be able to provide a detailed description of the pain. Nurses may deny or downplay the pain they observe in others (p. 410). Therefore, identifying your own personal attitude about pain and creating an effective nurse–client relationship is imperative for providing culturally competent care for clients in pain.

Developmental Stage

The age and developmental stage of a client is an important variable that will influence both the reaction to and the expression of pain. Age variations and related nursing interventions are presented in Table 44–3.

The field of pain management for infants and children has grown significantly. It is now accepted that anatomic, physiologic, and biochemical elements necessary for pain transmission are present in newborns, regardless of their gestational age. The American Academy of Pediatrics and the Canadian Paediatric Society (2000) recommend that environmental, non-pharmacologic, and pharmacologic interventions be used to prevent, reduce, or eliminate pain in neonates. Physiologic indicators may vary in infants, so behavioral observation is recommended for pain assessment (Ball & Bindler, 2003). Children may be less able than an adult to articulate their experience or needs related to pain, which may result in their pain being undertreated.

Elders constitute a major portion of the individuals within the health care system. The prevalence of pain in the older population is generally higher due to both acute and chronic dis-

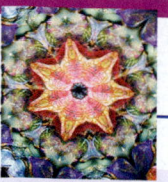

Providing Culturally Competent Care

CLIENTS IN PAIN

Nurses are in a position of power as they decide whether to believe the client's subjective report of pain. It is, therefore, important to develop an effective, positive relationship with the client, a relationship that incorporates the caring behaviors of
- Respecting clients as individuals by
  - Recognizing that clients can hold different beliefs about pain.
  - Inquiring about the client's beliefs and ways of coping with pain.
- Respecting the client's response to pain by
  - Recognizing that clients have the right to respond to pain in the way they learned is appropriate.
  - Recognizing that expressions of pain vary widely and no expression is good or bad.
- Never stereotyping a person on the basis of culture because expressions of pain vary between cultures and within cultures.

Note: From *Transcultural Concepts in Nursing Care,* 4th ed. (pp. 409–411), by M. M. Andrews and J. S. Boyle, 2003, Philadelphia: Lippincott Williams & Wilkins. Adapted with permission.

ease conditions. Pain threshold does not appear to change with aging, although the effect of analgesics may increase due to physiologic changes related to drug metabolism and excretion (Eliopoulos, 2001).

Environment and Support People

A strange environment such as a hospital, with its noises, lights, and activity, can compound pain. In addition, the lonely person who is without a support network may perceive pain as severe, whereas the person who has supportive people around may perceive less pain. Some people prefer to withdraw when they are in pain, whereas others prefer the distraction of people and activity around them. Family caregivers can be a significant support for a person in pain. With the increase in outpatient and home care, families are assuming an increased responsibility for the management of pain. Education related to the assessment and management of pain can positively affect the perceived quality of life for both clients and their caregivers (McCaffery & Pasero, 1999).

Expectations of significant others can affect a person's perceptions of and responses to pain. In some situations, for example, girls may be permitted to express pain more openly than boys. Family role can also affect how a person perceives or responds to pain. For instance, a single mother supporting three children may ignore pain because of her need to stay on the job. The presence of support people often changes a client's reaction to pain. For example, toddlers often tolerate pain more readily when supportive parents or nurses are nearby.

TABLE 44–3 Age Variations in the Pain Experience

Age Group	Pain Perception and Behavior	Selected Nursing Interventions
Infant	Perceives pain. Responds to pain with increased sensitivity. Older infant tries to avoid pain; for example, turns away and physically resists.	Give a glucose pacifier. Use tactile stimulation. Play music or tapes of a heartbeat.
Toddler and preschooler	Develops the ability to describe pain and its intensity and location. Often responds with crying and anger because child perceives pain as a threat to security. Reasoning with child at this stage is not always successful. May consider pain a punishment. Feels sad. May learn there are gender differences in pain expression. Tends to hold someone accountable for the pain.	Distract the child with toys, books, pictures. Involve the child in blowing bubbles as a way of "blowing away the pain." Appeal to the child's belief in magic by using a "magic" blanket or glove to take away pain. Hold the child to provide comfort. Explore misconceptions about pain.
School-age child	Tries to be brave when facing pain. Rationalizes in an attempt to explain the pain. Responsive to explanations. Can usually identify the location and describe the pain. With persistent pain, may regress to an earlier stage of development.	Use imagery to turn off "pain switches." Provide a behavioral rehearsal of what to expect and how it will look and feel. Provide support and nurturing.
Adolescent	May be slow to acknowledge pain. Recognizing pain or "giving in" may be considered weakness. Wants to appear brave in front of peers and not report pain.	Provide opportunities to discuss pain. Provide privacy. Present choices for dealing with pain. Encourage music or TV for distraction.
Adult	Behaviors exhibited when experiencing pain may be gender-based behaviors learned as a child. May ignore pain because to admit it is perceived as a sign of weakness or failure. Fear of what pain means may prevent some adults from taking action.	Deal with any misconceptions about pain. Focus on the client's control in dealing with the pain. Allay fears and anxiety when possible.
Elder	May have multiple conditions presenting with vague symptoms. May perceive pain as part of the aging process. May have decreased sensations or perceptions of the pain. Lethargy, anorexia, and fatigue may be indicators of pain. May withhold complaints of pain because of fear of the treatment, of any lifestyle changes that may be involved, or of becoming dependent. May describe pain differently, that is, as "ache," "hurt," or "discomfort." May consider it unacceptable to admit or show pain.	Thorough history and assessment is essential. Spend time with the client and listen carefully. Clarify misconceptions. Encourage independence whenever possible.

Past Pain Experiences

Previous pain experiences alter a client's sensitivity to pain. People who have personally experienced pain or who have been exposed to the suffering of someone close are often more threatened by anticipated pain than people without a pain experience. In addition, the success or lack of success of pain relief measures influences a person's expectations for relief. For example, a person who has tried several pain relief measures without success may have little hope about the helpfulness of nursing interventions.

Meaning of Pain

Some clients may accept pain more readily than others, depending on the circumstances and the client's interpretation of its significance. A client who associates the pain with a positive outcome may withstand the pain amazingly well. For example,

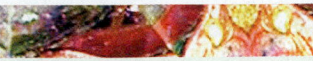

Lifespan Considerations

Elders

Elders often have multiple conditions that present with vague symptoms, making it difficult to determine the exact cause or causes of pain and the appropriate treatment. A thorough history and assessment by the nurse is important in providing information for a pain management program.

The old adage of "start low and go slow" is especially important when ordering dosages and pain medications for older adults. Decreased renal and liver function is a common change related to aging and increases the risk of toxicity from pain medications in older clients. In particular, risk of renal damage from NSAIDS increases, so dosages and lab work need to be carefully monitored related to renal function.

Changes in nerve transmission and vascular changes with aging may cause a variation in the pain sensation. Sometimes the pain is decreased and if neuropathy is present pain may increase or a different kind of pain may be experienced.

In some situations, pain presents itself with atypical symptoms, such as confusion, restlessness, or irritability. This is especially true in clients with dementia who cannot express themselves.

Maintaining optimal function is especially crucial for a high quality of life in older adults. If pain is not effectively controlled, the following areas are often affected in their daily lives:

- Activity tolerance
- Mobility
- Ability to socialize
- Sleep disturbance
- Ability to perform activities of daily living
- Ability to remain as independent as possible.

All efforts, pharmacologic and nonpharmacologic, should be used to help provide pain management and achieve and maintain functional ability. Involvement of the client and family is important when working with the physician, pharmacist, and nurse to plan which treatment is most appropriate and most acceptable to the client.

---

a woman giving birth to a child or an athlete undergoing knee surgery to prolong his career may tolerate pain better because of the benefit associated with it. These clients may view the pain as a temporary inconvenience rather than a potential threat or disruption to daily life.

By contrast, clients with unrelenting chronic pain may suffer more intensely. They may respond with despair, anxiety, and depression because they cannot attach a positive significance or purpose to the pain. In this situation, the pain may be looked on as a threat to body image or lifestyle and as a sign of possible impending death.

Anxiety and Stress

Anxiety often accompanies pain. The threat of the unknown and the inability to control the pain or the events surrounding it often augment the pain perception. Fatigue also reduces a person's ability to cope, thereby increasing pain perception. When pain interferes with sleep, fatigue and muscle tension often result and increase the pain; thus a cycle of pain–fatigue–pain develops. People in pain who believe that they have control of their pain have decreased fear and anxiety, which decreases their pain perception. A perception of lacking control or a sense of helplessness tends to increase pain perception. Clients who are able to express pain to an attentive listener and participate in pain management decisions can increase a sense of control and decrease pain perception.

NURSING MANAGEMENT

ASSESSING

Accurate pain assessment is essential for effective pain management. Many health facilities are making pain assessment the **fifth vital sign.** The strategy of linking pain assessment to routine vital sign assessment and documentation ensures pain

assessment for all clients. Because pain is subjective and experienced uniquely by each individual, nurses need to assess all factors affecting the pain experience—physiologic, psychologic, behavioral, emotional, and sociocultural.

The extent and frequency of the pain assessment varies according to the situation. For clients experiencing acute or severe pain, the nurse may focus only on location, quality, severity, and early intervention. Clients with less severe or chronic pain can usually provide a more detailed description of the experience. Frequency of pain assessment usually depends on the pain control measures being used and the clinical circumstances. For example, in the initial postoperative period, pain is often assessed whenever vital signs are taken, which may be as often as every 15 minutes and then extended to every 2 to 4 hours. Following pain management interventions, pain intensity should be reassessed at an interval appropriate for the intervention. For example, following the intravenous administration of morphine, the severity of pain should be reassessed in 20 to 30 minutes.

Because it has been found that many people will not voice their pain unless asked about it, pain assessments must be initiated by the nurse. Some of the many reasons clients may be reluctant to report pain are listed in Box 44–2. It is also essential that nurses listen to and rely on the client's perceptions of pain. Believing the person experiencing and conveying the perceptions is crucial in establishing a sense of trust.

Pain assessments consist of two major components: (a) a pain history to obtain facts from the client and (b) direct observation of behavioral and physiologic responses of the client. The goal of assessment is to gain an objective understanding of a subjective experience. Box 44–3 provides helpful mnemonics to make a complete pain assessment.

Pain History

While taking pain histories, the nurse must provide an opportunity for clients to express in their own words how they view the pain and the situation. This will help the nurse understand

BOX 44–2 ■ Why Clients May Be Reluctant to Report Pain

- Unwillingness to trouble staff who are perceived as busy
- Fear of the injectable route of analgesic administration—children in particular
- Belief that pain is to be expected as part of the recovery process
- Belief that pain is a normal part of aging or a necessary part of life—older adults in particular
- Belief that expressions of pain reveal weakness
- Difficulty expressing personal discomfort
- Concern about risks associated with opioid drugs (e.g., addiction)
- Fear about the cause of pain or that reporting pain will lead to further tests and expenses
- Concern about unwanted side effects, especially of opioid drugs
- Concern that use of drugs now will render the drug inefficient if or when the pain becomes worse

BOX 44–3 ■ Mnemonics for Pain Assessment

OLDCART mnemonic
O—onset
L—location
D—duration
C—characteristic
A—aggravating factors
R—radiation
T—treatment (what was previously ineffective and what has alleviated the pain)

PQRST mnemonic
P—provoked (what brought about pain)
Q—quality
R—region/radiation
S—severity
T—timing

Note: From "Undertreated Pain: Could It Land You in Court?" by S. LaDuke, 2002, *Nursing, 32,* p. 18. Reprinted with permission.

what the pain means to the client and how the client is coping with it. Remember that each person's pain experience is unique and that the client is the best interpreter of the pain experience. This history should be geared to the specific client: For example, questions asked of an accident victim would be different from those asked of a postoperative client or one suffering from chronic pain. The initial pain assessment for someone in severe acute pain may consist of only a few questions before intervention occurs. In addition, the nurse may focus on the following:

- Previous pain treatment and effectiveness
- When and what analgesics were last taken
- Other medications being taken
- Allergies to medications.

For the person with chronic pain, the nurse may focus on the client's coping mechanisms, effectiveness of current pain management, and ways in which the pain has affected activities of daily living (ADLs).

Data that should be obtained in a comprehensive pain history include pain location, intensity, quality, patterns, precipitating factors, alleviating factors, associated symptoms, effect on ADLs, past pain experiences, meaning of the pain to the person, coping resources, and affective responses. Questions to elicit this data are shown in the Assessment Interview.

Assessment Interview

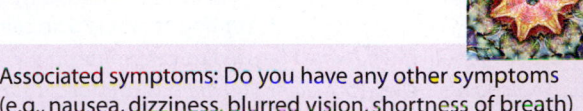

PAIN HISTORY

- Location: Where is your pain?
- Intensity: On a scale of 0 to 10 (with 1 representing the lowest pain level), how would you rate the degree of discomfort you are having?
- Quality: Tell me what your pain feels like.
- Pattern
  a. Time of onset: When did or does the pain start?
  b. Duration: How long have you had it, or how long does it usually last?
  c. Constancy: Do you have pain-free periods? When? And for how long?
- Precipitating factors: What triggers the pain or makes it worse?
- Alleviating factors: What measures or methods have you found helpful in lessening or relieving the pain? What pain medications do you use?

- Associated symptoms: Do you have any other symptoms (e.g., nausea, dizziness, blurred vision, shortness of breath) before, during, or after your pain?
- Effects on ADLs: How does the pain affect your daily life (e.g., eating, working, sleeping, and social and recreational activities)?
- Past pain experiences: Tell me about past pain experiences you have had and the effectiveness of pain relief measures.
- Meaning of pain: How do you interpret your pain? What outcomes (implications) do you anticipate from this pain? What do you fear most about your pain?
- Coping resources: What do you usually do to help cope with pain?
- Affective response: How does the pain make you feel? Anxious? Depressed? Frightened? Tired? Burdensome?

Location. To ascertain the specific location of the pain, ask the individual to point to the site of the discomfort. A chart consisting of drawings of the body can assist in identifying pain locations. The client marks the location of pain on the chart. This tool can be especially effective with clients who have more than one source of pain.

When assessing the location of a child's pain, the nurse needs to understand the child's vocabulary. For example, *tummy* might refer either to the abdomen or to part of the chest. Asking the child to point to the pain helps clarify the child's word usage to identify location. Again the use of figure drawings can assist in identifying pain locations. Parents can also be helpful in interpreting the meaning of a child's words.

When documenting pain location the nurse may use various body landmarks. Further clarification is possible with the use of terms such as *proximal, distal, medial, lateral,* and *diffuse.*

Pain Intensity or Rating Scales. *The single most important indicator of the existence and intensity of pain is the client's report of pain.* In practice, however, McCaffery, Ferrell, and Pasero (2000) found that nurses tend to use less reliable measures for assessing pain. The top factors identified by nurses were culturally influenced (e.g., facial expressions, verbalization, request for relief). In addition, studies have shown that health care providers may underrate or overrate the pain intensity (Bergh & Sjostrom, 1999). The use of pain intensity scales is an easy and reliable method of determining the client's pain intensity. Such scales provide consistency for nurses to communicate with the client and other health care providers. Most scales use either a 0 to 5 or 0 to 10 range with 0 indicating "no pain" and the highest number indicating the "worst pain possible" for that individual. A 10-point rating scale is shown in Figure 44–6 ■. The inclusion of word modifiers on the scale can assist some clients who find it difficult to apply a number level to their pain. The client is asked to indicate the scale point that best represents the pain intensity. The American Pain Society suggests that pain become the fifth vital sign, that is, that the nurse make pain intensity rating a part of the assessment and documentation of the client's vital signs (McCaffery & Pasero, 1999).

> ► **CLINICAL ALERT** *Perception is reality. The client's self-report of pain is what must be used to determine pain intensity. If you do not believe the client, you are basically accusing the client of lying, which is an adversarial rather than an advocacy relationship.* ■

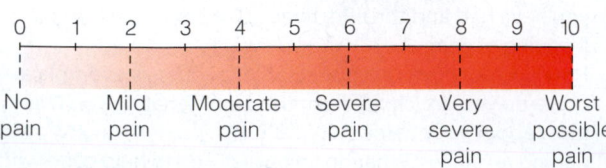

Figure 44–6 ■ A 10-point pain intensity scale with word modifiers.

When noting pain intensity it is important to determine any related factors that may be affecting the pain. When the intensity changes, the nurse needs to consider the possible cause. For example, the abrupt cessation of acute abdominal pain may indicate a ruptured appendix. Several factors affect the perception of intensity: (1) the amount of distraction, or the client's concentration on another event; (2) the client's state of consciousness; (3) the level of activity; and (4) the client's expectations.

Not all clients can understand or relate to numerical pain intensity scales. These include children who are unable to communicate discomfort verbally, elderly clients with impairments in cognition or communication, and people who do not speak English. For these clients the Wong-Baker FACES Rating Scale (Figure 44–7 ■) may be easier to use (Wong, Hockenberry-Eaton, Wilson, Winkelstein, & Schwartz, 2001). The face scale includes a number scale in relation to each expression so that the pain intensity can be documented. When it is not possible to use any kind of rating scale with a client, the nurse must rely on observation of behavior and any physiologic cues discussed later in this section. The input of the client's significant others, such as parents or caregivers, can assist the nurse in interpreting the observations. An objective description of the behavior and physiologic data is then documented.

For effective use of pain rating scales, clients need not only to understand the use of the scale but also to be educated about how the information will be used to determine changes in their condition and the effectiveness of pain management interventions. Clients should also be asked to indicate what level of comfort is acceptable so that they can perform specific activities (Acello, 2000). This will ensure that adequate pain management is achieved.

The use of a pain rating scale together with a pain flowsheet (Figure 44–8 ■) has been shown to be effective in improving pain management (McCaffery & Pasero, 1999). Documentation can be completed by the nurse, the client, or a caregiver and can be used in acute, outpatient, and home care settings.

> ► **CLINICAL ALERT** *A guideline based on studies: On a scale of 0 to 10, a pain rating of 3 or greater signals a need to revise the pain treatment plan (e.g., higher dose or different analgesia). A rating of 6 or more demands immediate attention (McCaffery & Pasero, 1999, pp. 74–75).* ■

Pain Quality. Descriptive adjectives help people communicate the quality of pain. A headache may be described as "hammerlike" or an abdominal pain as "piercing like a knife." Sometimes clients have difficulty describing pain because they have never experienced any sensation like it. Some of the terms commonly used to describe pain are listed in Table 44–4.

Nurses need to record the exact words clients use to describe pain. A client's words are more accurate and descriptive than an interpretation in the nurse's words. Exact information can be significant in both the diagnosis of the pain etiology and in the

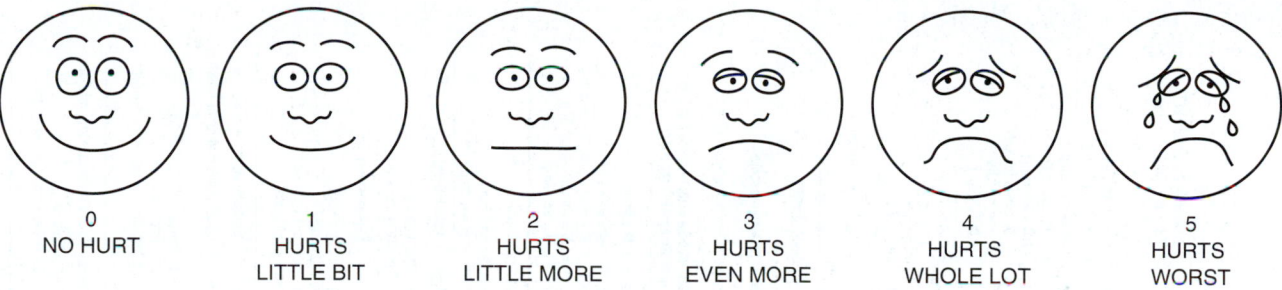

0
NO HURT

1
HURTS
LITTLE BIT

2
HURTS
LITTLE MORE

3
HURTS
EVEN MORE

4
HURTS
WHOLE LOT

5
HURTS
WORST

Explain to the person that each face is for a person who feels happy because he has no pain (hurt) or sad because he has some or a lot of pain. Face 0 is very happy because he doesn't hurt at all. Face 1 hurts just a little bit. Face 2 hurts a little more. Face 3 hurts even more. Face 4 hurts a whole lot. Face 5 hurts as much as you can imagine, although you don't have to be crying to feel this bad. Ask the person to choose the face that best describes how he is feeling.

Rating scale is recommended for persons age 3 years and older.

Brief word instructions: Point to each face using the words to describe the pain intensity. Ask the child to choose the face that best describes own pain and record the appropriate number.

Figure 44–7 ■ The Wong-Baker FACES Rating Scale. (*Note:* From *Wong's Essentials of Pediatric Nursing,* 6th ed. (p.1301), by D. L. Wong, M. Hockenserry-Eaton, D. Wilson, M. L. Winkelstein, and P. Schwartz, 2001, St. Louis, MO: Mosby. Reprinted with permission.)

treatment choices made. For example, pain described as hot, electrical, and sharp tends to be neuropathic in origin and will be more responsive to anticonvulsants (e.g., Tegretol) than an opioid (e.g., morphine).

Pattern. The pattern of pain includes time of onset, duration, and recurrence or intervals without pain. The nurse therefore determines when the pain began; how long the pain lasts; whether it recurs and, if so, the length of the interval without pain; and when the pain last occurred.

Precipitating Factors. Certain activities sometimes precede pain. For example, physical exertion may precede chest pain, or abdominal pain may occur after eating. These observations can help prevent pain and determine its cause.

Environmental factors such as extreme cold or heat and extremes of humidity can affect some types of pain. For example, sudden exercise on a hot day can cause muscle spasm.

Physical and emotional stressors can also precipitate pain. Emotional tension frequently brings on a migraine headache. Intense fear or physical exertion can cause angina.

Alleviating Factors. Nurses must ask clients to describe anything that they have done to alleviate the pain (e.g., home remedies such as herbal teas, medications, rest, applications of heat or cold, prayer, or distractions like TV). It is important to explore the effect any of these measures had on the pain, whether or not relief was obtained, or whether the pain became worse.

Associated Symptoms. Also included in the clinical appraisal of pain are associated symptoms such as nausea, vomiting, dizziness, and diarrhea. These symptoms may relate to the onset of the pain or they may result from the presence of the pain.

Effect on Activities of Daily Living. Knowing how ADLs are affected by chronic pain helps the nurse understand the client's perspective on the pain's severity. The nurse asks the client to describe how the pain has affected the following aspects of life:

- Sleep
- Appetite
- Concentration
- Work/school
- Interpersonal relationships
- Marital relations/sex
- Home activities
- Driving/walking
- Leisure activities
- Emotional status (mood, irritability, depression, anxiety).

Sunrise Hospital and Medical Center & Sunrise Children's Hospital
Pain Management Flow Sheet

SR-1420 (6/00)

*Monitoring Guidelines outlined on back of form

Patient's stated pain level goal: _____

Mode of Administration
A-PO opioid and nonopioid medications
B-PCA Infuser Basal with Patient Control
C-Continuous Infusion
D-Epidural Infuser Continuous Basal Only
E-Epidural Infuser Basal & Patient Control
F-Intermittent IV/IM Injection
G-Transdermal opioids
H-On-QPump
I-Per Rectum

Level of Pain Assessment Scales
Faces Pain Rating Scale
0   2   4   6   8   10

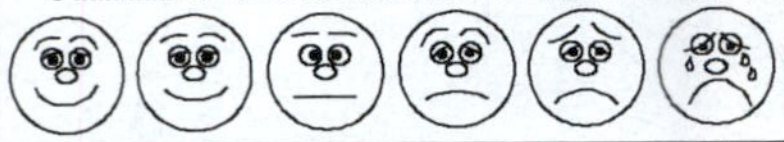

1-10 Pain Scale
0 -------------- 10
No pain or pain relieved   Worst pain imaginable

0-10 Sum Scale

A. Vocal
0 = Positive/ETT
1 = Whimpers
2 = Crying
3 = Screaming

C. Facial
0 = Smiling
1 = Neutral
2 = Frown/grimace
3 = Clenched teeth

B. Body Movement
0 = Moves easily
1 = Neutral shifting
2 = Tense/flailing limbs

D. Touching (localizing)
0 = Notouching
1 = Reaching/patting
2 = Grabbing

Location of Pain:
Right   Left   Left   Right

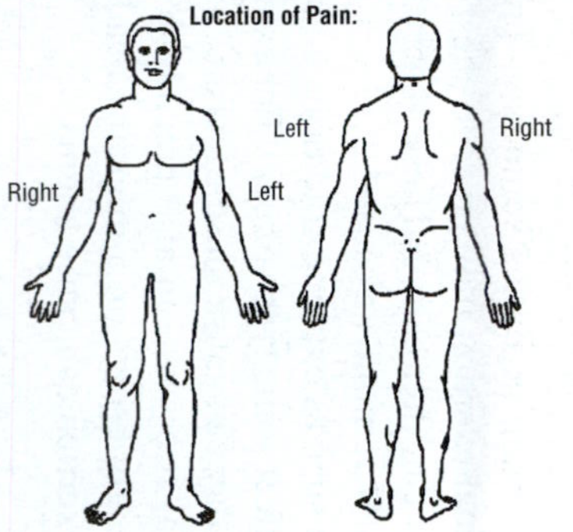

A = No pain
B-Z = Use letters to mark location of pain on graph

Frequency of Pain:
O = Occasional   F = Frequent   C = Constant

Type of Pain:
A = Burning   D = Sharp   G = Isolated
B = Stabbing   E = Shooting   H = Other
C = Radiating   F = Dull

Arousal Score:
0 = Alert   1 = Medically sedated/ETT
2 = Drowsy   3 = Somnolent
4 = Asleep

Non-Pharmacologic Interventions L
C = Cold   P = Pacifier
D = Distraction   PO = Positioning
H = Heat   R = Relaxation
HO = Holding   RO = Rocking
I = Imagery   S = Security/Object
M = Massage   T = Tens/Unit
MU = Music   O = Other

Analgesia Order:
1 = Increase in dosage/rate
2 = Decrease in doseage/rate
3 = Extra bolus
4 = PRN medication for break-through pain
5 = Discontinue

Reason for Analgesia Order:
1 = Unrelieved pain
2 = Decreased arousal/neuroscore
3 = Side effects (Seebelow)
4 = Discontinue therapy/change to oral route
5 = Adverse drug reactions
(Document all adverse drug reactions in Nsg notes and complete an ADR report)

Side Effects:
0 = None
A = Anxiety   N = Nausea
C = Confused   R = Respiratory Depression
Co = Constipation   U = Urinary Rentention
I = Itching   V = Vomiting

Sensory Function   Epidural Only
0 = Moves all extremities well
1 = Unable to move all extremities well

Motor Function   Epidural Only
0 = Able to feel tactile pressure
1 = Unable to feel tactile pressure

Neuro Score: Epidural Only
0 = No numbness, no weakness
1 = Medically sedated/ETT
2 = Numbness with out weakness
3 = Numbness and weakness

Catheter Site: Epidural Only
1 = No redness, drainage, inflammation or swelling
2 = Red, inflamed
3 = Visable clear drainage
4 = Visable purulent drainage
5 = Visable serosanguinous/sanguinous drainage
6 = Swelling

Catheter Integrity Upon Removal: Epidural Only
1 = Catheter tip visually intact
2 = Catheter NOT visually intact-See Nsg Notes

Date	
Time	
Initials	
Mode of Admin	
Level of Pain	
Location of Pain	
Frequency of Pain	
Type of Pain	
Arousal Score	
Non-Pharm. Intervent.	
Analgesia Order	
Reason for Order	
Side Effects	
Adverse Effects (Y/N)	
Sensory Function Epidural Only	
Motor Function Epidural Only	
Neuro Score Epidural Only	
Catheter Site Epidural Only	
Cath Integrity Epidural Only	
O2 Saturation	
Respirations	
Pulse	
Blood Pressure	
See Nursing Notes (Y/N)	

Initials	Signature

Patient Identification Label

Figure 44–8 ■ Pain Management Flow Sheet. (Courtesy of Aprille Ciaverella, RN and Lori Townsend, RN at Sunrise Hospital and Medical Center and Sunrise Children's Hospital, Las Vegas, Nevada.)

Research Note
Is There a Valid and Reliable Pain-Intensity Scale for Use with Black Older-Adults?

The authors point out that the older adult population experiences twice as much pain as the younger population. Additionally, the older adult population is growing and becoming more racially, ethnically, and culturally diverse. Studies have addressed the reliability and validity of various pain assessment tools; however, most did not include or included only a few minority subjects. The focus of the Taylor and Herr (2002) research was to evaluate the reliability and validity of the Faces Pain Scale (FPS) developed by Bieri, Reeve, Champion, Addicoat, and Ziegler (1990). The FPS is used with children and the authors tested to see whether it would be a useful tool for use with Black older adults. The FPS was chosen over other faces scales because the facial depictions were less childlike, the absence of tears avoided potential cultural bias, and a neutral face is used to represent no pain instead of a happy face.

The study focused on four psychometric analyses of construct validity, scale properties, concurrent validity, and test–retest reliability. The 39 Black older adults agreed that the faces represented pain. However, they also agreed that the faces represented other constructs such as sadness, anger, and sourness. Based on these findings the authors believe the FPS may measure overall pain as well as pain intensity.

Implications: Continued research is needed to validate the usefulness of the FPS and other pain-intensity measures. It is important for nurses to use valid and reliable assessment tools for all clients.

Note: From "Evaluation of the FACES Pain Scale with Minority Older Adults," by L. J. Taylor and K. Herr, 2002, *Journal of Gerontological Nursing, 27(4),* pp. 15–23.

TABLE 44–4 Commonly Used Pain Descriptors

Term	Sensory Words	Affective Words
Pain	Searing	Unbearable
	Scalding	Killing
	Sharp	Intense
	Piercing	Torturing
	Drilling	Agonizing
	Wrenching	Terrifying
	Shooting	Exhausting
	Burning	Suffocating
	Crushing	Frightful
	Penetrating	Punishing
		Miserable
Hurt	Hurting	Heavy
	Pricking	
	Pressing	
	Tender	Throbbing
Ache	Numb	Annoying
	Cold	Nagging
	Flickering	Tiring
	Radiating	Troublesome
	Dull	Gnawing
	Sore	Uncomfortable
	Aching	Sickening
	Cramping	Tender

A rating scale of none, a little, or a great deal or another range can be used to determine the degree of alteration.

Coping Resources. Each individual will exhibit personal ways of coping with pain. Strategies may relate to earlier pain experiences or the specific meaning of the pain; some may reflect religious or cultural influences. Nurses can encourage and support the client's use of methods known to have helped in modifying pain. Strategies may include withdrawal, distraction, prayer or other religious practices, and support from significant others.

Affective Responses. Affective responses vary according to the situation, the degree and duration of pain, the interpretation of it, and many other factors. The nurse needs to explore the client's feelings of anxiety, fear, exhaustion, depression, or a sense of failure. Because many people with chronic pain become depressed and potentially suicidal, it may also be necessary to assess the client's suicide risk. In such situations, the nurse needs to ask the client, "Do you ever feel so bad that you want to die? Do you feel that way now?"

Observation of Behavioral and Physiologic Responses

There are wide variations in nonverbal responses to pain. For clients who are very young, aphasic, confused, or disoriented, nonverbal expressions may be the only means of communicating pain. Facial expression is often the first indication of pain, and it may be the only one. Clenched teeth, tightly shut eyes, open somber eyes, biting of the lower lip, and other facial grimaces may be indicative of pain. Vocalizations like moaning and groaning or crying and screaming are sometimes associated with pain.

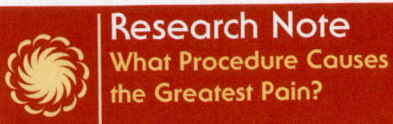

Research Note
What Procedure Causes the Greatest Pain?

Data were compiled from a multicenter study (Puntillo et al., 2001) in which more than 6,000 critically ill clients, ranging from 4 to 97, participated. Six procedures commonly experienced by acutely ill or critically ill clients were examined: turning, wound drain removal, tracheal suctioning, femoral catheter removal, placement of central venous catheter, and changing of nonburn wound dressings. Instruments included numerical rating scales for pain intensity and word lists for pain character.

The results showed that turning was the most painful to adults 18 and older, wound care was most distressing to adolescents (13 to 17 years old), and tracheal suctioning was most painful to children 8 to 12 years old. The authors noted that turning and suctioning were done frequently, and often without prior analgesia.

Implications: The intensity and distress caused by procedural pain varies depending on the specific procedure. The nurse can prevent or greatly reduce this kind of pain by providing preemptive pain control. The authors remark that because of the frequency with which procedures are done on acutely and critically ill clients, more directed, individualized attention to preparation for and control of procedural pain is warranted (p. 250).

Note: From "Patients' Perceptions and Reponses to Procedural Pain: Results from Thunder Project II," by K. A. Puntillo, et al., 2001, *American Journal of Critical Care, 10*, pp. 238–251.

Immobilization of the body or a part of the body may also indicate pain. The client with chest pain often holds the left arm across the chest. A person with abdominal pain may assume the position of greatest comfort, often with the knees and hips flexed, and moves reluctantly.

Purposeless body movements can also indicate pain—for example, tossing and turning in bed or flinging the arms about. Involuntary movements such as a reflexive jerking away from a needle inserted through the skin indicate pain. An adult may be able to control this reflex; however, a child may be unable or unwilling to do so.

Rhythmic body movements or rubbing may indicate pain. An adult or child may assume a fetal position and rock back and forth when experiencing abdominal pain. During labor a woman may massage her abdomen rhythmically with her hands.

It is important to note that behavioral responses can be controlled and so may not be very revealing. When pain is chronic there are rarely overt behavioral responses because the individual develops personal coping styles for dealing with pain, discomfort, or suffering.

Physiologic responses vary with the origin and duration of the pain. Early in the onset of acute pain the sympathetic nervous system is stimulated, resulting in increased blood pressure, pulse rate, respiratory rate, pallor, diaphoresis, and pupil dilation. The body does not sustain the increased sympathetic func-

tion over a prolonged period of time and, therefore, the sympathetic nervous system adapts, making the physiologic responses less evident or even absent. Physiologic responses are most likely to be absent in people with chronic pain because of central nervous system (CNS) adaptation. Thus, it is important that the nurse assess more than only physiologic responses, because they may be poor indicators of pain.

Daily Pain Diary

For clients who experience chronic pain, a daily diary may help the client and nurse identify pain patterns and factors that exacerbate or mediate the pain experience. In home care the family or other caregiver can be taught to complete the diary. The record can include

- Time or onset of pain
- Activity before pain
- Pain-related positions or behaviors
- Pain intensity level
- Use of analgesics or other relief measures
- Duration of pain
- Time spent in relief activities.

Recorded data can provide the basis for developing or modifying the plan for care. For this tool to be effective, it is important that the nurse educate the client and family about the value and use of the diary in achieving effective pain control. Determining the client's abilities to use the diary is essential.

DIAGNOSING

NANDA includes the following diagnostic labels for clients experiencing pain or discomfort:

- *Acute Pain*
- *Chronic Pain.*

When writing the diagnostic statement, the nurse should specify the location (e.g., right ankle pain, or left frontal headache). Related factors, when known, must also be part of the diagnostic statement and can include both physiologic and psychologic factors. For example, in addition to the injurious agent, related factors may include deficient knowledge of pain management techniques or fear of drug tolerance or addiction.

Examples of clinical application of these diagnoses using NANDA, NOC, and NIC designations are shown in Identifying Nursing Diagnoses, Outcomes, and Interventions.

Because the presence of pain can affect so many facets of a person's functioning, pain may be the etiology of other nursing diagnoses. Examples of such nursing diagnoses follow:

- *Ineffective Airway Clearance* related to weak cough secondary to postoperative incisional abdominal pain
- *Hopelessness* related to feelings of continual pain
- *Anxiety* related to past experiences of poor control of pain and to anticipation of pain
- *Ineffective Coping* related to prolonged continuous back pain, ineffective pain management, and inadequate support systems

IDENTIFYING NURSING DIAGNOSES, OUTCOMES, AND INTERVENTIONS

CLIENTS EXPERIENCING PAIN

DATA CLUSTER	NURSING DIAGNOSIS/ DEFINITION	SAMPLE DESIRED OUTCOMES [NOC#]/DEFINITION	INDICATORS	SELECTED INTERVENTIONS [NIC#]/DEFINITION	SAMPLE NIC ACTIVITIES
Mary Anderson, 75, fell and broke her right hip while shopping. She had surgery yesterday to repair the fracture. She rates her pain in the surgical site as 6 on a 0–10 scale and states the pain goes up to 9 when she is repositioned in bed. Morphine 10 mg Q4h prn is ordered. She received a dose 5 hours ago. She states, "I try to hold out as long as I can before asking for a pain killer."	Acute Pain/Unpleasant sensory and emotional experience arising from actual or potential tissue damage or described in terms of such damage (International Association for the Study of Pain); sudden or slow onset of any intensity from mild to severe with an anticipated or predictable end and a duration of less than 6 months	Pain Control [1605]/ Personal actions to control pain	Often demonstrated: • Recognizes causal factors • Uses analgesics appropriately • Reports symptoms to health care professional • Reports pain controlled	Analgesic Administration [2210]/Use of pharmacologic agents to reduce or eliminate pain	• Determine pain location, characteristics, quality, and severity before medicating client • Instruct to request prn pain medication before the pain is severe • Attend to comfort needs and other activities that assist relaxation to facilitate response to analgesia • Correct misconceptions/ myths client or family members may hold regarding analgesics, particularly opioids (e.g., addiction and risk of overdose)
Lan Nguyen, 51, was diagnosed with breast cancer 3 years ago and had a metastatic lung tumor removed 6 months ago. She describes prolonged post-thoracotomy pain as "hot, stabbing, and unbearable." Lan states that although she loves sewing and needlepoint she is unable to participate in these activities currently because of the pain.	Chronic Pain/Unpleasant sensory and emotional experience arising from actual or potential tissue damage or described in terms of such damage (International Association for the Study of Pain); sudden or slow onset of any intensity from mild to severe, constant or recurring without an anticipated or predictable end and a duration of greater than 6 months	Comfort Level [2100]/Physical and psychologic ease	Moderate to substantial: • Expressed satisfaction with pain control • Reported satisfaction with level of independence • Reported psychological well-being	Pain Management [1400]/Alleviation of pain or a reduction in pain to a level of comfort that is acceptable to the client	• Assure client attentive analgesic care • Determine the impact of the pain experience on quality of life (e.g., sleep, appetite, activity, cognition, mood, relationships, performance of job, and role responsibilities) • Select and implement a variety of measures (e.g., pharmacologic, non-pharmacologic, interpersonal) to facilitate pain relief, as appropriate • Collaborate with the client, significant other, and other health professionals to select and implement nonpharmacologic pain relief measures, as appropriate • Monitor client satisfaction with pain management at specified intervals

- *Ineffective Health Maintenance* related to chronic pain and fatigue
- *Self-Care Deficit (Specify)* related to poor control of pain
- *Deficient Knowledge (Pain Control Measures)* related to lack of exposure to information resources
- *Impaired Physical Mobility* related to arthritic pain in knee and ankle joints
- *Disturbed Sleep Pattern* related to increased pain perception at night

PLANNING

The established goals for the client will vary according to the diagnosis and its defining characteristics. Specific nursing interventions can be selected to meet the individual needs of the client. Examples of clinical application of NOC outcomes and NIC interventions are shown in Identifying Nursing Diagnoses, Outcomes, and Interventions.

Planning Independent of Setting

When planning, nurses need to choose pain relief measures appropriate for the client, based on the assessment data and input from the client or support persons. Nursing interventions may include a variety of pharmacologic and nonpharmacologic interventions. Developing a plan that incorporates a wide range of strategies is usually most effective. Whether in acute care or in home care, it is important for everyone involved in pain management to understand the plan of care. The plan should be documented in the client's record; in home care, a copy needs to be made available to the client, support persons, and caregivers. Involvement of the client and support persons is essential in pain management.

When the client's pattern and level of pain can be anticipated or is already known, regular or scheduled administration of analgesics can provide a steady serum level. With acute pain, this may be possible in the first 24 to 48 hours following surgery when the client is likely to have pain requiring opioid analgesics. Frequency of administration can be adjusted to prevent pain from recurring. When persistent, continuous pain exists, analgesics should be given around the clock (ATC), with additional as-needed (prn) doses available (Herr, 2002). Nonpharmacologic interventions should also be regularly scheduled. The additional advantage of scheduling measures is that the client spends less time in pain and does not experience the anxiety or fear of the pain recurring.

Planning for Home Care

In preparation for discharge, the nurse needs to determine the client's and family's needs, strengths, and resources. The accompanying Home Care Assessment describes the specific assessment data required when establishing a discharge plan. Using the assessment data, the nurse tailors a teaching plan for the client and family.

IMPLEMENTING

Pain management is the alleviation of pain or a reduction in pain to a level of comfort that is acceptable to the client. It includes two basic types of nursing interventions: pharmacologic and nonpharmacologic. Nursing management of pain consists of both independent and collaborative nursing actions. In general, noninvasive measures may be performed as an independent nursing function, whereas administration of analgesic medications requires a physician's order. However, the decision to administer the prescribed medication is frequently the nurse's, often requiring judgment as to the dose and the time of administration.

Generally speaking, a combination of strategies is best for the client in pain. Sometimes strategies need to be tried and changed until the client obtains effective pain relief. See the Practice Guidelines for individualizing care for clients with pain.

Barriers to Pain Management

Misconceptions and biases can affect pain management. These may involve attitudes of the nurse or the client as well as knowledge deficits. Clients respond to pain experiences based on their culture, personal experiences, and the meaning the pain has for them. For many people, pain is expected and

---

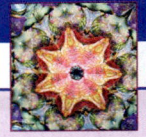

Home Care Assessment

PAIN

Client

- Level of knowledge: Pharmacologic and nonpharmacologic pain relief measures selected; adverse effects and measures to counteract these effects; warning signs to report to health care provider
- Self-care abilities for analgesic administration: Ability to use analgesics appropriately (e.g., to prepare correct dosages of analgesics and adhere to scheduled administration); physical dexterity to take pills or to administer intravenous medications and to store medications safely; and ability to obtain prescriptions or over-the-counter medications at the pharmacy

Family

- Caregiver availability, skills, and willingness: Primary and secondary persons able and willing to assist with pain management; shopping if the client has restricted activity; ability to comprehend selected therapies (e.g., infusion pumps, imagery, massage, positioning, and relaxation techniques) and perform them or assist the client with them as needed
- Family role changes and coping: Effect on financial status, parenting and spousal roles, sexuality, social roles

Community

- Resources: Availability of and familiarity with resources such as supplies, home health aid, or financial assistance

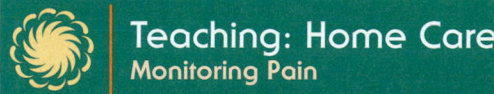

Teaching: Home Care
Monitoring Pain

- Teach client to keep a pain diary to monitor pain onset, activity before pain, pain intensity, use of analgesics or other relief measures, and so on.
- Instruct client to contact a health care professional if planned pain control measures are ineffective.

Pain Control

- Teach the use of preferred and selected nonpharmacologic techniques such as relaxation, guided imagery, distraction, music therapy, massage, and so on.
- Discuss the actions, side effects, dosages, and frequency of administration of prescribed analgesics.
- Suggest ways to handle side effects of medications.
- Provide accurate information about tolerance, physical dependence, and addiction if opioid analgesics are prescribed and these topics are of concern.
- Instruct the client to use pain control measures before the pain becomes severe.
- Inform the client of the effects of untreated pain.
- Demonstrate and have the client or caregiver return demonstrate appropriate skills to administer analgesics (e.g., skin patches, injections, infusion pumps, or patient-controlled analgesia). If a home infusion pump is being used, caregivers need to be able to
  a. Demonstrate stopping and starting the pump.
  b. Change the medication cartridge and tubing.
  c. Adjust the delivery dose.
  d. Demonstrate site care.
  e. Identify signs indicating the need to change an injection site.
  f. Describe care of the pump and insertion site when the client is ambulatory, bathing, sleeping, or traveling.
  g. Perform problem solving for pumps when alarms are activated.
  h. Change the battery.

Resources

- Provide appropriate information about how to access community resources, home care agencies, and associations that offer self-help groups and educational materials.

Practice Guidelines
Individualizing Care for Clients with Pain

- Establish a trusting relationship. Convey your concern, and acknowledge that you believe that the client is experiencing pain. A trusting relationship promotes expression of the client's thoughts and feelings and enhances effectiveness of planned pain therapies.
- Consider the client's ability and willingness to participate actively in pain relief measures. Some clients who are excessively fatigued, are sedated, or have altered levels of consciousness are less able to participate actively. For example, a client with an altered level of consciousness or altered thought processes may not be able to deal with patient-controlled analgesia. In contrast, a fatigued client may express a willingness to use pain-relief measures that require little effort, such as listening to music or performing relaxation techniques.
- Use a variety of pain relief measures. It is thought that using more than one measure has an additive effect in relieving pain. Two measures that should always be part of any pain relief plan are (a) establishing a client–nurse relationship and (b) client teaching. Because a client's pain may vary throughout a 24-hour period, different types of pain relief are often indicated during that time.
- Provide measures to relieve pain before it becomes severe. For example, providing an analgesic before the onset of pain is preferable to waiting for the client to complain of pain, when a larger dose may be required.
- Use pain-relieving measures that the client believes are effective. It has been recognized that clients are the authorities about their own pain. Thus, incorporating the client's measures into a pain relief plan is sensible unless they are harmful.
- Base the choice of pain relief measure on the client's report of the severity of the pain. If a client reports mild pain, an analgesic such as aspirin may be indicated, whereas a client who reports severe pain often requires a more potent relief measure.
- If a pain relief measure is ineffective, encourage the client to try it once or twice more before abandoning it. Anxiety may diminish the effects of a pain measure, and some approaches, such as distraction strategies, require practice before they are effective.
- Maintain an unbiased attitude (open mind) about what may relieve the pain. New ways to relieve pain are continually being developed. It is not always possible to explain pain relief measures; however, measures should be supported unless they are harmful.
- Keep trying. Do not ignore a client because pain persists in spite of measures. In these circumstances, reassess the pain, and consider other relief measures.
- Prevent harm to the client. Pain therapy should not increase discomfort or harm the client. Some pain relief measures may have adverse untoward effects, such as fatigue, but they should not disable the client.
- Educate the client and support people about pain. Clients and support people need to be informed about possible causes of pain, precipitating and alleviating factors, and alternatives to drug therapy. Misconceptions also need to be corrected.

TABLE 44-5 Common Misconceptions about Pain

Misconception	Correction
Clients experience severe pain only when they have had major surgery.	Even after minor surgery, clients can experience intense pain.
The nurse or other health care professionals are the authorities about a client's pain.	The person who experiences the pain is the only authority about its existence and nature.
Administering analgesics regularly for pain will lead to addiction.	Clients are unlikely to become addicted to an analgesic provided to treat pain.
The amount of tissue damage is directly related to the amount of pain.	Pain is a subjective experience, and the intensity and duration of pain vary considerably among individuals.
Visible physiologic or behavioral signs accompany pain and can be used to verify its existence.	Even with severe pain, periods of physiologic and behavioral adaptation can occur.

accepted as a normal aspect of illness. Clients and families may lack knowledge of the adverse effects of pain and may have misinformation regarding the use of analgesics. Clients may not report pain because they expect nothing can be done, they think it is not severe enough, or they feel it would distract or prejudice the health care provider. Other common misconceptions are shown in Table 44-5. Another barrier to effective pain management is the fear of becoming addicted, especially when long-term opioid use is prescribed. This fear is often held by both nurses and clients. It is important that all individuals know the difference between tolerance, dependence, and addiction (see Box 44-4).

BOX 44-4 ■ Definitions

The American Academy of Pain Medicine, the American Pain Society, and the American Society of Addiction Medicine recognize the following definitions and recommend their use.

Addiction
Addiction is a primary, chronic, neurobiologic disease, with genetic, psychosocial, and environmental factors influencing its development and manifestations. It is characterized by behaviors that include one or more of the following: impaired control over drug use, compulsive use, continued use despite harm, and craving.

Physical Dependence
Physical dependence is a state of adaptation that is manifested by a drug class specific withdrawal syndrome that can be produced by abrupt cessation, rapid dose reduction, decreasing blood level of the drug, and/or administration of an antagonist.

Tolerance
Tolerance is a state of adaptation in which exposure to a drug induces changes that result in a diminution of one or more of the drug's effects over time.

Note: From "Definitions Related to the Use of Opioids for the Treatment of Pain," *A Concensus Document from the American Academy of Pain Medicine, the American Pain Society, and the American Society of Addiction Medicine,* © 2001 American Academy of Pain Medicine, American Pain Society and the American Society of Addiction Medicine.

Key Factors in Pain Management

Key factors to strategies to reduce pain include acknowledging and accepting the client's pain, assisting support persons, reducing misconceptions about pain, reducing fear and anxiety, and preventing pain.

Acknowledging and Accepting Client's Pain. Basic to all strategies for reducing pain is that nurses convey to clients that they believe the client is having pain. Consider these four ways of communicating this belief:

1. Verbally acknowledge the presence of the pain. "I understand your leg is very painful. How do you feel about the pain?"
2. Listen attentively to what the client says about the pain.
3. Convey that you are assessing the client's pain to understand it better, not to determine whether the pain is real, for example, "How does your pain feel now?" or "Tell me how it feels compared to an hour ago."
4. Attend to the client's needs promptly.

Strategies to implement when the client's report of pain is not accepted are included in the Practice Guidelines.

> **CLINICAL ALERT** *So what if you are fooled by a client's self-report of pain? By believing everyone, you know that you have helped those who are in pain. You have shown respect by accepting the client's self-report and administered appropriate nursing care.* ■

Assisting Support Persons Support persons often need assistance to respond positively to the client experiencing pain. Nurses can help by giving them accurate information about the pain and providing opportunities for them to discuss their emotional reactions, which may include anger, fear, frustration, and feelings of inadequacy. Enlisting the aid of support persons in the provision of pain relief to the client, such as massaging the client's back, may diminish their feelings of helplessness and foster a more positive attitude toward the client's pain experi-

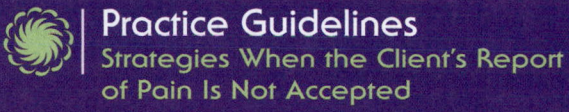

Practice Guidelines
Strategies When the Client's Report of Pain Is Not Accepted

What do we do if the health care team does not respond positively to the client's report of pain?

- Acknowledge that everyone is entitled to a personal opinion, but personal opinion does not form the basis for professional practice.
- Clarify that the sensation of pain is subjective and cannot be proved or disproved.
- Quote recommendations from clinical practice guidelines, especially the American Pain Society and the Agency for Health Care Policy and Research.
- Ask: Why is it so difficult to believe that this person hurts?

Note: From *Pain: Clinical Manual,* 2nd ed. (p. 41), by M. McCaffery and C. Pasero, 1999, St. Louis, MO: Mosby. Reprinted with permission from Elsevier Science.

ence. Support persons also may need the nurse's verbal recognition of their concern and participation in the client's care.

Reducing Misconceptions about Pain. Reducing a client's misconceptions about the pain and its treatment will often avoid intensifying the pain. The nurse should explain to the client that pain is a highly individual experience and that it is only the client who really experiences the pain, although others can understand and empathize. Misconceptions are also dealt with when nurse and client discuss why the pain has increased or decreased at certain times. For example, a client whose pain increases in the evening may mistakenly think this is the result of eating dinner rather than fatigue.

> **► CLINICAL ALERT** *Emphasize to the client the relationship between comfort (pain relief) and being able to function (e.g., cough and deep breathe, ambulate), which is needed to promote recovery. ■*

Reducing Fear and Anxiety. It is important to help relieve the emotional component, that is, anxiety or fear, associated with the pain. When clients have no opportunity to talk about their pain and associated fears, their perceptions and reactions to the pain can be intensified. The client may become angry or complain about the nurse's care when the problem really is a belief that the pain is not being treated. If the nurse is honest and sincere and promptly attends to the client's needs, the client is much more likely to know that the nurse does believe the client is in pain.

By providing accurate information, the nurse can also reduce many of the client's fears, such as a fear of addiction or a fear that the pain will always be present. It also helps many clients to have privacy when they are experiencing pain.

Preventing Pain. A preventive approach to pain management involves the provision of measures to treat the pain before it

occurs or before it becomes severe. **Preemptive analgesia** is the administration of analgesics prior to an invasive or operative procedure in order to treat pain before it occurs. For example, treating clients preoperatively with local infiltration of an anesthetic or parenteral administration of an opioid can reduce postoperative pain. Nurses can also use a preemptive approach by providing an analgesic around the clock (ATC), rather than as needed (prn).

Pharmacologic Pain Management

Pharmacologic pain management involves the use of opioids (narcotics), nonopioids/nonsteroidal anti-inflammatory drugs (NSAIDS), and adjuvants, or coanalgesic drugs (see Box 44–5).

Opioid Analgesics. Opioid (narcotic) analgesics include opium derivatives, such as morphine and codeine. McCaffery and Pasero (1999) state that the term *opioid* is now used rather than *narcotic,* which has become an obsolete term. Narcotic is used primarily in a legal context to refer to a wide variety of substances of potential abuse (p. 130).

Opioids relieve pain and provide a sense of euphoria largely by binding to opiate receptors and activating endogenous (i.e., arising from causes within the body) pain suppression in the CNS. There are several types of opiate receptors, including mu, delta, and kappa receptors. The mu receptor is most commonly associated with pain relief. Changes in mood and attitude and feelings of well-being make the person feel more comfortable even though the pain persists.

BOX 44–5 ■ Categories and Examples of Analgesics

Opioid Analgesics
- Butorphanol (Stadol)
- Fentanyl citrate (Sublimaze)
- Hydrocodone (Lortab, Vicodin)
- Hydromorphone hydrochloride (Dilaudid)
- Meperidine hydrochloride (Demerol)
- Codeine (Tylenol 3, Empirin 3)
- Morphine sulfate (morphine)
- Propoxyphene napsylate (Darvon-N, Darvocet-N)

Nonopioid Analgesics/NSAIDs
- Acetaminophen (Tylenol, Datril)
- Acetylsalicylic acid (aspirin)
- Choline magnesium trisalicylate (Trilisate)
- Diclofenac sodium (Voltaren)
- Ibuprofen (Motrin, Advil)
- Indomethacin sodium trihydrate (Indocin)
- Naproxen (Naprosyn)
- Naproxen sodium (Anaprox)
- Piroxicam (Feldene)
- Tolmetin sodium (Tolectin)

Adjuvant Analgesics
- Amitriptyline (Elavil)
- Chlorpromazine (Thorazine)
- Diazepam (Valium)
- Hydroxyzine (Vistaril)

There are three primary types of opioids:

1. *Full agonists.* These pure opioid drugs bind tightly to mu receptor sites, producing maximum pain inhibition, an agonist effect. A full **agonist analgesic** includes morphine, codeine, meperidine (Demerol), propoxyphene (Darvon), and hydromorphine (Dilaudid). There is no ceiling on the level of analgesia from these drugs; their dose can be steadily increased to relieve pain. There is also no maximum daily dose limit.

2. *Mixed agonists-antagonists.* **Agonist-antagonist analgesic** drugs can act like opioids and relieve pain (agonist effect) when given to a client who has not taken any pure opioids. However, they can block or inactivate other opioid analgesics when given to a client who has been taking pure opioids (antagonist effect). These drugs include dezocine (Dalgan), pentazocine hydrochloride (Talwin), butorphanol tartrate (Stadol), and nalbuphine hydrochloride (Nubain). They block the mu receptor site and activate a kappa receptor site. If a client has been receiving a mu agonist, such as morphine, for pain, the administration of a mixed agonist-antagonist will result in the inactivation of the morphine effect and increase pain. These drugs also have a ceiling dose level. They are not recommended for use with terminally ill clients.

3. *Partial agonists.* Partial agonists have a ceiling effect in contrast to a full agonist. These drugs such as buprenophrine (Buprenex) block the mu receptors or are neutral at that receptor but bind at a kappa receptor site.

When administering any analgesic, the nurse must review side effects. All opioids result in some initial drowsiness when first administered, but with regular administration, this side effect tends to decrease. Opioids also may cause nausea, vomiting, constipation, and respiratory depression. Opioids must be used cautiously in clients with respiratory problems.

> ► CLINICAL ALERT *Constipation is an almost universal adverse effect of opioid use. All clients should receive prophylactic stimulant laxative therapy, unless contraindicated. Inform clients about the following options to prevent constipation: increasing fiber intake, using a mild laxative (e.g., milk of magnesia) regularly, taking oral laxatives at bedtime, and using rectal suppositories in the morning. Remember, stool softeners are not useful in treating constipation unless they are used in combination with stimulant laxatives. ■*

If the client experiences significant respiratory depression (e.g., a drop from 18 to 12) or is overly sedated, the dosage is excessive. The nurse needs to assess a client's level of alertness and respiratory rate for baseline data before administering narcotics. An increasing sedation level can be an early warning sign of impending respiratory depression. (Pasero & McCaffery, 2002). See the sedation rating scale in Box 44–6. Often clients will manifest an increase in sedation *before* they manifest a decrease in respiratory rate and depth. The nurse should assess and document the client's level of sedation at the

---

BOX 44–6   ■ Sedation Scale

S = Sleep, easy to arouse
1 = Awake and alert
2 = Slightly drowsy, easily aroused
3 = Frequently drowsy, arousable, drifts off to sleep during conversation
4 = Somnolent, minimal or no response to physical stimulation

Note: From *Pain: Clinical Manual,* 2nd ed. (p. 267), by M. McCaffery and C. Pasero, 1999, St. Louis, MO: Mosby. Reprinted with permission from Elsevier Science.

---

same time respiratory status is checked. Early recognition of an increasing level of sedation or respiratory depression will enable the nurse to implement appropriate measures promptly (e.g., obtain an order to decrease the opioid dosage). Box 44–7 provides suggested measures to prevent and treat side effects of opioid analgesics.

> ► CLINICAL ALERT *Assessing for sedation and respiratory status is critical during the first 12 to 24 hours after starting opioid therapy. The longer the client receives opioids, the wider the safety margin as the client develops a tolerance to the sedative and respiratory depressive effects of the drug. ■*

Older clients are particularly sensitive to the analgesic properties of opioids and often require less medication than younger clients. This sensitivity may be related to reduced excretion of the drug in elderly clients.

Equianalgesic Dosing. According to McCaffery and Pasero (1999), the term **equianalgesia** means approximately equal analgesia and is used when referring to the doses of various opioid analgesics that provide approximately the same pain relief (p. 240). When individualizing the analgesic regimen it is sometimes beneficial to adjust the dose and the time interval of the doses as well as the route of administration and the exact medication. An equianalgesic chart can be used to help provide doses of approximately equal ability to relieve pain. For example, if a client is receiving Demerol 100 mg IM and experiencing adverse effects, the equianalgesic dose of parenteral morphine is 10 mg q3–4 hours. If a change to PO Dilaudid is indicated, the equianalgesic dose would be 7.5 mg q3–4 hours. It is important for doses and intervals between doses to be titrated according to individual responses. It is also important for the nurse to check the policy of the agency and physicians' orders regarding equianalgesic dosing.

> ► CLINICAL ALERT *Many health care professionals underestimate the effectiveness of ordinary aspirin and acetaminophen. Did you know that two regular aspirin or acetaminophen relieve as much pain as 5 mg of hydrocodone or meperidine 50 mg PO for mild to moderate pain? ■*

BOX 44–7	■ Common Opioid Side Effects, Preventive, and Treatment Measures

Constipation
- Increase fluid intake (e.g., 6 to 8 glasses daily).
- Increase fiber and bulk-forming agents to the diet (e.g., fresh fruits and vegetables).
- Increase exercise regimen.
- Administer stool softeners and if necessary provide a mild laxative.

Nausea and Vomiting
- Inform client that tolerance to this emetic effect generally develops after several days of opiate therapy.
- Provide an antiemetic as required.
- Change the analgesic as indicated.

Sedation
- Inform client that tolerance usually develops over 3 to 5 days.
- Administer a stimulant, such as dextroamphetamine sulfate (Dexedrine) or methylphenidate hydrochloride (Ritalin) each morning to clients who receive opiate therapy for chronic pain and do not develop tolerance.

Respiratory Depression
- Administer an opioid antagonist, such as naloxone hydrochloride (Narcan) until respirations return to an acceptable rate. Administer the medication slowly by intravenous route with 10 mL of saline. Monitor the client, and repeat the procedure as required.
- If the client is receiving intravenous patient-controlled analgesia, stop or slow the infusion.

Pruritus
- Apply cool packs, lotion, and diversional activity.
- Administer an antihistamine (e.g., diphenhydramine hydrochloride [Benadryl]).
- Inform the client that tolerance also develops to pruritus.

Urinary Retention
- May need to catheterize client.
- Administer narcotic antagonist (naloxone hydrochloride [Narcan]).

Nonopioids/NSAIDs. Nonopioids include acetaminophen and **nonsteroidal anti-inflammatory drugs (NSAIDs)** such as ibuprofen. NSAIDs have anti-inflammatory, analgesic, and antipyretic effects, whereas acetaminophen has only analgesic and antipyretic effects. They relieve pain by acting on peripheral nerve endings at the injury site and decreasing the level of inflammatory mediators and interfering with the production of prostaglandins at the site of injury. The mechanism of action for acetaminophen is different from that of aspirin and the other NSAIDSs. Analgesia appears to result primarily from a central mechanism rather than a peripheral one. Very little else is known about how acetaminophen relieves pain (McCaffery & Pasero, 1999, p. 130). In addition, several combinations of analgesic drugs are available, for example, an opioid and a nonopioid such as Tylenol 3, which combines acetaminophen with 30 mg of codeine.

Individual drugs in this category vary widely in their analgesic properties, metabolism, excretion, and side effects.

The most common side effect of nonopioid analgesics is gastrointestinal, such as heartburn or indigestion. Clients should be taught to take NSAIDs with food or a glass of water. Most NSAIDs also interfere with platelet aggregation. Acetaminophen, on the other hand, does not affect platelet function and rarely causes gastrointestinal distress. It can, however, cause hepatotoxicity and should be used cautiously in clients with liver problems.

The NSAIDs reduce the dose of opioids needed when the drugs are given together and provide better pain relief than use of either type separately. These drugs must be ordered by the physician; they all have a maximum daily dose limit. There are advantages to giving combination drugs such as NSAIDS and opioids for pain management but close attention must be paid not only to the physician's order but also to the amount that the client takes in a 24-hr period. For example, if a client is ordered to take Tylenol with codiene, the Tylenol part of the medication

has a ceiling and will cause toxicity if the recommended amount is exceeded in a 24-hr period. Opioids have no ceiling, so the codiene could be gradually increased as needed for pain management. The total intake of both Tylenol and codiene needs to be constantly evaluated and the physician notified if pain relief is not being safely obtained. A change in medication or dosage may be needed to provide pain relief while maintaining safe, nontoxic levels.

Pharmacologic management of mild to moderate pain should begin with NSAIDs, unless there is a specific contraindication (USDHHS, 1992, p. 16). NSAIDs are contraindicated, for example, in clients with impaired blood clotting, gastrointestinal bleeding or ulcer risk, renal disease, thromobocytopenia, and possibly infection (because NSAIDs will obscure fever). Table 44–6 lists common misconceptions about nonopioids.

Adjuvant Analgesics. An **adjuvant analgesic** is a medication that was developed for a use other than analgesia but has been found to reduce chronic pain and sometimes acute pain, in addition to its primary action. For example, mild sedatives or tranquilizers may help reduce anxiety, stress, and tension so that the client can obtain a good night's sleep. Antidepressants are used to treat underlying depression or mood disorders but may also enhance other pain strategies. Anticonvulsants, usually prescribed to treat seizures, can be useful in controlling painful neuropathies such as herpes zoster (shingles) and diabetic neuropathies.

WHO Three-Step Ladder Approach

The World Health Organization (WHO) recommends a three-step ladder approach to manage chronic cancer pain (Figure 44–9 ■). This approach focuses on the intensity of the pain, and clients do not necessarily progress through the three steps. Step 1 of the analgesic ladder suggests a nonopioid analgesic and the possibility of an adjuvant analgesic. If the client receives the maximum

TABLE 44-6 Misconceptions about Nonopioids

Misconception	Correction
Regular daily use of NSAIDs is much safer than taking opioids.	Side effects from long-term use of NSAIDs are considerably more severe and life threatening than the side effects from daily doses of oral morphine or other opioids. The most common side effect from long-term use of opioids is constipation, whereas NSAIDs can cause gastric ulcers, increased bleeding time, and renal insufficiency. Acetaminophen can cause hepatotoxicity.
A nonopioid should not be given at the same time as an opioid.	It is safe to administer a nonopioid and opioid at the same time. Giving a dose of nonopioid at the same time as a dose of opioid poses no more danger than giving the doses at different times. In fact, many opioids are compounded with a nonopioid (e.g., Percocet [oxycodone and acetaminophen]).
Administering antacids with NSAIDs is an effective method of reducing gastric distress.	Administering antacids with NSAIDs can lessen distress but may be counterproductive. Antacids reduce the absorption and therefore the effectiveness of the NSAID by releasing the drug in the stomach rather than in the small intestine where absorption occurs.
Nonopioids are not useful analgesics for severe pain.	Nonopioids alone are rarely sufficient to relieve severe pain, but they are an important part in the total analgesic plan. One of the basic principles of analgesic therapy is: Whenever pain is severe enough to require an opioid, adding a nonopioid should be considered.
Gastric distress (e.g., abdominal pain) is indicative of NSAID-induced gastric ulceration.	Most clients with gastric lesions have no symptoms until bleeding or perforation occurs.

Note: From Pain: Clinical Manual, 2nd ed., by M. McCaffery and C. Pasero, 1999, St. Louis, MO: Mosby. Reprinted with permission from Elsevier Science.

recommended dose of nonopioids and continues to experience pain, step 2 recommends adding an opioid. It appears that there is no difference between steps 2 and 3, however, in practice the difference is in the choice of analgesic. For example, opioid analgesics at step 3 should be available by a variety of routes (e.g., oral, rectal, subcutaneous). They should also have a short half-life in order to increase the dosage for severe, escalating (increasing) pain (McCaffery & Pasero, 1999, p. 117).

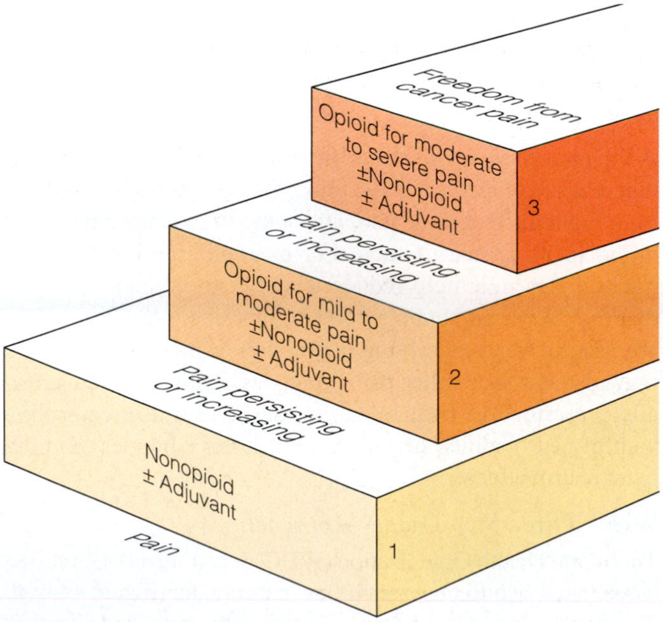

Some medications (e.g., Vicodin) contain both opioids and nonopioids. Nurses need to be aware of this in order to administer them safely and to complete proper discharge instructions related to these combination medications.

> **➤ CLINICAL ALERT** *Combining opioid and nonopioid analgesics is frequently overlooked. The method in which they relieve pain is different. Each has different side effects; they are two different analgesics. Alternating the two or giving them at the same time creates no danger. ∎*

Administration of Placebos

A **placebo** is "any medication or procedure, including surgery, that produces an effect in a client because of its implicit or explicit intent and not because of its specific physical or chemical properties." (McCaffery & Pasero, 1999). Placebos can be used as an effect in research to study the effects of a new medication. It is important to remember, however, that the subjects in a research study provide informed consent and know that a placebo may be given. On the other hand, the use of placebos to assess the presence or nature of pain raises serious ethical questions and challenges the nurse in relation to the American Nurses Association Code of Ethics (Tucker, 2001). A positive response to a placebo dose is not indicative of a lack of real pain but only of the reality of the placebo effect, which can be expected in 30% or more of any population (McCaffery & Pasero, 1999). Because placebos fail to relieve pain for many people it is recommended that the deceptive use of placebos be

Figure 44-9 ∎ The WHO three-step analgesic ladder. (*Note:* From *Cancer Pain Relief*, 2nd ed., by World Health Organization, 1996, Geneva: Author. Reprinted with permission.)

considered unacceptable in the management of pain (American Pain Society, 1999).

Routes for Opiate Delivery

Opioids have traditionally been administered by oral, subcutaneous, intramuscular, and intravenous routes. In addition, newer methods of delivering opiates have been developed to circumvent potential obstacles that occur with these traditional routes. Examples are transnasal and transdermal drug therapy, continuous subcutaneous infusions, and intraspinal infusion.

Oral. Oral administration of opiates remains the preferred route of delivery because of ease of administration. Because the duration of action of most opiates is approximately 4 hours, people with chronic pain have had to awaken several times during the night to medicate themselves for pain. To circumvent this problem, long-acting or sustained-release forms of morphine with a duration of 8 or more hours have been developed. Two examples of long-acting morphine are MS Contin and Oramorph SR. Clients receiving long-acting morphine also may need prn "rescue" doses of immediate-release analgesics such as short-acting oral transmucosal fentanyl citrate (Actiq) for acute breakthrough pain (Rhiner & Kedziera, 1999).

Another method of oral opiate delivery is high-concentration liquid morphine. This formulation enables clients who can swallow only small amounts to continue taking the drug orally.

Nasal. Transnasal administration has the advantage of rapid action of the medication because of direct absorption through the vascular nasal mucosa. A commonly used agent is a mixed agonist-antagonist butorphanol (Stadol) for acute headaches.

Transdermal. Transdermal drug therapy is advantageous in that it delivers a relatively stable plasma drug level and is noninvasive. Fentanyl (Duragesic) is an opioid currently available as a skin patch with various dosages. It provides drug delivery for up to 72 hours.

Rectal. Several opiates are now available in suppository form. The rectal route is particularly useful for clients who have dysphagia (difficulty swallowing) or nausea and vomiting. Oral analgesics, with the exception of sustained-release analgesics, may be crushed, dissolved in water, and given rectally (McCaffery & Pasero, 1999, p. 205). Sustained-release analgesics should not be crushed to be administered. Drugs such as oxycontin and MS Contin are made to last for 12 hours. If they are crushed and given to the client, the effects will be heightened in the first 1–2 hours, and then they may provide very little pain relief for the remainder of the 12-hour period.

Subcutaneous. Although the subcutaneous (SC) route has been used extensively to deliver opioids, another technique uses subcutaneous catheters and infusion pumps to provide continuous subcutaneous infusion (CSCI) of narcotics. CSCI is particularly helpful for clients (a) whose pain is poorly controlled by oral medications, (b) who are experiencing dysphagia or gastrointestinal obstruction, or (c) who have a need for prolonged use of parenteral narcotics. CSCI involves the use of

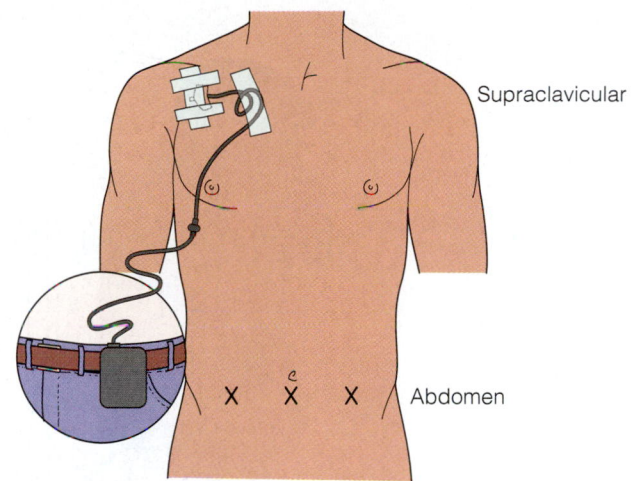

Figure 44–10 ■ Subcutaneous infusion needle placement. Figure shows sites for SC infusion needle placement, which may be attached to an ambulatory infusion pump. Other sites to consider include upper arms and thighs. Sites should be rotated. (*Note:* From *Pain: Clinical Manual*, 2nd ed. (p. 211), by M. McCaffery and C. Pasero, 1999, St. Louis, MO: Mosby, Copyright 1999, Mosby, Inc. Reprinted with permission from Elsevier Science.)

a small, light, battery-operated pump that administers the drug through a-23-or-25-gauge butterfly needle. The needle can be inserted into the anterior chest, the subclavicular region, the abdominal wall, the outer aspects of the upper arms, or the thighs. Client mobility is maintained with the application of a shoulder bag or holster to hold the pump (Figure 44–10 ■). The frequency of site change ranges from 3 to 7 days.

Because family caregivers must operate the pump and also change and care for the injection site, the nurse needs to provide appropriate instruction. Caregivers need to be able to

- Describe the basic parts and symbols of the system.
- Identify ways to determine whether the pump is working.
- Change the battery.
- Change the medication.
- Demonstrate stopping and starting the pump.
- Demonstrate tubing care, site care, and changing of the injection site.
- Identify signs indicating the need to change an injection site.
- Describe general care of the pump when the client is ambulatory, bathing, sleeping, or traveling.
- Identify actions to take to solve problems when the alarm signals.

Intramuscular. The intramuscular (IM) route is the least desirable route for opioid administration because of variable absorption, pain involved with administration, and the need to repeat administration every 3 to 4 hours.

Intravenous. The intravenous (IV) route provides rapid and effective pain relief with few side effects. The analgesic can be administered by IV bolus or by continuous infusion controlled by the client using a patient-controlled analgesia (PCA) machine at the bedside (see the discussion of PCA later in this chapter).

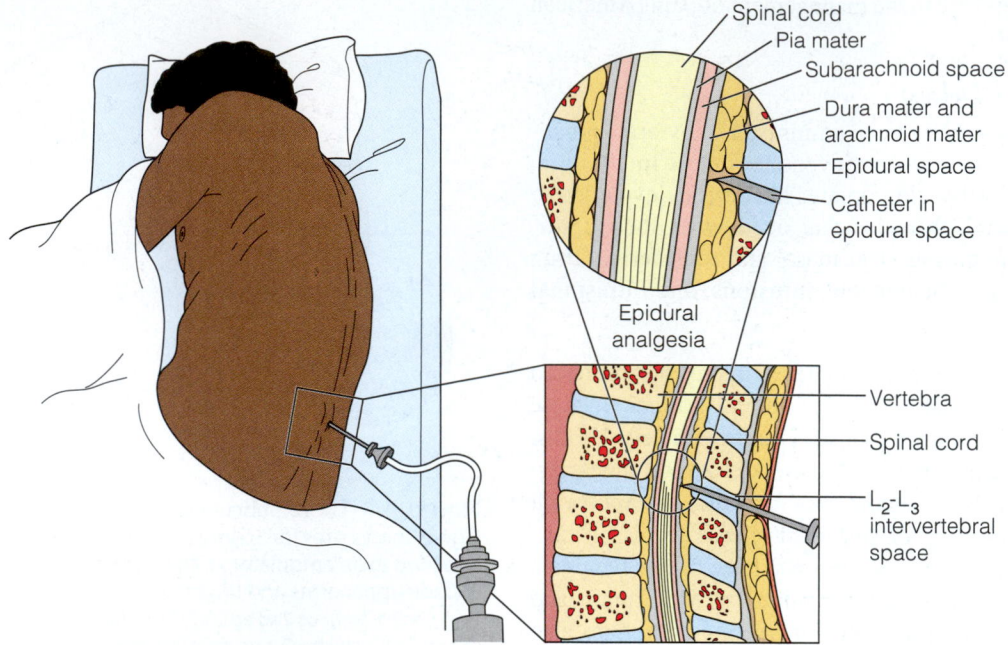

Figure 44–11 ■ Placement of intraspinal catheter in the epidural space.

Intraspinal. An increasingly popular method of delivery is the infusion of opiates into the epidural or intrathecal (subarachnoid) space (Figure 44–11 ■). Intraspinal analgesics act directly on opiate receptors in the dorsal horn of the spinal cord. Two commonly used medications are preservative-free morphine sulfate and fentanyl. The major benefit of intraspinal drug therapy is that it exerts a lesser sedative effect than do systemic opiates. The epidural space is most commonly used because the dura mater acts as a protective barrier against infection, including meningitis. Because the epidural catheter is in a space and not a blood vessel, a continuous epidural infusion may be stopped for hours and restarted without concern that the catheter has become occluded (McCaffery & Pasero, 1999, p. 37).

When the epidural space, rather than the intrathecal space, is used, a higher dosage of medication is required to achieve the same degree of analgesia. Because the intrathecal space contains cerebrospinal fluid (CSF) and directly surrounds the spinal cord, opiates act quickly on the dorsal horn. Very little drug is absorbed by blood vessels into the systemic circulation. In contrast, the epidural space is separated from the spinal cord by the dura mater, which acts as a barrier to drug diffusion. In addition, it is filled with fatty tissue and an extensive venous system. With this diffusion delay, some medication from the epidural space enters the systemic circulation via the venous plexus. Thus a higher dose of opiate is required to create the desired effect.

Intraspinal analgesia can be administered by three methods:

1. *Bolus.* For some surgical procedures (e.g., cesarean section), a single bolus may provide sufficient pain control for up to 24 hours. After this time, the client may be given oral or IV analgesics. Some agencies allow only the anesthesi-

ologist or nurse anesthetist to initiate an epidural infusion or administer a bolus. Check agency policy.

2. *Continuous infusion administered by pump.* The pump may be external (for acute or chronic pain) or implanted (for chronic pain).

3. *Patient-controlled epidural analgesia (PCEA).* Patient-controlled epidural analgesia is administered by the client using a pump. This is similar to patient-controlled analgesia in which a basal rate may meet the client's analgesic needs. If not, the client can push a button to deliver a preset dose. PCEA is often used to manage acute postoperative pain, chronic pain, and intractable cancer pain. The anesthesiologist or nurse anesthetist inserts a needle into the intrathecal or epidural space and threads a catheter through the needle. The catheter is connected to tubing that is then positioned along the spine and over the client's shoulder for the nurse to access. The entire catheter and tubing are taped securely to prevent dislodgement.

Temporary catheters, used for short-term acute pain management, are usually placed at the lumbar or thoracic vertebral level and often removed after 2 to 4 days. Permanent catheters, for clients with chronic pain, may be tunneled subcutaneously through the skin and exit at the client's side. Tunneling of the catheter reduces the risk of infection and displacement of the catheter. After the catheter is inserted, the nurse is responsible for monitoring the infusion and assessing the client. Nursing care of clients with intraspinal infusions is summarized in Table 44–7.

A common misconception is that there is a higher incidence of respiratory depression when opioids are administered by the epidural route and, therefore, clients receiving epidural analgesia should be monitored in an intensive care setting. The fact is

TABLE 44-7 Nursing Interventions for Clients Receiving Analgesics through an Epidural Catheter

Nursing Goals	Interventions
Maintain client safety	Label the tubing, the infusion bag, and the front of the pump with tape marked EPIDURAL to prevent confusion with similar-looking IV lines.
	Post sign above client's bed indicating epidural is in place.
	Secure all connections with tape.
	If there is no continuous infusion, apply tape over all injection ports on the epidural line to avoid the injection of substances intended for IV administration into the epidural catheter.
	Do not use alcohol in any care of catheter or insertion site as it can be neurotoxic.
	Ensure that any solution injected or infused intraspinally is sterile, preservative free, and safe for intraspinal administration.
Maintain catheter placement	Secure temporary catheters with tape.
	When bolus doses are used, gently aspirate prior to medication administration to determine catheter has not migrated into the subarachnoid space. (Expect <1 mL of fluid return in syringe.)
	Assist client in repositioning or moving out of bed.
	Teach client to avoid tugging on the catheter.
	Assess insertion site for leakage with each bolus dose or at least every 8–12 hours.
Prevent infection	Use strict aseptic techniques with all epidural-related procedures.
	Maintain sterile occlusive dressing over insertion site.
	Assess insertion site for signs of infection.
	Assess for increasing diffuse back pain or tenderness and/or paresthesia on intraspinal injection because these are cardinal signs of intraspinal infection (McCaffery & Pasero, 1999, p. 234).
Maintain urinary and bowel function	Monitor intake and output.
	Assess for bowel and bladder distention.
Prevent respiratory depression	Assess sedation level and respiratory status q1h for the first 24 hours and thereafter q4h.
	Do not administer other opioids or central nervous system depressants unless ordered.
	Keep an ampule of naloxone hydrochloride (0.4 mg) at the bedside.
	Notify the clinician in charge if the respiratory rate falls below 8 per minute or if the client is difficult to rouse.

that respiratory depression occurs less often with epidural analgesia than by the IM route but is closer in comparison to IV PCA (McCaffery & Pasero, 1999, 214). Clients who are receiving epidural analgesia do not require intensive care monitoring. The nurse who is outside the intensive care setting can safely monitor the respiratory and sedation status of a client receiving epidural analgesia.

> ► CLINICAL ALERT *As a precaution, have naloxone (Narcan), sodium chloride 0.9% diluent, and injection equipment on hand for each client receiving an opioid-containing epidural infusion (Cox, 2001).* ■

Continuous Local Anesthetics

Continuous subcutaneous administration of long-acting local anesthetics into or near the surgical site is a technique being used to provide postoperative pain control. This technique is being used for a variety of surgical procedures including knee arthroplasty, abdominal hysterectomy, hernia repair, and mastectomy (Pasero, 2000, p.22).

The surgeon inserts a catheter under the subcutaneous tissue and on top of the muscle near or in the surgical wound site. A transparent dressing secures the catheter. The client is given a loading dose of local anesthetic before the continuous infusion

is started. The catheter is connected to an infusion pump that is set at the rate ordered by the physician. The infusion pump may be similar to the type used for IV or epidural analgesia, or it may be a disposable pump if the client will be continuing the treatment at home after discharge from the hospital.

Nursing interventions for the client with infusion of a continuous local anesthetic include:

- Conduct pain assessment and documentation every 2 to 4 hours while the client is awake.
- Check the dressing every shift for intactness. The dressing is not usually changed in order to avoid dislodging the catheter. Contact the physician if the dressing becomes loose.
- Check the site of the catheter. It should be clean and dry.
- Assess the client for signs of local anesthetic toxicity (e.g., dizziness; ringing in the ears; a metallic taste; tingling or numbness of the lips, gums, or tongue) (Pasero, 2000, pp. 22–23).
- Notify the physician of signs of local anesthetic toxicity. If detected early, prompt treatment can be initiated and serious complications avoided.

Patient-Controlled Analgesia

Patient-controlled analgesia (PCA) is an interactive method of pain management that permits clients to treat their pain by self-administering doses of analgesics (McCaffery & Pasero,

1999). The oral route for PCA is most common, but the subcutaneous, intravenous, and epidural routes are increasingly being used. The PCA mode of therapy minimizes the roller-coaster effect of peaks of sedation and valleys of pain that occur with the traditional method of prn dosing. With the parenteral routes, the client administers a predetermined dose of a narcotic by an electronic infusion pump. This allows the client to maintain a more constant level of relief yet need less medication for pain relief. Patient-controlled analegias can be effectively used for clients with acute pain related to a surgical incision, traumatic injury, or labor and delivery, and for chronic pain as with cancer. In some settings PCAs are used even if the client is unable to initiate a dose by pushing the button, as long as a caregiver is willing to accept the responsibility; for example, when the client is an infant or toddler or is physically or cognitively impaired. This has been termed *family-controlled analgesia*.

The physician prescribes the analgesic dose, route, and frequency, with the client administering the medication. Whether in an acute hospital setting, an ambulatory clinic, or with home care, the nurse is responsible for the initial instruction regarding use of the PCA and for the ongoing monitoring of the therapy. The client's pain must be assessed at regular intervals and analgesic use is documented in the client's record.

Patient-controlled analgesia pumps are designed with built-in safety mechanisms to prevent client overdosage, abusive use, and narcotic theft. The most significant adverse effects are respiratory depression and hypotension; however, they occur rarely. Although PCA pumps vary in design, they all have the same protective features. The line of the PCA pump, a syringe-type pump, is usually introduced into the injection port of a primary IV fluid line (Figure 44–12 ■). When clients want a

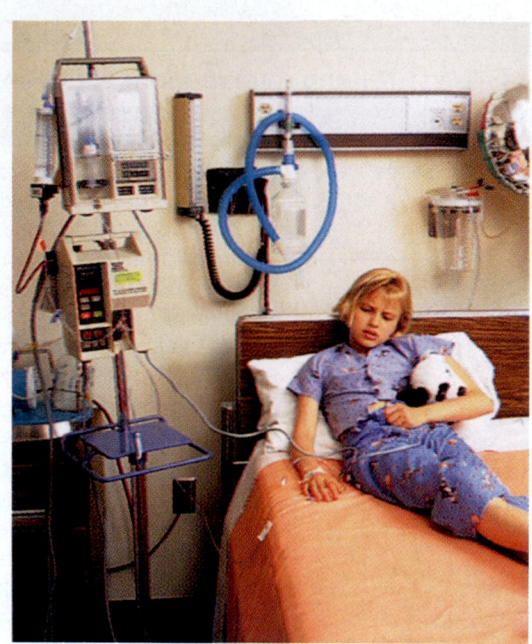

Figure 44–13 ■ The older child is able to regulate a PCA pump.

dose of analgesic, they can push a button attached to the infusion pump and the preset dose is delivered (Figure 44–13 ■). A programmable lockout interval (usually 10 to 15 minutes) follows the dose, when an additional dose cannot be given even if the client activates the button. It is also possible to program the maximum dose that can be delivered over a period of hours (usually four). Many pumps are capable of delivering a basal rate, or low continuous infusion, to provide sustained analgesia during times of rest and sleep. See Procedure 44–1.

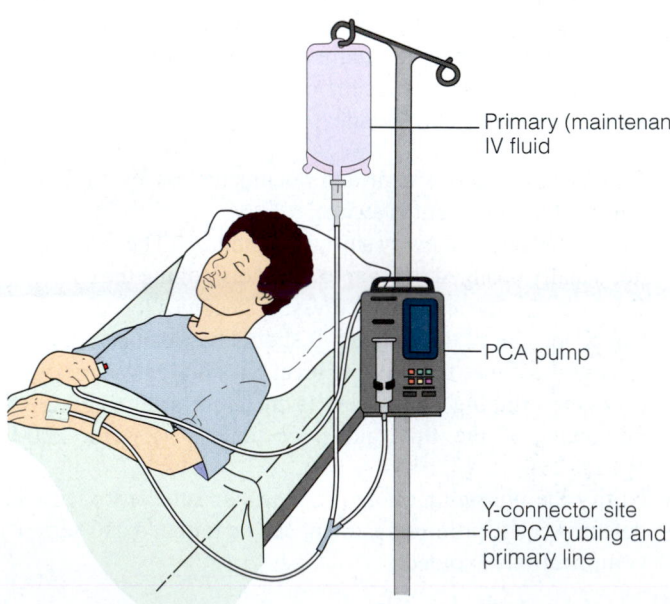

Primary (maintenan
IV fluid

PCA pump

Y-connector site
for PCA tubing and
primary line

Figure 44–12 ■ PCA line introduced into the injection port of a primary line.

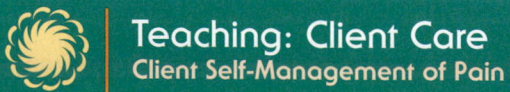

Teaching: Client Care
Client Self-Management of Pain

Choose a time to teach the client about pain management when the pain is controlled so that the client is able to focus on the teaching.

Teaching the client about self-management of pain can include the following:

- Demonstrate the operation of the PCA pump and explain that the client can safely push the button without fear of overmedicating.
- Describe the use of the pain scale and encourage the client to respond in order to demonstrate understanding.
- Explain to the client the need to notify staff when ambulation is desired (e.g., for bathroom use).

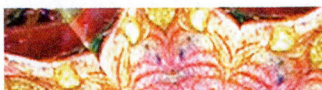

Procedure 44–1 Managing Pain with a Patient-Controlled Analgesia (PCA) Pump

Purposes
- To enhance pain control
- To decrease opioid requirements
- To facilitate client involvent in controlling pain

ASSESSMENT

Assess
- Pain (intensity, location, presence of radiation, associated factors, precipitating factors, and alleviating factors)
- Client's allergies
- Baseline vital signs
- Client's understanding of the pump

PLANNING

Delegation
Initiating and maintaining a PCA pump requires application of nursing knowledge, aseptic technique, critical thinking, and administration of a controlled substance and, therefore, is not delegated to unlicensed assistive personnel (UAP). The nurse can inform the UAP of the intended therapeutic effects and specific side effects of the medication and direct the UAP to report specific client observations (e.g., unrelieved pain) to the nurse for follow-up. The UAP must not administer a dose (push the button) for the client.

Equipment
- Clean gloves
- IV start kit
- IV catheter
- Primary line IV tubing
- Primary IV fluid (per orders)
- PCA pump and appropriate tubing
- Operational manual for specific pump to be used
- PCA flowsheet
- Premixed medication in appropriate syringe

IMPLEMENTATION

Preparation
Before initiating PCA therapy, determine factors that may contraindicate use (e.g., impaired mental status, impaired respiratory status), the amount of narcotic specified by the order, bolus and continuous infusion dosage parameters, type of primary fluid, and compatibility of the primary IV fluid and the PCA medication in the same line. Calculate:

- The initial bolus dose based on the number of milligrams of drug per milliliter of fluid
- The dose per intermittent bolus delivery
- The 4-hour lockout drug limit.

Confirm that the drug is premixed with the required amount of diluent.

Performance
1. Explain to the client the purpose and operation of the PCA.
2. Wash hands and observe other appropriate infection control procedures.
3. Provide for client privacy.
4. Prepare the client.
   - Check the client's identification band. *This ensures that the right client receives the medication.*

- If not previously assessed, take the baseline vital signs. If any of the findings are above or below the predetermined parameters, consult the physician before administering the medication.

5. Set up the primary IV line and fluid.
   - Put on clean gloves.
   - Start the IV line. *This will secure venous access.*
6. Set up the PCA infusion line according to the manufacturer's instructions.
   - Remove the protective caps from the injector (plunger) and premixed drug vial.
   - Connect (screw or twist) the injector into the drug vial.
   - Remove excess air from the vial by pushing the injector into the vial.
   - Connect the PCA tubing to the injector.
   - Prime the PCA tubing up to the point of the Y-connector.
   - Clamp the tubing above the Y-connector. *This prevents accidental bolusing and flushing of the primary line with the narcotic.*

- Place the injector with attached vial in the PCA machine according to the operational instructions.
7. Connect the PCA infusion line to the primary fluid line.
   - Connect the PCA tubing to the primary fluid line at the Y-connector site. (The clamps should still be closed on the primary IV line and the PCA line.)
8. Prime the line below the Y-connector with compatible primary IV fluid.
9. Deliver the loading dose.
   - Set the pump for a lockout time of zero minutes.
   - Set the volume to be delivered based on calculated dosage volume for the loading dose.
   - Inject the loading dose by pressing the loading dose control button.
10. Set the safety parameters for the infusion on the PCA pump according to the manufacturer's instructions. For example:
    - Dose volume limits. *This will limit the amount of drug that the client can receive when the client pushes the control button.*

continued on page 1160

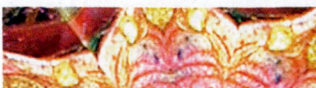

Procedure 44–1 Managing Pain with a Patient-Controlled Analgesia (PCA) Pump *continued*

IMPLEMENTATION *continued*

- Lockout interval between each dose. The lockout interval is generally between 5 and 12 minutes. *This sets the minimum time that must elapse before the client can receive another dose of the drug. Lockout time is based on the usual onset of the IV narcotic and the assessment of the client.*
- Four-hour limit. Set the 4-hour dosage limit as specified on the orders. *This is an additional safety feature to limit the amount of medication delivered over 4 hours.*

11. Lock the machine.
   - Close the door on the pump.
   - Look for any digital cues or alarms that may indicate the machine is

not set, and make corrections as needed.
   - Lock the machine with the key.
12. Begin the infusion.
   - Release the clamp on the Y-connector, and press the start button to begin the infusion.
   - Place the client control button within reach.
13. Monitor the client for vital signs, sedation level, pain control, and side effects.
   - Monitor the status of the client every 2 hours during the first 24 to 36 hours of infusion and regularly thereafter, depending on the client's health and agency protocol.

14. Monitor the infusion.
   - Verify correct PCA parameters.
   - Observe the IV site for signs of infiltration and phlebitis.
   - Inspect the tubing for kinks that may occlude the line.
   - Note the total number of doses and milligrams received.
15. Document all relevant information.
   - Record the initiation of PCA, the dose setting, the doses received, pain intensity, and all assessments. See agency protocol.

EVALUATION

Conduct appropriate follow-up:
- Pain status
- Respiratory rate and character
- Amount of medication used
- Frequency of use

- Side effects encountered and response to treatment of side effects

Relate to previous findings, if available, and report significant deviations from normal to the physician.

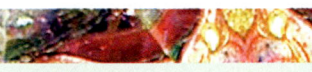

Lifespan Considerations

PCA Pump
Children
- Include the parents in teaching.
- Assess the child's ability to use the client control button.

Elders
- Carefully monitor for drug side effects.
- Use cautiously for individuals with impaired pulmonary or renal function.
- Assess the client's cognitive and physical ability to use the client control button.

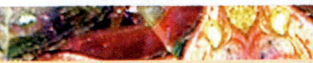

Home Care Considerations

PCA Pump
- Monitor for signs and symptoms of oversedation such as excessive drowsiness, slowed respiratory rate, or change in mental state.

- Do not adjust settings without consulting with the appropriate health care provider.

Nonpharmacologic Pain Management

Nonpharmacologic pain management consists of a variety of physical and cognitive-behavioral pain management strategies. Physical interventions include cutaneous stimulation, immobilization, transcutaneous electrical nerve stimulation (TENS), and acupuncture. Mind–body (cognitive-behavioral) interventions include distraction activities, relaxation techniques, imagery, meditation, biofeedback, hypnosis, and therapeutic

touch. Several physical interventions and distraction activities are discussed next. For information about the other mind–body interventions and acupuncture, see Chapter 14.

Physical Interventions. The goals of physical intervention include providing comfort, altering physiologic responses, and reducing fears associated with pain-related immobility or activity restriction.

Cutaneous Stimulation. Cutaneous stimulation can provide effective temporary pain relief. It distracts the client and focuses attention on the tactile stimuli, away from the painful sensations, thus reducing pain perception. Cutaneous stimulation is also believed to (a) create the release of endorphins that block pain stimuli transmission and (b) stimulate large-diameter A-beta sensory nerve fibers, thus decreasing the transmission of pain impulses through the smaller A-delta and C fibers. Cutaneous stimulation techniques include the following:

- Massage
- Application of heat or cold
- Acupressure
- Contralateral stimulation.

Cutaneous stimulation can be applied directly to the painful area, proximal to the pain, distal to the pain, and contralateral (opposite side) to the pain. Cutaneous stimulation is contraindicated in areas of skin breakdown.

Massage. Massage is a comfort measure that can aid relaxation, decrease muscle tension, and may ease anxiety because the physical contact communicates caring. It can also decrease pain intensity by increasing superficial circulation to the area. Massage can involve the back and neck, hands and arms, or feet. The use of ointments or liniments may provide localized pain relief with joint or muscle pain. Massage is contraindicated in areas of skin breakdown.

Heat and Cold Applications. A warm bath, heating pads, ice bags, ice massage, hot or cold compresses, and warm or cold sitz baths in general relieve pain and promote healing of injured tissues (See Chapter 34). 🔗

Acupressure. Acupressure developed from the ancient Chinese healing system of acupuncture. The therapist applies finger pressure to points that correspond to many of the points used in acupuncture. (see Chapter 14). 🔗

Contralateral Stimulation. Contralateral stimulation can be accomplished by stimulating the skin in an area opposite to the painful area (e.g., stimulating the left knee if the pain is in the right knee). The contralateral area may be scratched for itching, massaged for cramps, or treated with cold packs or analgesic ointments. This method is particularly useful when the painful area cannot be touched because it is hypersensitive, inaccessible by a cast or bandages, or when the pain is felt in a missing part (phantom pain).

Immobilization. Immobilizing or restricting the movement of a painful body part (e.g., arthritic joint, traumatized limb) may help to manage episodes of acute pain. Splints or supportive devices should hold joints in the position of optimal function and should be removed regularly in accordance with agency protocol to provide range-of-motion exercises. Prolonged immobilization can result in joint contracture, muscle atrophy, and cardiovascular problems. Therefore, clients should be encouraged to participate in self-care activities and remain as active as possible.

Transcutaneous Electrical Nerve Stimulation. **Transcutaneous electrical nerve stimulation (TENS)** is a method of applying low-

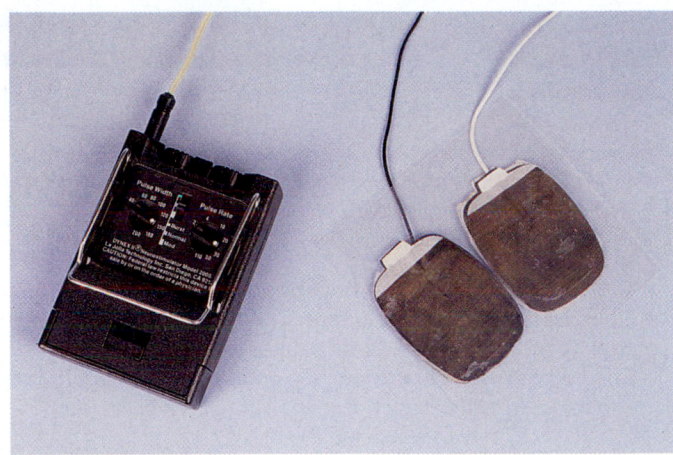

Figure 44–14 ■ A transcutaneous electric nerve stimulator.

voltage electrical stimulation directly over identified pain areas, at an acupressure point, along peripheral nerve areas that innervate the pain area, or along the spinal column. The TENS unit consists of a portable, battery-operated device with lead wire and electrode pads that are applied to the chosen area of skin (Figure 44–14 ■). Cutaneous stimulation from the TENS unit is thought to activate large-diameter fibers that modulate the transmission of the nociceptive impulse in the peripheral and central nervous system (closing the pain "gate"), resulting in pain relief. This stimulation may also cause a release of endorphins from the CNS centers. The use of TENS is contraindicated for clients with pacemakers, arrhythmias, or in areas of skin breakdown.

Distraction. Distraction draws the person's attention away from the pain and lessens the perception of pain. In some instances, distraction can make a client completely unaware of pain. For example, a client recovering from surgery may feel no pain while watching a football game on television, yet feel pain again when the game is over. Different types of distractions are shown in Box 44–8.

BOX 44–8 ■ **Types of Distraction**
Visual Distraction
■ Reading or watching TV
■ Watching a baseball game
■ Guided imagery
Auditory Distraction
■ Humor
■ Listening to music
Tactile Distraction
■ Slow, rhythmic breathing
■ Massage
■ Holding or stroking a pet or toy
Intellectual Distraction
■ Crossword puzzles
■ Card games (e.g., bridge)
■ Hobbies (e.g., stamp collecting, writing a story)

MediaLink | TREATING A CLIENT WITH STOMACH CANCER CASE STUDY

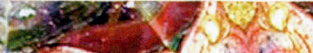

Lifespan Considerations

Pain Management

Infants

■ Giving an infant, particularly a very-low-birth-weight infant, a water and sucrose solution administered through a pacifier is effective in reducing pain during procedures that may be painful.

Children

■ Distract the child with toys, books, or pictures.
■ Hold the child to provide comfort.
■ Explore misconceptions about pain.
■ Children can use their imagination during guided imagery. To use the "pain switch," ask the child to imagine a pain switch

(even give it a color) and tell them to visualize turning the switch off in the area where there is pain. A "magic glove" or "magic blanket" is an imaginary object that the child applies on areas of the body (e.g., hand, thigh, back, hip) to lessen discomfort.

Elders

■ Focus on the client's control in dealing with the pain.
■ Spend time with the client and listen carefully.
■ Clarify misconceptions. Encourage independence whenever possible.

Home Care Considerations

Pain Management

■ Teach client to keep a pain diary to monitor pain onset, activity before pain, pain intensity, use of analgesics or other relief measures, and so on.
■ Instruct client to contact a health care professional if planned pain control measures are ineffective.
■ Teach the use of preferred and selected nonpharmacologic techniques such as relaxation, guided imagery, distraction, music therapy, massage, and so on.

■ Instruct the client to use pain control measures before the pain becomes severe.
■ Inform the client of the effects of untreated pain.
■ Provide appropriate information about how to access community resources, home care agencies, and associations that offer self-help groups and educational materials.

MediaLink TREATING CHRONIC BACK PAIN CARE PLAN ACTIVITY

Nonpharmacologic Invasive Therapies

A **nerve block** is a chemical interruption of a nerve pathway, effected by injecting a local anesthetic into the nerve. Nerve blocks are widely used during dental work. The injected drug blocks nerve pathways from the painful tooth, thus stopping the transmission of pain impulses to the brain. Nerve blocks are often used to relieve the pain of whiplash injury, lower back disorders, bursitis, and cancer. Sometimes alcohol blocks are used. These, however, destroy nerve fibers and as a result are generally used only for peripheral blocks, because peripheral nerve fibers regenerate.

Pain conduction pathways can be interrupted surgically. Because this disruption is permanent, surgery is performed only as a last resort, generally for intractable pain. Several surgical procedures may be performed. A **cordotomy** obliterates pain and temperature sensation below the level of the spinothalamic portion of the anterolateral tract severed, and is usually done for pain in the legs and trunk. **Rhizotomy** interrupts the anterior or posterior nerve root between the ganglion and the cord. Interruption of anterior motor nerve roots stops spasmodic movements that accompany paraplegia. Interruption of posterior sensory nerve roots eliminates pain in areas innervated by that specific nerve root. Rhizotomies are generally performed on cervical nerve roots to alleviate pain of the head and neck from cancer or neuralgia.

In **neurectomy,** peripheral or cranial nerves are interrupted to alleviate localized pain, such as pain in the lower leg or foot arising from a vascular occlusion. In a **sympathectomy,** pathways of the sympathetic division of the autonomic nervous system are

severed. This procedure eliminates vasospasm, improves peripheral blood supply, and thus is effective in treating painful vascular disorders such as angina and Raynaud's disease.

Spinal cord stimulation (SCS) is used with nonmalignant pain that has not been controlled with less invasive therapies. SCS involves the insertion of a cable that allows the placement of an electrode directly on the spinal cord. The cable is attached to a device that sends electric impulses to the spinal cord to control pain.

EVALUATING

The goals established in the planning phase are evaluated according to specific desired outcomes, also established in that phase (see the Identifying Nursing Diagnoses, Outcomes, and Interventions box earlier in this chapter). To assist in the evaluation process, flowsheet records or a client diary may be helpful. A weekly log or diary can be structured in a similar fashion for the individual client. For example, columns including day, time, onset of pain, activity before pain, pain relief measure, and duration of pain can be devised to help the client and nurse determine the effectiveness of pain relief strategies.

> ▶**CLINICAL ALERT** *The statement "Please tell me when your pain returns" helps to involve the client in pain management. It also gives permission to request relief for individuals whose culture may consider it inappropriate to report having pain.* ■

If outcomes are not achieved, the nurse and client need to explore the reasons before modifying the care plan. The nurse might consider the following questions:

- Is adequate analgesic being given? Would the client benefit from a change in dose or in the time interval between doses?
- Were the client's beliefs and values about pain therapy considered?
- Did the client understate the pain experience for some reason?
- Were appropriate instructions provided to allay misconceptions about pain management?
- Did the client and support people understand the instructions about pain management techniques?

- Is the client receiving adequate support from significant others?
- Has the client's physical condition changed, necessitating modifications in interventions?
- Should selected intervention strategies be reevaluated?

See the Nursing Care Plan and the Concept Map.

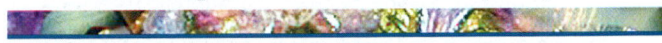

Focus on Critical Thinking

Mrs. Lundahl underwent abdominal surgery approximately 6 hours ago. She has a 15-cm midline incision that is covered with a dry and intact surgical dressing. Upon assessing Mrs. Lundahl you note that she is perspiring, lying in a rigid position, holding her abdomen, and grimacing. Her blood pressure is 150/90, heart rate 100, and respiratory rate 32. When asked to rate her pain on a scale of 1 to 10, Mrs. Lundahl rates her pain as 5.

1. What conclusions, if any, can be drawn about Mrs. Lundahl's pain status?

2. Does Mrs. Lundahl's rating her pain as 5 mean that she is not experiencing pain severe enough to warrant intervention?
3. What type of pain is Mrs. Lundahl experiencing?
4. What interventions, in addition to pain medication, may be useful in reducing Mrs. Lundahl's pain?
5. How will you know if your interventions have been effective in reducing Mrs. Lundahl's pain?

See Critical Thinking Possibilities in Appendix A.

NURSING CARE PLAN FOR ACUTE PAIN

ASSESSMENT DATA		*NURSING DIAGNOSIS*	DESIRED OUTCOMES [NOC #]/INDICATORS*
Nursing Assessment Mr. L. C. is a 57-year-old businessman who was admitted to the surgical unit for treatment of a possible strangulated inguinal hernia. Two days ago he had a partial bowel resection. Postoperative orders include NPO, intravenous infusion of D51/2 NS at 125 cc/hr left arm, nasogastric tube to low intermittent suction. Mr. C. is in a dorsal recumbent (supine) position and is attempting to draw up his legs. He appears restless and is complaining of abdominal pain (7 on a scale of 1–10).	**Physical Examination** Height: 188 cm (6'3") Weight: 90.0 kg (200 lb) Temperature: 37C (98.6F) Pulse: 90 BPM Respirations: 24/minute Blood pressure: 158/82 mm Hg Skin pale and moist, pupils dilated. Midline abdominal incision, sutures dry and intact. **Diagnostic Data** Chest x-ray and urinalysis negative, WBC 12,000	*Acute Pain* related to tissue injury secondary to surgical intervention (as evidenced by restlessness, pallor; elevated pulse, respirations, and systolic blood pressure, dilated pupils, and report of 7/10 abdominal pain)	**Comfort Level** [2100] as evidenced by • Substantial report of satisfaction with pain control • Turn, cough, and deep breathe with a minimum of discomfort by 2nd postop day **Pain Control** [1605] as evidenced by often demonstrating ability to • Use analgesics appropriately • Use nonanalgesic relief measures • Report symptoms to health care professional • Use preventive measures **Pain Level** [2102] As evidenced by slight to no • Reported pain • Protective body positioning • Restlessness • Pupil dilation • Perspiration • Change In BP, HR, R from normal baseline data

continued on page 1164

NURSING CARE PLAN FOR ACUTE PAIN *continued*

NURSING INTERVENTIONS [NIC #] / SELECTED ACTIVITIES*	RATIONALE
Pain Management [1400]	
• Perform a comprehensive assessment of pain to include location, characteristics, onset, duration, frequency, quality, intensity or severity, and precipitating factors of pain.	*Pain is a subjective experience and must be described by the client in order to plan effective treatment.*
• Consider cultural influences on pain response (e.g., cultural beliefs about pain may result in a stoic attitude).	*Each person experiences and expresses pain in an individual manner using a variety of sociocultural adaptation techniques.*
• Reduce or eliminate factors that precipitate or increase Mr. C's pain experience (e.g., fear, fatigue, monotony, and lack of knowledge).	*Personal factors can influence pain and pain tolerance. Those factors that may be precipitating or augmenting pain should be reduced or eliminated to enhance the overall pain management program.*
• Teach the use of nonpharmacologic techniques (e.g., relaxation, guided imagery, music therapy, distraction, and massage) before, after, and if possible during painful activities; before pain occurs or increases; and along with other pain relief measures.	*The use of noninvasive pain relief measures can increase the release of endorphins and enhance the therapeutic effects of pain relief medications.*
• Provide Mr. C. optimal pain relief with prescribed analgesics.	*Each client has a right to expect maximum pain relief. Optimal pain relief using analgesics includes determining the preferred route, drug, dosage, and frequency for each individual.*
• Medicate before an activity to increase participation, but evaluate the hazard of sedation.	*Turning and ambulation activities will be enhanced if pain is controlled or tolerable. Assessing level of sedation should precede the activity because many analgesics cause sedation and could compromise safety.*
• Evaluate the effectiveness of the pain control measures used through ongoing assessment of Mr. C's pain experience.	*Research shows that the most common reason for unrelieved pain is failure to routinely assess pain and pain relief. Many clients silently tolerate pain if not specifically asked about it.*
Analgesic Administration [2210]	
• Check the medical order for drug, dose, and frequency of analgesic prescribed.	*Ensures that the nurse has the right drug, right route, right dosage, right client, right frequency.*
• Determine analgesic selections (narcotic, nonnarcotic, or NSAID) based on type and severity of pain.	*Various types of pain (e.g., acute, chronic, neuropathic, arthritic) require different analgesic approaches. Some types of pain respond to nonopioid drugs alone, while others can be relieved by combining a low-dose opioid with a nonopioid.*
• Institute safety precautions as appropriate if Mr. C. receives narcotic analgesics.	*Side effects of opioid narcotics include drowsiness and sedation.*
• Instruct Mr. C. to request prn pain medication before the pain is severe.	*Severe pain is more difficult to control and increases the client's anxiety and fatigue. The preventive approach to pain management can reduce the total 24-hour analgesic dose.*
• Evaluate the effectiveness of analgesic at regular, frequent intervals after each administration and especially after the initial doses, also observing for any signs and symptoms of untoward effects (e.g., respiratory depression, nausea and vomiting, dry mouth, and constipation).	*The analgesic dose may not be adequate to raise the client's pain threshold or may be causing intolerable or dangerous side effects or both. Ongoing evaluation will assist in making necessary adjustments for effective pain management.*
• Document Mr. C's response to analgesics and any untoward effects.	*Documentation facilitates pain management by communicating effective and noneffective pain management strategies to the entire health care team.*
• Implement actions to decrease untoward effects of analgesics (e.g., constipation and gastric irritation).	*Constipation is a common side effect of opioid narcotics and a treatment plan to prevent occurrence should be instituted at the beginning of analgesic therapy.*

NURSING CARE PLAN FOR ACUTE PAIN *continued*

NURSING INTERVENTIONS [NIC #] / SELECTED ACTIVITIES*	RATIONALE
Simple Relaxation Therapy [6040]	
• Consider Mr. C's willingness and ability to participate, preference, past experiences, and contraindications before selecting a specific relaxation strategy.	*The client must feel comfortable trying a different approach to pain management. To avoid ineffective strategies, the client should be involved in the planning process.*
• Elicit behaviors that are conditioned to produce relaxation, such as deep breathing, yawning, abdominal breathing, or peaceful imaging.	*Relaxation techniques help reduce skeletal muscle tension, which will reduce the intensity of the pain.*
• Create a quiet, nondisruptive environment with dim lights and comfortable temperature when possible.	*Comfort and a quiet atmosphere promote a relaxed feeling and permit the client to focus on the relaxation technique rather than external distraction.*
• Individualize the content of the relaxation intervention (e.g., by asking for suggestions about what Mr. C. enjoys or finds relaxing).	*Each person may find different images or approaches to relaxation more helpful than others.*
• Demonstrate and practice the relaxation technique with Mr. C.	*Return demonstrations by the participant provide an opportunity for the nurse to evaluate the effectiveness of teaching sessions.*
• Evaluate and document his response to relaxation therapy.	*Conveys to the health care team effective strategies in reducing or eliminating pain.*

EVALUATION

Outcomes partially met. The client verbalizes pain and discomfort, requesting analgesics at onset of pain. States "the pain is a 2" (on a scale of 1–10) 30 minutes after analgesic administration. Requests analgesic 30 minutes before ambulation. Remains hesitant to cough and deep breathe even following analgesic administration on 2nd postop day. States willingness to try relaxation techniques, however, has not attempted to do so.

*Outcomes, interventions, and activities selected are only a sample of those suggested by NOC and NIC and should be further individualized for each client.

Applying Critical Thinking

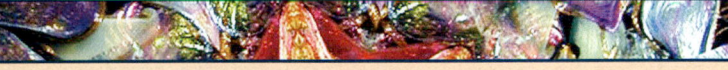

1. Is there any other assessment data you would want to gather to help plan Mr. C's pain management?
2. Mr. C. does not have a PCA. What nursing interventions are important?
3. What kind of data would cause you to discuss with the physician the possiblity of initiating a PCA pump?
4. Offer suggestions for ways to promote Mr. C's ability to cough and deep breathe.

See Critical Thinking Possibilities in Appendix A. 🔗

CONCEPT MAP 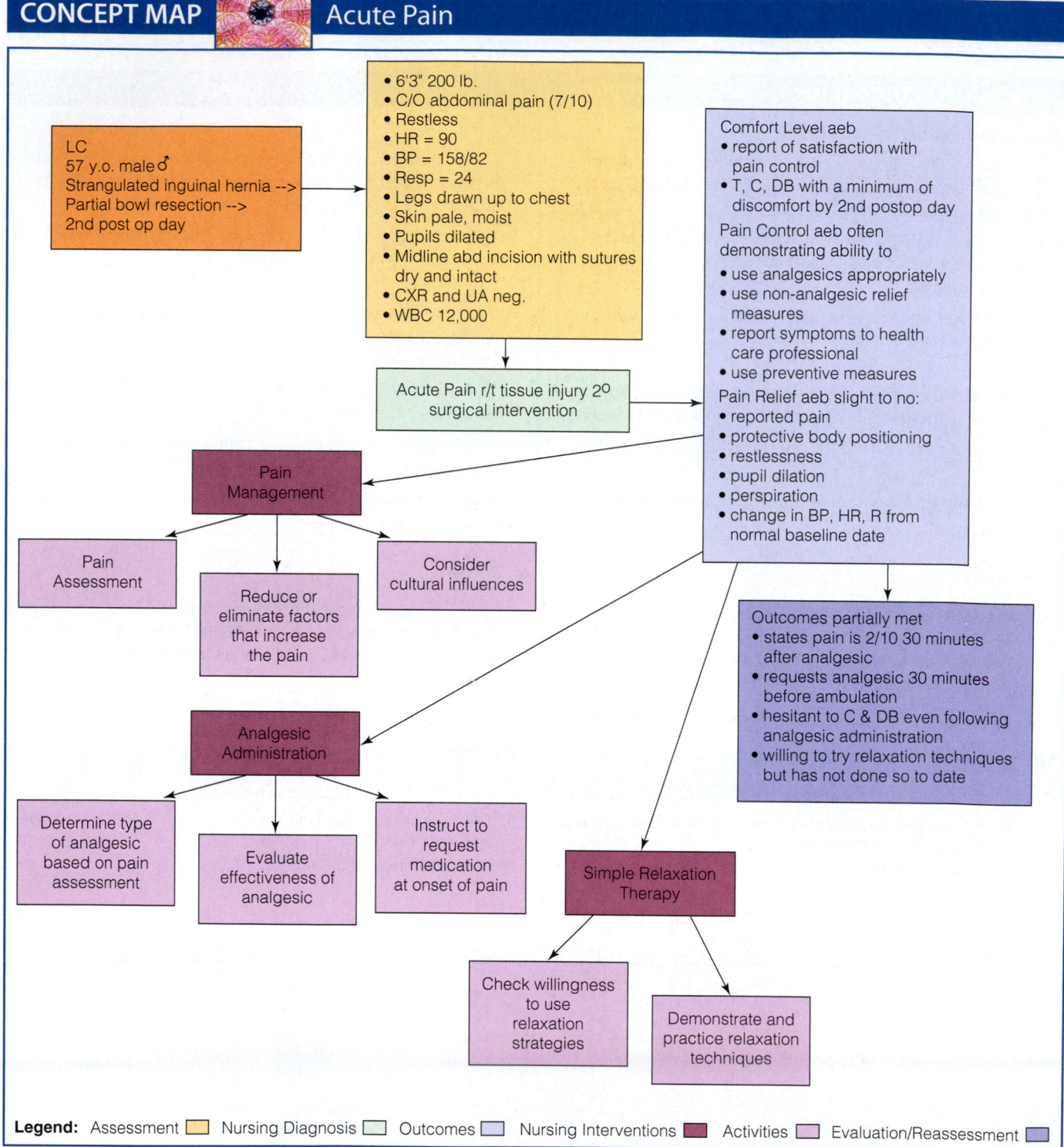 Acute Pain

LC
57 y.o. male ♂
Strangulated inguinal hernia -->
Partial bowl resection -->
2nd post op day

- 6'3" 200 lb.
- C/O abdominal pain (7/10)
- Restless
- HR = 90
- BP = 158/82
- Resp = 24
- Legs drawn up to chest
- Skin pale, moist
- Pupils dilated
- Midline abd incision with sutures dry and intact
- CXR and UA neg.
- WBC 12,000

Acute Pain r/t tissue injury 2° surgical intervention

Comfort Level aeb
- report of satisfaction with pain control
- T, C, DB with a minimum of discomfort by 2nd postop day

Pain Control aeb often demonstrating ability to
- use analgesics appropriately
- use non-analgesic relief measures
- report symptoms to health care professional
- use preventive measures

Pain Relief aeb slight to no:
- reported pain
- protective body positioning
- restlessness
- pupil dilation
- perspiration
- change in BP, HR, R from normal baseline date

Pain Management

Pain Assessment

Reduce or eliminate factors that increase the pain

Consider cultural influences

Outcomes partially met
- states pain is 2/10 30 minutes after analgesic
- requests analgesic 30 minutes before ambulation
- hesitant to C & DB even following analgesic administration
- willing to try relaxation techniques but has not done so to date

Analgesic Administration

Determine type of analgesic based on pain assessment

Evaluate effectiveness of analgesic

Instruct to request medication at onset of pain

Simple Relaxation Therapy

Check willingness to use relaxation strategies

Demonstrate and practice relaxation techniques

Legend: Assessment ▢ Nursing Diagnosis ▢ Outcomes ▢ Nursing Interventions ▢ Activities ▢ Evaluation/Reassessment ▢

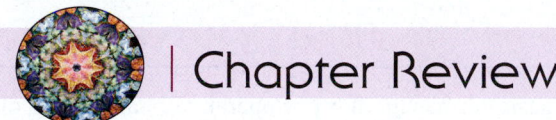

Chapter Review

EXPLORE MediaLink

NCLEX review questions, case studies, care plan activities, MediaLink applications, and other interactive resources for this chapter can be found on the Companion Website at www.prenhall.com/kozier. Click on Chapter 44 to select the activities for this chapter.

For more NCLEX review questions, and an audio glossary, access the Student CD-ROM accompanying this textbook.

Chapter Highlights

- Pain is a subjective sensation to which no two people respond in the same way. It can directly impair health and prolong recovery from surgery, disease, and trauma.
- Pain can be categorized according to its origin as cutaneous, deep somatic, or visceral—or according to its duration as acute pain or chronic pain.
- Pain threshold is generally similar in all people, but pain tolerance and response vary considerably.
- For pain to be perceived, nociceptors must be stimulated. Three types of pain stimuli are mechanical, thermal, and chemical.
- Nociception is comprised of the physiologic processes related to pain perception. It involves four processes: transduction, transmission, perception, and modulation.
- According to the gate control theory, peripheral nerve fibers carrying pain to the spinal cord can have their input modified at the spinal cord level before transmission to the brain. This theory is the basis of many pain intervention strategies.
- Numerous factors influence a person's perception and reaction to pain: ethnic and cultural values, developmental stage, environment and support people, earlier pain experiences, meaning of pain, and anxiety and stress.
- Pain is subjective, and the most reliable indicator of the presence or intensity of pain is the client's self-report. Assessment of a client who is experiencing pain should include a comprehensive pain history.
- Although the nursing diagnosis given to clients suffering pain is *Acute Pain* or *Chronic Pain,* the pain itself may be the etiology of many other nursing diagnoses.
- Overall client goals include preventing, modifying, or eliminating pain so that the client is able to partly or completely resume usual daily activities and to cope more effectively with the pain experience.
- When planning, nurses need to choose pain relief measures appropriate for the client.
- Pain management includes two basic types of nursing interventions: pharmacologic and nonpharmacologic.

- Scheduling measures to prevent pain is far more supportive of the client than trying to deal with pain once it is established.
- Major nursing strategies for all clients are to acknowledge and convey belief in the client's pain, assist support people, reduce misconceptions about pain, prevent pain, and reduce fear and anxiety associated with the pain.
- Pharmacologic interventions, ordered by the physician, include the use of opioids, nonopioids/NSAIDs, and adjuvant drugs.
- The World Health Organization recommends a three-step ladder approach to manage chronic cancer pain.
- Placebos fail to relieve pain for many people. Deceptive use of placebos is unacceptable practice.
- Analgesic medication can be delivered through a variety of routes and methods to meet the specific needs of the client. These routes include oral, nasal, rectal, transdermal, topical, subcutaneous or intravenous with a continuous infusion or a bolus dose, and intraspinal.
- Patient-controlled analgesia enables the client to exercise control and treat the pain by self-administering doses of analgesics.
- Physical nonpharmacologic pain interventions include such cutaneous stimulation as hot and cold applications, massage, acupressure, and contralateral stimulation; transcutaneous electrical nerve stimulation; immobilization; and acupuncture.
- Cognitive-behavioral interventions include distraction techniques, relaxation techniques, guided imagery, biofeedback, therapeutic touch, and hypnosis.
- Evaluation of the client's pain therapy includes the response of the client, the changes in the pain, and the client's perceptions of the effectiveness of the therapy. Ongoing verbal or written feedback from the client and family is integral to this process.

Review Questions

44–1. During the transduction phase of nociception, which method of pain control is most effective?
  a. tricyclic antidepressants
  b. opioids
  c. ibuprofen
  d. distraction

44–2. A client has arrived to the nursing unit from surgery. The nurse would most likely obtain which of the following information as a priority assessment?
  a. vital signs
  b. pain intensity
  c. location of pain
  d. pain history

44–3. A client who describes his pain as 6 on a scale of 1 to 10 is having
  a. severe pain.
  b. mild pain.
  c. very severe pain.
  d. moderate pain.

44–4. The client is 4 hours postop after abdominal surgery. She is receiving a continuous epidural infusion of an analgesic to manage her postoperative pain. Which of the following observations indicates a nursing intervention?
  a. drowsy; drifts off to sleep before completing a sentence
  b. respirations = 18/minute
  c. drowsy; easily aroused
  d. pain rating 1–2/10

44–5. The client has an order of morphine 2.5–5.0 mg IV every 4 hours. He received 2.5 mg IV 4 hours ago for pain rated at 3 on a scale of 0 to 10. He is now watching TV and visiting with family members. When you ask about his pain, he rates it as a 5. His VS are stable. What nursing intervention is the most appropriate?
  a. Give morphine 3.5 mg IV and inform him to continue watching TV because it is a distraction from the pain.
  b. Give 2.5 mg of morphine IV to avoid the client becoming addicted.
  c. Give nothing at this time because he is not exhibiting any signs of pain.
  d. Give morphine 5.0 mg IV and reassess in 20 minutes.

Readings and References

Suggested Readings

Loeb, J. L. (1999). Pain management in long-term care. *American Journal of Nursing, 99*(2), 48–52.
The author outlines three factors contributing to the incidence of inadequately controlled pain in long-term care: (a) underreporting by the residents because they may view pain as part of aging or they don't want to be viewed as complainers, (b) underdetection, especially with clients who have cognitive and physical impairments, and (c) undertreatment because of lack of knowledge. The author explains the implementation of a multidisciplinary pain management program and its positive outcomes.

McCaffery, M., & Robinson, E. S. (2002). Your patient is in pain. Here's how you respond. *Nursing, 32*(10), 36–45.
The authors reported the results of a survey asking nurses to self-evaluate their knowledge of pain management. The article provides the question, results of the survey, and rationale for the correct answer. The questions most often answered incorrectly related to pharmacology and addiction.

Panke, J. T. (2002). Difficulties in managing pain at the end of life. *American Journal of Nursing, 102*(7), 26–33.
This article provides a comprehensive overview of pain relief for nurses caring for dying clients and their families. The author focuses on three areas: difficulties in assessing clients who are nonverbal or cognitively impaired, differentiating pain from other symptoms, and the use of sedation.

Related Research

Howell, D., Butler, L., Vincent, L., Watt-Watson, J., & Stearns, N. (2002). Influencing nurses' knowledge, attitudes, and practice in cancer pain management. *Cancer Nursing, 23*(1), 55–63.

Kwekkeboom, K. L. (1999). A model for cognitive-behavioral interventions in cancer pain management. *Image: Journal of Nursing Scholarship, 31,* 151–155.

Parke, B. (1998). Realizing the presence of pain in cognitively impaired older adults: Gerontological nurses' ways of knowing. *Journal of Gerontological Nursing, 24*(6), 21–28.

Thomas, S. P. (2000). A phenomenologic study of chronic pain. *Western Journal of Nursing Research, 22,* 683–699.

Van Kooten, M. E. (1999). Non-pharmacologic pain management for postoperative coronary artery bypass graft surgery patients. *Image: Journal of Nursing Scholarship, 31*(2), 157.

References

Acello, B. (2000). Meeting JCAHO standards for pain control. *Nursing, 30*(3), 52–54.

American Academy of Pediatrics & Canadian Paediatric Society. (2000). Prevention and management of pain and stress in the neonate. *Pediatrics, 105*(2), 454–461.

American Pain Society. (1999). *Principles of analgesic use in the treatment of acute pain and cancer pain* (4th ed.). Glenview, IL: Author.

Andrews, M. M., & Boyle, J. S. (2003). *Transcultural concepts in nursing care* (4th ed.). Philadelphia: Lippincott Williams & Wilkins.

Ball, J. W., & Bindler, R. C. (2003). *Pediatric nursing: Caring for children* (3rd ed.). Upper Saddle River, NJ: Prentice Hall.

Bergh, I., & Sjostrom, B. (1999). A comparative study of nurses' and elderly patients' ratings of pain and pain tolerance. *Journal of Gerontological Nursing, 25*(5), 30–36.

Bieri, D., Reeve, R., Champion, G., Addicoat, L., & Ziegler, J. B. (1990). The Faces Pain Scale for the assessment of the severity of pain experienced by children: Development, initial validation, and preliminary investigation for ratio scale properties. *Pain, 41,* 139–150.

Cox, F. (2001). Clinical care of patients with epidural infusions. *The Professional Nurse, 16,* 1429–1432.

Eliopoulos, C. (2001). *Gerontological nursing* (5th ed.). Philadelphia: Lippincott.

Hawthorn, J., & Redmond, K. (1998). *Pain causes and management.* Oxford: Blackwell Science Ltd.

Herr, K. (2002). Chronic pain in the older patient: Management strategies. *Journal of Gerontological Nursing, 28*(2), 28–34.

LaDuke, S. (2002). Undertreated pain: Could it land you in court? *Nursing, 32*(9), 18.

Johnson, M., Maas, M., & Moorhead, S. (Eds.). (2000). *Nursing outcomes classification (NOC)* (2nd ed.). St. Louis, MO: Mosby.

McCaffery, M., Ferrell, B. R., & Pasero, C. (2000). Nurses' personal opinions about patients' pain and their effect on recorded assessments and titration of opioid doses. *Pain Management Nursing, 1*(3), 79–87.

McCaffery, M., & Pasero, C. (1999). *Pain: Clinical manual* (2nd ed.). St. Louis, MO: Mosby.

McCloskey, J. C., & Bulechek, G. M. (Eds.). (2000). *Nursing interventions classification (NIC)* (3rd ed.). St. Louis, MO: Mosby.

Melzack, R., & Wall, P. D. (1965). Pain mechanisms: A new theory. *Science, 150,* 971–979.

NANDA International. (2003). *NANDA nursing diagnoses: Definitions and classification 2003–2004.* Philadelphia: Author.

Paice, J. A. (2002). Controlling pain. Understanding nociceptive pain. *Nursing, 32*(3), 74–75.

Pasero, C. (2000). Continuous local anesthetics. *American Journal of Nursing, 100*(8), 22–23.

Pasero, C., & McCaffery, M. (2002). Pain control: Monitoring sedation. *American Journal of Nursing, 102*(2), 67–68.

Puntillo, K. A., White, C., Morris, A. B., Perdue, S. T., Stanik-Hutt, J., Thompson, C. L., et al. (2001). Patients' perceptions and responses to procedural pain: Results from Thunder Project II. *American Journal of Critical Care, 10,* 238–251.

Rhiner, M., & Kedziera, P. (1999). Managing breakthrough pain: A new approach. *American Journal of Nursing, 99*(3), Supplement 3–12.

Taylor, L. J., & Herr, K. (2002). Evaluation of the Faces Pain Scale with minority older adults. *Journal of Gerontological Nursing, 27*(4), 15–23.

Tucker, K. L. (2001). Deceptive placebo administration. *American Journal of Nursing, 101*(8), 55–56.

U.S. Department of Health and Human Services (1992). *Clinical practice guidelines: Acute pain management in adults: Operative procedures: Quick reference guide for clinicians.* (Publication No. 92-0019). Rockville, MD: Public Health Service Agency for Health Care Policy and Research.

Wong, D. L., Hockenberry-Eaton, M., Wilson, D., Winkelstein, M. L., & Schwartz, P. (2001). *Essentials of pediatric nursing* (6th ed.). St. Louis, MO: Mosby.

Selected Bibliography

Anonymous. (2001). Controlling pain. Taming pain with TENS. *Nursing, 31*(11), 84.

Gallagher, B. (2001). Controlling pain. Managing pain in elderly patients at home. *Nursing, 31*(8), 18.

Herr, K. (2002). Chronic pain. Challenges and assessment strategies. *Journal of Gerontological Nursing, 28*(1), 20–27.

Keefe, S. (2002). Children's drawings help diagnose migraines. *Nursing Spectrum Western Edition, 3*(11), 10–11.

Kingsley, C. (2001). Epidural analgesia. Your role. *RN, 64*(3), 53–57.

Kreger, C. (2001). Getting to the root of pain. Spinal anesthesia and analgesia. *Nursing, 31*(6), 36–41.

McCaffery, M. (2002). Controlling pain: Choosing a Faces pain scale. *Nursing, 32*(5), 68.

McCaffery, M., & Pasero, C. (2000). How to choose the best route for an opioid. *Nursing, 30*(12), 34–39.

McCaffery, M., & Pasero, C. (2001). Pain control. Assessment and treatment of patients with mental illness. *American Journal of Nursing, 101*(7), 69–70.

Merkel, S. (2002). Pain control. Pain assessment in infants and young children: The finger span scale. *American Journal of Nursing, 102*(11), 55–56.

Pasero, C., & McCaffery, M. (2001). Pain control: The lidocaine patch. *American Journal of Nursing, 101*(3), 22–23.

Pasero, C., & McCaffery, M. (2001). Pain control: The patient's report of pain. *American Journal of Nursing, 101*(12), 73–74.

Pasero, C., & McCaffery, M. (2001). Pain control: The undertreatment of pain. *American Journal of Nursing, 101*(11), 62–64.

Perkins, E. M. (2002). Less morphine, or more? *RN, 65*(11), 51–54.

Plaisance, L., & Ellis, J. A. (2002). Pain control: Opioid-induced constipation. *American Journal of Nursing, 102*(3), 72–73.

Salimbene, S. (2000). *What language does your patient hurt in? A practical guide to culturally competent patient care.* St. Paul, MN: EMC Paradigm.

Slaughter, A., Pasero, C., & Manworren, R. (2002). Pain control: Unacceptable pain levels. *American Journal of Nursing, 102*(5), 75–77.

U.S. Department of Health and Human Services (1992). *Clinical practice guidelines: Acute pain management in infants, children, and adolescents: Operative and medical procedures: Quick reference guide for clinicians* (Publication No. 92-0020). Rockville, MD: Public Health Service Agency for Health Care Policy and Research.

Wentz, J. D. (2001). Controlling pain. Assessing pain in cognitively impaired adults. *Nursing, 31*(7), 26.

World Health Organization (1999). *Cancer pain relief.* Geneva: Author.

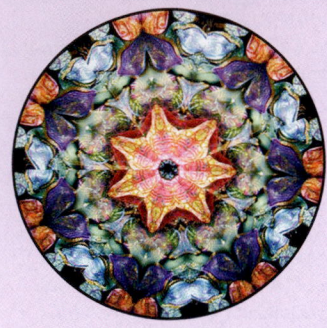

CHAPTER 45

NUTRITION

LEARNING OUTCOMES

After completing this chapter, you will be able to:

- Identify essential nutrients and dietary sources of each.
- Describe normal digestion, absorption, and metabolism of carbohydrates, proteins, and lipids.
- Explain essential aspects of energy balance.
- Discuss body weight and body mass standards.
- Identify factors influencing nutrition.
- Identify developmental nutritional considerations.
- Evaluate a diet using the food guide pyramid.
- Discuss essential components and purposes of nutritional screening and nutritional assessment.
- Identify risk factors for and clinical signs of malnutrition.
- Describe nursing interventions to promote optimal nutrition.
- Discuss nursing interventions to treat clients with nutritional problems.
- Plan, implement, and evaluate nursing care associated with nursing diagnoses related to nutritional problems.

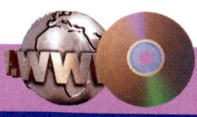

MediaLink

www.prenhall.com/kozier

Additional resources for this chapter can be found on the Student CD-ROM accompanying this textbook, and on the Companion Website at www.prenhall.com/kozier. Click on Chapter 45 to select the activities for this chapter.

CD-ROM
- Audio Glossary
- NCLEX Review
- Animations:
  - Carbohydrates
  - Proteins
  - Lipids
  - Inserting a Nasogastric Tube
  - A & P Review
    - Cellular Metabolism
    - Organic Compounds

Companion Website
- Additional NCLEX Review
- Case Study: Client with Percutaneous Endoscopic Gastrostomy Tube
- Care Plan Activity: Client Experiencing Loss of Appetite
- MediaLink Application: Vegetarian Nutrition
- Links to Resources

Nutrition is the sum of all the interactions between an organism and the food it consumes. In other words, nutrition is what a person eats and how the body uses it. **Nutrients** are organic and inorganic substances found in foods and are required for body functioning. People require the essential nutrients in food for the growth and maintenance of all body tissues and the normal functioning of all body processes.

An adequate food intake consists of a balance of essential nutrients: water, carbohydrates, proteins, fats, vitamins, and minerals. Foods differ greatly in their **nutritive value** (the nutrient content of a specified amount of food), and no one food provides all essential nutrients. Nutrients have three major functions: providing energy for body processes and movement, providing structural material for body tissues, and regulating body processes.

ESSENTIAL NUTRIENTS

The body's most basic nutrient need is water. Because every cell requires a continuous supply of fuel, the most urgent nutritional need, after water, is for nutrients that provide fuel, or energy. The energy-providing nutrients are carbohydrates, fats, and proteins. Hunger compels people to eat enough energy-providing nutrients to satisfy their energy needs, but no clear-cut body signals lead a person to ingest certain vitamins or minerals.

Carbohydrates

Carbohydrates are composed of the elements carbon (C), hydrogen (H), and oxygen (O) and are of two basic kinds: simple carbohydrates (sugars) and complex carbohydrates (starches and fiber).

Types of Carbohydrates

SUGARS. Sugars, the simplest of all carbohydrates, are water soluble and are produced naturally by both plants and animals. Sugars may be **monosaccharides** (single molecules) or **disaccharides** (double molecules). Of the three monosaccharides (glucose, fructose, and galactose), glucose is by far the most abundant.

Most sugars are produced naturally by plants, especially fruits, sugar cane, and sugar beets. However, lactose, a combination of glucose and galactose, is found in milk. Processed or refined sugars (e.g., table sugar, molasses, and corn syrup) are those that have been extracted and concentrated from natural sources. Processed sugars are added to foods such as soft drinks, cookies, candy, ice cream, and some cereals.

STARCHES. Starches are the insoluble, nonsweet forms of carbohydrate. They are **polysaccharides;** that is, they are composed of branched chains of dozens, sometimes hundreds, of glucose molecules. Like sugars, nearly all starches exist naturally in plants, such as grains, legumes, and potatoes. Starches are processed in various ways, for example, in making such foods as cereals, breads, flour, and puddings.

FIBER. Fiber, a complex carbohydrate derived from plants, cannot be digested by humans but supplies roughage, or bulk, to the diet. This bulk satisfies the appetite and helps the digestive tract to function effectively and to eliminate wastes. Fiber is present in the outer layer of grains, bran, and in the skin, seeds, and pulp of many vegetables and fruits.

Natural sources of carbohydrates also supply vital nutrients, such as protein, vitamins, and minerals that are not found in processed foods. Therefore, it is important that carbohydrate intake include natural foods. Processed carbohydrate foods are relatively low in nutrients in relation to the large number of calories they contain and thus are often referred to as "empty calories." Alcoholic beverages also may contain significant amounts of carbohydrate and are another source of empty calories.

Digestion

Major enzymes of carbohydrate digestion include ptyalin (salivary amylase), pancreatic amylase, and the disaccharidases: maltase, sucrase, and lactase. **Enzymes** are biologic catalysts that speed

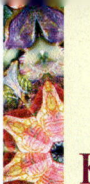
MediaLink | CARBOHYDRATES ANIMATION

1171

PROTEINS ANIMATION

MediaLink

up chemical reactions. The desired end products of carbohydrate digestion are monosaccharides. Some simple sugars are already monosaccharides and, therefore, require no digestion.

In healthy persons, essentially all monosaccharides are absorbed by the small intestine. Glucose transport through the cell membrane is augmented by insulin, a hormone secreted by the pancreas.

Carbohydrate Metabolism

Carbohydrate metabolism is a major source of body energy. After the body breaks carbohydrates down into glucose, some glucose continues to circulate in the blood to maintain blood glucose levels and to provide a readily available source of energy. The remainder is either used as energy or stored.

STORAGE AND CONVERSION. Carbohydrates are stored either as glycogen or as fat. **Glycogen** is a large polymer (compound molecule) of glucose. The process of glycogen formation is called **glycogenesis.** Almost all body cells are capable of storing glycogen; however, most is stored in the liver and skeletal muscles, where it is available for conversion back into glucose. Glucose that cannot be stored as glycogen is converted to fat.

Proteins

Proteins are organic substances composed of amino acids. Like carbohydrates, proteins contain carbon, hydrogen, and oxygen, but proteins also contain nitrogen. Every cell in the body contains some protein, and about three-quarters of body solids are proteins.

Amino acids are categorized as essential or nonessential. **Essential amino acids** are those that cannot be manufactured in the body and must be supplied as part of the protein ingested in the diet. Nine essential amino acids—threonine, leucine, isoleucine, valine, lysine, methionine, phenylalanine, tryptophan, and histidine—are necessary for tissue growth and maintenance. Arginine appears to have a role in the immune system.

Nonessential amino acids are those that the body can manufacture. The body takes apart amino acids derived from the diet and reconstructs new ones from their basic elements (carbohydrates and nitrogen). Nonessential amino acids include glycine, alanine, aspartic acid, glutamic acid, proline, hydroxyproline, cystine, tyrosine, and serine.

Proteins may be complete or incomplete. **Complete proteins** contain all of the essential amino acids plus many nonessential ones. Most animal proteins, including meats, poultry, fish, dairy products, and eggs, are complete proteins. Some animal proteins, however, contain less than the required amount of one or more essential amino acids and therefore cannot alone support continued growth. These proteins are sometimes referred to as **partially complete proteins.** Examples are gelatin, which has small amounts of tryptophan, and the milk protein casein, which has only a little arginine.

Incomplete proteins lack one or more essential amino acids (most commonly lysine, methionine, or tryptophan) and are usually derived from vegetables. If, however, an appropriate mixture of plant proteins is provided in the diet, a balanced ratio of essential amino acids can be achieved. For example, a combination of corn (low in tryptophan and lysine) and beans (low in methionine) is a complete protein. Such combinations of two or more vegetables are called *complementary proteins.* Another way to take full advantage of vegetable proteins is to eat them with a small amount of animal protein. Examples are spaghetti with cheese, rice with pork, noodles with tuna, and cereal with milk.

Digestion

Digestion of protein foods begins in the mouth, where the enzyme *pepsin* breaks protein down into smaller units. However, most protein is digested in the small intestine, where enzymes break it down into successively smaller molecules and finally into amino acids, the end products of protein digestion. The pancreas secretes the proteolytic enzymes trypsin, chymotrypsin, and carboxypeptidase; glands in the intestinal wall secrete aminopeptidase and dipeptidase.

Storage

Amino acids are absorbed by active transport through the small intestine into the portal blood circulation. The liver uses some amino acids to synthesize specific proteins (e.g., liver cells and the plasma proteins albumin, globulin, and fibrinogen). Plasma proteins are a storage medium that can rapidly be converted back into amino acids.

Other amino acids are transported to tissues and cells throughout the body, where they are used to make protein for cell structures. In a sense, protein is stored as body tissue. The body cannot actually store excess amino acids for future use. However, a limited amount is available in the "metabolic pool" that exists because of the constant breakdown and buildup of the protein in body tissues.

Protein Metabolism

Protein metabolism includes three activities: **anabolism** (building tissue), **catabolism** (breaking down tissue), and nitrogen balance.

ANABOLISM. All body cells synthesize proteins from amino acids. The types of proteins formed depend on the characteristics of the cell and are controlled by its genes.

CATABOLISM. Because a cell can accumulate only a limited amount of protein, excess amino acids are degraded for energy or converted to fat. Protein degradation occurs primarily in the liver.

NITROGEN BALANCE. Because nitrogen is the element that distinguishes protein from lipids and carbohydrates, nitrogen balance reflects the status of protein nutrition in the body. **Nitrogen balance** is a measure of the degree of protein anabolism and catabolism; it is the net result of intake and loss of nitrogen. When nitrogen intake equals nitrogen output, a state of nitrogen balance exists.

Lipids

Lipids are organic substances that are greasy and insoluble in water but soluble in alcohol or ether. **Fats** are lipids that are solid at room temperature; **oils** are lipids that are liquid at room temperature. In common use, the terms *fats* and *lipids* are used interchangeably. Lipids have the same elements (carbon, hydrogen, and oxygen) as carbohydrates, but they contain a higher proportion of hydrogen.

Fatty acids, made up of carbon chains and hydrogen, are the basic structural units of most lipids. Fatty acids are described as saturated or unsaturated, according to the relative number of hydrogen atoms they contain. **Saturated fatty acids** are those in which all carbon atoms are filled to capacity (i.e., saturated) with hydrogen; an example is butyric acid, found in butter. An **unsaturated fatty acid** is one that could accommodate more hydrogen atoms than it currently does. It has at least two carbon atoms that are not attached to a hydrogen atom; instead, there is a double bond between the two carbon atoms. Fatty acids with one double bond are called **monounsaturated fatty acids;** those with more than one double bond (or many carbons

not bonded to a hydrogen atom) are **polyunsaturated fatty acids.** An example of a polyunsaturated fatty acid is linoleic acid, found in vegetable oil.

Based on their chemical structure, lipids are classified as simple or compound. **Glycerides,** the simple lipids, are the most common form of lipids. They consist of a glycerol molecule with up to three fatty acids attached. **Triglycerides** (which have three fatty acids) account for more than 90% of the lipids in food and in the body. Triglycerides may contain saturated or unsaturated fatty acids. Saturated triglycerides are found in animal products, such as butter, and are usually solid at room temperature. Unsaturated triglycerides are usually liquid at room temperature and are found in plant products, such as olive oil and corn oil.

Cholesterol is a fatlike substance that is both produced by the body and found in foods of animal origin. Most of the body's cholesterol is synthesized in the liver; however, some is absorbed from the diet (e.g., from milk, egg yolk, and organ meats). Cholesterol is needed to create bile acids and to synthesize steroid hormones. Along with phospholipids, large quantities of cholesterol are present in cell membranes as well as other cell structures.

Digestion

Although chemical digestion of lipids begins in the stomach, they are digested mainly in the small intestine, primarily by bile, pancreatic lipase, and enteric lipase, an intestinal enzyme. The end products of lipid digestion are glycerol, fatty acids, and cholesterol. These are immediately reassembled inside the intestinal cells into triglycerides and cholesterol esters (cholesterol with a fatty acid attached to it), which are not water soluble. For these reassembled products to be transported and used, the small intestine and the liver must convert them into soluble compounds called lipoproteins. **Lipoproteins** are made up of various lipids and a protein.

Micronutrients

A **vitamin** is an organic compound that cannot be manufactured by the body and is needed in small quantities to catalyze metabolic processes. Thus, when vitamins are lacking in the diet, metabolic deficits result. Vitamins are generally classified as fat soluble or water soluble. **Water-soluble vitamins** include C and the B-complex vitamins: B_1 (thiamine), B_2 (riboflavin), B_3 (niacin or nicotinic acid), B_6 (pyridoxine), B_9 (folic acid), B_{12} (cobalamin), pantothenic acid, and biotin. The body cannot store water-soluble vitamins; thus, people must get a daily supply in the diet. Water-soluble vitamins can be affected by food processing, storage, and preparation.

Fat-soluble vitamins include A, D, E, and K. The body can store these vitamins, although there is a limit to the amounts of vitamins E and K the body can store. Therefore, a daily supply of fat-soluble vitamins is not absolutely necessary. Vitamin content is highest in fresh foods that are consumed as soon as possible after harvest.

Minerals are found in organic compounds, as inorganic compounds, and as free ions. On oxidation, minerals leave an ash, which can be acid or alkaline. Calcium and phosphorus make up 80% of all mineral elements in the body. The two categories of minerals are macrominerals and microminerals. **Macrominerals** are those that people require daily in amounts over 100 mg. They include calcium, phosphorus, sodium, potassium, magnesium, chloride, and sulfur. **Microminerals** are those that people require daily in amounts less than 100 mg. They include iron, zinc, manganese, iodine, fluoride, copper, cobalt, chromium, and selenium.

Common problems associated with the mineral nutrients are iron deficiency resulting in anemia, and osteoporosis resulting from loss of bone calcium. Additional information about major minerals associated with the body's fluid and electrolyte balance is given in Chapter 50. ∞

ENERGY BALANCE

Energy balance is the relationship between the energy derived from food and the energy used by the body. The body obtains energy in the form of calories from carbohydrates, protein, fat, and alcohol. The body uses energy for voluntary activities such as walking and talking and for involuntary activities such as breathing and secreting enzymes. A person's energy balance is determined by comparing his or her energy intake with energy output.

Energy Intake

The amount of energy that nutrients or foods supply to the body is their **caloric value. A calorie (c, cal, kcal)** is a unit of heat energy. A **small calorie** is the amount of heat required to raise the temperature of 1 gram of water 1 degree Celsius. This unit of measure is used in chemistry and physics. A **large calorie [Calorie, kilocalorie (Kcal)]** is the amount of heat required to raise the temperature of 1 gram of water 15 to 16 degrees Celsius and is the unit used in nutrition (although it is not universally capitalized). It was recommended in 1970 that the unit kilojoule (kJ), a metric measurement, replace the kilocalorie. However, to date, the United States and Canada have not made the change. A **kilojoule (kJ)** is the amount of energy required when a force of 1 newton (N) moves 1 kilogram of weight 1 meter distance.

One Calorie (Kcal) equals 4.18 kilojoules. The energy liberated from the metabolism of food has been determined to be:

- 4 Calories/gram (17 kJ) of carbohydrates
- 4 Calories/gram (17 kJ) of protein
- 9 Calories/gram (38 kJ) of fat
- 7 Calories/gram (29 kJ) of alcohol.

Energy Output

Metabolism refers to all biochemical and physiologic processes by which the body grows and maintains itself. Metabolic rate is normally expressed in terms of the rate of heat liberated during these chemical reactions. The **basal metabolic rate (BMR)** is the rate at which the body metabolizes food to maintain the energy requirements of a person who is awake and at rest. The energy in food maintains the basal metabolic rate of

the body and provides energy for activities such as running and walking.

Resting energy expenditure (REE) is the amount of energy required to maintain basic body functions; in other words, the calories required to maintain life. The resting expenditure of energy of healthy persons is generally about 1 cal/kg of body weight/hr for men and 0.9 cal/kg/hr for women although there is great variation among individuals. BMR is calculated by measuring the REE in the early morning, 12 hours after eating.

The actual daily expenditure of energy depends on the degree of activity of the individual. Approximate caloric expenditures compared to the REE are

Sleeping	90%
Light housework	210%
Walking steadily	350%
Heavy housework	400%
Laboring	500%
Average jogging/cycling/energetic swimming	700%

BODY WEIGHT AND BODY MASS STANDARDS

Maintaining a healthy or ideal body weight requires a balance between the expenditure of energy and the intake of nutrients. Generally, when energy requirements of an individual equate with the daily caloric intake, the body weight remains stable. **Ideal body weight (IBW)** is the optimal weight recommended for optimal health. To determine an individual's approximate IBW, the nurse can consult standardized tables or can quickly calculate a value using the Rule of 5 for women and the Rule of 6 for men (see Box 45–1). Many standardized tables and formulas were developed many years ago and are based on limited samples (Pai & Paloucek, 2000). The nurse should use great caution in suggesting that these weights apply to all clients.

Many health professionals consider the body mass index to be a more reliable indicator of a person's healthy weight. For people older than 18 years, the **body mass index (BMI)** is an indicator of changes in body fat stores and whether a person's weight is appropriate for height, and may provide a useful estimate of malnutrition. However, the results must be used with caution in people who have fluid retention (e.g., ascites or edema), athletes, or elders. To calculate the BMI:

1. Measure the person's height in meters (e.g., 1.5 m) (1 meter = 3.3 ft, or 39.6 in)
2. Measure the weight in kilograms (e.g., 60 kg) (1 kg = 2.2 pounds)
3. Calculate the BMI using the following formula

$$BMI = \frac{\text{Weight in kilograms}}{(\text{Height in meters})^2}$$

or

$$\frac{60 \text{ kilograms}}{1.5 \times 1.5 \text{ (meters)}^2} = 26.6$$

Box 45–2 provides an interpretation of the results.

BOX 45–1   ■ Approximating Ideal Body Weight

Rule of 5 for females:
   100 lbs for 5 ft of height
   + 5 lbs for each inch over 5 ft
   ±10% for body-frame size*

Rule of 6 for males:
   106 lbs for 5 ft of height
   + 6 lbs for each inch over 5 ft
   ±10% for body-frame size*

*Determine body-frame size by measuring the client's wrist circumference and applying to the tables below add 10% for large body-frame and subtract 10% for small body-frame size.

Female Wrist Measurements			
	Height less than 5′ 2″ (Less than 155 cms)	**Height 5′ 2″ – 5′ 5″ (155 cms – 163 cms)**	**Height more than 5′ 5″ (More than 163 cms)**
Small	Less than 5.5″ (140 mm)	Less than 6.0″ (152 mm)	Less than 6.25″ (159 mm)
Medium	5.5″ – 5.75″ (140 – 146 mm)	6″ – 6.25″ (152 – 159 mms)	6.25″ – 6.5″ (159 – 165 mm)
Large	More than 5.75″ (146 mm)	More than 6.25″ (159 mm)	More than 6.5″ (165 mm)

Male Wrist Measurements	
	Height more than 5′ 5″ (More than 163 cms)
Small	5.5″ – 6.5″ (140 - 165 mm)
Medium	6.5″ – 7.5″ (165 – 191 mm)
Large	More than 7.5≤ (191 mm)

BOX 45–2   ■ Guide for BMI Evaluation

<16	Malnourished
16–19	Underweight
20–25	Normal
26–30	Overweight
31–40	Moderately to severely obese
>40	Morbidly obese

Note: From "Know How: Nutritional Assessment," by E. Walters, 1998, *Nursing Times, 94*(8), pp. 68–69. Copyright Emap Healthcare, reproduced with permission.

Another measure of body mass is percent body fat. Because BMI uses only height and weight, it can give misleading results for certain groups of clients such as athletes, the frail elderly, and children. Percent of body fat can be measured by underwater weighing and dual-energy x-ray absorptiometry (DEXA) but these methods are time consuming and expensive. Other indirect, but more practical measures include the waist-to-hip ratio, skinfold testing, bioelectrical impedance analysis (used by

BOX 45–3   ■ Healthy Range of Body Fat

Age (Years)	Females (%)	Males (%)
18–39	21–32	8–19
40–59	23–33	11–21
60–79	24–35	13–24

some modern weight scales), and near-infrared interactance using a fiber-optic probe on the center of the biceps of the dominant arm, which measures tissue composition (Schnirring, 2001). Ranges considered healthy for percent body weight are shown in Box 45–3.

FACTORS AFFECTING NUTRITION

Although the nutritional content of food is an important consideration when planning a diet, an individual's food preferences and habits are often a major factor affecting actual food intake. Habits about eating are influenced by developmental considerations, gender, ethnicity and culture, beliefs about food, personal preferences, religious practices, lifestyle, medications and therapy, health, alcohol consumption, advertising, and psychologic factors.

Development

People in rapid periods of growth (i.e., infancy and adolescence) have increased needs for nutrients. Older people, on the other hand, need fewer calories and dietary changes in view of the risk of coronary heart disease, osteoporosis, and hypertension.

Gender

Nutrient requirements are different for men and women because of body composition and reproductive functions. The larger muscle mass of men translates into a greater need for calories and proteins. Because of menstruation, women require more iron than men do prior to menopause. Pregnant and lactating women have increased caloric and fluid needs.

Ethnicity and Culture

Ethnicity often determines food preferences. Traditional foods (e.g., rice for Asians, pasta for Italians, curry for Indians) are eaten long after other customs are abandoned.

Nurses should not use a "good food, bad food" approach, but rather should realize that variations of intake are acceptable under different circumstances. The only "universally" accepted guidelines are (a) to eat a wide variety of foods to furnish adequate nutrients and (b) to eat moderately to maintain correct body weight. Food preference probably differs as much among individuals of the same cultural background as it does generally between cultures. Not all Italians like pizza, for example, and many undoubtedly enjoy Mexican food.

Beliefs about Food

Beliefs about effects of foods on health and well-being can affect food choices. Many people acquire their beliefs about food from television, magazines, and other media. For example, some people are reducing their intake of animal fats in response to published evidence that excessive consumption of animal fats is a major risk factor in cardiovascular disease.

Food fads that involve nontraditional food practices are relatively common. A **fad** is a widespread but short-lived interest or a practice followed with considerable zeal. It may be based either on the belief that certain foods have special powers or on the notion that certain foods are harmful. Examples of some food fads are given in Box 45–4. Food fads appeal to the individual seeking a miracle cure for a disease, the person who desires superior health, or one who wants to delay aging. Some fad diets are harmless, but others are potentially dangerous. Determining the needs a fad diet fills for the client enables the nurse both to support these needs and to suggest a more nutritious diet.

Personal Preferences

People develop likes and dislikes based on associations with a typical food. A child who loves to visit his grandparents may

---

BOX 45–4 ■ Examples of Food Fads and Myths

- Eating large amounts of yogurt and vitamin E retards aging.
- Honey is healthier than sugar, more readily digested, and a cure for the common cold.
- Cabbage and onions turn breast milk sour.
- Raw eggs, rare lean beef, and oysters increase sexual potency or fertility.
- Organic foods are always healthier than those exposed to pesticides.
- Stomach enzymes cannot work on vegetables and fish at the same time and therefore these foods should not be eaten together.

---

love pickled crabapples because they are served in the grandparents' home. Another child who dislikes a very strict aunt grows up to dislike the chicken casserole she often prepares. People often carry such preferences into adulthood.

Individual likes and dislikes can also be related to familiarity. Children often say they dislike a food before they sample it. Some adults are very adventuresome and eager to try new foods. Others prefer to eat the same foods repeatedly. Preferences in the tastes, smells, flavors (blends of taste and smell), temperatures, colors, shapes, and sizes of food influence a person's food choices. For example, some people may prefer sweet and sour tastes to bitter or salty tastes. Textures play a great role in food preferences. Some people prefer crisp food to limp food, firm to soft, tender to tough, smooth to lumpy, or dry to soggy.

Religious Practices

Religious practice also affects diet. Some Roman Catholics avoid meat on certain days, and some Protestant faiths prohibit meat, tea, coffee, or alcohol. Both Orthodox Judaism and Islam prohibit pork. Orthodox Jews observe kosher customs, eating certain foods only if they are inspected by a rabbi and prepared according to dietary laws. The nurse must be sensitive to such religious dietary practices.

Lifestyle

Certain lifestyles are linked to food-related behaviors. People who are always in a hurry probably buy convenience grocery items or eat restaurant meals. People who spend many hours at home may take time to prepare more meals "from scratch." Individual differences also influence lifestyle patterns (e.g., cooking skills, concern about health). Some people work at different times, such as evening or night shifts. They might need to adapt their eating habits to this and also make changes in their medication schedules if they are related to food intake.

Muscular activity affects metabolic rate more than any other factor; the more strenuous the activity, the greater the stimulation of the metabolism. Mental activity, which requires only about 4 Kcal per hour, provides very little metabolic stimulation.

TABLE 45-1 Selected Drug–Nutrient Interactions

Drug	Effect on Nutrition
Acetylsalicylic acid	Decreases serum folate and folacin nutrition
	Increases excretion of vitamin C, thiamine, potassium, amino acids, and glucose
	May cause nausea and gastritis
Antacids containing aluminum or magnesium hydroxide	Decrease absorption of phosphate and vitamin A
	Inactivate thiamine
	May cause deficiency of calcium and vitamin D
Thiazide diuretics	Increase excretion of sodium, potassium, chloride, calcium, magnesium, zinc, and riboflavin
	May cause anorexia, nausea, vomiting, diarrhea, or constipation
	Decreases absorption of vitamin B_{12}
	May cause diarrhea, nausea, or vomiting
Potassium chloride	Increases excretion of potassium, magnesium, and calcium
	May cause anorexia, nausea, or vomiting
	Is incompatible with protein hydrolysates
Laxatives	May cause calcium and potassium depletion
	Mineral oil and phenolphthalein (Ex-Lax) decrease absorption of vitamins, A, D, E, and K
Antihypertensives	Hydralazine (Apresoline) may cause anorexia, vomiting, nausea, and constipation
	Methyldopa (Aldomet) increases need for vitamin B_{12} and folate
	May cause dry mouth, nausea, vomiting, diarrhea, constipation
Anti-inflammatory agents	Colchicine decreases absorption of vitamin B_{12}, carotene, fat, lactose, sodium, potassium, protein, and cholesterol
	Prednisone decreases absorption of calcium and phosphorus
Antidepressants	Amitriptyline (Elavil) increases food intake (large amounts may suppress intake)
Antineoplastics	Can cause nausea, vomiting, malabsorption, diarrhea

Nutrient	Effect on Drugs
Grapefruit	Can cause toxicity when taken with amlodipine (Norvasc), nifedipine (Procardia, Adalat), cisapride (Propulsid) carbamazepine (Tegretol), cyclosporine (Neoral), saquinavir (Fortovase), verapamil (Calan), sirolimus (Rapamune), tacrolimus (Prograf)
Vitamin K	Can decrease the effectiveness of warfarin (Coumadin)
Tyramine (found in aged cheeses, tap beer, dried sausages, fermented soy, sauerkraut)	Monoamine oxidase inhibitor (MAOI) medications, e.g., phenelzine (Nardil), tranylcypromine (Parnate), isocarboxazid (Marplan)
Milk	Interferes with absorption of tetracycline antibiotics

What, how much, and how often a person eats are frequently affected by socioeconomic status. For example, people with limited income, including some older people, may not be able to afford meat and fresh vegetables. In contrast, people with higher incomes may purchase more proteins and fats and fewer complex carbohydrates.

Medications and Therapy

The effects of drugs on nutrition vary considerably. They may alter appetite, disturb taste perception, or interfere with nutrient absorption or excretion. Nurses need to be aware of the nutritional effects of specific drugs when evaluating a client for nutritional problems. The nursing history interview should include questions about the medications the client is taking. Conversely, nutrients can affect drug utilization. Some nutri-

ents can decrease drug absorption; others enhance absorption. For example, the calcium in milk hinders absorption of the antibiotic tetracycline but enhances the absorption of the antibiotic erythromycin. Selected drug and nutrient interactions are shown in Table 45–1.

Therapies (e.g., chemotherapy and radiation) prescribed for certain diseases may also adversely affect eating patterns and nutrition. Normal cells of the bone marrow and the gastrointestinal mucosa are naturally very active and particularly susceptible to antineoplastic agents. Oral ulcers, intestinal bleeding, or diarrhea resulting from the toxicity of antineoplastic agents used in chemotherapy can diminish a person's nutritional status seriously.

The effects of radiotherapy depend on the area that is treated. For example, radiotherapy of the head and neck may cause decreased salivation, taste distortions, and swallowing difficulties; radiotherapy of the abdomen and pelvis may cause malabsorption, nausea, vomiting, and diarrhea. Many clients feel profound fatigue and anorexia.

Health

An individual's health status greatly affects eating habits and nutritional status. The lack of teeth, ill-fitting teeth, or a sore mouth makes chewing food difficult. Difficulty swallowing (**dysphagia**) due to a painfully inflamed throat or a stricture of the esophagus can prevent a person from obtaining adequate nourishment. Disease processes and surgery of the gastrointestinal tract can affect digestion, absorption, metabolism, and excretion of essential nutrients. Gastrointestinal and other diseases also create anorexia, nausea, vomiting, and diarrhea, all of which can adversely affect a person's appetite and nutritional status. Gallstones, which can block the flow of bile, are a common cause of impaired lipid digestion. Metabolic processes can be impaired by diseases of the liver. Diseases of the pancreas can affect glucose metabolism or fat digestion.

Between 30 and 50 million Americans have lactose intolerance, a shortage of the enzyme lactase which is needed to break down the sugar in milk. Certain populations are more widely affected: As many as 75% of African Americans and American Indians and 90% of Asian Americans are lactose intolerant (National Institute of Diabetes and Digestive and Kidney Diseases, 2002).

Alcohol Consumption

The calories contained in alcoholic drinks include both those of the alcohol itself and of the juices or other beverages added to the drink. In total, these can constitute large numbers of calories, for example, 150 calories for a regular 12-ounce beer, 160 calories for a "screwdriver" (1.5 ounces vodka plus four ounces orange juice). Drinking alcohol can lead to weight gain through the addition of these calories to the regular diet plus the effect of alcohol on fat metabolism. A small amount of the alcohol is converted directly to fat. However, the greater effect is that the remainder of the alcohol is converted into acetate by the liver. The acetate released to the bloodstream is used for energy instead of fat and the fat is then stored. In one study, the rate of fat metabolism fell 73% after two alcoholic drinks (Siler, Neese, & Hellerstein, 1999).

Excessive alcohol use contributes to nutritional deficiencies in a number of ways. Alcohol may replace food in a person's diet, and it can depress the appetite. Excessive alcohol can have a toxic effect on the intestinal mucosa, thereby decreasing the absorption of nutrients. The need for vitamin B increases, because it is used in alcohol metabolism. Alcohol can impair the storage of nutrients and increase nutrient catabolism and excretion.

Advertising

Food producers try to persuade people to change from the product they currently use to the brand of the producer. Popular actors and actresses are often used to influence television viewers' or radio listeners' choices. Advertising is thought to influence people's food choices and eating patterns to a certain extent. Of note is that such products as alcoholic beverages, cake and other dessert mixes, soups, tea, coffee, frozen dinners, and soft drinks are more heavily advertised than such products as milk, canned seafood, bread, cheese, poultry, vegetables, and fruits.

There has been an increase in advertising that targets elders in particular and encourages use of herbs and supplements. Some products are nutritionally safe while others are not and can cause interactions with medications they might be taking or cause unexpected side effects. The cost of some of these supplements is also usually high and may take money that the person could spend for healthier food.

Psychologic Factors

Although some people overeat when stressed, depressed, or lonely, others eat very little under the same conditions. Anorexia and weight loss can indicate severe stress or depression. Anorexia nervosa and bulimia are severe psychophysiologic conditions seen most frequently in female adolescents.

NUTRITIONAL VARIATIONS THROUGHOUT THE LIFE CYCLE

Nutritional requirements vary throughout the life cycle. Guidelines follow for the major developmental stages.

Neonate to 1 Year

The neonate's fluid and nutritional needs are met by breast milk or formula. Fluid needs of infants are proportionally greater than those of adults because of a higher metabolic rate, immature kidneys, and greater water losses through the skin and the lungs. The last is largely due to rapid respirations. Therefore, fluid balance is a critical factor. Under normal environmental conditions, infants do not need additional water; however, neonates in very warm environments may require additional fluids.

The total daily nutritional requirement of the newborn is about 80 to 100 mL of breast milk or formula per kilogram of body weight. The newborn infant's stomach capacity is about 90 mL, and feedings are required every 2 1/2 to 4 hours.

The newborn infant is usually fed "on demand." **Demand feeding** usually means that the child is fed when hungry. This method tends to decrease the problem of overfeeding or underfeeding the infant. The newborn who is hungry usually cries and exhibits tension in the entire body. During feeding, the infant sucks readily and needs burping after each ounce of formula or after 5 minutes of breast-feeding. Parents should be warned that infant bottles should never be propped up for feeding. There is a real danger that aspiration or choking could result.

Infants demonstrate satisfaction by slowing their sucking activity or by falling asleep. Once satisfaction has been demonstrated, infants should not be coaxed into finishing the feeding. This could lead to discomfort or overfeeding. When feeding is completed, healthy infants can be placed in a lateral or supine position for sleep during the first 6 months of life to reduce the risk of sudden infant death syndrome, or SIDS.

Regurgitation, or spitting up, during or after a feeding is a common occurrence during the first year. Although this may be of concern to parents, it does not usually result in nutritional deficiency. Demonstration of adequate weight gain should reassure parents that the infant is receiving adequate nutrition.

The addition of solid food to the diet usually takes place between 4 and 6 months of age. Six-month-old infants can consume solid food more readily because they can sit up, can hold a spoon, and have a decreased sucking reflex. Solid foods (strained or pureed) are generally introduced in the following order: cereals (rice), fruits, vegetables (yellow before green), and strained meats. Foods are introduced one at a time, usually with only one new food introduced every 5 days to ensure that the infant tolerates the food and demonstrates no allergy to it. This sequence can vary according to cultural preferences. With the eruption of teeth at about 7 to 9 months, the infant is ready to chew and can begin to experience different textures of food. At this time, the infant enjoys finger foods, such as skinless fruit cut into small pieces to prevent choking, dry cereal, or toast.

At about 6 months of age, infants require iron supplementation to prevent **iron deficiency anemia.** Iron deficiency anemia is a form of anemia caused by inadequate supply of iron for synthesis of hemoglobin. Iron-fortified cereals are usually recommended by 6 months of age and are continued until the child reaches 18 months.

Weaning from the breast or bottle to the cup takes place gradually and is usually achieved by age 1. Some infants have difficulty giving up the bottle, particularly at nap time or bedtime. Parents should be warned that having the bottle in bed can lead to **bottle mouth syndrome.** The term describes decay of the teeth caused by constant contact with sweet liquid from the bottle. Some dentists advocate brushing or cleaning the infant's teeth to prevent bottle mouth syndrome, especially for the infant who requires a bottle only at nap or bedtime. Weaning from the bottle can be facilitated by diluting the formula with water increasingly until the infant is drinking plain water. By the age of 1, most infants can be completely fed on table food, and milk intake is about 20 ounces per day.

Toddler

Because of a maturing gastrointestinal tract, toddlers can eat most foods and adjust to three meals each day. Toddlers' manipulative skills are sufficiently well developed for them to learn how to feed themselves. Before the age of 20 months, most toddlers require help with glasses and cups because their wrist control is limited. By age 3, when most of the deciduous teeth have emerged, the toddler is able to bite and chew adult table food.

Developing independence may be exhibited through the toddler's refusal of certain foods. Meals should be short because of the toddler's brief attention span and environmental distractions. Often toddlers display their liking of rituals by eating foods in a certain order, cutting foods a specific way, or accompanying certain foods with a particular drink.

The toddler is less likely to have fluid imbalances than the infant. The toddler's gastrointestinal function is more mature, and the percentage of fluid body weight is lower. A healthy toddler weighing 15 kg (33 lb) needs about 1,250 mL of fluid per 24 hours.

During the toddler stage, the caloric requirement decreases to 900 to 1,800 Kcal per day because of a decrease in the rate of growth. From 1 to 2 years of age, the toddler may be eating a combination of prepared toddler foods and some table foods. Parents should be instructed to read labels carefully and be aware that table foods offer more variety and are less expensive and more nutritious than prepared toddler foods. The Food Guide Pyramid discussed later in this chapter should be used as a guide in discussing the toddler's diet with parents. The need for adequate iron, calcium, and vitamins C and A, which are common toddler deficiencies, should also be discussed.

The following suggestions may help parents meet the child's nutritional needs and promote effective parent–child interactions: (a) Make mealtime a pleasant time by avoiding tensions at the table and discussions of bad behavior; (b) offer a variety of simple, attractive foods in small portions, and avoid meals that combine foods into one dish, such as a stew; (c) do not use food as a reward or punish a child who does not eat; (d) schedule meals, sleep, and snack times that will allow for optimum appetite and behavior; and (e) avoid the routine use of sweet desserts.

Preschooler

The preschooler eats adult foods. Parents should become informed about the diet of their child in day-care or preschool settings so that they can be sure of meeting the child's total nutritional needs. Children at this age are very active and may rush through meals to return to playing. The 4-year-old still requires parents' help in cutting meat and may spill milk when pouring from a large container. Parents also need to teach the preschooler how to use utensils and should provide them with the opportunity to practice (e.g., buttering bread). However, 4- and 5-year-olds often use their fingers to pick food up. Table manners are marginal at best. Active children often require snacks between meals. Cheese, fruits, yogurt, raw vegetables, and milk are good choices. Children at this age may enjoy helping in the kitchen, and both girls and boys should be encouraged to do so.

The preschooler is even less susceptible than the toddler to fluid imbalances. The average 5-year-old weighing 20 kg (45 lb) requires at least 75 mL of liquid per kilogram of body weight per day, or 1,500 mL every 24 hours.

School-Age Child

Nutrition continues to be a high priority for growing children. School-age children require a balanced diet including 2,400 kcal per day. School-age children eat three meals a day and one or two nutritious snacks. Children need a protein-rich food at breakfast to sustain the prolonged physical and mental effort required at school. Studies have shown that children who skip breakfast become inattentive and restless by late morning and have decreased problem-solving ability. Undernourished children become fatigued easily and face a greater risk of infection, resulting in frequent absences from school.

The average healthy 8-year-old weighing 30 kg (66 lb) requires about 1,750 mL of fluid per day. Many school-age children have only one meal a day with their family, at dinner. Mealtime should be a social time enjoyed by all, and parents should refrain from discussing a child's poor eating habits at this time. Parents should be aware that children learn many of their food habits by observing their parents. Eating a balanced diet should be the norm for both parent and child.

The school-age child generally eats lunch at school. The child may bring lunch from home or buy lunch at the school. Many dietary problems stem from this independence in food choices. The children may trade their food, not eat lunch at all, or buy sweets or junk food with their lunch money. Parents should discuss with the child the foods that they should eat and continue to provide a balanced diet in the home setting.

Poor eating habits may result in obesity. Obesity in school-age children tends to result in decreased activity as well as psychosocial problems. Obese children may be ridiculed and discriminated against by peers. Such behavior reinforces low self-esteem. Counseling should include the following:

- Reviewing the child's eating habits, including snacks
- Altering meal content
- Using rewards other than food
- Promoting regular exercise.

Adolescent

The adolescent's need for nutrients and calories increases, particularly during the growth spurt. In particular, the need for protein, calcium, vitamin D, iron, and B vitamins increases during adolescence. An adequate diet for an adolescent is 1 quart of milk per day as well as appropriate amounts of meat, vegetables, fruits, breads, and cereals. Calcium intake during adolescent years (1,200 to 1,500 mg/day) may help decrease osteoporosis (a decrease in bone density) in later life (Committee on Nutrition, American Academy of Pediatrics, 1999).

Many parents may observe that teenagers, particularly boys, seem to be eating all the time. Teenagers have active lifestyles and irregular eating patterns. They tend to diet or snack frequently, often eating high-calorie foods such as doughnuts, soft drinks, ice cream, and fast foods. Parents and nurses can promote better lifelong eating habits by encouraging teenagers to eat healthy snacks. Parents can provide healthy snacks such as fruits and cheese and at the same time limit the amount of "junk food" available in the home. The teenager's food choices relate to physical, social, and emotional factors and impulses and may not be influenced by teaching. Nurses need to advise parents that adolescents must take responsibility for their decisions in many areas of life, and parents should avoid conflicts that relate to food.

Common problems related to nutrition and self-esteem among adolescents include obesity, anorexia nervosa, and bulimia. Obesity is a common problem of the preadolescent period and continues to be a problem in the adolescent period. Many obese adolescents feel ugly and socially unacceptable. Depression is not unusual among obese adolescents. Treatment of obesity in this age group includes education on nutrition as well as assessment of psychosocial problems that may produce overeating.

Under social pressure to be slim, some adolescents severely limit their food intake to a level significantly below that required to meet the demands of normal growth. In some instances, the adolescent may develop an eating disorder, such as anorexia or bulimia. Anorexia nervosa and bulimia are severe psychophysiologic conditions usually seen in adolescent girls and young women. **Anorexia nervosa** is characterized by a prolonged inability or refusal to eat, rapid weight loss, and emaciation in persons who continue to believe they are fat. Anorexics may also induce vomiting and use laxatives and diuretics to remain thin. **Bulimia** is an uncontrollable compulsion to consume enormous amounts of food and then expel it by self-induced vomiting or by taking laxatives. These illnesses are most effectively treated in the early stages by psychotherapy. Hospitalization may be necessary when the effects of starvation become life threatening.

Young Adult

The nutritional habits established during young adulthood often lay the foundation for the patterns maintained throughout a person's life. Many young adults are aware of the food groups but may not be knowledgeable about how many servings of each group they need or how much constitutes a serving. The nurse should provide the young adult client with resources such as a chart or list that contains the foods and the amounts needed in each category.

Young adult females need to maintain adequate iron intake. A substantial number of women do not ingest sufficient dietary iron each day. **Anemia** is defined as a condition characterized by a decrease in circulating red blood cells. To prevent anemia, menstruating females should ingest 18 mg of iron daily. The nurse should instruct the female client to include iron-rich foods, such as organ meats (liver and kidneys), eggs, fish, poultry, leafy vegetables, and dried fruits, in her daily diet.

Calcium is needed in young adulthood to maintain bones and help decrease the chances of developing osteoporosis in later life. Along with calcium, the person must have adequate vitamin D, necessary for the calcium to enter the bloodstream. Vitamin D is made in the skin on exposure to the sun. If the person does not get sufficient sun exposure (15 minutes three times each week), supplements may be indicated.

Obesity may occur during the young adult years as the active teen becomes the sedentary adult but does not decrease caloric intake. The overweight or obese young adult is at risk for hypertension, a major health problem for this age group.

Hypertension and obesity are 2 of more than 40 risk factors that have been identified in the development of cardiovascular (CV) disease. Preventing these risk factors and lowering the risk of CV disease are critical. Low-fat and/or low-cholesterol diets play a significant role in both the prevention and treatment of CV disease.

Middle-Aged Adult

The middle-aged adult should continue to eat a healthy diet, following the recommended portions of the five food groups, with special attention to protein, calcium, and limiting cholesterol and caloric intake. Two or three liters of fluid should be included in the daily diet. Postmenopausal women need to ingest sufficient calcium and vitamin D to reduce osteoporosis, and antioxidants such as vitamins A, C, and E may be helpful in reducing the risks of heart disease in women.

Middle-aged adults who gain weight may not be aware of some common facts about this age period. Decreased metabolic activity and decreased physical activity mean a decrease in caloric need. The nurse's role in nutritional health promotion is to counsel clients to prevent obesity by reducing caloric intake and participating in regular exercise. Clients should also be warned that being overweight is a risk factor for many chronic diseases, such as diabetes and hypertension, and for problems of mobility, such as arthritis.

For the client who requires additional management resources, a variety of programs is frequently available. Most programs use behavior modification techniques and group support to assist clients in reaching their goals. Clients should seek medical advice before considering any major changes in their diets.

During late middle age, gastric juice secretions and free acid gradually decline. As a result, some individuals may complain of "heartburn" (acid indigestion) or an increase in belching. They may determine that certain foods disagree with them. Clients should be advised to develop sensible eating habits and avoid fried or fatty foods.

Elder

The older adult requires the same basic nutrition as the younger adult. However, fewer calories are needed by elders because of the lower metabolic rate and the decrease in physical activity.

Some elders may need more carbohydrates for fiber and bulk, but most nutrient requirements remain relatively unchanged. Such physical changes as tooth loss and impaired sense of taste and smell may affect eating habits. Decreased saliva and gastric juice secretion may also affect a person's nutrition

Psychosocial factors may also contribute to nutritional problems. Some elders who live alone do not want to cook for themselves or eat alone. As a result, they may adopt poor dietary habits. Other factors, such as lack of transportation, poor access to stores, and inability to prepare the food also affect nutritional status. Loss of spouse, anxiety, depression, dependence on others, and lowered income all affect eating habits (see Table 45–2). Guidelines for the inclusion of high-nutrient foods that are compatible with the nutritional needs of elders are summarized in Teaching: Wellness Care and in the Nutritional Reference Guide on pages 1182–1185. Also see Lifespan Considerations: Nutritional Considerations for Elders on page 1186.

STANDARDS FOR A HEALTHY DIET

Various daily food guides have been developed to help healthy people meet the daily requirements of essential nutrients and to facilitate meal planning. Food group plans emphasize the general types or groups of foods rather than the specific foods, because related foods are similar in composition and often have similar nutrient values. For example, all grains, whether wheat or oats, are significant sources of carbohydrate, iron, and the B vitamin thiamine. Daily food guides that are currently used include *Dietary Guidelines for Americans,* the Food Guide Pyramid, and *Canada's Food Guide to Healthy Eating.*

TABLE 45–2 Problems Associated with Nutrition in Older Adults

Problems	Nursing Interventions
Difficulty chewing	Encourage regular visits to the dentist to have dentures repaired, refitted, or replaced.
	Chop fruits and vegetables finely; shred green, leafy vegetables; select ground meat, poultry, or fish.
Lowered glucose tolerance	Eat more complex carbohydrates (e.g., breads, cereals, rice, pasta, potatoes, and legumes) rather than sugar-rich foods.
Decreased social interaction, loneliness	Promote appropriate social interaction at meals, when possible.
	Encourage the client and spouse to take an interest in food preparation and serving, perhaps as an activity they can do together.
	If food preparation is not possible, suggest community resources, such as Meals on Wheels.
	Suggest picnics in the yard or inviting friends over for meals.
Loss of appetite and senses of smell and taste	Eat essential, nutrient-dense foods first; follow with desserts and low-nutrient-density foods.
	Review dietary restrictions, and find ways to make meals appealing within these guidelines.
	Eat small meals frequently instead of three large meals a day.
Limited income	Suggest using generic brands and coupons.
	Substitute milk, dairy products, and beans for meat.
	Avoid convenience foods if able to cook. Buy foods that are on sale and freeze for future use.
	Suggest community resources and nutrition programs.
Difficulty sleeping at night	Have the major meal at noon instead of in the evening.
	Avoid tea, coffee, or other stimulants in the evening.

Teaching: Wellness Care
Nutrition for Elders

■ Include at least the minimal number of servings from each group on the Food Guide Pyramid:

Bread, cereal, grains, and pasta	6 servings
Vegetables	3 servings
Fruits	2 servings
Milk, yogurt, and cheese	2 servings
Meat, poultry, fish, beans, eggs, and nuts	2 servings

■ Reduce caloric intake. Caloric needs generally decrease in elders often because of decreased activity. Elders need to consume nutrient-dense foods and avoid foods that are high in calories but have few nutrients ("empty-calorie" foods).

■ Reduce fat consumption. Use leaner cuts of meat, and limit portions to 4 to 6 oz per day. (But be sure intake of meat group is sufficient, because elders often consume inadequate amounts of these foods.) Broil, boil, or bake foods instead of frying them. Use low-fat milk and cheese; limit intake of butter, margarine, and salad dressings.

■ Reduce consumption of empty calories. Substitute fruit or puddings made with low-fat milk in place of pastry, cookies, and rich desserts.

■ Reduce sodium consumption for clients who have hypertension or other cardiac problems. Avoid canned soups, ketchup, mustard. Avoid salted, smoked, cured, and pickled meats (e.g., ham and bacon), poultry, and fish. Do not add salt when cooking foods or at the table.

■ Ensure adequate calcium intake (at least 800 mg) to prevent bone loss. Milk, cheese, yogurt, cream soups, puddings, and frozen milk products are good sources. See the Major Food Sources of Calcium table below.

■ Ensure adequate vitamin D intake. Vitamin D is essential to maintain calcium homeostasis. Include some milk, because other dairy products are not usually fortified with vitamin D. If milk cannot be tolerated because of a lactose deficiency, provide vitamin supplements.

■ Ensure adequate iron intake. Iron intake in older people may be compromised by such factors as increased incidence of gastrointestinal disturbance, chronic diarrhea, regular aspirin use, and possible reduction in meat consumption. See the Major Food Sources of Iron table on page 1183.

■ Consume fiber-rich foods to prevent constipation and minimize use of laxatives. See the Fiber-Rich Foods table on page 1183. Because fiber-rich foods provide bulk and feeling of fullness, they help people control their appetites and lose weight.

Nutritional Reference Guide

Major Food Sources of Calcium

Foods	Household Measure	Calcium (mg)	Foods	Household Measure	Calcium (mg)
Dairy Products			**Fish, Meat, and Poultry**		
Cheese, cheddar	1 oz	213	Salmon (canned)	1 oz	91
Cheese, cottage, 4% milk fat	1 oz	27	Sardines	1 oz	124
Cheese, processed	1 oz (1 slice)	198	Shellfish	1 oz	35
Cheese, Swiss	1 oz	262			
Custard	1/2 cup	148	**Vegetables**		
Ice cream	1/2 cup	97	Beet greens	1/2 cup	72
Milk, nonfat dry (reconstituted)	1 cup	240	Broccoli (cooked)	1 medium stalk	158
Milk, skim (1% fat)	1 cup	296	Greens, collards	1/2 cup	179
Milk, whole	1 cup	288	Okra	10 pods	98
Yogurt	1 cup	295			
			Fruits		
			Blackberries	1 cup	46
			Dates	10	45
			Orange	1 medium	54
			Rhubarb (sweetened)	1/2 cup	105

Nutritional Reference Guide

Major Food Sources of Iron

Foods	Household Measure	Iron (mg)	Foods	Household Measure	Iron (mg)
Meat, Fish, Poultry			**Grain Products**		
Beef (ground)	3 oz	3.2	Bread		
Beef liver	3 oz	5.1	white	1 slice	0.6
Beef heart	3 1/2 oz	5.9	whole-wheat	1 slice	0.8
Beef kidneys	3 1/2 oz	7.4	Cereal (bran flakes)	1 oz	5.3
Chicken (breast)	3 oz	1.3	Cereal (oat flakes)	1 oz	5.4
Oysters	5 to 8 medium	5.5	Enriched pasta	1/2 cup	2.0
Scallops	3 1/2 oz	3.0	Spaghetti (enriched)	1/2 cup	0.3
Shrimp	3 1/2 oz	3.1			
Tuna (canned)	3 oz	1.5	**Other**		
			Corn syrup	1/3 cup	4.1
Vegetables and Fruits			Eggs	2 medium	2.3
Beet greens	2/3 cup	1.9	Molasses	1 T	0.9
Chick peas	1/2 cup	3	Peanuts	2/3 cup	2.1
Dates (pitted)	1/2 cup	3	Tofu (soybean curd)	1/2 cup	1.9
Kidney beans	1/2 cup	3			
Prune juice	1/2 cup	4.1			
Raisins	2/3 cup	3.5			
Soybeans	3 1/2 oz	2.8			
Spinach					
raw	1/2 cup	2			
cooked	1/2 cup	2.2			

Fiber-Rich Foods

Food	Portion	Insoluble Dietary Fiber Content (g)
Apple	1 medium	3.3
Banana	1	2.1
Beans, green	1/2 cup	1.8–2.2
Broccoli	1 cup	4.8
Cereal, all bran	1/3 cup	7.8
Cereal, bran flakes	1 cup	6.8
Fresh pear	1 medium	4.2
Kidney beans	1/2 cup	5.6
Lima beans	1/2 cup	3.2
Peas	1 cup	5.0

Types of Vegetarian Diets

Kind	Description
Vegans	Strict vegetarians; avoid all foods of animal origin.
Lacto-ovo-vegetarians	Use dairy products and eggs but avoid eating flesh.
Lacto-vegetarians	Use dairy products but avoid eating flesh and eggs.
Ovo-vegetarians	Use eggs but avoid dairy products and flesh.
Pesco-vegetarians	Use dairy products, eggs, and fish but avoid all other meat products.
Partial vegetarians (semivegetarians)	Avoid selected meats (e.g., red meat).
Fruitarians	Use only fresh (raw) fruits, juices, nuts, honey, and/or olive oil.
Macrobiotic vegetarians	Progress through 10 dietary stages from a widely inclusive selection to a restrictive selection.

Nutritional Reference Guide

Daily Food Guide

Food Groups and Servings	Foods and Sizes of Servings	Major Nutrients
Bread, Cereal, Rice and Pasta 6 to 11 servings, including several whole grains and enriched products. Limit fats and sugar (e.g., pastries, cookies).	1 serving = 1 slice bread, 1 oz ready-to-eat cereal, or 1/2 cup of the following: cooked cereal, cornmeal, grits, spaghetti, macaroni, noodles, popcorn, tortillas, or rice.	Complex carbohydrate; thiamine; niacin; iron; some protein; fiber

Vegetable Group
 	
3 to 5 servings, including
 	
    a. 1 to 2 servings of good sources of vitamin C.
 	
    b. 1 good source of vitamin A at least every other day.
 	
(Choose dark green and orange vegetables often.)
	1 serving = 1 cup raw leafy vegetables; 1/2 cup other fresh, frozen, or canned vegetables; 3/4 cup fresh, frozen, or canned juice; 1/4 cup dried vegetables.
	
	Broccoli, Brussels sprouts, green pepper, asparagus, cabbage, cauliflower, collards, potatoes, spinach, tomatoes.
	
	Broccoli, carrots, chard, collards, kale, pumpkin, spinach, sweet potatoes, turnip greens, winter squash.
		Carbohydrate; vitamin C; vitamin A; iron; folacin; calcium; fiber (naturally low in fat)

Fruit Group
 	
2 to 4 servings, including
 	
    a. 1 to 2 good sources of vitamin C.
 	
    b. Good sources of vitamin A.
(Choose orange fruits often.)
	1 serving = 1 medium apple, banana, or orange; 1/2 cup of raw, cooked, or canned fruit; 3/4 cup of fruit juice; 1/4 cup of dried fruit.
	
	Grapefruit or grapefruit juice; orange or orange juice; cantaloupe; raw strawberries.
	
	Apricots, cantaloupe.
		Vitamins A and C; potassium; folacin; fiber (naturally low in sodium)

Meat, Poultry, Fish, Beans, Eggs, and Nuts 2 to 3 servings. (Choose lean meat; poultry without skin; limit egg yolks, but not whites.)	1 serving = 1 egg; 1/2 cup cooked legumes (e.g., garbonzo, kidney, lima, pinto, or navy beans; lentils, split peas); 3 oz tofu; 2 T peanut butter; 1/4 cup nuts or seeds; 2 to 3 oz lean beef, pork, lamb, veal, poultry, or fish (no bone).	Protein; vitamin B; iron; zinc; niacin; fats (in meats, nuts, and seeds)
Milk, Yogurt, and Cheese Servings: Child under 9: 2 to 3 Child 9 to 12: 3 or more Teenager: 4 or more Adult: 2 or more Pregnant: 3 or more Lactating: 4 or more (Choose skim and low-fat milk and yogurt often. Limit high-fat cheese and ice cream.)	1 serving = 1 cup (8 oz) milk or yogurt, 11/2 oz natural cheese, 2 oz processed cheese food, 2 cups cottage cheese, 1 cup sauces or puddings, 12/3 cups ice cream. (Servings are based on calcium content.)	Protein; fat; vitamins A and D; riboflavin; B$_{12}$; calcium; phosphorus
Fats, Oils, and Sweets Use sparingly	Butter, salad oils, margarine, lard. Table sugar, brown sugar, confectioner's sugar, honey, molasses, maple syrup, corn syrup, jams, jellies, colas, and soft drinks.	Fat, carbohydrate (very high in calories)

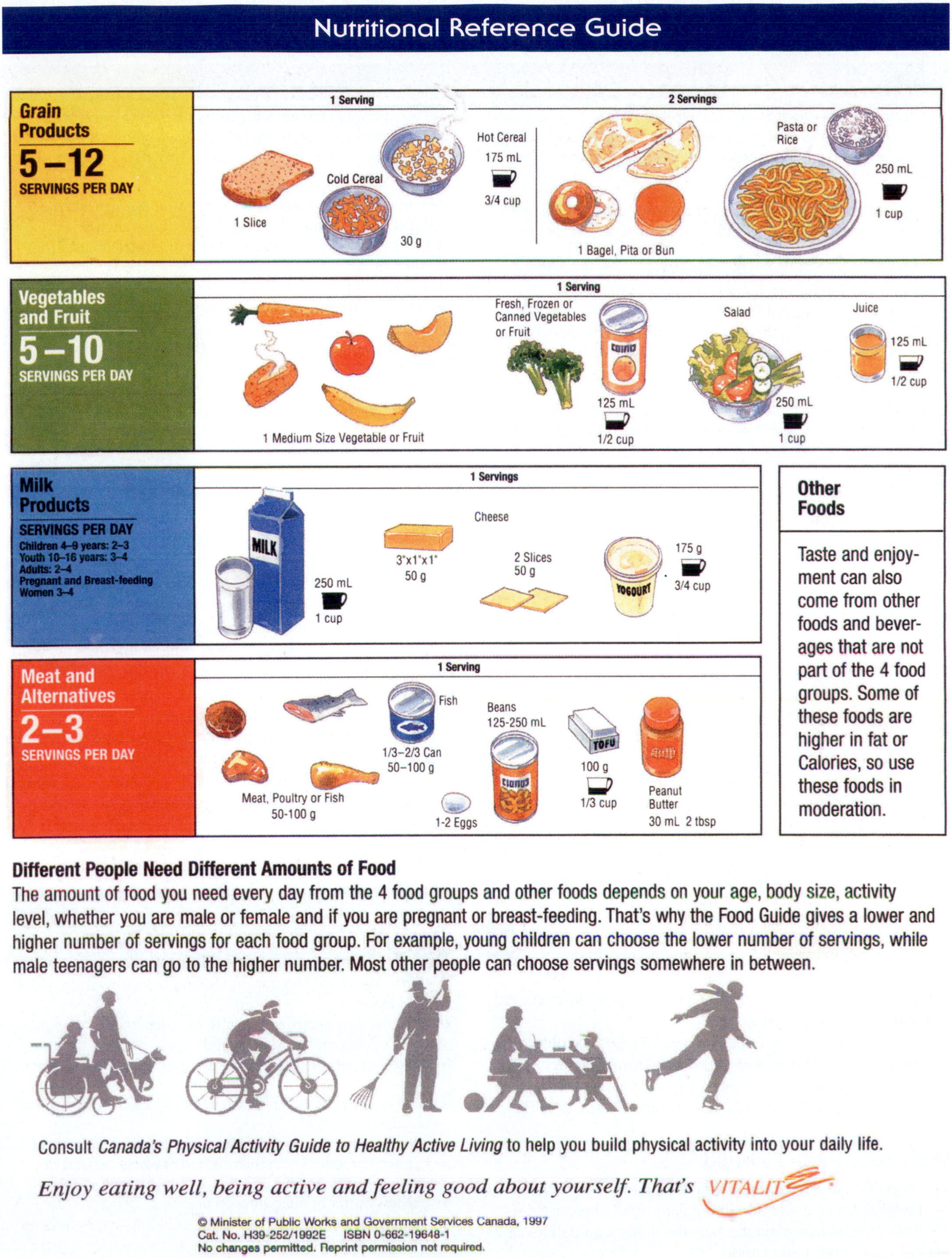
Nutritional Reference Guide
Grain Products
5–12
SERVINGS PER DAY
1 Serving
1 Slice
Cold Cereal
30 g
Hot Cereal
175 mL
3/4 cup
2 Servings
1 Bagel, Pita or Bun
Pasta or Rice
250 mL
1 cup
Vegetables and Fruit
5–10
SERVINGS PER DAY
1 Serving
1 Medium Size Vegetable or Fruit
Fresh, Frozen or Canned Vegetables or Fruit
125 mL
1/2 cup
Salad
250 mL
1 cup
Juice
125 mL
1/2 cup
Milk Products
SERVINGS PER DAY
Children 4–9 years: 2–3
Youth 10–16 years: 3–4
Adults: 2–4
Pregnant and Breast-feeding Women 3–4
1 Servings
MILK
250 mL
1 cup
Cheese
3"x1"x1"
50 g
2 Slices
50 g
YOGOURT
175 g
3/4 cup
Meat and Alternatives
2–3
SERVINGS PER DAY
1 Serving
Meat, Poultry or Fish
50-100 g
Fish
1/3–2/3 Can
50–100 g
1-2 Eggs
Beans
125-250 mL
TOFU
100 g
1/3 cup
Peanut Butter
30 mL 2 tbsp
Other Foods
Taste and enjoyment can also come from other foods and beverages that are not part of the 4 food groups. Some of these foods are higher in fat or Calories, so use these foods in moderation.
Different People Need Different Amounts of Food
The amount of food you need every day from the 4 food groups and other foods depends on your age, body size, activity level, whether you are male or female and if you are pregnant or breast-feeding. That's why the Food Guide gives a lower and higher number of servings for each food group. For example, young children can choose the lower number of servings, while male teenagers can go to the higher number. Most other people can choose servings somewhere in between.
Consult Canada's Physical Activity Guide to Healthy Active Living to help you build physical activity into your daily life.
Enjoy eating well, being active and feeling good about yourself. That's VITALITE
© Minister of Public Works and Government Services Canada, 1997
Cat. No. H39-252/1992E ISBN 0-662-19648-1
No changes permitted. Reprint permission not required.

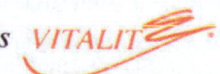

Figure 45–1 ■ Canada's Food Guide for Healthy Eating (1997) (*Note:* From *Canada's Food Guide to Healthy Eating,* Health Canada, 1992. Reproduced with the permission of the Minister of Public Works and Government Services: Canada, 2003.)

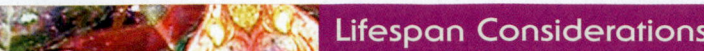

Lifespan Considerations

Nutritional Considerations for Elders

Most elders take several medications as a result of having an increase in the number of chronic illnesses. Considerations for potential problems include:

- Some foods interact adversely or decrease the effectiveness of certain medications, such as foods high in vitamin K and the anticoagulant coumadin.
- Some medications increase appetite, such as glucocorticoids.
- Some medications decrease appetite by their actions or by causing an unpleasant taste.
- Certain medications should not be crushed to be given by mouth or by gastric tubes, such as enteric coated or slow-release medications.

Conditions such as neuromuscular disorders and dementia can make it difficult for elders to eat or to be fed. Safety should al-

ways be a priority concern with attention paid to prevent aspiration. All health care personnel and family caregivers should be taught proper techniques to reduce this risk. Effective techniques include:

- Use the chin-tuck method when feeding clients with dysphagia. Having them flex their head toward their chest when swallowing decreases the risk of aspiration into the lungs.
- Use foods of prescribed consistency. Many elders can swallow foods with thicker consistency more easily than thin liquids.
- Try to focus on food preferences—the family can help provide this information.
- Try to maintain mealtime as a positive social occasion with conversations and extra attention paid to having a pleasant environment.

Dietary Guidelines for Americans

This guide is published by the U.S. Department of Agriculture (USDA, 2000a), and the 2000 revision contains recommendations for food choices to help promote health and prevent certain diseases. Key points of the dietary guidelines follow:

- Eat a variety of foods.
- Balance food with physical activity to maintain or improve weight.
- Eat plenty of grain products, vegetables, and fruits.
- Eat a diet low in fat, saturated fat, and cholesterol.
- Use sugars in moderation.
- Use salt and sodium in moderation.
- If you drink alcohol, do so in moderation.

These dietary recommendations are intended to help achieve the nutritional goals stated in *Healthy People 2010*. In that report, the U.S. surgeon general identified 25 specific nutritional objectives, such as the following (U.S. Department of Health and Human Services, 2000b):

- Reduce the incidence of overweight adults (target = 15%) and children (target = 5%).
- Reduce growth retardation among low-income children aged 5 and younger to less than 5%.
- Increase the proportion of persons aged 2 years and older who consume no more than 30% of calories from total fat to 75%.
- Increase the proportion of persons aged 2 years and older who consume no more than 2,400 mg of sodium daily to 65%.

The Food Guide Pyramid

The Food Guide Pyramid is a graphic aid that was developed by the USDA as a guide in making daily food choices (Figure 45–2 ■). The pyramid synthesizes the dietary guidelines and the old Basic Four Food Guide.

The pyramid suggests that people eat a variety of foods to obtain the nutrients they need. It divides foods into five groups,

each rich in certain nutrients. The groups are assigned to blocks of different sizes; the foods needed in the largest amounts (i.e., the bread, cereal, rice, and pasta group) appear in the largest block. Beside each block is the recommended number of daily servings. These are not listed as minimums, but as ranges to meet the nutrient needs of a variety of people. Because individuals differ in size, activity level, and so on, they need different amounts of food to meet their various nutrient needs. Numbers and sizes of servings are listed for each group in the Daily Food Guide table on page 1184.

The pyramid is designed to help people reduce their intake of fat and concentrated sugars. In the smallest box, at the top of the pyramid, is a fats, oils, and sweets category; it is labeled "Use Sparingly." See also Teaching: Wellness Care for ways to reduce fat intake.

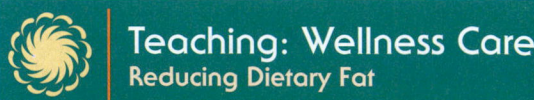

Teaching: Wellness Care
Reducing Dietary Fat

- Cook meat by grilling, baking, broiling, or microwaving rather than frying.
- Substitute popcorn or pretzels for such snacks as potato chips, cheese puffs and corn chips.
- Read labels. Some crackers, for example, are high in fat; others are not.
- Limit desserts high in fat, such as candy, ice cream, cake, and cookies.
- Substitute hard candies for chocolate bars.
- Use skim or reduced-fat milk instead of whole milk, for drinking as well as in recipes.
- Use less butter or margarine on breads.
- Remove fat from meat and skin from chicken before cooking.
- Eat less meat; eat more fish.
- Use less dressing, or use low-fat dressings, on salads.
- Eat plant sources of protein (e.g., kidney, lima, and navy beans).

Food Guide Pyramid
A Guide to Daily Food Choices

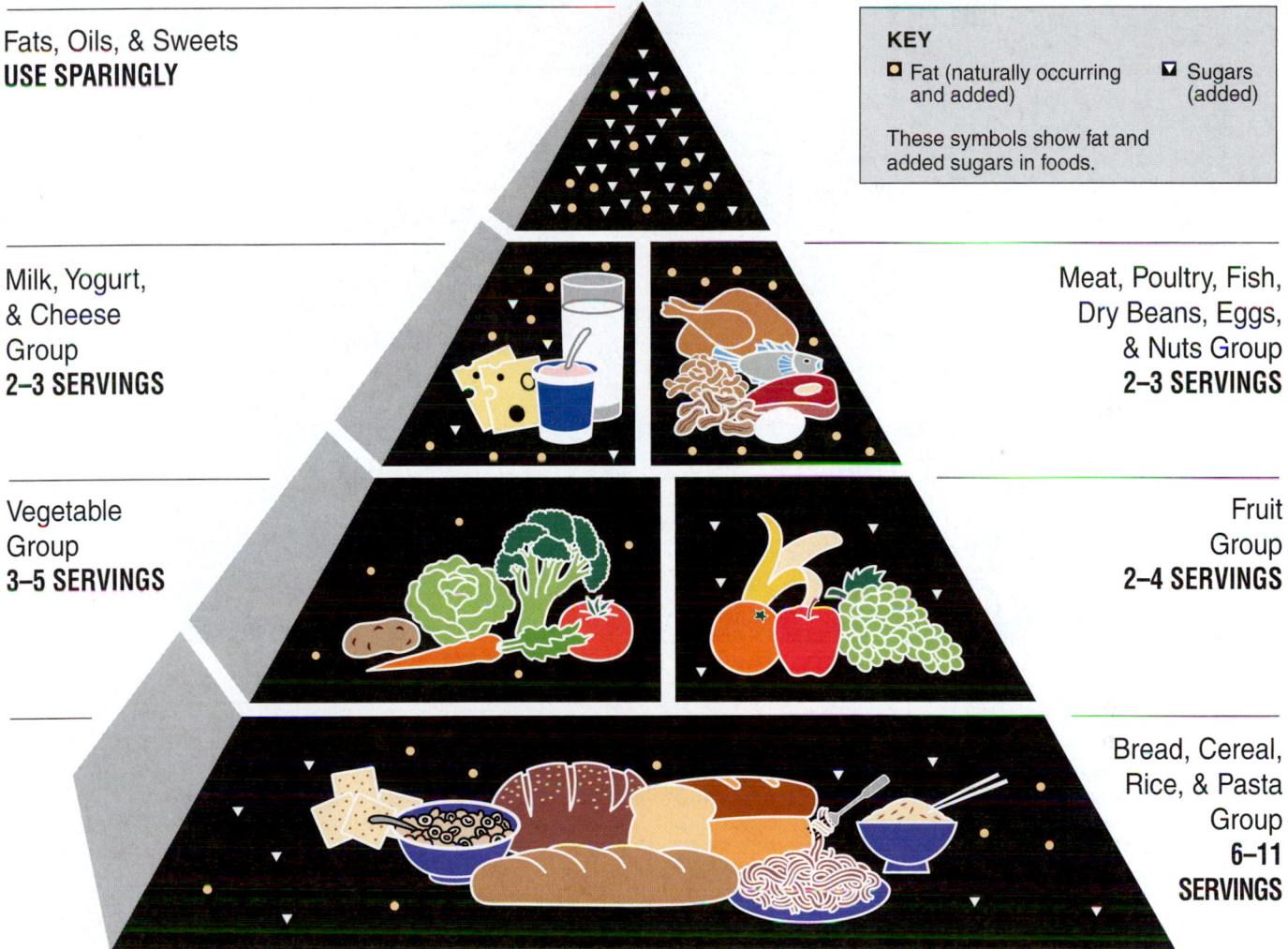

Fats, Oils, & Sweets
USE SPARINGLY

KEY
☐ Fat (naturally occurring and added)   ☑ Sugars (added)

These symbols show fat and added sugars in foods.

Milk, Yogurt, & Cheese Group
2–3 SERVINGS

Meat, Poultry, Fish, Dry Beans, Eggs, & Nuts Group
2–3 SERVINGS

Vegetable Group
3–5 SERVINGS

Fruit Group
2–4 SERVINGS

Bread, Cereal, Rice, & Pasta Group
6–11 SERVINGS

Figure 45–2 ■ The Food Guide Pyramid. (*Note:* From U.S. Department of Agriculture and U.S. Department of Health and Human Services, 1996.)

Using and following this guide does not guarantee that a person will consume the necessary levels of all essential nutrients. For example, someone who chooses cooked and low-fiber fruits and vegetables might have an inadequate intake of dietary fiber even though the recommended number of servings is eaten. However, the food guide is easy to follow, and people who eat a variety of foods from each group, in the suggested amounts, are likely to come close to recommended nutrient levels. The Food Guide Pyramid does not address fluid intake or provide guidelines about combination foods (such as chili, which contains meat, beans, and a vegetable) or about convenience foods (such as hamburgers, milk shakes, and pizzas), which are a large part of the North American diet.

There are many variations of the standard food pyramid. Examples include the pyramid for young children (Figure 45–3 ■) and the pyramid for elders (Figure 45–4 ■). There are pyramids or other shaped diagrams for food guides in many countries and Georgia State University has translated the pyramid into more than 37 languages (http://monarch.gsu.edu/nutrition/download.htm).

Canada's Food Guide to Healthy Eating

Canada's Food Guide to Healthy Eating is a booklet of dietary guidelines for Canadians 4 years old and over. It stresses the

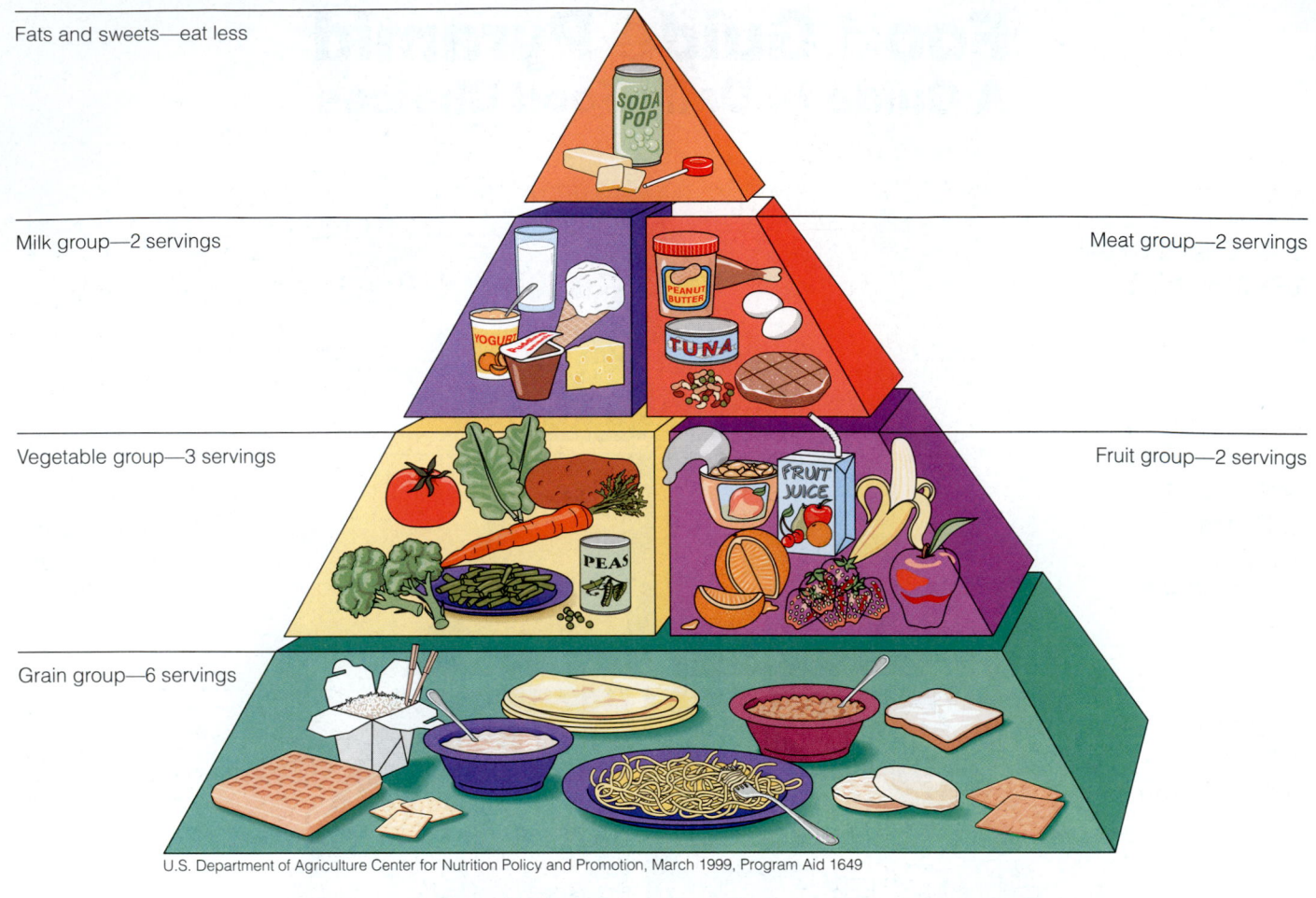

Fats and sweets—eat less

Milk group—2 servings

Meat group—2 servings

Vegetable group—3 servings

Fruit group—2 servings

Grain group—6 servings

U.S. Department of Agriculture Center for Nutrition Policy and Promotion, March 1999, Program Aid 1649

WHAT COUNTS AS ONE SERVING

GRAIN GROUP
1 slice of bread
1/2 cup of cooked rice or pasta
1/2 cup of cooked cereal
1 ounce of ready-to-eat cereal

VEGETABLE GROUP
1/2 cup of chopped raw
 or cooked vegetables
1 cup of raw leafy vegetables

FRUIT GROUP
1 piece of fruit or melon wedge
3/4 cup of juice
1/2 cup of canned fruit
1/4 cup of dried fruit

MILK GROUP
1 cup of milk or yogurt
2 ounces of cheese

MEAT GROUP
2 to 3 ounces of cooked lean
 meat, poultry, or fish

1/2 cup of cooked dry beans, or
1 egg counts as 1 ounce of lean
meat. 2 tablespoons of peanut
butter count as 1 ounce of
meat.

FATS AND SWEETS
Limit calories from these.

**Four- to 6-year-olds can eat these serving sizes. Offer 2- to 3-year-olds less, except for milk.
Two- to 6 year-old children need a total of 2 servings from the milk group each day.**

Figure 45–3 ■ Food guide pyramid for young children. (*Note:* From U.S. Department of Agriculture and U.S. Department of Health and Human Services, 1996.)

need to choose a variety of foods from within each of its four groups. Foods selected according to the guide supply 1,000 to 1,400 kilocalories. Those who need more calories or nutrients should increase the number and size of servings from the various groups and/or add other foods. Recommendations also include a decrease in fat consumption and limited use of salt, alcohol, and caffeine. See nutrition recommendations for Canadians in the *Canada's Food Guide to Healthy Eating* box (Figure 45–1 ■) on page 1185.

Recommended Dietary Intake

The Committee on Dietary Allowances of the Food and Nutrition Board of the National Academy of Sciences in Washington, DC, publishes the Dietary Reference Intakes (DRI) tables, which contain four sets of reference values: estimated average requirements (EAR), recommended dietary allowances (RDAs), adequate intakes (AI), and tolerable upper intake levels (UL). Definitions of these terms are found in Box

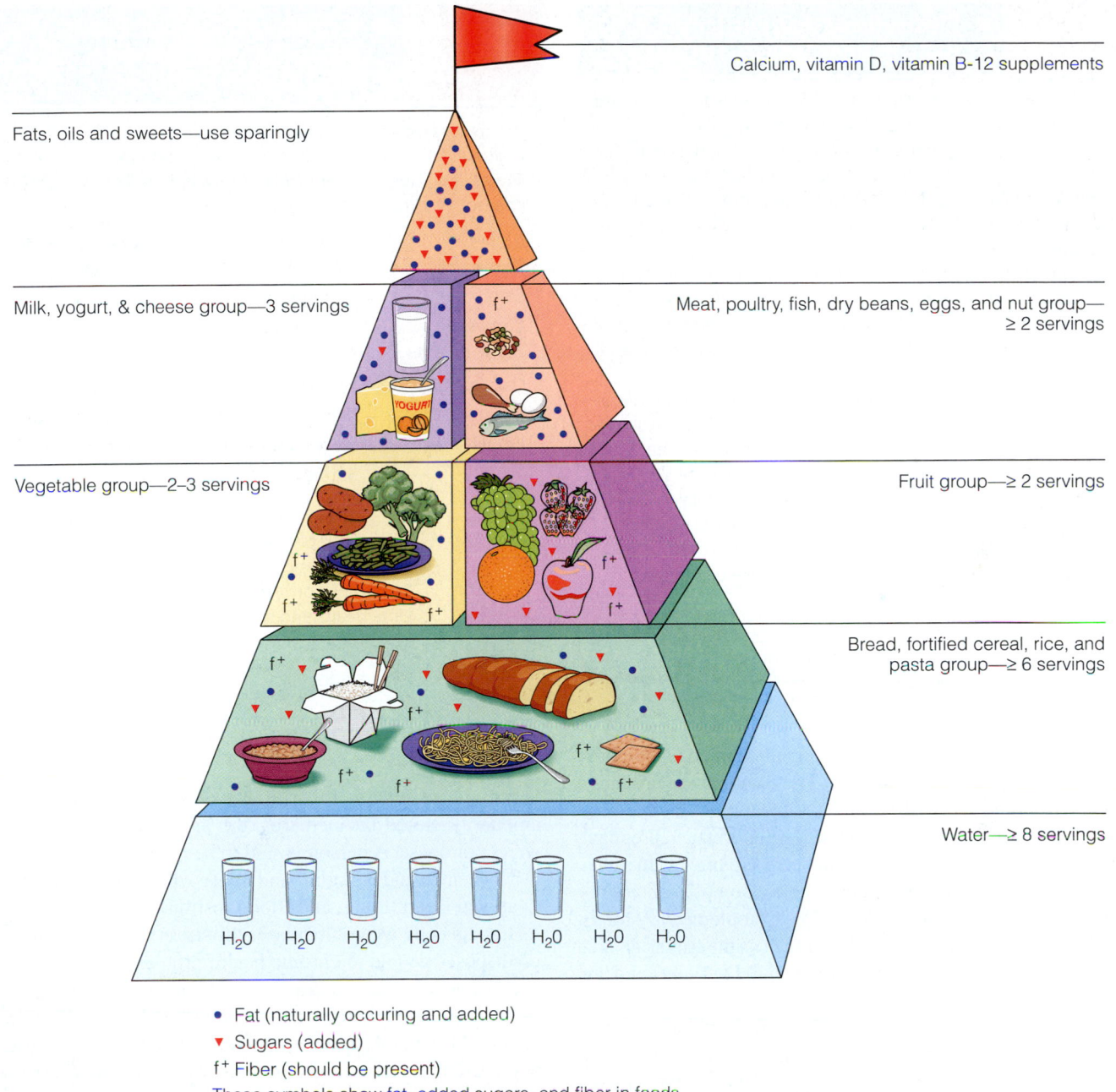

Calcium, vitamin D, vitamin B-12 supplements

Fats, oils and sweets—use sparingly

Milk, yogurt, & cheese group—3 servings

Meat, poultry, fish, dry beans, eggs, and nut group— ≥ 2 servings

Vegetable group—2–3 servings

Fruit group—≥ 2 servings

Bread, fortified cereal, rice, and pasta group—≥ 6 servings

Water—≥ 8 servings

H₂O H₂O H₂O H₂O H₂O H₂O H₂O H₂O

- Fat (naturally occuring and added)
- ▼ Sugars (added)
- f⁺ Fiber (should be present)
  These symbols show fat, added sugars, and fiber in foods.

Figure 45–4 ■ A modified food guide pyramid for people older than 70 years of age. (Copyright © 2002 From Tufts University School of Nutrition Science and Policy. Reprinted with permission.)

45–5. The values for RDAs and AIs in the tables are modified for different age groups and according to gender. As of 2003, the Canadian Department of National Health and Welfare has also adopted the DRIs. The effect of illness or injury (increasing the need for nutrients) and the variability among individuals within any given subgroup are not taken into account in the DRIs.

Vegetarian Diets

People may become vegetarians for economic, health, religious, ethical, or ecologic reasons. There are two basic vege-

tarian diets: those that use only plant foods (vegan) and those that include milk, eggs, or dairy products. Some people eat fish and poultry but not beef, lamb, or pork; others eat only fresh fruit, juices, and nuts; and still others eat plant foods and dairy products but not eggs. See the Types of Vegetarian Diets table on page 1183.

Vegetarian diets can be nutritionally sound if they include a wide variety of foods and if proper protein and vitamin and mineral supplementation are provided. Because the proteins found in plant foods are incomplete proteins, vegetarians must eat complementary protein foods to obtain all the essential

BOX 45-5	■ Definitions for Dietary Reference Value Tables

Dietary reference intakes (DRIs): The new standards for nutrient recommendations that include the following values:

Estimated average requirement (EAR): A nutrient intake value that is estimated to meet the requirement of half the healthy individuals in a group. It is used to assess nutritional adequacy of intakes of population groups. In addition, EARs are used to calculate RDAs.

Recommended dietary allowance (RDA): This value is a goal for individuals that is based on the EAR. It is the daily dietary intake level that is sufficient to meet the nutrient requirement of 97% to 98% of all healthy individuals in a group. If an EAR cannot be set, no RDA value can be proposed.

Adequate intake (AI): This is used when a RDA cannot be determined. It is a recommended daily intake level based on an observed or experimentally determined approximation of nutrient intake for a group (or groups) of healthy people.

Tolerable upper intake level (UL): The highest level of daily nutrient intake that is likely to pose no risks of adverse heath effects to almost all individuals in the general population. As intake increases above the UL, the risk of adverse effects increases.

Note: From *Dietary Reference Intakes: Applications in Dietary Assessment* (pp. 2–5), by the National Academy of Sciences, 2001, Washington, DC: National Academy Press. Reprinted with permission.

BOX 45-6	■ Combinations of Plant Proteins that Provide Complete Proteins

Grains plus legumes = complete protein.
Legumes plus nuts or seeds = complete protein.
Grains, legumes, nuts, or seeds plus milk or milk products (e.g., cheese) = complete protein.

Grains	Legumes	Nuts and Seeds
Brown rice	Black beans	Almonds
Barley	Kidney beans	Brazil nuts
Corn meal	Lima beans	Cashews
Millet	Soybeans	Pecans
Oats/oatmeal	Lentils	Walnuts
Rye	Tofu	Pumpkin seeds
Whole wheat	Black-eyed peas	Sesame seeds
	Sunflower seeds	
	Split peas	

Examples	Black-eyed peas and rice
	Lentil soup and whole wheat bread
	Beans and tortillas
	Lima beans and sesame seeds
	or
	Cereal with milk
	Macaroni with cheese

VEGETARIAN NUTRITION APPLICATION   MediaLink

amino acids. A plant protein can be complemented by combining it with a different plant protein. The combination produces a complete protein (see Box 45–6). Obtaining complete proteins is especially important for growing children and pregnant and lactating women, whose protein needs are high. Generally, legumes (starchy beans, peas, lentils) have complementary relationships with grains, nuts, and seeds. Complementary foods must be eaten in the same meal. Diets such as the fruitarian diet do not provide sufficient amounts of essential nutrients and are not recommended for long-term use.

Foods of animal origin are the best source of vitamin B_{12}. Therefore, vegans need to obtain this vitamin from other sources: brewer's yeast, foods fortified with vitamin B_{12}, or a vitamin supplement. Because iron from plant sources is not absorbed as efficiently as iron from meat, vegans should eat iron-rich foods (e.g., green leafy vegetables, whole grains, raisins, and molasses) and iron-enriched foods. They should eat a food rich in vitamin C at each meal to enhance iron absorption. Calcium deficiency is a concern only for strict vegetarians. It can be prevented by including in the diet soybean milk and tofu (soybean curd) fortified with calcium and leafy green vegetables. Figure 45–5 ■ shows a food guide pyramid for vegetarians.

ALTERED NUTRITION

Malnutrition is commonly defined as the lack of necessary or appropriate food substances but in practice includes both undernutrition and overnutrition. **Overnutrition** refers to a caloric intake in excess of daily energy requirements, resulting

in storage of energy in the form of adipose tissue. As the amount of stored fat increases, the individual becomes overweight or obese. A person is said to be **overweight** when BMI is between 26 and 30 kg/m^2 and **obese** when BMI is >30 kg/m^2 (National Heart, Lung, and Blood Institute, 1998).

Excess body weight increases the stress on body organs and predisposes people to chronic health problems such as hypertension and diabetes mellitus. Obesity that interferes with mobility or breathing is referred to as morbid obesity. Obese people may also manifest undernourishment in important nutrients (e.g., essential vitamins or minerals) even though excess calories are ingested.

Undernutrition refers to an intake of nutrients insufficient to meet daily energy requirements because of inadequate food intake or improper digestion and absorption of food. An inadequate food intake may be caused by the inability to acquire and prepare food, inadequate knowledge about essential nutrients and a balanced diet, discomfort during or after eating, dysphagia, **anorexia** (loss of appetite), nausea or vomiting, and so on. Improper digestion and absorption of nutrients may be caused by an inadequate production of hormones or enzymes or by medical conditions resulting in inflammation or obstruction of the gastrointestinal tract.

Inadequate nutrition is associated with marked weight loss, generalized weakness, altered functional abilities, delayed wound healing, increased susceptibility to infection, decreased immunocompetence, impaired pulmonary function, and prolonged length of hospitalization. In response to undernutrition,

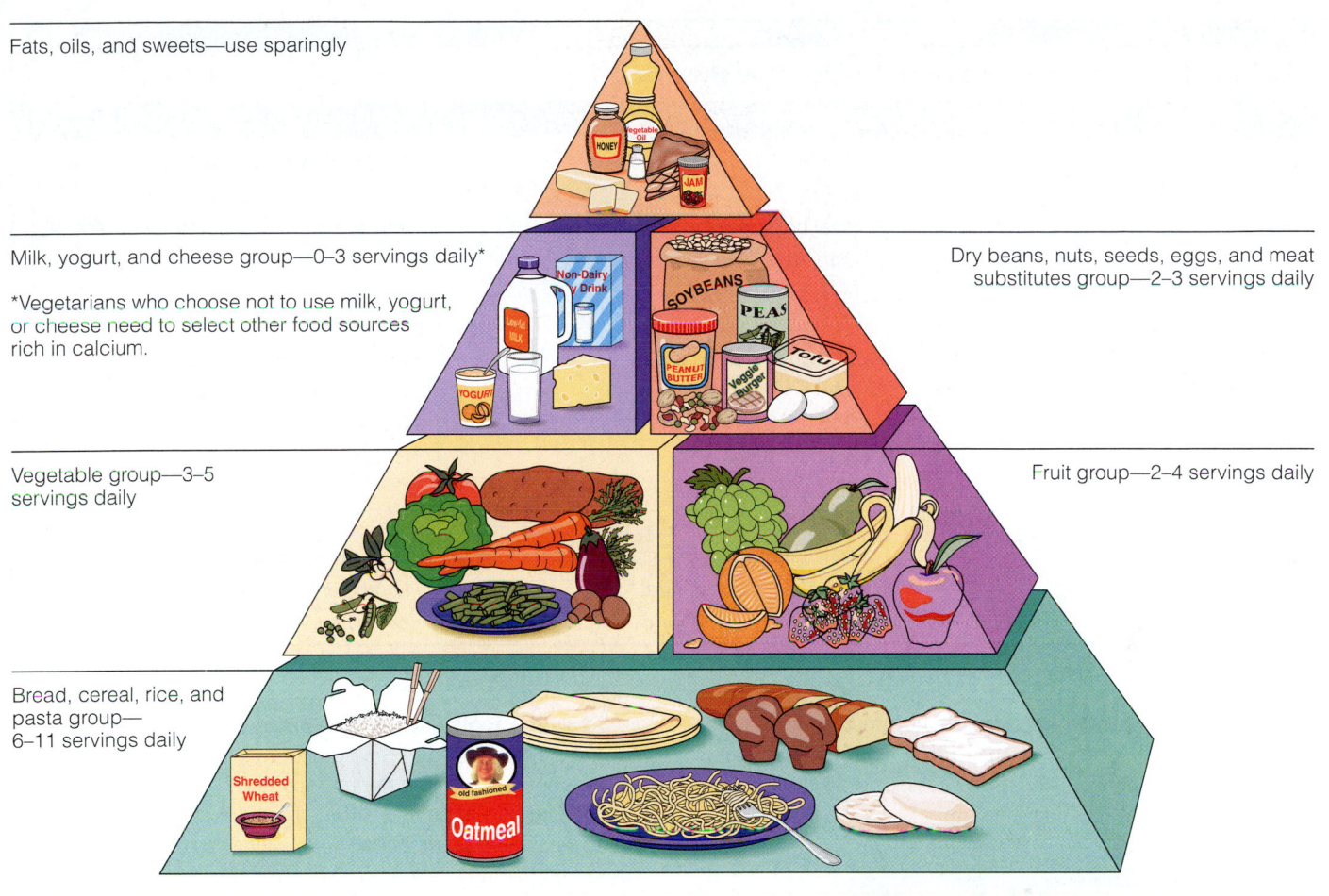

Fats, oils, and sweets—use sparingly

Milk, yogurt, and cheese group—0–3 servings daily*

*Vegetarians who choose not to use milk, yogurt, or cheese need to select other food sources rich in calcium.

Dry beans, nuts, seeds, eggs, and meat substitutes group—2–3 servings daily

Vegetable group—3–5 servings daily

Fruit group—2–4 servings daily

Bread, cereal, rice, and pasta group— 6–11 servings daily

WHAT COUNTS AS ONE SERVING

GRAIN GROUP
1 slice of bread
1 ounce of ready-to-eat cereal
1/2 cup of cooked cereal
1/2 cup of cooked rice, pasta, or other grains
1/2 bagel

VEGETABLE GROUP
1/2 cup of chopped raw or cooked vegetables
1 cup of raw leafy vegetables

FRUIT GROUP
3/4 cup of juice
1/4 cup of dried fruit
1/2 cup of chopped raw fruit
1/2 cup of canned fruit
1 medium-size piece of fruit, such as banana, apple, or orange

MILK GROUP
1 cup of milk or yogurt
1 2/3 ounces of natural cheese

DRY BEANS, NUTS, SEEDS, EGGS, AND MEAT SUBSTITUTES GROUP
1 cup of soy milk
1/2 cup cooked dry beans or peas
1 egg or 2 egg whites
2 tbsp nuts or seeds
1/4 cup tofu or tempeh
2 tbsp peanut butter

FATS AND SWEETS
Use sparingly.

Figure 45–5 ■ A food guide pyramid for vegetarian meal planning. (*Note:* From "Position of the American Dietetic Association: Vegetarian Diets," by V. K. Messina and K. I. Burke, 1997, *Journal of the American Dietetic Association, 97*(11). Reprinted with permission from Elsevier Science.)

carbohydrate reserves, stored as liver and muscle glycogen, are mobilized. However, these reserves can only meet energy requirements for a short time (e.g., 24 hours) and then body protein is mobilized.

Protein-calorie malnutrition (PCM), once associated with the manifestation of malnutrition seen in starving children of third world countries, is now recognized as a significant problem of clients with long-term deficiencies in caloric intake (e.g., those with cancer and chronic disease). Characteristics of

PCM are depressed visceral proteins (e.g., albumin), weight loss, and visible muscle and fat wasting.

Protein stores in the body are generally divided into two compartments: somatic and visceral. Somatic protein consists largely of skeletal muscle mass; it is assessed most commonly by conducting anthropometric measurements such as the mid-arm circumference (MAC) and the mid-arm muscle circumference (MAMC). (See the "Anthropometric Measurements" section on page 1196.) Visceral protein includes plasma protein,

TABLE 45–3 Components of a Nutritional Assessment

	Screening Data	Additional In-Depth Data
Anthropometric Data	• Height • Weight • Ideal body weight • Usual body weight • Body mass index	• Triceps skinfold (TSF) • Mid-arm circumference (MAC) • Mid-arm muscle circumference (MAMC)
Biochemical Data	• Hemoglobin • Serum albumin • Total lymphocyte count	• Serum transferrin level • Urinary urea nitrogen • Urinary creatinine excretion
Clinical	• Skin • Hair and nails • Mucous membranes • Activity level	• Hair analysis • Neurological testing
Dietary Data	• 24-Hour food recall • Food frequency record	• Selective food frequency record • Food diary • Diet history

hemoglobin, several clotting factors, hormones, and antibodies. It is usually assessed by measuring serum protein levels such as albumin and transferrin discussed in the "Laboratory Data" section of "Assessing," below.

NURSING MANAGEMENT

ASSESSING

The purpose of a nutritional assessment is to identify clients at risk for malnutrition and those with poor nutritional status. In most health care facilities, the responsibility for nutritional assessment and support is shared by the physician, the dietitian, and the nurse. Because a comprehensive nutritional assessment is time consuming and expensive, various levels and types of assessment are available. Generally, nurses perform a nutritional screen. A comprehensive nutritional assessment is often performed by a nutritionist, or a dietitian, and the physician. Components of a nutritional assessment are shown in Table 45–3 and may be remembered as ABCD data: anthropometric, biochemical, clinical, and dietary.

Nutritional Screening

A nutritional screen is an assessment performed to identify clients at risk for malnutrition or those who are malnourished. Clients who are found to be at moderate or high risk are followed with a comprehensive assessment by a dietitian (see Box 45–7).

Nurses carry out nutritional screens through routine nursing histories and physical examinations. Custom-designed screens for a particular population (e.g., elders and pregnant women) and specific disorders (e.g., cardiac disease) are available.

Screening tools such as the Patient Generated Subjective Global Assessment and the Nutrition Screening Initiative can be incorporated into the nursing history.

The Patient Generated Subjective Global Assessment (PG-SGA) is a method of classifying clients as either well nourished, moderately malnourished, or severely malnourished based on a dietary history and physical examination (McCallum, 2000). It was established primarily for use with cancer patients but has been widely tested and is appropriate for both inpatient and outpatient clients with various diagnoses. A version of the instrument (Figure 45–6 ■) can be completed and analyzed online by the client without a health care provider (http://www.unr.edu/nerp/pgsga.html).

The Nutrition Screening Initiative (NSI) is an ongoing project of the American Academy of Family Physicians, the American Dietetic Association, the National Council of Aging, and other organizations to promote nutrition screening and improved nutritional care for elders. The NSI screens elders using a nutrition checklist that contains nine warning signs of conditions that can interfere with good nutrition (see Box 45–8 on page 1196). Elders can also complete the tool online and have a risk score calculated (http://www.aafp.org/x16138.xml). The booklet *A Physician's Guide to Nutrition in Chronic Disease Management for Older Adults* contains information for physicians and handouts for clients and is also available online at http://www.eatright.org/nsi.html (Mathieu, 2002).

Nursing History

As mentioned earlier, nurses obtain considerable nutrition-related data in the routine admission nursing history. Data include but are not limited to

• Age, sex, and activity level
• Difficulty eating (e.g., impaired chewing or swallowing)

BOX 45–7 ■ Summary of Risk Factors for Nutritional Problems

Diet History

- Chewing or swallowing difficulties (including ill-fitting dentures, dental caries, and missing teeth)
- Inadequate food budget
- Inadequate food intake
- Inadequate food preparation facilities
- Inadequate food storage facilities
- Intravenous fluids (other than total parenteral nutrition for 10 or more days)
- Living and eating alone
- No intake for 10 or more days
- Physical disabilities
- Restricted or fad diets

Medical History

- Adolescent pregnancy or closely spaced pregnancies
- Alcohol or substance abuse
- Catabolic or hypermetabolic condition: burns, trauma
- Chronic illness: end-stage renal disease, liver disease, HIV, pulmonary disease (COPD), cancer

- Dental problems: difficulty chewing, ill-fitting dentures
- Fluid and electrolyte imbalance
- Gastrointestinal problems: anorexia, dysphagia, nausea, vomiting, diarrhea, constipation
- Neurologic or cognitive impairment
- Oral and gastrointestinal surgery
- Unintentional weight loss or gain of 10% within 6 months

Medication History*

- Antacid
- Antidepressants
- Antihypertensives
- Anti-inflammatory agents
- Antineoplastic agents
- Aspirin
- Digitalis
- Diuretics (thiazides)
- Laxatives
- Potassium chloride

*The potential effects of some medications on nutrition are shown in Table 45–1 on page 1177.

- Changes in appetite
- Changes in weight
- Physical disabilities that affect, purchasing, preparing, and eating food
- Cultural and religious beliefs that affect food choices
- Living arrangements (e.g., living alone) and economic status
- General health status and medical condition
- Medication history.

Physical Examination

Physical examination reveals nutritional deficiencies and excesses in addition to obvious weight changes. Assessment focuses on rapidly proliferating tissues such as skin, hair, nails, eyes, and mucosa but also includes a systematic review comparable to any routine physical examination. Clinical signs associated with malnutrition are provided in Table 45–4 on page 1196. These signs of malnutrition must be viewed as suggestive of malnutrition because the signs are nonspecific. For example, a red conjunctiva may indicate an infection rather than a nutritional deficit, and dry, dull hair may be related to excessive exposure to the sun rather than kwashiorkor (severe protein depletion). To confirm malnutrition, clinical findings need to be substantiated with laboratory tests and dietary data.

Calculating Percentage of Weight Loss

Accurate assessment of the client's height, current body weight (CBW), and usual body weight (UBW) is essential. Although the client's current body weight can be compared with an ideal body weight discussed earlier, the IBW is based on healthy people and does not account for changes in the client's body composition that accompany illness or reflect any changes in

weight. The client's usual body weight better reflects weight change and the possibility of malnutrition. Calculation and interpretation of the percent of deviation from UBW and the percent of weight loss are shown in Box 45–9 on page 1197. An important aspect of weight assessment, obtained in the nursing history, is a description of weight change. The nurse should describe any weight loss or gain, the duration of the change, and whether the weight change was intentional or unintentional.

Dietary History

A dietary history includes data about the client's usual eating patterns and habits; food preferences, allergies, and intolerances; frequency, types, and quantities of foods consumed; and social, economic, ethnic, or religious factors influencing nutrition. Factors may include, but are not limited to, living and eating alone, ability to purchase and prepare food, availability of refrigeration and cooking facilities, income, and effect of religion and ethnicity on food choices.

Four possible methods for collecting dietary data are a 24-hour food recall, a food frequency record, a food diary, and a diet history.

For a **24-hour food recall,** the nurse asks the client to recall all the food and beverages the client consumes during a typical 24-hour period. The data obtained are then generally evaluated according to the Food Guide Pyramid to judge overall adequacy.

A **food frequency record** is a checklist that indicates how often general food groups or specific foods are eaten. Frequency may be categorized as times/day, times/week, times/month, or frequently, seldom, never. This record, like the 24-hour food recall, provides information about the types of foods eaten but not the quantities. When specific foods or nutrients are suspected of being deficient or excessive, the health

Scored Patient-Generated Subjective Global Assessment (PG-SGA)
History (Boxes 1–4 are designed to be completed by the patient.)

Patient ID Information

---

1. Weight (*See Worksheet 1*)

In summary of my current and recent weight:

I currently weigh about _____ pounds
I am about _____ feet _____ tall

One month ago I weighed about _____ pounds
Six months ago I weighed about _____ pounds

During the past two weeks my weight has:

☐ decreased $_{(1)}$ ☐ not changed $_{(0)}$ ☐ increased $_{(0)}$

Box 1 ☐

---

2. Food Intake: As compared to my normal intake, I would rate my food intake during the past month as:

☐ unchanged $_{(0)}$
☐ more than usual $_{(0)}$
☐ less than usual $_{(1)}$
  I am now taking:
  ☐ *normal food* but less than normal amount $_{(1)}$
  ☐ little solid food $_{(2)}$
  ☐ only liquids $_{(3)}$
  ☐ only nutritonal supplements $_{(3)}$
  ☐ very little of anything $_{(4)}$
  ☐ only tube feedings or only nutrition by vein $_{(0)}$

Box 2 ☐

---

3. Symptoms: I have had the following problems that have kept me from eating enough during the past two weeks (check all that apply):

☐ no problems eating $_{(0)}$

☐ no appetite, just did not feel like eating $_{(3)}$

☐ nausea $_{(1)}$ ☐ vomiting $_{(3)}$
☐ constipation $_{(1)}$ ☐ diarrhea $_{(3)}$
☐ mouth sores $_{(2)}$ ☐ dry mouth $_{(1)}$
☐ things taste funny or have no taste $_{(1)}$ ☐ smells bother me $_{(1)}$
☐ problems swallowing $_{(2)}$ ☐ feel full quickly $_{(1)}$

☐ pain; where? $_{(3)}$_____

☐ other** $_{(1)}$ _____

** Examples: depression, money, or dental problems

Box 3 ☐

---

4. Activities and Function: Over the past month, I would generally rate my activity as:

☐ normal with no limitations $_{(0)}$

☐ not my normal self, but able to be up and about with fairly normal activities $_{(1)}$

☐ not feeling up to most things, but in bed or chair less than half the day $_{(2)}$

☐ able to do little activity and spend most of the day in bed or chair $_{(3)}$

☐ pretty much bedridden, rarely out of bed $_{(3)}$

Box 4 ☐

Additive Score of the Boxes 1–4 ☐ A

The remainder of this form will be completed by your doctor, nurse, or therapist. Thank you.

---

5. Disease and its relation to nutritional requirements (*See Worksheet 2*)

All relevant diagnoses (specify) _____

Primary disease stage (circle if known or appropriate)   I   II   III   IV   Other _____

Age _____

Numerical score from Worksheet 2 ☐ B

6. Metabolic Demand (*See Worksheet 3*)

Numerical score from Worksheet 3 ☐ C

7. Physical (*See Worksheet 4*)

Numerical score from Worksheet 4 ☐ D

Global Assessment (*See Worksheet 5*)

☐ Well-nourished or anabolic (SGA-A)
☐ Moderate or suspected malnutrition (SGA-B)
☐ Severely malnourished (SGA-C)

Total PG-SGA score

(Total numerical score of A+B+C+D above) ☐
(See triage recommendations below)

Clinician Signature _____ RD RN PA MD DO Other ___   Date _____

Nutritional Triage Recommendations: Additive score is used to define specific nutritional interventions including patient & family education, symptom management including pharmacologic intervention, and appropriate nutrient intervention (food, nutritional supplements, enteral, or parenteral triage). First line nutrition intervention includes optimal symptom management.

0–1 No intervention required at this time. Re-assessment on routine and regular basis during treatment.
2–3 Patient & family education by dietitian, nurse, or other clinician with pharmacologic intervention as indicated by symptom survey (Box 3) and laboratory values as appropriate.
4–8 Requires intervention by dietitian, in conjunction with nurse or physician as indicated by symptoms survey (Box 3).
≥ 9 Indicates a critical need for improved symptom management and/or nutrient intervention options.

Figure 45–6 ■ Scored Patient-Generated Subjective Global Assessment (PG-SGA). (*Note:* © FD Ottery, 2001, email: fottery@noat.org. Reprinted with permission.)

Worksheets for PG-SGA Scoring

Boxes 1–4 of the PG-SGA are designed to be completed by the patient. The PG-SGA numerical score is determined using 1) the parenthetical points noted in boxes 1–4 and 2) the worksheets below for items not marked with parenthetical points. Scores for boxes 1 and 3 are additive within each box and scores for boxes 2 and 4 are based on the highest scored item checked off by the patient.

Worksheet 1 — Scoring Weight (Wt) Loss

To determine score, use 1 month weight data if available. Use 6 month data only if there is no 1 month weight data. Use points below to score weight change and add one extra point if patient has lost weight during the past 2 weeks. Enter total point score in Box 1 of the PG-SGA.

Wt loss in 1 month	Points	Wt loss in 6 months
10% or greater	4	20% or greater
5–9.9%	3	10–19.9%
3–4.9%	2	6–9.9%
2–2.9%	1	2–5.9%
0–1.9%	0	0–1.9%

Score for Worksheet 1 [ ]
Record in Box 1

Worksheet 2 — Scoring Criteria for Condition

Score is derived by adding 1 point for each of the conditions listed below that pertain to the patient.

Category Points

Cancer	1
AIDS	1
Pulmonary or cardiac cachexia	1
Presence of decubitus, open wound, or fistula	1
Presence of trauma	1
Age greater than 65 years	1

Score for Worksheet 2 = [ ]
Record in Box B

Worksheet 3 — Scoring Metabolic Stress

Score for metabolic stress is determined by a number of variables known to increase protein & calorie needs. The score is additive so that a patient who has a fever of > 102 degrees (3 points) and is on 10 mg of prednisone chronically (2 points) would have an additive score for this section of 5 points.

Stress	none (0)	low (1)	moderate (2)	high (3)
Fever	no fever	>99 and <101	≥101 and <102	≥102
Fever duration	no fever	<72 hrs	72 hrs	> 72 hrs
Corticoteroids	no corticosteroids	low dose (<10mg prednisone equivalents/day)	moderate dose (≥10 and <30mg prednisone equivalents/day)	high dose steroids (≥30mg prednisone equivalents/day)

Score for Worksheet 3 = [ ]
Record in Box C

Worksheet 4 — Physical Examination

Physical exam includes a subjective evaluation of 3 aspects of body composition: fat, muscle, & fluid status. Since this is subjective, each aspect of the exam is rated for degree of deficit. Muscle deficit impacts point score more than fat deficit. Definition of categories: 0 = no deficit, 1+ = mild deficit, 2+ = moderate deficit, 3+ = severe deficit. Rating of deficit in these categories are *not* additive but are used to clinically assess the degree of deficit (or presence of excess fluid).

Fat Stores:

orbital fat pads	0	1+	2+	3+
triceps skin fold	0	1+	2+	3+
fat overlying lower ribs	0	1+	2+	3+
Global fat deficit rating	**0**	**1+**	**2+**	**3+**

Muscle Status:

temples (temporalis muscle)	0	1+	2+	3+
clavicles (pectoralis & deltoids)	0	1+	2+	3+
shoulders (deltoids)	0	1+	2+	3+
interosseous muscles	0	1+	2+	3+
scapula (latissimus dorsi, trapezius, deltoids)	0	1+	2+	3+
thigh (quadriceps)	0	1+	2+	3+
calf (gastrocnemius)	0	1+	2+	3+
Global muscle status rating	**0**	**1+**	**2+**	**3+**

Fluid Status:

ankle edema	0	1+	2+	3+
sacral edema	0	1+	2+	3+
ascites	0	1+	2+	3+
Global fluid status rating	**0**	**1+**	**2+**	**3+**

Point score for the physical exam is determined by the overall subjective rating of total body deficit.

No deficit	score = 0 points
Mild deficit	score = 1 point
Moderate deficit	score = 2 points
Severe deficit	score = 3 points

Score for Worksheet 4 = [ ]
Record in Box D

Worksheet 5 — PG-SGA Global Assessment Categories

	Stage A	Stage B	Stage C
Category	Well-nourished	Moderately malnourished or suspected malnutrition	Severely malnourished
Weight	No wt loss OR Recent non-fluid wt gain	~5% wt loss within 1 month (or 10% in 6 months) OR No wt stabilization or wt gain (i.e., continued wt loss)	> 5% wt loss in 1 month (or >10% in 6 months) OR No wt stabilization or wt gain (i.e., continued wt loss)
Nutrient Intake	No deficit OR Significant recent improvement	Definite decrease in intake	Severe deficit in intake
Nutrition Impact Symptoms	None OR Significant recent improvement allowing adequate intake	Presence of nutrition impact symptoms (Box 3 of PG-SGA)	Presence of nutrition impact symptoms (Box 3 of PG-SGA)
Functioning	No deficit OR Significant recent improvement	Moderate functional deficit OR Recent deterioration	Severe functional deficit OR recent significant deterioration
Physical Exam	No deficit OR Chronic deficit but with recent clinical improvement	Evidence of mild to moderate loss of SQ fat &/or muscle mass &/or muscle tone on palpation	Obvious signs of malnutrition (e.g., severe loss of SQ tissues, possible edema)

Global PG-SGA rating (A, B, or C) = [ ]

Figure 45–6 ■ *continued*

BOX 45–8   ■ Nutritional Screening Tool

Read the statement. Circle the number in the Yes column for those that apply to you. Total your nutritional assessment.

Nutritional Assessment Statements	Yes
I have an illness or condition that made me change the kind or amount of food I eat.	2
I eat fewer than two meals per day.	3
I eat few fruits, vegetables, or milk products.	2
I have three or more drinks of beer, liquor, or wine almost every day.	2
I have tooth or mouth problems that make it hard for me to eat.	2
I do not always have enough money to buy the food I need.	4
I eat alone most of the time.	1
I take three or more different prescribed or over-the-counter drugs a day.	1
Without wanting to, I have lost or gained 10 pounds in the last 6 months.	2
I am not always physically able to shop, cook, or feed myself	2
Total	____

If you scored 0–2: Good! Recheck your nutritional score in 6 months.

If you scored 3–5: You are at moderate nutritional risk. See what can be done to improve your eating habits and lifestyle. Recheck your score in 3 months.

If you score 6 or above: You are at high nutritional risk. Take this checklist to your doctor, nurse practitioner, or home health nurse. Ask for help to improve your nutritional health.

Note: From "Determine Your Nutritional Health," by the Nutrition Screening Initiative, 2003, Washington, DC: National Council on Aging. Reprinted with permission by the Nutrition Screening Initiative, a project of the American Dietetic Association, funded in part by a grant from Ross Products Division, Abbott Laboratories, Inc.

care professional may use a selective food frequency that focuses, for example, on fat, fruit, vegetable, and fiber intake.

A **food diary** is a detailed record of measured amounts (portion sizes) of all food and fluids a client consumes during a specified period, usually 3 to 7 days.

A **diet history** is a comprehensive time-consuming assessment of a client's food intake that involves an extensive interview by a nutritionist or dietitian. It includes characteristics of foods usually eaten as well as the frequency and amount of food consumed. Thus, it may include a 24-hour recall, a food frequency record, and a food diary. Medical and psychosocial factors are also assessed to evaluate their impact on nutritional requirements, food habits, and choices. Data obtained are analyzed by computer and translated into caloric and nutrient intake. Results are compared with the DRIs that are appropriate for the client's age, sex, and condition.

Anthropometric Measurements

Anthropometric measurements are noninvasive techniques that aim to quantify changes in body composition. A **skinfold measurement** is performed to determine fat stores. The most common site for skinfold measurement is the triceps skinfold. The fold of skin measured includes subcutaneous tissue but not the underlying muscle. It is measured in millimeters using special

TABLE 45–4   Clinical Signs of Malnutrition

Area of Examination	Signs Associated with Malnutrition
General appearance and vitality	Apathetic, listless, looks tired, easily fatigued
Weight	Overweight or underweight
Skin	Dry, flaky, or scaly; pale or pigmented; presence of petechiae or bruises; lack of subcutaneous fat
Nails	Brittle, pale, ridged, or spoon shaped
Hair	Dry, dull, sparse, loss of color, brittle
Eyes	Pale or red conjunctiva, dryness, soft cornea, dull cornea
Lips	Swollen, red cracks at side of mouth, vertical fissures
Tongue	Swollen, beefy red or magenta colored; smooth appearance; decrease or increase in size
Gums	Spongy, swollen, inflamed; bleed easily
Muscles	Underdeveloped, flaccid, wasted, soft
Gastrointestinal system	Anorexia, indigestion, diarrhea, constipation, enlarged liver, protruding abdomen
Nervous	Decreased reflexes, sensory loss, burning and tingling of hands and feet, mental confusion or irritability

BOX 45–9	■ Calculating and Interpreting the Percent of Deviation from Usual Body Weight and the Percent of Weight Loss

Calculating Percent of Usual Body Weight

$$\% \text{ usual body weight} = \frac{\text{Current weight}}{\text{Usual body weight}} \times 100$$

Mild malnutrition	85–90%
Moderate malnutrition	75–84%
Severe malnutrition	Less than 74%

Calculating Percent of Weight Loss

$$\% \text{ weight loss} = \frac{\text{Usual weight} - \text{current weight}}{\text{Usual weight}} \times 100$$

Significant weight loss	**Severe weight loss**
5% over 1 mo	> 5% over 1 mo
7.5% over 3 mo	> 7.5% over 3 mo
10% over 6 mo	> 10% over 6 mo

calipers. To measure the triceps skinfold (TSF), locate the midpoint of the upper arm (halfway between the acromion process and the olecranon process), then grasp the skin on the back of the upper arm along the long axis of the humerus (Figure 45–7 ■). Placing the calipers 1 cm (0.4 in.) below the fingers, measure the thickness of the fold to the nearest millimeter.

The **mid-arm circumference (MAC)** is a measure of fat, muscle, and skeleton. To measure the MAC, ask the client to sit or stand with the arm hanging freely and the forearm flexed to horizontal. Measure the circumference at the midpoint of the arm, recording the measurement in centimeters, to the nearest millimeter (e.g., 24.6 cm) (Figure 45–8 ■).

The **mid-arm muscle circumference (MAMC)** is then calculated by using reference tables or by using a formula that incorporates the triceps skinfold and the MAC. The MAMC is an estimate of lean body mass, or skeletal muscle reserves. If tables are not available, the nurse uses the following formula to calculate the MAMC from the triceps skinfold and MAC direct measurements:

$$\text{MAMC (cm)} = \frac{\text{MAC (cm)} - 3.143 \text{ TSF (mm)}}{10}$$

Standard values for anthropometric measurements for adults are shown in Table 45–5.

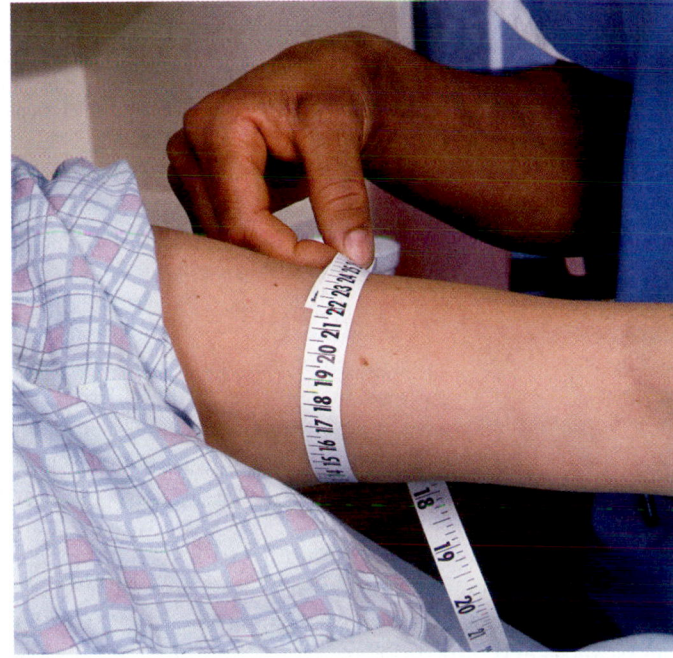

Figure 45–8 ■ Measuring the mid-arm circumference.

Changes in anthropometric measurements often occur slowly and reflect chronic rather than acute changes in nutritional status. They are, therefore, used to monitor the client's progress for months to years rather than days to weeks. Ideally, initial and subsequent measurements need to be taken by the same clinician. In

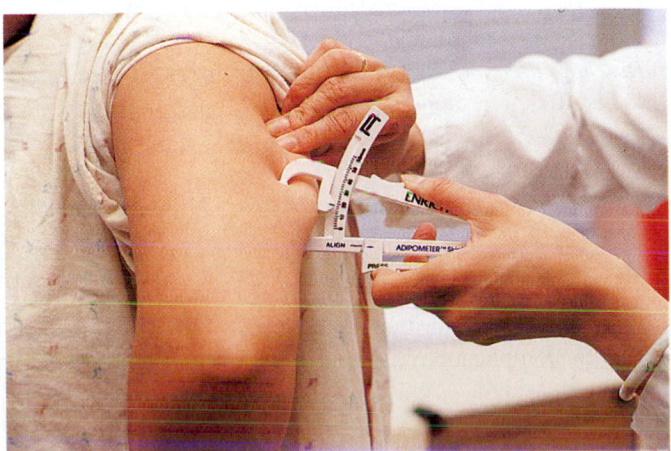

Figure 45–7 ■ Measuring the triceps skinfold.

TABLE 45–5 Standard Values for Anthropometric Measurements for Adults

Measurement	Male	Female
Triceps skinfold (mm)	12.5	16.5
Mid-arm circumference (cm)	29.3	28.5
Mid-arm muscle circumference (cm)	25.3	23.2

Note: From *Nutrition Handbook for Nursing Practice*, 3rd ed. (p. 239), by S. G. Dudek, 1997, Philadelphia: Lippincott. Adapted with permission.

addition, measurements obtained need to be interpreted with caution. Fluctuations in hydration status that often occur during illness can influence the accuracy of results. In addition, normal standards often do not account for normal changes in body composition such as those that occur with aging.

Laboratory Data

Laboratory tests provide objective data to the nutritional assessments, but because many factors can influence these tests, no single test specifically predicts nutritional risk or measures the presence or degree of a nutritional problem. The tests most commonly used are serum proteins, urinary urea nitrogen and creatinine, and total lymphocyte count.

Serum Proteins. Serum protein levels provide an estimate of visceral protein stores. Tests commonly include hemoglobin, albumin, transferrin, and total iron-binding capacity. A low hemoglobin level may be evidence of iron deficiency anemia. However, abnormal blood loss or a pathologic process such as gastrointestinal cancer must be ruled out before iron deficiency related to diet is confirmed.

Albumin, which accounts for more than 50% of the total serum proteins, is one of the most common visceral proteins evaluated as part of the nutritional assessment. Because there is so much albumin in the body and because it is not broken down very quickly [i.e., it has a long half-life (18–20 days)], albumin concentrations change slowly. Thus, a low serum albumin level is a useful indicator of prolonged protein depletion rather than acute or short-term changes in nutritional status. However, many conditions besides malnutrition can depress albumin concentration, such as altered liver function, hydration status, and losses from open wounds and burns.

Transferrin is a protein that binds and carries iron from the intestine through the serum. Because it has a shorter half-life than albumin (8–9 days), transferrin is likely to respond more quickly to protein depletion than albumin. Serum transferrin can be measured directly or by a total iron-binding capacity (TIBC) test, which indicates the amount of iron in the blood to which transferrin can bind. Transferrin levels below normal indicate protein loss, iron deficiency anemia, pregnancy, hepatitis, and liver dysfunction. An increase in TIBC can indicate iron deficiency; a decrease, anemia.

Prealbumin (PAB), also referred to as thyroxine-binding albumin and transthyretin, has the shortest half-life and smallest body pool, and is, therefore, the most responsive serum protein to rapid changes in nutritional status but unfortunately is expensive to measure.

Urinary Tests. Urinary urea nitrogen and urinary creatinine are measures of protein catabolism and the state of nitrogen balance. **Urea,** the chief end product of amino acid metabolism, is formed from ammonia detoxified by the liver, circulated in the blood (BUN), and transported to the kidneys for excretion in urine. Urea concentrations in the blood and urine, therefore, directly reflect the intake and breakdown of dietary protein, the rate of urea production in the liver, and the rate of urea removal by the kidneys.

The state of nitrogen balance is determined by comparing the nitrogen intake (grams of protein) to the nitrogen output over a 24-hour period. A positive nitrogen balance exists when intake exceeds nitrogen output; a negative nitrogen balance occurs when output exceeds nitrogen intake. Protein intake must be accurately recorded and kidney function must be normal to ensure the validity of a UUN (urinary urea nitrogen) test.

Urinary creatinine reflects a person's total muscle mass because creatinine is the chief end product of the creatine produced when energy is released during skeletal muscle metabolism. The rate of creatinine formation is directly proportional to the total muscle mass. Creatinine is removed from the bloodstream by the kidneys and excreted in the urine at a rate that closely parallels its formation. The greater the muscle mass, the greater the excretion of creatinine. As skeletal muscle atrophies during malnutrition, creatinine excretion decreases. Standards for creatinine excretion are developed based on gender and height. Urinary creatinine is also influenced by protein intake, exercise, age, renal function, and thyroid function.

Total Lymphocyte Count. Certain nutrient deficiencies and forms of PCM can depress the immune system. The total number of lymphocytes decreases as protein depletion occurs.

DIAGNOSING

NANDA (2003) includes the following diagnostic labels for nutritional problems:

- *Imbalanced Nutrition: More Than Body Requirements*
- *Imbalanced Nutrition: Less Than Body Requirements*
- *Risk for Imbalanced Nutrition: More Than Body Requirements*

Clinical examples of assessment data clusters and related nursing diagnoses are shown in Identifying Nursing Diagnoses, Outcomes, and Interventions.

Many other NANDA nursing diagnoses may apply to certain individuals, because nutritional problems often affect other areas of human functioning. In this case, the nutritional diagnostic label may be used as the etiology of other diagnoses. Examples include

- *Activity Intolerance* related to inadequate intake of iron-rich foods resulting in iron-deficiency anemia
- *Constipation* related to inadequate fluid intake and fiber intake
- *Low Self-Esteem* related to obesity
- *Risk for Infection* related to immunosuppression secondary to insufficient protein intake.

PLANNING

Major goals for clients with or at risk for nutritional problems include

- Maintain or restore optimal nutritional status.
- Promote healthy nutritional practices.
- Prevent complications associated with malnutrition.
- Decrease weight.
- Regain specified weight.

Examples of NOC outcomes and NIC interventions related to some of these goals, are shown in Identifying Nursing

IDENTIFYING NURSING DIAGNOSES, OUTCOMES, AND INTERVENTIONS
CLIENTS WITH NUTRITIONAL DISORDERS

DATA CLUSTER	NURSING DIAGNOSIS/ DEFINITION	SAMPLE DESIRED OUTCOMES [NOC#]/DEFINITION	INDICATORS	SELECTED INTERVENTIONS [NIC#]/DEFINITION	SAMPLE NIC ACTIVITIES
Mark Malakoff, 71 years old, has chronic obstructive lung disease. His wife died 2 years ago. He says, "I'm not interested in food. Even if I were, I don't have the energy to buy food. It's too much bother to fix meals for just me." He is 5' 10" (178 cm) tall and weighs 135 lbs. (61.2 kg). His triceps skinfold measurement is 9.2 mm; arm muscle circumference is 20.4 mm. Dietary assessment indicates that he eats mostly bread, cereal, whole milk, and canned fish and meats. He eats almost no fruits and vegetables.	*Imbalanced Nutrition: Less Than Body Requirements/ Intake of nutrients insufficient to meet metabolic needs*	Nutritional Status: Nutrient Intake [1009]/*Adequacy of nutrients taken into the body*	Substantially adequate • Caloric intake • Vitamin intake	Nutrition Therapy [1120]/*Administration of food and fluids to support metabolic processes of a client who is malnourished or at high risk of becoming malnourished*	• Determine food preferences with consideration of cultural and religious preferences • Determine number of calories and types of nutrients needed • Ensure availability of appropriate nutritional foods. • Structure the environment to support healthy eating patterns
Rose Rosenthal, a 27-year-old taxi dispatcher, says that her parents, who are both pastry cooks, are "fat." "I love Dad's doughnuts and often bring some to work to munch on through the day. I hate exercise, but at this rate, I'm going to have to do something, or I'll end up looking like Mum and Dad." Height, 5' 1" (155 cm); weight 130 lbs. (58.5 kg).	*Risk for Imbalanced Nutrition: More Than Body Requirements/At risk for an intake of nutrients that exceeds metabolic needs*	Nutritional Status: Body Mass [1006]/*Congruence of body weight, muscle, and fat to height, frame, and gender*	Mild deviation from expected range • Weight • Waist/hip circumference ratio	Nutrition Monitoring [1160]/*Collection and analysis of patient data to prevent or minimize malnourishment*	• Weigh patient at specified intervals • Monitor type and amount of usual exercise • Monitor environment where eating occurs • Determine if patient requires nutrition education.

Diagnoses, Outcomes, and Interventions. Specific nursing activities associated with each of these interventions can be selected to meet the individual needs of the client. See the Nursing Care Plan and Concept Map at the end of this chapter.

Planning for Home Care

To provide for continuity of care, the nurse must consider the client's need for assistance with nutrition. Some clients will need help with eating, purchasing food, and preparing meals; others will need instructions about enteral and parenteral nutrition therapy.

Home care planning incorporates an assessment of the client and family's abilities for self-care, financial resources, and the need for referrals and home health services. The Home Care Assessment box outlines a home care assessment about nutritional problems and needs. A major aspect of discharge planning involves instructional needs of the client and family (see Teaching: Home Care.)

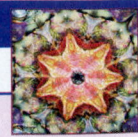

Home Care Assessment
NUTRITION

Client/Environment

- **Self-care abilities:** Assess ability to feed self, to purchase food, and to prepare meals.
- **Adaptive feeding aids required:** Determine need for special drinking cups, plates, or feeding utensils.
- **Instructional needs:** Consider nutritional requirements (e.g., Food Guide Pyramid, dietary guidelines, special diet), adaptive aids available, recommended lifestyle variations, management of enteral/parenteral nutrition.
- **Physical environment:** Assess adequacy of water, electricity, refrigeration, and telephone facilities; and presence of clean, secure area to store and set up enteral/parenteral equipment as needed.

Family

- **Caregiver availability, skills, and willingness:** Primary and secondary persons able to assist with food purchase, meal preparation, and feeding and able to comprehend and administer special diets or enteral/parenteral nutrition required.

- **Family role changes and coping:** Effect on parenting and spousal roles, financial resources, and social roles.
- **Alternate potential primary or respite caregivers:** For example, other family members, volunteers, church members, paid caregivers, or housekeeping services; available community respite care (adult day care, senior centers) and so on.

Community

- **Current knowledge, use, and experience with community resources:** Nutritional counseling services; home health agencies for enteral/parenteral nutrition support; dietitian or nutritionist for planning appropriate meals for prescribed diet, ways to include ethnic food preferences into the diet, and providing written meal plans; medical equipment and supply companies; financial assistance services; support and educational services such as
  - Weight management programs (e.g., Weight Watchers)
  - National Center for Nutrition and Dietetics for information on all nutrition topics
  - National Eating Disorder Information Center
  - Meals on Wheels.

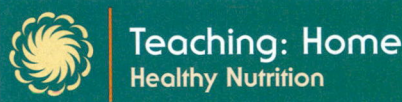

Teaching: Home Care
Healthy Nutrition

- Instruct clients about the content of a healthy diet based on the Food Guide Pyramid, *Dietary Guidelines for Americans,* or *Canada's Food Guide to Healthy Eating.*
- Encourage clients, particularly older clients, to reduce dietary fat (see Teaching: Wellness on reducing dietary fat, page 1186).
- Instruct strict vegetarians as needed about proper protein complementation and additional vitamin and mineral supplementation.
- Discuss foods high in specific nutrients required such as protein, iron, calcium, vitamin C, and fiber.
- Discuss importance of properly fitted dentures and dental care.
- Discuss safe food preparation and preservation techniques as appropriate.

Dietary Alterations

- Explain the purpose of the diet.
- Discuss allowed and prohibited foods.
- Explain the importance of reading food labels when selecting foods.
- Include family or significant others as appropriate.
- Reinforce information provided by the dietitian or nutritionist as appropriate.
- Discuss herbs and spices as alternatives to salt and substitutes for sugar.

For Overweight Clients

- Discuss physiologic, psychologic, and lifestyle factors that predispose to weight gain.
- Provide information about normal weight range and recommended calorie intake.

- Discuss principles of a well-balanced diet and high- and low-calorie foods.
- Encourage intake of low-calorie, caffeine-free beverages and plenty of water.
- Discuss ways to adapt eating practices by using smaller plates, smaller servings, chewing each bit a specified number of times, and putting fork down between bites.
- Discuss ways to control the desire to eat by taking a walk, drinking a glass of water, or doing slow deep-breathing exercises.
- Discuss the importance of exercise and help the client plan an exercise program.
- Discuss stress-reduction techniques.
- Provide information about available community resources (e.g., weight-loss groups, dietary counseling, exercise programs, self-help groups).

For Underweight Clients

- Discuss factors contributing to inadequate nutrition and weight loss.
- Discuss recommended calorie intake and normal weight range.
- Provide information about the content of a balanced diet.
- Provide information about ways to increase calorie intake (e.g., high-protein or high-calorie foods and supplements).
- Discuss ways to manage, minimize, or alter the factors contributing to malnourishment.
- If appropriate, discuss ways to purchase low-cost nutritious foods.
- Provide information about community agencies that can assist in providing food (e.g., Meals on Wheels).

IMPLEMENTING

Nursing interventions to promote optimal nutrition for hospitalized clients are often provided in collaboration with the physician who writes the diet orders and the dietitian who informs clients about special diets. The nurse reinforces this instruction and, in addition, creates an atmosphere that encourages eating, provides assistance with eating, monitors the client's appetite and food intake, administers enteral and parenteral feedings, and consults with the physician and dietitian about nutritional problems that arise.

In the community setting, the nurse's role is largely educational. For example, nurses promote optimal nutrition at health fairs, in schools, at prenatal classes, and with well or ill clients and support people in their homes. In the home setting, nurses also initiate nutritional screens, refer clients at risk to appropriate resources, instruct clients about enteral and parenteral feedings, and offer nutrition counseling as needed. Nutrition counseling involves more than simply providing information. The nurse must help clients integrate diet changes into their lifestyles and provide strategies to motivate them to change their eating habits.

Assisting with Special Diets

Alterations in the client's diet are often needed to treat a disease process such as diabetes mellitus, to prepare for a special examination or surgery, to increase or decrease weight, to restore nutritional deficits, or to allow an organ to rest and promote healing. Diets are modified in one or more of the following aspects: texture, kilocalories, specific nutrients, seasonings, or consistency.

Hospitalized clients who do not have special needs eat the regular (standard or house) diet, a balanced diet that supplies the metabolic requirements of a sedentary person (about 2,000 Kcal). Most agencies offer clients a daily menu from which to select their meals for the next day; others provide standard meals to each client on the general diet. Certain foods (e.g., cabbage, which tends to produce flatus, and highly seasoned and fried foods, which are difficult for some people to digest) are usually omitted from the regular diet.

A variation of the regular diet is the light diet, designed for postoperative and other clients who are not ready for the regular diet. Foods in the light diet are plainly cooked and fat is usually omitted, as are bran and foods containing a great deal of fiber.

Temporary Consistency Modifications. Diets that are modified in consistency are often given to clients before and after surgery or to promote healing in clients with gastrointestinal distress. These diets include clear liquid, full liquid, soft, and diet as tolerated.

Clear Liquid Diet. This diet is limited to water, tea, coffee, clear broths, ginger ale, or other carbonated beverages, strained and clear juices, and plain gelatin. This diet provides the client with fluid and carbohydrate (in the form of sugar) but does not supply adequate protein, fat, vitamins, minerals, or calories. It is a short-term diet (24–36 hours) provided for clients after certain surgeries or in the acute stages of infection, particularly of the gastrointestinal tract. The major objectives of this diet are to relieve thirst, prevent dehydration, and minimize stimulation of the gastrointestinal tract. Examples of foods allowed in clear liquid, full liquid, and soft diets are shown in Box 45–10.

Full Liquid Diet. This diet contains only liquids or foods that turn to liquid at body temperature, such as ice cream (see Box 45–10). Full liquid diets are often eaten by clients who have gastrointestinal disturbances or are otherwise unable to tolerate solid or semisolid foods. This diet is not recommended for long-term use because it is low in iron, protein, and calories. In addition, its cholesterol content is high because of the amount

---

BOX 45–10 ■ Examples of Foods for Clear Liquid, Full Liquid, and Soft Diets

Clear Liquid	Full Liquid	Soft
Coffee, regular and de-caffeinated	All foods on clear liquid diet plus:	All foods on full and clear liquid diets, plus:
Tea	Milk and milk drinks	Meat: All lean, tender meat, fish, or poultry (chopped, shredded); spaghetti sauce with ground meat over pasta
Carbonated beverages	Puddings, custards	Meat alternatives: Scrambled eggs, omelet, poached eggs; cottage cheese and other mild cheese
Bouillon, fat-free broth	Ice cream, sherbet	
Clear fruit juices (apple, cranberry, grape)	Vegetable juices	Vegetables: Mashed potatoes, sweet potatoes, or squash; vegetables in cream or cheese sauce; other cooked vegetables as tolerated (e.g., spinach, cauliflower, asparagus tips), chopped and mashed as needed; avocado
Other fruit juices, strained	Refined or strained cereals (e.g., cream of rice)	
Popsicles	Cream, butter, margarine	Fruits: Cooked or canned fruits; bananas, grapefruit and orange sections without membranes, applesauce
Gelatin	Eggs (in custard and pudding)	
Sugar, honey	Smooth peanut butter	Breads and cereals: Enriched rice, barley, pasta; all breads; cooked cereals (e.g., oatmeal)
Hard candy	Yogurt	Desserts: Soft cake, bread pudding

of milk offered. Clients who must receive only liquids for long periods are usually given a nutritionally balanced oral supplement, such as Ensure or Sustacal. The full liquid diet is monotonous and difficult for clients to accept. Planning six or more feedings per day may encourage a more adequate intake.

Soft Diet. The soft diet is easily chewed and digested. It is often ordered for clients who have difficulty chewing and swallowing. It is a low-residue (low-fiber) diet containing very few uncooked foods; however, restrictions vary among agencies and according to individual tolerance. Examples of foods that can be included in a soft or semisoft diet are shown in Box 45–10. The **pureed diet** is a modification of the soft diet. Liquid may be added to the food, which is then blended to a semisolid consistency.

Diet as Tolerated. Diet as tolerated is ordered when the client's appetite, ability to eat, and tolerance for certain foods may change. For example, on the first postoperative day a client may be given a clear liquid diet. If no nausea occurs, normal intestinal motility has returned, and the client feels like eating, the diet may be advanced to a full liquid, light, or regular diet.

Modification for Disease. Many special diets may be prescribed to meet requirements for disease process or altered metabolism. For example, a client with diabetes mellitus may need a diet recommended by the National Diabetic Association, on obese client may need a calorie restricted diet, a cardiac client may need sodium and cholesterol restrictions, and a client with allergies will need a hypoallergenic diet.

Some clients may have no difficulty with choosing a healthy diet, but be at risk for nutritional problems due to dysphagia. These clients may have inadequate solid or fluid intake, be unable to swallow their medications, or aspirate food or fluids into the lungs—causing pneumonia. Clients at risk for dysphagia include elders, those who have experienced a stroke, cancer patients who have had radiation therapy to the head and neck, and others with cranial nerve dysfunction. Nurses may be the first persons to detect dysphagia and are in an excellent position to recommend further evaluation; implement specialized feeding techniques and diets; and work with clients, family members, and other health care professionals to develop a plan to assist the client with difficulties (Terrado, Russell, & Bowman, 2001). If the client condition suggests dysphagia, the nurse should review the history in detail; interview the client or family; assess the mouth, throat, and chest; and observe the client swallowing. Presence of the gag reflex, often thought to indicate that the client can swallow safely, has not been shown to be a reliable indicator (Williams & Waxman, 2002).

A multidisciplinary group has developed the National Dysphagia Diet (NDD) that delineates standards of food textures (American Dietetic Association, 2002). The four levels of liquid foods are thin, nectar-like, honey-like, and spoon-thick liquids. The four levels of semisolid/solid foods are pureed, mechanically altered, advanced/mechanically soft, and regular/general. In consultation with the dietitian, occupational therapist, swallowing specialist, and/or physician, these levels can be used to determine a consistent approach to a particular

client's dysphagia. For example, a mechanically soft diet has been shown to result in lower pneumonia rates than pureed diet in stroke patients with a history of aspiration pneumonia (Agency for Health Care Policy and Research, 1999). Early detection and intervention can prevent the adverse outcomes of dysphagia in most clients.

Some clients must follow certain diets (e.g., the diabetic diet) for a lifetime. If the diet is long term, the client must not only understand the diet but also develop a healthy, positive attitude toward it. Assisting clients and support persons with special diets is a function shared by the dietitian or nutritionist and the nurse. The dietitian informs the client and support persons about the specific foods allowed and not allowed and assists the client with meal planning. The nurse reinforces this instruction, assists the client to make changes, and evaluates the client's responses.

All dietary instructions must be individually designed to meet the client's intellectual ability, motivation level, lifestyle, culture, and economic status. Both nutritionists and dietitians can often help to adapt a diet to suit the client. Simple verbal instructions need to be given and reinforced with written material. Family and support people must be included in the dietary instruction.

Stimulating the Appetite

Physical illness, unfamiliar or unpalatable food, environmental and psychologic factors, and physical discomfort or pain may depress the appetites of many clients. A short-term decrease in food intake usually is not a problem for adults; over time, however, it leads to weight loss, decreased strength and stamina, and other nutritional problems. A decreased food intake is often accompanied by a decrease in fluid intake, which may cause fluid and electrolyte problems. Stimulating a person's appetite requires the nurse to determine the reason for the lack of appetite and then deal with the problem. Some interventions for improving the client's appetite are summarized in Box 45–11.

BOX 45–11 ■ Improving Appetite

- Provide familiar food that the person likes. Often the relatives of clients are pleased to bring food from home but may need some guidance about special diet requirements.
- Select small portions so as not to discourage the anorexic client.
- Avoid unpleasant or uncomfortable treatments immediately before or after a meal.
- Provide a tidy, clean environment that is free of unpleasant sights and odors. A soiled dressing, a used bedpan, an uncovered irrigation set, or even used dishes can negatively affect the appetite.
- Encourage or provide oral hygiene before mealtime. This improves the client's ability to taste.
- Relieve illness symptoms that depress appetite before mealtime; for example, give an analgesic for pain or an antipyretic for a fever or allow rest for fatigue.
- Reduce psychologic stress. A lack of understanding of therapy, the anticipation of an operation, and fear of the unknown can cause anorexia. Often, the nurse can help by discussing feelings with the client, giving information and assistance, and allaying fears.

Assisting Clients with Meals

Because clients in health care agencies are frequently confined to their beds, meals are often brought to the client. The client receives a tray that has been assembled in a central kitchen. Nursing personnel may be responsible for giving out and collecting the trays; however, in most settings this is done by special dietary personnel. Long-term care facilities and some hospitals serve meals to ambulatory clients in a special dining area. Guidelines for providing meals to clients are summarized in Box 45–12.

Two groups of people frequently require help with their meals: older adults who are weakened; and persons with handicaps, such as blind clients, those who must remain in a back-lying position, or those who cannot use their hands. The client's nursing care plan will indicate that assistance is required with meals.

The nurse must be sensitive to clients' feelings of embarrassment, resentment, and loss of autonomy. Whenever possible, the nurse should help incapacitated clients feed themselves rather than feed them. Some clients become depressed because they require help and because they believe they are burdensome to busy nursing personnel. Although feeding a client is time consuming, nurses should try to appear unhurried and convey that they have ample time. Sitting at the bedside is one way to convey this impression.

When feeding a client, ask in which order the client would like to eat the food. If the client cannot see, tell the client which food is being given. Always allow ample time for the client to chew and swallow the food before offering more. Also, provide fluids as requested, or, if the client is unable to communicate, offer fluids after every three or four mouthfuls of solid food. It is important to make the time a pleasant one, choosing topics of conversation that are of interest to clients who want to talk.

Although normal utensils should be used whenever possible, special utensils may be needed to assist a client to eat. For clients who have difficulty drinking from a cup or glass, a straw often permits them to obtain liquids with less effort and less spillage. Special drinking cups are also available. One model has a spout; another is specially designed to permit drinking with less tipping of the cup than is normally required.

Many adaptive feeding aids are available to help clients maintain independence. A standard eating utensil with a built-up or widened handle helps clients who cannot grasp objects easily. Utensils with wide handles can be purchased, or a regular eating utensil can be modified by taping foam around the handle. The foam increases friction and thus steadies the client's grasp. Handles may be bent or angled to compensate for limited motion. Collars or bands that prevent the utensil from being dropped can be attached to the end of the handle and fit over the client's hand. Clients requiring pureed or liquid diets are sometimes fed with a feeding syringe.

Plates with rims and plastic or metal plate guards enable the client to pick up the food by first pushing it against this raised edge. A suction cup or damp sponge or cloth may be placed under the dish to keep it from moving while the client is eating. No-spill mugs and two-handled drinking cups are especially useful for persons with impaired hand coordination. Stretch

---

BOX 45–12 ■ Providing Client Meals

- Offer the client assistance with hand washing and oral hygiene before a meal.
- Most people sit during a meal; if it is permitted, assist the client to a comfortable position in bed or in a chair, whichever is appropriate.
- Clear the overbed table so that there is space for the tray. If the client must remain in a lying position in bed, arrange the overbed table close to the bedside so that the client can see and reach the food.
- Check each tray for the client's name, the type of diet, and completeness. Do not leave an incorrect diet for a client to eat.
- Assist the client as required to remove the food covers, butter the bread, pour the tea, and cut the meat.
- For a blind person, identify the placement of the food as you would describe the time on a clock (Figure 45–9 ■). For instance, the nurse might say, "The potatoes are at eight o'clock, the chicken at 12 o'clock, and the green beans at 4 o'clock."
- After the client has completed the meal, observe how much and what the client has eaten and the amount of fluid taken. Record fluid intake and calorie count as required.
- If the client is on a special diet or is having problems eating, record the amount of food eaten and any pain, fatigue, or nausea experienced.
- If the client is not eating, document this so that changes can be made, such as rescheduling the meals, providing smaller, more frequent meals, or obtaining special self-feeding aids.

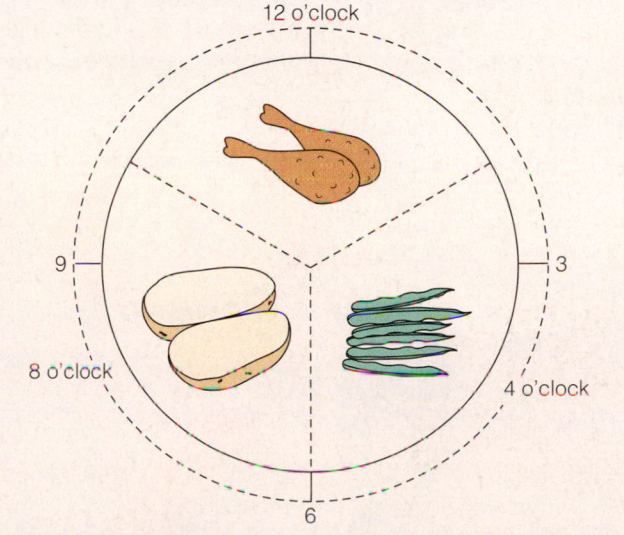

Figure 45–9 ■ For a client who is blind, the nurse can use the clock system to describe the location of food on the plate.

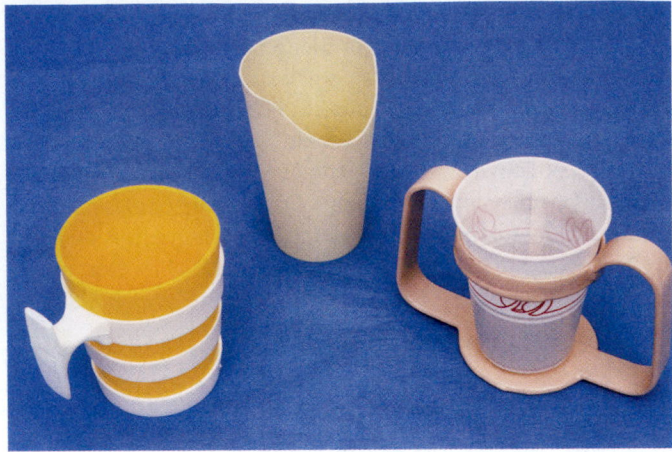

Figure 45–10 ■ Left to right: glass holder, cup with hole for nose, two-handled cup holder.

terry cloth and knitted or crocheted glass covers enable the client to keep a secure grasp on a glass. Lidded tip-proof glasses are also available. Figures 45–10 ■ and 45–11 ■ show some of these aids.

Special Community Nutritional Services

In many places community programs have been developed to help special groups of the population meet their nutritional needs. For older people who cannot prepare meals or leave their homes, ready-to-eat meals or frozen dinners are delivered to the home by local organizations. Meals on Wheels is one such well-known organization. For people who can prepare meals but are physically handicapped and unable to shop for groceries, some organizations provide grocery delivery services.

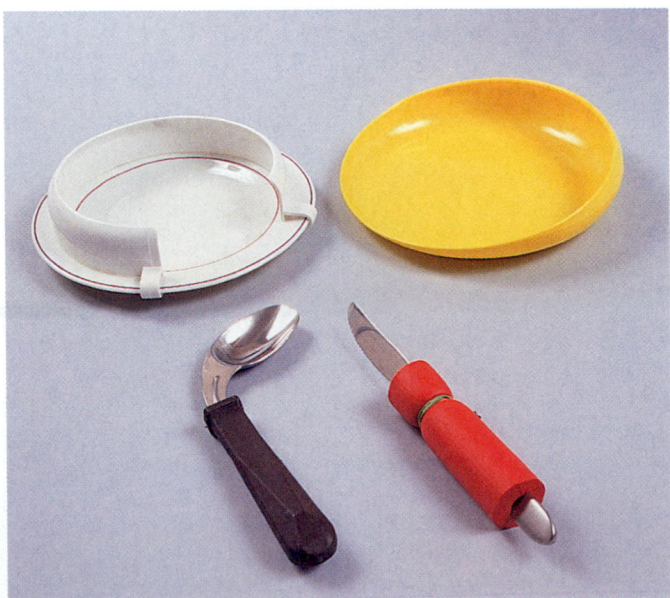

Figure 45–11 ■ Dinner plate with guard attached and lipped plate facilitate scooping; wide-handled spoon and knife facilitate grip.

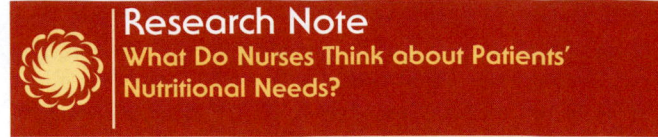

Research Note
What Do Nurses Think about Patients' Nutritional Needs?

The purposes of this study by Crogan, Shultz, Adams, and Massey (2001) were to determine and compare how nurses and nursing assistants view their roles in relation to assisting nursing home residents with their meals. Using the Health Belief Model, the researchers created a questionnaire examining role, attitudes, and beliefs about barriers to helping the residents with meals. The sample included 99 nursing assistants and 44 nurses. Although the nurses and nursing assistants agreed on certain issues, nurses felt more strongly that communication between the team members was adequate to helping them meet the residents' nutritional needs. Both agreed that quality of food and short staffing were barriers to residents eating.

Implications: The researchers concluded that education of the nursing assistants, communication between nurses and assistants, and nurse participation in observing client eating were indicated. In situations where the client may be in a nursing home for an extended period, their susceptibility to malnutrition as a result of the barriers can be significant. Programs should be implemented in long-term care facilities to highlight these findings and to develop methods of preventing adverse client outcomes.

Note: From "Barriers to Nutrition Care for Nursing Home Residents," by N. L. Crogan, J. A. Shultz, C. E. Adams, and L. K. Massey, 2001, *Journal of Gerontological Nursing, 27*(12), pp. 25–31.

For the impoverished in the United States, the USDA funds a food stamp program. People with low incomes can use stamps to purchase food at any approved grocery store. The value of the food stamps provided depends on the size and income of the family.

Enteral Nutrition

An alternative feeding method to ensure adequate nutrition includes **enteral** (through the gastrointestinal system) methods. Enteral nutrition (EN), also referred to as total enteral nutrition (TEN), is provided when the client is unable to ingest foods or the upper gastrointestinal tract is impaired and the transport of food to the small intestine is interrupted. Enteral feedings are administered through nasogastric and small-bore feeding tubes or through gastrostomy or jejunostomy tubes.

Enteral Access Devices. Enteral access is achieved by means of nasogastric or nasointestinal (nasoenteric) tubes, or gastrostomy or jejunostomy tubes.

A **nasogastric tube** is inserted through one of the nostrils, down the nasopharynx, and into the alimentary tract. In some instances, the tube is passed through the mouth and pharynx, although this route may be more uncomfortable for the adult client and cause gagging. This approach is often used for infants who are obligatory nose breathers (who must breathe through the nose) and premature infants who have no gag reflex.

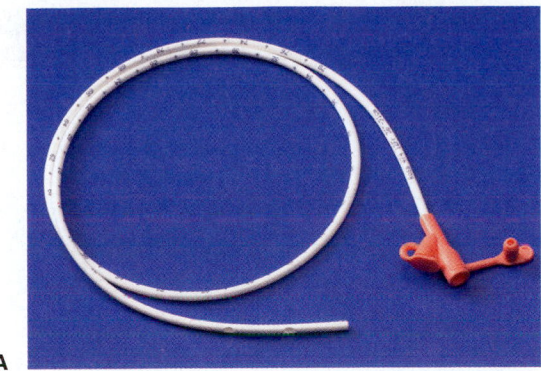

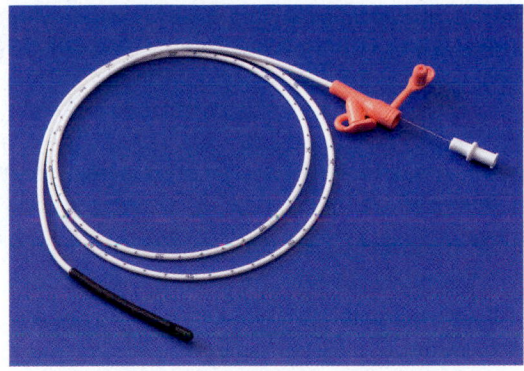

Figure 45–12 ■ Nasoenteric feeding tubes. *A,* 12 Fr 36 in.; *B,* 8 Fr opaque, 45 in., stylet, weighted tip. Note that both have a Y-port connector to permit irrigation and medication administration without disconnecting feeding device. (Courtesy of Ross Products Division of Abbott Laboratories, Columbus, Ohio.)

Traditional firm, large-bore nasogastric tubes (i.e., those larger than 12 Fr in diameter) are placed in the stomach. Examples are the Levin tube, a flexible rubber or plastic, single-lumen tube with holes near the tip, and the Salem sump tube, with a double lumen. The larger tube of the Salem sump tube drains gastric contents; the smaller tube allows for an inflow of atmospheric air, which prevents a vacuum if the gastric tube adheres to the wall of the stomach. Irritation of the gastric mucosa is thereby avoided. Softer, more flexible and less irritating small-bore tubes (smaller than 12 Fr in diameter) are frequently used (Figure 45–12 ■).

Nasogastric tubes are used for clients who have intact gag and cough reflexes, who have adequate gastric emptying, and who require short-term feedings. Procedure 45–1 provides guidelines for inserting a nasogastric tube. Procedure 45–2 outlines the steps for removing a nasogastric tube.

Although the focus of this chapter is nutrition, nasogastric tubes may be inserted for reasons other than to provide a route for feeding the client, including these:

- To prevent nausea, vomiting, and gastric distention following surgery. In this case, the tube is attached to a suction source.
- To remove stomach contents for laboratory analysis.
- To lavage (wash) the stomach in cases of poisoning or overdose of medications.

A **nasoenteric tube,** a longer tube than the nasogastric tube (at least 40 inches for an adult) is inserted through one nostril down into the upper small intestine. Some agencies may require specially trained nurses or physicians for this procedure. Nasoenteric tubes are used for clients who are at risk for aspiration. Clients at risk for aspiration are those who manifest the following:

- Decreased level of consciousness
- Poor cough or gag reflexes
- Endotracheal intubation
- Recent extubation
- Inability to cooperate with the procedure
- Restlessness or agitation.

MediaLink | INSERTING A NASOGASTRIC TUBE ANIMATION

Procedure 45–1 Inserting a Nasogastric Tube

Purposes

- To administer tube feedings and medications to clients unable to eat by mouth or swallow a sufficient diet without aspirating food or fluids into the lungs
- To establish a means for suctioning stomach contents to prevent gastric distention, nausea, and vomiting
- To remove stomach contents for laboratory analysis
- To lavage (wash) the stomach in case of poisoning or overdose of medications

ASSESSMENT

Assess

- Check patency of nares and intactness of nasal tissues. Check for history of nasal surgery or deviated septum.
- Determine presence of gag reflex.
- Assess mental status or ability to cooperate with procedure.

PLANNING

Before inserting a nasogastric tube, determine the size of tube to be inserted and whether or not the tube is to be attached to suction.

Delegation

Insertion of a nasogastric tube is an invasive procedure requiring application of knowledge (e.g., anatomy and physiology, risk factors,

continued on page 1206

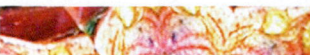

Procedure 45–1   Inserting a Nasogastric Tube *continued*

PLANNING *continued*

etc.) and problem solving. Delegation of this skill to UAP is not appropriate. The UAP, however, can assist with the oral hygiene needs of a client with a nasogastric tube.

Equipment
- Large- or small-bore tube
- Guidewire or stylet for small-bore tube
- Solution basin filled with warm water (if a plastic tube is being used) or ice (if a rubber tube is being used)
- Nonallergenic adhesive tape, 2.5 cm (1 in.) wide
- Clean gloves
- Water-soluble lubricant

- Facial tissues
- Glass of water and drinking straw
- 20- to 50-mL syringe with an adapter
- Basin
- pH test strip or meter
- Stethoscope
- Disposable pad or towel
- Clamp or plug (optional)
- Suction apparatus if required
- Gauze square or plastic specimen bag and elastic band
- Safety pin and elastic band

IMPLEMENTATION

Preparation

Assist the client to a high-Fowler's position if his or her health condition permits, and support the head on a pillow. *It is often easier to swallow in this position and gravity helps the passage of the tube.*

Place a towel or disposable pad across the chest.

Performance

1. Explain to the client what you plan to do. The passage of a gastric tube is not painful, but it is unpleasant because the gag reflex is activated during insertion. Establish a method for the client to indicate distress and a desire for you to pause the insertion. Raising a finger or hand is often used for this.
2. Wash hands and observe other appropriate infection control procedures (e.g., clean gloves).
3. Provide for client privacy.
4. Assess the client's nares.
   - Ask the client to hyperextend the head, and, using a flashlight, observe the intactness of the tissues of the nostrils, including any irritations or abrasions.
   - Examine the nares for any obstructions or deformities by asking the client to breathe through one nostril while occluding the other.
   - Select the nostril that has the greater airflow.
5. Prepare the tube.
   - If a rubber tube is being used, place it on ice for 5 to 10 minutes. *This stiffens the tube, facilitating insertion.* If a plastic tube is being used, place it in warm water until the tube is softer and more flexible. *This facilitates insertion.*

- If a small-bore tube is being used, insert stylet or guidewire into the tube making sure that it is secured in position. *An improperly positioned stylet or guidewire can traumatize the nasopharynx, esophagus, and stomach.*
6. Determine how far to insert the tube.
   - Use the tube to mark off the distance from the tip of the client's nose to the tip of the earlobe and then from the tip of the earlobe to the tip of the xiphoid (Figure 45–13 ■). *This length approximates the distance from the nares to the stomach. This distance varies among individuals.*
   - Mark this length with adhesive tape if the tube does not have markings.

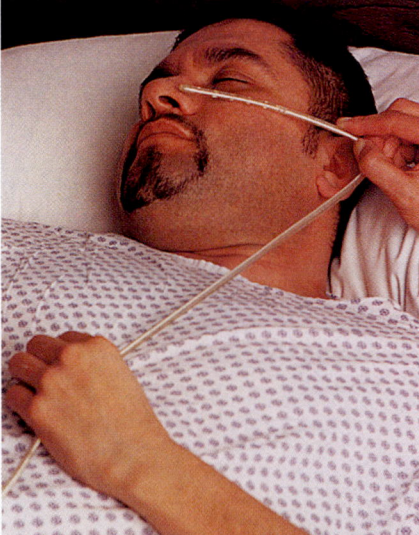

Figure 45–13 ■ Measuring the appropriate length to insert a nasogastric tube.

7. Insert the tube.
   - Put on gloves.
   - Lubricate the tip of the tube well with water-soluble lubricant or water to ease insertion. A water-soluble lubricant dissolves if the tube accidentally enters the lungs. An oil-based lubricant, such as petroleum jelly, will not dissolve and could cause respiratory complications if it enters the lungs.
   - Insert the tube, with its natural curve toward the client, into the selected nostril. Ask the client to hyperextend the neck, and gently advance the tube toward the nasopharynx. *Hyperextension of the neck reduces the curvature of the nasopharyngeal junction.*
   - Direct the tube along the floor of the nostril and toward the ear on that side. Directing the tube along the floor avoids the projections (turbinates) along the lateral wall.
   - Slight pressure is sometimes required to pass the tube into the nasopharynx, and some clients eyes may water at this point. *Tears are a natural body response.* Provide the client with tissues as needed.
   - If the tube meets resistance, withdraw it, relubricate it, and insert it in the other nostril. *The tube should never be forced against resistance because of the danger of injury.*
   - Once the tube reaches the oropharynx (throat), the client will feel the tube in the throat and may gag and retch. Ask the client to tilt the head forward, and encourage the client to drink and swallow. *Tilting the*

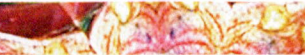

Procedure 45–1 Inserting a Nasogastric Tube *continued*

IMPLEMENTATION *continued*

head forward facilitates passage of the tube into the posterior pharynx and esophagus rather than into the larynx; swallowing moves the epiglottis over the opening to the larynx (Figure 45–14 ■).

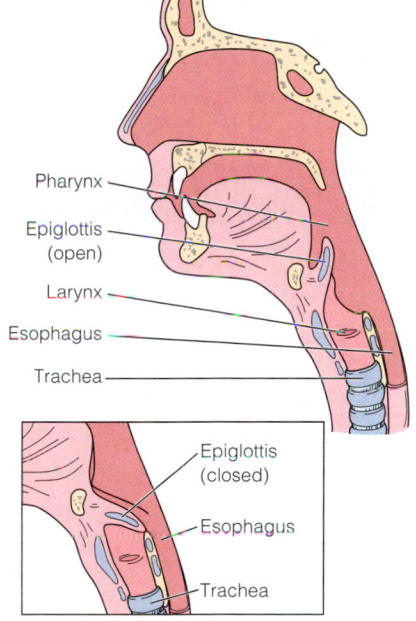

Figure 45–14 ■ Swallowing closes the epiglottis.

- If the client gags, stop passing the tube momentarily. Have the client rest, take a few breaths, and take sips of water to calm the gag reflex.
- In cooperation with the client, pass the tube 5 to 10 cm (2 to 4 in.) with each swallow, until the indicated length is inserted.
- If the client continues to gag and the tube does not advance with each swallow, withdraw it slightly, and inspect the throat by looking through the mouth. *The tube may be coiled in the throat.* If so, withdraw it until it is straight, and try again to insert it.

8. Ascertain correct placement of the tube.
   - Aspirate stomach contents, and check the pH, which should be acidic. Research indicates that testing pH is a reliable way to determine location of a feeding tube.

- Auscultate air insufflation by placing a stethoscope over the client's epigastrium and injecting 10 to 30 mL of air into the tube while listening for a whooshing sound. Do not use this method as the primary method for determining placement of the feeding tube *because it is often unreliable.*
- If the signs do not indicate placement in the stomach, advance the tube 5 cm (2 in.), and repeat the tests.
- If a small-bore tube is used, leave the stylet or guidewire in place until correct position is verified by x-ray.

9. Secure the tube by taping it to the bridge of the client's nose.
   - If the client has oily skin, wipe the nose first with alcohol.
   - Cut 7.5 cm (3 in.) of tape, and split it lengthwise at one end, leaving a 2.5-cm (1-in.) tab at the end.
   - Place the tape over the bridge of the client's nose, and bring the split ends either under and around the tubing, or under the tubing and back up over the nose (Figure 45–15 ■). *Taping in this manner prevents the tube from pressing against and irritating the edge of the nostril.*

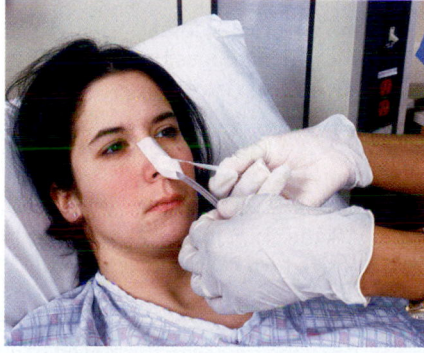

Figure 45–15 ■ Taping a nasogastric tube to the bridge of the nose.

10. Attach the tube to a suction source or feeding apparatus as ordered, or clamp the end of the tubing.
    - The tube, if inserted preoperatively, is usually clamped or plugged; or it may be covered with a gauze square or plastic specimen bag and an elastic band.

11. Secure the tube to the client's gown.
    - Loop an elastic band around the end of the tubing, and attach the elastic band to the gown with a safety pin.
    or
    - Attach a piece of adhesive tape to the tube, and pin the tape to the gown. *The tube is attached to prevent it from dangling and pulling.*

12. Document relevant information: the insertion of the tube, the means by which correct placement was determined, and client responses (e.g., discomfort or abdominal distention).

13. Establish a plan for providing daily nasogastric tube care.
    - Inspect the nostril for discharge and irritation.
    - Clean the nostril and tube with moistened, cotton-tipped applicators.
    - Apply water-soluble lubricant to the nostril if it appears dry or encrusted.
    - Change the adhesive tape as required.
    - Give frequent mouth care. The client may breathe through the mouth and cannot drink.

14. If suction is applied, ensure that the patency of both the nasogastric and suction tubes is maintained.
    - Irrigations of the tube with 30 mL of normal saline may be required at regular intervals. In some agencies, irrigations must be ordered by the physician.
    - Keep accurate records of the client's fluid intake and output, and record the amount and characteristics of the drainage.
    - Document the type of tube inserted, date and time of tube insertion, type of suction used, color and amount of gastric contents, and the client's tolerance of the procedure.

VARIATION: INSERTING A NASOINTESTINAL TUBE

- Add 3 to 4 cm (1-1.5 in.) to the length measured for the nasogastric tube and mark it with tape.
- After inserting the tube into the stomach, position the client on his or her right side to enable advancement of the tube through the pyloric sphincter. This may take up to 24 hours.

continued on page 1208

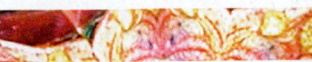

Procedure 45–1 Inserting a Nasogastric Tube *continued*

IMPLEMENTATION *continued*

- When the tube has advanced to the premarked point, test the pH of the aspirate to determine placement in the intestine.

- Have proper placement confirmed by x-ray and tape the tube in place when confirmation is received.

EVALUATION

Conduct appropriate follow-up, such as degree of client comfort, client tolerance of the nasogastric tube, correct placement of nasogastric tube in stomach, client understanding of restrictions, color and amount of gastric contents if attached to suction, or stomach contents aspirated.

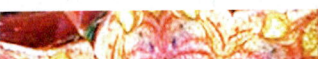

Procedure 45–2 Removing a Nasogastric Tube

ASSESSMENT

Assess

- For the presence of bowel sounds.
- For the absence of nausea or vomiting when tube is clamped.

PLANNING

Delegation

The skill of removing a nasogastric tube is not delegated to a UAP.

Equipment

- Disposable pad
- Tissues
- Clean gloves
- 50-mL syringe (optional)
- Plastic disposable bag

IMPLEMENTATION

Preparation

- Confirm the physician's order to remove the tube.
- Assist the client to a sitting position if health permits.
- Place the disposable pad across the client's chest to collect any spillage of mucous and gastric secretions from the tube.
- Provide tissues to the client to wipe the nose and mouth after tube removal.

Performance

1. Explain to the client what you are going to do, why it is necessary, and how he or she can cooperate. Explain that the procedure will cause no discomfort.
2. Wash hands and observe other appropriate infection control procedures (e.g., clean gloves).
3. Provide for client privacy.
4. Detach the tube.
   - Disconnect the nasogastric tube from the suction apparatus, if present.
   - Unpin the tube from the client's gown.
   - Remove the adhesive tape securing the tube to the nose.
5. Remove the nasogastric tube.
   - Put on disposable gloves.
   - (Optional) Instill 50 mL of air into the tube. *This clears the tube of any contents such as feeding or gastric drainage.*
   - Ask the client to take a deep breath and to hold it. *This closes the glottis, thereby preventing accidental aspiration of any gastric contents.*
   - Pinch the tube with the gloved hand. *Pinching the tube prevents any contents inside the tube from draining into the client's throat.*
   - Quickly and smoothly, withdraw the tube.
   - Place the tube in the plastic bag. *Placing the tube immediately into the bag prevents the transference of microorganisms from the tube to other articles or people.*
   - Observe the intactness of the tube.
6. Ensure client comfort.
   - Provide mouth care if desired.
   - Assist the client as required to blow the nose. *Excessive secretions may have accumulated in the nasal passages.*
7. Dispose of the equipment appropriately.
   - Place the pad, bag with tube, and gloves in the receptacle designated by the agency. *Correct disposal prevents the transmission of microorganisms.*
8. Assess the nasogastric drainage if suction was used.
   - Measure the amount of gastric drainage and record it on the client's fluid output record.
   - Inspect the drainage for appearance and consistency.
9. Document all relevant information.
   - Record the removal of the tube, the amount and appearance of any drainage if connected to suction, and any relevant assessments of the client.

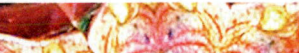

Procedure 45–2 Removing a Nasogastric Tube *continued*

EVALUATION

- Perform a follow-up examination, such as presence of bowel sounds, absence of nausea or vomiting when tube is removed, and intactness of tissues of the nares.

- Relate findings to previous assessment data if available.
- Report significant deviations from normal to the physician.

Gastrostomy and **jejunostomy** devices are used for long-term nutritional support, generally more than 6 to 8 weeks. Conventional tubes are placed surgically or by laparoscopy through the abdominal wall into the stomach (gastrostomy) or into the jejunum (jejunostomy).

The surgical opening is sutured tightly around the tube or catheter to prevent leakage. Care of this opening before it heals requires surgical asepsis. When the incision heals (10 to 14 days), the tube or catheter can be removed and reinserted for each feeding. Between feedings, a prosthesis may be used to close the ostomy opening. It consists of a shaft 3 to 5 cm (11/2 to 2 in.) long, with internal and external flanges and a screw cap.

A **percutaneous endoscopic gastrostomy (PEG)** (Figure 45–16 ■) or **percutaneous endoscopic jejunostomy (PEJ)** (Figure 45–17 ■) is created by using an endoscope to visualize the inside of the stomach, making a puncture through the skin and subcutaneous tissues of the abdomen into the stomach, and

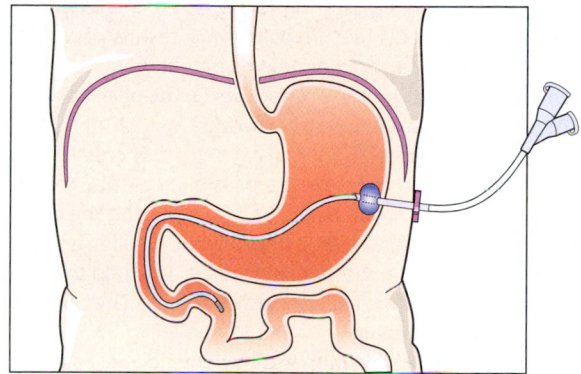

Figure 45–17 ■ Percutaneous endoscopic jejunostomy (PEJ) tube.

inserting the PEG or PEJ catheter through the puncture. The catheter has internal and external bumpers and an inflatable retention balloon to maintain placement. Once the opening has healed, replacement tubes can be inserted without the use of endoscopy.

Testing Feeding Tube Placement. Before feedings are introduced, tube placement is confirmed by radiography, particularly when a small-bore tube has been inserted or when the client is at risk for aspiration. After placement is confirmed, the nurse marks the tube with indelible ink or tape at its exit point from the nose and documents the length of visible tubing for baseline data. The nurse is responsible, however, for verifying tube placement (i.e., gastrointestinal placement versus respiratory placement) before each intermittent feeding and at regular intervals (e.g., at least once per shift) when continuous feedings are being administered.

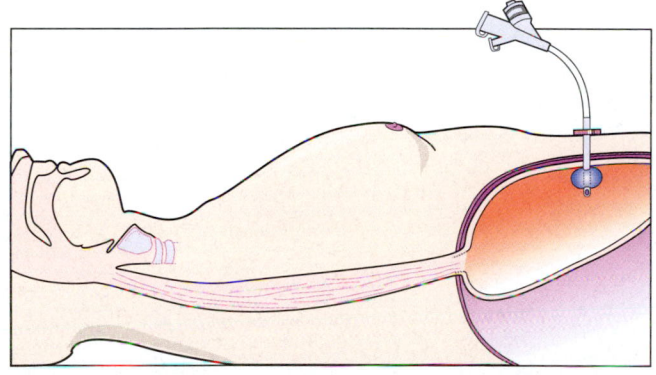

Figure 45–16 ■ Percutaneous endoscopic gastrostomy (PEG) tube.

Lifespan Considerations

Inserting a Nasogastric Tube
Infants and Young Children

- Restraints may be necessary during tube insertion and throughout therapy. *Restraints will prevent accidental dislodging of the tube.*
- Place the infant in an infant seat or position the infant with a rolled towel or pillow under the head and shoulders.
- When assessing the nares, obstruct one of the infant's nares and feel for air passage from the other. If the nasal passageway is very small or is obstructed, an orogastric tube may be more appropriate.

- Measure appropriate nasogastric tube length from the nose to the tip of the earlobe and then to the point midway between the umbilicus and the xiphoid process.
- If an orogastric tube is used, measure from the tip of the earlobe to the corner of the mouth to the xiphoid process.
- Do not hyperextend or hyperflex an infant's neck. *Hyperextension or hyperflexion of the neck could occlude the airway.*
- Tape the tube to the area between the end of the nares and the upper lip as well as to the cheek.

Practice Guidelines
Aspirating Gastrointestinal Secretions from Small-Bore Tubes

- Using a 30- to 60-mL syringe, inject 20 mL of air into the tube. This clears the tube of fluid and residual feeding, and moves the tip of the tube away from the mucosal lining.
- Aspirate the air and gastrointestinal fluid. Removing the air prevents gastric distention. Avoid exerting excessive negative pressure when aspirating to prevent tube collapse.
- If fluid is aspirated, measure its volume, test its pH, and flush the tube with water to maintain its patency.
- If fluid is not aspirated, inject another 20 mL of air and replace the larger syringe with a smaller syringe (e.g., 10 mL) before attempting to aspirate. The smaller syringe may create less negative pressure and decrease the possibility of tube collapse.
- If still unsuccessful, repeat the above step using the larger syringe to instill air and then attaching the smaller syringe, except this time leave the smaller syringe attached to the tube for 15 minutes before aspirating air and fluid. This allows time for fluid to accumulate.
- Change the client's position from side to side or raise or lower the head of the bed. These actions may make the tube move to an area where fluid has collected.

Methods nurses use to check tube placement include the following:

1. Aspirate 20 to 30 mL of gastrointestinal secretions. Small-bore tubes offer more resistance during aspirations than large-bore tubes and are more likely to collapse when negative pressure is applied. An effective method for aspirating fluid from small-bore tubes is outlined in the accompanying Practice Guidelines. Gastric secretions tend to be a grassy-green, off-white, or tan color; intestinal fluid is stained with bile and has a golden yellow or brownish-green color.
2. Measure the pH of aspirated fluid. This is the recommended method to determine tube placement. Testing the pH of aspirates can help distinguish gastric from respiratory and intestinal placement (Metheny & Titler, 2001; Metheny, Wehrle, Wiersema, & Clark, 1998) as follows:
   - Gastric aspirates tend to be acidic and have a pH of 1 to 4 but may be as high as 6 if the client is receiving medications that control gastric acid.
   - Small intestine aspirates generally have a pH equal to or higher than 6.
   - Respiratory secretions are more alkaline with values of 7 or higher. However, there is a slight possibility of respiratory placement when the pH reading is as low as 6. Therefore, when pH readings are 6 or higher, radiographic confirmation of tube location needs to be considered, especially in clients with diminished cough and gag reflexes.
3. Auscultate the epigastrium while injecting 5 to 20 mL of air. Air injected into the stomach produces whooshing, gurgling, or bubbling sounds over the epigastrium and the upper left quadrant. Accuracy of this method in predicting placement is less reliable than pH testing.

Currently, the most effective method appears to be radiographic verification of tube placement. Repeated x-ray studies, however, are not feasible in terms of cost and radiation risk. More research is required to devise effective alternatives, especially for placement of small-bore tubes. In the meantime, nurses should (a) ensure initial radiographic verification of small-bore tubes, (b) aspirate contents when possible and check their acidity, (c) closely observe the client for signs of obvious distress, and (d) suspect tube dislodgement after episodes of coughing, sneezing, and vomiting.

Enteral Feedings. The frequency of feedings and amounts to be administered are ordered by the physician. Liquid feeding mixtures are available commercially or may be prepared by the dietary department in accordance with the physician's orders. A standard formula provides 1 Kcal per milliliter of solution with protein, fat, carbohydrate, minerals, and vitamins in specified proportions.

Enteral feedings can be given intermittently or continuously. Intermittent feedings are the administration of 300 to 500 mL of enteral formula several times per day. The stomach is the preferred site for these feedings, which are usually administered over at least 30 minutes. Bolus intermittent feedings

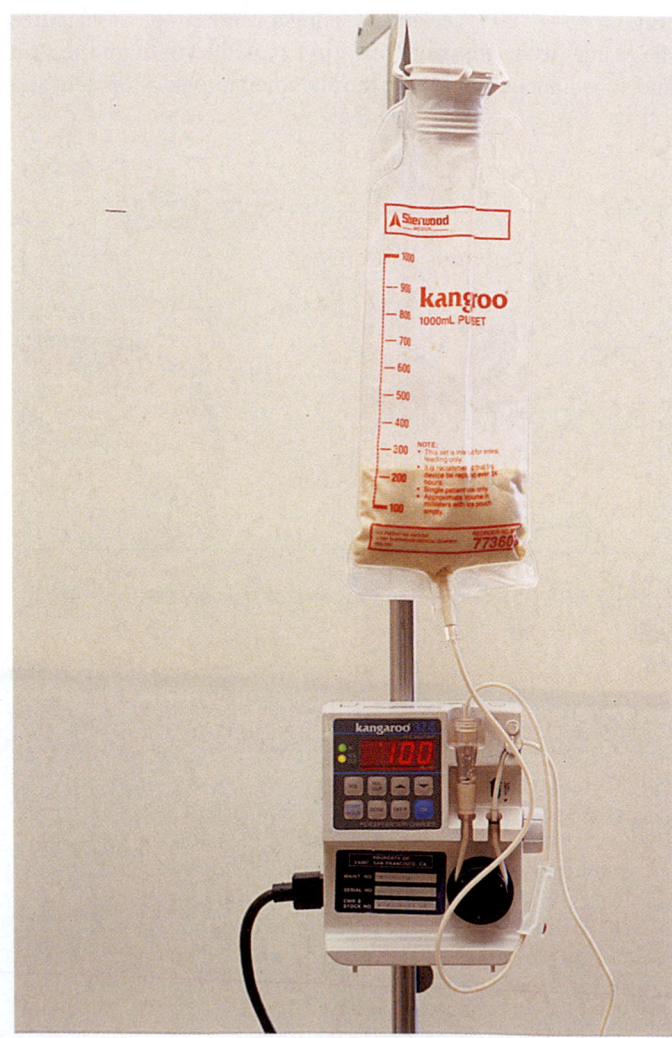

Figure 45–18 ■ An enteric feeding pump.

are those that use a syringe to deliver the formula into the stomach. Because the formula is delivered rapidly by this method, it is not usually recommended but may be used in long-term situations if the client tolerates them. These feedings must be given only into the stomach; the client must be monitored closely for distention and aspiration.

Continuous feedings are generally administered over a 24-hour period using an infusion pump that guarantees a constant flow rate (Figure 45–18 ■). Continuous feedings are essential when feedings are administered in the small bowel. They are also used when smaller bore gastric tubes are in place or when gravity flow is insufficient to instill the feeding.

Cyclic feedings are continuous feedings that are administered in less than 24 hours (e.g., 12 to 16 hours). These feedings, often administered at night and referred to as nocturnal feedings, allow the client to attempt to eat regular meals through the day. Because nocturnal feedings may use higher nutrient densities and higher infusion rates than the standard continuous feeding, particular attention needs to be given to monitoring fluid status and circulating volume overload.

Enteral feedings are administered to clients through open or closed systems. Open systems use an open-top container or a syringe for administration. Enteral feedings for use with open systems are provided in flip-top cans or powdered formulas that are reconstituted with sterile water. Sterile water, rather than tap water, is used to reduce the risk of microbial contamination. Closed systems consist of a prefilled container that is spiked with enteral tubing and attached to the enteral access device. Prefilled containers generally have 1 liter of formula and can hang safely for 24 to 36 hours if sterile technique is used.

Procedure 45–3 provides the essential steps involved in administering a tube feeding, and Procedure 45–4 indicates the steps involved in administering a gastrostomy or jejunostomy tube feeding.

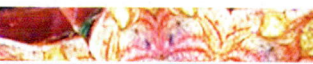

Procedure 45–3 Administering a Tube Feeding

Purposes

- To restore or maintain nutritional status
- To administer medications

ASSESSMENT

Assess

- For any clinical signs of malnutrition or dehydration.
- Check for allergies to any food in the feeding.
- For the presence of bowel sounds.
- Note any problems that suggest lack of tolerance of previous feedings (e.g., delayed gastric emptying, abdominal distention, dumping syndrome, constipation, or dehydration).

PLANNING

Before commencing a nasogastric or orogastric feeding, determine the type, amount, and frequency of feedings and tolerance of previous feedings.

Delegation

Administering a tube feeding requires application of knowledge and problem solving and it is not usually delegated to UAP. Some agencies, however, may allow a trained UAP to administer a feeding. In this case, it is the responsibility of the nurse to assess tube placement and determine that the tube is patent. The nurse should reinforce major points, such as making sure the client is sitting upright, and instruct the UAP to report any difficulty administering the feeding or any complaints voiced by the client.

Equipment

- Correct amount of feeding solution
- 20- to 50-mL syringe with an adapter
- Emesis basin
- Clean gloves
- Large syringe with plunger or calibrated plastic feeding bag with tubing that can be attached to the feeding tube or prefilled bottle with a drip chamber, tubing, and a flow-regulator clamp
- pH test strip or meter
- Measuring container from which to pour the feeding (if using open system)
- Water (60 mL unless otherwise specified) at room temperature
- Feeding pump as required

IMPLEMENTATION

Preparation

Assist the client to a Fowler's position in bed or a sitting position in a chair, the normal position for eating. If a sitting position is contraindicated, a slightly elevated right side-lying position is acceptable. *These positions enhance the gravitational flow of the solution and prevent aspiration of fluid into the lungs.*

Performance

1. Explain to the client what you are going to do, why it is necessary, and how he or she can cooperate. Inform client that the feeding should not cause any discomfort but may cause a feeling of fullness. For an adult, the usual intermittent feeding will take about 30 minutes; the exact length of time depends largely on the volume of the feeding.

2. Wash hands and observe appropriate infection control procedures (e.g., clean gloves).

continued on page 1212

Procedure 45–3 Administering a Tube Feeding *continued*

IMPLEMENTATION *continued*

3. Provide privacy for this procedure if the client desires it. Nasogastric or nasoenteric feedings are embarrassing to some people.

4. Assess tube placement.
   - Attach the syringe to the open end of the tube and aspirate alimentary secretions. Check the pH.
   - Allow 1 hour to elapse before testing the pH if the client has received a medication.
   - Use a pH meter rather than pH paper if the client is receiving a continuous feeding or if food coloring has been added to the formula.

5. Assess residual feeding contents.
   - Aspirate all stomach contents and measure the amount before administering the feeding. *This is done to evaluate absorption of the last feeding; that is, whether undigested formula from a previous feeding remains.*
   - If 100 mL (or more than half the last feeding) is withdrawn, check with the nurse in charge or refer to agency policy before proceeding. The precise amount is usually determined by the physician's order or by agency policy. *At some agencies, a feeding is withheld when the specified amount or more of formula remains in the stomach. In other agencies, the amount withdrawn is subtracted from the total feeding and that volume (less the undigested portion) is administered slowly.*
     or
   - Reinstill the gastric contents into the stomach if this is the agency policy or physician's order. Remove the syringe bulb or plunger, and pour the gastric contents via the syringe into the nasogastric tube. *Removal of the contents could disturb the client's electrolyte balance.*
   - If the client is on a continuous feeding, check the gastric residual every 4 to 6 hours or according to agency protocol.

6. Administer the feeding.
   - Before administering feeding: Check the expiration date of the feeding.
     Warm the feeding to room temperature. *An excessively cold feeding may cause cramps.*

- When an open system is used, clean the top of the feeding container with alcohol before opening it. *This minimizes the risk of contaminants entering the feeding syringe or feeding bag.*

FEEDING BAG (OPEN SYSTEM)

- Hang the bag from an infusion pole about 30 cm (12 in.) above the tube's point of insertion into the client.
- Clamp the tubing and add the formula to the bag.
- Open the clamp, run the formula through the tubing, and reclamp the tube. The formula will displace the air in the tubing, thus preventing the instillation of excess air into the client's stomach or intestine.
- Attach the bag to the nasogastric/nasoenteric tube (Figure 45–19 ■) and regulate the drip by adjusting the clamp to the drop factor on the bag (e.g., 20 drops/mL).

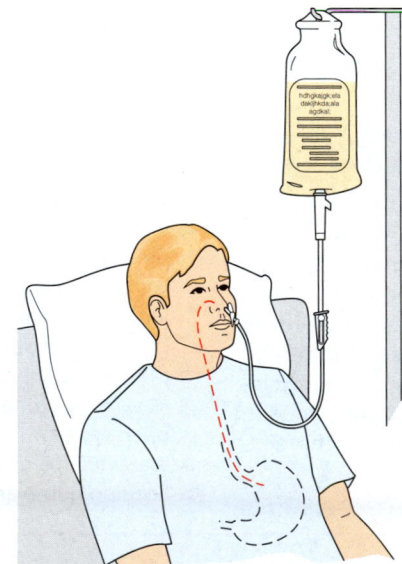

Figure 45–19 ■ Using a calibrated plastic bag to administer a tube feeding.

SYRINGE (OPEN SYSTEM)

- Remove the plunger from the syringe and connect the syringe to a pinched or clamped nasogastric tube. *Pinching or clamping the tube prevents excess air from entering the stomach and causing distention.*

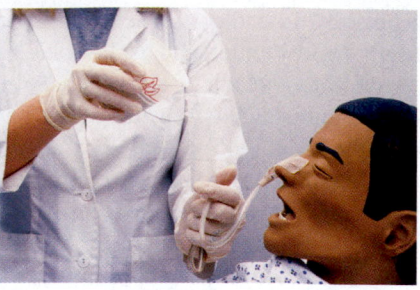

Figure 45–20 ■ Using a syringe to administer a tube feeding.

- Add the feeding to the syringe barrel (Figure 45–20 ■).
- Permit the feeding to flow in slowly at the prescribed rate. Raise or lower the syringe to adjust the flow as needed. Pinch or clamp the tubing to stop the flow for a minute if the client experiences discomfort. *Quickly administered feedings can cause flatus, cramps, and/or reflux vomiting.*

PREFILLED BOTTLE WITH DRIP CHAMBER (CLOSED SYSTEM)

- Remove the screw-on cap from the container and attach the administration set with the drip chamber and tubing (Figure 45–21 ■).

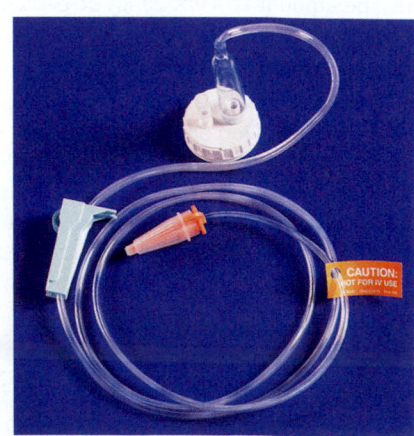

Figure 45–21 ■ Feeding set tubing with drip chamber. (Ross Products Division, Abbott Laboratories. Used with permission.)

- Close the clamp on the tubing.
- Hang the container on an intravenous pole about 30 cm (12 in.) above the tube's insertion point into the client. *At this height, the formula*

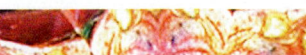

Procedure 45–3 Administering a Tube Feeding *continued*

IMPLEMENTATION *continued*

should run at a safe rate into the stomach or intestine.

- Squeeze the drip chamber to fill it to one-third to one-half of its capacity.
- Open the tubing clamp, run the formula through the tubing, and reclamp the tube. *The formula will displace the air in the tubing, thus preventing the instillation of excess air.*
- Attach the feeding set tubing to the feeding tube and regulate the drip rate to deliver the feeding over the desired length of time. Prefilled tube-feeding sets can be attached to a feeding pump to regulate the flow.

7. Rinse the feeding tube immediately before all of the formula has run through the tubing.
   - Instill 50 to 100 mL of water through the feeding tube. Water flushes the lumen of the tube, preventing future blockage by sticky formula.
   - Be sure to add the water before the feeding solution has drained from the neck of a syringe or from the tubing of an administration set. Before adding water to a feeding bag or prefilled tubing set, first clamp and disconnect both feeding and administration tubes. *Adding the water before the syringe or tubing is empty prevents the instillation of air into the stomach or intestine and thus prevents unnecessary distention.*

8. Clamp and cover the feeding tube.
   - Clamp the feeding tube before all of the water is instilled. *Clamping prevents leakage and air from entering the tube if done before water is instilled.*

- Cover the end of the feeding tube with gauze held by an elastic band. *Covering the tube end prevents leakage from it.*

9. Ensure client comfort and safety.
   - Pin the tubing to the client's gown. *This minimizes pulling of the tube, thus preventing discomfort and dislodgement.*
   - Ask the client to remain sitting upright in Fowler's position or in a slightly elevated right lateral position for at least 30 minutes. *These positions facilitate digestion and movement of the feeding from the stomach along the alimentary tract, and prevent the potential aspiration of the feeding into the lungs.*
   - Check the agency's policy on the frequency of changing the nasogastric tube and the use of smaller lumen tubes if a large-bore tube is in place. *These measures prevent irritation and erosion of the pharyngeal and esophageal mucous membranes.*

10. Dispose of equipment appropriately.
    - If the equipment is to be reused, wash it thoroughly with soap and water so that it is ready for reuse.
    - Change the equipment every 24 hours or according to agency policy.

11. Document all relevant information.
    - Document the feeding, including amount and kind of solution taken, duration of the feeding, and assessments of the client.
    - Record the volume of the feeding and water administered on the client's intake and output record.

12. Monitor the client for possible problems.
    - Carefully assess clients receiving tube feedings for problems.

- To prevent dehydration, give the client supplemental water in addition to the prescribed tube feeding as ordered.

VARIATION: CONTINUOUS-DRIP FEEDING

- If the feeding is a continuous-drip tube feeding, place a label on the container.
- Clamp the tubing at least every 4 to 6 hours, or as indicated by agency protocol or the manufacturer, and aspirate and measure the gastric contents. Then flush the tubing with 30 to 50 mL of water. *This determines adequate absorption and verifies correct placement of the tube. If placement of a small-bore tube is questionable, a repeat x-ray should be done.*
- Determine agency protocol regarding withholding a feeding. Many agencies withhold the feeding if more than 75 to 100 mL of feeding is aspirated.
- To prevent spoilage or bacterial contamination, do not allow the feeding solution to hang longer than 4 to 8 hours. *Check agency policy or manufacturer's recommendations regarding time limits.*
- Follow agency policy regarding how frequently to change the feeding bag and tubing. Changing the feeding bag and tubing every 24 hours reduces the risk of contamination.

EVALUATION

Perform a follow-up examination of the following:
- Tolerance of feeding
- Regurgitation and feelings of fullness after feedings
- Weight gain or loss
- Fecal elimination pattern (e.g., diarrhea, flatulence, constipation)
- Skin turgor
- Urine output
- Glucose and acetone in urine
- Relate findings to previous assessment data if available. Report significant deviations from normal to the physician.

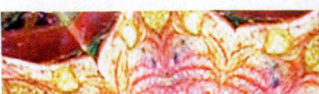

Procedure 45–4 Administering a Gastrostomy or Jejunostomy Feeding

Purposes

See Procedure 45–3.

See Procedure 45–3.

Before commencing a gastrostomy or jejunostomy feeding, determine the type and amount of feeding to be instilled, frequency of feedings, and any pertinent information about previous feedings (e.g., the positioning which the client best tolerates the feeding).

Delegation
See Procedure 45–3.

Equipment
- Correct amount of feeding solution
- Graduated container to hold the feeding
- Large bulb syringe
- Graduated container with 60 mL of water to flush the tubing
- Graduated container to measure residual formula

FOR A TUBE SUTURED IN PLACE
- 4-in. × 4-in. gauze squares to cover the end of the tube
- Elastic band

FOR TUBE INSERTION
- Clean gloves
- Moisture-proof bag
- Water-soluble lubricant
- 18 Fr whistle-tip catheter or other feeding tube
- Tubing clamp

FOR CLEANING THE PERISTOMAL SKIN AND DRESSING THE STOMA
- Mild soap and water
- Clean gloves
- Petrolatum, zinc oxide ointment, or other skin protectant
- Precut 4-in. × 4-in. gauze squares
- Uncut 4-in. × 4-in. gauze squares
- Abdominal pads
- Abdominal binder or Montgomery straps

Preparation
See Procedure 45–3.

Performance
1. Explain to the client what you are going to do, why it is necessary, and how he or she can cooperate.
2. Wash hands and observe other appropriate infection control procedures.
3. Provide for client privacy.
4. Assess and prepare the client. See Procedure 45–3.
5. Insert a feeding tube, if one is not already in place.
   - Wearing gloves, remove the ostomy dressing. Then discard the dressing and gloves in the moisture-proof bag.
   - Lubricate the end of the tube, and insert it into the ostomy opening 10 to 15 cm (4 to 6 in.).
6. Check the patency of a tube that is sutured or secured in place.
   - Determine correct placement of the tube by aspirating secretions and checking the pH.
   - Pour 15 to 30 mL of water into the syringe, remove the tube clamp, and allow the water to flow into the tube. *This determines the patency of*

the tube. *If water flows freely, the tube is patent.*
   - If the water does not flow freely, notify the nurse in charge and/or physician.
7. Check for residual formula.
   - Attach the bulb to the syringe and compress the bulb. *Compressing the bulb before the syringe is attached to the feeding tube prevents the instillation of air into the stomach or jejunum.*
   - Attach the syringe to the end of the feeding tube, and withdraw and measure the stomach or jejunal contents.
   - Follow agency practice if there is no more than 50 mL of undigested formula. Hold the feeding if there is more than 150 mL, and recheck in 3 to 4 hours or according to agency policy. Notify the physician if a large residual still remains.
   - For continuous feedings, check the residual every 4 to 6 hours and hold feedings according to agency policy. The physician should be notified if a large residual persists.

8. Administer the feeding.
   - Hold the barrel of the syringe 7 to 15 cm (3 to 6 in.) above the ostomy opening.
   - Slowly pour the solution into the syringe and allow it to flow through the tube by gravity.
   - Just before all the formula has run through and the syringe is empty, add 30 mL of water. *Water flushes the tube and preserves its patency.*
   - If the tube is sutured in place, hold it upright, remove the syringe, and then clamp or plug the tube to prevent leakage. Cover the end of the tube with a 4-in. × 4-in. gauze, and secure the gauze with a rubber band.
   - If a catheter was inserted for the feeding, remove it.
9. Ensure client comfort and safety.
   - After the feeding, ask the client to remain in the sitting position or a slightly elevated right lateral position for at least 30 minutes. *This minimizes the risk of aspiration.*
   - Assess status of peristomal skin. Gastric or jejunal drainage contains digestive enzymes that can irritate

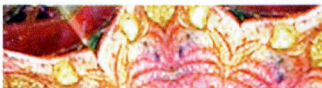

Procedure 45–4 Administering a Gastrostomy or Jejunostomy Feeding *continued*

IMPLEMENTATION *continued*

the skin. Document any redness and broken skin areas.

- Check orders about cleaning the peristomal skin, applying a skin protectant, and applying appropriate dressings. Generally, the peristomal skin is washed with mild soap and water at least once daily. Petrolatum, zinc oxide ointment, or other skin protectant may be applied around the stoma, and precut 4-in. × 4-in. gauze squares may be placed around the tube. The precut squares are then covered with regular 4-in. × 4-in. gauze squares, and the tube is coiled over them. The coiled tube is covered with abdominal pads and secured with either an abdominal binder or Montgomery straps.

- Observe for common complications of enteral feedings: aspiration, hyperglycemia, abdominal distention, diarrhea, and fecal impaction. Report findings to physician. Often, a change in formula or rate of administration can correct problems.

- When appropriate, teach the client how to administer feedings and when to notify the health care provider concerning problems.

VARIATION: PERCUTANEOUS ENDOSCOPIC GASTROSTOMY (PEG)

A PEG is kept in place with a short crosspiece or bolster near the skin level at the stoma.

- Clean the stoma daily with soap and water using a cotton swab or small piece of gauze in a circular motion.
- Rotate the bolster and clean the skin under it.
- Rotate the tube in a full circle between the thumb and forefinger daily.
- After cleaning, allow the skin to air dry.
- Report any signs of redness, pain, soreness, swelling, or drainage to the health care provider.
- Do not apply a dressing over the PEG. *A dressing and tape may result in skin excoriation and breakdown.*

10. Document all assessments and interventions.

EVALUATION

See Procedure 45–3.

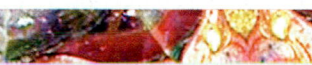

Lifespan Considerations

Administering a Tube Feeding

Infants
- Feeding tubes may be reinserted at each feeding to prevent irritation of the mucous membrane, nasal airway obstruction, and stomach perforation that may occur if the tube is left in place continuously. Check agency practice.

Children
- Position a small child or infant in your lap, provide a pacifier, and hold and cuddle the child during feedings. This promotes comfort, supports the normal sucking instinct of the infant, and facilitates digestion.

Elders
- Physiologic changes associated with aging may make the elder more vulnerable to complications associated with enteral feedings. Decreased gastric emptying may necessitate checking frequently for gastric residual. Diarrhea from administering the feeding too fast or at too high a concentration may cause dehydration. If the feeding has a high concentration of glucose, assess for hyperglycemia because with aging, the body has a decreased ability to handle increased glucose levels.

- Conditions such as hiatal hernia and diabetes mellitus may cause the stomach to empty more slowly. This increases the risk of aspiration in a client receiving a tube feeding. Checking for gastric residual more frequently can help document this if it is an ongoing problem. Changing the formula or the rate of administration, repositioning the client, or obtaining a physician's order for a medication to increase stomach emptying may resolve this problem.

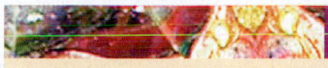

Home Care Considerations

Administering a Tube Feeding
- Teach the client or caregiver how to assess for tube placement using pH measurement before administering the feeding.
- Provide instructions for care of the tube and insertion site.
- Teach signs and symptoms to report to the doctor or home health nurse.

TABLE 45–6 Assessing Clients Receiving Tube Feedings

Assessments	Rationale
Allergies to any food in the feeding	Common allergenic foods include milk, sugar, water, eggs, and vegetable oil.
Bowel sounds before each feeding or, for continuous feedings, every 4 to 8 hours	To determine intestinal activity.
Correct placement of tube, before feedings	To prevent aspiration of feedings
Presence of regurgitation and feelings of fullness after feedings	May indicate delayed gastric emptying, need to decrease quantity or rate of the feeding, or high fat content of the formula.
Dumping syndrome: nausea, vomiting, diarrhea, cramps, pallor, sweating, heart palpitations, increased pulse rate, and fainting after a feeding	Jejunostomy clients may experience these symptoms, which result when hypertonic foods and liquids suddenly distend the jejunum. To make the intestinal contents isotonic, body fluids shift rapidly from the client's vascular system.
Abdominal distention, at least daily. Measure abdominal girth at the umbilicus	Abdominal distention may indicate intolerance to a previous feeding.
Diarrhea, constipation, or flatulence	The lack of bulk in liquid feedings may cause constipation. The presence of hypertonic or concentrated ingredients may cause diarrhea and flatulence.
Urine for sugar and acetone	Hyperglycemia may occur if the sugar content is too high.
Hematocrit and urine specific gravity	Both increase as a result of dehydration.
Serum BUN and sodium levels	Feeding formula may have a high protein content. If a high protein intake is combined with an inadequate fluid intake, the kidneys may not be able to excrete nitrogenous wastes adequately.

Before administering a tube feeding, the nurse must determine any food allergies of the client and assess tolerance to previous feedings. Table 45–6 lists essential assessments to conduct before administering tube feedings. The nurse must also check the expiration date on a commercially prepared formula or the preparation date and time of agency-prepared solution, discarding any formula that has passed the expiration date or solution more than 24 hours old.

Feedings are usually administered at room temperature unless the order specifies otherwise. The nurse warms the specified amount of solution in a basin of warm water or leaves it to stand for a while until it reaches room temperature. Because a formula that is warmed can grow microorganisms, it should not hang longer than the manufacturer recommends. If it will hang longer, it should be kept cool with ice chips. Continuous-feeding formulas should be kept cold; excessive heat coagulates feedings of milk and egg, and hot liquids can irritate the mucous membranes.

However, excessively cold feedings can reduce the flow of digestive juices by causing vasoconstriction and may cause cramps.

Parenteral Nutrition

Parenteral nutrition (PN), also referred to as total parenteral nutrition (TPN) or intravenous hyperalimentation (IVH), is provided when the gastrointestinal tract is nonfunctional because of an interruption in its continuity or because its absorptive capacity is impaired. **Parenteral** nutrition is administered intravenously such as through a central venous catheter into the superior vena cava.

Parenteral feedings are solutions of dextrose, water, fat, proteins, electrolytes, vitamins, and trace elements; they provide all needed calories. Because TPN solutions are hypertonic (highly concentrated in comparison to the solute concentration of blood), they are injected only into high-flow central veins, where they are diluted by the client's blood.

TPN is a means of achieving an anabolic state in clients who are unable to maintain a normal nitrogen balance. Such clients may include those with severe malnutrition, severe burns, bowel disease disorders (e.g., ulcerative colitis or enteric fistula), acute renal failure, hepatic failure, metastatic cancer, or major surgeries where nothing may be taken by mouth for more than 5 days.

TPN is not risk free. Infection control is of utmost importance during TPN therapy. The nurse must always observe surgical aseptic technique when changing solutions, tubing, dressings, and filters. Clients are at increased risk of fluid, electrolyte, and glucose imbalances and require frequent evaluation and modification of the TPN mixture.

TPN solutions are 10% to 50% dextrose in water, plus a mixture of amino acids and special additives such as vitamins (e.g., B complex, C, D, K), minerals (e.g., potassium, sodium, chloride, calcium, phosphate, magnesium), and trace elements (e.g., cobalt, zinc, manganese). Additives are modified to each client's nutritional needs. Fat emulsions may be given to provide essential fatty acids to correct and/or prevent essential fatty acid deficiency or to supplement the calories for clients who, for example, have high calorie needs or cannot tolerate glucose as the only calorie source. Note that 1,000 mL of 5% glucose or dextrose contains 50 grams of sugar. Thus, a liter of this solution provides less than 200 calories!

Because TPN solutions are high in glucose, infusions are started gradually to prevent hyperglycemia. The client needs to adapt to TPN therapy by increasing insulin output from the pancreas. For example, an adult client may be given 1 liter (40 mL/hr) of TPN solution the first day, if the infusion is tolerated; the amount may be increased to 2 liters (80 mL/hr) for 24 to 48 hours, and then to 3 liters (120 mL/hr) within 3 to 5 days. Glucose levels are monitored during the infusion.

When TPN therapy is to be discontinued, the TPN infusion rates are decreased slowly to prevent hyperinsulinemia and hypoglycemia. Weaning a client from TPN may take up to 48 hours but can occur in 6 hours as long as the client receives adequate carbohydrates either orally or intravenously.

Enteral or parenteral feedings may be continued beyond hospital care in the client's home or may be initiated in the home.

EVALUATING

The goals established in the planning phase are evaluated according to specific desired outcomes, also established in that phase (see Identifying Nursing Diagnoses, Outcomes, and Interventions).

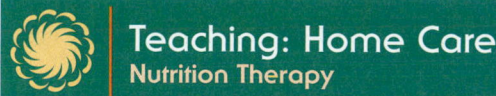

Teaching: Home Care
Nutrition Therapy

Clients and caregivers need the following instructions to manage these feedings:

- Preparation of the formula. Include name of the formula and how much and how often it is to be given; the need to inspect the formula for expiration date and leaks and cracks in bags or cans; how to mix or prepare the formula, if needed; and aseptic techniques such as swabbing the container's top with alcohol before opening it, and changing the syringe administration set and reservoir every 24 hours.
- Proper storage of the formula. Include the need to refrigerate diluted or reconstituted formula and formula that contains additives.
- Administration of the feeding. Include proper hand-washing technique, how to fill and hang the feeding bag, operation of an infusion pump if indicated, the feeding rate, and client positioning during and after the feeding.
- Management of the enteral or parenteral access device. Include site care, aseptic precautions, dressing change, as indicated, how the site should look normally, and flushing protocols (e.g., type of irrigant and schedule).
- Daily monitoring needs. Include temperature, weight, and intake and output.
- Signs and symptoms of complications to report. Include fever, increased respiratory rate, decrease in urine output, increased stool frequency, and altered level of consciousness.
- Whom to contact regarding questions or problems. Include emergency telephone numbers of home care agency, nursing clinician and/or physician, or other 24-hour on-call emergency number.

If the outcomes are not achieved, the nurse should explore the reasons. The nurse might consider the following questions:

- Was the cause of the problem correctly identified?
- Was the family included in the teaching plan? Are family members supportive?
- Is the client experiencing symptoms that cause loss of appetite (e.g., pain, nausea, fatigue)?
- Were the outcomes unrealistic for this person?
- Were the client's food preferences considered?
- Is anything interfering with digestion or absorption of nutrients (e.g., diarrhea)?

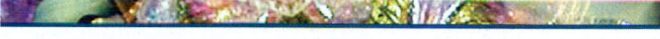

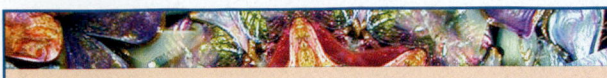

NURSING CARE PLAN FOR NUTRITION

ASSESSMENT DATA		*NURSING DIAGNOSIS*	DESIRED OUTCOMES [NOC #]/INDICATORS*
Nursing Assessment Mrs. Rose Santini, a 59-year-old homemaker, attends a community hospital–sponsored health fair. She approaches the nutrition information booth, and the clinical specialist in nutritional support gathers a nutritional history. Mrs. Santini is very upset about her 9-kg (20-lb) weight gain. She relates to the nurse clinician that since the death of her husband 1 month ago she has lost interest in many of her usual physical and social activities. She no longer attends YMCA exercise and swimming sessions and has lost contact with her couple's bridge group. Mrs. Santini states she is bored, depressed, and very unhappy about her appearance. She has a small frame and has always prided herself on her petite figure. She says her eating habits have changed considerably. She snacks while watching TV and rarely prepares a complete meal.	**Physical Examination** Height: 162.6 cm (5'4") Weight: 63.6 kg (140 lb) Temperature: 37C (98.6F) Pulse: 76 BPM Respirations: 16/minute Blood pressure: 144/84 mm Hg Triceps skinfold: 21 mm Small frame, weight in excess of 10% over ideal for height and frame **Diagnostic Data** CBC normal, urinalysis negative, chest x-ray negative, thyroid profile within normal limits	*Imbalanced Nutrition: More than body requirements* related to excess intake and decreased activity expenditure (as evidenced by weight gain of 20 lbs, triceps skin fold greater than normal, undesirable eating patterns).	Weight Control [1612] as evidenced by • Eats three meals each day that result in a 500-calorie reduction in intake. • Develops a physical exercise plan that engages her in 15 to 20 minutes of exercise by day 5. • Identifies eating habits that contribute to weight gain by day 2.

NURSING INTERVENTIONS [NIC#]/SELECTED ACTIVITIES*	*RATIONALE*
Weight Reduction Assistance [1280]	
• Determine current eating patterns by having Mrs. Santini keep a diary of what, when, and where she eats	*Increases awareness of activities and foods that contribute to excessive intake.*
• Set a weekly goal for weight loss	*The desirable weight loss rate is 1–2 pounds per week.*
• Encourage use of internal reward systems when goals are accomplished	*Goal setting provides motivation, which is essential for a successful weight-loss program.*
• Set a realistic plan with Mrs. Santini to include reduced food intake and increased energy expenditure	*A combined plan of calorie reduction and exercise can enhance weight loss since exercise increases caloric utilization.*
• Assist client to identify motivation for eating and internal and external cues associated with eating	*Awareness of factors that contribute to overeating will assist the individual in planning behavior modification techniques to avoid situations that prompt excess food consumption.*
• Encourage attendance at support groups for weight loss and or refer to a community weight control program	*Overweight people are often nutritionally deprived. Intake must be reduced by 500 calories per day to obtain a one-pound-per-week weight loss.*
• Develop a daily meal plan with a well-balanced diet, reduced calories, and reduced fat	*Support groups can provide companionship, increase motivation, and offer practical solutions to problems associated with dieting.*
Nutritional Counseling [5246]	
• Facilitate identification of eating behaviors to be changed	*Increases individual's awareness of those actions that contribute to excessive intake.*
• Use accepted nutritional standards to assist Mrs. Santini in evaluating adequacy of dietary intake	*Comparing the individual's dietary history with nutritional standards will facilitate identification of nutritional deficiencies and/or excesses.*

NURSING CARE PLAN FOR NUTRITION *continued*

NURSING INTERVENTIONS [NIC #] / SELECTED ACTIVITIES*	RATIONALE
• Help Mrs. Santini to consider factors of age, past eating experiences, culture, and finances in planning ways to meet nutritional requirements	*Social, economic, physical, and psychological factors play a role in nutrition and/or malnutrition.*
• Discuss Mrs. Santini's knowledge of the basic four food groups, as well as perceptions of the needed diet modification	*Helps to determine the patient's knowledge base and identify misconceptions and/or gaps in understanding.*
• Discuss food likes and dislikes.	*Incorporating Mrs. Santini's food preferences into the dietary plan will promote adherence to the weight loss program.*
• Assist Mrs. Santini in stating her feelings and concerns about goal achievement	*Fear of success, failure, or other concerns may block goal achievement.*

Behavior Modification [4360]

• Assist Mrs. Santini to identify strengths and reinforce these	*Reinforcing strengths enhances self-esteem and encourages the individual to draw on these assets during the weight-loss program.*
• Encourage her to examine her own behavior	*Involving Mrs. Santini in self-appraisal will promote identification of behaviors that may be contributing to excessive caloric intake.*
• Identify the behavior to be changed in specific, concrete terms (e.g., stop snacking in front of the TV)	*Identification of specific behaviors is essential for planning behavior modification.*
• Consider that it is easier to increase a behavior than to decrease a behavior (e.g., increase activities or hobbies that involve the hands such as sewing versus decreasing TV snacking)	*Habitual behaviors are difficult to change. Breaking old habits may be easier if viewed from the standpoint of increasing an enjoyable, healthy activity.*
• Choose reinforcers that are meaningful to Mrs. Santini	*Positive reinforcement is not likely to be an effective part of behavior modification if the reinforcer is meaningless to the individual.*

EVALUATION

Outcome met. Mrs. Santini kept a dietary log for 5 days and has eaten balanced meals each day, resulting in a daily deficit of 400 to 500 calories. She is aware that she eats excessively because she is bored and depressed. She has reestablished her former social contacts including her church bridge club. Mrs. Santini has purchased a stationary bicycle and exercises 20 minutes daily. She enrolled in a knitting class that meets two nights per week. She has lost 1½ lbs in the past week. As a reward, Mrs. Santini renewed her membership to the YMCA.

---

*Outcomes, interventions, and activities selected are only a sample of those suggested by NOC and NIC and should be further individualized for each client.

Applying Critical Thinking

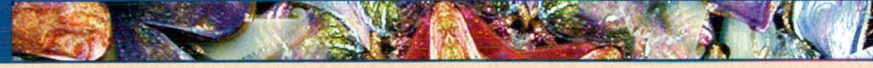

1. How do Mrs. Santini's personal characteristics influence her nutritional needs?
2. What further information do you need regarding Mrs. Santini's present diet?
3. Offer suggestions for ways to modify Mrs. Santini's tendency to snack.
4. Mrs. Santini asks what her weight should be. How do you respond?

See Critical Thinking Possibilities in Appendix A.

RS
59 y.o. ♀

- Homemaker, 9 kg weight gain
- Since death of her husband 1 month ago, lost interest in many usual physical & social activities, no longer attends YMCA exercise and swimming, lost contact with couples bridge group
- States is bored, depressed, & very unhappy about her appearance
- Has small frame & always prided herself on petite figure

- Eating habits have changed: snacks watching TV, rarely prepares complete meal
- Height: 162.6 cm (5'4")
- Weight: 63.6 kg (140 lb)
- T: 37C (98.6F) P: 76 BPM R: 16 BP: 144/84
- Triceps skinfold: 21 mm
- Small frame, weight > 10% over ideal for height and frame
- CBC, UA, CXR, thyroid panel negative

Imbalanced Nutrition: More than Body Requirements r/t excess intake and decreased activity expenditure (aeb weight gain of 20 lbs, triceps skin fold greater than normal, undesirable eating patterns)

Weight Reduction Assistance

- Set a realistic plan with her to include reduced food intake and increased energy expenditure

- Encourage use of internal reward systems when goals are accomplished

- Determine current eating patterns by having her keep a diary of what, when, and where she eats

- Set a weekly goal for weight loss

- Assist her to identify motivation for eating and internal and external cues associated with eating

Weight Control aeb
- eats three meals each day that result in a 500-calorie reduction in intake
- develops a physical exercise plan that engages her in 15 to 20 minutes of exercise by day 5
- identifies eating habits that contribute to weight gain by day 2

Outcome met
- kept dietary log for 5 days
- planned balanced meals each day, → daily deficit 400 to 500 cals.
- is aware eats excessively because is bored and depressed
- has reestablished social contacts incl. church bridge club
- purchased stationary bicycle & exercises 20 minutes/day
- enrolled in knitting class two nights/week
- has lost 1 1/2 lbs in past week. As a reward, renewed membership in YMCA

Nutritional Counseling

- Discuss food likes and dislikes

- Facilitate identification of eating behaviors to be changed

- Assist her in stating her feelings and concerns about goal achievement

- Use accepted nutritional standards to assist her in evaluating adequacy of dietary intake

- Discuss her knowledge of the basic four food groups, as well as perceptions of the needed diet modification

- Help her to consider factors of age, past eating experiences, culture, and finances in planning ways to meet nutritional requirements

Behavior Modification

- Assist her to identify strength and reinforce these

- Encourage her to examine her own behavior

- Choose reinforcers that are meaningful to her

- Consider that it is easier to increase a behavior than to decrease a behavior (e.g., increase activities or hobbies that involve the hands such as sewing versus decreasing TV snacking)

- Identify the behavior to be changed in specific, concrete terms (e.g., stop snacking in front of the TV)

Legend: Assessment ▢   Nursing Diagnosis ▢   Outcomes ▢   Nursing Interventions ▢   Activities ▢   Evaluation/Reassessment ▢

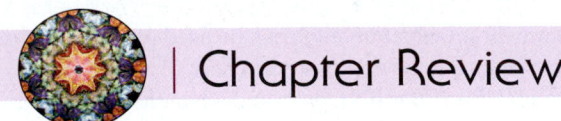

Chapter Review

 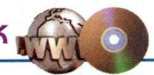

NCLEX review questions, case studies, care plan activities, MediaLink applications, and other interactive resources for this chapter can be found on the Companion Website at www.prenhall.com/kozier. Click on Chapter 45 to select the activities for this chapter.

For animations, more NCLEX review questions, and an audio glossary, access the Student CD-ROM accompanying this textbook.

Chapter Highlights

- Although people are bombarded with information about what to eat and what not to eat, each person is responsible for selecting foods that provide essential nutrients. Nurses assist people to evaluate the information they receive about nutrients.
- Essential nutrients are grouped into six categories: water, carbohydrates, fats, proteins, vitamins, and minerals.
- Nutrients serve three basic purposes: forming body structures (such as bones and blood), providing energy, and helping to regulate the body's biochemical reactions.
- Energy balance is the relationship between the energy derived from food and the energy used by the body.
- The amount of energy that nutrients or foods supply to the body is their caloric value. The amount of energy required to maintain basic body functions is referred to as the resting energy expenditure (REE). The basal metabolic rate (BMR) is the rate at which the body metabolizes food to maintain the energy and requirements of a person who is awake and at rest.
- A person's state of energy balance can be determined by comparing caloric intake with caloric expenditure.
- Ideal body weight (IBW) is the optimal weight recommended for optimal health and can be approximated by the Rule of 5 for females and the Rule of 6 for males.
- Body mass index (BMI) or percent body fat are indicators of changes in body fat stores, whether a person's weight is appropriate for height, and may provide a useful estimate of nutrition.
- Factors influencing a person's nutrition include development, gender, ethnicity and culture, beliefs about foods, personal preferences, religious practices, lifestyle, medications and medical therapy, health status, alcohol abuse, advertising, and psychologic factors such as stress, isolation, and depression.
- Nutritional needs vary considerably according to age, growth, and energy requirements. Adolescents have high energy requirements due to their rapid growth; a diet plentiful in milk, meats, green and yellow vegetables, and fresh fruits is required. Middle-aged adults and older adults often need to reduce their caloric intake because of decreases in metabolic rate and activity levels. Fats, sugary foods, and sodium must often be limited.
- Various daily food guides have been developed to help healthy people meet the daily requirements of essential nutrients and to facilitate meal planning. These include the *Dietary Guidelines for Americans,* the Food Guide Pyramid, and *Canada's Food Guide to Healthy Eating.*
- Both inadequate and excessive intakes of nutrients result in malnutrition. The effects of malnutrition can be general or specific, depending on which nutrients and what level of deficiency or excess are involved.
- Some of the long-range effects of certain nutrient excesses are among the many factors involved in certain diseases, such as coronary artery disease and cancer.
- Assessment of nutritional status may involve all or some of the following: nursing history data, nutritional screening, physical examination, calculation of the percentage of weight loss, a dietary history, anthropometric measurements, and laboratory data.
- Nursing diagnoses for clients with nutritional problems may be broadly stated as *Imbalanced Nutrition: Less Than Body Requirements, More Body Than Requirements,* or *Risk for Imbalanced Nutrition: More Than Body Requirements.* Because nutritional problems may affect many other areas of human functioning, the nutritional problem may be the etiology of other diagnoses, such as *Activity Intolerance* and *Low Self-Esteem.*
- Major goals for clients with or at risk for nutritional problems include the following: maintain or restore optimal nutritional status, decrease or regain specified weight, promote healthy nutritional practices, and prevent complications associated with malnutrition.
- Assisting clients and support persons with therapeutic diets is a function shared by the nurse and the dietitian. The nurse reinforces the dietitian's instructions, assists the client to make beneficial changes, and evaluates the client's response to planned changes.
- Because many hospitalized clients have poor appetites, a major responsibility of the nurse is to provide nursing interventions that stimulate their appetites.
- Whenever possible, the nurse should help incapacitated clients to feed themselves; a number of self-feeding aids help clients who have difficulty handling regular utensils.
- The nurse can refer clients to various community programs that help special subgroups of the population meet their nutritional needs.

- Enteral feedings, administered through nasogastric, nasointestinal, gastrostomy, or jejunostomy tubes, are provided when the client is unable to ingest foods or the upper gastrointestinal tract is impaired.
- A nasogastric or nasointestinal tube is used to provide enteral nutrition for short-term use (less than 6 weeks) while a gas-

trostomy or jejunostomy tube can be used to supply nutrients via the enteral route for long-term use.
- Parenteral nutrition (PN), provided when the gastrointestinal tract is nonfunctional (e.g., absorptive capacity impaired), is given intravenously into a large central vein (e.g., the superior vena cava).

Review Questions

45–1. A client with a BMI of 35 would likely have which of the following nursing diagnoses?
 a. *Imbalanced Nutrition:* Less *than body requirements*
 b. *Imbalanced Nutrition:* More *than body requirements*
 c. *Risk for Imbalanced Nutrition*
 d. *Deficient Knowledge*

45–2. An adult reports eating, on average, the following each day: 2 servings dairy, 3 servings fruit, 4 servings vegetables, and 5 servings grains. The nurse would counsel the client to
 a. maintain the diet, the servings are adequate.
 b. increase the number of servings of dairy.
 c. decrease the number of servings of vegetables.
 d. increase the number of servings of grains.

45–3. Which of the following is *NOT* allowed on a full liquid diet?
 a. scrambled eggs
 b. chocolate pudding
 c. tomato juice
 d. hard candy

45–4. Which of the following is the best indication of proper placement of a nasogastric tube in the stomach?
 a. Client is unable to speak.
 b. Client gags during insertion.
 c. pH of the aspirate is less than 5.
 d. Fluid is easily instilled into the tube.

45–5. What is the proper technique with gravity tube feeding?
 a. Feeding bag is hung 1 foot higher than the tube's insertion point into the client.
 b. Nurse administers the next feeding only if there is less than 25 mL of residual volume from the previous feeding.
 c. Client is placed in the left lateral position to promote feeding flow into the intestines.
 d. Feeding is administered at refrigerated temperature to reduce bacterial growth during feeding.

Readings and References

Suggested Readings

Loan, T., Magnuson, B., & Williams, S. (1998). Debunking six myths about enteral feeding. *Nursing 98, 28*(8), 43–48.
 This continuing education article, with tests included, outlines six misconceptions about enteral feeding that could be doing clients a disservice. They include myths about bowel sounds, feeding tube locations, aspiration of feedings, and stopping feedings.

Related Research

Biggs, A. J., & Freed, P. E. (2000). Nutrition and older adults. *Journal of Gerontological Nursing, 26*(8), 6–14.

Blaum, C. S., O'Neill, E. F., Clements, K. M., Fries, B. E., & Fiatarone, M. A. (1999). Validity of the Minimum Data Set for assessing nutritional status in nursing home residents. *American Journal of Clinical Nutrition, 66*(4), 787–794.

References

Agency for Health Care Policy and Research. (1999). *Diagnosis and treatment of swallowing disorders (dysphagia) in acute-care stroke patients.* Rockville, MD: Author. Retrieved

May 19, 2003, from http://www.ahrq.gov/clinic/ epcsums/dysphsum.htm

American Dietetic Association. (2002). *The national dysphagia diet (NDD: Standardization for optimal care).* Chicago: Author.

Canada's Food Guide to Healthy Eating. (1992). Ottawa, Ontario: Minister of Public Works and Government Services Canada.

Committee on Nutrition, American Academy of Pediatrics. (1999). Calcium requirements of infants, children, and adolescents. *Pediatrics, 104,* 1152–1157.

Crogan, N. L., Shultz, J. A., Adams, C. E., & Massey, L. K. (2001). Barriers to nutrition care for nursing home residents. *Journal of Gerontological Nursing, 27*(12), 25–31.

Dudek, S. G. (1997). *Nutrition handbook for nursing practice* (3rd ed.). Philadelphia: Lippincott.

Institute of Medicine. (2001). *Dietary reference intakes: Applications in dietary assessment.* Washington, DC: National Academy Press.

Johnson, M., Maas, M., & Moorhead, S. (Eds.). (2000). *Nursing outcomes classification (NOC)* (2nd ed.). St. Louis, MO: Mosby.

Mathieu, J. (2002). NSI: Providing simple tools for our nation's health. *Journal of the American Dietetic Association, 102,* 1394.

McCallum, P. D. (2000). Patient generated subjective global assessment. In P. D. McCallum & C. G. Polisena (Eds.), *The clinical guide to oncology nutrition.* Chicago, IL: American Dietetic Association.

McCloskey, J.C., & Bulechek, G. M. (Eds.). (2000). *Nursing interventions classification (NIC)* (3rd ed.). St. Louis, MO: Mosby.

Messina, V. K., & Burke, K. I. (1997). Position of the American Dietetic Association: Vegetarian diets. *Journal of the American Dietetic Association, 97*(11). Retrieved May 19, 2003, from http://www.vrg.org/nutrition/adapaper.htm

Metheny, N., Wehrle, M. A., Wiersema, L., & Clark, J. (1998). Testing feeding tube placement: Auscultation vs. pH method. *American Journal of Nursing, 98*(5), 37–42.

Metheny, N. A., & Titler, M. G. (2001). Assessing placement of feeding tubes. *American Journal of Nursing, 101*(5), 36–46.

National Heart, Lung, and Blood Institute. (1998). *Clinical guidelines on the identification, evaluation, and treatment of overweight and obesity in adults: The evidence report.* Washington, DC: U.S. Department of Health & Human Services.

National Institute of Diabetes and Digestive and Kidney Diseases. (2002). *Lactose intolerance* (NIH Publication No. 02-2751). Bethesda, MD: Author.

NANDA International. (2003). *NANDA nursing diagnoses: Definitions and classification 2003–2004*. Philadelphia: Author.

Nutrition Screening Initiative. (2003). *Determine your nutritional health*. Washington, DC: National Council on Aging.

Pai, M. P., & Paloucek, F. P. (2000). The origin of the "ideal" body weight equations. *The Annals of Pharmacotherapy, 34,* 1066–1069.

Schnirring, L. (2001). Body fat testing: Evaluating the options. *The Physician and Sportsmedicine, 29*(5), 13–16.

Siler, S. Q., Neese, R. A., & Hellerstein, M. K. (1999). *De novo* lipogenesis, lipid kinetics, and whole-body lipid balances in humans after acute alcohol consumption. *American Journal of Clinical Nutrition, 70,* 928–936.

Terrado, M., Russell, C., & Bowman, J. B. (2001). Dysphagia: An overview. *MEDSURG Nursing, 10,* 233–250.

U.S. Department of Agriculture. (2000). *Dietary guidelines for Americans* (5th ed.). Washington, DC: Author.

U.S. Department of Health and Human Services. (2000). *Healthy people 2010: Understanding and improving health* (2nd ed.). Washington, DC: U.S. Government Printing Office.

Walters, E. (1998). Know how: Nutritional assessment. *Nursing Times, 94*(8), 68–69.

Williams, M. P., & Waxman, J. (2002). How to assess swallowing after a stroke. *Nursing, 32*(8), HN5–HN6.

Selected Bibliography

Bond, S. (1998). Why eating matters. *Nursing Standard, 12*(50), 26–27.

Bowers, S. (2000). All about tubes. *Nursing, 30*(12), 41–48.

Cason, K. L. (1998). Maintaining nutrition during drug therapy. *Nursing, 28*(9), 54–55.

Dudek, S. G. (2000). *Nutrition essentials for nursing practice* (4th ed.). Philadelphia: Lippincott Williams & Wilkins.

Gary, R., & Fleury, J. (2002). Nutritional status: Key to preventing functional decline in hospitalized older adults. *Topics in Geriatric Rehabilitation, 17*(3), 40–71.

Hamilton, S. (2001). Detecting dehydration and malnutrition in the elderly. *Nursing, 31*(12), 56–57.

Holmes, S. (1998). Food for thought. *Nursing Standard, 12*(46), 23–26.

Jeffery, R. W., & French, S. A. (1998). Epidemic obesity in the United States: Are fast foods and television viewing contributing? *American Journal of Public Health, 88*(2), 277–280.

Kayser-Jones, J. (2001). Starved for attention. *Reflections on Nursing Leadership, 27*(1), 10–14, 45.

Kohn-Keeth, C. (2000). How to keep feeding tubes flowing freely. *Nursing, 30*(3), 58–59.

Koschel, M. J. (2001). Inserting an NG tube. *American Journal of Nursing, 101*(6), 75.

Krupp, K. B., & Heximer, B. (1998). Going with the flow: How to prevent feeding tubes from clogging. *Nursing, 28*(4), 54–55.

Laporte, M., Villalon, L., & Payette, H. (2001). Simple nutrition screening tools for healthcare facilities: Development and validity assessment. *Canadian Journal of Dietetic Practice and Research, 62*(1), 26–34.

Lord, L. (2001). How to insert a large-bore nasogastric tube. *Nursing, 31*(9), 46–48.

McConnell, E. A. (2001). Myths and facts about dysphagia. *Nursing, 31*(7), 29.

McLaren, S., & Green, S. (1998). Nutritional screening and assessment. *Nursing Standard, 12*(48), 28–29.

Miceli, B. V. (1999). Nursing unit meal management maintenance program: Continuation of safe swallowing and feeding beyond skilled therapeutic intervention. *Journal of Gerontological Nursing, 25*(8), 22–36.

Moore, J. (1998). Vitamins and health: The role of a balanced diet. *Community Nurse, 4*(4), 15–17.

O'Brien, B., Davis, S., & Erwin-Toth, P. (1999). G-tube site care: A practical guide. *RN, 62*(2), 52–56.

Scott, A., & Hamilton, K. (1998). Nutritional screening: An audit. *Nursing Standard, 12*(48), 46–47.

White, S. (1998). Percutaneous endoscopic gastrostomy (PEG). *Nursing Standard, 12*(28), 41–47.

World Health Organization and Food and Agricultural Organization. (1998). Carbohydrate and nutrition. *Nursing Standard, 12*(45), 32–33.

Williams, S. R., & Schlenker, E. (2003). *Essentials of nutrition and diet therapy* (8th ed.). St. Louis, MO: Mosby.

Wilson, J. M. (1998). Nutritional assessment and its application. *Journal of Intravenous Nursing, 19*(6), 307–314.

Wood, P., & Vogen, B. D. (1998). Feeding the anorectic client: Comfort foods and happy hour. *Geriatric Nursing, 19*(4), 192–194.

Yen, P. K. (1998). Adding calories to medications. *Geriatric Nursing, 19*(3), 168–169.

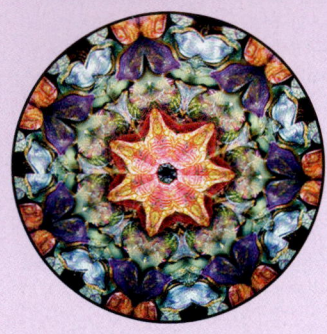

CHAPTER 46

FECAL ELIMINATION

LEARNING OUTCOMES

After completing this chapter, you will be able to:

- Understand the physiology of defecation.

- Identify factors that influence fecal elimination and patterns of defecation.

- Distinguish normal from abnormal characteristics and constituents of feces.

- Describe methods used to assess the intestinal tract.

- Identify common causes and effects of selected fecal elimination problems.

- Identify examples of nursing diagnoses, outcomes, and interventions for clients with elimination problems.

- Identify measures that maintain normal fecal elimination patterns.

- Describe essentials of fecal stoma care for clients with ostomies.

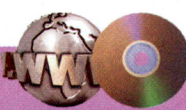

MediaLink

www.prenhall.com/kozier

Additional resources for this chapter can be found on the Student CD-ROM accompanying this textbook, and on the Companion Website at www.prenhall.com/kozier. Click on Chapter 46 to select the activities for this chapter.

CD-ROM
- Audio Glossary
- NCLEX Review
- Animations:
    The Digestive System 3D
    Performing an Enema
    A & P Review
       The Digestive System
       The Intestinal Wall

Companion Website
- Additional NCLEX Review
- Case Study: Client Who Had Abdominal Surgery
- Care Plan Activity: Client Who Had a Stroke
- MediaLink Application: The United Ostomy Association
- Links to Resources

Nurses frequently are consulted or involved in assisting clients with elimination problems. These problems can be embarrassing to clients and can cause considerable discomfort. The elimination of feces is a prominent public topic in North America. Laxative advertisements, describing such feelings as tiredness due to irregularity, keep the subject in the public consciousness. Some elders are preoccupied with their bowels. People who have had a bowel movement once a day for 75 years can view missing 1 day as a serious problem.

PHYSIOLOGY OF DEFECATION

Elimination of the waste products of digestion from the body is essential to health. The excreted waste products are referred to as **feces** or **stool.**

Large Intestine

The large intestine extends from the ileocecal (ileocolic) valve, which lies between the small and large intestines, to the anus. The colon (large intestine) in the adult is generally about 125 to 150 cm (50 to 60 in.) long. It has seven parts: the cecum; ascending, transverse, and descending colons; sigmoid colon; rectum; and anus (Figure 46–1 ■).

The large intestine is a muscular tube lined with mucous membrane. The muscle fibers are both circular and longitudinal, permitting the intestine to enlarge and contract in both width and length. The longitudinal muscles are shorter than the colon and therefore cause the large intestine to form pouches, or **haustra.**

The colon's main functions are the absorption of water and nutrients, the mucal protection of the intestinal wall, and fecal elimination. The contents of the colon normally represent foods ingested over the previous 4 days, although most of the waste products are excreted within 48 hours of **ingestion** (the act of taking food). The waste products leaving the stomach through the small intestine and then passing through the ileocecal valve are called **chyme.** As much as 1,500 mL of chyme passes into the large intestine daily, and all but about 100 mL is reabsorbed in the proximal half of the colon. The 100 mL of fluid is excreted in the feces.

The colon also serves a protective function in that it secretes mucus. This mucus contains large amounts of bicarbonate ions. The mucus secretion is stimulated by excitation of parasympathetic nerves. During extreme stimulation—for example, as a result of emotions—large amounts of mucus are secreted, resulting in the passage of stringy mucus with little or no feces. Mucus serves to protect the wall of the large intestine from trauma by the acids formed in the feces, and it serves as an adherent for holding the fecal material together. Mucus also protects the intestinal wall from bacterial activity.

The colon acts to transport along its lumen the products of digestion, which are eventually eliminated through the anal canal. These products are flatus and feces. **Flatus** is largely air and the by-products of the digestion of carbohydrates. Three types of movements occur in the large intestine: haustral churning, colon peristalsis, and mass peristalsis. **Haustral churning** involves

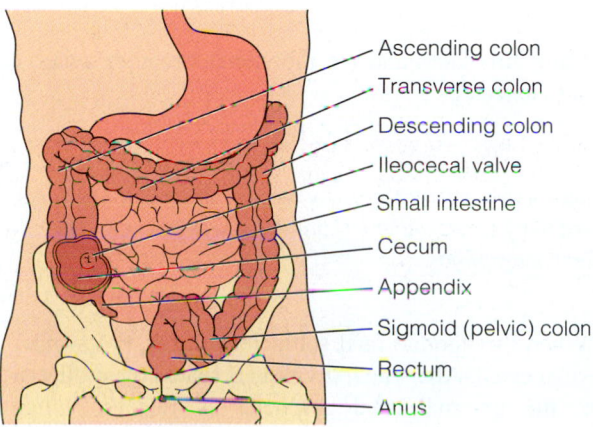

- Ascending colon
- Transverse colon
- Descending colon
- Ileocecal valve
- Small intestine
- Cecum
- Appendix
- Sigmoid (pelvic) colon
- Rectum
- Anus

Figure 46–1 ■ The large intestine and rectum.

movement of the chyme back and forth within the haustra. In addition to mixing the contents, this action aids in the absorption of water and moves the contents forward to the next haustra. **Peristalsis** is wavelike movement produced by the circular and longitudinal muscle fibers of the intestinal walls; it propels the intestinal contents forward. Colon peristalsis is very sluggish and is thought to move the chyme very little along the large intestine. **Mass peristalsis,** the third type of colonic movement, involves a wave of powerful muscular contraction that moves over large areas of the colon. Usually mass peristalsis occurs after eating, stimulated by the presence of food in the stomach and small intestine. In adults, mass peristaltic waves occur only a few times a day.

Rectum and Anal Canal

The rectum in the adult is usually 10 to 15 cm (4 to 6 in.) long; the most distal portion, 2.5 to 5 cm (1 to 2 in.) long, is the anal canal. In the rectum are folds that extend vertically. Each of the vertical folds contains a vein and an artery. It is believed that these folds help retain feces within the rectum. When the veins become distended, as can occur with repeated pressure, a condition known as **hemorrhoids** occurs (Figure 46–2 ■).

The anal canal is bounded by an internal and an external sphincter muscle (Figure 46–3 ■). The internal sphincter is under involuntary control, and the external sphincter normally is voluntarily controlled. The internal sphincter muscle is innervated by the autonomic nervous system; the external sphincter is innervated by the somatic nervous system.

Defecation

Defecation is the expulsion of feces from the anus and rectum. It is also called a *bowel movement*. The frequency of defecation is highly individual, varying from several times per day to two or three times per week. The amount defecated also varies from person to person. When peristaltic waves move the feces into the sigmoid colon and the rectum, the sensory nerves in the rec-

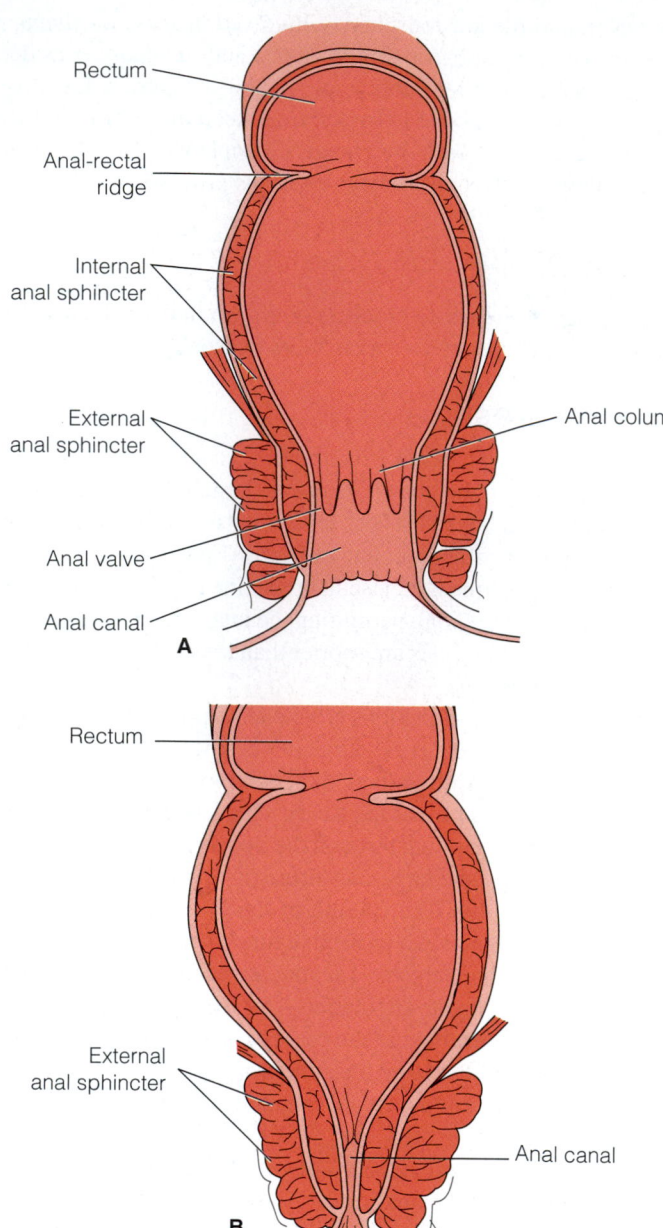

Figure 46–3 ■ The rectum, anal canal, and anal sphincters: *A,* open; *B,* closed.

tum are stimulated and the individual becomes aware of the need to defecate.

> ► **CLINICAL ALERT** *Individuals (especially children) may use very different terms for a bowel movement. The nurse may need to try several different common words before finding one the client understands.* ■

When the internal anal sphincter relaxes, feces move into the anal canal. After the individual is seated on a toilet or bedpan, the external anal sphincter is relaxed voluntarily. Expulsion of the feces is assisted by contraction of the abdominal muscles and the diaphragm, which increases abdominal

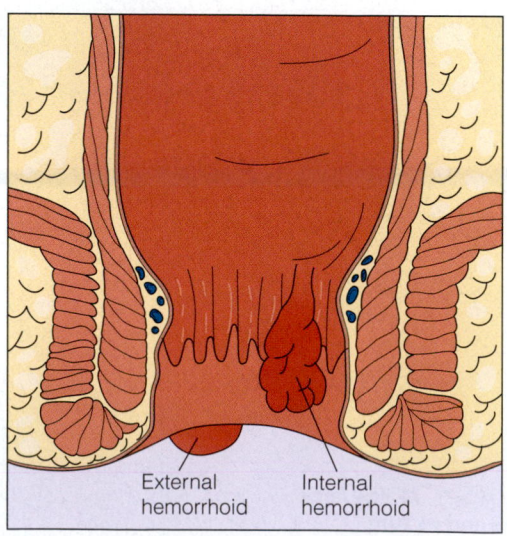

Figure 46–2 ■ Internal and external hemorrhoids.

pressure, and by contraction of the muscles of the pelvic floor, which moves the feces through the anal canal. Normal defecation is facilitated by (a) thigh flexion, which increases the pressure within the abdomen, and (b) a sitting position, which increases the downward pressure on the rectum.

If the defecation reflex is ignored, or if defecation is consciously inhibited by contracting the external sphincter muscle, the urge to defecate normally disappears for a few hours before occurring again. Repeated inhibition of the urge to defecate can result in expansion of the rectum to accommodate accumulated feces and eventual loss of sensitivity to the need to defecate. Constipation can be the ultimate result.

Feces

Normal feces are made of about 75% water and 25% solid materials. They are soft but formed. If the feces are propelled very quickly along the large intestine, there is not time for most of the water in the chyme to be reabsorbed and the feces will be more fluid, containing perhaps 95% water. Normal feces require a normal fluid intake; feces that contain less water may be hard and difficult to expel.

Feces are normally brown, chiefly due to the presence of stercobilin and urobilin, which are derived from bilirubin (a red pigment in bile). Another factor that affects fecal color is the action of bacteria such as *Escherichia coli* or staphylococci, which are normally present in the large intestine. The action of microorganisms on the chyme is also responsible for the odor of feces. Table 46–1 lists the characteristics of normal and abnormal feces.

An adult usually forms 7 to 10 L of flatus (gas) in the large intestine every 24 hours. The gases include carbon dioxide, methane, hydrogen, oxygen, and nitrogen. Some are swallowed

TABLE 46–1 Characteristics of Normal and Abnormal Feces

Characteristic	Normal	Abnormal	Possible Cause
Color	Adult: brown	Clay or white	Absence of bile pigment (bile obstruction); diagnostic study using barium
	Infant: yellow	Black or tarry	Drug (e.g., iron); bleeding from upper gastrointestinal tract (e.g., stomach, small intestine); diet high in red meat and dark green vegetables (e.g., spinach)
		Red	Bleeding from lower gastrointestinal tract (e.g., rectum); some foods (e.g., beets)
		Pale	Malabsorption of fats; diet high in milk and milk products and low in meat
		Orange or green	Intestinal infection
Consistency	Formed, soft, semisolid, moist	Hard, dry	Dehydration; decreased intestinal motility resulting from lack of fiber in diet, lack of exercise, emotional upset, laxative abuse
		Diarrhea	Increased intestinal motility (e.g., due to irritation of the colon by bacteria)
Shape	Cylindrical (contour of rectum) about 2.5 cm (1 in.) in diameter in adults	Narrow, pencil-shaped, or stringlike stool	Obstructive condition of the rectum
Amount	Varies with diet (about 100–400 g per day)		
Odor	Aromatic: affected by ingested food and person's own bacterial flora	Pungent	Infection, blood
Constituents	Small amounts of undigested roughage, sloughed dead bacteria and epithelial cells, fat, protein, dried constituents of digestive juices (e.g., bile pigments, inorganic matter)	Pus Mucus Parasites Blood Large quantities of fat Foreign objects	Bacterial infection Inflammatory condition Gastrointestinal bleeding Malabsorption Accidental ingestion

with food and fluids taken by mouth, others are formed through the action of bacteria on the chyme in the large intestine, and other gas diffuses from the blood into the gastrointestinal tract.

FACTORS THAT AFFECT DEFECATION

Defecation patterns vary at different stages of life. Circumstances of diet, fluid intake and output, activity, psychologic factors, lifestyle, medications and medical procedures, and disease also affect defecation.

Development

Newborns and infants, toddlers, children, and elders are groups within which members have similarities in elimination patterns.

Newborns and Infants

Meconium is the first fecal material passed by the newborn, normally up to 24 hours after birth. It is black, tarry, odorless, and sticky. Transitional stools, which follow for about a week, are generally greenish yellow; they contain mucus and are loose.

Infants pass stool frequently, often after each feeding. Because the intestine is immature, water is not well absorbed and the stool is soft, liquid, and frequent. When the intestine matures, bacterial flora increase. After solid foods are introduced, the stool becomes less frequent and firmer.

Infants who are breastfed have bright yellow to golden feces and infants who are taking cow's milk formula will have dark yellow or tan stool that is more formed.

Toddlers

Some control of defecation starts at 1½ to 2 years of age. By this time, children have learned to walk, and the nervous and muscular systems are sufficiently well developed to permit bowel control. A desire to control daytime bowel movements and to use the toilet generally starts when the child becomes aware of (a) the discomfort caused by a soiled diaper and (b) the sensation that indicates the need for a bowel movement. Daytime control is normally attained by age 2½, after a process of toilet training.

School-Age Children and Adolescents

School-age children and adolescents have bowel habits similar to those of adults. Patterns of defecation vary in frequency, quantity, and consistency. Some school-age children may delay defecation because of an activity such as play.

Elders

Constipation is a common problem in the elder population. This is due, in part, to reduced activity levels, inadequate amounts of fluid and fiber intake, and muscle weakness. Many older people believe that "regularity" means a bowel movement every day. Those who do not meet this criterion often seek over-the-counter preparations to relieve what they believe to be constipation. Elders should be advised that normal patterns of bowel elimination vary considerably. For some, a normal pattern may be every other day; for others, twice a day. Adequate roughage in the diet, adequate exercise, and 6 to 8 glasses of fluid daily are essential preventive measures for constipation. A cup of hot water or tea at a regular time in the morning is helpful for some. Responding to the **gastrocolic reflex** (increased peristalsis of the colon after food has entered the stomach) is also an important consideration.

The older adult should be warned that consistent use of laxatives inhibits natural defecation reflexes and is thought to cause rather than cure constipation. The habitual user of laxatives eventually requires larger or stronger doses because the effect is progressively reduced with continual use. Laxatives may also interfere with the body's electrolyte balance and decrease the absorption of certain vitamins. The reasons for constipation can range from lifestyle habits (e.g., lack of exercise) to serious malignant disorders. The nurse should evaluate any complaints of constipation carefully for each individual. A change in bowel habits over several weeks with or without weight loss, pain, or fever should be referred to a physician for a complete medical evaluation.

Diet

Sufficient bulk (cellulose, fiber) in the diet is necessary to provide fecal volume. Bland diets and low-fiber diets are lacking

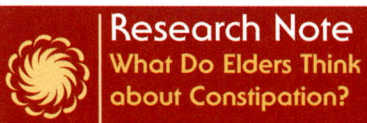

Research Note
What Do Elders Think about Constipation?

Concerned that the definitions and treatment of constipation were different between older adults and health care providers, Koch and Hudson (2000) designed a pilot study to explore the issues. A variety of detailed questions on the survey inquired about elders' definitions of terms, their use of remedies including home-designed ones, and their belief systems. Researchers followed the survey with individual interviewing of elders who self-identified as constipated. An obviously undesirable situation, elders reported noxious symptoms from both the constipation and the treatment that would lead to nursing diagnoses such as loneliness, low self-esteem, and anxiety. The also article reviews existing literature on laxative use.

Implications: Assisting clients with problems surrounding fecal elimination, although common, is not necessarily easy. It is important that nurses begin from a perspective congruent with the one the client has so that teaching and intervention can be appropriately planned. People's perceptions of their daily functioning evolve over decades and older adults are likely to have some very deep-rooted beliefs about what is acceptable. More research such as this is needed in order to have a global understanding of constipation as a concern of elders, from which care can be individualized.

Note: From "Older People and Laxative Use: Literature Review and Pilot Study Report," by T. Koch and S. Hudson, 2000, *Journal of Clinical Nursing, 9,* pp. 516–525.

in bulk and therefore create insufficient residue of waste products to stimulate the reflex for defecation. Low-residue foods, such as rice, eggs, and lean meats, move more slowly through the intestinal tract. Increasing fluid intake with such foods increases their rate of movement.

Certain foods are difficult or impossible for some people to digest. This inability results in digestive upsets and, in some instances, the passage of watery stools. Irregular eating can also impair regular defecation. Individuals who eat at the same times every day usually have a regularly timed, physiologic response to the food intake and a regular pattern of peristaltic activity in the colon.

Spicy foods can produce diarrhea and flatus in some individuals. Excessive sugar can also cause diarrhea. Other foods that may influence bowel elimination include the following:

- Gas-producing foods, such as cabbage, onions, cauliflower, bananas, and apples
- Laxative-producing foods, such as bran, prunes, figs, chocolate, and alcohol
- Constipation-producing foods, such as cheese, pasta, eggs, and lean meat

Fluid

Even when fluid intake is inadequate or output (urine or vomitus, for example) is excessive for some reason, the body continues to reabsorb fluid from the chyme as it passes along the colon. The chyme becomes drier than normal, resulting in hard feces. In addition, reduced fluid intake slows the chyme's passage along the intestines, further increasing the reabsorption of fluid from the chyme. Healthy fecal elimination usually requires a daily fluid intake of 2,000 to 3,000 mL. If chyme moves abnormally quickly through the large intestine, however, there is less time for fluid to be absorbed into the blood; as a result, the feces are soft or even watery.

Activity

Activity stimulates peristalsis, thus facilitating the movement of chyme along the colon. Weak abdominal and pelvic muscles are often ineffective in increasing the intra-abdominal pressure during defecation or in controlling defecation. Weak muscles can result from lack of exercise, immobility, or impaired neurologic functioning. Clients confined to bed are often constipated.

Psychologic Factors

Some people who are anxious or angry experience increased peristaltic activity and subsequent nausea or diarrhea. In contrast, people who are depressed may experience slowed intestinal motility, resulting in constipation. How a person responds to these emotional states is the result of individual differences in the response of the enteric nervous system to vagal stimulation from the brain.

Defecation Habits

Early bowel training may establish the habit of defecating at a regular time. Many people defecate after breakfast, when the gastrocolic reflex causes mass peristaltic waves in the large intestine. If a person ignores this urge to defecate, water continues to be reabsorbed, making the feces hard and difficult to expel. When the normal defecation reflexes are inhibited or ignored, these conditioned reflexes tend to be progressively weakened. When habitually ignored, the urge to defecate is ultimately lost. Adults may ignore these reflexes because of the pressures of time or work. Hospitalized clients may suppress the urge because of embarrassment about using a bedpan, lack of privacy, or because defecation is too uncomfortable.

Medications

Some drugs have side effects that can interfere with normal elimination. Some cause diarrhea; others, such as large doses of certain tranquilizers and repeated administration of morphine and codeine, cause constipation because they decrease gastrointestinal activity through their action on the central nervous system. Iron tablets, which have an astringent effect, act more locally on the bowel mucosa to cause constipation.

Some medications directly affect elimination. **Laxatives** are medications that stimulate bowel activity and so assist fecal elimination. Other medications soften stool, facilitating defecation. Certain medications suppress peristaltic activity and may be used to treat diarrhea.

Medications also affect the appearance of the feces. Any drug that causes gastrointestinal bleeding (e.g., aspirin products) can cause the stool to be red or black. Iron salts lead to black stool because of the oxidation of the iron; antibiotics may cause a gray-green discoloration; and antacids can cause a whitish discoloration or white specks in the stool. Pepto-Bismol, a common over-the-counter drug, causes stools to be black.

Diagnostic Procedures

Before certain diagnostic procedures, such as visualization of the colon (colonoscopy or sigmoidoscopy), the client is restricted from ingesting food or fluid. The client may also be given a cleansing enema prior to the examination. In these instances normal defecation usually will not occur until eating resumes.

Anesthesia and Surgery

General anesthetics cause the normal colonic movements to cease or slow by blocking parasympathetic stimulation to the muscles of the colon. Clients who have regional or spinal anesthesia are less likely to experience this problem.

Surgery that involves direct handling of the intestines can cause temporary cessation of intestinal movement. This condition, called ileus, usually lasts 24 to 48 hours. Listening for bowel sounds that reflect intestinal motility is an important nursing assessment following surgery.

Pathologic Conditions

Spinal cord injuries and head injuries can decrease the sensory stimulation for defecation. Impaired mobility may limit the client's ability to respond to the urge to defecate and the client may experience constipation. Or, a client may experience fecal incontinence because of poorly functioning anal sphincters.

Pain

Clients who experience discomfort when defecating (e.g., following hemorrhoid surgery) often suppress the urge to defecate to avoid the pain. Such clients can experience constipation as a result. Clients taking narcotic analgesics for pain may also experience constipation as a side effect of the medication.

FECAL ELIMINATION PROBLEMS

Four common problems are related to fecal elimination: constipation, diarrhea, bowel incontinence, and flatulence.

Constipation

Constipation may be defined as fewer than three bowel movements per week. This infers the passage of dry, hard stool or the passage of no stool. It occurs when the movement of feces through the large intestine is slow, thus allowing time for additional reabsorption of fluid from the large intestine. Associated with constipation are difficult evacuation of stool and increased effort or straining of the voluntary muscles of defecation. The person may also have a feeling of incomplete stool evacuation after defecation. However, it is important to define constipation in relation to the person's regular elimination pattern. Some people normally defecate only a few times a week; other people defecate more than once a day. Careful assessment of the person's habits is necessary before a diagnosis of constipation is made. Box 46–1 lists the frequent defining characteristics of constipation.

Many causes and factors contribute to constipation. Among them are the following:

- Insufficient fiber intake
- Insufficient fluid intake
- Insufficient activity or immobility
- Irregular defecation habits
- Change in daily routine
- Lack of privacy

BOX 46–1	■ Sample Defining Characteristics for Constipation

- Decreased frequency of defecation
- Hard, dry, formed stools
- Straining at stool; painful defecation
- Reports of rectal fullness or pressure or incomplete bowel evacuation
- Abdominal pain, cramps, or distention
- Use of laxatives
- Decreased appetite
- Headache

- Chronic use of laxatives or enemas
- Emotional disturbances such as depression or mental confusion
- Medications such as opiates or iron salts

Constipation can be hazardous to some clients. Straining associated with constipation often is accompanied by holding the breath. This Valsalva maneuver can present serious problems to people with heart disease, brain injuries, or respiratory disease. Holding the breath increases the intrathoracic and the intracranial pressures.

Fecal Impaction

Fecal impaction is a mass or collection of hardened feces in the folds of the rectum. Impaction results from prolonged retention and accumulation of fecal material. In severe impactions the feces accumulate and extend well up into the sigmoid colon and beyond. Fecal impaction can be recognized by the passage of liquid fecal seepage (diarrhea) and no normal stool. The liquid portion of the feces seeps out around the impacted mass. Impaction can also be assessed by digital examination of the rectum, during which the hardened mass can often be palpated.

Along with fecal seepage and constipation, symptoms include frequent but nonproductive desire to defecate and rectal pain. A generalized feeling of illness results; the client becomes anorexic, the abdomen becomes distended, and nausea and vomiting may occur.

The causes of fecal impaction are usually poor defecation habits and constipation. The barium used in radiologic examinations of the upper and lower gastrointestinal tracts can also be a causative factor. Therefore, after these examinations, laxatives or enemas are usually taken to ensure removal of the barium.

Digital examination of the impaction through the rectum should be done gently and carefully. Although digital rectal examination is within the scope of nursing practice, some agency policies require a physician's order for digital manipulation and removal of a fecal impaction.

Although fecal impaction can generally be prevented, treatment of impacted feces is sometimes necessary. When fecal impaction is suspected, the client is often given an oil retention enema, a cleansing enema 2 to 4 hours later, and daily additional cleansing enemas, suppositories, or stool softeners. If these measures fail, manual removal is often necessary.

Diarrhea

Diarrhea refers to the passage of liquid feces and an increased frequency of defecation. It is the opposite of constipation and results from rapid movement of fecal contents through the large intestine. Rapid passage of chyme reduces the time available for the large intestine to reabsorb water and electrolytes. Some people pass stool with increased frequency, but diarrhea is not present unless the stool is relatively unformed and excessively liquid. The person with diarrhea finds it difficult or impossible to control the urge to defecate for very long. Diarrhea and the

TABLE 46–2 Major Causes of Diarrhea

Cause	Physiologic Effect
Psychologic stress (e.g., anxiety)	Increased intestinal motility and mucus secretion
Medications	
Antibiotics	Inflammation and infection of mucosa due to overgrowth of pathogenic intestinal microorganisms
Iron	Irritation of intestinal mucosa
Cathartics	Irritation of intestinal mucosa
Allergy to food, fluid, drugs	Incomplete digestion of food or fluid
Intolerance of food or fluid	Increased intestinal motility and mucus secretion
Diseases of the colon (e.g.,	
Malabsorption syndrome	Reduced absorption of fluids
Crohn's disease)	Inflammation of the mucosa often leading to ulcer formation

threat of incontinence are sources of concern and embarrassment. Often, spasmodic cramps are associated with diarrhea. Bowel sounds are increased. With persistent diarrhea, irritation of the anal region extending to the perineum and buttocks generally results. Fatigue, weakness, malaise, and emaciation are the results of prolonged diarrhea.

When the cause of diarrhea is irritants in the intestinal tract, diarrhea is thought to be a protective flushing mechanism. It can create serious fluid and electrolyte losses in the body, however, that can develop within frighteningly short periods of time, particularly in infants, small children, and elders. Table 46–2 lists some of the major causes of diarrhea and the physiologic responses of the body.

Feces are acidic and contain digestive enzymes that are highly irritating to skin. Therefore, the area around the anal region should be kept clean and dry and be protected with zinc oxide or other ointment. In addition, a fecal collector can be used (see page 1245).

Bowel Incontinence

Bowel incontinence, also called **fecal incontinence,** refers to the loss of voluntary ability to control fecal and gaseous discharges through the anal sphincter. The incontinence may occur at specific times, such as after meals, or it may occur irregularly. Two types of bowel incontinence are described: partial and major. Partial incontinence is the inability to control flatus or to prevent minor soiling. Major incontinence is the inability to control feces of normal consistency.

Fecal incontinence is generally associated with impaired functioning of the anal sphincter or its nerve supply, such as in some neuromuscular diseases, spinal cord trauma, and tumors of the external anal sphincter muscle.

Fecal incontinence is an emotionally distressing problem that can ultimately lead to social isolation. Afflicted persons withdraw into their homes or, if in the hospital, the confines of their room to minimize the embarrassment associated with soiling. Several surgical procedures are used for the treatment of fecal incontinence. These include repair of the sphincter and fecal diversion or colostomy.

Flatulence

There are three primary sources of flatus: (a) action of bacteria on the chyme in the large intestine, (b) swallowed air, and (c) gas that diffuses between the bloodstream and the intestine.

Most gases that are swallowed are expelled through the mouth by eructation (belching). However, large amounts of gas can accumulate in the stomach, resulting in gastric distention. The gases formed in the large intestine are chiefly absorbed through the intestinal capillaries into the circulation. **Flatulence** is the presence of excessive flatus in the intestines and leads to stretching and inflation of the intestines (intestinal distention). Flatulence can occur in the colon from a variety of causes, such as foods (e.g., cabbage, onions), abdominal surgery, or narcotics. If the gas is propelled by increased colon activity before it can be absorbed, it may be expelled through the anus. If excessive gas cannot be expelled through the anus, it may be necessary to insert a rectal tube to remove it.

BOWEL DIVERSION OSTOMIES

An **ostomy** is an opening for the gastrointestinal, urinary, or respiratory tract onto the skin. There are many types of intestinal ostomies. A **gastrostomy** is an opening through the abdominal wall into the stomach. A **jejunostomy** opens through the abdominal wall into the jejunum, an **ileostomy** opens into the ileum (small bowel), and a **colostomy** opens into the colon (large bowel). Gastrostomies and jejunostomies are generally performed to provide an alternate feeding route. The purpose of bowel ostomies is to divert and drain fecal material. Bowel diversion ostomies are often classified according to (a) their status as permanent or temporary, (b) their anatomic location, and (c) the construction of the **stoma,** the opening created in the abdominal wall by the ostomy.

Permanence

Colostomies can be either temporary or permanent. Temporary colostomies are generally performed for traumatic injuries or inflammatory conditions of the bowel. They allow the distal

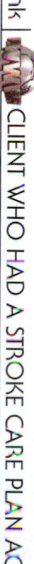

MediaLink | CLIENT WHO HAD A STROKE CARE PLAN ACTIVITY

Lifespan Considerations

Factors in Potential Bowel Elimination Problems
Elders

- Poor fluid intake and inability to eat a high-fiber diet, due to swallowing or chewing difficulties, are often causes of constipation.
- Medications that are commonly taken by elders such as antacids, many antihypertensives, antidepressants, diuretics, and narcotics for pain also contribute to constipation.
- Clients receiving tube feedings can experience diarrhea. To alleviate it, they require a change of formula, a change in its strength, or a change in the speed or temperature of tube feeding administration.

- Clients receiving laxative preparation for x-rays or other procedures may experience fluid and electrolyte imbalances due to diarrhea.
- Persons with cognitive impairment, such as Alzheimer's disease, may be unaware of what and when they eat or drink or of their bowel habits. These should be monitored by the caregiver, whether the person is being cared for at home or in an institution, to note any special needs or concerns.
- Persons with impaired mobility may have difficulty getting to the bathroom or using a regular toilet. A raised toilet seat and other devices, such as bars to assist in ambulation, may be very helpful. The decrease in activity may also contribute to constipation.

---

diseased portion of the bowel to rest and heal. Permanent colostomies are performed to provide a means of elimination when the rectum or anus is nonfunctional as a result of a birth defect or a disease such as cancer of the bowel.

> **► CLINICAL ALERT** *Surgery to reconnect the ends of the bowel of a temporary ostomy may be called a* take-down. ■

Anatomic Location

An ileostomy generally empties from the distal end of the small intestine. A cecostomy empties from the cecum (the first part of the ascending colon). An ascending colostomy empties from the ascending colon, a transverse colostomy from the transverse colon, a descending colostomy from the descending colon, and a sigmoidostomy from the sigmoid colon (Figure 46–4 ■).

The location of the ostomy influences the character and management of the fecal drainage. The farther along the bowel, the more formed the stool (because the large bowel reabsorbs water from the fecal mass) and the more control over the frequency of stomal discharge can be established. For example:

- An ileostomy produces liquid fecal drainage. Drainage is constant and cannot be regulated. Ileostomy drainage contains some digestive enzymes, which are damaging to the skin. For this reason, ileostomy clients must wear an appliance continuously and take special precautions to prevent skin breakdown. Compared to colostomies, however, odor is minimal because fewer bacteria are present.
- An ascending colostomy is similar to an ileostomy in that the drainage is liquid and cannot be regulated, and digestive enzymes are present. Odor, however, is a problem requiring control.
- A transverse colostomy produces a malodorous, mushy drainage because some of the liquid has been reabsorbed. There is usually no control.
- A descending colostomy produces increasingly solid fecal drainage. Stools from a sigmoidostomy are of normal or formed consistency, and the frequency of discharge can be regulated. People with a sigmoidostomy may not have to wear an appliance at all times, and odors can usually be controlled.

The length of time that an ostomy is in place also helps to determine the consistency of the stool, particularly with transverse and descending colostomies. Over time, the stool becomes more formed because the remaining functioning portions of the colon tend to compensate by increasing water reabsorption.

Construction of the Stoma

Stoma constructions are described as single, loop, divided, or double-barreled colostomies. The *single* stoma is created when one end of bowel is brought out through an opening onto the anterior abdominal wall. This is referred to as an *end* or *terminal colostomy;* the stoma is permanent (Figure 46–5 ■).

In the *loop colostomy,* a loop of bowel is brought out onto the abdominal wall and supported by a plastic bridge, a glass rod, or a piece of rubber tubing (Figure 46–6 ■). A loop stoma has two openings: the proximal or afferent end, which is active, and the distal or efferent end, which is inactive. The loop colostomy is usually performed in an emergency procedure and is often situated on the right transverse colon. It is a bulky stoma that is more difficult to manage than a single stoma.

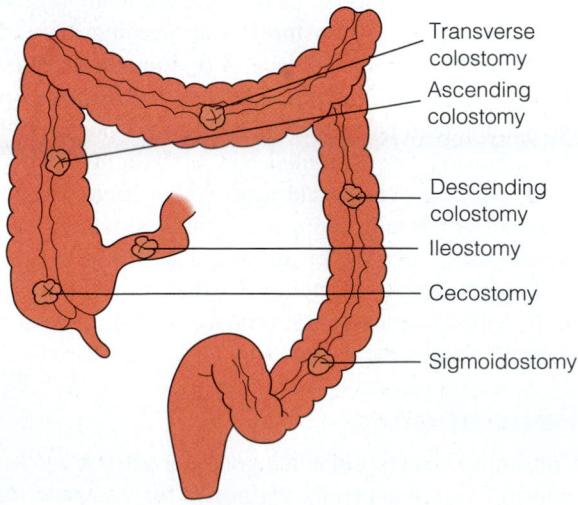

Transverse colostomy

Ascending colostomy

Descending colostomy

Ileostomy

Cecostomy

Sigmoidostomy

Figure 46–4 ■ The locations of bowel diversion ostomies.

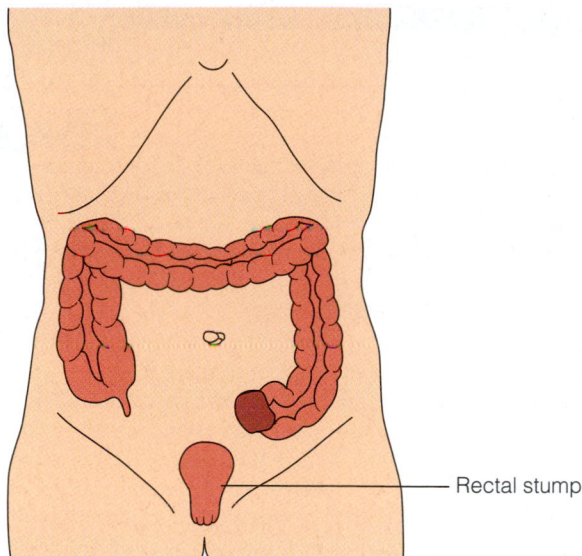

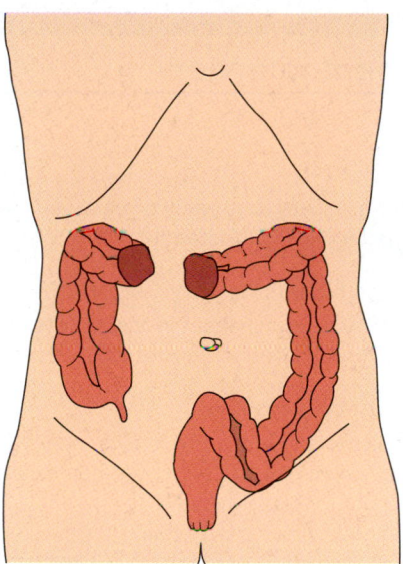

Figure 46–5 ■ End colostomy: the diseased portion of bowel is removed and a rectal pouch remains.

Figure 46–7 ■ Divided colostomy with two separated stomas.

Rectal stump

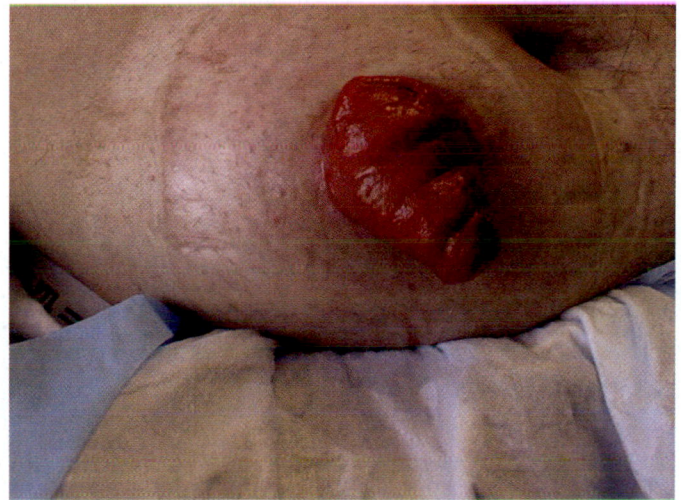

Figure 46–6 ■ Loop colostomy. (Courtesy of Cory Patrick Hartley, San Ramon Regional Medical Center, San Ramon, CA.)

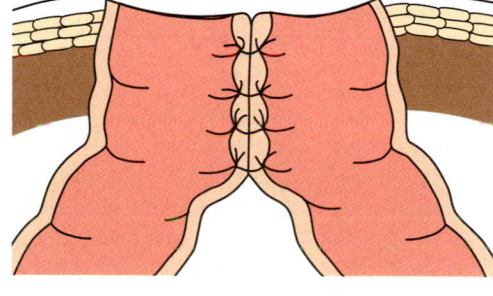

Figure 46–8 ■ Double-barreled colostomy.

NURSING MANAGEMENT

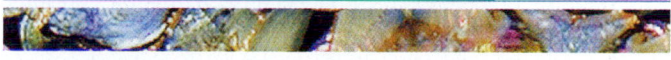

ASSESSING

Assessment of fecal elimination includes taking a nursing history; performing a physical examination of the abdomen, rectum, and anus; and inspecting the feces. The nurse also should review any data obtained from relevant diagnostic tests.

Nursing History

A nursing history for fecal elimination helps the nurse ascertain the client's normal pattern. The nurse elicits a description of usual feces and any recent changes and collects information about any past or current problems with elimination, the presence of an ostomy, and factors influencing the elimination pattern.

Examples of questions to elicit this information are shown in the Assessment Interview. The number of questions to ask is adapted to the individual client, according to the client's responses in the first three categories. For example, questions

The *divided colostomy* consists of two edges of bowel brought out onto the abdomen but separated from each other (Figure 46–7 ■). The opening from the digestive or proximal end is the colostomy. The distal end in this situation is often referred to as a mucous fistula, since this section of bowel continues to secrete mucus. The divided colostomy is often used in situations where spillage of feces into the distal end of the bowel needs to be avoided.

The *double-barreled colostomy* resembles a double-barrelled shotgun (Figure 46–8 ■). In this type of colostomy, the proximal and distal loops of bowel are sutured together for about 10 cm (4 in.) and both ends are brought up onto the abdominal wall.

Assessment Interview

FECAL ELIMINATION

Defecation Pattern

- When do you usually have a bowel movement?
- Has this pattern changed recently?

Description of Feces and Any Changes

- Have you noticed any changes in the color, texture (hard, soft, watery), shape, or odor of your stool recently?

Fecal Elimination Problems

- What problems have you had or do you now have with your bowel movements (constipation, diarrhea, excessive flatulence, seepage, or incontinence)?
- When and how often does it occur?
- What do you think causes it (food, fluids, exercise, emotions, medications, disease, surgery)?
- What have you tried to solve the problem, and how effective was it?

Factors Influencing Elimination

- Use of elimination aids. What routines do you follow to maintain your usual defecation pattern? Do you use natural aids such as specific foods or fluids (e.g., a glass of hot lemon juice before breakfast), laxatives, or enemas to maintain elimination?
- Diet. What foods do you believe affect defecation? What foods do you typically eat? What foods do you avoid? Do you take meals at regular times?
- Fluid. What amount and kind of fluid do you take each day (e.g., 6 glasses of water, 2 cups of coffee)?
- Exercise. What is your usual daily exercise pattern? (Obtain specifics about exercise rather than asking whether it is sufficient; ideas of what is sufficient vary among individuals.)
- Medications. Have you taken any medications that could affect the intestinal tract (e.g., iron, antibiotics)?
- Stress. Are you experiencing any stress? Do you think this affects your defecation pattern? How?

Presence and Management of Ostomy

- What is your usual routine with your colostomy/ileostomy?
- What problems, if any, do you have with it?
- How can the nurses help you manage your colostomy/ileostomy?

about factors influencing elimination might be addressed only to clients who are experiencing problems.

When eliciting data about the client's defecation pattern, the nurse needs to understand that the time of defecation and the amount of feces expelled are as individual as the frequency of defecation. Often, the patterns individuals follow depend largely on early training and on convenience.

Physical Examination

Physical examination of the abdomen in relation to fecal elimination problems includes inspection, auscultation, percussion, and palpation with specific reference to the intestinal tract. Auscultation precedes palpation because palpation can alter peristalsis. Examination of the rectum and anus includes inspection and palpation. Physical examination of the abdomen, rectum, and anus is discussed in Chapter 28. 🔗

Inspecting the Feces

Observe the client's stool for color, consistency, shape, amount, odor, and the presence of abnormal constituents. Table 46–1, earlier in this chapter, summarizes normal and abnormal characteristics of stool and possible causes.

Diagnostic Studies

Diagnostic studies of the gastrointestinal tract include direct visualization techniques, indirect visualization techniques, and laboratory tests for abnormal constituents (see Chapter 32). 🔗

DIAGNOSING

NANDA includes the following diagnostic labels for fecal elimination problems:

- *Bowel Incontinence*
- *Constipation*
- *Risk for Constipation*
- *Perceived Constipation*
- *Diarrhea.*

Clinical application of selected diagnoses is shown in Identifying Nursing Diagnoses, Outcomes, and Interventions, and at the end of the chapter in the Nursing Care Plan and the Concept Map.

Fecal elimination problems may affect many other areas of human functioning and as a consequence may be the etiology of other NANDA diagnoses. Examples follow:

- *Risk for Deficient Fluid Volume* related to
  a. Prolonged diarrhea
  b. Abnormal fluid loss through ostomy
- *Risk for Impaired Skin Integrity* related to
  a. Prolonged diarrhea
  b. Bowel incontinence
  c. Bowel diversion ostomy
- *Low Self-Esteem* related to
  a. Ostomy
  b. Fecal incontinence
  c. Need for assistance with toileting
- *Deficient Knowledge (Bowel Training, Ostomy Management)* related to lack of previous experience
- *Anxiety* related to
  a. Lack of control of fecal elimination secondary to ostomy
  b. Response of others to ostomy.

IDENTIFYING NURSING DIAGNOSES, OUTCOMES, AND INTERVENTIONS
CLIENTS WITH FECAL ELIMINATION PROBLEMS

DATA CLUSTER	NURSING DIAGNOSIS/ DEFINITION	SAMPLE DESIRED OUTCOMES [NOC#]/DEFINITION	INDICATORS	SELECTED INTERVENTIONS [NIC#]/DEFINITION	SAMPLE NIC ACTIVITIES
Marvin Lombardi reports having loose, liquid, light brown stools for 2 days. Passage of stools is associated with cramping abdominal pain. Bowel sounds are increased. Temperature is 38C (100.4F). Has not taken any medications but reports a feeling of general malaise. States he "ate at a fast-food restaurant 2 nights ago."	*Diarrhea/Passage of loose, unformed stools*	Bowel Elimination [0501]/*Ability of the gastrointestinal tract to form and evacuate stool effectively.*	Not compromised • Diarrhea not present • Painful cramps not present	Diarrhea Management [0460]/ *Management and alleviation of diarrhea*	• Stool for culture and sensitivity if diarrhea continues • Observe skin turgor • Monitor skin in perianal region for irritation or ulceration • Consult physician if signs and symptoms of diarrhea persist
Mary Kuoko has had involuntary leakage of stool. States her clothing is soiled several times a day. Says she is too embarrassed to go out with her friends because of the fecal odor. Last bowel movement was more than 3 days ago. Digital examination reveals impaction.	*Bowel Incontinence/ Change in normal bowel habits, characterized by involuntary passage of stool*	Bowel Continence [0500]/*Control of passage of stool from the bowel*	Consistently demonstrated • Regular evacuation of stool at least q 3 days • Responds to urge in a timely manner • Knows relationship of intake to evacuation pattern	Constipation/ Impaction Management [0450]/*Prevention and alleviation of constipation/ impaction*	• Administer laxative or enema as indicated • Inform patient of procedure for manual removal of impaction of stool if necessary
				Bowel Incontinence Care [0410]/ *Promotion of bowel continence and maintenance of perianal skin integrity*	• Wash perianal area with soap and water and dry it thoroughly after each stool • Monitor for adequate bowel evacuation • Monitor for diet and fluid requirements

PLANNING

The major goals for clients with fecal elimination problems are to

- Maintain or restore normal bowel elimination pattern.
- Maintain or regain normal stool consistency.
- Prevent associated risks such as fluid and electrolyte imbalance, skin breakdown, abdominal distention, and pain.

Appropriate preventive and corrective nursing interventions that relate to these must be identified. Specific nursing activities associated with each of these interventions can be selected to meet the client's individual needs. Examples of clinical applications of these using NANDA, NIC, and NOC designations are shown in Identifying Nursing Diagnoses, Outcomes, and Interventions and in the Nursing Care Plan.

Planning for Home Care

Clients who have bowel diversion ostomies, who require fecal incontinence pouches, or who have other ongoing elimination problems will need continuing care in the home setting. In preparation for discharge, the nurse needs to assess the client's and family's ability to meet specific care needs. The Home Care Assessment outlines the specific assessment data required before developing a home care plan. Using the assessment data, the nurse designs a teaching plan for the client and family (see Teaching: Home Care).

IMPLEMENTING

Promoting Regular Defecation

The nurse can help clients achieve regular defecation by attending to (a) the provision of privacy, (b) timing, (c) nutrition and fluids, (d) exercise, and (e) positioning. See Teaching: Wellness Care for healthy habits related to bowel elimination.

Privacy. Privacy during defecation is extremely important to many people. The nurse should therefore provide as much privacy as possible for such clients but may need to stay with those who are too weak to be left alone. Some clients also prefer to wipe, wash, and dry themselves after defecating. A nurse may need to provide water and a washcloth and towel for this purpose.

Timing. A client should be encouraged to defecate when the urge is recognized. To establish regular bowel elimination, the client and nurse can discuss when mass peristalsis normally occurs and provide time for defecation. Many people have well-established routines. Other activities, such as bathing and ambulating, should not interfere with the defecation time.

Nutrition and Fluids. The diet a client needs for regular normal elimination varies, depending on the kind of feces the client currently has, the frequency of defecation, and the types of foods that the client finds assist with normal defecation.

For Constipation. Increase daily fluid intake, and instruct the client to drink hot liquids and fruit juices, especially prune juice. Include fiber in the diet, that is, foods such as raw fruit, bran products, and whole-grain cereals and bread.

For Diarrhea. Encourage oral intake of fluids and bland food. Eating small amounts can be helpful because it is more easily absorbed. Excessively hot or cold fluids should be avoided because they stimulate peristalsis. In addition, highly spiced foods and high-fiber foods can aggravate diarrhea. See Teaching: Client Care for details about managing diarrhea.

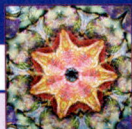

Home Care Assessment

FECAL ELIMINATION

Client and Environment

- Self-care abilities for toileting: Ability to get to the toilet, to manipulate clothing for toileting, to perform toilet hygiene, and to flush the toilet
- Mechanical aids required: Walker, cane, wheelchair, raised toilet seat, grab bars, bedpan, commode
- Mechanical barriers that limit access to the toilet or are unsafe: Poor lighting, cluttered pathway to bathroom, narrow doorway for wheelchair, and so on
- Bowel elimination problem: Alterations in characteristics of feces, diarrhea, constipation, incontinence, presence of ostomy, and methods of handling these
- Level of knowledge: Planned bowel management or training program, prescribed medications, ostomy care, dietary alterations, and fluid and exercise requirements or restrictions

- Facilities: Adequacy of bathroom facilities to facilitate toilet hygiene and ostomy care and to contain potentially infectious fecal effluent or stool

Family

- Caregiver availability and skills: People able to assist with toileting, medications, ostomy care, or other prescribed therapeutic measures
- Family role changes and coping: Effect on financial status, parenting and spousal roles, sexuality, social roles
- Alternate potential primary or respite caregivers: For example, other family members, volunteers, church members, paid caregivers or housekeeping services; available community respite care (adult day care, senior centers)

Community

- Availability of and familiarity with possible sources of assistance: Equipment and supply companies, financial assistance, home health agencies

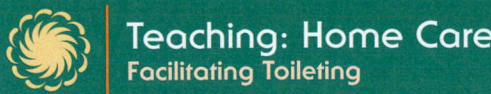

Teaching: Home Care
Facilitating Toileting

- Ensure safe and easy access to the toilet. Make sure lighting is appropriate, scatter rugs are removed or securely fastened, and so on.
- Facilitate instruction as needed about transfer techniques.
- Suggest ways that garments can be adjusted to make disrobing easier for toileting (e.g., Velcro closing on clothing).

Monitoring Bowel Elimination Pattern

- If appropriate, instruct the client to keep a record of time and frequency of stool passage, any associated pain, and color and consistency of the stool.

Dietary Alterations

- Provide information about required food and fluid alterations to promote defecation or to manage diarrhea.

Medications

- Discuss problems associated with overuse of laxatives, if appropriate, and the use of alternatives to laxatives, suppositories, and enemas.
- If the client is taking a constipating medication, discuss the addition of a fiber supplement.

Measures Specific to Elimination Problem

- Provide instructions associated with specific elimination problems and treatment, such as
  a. Constipation
  b. Diarrhea
  c. Ostomy care

Community Agencies and Other Sources of Help

- Make appropriate referrals to home care or community care for assistance with resources such as installation of grab bars and raised toilet seats, structural alterations for wheelchair access, homemaker or home health aide services to assist with ADLs, and enterostomal therapy nurse for assistance with stoma care and selection of ostomy appliances.
- Provide information about companies where durable medical equipment (e.g., raised toilet seats, commodes, bedpans, urinals) can be purchased, rented, or obtained free of charge, and where medical supplies such as incontinence pads or ostomy irrigating supplies and appliances can be obtained.
- Suggest additional sources of information and help such as ostomy self-help and support groups or clubs.

For Flatulence. Limit carbonated beverages, the use of drinking straws, and chewing gum—all of which increase the ingestion of air. Gas-forming foods, such as cabbage, beans, onions, and cauliflower, should also be avoided.

Exercise. Regular exercise helps clients develop a regular defecation pattern. A client with weak abdominal and pelvic muscles (which impede normal defecation) may be able to strengthen them with the following isometric exercises:

- In a supine position, the client tightens the abdominal muscles as though pulling them inward, holding them for about 10 seconds and then relaxing them. This should be repeated 5 to 10 times, four times a day, depending on the client's health.
- Again in a supine position, the client can contract the thigh muscles and hold them contracted for about 10 seconds, repeating the exercise 5 to 10 times, four times a day. This

helps the client confined to bed gain strength in the thigh muscles, thereby making it easier to use a bedpan.

Positioning. Although the squatting position best facilitates defecation, on a toilet seat the best position for most people seems to be leaning forward.

Teaching: Wellness Care
Healthy Defecation

- Establish a regular exercise regimen.
- Include high-fiber foods, such as vegetables, fruits, and whole grains, in the diet.
- Maintain fluid intake of 2,000 to 3,000 mL a day.
- Do not ignore the urge to defecate.
- Allow time to defecate, preferably at the same time each day.
- Avoid over-the-counter medications to treat constipation and diarrhea.

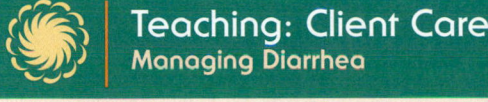

Teaching: Client Care
Managing Diarrhea

- Drink at least 8 glasses of water per day to prevent dehydration.
- Ingest foods with sodium and potassium. Most foods contain sodium. Potassium is found in meats, and many vegetables and fruits, especially tomatoes, potatoes, bananas, peaches, and apricots.
- Increase foods containing soluble fiber, such as oatmeal and skinless fruits and potatoes.
- Avoid alcohol and beverages with caffeine, which aggravate the problem.
- Limit foods containing insoluble fiber, such as whole-wheat and whole-grain breads and cereals, and raw fruits and vegetables.
- Limit fatty foods.
- Thoroughly clean and dry the perianal area after passing stool to prevent skin irritation and breakdown. Use soft toilet tissue to clean and dry the area. Apply a moisture-barrier cream or ointment, such as zinc oxide or petrolatum, as needed.
- If possible, discontinue medications that cause diarrhea.
- When diarrhea has stopped, reestablish normal bowel flora by taking fermented dairy products, such as yogurt or buttermilk.

For clients who have difficulty sitting themselves down and getting up from the toilet, an elevated toilet seat can be attached to a regular toilet. Clients then do not have to lower themselves as far onto the seat and do not have to lift as far off the seat. Elevated toilet seats can be purchased for use in the home.

A bedside **commode,** a portable chair with a toilet seat and a receptacle beneath that can be emptied, is often used for the adult client who can get out of bed but is unable to walk to the bathroom. Some commodes have wheels and can slide over the base of a regular toilet when the waste receptacle is removed, thus providing clients the privacy of a bathroom. Some commodes have a seat and can be used as a chair (Figure 46–9 ■). Potty chairs are available for children.

Clients restricted to bed may need to use a **bedpan,** a receptacle for urine and feces (Figure 46–10 ■). Female clients use a bedpan for both urine and feces; male clients use a bedpan for feces and a urinal for urine.

There are two main types of bedpans, the regular high-back pan and the slipper, or fracture, pan (see Figure 46–10). The slipper pan has a low back and is used for clients unable to raise their buttocks because of physical problems or therapy that contraindicates such movement. Many older adults benefit from the use of a slipper pan. See Practice Guidelines for the techniques of giving and removing a bedpan.

Teaching about Medications

The most common categories of medications affecting fecal elimination are cathartics and laxatives, antidiarrheals, and antiflatulents.

Cathartics and Laxatives. **Cathartics** are drugs that induce defecation. They can have a strong, purgative effect. A laxative

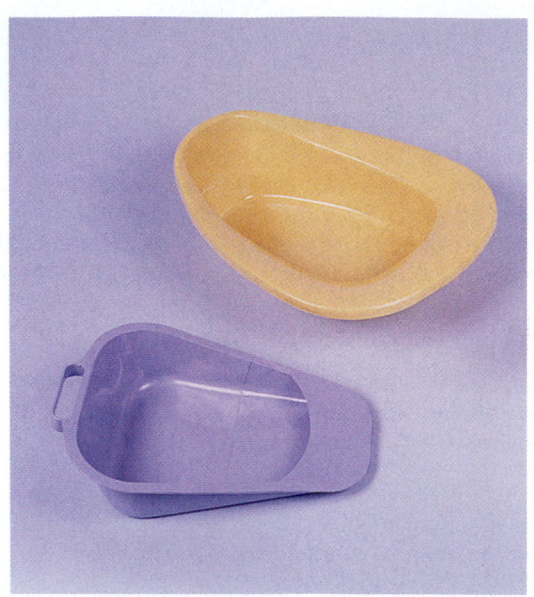

Figure 46–10 ■ *Top,* the high-back or regular bedpan; *Bottom,* the slipper or fracture pan.

is mild in comparison to a cathartic, and it produces soft or liquid stools that are sometimes accompanied by abdominal cramps. Examples of cathartics are castor oil, cascara, phenolphthalein, and bisacodyl. Table 46–3 describes the different types of laxatives.

Laxatives are contraindicated in the client who has nausea, cramps, colic, vomiting, or undiagnosed abdominal pain. Clients need to be informed about the dangers of laxative use. Continual use of laxatives to encourage bowel evacuation weakens the bowel's natural responses to fecal distention, resulting in chronic constipation. To eliminate chronic laxative use, it is usually necessary to teach the client about dietary fiber, regular exercise, taking sufficient fluids, and establishing regular defecation habits. In addition, any medication regimen should be examined to see whether it could cause constipation.

Some laxatives are given in the form of **suppositories.** These act in various ways: by softening the feces, by releasing gases such as carbon dioxide to distend the rectum, or by stimulating the nerve endings in the rectal mucosa. The best results can be obtained by inserting the suppository 30 minutes before the client's usual defecation time or when the peristaltic action is greatest, such as after breakfast.

Antidiarrheal Medications. These medications slow the motility of the intestine or absorb excess fluid in the intestine. Guidelines for using antidiarrheals are shown in Box 46–2.

Antiflatulent Medications. Antiflatulent agents such as simethicone do not decrease the formation of flatus but they do coalesce the gas bubbles and facilitate their passage by belching through the mouth or expulsion through the anus. These agents are frequently combined with an antacid. **Carminatives** are herbal oils known to act as agents that help expel gas from the stomach and intestines. Suppositories can also be given to relieve flatus by increasing intestinal motility.

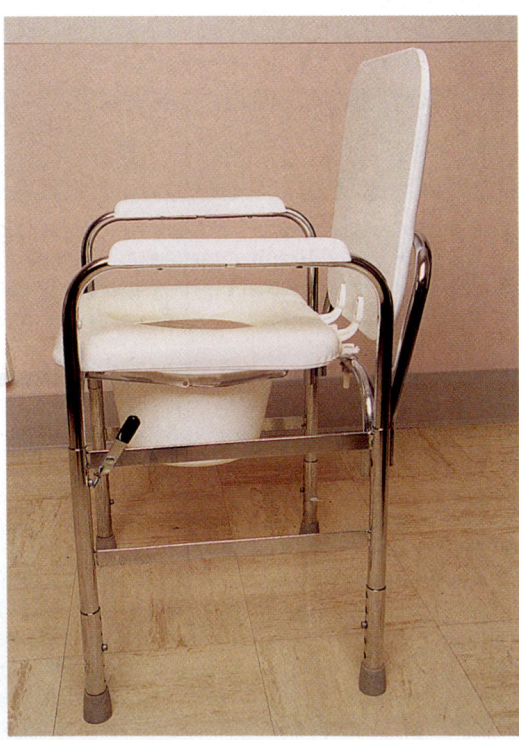

Figure 46–9 ■ A commode with overlying seat.

Practice Guidelines
Giving and Removing a Bedpan

- Provide privacy.
- Wear disposable gloves.
- If the bedpan is metal, warm it by rinsing it with warm water.
- Adjust the bed to a height appropriate to prevent back strain.
- Elevate the side rail on the opposite side to prevent the client from falling out of bed.
- Ask the client to assist by flexing the knees, resting the weight on the back and heels, and raising the buttocks, or by using a trapeze bar, if present.
- Help lift the client as needed by placing one hand under the lower back, resting your elbow on the mattress, and using your forearm as a lever.
- Place a regular bedpan so that the client's buttocks rest on the smooth, rounded rim. Place a slipper pan with the flat, low end under the client's buttocks (Figure 46–11 ■).
- For the client who cannot assist, obtain the assistance of another nurse to help lift the client onto the bedpan or place the client on his or her side, place the bedpan against the buttocks (Figure 46–12 ■), and roll the client back onto the bedpan.
- To provide a more normal position for the client's lower back, elevate the client's bed to a semi-Fowler's position, if permitted. If elevation is contraindicated, support the client's back with pillows as needed to prevent hyperextension of the back.
- Cover the client with bed linen to maintain comfort and self-dignity.

- Provide toilet tissue, place the call light within reach, lower the bed to the low position, elevate the side rail if indicated, and leave the client alone.
- Answer the call bell promptly.
- When removing the bedpan, return the bed to the position used when giving the bedpan, hold the bedpan steady to prevent spillage of its contents, cover the bedpan, and place it on the adjacent chair.
- If the client needs assistance, don gloves and wipe the client's perineal area with several layers of toilet tissue. If a specimen is to be collected, discard the soiled tissue into a moisture-proof receptacle other than the bedpan. For female clients, clean from the urethra toward the anus to prevent transferring rectal microorganisms into the urinary meatus.
- Wash the perineal area of dependent clients with soap and water as indicated and thoroughly dry the area.
- For all clients, offer warm water, soap, a washcloth, and a towel to wash the hands.
- Assist the client to a comfortable position, empty and clean the bedpan, and return it to the bedside.
- Remove and discard your gloves and wash your hands.
- Spray the room with air freshener as needed to control odor unless contraindicated because of respiratory problems or allergies.
- Document color, odor, amount, and consistency of urine and feces, and the condition of the perineal area.

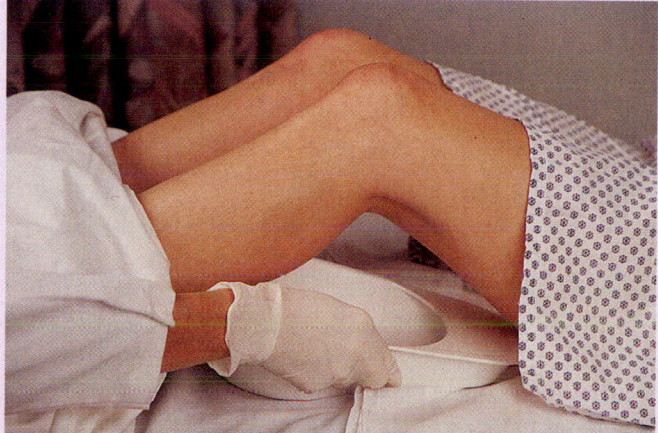

Figure 46–11 ■ Placing a slipper pan under the buttocks.

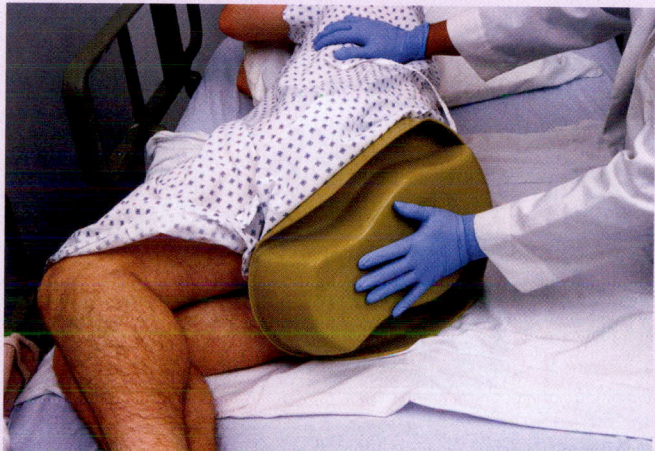

Figure 46–12 ■ Placing a regular bedpan against the client's buttocks.

Decreasing Flatulence

There are a number of ways to reduce or expel flatus, including avoiding gas-producing foods, exercise, moving in bed, and ambulation. Movement stimulates peristalsis and the escape of flatus and reabsorption of gases in the intestinal capillaries. One method of treating flatulence involves the insertion of a rectal tube. This generally requires a physician's order. Guidelines for rectal tube insertion include these:

1. Use a rectal tube (size 22 to 30 French) for adults and a smaller size for children.
2. Have the client assume a side-lying position.
3. Lubricate the rectal tube to reduce mucous membrane irritation.
4. Expose the anus and insert the rectal tube into the rectum 10 cm (4 in.). The rectal tube will stimulate peristalsis. If no flatus is expelled, insert the tube another inch or so. Do not force the tube if it does not insert easily.

TABLE 46–3 Types of Laxatives

Type	Action	Examples	Pertinent Teaching Information
Bulk-forming	Increases the fluid, gaseous, or solid bulk in the intestines	Psyllium hydrophilic mucilloid (Metamucil), methylcellulose (Citrucel)	May take 12 or more hours to act. Sufficient fluid must be taken. Safe for long-term use.
Emollient/stool softener	Softens and delays the drying of the feces; permits fat and water to penetrate feces	Docusate sodium (Colace)	Slow-acting, may take several days.
Stimulant/irritant	Irritates the intestinal mucosa or stimulates nerve endings in the wall of the intestine, causing rapid propulsion of the contents	Bisacodyl (Dulcolax, Correctol), senna (Senokot, Ex-lax), cascara, castor oil	Acts more quickly than bulk-forming agents. Fluid is passed with the feces. May cause cramps. Prolonged use may cause fluid and electrolyte imbalance.
Lubricant	Lubricates the feces in the colon	Mineral oil (Haley's M-O)	Prolonged use inhibits the absorption of some fat-soluble vitamins.
Saline/osmotic	Draws water into the intestine by osmosis, distends bowel, and stimulates peristalsis	Epsom salts, magnesium hydroxide (milk of magnesia), magnesium citrate, sodium phosphate (Fleet phospho-soda)	May be rapid acting. Can cause fluid and electrolyte imbalance, particularly in elderly people and children with cardiac and renal disease. Should not be used by elderly clients. Prolonged use inhibits the absorption of some fat-soluble vitamins.

5. Wrap an abdominal or incontinence pad around the end of the rectal tube to catch any liquid that may be expelled. Some nurses suggest inserting the rectal tube and then placing the end into a receptacle filled with water. The passage of flatus will be seen as bubbles are produced.

6. Leave the tube in no longer than 30 minutes to avoid irritation of the rectal mucosa. If abdominal distention is not relieved, the tube may be inserted every 2 to 3 hours.
7. Encourage the client to assume various positions in bed.

If a rectal tube does not relieve flatus, consult with the physician about a suppository, enema, or medication.

Administering Enemas

An **enema** is a solution introduced into the rectum and large intestine. The action of an enema is to distend the intestine and sometimes to irritate the intestinal mucosa, thereby increasing peristalsis and the excretion of feces and flatus.

Types of Enemas. Enemas are classified into four groups: cleansing, carminative, retention, and return-flow enemas.

Cleansing Enemas. Cleansing enemas are intended to remove feces. They are given chiefly to

- Prevent the escape of feces during surgery.
- Prepare the intestine for certain diagnostic tests such as x-ray or visualization tests (e.g., colonoscopy).
- Remove feces in instances of constipation or impaction.

Cleansing enemas use a variety of solutions. Table 46–4 lists commonly used solutions.

Hypertonic solutions (e.g., saline) exert osmotic pressure, which draws fluid from the interstitial space into the colon.

BOX 46–2 ■ Guidelines for Using Antidiarrheal Medications

- If the diarrhea persists for more than 3 or 4 days, determine the underlying cause. Using a medication such as an opiate when the cause is an infection, toxin, or poison may prolong diarrhea.
- Long-term use of over-the-counter medications (e.g., loperamide hydrochloride [Imodium]) can produce dependence.
- Some antidiarrheal agents can cause drowsiness (e.g., diphenoxylate hydrochloride [Lomotil]) and should not be used when driving an automobile or running machinery.
- Kaolin-pectin preparations (e.g., Kaopectate) may absorb nutrients.
- Bulk laxatives and other absorbents may be used to help bind toxins and absorb excess bowel liquid.
- Bismuth preparations (e.g., Pepto-Bismol), often used to treat "traveler's diarrhea," may contain aspirin and should not be given to children and teenagers with chicken pox, influenza, and other viral infections.

TABLE 46-4 Commonly Used Enema Solutions

Solution	Constituents	Action	Time to Take Effect	Adverse Effects
Hypertonic	90–120 mL of solution (e.g., sodium phosphate)	Draws water into the colon	5–10 min	Retention of sodium
Hypotonic	500–1,000 mL of tap water	Distends colon, stimulates peristalsis, and softens feces	15–20 min	Fluid and electrolyte imbalance; water intoxication
Isotonic	500–1,000 mL of normal saline (9 mL NaCl to 1,000 mL water)	Distends colon, stimulates peristalsis, and softens feces	15–20 min	Possible sodium retention
Soapsuds	500–1,000 mL (3–5 mL soap to 1,000 mL water)	Irritates mucosa, distends colon	10–15 min	Irritates and may damage mucosa
Oil (mineral, olive, cottonseed)	90–120 mL	Lubricates the feces and the colonic mucosa	$\frac{1}{2}$–3 hrs	

The increased volume in the colon stimulates peristalsis and hence defecation. A commonly used hypertonic enema is the commercially prepared Fleet phosphate enema. Hypotonic solutions (e.g., tap water) exert a lower osmotic pressure than the surrounding interstitial fluid, causing water to move from the colon into the interstitial space. Before the water moves from the colon, it stimulates peristalsis and defecation. Because the water moves out of the colon, the tap water enema should not be repeated because of danger of circulatory overload when the water moves from the interstitial space into the circulatory system.

Isotonic solutions, such as physiologic (normal) saline, are considered the safest enema solutions to use. They exert the same osmotic pressure as the interstitial fluid surrounding the colon. Therefore, there is no fluid movement into or out of the colon. The instilled volume of saline in the colon stimulates peristalsis. Soapsuds enemas stimulate peristalsis by increasing the volume in the colon and irritating the mucosa. Only pure soap (i.e., castile soap) should be used in order to minimize mucosa irritation.

Some enemas are large volume (i.e., 500 to 1,000 mL) for an adult and others are small volume, including hypertonic solutions. The amount of solution administered for a high-volume enema will depend on the age and medical condition of the individual. For example, clients with certain cardiac or renal diseases would be adversely affected by significant fluid retention that might result from large-volume hypotonic enemas.

Cleansing enemas may also be described as high or low. A high enema is given to cleanse as much of the colon as possible. The client changes from the left lateral position to the dorsal recumbent position and then to the right lateral position during administration so that the solution can follow the large intestine. The low enema is used to clean the rectum and sigmoid colon only. The client maintains a left lateral position during administration.

The force of flow of the solution is governed by (a) the height of the solution container, (b) size of the tubing, (c) viscosity of the fluid, and (d) resistance of the rectum. The higher the solution container is held above the rectum, the faster the flow and the greater the force (pressure) in the rectum. During most adult enemas, the solution container should be no higher than 30 cm (12 in.) above the rectum. During a high cleansing enema, the solution container is usually held 30 to 46 cm (12 to 18 in.) above the rectum because the fluid is instilled farther to clean the entire bowel.

Carminative Enema. A carminative enema is given primarily to expel flatus. The solution instilled into the rectum releases gas, which in turn distends the rectum and the colon, thus stimulating peristalsis. For an adult, 60 to 80 mL of fluid is instilled.

Retention Enema. A retention enema introduces oil or medication into the rectum and sigmoid colon. The liquid is retained for a relatively long period (e.g., 1 to 3 hours). An oil retention enema acts to soften the feces and to lubricate the rectum and anal canal, thus facilitating passage of the feces. Antibiotic enemas are used to treat infections locally, anthelmintic enemas to kill helminths such as worms and intestinal parasites, and nutritive enemas to administer fluids and nutrients to the rectum.

Return-Flow Enema. A return-flow enema is used occasionally to expel flatus. Alternating flow of 100 to 200 mL of fluid into and out of the rectum and sigmoid colon stimulates peristalsis. This process is repeated five or six times until the flatus is expelled and abdominal distention is relieved.

Procedure 46–1 describes how to administer an enema.

> ➤ **CLINICAL ALERT**   *Some clients may wish to administer their own enemas. If this is appropriate, the nurse validates the client's knowledge of correct technique and assists as needed.* ■

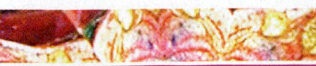

Procedure 46–1 Administering an Enema

Purposes

■ To achieve one or more of the actions described above

ASSESSMENT

Assess

■ When the client last had a bowel movement and the amount, color, and consistency of the feces
■ Presence of abdominal distention (the distended abdomen appears swollen and feels firm rather than soft when palpated)

■ Whether the client has sphincter control
■ Whether the client can use a toilet or commode or must remain in bed and use a bedpan

---

PLANNING

Before administering an enema, determine whether a physician's order is required. At some agencies, a physician must order the kind of enema and the time to give it, for example, the morning of an examination. When the client has rectal disease, the physician may also specify the size of the rectal tube to use. At other agencies, enemas are given at the nurses' discretion (i.e., as necessary on a prn order). In addition, determine the presence of kidney or cardiac disease that contraindicates the use of a hypotonic solution.

Delegation

Administration of some enemas may be delegated to unlicensed assistive personnel (UAP). However, the nurse must ensure the personnel are competent in the use of standard precautions. Abnormal findings such as inability to insert the rectal tip, client inability to retain the solution, or unusual return from the enema must be validated and interpreted by the nurse.

Equipment

■ Disposable linen-saver pad
■ Bath blanket
■ Bedpan or commode
■ Clean gloves
■ Water-soluble lubricant if tubing not prelubricated
■ Paper towel

LARGE-VOLUME ENEMA

■ Solution container with tubing of correct size and tubing clamp
■ Correct solution, amount, and temperature
■ IV pole

SMALL-VOLUME ENEMA

■ Prepackaged container of enema solution with lubricated tip

---

IMPLEMENTATION

Preparation

■ Lubricate about 5 cm (2 in.) of the rectal tube (some commercially prepared enema sets already have lubricated nozzles). Lubrication facilitates insertion through the sphincters and minimizes trauma.
■ Run some solution through the connecting tubing of a large-volume enema set and the rectal tube to expel any air in the tubing; then close the clamp. *Air instilled into the rectum, although not harmful, causes unnecessary distention.*

Performance

1. Explain to the client what you are going to do, why it is necessary, and how he or she can cooperate. Discuss how the results will be used in planning further care or treatments. Indicate that the client may experience a feeling of fullness while the solution is being administered.
2. Wash hands, apply clean gloves, and observe appropriate infection control procedures.
3. Provide for client privacy.

4. Assist the adult client to a left lateral position, with the right leg as acutely flexed as possible (Figure 46–13 ■), and the linen-saver pad under the buttocks. *This position facilitates the flow of solution by gravity into the sigmoid and descending colon, which are on the left side. Having the right leg acutely flexed provides for adequate exposure of the anus.*

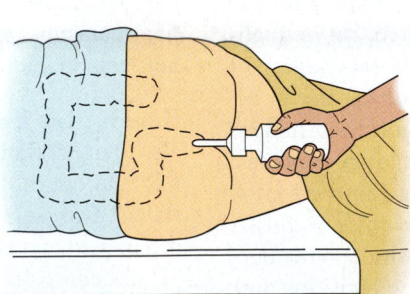

Figure 46–13 ■ Assuming a left lateral position for an enema. Note the commercially prepared enema.

5. Insert the rectal tube.
   • For clients in the left lateral position, lift the upper buttock *to ensure good visualization of the anus.*
   • Insert the tube smoothly and slowly into the rectum, directing it toward the umbilicus (Figure 46–14 ■). *The angle follows the normal contour of*

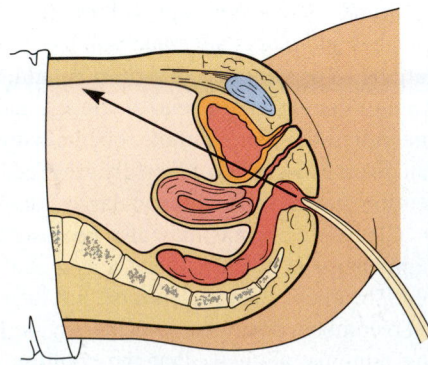

Figure 46–14 ■ Inserting the rectal tube following the direction of the rectum.

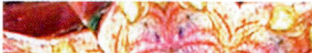

Procedure 46–1 Administering an Enema *continued*

IMPLEMENTATION *continued*

the rectum. *Slow insertion prevents spasm of the sphincter.*
- Insert the tube 7 to 10 cm (3 to 4 in.). *Because the anal canal is about 2.5 to 5 cm (1 to 2 in.) long in the adult, insertion to this point places the tip of the tube beyond the anal sphincter into the rectum.*
- If resistance is encountered at the internal sphincter, ask the client to take a deep breath, then run a small amount of solution through the tube *to relax the internal anal sphincter.*
- Never force tube or solution entry. If instilling a small amount of solution does not permit the tube to be advanced or the solution to freely flow, withdraw the tube. Check for any stool that may have blocked the tube during insertion. If present, flush it and retry the procedure. You may also perform a digital rectal examination to determine if there is an impaction or other mechanical blockage. If resistance persists, end the procedure and report the resistance to the physician and nurse in charge.
6. Slowly administer the enema solution.
   - Raise the solution container, and open the clamp to allow fluid flow.
   or
   - Compress a pliable container by hand.
   - During most low enemas, hold or hang the solution container no higher than 30 cm (12 in.) above the rectum. *The higher the solution container is held above the rectum, the faster the flow and the greater the force (pressure) in the rectum.* During a high enema, hang the solution container about 45 cm (18 in.). *The fluid must be instilled farther to clean the entire bowel.* See agency protocol.
   - Administer the fluid slowly. If the client complains of fullness or pain,

use the clamp to stop the flow for 30 seconds, and then restart the flow at a slower rate. *Administering the enema slowly and stopping the flow momentarily decrease the likelihood of intestinal spasm and premature ejection of the solution.*
- If you are using a plastic commercial container, roll it up as the fluid is instilled. This prevents subsequent suctioning of the solution (Figure 46–15 ■).
- After all the solution has been instilled or when the client cannot

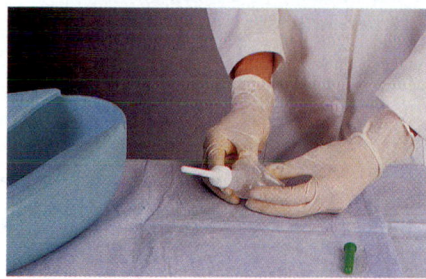

Figure 46–15 ■ Rolling up a commercial enema container.

hold any more and feels the desire to defecate (the urge to defecate usually indicates that sufficient fluid has been administered), close the clamp, and remove the rectal tube from the anus.
- Place the rectal tube in a disposable towel as you withdraw it.
7. Encourage the client to retain the enema.
   - Ask the client to remain lying down. It is easier for the client to retain the enema when lying down than when sitting or standing, because gravity promotes drainage and peristalsis.
   - Request that the client retain the solution for the appropriate amount of time, for example, 5 to 10 minutes for a cleansing enema or at least 30 minutes for a retention enema.

8. Assist the client to defecate.
   - Assist the client to a sitting position on the bedpan, commode, or toilet. A sitting position facilitates the act of defecation.
   - Ask the client who is using the toilet not to flush it. The nurse needs to observe the feces.
   - If a specimen of feces is required, ask the client to use a bedpan or commode.

VARIATION: ADMINISTERING AN ENEMA TO AN INCONTINENT CLIENT
Occasionally a nurse needs to administer an enema to a client who is unable to control the external sphincter muscle and thus cannot retain the enema solution for even a few minutes. In that case, after the rectal tube is inserted, the client assumes a supine position on a bedpan. The head of the bed can be elevated slightly, to 30 degrees if necessary for easier breathing, and pillows support the client's head and back.

VARIATION: ADMINISTERING A RETURN-FLOW ENEMA
For a return-flow enema, the solution (100 to 200 mL for an adult) is instilled into the client's rectum and sigmoid colon. Then the solution container is lowered so that the fluid flows back out through the rectal tube into the container, pulling the flatus with it. The inflow–outflow process is repeated five or six times (to stimulate peristalsis and the expulsion of flatus), and the solution is replaced several times during the procedure if it becomes thick with feces.
9. Document type of solution; length of time solution was retained; the amount, color, and consistency of the returns; and the relief of flatus and abdominal distention in the client record using forms or checklists supplemented by narrative notes when appropriate.

EVALUATION

- Perform a detailed follow-up based on findings that deviated from expected or normal for the client. Relate findings to previous assessment data if available. Report significant deviations from expected to the physician.

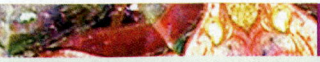

Lifespan Considerations

Administering an Enema
Infants/Children

- Provide a careful explanation to the parents and child before procedure.
- The enema solution should be isotonic (usually normal saline). Some hypertonic commercial solutions (e.g., Fleet phosphate enema) can lead to hypovolemia and electrolyte imbalances. In addition, the osmotic effect of the enema may produce diarrhea and subsequent metabolic acidosis.
- Infants and small children do not exhibit sphincter control and need to be assisted in retaining the enema. The nurse administers the enema while the infant or child is lying with the buttocks over the bedpan and the nurse firmly presses the buttocks together to prevent the immediate expulsion of the solution. Older children can usually hold the solution if they understand what to do and are not required to hold it for too long a period. It may be necessary to ensure that the bathroom is available for an ambulatory child before starting the procedure or to have a bedpan ready.
- Enema temperature should be 37.7C (100F) unless otherwise ordered.
- Large-volume enemas consist of 50 to 200 mL in children less than 18 months old; 200 to 300 mL in children 18 months to 5 years; 300 to 500 mL in children 5 to 12 years old.

- Careful explanation is especially important for the preschool child. An enema is an intrusive procedure and therefore threatening.
- For infants and small children, the dorsal recumbent position is frequently used. Position them on a small padded bedpan with support for the back and head. Secure the legs by placing a diaper under the bedpan and then over and around the thighs. Place the underpad under the client's buttocks to protect the bed linen, and drape the client with the bath blanket.
- Insert the tube 5 to 7.5 cm (2 to 3 in.) in the child and only 2.5 to 3.75 cm (1 to 1.5 in.) in the infant.
- For children, lower the height of the solution container appropriately for the age of the child. See agency protocol.
- To assist a small child in retaining the solution, apply firm pressure over the anus with tissue wipes, or firmly press the buttocks together.

Elders
- Elders may fatigue easily.
- Elders may be more susceptible to fluid and electrolyte imbalances. Use tap water enemas with great caution.
- Monitor the client's tolerance during the procedure, watching for vagal episodes and dysrhythmias.
- Protect older adults' skin from prolonged exposure to moisture.
- Assist older clients with perineal care as indicated.

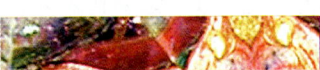

Home Care Considerations

Administering an Enema
Teach the caregiver or client the following:
- To make saline solution, mix 1 teaspoon of table salt with 500 mL of tap water.

- Use enemas only as directed. Do not rely on them for regular bowel evacuation.
- Prior to administration, make sure a bedpan, commode, or toilet is nearby.

Digital Removal of a Fecal Impaction

Digital removal involves breaking up the fecal mass digitally and removing it in portions. Because the bowel mucosa can be injured during this procedure, some agencies restrict and specify the personnel permitted to conduct digital disimpactions. Rectal stimulation is also contraindicated for some people because it may cause an excessive vagal response resulting in cardiac arrhythmia. Before disimpaction it is suggested an oil retention enema be given and held for 30 minutes. After a disimpaction, the nurse can use various interventions to remove remaining feces, such as a cleansing enema or the insertion of a suppository.

Because manual removal of an impaction can be painful, the nurse may use 1 to 2 mL of lidocaine (Xylocaine) gel on a gloved finger inserted into the anal canal as far as the nurse can reach. The lidocaine will anesthetize the anal canal and rectum and should be inserted 5 minutes before the disimpaction.

For digital removal of a fecal impaction:

1. If indicated, obtain assistance from a second person who can comfort the client during the procedure.

2. Ask the client to assume a left side-lying position, with the knees flexed and the back toward the nurse.
3. Place a bedpad under the client's buttocks and a bedpan nearby to receive stool.
4. Drape the client for comfort and to avoid unnecessary exposure of the body.
5. Put on a pair of clean gloves and liberally lubricate the index finger to be inserted.
6. Gently insert the index finger into the rectum and move the finger along the length of the rectum.
7. Loosen and dislodge stool by gently massaging around it. Break up stool by working the finger into the hardened mass, taking care to avoid injury to the mucosa of the rectum.
8. Carefully work stool downward to the end of the rectum and remove it in small pieces. Continue to remove as much fecal material as possible. Periodically assess the client for signs of fatigue, such as facial pallor, diaphoresis, or change in pulse rate. Manual stimulation should be minimal.
9. Following disimpaction, assist the client to clean the anal area and buttocks. Then assist the client onto a bedpan or commode for a short time because digital stimulation of the rectum often induces the urge to defecate.

Bowel Training Programs

For clients who have chronic constipation, frequent impactions, or fecal incontinence, bowel training programs may be helpful. The program is based on factors within the client's control and is designed to help the client establish normal defecation. Such matters as food and fluid intake, exercise, and defecation habits are all considered. Before beginning such a program, clients must understand it and want to be involved. The major phases of the program are as follows:

- Determine the client's usual bowel habits and factors that help and hinder normal defecation.
- Design a plan with the client that includes the following:
  a. Fluid intake of about 2,500 to 3,000 mL per day
  b. Increase in fiber in the diet
  c. Intake of hot drinks, especially just before the usual defecation time
  d. Increase in exercise.
- Maintain the following daily routine for 2 to 3 weeks:
  a. Administer a cathartic suppository (e.g., Dulcolax) 30 minutes before the client's defecation time to stimulate peristalsis.
  b. When the client experiences the urge to defecate, assist the client to the toilet or commode or onto a bedpan. Note the length of time between the insertion of the suppository and the urge to defecate.
  c. Provide the client with privacy for defecation and a time limit; 30 to 40 minutes is usually sufficient.
  d. Teach the client to lean forward at the hips, to apply pressure on the abdomen with the hands, and to bear down for defecation. These measures increase pressure on the colon. Straining should be avoided because it can cause hemorrhoids.
- Provide positive feedback when the client successfully defecates. Refrain from negative feedback if the client fails to defecate.
- Offer encouragement to the client and convey that patience is often required. Many clients require weeks or months of training to achieve success.

Fecal Incontinence Pouch

To collect and contain large volumes of feces, the nurse may place a fecal incontinence pouch (rectal pouch) around the anal area. The purpose of the pouch is to prevent progressive perianal skin irritation and breakdown and frequent linen changes necessitated by incontinence. In many agencies, the pouch is replacing the traditional approach to this problem, that is, inserting a large Foley catheter into the client's rectum and inflating the balloon to keep it in place—a practice that may damage the rectal sphincter and rectal mucosa. A rectal catheter also increases peristalsis and incontinence by stimulating sensory nerve fibers in the rectum.

A rectal pouch is secured around the anal opening and may or may not be attached to drainage. Pouches are best applied before the perianal skin becomes excoriated. If perianal skin excoriation is present, the nurse either (a) applies a moisture-barrier cream to the skin to protect it from feces until it heals

and then applies the pouch, or (b) applies a protective powder, skin barrier, or hydrocolloid wafer such as Duoderm underneath the pouch to achieve the best possible seal.

Nursing responsibilities for clients with a rectal pouch include (a) regular assessment and documentation of the perianal skin status, (b) changing the bag every 72 hours or sooner if there is leakage, (c) maintaining the drainage system, and (d) providing explanations and support to the client and support people.

Some clients may be treated surgically for fecal incontinence with surgical repair of a damaged sphincter or an artificial bowel sphincter. The artificial sphincter consists of three parts: a cuff around the anal canal, a pressure-regulating balloon, and a pump that inflates the cuff (Figure 46–16 ■). The cuff is inflated to close the sphincter, maintaining continence. To have a bowel movement, the client deflates the cuff. The cuff automatically reinflates in 10 minutes.

Ostomy Management

Clients with fecal diversions need considerable psychologic support, instruction, and physical care. This section is limited to the nurse's physical interventions of stoma assessment, application of an appliance to collect feces, and promotion of predictable evacuation with colostomy irrigation. Many agencies have wound, ostomy, continence nurses (WOCN) to assist these clients.

Stoma and Skin Care. Care of the stoma and skin is important for all clients who have ostomies. The fecal material from a colostomy or ileostomy is irritating to the peristomal skin. This is particularly true of ileal effluent, which contains digestive enzymes. It is important to assess the peristomal skin for irritation each time the appliance is changed. Any irritation or skin breakdown needs to be treated immediately. The skin is kept clean by washing off any excretion and drying thoroughly. A barrier such as karaya gum is applied over the skin around the stoma to prevent contact with any excretion. An appliance (bag) is then fitted to the stoma so that there is no leakage

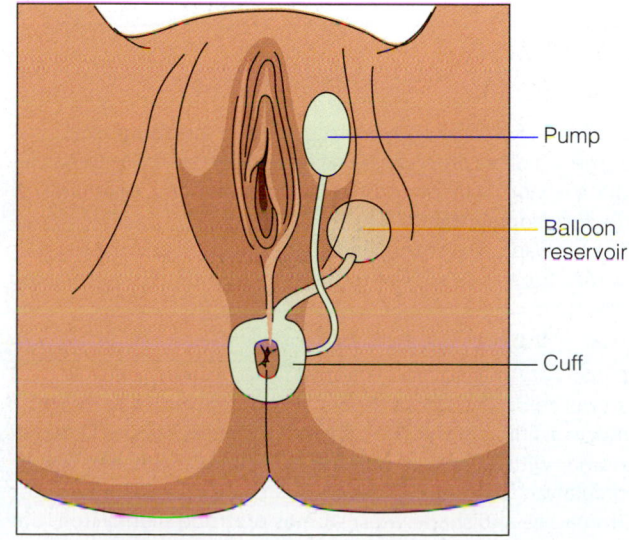

Figure 46–16 ■ Inflatable artificial sphincter.

around it. It is exceedingly important to dry the skin before attaching the appliance. The pouch will not adhere to moist skin, causing effluent to leak onto the skin. Numerous pouch systems are commercially available. All appliances have three features in common: a pouch to collect the effluent, an outlet at the bottom for easy emptying, and a faceplate. Temporary, disposable pouches are made of transparent plastic and have a peel-off adhesive square into which a hole the size of the stoma is cut. Permanent pouches may be clear or opaque, rubber or vinyl, and have a solid ring faceplate that fits around the stoma (Figure 46–17 ■).

Odor control is essential to clients' self-esteem. As soon as clients are ambulatory, they can learn to work with the ostomy in the bathroom to avoid odors at the bedside. Selecting the appropriate kind of appliance promotes odor control. An intact appliance contains odors. The appliance should be rinsed thoroughly when it is emptied. Deodorizers can be placed in the pouch of the appliance, or pouches with charcoal filter discs are available.

Disposable ostomy appliances can be applied for up to 7 days (and emptied whenever ⅓ to ½ full). They need to be changed whenever the effluent leaks onto the peristomal skin. Many people prefer to change them daily or whenever they become soiled, but this practice can be detrimental to the integrity of the peristomal skin and is expensive. Check agency practice in this regard. Some people recommend removing the pouch and skin barrier twice a week to clean and inspect the peristomal skin. If the skin is erythematous, eroded, denuded, or ulcerated, the pouch should be changed every 24 to 48 hours to

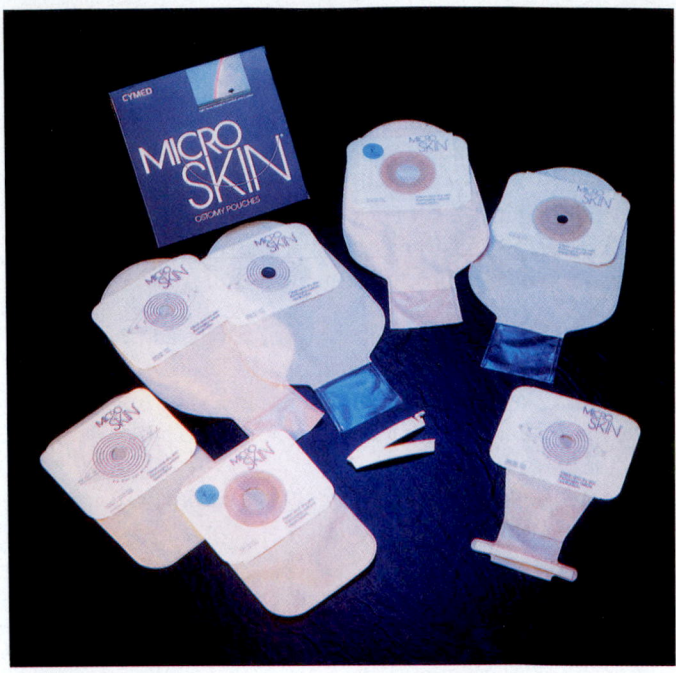

Figure 46–17 ■ Ostomy appliances. (Courtesy of Cymed Ostomy Co., Princeton, NJ.)

allow appropriate treatment of the skin. More frequent changes are recommended if the client complains of pain or discomfort. Procedure 46–2 explains how to change a bowel diversion ostomy appliance.

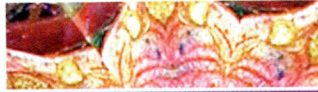 ## Procedure 46–2 Changing a Bowel Diversion Ostomy Appliance

Purposes

- To assess and care for the peristomal skin
- To collect effluent for assessment of the amount and type of output
- To minimize odors for the client's comfort and self-esteem

ASSESSMENT

Determine

- The kind of ostomy and its placement on the abdomen. Surgeons often draw diagrams when there are two stomas. If there is more than one stoma, it is important to confirm which is the functioning stoma.
- The type and size of appliance currently used and the special barrier substance applied to the skin, according to the nursing care plan.
- Tape allergy.

Assess

- Stoma color: The stoma should appear red, similar in color to the mucosal lining of the inner cheek. Very pale or darker-colored stomas with a bluish or purplish hue indicate impaired blood circulation to the area.
- Stoma size and shape: Most stomas protrude slightly from the abdomen. New stomas normally appear swollen, but swelling

generally decreases over 2 or 3 weeks or for as long as 6 weeks. Failure of swelling to recede may indicate a problem, for example, blockage.
- Stomal bleeding: Slight bleeding initially when the stoma is touched is normal, but other bleeding should be reported.
- Status of peristomal skin: Any redness and irritation of the peristomal skin—the 5 to 13 cm (2 to 5 in.) of skin surrounding the stoma—should be noted. Transient redness after removal of adhesive is normal.
- Amount and type of feces: For ileal effluent and feces (colostomy effluent), assess the amount, color, odor, and consistency. Inspect for abnormalities, such as pus or blood.
- Complaints: Complaints of burning sensation under the faceplate may indicate skin breakdown. The presence of abdominal discomfort and/or distention also needs to be determined.

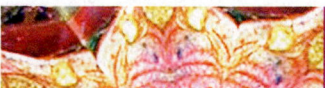

Procedure 46–2 Changing a Bowel Diversion Ostomy Appliance *continued*

ASSESSMENT *continued*

- The client's and family members' learning needs regarding the ostomy and self-care.
- The client's emotional status, especially strategies used to cope with the ostomy.

PLANNING

Review features of the appliance to ensure that all parts are present and function correctly.

Delegation

Care of a new ostomy is not delegated to UAP. However, aspects of ostomy function are observed during usual care and may be recorded by persons other than the nurse. Abnormal findings must be validated and interpreted by the nurse. In some agencies, UAP may remove and replace well-established ostomy appliances.

Equipment
- Clean gloves
- Electric or safety razor
- Bedpan

- Solvent (presaturated sponges or liquid)
- Moisture-proof bag (for disposable pouches)
- Cleaning materials, including tissues, warm water, mild soap (optional), washcloth or cotton balls, towel
- Tissue or gauze pad
- Skin barrier (paste, powder, water, or liquid skin sealant)
- Stoma measuring guide
- Pen or pencil and scissors
- Clean ostomy appliance, with optional belt
- Tail closure clamp
- Special adhesive, if needed
- Stoma guidestrip, if needed
- Deodorant (liquid or tablet) for a nonodorproof colostomy bag

IMPLEMENTATION

Preparation

1. Determine the need for an appliance change.
   - Assess the used appliance for leakage of effluent. *Effluent can irritate the peristomal skin.*
   - Ask the client about any discomfort at or around the stoma. *A burning sensation may indicate breakdown beneath the faceplate of the pouch.*
   - Assess the fullness of the pouch. *The weight of an overly full bag may loosen the faceplate and separate it from the skin, causing the effluent to leak and irritate the peristomal skin.*
2. If there is pouch leakage or discomfort at or around the stoma, change the appliance.
3. Select an appropriate time to change the appliance.
   - Avoid times close to meal or visiting hours. *Ostomy odor and effluent may reduce appetite or embarrass the client.*
   - Avoid times immediately after meals or the administration of any medications that may stimulate bowel evacuation. *It is best to change the pouch when drainage is least likely to occur.*

Performance

1. Explain to the client what you are going to do, why it is necessary, and how he or she can cooperate. Discuss how

the results will be used in planning further care or treatments. Changing an ostomy appliance should not cause discomfort, but it may be distasteful to the client. Communicate acceptance and support to the client. It is important to change the appliance competently and quickly. Include support persons as appropriate.

2. Wash hands, apply clean gloves, and observe appropriate infection control procedures.
3. Provide for client privacy preferably in the bathroom, where clients can learn to deal with the ostomy as they would at home.
4. Assist the client to a comfortable sitting or lying position in bed or preferably a sitting or standing position in the bathroom. *Lying or standing positions may facilitate smoother pouch application, that is, avoid wrinkles.*
5. Unfasten the belt if the client is wearing one.
6. Shave the peristomal skin of well-established ostomies as needed.
   - Use an electric or safety razor on a regular basis to remove excessive hair. *Hair follicles can become irritated or infected by repeated pulling out of hairs during removal of the appliance and skin barrier. Excessive hair can interfere with adhesive action.*

7. Empty and remove the ostomy appliance.
   - Empty the contents of the pouch through the bottom opening into a bedpan. *Emptying before removing the pouch prevents spillage of effluent onto the client's skin.*
   - Assess the consistency and the amount of effluent.
   - Peel the bag off slowly while holding the client's skin taut. *Holding the skin taut minimizes client discomfort and prevents abrasion of the skin.*
   - If the appliance is disposable, discard it in a moisture-proof bag.
8. Clean and dry the peristomal skin and stoma.
   - Use toilet tissue to remove excess stool.
   - Use warm water, mild soap (optional), and cotton balls or a washcloth and towel to clean the skin and stoma (Figure 46–18 ■). Check agency practice on the use of soap. *Soap is sometimes not advised because it can be irritating to the skin.*
   - Use a special skin cleanser to remove dried, hard stool. *This emulsifies the stool, making removal less damaging to the skin.*
   - Dry the area thoroughly by patting with a towel or cotton balls. *Excess rubbing can abrade the skin.*

continued on page 1248

Procedure 46–2 Changing a Bowel Diversion Ostomy Appliance *continued*

IMPLEMENTATION *continued*

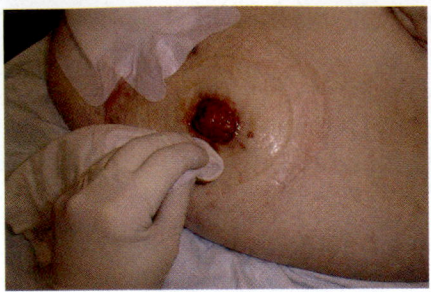

Figure 46–18 ■ Cleaning the skin. (Cory Patrick Hartley, San Ramon Regional Medical Center, San Ramon, CA. Reprinted with permission)

9. Assess the stoma and peristomal skin.
   • Inspect the stoma for color, size, shape, and bleeding.
   • Inspect the peristomal skin for any redness, ulceration, or irritation. Transient redness after the removal of adhesive is normal.
   • Place a piece of tissue or gauze pad over the stoma, and change it as needed. This absorbs any seepage from the stoma.
10. Apply paste-type skin barrier if needed.
    • Fill in abdominal creases or dimples with paste. *This establishes a smooth surface for application of the skin barrier and pouch.*
    • Allow the paste to dry for 1 to 2 minutes or as recommended by the manufacturer.
11. Prepare and apply the skin barrier (peristomal seal).

FOR A SOLID WAFER OR DISC SKIN BARRIER
   • Use the guide (Figure 46–19 ■) to measure the size of the stoma.

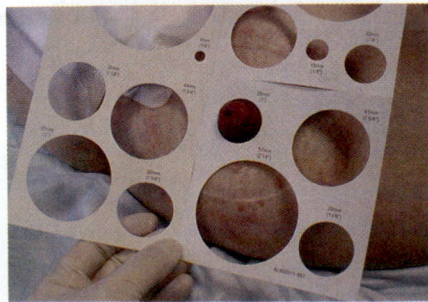

Figure 46–19 ■ A guide for measuring the stoma. (Cory Patrick Hartley, San Ramon Regional Medical Center, San Ramon, CA. Reprinted with permission.)

• On the backing of the skin barrier, trace a circle the same size as the stomal opening.
• Cut out the traced stoma pattern to make an opening in the skin barrier. Make the opening no more than 0.3 to 0.4 cm (1/8 to 1/6 in.) larger than the stoma. *This allows space for the stoma to expand slightly when functioning and minimizes the risk of effluent contacting peristomal skin.*
• Remove the backing to expose the sticky adhesive side.
• Center the skin barrier over the stoma, and gently press it onto the client's skin, smoothing out any wrinkles or bubbles (Figure 46–20 ■).

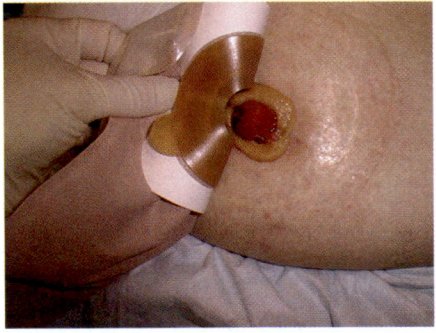

Figure 46–20 ■ Centering the skin barrier over the stoma. (Cory Patrick Hartley, San Ramon Regional Medical Center, San Ramon, CA. Reprinted with permission.)

FOR LIQUID SKIN SEALANT
   • Cover the stoma with a gauze pad. *This prevents contact with the skin sealant.*
   • Either wipe or apply the product evenly around the peristomal skin to form a thin layer of the liquid plastic coating to the same area.
   • Allow the skin sealant to dry until it no longer feels tacky.
12. Fill in any exposed skin around an irregularly shaped stoma.
    • Apply paste to any exposed skin areas. Use a non-alcohol-based product if the skin is excoriated. *Alcohol may cause stinging and burning.*
    or
    • Sprinkle peristomal powder on the skin, wipe off the excess, and dab the powder with a slightly moist gauze or an applicator moistened with a liquid skin barrier. *This creates a barrier or seal.*

13. Prepare and apply the clean appliance.
    • Remove the tissue over the stoma before applying the pouch.

FOR A DISPOSABLE POUCH WITH ADHESIVE SQUARE
   • If the appliance does not have a precut opening, trace a circle 0.3 to 0.4 cm (1/8 to 1/6 in.) larger than the stoma size on the appliance's adhesive square. *The opening is made slightly larger than the stoma to prevent rubbing, cutting, or trauma to the stoma.*
   • Cut out a circle in the adhesive. Take care not to cut any portion of the pouch (Figure 46–21 ■).

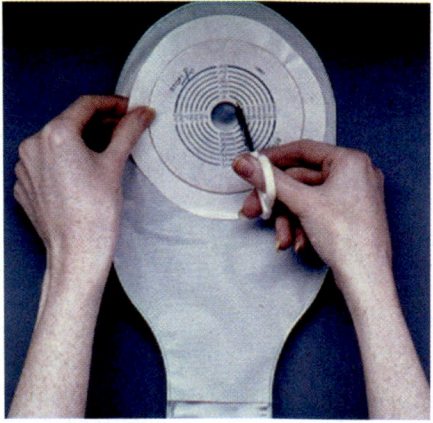

Figure 46–21 ■ Cutting the wafer. (Courtesy of Convatec, a Bristol-Meyers Squibb Company.)

   • Peel off the backing from the adhesive seal.
   • Center the opening of the pouch over the client's stoma and apply it directly onto the skin barrier (Figure 46–22 ■).

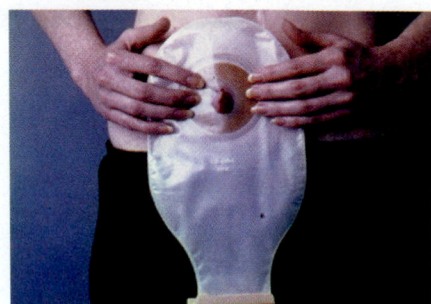

Figure 46–22 ■ Applying the disposable pouch. (Courtesy of Convatec, a Bristol-Meyers Squibb Company.)

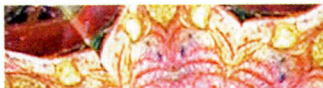

Procedure 46–2 Changing a Bowel Diversion Ostomy Appliance *continued*

IMPLEMENTATION *continued*

- Gently press the adhesive backing onto the skin and smooth out any wrinkles, working from the stoma outward. *Wrinkles allow seepage of effluent, which can irritate the skin or soil clothing.*
- Remove the air from the pouch. *Removing the air helps the pouch lie flat against the abdomen.*
- Place a deodorant on the pouch (optional).
- Close the pouch by turning up the bottom a few times, fanfolding its end lengthwise, and securing it with a tail closure clamp.

FOR A REUSABLE POUCH WITH FACEPLATE ATTACHED
- Apply either adhesive cement or a double-faced adhesive disc to the faceplate of the appliance, depending on the type of appliance being used. Follow the manufacturer's directions.
- Insert a coiled paper guidestrip [15-cm (6-in.) strip of 1.3-cm (1/2-in.) wide paper] into the faceplate opening (Figure 46–23 ■). The strip should protrude slightly from the opening and expand to fit it. *The guidestrip helps the nurse center the appliance over the stoma and prevents pressure or irritation to the stoma due to an ill-fitting appliance.*

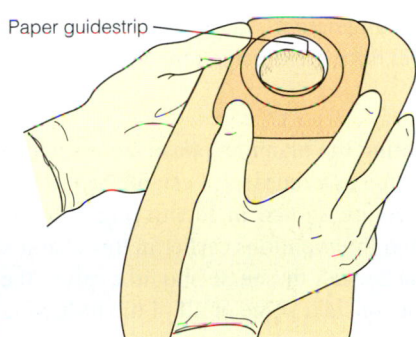

Paper guidestrip

Figure 46–23 ■ The coiled paper guidestrip in the faceplate opening.

- Using the guidestrip, center the faceplate over the stoma.
- Firmly press the adhesive seal to the peristomal skin. The guidestrip will fall into the pouch; commercially

prepared guidestrips will dissolve in the pouch.
- Place a deodorant in the bag if the bag is not odorproof. Most pouches are odorproof.
- Close the end of the pouch with the designated clamp.
- Attach the pouch belt, and fasten it around the client's waist (optional).

VARIATION: APPLYING A REUSABLE POUCH WITH DETACHABLE FACEPLATE
Some nurses recommend applying a skin sealant (e.g., Skin Prep) to the faceplate before attaching the adhesive disc. *This makes it easier to remove the adhesive disc from the faceplate.*

- Remove the protective paper strip from one side of the double-faced adhesive disc.
- Apply the sticky side to the back of the faceplate.
- Remove the remaining protective paper strip from the other side of the adhesive disc.
- Center the faceplate over the stoma and skin barrier, then press and hold the faceplate against the client's skin for a few minutes to secure the seal.
- Press the adhesive around the circumference of the adhesive disc.
- Tape the faceplate to the client's abdomen using four or eight 7.5-cm (3-in.) strips of hypoallergenic tape. Place the strips around the faceplate in a "picture-framing" manner, one strip down each side, one across the top, and one across the bottom (Figure 46–24 ■). The additional four strips can be placed diagonally over the other tapes to secure the seal.

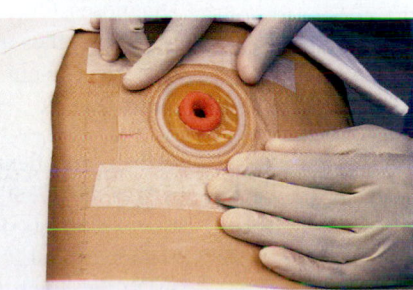

Figure 46–24 ■ Taping the faceplate to the client's abdomen.

- Stretch the opening on the back of the pouch, and position it over the base of the faceplate. Ease it over the faceplate flange.
- Place the lock ring between the pouch and the faceplate flange (Figure 46–25 ■) to seal the pouch against the faceplate.
- Close the base of the pouch with the appropriate clamp.
- Attach the pouch belt and fasten it around the client's waist (optional).

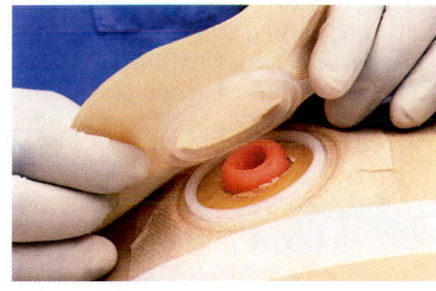

Figure 46–25 ■ Sealing the pouch against the face plate.

14. Dispose of equipment or clean any reusable equipment.
- Discard a disposable bag in a plastic bag before placing in the waste container.
- If feces are liquid, measure the volume. Note the feces' character, consistency, and color before emptying the feces into a toilet or hopper.
- Wash reusable bags with cool water and mild soap, rinse, and dry.
- Wash a soiled belt with warm water and mild soap, rinse, and dry.
- Remove and discard gloves.

VARIATION: APPLYING THE SKIN BARRIER AND APPLIANCE AS ONE UNIT
If a disc- or wafer-type skin barrier is used, the skin barrier and appliance can be applied as one unit. Applying the skin barrier and the appliance together not only is quicker but also is thought to reduce the chance of wrinkles. It also is easier for the client to apply without help.
- Prepare the skin barrier by measuring the size of the stoma, tracing a circle on the backing of the skin barrier, and cutting out the traced stoma pattern to make an opening in the skin barrier.

continued on page 1250

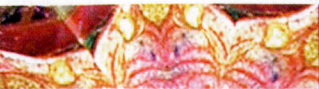

Procedure 46–2 Changing a Bowel Diversion Ostomy Appliance *continued*

IMPLEMENTATION *continued*

- Prepare the appliance by cutting an opening 0.3 to 0.4 cm (1/8 to 1/6 in.) larger than the stoma size (if not already present) and peeling off the backing from the adhesive seal.
- Center the opening of the pouch over the skin barrier.
- Remove the skin barrier backing to expose the sticky adhesive side.

- Center the skin barrier and appliance over the stoma, and press it onto the client's skin.
15. Document the procedure in the client record using forms or checklists supplemented by narrative notes when appropriate. Report and record pertinent assessments and interventions. Report any increase in stoma size,

change in color indicative of circulatory impairment, and presence of skin irritation or erosion. Record on the client's chart discoloration of the stoma, the appearance of the peristomal skin, the amount and type of drainage, the client reaction to the procedure, the client's experience with the ostomy, and skills learned by the client.

EVALUATION

- Relate findings to previous data if available. Adjust the teaching plan and nursing care plan as needed. Include on the teaching plan the equipment and procedure used. *Client learning is facilitated by consistent nursing interventions.*

- Perform detailed follow-up based on findings that deviated from expected or normal for the client. Report significant deviations from normal to the physician.

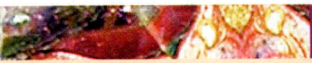

Home Care Considerations

Changing an Ostomy Appliance

- Provide the client with the names and phone numbers of a WOCN, supply vendor, and other resource people to contact when needed.
- Inform the client of signs to report to a health care provider (e.g., peristomal redness, skin breakdown, and changes in stomal color).
- Provide client and family education regarding care of the ostomy and appliance when traveling.

- Educate the client and family regarding infection control precautions, including proper disposal of used pouches since these cannot be flushed down a toilet.
- Younger clients may have special concerns about odor and appearance. Provide information about ostomy care and community support groups. A visit from someone who has had an ostomy under similar circumstances may be helpful.

Colostomy Irrigation. A colostomy irrigation, similar to an enema, is a form of stoma management used only for clients who have a sigmoid or descending colostomy. The purpose of irrigation is to distend the bowel sufficiently to stimulate peristalsis, which stimulates evacuation. When a regular evacuation pattern is achieved, the wearing of a colostomy pouch is unnecessary. Currently, colostomy irrigations are not routinely taught to most clients. Routine daily irrigations for control of the time of elimination ultimately become the client's decision. Some clients prefer to control the time of elimination through rigid dietary regulation and not be bothered with irrigations, which can take up to an hour to complete. When regulation by irrigation is chosen, it should be done at the same time each day. Control by irrigations also necessitates some control of the diet. For example, laxative foods that might cause an unexpected evacuation need to be avoided.

For most clients, a relatively small amount of fluid (300 to 500 mL) stimulates evacuation. For others, up to 1,000 mL may be needed because a colostomy has no sphincter and the fluid tends to return as it is instilled. This problem is reduced by the

use of a cone on the irrigating catheter. The cone helps to hold the fluid within the bowel during the irrigation.

EVALUATING

The goals established during the planning phase are evaluated according to specific desired outcomes, also established in that phase. Examples of these are shown in Identifying Nursing Diagnoses, Outcomes, and Interventions earlier in this chapter.

If outcomes are not achieved, the nurse should explore the reasons. The nurse might consider some or all of the following questions:

- Were the client's fluid intake and diet appropriate?
- Was the client's activity level appropriate?
- Are prescribed medications or other factors affecting the gastrointestinal function?
- Do the client and family understand the provided instructions well enough to comply with the required therapy?
- Were sufficient physical and emotional support provided?

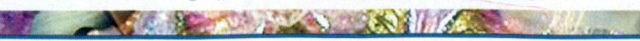

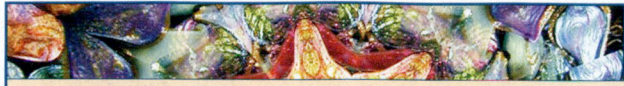

ASSESSMENT DATA	NURSING DIAGNOSIS	DESIRED OUTCOMES [NOC #]/INDICATORS*
Nursing Assessment Mrs. Emma Brown is a 78-year-old widow of 9 months. She lives alone in a low-income housing complex for elders. Her two children live with their families in a city approximately 150 miles away. She has always enjoyed cooking for her family; however, now that she is alone, she does not cook for herself. As a result, she has developed irregular eating patterns and tends to prepare soup-and-toast meals. She gets little exercise and has had bouts of insomnia since her husband's death. For the past month, Mrs. Brown has been having a problem with constipation. She states she has a bowel movement about every 3 to 4 days and her stools are hard and painful to excrete. Mrs. Brown decides to attend the health fair sponsored by the housing complex and seeks assistance from the county public health nurse. **Physical Examination** Height: 162 cm (5'4") Weight: 65 kg (143 lb) Temperature: 36.2C (97.2F) Pulse: 82 BPM Respirations: 20/minute Blood pressure: 128/74 mm Hg Active bowel sounds, abdomen slightly distended **Diagnostic Data** CBC: Hgb 10.8 Urinalysis negative	*Constipation* related to low-fiber diet and inactivity (as evidenced by infrequent, hard stools; painful defecation; abdominal distention)	Bowel Elimination [0501], as evidenced by • Comfort of stool passage. • Ingests adequate fiber. • Exercises adequate amount

NURSING INTERVENTIONS [NIC#]/SELECTED ACTIVITIES*

RATIONALE

Constipation/Impaction Management [0450]

• Identify factors (e.g., medications, bed rest, diet) that may cause or contribute to constipation.

• Encourage increased fluid intake, unless contraindicated.

• Evaluate medication profile for gastrointestinal side effects.

• Teach Mrs. Brown how to keep a food diary.

• Instruct Mrs. Brown on a high-fiber diet, as appropriate.

• Instruct her on the relationship of diet, exercise, and fluid intake to constipation and impaction.

Exercise Promotion [0200]

• Encourage verbalization of feelings about exercise or need for exercise.

• Assist in identifying a positive role model for maintaining the exercise program.

• Inform Mrs. Brown about the health benefits and physiologic effects of exercise.

• Instruct her about appropriate types of exercise for her level of health, in collaboration with a physician.

• Assist Mrs. Brown to set short-term and long-term goals for the exercise program.

Assessing causative factors is an essential first step in teaching and planning for improved bowel elimination.

Sufficient fluid intake is necessary for the bowel to absorb sufficient amounts of liquid to promote proper stool consistency.

Constipation is a common side effect of many drugs including narcotics and antacids.

An appraisal of food intake will help identify if Mrs. Brown is eating a well-balanced diet and consuming adequate amounts of fluid and fiber. Excessive meat or refined food intake will produce small, hard stools.

Fiber absorbs water, which adds bulk and softness to the stool and speeds up passage through the intestines.

Fiber without adequate fluid can aggravate, not facilitate, bowel function.

Perceptions of the need for exercise may be influenced by misconceptions, cultural and social beliefs, fears, or age.

Individuals who have been successful in an exercise program can assist Mrs. Brown by providing incentive and enhancing motivation. For example, a walking partner may be beneficial.

Activity influences bowel elimination by improving muscle tone and stimulating peristalsis.

Any individual beginning an exercise program should consult a physician primarily for a cardiac evaluation. Mrs. Brown's age and lack of activity should be considered in planning the level of activity.

Realistic goal-setting provides direction and motivation.

continued on page 1252

NURSING CARE PLAN FOR ALTERED BOWEL ELIMINATION *continued*

EVALUATION

Outcome not met. Mrs. Brown has kept a food diary and is able to identify the need for more fluid and fiber but has not consistently included fiber in her diet. She has started a walking program with a neighbor but is only able to walk for 10 minutes at a time twice a week. She states her last bowel movement was 3 days ago.

*Outcomes, interventions, and activities selected are only a sample of those suggested by NOC and NIC and should be further individualized for each client.

Applying Critical Thinking

1. You learn that Mrs. Brown's stools have been liquid, in very small amounts, and at infrequent intervals, generally occurring when she feels the urge to defecate. What additional data are important to obtain from her?

2. What nursing intervention is most appropriate before making suggestions to correct or prevent the problem she is experiencing?

3. What suggestions can you give her about maintaining a regular bowel pattern?

4. Explain why cathartics and laxatives are generally contraindicated for people in Mrs. Brown's situation.

See Critical Thinking Possibilities in Appendix A.

CONCEPT MAP 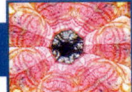 Altered Bowel Elimination

EB 78 y.o. ♀

→

- Recent widow, lives alone. C/O hard, painful stools q3–4 days x 1 month. Irregular eating pattern.
- Height: 162 cm (5'4")
- Weight: 65 kg (143 lb)
- Temperature: 36.2C (97.2F)
- Pulse: 82 BPM
- Respirations: 20/minute
- Blood pressure: 128/74 mm Hg
- Active bowel sounds, abdomen slightly distended
- CBC: Hgb 10.8
- Urinalysis negative

Constipation r/t low-fiber diet and inactivity (aeb infrequent, hard stools; painful defecation; abdominal distension)

Bowel Elimination aeb
- comfort of stool passage
- ingests adequate fiber
- exercises adequate amount

Constipation/Impaction Management

- Encourage increased fluid intake, unless contraindicated
- Identify factors (e.g., medications, bed rest, diet) that may cause or contribute to constipation
- Evaluate medication profile for gastrointestinal side effects
- Instruct Mrs. B. on a high-fiber diet, as appropriate
- Teach Mrs. B. how to keep a food diary
- Instruct her on the relationship of diet, exercise, and fluid intake to constipation and impaction

Exercise Promotion

- Assist in identifying a positive role model for maintaining the exercise program
- Encourage verbalization of feelings about exercise or need for exercise
- Instruct her about appropriate types of exercise for her level of health, in collaboration with a physician
- Assist Mrs. B. to set short-term and long-term goals for the exercise program
- Inform Mrs. B. about the health benefits and physiologic effects of exercise

Outcome not met
- Mrs. B. has kept a food diary and is able to identify the need for more fluid and fiber but has not consistently included fiber in her diet
- she has started a walking program with a neighbor but is only able to walk for 10 minutes at a time twice a week
- she states her last bowel movement was 3 days ago

Legend: Assessment ☐ Nursing Diagnosis ☐ Outcomes ☐ Nursing Interventions ☐ Activities ☐ Evaluation/Reassessment ☐

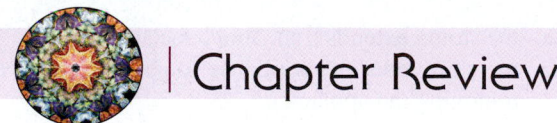

Chapter Review

EXPLORE MediaLink

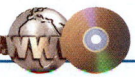

NCLEX review questions, case studies, care plan activities, MediaLink applications, and other interactive resources for this chapter can be found on the Companion Website at www.prenhall.com/kozier. Click on Chapter 46 to select the activities for this chapter.

For animations, more NCLEX review questions, and an audio glossary, access the Student CD-ROM accompanying this textbook.

Chapter Highlights

- Primary functions of the large intestine are the excretion of digestive waste products and the maintenance of fluid balance.
- Patterns of fecal elimination vary greatly among people, but a regular pattern of fecal elimination with formed, soft stools is essential to health and a sense of well-being.
- A variety of factors affects defecation: developmental level, diet, fluid intake, activity and exercise, psychologic factors, regular defecation, medications, diagnostic procedures, anesthesia, and pathologic conditions.
- Normal defecation is often facilitated in both well and ill clients by providing privacy, teaching clients to attend to defecation urges promptly, assisting clients to normal sitting positions whenever possible, encouraging appropriate food and fluid intake, and scheduling regular exercise.
- Common fecal elimination problems include constipation, diarrhea, bowel incontinence, and flatulence. Each has specific defining characteristics and contributing causes that often relate to or are identical to the factors that affect defecation.
- Lack of exercise, irregular defecation habits, bland diets, and overuse of laxatives are all thought to contribute to constipation. Sufficient fluid and fiber intake are required to keep feces soft.
- An adverse effect of constipation is straining during defecation, during which the Valsalva maneuver may be used. Cardiac problems may ensue.
- An adverse effect of prolonged diarrhea is fluid and electrolyte imbalance.
- Assessment relative to fecal elimination includes a nursing history; physical examination of the abdomen, rectum, and anus; and in some situations, visualization studies and inspection and analysis of stool for abnormal constituents such as blood.

- A nursing history includes data about the client's defecating pattern, description of feces and any changes, problems associated with elimination, and data about possible factors altering bowel elimination.
- When inspecting the client's stool, the nurse must observe its color, consistency, shape, amount, odor, and the presence of abnormal constituents.
- A function of the nurse is to assist clients with diet and bowel preparation before endoscopic and radiographic studies of the large intestine.
- NANDA-approved nursing diagnoses that relate specifically to altered bowel elimination include *Risk for Constipation, Constipation, Perceived Constipation, Diarrhea,* and *Bowel Incontinence.* However, because altered elimination patterns affect several areas of human functioning, diagnoses such as *Risk for Deficient Fluid Volume, Low Self-Esteem,* and *Risk for Impaired Skin Integrity* may also apply.
- Nursing strategies include administering cathartics and antidiarrheals; administering cleansing, carminative, or retention enemas; inserting rectal tubes to decrease flatulence; applying protective skin agents; monitoring fluid and electrolyte balance; and instructing clients in ways to promote normal defecation.
- Digital removal of an impaction should be carried out gently because of vagal nerve stimulation and subsequent depressed cardiac rate. A physician's order is often necessary.
- Clients who have bowel diversion ostomies require special care, with attention to psychologic adjustment, diet, and stoma and skin care. A variety of stomal management methods is available to these clients, depending on the type and position of the ostomy.

Review Questions

46–1. Clients should be taught that repeatedly ignoring the sensation of needing to defecate could result in
  a. constipation.
  b. diarrhea.
  c. incontinence.
  d. hemorrhoids.

46–2. Which of the following statements from an older adult who is prone to constipation indicates a need for increased teaching?
  a. "I need to drink one and a half to two quarts of liquids each day."

b. "I should take a laxative such as milk of magnesia if I don't have a stool in 24 hours."

c. "If my bowel pattern changes on its own, I should call you."

d. "Eating my meals at the same time every day increases the chance that I will have regular bowel movements."

46–3. A client will be undergoing a sigmoidoscopy requiring visualization of the anus, rectum, and sigmoid colon. The nurse expects the preparation to include which type of enema?

a. oil retention

b. return flow

c. high, large volume

d. low, small volume

46–4. While assessing an established colostomy, the nurse reports it as an unusual finding if

a. the stoma extends ½ in. above the abdomen.

b. the skin under the appliance looks red briefly after removing the appliance.

c. the stoma color is a deep red-purple.

d. an ascending colostomy delivers liquid feces.

46–5. An appropriate goal for clients with diarrhea thought to be a result of an antibiotic given to treat an upper respiratory infection would be which of the following?

a. The client will wear a medic-alert bracelet for antibiotic allergy.

b. The client will return to his or her previous fecal elimination pattern.

c. The client verbalizes the need to take an antidiarrheal medication every 4 hours around the clock.

d. The client verbalizes the need to increase intake of insoluble fiber such as grains and cereals.

Readings and References

Suggested Readings

Nyam, D. C. N. K. (2000). Fecal incontinence: Hope for an underdiagnosed condition. *Singapore Medical Journal, 41*(4), 188–192.
The physician author of this article reviews the epidemiology of fecal incontinence and presents a very systematic method of assessing and managing incontinence. Although a few interventions are medical in nature, the majority involve diet, over-the-counter medications, bowel exercise programs, and teaching. A very practical and useful review.

Ross, H. (1998). Constipation: Cause and control in an acute hospital setting. *British Journal of Nursing, 7*, 907–913.
In this article, the author reviews the existing literature on causes of constipation plus treatment availability, advantages, and disadvantages. It is intended to assist hospital nurses in establishing a systematic bowel program.

Thompson, J. (2000). A practical ostomy guide. *RN, 63*(11), 61–64, 66, 68, 71–73.
This is a very useful article that contains information for nurses assisting clients with ostomies from preop to recovery. Tables describe both fecal and urinary diversion surgeries. A list of patient support organizations is included.

Related Research

Annells, M., & Koch, T. (2002). Faecal impaction: Older people's experiences and nursing practice. *British Journal of Community Nursing, 7*(3), 118, 120–122, 124–126.

Hinrichs, M. D., & Huseboe, J. (2001). Research-based protocol: Management of constipation. *Journal of Gerontological Nursing, 27*(2), 17–28.

Schmelzer, M., Case, P., Chappell, S. M., & Wright, K. B. (2000). Colonic cleansing, fluid absorption, and discomfort following tap water and soapsuds enemas. *Applied Nursing Research, 13*, 83–91.

References

Johnson, M., Maas, M., & Moorhead, S. (Eds.). (2000). *Nursing outcomes classification (NOC)* (2nd ed.). St. Louis, MO: Mosby.

Koch, T., & Hudson, S. (2000). Older people and laxative use: Literature review and pilot study report. *Journal of Clinical Nursing, 9*, 516–525.

McCloskey, J. C., & Bulechek, G. M. (Eds.). (2000). *Nursing interventions classification (NIC)* (3rd ed.). St. Louis, MO: Mosby.

NANDA International. (2003). *NANDA nursing diagnoses: Definitions and classification 2003-2004*. Philadelphia: Author.

Selected Bibliography

Addison, R., Ness. W., Abulafi, M., & Swift, I. (2000). How to administer enemas and suppositories. *Nursing Times, 96*(6), 3–4.

Anonymous. (2000). Quick reference guide 13: Protocols for stoma care. *Nursing Standard, 14*(20), insert 2p.

Arnold, M. (2002). Ostomy care. *Advance for Providers of Post-Acute Care, 5*(2), 18–19.

Ball, E. M. (2000). A teaching guide for continent ileostomy. *RN, 63*(12), 35–36, 38, 40.

Butler, M. (1998). Laxatives and rectal preparations. *Nursing Times, 94*(3), 56–58.

Fries, C. F. (1999). Wound care: Managing an ostomy. *Nursing, 29*(8), 26.

Kenny, K. A., & Skelly, J. M. (2001). Dietary fiber for constipation in older adults: A systematic review. *Clinical Effectiveness in Nursing, 5*(3), 120–128.

Moppett, S. (1999). Practical procedures for nurses: Administration of an enema. *Nursing Times, 95*(22), insert 2p.

O'Brien, B. K. (1999). Coming of age with an ostomy: Life with a stoma may be especially difficult for teens. *American Journal of Nursing, 99*(8), 71–74, 76.

Plaisance, L., & Ellis, J. A. (2002). Opioid-induced constipation. *American Journal of Nursing, 102*(3), 72–73.

Selig, H., & Boyle, J. (2001). Bowel care and maintenance in long-term care. *Canadian Nurse, 97*(8), 28–33.

Vaccari, J. A. (1998). Making it easy for patients to clean colostomy pouches. . . . This practice may actually harm patients. *RN, 61*(12), 9–10.

CHAPTER 47

URINARY ELIMINATION

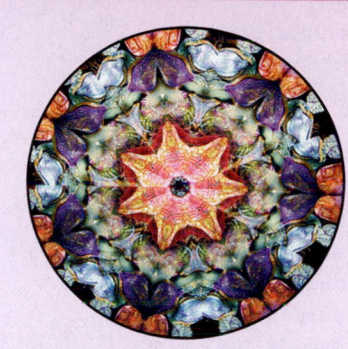

LEARNING OUTCOMES

After completing this chapter, you will be able to:

- Describe the process of urination, from urine formation through micturition.

- Identify factors that influence urinary elimination.

- Identify common causes of selected urinary problems.

- Describe nursing assessment of urinary function including subjective and objective data.

- Identify normal and abnormal characteristics and constituents of urine.

- Develop nursing diagnoses, desired outcomes, and interventions related to urinary elimination.

- Delineate ways to prevent urinary infection.

- Explain the care of clients with retention catheters or urinary diversions.

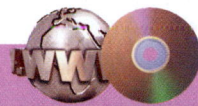

MediaLink

www.prenhall.com/kozier

Additional resources for this chapter can be found on the Student CD-ROM accompanying this textbook, and on the Companion Website at www.prenhall.com/kozier. Click on Chapter 47 to select the activities for this chapter.

CD-ROM
- Audio Glossary
- NCLEX Review
- Animations:
   Renal Function
   Furosemide Drug
   Catheterization
   A & P Review

Companion Website
- Additional NCLEX Review
- Case Study: Intermittent Self-Catheterization
- Care Plan Activity: Client Who Just Had Urinary Catheter Removed
- MediaLink Application: Urinary Incontinence
- Links to Resources

Elimination from the urinary tract is usually taken for granted. Only when a problem arises do most people become aware of their urinary habits and any associated symptoms.

A person's urinary habits depend on social culture, personal habits, and physical abilities. In North America, most people are accustomed to privacy and clean (even decorative) surroundings while they urinate.

Personal habits regarding urination are affected by the social propriety of leaving to urinate, the availability of a private clean facility, and initial bladder training. Urinary elimination is essential to health, and voiding can be postponed for only so long before the urge normally becomes too great to control.

PHYSIOLOGY OF URINARY ELIMINATION

Urinary elimination depends on effective functioning of four urinary tract organs: kidneys, ureters, bladder, and urethra (Figure 47–1 ■).

Kidneys

The paired kidneys are situated on either side of the spinal column, behind the peritoneal cavity. They are the primary regulators of fluid and acid–base balance in the body. The functional units of the kidneys, the nephrons, filter the blood and remove metabolic wastes. In the average adult 1,200 mL of blood, or about 21% of the cardiac output, passes through the kidneys every minute. Each kidney contains approximately 1 million nephrons. Each nephron has a **glomerulus,** a tuft of capillaries surrounded by Bowman's capsule (Figure 47–2 ■). The endothelium of glomerular capillaries is porous, allowing fluid and solutes to readily move across this membrane into the capsule. Plasma proteins and blood cells, however, are too large to cross the membrane normally. Glomerular filtrate is similar in composition to plasma, made up of water, electrolytes, glucose, amino acids, and metabolic wastes.

From Bowman's capsule the filtrate moves into the tubule of the nephron. In the proximal convoluted tubule, most of the water and electrolytes are reabsorbed. Solutes such as glucose are re-

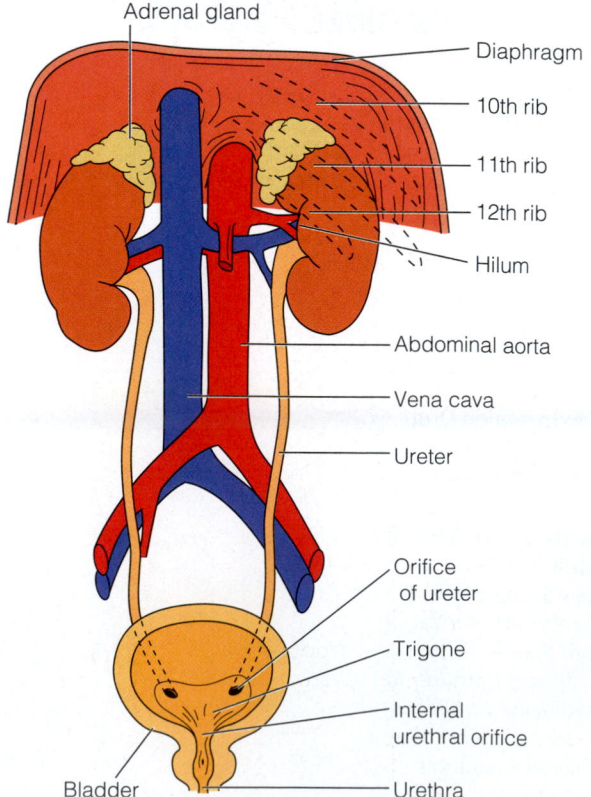

Figure 47–1 ■ Anatomic structures of the urinary tract.

Labels: Adrenal gland, Diaphragm, 10th rib, 11th rib, 12th rib, Hilum, Abdominal aorta, Vena cava, Ureter, Orifice of ureter, Trigone, Internal urethral orifice, Bladder, Urethra

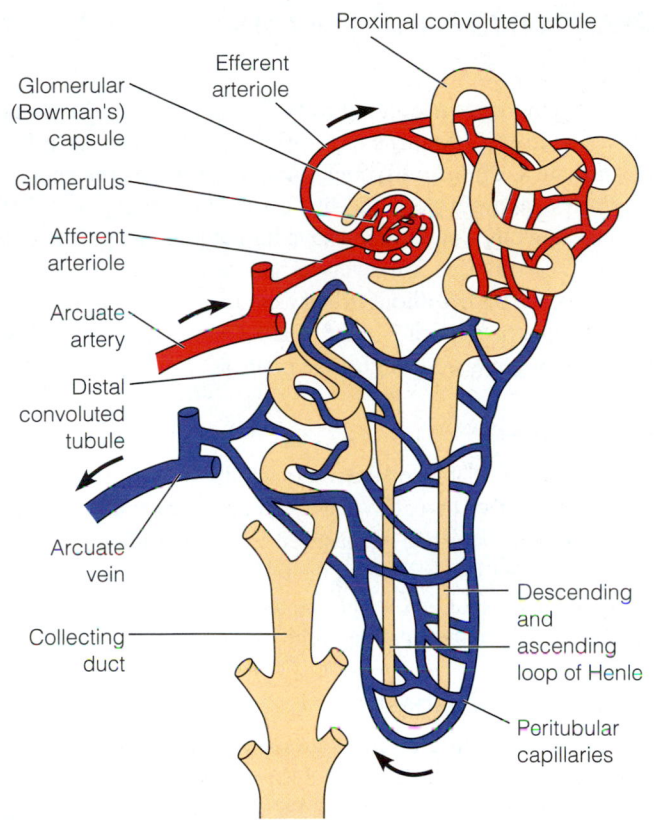

Figure 47–2 ■ The nephrons of the kidney are composed of six parts: the glomerulus, Bowman's capsule, proximal convoluted tubule, loop of Henle, distal convoluted tubule, and collecting duct.

absorbed in the loop of Henle, but in the same area, other substances are secreted into the filtrate, concentrating the urine. In the distal convoluted tubule, additional water and sodium are reabsorbed under the control of hormones such as antidiuretic hormone (ADH) and aldosterone. This controlled reabsorption allows fine regulation of fluid and electrolyte balance in the body. When fluid intake is low or the concentration of solutes in the blood is high, ADH is released from the anterior pituitary, more water is reabsorbed in the distal tubule, and less urine is excreted. By contrast, when fluid intake is high or the blood solute concentration is low, ADH is suppressed. Without ADH, the distal tubule becomes impermeable to water, and more urine is excreted. Aldosterone also affects the tubule. When aldosterone is released from the adrenal cortex, sodium and water are reabsorbed in greater quantities, increasing the blood volume and decreasing urinary output.

Ureters

Once the urine is formed in the kidneys, it moves through the collecting ducts into the calyces of the renal pelvis and from there into the ureters. The ureters are from 25 to 30 cm (10 to 12 in.) long in the adult and about 1.25 cm (0.5 in.) in diameter. The upper end of each ureter is funnel shaped as it enters the kidney. The lower ends of the ureters enter the bladder at the posterior corners of the floor of the bladder (see Figure 47–1). At the junction

between the ureter and the bladder, a flaplike fold of mucous membrane acts as a valve to prevent **reflux** (backflow) of urine up the ureters.

Bladder

The urinary bladder is a hollow, muscular organ that serves as a reservoir for urine and as the organ of excretion. When empty, it lies behind the symphysis pubis. In men, the bladder lies in front of the rectum and above the prostate gland (Figure 47–3 ■); in women it lies in front of the uterus and vagina (Figure 47–4 ■). The wall of the bladder is made up of four layers: (a) an inner mucous layer, (b) a connective tissue layer, (c) three layers of smooth muscle fibers, some of which extend lengthwise, some obliquely, and some more or less circularly, and (d) an outer serous layer. The smooth muscle layers are collectively called the **detrusor muscle.** The **trigone** at the base of the bladder is a triangular area marked by the ureter openings at the posterior corners and the opening of the urethra at the anterior inferior corner.

The bladder is capable of considerable distention because of rugae (folds) in the mucous membrane lining and because of the elasticity of its walls. When full, the dome of the bladder

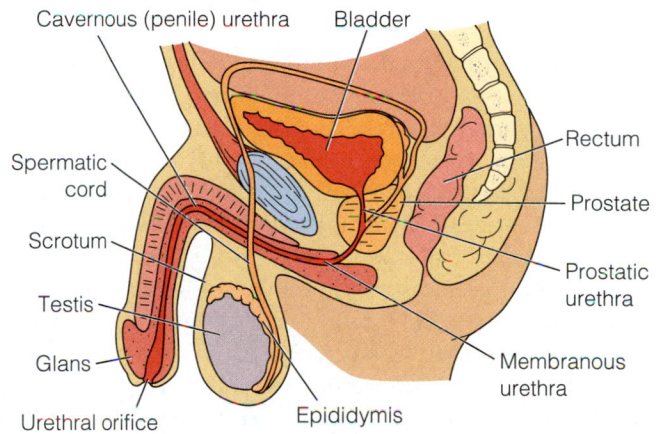

Figure 47–3 ■ The male urogenital system.

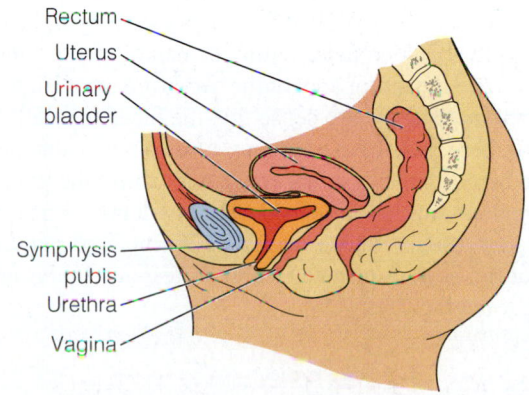

Figure 47–4 ■ The female urogenital system.

may extend above the symphysis pubis; in extreme situations, it may extend as high as the umbilicus.

Urethra

The urethra extends from the bladder to the urinary **meatus** (opening). In the adult woman, the urethra lies directly behind the symphysis pubis, anterior to the vagina, and is about 3.7 cm (1.5 in.) long (see Figure 47–4). The urethra serves only as a passageway for the elimination of urine. The urinary meatus is located between the labia minora, in front of the vagina and below the clitoris. The male urethra is about 20 cm (8 in.) long and serves as a passageway for semen as well as urine (see Figure 47–3). The meatus is located at the distal end of the penis.

The internal sphincter muscle situated at the base of the urinary bladder is under involuntary control. The external sphincter muscle is under voluntary control, allowing the individual to choose when urine is eliminated.

In both men and women, the urethra has a mucous membrane lining that is continuous with the bladder and the ureters. Thus, an infection of the urethra can extend through the urinary tract to the kidneys. Women are particularly prone to urinary tract infections because of their short urethra and the proximity of the urinary meatus to the vagina and anus.

Urination

Micturition, voiding, and **urination** all refer to the process of emptying the urinary bladder. Urine collects in the bladder until pressure stimulates special sensory nerve endings in the bladder wall called stretch receptors. This occurs when the adult bladder contains between 250 and 450 mL of urine. In children, a considerably smaller volume, 50 to 200 mL, stimulates these nerves.

The stretch receptors transmit impulses to the spinal cord, specifically to the voiding reflex center located at the level of the second to fourth sacral vertebrae, causing the internal sphincter to relax and stimulating the urge to void. If the time and place are appropriate for urination, the conscious portion of the brain relaxes the external urethral sphincter muscle and urination takes place. If the time and place are inappropriate, the micturition reflex usually subsides until the bladder becomes more filled and the reflex is stimulated again.

Voluntary control of urination is possible only if the nerves supplying the bladder and urethra, the neural tracts of the cord and brain, and the motor area of the cerebrum are all intact. The individual must be able to sense that the bladder is full. Injury to any of these parts of the nervous system—for example, by a cerebral hemorrhage or spinal cord injury above the level of the sacral region—results in intermittent involuntary emptying of the bladder. Elders whose cognition is impaired may not be aware of the need to urinate or able to respond to this urge by seeking toilet facilities.

FACTORS AFFECTING VOIDING

Numerous factors affect the volume and characteristics of the urine produced and the manner in which it is excreted.

Developmental Factors

Infants

Urine output varies according to fluid intake but gradually increases to 250 to 500 mL a day during the first year. An infant may urinate as often as 20 times a day. The urine of the neonate is colorless and odorless and has a specific gravity of 1.008. Because newborns and infants have immature kidneys, they are unable to concentrate urine very effectively.

Infants are born without urinary control. Most will develop this between the ages of 2 and 5 years. Control during the daytime normally precedes nighttime control.

Preschoolers

The preschooler is able to take responsibility for independent toileting. Parents need to realize that accidents do occur and the child should never be punished or chastised for this. Children often forget to wash their hands or flush the toilet and need instruction in wiping themselves. Girls should be taught to wipe from front to back to prevent contamination of the urinary tract by feces.

School-Age Children

The school-age child's elimination system reaches maturity during this period. The kidneys double in size between ages 5 and 10 years. During this period, the child urinates six to eight times a day. **Enuresis,** which is defined as the involuntary passing of urine when control should be established (about 5 years of age), can be a problem for some school-age children. About 10% of all 6-year-olds experience difficulty controlling the bladder. **Nocturnal enuresis,** or bed-wetting, is the involuntary passing of urine during sleep. Bed-wetting should not be considered a problem until after the age of 6. Nocturnal enuresis may be referred to as primary when the child has never achieved nighttime urinary control. The most common causes include genetic predisposition and delay of maturation (Cendron, 1999). The incidence of nocturnal enuresis declines as the child matures. Secondary enuresis is that which appears related to another physical problem such as stress or illness and resolves when the cause is eliminated.

Elders

The excretory function of the kidney diminishes with age, but usually not significantly below normal levels unless a disease process intervenes. Blood flow can be reduced by arteriosclerosis, impairing renal function. With age, the number of functioning nephrons decreases to some degree, impairing the kidney's filtering abilities. Conditions that alter normal fluid intake and output, such as having influenza or having surgery, can compromise the kidney's ability to filter, maintain acid–base balance, and maintain electrolyte balance in elders. It also takes a much longer time for these processes to return to normal functioning. The decrease in kidney function also places the elder at higher risk for toxicity from medications if excretion rates are longer.

The more noticeable changes with age are those related to the bladder. Complaints of urinary urgency and urinary fre-

TABLE 47-1 Changes in Urinary Elimination through the Life Span

Stage	Variations
Fetuses	The fetal kidney begins to excrete urine between the 11th and 12th week of development.
Infants	Ability to concentrate urine is minimal; therefore, urine appears light yellow.
	Because of neuromuscular immaturity, voluntary urinary control is absent.
Children	Kidney function reaches maturity between the first and second year of life; urine is concentrated effectively and appears a normal amber color.
	Between 18 and 24 months of age, the child starts to recognize bladder fullness and is able to hold urine beyond the urge to void.
	At approximately 2 1/2 to 3 years of age, the child can perceive bladder fullness, hold urine after the urge to void, and communicate the need to urinate.
	Full urinary control usually occurs at age 4 or 5 years; daytime control is usually achieved by age 3 years.
	The kidneys grow in proportion to overall body growth.
Adults	The kidneys reach maximum size between 35 and 40 years of age.
	After 50 years, the kidneys begin to diminish in size and function. Most shrinkage occurs in the cortex of the kidney as individual nephrons are lost.
Elders	An estimated 30% of nephrons are lost by age 80.
	Renal blood flow decreases because of vascular changes and a decrease in cardiac output.
	The ability to concentrate urine declines.
	Bladder muscle tone diminishes, causing increased frequency of urination and nocturia (awakening to urinate at night).
	Diminished bladder muscle tone and contractibility may lead to residual urine in the bladder after voiding, increasing the risk of bacterial growth and infection.
	Urinary incontinence may occur due to mobility problems or neurologic impairments.

quency are common. In men, these changes are often due to an enlarged prostate gland and in women to weakened muscles supporting the bladder or weakness of the urethral sphincter. The capacity of the bladder and its ability to completely empty diminish with age. This explains the need for elders to arise during the night to void (**nocturnal frequency**) and the retention of residual urine, predisposing the elder to bladder infections.

See Table 47–1 for a summary of the developmental changes affecting urinary output and the Lifespan Considerations feature.

Psychosocial Factors

For many people, a set of conditions helps stimulate the micturition reflex. These conditions include privacy, normal position, sufficient time, and, occasionally, running water. Circumstances that counter the client's accustomed conditions may produce anxiety and muscle tension. As a result, the person is unable to relax abdominal and perineal muscles and the external urethral sphincter and voiding is inhibited. People also may voluntarily suppress urination because of perceived time pressures; for example, nurses often ignore the urge to void until they are able to take a break. This behavior can increase the risk of urinary tract infections.

Fluid and Food Intake

The healthy body maintains a balance between the amount of fluid ingested and the amount of fluid eliminated. When the amount of fluid intake increases, therefore, the output normally increases. Certain fluids, such as alcohol, increase fluid output by inhibiting the production of antidiuretic hormone. Fluids that contain caffeine (e.g., coffee, tea, and cola drinks) also increase urine production. By contrast, food and fluids high in sodium can cause fluid retention because water is retained to maintain the normal concentration of electrolytes.

Some foods and fluids can change the color of urine. For example, beets can cause urine to appear red; foods containing carotene can cause the urine to appear yellower than usual.

Medications

Many medications, particularly those affecting the autonomic nervous system, interfere with the normal urination process and may cause retention (see Box 47–1). **Diuretics** (e.g., chlorothiazide and furosemide) increase urine formation by preventing the reabsorption of water and electrolytes from the tubules of the kidney into the bloodstream. Some medications may alter the color of the urine.

Muscle Tone

Good muscle tone is important to maintain the stretch and contractility of the detrusor muscle so the bladder can fill adequately and empty completely. Clients who require a retention catheter for a long period may have poor bladder muscle tone because continuous drainage of urine prevents the bladder from filling and emptying normally. Abdominal and pelvic muscle tone also contribute: Abdominal muscle contraction assists in

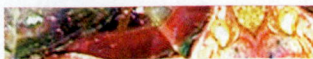

Lifespan Considerations

Factors Affecting Voiding
Infants and Children

- Urinary tract infections are the second most common infection in children; occurring more frequently in newborn and young infant boys due to obstructions and more frequently in older infant girls due to contamination of the urethra with stool (Ball & Bindler, 2003).
- Teaching proper perineal hygiene can reduce infection. Girls should learn to wipe from front to back and wear cotton underwear.
- Teach children and parents that they should go to the bathroom as soon as the sensation to void is felt and not try to hold the urine in.

Elders

Many changes of aging, cause specific problems in urinary elimination in the older adult. Many conditions can be treated and interventions can be used to either resolve or decrease the problem. Some of the following conditions are etiological factors in problems with urinary elimination:

- Many older men have enlarged prostate glands, which can cause retention and incontinence of urine.

- Women past menopause have decreased estrogen, which results in a decrease in perineal tone and support of bladder, vagina, and supporting tissues. This often results in urgency and stress incontinence and can even increase the incidence of urinary tract infections.
- Increased stiffness and pain in joints, previous joint surgery, and neuromuscular problems can impair mobility and often make it difficult to get to the bathroom.
- Cognitive impairment, such as in dementia, often prevents the person from understanding the need to urinate and the actions needed to perform the activity.
   Interventions that may improve these conditions are:
- Medications or surgery to relieve obstructions in men and strengthen support in the urogenital area in women.
- Behavioral training for better bladder control
- Providing safe, easy access to the bathroom or bedside commode, whether at home or in an institution. Make sure the room is well lit, the environment is safe, and the proper assistive devices are within reach (such as walkers, canes).
- Habit training, such as taking the person to the bathroom at a regular, scheduled time can often work very well with cognitively impaired persons.

BOX 47–1 ■ Medications that May Cause Urinary Retention

- Anticholinergic and antispasmodic medications, such as atropine and papaverine
- Antidepressant and antipsychotic agents, such as phenothiazines and MAO inhibitors
- Antihistamine preparations, such as pseudoephedrine (Actifed and Sudafed)
- Antihypertensives, such as hydralazine (Apresoline) and methyldopate (Aldomet)
- Antiparkinsonism drugs, such as levodopa, trihexyphenidyl (Artane), and benztropine mesylate (Cogentin)
- Beta-adrenergic blockers, such as propranolol (Inderal)
- Opioids, such as hydrocodone (Vicodin)

---

bladder emptying; pelvic muscle tone is a factor in being able to retain urine voluntarily once the urge to urinate is perceived.

Pathologic Conditions

Some diseases and pathologies can affect the formation and excretion of urine. Diseases of the kidneys may affect the ability of the nephrons to produce urine. Abnormal amounts of protein or blood cells may be present in the urine, or the kidneys may virtually stop producing urine altogether, a condition known as renal failure. Heart and circulatory disorders such as heart failure, shock, or hypertension can affect blood flow to the kidneys, interfering with urine production. If abnormal amounts of fluid are lost through another route (e.g., vomiting or high fever), water is retained by the kidneys and urinary output falls.

Processes that interfere with the flow of urine from the kidneys to the urethra affect urinary excretion. A urinary stone (calculus) may obstruct a ureter, blocking urine flow from the kidney to the bladder. Hypertrophy of the prostate gland, a common condition affecting older men, may obstruct the urethra, impairing urination and bladder emptying.

Surgical and Diagnostic Procedures

Some surgical and diagnostic procedures affect the passage of urine and the urine itself. The urethra may swell following a cystoscopy, and surgical procedures on any part of the urinary tract may result in some postoperative bleeding; as a result, the urine may be red or pink tinged for a time.

Spinal anesthetics can affect the passage of urine because they decrease the client's awareness of the need to void. Surgery on structures adjacent to the urinary tract (e.g., the uterus) can also affect voiding because of swelling in the lower abdomen.

ALTERED URINE PRODUCTION

Although people's patterns of urination are highly individual, most people void about five times a day. People usually void when they first awaken in the morning, before they go to bed, and around mealtimes. Table 47–2 shows the average urinary output per day at different ages.

Polyuria

Polyuria (or **diuresis**) refers to the production of abnormally large amounts of urine by the kidneys, often several liters more

TABLE 47–2 Average Daily Urine Output by Age

Age	Amount (mL)
1 to 2 days	15–60
3 to 10 days	100–300
10 days to 2 months	250–450
2 months to 1 year	400–500
1 to 3 years	500–600
3 to 5 years	600–700
5 to 8 years	700–1000
8 to 14 years	800–1400
14 years through adulthood	1,500
Older adulthood	1,500 or less

than the client's usual daily output. Polyuria can follow excessive fluid intake, a condition known as **polydipsia,** or may be associated with diseases such as diabetes mellitus, diabetes insipidus, and chronic nephritis. Polyuria can cause excessive fluid loss, leading to intense thirst, dehydration, and weight loss.

Oliguria and Anuria

The terms oliguria and anuria are used to describe decreased urinary output. **Oliguria** is low urine output, usually less than 500 mL a day or 30 mL an hour. Although oliguria may occur because of abnormal fluid losses or a lack of fluid intake, it often indicates impaired blood flow to the kidneys or impending renal failure and should be promptly reported to the primary care provider. Restoring renal blood flow and urinary output promptly can prevent renal failure and its complications. **Anuria** refers to a lack of urine production.

Should the kidneys become unable to adequately function, some mechanism of filtering the blood is necessary to prevent illness and death. This filtering is done though the use of renal **dialysis,** a technique by which fluids and molecules pass through a semipermeable membrane according to the rules of osmosis. The two most common methods of dialysis are hemodialysis and peritoneal dialysis. In hemodialysis, the client's blood flows through vascular catheters, passes by the dialysis solution in an external machine, and then returns to the client. In peritoneal dialysis, the dialysis solution is instilled into the abdominal cavity through a catheter, allowed to rest there while the fluid and molecules exchange, and then removed through the catheter. Both hemodialysis and peritoneal dialysis must be performed at frequent intervals until the client's kidneys can resume the filtering function.

ALTERED URINARY ELIMINATION

Despite normal urine production, a number of factors or conditions can affect urinary elimination. Frequency, nocturia, urgency, and dysuria often are manifestations of underlying conditions such as a urinary tract infection. Enuresis, incontinence, retention, and neurogenic bladder may be either a manifestation or the primary problem affecting urinary elimination.

Selected factors associated with altered patterns of urine elimination are identified in Table 47–3.

Frequency and Nocturia

Urinary frequency is voiding at frequent intervals, that is, more often than usual. An increased intake of fluid causes some increase in the frequency of voiding. Conditions such as urinary tract infection, stress, and pregnancy can cause frequent voiding of small quantities (50 to 100 mL) of urine. Total fluid intake and output may be normal.

Nocturia is voiding two or more times at night. Like frequency, it is usually expressed in terms of the number of times the person gets out of bed to void, for example, "nocturia $\times$ 4."

Urgency

Urgency is the feeling that the person must void. There may or may not be a great deal of urine in the bladder, but the person feels a need to void immediately. Urgency accompanies psychologic stress and irritation of the trigone and urethra. It is also common in young children who have poor external sphincter control.

Dysuria

Dysuria means voiding that is either painful or difficult. It can accompany a stricture (decrease in caliber) of the urethra, urinary infections, and injury to the bladder and urethra. Often clients will say they have to push to void or that burning accompanies or follows voiding. The burning may be described as severe, like a hot poker, or more subdued, like a sunburn. Often, **urinary hesitancy** (a delay and difficulty in initiating voiding) is associated with dysuria.

Enuresis

Enuresis is involuntary urination in children beyond the age when voluntary bladder control is normally acquired, usually 4 or 5 years of age. Nocturnal enuresis often is irregular in occurrence and affects boys more often than girls. Diurnal (daytime) enuresis may be persistent and pathologic in origin. It affects women and girls more frequently.

Urinary Incontinence

Urinary incontinence, or involuntary urination, is a symptom, not a disease. It can have a significant impact on the client's life, creating physical problems such as skin breakdown and possibly leading to psychosocial problems such as embarrassment, isolation, and social withdrawal. Although incontinence is common in elders, it is not a normal consequence of aging and can often be treated. All clients should be asked about their voiding patterns. If incontinence is described, a thorough history and assessment is indicated. Clients at highest risk for developing incontinence include those with a history of urinary tract infections, surgery, or trauma; sexually transmitted diseases; multiple vaginal births; and musculoskeletal, endocrine, or neurological disorders (Shultz, 2002). NANDA categorizes five types of incontinence (see "Diagnosing" on page 1265). Treatment may include surgery, medication, or behavioral therapies.

TABLE 47–3 Selected Factors Associated with Altered Urinary Elimination

Pattern	Selected Associated Factors
Polyuria	Ingestion of fluids containing caffeine or alcohol
	Prescribed diuretic
	Presence of thirst, dehydration, and weight loss
	History of diabetes mellitus, diabetes insipidus, or kidney disease
Oliguria, anuria	Decrease in fluid intake
	Signs of dehydration
	Presence of hypotension, shock, or heart failure
	History of kidney disease
	Signs of renal failure such as elevated blood urea nitrogen (BUN) and serum creatinine, edema, hypertension
Frequency or nocturia	Pregnancy
	Increase in fluid intake
	Urinary tract infection
Urgency	Presence of psychologic stress
	Urinary tract infection
Dysuria	Urinary tract inflammation, infection, or injury
	Hesitancy, hematuria, pyuria (pus in the urine), and frequency
Enuresis	Family history of enuresis
	Difficult access to toilet facilities
	Home stresses
Incontinence	Bladder inflammation or other disease
	Difficulties in independent toileting (mobility impairment)
	Leakage when coughing, laughing, sneezing
	Cognitive impairment
Retention	Distended bladder on palpation and percussion
	Associated signs, such as pubic discomfort, restlessness, frequency, and small urine volume
	Recent anesthesia
	Recent perineal surgery
	Presence of perineal swelling
	Medications prescribed
	Lack of privacy or other factors inhibiting micturition

Urinary Retention

When emptying of the bladder is impaired, urine accumulates and the bladder becomes overdistended, a condition known as **urinary retention.** Overdistention of the bladder causes poor contractility of the detrusor muscle, further impairing urination. Common causes of urinary retention include prostatic hypertrophy (enlargement), surgery, and some medications (see Box 47–1).

Clients with urinary retention may experience overflow voiding or incontinence, eliminating 25 to 50 mL of urine at frequent intervals. The bladder is firm and distended on palpation and may be displaced to one side of midline.

Neurogenic Bladder

Impaired neurologic function can interfere with the normal mechanisms of urine elimination, resulting in a **neurogenic bladder.** The client with a neurogenic bladder does not per-

ceive bladder fullness and is unable to control the urinary sphincters. The bladder may become flaccid and distended or spastic, with frequent involuntary urination.

NURSING MANAGEMENT

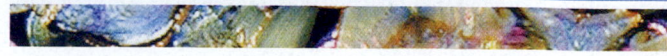

ASSESSING

A complete assessment of a client's urinary function includes the following:

- Nursing history
- Physical assessment of the genitourinary system, hydration status, and examination of the urine
- Relating the data obtained to the results of any diagnostic tests and procedures.

Assessment Interview

URINARY ELIMINATION

Voiding Pattern

- How many times do you urinate during a 24-hour period?
- Has this pattern changed recently?
- Do you need to get out of bed to void at night? How often?

Description of Urine and Any Changes

- How would you describe your urine in terms of color, clarity (clear, transparent, or cloudy), and odor (faint or strong)?

Urinary Elimination Problems

- What problems have you had or do you now have with passing your urine?
- Passage of small amounts of urine?
- Voiding at intervals that are more frequent?
- Trouble getting to the bathroom in time or feeling an urgent need to void?
- Painful voiding?
- Difficulty starting urine stream?
- Frequent dribbling of urine or feeling of bladder fullness associated with voiding small amounts of urine?
- Reduced force of stream?
- Accidental leakage of urine? If so, when does this occur (e.g., when coughing, laughing, or sneezing; at night; during the day)?

- Past urinary tract illness such as infection of the kidney, bladder, or urethra; urinary calculi; surgery of kidney, ureters, or bladder?

Factors Influencing Urinary Elimination

- Medications. Do you take any medications that could increase urinary output or cause retention of urine? Note specific medication and dosage.
- Fluid intake. What amount and kind of fluid do you take each day (e.g., six glasses of water, two cups of coffee, three cola drinks with or without caffeine)?
- Environmental factors. Do you have any problems with toileting (mobility, removing clothing, toilet seat too low, facility without grab bar)?
- Stress. Are you experiencing any major stress? If so, what are the stressors? Do you think these affect your urinary pattern?
- Disease. Have you had or do you have any illnesses that may affect urinary function, such as hypertension, heart disease, neurologic disease, cancer, prostatic enlargement, diabetes?
- Diagnostic procedures. Have you recently had a cystoscopy or anesthetic?

Nursing History

The nurse determines the client's normal voiding pattern and frequency, appearance of the urine and any recent changes, any past or current problems with urination, the presence of an ostomy, and factors influencing the elimination pattern.

Examples of interview questions to elicit this information are shown in the Assessment Interview. The number of questions asked depends on the individual and the responses to the first three categories.

Physical Assessment

Complete physical assessment of the urinary tract usually includes percussion of the kidneys to detect areas of tenderness. Palpation and percussion of the bladder are also performed. If the client's history or current problems indicate a need for it, the urethral meatus of both male and female clients is inspected for swelling, discharge, and inflammation.

Because problems with urination can affect the elimination of wastes from the body, it is important that the nurse assess the skin for color, texture, and tissue turgor as well as the presence of edema. If incontinence, dribbling, or dysuria is noted in the history, the skin of the perineum should be inspected for irritation because contact with urine can excoriate the skin.

Assessing Urine

Normal urine consists of 96% water and 4% solutes. Organic solutes include urea, ammonia, creatinine, and uric acid. Urea

is the chief organic solute. Inorganic solutes include sodium, chloride, potassium, sulfate, magnesium, and phosphorus. Sodium chloride is the most abundant inorganic salt. Characteristics of normal and abnormal urine are shown in Table 47–4.

Measuring Urinary Output. Normally, the kidneys produce urine at a rate of approximately 60 mL per hour or about 1,500 mL per day. Urine output is affected by many factors, including fluid intake, body fluid losses through other routes such as perspiration and breathing or diarrhea, and the cardiovascular and renal status of the individual.

Urine outputs below 30 mL per hour may indicate low blood volume or kidney malfunction and must be reported. To measure fluid output the nurse follows these steps:

- Wear clean gloves to prevent contact with microorganisms or blood in urine.
- Ask the client to void in a clean urinal, bedpan, commode, or toilet collection device ("hat").
- Instruct the client to keep urine separate from feces and to avoid putting toilet paper in the urine collection container.
- Pour the voided urine into a calibrated container.
- Holding the container at eye level, read the amount in the container. Containers usually have a measuring scale on the inside.
- Record the amount on the fluid intake and output sheet, which may be at the bedside or in the bathroom.
- Rinse the urine collection and measuring containers with cool water and store appropriately.

TABLE 47–4 Characteristics of Normal and Abnormal Urine

Characteristic	Normal	Abnormal	Nursing Considerations
Amount in 24 hours (adult)	1,200–1,500 mL	Under 1,200 mL A large amount over intake	Urinary output normally is approximately equal to fluid intake. Output of less than 30 mL/hr may indicate decreased blood flow to the kidneys and should be immediately reported.
Color, clarity	Straw, amber Transparent	Dark amber Cloudy Dark orange Red or dark brown Mucous plugs, viscid, thick	Concentrated urine is darker in color. Dilute urine may appear almost clear, or very pale yellow. Some foods and drugs may color urine. Red blood cells in the urine (hematuria) may be evident as pink, bright red, or rusty brown urine. Menstrual bleeding can also color urine but should not be confused with hematuria. White blood cells, bacteria, pus, or contaminants such as prostatic fluid, sperm, or vaginal drainage may cause cloudy urine.
Odor	Faint aromatic	Offensive	Some foods (e.g., asparagus) cause a musty odor; infected urine can have a fetid odor; urine high in glucose has a sweet odor.
Sterility	No microorganisms present	Microorganisms present	Urine specimens may be contaminated by bacteria from the perineum during collection.
pH	4.5–8	Over 8 Under 4.5	Freshly voided urine is normally somewhat acidic. Alkaline urine may indicate a state of alkalosis, urinary tract infection, or a diet high in fruits and vegetables. More acidic urine (low pH) is found in starvation, diarrhea, or with a diet high in protein foods or cranberries.
Specific gravity	1.010–1.025	Over 1.025 Under 1.010	Concentrated urine has a higher specific gravity; diluted urine has a lower specific gravity.
Glucose	Not present	Present	Glucose in the urine indicates high blood glucose levels (>180 mg/dL) and may be indicative of undiagnosed or uncontrolled diabetes mellitus.
Ketone bodies (acetone)	Not present	Present	Ketones, the end product of the breakdown of fatty acids, are not normally present in the urine. They may be present in the urine of clients who have uncontrolled diabetes mellitus, are in a state of starvation, or who have ingested excessive amounts of aspirin.
Blood	Not present	Occult (microscopic) Bright red	Blood may be present in the urine of clients who have urinary tract infection, kidney disease, or bleeding from the urinary tract.

- Remove gloves and wash hands.
- Calculate and document the total output at the end of each shift and at the end of 24 hours on the client's chart.

Many clients can measure and record their own urine output when the procedure is explained to them.

When measuring urine from a client who has an indwelling catheter, the nurse follows these steps:

- Don clean gloves.
- Take the calibrated container to the bedside.
- Place the container under the urine collection bag so that the spout of the bag is above the container but not touching it. The calibrated container is not sterile, but the inside of the collection bag is sterile.

- Open the spout and permit the urine to flow into the container.
- Close the spout, then proceed as described in the previous list.

Measuring Residual Urine. **Residual urine** (urine remaining in the bladder following the voiding) is normally not present or consists of only a few milliliters. However, a bladder outlet obstruction (e.g., enlargement of the prostate gland) or loss of bladder muscle tone may interfere with complete emptying of the bladder during urination. Manifestations of urine retention may include frequent voiding of small amounts (e.g., less than 100 mL in an adult). Urinary stasis and urinary tract infection are possible consequences of incomplete bladder emptying. Residual urine is measured to assess the amount of retained urine after voiding and determine the need for interventions (e.g., medications to promote detrusor muscle contraction).

To measure residual urine, the nurse catheterizes the client immediately after voiding. The amount of urine voided and the amount obtained by catheterization are measured and recorded. An indwelling catheter may be inserted if the residual urine exceeds a specified amount.

Diagnostic Tests

Blood levels of two metabolically produced substances, urea and creatinine, are routinely used to evaluate renal function. Both are normally eliminated by the kidneys through filtration and tubular secretion. Urea, the end product of protein metabolism, is measured as **blood urea nitrogen (BUN).** Creatinine is produced in relatively constant quantities by the muscles. The **creatinine clearance** test uses 24-hour urine and serum creatinine levels to determine the glomerular filtration rate, a sensitive indicator of renal function. Description of other tests related to urinary functions such as collecting urine specimens, measuring specific gravity, and visualization procedures are described in Chapter 32. ∞

DIAGNOSING

NANDA (2003) includes one general diagnostic label for urinary elimination problems and several labels that are more specific:

- *Impaired Urinary Elimination:* disturbance in urine elimination.

Other NANDA nursing diagnoses related to urinary elimination are subcategories of this diagnosis, and include

- *Functional Urinary Incontinence*
- *Reflex Urinary Incontinence*
- *Stress Urinary Incontinence*
- *Total Urinary Incontinence*
- *Urge Urinary Incontinence*
- *Urinary Retention*

Clinical examples of assessment data clusters and related nursing diagnoses, outcomes, and interventions are shown in Identifying Nursing Diagnosis, Outcomes, and Interventions and in the Nursing Care Plan and the Concept Map at the end of this chapter.

Problems of urinary elimination also may become the etiology for other problems experienced by the client. Examples include the following:

- *Risk for Infection* if the client has urinary retention or undergoes an invasive procedure such as catheterization or cystoscopic examination.
- *Low Self-Esteem* or *Social Isolation* if the client is incontinent. Incontinence can be physically and emotionally distressing to clients because it is considered socially unacceptable. Often the client is embarrassed about dribbling or having an accident and may restrict normal activities for this reason.
- *Risk for Impaired Skin Integrity* if the client is incontinent. Bed linens and clothes saturated with urine irritate and exco-

riate the skin. Prolonged skin dampness leads to dermatitis (inflammation of the skin) and subsequent formation of decubitus ulcers.

- *Self-Care Deficit:* Toileting if the client has functional incontinence.
- *Risk for Deficient Fluid Volume* or *Excess Fluid Volume* if the client has impaired urinary function associated with a disease process.
- *Disturbed Body Image* if the client has a urinary diversion ostomy.
- *Deficient Knowledge* if the client requires self-care skills to manage (e.g., a new urinary diversion ostomy).
- *Risk for Caregiver Role Strain* if the client is incontinent and being cared for by a family member for extended periods.

PLANNING

The goals established will vary according to the diagnosis and defining characteristics. Examples of overall goals for clients with urinary elimination problems may include the following:

- Maintain or restore a normal voiding pattern.
- Regain normal urine output.
- Prevent associated risks such as infection, skin breakdown, fluid and electrolyte imbalance, and lowered self-esteem.
- Perform toilet activities independently with or without assistive devices.

Appropriate preventive and corrective nursing interventions that relate to these must be identified. Specific nursing activities associated with each of these interventions can be selected to meet the client's individual needs. Examples of clinical applications of these using NANDA, NIC, and NOC designations are shown in Identifying Nursing Diagnoses, Outcomes, and Interventions and in the Nursing Care Plan and Concept Map at the end of the chapter.

Planning for Home Care

To provide for continuity of care, the nurse needs to consider the client's needs for teaching and assistance with care in the home. Discharge planning includes assessment of the client's and family's resources and abilities for self-care, available financial resources, and the need for referrals and home health services. The Home Care Assessment on page 1267 outlines an assessment of home care capabilities related to urinary elimination problems and needs. Teaching: Home Care on page 1268 addresses the learning needs of the client and family.

IMPLEMENTING
Maintaining Normal Urinary Elimination

Most interventions to maintain normal urinary elimination are independent nursing functions. These include promoting adequate fluid intake, maintaining normal voiding habits, and assisting with toileting.

Promoting Fluid Intake. Increasing fluid intake increases urine production, which in turn stimulates the micturition reflex. A normal daily intake averaging 1,500 mL of measurable fluids is adequate for most adult clients.

IDENTIFYING NURSING DIAGNOSES, OUTCOMES, AND INTERVENTIONS

CLIENTS WITH URINARY ELIMINATION DISORDERS

DATA CLUSTER	NURSING DIAGNOSIS/ DEFINITION	SAMPLE DESIRED OUTCOMES [NOC#]/DEFINITION	INDICATORS	SELECTED INTERVENTIONS [NIC#]/DEFINITION	SAMPLE NIC ACTIVITIES
Mrs. Amy Brown, 75, reports accidental loss of urine before she is able to reach the toilet. She is aware of the urge to void but states, "Because of my stroke I sometimes can't get there soon enough."	Functional Urinary Incontinence/Involuntary, unpredictable passage of urine	Urinary Continence [0502]/Control of the elimination of urine	Consistently demonstrates • Responds in timely manner to urge • Voids >150 mL each time • Absence of postvoid residual >100 mL	Prompted Voiding [0640]/Promotion of urinary continence through the use of timed verbal toileting reminders and positive social feedback for successful toileting	• Determine patient awareness of continence status by asking if wet or dry • Prompt up to three times to use toilet or substitute, regardless of continence status • Give positive feedback by praising desired toileting behavior • Document outcomes of toileting session
Anthony Cherry, a teenager with a spinal cord injury, has no awareness of bladder filling, the urge to void, or feelings of bladder fullness. He reports loss of urine at fairly regular intervals.	Reflex Urinary Incontinence/Involuntary loss of urine at somewhat predictable intervals when a specific bladder volume is reached	Urinary Elimination [0503]/Ability of the urinary system to filter wastes, conserve solutes, and collect and discharge urine in a healthy pattern	Not compromised: • 24-hour intake and output balance • Empties bladder completely • Urinary continence • Serum BUN, creatinine WNL	Urinary Catheterization: Intermittent [0582]/Regular periodic use of a catheter to empty the bladder	• Teach patient/ family purpose, supplies, method, and rationale of intermittent catheterization • Demonstrate procedure and have a return demonstration • Determine catheterization schedule based on a comprehensive assessment
Tammy Tyndale reports dribbling whenever she laughs, coughs, or sneezes. She is 8 months pregnant.	Stress Urinary Incontinence/Loss of less than 50 mL of urine occurring with increased abdominal pressure	Symptom Control [1608]/Personal actions to minimize perceived adverse changes in physical and emotional functioning	Consistently demonstrated • Uses preventive measure • Uses available resources	Pelvic Muscle Exercise [0560]/Strengthening and training the levator ani and urogenital muscles through voluntary repetitive contraction to decrease stress, urge, or mixed types of urinary incontinence	• Instruct patient to tighten, then relax, the ring of muscle around urethra and anus, as if trying to prevent urination or bowel movement • Assist to select appropriate incontinence garment/ pad for short-term management • Cleanse genital skin area at regular intervals

IDENTIFYING NURSING DIAGNOSES, OUTCOMES, AND INTERVENTIONS *continued*

CLIENTS WITH URINARY ELIMINATION DISORDERS

DATA CLUSTER	*NURSING DIAGNOSIS/ DEFINITION*	SAMPLE DESIRED OUTCOMES [NOC#]/*DEFINITION*	INDICATORS	SELECTED INTERVENTIONS [NIC#]/*DEFINITION*	SAMPLE NIC ACTIVITIES
Mrs. Gail Brady reports urinary urgency, difficulty in getting to the bathroom in time, frequency (more often than every 2 hours), and leakage of urine when unable to reach the toilet in time.	*Urge Urinary Incontinence/Involuntary passage of urine occurring soon after a strong sense of urgency to void*	Tissue Integrity: Skin and Mucous Membranes [1101]/ *Structural intactness and normal physiological function of skin and mucous membranes*	Not compromised: • Skin intactness	Urinary Bladder Training [0570]/ *Improving bladder function for those with urge incontinence by increasing the bladder's ability to hold urine and the patient's ability to suppress urination*	• Keep a continence record to establish voiding pattern • Establish interval for toileting, preferably more than 2 hours • Reduce toileting interval by 1/2 hour if more than 3 incontinence episodes in 24 hours • Increase interval by 1/2 hour if no incontinence episodes for 3 days until optimal 4-hour interval is reached

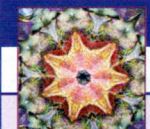

Home Care Assessment

URINARY ELIMINATION

Client and Environment

- Self-care abilities: Ability to consume adequate fluids, to perceive bladder fullness, to ambulate and get to the toilet, to manipulate clothing for toileting, and to perform hygiene measures after toileting
- Current level of knowledge: Fluid and dietary intake modifications to promote normal patterns of urinary elimination bladder training methods and specific techniques to promote voiding care for indwelling catheter or ostomy (if appropriate)
- Assistive devices required: Ambulatory aids such as walker, cane, or wheelchair; safety devices such as grab bars; toileting aids such as raised toilet seat, urinal, commode, or bedpan; presence of a urinary catheter
- Home environment factors that interfere with toileting: Distance to the bathroom from living areas or bedrooms; barriers such as stairways, scatter rugs, clutter, or narrow doorways that interfere with bathroom access; lighting (including night lighting)
- Urinary elimination problems: Type of incontinence and precipitating factors; manifestations of urinary tract infection such as dysuria, frequency, urgency; evidence of prostatic hypertrophy and effect on urination; ability to perform self-catheterization and care for other urinary elimination devices

such as indwelling catheter, urinary diversion ostomy, or condom drainage

Family

- Caregiver availability, skills, and responses: Ability and willingness to assume responsibilities for care, including assisting with toileting, intermittent catheterization, indwelling catheter care, urinary drainage devices or ostomy care; ready access to laundry facilities; access to and willingness to use respite or relief caregivers
- Family role changes and coping: Effect on spousal and family roles, sleep/rest patterns, sexuality, and social interactions
- Financial resources: Ability to purchase protective pads and garments, supplies for catheterization or ostomy care

Community

- Environment: Access to public restrooms and sanitary facilities
- Current knowledge of and experience with community resources: Medical and assistive equipment and supply companies, home health agencies, local pharmacies, available financial assistance, support and educational organizations

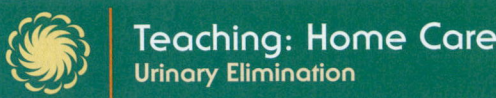

Teaching: Home Care
Urinary Elimination

Facilitating Urinary Elimination Self-Care

- Teach the client and family to maintain easy access to toilet facilities, including removing scatter rugs and ensuring that halls and doorways are free of clutter.
- Suggest graduated lighting for nighttime voiding: a dim night-light in the bedroom and low-wattage hallway lighting.
- Advise the client and family to install grab bars and elevated toilet seats as needed.
- Provide for instruction in safe transfer techniques. Contact physical therapy to provide training as needed.
- Suggest clothing that is easily removed for toileting, such as elastic waist pants or Velcro closures.

Promoting Urinary Elimination

- Instruct the client to respond to the urge to void as soon as possible; avoid voluntary urinary retention.
- Teach the client to empty the bladder completely at each voiding.
- Emphasize the importance of drinking eight to ten 8-ounce glasses of water daily.
- Teach female clients about Kegel exercises to strengthen perineal muscles.
- Inform the client about the relationship between tobacco use and bladder cancer and provide information about smoking cessation programs as indicated.
- Teach the client to promptly report any of the following to the primary care provider: pain or burning on urination, changes in urine color or clarity, malodorous urine, or changes in voiding patterns (e.g., nocturia, frequency, dribbling).

Asepsis

- Teach the client to maintain perineal-genital cleanliness, washing with soap and water daily and cleansing the anal and perineal area after defecating.
- Instruct female clients to wipe from front to back (from the urinary meatus toward the anus) after voiding, and to discard toilet paper after each swipe.
- Provide information about products to protect the skin, clothing, and furniture for clients who are incontinent. Emphasize the importance of cleaning and drying the perineal area after incontinence episodes. Instruct in the use of protective skin barrier products as needed.
- Teach clients with an indwelling catheter and their family about care measures such as cleaning the urinary meatus, managing and emptying the collection device, maintaining a closed system, and bladder irrigation or flushing if ordered.
- For clients with a urinary diversion, teach about care of the stoma, drainage devices, and surrounding skin. For continent diversions, teach the client how to catheterize the stoma to drain urine.
- For clients with an indwelling catheter or urinary diversion, emphasize the importance of maintaining a generous fluid intake (2.5 to 3 quarts daily) and of promptly reporting changes in urinary output, signs of urinary retention such as abdominal pain, and manifestations of urinary tract infection such as malodorous urine, abdominal discomfort, fever, or confusion.

Medications

- Emphasize the importance of taking medications as prescribed. Instruct the client to take the full course of antibiotics ordered to treat a urinary tract infection, even though symptoms are relieved.
- Inform the client and family about any expected changes in urine color or odor associated with prescribed medications.
- For clients with urinary retention, emphasize the need to contact the primary care provider before taking any medication (even over-the-counter medications such as antihistamines) that may exacerbate symptoms.
- For clients taking medications that may damage the kidneys (e.g., aminoglycoside antibiotics), stress the importance of maintaining a generous fluid intake while taking the medication.
- Suggest measures to reduce anticipated side effects of prescribed medications, such as increasing intake of potassium-rich foods when taking a potassium-depleting diuretic such as furosemide.

Dietary Alterations

- Teach the client about dietary changes to promote urinary function, such as consuming cranberry juice and foods that acidify the urine to reduce the risk of repeated urinary tract infections or forming calcium-based urinary stones. See "Dietary Measures" on page 1279.
- Instruct clients with stress or urge incontinence to limit their intake of caffeine, alcohol, citrus juices, and artificial sweeteners because these are bladder irritants that may increase incontinence. Also, teach clients to limit their evening fluid intake to reduce the risk of nighttime incontinence episodes.

Measures Specific to Urinary Problems

- Provide instructions for clients with specific urinary problems or treatments such as
  a. Timed urine specimens (see Chapter 32)
  b. Urinary incontinence
  c. Urinary retention
  d. Retention catheters.

Referrals

- Make appropriate referrals to home health agencies, community agencies, or social services for assistance with resources such as grab bars and raised toilet seats, providing wheelchair access to bathrooms, obtaining toileting aids such as commodes, urinals, or bedpans, and services such as home health aides for assistance with activities of daily living.

Community Agencies and Other Resources

- Provide information about resources for durable medical equipment such as commodes or raised toilet seats, possible financial assistance, and medical supplies such as drainage bags, incontinence briefs, or protective pads.
- Suggest additional sources of information and help such as the National Council of Independent Living; United Ostomy Association, Inc.; National Association for Continence; Simon Foundation for Continence.

Practice Guidelines
Maintaining Normal Voiding Habits

Positioning

■ Assist the client to a normal position for voiding: standing for males clients; for female clients, squatting or leaning slightly forward when sitting. These positions enhance movement of urine through the tract by gravity.

■ If the client is unable to ambulate to the lavatory, use a bed-side commode for females and a urinal for males standing at the bedside.

■ If necessary, encourage the client to push over the pubic area with the hands or to lean forward to increase intra-abdominal pressure and external pressure on the bladder.

Relaxation

■ Provide privacy for the client. Many people cannot void in the presence of another person.

■ Allow the client sufficient time to void.

■ Suggest the client read or listen to music.

■ Provide sensory stimuli that may help the client relax. Pour warm water over the perineum of a female or have the client sit in a warm bath to promote muscle relaxation. Applying a hot water bottle to the lower abdomen of both men and women may also foster muscle relaxation.

■ Turn on running water within hearing distance of the client to stimulate the voiding reflex and to mask the sound of voiding for people who find this embarrassing.

■ Provide ordered analgesics and emotional support to relieve physical and emotional discomfort to decrease muscle tension.

Timing

■ Assist clients who have the urge to void immediately. Delays only increase the difficulty in starting to void, and the desire to void may pass.

■ Offer toileting assistance to the client at usual times of voiding, for example, on awakening, before or after meals, and at bedtime.

For Bed-Confined Clients

■ Warm the bedpan. A cold bedpan may prompt contraction of the perineal muscles and inhibit voiding.

■ Elevate the head of the client's bed to Fowler's position, place a small pillow or rolled towel at the small of the back to increase physical support and comfort, and have the client flex the hips and knees. This position simulates the normal voiding position as closely as possible.

Many clients have increased fluid requirements, necessitating a higher daily fluid intake. For example, clients who are perspiring excessively (have diaphoresis) or who are experiencing abnormal fluid losses through vomiting, gastric suction, diarrhea, or wound drainage require fluid to replace these losses in addition to their normal daily intake requirements.

Clients who are at risk for urinary tract infection or urinary calculi (stones) should consume 2,000 to 3,000 mL of fluid daily. Dilute urine and frequent urination reduce the risk of urinary tract infection as well as stone formation.

Increased fluid intake may be contraindicated for some clients such as people with kidney failure or heart failure. For these clients, a fluid restriction may be necessary to prevent fluid overload and edema.

Maintaining Normal Voiding Habits. Prescribed medical therapies often interfere with a client's normal voiding habits. When a client's urinary elimination pattern is adequate, the nurse helps the client adhere to normal voiding habits as much as possible (see Practice Guidelines.)

Assisting with Toileting. Clients who are weakened by a disease process or impaired physically require assistance to toilet. The nurse should assist these clients to the bathroom and remain with them if the client is at risk for falling. The bathroom should contain an easily accessible call signal to summon help if needed. Clients also need to be encouraged to use handrails placed near the toilet.

For clients unable to use bathroom facilities, the nurse provides urinary equipment close to the bedside (e.g., urinal, bedpan, commode) and provides the necessary assistance to use them.

> **► CLINICAL ALERT** *Stress incontinence in women may be successfully treated by insertion (under local anesthesia) of a transvaginal mesh tape sling to support the urethra.* ■

Preventing Urinary Tract Infections

The rate of urinary tract infection (UTI) in women is about 20% yearly compared with a rate of 0.1% in men, and it accounts for 40% of all nosocomial infections (Marchiondo, 1998). Most UTIs are caused by bacteria common to the intestinal environment (e.g., *Escherichia coli*). These gastrointestinal bacteria can colonize the perineal area and move into the urethra, especially when there is urethral trauma, irritation, or manipulation. Women are particularly at risk because of the short urethra and its proximity to the anal and vaginal areas.

For women who have experienced a UTI, nurses need to provide instructions about ways to prevent a recurrence. Marchiondo (1998) provides the following guidelines that are useful for anyone:

• Drink eight 8-ounce glasses of water per day to flush bacteria out of the urinary system.

• Practice frequent voiding (every 2 to 4 hours) to flush bacteria out of the urethra and prevent organisms from ascending into the bladder. Void immediately after intercourse.

• Avoid use of harsh soaps, bubble bath, powder, or sprays in the perineal area. These substances can be irritating to the urethra and encourage inflammation and bacterial infection.

• Avoid tight-fitting pants or other clothing that creates irritation to the urethra and prevents ventilation of the perineal area.

- Wear cotton rather than nylon underclothes. Accumulation of perineal moisture facilitates bacterial growth and cotton enhances ventilation of the perineal area.
- Girls and women should always wipe the perineal area from front to back following urination or defecation in order to prevent introduction of gastrointestinal bacteria into the urethra.
- If recurrent urinary infections are a problem, take showers rather than baths. Bacteria present in bathwater can readily enter the urethra.
- Increase the acidity of urine through regular intake of vitamin C and drinking two to three glasses of cranberry juices daily.

Managing Urinary Incontinence

It is important to remember that urinary incontinence is not a normal part of aging and often is treatable. Independent nursing interventions for clients with urinary incontinence (UI) include (a) a behavior-oriented continence training program that may consist of bladder training, habit training, prompted voiding, pelvic muscle exercises, and positive reinforcement; (b) meticulous skin care; and (c) for males, application of an external drainage device (condom-type catheter device).

Continence (Bladder) Training. A continence training program requires the involvement of the nurse, the client, and support people. Clients must be alert and physically able to follow a program. A bladder training program may include the following:

- Education of the client and support people.
- **Bladder training,** which requires that the client postpone voiding, resist or inhibit the sensation of urgency, and void according to a timetable rather than according to the urge to void. The goals are to gradually lengthen the intervals between urination to correct the client's frequent urination, to stabilize the bladder, and to diminish urgency. This form of training may be used for clients who have bladder instability

and urge incontinence. Delayed voiding provides larger voided volumes and longer intervals between voiding. Initially, voiding may be encouraged every 2 to 3 hours except during sleep and then every 4 to 6 hours. A vital component of bladder training is inhibiting the urge-to-void sensation. To do this, the nurse instructs the client to practice deep, slow breathing until the urge diminishes or disappears. This is performed every time the client has a premature urge to void.

- **Habit training,** also referred to as timed voiding or scheduled toileting, attempts to keep clients dry by having them void at regular intervals. With habit training, there is no attempt to motivate the client to delay voiding if the urge occurs.
- **Prompted voiding** supplements habit training by encouraging the client to try to use the toilet (prompting) and reminding the client when to void.

Pelvic Muscle Exercises. Pelvic muscle exercises, referred to as Kegel exercises, strengthen pelvic floor muscles in women and can reduce episodes of incontinence. The client can identify perineal muscles by stopping urination midstream or by tightening the anal sphincter as if to hold a bowel movement.

The following technique is sometimes used to teach Kegel exercises. Ask the client to think of her perineal muscles as an elevator. When the client relaxes, the elevator is on the first floor. To perform the exercise, contract the perineal muscles, bringing the elevator to the second, third, and fourth floors. Keep the elevator on the fourth floor for a few seconds, and then gradually relax the area. When the exercise is properly performed, contraction of the muscles of the buttocks and thighs is avoided.

Kegel exercises can be performed anytime, anywhere, sitting or standing—even when voiding. Specific client instructions for performing Kegel exercises are summarized in Teaching: Client Care.

Practice Guidelines
Bladder Training

- Determine the client's voiding pattern and encourage voiding at those times, or establish a regular voiding schedule and help the client to maintain it, whether the client feels the urge or not (e.g., on awakening, every 1 or 2 hours during the day and evening, before retiring at night, every 4 hours at night). The stretching-relaxing sequence of such a schedule tends to increase bladder muscle tone and promote more voluntary control. Encourage the client to inhibit the urge-to-void sensation when a premature urge to void is experienced. Instruct the client to practice slow, deep breathing until the urge diminishes or disappears.
- When the client finds that voiding can be controlled, the intervals between voiding can be lengthened slightly without loss of continence.
- Regulate fluid intake, particularly during evening hours, to help reduce the need to void during the night.
- Encourage fluids about half an hour before the voiding time between the hours of 0600 and 1800.

- Avoid excessive consumption of citrus juices, carbonated beverages (especially those containing artificial sweeteners), alcohol, and drinks containing caffeine because these irritate the bladder, increasing the risk of incontinence.
- Schedule diuretics early in the morning.
- Explain to clients that adequate fluid intake is required to ensure adequate urine production that stimulates the micturition reflex.
- Apply protector pads to keep the bed linen dry and provide specially made waterproof underwear to contain the urine and decrease the client's embarrassment. Avoid using diapers, which are demeaning and also suggest that incontinence is permissible.
- Assist the client with an exercise program to increase the tone of abdominal and pelvic muscles.
- Provide positive reinforcements to encourage continence. Praise clients for attempting to toilet and for maintaining continence.

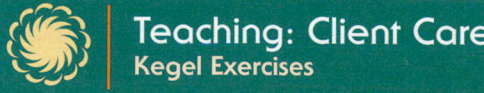

Teaching: Client Care
Kegel Exercises

- First, sit or stand with the legs apart.
- Pull your rectum, urethra, and vagina up inside, and hold for a count of 3 to 5 seconds. The pull should be felt at the cleft of your buttocks.
- Initially perform each contraction 10 times, five times daily.
- Develop a schedule that will help remind you to do these exercises, for example, while driving to work, when working at the kitchen sink, or at scheduled times (e.g., 0700, 1000, 1300, 1600, and 1900 hours).
- Try to start and stop your stream of urine.
- To control episodes of stress incontinence, brace the muscles and use the Kegel maneuver when doing any activity that increases intra-abdominal pressure, such as coughing, laughing, sneezing, or lifting.

Maintaining Skin Integrity. Skin that is continually moist becomes macerated (softened). Urine that accumulates on the skin is converted to ammonia, which is very irritating to the skin. Because both skin irritation and maceration predispose the client to skin breakdown and ulceration, the incontinent person requires meticulous skin care. To maintain skin integrity, the nurse washes the client's perineal area with soap and water after episodes of incontinence, rinses it thoroughly, dries it gently and thoroughly, and provides clean, dry clothing

or bed linen. If the skin is irritated, the nurse applies barrier creams such as zinc oxide ointment to protect it from contact with urine. If it is necessary to pad the client's clothes for protection, the nurse should use products that absorb wetness and leave a dry surface in contact with the skin.

Specially designed incontinence drawsheets may be used that provide significant advantages over standard drawsheets for incontinent clients confined to bed. These sheets are like a drawsheet but are double layered, with a quilted upper nylon or polyester surface and an absorbent viscose rayon layer below. The rayon soaker layer generally has a waterproof backing on its underside. Fluid (i.e., urine) passes through the upper quilted layer and is absorbed and dispersed by the viscose rayon, leaving the quilted surface dry to the touch. This absorbent sheet helps maintain skin integrity; it does not stick to the skin when wet, decreases the risk of bedsores, and reduces odor.

Applying External Urinary Drainage Devices. The application of a condom or external catheter connected to a urinary drainage system is commonly prescribed for incontinent males. Use of a condom appliance is preferable to insertion of a retention catheter because the risk of urinary tract infection is minimal.

Methods of applying condoms vary. The nurse needs to follow the manufacturer's instructions when applying a condom. First the nurse determines when the client experiences incontinence. Some clients may require a condom appliance at night only, others continuously. Procedure 47–1 describes how to apply and remove an external catheter.

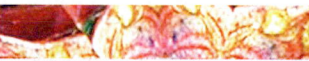

Procedure 47–1 Applying an External Catheter

Purposes

- To collect urine and control urinary incontinence
- To permit the client physical activity without fear of embarrassment because of leaking urine
- To prevent skin irritation as a result of urine incontinence

ASSESSMENT

- Review the client record to determine a pattern to voiding and other pertinent data.
- Apply clean gloves and examine the client's penis for swelling or excoriation that would contraindicate use of the condom catheter.

PLANNING

Determine if the client has had an external catheter previously and any difficulties with it. Perform any procedures that are best completed without the catheter in place, for example, weighing the client would be easier without the tubing and bag.

Delegation
Applying a condom catheter may be delegated to unlicensed assistive personnel (UAP). However, the nurse must determine if the specific client has unique needs that would require special training of the UAP in the use of the condom catheter.

Equipment
- Leg drainage bag with tubing or urinary drainage bag with tubing
- Condom sheath
- Bath blanket or similar drape
- Clean gloves
- Basin of warm water and soap
- Washcloth and towel
- Elastic tape or Velcro strap

continued on page 1272

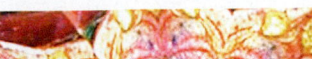

Procedure 47–1 Applying an External Catheter *continued*

IMPLEMENTATION

Preparation

- Assemble the leg drainage bag or urinary drainage bag for attachment to the condom sheath.
- Roll the condom outward onto itself to facilitate easier application (Figure 47–5 ■). On some models, an inner flap will be exposed. This flap is applied around the urinary meatus to prevent the reflux of urine.
- Position the client in either a supine or a sitting position.

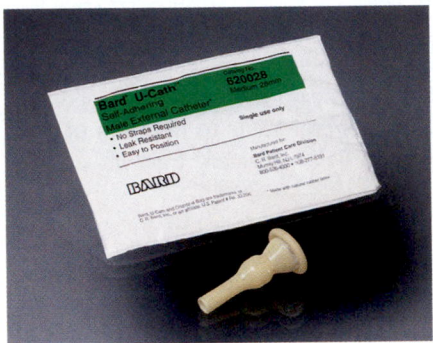

Figure 47–5 ■ Before application, roll the condom outward onto itself. (Courtesy of Bard Medical Division.)

Performance

1. Explain to the client what you are going to do, why it is necessary, and how he can cooperate.
2. Discuss if using a condom catheter will impact further care or treatments.
3. Wash hands, apply clean gloves, and observe appropriate infection control procedures.
4. Provide for client privacy.
   - Drape the client appropriately with the bath blanket, exposing only the penis.
5. Inspect and clean the penis.
   - Clean the genital area and dry it thoroughly. *This minimizes skin irritation and excoriation after the condom is applied.*
6. Apply and secure the condom.
   - Roll the condom smoothly over the penis, leaving 2.5 cm. (1 in.) between the end of the penis and the

rubber or plastic connecting tube (Figure 47–6 ■) . *This space prevents*

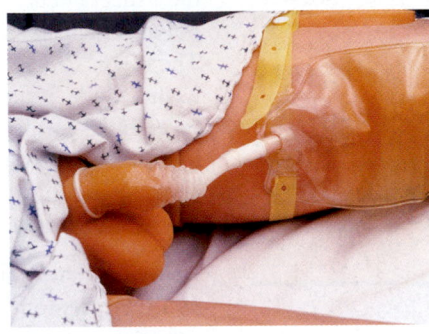

Figure 47–6 ■ The condom rolled over the penis.

irritation of the tip of the penis and provides for full drainage of urine.
   - Secure the condom firmly, but not too tightly, to the penis. Some condoms have an adhesive inside the proximal end that adheres to the skin of the base of the penis. Many condoms are packaged with special tape. If neither is present, use a strip of elastic tape or Velcro around the base of the penis over the condom. Ordinary tape is contraindicated because it is not flexible and can stop blood flow.
7. Securely attach the urinary drainage system.
   - Make sure that the tip of the penis is not touching the condom and that the condom is not twisted. *A twisted condom could obstruct the flow of urine.*
   - Attach the urinary drainage system to the condom.
   - Remove the gloves and wash your hands.
   - If the client is to remain in bed, attach the urinary drainage bag to the bed frame.
   - If the client is ambulatory, attach the bag to the client's leg (Figure 47–7 ■). *Attaching the drainage bag to the leg helps control the movement of the tub-*

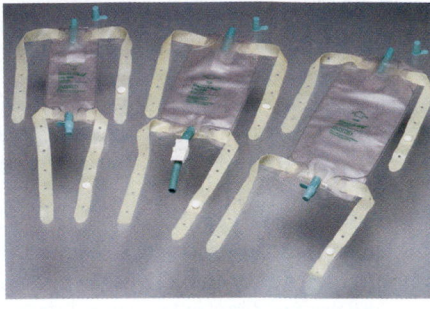

Figure 47–7 ■ Urinary drainage leg bags. (Courtesy of Bard Medical Division.)

ing and prevents twisting of the thin material of the condom appliance at the tip of the penis.
8. Teach the client about the drainage system.
   - Instruct the client to keep the drainage bag below the level of the condom and to avoid loops or kinks in the tubing.
9. Inspect the penis 30 minutes following the condom application, and check urine flow. Document these findings.
   - Assess the penis for swelling and discoloration, *which indicates that the condom is too tight.*
   - Assess urine flow if the client has voided. Normally, some urine is present in the tube if the flow is not obstructed.
10. Change the condom daily and provide skin care.
   - Remove the elastic or Velcro strip, apply clean gloves, and roll off the condom.
   - Wash the penis with soapy water, rinse, and dry it thoroughly.
   - Assess the foreskin for signs of irritation, swelling, and discoloration.
   - Reapply a new condom.
11. Document in the client record using forms or checklists supplemented by narrative notes when appropriate. Record the application of the condom, the time, and pertinent observations, such as irritated areas on the penis.

EVALUATION

- Perform a detailed follow-up based on findings that deviated from expected or normal for the client. Relate findings to previous assessment data if available.
- Report significant deviations from normal to the primary care provider.

Managing Urinary Retention

Interventions that assist the client to maintain a normal voiding pattern, discussed earlier, also apply when dealing with urinary retention. If these actions are unsuccessful, the primary care provider may order a cholinergic drug such as bethanechol chloride (Urecholine) to stimulate bladder contraction and facilitate voiding. Clients who have a **flaccid** bladder (weak, soft, and lax bladder muscles) may use manual pressure on the bladder to promote bladder emptying. This is known as **Credé's maneuver** or Credé's method. It is not advised without a physician or nurse practitioner's order and is used only for clients who have lost and are not expected to regain voluntary bladder control. When all measures fail to initiate voiding, urinary catheterization may be necessary to empty the bladder completely. An indwelling Foley catheter may be inserted until the underlying cause is treated. Alternatively, intermittent straight catheterization (every 3 to 4 hours) may be performed because the risk of urinary tract infection may be less than with an indwelling catheter.

Urinary Catheterization

Urinary catheterization is the introduction of a catheter through the urethra into the urinary bladder. This is usually performed only when absolutely necessary, because the danger exists of introducing microorganisms into the bladder. Clients who have lowered immune resistance are at the greatest risk. Once an infection is introduced into the bladder, it can ascend the ureters and eventually involve the kidneys. The hazard of infection remains after the catheter is in place because normal defense mechanisms such as intermittent flushing of microorganisms from the urethra through voiding are bypassed. Thus, strict sterile technique is used for catheterization.

> ➤ **CLINICAL ALERT** *More than 5 million urinary catheters are inserted annually. They are the most common cause of hospital-acquired infections (Maki & Tambyah, 2001).* ■

Another hazard is trauma, particularly in the male client, whose urethra is longer and more tortuous. It is important to insert a catheter along the normal contour of the urethra. Damage to the urethra can occur if the catheter is forced through strictures or at an incorrect angle. In males, the urethra is normally curved, but it can be straightened by elevating the penis to a position perpendicular to the body.

Catheters are commonly made of rubber or plastics although they may be made from latex, silicone, or polyvinyl chloride (PVC). They are sized by the diameter of the lumen using the French (Fr) scale: the larger the number, the larger the lumen. Either straight catheters, inserted to drain the bladder and then immediately removed, or retention catheters, which remain in the bladder to drain urine, may be used.

The straight catheter is a single-lumen tube with a small eye or opening about 1¼ cm (1/2 in.) from the insertion tip (Figure 47–8 ■). The coudé catheter is a variation of the straight catheter. It is more rigid than other straight catheters

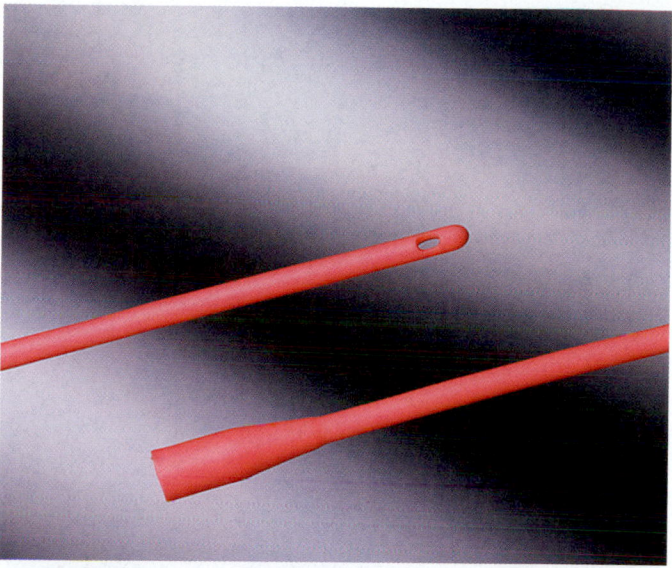

A

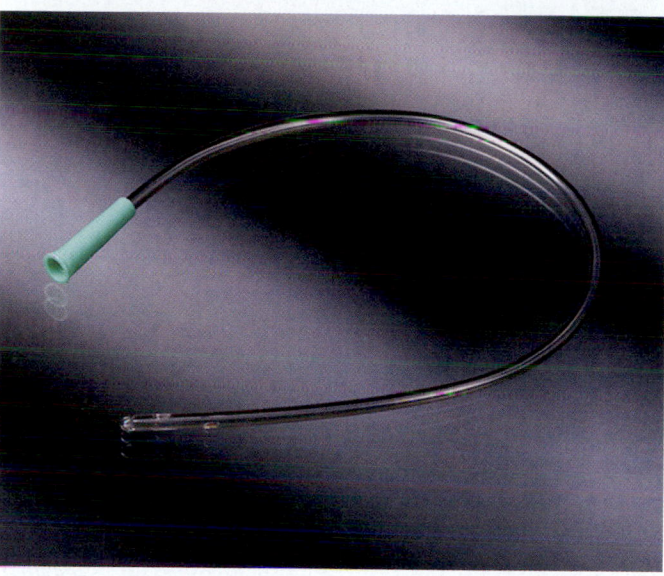

B

Figure 47–8 ■ Red-rubber or plastic Robinson straight catheters. (Courtesy of Bard Medical Division.)

and has a tapered, curved tip (Figure 47–9 ■). This catheter may be used for men with prostatic hypertrophy because it is more easily controlled and less traumatic on insertion.

The retention, or Foley, catheter is a double-lumen catheter. The larger lumen drains urine from the bladder. A second, smaller lumen is used to inflate a balloon near the tip of the catheter to hold the catheter in place within the bladder (Figure 47–10 ■). Clients who require continuous or intermittent bladder irrigation may have a three-way Foley catheter (Figure 47–11 ■). The three-way catheter has a third lumen through which sterile irrigating fluid can flow into the bladder. The fluid then exits the bladder through the drainage lumen, along with the urine.

The balloons of retention catheters are sized by the volume of fluid used to inflate them. The two commonly used sizes are 5-mL and 30-mL balloons. The size of the balloon is indicated

MediaLink | CATHETERIZATION ANIMATION

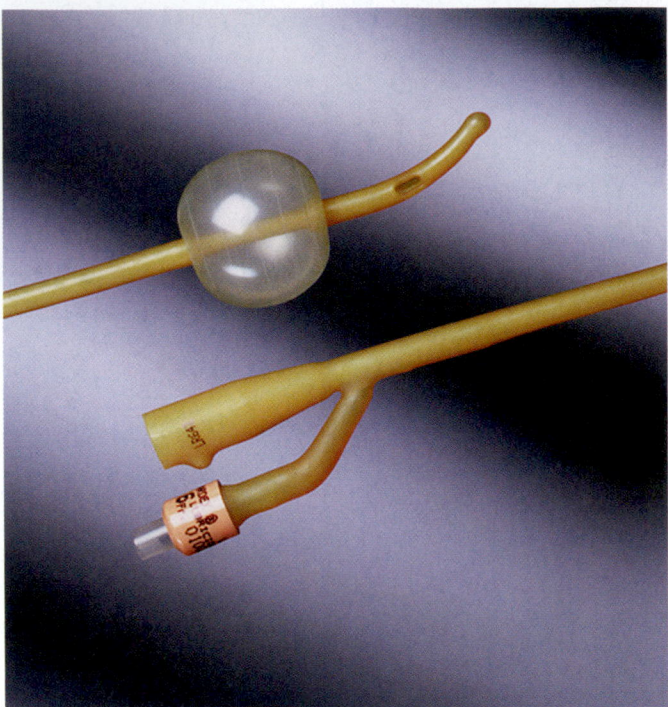

Figure 47–9 ■ A coudé catheter. (Courtesy of Bard Medical Division.)

on the catheter along with the diameter, for example, "#18 Fr— 5 mL." Box 47–2 provides guidelines for catheter selection.

Retention catheters usually are connected to a closed gravity drainage system. This system consists of the catheter, drainage tubing, and a collecting bag for the urine. A closed system cannot be opened anywhere along the system, from catheter to collecting bag. Closed systems reduce the risk of microorganisms entering the system and infecting the urinary

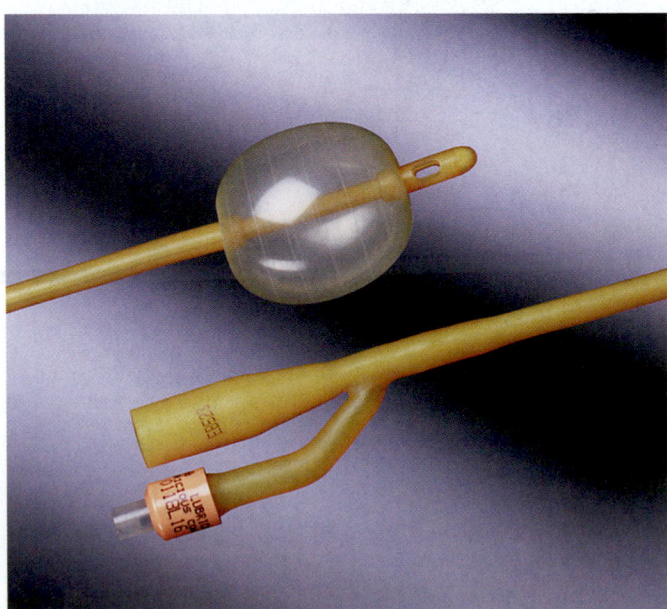

Figure 47–10 ■ A retention (Foley) catheter with the balloon inflated. (Courtesy of Bard Medical Division.)

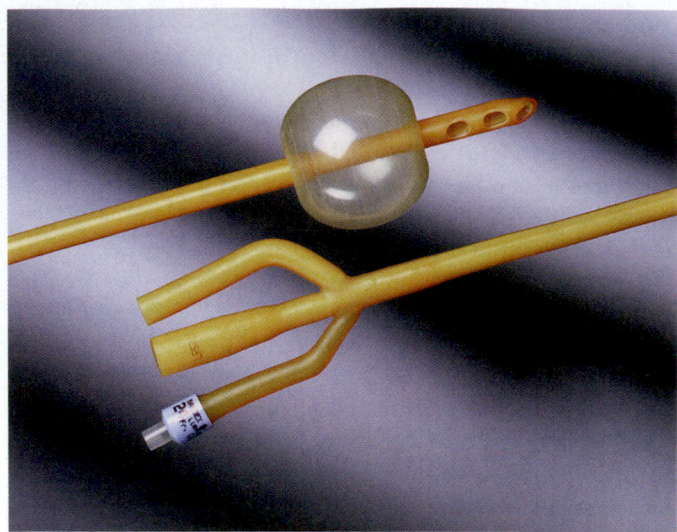

Figure 47–11 ■ A three-way Foley catheter. (Courtesy of Bard Medical Division.)

tract. Urinary drainage systems typically depend on the force of gravity to drain urine from the bladder to the collecting bag.

Procedure 47–2 describes catheterization of females and males, using straight and retention catheters.

BOX 47–2   ■ Selecting an Appropriate Catheter

■ Select the type of material in accordance with the estimated length of the catheterization period. Antimicrobial-impregnated or hydrogel/silver-coated catheters may also be used to reduce the risk of infection.
   a. Use plastic catheters for short periods only (e.g., 1 week or less), because they are inflexible.
   b. Use a rubber or silastic catheter for periods of 2 or 3 weeks. Latex may be used for clients with no known latex allergy. However, because of these allergies, latex is being phased out of health care products.
   c. Use silicone catheters for long-term use (e.g., 2 to 3 months) because they create less encrustation at the urethral meatus. However, they are expensive.
   d. Use PVC catheters for 4- to 6-week periods. They soften at body temperature and conform to the urethra.
■ Determine appropriate catheter length by the client's gender. For adult female clients, use a 22-cm catheter; for adult male clients, a 40-cm catheter.
■ Determine appropriate catheter size by the size of the urethral canal. Use sizes such as #8 or #10 for children, #14 or #16 for adults. Men frequently require a larger size than women, for example, #18.
■ Select the appropriate balloon size. For adults, use a 5-mL balloon to facilitate optimal urine drainage. The smaller balloons allow more complete bladder emptying because the catheter tip is closer to the urethral opening in the bladder. However, a 30-mL balloon is commonly used to achieve hemostasis of the prostatic area following a prostatectomy. Use 3-mL balloons for children.

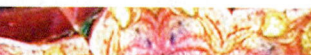

Procedure 47-2 Performing Urinary Catheterization

Purposes

- To relieve discomfort due to bladder distention or to provide gradual decompression of a distended bladder
- To assess the amount of residual urine if the bladder empties incompletely
- To obtain a urine specimen
- To empty the bladder completely prior to surgery

- To facilitate accurate measurement of urinary output for critically ill clients whose output needs to be monitored hourly
- To provide for intermittent or continuous bladder drainage and irrigation
- To prevent urine from contacting an incision after perineal surgery
- To manage incontinence when other measures have failed

ASSESSMENT

- Determine the most appropriate method of catheterization based on the purpose and any criteria specified in the order such as total amount of urine to be removed or size of catheter to be used.
- Use a straight catheter if only a spot urine specimen is needed, if amount of residual urine is being measured, or if temporary decompression/emptying of the bladder is required.

- Use an indwelling/retention catheter if the bladder must remain empty or continuous urine measurement/collection is needed.
- Assess the client's overall condition. Determine if the client is able to cooperate and hold still during the procedure and if the client can be positioned supine with head relatively flat.
- Determine when the client last voided or was last catheterized.
- Percuss the bladder to check for fullness or distension.

PLANNING

Allow adequate time to perform the catheterization. Although the entire procedure can require as little as 15 minutes, several sources of difficulty could result in a much longer time. If possible, it should not be performed just prior to or after the client eats.

Delegation

Due to the need for sterile technique and detailed knowledge of anatomy, insertion of a urinary catheter is not delegated to UAP.

Equipment

- Sterile catheter of appropriate size (An extra catheter should also be at hand.)
- Catheterization kit (Figure 47–12 ■) or individual sterile items:
  - 1–2 pair sterile gloves
  - Waterproof drape(s)
  - Antiseptic solution

  - Cleansing balls
  - Forceps
  - Water soluble lubricant
  - Urine receptacle
  - Specimen container
- For an indwelling catheter:
  - Syringe prefilled with sterile water in amount specified by catheter manufacturer
  - Collection bag and tubing
- 2% Xylocaine gel (if agency permits)
- Disposable clean gloves
- Supplies for performing perineal cleansing
- Bath blanket or sheet for draping the client
- Adequate lighting; (Obtain a flashlight or lamp if necessary.)

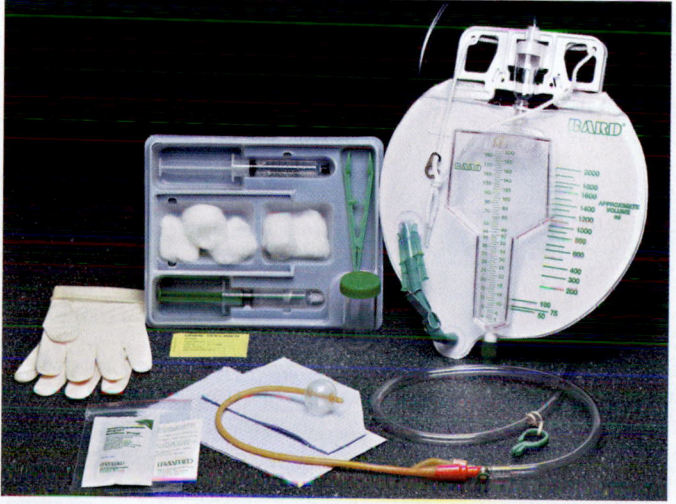
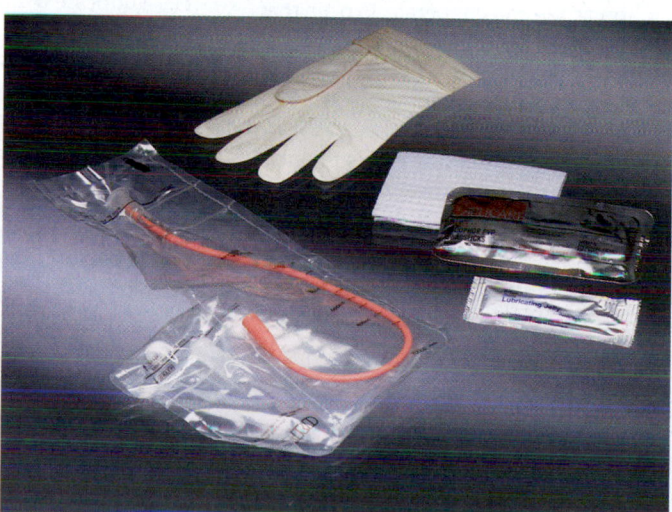

A   B

Figure 47–12 ■ Catheter insertion kits: *A,* indwelling; *B,* straight. (Courtesy of Bard Medical Division.)

continued on page 1276

Procedure 47-2 Performing Urinary Catheterization *continued*

IMPLEMENTATION

Preparation

If using a catheterization kit, read the label carefully to be sure all necessary items are included. Perform routine perineal care to cleanse the meatus from gross contamination. For women, use this time to locate the urinary meatus relative to surrounding structures (47–13 ■).

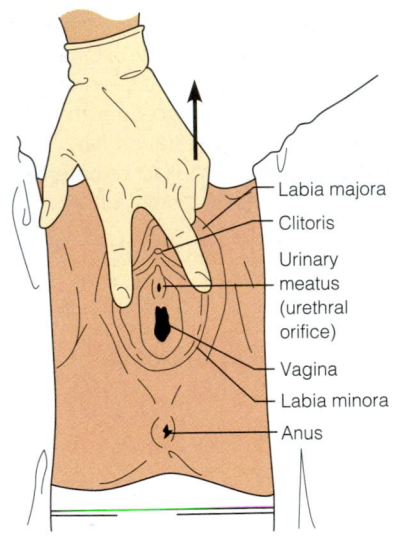

Figure 47–13 ■ To expose the urinary meatus, separate the labia minora and retract the tissue upward.

- Labia majora
- Clitoris
- Urinary meatus (urethral orifice)
- Vagina
- Labia minora
- Anus

Performance

1. Explain to the client what you are going to do, why it is necessary, and how he or she can cooperate. Explain that catheter insertion causes the sensation of voiding and, possibly, a burning feeling. Discuss how the results of the catheterization will be used in planning further care or treatments.
2. Wash hands and observe appropriate infection control procedures.
3. Provide for client privacy.
4. Place the client in the appropriate position and drape all areas except the perineum.
   a. Female: supine with knees flexed and externally rotated
   b. Male: supine, legs slightly abducted
5. Establish adequate lighting. Stand on the client's right if you are right-handed, on the client's left if you are left-handed.

6. If using a collecting bag and it is not contained within the catheterization kit, open the drainage package and place the end of the tubing within reach. *Since one hand is needed to hold the catheter once it is in place, open the package while two hands are still available.*
7. If agency policy permits, apply clean gloves and inject 10 to 15 mL Xylocaine gel into the urethra. In the male client, wipe the underside of the shaft to distribute the gel up the urethra. Wait at least 5 minutes for the gel to take effect before inserting the catheter. Remove gloves.
8. Open the catheterization kit. Place a waterproof drape under the buttocks (female) or penis (male) without contaminating the center of the drape with your hands.
9. Apply sterile gloves.
10. Organize the remaining supplies:
    - Saturate the cleansing balls with the antiseptic solution.
    - Open the lubricant package.
    - Remove the specimen container and place it nearby with the lid loosely on top.
11. Attach the prefilled syringe to the indwelling catheter inflation hub and test the balloon. *If the balloon malfunctions, it is important to replace it prior to use.*
12. Lubricate the catheter (1 to 2 in. for females, 6 to 7 in. for males) and place it with the drainage end inside the collection container.
13. If desired, place the fenestrated drape over the perineum, exposing the urinary meatus.
14. Cleanse the meatus. *Note:* The nondominant hand is considered contaminated once it touches the client's skin.
    a. Women:
       Use your nondominant hand to spread the labia. Establish a firm but gentle position. The antiseptic may make the tissues slippery but the labia must not be allowed to return over the cleaned meatus. Pick up a cleansing ball with the forceps in your dominant hand

and wipe one side of the labia majora in an anteroposterior direction (Figure 47–14 ■). Use great care that wiping the client does not contaminate this sterile hand. Use a new ball for the opposite side. Repeat for the labia minora. Use the last ball to cleanse directly over the meatus.

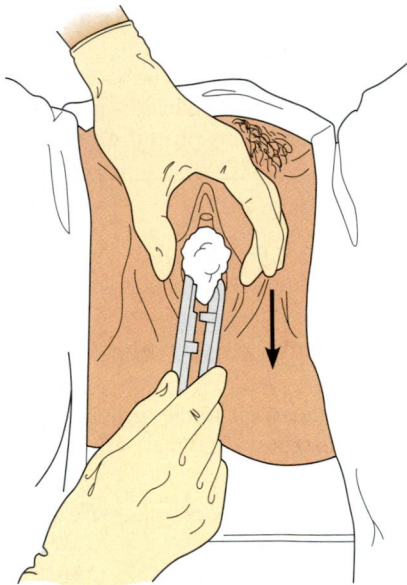

Figure 47–14 ■ When cleaning the urinary meatus, move the swab downward.

    b. Men:
       Use your nondominant hand to grasp the penis just below the glans. If necessary, retract the foreskin. Hold the penis firmly upright, with slight tension. *Lifting the penis in this manner helps straighten the urethra.* Pick up a cleansing ball with the forceps in your dominant hand and wipe from the center of the meatus in a circular motion around the glans. Use great care that wiping the client does not contaminate this sterile hand. Use a new ball and repeat three more times. The antiseptic may make the tissues slippery but the foreskin must not be allowed to return over the cleaned meatus nor the penis be dropped.

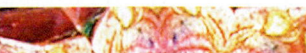

Procedure 47-2 Performing Urinary Catheterization *continued*

IMPLEMENTATION *continued*

15. Insert the catheter.
    - Grasp the catheter firmly 2 to 3 in. from the tip. Ask the client to take a slow deep breath and insert the catheter as the client exhales. Slight resistance is expected as the catheter passes through the sphincters. If necessary, twist the catheter or hold pressure on the catheter until the sphincter relaxes.
    - Advance the catheter 2 inches further after the urine begins to flow through it, *to be sure it is fully in the bladder.*
    - If the catheter accidentally contacts the labia or slips into the vagina, it is considered contaminated and a new, sterile catheter must be used. The contaminated catheter may be left in the vagina until the new catheter is inserted to help avoid mistaking the vaginal opening for the urethral meatus.
16. Hold the catheter with the nondominant hand. In males, lay the penis down onto the drape, being careful that the catheter does not pull out.
17. For an indwelling catheter, inflate the retention balloon with the designated volume.
    - Without releasing the catheter, hold the inflation valve between two fingers of your nondominant hand while you attach the syringe (if not left attached earlier when testing the balloon) and inflate with your dominant hand. If the client complains of discomfort, immediately withdraw the instilled fluid, advance the catheter further, and attempt to inflate the balloon again.
    - Pull gently on the catheter until resistance is felt to ensure that the balloon has inflated and to place it in the trigone of the bladder (Figure 47–15 ■, *A* and *B*).
18. Collect a urine specimen if needed. Allow 20 to 30 mL to flow into the bottle without touching the catheter to the bottle.
19. Allow the straight catheter to continue draining. If necessary, attach the drainage end of an indwelling catheter to the collecting tubing and bag.

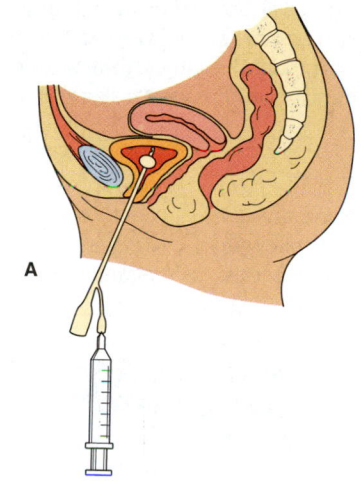

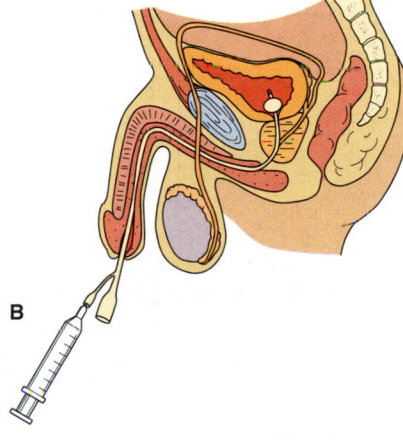

Figure 47–15 ■ Placement of retention catheter and inflated balloon in *A,* female client; and *B,* male client.

20. Examine and measure the urine. In some cases, only 750 to 1,000 mL of urine are to be drained from the bladder at one time. Check agency policy for further instructions if this should occur.
21. Remove the straight catheter when urine flow stops. For an indwelling catheter, secure the catheter tubing to the inner thigh for female clients (Figure 47–16 ■)or the upper thigh/abdomen for male clients (Figure 47–17 ■)with enough slack to allow usual movement. Also secure the collecting tubing to the bed linens and hang the bag below the level of the bladder. No tubing should fall below the top of the bag (Figure 47–18 ■).

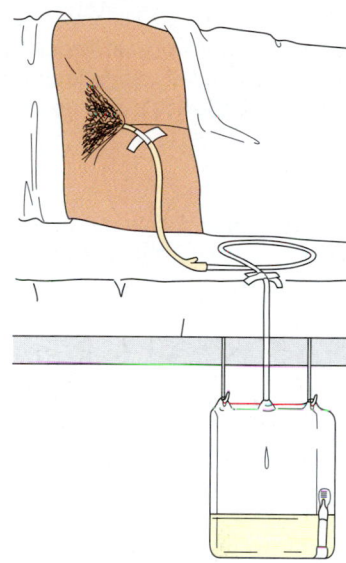

Figure 47–16 ■ Tape the catheter to the inside of a female client's thigh.

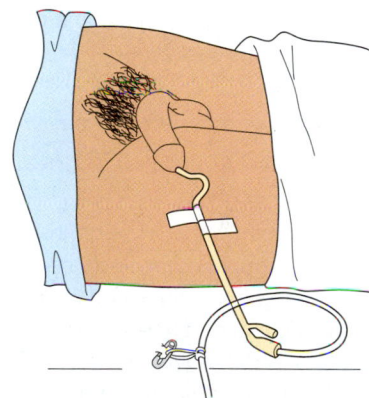

Figure 47–17 ■ Tape the catheter to the thigh or abdomen of a male client.

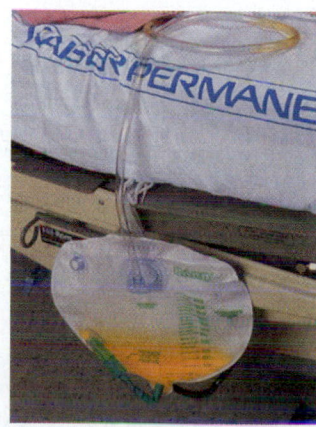

Figure 47–18 ■ Correct position for urine drainage bag and tubing.

continued on page 1278

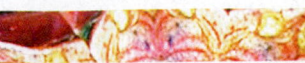

Procedure 47-2 Performing Urinary Catheterization *continued*

IMPLEMENTATION *continued*

22. Wipe the perineal area of any remaining antiseptic or lubricant. Replace the foreskin if retracted earlier. Return the client to a comfortable position.

23. Discard all used supplies in appropriate receptacles and wash your hands.
24. Document the catheterization procedure including catheter size and results in the client record using forms or checklists supplemented by narrative notes when appropriate.

EVALUATION

Conduct appropriate follow-up such as notifying the primary care provider of the catheterization results. Perform a detailed follow-up based on findings that deviated from expected or normal for the client. Relate findings to previous assessment data if available. Teach the client how to care for the indwelling catheter, to drink more fluids, and other appropriate instructions.

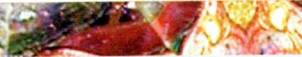

Lifespan Considerations

Catheterization
Infants and Children
- Adapt the size of the catheter for pediatric clients.
- Ask a family member to assist in holding the child during catheterization, if appropriate.

Elders
When catheterizing older adults, be very attentive to problems of limited movement, especially in the hips. Arthritis, or previous hip or knee surgery, may limit their movement and cause discomfort. Modify the position e.g., slide-lying, as needed to perform the procedure safely, and comfortably. For women, obtain the assistance of another nurse to flex and hold client's knees and hips as necessary or place her in a modified Sims' position.

Home Care Considerations

Catheterization
For intermittent catheterization, instruct the client to
- Follow instructions for clean technique.
- Wash hands well with warm water and soap prior to handling equipment or performing catheterization.
- Monitor for signs and symptoms of urinary tract infection including burning, urgency, abdominal pain, and cloudy urine; in elders, confusion may be an early sign.
- Ensure adequate oral intake of fluids.
- After each catheterization, assess the urine for color, odor, clarity, and the presence of blood.
- Wash rubber catheters thoroughly with soap and water after use, dry, and store in a clean place.

For indwelling catheters, instruct the client to
- Never pull on the catheter.
- Ensure that there are no kinks or twists in the tubing.
- Keep the urine drainage bag below the level of the bladder (Figure 47–19 ■). A leg bag may substitute for a hanging bag for those who are upright.
- Empty the drainage bag regularly.
- Take a shower rather than a tub bath; *sitting in a tub allows bacteria easier access into the urinary tract.*
- Monitor for signs and symptoms of urinary tract infection including burning, urgency, abdominal pain, cloudy urine; in older adults confusion may be an early sign.
- Ensure adequate oral intake of fluids.

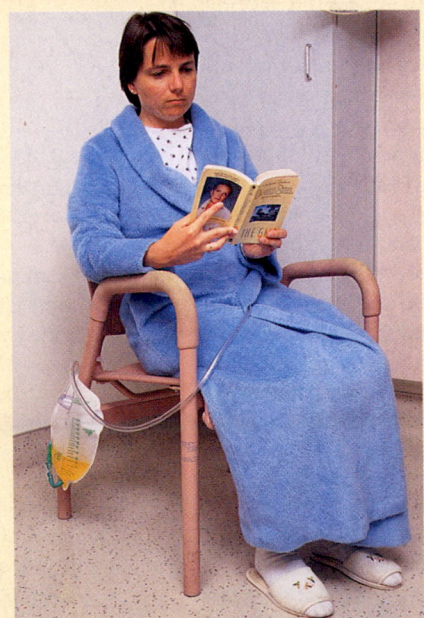

Figure 47–19 ■ Positioning the collecting bag and tubing when sitting in a chair.

- Clients who have indwelling catheters for lengthy periods of time need to have the catheter and bag changed at regular intervals. Changing equipment once a month is often the standard although agency policy may differ.

BOX 47–3 ■ Ongoing Assessment of Clients with Retention Catheters

- Ensure that there are no obstructions in the drainage. Check that there are no kinks in the tubing, the client is not lying on the tubing, and the tubing is not clogged with mucus or blood.
- Check that there is no tension on the catheter or tubing, that the catheter is securely taped to the thigh or abdomen, and that the tubing is fastened appropriately to the bedclothes.
- Ensure that gravity drainage is maintained. Make sure there are no loops in the tubing below its entry to the drainage recepta-

cle and that the drainage receptacle is below the level of the client's bladder.
- Ensure that the drainage system is well sealed or closed. Check that there are no leaks at the connection sites in open systems. Apply waterproof tape around the connection site of the catheter and tubing.
- Observe the flow of the urine every 2 or 3 hours, and note color, odor, and any abnormal constituents. If sediment is present, check the catheter more frequently to ascertain whether it is plugged.

Nursing Interventions for Clients with Retention Catheters

Nursing care of the client with an indwelling catheter and continuous drainage is largely directed toward preventing infection of the urinary tract and encouraging urinary flow through the drainage system. It includes encouraging large amounts of fluid intake, accurately recording the fluid intake and output, changing the retention catheter and tubing, maintaining the patency of the drainage system, preventing contamination of the drainage system, and teaching these measures to the client.

Fluids. The client with a retention catheter should drink up to 3,000 mL per day if permitted. Large amounts of fluid ensure a large urine output, which keeps the bladder flushed out and decreases the likelihood of urinary stasis and subsequent infection. Large volumes of urine also minimize the risk of sediment or other particles obstructing the drainage tubing.

Dietary Measures. Acidifying the urine of clients with a retention catheter may reduce the risk of urinary tract infection and calculus formation. Foods such as eggs, cheese, meat and poultry, whole grains, cranberries, plums and prunes, and tomatoes tend to increase the acidity of urine. Conversely, most fruits and vegetables, legumes, and milk and milk products result in alkaline urine.

Perineal Care. No special cleaning other than routine hygienic care is necessary for clients with retention catheters, nor is special meatal care recommended. Agency practices regarding catheter care vary considerably. The nurse should check agency practice in this regard.

Changing the Catheter and Tubing. Routine changing of catheter and tubing is not recommended. Collection of sediment in the catheter or tubing or impaired urine drainage are indicators for changing the catheter and drainage system. When this occurs the catheter and drainage system are removed and discarded, and a new sterile catheter with a closed drainage system is inserted.

Guidelines to prevent catheter-associated urinary tract infections are given in Practice Guidelines. Ongoing assessment of clients with retention catheters is a high priority (see Box 47–3).

Removing Retention Catheters. Retention catheters are removed after their purpose has been achieved, usually on the order of the primary care provider. If the catheter has been in

place for a short time (e.g., a few days), the client usually has little difficulty regaining normal urinary elimination patterns. Swelling of the urethra, however, may initially interfere with voiding, so the nurse should regularly assess the client for urinary retention until voiding is reestablished.

Clients who have had a retention catheter for a prolonged period may require bladder retraining to regain bladder muscle tone. With an indwelling catheter in place, the bladder muscle does not stretch and contract regularly as it does when the bladder fills and empties by voiding. A few days before removal, the catheter may be clamped for specified periods of time (e.g., 2 to 4 hours), then released to allow the bladder to empty. This allows the bladder to distend and stimulates its musculature. Check agency policy regarding bladder training procedures.

To remove a retention catheter, the nurse follows these steps:

- Obtain a receptacle for the catheter (e.g., a disposable basin); a clean, disposable towel; clean gloves; and a sterile syringe to deflate the balloon. The syringe should be large enough to withdraw all the solution in the catheter balloon. The size of the balloon is indicated on the label at the end of the catheter.
- Ask the client to assume a supine position as for a catheterization.
- *Optional:* Obtain a sterile specimen before removing the catheter. Check agency protocol.

Practice Guidelines
Preventing Catheter-Associated Urinary Infections

- Have an established infection control program.
- Catheterize clients only when necessary, by using aseptic technique, sterile equipment, and trained personnel.
- Maintain a sterile closed-drainage system.
- Do not disconnect the catheter and drainage tubing unless absolutely necessary.
- Remove the catheter as soon as possible.
- Follow and reinforce good hand washing technique.
- Provide routine perineal hygiene, including cleansing with soap and water after defecation.
- Prevent contamination of the catheter with feces in the incontinent client.

Research Note
What Time Is Best to Remove an Indwelling Catheter?

For many years, once the physician's order has been received, it has been common practice to remove an indwelling urinary catheter first thing in the morning—usually by the night shift nurse just prior to the arrival of the day shift staff. However, no research had previously been conducted to indicate that this time was any more or less beneficial than any other time. Research by Kelleher (2002) compared the time from catheter removal to the first and second voids, volume of urine in first and second voids, need for re-catheterization after removal, and time of discharge between two groups of 80 patients—one group had catheters removed at 0600 (group 1) and the other had catheters removed at midnight (group 2). The surgical procedures necessitating the catheter were similar for both groups. Statistically significant findings were as follows: (a) Group 2 had longer time to first void (3.65 hours versus 2.97 hours) and (b) Group 2 had larger first and second voids (286 mL versus 177 mL for first and 322 mL versus 195 mL for second). In addition, while 93% of the midnight group's catheters were actually removed within 30 minutes of the designated time, this occurred in only 65% of the 0600 group. Because the midnight group voided earlier in the day (80% at least once before 0600), they were more likely than group 1 to be able to be discharged the same day.

Implications: Many nursing practices are based on tradition and nurse convenience rather than on research evidence. This study demonstrated advantages to the patient of changing a routine—removing indwelling catheters at midnight rather than at 0600. The results suggest that the midnight group began to return to more normal voiding patterns (time between voids and volume of urine) than the 0600 group. In addition, since for one-third of the 0600 patients, the nurse was unable to remove the catheter "on time," the usual practice might not be the most opportune for the staff as may have been previously thought. Although further research is needed to verify these beneficial results in other settings, a change in practice was initiated at the hospital in which the study was conducted. Nurses should continue to investigate the evidence supporting or refuting common practices, especially when a change may be advantageous to both patients and caregivers.

Note: From "Removal of Urinary Catheters: Midnight vs. 0600 Hours," by M. M. B. Kelleher, 2002, *British Journal of Nursing, 11,* pp. 84, 86, 88–90.

- Remove the tape attaching the catheter to the client, don gloves, and then place the towel between the legs of the female client or over the thighs of the male.
- Insert the syringe into the injection port of the catheter, and withdraw the fluid from the balloon. If not all of the fluid can be removed, report this fact to the nurse in charge before proceeding.
- Do not pull the catheter while the balloon is inflated; doing so may injure the urethra.
- After all of the fluid is withdrawn from the balloon, gently withdraw the catheter and place it in the waste receptacle.
- Dry the perineal area with a towel.
- Remove gloves.
- Measure the urine in the drainage bag, and record the removal of the catheter. Include in the recording (a) the time the catheter was removed; (b) the amount, color, and clarity of the urine; (c) the intactness of the catheter; and (d) instructions given to the client.
- Following removal of the catheter, determine the time of the first voiding and the amount voided during the first 8 hours. Compare this output to the client's intake.

Clean Intermittent Self-Catheterization

Clean intermittent self-catheterization (CISC) is performed by many clients who have some form of neurogenic bladder dysfunction, such as that caused by spinal cord injury. Clean or medical aseptic technique is used. Intermittent self-catheterization

- Enables the client to retain independence and gain control of the bladder.
- Reduces incidence of urinary tract infection.
- Protects the upper urinary tract from reflux.
- Allows normal sexual relations without incontinence.
- Reduces the use of aids and appliances.
- Frees the client from embarrassing dribbling.

The procedure for self-catheterization is similar to that used by the nurse to catheterize a client. Essential steps are outlined in the accompanying Teaching: Client Care feature. Because the procedure requires physical and mental preparation, client assessment is important. The client should have

- Sufficient manual dexterity to manipulate a catheter
- Sufficient mental ability
- Motivation and acceptance of the procedure
- For women, reasonable agility to access the urethra
- Bladder capacity greater than 100 mL.

Before teaching CISC, the nurse should establish the client's voiding patterns, the volume voided, fluid intake, and residual amounts. CISC is easier for males to learn because of the visibility of the urinary meatus. Females need to learn initially with the aid of a mirror but eventually should perform the procedure by using only the sense of touch (as described in Teaching: Client Care).

Urinary Irrigations

An **irrigation** is a flushing or washing-out with a specified solution. Bladder irrigation is carried out on a physician or nurse practitioner's order, usually to wash out the bladder and sometimes to apply a medication to the bladder lining. Catheter irrigations may be performed to maintain or restore the patency of

Teaching: Client Care
Clean Intermittent Self-Catheterization

- Catheterize as often as needed to maintain. At first, catheterization may be necessary every 2 to 3 hours, increasing to 4 to 6 hours.
- Attempt to void before catheterization; insert the catheter to remove residual urine if unable to void or if amount voided is insufficient (e.g., less than 100 mL).
- Assemble all needed supplies ahead of time. Good lighting is essential, especially for women.
- If a woman, remove a tampon before catheterizing. *A tampon can inhibit catheterization.*
- Wash your hands.
- Clean the urinary meatus with either a towelette or soapy washcloth, then rinse with a wet washcloth. Women should clean the area from front to back.
- Assume a position that is comfortable and that facilitates passage of the catheter, such as a semireclining position in bed or sitting on a chair or the toilet. Men may prefer to stand over the toilet; women may prefer to stand with one foot on the side of the bathtub.
- Apply lubricant to the catheter tip [1 in. (2.5 cm) for women; 2 to 6 in. (5 to 15 cm) for men].
- Insert the catheter until urine flows through.
  - a. If a woman, locate the meatus using a mirror or other aid, or use the "touch" technique as follows:
    - Place the index finger of your nondominant hand on your clitoris.
    - Place the third and fourth fingers at the vagina.
    - Locate the meatus between the index and third fingers.
    - Direct the catheter through the meatus and then upward and forward.
  - b. If a man, hold the penis with a slight upward tension at a 60- to 90-degree angle to insert the catheter. Return the penis to its natural position when urine starts to flow.
- Hold the catheter in place until all urine is drained.
- Withdraw the catheter slowly *to ensure complete drainage of urine.*
- Wash the catheter with soap and water; store in a clean container. Replace the catheter when it becomes difficult to clean, or too soft or hard to insert easily.
- Contact your care provider if your urine becomes cloudy or contains sediment; if you have bleeding, difficulty, or pain when passing the catheter; or if you have a fever.
- Drink at least 2,000 to 2,500 mL of fluid a day *to ensure adequate bladder filling and flushing.* To keep your urine acidic and reduce the risk of bladder infections, drink cranberry and prune juices.

---

a catheter, for example, to remove pus or blood clots blocking the catheter.

The closed method is the preferred technique for catheter or bladder irrigation because it is associated with a lower risk of urinary tract infection. Closed catheter irrigations may be either continuous or intermittent. A three-way, or triple lumen, catheter (see Figure 47–11) generally is used for closed irrigations. The irrigating solution flows into the bladder through the irrigation port of the catheter and out through the urinary drainage lumen of the catheter.

Occasionally an open irrigation may be necessary to restore catheter patency. The risk of injecting microorganisms into the urinary tract is greater with open irrigations, because the connection between the indwelling catheter and the drainage tubing is broken. Strict precautions to maintain the sterility of the drainage tubing connector and interior of the indwelling catheter must be taken to minimize this risk.

The open method of catheter or bladder irrigation is performed with double-lumen indwelling catheters. It may be necessary for clients who develop blood clots and mucous fragments that occlude the catheter and when it is undesirable to change the catheter. Techniques for catheter irrigation are outlined in Procedure 47–3.

Procedure 47–3 Performing Bladder Irrigation

Purposes

- To maintain the patency of a urinary catheter and tubing (continuous irrigation)
- To free a blockage in a urinary catheter or tubing (intermittent irrigation)

ASSESSMENT

- Determine the client's current urinary drainage system. Review the client record for recent intake and output and any difficulties the client has been experiencing with the system. Review the results of previous irrigations.
- Assess the client for any discomfort, bladder spasms, or distended bladder.

continued on page 1282

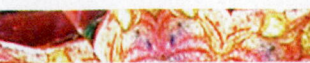

Procedure 47–3 Performing Bladder Irrigation *continued*

PLANNING

Before irrigating a catheter or bladder, check (a) the reason for the irrigation; (b) the order authorizing the continuous or intermittent irrigation (in most agencies, a physician or nurse practitioner's order is required); (c) the type of sterile solution, the amount, and strength to be used, and the rate (if continuous); and (d) the type of catheter in place. If these are not specified on the client's chart, check agency protocol.

Delegation

Due to the need for sterile technique, urinary irrigation is generally not delegated to UAP. If the client has continuous irrigation, the UAP may care for the client and note abnormal findings. These must be validated and interpreted by the nurse.

Equipment

- Clean gloves (2 pairs)
- Retention catheter in place
- Drainage tubing and bag (if not in place)
- Drainage tubing clamp
- Antiseptic swabs
- Sterile receptacle
- Sterile irrigating solution warmed or at room temperature (Label the irrigant clearly with the words *Bladder Irrigation,* including the information about any medications that have been added to the original solution.)
- Infusion tubing
- IV pole

IMPLEMENTATION

Performance

1. Explain to the client what you are going to do, why it is necessary, and how he or she can cooperate. The irrigation should not be painful or uncomfortable. Discuss how the results will be used in planning further care or treatments.
2. Wash hands and observe appropriate infection control procedures.
3. Provide for client privacy.
4. Apply clean gloves.
5. Empty, measure, and record the amount and appearance of urine present in the drainage bag. Discard urine and gloves. *Emptying the drainage bag allows more accurate measurement of urinary output after the irrigation is in place or completed. Assessing the character of the urine provides baseline data for later comparison.*
6. Prepare the equipment.
   - Wash hands.
   - Connect the irrigation infusion tubing to the irrigating solution and flush the tubing with solution, keeping the tip sterile. *Flushing the tubing removes air and prevents it from being instilled into the bladder.*
   - Apply clean gloves and cleanse the port with antiseptic swabs.
   - Connect the irrigation tubing to the input port of the three-way catheter.
   - Connect the drainage bag and tubing to the urinary drainage port if not already in place.
   - Remove the gloves and wash your hands.

7. Irrigate the bladder.
   a. For continuous irrigation, open the flow clamp on the urinary drainage tubing (if present). *This allows the irrigating solution to flow out of the bladder continuously.*
      - Open the regulating clamp on the irrigating tubing and adjust the flow rate as prescribed by the primary care provider or to 40 to 60 drops per minute if not specified.
      - Assess the drainage for amount, color, and clarity. The amount of drainage should equal the amount of irrigant entering the bladder plus expected urine output.
   b. For intermittent irrigation, determine whether the solution is to remain in the bladder for a specified time.
      - If the solution is to remain in the bladder (a bladder irrigation or instillation), apply the flow clamp to the urinary drainage tubing. *Closing the flow clamp allows the solution to be retained in the bladder and in contact with bladder walls.*
      - If the solution is being instilled to irrigate the catheter, open the flow clamp on the urinary drainage tubing. *Irrigating solution will flow through the urinary drainage port and tubing, removing mucous shreds or clots.*

   - Open the flow clamp on the irrigating tubing, allowing the specified amount of solution to infuse. Clamp the tubing.
   - After the specified period the solution is to be retained, open the drainage tubing flow clamp and allow the bladder to empty.
   - Assess the drainage for amount, color, and clarity. The amount of drainage should equal the amount of irrigant entering the bladder plus expected urine output.

8. Assess the client and the urinary output.
   - Assess the client's comfort.
   - Empty the drainage bag and measure the contents. Subtract the amount of irrigant instilled from the total volume of drainage to obtain the volume of urine output.

9. Document the procedure and results in the client record using forms or checklists supplemented by narrative notes when appropriate.
   - Note any abnormal constituents such as blood clots, pus, or mucous shreds.

VARIATION: CLOSED IRRIGATION USING A TWO-WAY INDWELLING CATHETER

1. Assemble the equipment. Use an irrigation tray (Figure 47–20 ■) or assemble individual items, including
   - Clean gloves
   - Disposable water-resistant towel
   - Sterile irrigating solution

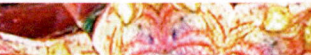

Procedure 47–3 Performing Bladder Irrigation *continued*

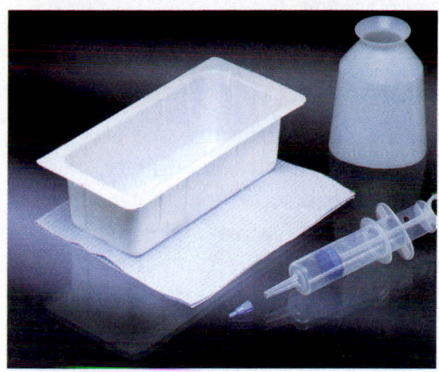

Figure 47–20 ■ An irrigation set.
(Courtesy of Bard Medical Division.)

- Sterile basin
- Sterile 30- to 50-mL syringe with a #18- or #19-gauge needle
- Antiseptic swabs

2. Prepare the client (see steps 1–5 of main procedure for catheter irrigation).

3. Prepare the equipment.
   - Wash hands and don gloves.
   - Place the disposable water-resistant towel under the catheter.
   - Clamp the drainage tubing distal to the injection port on the tubing or catheter. *Clamping prevents the urine and solution from draining into the drainage bag.*

- Using aseptic technique, open supplies and pour the irrigating solution into the sterile basin or receptacle. *Aseptic technique is vital to reduce the risk of instilling microorganisms into the urinary tract during the irrigation.*
- Remove the cap from the needle and draw the prescribed amount of irrigating solution into the syringe, maintaining the sterility of the syringe and solution.
- Using the antiseptic swab, clean the port on the catheter or drainage tubing through which the solution will be instilled.

4. Irrigate the bladder.
   - Insert the needle into the port.
   - Gently inject the solution into the catheter. In adults, about 30 to 40 mL generally is instilled for catheter irrigations; 100 to 200 mL may be instilled for bladder irrigation or instillation. *Gentle instillation reduces the risks of injury to bladder mucosa and of bladder spasms.*
   - For catheter irrigation, open the drainage tubing clamp *to allow the irrigant to flow back through the catheter.*

- When the total amount to be instilled has been injected (or for catheter irrigation, when urine is flowing freely), remove the needle from the port and discard the syringe and needle in an appropriate receptacle (sharps container). *Safe disposal of the syringe and needle is important to minimize the risk of needlestick injury.*
- Remove gloves and wash your hands.
- After the prescribed dwelling time for bladder irrigation, remove the clamp from the drainage tubing and allow the urine and irrigating solution to drain into the drainage bag.
- Assess the drainage for amount, color, and clarity. The amount of drainage should equal the amount of irrigant entering the bladder plus expected urine output.

5. Assess the client and the urinary output and document the procedure as in steps 8 and 9 above.

EVALUATION

- Perform detailed follow-up based on findings that deviated from expected or normal for the client. Relate findings to previous assessment data if available.

- Report significant deviations from normal to the primary care provider.

Urinary Diversions

A urinary diversion is the surgical rerouting of urine from the kidneys to a site other than the bladder. Urinary diversions are usually created when the bladder must be removed, for example, because of cancer or trauma. The ureters may be brought directly to the surface of the skin to form small stomas (cutaneous ureterostomy). This procedure, however, has some disadvantages in that the stomas provide direct access for microorganisms from the skin to the kidneys, the small stomas are difficult to fit with an appliance to collect the urine, and they may narrow, impairing urine drainage.

The most common urinary diversion is the ileal conduit or ileal loop (Figure 47–21 ■). In this procedure, a segment of the ileum is removed and the intestinal ends are reattached. One end of the portion removed is closed with sutures to create a pouch, and the other end is brought out through the abdominal

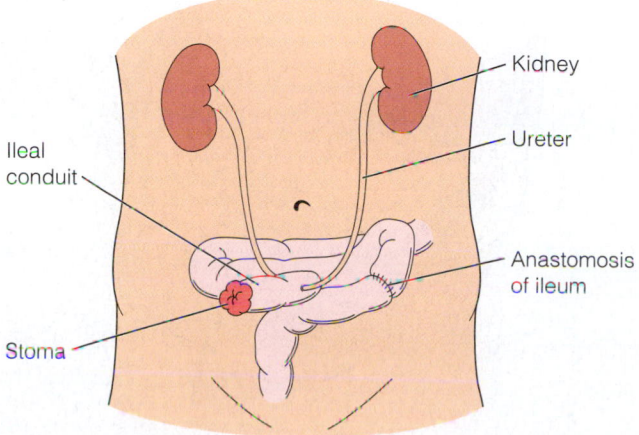

Figure 47–21 ■ An ileal conduit.

wall to create a stoma. The ureters are implanted into the ileal pouch. The ileal stoma is more readily fitted with an appliance than ureterostomies because of its larger size. The mucous membrane lining of the ileum also provides some protection from ascending infection. Urine drains continuously from the ileal pouch.

Highly motivated clients may be candidates for a continent urinary diversion. The Kock pouch, or continent ileal bladder conduit, also uses a portion of the ileum to form a reservoir for urine. In this procedure, nipple valves are formed by doubling the tissue backward into the reservoir where the pouch connects to the skin and the ureters connect to the pouch. These valves close as the pouch fills with urine, preventing leakage and reflux of urine back toward the kidneys. The client empties the pouch by inserting a clean catheter approximately every 4 hours. Between catheterizations, a small dressing is worn to protect the stoma and clothing.

A continent vesicostomy (sometimes also known as a Kock pouch) may be formed when the bladder is left intact but voiding through the urethra is not possible (e.g., due to an obstruction or a neurogenic bladder). The ureters remain connected to the bladder, and the bladder wall is sutured to the abdominal wall, forming a stoma (Figure 47–22 ■).

When caring for clients with a urinary diversion, the nurse must accurately assess intake and output, note any changes in urine color, odor, or clarity (mucous shreds are commonly seen in the urine of clients with an ileal diversion), and frequently assess the condition of the stoma and surrounding skin. Clients who must wear a urine collection appliance are at risk for impaired skin integrity because of irritation by urine. Well-fitting appliances are vital. The nurse should consult with an enterostomal therapist/wound, ostomy, continence nurse to identify the most appropriate appliance for the client's needs.

Clients with urinary diversions may experience problems with their body image and sexuality and may require assistance in coping with these changes and managing the stoma. Most clients are able to resume their normal activities and lifestyle.

► CLINICAL ALERT *As opposed to the vesicostomy, a neobladder or Suder pouch replaces a diseased or damaged bladder with a piece of ileum that is sutured to the functional urethra. Clients with these can control voiding.* ■

Suprapubic Catheter Care

A **suprapubic catheter** is inserted through the abdominal wall above the symphysis pubis into the urinary bladder (Figure 47–23 ■). The physician inserts the catheter using local anesthesia or during bladder or vaginal surgery. The catheter may be secured in place with sutures if a retention balloon is not used and is then attached to a closed drainage system. The suprapubic catheter may be placed for temporary bladder drainage until the client is able to resume normal voiding or may be a permanent device.

Care of clients with a suprapubic catheter includes regular assessments of the client's urine, fluid intake, and comfort; maintenance of a patent drainage system; skin care around the insertion site; and periodic clamping of the catheter preparatory to removing it if it is not a permanent appliance. If the catheter is temporary, orders generally include leaving the catheter open to drainage for 48 to 72 hours, then clamping the catheter for 3- to 4-hour periods during the day until the client can void satisfactory amounts. Satisfactory voiding is determined by measuring the client's residual urine after voiding.

Care of the catheter insertion site involves sterile technique. Dressings around the newly placed suprapubic catheter are changed whenever they are soiled with drainage to prevent bacterial growth around the insertion site and reduce the potential for infection. A small amount of povidone-iodine ointment is frequently applied around the insertion site and the site covered with gauze dressings. For catheters that have been in

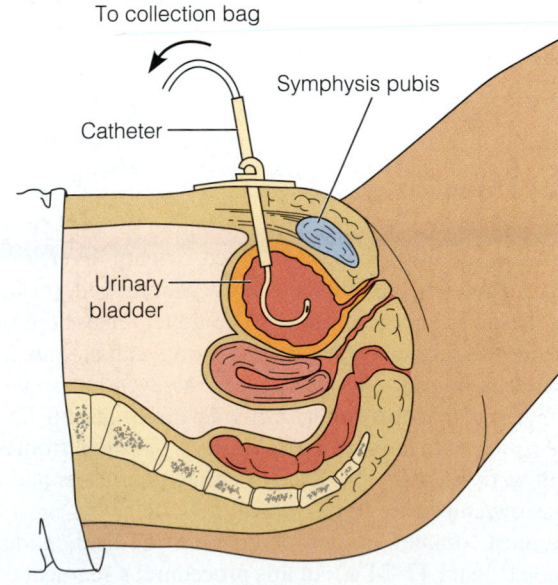

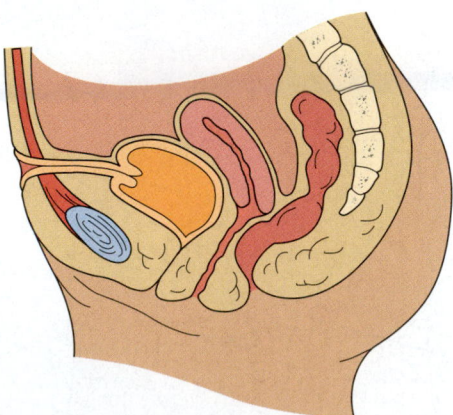

Figure 47–22 ■ A continent vesicostomy (Kock pouch).

Figure 47–23 ■ A suprapubic catheter in place.

place for an extended period, no dressing may be needed and the healed insertion tract enables removal and replacement of the catheter as needed. The nurse assesses the insertion area at regular intervals. If abdominal hair invades the insertion site, it may be carefully shaved. Any redness or discharge at the skin around the insertion site must be reported.

EVALUATING

Using the overall goals and desired outcomes identified in the planning stage, the nurse collects data to evaluate the effectiveness of nursing activities. Examples of desired outcomes for the identified goals are listed in the Identifying Nursing Diagnoses, Interventions, and Outcomes box earlier in this chapter.

If the desired outcomes are not achieved, explore the reasons before modifying the care plan. For example, if the outcome "Remains dry between voidings and at night" is not met, examples of questions that need to be considered include:

- What is the client's perception of the problem?
- Does the client understand and comply with the health care instructions provided?

- Is access to toilet facilities a problem?
- Can the client manipulate clothing for toileting? Are there adjustments that can be made to allow easier disrobing?
- Are scheduled toileting times appropriate?
- Is there adequate transition lighting for nighttime toileting?
- Are mobility aids such as a walker, elevated toilet seat, or grab bar needed? If currently used, are they appropriate or adequate?
- Is the client performing pelvic floor muscle exercises appropriately as scheduled?
- Is the client's fluid intake adequate? Does the timing of fluid intake need to be adjusted (e.g., restricted after dinner)?
- Is the client restricting caffeine, citrus juice, carbonated beverages, and artificial sweetener intake?
- Is the client taking a diuretic? If so, when is the medication taken? Do the times need to be adjusted (e.g., taking second dose no later than 4 PM)?
- Should continence aids such as a condom catheter or absorbent pads be considered or used?

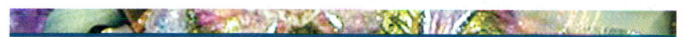

NURSING CARE PLAN FOR URINARY ELIMINATION

ASSESSMENT DATA		*NURSING DIAGNOSIS*	DESIRED OUTCOMES [NOC#]/INDICATORS*
Nursing Assessment Mr. John Baker is a 68-year-old shopkeeper who was admitted to the hospital with urinary retention, hematuria, and fever. The admitting nurse gathers the following information when taking a nursing history. Mr. Baker states he has noticed urinary frequency during the day for the past 2 weeks, and that he doesn't feel he has emptied his bladder after urinating. He also has to get up two or three times during the night to urinate. During the past few days, he has had difficulty starting urination and dribbles afterward. He verbalizes the embarrassment his urinary problems cause in his dealings with the public. Mr. Baker is concerned about the cause of this urinary problem. He is diagnosed with benign prostatic hypertrophy (BPH) and referred to a urologist who suggests a transurethral resection of the prostate (TURP) in several months. He is placed on antibiotic therapy.	**Physical Examination** Height: 185.4 cm (6'2") Weight: 85.7 kg (189 lb) Temperature: 38.1C (100.6F) Pulse: 88 BPM Respirations: 20/minute Blood pressure: 146/86 mm Hg Catheterization for urinary retention yielded 300 mL amber urine Foley left in place for 2 days **Diagnostic Data** CBC normal; urinalysis: amber, clear, pH 6.5, specific gravity 1.025, negative for glucose, protein, ketone, RBCs, and bacteria; IVP: evidence of enlarged prostate gland	*Altered Urinary Elimination* (retention and overflow incontinence) related to bladder neck obstruction by enlarged prostate gland (as evidenced by dysuria, frequency, nocturia, dribbling, hesitancy, and bladder distention)	Urinary Continence [0502] as evidenced by • Able to start and stop stream • Empties bladder completely Knowledge: Treatment Regimen [1813] as evidenced by substantial • Description of self-care responsibilities for ongoing care • Performance of treatment procedure

continued on page 1286

NURSING CARE PLAN FOR URINARY ELIMINATION *continued*

NURSING INTERVENTIONS [NIC#]/SELECTED ACTIVITIES*	RATIONALE
Urinary Incontinence Care [0610]	
• Monitor urinary elimination, including consistency, odor, volume, and color.	*These parameters help determine adequacy of urinary tract function.*
• Help the client select appropriate incontinence garment or pad for short-term management while more definitive treatment is designed.	*Appropriate undergarments can help diminish the embarrassing aspects of urinary incontinence.*
• Instruct Mr. Baker to limit fluids for 2 to 3 hours before bedtime.	*Decreased fluid intake several hours before bedtime will decrease the incidence of urinary retention and overflow incontinence, and promote rest.*
• Instruct him to drink a minimum of 1500 mL (six 8-ounce glasses fluids per day).	*Increased fluids during the day will increase urinary output and discourage bacterial growth.*
• Limit ingestion of bladder irritants (e.g., colas, coffee, tea, and chocolate).	*Alcohol, coffee, and tea have a natural diuretic effect and are bladder irritants.*
Urinary Retention Care [0620]	
• Instruct Mr. Baker or a family member to record urinary output.	*Serves as an indicator of urinary tract and renal function and of fluid balance.*
• Catheterize for residual urine, as appropriate.	*An enlarged prostate compresses the urethra so that urine is retained. Checking for residual urine provides information about bladder emptying.*
• Implement intermittent catheterization, as appropriate.	*Helps maintain tonicity of the bladder muscle by preventing overdistention and providing for complete emptying.*
• Provide enough time for bladder emptying (10 minutes).	*In addition to the effect of an enlarged prostate on the bladder, stress or anxiety can inhibit relaxation of the urinary sphincter. Sufficient time should be allowed for micturition.*
• Instruct the client in ways to avoid constipation or stool impaction.	*Impacted stool may place pressure on the bladder outlet, causing urinary retention.*
Teaching: Disease Process [5602]	
• Appraise Mr. Baker's current level of knowledge about benign prostatic hypertrophy.	*Assessing the client's knowledge will provide a foundation for building a teaching plan based on his present understanding of his condition.*
• Explain the pathophysiology of the disease and how it relates to urinary anatomy and function.	*In this case, urinary retention and overflow incontinence are caused by obstruction of the bladder neck by an enlarged prostate gland.*
• Describe the rationale behind management, therapy, and treatment recommendations.	*Adequate information about treatment options is important to diminish anxiety, promote compliance, and enhance decision making.*
• Instruct Mr. Baker on which signs and symptoms to report to the health care provider (e.g., burning on urination, hematuria, oliguria).	*In the individual with prostatic hypertrophy, urinary retention and an overdistended bladder reduce blood flow to the bladder wall, making it more susceptible to infection from bacterial growth. Monitoring for these manifestations of urinary tract infection is essential to prevent urosepsis.*

EVALUATION

Outcomes partially met. Following removal of the Foley catheter, Mr. Baker reported continued difficulty initiating a urinary stream but experienced less dribbling and nocturia. He and his wife selected an undergarment that was acceptable to Mr. Baker and he reports that he feels more confident. Intermittent catheterization not indicated. Intake is approximately 200 mL in excess of output. He is able to discuss the correlation between his enlarged prostate and urinary difficulties. A transurethral resection of the prostate is scheduled in 2 weeks.

*Outcomes, interventions, and activities selected are only a sample of those suggested by NOC and NIC and should be further individualized for each client.

continued on page 1287

NURSING CARE PLAN FOR URINARY ELIMINATION *continued*

Applying Critical Thinking

1. Considering Mr. Baker's history and assessment data, what other physical conditions could explain his symptoms?

2. The physician has recommended surgery. What assumptions will the nurse need to validate in helping prepare Mr. and Mrs. Baker for this surgery?

3. It does not appear that other alternatives have been considered. Why might this be so?

4. Incontinence can lead to client decisions to limit social interactions. What would be an appropriate response if Mr. Baker states that he will just stay home until he has his surgery?

See Critical Thinking Possibilities in Appendix A.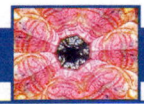

CONCEPT MAP   Urinary Elimination

JB 68 y.o. ♂ BPH

- Shopkeeper, c/o urinary frequency 2 weeks, nocturia 2–3x/night, difficulty starting stream, dribbles, c/o not feeling like bladder is emptied

- Height: 185.4 cm (6'2")
- Weight: 85.7 kg (189 lb)
- Temperature: 38.1C (100.6F)
- Pulse: 88 BPM
- Respirations: 20/minute
- Blood pressure: 146/86 mm Hg

- Catheterization for residual: 300mL amber urine
- Foley left in place for 2 days
- CBC normal; UA: amber, clear, pH 6.5, SpGr 1.025, glucose, protein, ketones, RBCs, & bacteria = neg; IVP: enlarged prostate gland

Altered Urinary Elimination (Retention and Overflow Incontinence) r/t bladder neck obstruction by enlarged prostate gland (aeb dysuria, frequency, nocturia, dribbling, hesitancy, and bladder distention)

Urinary Continence aeb
- able to start and stop stream
- empties bladder completely

Knowledge: Treatment Regimen aeb substantial
- description of self-care responsibilities for ongoing care
- performance of treatment procedure

Urinary Continence Care

Instruct client to limit fluids for 2 to 3 hours before bedtime

Monitor urinary elimination, including consistency, odor, volume, and color

Limit ingestion of bladder irritants (e.g., colas, coffee, tea, and chocolate)

Help the client select appropriate incontinence garment or pad for short-term management while more definitive treatment is designed

Instruct him to drink a minimum of 1,500 mL (six 8–ounce glasses fluids per day)

Urinary Retention Care

Instruct client or a family member to record urinary output

Provide enough time for bladder emptying (10 minutes)

Catheterize for residual urine, as appropriate

Instruct the client in ways to avoid constipation or stool impaction

Implement intermittent catheterization, as appropriate

Teaching: Disease Process

Explain the pathophysiology of the disease and how it relates to urinary anatomy and function

Describe the rationale behind management, therapy, and treatment recommendations

Instruct client on which signs and symptoms to report to the health care provider (e.g., burning on urination, hematuria, oliguria)

Appraise client's current level of knowledge about benign prostatic hypertrophy

Outcomes partially met
- following removal of the Foley catheter, client reported continued difficulty initiating a urinary stream but less dribbling and nocturia
- selected an acceptable undergarment and he reports more confident
- intermittent catheterization not indicated
- intake is ~200 mL > output
- able to discuss the correlation between enlarged prostate and urinary difficulties
- TURP scheduled in 2 weeks

Legend: Assessment ☐   Nursing Diagnosis ☐   Outcomes ☐   Nursing Interventions ☐   Activities ☐   Evaluation/Reassessment ☐

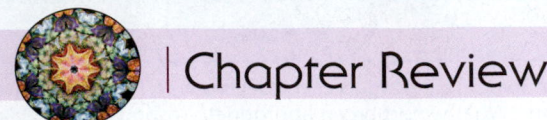

Chapter Review

EXPLORE MediaLink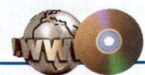

NCLEX review questions, case studies, care plan activities, MediaLink applications, and other interactive resources for this chapter can be found on the Companion Website at www.prenhall.com/kozier. Click on Chapter 47 to select the activities for this chapter.

For animations, more NCLEX review questions, and an audio glossary, access the Student CD-ROM accompanying this textbook.

Chapter Highlights

- Urinary elimination depends on normal functioning of the urinary, cardiovascular, and nervous systems.
- Urine is formed in the nephron, the functional unit of the kidney, through a process of filtration, reabsorption, and secretion. Hormones such as antidiuretic hormone (ADH) and aldosterone affect the reabsorption of sodium and water, thus affecting the amount of urine formed.
- The normal process of urination is stimulated when sufficient urine collects in the bladder to stimulate stretch receptors. Impulses from stretch receptors are transmitted to the spinal cord and the brain, causing relaxation of the internal sphincter (unconscious control) and, if appropriate, relaxation of the external sphincter (conscious control).
- In the adult, urination generally occurs after 250 to 450 mL of urine has collected in the bladder.
- Many factors influence a person's urinary elimination including growth and development, fluid intake, stress, activity, medications, and various diseases.
- Alterations in urine production and elimination include polyuria, oliguria, anuria, frequency, nocturia, urgency, dysuria, enuresis, hematuria, incontinence, and retention. Each may have various influencing and associated factors that need to be identified.
- Assessment of a client's urinary function includes (a) nursing history that identifies voiding patterns, recent changes, past and current problems with urination, and factors influencing the elimination pattern; (b) a physical assessment of the genitourinary system; (c) inspection of the urine for amount, color, clarity, and odor; and, if indicated, (d) testing of urine for specific gravity, pH, and the presence of glucose, ketone bodies, protein, and occult blood.
- Many NANDA-approved nursing diagnoses may apply to clients with altered urinary elimination patterns, for example, *Functional Incontinence, Urinary Retention,* and related diagnoses such as *Risk for Infection.*
- Incontinence can be physically and emotionally distressing to clients because it is considered socially unacceptable.
- Bladder training can often reduce episodes of incontinence.

- Clients with urinary retention not only experience discomfort but also are at risk of urinary tract infection.
- The most common cause of urinary tract infection is invasive procedures such as catheterization and cystoscopic examination. Women in particular are prone to ascending urinary tract infections because of their short urethras.
- Goals for the client with problems with urinary elimination include maintaining or restoring normal elimination patterns and preventing associated risks such as skin breakdown.
- In planning for home care, the nurse considers the client's needs for teaching and assistance or assistive devices in the home.
- Nursing interventions related to urinary elimination are generally directed toward facilitating the normal functioning of the urinary system or toward assisting the client with particular problems.
- Interventions include (a) assisting the client to maintain an appropriate fluid intake, (b) assisting the client to maintain normal voiding patterns, (c) monitoring the client's daily fluid intake and output, and (d) maintaining cleanliness of the genital area.
- Urinary catheterization is frequently required for clients with urinary retention but is only performed when all other measures to facilitate voiding fail. Sterile technique is essential to prevent ascending urinary infections.
- Care of clients with indwelling catheters is directed toward preventing infection of the urinary tract and encouraging urinary flow through the drainage system.
- Clients with urinary retention may be taught to perform clean intermittent self-catheterization to enhance their independence, reduce the risk of infection, and eliminate incontinence.
- Bladder or catheter irrigations may be used to apply medication to bladder walls or maintain catheter patency.
- When the urinary bladder is removed, a urinary diversion is formed to allow urine to be eliminated from the body. The ileal conduit or ileal loop is the most common diversion and requires that the client wear a urine collection device continually over the stoma.

Review Questions

47–1. The nurse recognizes that urinary elimination changes may occur even in healthy elders because
a. the bladder distends and its capacity increases.
b. elders ignore the need to void.
c. urine becomes more concentrated.
d. the amount of urine retained after voiding increases.

47–2. During assessment of the client with urinary incontinence, the nurse anticipates finding any of the following EXCEPT
a. perineal skin irritation.
b. fluid intake of less than 1,500 mL/day.
c. history of antihistamine intake.
d. history of frequent urinary tract infections.

47–3. Which of the following represents correct condom catheter nursing care?
a. Ensure that the tip of the penis fits snugly against the end of the condom.
b. Check the penis for adequate circulation 30 minutes after applying.
c. Change the condom every 8 hours.
d. Tape the collecting tubing to the lower abdomen.

47–4. During the straight catheterization of a female client, if the catheter slips into the vagina, the nurse should
a. leave the catheter in place and get a new sterile catheter.
b. leave the catheter in place and ask another nurse to attempt the procedure.
c. remove the catheter and redirect it to the urinary meatus.
d. remove the catheter, wipe it with a sterile gauze, and redirect it to the urinary meatus.

47–5. Which of the following statements indicates a need for further teaching of the home care client with a long-term indwelling catheter?
a. "I will keep the collecting bag below the level of the bladder at all times."
b. "Intake of cranberry juice may help decrease the chances of developing an infection."
c. "Soaking in warm tub bath may ease the irritating feeling from having a catheter."
d. "I should use clean technique when emptying the collecting bag."

Readings and References

Suggested Readings

Association of Women's Health, Obstetric and Neonatal Nurses (AWHONN). (2000). *Evidence-based clinical practice guideline: Continence for women.* Washington, DC: Author. This document provides research-based guidelines for screening for urinary incontinence, basic evaluation and physical assessment of the woman with incontinence, steps in the decision-making process for treatment, possible interventions, and principles for referral to other healthcare providers.

Bates, F., & Porter, G. (2002). The role of the nurse continence advisor in a urology wellness clinic. *Urologic Nursing, 22*(1), 23–26. Urinary incontinence is both a social and a medical problem. This article describes the role of the nurse continence advisor, who has the potential to contribute significantly to resolving incontinence and in decreasing the cost of incontinence management in home care programs.

Related Research

Tambyah, P. A., Knasinski, V., & Maki, D. G. (2002). The direct costs of nosocomial catheter-associated urinary tract infections in the era of managed care. *Infection Control and Hospital Epidemiology, 23,* 27–31.

Webster, J., Hood, R. H., Burridge, C. A., Doidge, M. L., Phillips, K. M., & George, N. (2001). Water or antiseptic for periurethral cleaning for urinary catheterization: A randomized controlled trial. *American Journal of Infection Control, 29,* 389–394.

References

Ball, J. W., & Bindler, R. C. (2003). *Pediatric nursing: Caring for children* (3rd ed.). Upper Saddle River, NJ: Prentice Hall.

Cendron, M. (1999). Primary nocturnal enuresis: Current concepts. *American Family Physician, 59,* 1205–1214, 1219–1220.

Johnson, M., Maas, M., & Moorhead, S. (Eds.). (2000). *Nursing outcomes classification (NOC)* (2nd ed.). St. Louis, MO: Mosby.

Kelleher, M. M. B. (2002). Removal of urinary catheters: Midnight vs. 0600 hours. *British Journal of Nursing, 11,* 84, 86, 88–90.

Maki, D. G., & Tambyah, P. A. (2001). Engineering out the risk of infection with urinary catheters. *Emerging Infectious Diseases, 7*(2), 1–6.

Marchiondo, K. (1998). A new look at urinary tract infection. *American Journal of Nursing, 98*(3), 34–39.

McCloskey, J. C., & Bulechek, G. M. (Eds.). (2000). *Nursing interventions classification (NIC)* (3rd ed.). St. Louis, MO: Mosby.

NANDA International. (2003). *NANDA Nursing diagnoses: Definitions and classification 2003-2004.* Philadelphia: Author.

Shultz, J. M. (2002). Urinary incontinence: Solving a secret problem. *Nursing, 32*(11), 53–55.

Selected Bibliography

Archer, C. L., & Foote, J. E. (2000). Urinary incontinence in the elderly female. *Urologic Nursing, 20,* 301–305.

Brennan, M. L., & Evans, A. (2001). Why catheterize? Audit findings on the use of catheters. *British Journal of Nursing, 10,* 580, 582, 584, 588, 590.

Dougherty, M. C., Dwyer, J. W., Pendergast, J. F., Boyington, A. R., Tomlinson, B. U., Coward, R. T., et al. (2002). Urinary incontinence in older rural women. *Research in Nursing & Health, 25,* 3–13.

Fillingham, S. (1999). Caring for patients with urological stomas. *Journal of Community Health Nursing, 13*(12), 29–30, 32, 34.

Gray, M. (2000). Urinary retention: Management in the acute care setting, Part 1. *American Journal of Nursing, 100*(7), 40–48.

Gray, M. (2000). Urinary retention: Management in the acute care setting, Part 2. *American Journal of Nursing, 100*(8), 36–44.

Gray, M., Ratliff, C., & Donovan, A. (2002). Tender mercies: Providing skin care for an incontinent patient. *Nursing, 32*(7), 51–54.

Kane, A. M. (2000). Criteria for successful neobladder surgery: Patient selection and surgical construction. *Urologic Nursing, 20,* 182, 187–188, 198.

Kane, A. M. (2000). Nursing management of neobladder surgery: The Studer pouch. *Urologic Nursing, 20,* 189–193, 197.

Matthews, S. D. (2001). Orthotopic neobladder surgery. *American Journal of Nursing, 101*(7), 24AA–24EE.

McConnell, E. A. (2000). New catheters decrease nosocomial infections. *Nursing Management, 31*(6), 52, 55.

McConnell, E. A. (2001). Applying a condom catheter. *Nursing, 31*(1), 70.

Muller, N. (2001). The impact of incontinence. *Advance for Providers of Post-Acute Care, 4*(6), 26, 79.

Newman, D. K., & Giovannini, D. (2002). The overactive bladder: A nursing perspective. *American Journal of Nursing, 102*(6), 36–46.

Reilly, N. J. (2000). Nursing management of older women with urinary incontinence. *Urologic Nursing, 20,* 307–311, 315.

Rosto, L. (2001). Slowing the flow. *Advance for Providers of Post-Acute Care, 4*(2), 59–62.

Taylor, P. (2001). Choosing the right stoma appliance for a urostomy. *Community Nurse, 7*(2), 35–36.

Winder, A. (1999). Female urinary catheterization. *Community Nurse, 5*(10), 33–34, 36.

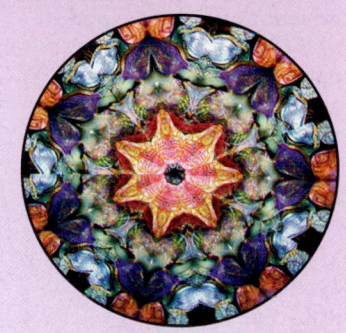

CHAPTER 48

OXYGENATION

LEARNING OUTCOMES

After completing this chapter, you will be able to:

- Outline the structure and function of the respiratory system.
- Describe the processes of breathing (ventilation) and gas exchange (respiration).
- Explain the role and function of the respiratory system in transporting oxygen and carbon dioxide to and from body tissues.
- Identify factors influencing respiratory function.
- Identify common manifestations of impaired respiratory function.
- Identify and describe nursing measures to promote respiratory function and oxygenation.
- Explain the use of therapeutic measures such as medications, inhalation therapy, oxygen therapy, artificial airways, pharyngeal suction, and chest drainage to promote respiratory function.
- State outcome criteria for evaluating client responses to measures that promote adequate oxygenation.

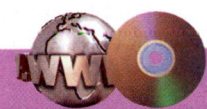

MediaLink

www.prenhall.com/kozier

Additional resources for this chapter can be found on the Student CD-ROM accompanying this textbook, and on the Companion Website at www.prenhall.com/kozier. Click on Chapter 48 to select the activities for this chapter.

CD-ROM
- Audio Glossary
- NCLEX Review
- Animations:
   Gas Exchange in the Lung
   Carbon Dioxide Transport
   Oxygen Transport
   A & P Review
- Videos:
   Humidifier
   Face Mask

Companion Website
- Additional NCLEX Review
- Case Study: Coping With Emphysema
- Care Plan Activity: Deep Breathing and Coughing
- MediaLink Application: Learning About Lung Disease
- Links to Resources

Oxygen, a clear, odorless gas that constitutes approximately 21% of the air we breathe, is necessary for all living cells. The absence of oxygen can lead to death. Although the delivery of oxygen to body tissues is affected at least indirectly by all body systems, the respiratory system is most directly involved in this process. Impaired function of the system can significantly affect our ability to breathe, transport gases, and participate in everyday activities.

Respiration is the process of gas exchange between the individual and the environment. The process of respiration involves two components:

1. Pulmonary ventilation or breathing; the movement of air between the atmosphere and the alveoli of the lungs
2. Diffusion of oxygen and carbon dioxide between the alveoli and pulmonary capillaries.

PHYSIOLOGY OF THE RESPIRATORY SYSTEM

The function of the respiratory system is gas exchange. Oxygen from inspired air diffuses from alveoli in the lungs into the blood in pulmonary capillaries. Carbon dioxide produced during cell metabolism diffuses from the blood into the alveoli and is exhaled. The organs of the respiratory system facilitate this gas exchange and protect the body from foreign matter such as particulates and pathogens.

Structure of the Respiratory System

The respiratory system (Figure 48–1 ■) is divided structurally into the upper respiratory system and the lower respiratory system. The mouth, nose, pharynx, and larynx compose the upper respiratory system. The lower respiratory system includes the trachea and lungs, with the bronchi, bronchioles, alveoli, pulmonary capillary network, and pleural membranes.

Air enters through the nose, where it is warmed, humidified, and filtered. Large particles in the air are trapped by the hairs at the entrance of the nares, and smaller particles are filtered and trapped as air changes direction on contact with the nasal turbinates and septum. The sneeze reflex is initiated by irritants in nasal passages. A large volume of air rapidly exits through the nose and mouth during a sneeze, helping to clear nasal passages.

Inspired air passes from the nose through the pharynx. The pharynx is a shared pathway for air and food. It includes both the nasopharynx and the oropharynx, which are richly supplied with lymphoid tissue that traps and destroys pathogens entering with the air.

The larynx is a cartilaginous structure that can be identified externally as the Adam's apple. In addition to its role in providing for speech, the larynx is important for maintaining airway patency and protecting the lower airways from swallowed food and fluids. During swallowing, the inlet to the larynx (the epiglottis) closes, routing food to the esophagus. The epiglottis is open during breathing, allowing air to move freely into the lower airways.

Below the larynx, the trachea leads to the right and left main bronchi (primary bronchi) and the conducting airways of the lungs. Within the lungs, the primary bronchi divide repeatedly into smaller and smaller bronchi, ending with the terminal bronchioles. Together these airways are known as the bronchial tree. The trachea and bronchi are lined with mucosal epithelium. These cells produce a thin layer of mucus, the "mucous blanket," that traps pathogens and microscopic particulate matter. These foreign particles are then swept upward toward the larynx and throat by cilia, tiny hairlike projections on the epithelial cells. The cough reflex is triggered by irritants in the larynx, trachea, or bronchi and is described in Box 48–1.

Until air passes through the terminal bronchioles and enters the respiratory bronchioles and alveoli, no gas exchange occurs. The respiratory zone of the lungs includes the respiratory bronchioles (which have scattered air sacs in their walls), the alveolar ducts, and the alveoli (Figure 48–1). Alveoli have very thin walls, composed of a single layer of epithelial cells covered by a thick mesh of pulmonary capillaries. The alveolar and capillary walls form the **respiratory membrane,** where gas exchange occurs between the air on the alveolar side and the blood on the capillary side. The airways move air to and from the alveoli; the right ventricle and pulmonary vascular system transport blood to the capillary side of the membrane.

The outer surface of the lungs is covered by a thin, double layer of tissue known as the pleura. The parietal pleura lines the thorax and surface of the diaphragm. It doubles back to form the visceral pleura, covering the external surface of the lungs. Between these pleural layers is a potential

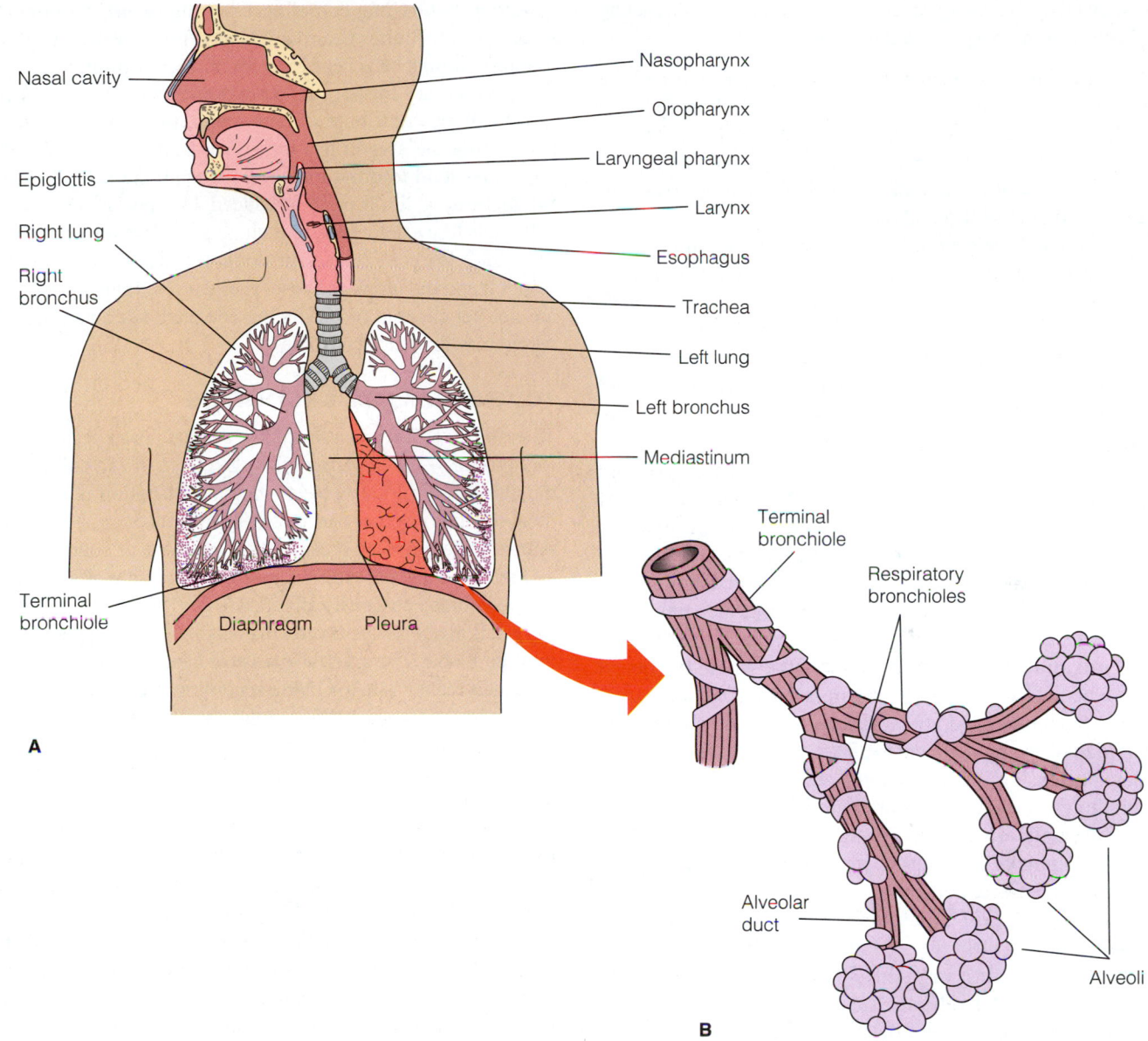

Figure 48–1 ■ *A*, Organs of the respiratory tract. *B*, Respiratory bronchioles, alveolar ducts, and alveoli.

- Nerve impulses are sent through the vagus nerve to the medulla.
- A large inspiration of approximately 2.5 L occurs.
- The epiglottis and glottis (vocal cords) close.
- A strong contraction of abdominal and internal intercostal muscles dramatically raises the pressure in the lungs.
- The epiglottis and glottis open suddenly.
- Air rushes outward with great velocity.
- Mucus and any foreign particles are dislodged from the lower respiratory tract and are propelled up and out.

space that contains a small amount of pleural fluid, a serous lubricating solution. This fluid prevents friction during the movements of breathing and serves to keep the layers adherent through its surface tension.

Pulmonary Ventilation

Ventilation of the lungs is accomplished through the act of breathing: **inspiration (inhalation)** when air flows into the lungs and **expiration (exhalation)** as air moves out of the lungs. Adequate ventilation depends on several factors:

- Clear airways
- An intact central nervous system and respiratory center

- An intact thoracic cavity capable of expanding and contracting
- Adequate pulmonary compliance and recoil.

A number of mechanisms including ciliary action and the cough reflex work to keep airways open and clear. In some cases, however, these defenses may be overwhelmed. The inflammation, edema, and excess mucous production that occur with some types of pneumonia may clog small airways, impairing ventilation of distal alveoli.

The respiratory centers of the medulla and pons in the brain stem control breathing. Severe head injury or drugs that depress the central nervous system (e.g., opiates or barbiturates) can affect the respiratory centers, impairing the drive to breathe.

Expansion and recoil of the lungs occurs passively in response to changes in pressures within the thoracic cavity and the lungs themselves. The **intrapleural pressure** (pressure in the pleural cavity surrounding the lungs) is always slightly negative in relation to atmospheric pressure. This negative pressure is essential because it creates the suction that holds the visceral pleura and the parietal pleura together as the chest cage expands and contracts. The recoil tendency of the lungs is a major factor in creating this negative pressure. The intrapleural fluid also contributes by causing the pleura to adhere together, much as a film of water can cause two glass slides to adhere together.

The **intrapulmonary pressure** (pressure within the lungs) always equalizes with atmospheric pressure. Inspiration occurs when the diaphragm and intercostal muscles contract, increasing the size of the thoracic cavity. The volume of the lungs increases, decreasing intrapulmonary pressure. Air then rushes into the lungs to equalize this pressure with atmospheric pressure. Conversely, when the diaphragm and intercostal muscles relax, the volume of the lungs decreases, intrapulmonary pressure rises, and air is expelled.

The degree of chest expansion during normal breathing is minimal, requiring little energy expenditure. In adults, approximately 500 mL of air is inspired and expired with each breath. This is known as **tidal volume.** Breathing during strenuous exercise or some types of heart disease require greater chest expansion and effort. At this time, more than 1,500 mL of air may be moved with each breath. Accessory muscles of respiration, including the anterior neck muscles, intercostal muscles, and muscles of the abdomen, are employed. Active use of these muscles and noticeable effort in breathing are seen in clients with obstructive pulmonary disease.

Diseases such as muscular dystrophy, or trauma such as spinal cord injury can affect the muscles of respiration, impairing the ability of the thoracic cavity to expand and contract. A gunshot wound or other trauma to the chest wall may allow intrapleural pressure to equalize with the atmosphere, causing the lung to collapse.

Lung compliance, the expansibility or stretchability of lung tissue, plays a significant role in the ease of ventilation. At birth, the fluid-filled lungs are stiff and resistant to expansion, much as a new balloon is difficult to inflate. With each subsequent breath, the alveoli become more compliant and easier to inflate, just as a balloon becomes easier to inflate after several tries. Lung compliance tends to decrease with aging, making it more difficult to expand alveoli and increasing risk of **atelectasis,** or collapse of a portion of the lung.

In contrast to lung compliance is **lung recoil,** the continual tendency of the lungs to collapse away from the chest wall. Just as lung compliance is necessary for normal inspiration, lung recoil is necessary for normal expiration. Although elastic fibers in lung tissue contribute to lung recoil, the surface tension of fluid lining the alveoli has the greatest effect on recoil. Fluid molecules tend to draw together, reducing the size of alveoli. **Surfactant,** a lipoprotein produced by specialized alveolar cells, acts like a detergent, reducing the surface tension of alveolar fluid. Without surfactant, lung expansion is exceedingly difficult and the lungs collapse. Premature infants whose lungs are not yet capable of producing adequate surfactant develop respiratory distress syndrome.

Alveolar Gas Exchange

After the alveoli are ventilated, the second phase of the respiratory process—*the diffusion of* oxygen from the alveoli and into the pulmonary blood vessels—begins. **Diffusion** is the movement of gases or other particles from an area of greater pressure or concentration to an area of lower pressure or concentration.

Pressure differences in the gases on each side of the respiratory membrane obviously affect diffusion. When the pressure of oxygen is greater in the alveoli than in the blood, oxygen diffuses into the blood. The **partial pressure** (the pressure exerted by each individual gas in a mixture according to its concentration in the mixture) of oxygen (PO_2) in the alveoli is about 100 mm Hg (sometimes referred to as **torr** which is the same as millimeters of mercury), whereas the PO_2 in the venous blood of the pulmonary arteries is about 60 mm Hg. These pressures rapidly equalize, however, so that the arterial oxygen pressure also reaches about 100 mm Hg. By contrast, carbon dioxide in the venous blood entering the pulmonary capillaries has a partial pressure of about 45 mm Hg (PCO_2), whereas that in the alveoli has a partial pressure of about 40 mm Hg. Therefore, carbon dioxide diffuses from the blood into the alveoli, where it can be eliminated with expired air. When referring to the pressure of oxygen in the arterial blood the abbreviation is PaO_2. When referring to partial pressure in venous blood there is no "a," that is, PO_2.

Transport of Oxygen and Carbon Dioxide

The third part of the respiratory process involves the transport of respiratory gases. Oxygen needs to be transported from the lungs to the tissues, and carbon dioxide must be transported from the tissues back to the lungs. Normally most of the oxygen (97%) combines loosely with **hemoglobin** (oxygen-carrying red pigment) in the red blood cells and is carried to the tissues as **oxyhemoglobin** (the compound of oxygen and hemoglobin). The remaining oxygen is dissolved and transported in the fluid of the plasma and cells.

Several factors affect the rate of oxygen transport from the lungs to the tissues:

1. Cardiac output
2. Number of erythrocytes and blood hematocrit
3. Exercise.

The **hematocrit** is the percentage of the blood that is erythrocytes.

Any pathologic condition that decreases cardiac output (e.g., damage to the heart muscle, blood loss, or pooling of blood in the peripheral blood vessels) diminishes the amount of oxygen delivered to the tissues. The heart compensates for inadequate output by increasing its pumping rate; however, with severe damage or blood loss, this compensatory mechanism may not restore adequate blood flow and oxygen to the tissues.

The second factor influencing oxygen transport is the number of **erythrocytes** (red blood cells, or RBCs) and the hematocrit. In men, the number of circulating erythrocytes normally averages about 5 million per cubic milliliter of blood, and in women, about 4 1/2 million per cubic milliliter. Normally the hematocrit is about 40% to 54% in men and 37% to 48% in women. Excessive increases in the blood hematocrit raise the blood viscosity, reducing the cardiac output and therefore reducing oxygen transport. Excessive reductions in the blood hematocrit, such as occur in anemia, reduce oxygen transport.

Exercise also has a direct influence on oxygen transport. In well-trained athletes, oxygen transport can be increased up to 20 times the normal rate, due in part to an increased cardiac output and to increased use of oxygen by the cells.

Carbon dioxide, continually produced in the processes of cell metabolism, is transported from the cells to the lungs in three ways. The majority (about 65%) is carried inside the red blood cells as bicarbonate (HCO_3^-) and is an important component of the bicarbonate buffer system (see Chapter 50). A moderate amount of carbon dioxide (30%) combines with hemoglobin as carbhemoglobin (also known as carbaminohemoglobin) for transport. Smaller amounts (5%) are transported in solution in the plasma and as carbonic acid (the compound formed when carbon dioxide combines with water).

RESPIRATORY REGULATION

Respiratory regulation includes both neural and chemical controls to maintain the correct concentrations of oxygen, carbon dioxide, and hydrogen ions in body fluids. The nervous system of the body adjusts the rate of alveolar ventilations to meet the needs of the body so that PO_2 and PCO_2 remain relatively constant. The body's "respiratory center" is actually a number of groups of neurons located in the medulla oblongata and pons of the brain.

A chemosensitive center in the medulla oblongata is highly responsive to increases in blood CO_2 or hydrogen ion concentration. By influencing other respiratory centers, this center can increase the activity of the inspiratory center and the rate and depth of respirations. In addition to this direct chemical stimulation of the respiratory center in the brain, special neural receptors sensitive to decreases in O_2 concentration are located outside the central nervous system in the carotid bodies (just above the bifurcation of the common carotid arteries) and aortic bodies. Decreases in arterial oxygen concentrations stimulate these chemoreceptors, and they in turn stimulate the respiratory center to increase ventilation. Of the three blood gases (hydrogen, oxygen, and carbon dioxide) that can trigger chemoreceptors, increased carbon dioxide concentration normally stimulates respiration most strongly.

However, in clients with certain chronic lung ailments such as **emphysema,** oxygen concentrations, not carbon dioxide concentrations, play a major role in regulating respiration. For such clients, decreased oxygen concentrations are the main stimuli for respiration. This is sometimes called the hypoxic drive. Increasing the concentration of oxygen depresses the respiratory rate. Thus, only low concentrations of supplemental oxygen are administered to these clients.

> **CLINICAL ALERT** *In clients with chronic obstructive lung disease, administering supplemental oxygen can actually cause the client to stop breathing.* ■

FACTORS AFFECTING RESPIRATORY FUNCTION

Factors that influence oxygenation affect the cardiovascular system as well as the respiratory system. These factors include age, environment, lifestyle, health status, medications, and stress.

Age

Developmental factors are important influences on respiratory function. At birth, profound changes occur in the respiratory systems. The fluid-filled lungs drain, the PCO_2 rises, and the neonate takes a first breath. The lungs gradually expand with each subsequent breath, reaching full inflation by 2 weeks of age. Changes of aging that affect the respiratory system of elders become especially important if the system is compromised by changes such as infection, physical or emotional stress, surgery, anesthesia, or other procedures. Changes are:

* Chest wall and airways become more rigid and less elastic.
* The amount of exchanged air is decreased.
* The cough reflex and cilia action are decreased.
* Mucous membranes become drier and more fragile.
* Decreases in muscle strength and endurance occur.
* If osteoporosis is present, adequate lung expansion may be compromised.
* A decrease in efficiency of the immune system occurs.
* Gastroesophageal reflux disease is more common in older adults and increases the risk of aspiration. The aspiration of stomach contents into the lungs often causes bronchospasm by setting up an inflammatory response.

Environment

Altitude, heat, cold, and air pollution affect oxygenation. The higher the altitude, the lower the PO_2 an individual breathes. As a result, the person at high altitudes has increased respiratory and cardiac rates and increased respiratory depth, which usually become most apparent when the individual exercises.

Healthy people exposed to air pollution, such as smog, often experience stinging of the eyes, headache, dizziness, coughing, and choking. People who have a history of existing lung disease and altered respiratory function experience varying degrees of

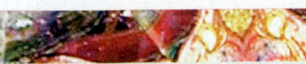

Lifespan Considerations

Respiratory Development

Infants

■ Respiratory rates are highest and most variable in newborns. The respiratory rate of a neonate is 40 to 80 breaths per minute

■ Infant respiratory rates average about 30 per minute.

■ Because of rib cage structure, infants rely almost exclusively on diaphragmatic movement for breathing. This is seen as abdominal breathing, as the abdomen rises and falls with each breath.

Children

■ The respiratory rate gradually decreases, averaging around 25 per minute in the preschooler and reaching the adult rate of 12 to 18 per minute by late adolescence.

■ During infancy and childhood, upper respiratory infections are common and, fortunately, usually not serious. Infants and preschoolers also are at risk for airway obstruction by foreign objects such as coins and small toys. Cystic fibrosis is a congenital disorder that affects the lungs, causing them to become congested with thick, tenacious (sticky) mucus. Asthma is another chronic disease often identified in childhood. The airways of the asthmatic child respond to stimuli such as allergens, exercise, or cold air by constricting, becoming edematous, and producing excessive mucus. Airflow is impaired, and the child may wheeze as air moves through narrowed air passages.

Elders

■ Elders are at increased risk for acute respiratory diseases such as pneumonia and chronic diseases such as emphysema and chronic bronchitis. Chronic obstructive pulmonary disease (COPD) may affect elders, particularly after years of exposure to cigarette smoke or industrial pollutants.

■ Pneumonia may not present with the usual symptoms of a fever, but will present with atypical symptoms, such as confusion, weakness, loss of appetite, and increase in heart rate and respirations.

Nursing interventions should be directed toward achieving optimal respiratory effort and gas exchange:

■ Always encourage wellness and prevention of disease by reinforcing the need for good nutrition, exercise, and immunizations, such as for influenza and pneumonia.

■ Increase fluid intake, if not contraindicated by other problems, such as cardiac or renal impairment.

■ Proper positioning and frequent changing of positions allow for better lung expansion and air and fluid movement.

■ Teach client to use breathing techniques for better air exchange (see Teaching: Client Care boxes throughout this chapter).

■ Pace activities to conserve energy.

■ Encourage the client to eat more frequent, smaller meals to decrease gastric distention, which can cause pressure on the diaphragm.

■ Teach client to avoid extreme hot or cold temperatures that will further tax the respiratory system.

■ Teach actions and side effects of drugs, inhalers, and treatments.

---

respiratory difficulty in a polluted environment. Some are unable to perform self-care in such an environment.

Lifestyle

Physical exercise or activity increases the rate and depth of respirations and hence the supply of oxygen in the body. Sedentary people, by contrast, lack the alveolar expansion and deep breathing patterns of people with regular activity and are less able to respond effectively to respiratory stressors.

Certain occupations predispose an individual to lung disease. For example, silicosis is seen more often in sandstone blasters and potters than in the rest of the population; asbestosis in asbestos workers; anthracosis in coal miners; and organic dust disease in farmers and agricultural employees who work with moldy hay.

Health Status

In the healthy person, the respiratory system can provide sufficient oxygen to meet the body needs. Diseases of the respiratory system, however, can adversely affect the oxygenation of the blood.

Medications

A variety of medications can decrease the rate and depth of respirations. The most common medications with this effect are the benzodiazepine sedative-hypnotics and antianxiety drugs [e.g., diazepam (Valium), flurazepam (Dalmane), midazolam (Versed)], barbiturates (e.g., phenobarbital), and narcotics such as morphine and meperidine hydrochloride (Demerol). When administering these, the nurse must carefully monitor respiratory status, especially when the medication is begun or when the dose is increased. Although this is a safety concern, often the importance of the medication outweighs the risk of respiratory depression.

Stress

When stress and stressors are encountered, both psychologic and physiologic responses can affect oxygenation. Some people may hyperventilate in response to stress. When this occurs, arterial PO_2 rises and PCO_2 falls. The person may experience light-headedness and numbness and tingling of the fingers, toes, and around the mouth as a result.

Physiologically, the sympathetic nervous system is stimulated and epinephrine is released. Epinephrine causes the bronchioles to dilate, increasing blood flow and oxygen delivery to active muscles. Although these responses are adaptive in the short term, when stress continues they can be destructive, increasing the risk of cardiovascular disease.

ALTERATIONS IN RESPIRATORY FUNCTION

Respiratory function can be altered by conditions that affect

• The movement of air into or out of the lungs
• The diffusion of oxygen and carbon dioxide between the alveoli and the pulmonary capillaries

- The transport of oxygen and carbon dioxide via the blood to and from the tissue cells

Three major alterations in respiration are hypoxia, altered breathing patterns, and obstructed or partially obstructed airway.

Hypoxia

Hypoxia is a condition of insufficient oxygen anywhere in the body, from the inspired gas to the tissues. It can be related to any of the parts of respiration—ventilation, diffusion of gases, or transport of gases by the blood—and can be caused by any condition that alters one or more parts of the process.

Hypoventilation, that is, inadequate alveolar ventilation, can lead to hypoxia. Hypoventilation may occur because of diseases of the respiratory muscles, drugs, or anesthesia. With hypoventilation, carbon dioxide often accumulates in the blood, a condition called **hypercarbia (hypercapnia).**

Hypoxia can also develop when the diffusion of oxygen from alveoli into the arterial blood decreases, as with pulmonary edema, or it can result from problems in the delivery of oxygen to the tissues (e.g., anemia, heart failure, and embolism). The term **hypoxemia** refers to reduced oxygen in the blood and is characterized by a low partial pressure of oxygen in arterial blood or a low hemoglobin saturation. Box 48–2 lists signs of hypoxia.

Cyanosis (bluish discoloration of the skin, nailbeds, and mucous membranes, due to reduced hemoglobin-oxygen saturation) may also be present. Cyanosis requires these two conditions: The blood must contain about 5 g or more of unoxygenated hemoglobin per 100 mL of blood, and the surface blood capillaries must be dilated. Factors that interfere with either of these conditions (e.g., severe anemia or the administration of epinephrine) will eliminate cyanosis as a sign even if the client is experiencing hypoxia.

Adequate oxygenation is essential for cerebral functioning. The cerebral cortex can tolerate hypoxia for only 3 to 5 minutes before permanent damage occurs. The face of the acutely hypoxic person usually appears anxious, tired, and drawn. The person usually assumes a sitting position, often leaning forward slightly to permit greater expansion of the thoracic cavity.

With chronic hypoxia, the client often appears fatigued and is lethargic. The client's fingers and toes may be clubbed as a result of long-term lack of oxygen in the arterial blood supply. With clubbing, the base of the nail becomes swollen and the ends of the fingers and toes increase in size. The angle between the nail and the base of the nail increases to more than 180 degrees. See Figure 28–12, page 542.

Altered Breathing Patterns

Breathing patterns refer to the rate, volume, rhythm, and relative ease or effort of respiration. Normal respiration (**eupnea**) is quiet, rhythmic, and effortless. **Tachypnea** (rapid rate) is seen with fevers, metabolic acidosis, pain, and with hypercapnia or hypoxemia. **Bradypnea** is an abnormally slow respiratory rate, which may be seen in clients who have taken drugs such as morphine, who have metabolic alkalosis, or who have increased intracranial pressure (e.g., from brain injuries). **Apnea** is the cessation of breathing.

Hyperventilation, often called *alveolar hyperventilation,* is an increased movement of air into and out of the lungs. During hyperventilation, the rate and depth of respirations increase, and more CO_2 is eliminated than is produced. One particular type of hyperventilation that accompanies metabolic acidosis is **Kussmaul's breathing,** by which the body attempts to compensate (give off excess body acids) by blowing off the carbon dioxide through deep and rapid breathing. Hyperventilation can also occur in response to stress, as mentioned earlier.

Abnormal respiratory rhythms create an irregular breathing pattern. Two abnormal respiratory rhythms are

- **Cheyne-Stokes respirations.** Marked rhythmic waxing and waning of respirations from very deep to very shallow breathing and temporary apnea; common causes include congestive heart failure, increased intracranial pressure, and drug overdose
- **Biot's (cluster) respirations.** Shallow breaths interrupted by apnea; may be seen in clients with central nervous system disorders.

Orthopnea is the inability to breathe except in an upright or standing position. Difficult or uncomfortable breathing is called **dyspnea.** The dyspneic person often appears anxious and may experience *shortness of breath* (SOB), a feeling of being unable to get enough air (breathlessness). Often the nostrils are flared because of the increased effort of inspiration. The skin may appear dusky; heart rate is increased. Dyspnea may have many causes, most of which stem from cardiac or respiratory disorders. It is a subjective feeling; that is, dyspnea may not be directly observed or measured but is reported by the client. Since treatment is aimed at removing the underlying cause, it is important for the nurse to conduct a thorough history of the onset, duration, and precipitating and relieving factors of the client's dyspnea plus a comprehensive physical examination.

Obstructed Airway

A completely or partially obstructed airway can occur anywhere along the upper or lower respiratory passageways. An upper airway obstruction—that is, in the nose, pharynx, or larynx—can arise because of a foreign object such as food, because the tongue falls back into the oropharynx when a person is unconscious, or when secretions collect in the passageways. In the latter instance,

BOX 48–2 ■ Signs of Hypoxia

- Rapid pulse
- Rapid, shallow respirations and dyspnea
- Increased restlessness or light-headedness
- Flaring of the nares
- Substernal or intercostal retractions
- Cyanosis

the respirations will sound gurgly or bubbly as the air attempts to pass through the secretions. Lower airway obstruction involves partial or complete occlusion of the passageways in the bronchi and lungs.

Maintaining an open (patent) airway is a nursing responsibility, one that often requires immediate action. Partial obstruction of the upper airway passages is indicated by a low-pitched snoring sound during inhalation. Complete obstruction is indicated by extreme inspiratory effort that produces no chest movement. Such a client, in an effort to obtain air, may also exhibit marked sternal and intercostal retractions. Lower airway obstruction is not always as easy to observe. **Stridor,** a harsh, high-pitched sound, may be heard during inspiration. The client may have altered arterial blood gas levels, restlessness, dyspnea, and **adventitious breath sounds** (abnormal breath sounds). See Table 28–8, page 575.

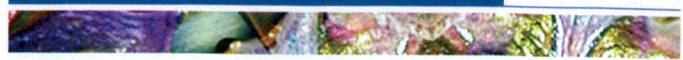

NURSING MANAGEMENT

ASSESSING

Nursing assessment of oxygenation status includes a history, physical examination, and review of relevant diagnostic data.

Nursing History

A comprehensive nursing history relevant to oxygenation status should include data about current and past respiratory problems; lifestyle; presence of cough, **sputum** (coughed-up material), pain; medications for breathing; and presence of risk factors for impaired oxygenation status. Examples of interview questions to elicit this information are shown in the Assessment Interview.

Assessment Interview

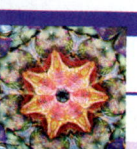

OXYGENATION

Current Respiratory Problems

- Have you noticed any changes in your breathing pattern (e.g., shortness of breath, difficulty in breathing, need to be in upright position to breathe, or rapid and shallow breathing)?
- If so, which of your activities might cause these symptom(s) to occur?
- How many pillows do you use to sleep at night?

History of Respiratory Disease

- Have you had colds, allergies, asthma, tuberculosis, bronchitis, pneumonia, or emphysema?
- How frequently have these occurred? How long did they last? And how were they treated?
- Have you been exposed to any pollutants?

Lifestyle

- Do you smoke? If so, how much? If not, did you smoke previously, and when did you stop?
- Does any member of your family smoke?
- Is there cigarette smoke or other pollutants (e.g., fumes, dust, coal, asbestos) in your workplace?
- Do you use alcohol? If so, how many drinks (mixed drinks, glasses of wine, or beers) do you usually have per day or per week?
- Describe your exercise patterns. How often do you exercise and for how long?

Presence of Cough

- How often and how much do you cough?
- Is it productive, that is, accompanied by sputum, or nonproductive, that is, dry?
- Does the cough occur during certain activity or at certain times of the day?

Description of Sputum

- When is the sputum produced?
- What is the amount, color, thickness, odor?
- Is it ever tinged with blood?

Presence of Chest Pain

- Do you experience any pain with breathing or activity?
- Where is the pain located?
- Describe the pain. How does it feel?
- Does it occur when you breathe in or out?
- How long does it last, and how does it affect your breathing?
- Do you experience any other symptoms when the pain occurs (e.g., nausea, shortness of breath or difficulty breathing, light-headedness, palpitations)?
- What activities precede your pain?
- What do you do to relieve the pain?

Presence of Risk Factors

- Do you have a family history of lung cancer, cardiovascular disease (including strokes), or tuberculosis?
- The nurse should also note the client's weight, activity pattern, and dietary assessment. Risk factors include obesity, sedentary lifestyle, and diet high in saturated fats.

Medication History

- Have you taken or do you take any over-the-counter or prescription medications for breathing (e.g., bronchodilator, inhalant, narcotic)?
- If so, which ones? And what are the dosages, times taken, and results, including side effects?

Physical Examination

In assessing a client's oxygenation status, the nurse uses all four physical examination techniques: inspection, palpation, percussion, and auscultation. The nurse first observes the rate, depth, rhythm, and quality of respirations, noting the position the client assumes for breathing. Some clients with chronic respiratory problems prefer to bend forward at the waist to ease breathing or to sit leaning over a table because these positions permit greater lung expansion. Lying on the back or on either side restricts expansion of part of the thorax (the underlying portion). This relatively small increase in expansion may be important to a dyspneic client.

Variations in the shape of the thorax may indicate adaptation to chronic respiratory conditions. For example, clients with emphysema frequently develop a *barrel chest*.

Diagnostic Studies

The physician may order various diagnostic tests to assess respiratory status, function, and oxygenation. Included are sputum specimens, throat cultures and, visualization procedures (see Chapter 32 ⊙), venous and arterial blood specimens, and pulmonary function tests.

Measurement of arterial blood gases is an important diagnostic procedure (see Chapter 50). ⊙ Specimens of arterial blood are normally taken by specialty nurses, respiratory therapists, or medical technicians. Blood for these tests is taken directly from the radial, brachial, or femoral arteries or from central catheters placed in large arteries. Because of the relatively great pressure of the blood in these arteries, it is important to prevent hemorrhaging by applying pressure to the puncture side for about 5 minutes after removing the needle.

Pulmonary Function Tests. Pulmonary function tests measure lung volume and capacity. Clients undergoing pulmonary function tests, which are usually carried out by a respiratory therapist, do not require an anesthetic. The client breathes into a machine. The tests are painless, but the client's cooperation is essential. Nurses need to explain the tests to people beforehand and help clients to get rest afterward because the tests are often tiring. Table 48–1 describes the measurements taken, and Figure 48–2 ■ shows their relationships and normal adult values.

DIAGNOSING

NANDA includes the following diagnostic labels for clients with oxygenation problems:

- *Ineffective Airway Clearance:* Inability to clear secretions or obstructions from the respiratory tract to maintain a clear airway. A clinical example using this nursing diagnosis is shown in the Nursing Care Plan and the Concept Map later in the chapter.
- *Ineffective Breathing Pattern:* Inspiration and/or expiration that does not provide adequate ventilation
- *Impaired Gas Exchange:* Excess or deficit in oxygenation and/or carbon dioxide elimination at the alveolar-capillary membrane
- *Activity Intolerance:* Insufficient physiological or psychological energy to endure or complete required or desired daily activities.

The preceding nursing diagnoses may also be the etiology of several other nursing diagnoses. Examples follow:

- *Anxiety* related to ineffective airway clearance and feeling of suffocation
- *Fatigue* related to ineffective breathing pattern
- *Fear* related to chronic disabling respiratory illness
- *Powerlessness* related to inability to maintain independence in self-care activities because of ineffective breathing pattern
- *Disturbed Sleep Pattern* related to orthopnea and required O_2 therapy
- *Social Isolation* related to activity intolerance and inability to travel to usual social activities.

TABLE 48–1 Pulmonary Volumes and Capacities

Measurement	Description
Tidal volume (V_T)	Volume inhaled and exhaled during normal quiet breathing
Inspiratory reserve volume (IRV)	Maximum amount of air that can be inhaled over and above a normal breath
Expiratory reserve volume (ERV)	Maximum amount of air that can be exhaled following a normal exhalation
Residual volume (RV)	The amount of air remaining in the lungs after maximal exhalation
Total lung capacity (TLC)	The total volume of the lungs at maximum inflation; calculated by adding the V_T, IRV, ERV, and RV
Vital capacity (VC)	Total amount of air that can be exhaled after a maximal inspiration; calculated by adding the V_T, IRV, and ERV
Inspiratory capacity	Total amount of air that can be inhaled following normal quiet exhalation; calculated by adding the V_T and IRV
Functional residual capacity (FRC)	The volume left in the lungs after normal exhalation; calculated by adding the ERV and RV
Minute volume (MV)	The total volume or amount of air breathed in 1 minute

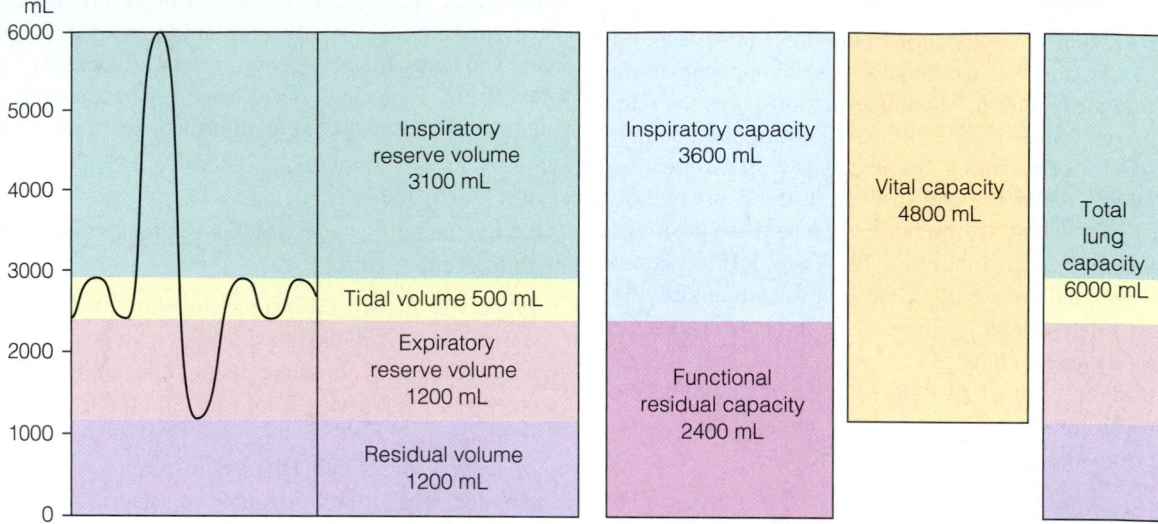

Figure 48–2 ■ The relationship of lung volumes and capacities. Volumes (mL) shown are for an average adult male; female volumes are 20% to 25% smaller.

PLANNING

The overall goals for a client with oxygenation problems are to

- Maintain a patent airway.
- Improve comfort and ease of breathing.
- Maintain or improve pulmonary ventilation and oxygenation.
- Improve ability to participate in physical activities.

- Prevent risks associated with oxygenation problems such as skin and tissue breakdown, syncope, acid–base imbalances, and feelings of hopelessness and social isolation.

Examples of nursing interventions to facilitate pulmonary ventilation may include ensuring a patent airway, positioning, encouraging deep breathing and coughing, and ensuring ade-

---

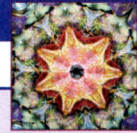

Home Care Assessment

OXYGENATION

Client

- Self-care abilities: Ability to ambulate and perform ADLs independently
- Exercise and activity pattern: Type and regularity of usual exercise, perceived and actual energy for desired and required leisure activities
- Assistive devices required: Supplemental oxygen, humidifier, nebulizer treatments or inhalers; walker, cane, or wheelchair; grab bars, shower chair, and other devices to promote safety and minimize energy expenditure; scale to monitor weight on a regular basis
- Home environment for factors that impair airway clearance, gas exchange, or activity tolerance: Indoor pollutants such as cigarette smoke, dust, and allergens such as pets; lack of humidity in the air; and barriers such as stairs
- Current level of knowledge: Importance of avoiding smoking and other pollutants; dietary salt and other restrictions (if appropriate); recommended activities; medications; need to limit exposure to respiratory infections; use of prescribed nebulizer, inhaler, home oxygen; activity level

Family

- Caregiver availability, skills, and responses: Ability and willingness to provide care as needed (help with ADLs, providing

meals, assisting with transportation and shopping, caring for dependents; performing treatments such as percussion and postural drainage)
- Family role changes and coping: Effect on financial status, parenting and spousal roles, sexuality, social roles
- Alternate potential primary or respite caregivers: For example, other family members, volunteers, church members, paid caregivers or housekeeping services; available community respite care (e.g., adult day care, senior centers)

Community

- Environment: Usual temperature and humidity, presence of air pollutants such as automobile exhaust, industrial smoke and pollutants, smoke from field burning
- Current knowledge of and experience with community resources: Medical and assistive equipment and supply companies, respiratory and physical therapy services, home health agencies, local pharmacies, available financial assistance, support and educational organizations such as the local lung association, COPD support groups.

quate hydration. Other nursing interventions helpful to ventilation are suctioning, lung inflation techniques, administration of analgesics before deep breathing and coughing, postural drainage, and percussion and vibration. Nursing strategies to facilitate the diffusion of gases through the alveolar membrane include encouraging coughing, deep breathing, and suitable activity. A client's nursing care plan should also include appropriate dependent nursing interventions such as oxygen therapy, tracheostomy care, and maintenance of a chest tube.

A clinical example of desired outcomes, interventions, and activities are provided in the Nursing Care Plan and the Concept Map later in the chapter.

Planning for Home Care

To provide for continuity of care, the nurse needs to consider the client's learning needs and needs for assistance with care in the home. Planning incorporates an assessment of the client's and family's knowledge and abilities for self-care, financial resources, and evaluation of the need for referrals and for home health services. The Home Care Assessment outlines a home care assessment related to the client's oxygenation problems and needs. Teaching: Home Care addresses the learning needs of the client and family.

IMPLEMENTING

Promoting Oxygenation

Most people in good health give little thought to their respiratory function. Changing position frequently, ambulating, and exercising usually maintain adequate ventilation and gas exchange. Teaching: Wellness Care lists other ways to promote healthy breathing.

When people become ill, however, their respiratory functions may be inhibited for such reasons as pain and immobility. Shallow respirations inhibit both diaphragmatic excursion and lung distensibility. The result of inadequate chest expansion is pooling of respiratory secretions, which ultimately harbor microorganisms and promote infection. This situation is often compounded by giving narcotics for pain, because narcotics further depress the rate and depth of respiration.

Interventions by the nurse to maintain the normal respirations of clients include

- Positioning the client to allow for maximum chest expansion
- Encouraging or providing frequent changes in position
- Encouraging ambulation
- Implementing measures that promote comfort, such as giving pain medications.

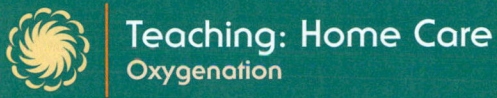

Teaching: Home Care
Oxygenation

Maintaining Airway Clearance and Effective Gas Exchange

- Emphasize to the client and family the importance of not smoking. Refer them to smoking cessation programs as needed. For family members resistant to not smoking, emphasize the need to avoid smoking inside the home.
- Instruct the client in effective coughing techniques such as controlled coughing or "huff" coughing (see "Deep Breathing and Coughing" in the "Implementing" section).
- Discuss the significance of changes in sputum, including the amount and characteristics such as color, viscosity, and odor. Instruct the client when to contact a health care provider.
- Teach the client to maintain a fluid intake of 2,500 mL (2.5 qt) to 3,000 mL (3 qt) per day.
- Instruct the client on how to use nebulizers or inhalers if prescribed; see Chapter 33 ☞, pages 849–851.
- Teach the client and family how to use home oxygen delivery systems.

Promoting Effective Breathing

- Teach relaxation techniques such as progressive muscle relaxation, meditation, and visualization. Use prerecorded tapes as needed.
- Help the client identify specific factors that affect breathing such as stress, exposure to allergens or air pollution, exposure to cold. Assist with identifying possible interventions and measures to avoid these factors.

Medications

- Teach the client about prescribed medications, including the dose, the desired and possible adverse effects, and any precautions about using a medication with food, beverages, or other medications.

Specific Measures for Oxygenation Problems

- Provide instructions for specific procedures and problems such as
  a. Suctioning oropharyngeal and nasopharyngeal cavities
  b. Caring for a temporary or permanent tracheostomy
  c. Preventing the spread of tuberculosis and other respiratory infections to family members and others

Referrals

- Make appropriate referrals to home health agencies or community social services for assistance in obtaining medical and assistive equipment such as grab bars, respiratory and physical therapy services, and home health or housekeeping services to assist with ADLs.

Community Agencies and Other Sources of Help

- Provide information about where durable medical equipment can be purchased, rented, or obtained free of charge; how to access home oxygen equipment and support services; physical and occupational therapy services; and where to obtain supplies such as tracheostomy supplies, or nutritional supplements.
- Suggest additional sources of information such as the American Lung Association and the Asthma and Allergy Foundation of America.

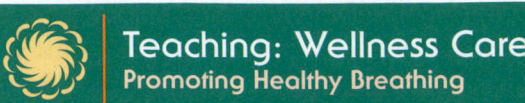

Teaching: Wellness Care
Promoting Healthy Breathing

- Sit straight and stand erect to permit full lung expansion.
- Exercise regularly.
- Breathe through the nose.
- Breathe in to expand the chest fully.
- Do not smoke cigarettes, cigars, or pipes.
- Eliminate or reduce the use of household pesticides and irritating chemical substances.
- Do not incinerate garbage in the house.
- Avoid exposure to second-hand smoke.
- Use building materials that do not emit vapors.
- Make sure furnaces, ovens, and wood stoves are correctly ventilated.
- Support a pollution-free environment.

The semi-Fowler's or high-Fowler's position allows maximum chest expansion in bed-confined clients, particularly dyspneic clients. The nurse also encourages clients to turn from side to side frequently, so that alternate sides of the chest are permitted maximum expansion. Dyspneic clients often sit in bed and lean over their overbed tables (which are raised to a suitable height), usually with a pillow for support. This orthopneic position is an adaptation of the high-Fowler's position. It has a further advantage in that, unlike in high-Fowler's, the abdominal organs are not pressing on the diaphragm. Also, a client in the orthopneic position can press the lower part of the chest against the table to help in exhaling (Figure 48–3 ■).

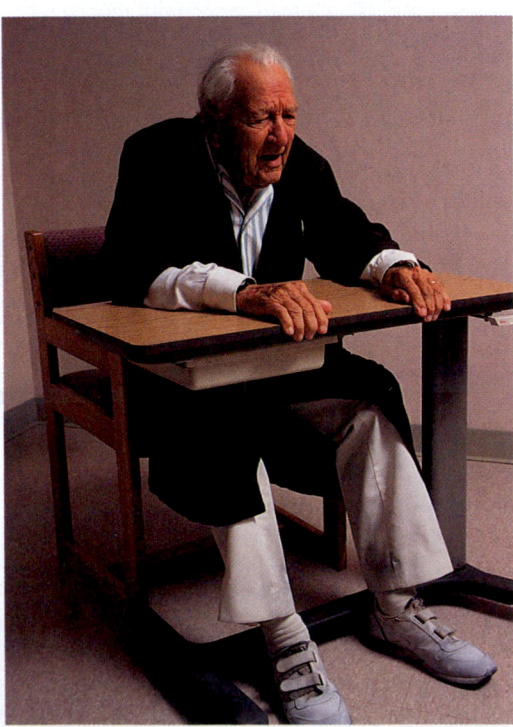

Figure 48–3 ■ A client using the overbed table to assist with breathing.

Deep Breathing and Coughing

The nurse can facilitate respiratory functioning by encouraging deep breathing exercises and coughing to remove secretions from the airways. When coughing raises secretions high enough, the client may either **expectorate** (spit out) or swallow them. Swallowing the secretions is not harmful but does not allow the nurse to view the secretions for documentation purposes or to obtain a specimen for testing.

Breathing exercises are frequently indicated for clients with restricted chest expansion, such as people with chronic obstructive pulmonary disease (COPD) or clients recovering from thoracic surgery.

A commonly employed breathing exercise is *abdominal (diaphragmatic)* and pursed-lip breathing. Abdominal breathing permits deep full breaths with little effort. Pursed-lip breathing helps the client develop control over breathing. The pursed lips create a resistance to the air flowing out of the lungs, thereby prolonging exhalation and preventing airway collapse by maintaining positive airway pressure. The client purses the lips as if about to whistle and breathes out slowly and gently, tightening the abdominal muscles to exhale more effectively. The client usually inhales to a count of 3 and exhales to a count of 7.

Forceful coughing often is less effective than using controlled or huff coughing techniques. Instructions for abdominal (diaphragmatic) and pursed-lip breathing and coughing techniques are provided in Teaching: Client Care.

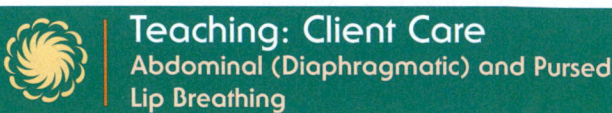

Teaching: Client Care
Abdominal (Diaphragmatic) and Pursed-Lip Breathing

- Assume a comfortable semi-sitting position in bed or a chair or a lying position in bed with one pillow.
- Flex your knees to relax the muscles of the abdomen.
- Place one or both hands on your abdomen, just below the ribs.
- Breathe in deeply through the nose, keeping the mouth closed.
- Concentrate on feeling your abdomen rise as far as possible; stay relaxed, and avoid arching your back. If you have difficulty raising your abdomen, take a quick, forceful breath through the nose.
- Then purse your lips as if about to whistle, and breathe out slowly and gently, making a slow "whooshing" sound without puffing out the cheeks. This pursed-lip breathing creates a resistance to air flowing out of the lungs, increases pressure within the bronchi (main air passages), and minimizes collapse of smaller airways, a common problem for people with COPD.
- Concentrate on feeling the abdomen fall or sink, and tighten (contract) the abdominal muscles while breathing out to enhance effective exhalation. Count to seven during exhalation.
- Use this exercise whenever feeling short of breath, and increase gradually to 5 to 10 minutes four times a day. Regular practice will help you do this type of breathing without conscious effort. The exercise, once learned, can be performed when sitting upright, standing, and walking.

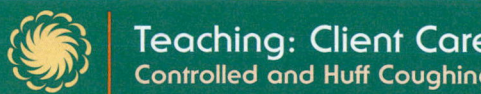

Teaching: Client Care
Controlled and Huff Coughing

- After using a bronchodilator treatment (if prescribed), inhale deeply and hold your breath for a few seconds.
- Cough twice. The first cough loosens the mucus; the second expels secretions.
- For huff coughing, lean forward and exhale sharply with a "huff" sound. This technique helps keep your airways open while moving secretions up and out of the lungs.
- Inhale by taking rapid short breaths in succession ("sniffing") to prevent mucus from moving back into smaller airways.
- Rest.
- Try to avoid prolonged episodes of coughing because these may cause fatigue and hypoxia.

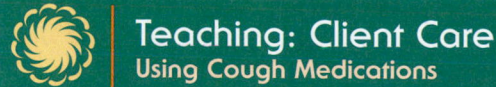

Teaching: Client Care
Using Cough Medications

- Do not take cough medications in excessive amounts because of adverse side effects.
- If you have diabetes mellitus, avoid cough syrups that contain sugar or alcohol; these can disturb metabolism.
- When a cough medicine does not act as expected, consult a health care professional.
- Be aware of side effects (e.g., drowsiness) that can make the operation of machinery dangerous.

Hydration

Adequate hydration maintains the moisture of the respiratory mucous membranes. Normally, respiratory tract secretions are thin and are therefore moved readily by ciliary action. However, when the client is dehydrated or when the environment has a low humidity, the respiratory secretions can become thick and tenacious. Fluid intake should be as great as the client can tolerate. See Chapter 50 🔗 for normal daily fluid intake.

Humidifiers are devices that add water vapor to inspired air. Room humidifiers provide cool mist to room air. Nebulizers are used to deliver humidity and medications. They also are used with oxygen delivery systems to provide moistened air directly to the client. Their purposes are to prevent mucous membranes from drying and becoming irritated and to loosen secretions for easier expectoration.

Medications

A number of types of medications can be used for clients with oxygenation problems.

Bronchodilators, anti-inflammatory drugs, expectorants, and cough suppressants are some medications that may be used to treat respiratory problems. Bronchodilators, including sympathomimetic drugs and xanthines, reduce bronchospasm, opening tight or congested airways and facilitating ventilation. These drugs may be administered orally or intravenously, but the preferred route is by inhalation to prevent many systemic side effects.

Since drugs used to dilate the bronchioles and improve breathing are usually drugs that enhance the sympathetic nervous system, clients must be monitored for side effects of increased heart rate, blood pressure, anxiety, and restlessness. This is especially important in elders, who may also have cardiac problems. Some over-the-counter drugs for respiratory problems have these same effects, so clients should be cautioned about taking them without checking with their physician. Another class of drugs used is the *anti-inflammatory drugs,* such as glucocorticoids. They can be given orally, intravenously, or by inhaler. They work by decreasing the edema and inflammation in the airways and allowing a better air exchange. If both bronchodilators and anti-inflammatory drugs

are ordered by inhaler, the client should be instructed to use the bronchodilator inhaler first and then the anti-inflammatory inhaler. If the bronchioles are dilated first, more tissue is exposed for the anti-inflammatory drugs to act upon.

Expectorants help "break up" mucus, making it more liquid and easier to expectorate. Guaifenesin is a common expectorant found in many prescription and nonprescription cough syrups. When frequent or prolonged coughing interrupts sleep, a cough suppressant such as codeine may be prescribed.

Other medications can be used to improve oxygenation by improving cardiovascular function. The *digitalis glycosides* act directly on the heart to improve the strength of contraction and slow the heart rate. *Beta-adrenergic blocking agents* such as propranolol affect the sympathetic nervous system to reduce the workload of the heart. These drugs, however, can negatively affect people with asthma or COPD as they may constrict airways.

Incentive Spirometry

Incentive spirometers (Figure 48–4 ■), also referred to as *sustained maximal inspiration devices* (SMIs), measure the flow of air inhaled through the mouthpiece and are used to

- Improve pulmonary ventilation.
- Counteract the effects of anesthesia or hypoventilation.
- Loosen respiratory secretions.
- Facilitate respiratory gaseous exchange.
- Expand collapsed alveoli.

They offer an incentive to improve inhalation. When using an SMI, the client should be assisted into a position, preferably an upright sitting position in bed or a chair, that facilitates maximum ventilation. Teaching: Client Care lists instructions for clients in the use of incentive spirometers.

Percussion, Vibration, and Postural Drainage

Percussion, vibration, and postural drainage (PVD) are dependent nursing functions performed according to a physician's order. **Percussion,** sometimes called *clapping,* is forceful striking of the skin with cupped hands. Mechanical percussion cups and vibrators are also available. When the hands are used, the fingers and thumb are held together and flexed slightly to form a cup, as one would to scoop up water. Percussion over congested lung areas can mechanically dislodge tenacious secretions from

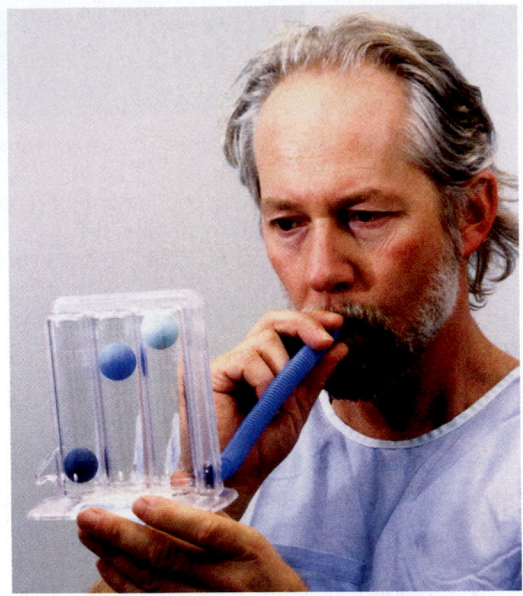

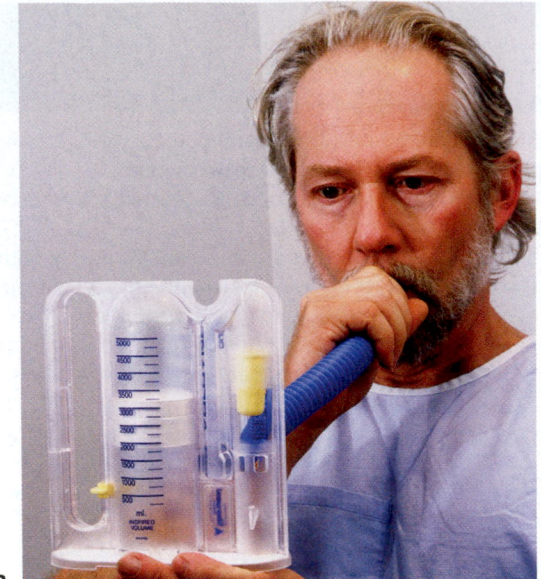

Figure 48–4 ■ *A*, Flow-oriented SMI; *B*, volume-oriented SMI.

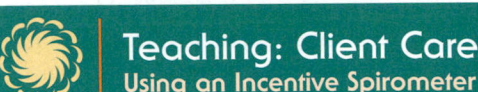

Teaching: Client Care
Using an Incentive Spirometer

■ Hold or place the spirometer in an upright position. A tilted *flow-oriented* device requires less effort to raise the balls or discs; a *volume-oriented* device will not function correctly unless upright.

■ Exhale normally.

■ Seal the lips tightly around the mouthpiece.

■ Take in a slow, deep breath to elevate the balls or cylinder, and then hold the breath for 2 seconds initially, increasing to 6 seconds (optimum), to keep the balls or cylinder elevated if possible.

■ For a flow-oriented device, avoid brisk, low-volume breaths that snap the balls to the top of the chamber. Greater lung expansion is achieved with a very slow inspiration than with a brisk, shallow breath, even though it may not elevate the balls or keep them elevated while you hold your breath. Sustained elevation of the balls or cylinder ensures adequate ventilation of the alveoli (lung air sacs).

■ If you have difficulty breathing only through the mouth, a nose clip can be used.

■ Remove the mouthpiece and exhale normally.

■ Cough after the incentive effort. Deep ventilation may loosen secretions, and coughing can facilitate their removal.

■ Relax and take several normal breaths before using the spirometer again.

■ Repeat the procedure several times and then four or five times hourly. Practice increases inspiratory volume, maintains alveolar ventilation, and prevents atelectasis (collapse of the air sacs).

■ Clean the mouthpiece with water and shake it dry.

the bronchial walls. Cupped hands trap the air against the chest. The trapped air sets up vibrations through the chest wall to the secretions.

To percuss a client's chest, the nurse follows these steps:

• Cover the area with a towel or gown to reduce discomfort.
• Ask the client to breathe slowly and deeply to promote relaxation.
• Alternately flex and extend the wrists rapidly to slap the chest (Figure 48–5 ■).
• Percuss each affected lung segment for 1 to 2 minutes.

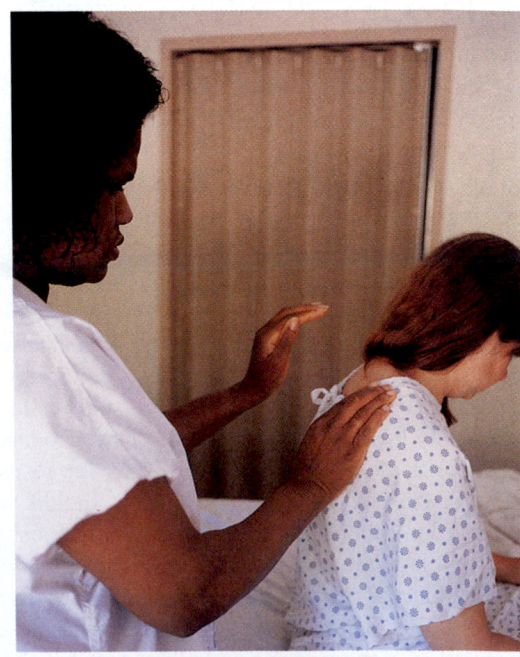

Figure 48–5 ■ Percussing the upper posterior chest.

When done correctly, the percussion action should produce a hollow, popping sound. Percussion is avoided over the breasts, sternum, spinal column, and kidneys.

Vibration is a series of vigorous quiverings produced by hands that are placed flat against the client's chest wall. Vibration is used after percussion to increase the turbulence of the exhaled air and thus loosen thick secretions. It is often done alternately with percussion.

To vibrate the client's chest, the nurse follows these steps:

- Place hands, palms down, on the chest area to be drained, one hand over the other with the fingers together and extended (Figure 48–6 ■). Alternatively, the hands may be placed side by side.
- Ask the client to inhale deeply and exhale slowly through the nose or pursed lips.
- During the exhalation, tense all the hand and arm muscles, and using mostly the heel of the hand, vibrate (shake) the hands, moving them downward. Stop the vibrating when the client inhales.
- Vibrate during five exhalations over one affected lung segment.
- After each vibration, encourage the client to cough and expectorate secretions into the sputum container.

Postural drainage is the drainage by gravity of secretions from various lung segments. Secretions that remain in the lungs or respiratory airways promote bacterial growth and subsequent infection. They also can obstruct the smaller airways and cause atelectasis. Secretions in the major airways, such as the trachea and the right and left main bronchi, are usually coughed into the pharynx, where they can be expectorated, swallowed, or effectively removed by suctioning.

A wide variety of positions is necessary to drain all segments of the lungs, but not all positions are required for every client.

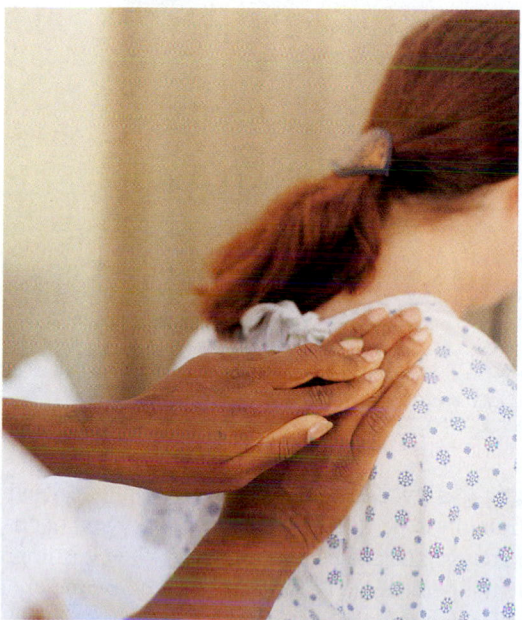

Figure 48–6 ■ Vibrating the upper posterior chest.

Only those positions that drain specific affected areas are used. The lower lobes require drainage most frequently because the upper lobes drain by gravity. Before postural drainage, the client may be given a bronchodilator medication or nebulization therapy to loosen secretions. Postural drainage treatments are scheduled two or three times daily, depending on the degree of lung congestion. The best times include before breakfast, before lunch, in the late afternoon, and before bedtime. It is best to avoid hours shortly after meals because postural drainage at these times can be tiring and can induce vomiting.

The nurse needs to evaluate the client's tolerance of postural drainage by assessing the stability of the client's vital signs, particularly the pulse and respiratory rates, and by noting signs of intolerance, such as pallor, diaphoresis, dyspnea, and fatigue. Some clients do not react well to certain drainage positions, and the nurse must make appropriate adjustments. For example, some become dyspneic in Trendelenburg's position and require only a moderate tilt or a shorter time in that position.

The sequence for PVD is usually as follows: positioning, percussion, vibration, and removal of secretions by coughing or suction. Each position is usually assumed for 10 to 15 minutes, although beginning treatments may start with shorter times and gradually increase.

Following PVD, the nurse should auscultate the client's lungs, compare the findings to the baseline data, and document the amount, color, and character of expectorated secretions.

Oxygen Therapy

Clients who have difficulty ventilating all areas of their lungs, those whose gas exchange is impaired, or people with heart failure may require oxygen therapy to prevent hypoxia.

Oxygen therapy is prescribed by the physician, who specifies the concentration, method of delivery, and liter flow per minute. The concentration is of more importance than the liter flow per minute. When administering oxygen is an emergency measure, the nurse may initiate the therapy. For clients who have COPD, a low-flow oxygen system is essential.

Safety precautions are essential during oxygen therapy (see Box 48–3). Although oxygen by itself will not burn or explode, it does facilitate combustion. For example, a bed sheet ordinarily burns slowly when ignited in the atmosphere; however, if saturated with free-flowing oxygen and ignited by a spark, it will burn rapidly and explosively. The greater the concentration of oxygen, the more rapidly fires start and burn, and such fires are difficult to extinguish. Because oxygen is colorless, odorless, and tasteless, people are often unaware of its presence.

Oxygen is supplied in several different ways. In hospitals and long-term care facilities, it is usually piped into wall outlets at the client's bedside, making it readily available for use at all times. Tanks or cylinders of oxygen under pressure are also frequently available for use when wall oxygen either is unavailable or impractical (e.g., for transporting oxygen-dependent clients between treatment areas).

Clients who require oxygen therapy in the home may use small cylinders of oxygen, oxygen in liquid form, or an oxygen concentrator. Portable oxygen delivery systems are available to increase the client's independence. Home oxygen

BOX 48-3   ■ Oxygen Therapy Safety Precautions

- For home oxygen use or when the facility permits smoking, teach family members and roommates to smoke only outside or in provided smoking rooms away from the client.
- Place cautionary signs reading "No Smoking: Oxygen in Use" on the client's door, at the foot or head of the bed, and on the oxygen equipment.
- Instruct the client and visitors about the hazard of smoking with oxygen in use.
- Make sure that electric devices (such as razors, hearing aids, radios, televisions, and heating pads) are in good working order to prevent the occurrence of short-circuit sparks.

- Avoid materials that generate static electricity, such as woolen blankets and synthetic fabrics. Cotton blankets should be used, and clients and caregivers should be advised to wear cotton fabrics.
- Avoid the use of volatile, flammable materials, such as oils, greases, alcohol, ether, and acetone (e.g., nail polish remover), near clients receiving oxygen.
- Ground electric monitoring equipment, suction machines, and portable diagnostic machines.
- Make known the location of fire extinguishers, and make sure personnel are trained in their use.

therapy services are readily available in most communities. These services generally supply the oxygen and delivery devices, training for the client and family, equipment maintenance, and emergency services should a problem occur.

Oxygen administered from a cylinder or wall-outlet system is dry. Dry gases dehydrate the respiratory mucous membranes. Humidifying devices that add water vapor to inspired air are thus an essential adjunct of oxygen therapy, particularly for liter flows over 2 L per minute (Figure 48–7 ■). These devices provide 20% to 40% humidity. The oxygen passes through sterile distilled water or tap water and then along a line to the device through which the moistened oxygen is inhaled (e.g., a cannula, nasal catheter, or oxygen mask).

Humidifiers prevent mucous membranes from drying and becoming irritated and loosen secretions for easier expectoration. Oxygen passing through water picks up water vapor before it reaches the client. The more bubbles created during this process, the more water vapor is produced. Very low liter flows (e.g., 1 to 2 L per minute by nasal cannula) do not require humidification.

Oxygen cylinders need to be handled and stored with caution and strapped securely in wheeled transport devices or stands to prevent possible falls and outlet breakages. They should be placed away from traffic areas and heaters.

To use an oxygen wall outlet, the nurse carries out these steps:

- Attach the flow meter to the wall outlet, exerting firm pressure. The flow meter should be in the off position.
- Fill the humidifier bottle with distilled or tap water in accordance with agency protocol. This can be done before coming to the bedside. Some humidifier bottles come prefilled by the manufacturer.
- Attach the humidifier bottle to the base of the flow meter.
- Attach the prescribed oxygen tubing and delivery device to the humidifier.
- Regulate the flow meter to the prescribed level.

Oxygen Delivery Systems

A number of systems are available to deliver oxygen to the client. The choice of system depends on the client's oxygen needs, comfort, and developmental considerations. With many systems, the oxygen delivered mixes with room air before being inspired. The amount of oxygen delivered is determined by

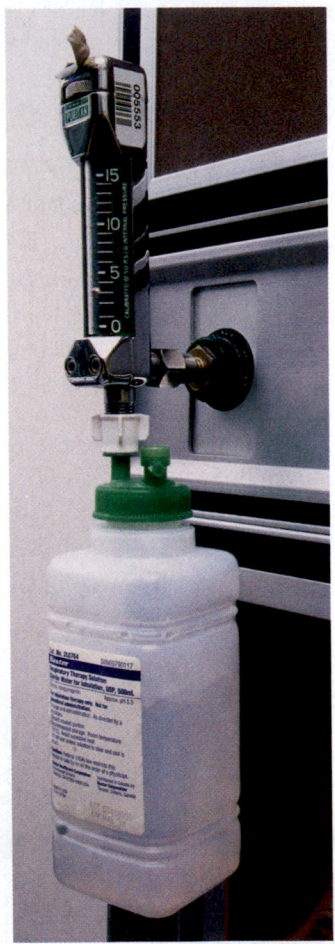

Figure 48–7 ■ An oxygen humidifier attached to a wall outlet oxygen flow meter.

regulating its flow rate (e.g., 2 to 6 L per minute), and precise regulation of the percentage of inspired oxygen, or fraction of inspired oxygen (FiO_2), is not possible. When it is important to regulate the percentage of oxygen received by the client more precisely, a device such as a Venturi mask may be used.

Cannula. The nasal cannula (nasal prongs) is the most common inexpensive device used to administer oxygen (Figure 48–8 ■).

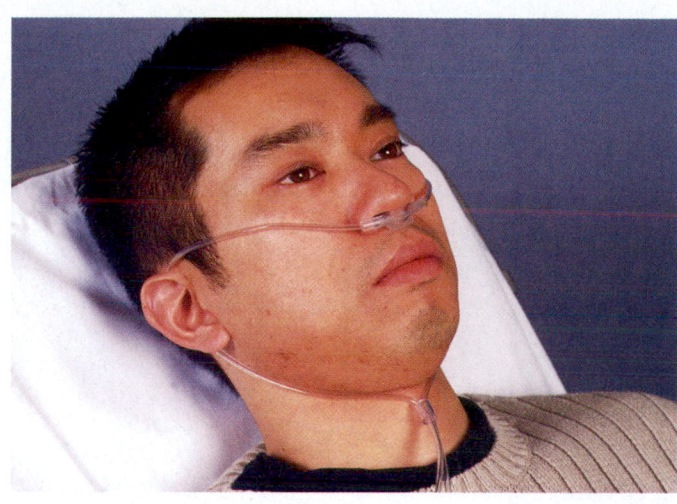

Figure 48–8 ■ A nasal cannula.

The nasal cannula is easy to apply and does not interfere with the client's ability to eat or talk. It also is relatively comfortable, permits some freedom of movement, and is well tolerated by the client. It delivers a relatively low concentration of oxygen (24% to 45%) at flow rates of 2 to 6 L per minute. Above 6 L per minute, the client tends to swallow air and the FiO_2 is not increased.

Administering oxygen by cannula is detailed in Procedure 48–1.

Face Mask. Face masks that cover the client's nose and mouth may be used for oxygen inhalation. Exhalation ports on the sides of the mask allow exhaled carbon dioxide to escape. A variety of oxygen masks are marketed:

- The simple face mask delivers oxygen concentrations from 40% to 60% at liter flows of 5 to 8 L per minute, respectively (Figure 48–9 ■).
- The partial rebreather mask delivers oxygen concentrations of 60% to 90% at liter flows of 6 to 10 L per minute, respec-

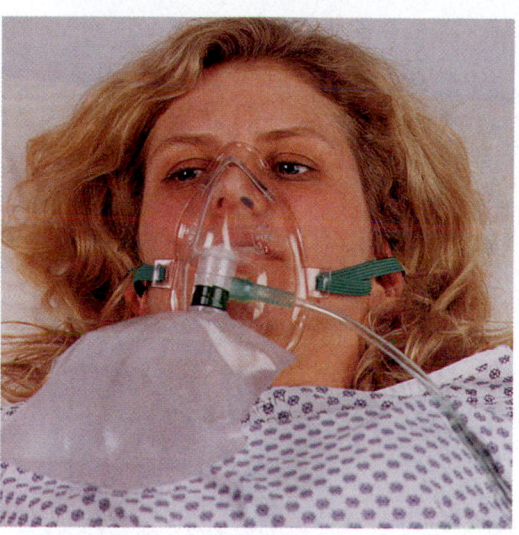

Figure 48–10 ■ A partial rebreather mask.

tively. The oxygen reservoir bag that is attached allows the client to rebreathe about the first third of the exhaled air in conjunction with oxygen (Figure 48–10 ■). Thus, it increases the FiO_2 by recycling expired oxygen. The partial rebreather bag must not totally deflate during inspiration to avoid carbon dioxide buildup. If this problem occurs, the nurse increases the liter flow of oxygen.

- The nonrebreather mask delivers the highest oxygen concentration possible—95% to 100%—by means other than intubation or mechanical ventilation, at liter flows of 10 to 15 L per minute. One-way valves on the mask and between the reservoir bag and the mask prevent the room air and the client's exhaled air from entering the bag so only the oxygen in the bag is inspired (Figure 48–11 ■). To prevent carbon

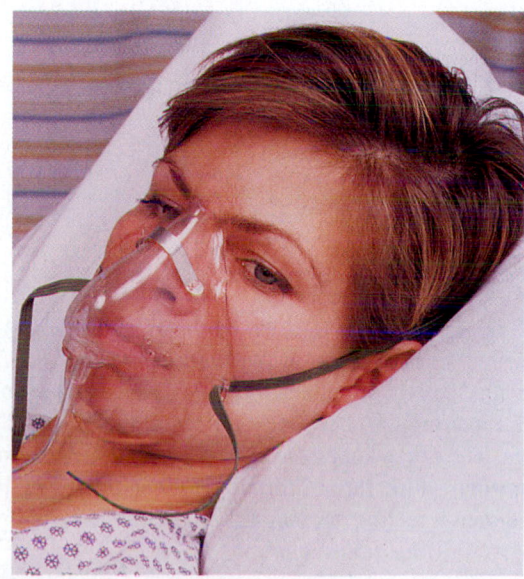

Figure 48–9 ■ A simple face mask.

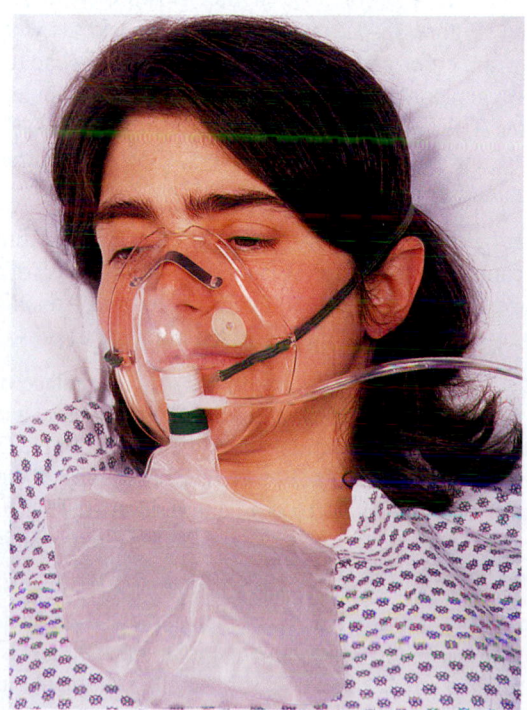

Figure 48–11 ■ A nonrebreather mask.

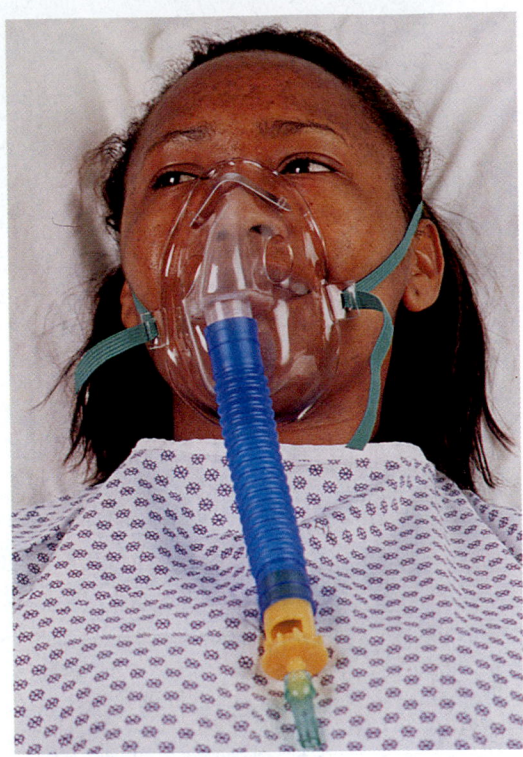

Figure 48–12 ■ A Venturi mask.

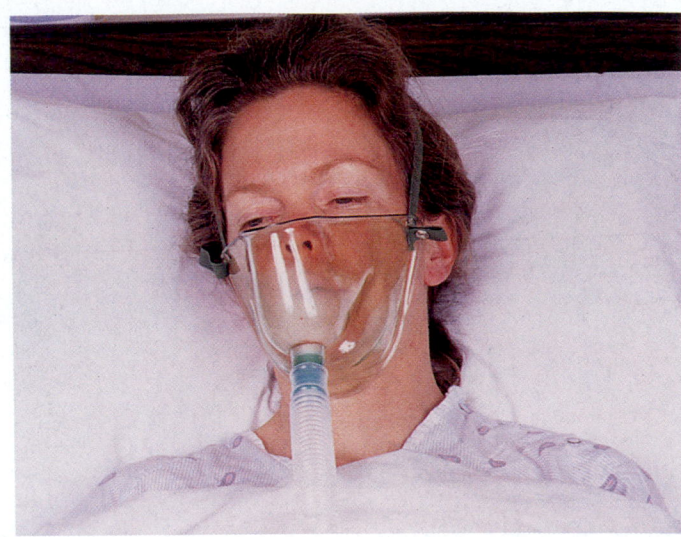

Figure 48–13 ■ An oxygen face tent.

dioxide buildup, the nonrebreather bag must not totally deflate during inspiration. If it does, the nurse can correct this problem by increasing the liter flow of oxygen.

- The Venturi mask delivers oxygen concentrations varying from 24% to 40% or 50% at liter flows of 4 to 10 L per minute (Figure 48–12 ■). The Venturi mask has wide-bore tubing and color-coded jet adapters that correspond to a precise oxygen concentration and liter flow. For example, a blue adapter delivers a 24% concentration of oxygen at 4 L per minute, and a green adapter delivers a 35% concentration of oxygen at 8 L per minute.

Initiating oxygen by mask is much the same as initiating oxygen by cannula, except that the nurse must find a mask of appropriate size. Smaller sizes are available for children. Administering oxygen by mask or face tent is detailed in Procedure 48–1.

Face Tent. Face tents (Figure 48–13 ■) can replace oxygen masks when masks are poorly tolerated by clients. Face tents provide varying concentrations of oxygen, for example, 30% to 50% concentration of oxygen at 4 to 8 L per minute. Frequently inspect the client's facial skin for dampness or chafing, and dry and treat as needed. As with face masks, the client's facial skin must be kept dry.

Transtracheal Oxygen Delivery. Transtracheal oxygen delivery may be used for oxygen-dependent clients. Oxygen is delivered through a small, narrow plastic cannula surgically inserted

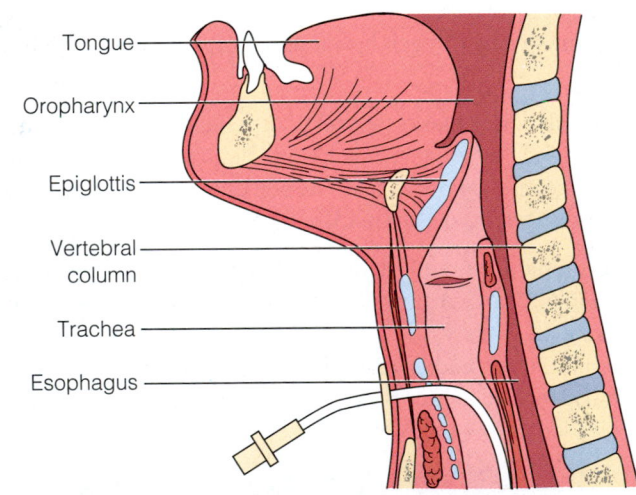

Tongue
Oropharynx
Epiglottis
Vertebral column
Trachea
Esophagus

Figure 48–14 ■ A transtracheal oxygen catheter in place.

through the skin directly into the trachea (Figure 48–14 ■). A chain around the neck holds the catheter in place.

With this delivery system, the client requires less oxygen (0.5 to 2 L per minute) because all of the flow delivered enters the lungs. The nurse keeps the catheter patent by injecting 1.5 mL of normal saline into it, moving a cleaning rod in and out of it, and then injecting another 1.5 mL of saline solution. This is done two or three times a day.

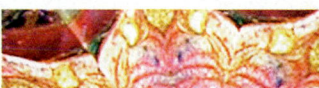

Procedure 48–1 Administering Oxygen by Cannula, Face Mask, or Face Tent

Before administering oxygen, check (a) the order for oxygen, including the administering device and the liter flow rate (L/min) or the percentage of oxygen; (b) the levels of oxygen (PO_2) and carbon dioxide ($PaCO_2$) in the client's arterial blood (PaO_2 is normally 80 to 100 mm Hg; $PaCO_2$ is normally 35 to 45 mmHg); and (c) whether the client has COPD.

Purposes

CANNULA

■ To deliver a relatively low concentration of oxygen when only minimal O_2 support is required

■ To allow uninterrupted delivery of oxygen while the client ingests food or fluids

FACE MASK

■ To provide moderate O_2 support and a higher concentration of oxygen and/or humidity than is provided by cannula

FACE TENT

■ To provide high humidity
■ To provide oxygen when a mask is poorly tolerated
■ To provide a high flow of O_2 when attached to a Venturi system

---

ASSESSMENT

See also Procedure 28–11, Assessing the Thorax and Lungs on page 575.

Assess

■ Skin and mucous membrane color: Note whether cyanosis is present
■ Breathing patterns: Note depth of respirations and presence of tachypnea, bradypnea, orthopnea
■ Chest movements: Note whether there are any intercostal, substernal, suprasternal, supraclavicular, or tracheal retractions during inspiration or expiration
■ Chest wall configuration (e.g., kyphosis)
■ Lung sounds audible by auscultating the chest and by ear
■ Presence of clinical signs of hypoxemia: tachycardia, tachypnea, restlessness, dyspnea, cyanosis, and confusion. Tachycardia and tachypnea are often early signs. Confusion is a later sign of severe oxygen deprivation
■ Presence of clinical signs of hypercarbia (hypercapnia): restlessness, hypertension, headache, lethargy, tremor

■ Presence of clinical signs of oxygen toxicity: tracheal irritation and cough, dyspnea, and decreased pulmonary ventilation

Determine

■ Vital signs, especially pulse rate and quality, and respiratory rate, rhythm, and depth
■ Whether the client has COPD. A high carbon dioxide level in the blood is the normal stimulus to breathe. However, people with COPD may have a chronically high carbon dioxide level, and their stimulus to breathe is hypoxemia. Low flows of oxygen (2 L/min) stimulate breathing for such persons by maintaining slight hypoxemia. During continuous oxygen administration, arterial blood gas levels of oxygen (PO_2) and carbon dioxide (PCO_2) are measured periodically to monitor hypoxemia
■ Results of diagnostic studies
■ Hemoglobin, hematocrit, complete blood count
■ Arterial blood gases
■ Pulmonary function tests

PLANNING

Consult with a respiratory therapist as needed in the beginning and during ongoing care of clients receiving oxygen therapy. In many agencies, the therapist establishes the initial equipment and client teaching.

Delegation

Initiating the administration of oxygen is considered similar to administering a medication and is not delegated to unlicensed assistive personnel (UAP). However, reapplying the oxygen delivery device may be performed by the UAP and many aspects of the client's response to oxygen therapy are observed during usual care and may be recorded by persons other than the nurse. Abnormal findings must be validated and interpreted by the nurse. The nurse is also responsible for ensuring that the correct delivery method is being used.

Equipment
CANNULA

■ Oxygen supply with a flow meter and adapter
■ Humidifier with distilled water or tap water according to agency protocol

■ Nasal cannula and tubing
■ Tape
■ Padding for the elastic band

FACE MASK

■ Oxygen supply with a flow meter and adapter
■ Humidifier with distilled water or tap water according to agency protocol
■ Prescribed face mask of the appropriate size
■ Padding for the elastic band

FACE TENT

■ Oxygen supply with a flow meter and adapter
■ Humidifier with distilled water or tap water according to agency protocol
■ Face tent of the appropriate size

---

continued on page 1310

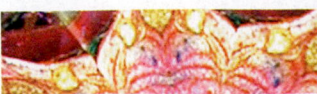

Procedure 48–1 Administering Oxygen by Cannula, Face Mask, or Face Tent *continued*

IMPLEMENTATION

Preparation

1. Determine the need for oxygen therapy, and verify the order for the therapy.
   - Perform a respiratory assessment to develop baseline data if not already available.
2. Prepare the client and support people.
   - Assist the client to a semi-Fowler's position if possible. *This position permits easier chest expansion and hence easier breathing.*
   - Explain that oxygen is not dangerous when safety precautions are observed. Inform the client and support people about the safety precautions connected with oxygen use.

Performance

1. Explain to the client what you are going to do, why it is necessary, and how he or she can cooperate. Discuss how the effects of the oxygen therapy will be used in planning further care or treatments.
2. Wash hands and observe appropriate infection control procedures.
3. Provide for client privacy, if appropriate.
4. Set up the oxygen equipment and the humidifier.
   - Attach the flow meter to the wall outlet or tank. The flow meter should be in the off position.
   - If needed, fill the humidifier bottle. (This can be done before coming to the bedside.)
   - Attach the humidifier bottle to the base of the flow meter.
   - Attach the prescribed oxygen tubing and delivery device to the humidifier.

5. Turn on the oxygen at the prescribed rate and ensure proper functioning.
   - Check that the oxygen is flowing freely through the tubing. There should be no kinks in the tubing, and the connections should be airtight. There should be bubbles in the humidifier as the oxygen flows through. You should feel the oxygen at the outlets of the cannula, mask, or tent.
   - Set the oxygen at the flow rate ordered.
6. Apply the appropriate oxygen delivery device.

CANNULA
   - Put the cannula over the client's face, with the outlet prongs fitting into the nares and the elastic band around the head (see Figure 48–8). Some models have a strap to adjust under the chin.
   - If the cannula will not stay in place, tape it at the sides of the face.
   - Pad the tubing and band over the ears and cheekbones as needed.

FACE MASK
   - Guide the mask toward the client's face, and apply it from the nose downward.
   - Fit the mask to the contours of the client's face (see Figure 48–9). *The mask should mold to the face, so that very little oxygen escapes into the eyes or around the cheeks and chin.*
   - Secure the elastic band around the client's head so that the mask is comfortable but snug.
   - Pad the band behind the ears and over bony prominences. *Padding will prevent irritation from the mask.*

FACE TENT
   - Place the tent over the client's face, and secure the ties around the head (Figure 48–13).
7. Assess the client regularly.
   - Assess the client's vital signs, level of anxiety, color, and ease of respirations, and provide support while the client adjusts to the device.
   - Assess the client in 15 to 30 minutes, depending on the client's condition, and regularly thereafter.
   - Assess the client regularly for clinical signs of hypoxia, tachycardia, confusion, dyspnea, restlessness, and cyanosis. Review arterial blood gas results if they are available.

NASAL CANNULA
   - Assess the client's nares for encrustations and irritation. Apply a water-soluble lubricant as required to soothe the mucous membranes.

FACE MASK OR TENT
   - Inspect the facial skin frequently for dampness or chafing, and dry and treat it as needed.
8. Inspect the equipment on a regular basis.
   - Check the liter flow and the level of water in the humidifier in 30 minutes and whenever providing care to the client.
   - Make sure that safety precautions are being followed.
9. Document findings in the client record using forms or checklists supplemented by narrative notes when appropriate.

EVALUATION

- Perform follow-up based on findings that deviated from expected or normal for the client. Relate findings to previous data if available.

- Report significant deviations from normal to the physician.

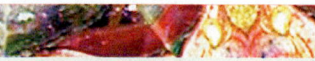

Lifespan Considerations

Oxygen Delivery Equipment
Infants
Oxygen Hood
- An oxygen hood is a rigid plastic dome that encloses an infant's head. It provides precise oxygen levels and high humidity.
- The gas should not be allowed to blow directly into the infant's face, and the hood should not rub against the infant's neck, chin, or shoulder.

Children
Oxygen Tent (Figure 48–15 ■)
- The tent consists of a rectangular, clear, plastic canopy with outlets that connect to an oxygen or compressed air source and to a humidifier that moisturizes the air or oxygen.
- Because the enclosed tent becomes very warm, some type of cooling mechanism such as an ice chamber or a refrigeration unit is provided to maintain the temperature at 20 to 21C (68 to 70F).
- Cover the child with a gown or a cotton blanket. Some agencies provide gowns with hoods, or a small towel may be wrapped around the head. *The child needs protection from chilling and from the dampness and condensation in the tent.*
- Flood the tent with oxygen by setting the flow meter at 15 L/min for about 5 minutes. Then, adjust the flow meter

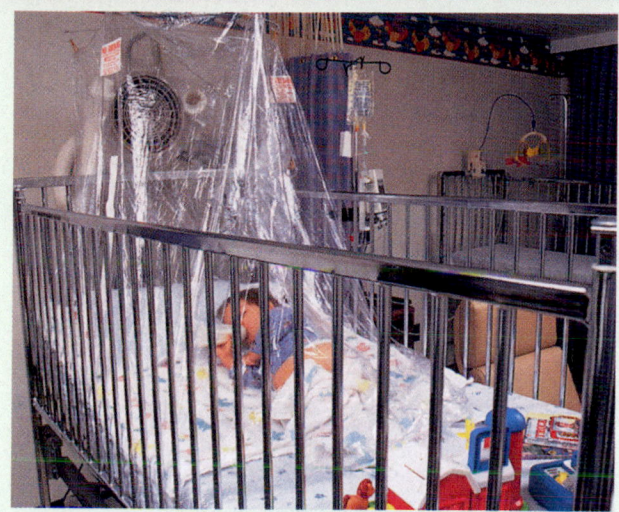

Figure 48–15 ■ Pediatric oxygen tent.

according to orders (e.g., 10 to 15 L/min). *Flooding the tent quickly increases the oxygen to the desired level.*
- The tent can deliver approximately 30% oxygen.

Home Care Considerations

Home Care Oxygen Equipment
Three major oxygen systems for home care use are available in most communities: cylinders or tanks of compressed gas, liquid (cryogenic) oxygen, and oxygen concentrators.

1. Cylinders ("green tanks"): These are the system of choice for clients who need oxygen episodically (e.g., on a prn basis). Advantages are that cylinders deliver all liter flows (1 to 15 L/min), and oxygen evaporation does not occur during storage. Disadvantages are that the cylinders are heavy and awkward to move, the supply company must be notified when a refill is needed, and they are costly for the high-use client. A size "D" tank weighs about 8 pounds and stores 425 L of oxygen; an "E" tank holds 680 L and is transported on wheels (Figure 48–16 ■). The large "H" tank weighs 150 pounds. The gauge on a full tank reads a pressure of at least 2,000 pounds per square inch (psi), and a tank is considered empty when it reads less than 500 psi.

2. Liquid oxygen: Liquid systems have two parts—a large stationary container and a portable unit with a small lightweight tank that is refilled from the stationary unit. Liquid reservoirs store oxygen at −212C (−350F) in a smaller amount of space than compressed gas. Advantages are that these reservoirs are lighter in weight and cleaner in appearance than cylinders and they are not as difficult to operate. Disadvantages of liquid oxygen are that many home care medical supply and service companies are not able to handle

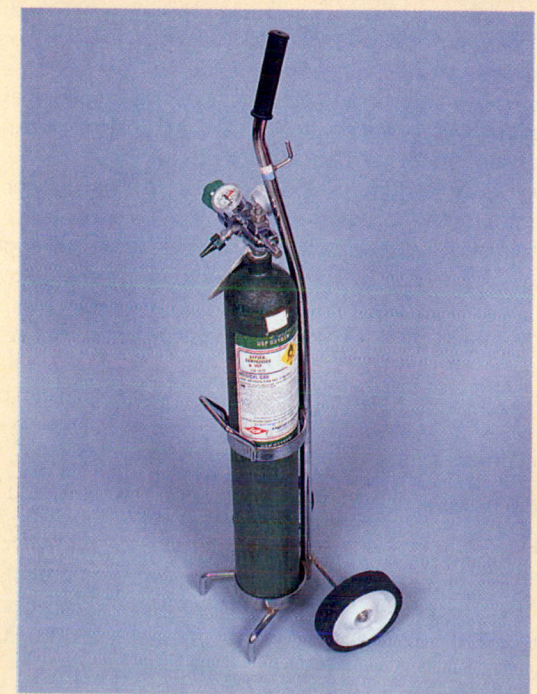

Figure 48–16 ■ An "E" cylinder oxygen tank on a wheeled stand.

continued on page 1312

Home Care Considerations *continued*

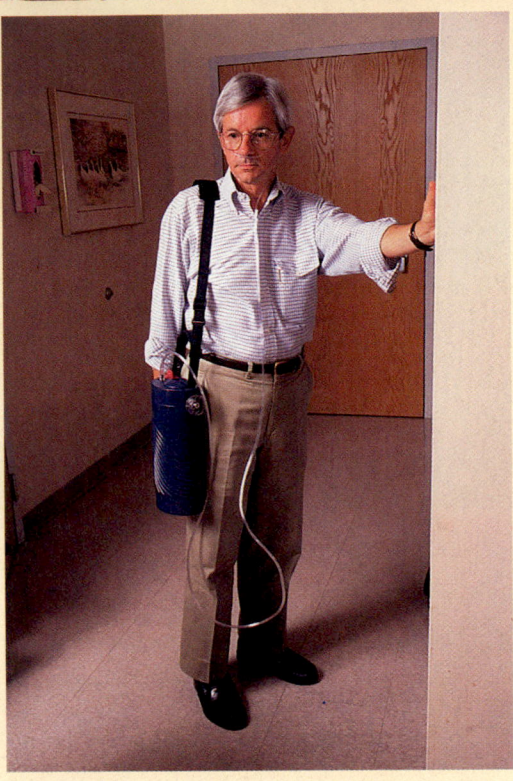

Figure 48–17 ■ A portable liquid oxygen supply.

it, oxygen evaporation occurs when the unit is not used, only low flows (1 to 4 L/min) can be used or freezing occurs, and the portable unit designed to be carried over the shoulder weighs 8 to 10 pounds, a possible burden to the typical COPD client (Figure 48–17 ■). A wheeled cart can be used to carry the unit but may be awkward.

3. Oxygen concentrators: Concentrators are electrically powered systems that manufacture oxygen from room air. At 1 L/min, such a system can deliver a concentration of about 95% oxygen, but the concentration drops when the flow rate increases (e.g., 75% concentration at 4 L/min). Advantages are that they are more attractive in appearance, resembling furniture rather than medical equipment; they eliminate the need for regular delivery of oxygen or

refilling of cylinders; because the supply of oxygen is constant, they alleviate the client's anxiety about running out of oxygen; and they are the most economical system when continuous use is required. Major disadvantages of a concentrator are that it is expensive; lacks real portability (small units weigh 28 pounds); tends to be noisy; is powered by electricity (an emergency backup unit, for example, an oxygen tank, must be provided for clients for whom a power failure could be life threatening); and heat produced by the concentrator motor is a problem for those who live in trailers, small houses, or warm climates, where air conditioners are required. The oxygen concentrator must also be checked periodically with an O_2 analyzer to ensure that it is providing an adequate delivery of oxygen.

Another type of oxygen concentrator is the *oxygen enricher*. It uses a plastic membrane that allows water vapor to pass through with the oxygen, thus eliminating the need for a humidifying device. It is also thought to filter out bacteria present in the air. The enricher provides an O_2 concentration of 40% at all flow rates, it tends to be quieter than the concentrator, there is less chance of combustion (since the gas is only 40% oxygen), it has only two moving parts (thus decreasing the risk of something going wrong), and a nebulizer can be operated off the enricher because of the high flow rate.

The nurse needs to ensure that the client has appropriate help in choosing a reputable home oxygen vendor. Services furnished should include

- A 24-hour emergency service
- Trained personnel to make the initial delivery and instruct the client in safe, appropriate use of the oxygen and maintenance of the equipment
- At least monthly follow-up visits to check the equipment and reinstruct the client as necessary
- A regular cost review to ensure that the system is the most cost effective one for that client, with routine notification of the physician or home care professional if it seems that another system is more appropriate

The nurse needs to also ensure that the client knows about the financial reimbursements available from Medicare and Medicaid or other insurance agencies. In Canada's system of socialized health care, the cost of home oxygen therapy is fully covered.

Artificial Airways

Artificial airways are inserted to maintain a patent air passage for clients whose airway has become or may become obstructed. A patent airway is necessary so that air can flow to and from the lungs. Four of the more common types of airways are oropharyngeal, nasopharyngeal, endotracheal, and tracheostomy.

Oropharyngeal and Nasopharyngeal Airways. Oropharyngeal and nasopharyngeal airways are used to keep the upper air passages open when they may become obstructed by secretions or the tongue. These airways are easy to insert and have a low risk of complications. Sizes vary and should be appropriate to the size and age of the client. The airway should be well lubricated with water-soluble gel prior to inserting.

Oropharyngeal airways (Figure 48–18 ■) stimulate the gag reflex and are only used for clients with altered levels of consciousness (e.g., because of general anesthesia, overdose, or head injury). To insert the airway:

- Place the client in supine or semi-Fowler's position.
- Put on clean gloves.
- Hold the lubricated airway by the outer flange, with the distal end pointing up.
- Open the client's mouth and insert the airway along the top of the tongue.
- When the distal end of the airway reaches the soft palate at the back of the mouth, rotate the airway 180 degrees downward, and slip it past the uvula into the oral pharynx.

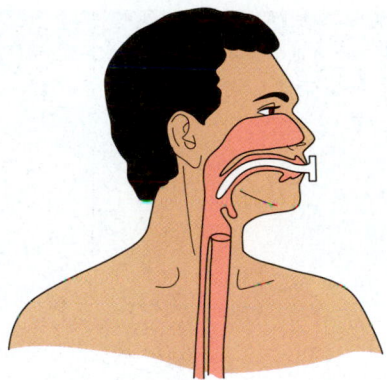

Figure 48–18 ■ An oropharyngeal airway in place.

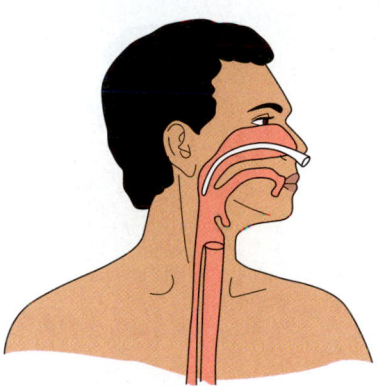

Figure 48–19 ■ A nasopharyngeal airway in place.

- If not contraindicated, place the client in a side-lying position or with the head turned to the side to allow secretions to drain out of the mouth.
- The oropharynx may be suctioned as needed by inserting the suction catheter alongside the airway.
- Do not tape the airway in place; remove it when the client begins to cough or gag.
- Provide mouth care at least every 2 to 4 hours, keeping suction available at the bedside.

Nasopharyngeal airways are tolerated better by alert clients. They are inserted through the nares, terminating in the oropharynx (Figure 48–19 ■). When caring for a client with a nasopharyngeal airway, provide frequent oral and nares care, repositioning the airway in the other naris every 8 hours or as ordered to prevent necrosis of the mucosa.

Endotracheal Tubes. Endotracheal tubes are most commonly inserted for clients who have had general anesthetics or for those in emergency situations where mechanical ventilation is required. An endotracheal tube is inserted by the physician or nurse with specialized education through either the mouth or the nose and into the trachea with the guide of a

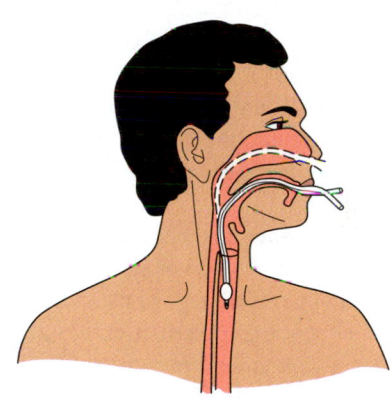

Figure 48–20 ■ An endotracheal tube in place.

laryngoscope (Figure 48–20 ■). The tube terminates just superior to the bifurcation of the trachea into the bronchi. The tube may have an air-filled cuff to prevent air leakage around it. Because an endotracheal tube passes through the epiglottis and glottis, the client is unable to speak while it is in place. Nursing interventions for clients with endotracheal tubes are shown in Box 48–4.

BOX 48–4   ■ Nursing Interventions for Clients with Endotracheal Tubes

- Assess the client's respiratory status at least every 4 hours, or more frequently if indicated. Include respiratory rate, rhythm, depth, equality of chest excursion, and lung sounds; level of consciousness; and skin color in your assessment.
- Frequently assess nasal and oral mucosa for redness and irritation. Report any abnormal findings to the physician.
- Secure the endotracheal tube with tape to prevent accidental movement of the tube further into or out of the trachea. Assess the position of the tube frequently. Notify the physician immediately if the tube is dislodged out of the airway. If the tube advances into a main bronchus, it may need to be slightly withdrawn to ensure ventilation of both lungs.
- Unless contraindicated, place the client in a side-lying or semiprone position as tolerated to prevent aspiration of oral secretions.
- Using sterile technique, suction the endotracheal tube as needed to remove excessive secretions.

- Closely monitor cuff pressure, maintaining a pressure of 20 to 25 mm Hg (or as recommended by the tube manufacturer) to minimize the risk of tracheal tissue necrosis. If recommended, deflate the cuff periodically.
- Provide oral and nasal care every 2 to 4 hours. Use an oropharyngeal airway to prevent the client from biting down on an oral endotracheal tube. Move oral endotracheal tubes to the opposite side of the mouth every 8 hours or per agency protocol, taking care to maintain the position of the tube in the trachea.
- Provide humidified air or oxygen because the endotracheal tube bypasses the upper airways, which normally moisten the air.
- If the client is on mechanical ventilation, ensure that all alarms are enabled at all times because the client cannot call for help should an emergency occur.
- Communicate frequently with the client, providing a note pad or picture board for the client to use in communicating.

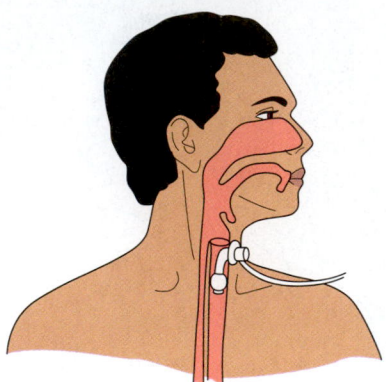

Figure 48–21 ■ A tracheostomy tube in place.

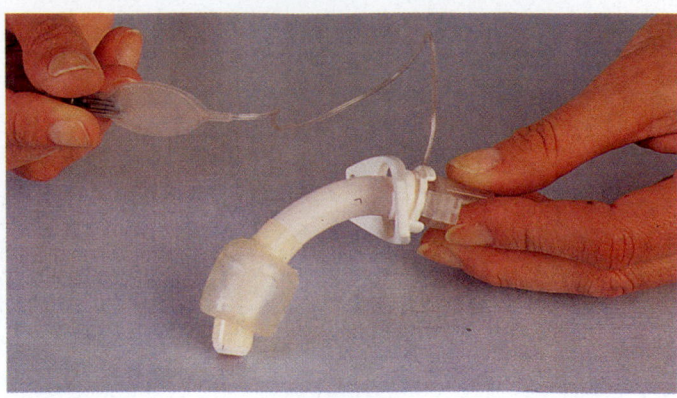

Figure 48–23 ■ A tracheostomy tube with a low-pressure cuff.

Tracheostomy Clients who need long-term airway support may have a tracheostomy, a surgical incision in the trachea just below the larynx. A curved tracheostomy tube is inserted to extend through the stoma into the trachea (Figure 48–21 ■). Tracheostomy tubes may be either plastic or metal and are available in different sizes.

Tracheostomy tubes have an outer cannula that is inserted into the trachea and a flange that rests against the neck and allows the tube to be secured in place with tape or ties (Figure 48–22 ■). All tubes also have an obturator, used to insert the outer cannula and then removed. The obturator is kept at the client's bedside in case the tube becomes dislodged and needs to be reinserted. Some tracheostomy tubes have an inner cannula that may be removed for periodic cleaning.

Cuffed tracheostomy tubes are surrounded by an inflatable cuff that produces an airtight seal between the tube and the trachea. This seal prevents aspiration of oropharyngeal secretions and air leakage between the tube and the trachea. Cuffed tubes are often used immediately after a tracheostomy and are essential when ventilating a tracheostomy client with a mechanical ventilator. Children do not require cuffed tubes, because their tracheas are resilient enough to seal the air space around the tube.

Low-pressure cuffs (Figure 48–23 ■) are commonly used to distribute a low, even pressure against the trachea, thus decreasing the risk of tracheal tissue necrosis. They do not need to be deflated periodically to reduce pressure on the tracheal

wall. Foam cuffed tracheostomy tubes (Figure 48–24 ■) do not require injected air; instead, when the port is opened, ambient air enters the balloon, which then conforms to the client's trachea. Air is removed from the cuff prior to insertion or removal of the tube.

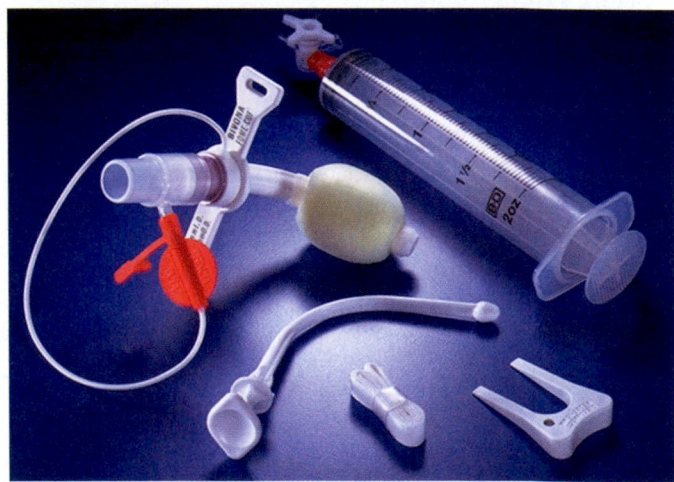

Figure 48–24 ■ A tracheostomy tube with a foam cuff.
(Courtesy of Portex Inc., Keene, NH.)

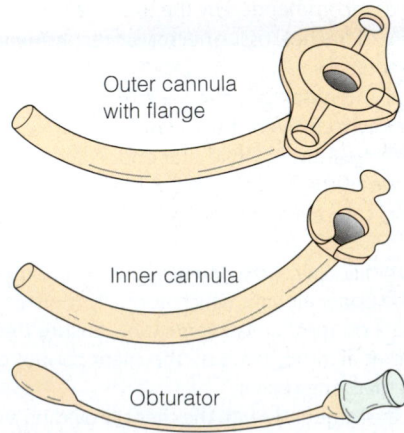

Figure 48–22 ■ Components of a tracheostomy tube.

Outer cannula with flange

Inner cannula

Obturator

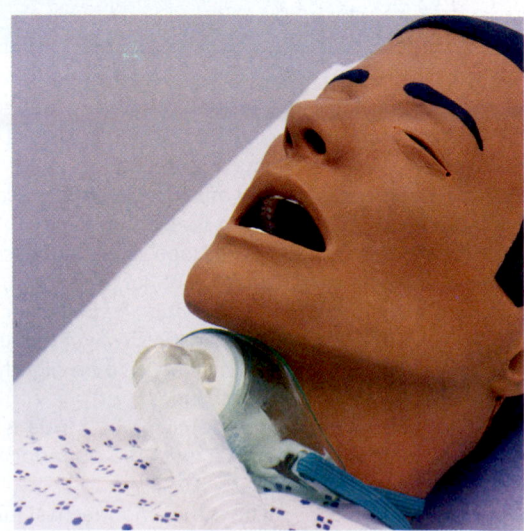

Figure 48–25 ■ A tracheostomy mist collar.

The nurse provides tracheostomy care for the client with a new or recent tracheostomy to maintain patency of the tube and reduce the risk of infection. Initially a tracheostomy may need to be suctioned (see the section on suctioning that follows) and cleaned as often as every 1 to 2 hours. After the initial inflammatory response subsides, tracheostomy care may only need to be done once or twice a day, depending on the client. Procedure 48–2 describes tracheostomy care.

When the client breathes through a tracheostomy, air is no longer filtered and humidified as it is when passing through the upper airways; therefore, special precautions are necessary. Humidity may be provided with a mist collar (Figure 48–25 ■). Clients with long-term tracheostomies may wear a light scarf or a 4-in. × 4-in. gauze held in place with a cotton tie over the stoma to filter air as it enters the tracheostomy.

Procedure 48–2 Providing Tracheostomy Care

Purposes

- To maintain airway patency
- To maintain cleanliness and prevent infection at the tracheostomy site
- To facilitate healing and prevent skin excoriation around the tracheostomy incision
- To promote comfort

ASSESSMENT

Assess

- Respiratory status including ease of breathing, rate, rhythm, depth, and lung sounds
- Pulse rate
- Character and amount of secretions from tracheostomy site
- Presence of drainage on tracheostomy dressing or ties
- Appearance of incision (note any redness, swelling, purulent discharge, or odor)

PLANNING

Delegation

Tracheostomy care involves application of scientific knowledge, sterile technique, and problem solving, and therefore needs to be performed by a nurse.

Equipment

- Sterile disposable tracheostomy cleaning kit or supplies including sterile containers, sterile nylon brush and/or pipe cleaners, sterile applicators, gauze squares
- Towel or drape to protect bed linens
- Sterile suction catheter kit (suction catheter and sterile container for solution)
- Hydrogen peroxide and sterile normal saline
- Sterile gloves (2 pairs)
- Clean gloves
- Moisture-proof bag
- Commercially prepared sterile tracheostomy dressing or sterile 4-in. × 4-in. gauze dressing
- Cotton twill ties
- Clean scissors

IMPLEMENTATION

Performance

1. Explain to the client what you are going to do, why it is necessary, and how he or she can cooperate. Provide for a means of communication, such as eye blinking or raising a finger, to indicate pain or distress.
2. Wash hands and observe other appropriate infection control procedures.
3. Provide for client privacy.
4. Prepare the client and the equipment.
   - Assist the client to a semi-Fowler's or Fowler's position *to promote lung expansion.*
   - Open the tracheostomy kit or sterile basins. Pour hydrogen peroxide and sterile normal saline into separate containers.
   - Establish a sterile field.
   - Open other sterile supplies as needed including sterile applicators, suction kit, and tracheostomy dressing.
5. Suction the tracheostomy tube.
   - Put a clean glove on your nondominant hand and a sterile glove on your dominant hand (or put on a pair of sterile gloves).
   - Suction the full length of the tracheostomy tube to remove secretions and ensure a patent airway (see Procedure 48–3).
   - Rinse the suction catheter and wrap the catheter around your hand, and peel the glove off so that it turns inside out over the catheter.
   - Using the gloved hand, unlock the inner cannula (if present) and remove it by gently pulling it out toward you in line with its curvature. Place the inner cannula in the hydrogen peroxide solution. *This moistens and loosens dried secretions.*
   - Remove the soiled tracheostomy dressing. Place the soiled dressing in your gloved hand and peel the glove off so that it turns inside out over the dressing. Discard the glove and the dressing.
   - Put on sterile gloves. Keep your dominant hand sterile during the procedure.

continued on page 1316

IMPLEMENTATION *continued*

6. Clean the inner cannula.
   - Remove the inner cannula from the soaking solution.
   - Clean the lumen and entire inner cannula thoroughly using the brush or pipe cleaners moistened with sterile normal saline (Figure 48–26 ■). Inspect the cannula for cleanliness by holding it at eye level and looking through it into the light.

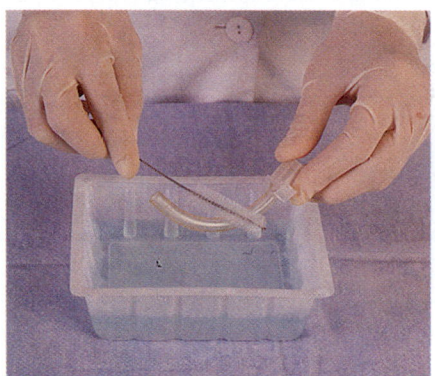

Figure 48–26 ■ Cleaning the inner cannula with a brush.

   - Rinse the inner cannula thoroughly in the sterile normal saline. *Thorough rinsing is important to remove the hydrogen peroxide from the inner cannula.*
   - After rinsing, gently tap the cannula against the inside edge of the sterile saline container. Use a pipe cleaner folded in half to dry only the inside of the cannula; do not dry the outside. *This removes excess liquid from the cannula and prevents possible aspiration by the client, while leaving a film of moisture on the outer surface to lubricate the cannula for reinsertion.*
   - Using sterile technique, suction the outer cannula. *Suctioning removes secretions from the outer cannula.*

7. Replace the inner cannula, securing it in place.
   - Insert the inner cannula by grasping the outer flange and inserting the cannula in the direction of its curvature.
   - Lock the cannula in place by turning the lock (if present) into position to secure the flange of the inner cannula to the outer cannula.

8. Clean the incision site and tube flange.
   - Using sterile applicators or gauze dressings moistened with normal saline, clean the incision site (Figure 48–27 ■). Handle the sterile supplies with your dominant hand. Use each applicator or gauze dressing only once and then discard. *This avoids contaminating a clean area with a soiled gauze dressing or applicator.*

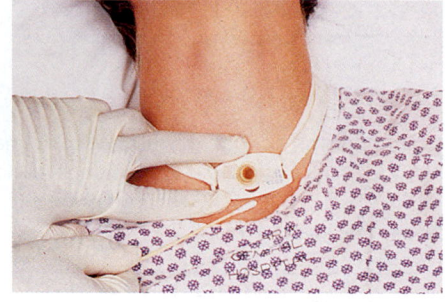

Figure 48–27 ■ Using an applicator stick to clean the tracheostomy site.

   - Hydrogen peroxide may be used (usually in a half-strength solution mixed with sterile normal saline; use a separate sterile container if this is necessary) to remove crusty secretions. Thoroughly rinse the cleaned area using gauze squares moistened with sterile normal saline. *Hydrogen peroxide can be irritating to the skin and inhibit healing if not thoroughly removed.*
   - Clean the flange of the tube in the same manner.
   - Thoroughly dry the client's skin and tube flanges with dry gauze squares.

9. Apply a sterile dressing
   - Use a commercially prepared tracheostomy dressing of nonraveling material or open and refold a 4-in. 4-in. gauze dressing into a V shape as shown in Figure 48–28 ■, *A* through *D*. Avoid using cotton-filled gauze squares or cutting the 4-in. × 4-in. gauze. *Cotton lint or gauze fibers can be aspirated by the client, potentially creating a tracheal abscess.*

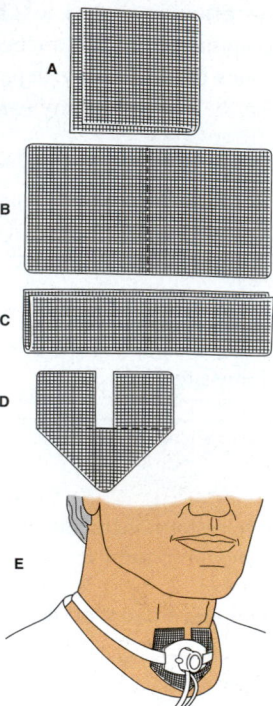

Figure 48–28 ■ Folding a 4-in. × 4-in. gauze to make a tracheostomy dressing.

   - Place the dressing under the flange of the tracheostomy tube as shown in Figure 48–28, *E.*
   - While applying the dressing, ensure that the tracheostomy tube is securely supported. *Excessive movement of the tracheostomy tube irritates the trachea.*

10. Change the tracheostomy ties.

TWO-STRIP METHOD

   - Cut two unequal strips of twill tape, one approximately 25 cm (10 in.) long and the other about 50 cm (20 in.) long. *Cutting one tape longer than the other allows them to be fastened at the side of the neck for easy access and to avoid the pressure of a knot on the skin at the back of the neck.*
   - Cut a 1-cm (0.5-in.) lengthwise slit approximately 2.5 cm (1 in.) from one end of each strip. To do this, fold the end of the tape back onto itself about 2.5 cm (1 in.), then cut a slit in the middle of the tape from its folded edge.

Procedure 48–2 Providing Tracheostomy Care *continued*

IMPLEMENTATION *continued*

- Leaving the old ties in place, thread the slit end of one clean tape through the eye of the tracheostomy flange from the bottom side; then thread the long end of the tape through the slit, pulling it tight until it is securely fastened to the flange. *Leaving the old ties in place while securing the clean ties prevents inadvertent dislodging of the tracheostomy tube. Securing tapes in this manner avoids the use of knots, which can come untied or cause pressure and irritation.*
- If old ties are very soiled or it is difficult to thread new ties onto the tracheostomy flange with old ties in place, have an assistant put on a sterile glove and hold the tracheostomy in place while you replace the ties.
- Repeat the process for the second tie.
- Ask the client to flex the neck. Slip the longer tape under the client's neck, place two fingers between the tape and the client's neck (Figure 48–29 ■), and tie the tapes together at the side of the neck.

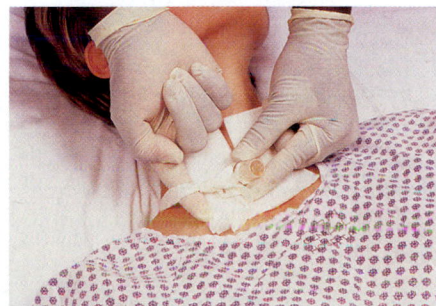

Figure 48–29 ■ Placing a finger underneath the tie tape before tying it.

Flexing the neck increases its circumference the way coughing does. Placing two fingers under the ties prevents making the ties too tight, which could interfere with coughing or place pressure on the jugular veins.
- Tie the ends of the tapes using square knots. Cut off any long ends, leaving approximately 1 to 2 cm (0.5 in.). *Square knots prevent slippage and loosening. Adequate ends beyond the knot prevent the knot from inadvertently untying.*
- Once the clean ties are secured, remove the soiled ties and discard.

ONE-STRIP METHOD

- Cut a length of twill tape 2.5 times the length needed to go around the client's neck from one tube flange to the other.
- Thread one end of the tape into the slot on one side of the flange.
- Bring both ends of the tape together, take them around the clients neck, keeping them flat and untwisted.
- Thread the end of the tape next to the client's neck through the slot from the back to the front.
- Have the client flex the neck. Tie the loose ends with a square knot at the side of the client's neck, allowing for slack by placing two fingers under the ties as with the two-strip method. Cut off long ends.
11. Tape and pad the tie knot.
   - Place a folded 4-in. × 4-in. gauze square under the tie knot, and apply tape over the knot. *This reduces skin irritation from the knot and prevents confusing the knot with the clients gown ties.*
12. Check the tightness of the ties.

- Frequently check the tightness of the tracheostomy ties and position of the tracheostomy tube. *Swelling of the neck may cause the ties to become too tight, interfering with coughing and circulation. Ties can loosen in restless clients, allowing the tracheostomy tube to extrude from the stoma.*
13. Document all relevant information.
   - Record suctioning, tracheostomy care, and the dressing change, noting your assessments.

VARIATION: USING A DISPOSABLE INNER CANNULA

- Check policy for frequency of changing inner cannula *because standards vary among institutions.*
- Open a new cannula package.
- Using a gloved hand, unlock the current inner cannula (if present) and remove it by gently pulling it out toward you in line with its curvature.
- Check the cannula for amount and type of secretions and discard properly.
- Pick up the new inner cannula touching only the outer locking portion.
- Insert the new inner cannula into the tracheostomy.
- Lock the cannula in place by turning the lock (if present).

EVALUATION

- Perform appropriate follow-up such as determining character and amount of secretions, drainage from the tracheostomy, appearance of the tracheostomy incision, pulse rate and respiratory status compared to baseline data, complaints of pain or discomfort at the tracheostomy site.
- Relate findings to previous assessment data if available.
- Report significant deviations from normal to the physician.

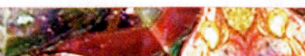

Lifespan Considerations

Tracheostomy Care

Infants and Children

- An assistant should *always* be present while tracheostomy care is performed.
- Always keep a sterile, packaged tracheostomy tube taped to the child's bed so that if the tube dislodges, a new one is

available for immediate reintubation (Bindler & Ball, 2003, p. 95).

Elders

- Older adult skin is more fragile and prone to breakdown. Care of the skin at the tracheostomy stoma is very important.

Home Care Considerations

Tracheostomy Care

- For tracheostomies older than 1 month, clean technique is used for tracheostomy care (Humphrey, 1998).
- Stress the importance of good hand washing technique to the caregiver.
- Tap water may be used for rinsing the inner cannula.
- Teach the caregiver the tracheostomy care procedure and observe a return demonstration.

- Inform the caregiver of the signs and symptoms that may indicate an infection of the stoma site or lower airway.
- Names and telephone numbers of health care personnel who can be reached for emergencies or advice must be available to the client and/or caregiver.

Suctioning

When clients have difficulty handling their secretions or an airway is in place, suctioning may be necessary to clear air passages. **Suctioning** is aspirating secretions through a catheter connected to a suction machine or wall suction outlet. Even though the upper airways (the oropharynx and nasopharynx) are not sterile, sterile technique is recommended for all suctioning to avoid introducing pathogens into the airways.

Suction catheters may be either open tipped or whistle tipped (Figure 48–30 ■). The whistle-tipped catheter is less irritating to respiratory tissues, although the open-tipped catheter may be more effective for removing thick mucous plugs. An oral suction tube, or Yankauer device, is used to suction the oral cavity (Figure 48–31 ■). Most suction catheters have a thumb port on the side to control the suction. The catheter is connected to suction tubing, which in turn is connected to a collection chamber and suction control gauge (Figure 48–32 ■).

Oropharyngeal or nasopharyngeal suctioning removes secretions from the upper respiratory tract. Endotracheal suctioning is used to remove secretions from the trachea and bronchi. The nurse decides when suctioning is needed by assessing the client for signs of respiratory distress or evidence that the client is unable to cough up and expectorate secretions. Dyspnea,

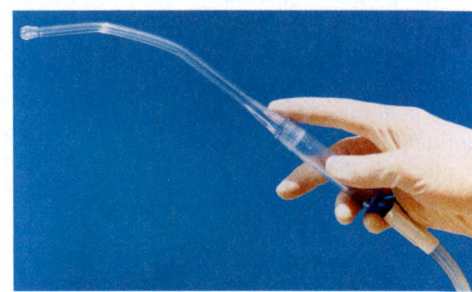

Figure 48–31 ■ Oral (Yankauer) suction tube.

bubbling or rattling breath sounds, poor skin color (cyanosis), or decreased SaO_2 levels (also called O_2 sat) may indicate the need for suctioning. Good nursing judgment is necessary, because suctioning irritates mucous membranes and can increase secretions if performed too frequently. Procedure 48–3 outlines oropharyngeal and nasopharyngeal suctioning.

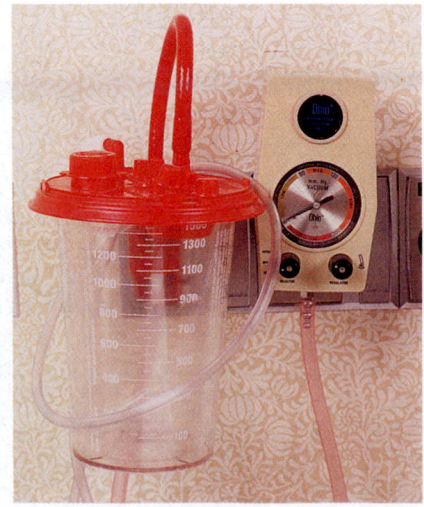

Figure 48–32 ■ A wall suction unit.

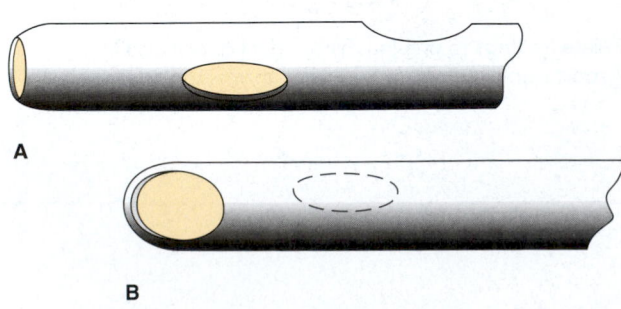

Figure 48–30 ■ Types of suction catheters: *A,* open tipped; *B,* whistle tipped.

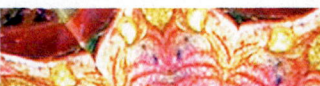

Procedure 48–3 Suctioning Oropharyngeal and Nasopharyngeal Cavities

Purposes

- To remove secretions that obstruct the airway
- To facilitate ventilation
- To obtain secretions for diagnostic purposes
- To prevent infection that may result from accumulated secretions

ASSESSMENT

Assess for clinical signs indicating the need for suctioning:

- Restlessness
- Gurgling sounds during respiration
- Adventitious breath sounds when the chest is auscultated
- Change in mental status
- Skin color
- Rate and pattern of respirations
- Pulse rate and rhythm

PLANNING

Delegation

Oral or oropharyngeal suctioning using a Yankauer suction tube can be delegated to UAP and to the client or family, if appropriate, since this is not a sterile procedure. The nurse needs to review the procedure and important points such as not applying suction during insertion of the tube to avoid trauma to the mucous membrane. In contrast, nasopharyngeal suction or oropharyngeal suction that uses sterile technique requires application of knowledge and problem solving and should be performed by the nurse.

Equipment

- Towel or moisture-resistant pad
- Portable or wall suction machine with tubing and collection receptacle
- Sterile disposable container for fluids
- Sterile normal saline or water
- Sterile gloves
- Goggles or face shield, if appropriate
- Sterile suction catheter kit (#12 to #18 Fr for adults; #8 to #10 Fr for children, and #5 to #8 Fr for infants); if both the oropharynx and the nasopharynx are to be suctioned, one sterile catheter is required for each
- Water-soluble lubricant (for nasopharyngeal suctioning)
- Y-connector
- Sterile gauzes
- Moisture-resistant disposal bag
- Sputum trap, if specimen is to be collected

IMPLEMENTATION

Performance

1. Explain to the client what you are going to do, why it is necessary, and how he or she can cooperate. Inform the client that suctioning will relieve breathing difficulty and that the procedure is painless but may be uncomfortable and stimulate the cough, gag, or sneeze reflex. *Knowing that the procedure will relieve breathing problems is often reassuring and enlists the client's cooperation.*
2. Wash hands and observe other appropriate infection control procedures.
3. Provide for client privacy.
4. Prepare the client.
   - Position a conscious person who has a functional gag reflex in the semi-Fowler's position with the head turned to one side for oral suctioning or with the neck hyperextended for nasal suctioning. *These positions facilitate the insertion of the catheter and help prevent aspiration of secretions.*
   - Position an unconscious client in the lateral position, facing you. *This position allows the tongue to fall forward, so that it will not obstruct the catheter on insertion. The lateral posi-*

tion also facilitates drainage of secretions from the pharynx and prevents the possibility of aspiration.
   - Place the towel or moisture-resistant pad over the pillow or under the chin.
5. Prepare the equipment.
   - Set the pressure on the suction gauge, and turn on the suction. Many suction devices are calibrated to three pressure ranges:
   - *Wall Unit*
     Adult: 100 to 120 mm Hg
     Child: 95 to 110 mm Hg
     Infant: 50 to 95 mm Hg
   - *Portable Unit*
     Adult: 10 to 15 mm Hg
     Child: 5 to 10 mm Hg
     Infant: 2 to 5 mm Hg
   - Open the lubricant if performing nasopharyngeal suctioning
   - Open the sterile suction package.
     a. Set up the cup or container, touching only the outside.
     b. Pour sterile water or saline into the container.
     c. Put on the sterile gloves, or put on a nonsterile glove on the

nondominant hand and then a sterile glove on the dominant hand. *The sterile gloved hand maintains the sterility of the suction catheter, and the unsterile glove prevents the transmission of the microorganisms to the nurse.*
   - With your sterile gloved hand, pick up the catheter and attach it to the suction unit (Figure 48–33 ■).

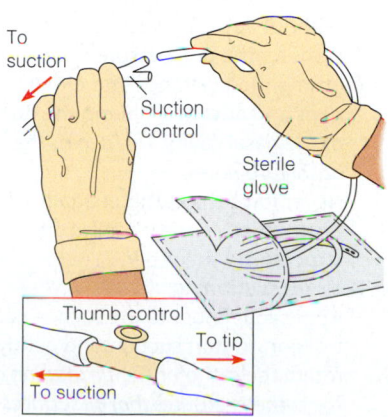

To suction

Suction control

Sterile glove

Thumb control

To tip

To suction

Figure 48–33 ■ Attaching the catheter to the suction unit.

continued on page 1320

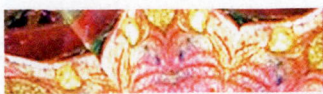

Procedure 48–3 Suctioning Oropharyngeal and Nasopharyngeal Cavities *continued*

IMPLEMENTATION *continued*

6. Make an approximate measure of the depth for the insertion of the catheter and test the equipment.
   - Measure the distance between the tip of the client's nose and the ear-lobe, or about 13 cm (5 in.) for an adult.
   - Mark the position on the tube with the fingers of the sterile gloved hand.
   - Test the pressure of the suction and the patency of the catheter by applying your sterile gloved finger or thumb to the port or open branch of the Y-connector (the suction control) to create suction.
7. Lubricate and introduce the catheter.
   - For nasopharyngeal suction, lubricate the catheter tip with sterile water, saline, or water-soluble lubricant; for oropharyngeal suction, moisten the tip with sterile water or saline. *This reduces friction and eases insertion.*

FOR OROPHARYNGEAL SUCTION
   - Pull the tongue forward, if necessary, using gauze.
   - Do not apply suction (that is, leave your finger off the port) during insertion. *Applying suction during insertion causes trauma to the mucous membrane.*
   - Advance the catheter about 10 to 15 cm (4 to 6 in.) along one side of the mouth into the oropharynx. *Directing the catheter along the side prevents gagging.*

FOR NASOPHARYNGEAL SUCTION
   - Without applying suction, insert the catheter the premeasured or recommended distance into either naris and advance it along the floor of the nasal cavity. *This avoids the nasal turbinates.*
   - Never force the catheter against an obstruction. If one nostril is obstructed, try the other.
8. Perform suctioning.
   - Apply your finger to the suction control port to start suction, and gently rotate the catheter. *Gentle rotation of the catheter ensures that all surfaces are reached and prevents trauma to any one area of the respiratory mucosa due to prolonged suction.*

   - Apply suction for 5 to 10 seconds while slowly withdrawing the catheter, then remove your finger from the control and remove the catheter.
   - A suction attempt should last only 10 to 15 seconds. During this time, the catheter is inserted, the suction applied and discontinued, and the catheter removed.
   - It may be necessary during oropharyngeal suctioning to apply suction to secretions that collect in the vestibule of the mouth and beneath the tongue.
9. Clean the catheter and repeat suctioning as above.
   - Wipe off the catheter with sterile gauze if it is thickly coated with secretions. Dispose of the used gauze in a moisture-resistant bag.
   - Flush the catheter with sterile water or saline.
   - Relubricate the catheter, and repeat suctioning until the air passage is clear.
   - Allow 20- to 30-second intervals between each suction and limit suctioning to 5 minutes in total. *Applying suction for too long may cause secretions to increase or decrease the client's oxygen supply.*
   - Alternate nares for repeat suctioning.
   - Encourage the client to breathe deeply and to cough between suctions. *Coughing and deep breathing help carry secretions from the trachea and bronchi into the pharynx, where they can be reached with the suction catheter.*
10. Obtain a specimen if required. Use a sputum trap (Figure 48–34 ■) as follows:
    - Attach the suction catheter to the tubing of the sputum trap.
    - Attach the suction tubing to the sputum trap air vent.
    - Suction the client's nasopharynx or oropharynx. The sputum trap will collect the mucus during suctioning.
    - Remove the catheter from the client. Disconnect the sputum trap tubing from the suction catheter. Remove the suction tubing from the trap air vent.

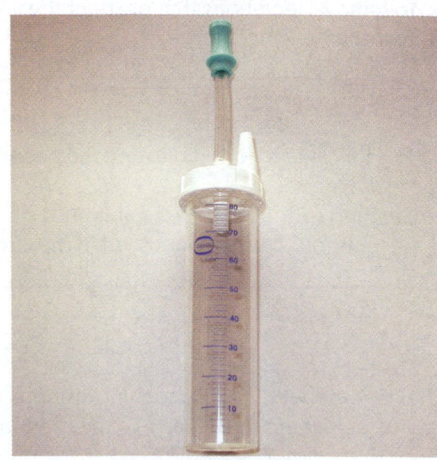

Figure 48–34 ■ A sputum collection trap.

   - Connect the tubing of the sputum trap to the air vent. *This retains any microorganisms in the sputum trap.*
   - Connect the suction catheter to the tubing.
   - Flush the catheter to remove secretions from the tubing.
11. Promote client comfort.
    - Offer to assist the client with oral or nasal hygiene.
    - Assist the client to a position that facilitates breathing.
12. Dispose of equipment and ensure availability for the next suction.
    - Dispose of the catheter, gloves, water, and waste container. Wrap the catheter around your sterile gloved hand and hold the catheter as the glove is removed over it for disposal.
    - Rinse the suction tubing as needed by inserting the end of the tubing into the used water container. Empty and rinse the suction collection container as needed or indicated by protocol. Change the suction tubing and container daily.
    - Ensure that supplies are available for the next suctioning (suction kit, gloves, water or normal saline).
13. Assess the effectiveness of suctioning.
    - Auscultate the client's breath sounds to ensure they are clear of secretions. Observe skin color, dyspnea, and level of anxiety.
14. Document relevant data.
    - Record the procedure: the amount, consistency, color, and odor of spu-

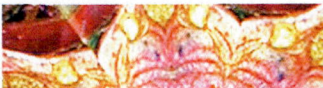

Procedure 48–3 Suctioning Oropharyngeal and Nasopharyngeal Cavities *continued*

IMPLEMENTATION *continued*

tum (e.g., foamy, white mucus; thick, green-tinged mucus; or blood-flecked mucus) and the client's breathing status before and after the procedure.

- If the procedure is carried out frequently (e.g., every hour), it may be appropriate to record only once, at

the end of the shift; however, the frequency of the suctioning must be recorded.

EVALUATION

- Conduct appropriate follow-up, such as appearance of secretions suctioned; breath sounds; respiratory rate, rhythm, and depth; pulse rate and rhythm; and skin color.

- Compare findings to previous assessment data if available.
- Report significant deviations from normal to the physician.

Following endotracheal intubation or a tracheostomy, the trachea and surrounding respiratory tissues are irritated and react by producing excessive secretions. Suctioning is necessary to remove these secretions and maintain a patent airway. The frequency of suctioning depends on the client's health and how recently the intubation was done.

Suctioning is associated with several complications: hypoxemia, trauma to the airway, nosocomial infection, and cardiac dysrhythmia, which is related to the hypoxemia. The following techniques are used to minimize or decrease these complications:

- **Hyperinflation.** This involves giving the client breaths that are 1 to 1.5 times the tidal volume set on the ventilator through the ventilator circuit or via a manual resuscitation bag. Three to five breaths are delivered before and after each pass of the suction catheter.
- **Hyperoxygenation.** This can be done with a manual resuscitation bag or through the ventilator and is performed by increasing the oxygen flow (usually to 100%) before suctioning and between suction attempts.

For tracheostomy and endotracheal suctioning, the diameter of the suction catheter should be about half the inside diameter of the tracheostomy or endotracheal tube so that hypoxia can be prevented. The nurse uses sterile techniques to prevent infection of the respiratory tract (see Procedure 48–4.) The traditional method of suctioning an endotracheal tube or tracheostomy is sometimes referred to as the *open method*. If a client is connected to a ventilator, the nurse disconnects the client from the ventilator, suctions the airway, reconnects the client to the ventilator, and discards the suction catheter. Drawbacks to the open airway suction system include the nurse needing to wear personal protective equipment (e.g., goggles or face shield, gown) to avoid exposure to the client's sputum and the potential cost of one-time catheter use, especially if the client requires frequent suctioning.

With the alternative *closed airway/tracheal suction system (in-line suctioning)* (Figure 48–35 ■), the suction catheter attaches to the ventilator tubing and the client does not need to be disconnected from the ventilator. The nurse is not exposed to

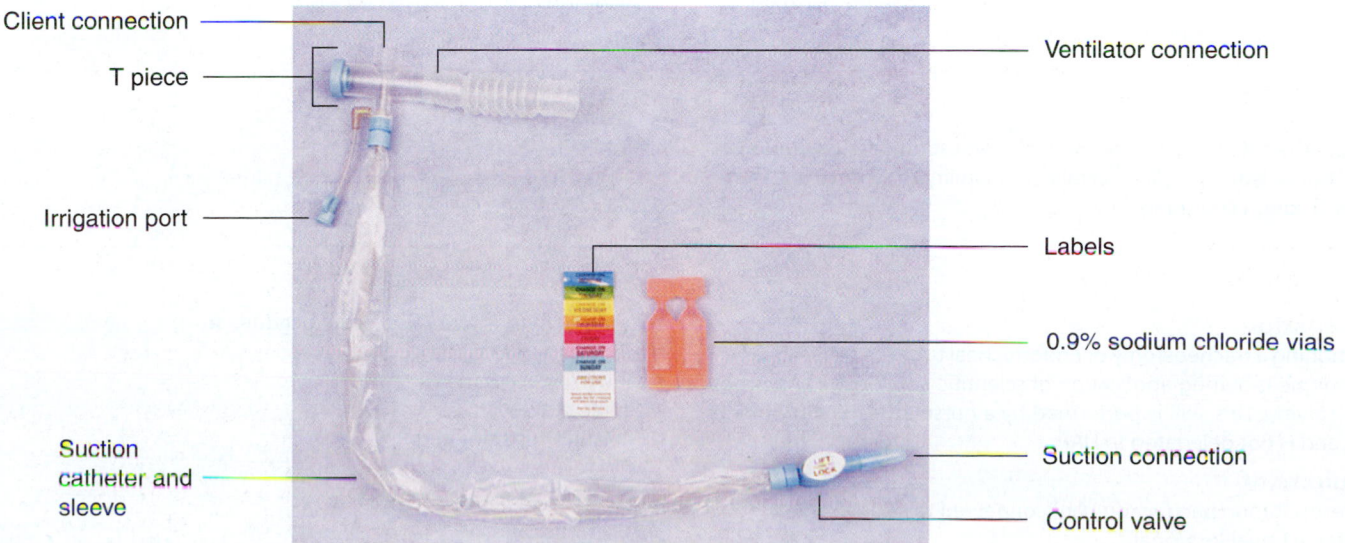

Client connection —
T piece —
Irrigation port —
Suction catheter and sleeve —

Ventilator connection
Labels
0.9% sodium chloride vials
Suction connection
Control valve

Figure 48–35 ■ A closed airway suction (in-line) system.

any secretions because the suction catheter is enclosed in a plastic sheath. The catheter can be reused as many times as necessary until the system is changed. Manufacturers recommend changing closed suction catheter systems on a daily basis. Some studies, however, challenge this recommendation with showing no difference in specified factors such as ventilator-associated pneumonia and length of hospital stay for clients who had the closed system changed daily versus once a week (Hess, 1999)

or the system changed on an as-needed basis (Little, 1998). The closed catheter system costs many times more than a conventional suction catheter. However, closed suctioning is becoming more common in health care settings given the benefit of using the catheter multiple times along with other recent studies indicating a cost saving with weekly or as-needed changing of the system. The nurse needs to inquire about the agency's policy for changing the closed suction system.

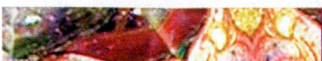

Lifespan Considerations

Suctioning
Infants
- A bulb syringe is used to remove secretions from an infant's nose or mouth. Care needs to be taken to avoid stimulating the gag reflex.

Children
- A catheter is used to remove secretions from an older child's mouth or nose.

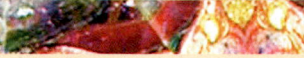

Home Care Considerations

Suctioning
- Teach clients and families that the most important aspect of infection control is frequent hand washing.
- Airway suctioning in the home is considered a clean procedure (Humphrey, 1998).
- The catheter or Yankauer should be flushed by suctioning recently boiled or distilled water to rinse away mucus, followed by the suctioning of air through the device to dry the internal surface and, thus, discourage bacterial growth. The

outer surface of the device may be wiped with alcohol or hydrogen peroxide. The suction catheter or Yankauer should be allowed to dry and then be stored in a clean, dry area (American Association for Respiratory Care [AARC], 1999, p. 100).
- Suction catheters treated in the manner described above may be reused. It is recommended that catheters be discarded after 24 hours. Yankauer suction tubes may be cleaned, boiled, and reused indefinitely (AARC, 1999, p. 100).

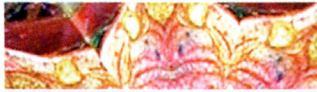

Procedure 48–4   Suctioning a Tracheostomy or Endotracheal Tube

Purposes
- To maintain a patent airway and prevent airway obstructions
- To promote respiratory function (optimal exchange of oxygen and carbon dioxide into and out of the lungs)
- To prevent pneumonia that may result from accumulated secretions

ASSESSMENT

Assess the client for the presence of congestion on auscultation of the thorax. Note the client's ability or inability to remove the secretions through coughing.

PLANNING

Delegation
Suctioning a tracheostomy or endotracheal tube is a sterile, invasive technique requiring application of scientific knowledge and problem solving. This skill is performed by a nurse or respiratory therapist and is not delegated to UAP.

Equipment
- Resuscitation bag (Ambu bag) connected to 100% oxygen
- Sterile towel (optional)

- Equipment for suctioning (see Procedure 48–3)
- Goggles and mask if necessary
- Gown (if necessary)
- Sterile gloves
- Moisture-resistant bag

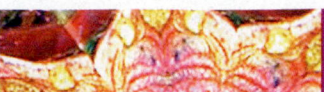

IMPLEMENTATION

Preparation

Determine if the client has been suctioned previously and, if so, review the documentation of the procedure. This information can be very helpful in preparing the nurse for both the physiologic and psychologic impact of suctioning on the client.

Performance

1. Explain to the client what you are going to do, why it is necessary, and how he or she can cooperate. Inform the client that suctioning usually causes some intermittent coughing and that this assists in removing the secretions.
2. Wash hands and observe other appropriate infection control procedures (e.g., gloves, goggles).
3. Provide for client privacy.
4. Prepare the client.
   - If not contraindicated because of health, place the client in the semi-Fowler's position to promote deep breathing, maximum lung expansion, and productive coughing. *Deep breathing oxygenates the lungs, counteracts the hypoxic effects of suctioning, and may induce coughing. Coughing helps to loosen and move secretions.*
   - If necessary, provide analgesia before suctioning. Endotracheal suctioning stimulates the cough reflex, which can cause pain for clients who have had thoracic or abdominal surgery or who have experienced traumatic injury. *Premedication can increase the client's comfort during the suctioning procedure.*
5. Prepare the equipment.
   - Attach the resuscitation apparatus to the oxygen source (Figure 48–36 ■).

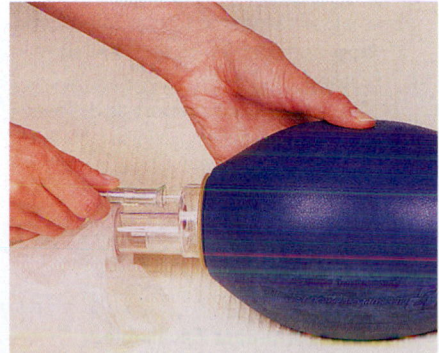

Figure 48–36 ■ Attaching the resuscitation apparatus to the oxygen source.

Adjust the oxygen flow to 100% flush.
- Open the sterile supplies in readiness for use.
- Place the sterile towel, if used, across the client's chest below the tracheostomy.
- Turn on the suction, and set the pressure in accordance with agency policy. For a wall unit, a pressure setting of about 100 to 120 mm Hg is normally used for adults, 50 to 95 mm Hg for infants and children.
- Put on goggles, mask, and gown if necessary.
- Put on sterile gloves. Some agencies recommend putting a sterile glove on the dominant hand and an unsterile glove on the nondominant hand to protect the nurse.
- Holding the catheter in the dominant hand and the connector in the nondominant hand, attach the suction catheter to the suction tubing (see Figure 48–33).
6. Flush and lubricate the catheter.
   - Using the dominant hand, place the catheter tip in the sterile saline solution.
   - Using the thumb of the nondominant hand, occlude the thumb control and suction a small amount of the sterile solution through the catheter. *This determines that the suction equipment is working properly and lubricates the outside and the lumen of the catheter. Lubrication eases insertion and reduces tissue trauma during insertion. Lubricating the lumen also helps prevent secretions from sticking to the inside of the catheter.*
7. If the client does not have copious secretions, hyperventilate the lungs with a resuscitation bag before suctioning.
   - Summon an assistant, if one is available, for this step.
   - Using your nondominant hand, turn on the oxygen to 12 to 15 L/min.
   - If the client is receiving oxygen, disconnect the oxygen source from the tracheostomy tube using your nondominant hand.
   - Attach the resuscitator to the tracheostomy or endotracheal tube (Figure 48–37 ■).
   - Compress the Ambu bag three to five times, as the client inhales. This

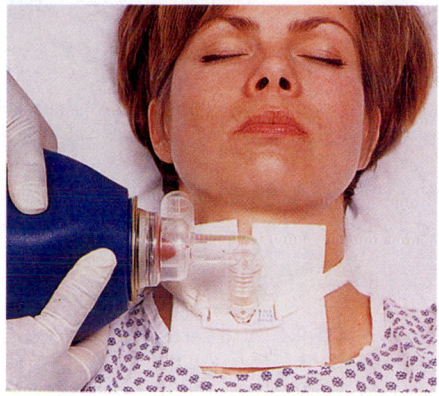

Figure 48–37 ■ Attaching the resuscitator to the tracheostomy.

is best done by a second person who can use both hands to compress the bag, thus, providing a greater inflation volume.
- Observe the rise and fall of the client's chest to assess the adequacy of each ventilation.
- Remove the resuscitation device and place it on the bed or the client's chest with the connector facing up.

VARIATION -USING A VENTILATOR TO PROVIDE-HYPERVENTILATION.

If the client is on a ventilator, use the ventilator for hyperventilation and hyperoxygenation. Newer models have a mode that provides 100% oxygen for 2 minutes and then switches back to the previous oxygen setting as well as a manual breath or sigh button. *The use of ventilator settings provides more consistent delivery of oxygenation and hyperinflation than a resuscitation device.*

8. If the client has copious secretions, do not hyperventilate with a resuscitator. *Instead:*
   - Keep the regular oxygen delivery device on and increase the liter flow or adjust the FiO_2 to 100% for several breaths before suctioning. *Hyperventilating a client who has copious secretions can force the secretions deeper into the respiratory tract.*
9. Quickly but gently insert the catheter *without* applying any suction.
   - With your nondominant thumb off the suction port, quickly but gently insert the catheter into the trachea through the tracheostomy tube (Figure 48–38 ■). *To prevent tissue trauma and oxygen loss, suction is not*

continued on page 1324

IMPLEMENTATION *continued*

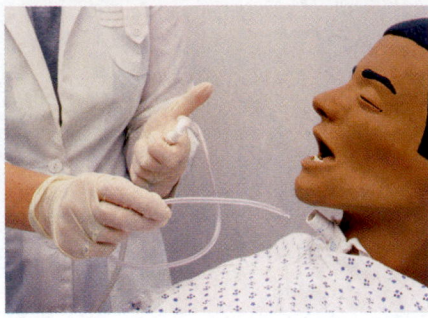

Figure 48–38 ■ Inserting the catheter into the trachea through the tracheostomy tube. *Note:* Suction is not applied while inserting the catheter.

applied during insertion of the catheter.
- Insert the catheter about 12.5 cm (5 in.) for adults, less for children, or until the client coughs or you feel resistance. *Resistance usually means that the catheter tip has reached the bifurcation of the trachea. To prevent damaging the mucous membranes at the bifurcation, withdraw the catheter about 1 to 2 cm (0.4 to 0.8 in.) before applying suction.*
10. Perform suctioning.
    - Apply intermittent suction for 5 to 10 seconds by placing the nondominant thumb over the thumb port. *Suction time is restricted to 10 seconds or less to minimize oxygen loss.*
    - Rotate the catheter by rolling it between your thumb and forefinger while slowly withdrawing it. *This prevents tissue trauma by minimizing the suction time against any part of the trachea.*
    - Withdraw the catheter completely, and release the suction.
    - Hyperventilate the client.
    - Then suction again.
11. Reassess the client's oxygenation status and repeat suctioning.
    - Observe the client's respirations and skin color. Check the client's pulse if necessary, using your nondominant hand.

- Encourage the client to breathe deeply and to cough between suctions.
- Allow 2 to 3 minutes between suctions when possible. *This provides an opportunity for reoxygenation of the lungs.*
- Flush the catheter and repeat suctioning until the air passage is clear and the breathing is relatively effortless and quiet.
- After each suction, pick up the resuscitation bag with your nondominant hand and ventilate the client with no more than three breaths.
12. Dispose of equipment and ensure availability for the next suction.
    - Flush the catheter and suction tubing.
    - Turn off the suction and disconnect the catheter from the suction tubing.
    - Wrap the catheter around your sterile hand and peel the glove off so that it turns inside out over the catheter.
    - Discard the glove and the catheter in the moisture-resistant bag.
    - Replenish the sterile fluid and supplies so that the suction is ready for use again. *Clients who require suctioning often require it quickly, so it is essential to leave the equipment at the bedside ready for use.*
13. Provide for client comfort and safety.
    - Assist the client to a comfortable, safe position that aids breathing. If the person is conscious, a semi-Fowler's position is frequently indicated. If the person is unconscious, Sims' position aids in the drainage of secretions from the mouth.
14. Document relevant data.
    - Record the suctioning, including the amount and description of suction returns and any other relevant assessments.

VARIATION: CLOSED AIRWAY/TRACHEAL SUCTION SYSTEM (IN-LINE CATHETER)
- If a catheter is not attached, put on clean gloves, aseptically open a new

closed catheter set, and attach the ventilator connection on the T piece to the ventilator tubing. Attach the client connection to the endotracheal tube or tracheostomy.
- Attach one end of the suction connecting tubing to the suction connection port of the closed system and the other end of the connecting tubing to the suction device.
- Turn suction on, occlude or kink tubing, and depress the suction control valve (on the closed catheter system) to set suction to the appropriate level. Release the suction control valve.
- Use the ventilator to hyperoxygenate and hyperinflate the client's lungs.
- Unlock the suction control mechanism if required by the manufacturer.
- Advance the suction catheter enclosed in its plastic sheath with the dominant hand. Steady the T piece with the nondominant hand.
- Depress the suction control valve and apply suction for no more than 10 seconds and gently withdraw the catheter.
- Repeat as needed remembering to provide hyperoxygenation and hyperinflation as needed.
- When completed suctioning, withdraw the catheter into its sleeve and close the access valve, if appropriate. *If the system does not have an access valve on the client connector, the nurse needs to observe for the potential of the catheter migrating into the airway and partially obstructing the artificial airway.*
- Flush the catheter by instilling normal saline into the irrigation port and applying suction. Repeat until the catheter is clear.
- Close the irrigation port and close the suction valve.

EVALUATION
- Perform a follow-up examination of the client to determine the effectiveness of the suctioning (e.g., respiratory rate, depth, and character; breath sounds; color of skin and nailbeds; character and amount of secretions suctioned; changes in vital signs).
- Relate findings to previous assessment data if available.
- Report significant deviations from normal to the physician.

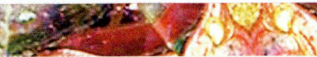

Lifespan Considerations

Suctioning a Tracheostomy or Endotracheal Tube
Infants and Children

- Have an assistant gently restrain the child to keep the child's hands out of the way. The assistant will need to keep the child's head in the midline position (Bindler & Ball, 2003, p. 107).

Elders

- Elders often have cardiac and/or pulmonary disease, thus increasing their susceptibility to hypoxemia related to suctioning. Watch closely for signs of hypoxemia. If noted, stop suctioning and hyperoxygenate.
- Do a thorough lung assessment before and after suctioning to determine effectiveness of suctioning and to be aware of any special problems.

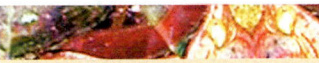

Home Care Considerations

Suctioning a Tracheostomy or Endotracheal Tube

- Whenever possible, the client should be encouraged to clear the airway by coughing.
- Clients may need to learn to suction their secretions if they cannot cough effectively.
- Clean gloves should be used when endotracheal suctioning is performed in the home environment (AARC, 1999).

- The nurse needs to instruct the caregiver on how to determine the need for suctioning and the correct process of suctioning to avoid potential complications of suctioning.
- Stress the importance of adequate hydration as it thins secretions, which can aid in the removal of secretions by coughing or suctioning.

Research Note
How Well Do Nurses Use Current Knowledge about Closed-System Suctioning Techniques?

The purposes of a study by Paul-Allen and Ostrow (2000) were to determine the frequency of use of closed and open suctioning systems and the nurses' knowledge about proper techniques for using the closed system. Critical care nurses were surveyed and 120 responses analyzed. Almost all of the nurses reported using the closed system all or some of the time. The majority of the nurses who used the closed system reported using hyperoxygenation although a few of those only used it before the first catheter insertion or between passes rather than before, between, and after. Only about half of the nurses used hyperinflation and, again, some used it only before or after suctioning rather than at both times.

Implications: In this sample, more than half of the nurses never use the open system of suctioning. It suggests that this may be a trend that will continue. However, not all of the nurses properly oxygenated their clients. More research is needed to quantify the suspected positive impact of hyperoxygenation and hyperinflation as a well as the potential negative effects. In addition, the best mechanism for informing practicing nurses of this evidence must be established.

Note: From "Survey of Nursing Practices with Closed-System Suctioning," by J. Paul-Allen and C. L. Ostrow, 2000, *American Journal of Critical Care, 9(1),* pp. 9–17.

Chest Tubes and Drainage Systems

If the thin, double-layered pleural membrane is disrupted by lung disease, surgery, or trauma, the negative pressure between the pleural layers may be lost. The lung then collapses because it is no longer drawn outward as the diaphragm and intercostal muscles contract during inhalation. When air collects in the pleural space, it is known as a **pneumothorax.** Blood or fluid in the pleural space, a **hemothorax,** places pressure on lung tissue and interferes with lung expansion. Chest tubes may be inserted into the pleural cavity to restore negative pressure and drain collected fluid or blood. Because air rises, chest tubes for pneumothorax often are placed in the upper anterior thorax, whereas chest tubes used to drain fluid generally are placed in the lower lateral chest wall.

When chest tubes are inserted, they must be connected to a sealed drainage system or a one-way valve that allows air and fluid to be removed from the chest cavity but prevents air from entering from the outside. Sterile disposable drainage systems are used to prevent outside air from entering the chest tube. These systems typically have a closed collection chamber for drainage that is connected to a wet or dry seal chamber (Figure 48–39 ■). With the water-seal system, when the client inhales, the water prevents air from entering the system from the atmosphere. During exhalation, however, air can exit the chest cavity, bubbling up through the water. Suction can be added to the system to facilitate removing air and secretions from the chest cavity. The drainage system should always be kept below the level of the client's chest to prevent fluid and drainage from being drawn back into the chest cavity.

A Heimlich valve or comparable system may be used for ambulatory clients who have a pneumothorax. These valves allow air to escape from the chest cavity, but they close during inhalation to prevent air from entering.

Chest tube insertion and removal require sterile technique and must be done without introducing air or microorganisms into the pleural cavity.

Nursing responsibilities regarding drainage systems include the following:

- Monitor and maintain the patency and integrity of the drainage system.

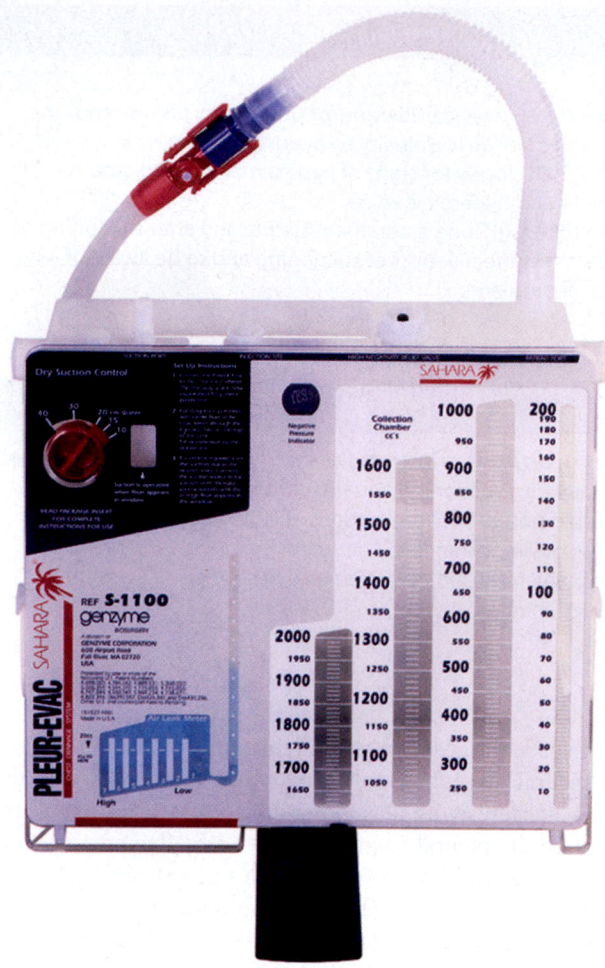

Figure 48–39 ■ A disposable chest drainage system. (Pleur-evac® Chest Drainage System. Reprinted with permission from Genzyme Biosurgery, Cardiothoracic Division, Fall River, MA.)

- Assess the client's vital signs, oxygen saturation, cardiovascular status, and respiratory status.
- Keep rubber-tipped clamps and a sterile occlusive dressing near the client. If the tube becomes disconnected from the collecting system, submerge the end in 1 in. of sterile saline or water *to maintain the seal.* If the chest tube is inadvertently pulled out, the wound should be immediately covered with a dry sterile dressing. If you can hear air leaking out the site, ensure that the dressing is not occlusive. *If the air cannot escape, this would lead to pneumothorax.*
- Use standard precautions and personal protective equipment while manipulating the system and assisting with insertion or removal.
- Observe the dressing site at least every 4 hours. Inspect the dressing for excessive and abnormal drainage, such as bleeding or foul-smelling discharge. Palpate around the dressing site, and listen for a crackling sound indicative of subcutaneous emphysema. *Subcutaneous emphysema can result from a poor seal at the chest tube insertion site.*
- Determine level of discomfort with and without activity and medicate the client for pain if indicated.
- Encourage deep breathing and coughing exercises every 2 hours (this may be contraindicated in clients who have had a

lung removed). Have the client sit upright to perform the exercises, and splint the chest around the tube insertion site with a pillow or with a hand to minimize discomfort.
- Reposition the client every 2 hours. When the client is lying on the affected side, place rolled towels beside the tubing. *Frequent position changes promote drainage, prevent complications, and provide comfort. Rolled towels prevent occlusion of the chest tube by the client's weight.*
- Assist the client with range-of-motion exercises of the affected shoulder three times per day to maintain joint mobility.
- When transporting and ambulating the client:
  a. Attach rubber-tipped forceps to the client's gown for emergency use.
  b. Keep the water-seal unit below chest level and upright.
  c. Disconnect the drainage system from the suction apparatus before moving the client and make sure the air vent is open.

Removal of a chest tube is a brief but quite painful procedure. Medicate the client before the removal. Remove the dressing around the tube and prepare the dressing that will cover the insertion site. This will be an occlusive dressing if there is no purse-string suture around the insertion site to prevent air from entering the chest. Generally, the physician performs the removal but, in some areas, specially trained nurses may be permitted to do so.

EVALUATING

Using the goals and desired outcomes identified in the planning stage of the nursing process, the nurse collects data to evaluate the effectiveness of interventions. If outcomes are not achieved, the nurse, client, and support person if appropriate need to explore the reasons before modifying the care plan. For example, if the outcome "Respirations unlabored and rate is within expected range" is not met, examples of questions that need to be considered include the following:

- What is the client's perception of the problem?
- Is the client complaining of shortness of breath or difficulty breathing?
- Is the client taking medications or performing treatments such as percussion, vibration, and postural drainage as prescribed?
- Has the client been exposed to an upper respiratory infection that is affecting breathing?
- Do other factors need to be considered, such as the client's psychologic stress level?

Examples of questions to consider if the outcome "Able to complete ADLs without fatigue" is not met include the following:

- What other factors may be affecting the client's ability to complete ADLs?
- Is the client getting adequate sleep? If not, what is interfering with the client's rest?
- Are there assistive devices (e.g., a shower chair, clothing that is easy to put on) that could help the client achieve this goal?
- Does the client need help with housework and other ADLs?
- Is the client's diet adequate to meet nutritional needs?

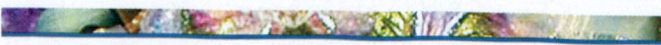

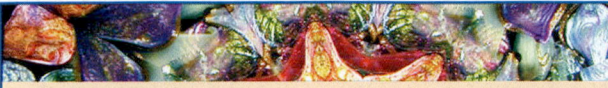

NURSING CARE PLAN FOR INEFFECTIVE AIRWAY CLEARANCE

ASSESSMENT DATA		NURSING DIAGNOSIS	DESIRED OUTCOMES [NOC #]/INDICATORS*

Nursing Assessment

Johti Singh is a 39-year-old secretary who was admitted to the hospital with an elevated temperature, fatigue, rapid, labored respirations; and mild dehydration. The nursing history reveals that Ms. Singh has had a "bad cold" for several weeks that just wouldn't go away. She has been dieting for several months and skipping meals. Ms. Singh mentions that in addition to her full-time job as a secretary she is attending college classes two evenings a week. She has smoked one package of cigarettes per day since she was 18 years old. Chest x-ray confirms pneumonia.

Physical Examination

Height: 167.6 cm (5′6″)
Weight: 54.4 kg (120 lb)
Temperature: 39.4C (103F)
Pulse: 68 BPM
Respirations: 24/minute
Blood pressure:
118/70 mm Hg

Skin pale; cheeks flushed; chills; nasal flaring; use of accessory muscles; inspiratory crackles with diminished breath sounds right base; thick, yellow sputum

Diagnostic Data

Chest x-ray: right lobar infiltration
WBC: 14,000
pH: 7.49
$PaCO_2$: 33 mm Hg
HCO_3^-: 20 mEq/L
PaO_2: 80 mm Hg

Ineffective Airway Clearance related to thick sputum, secondary to pneumonia, and fatigue (as evidenced by rapid respirations, nasal flaring, and adventitious breath sounds)

Respiratory Status: Airway Patency [0410] as evidenced by not compromised
• Fever is not present
• Respiratory rate is in expected range
• Moves sputum out of airway
• Is free of adventitious breath sounds

NURSING INTERVENTIONS [NIC#]/SELECTED ACTIVITIES*	RATIONALE

Cough Enhancement [3250]

• Assist Ms. Singh to a sitting position with head slightly flexed, shoulders relaxed, and knees flexed.

• Encourage her to take several deep breaths.

• Encourage her to take a deep breath, hold for 2 seconds, and cough two or three times in succession.

• Encourage use of incentive spirometry, as appropriate.

• Promote systemic fluid hydration, as appropriate.

Respiratory Monitoring [3350]

• Monitor rate, rhythm, depth, and effort of respirations.

• Note chest movement, watching for symmetry, use of accessory muscles, and supraclavicular and intercostal muscle retractions.

• Auscultate breath sounds, noting areas of decreased or absent ventilation and presence of adventitious sounds.

• Auscultate lung sounds after treatments to note results.

• Monitor client's ability to cough effectively.

Lying flat causes the abdominal organs to shift toward the chest, crowding the lungs and making it more difficult to breathe.

Deep breathing promotes oxygenation before controlled coughing.

Controlled coughing is accomplished by closure of the glottis and the explosive expulsion of air from the lungs by the work of abdominal and chest muscles.

Breathing exercises help maximize ventilation.

Adequate fluid intake enhances liquefaction of pulmonary secretions and facilitates expectoration of mucus.

Provides a basis for evaluating adequacy of ventilation.

Presence of nasal flaring and use of accessory muscles of respirations may occur in response to ineffective ventilation.

As fluid and mucus accumulate, abnormal breath sounds can be heard including crackles and diminished breath sounds owing to fluid-filled air spaces and diminished lung volume.

Assists in evaluating prescribed treatments and client outcomes.

Respiratory tract infections alter the amount and character of secretions. An ineffective cough compromises airway clearance and prevents mucus from being expelled.

continued on page 1328

NURSING CARE PLAN FOR INEFFECTIVE AIRWAY CLEARANCE *continued*

NURSING INTERVENTIONS [NIC#]/SELECTED ACTIVITIES*	RATIONALE
• Monitor client's respiratory secretions.	*People with pneumonia commonly produce rust-colored, purulent sputum.*
• Institute respiratory therapy treatments (e.g., nebulizer) as needed.	*A variety of respiratory therapy treatments may be used to open constricted airways and liquefy secretions.*
• Monitor for increased restlessness, anxiety, and air hunger.	*These clinical manifestations would be early indicators of hypoxia.*
• Note changes in SaO_2, and tidal CO_2, and changes in arterial blood gas values, as appropriate.	*Evaluates the status of oxygenation, ventilation, and acid–base balance.*
Oxygen Therapy [3320]	
• Instruct Ms. Singh about importance of leaving oxygen delivery device on.	*Oxygen demand is greater during febrile illness and physical stress. At low P_{O_2} levels in the atmosphere, oxygen saturation falls rapidly; therefore, oxygen should be maintained, especially during activity.*
• Periodically check oxygen delivery device to ensure that the prescribed concentration is being delivered.	*Too much or too little oxygen can be detrimental, especially in the client with a history of smoking.*
• Observe for signs of oxygen-induced hypoventilation.	*In individuals with chronic lung disease, the stimulus for breathing is low oxygen levels rather than elevated carbon dioxide. This client is at risk for COPD because of smoking. Administration of high level of oxygen could lead to hypoventilation.*

EVALUATION

Outcome partially met. Ms. Singh coughs and deep breathes purposefully q1–2h during the day. Her fluid intake is approximately 1,500 mL each day. Cough continues to be productive of moderately thick, rusty-colored sputum. Inspiratory crackles remain present in right lower lobe. Her PaO_2 is 85 mm Hg.

---

*Outcomes, interventions, and activities selected are only a sample of those suggested by NOC and NIC and should be further individualized for each client.

Applying Critical Thinking

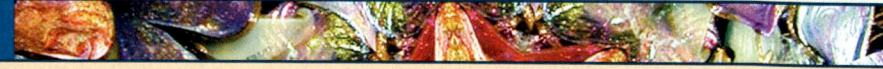

1. What factors may have led the medical staff to suspect that Ms. Singh had more than a very bad cold? Would you have come to the same conclusion?

2. The care plan appropriately focuses on the acute care of this client. Once she is significantly improved, the nurse will perform discharge teaching. What areas should be included?

3. The client already has some signs of respiratory distress. What signs might indicate that her condition was deteriorating into a more emergency situation? How would you handle this?

4. It appears that the client's sputum has not been cultured. In caring for this client, what infection control guidelines would be needed?

5. Ms. Singh's oxygen order is for a face mask at 6 L/minute. She repeatedly pulls it off and you find it lying in the sheets. How might you intervene?

See Critical Thinking Possibilities in Appendix A.

CONCEPT MAP Ineffective Airway Clearance

JS
39 y.o. ♀
Pneumonia

- ↑ Temperature; fatigue; rapid, labored respirations; mild dehydration. "Bad cold" x several weeks. Dieting for several months & skipping meals. Works full-time job as secretary, college classes 2x/week. Smokes, 21 pack/years.

- Height: 167.6 cm (5'6")
- Weight: 54.4 kg (120 lb)
- TPR: 39.4C (103F), 68, 24, BP: 118/70
- Skin pale; cheeks flushed; chills; nasal flaring; use of accessory muscles; inspiratory crackles with diminished breath sounds right base; thick, yellow sputum

- Chest x-ray: right lobar infiltration
- WBC: 14,000
- pH: 7.49
- $PaCO_2$: 33 mm Hg
- HCO_3^-: 20 mEq/L
- PaO_2: 80 mm Hg

Cough Enhancement

Assist to a sitting position with head slightly flexed, shoulders relaxed, and knees flexed

Encourage use of incentive spirometry, as appropriate

Promote systemic fluid hydration, as appropriate

Encourage her to take several deep breaths

Encourage her to take a deep breath, hold for 2 seconds, and cough two or three time in succession

---

Ineffective Airway Clearance r/t thick sputum, secondary to pneumonia, and fatigue (aeb rapid respirations, nasal flaring, and adventitious breath sounds)

Respiratory Status: Airway Patency aeb not compromised
- fever not present
- respiratory rate in expected range
- moves sputum out of airway
- free of adventitious breath sounds

Respiratory Monitoring

Institute respiratory therapy treatments (e.g., nebulizer) as needed

Monitor rate, rhythm, depth, and effort of respirations

Monitor for increased restlessness, anxiety, and air hunger

Note chest movement, watching for symmetry, use of accessory muscles, and supraclavicular and intercostal muscle retractions

Auscultate lung sounds after treatments to note results

Monitor client's respiratory secretions

Monitor client's ability to cough effectively

Note changes in SaO_2, and tidal CO_2, and changes in arterial blood gas values, as appropriate

Auscultate breath sounds, noting areas of decreased or absent ventilation and presence of adventitious sounds

---

Oxygen Therapy

Instruct about importance of leaving oxygen delivery device on

Observe for signs of oxygen-induced hypoventilation

Periodically check oxygen delivery device to ensure that the prescribed concentration is being delivered

---

Outcome partially met
- coughs and deep breaths purposefully q1–2hr during the day
- fluid intake ~1500 mL/day
- cough productive of moderately thick, rusty-colored sputum
- inspiratory crackles remain present in right lower lobe
- PaO_2 is 85 mm Hg

Legend: Assessment ☐ Nursing Diagnosis ☐ Outcomes ☐ Nursing Interventions ☐ Activities ☐ Evaluation/Reassessment ☐

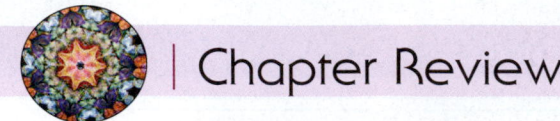

Chapter Review

EXPLORE MediaLink

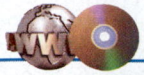

NCLEX review questions, case studies, care plan activities, MediaLink applications, and other interactive resources for this chapter can be found on the Companion Website at www.prenhall.com/kozier. Click on Chapter 48 to select the activities for this chapter.

For animations, video clips, more NCLEX review questions, and an audio glossary, access the Student CD-ROM accompanying this textbook.

Chapter Highlights

- Respiration is the process of gas exchange between the individual and the environment.
- The respiratory system contributes to effective respiration through pulmonary ventilation (the movement of air between the atmosphere and the lungs) and the diffusion of oxygen and carbon dioxide across the pulmonary membrane.
- Alveoli and the capillaries that surround them form the respiratory membrane, where gas exchange between the lungs and the blood occurs.
- Effective pulmonary ventilation, or breathing, requires clear airways, an intact central nervous system and respiratory center, an intact thoracic cavity and musculature, and adequate pulmonary compliance (stretch) and recoil.
- Gas exchange occurs by diffusion, as gas molecules move from an area of higher concentration to an area of lower concentration. At the respiratory membrane, oxygen moves from the alveolus into the blood, while carbon dioxide moves from the blood into the alveolus.
- Most oxygen (97%) is carried to the tissues loosely combined with hemoglobin in red blood cells (RBCs). Anemia, which is too few RBCs or low hemoglobin levels, impairs oxygen transportation.
- Respiratory rates normally are highest in neonates and infants, gradually slowing to adult ranges.
- Aging affects the respiratory system: The chest wall becomes more rigid and lungs less elastic.
- Other factors affecting oxygenation include the environment, lifestyle, health status, narcotic analgesics, and stress and coping.
- Hypoxia, insufficient oxygen in the tissues, can result from impaired ventilation (hypoventilation) or diffusion, or from impaired oxygen transportation to the tissues because of anemia or decreased cardiac output.
- Normal respirations are quiet and unlabored; altered respiratory patterns include tachypnea, bradypnea, hyperventilation, hypoventilation, and dyspnea. Shortness of breath is a subjective sensation of not getting enough air.
- Airway obstruction interferes with ventilation. A low-pitched snoring sound, stridor, and abnormal breath sounds may accompany partial airway obstruction. Extreme inspiratory effort with no chest movement indicates complete upper airway obstruction.

- The nursing history includes questions about current or past respiratory problems and about lifestyle, presence of symptoms such as cough or shortness of breath, smoking and other risk factors, and medications.
- Physical assessment should include a general assessment, as well as specific examination of the respiratory system.
- Diagnostic tests that may be performed to assess oxygenation include sputum and throat culture specimens; blood tests such as arterial blood gases; pulmonary function tests; and visualization procedures such as x-rays, lung scans, laryngoscopy, and bronchoscopy.
- Nursing diagnoses for the client with problems of oxygenation include *Ineffective Airway Clearance, Ineffective Breathing Pattern, Impaired Gas Exchange,* and *Activity Intolerance.* These problems also may be the etiology for several other nursing diagnoses, including *Anxiety, Fatigue, Fear, Powerlessness, Sleep Pattern Disturbance,* and *Social Isolation.*
- In discharge and home care planning, the nurse assesses the client's self-care abilities and need for assistive devices, home environment, compliance with medical regimen, and knowledge level. The ability of the family or support people to provide assistance and financial support and to cope with the changes is also assessed, as are community factors like the environment and resources.
- The nurse teaches the client about home care activities to maintain a patent airway and gas exchange and to promote healthy breathing. Dietary modifications, prescribed medications, and specific procedures also are taught, and the nurse makes referrals to community agencies as needed.
- Nursing interventions to promote oxygenation include promoting healthy breathing and a healthy heart, deep breathing and coughing, and hydration; administering medications; implementing measures to clear secretions (e.g., incentive spirometry, percussion, vibration, and postural drainage); initiating and monitoring oxygen therapy; initiating or assisting with procedures to maintain the airway (e.g., artificial airways and suctioning); providing tracheostomy care; and monitoring chest drainage systems.
- The effectiveness of nursing interventions is evaluated by using the goals and desired outcomes identified in the planning stage of the nursing process. If a goal is not met, the nurse asks pertinent questions to assess the reason for not meeting the goal.

Review Questions

48–1. A client with chronic pulmonary disease has a bluish tinge around the lips. This would most accurately be documented as
   a. hypoxia.
   b. hypoxemia.
   c. dyspnea.
   d. cyanosis.

48–2. The nurse is to assist the client with coughing and deep breathing exercises to prevent postoperative complications. This is best accomplished by planning
   a. coughing exercises 1 hour before meals and deep breathing 1 hour after meals.
   b. forceful coughing as many times as tolerated.
   c. huff coughing every 2 hours and as needed.
   d. diaphragmatic and purse-lip breathing 5 to 10 times four times a day.

48–3. A client with a chronic lung disorder requires some supplemental oxygen. The nurse anticipates that safe delivery would be oxygen
   a. 2 L/min per nasal cannula.
   b. 6 L/min per face mask.
   c. 8 L/min per partial rebreathing mask.
   d. 10 L/min per nonrebreathing mask.

48–4. Which of the following represents proper nasopharyngeal/nasotracheal suction technique?
   a. Lubricate the suction catheter with Vaseline before and between insertions.
   b. Apply suction intermittently while inserting the suction catheter.
   c. Rotate the catheter while applying suction.
   d. Hyperoxygenate the client with 100% oxygen for 30 minutes before and after suctioning.

48–5. Which of the following statements by the client indicates successful teaching regarding the proper use of an incentive spirometer?
   a. "I should breathe out as fast and hard as possible into the device."
   b. "I should inhale slowly and steadily to keep the balls up."
   c. "I should use the device three times a day, after meals."
   d. "The entire device should be washed thoroughly in sudsy water once a week."

Readings and References

Suggested Readings

Lazzara, D. (2002). Eliminate the air of mystery from chest tubes. *Nursing, 32*(6), 36–43. This in-depth article describes the reasons for chest tube placement and the various types of catheters, valves, and collecting systems used. It includes steps for the nurse to assist with chest tube insertion and care of the client after insertion.

Related Research

Belza, B., Steele, B. G., Hunziker, J., Lakshminaryan, S., Holt, L., & Buchner, D. M. (2001). Correlates of physical activity in chronic obstructive pulmonary disease. *Nursing Research, 50*, 195–202.

Kinloch, D. (1999). Instillation of normal saline during endotracheal suctioning: Effects on mixed venous oxygen saturation. *American Journal of Critical Care, 8*, 231–242.

References

American Association for Respiratory Care. (1999). AARC clinical practice guideline: Suctioning of the patient in the home. *Respiratory Care, 44*(1), 99–104.

Bindler, R. C., & Ball, J. W. (2003). *Clinical skills manual for pediatric nursing: Caring for children* (3rd ed.). Upper Saddle River, NJ: Prentice Hall Health.

Hess, D. R. (1999). Managing the artificial airway. *Respiratory Care, 44*, 759–776.

Humphrey, C. J. (1998). *Home care nursing handbook* (3rd ed.). Gaithersburg, MD: Aspen.

Johnson, M., Maas, M., & Moorhead, S. (Eds.). (2000). *Nursing outcomes classification (NOC)* (2nd ed.). St. Louis, MO: Mosby.

Little, K. (1998). As needed in line suction catheter changes were as safe as and less expensive than daily scheduled catheter changes during mechanical ventilation. *Evidence Based Nursing, 1*(3), 82.

McCloskey, J. C., & Bulechek, G. M. (Eds.). (2000). *Nursing interventions classification (NIC)* (3rd ed.). St. Louis, MO: Mosby.

NANDA International. (2003). *NANDA Nursing diagnoses: Definitions and classification 2003-2004.* Philadelphia: Author.

Paul-Allen J., & Ostrow, C. L. (2000). Survey of nursing practices with closed-system suctioning. *American Journal of Critical Care, 9*(1), 9–17.

Selected Bibliography

Anonymous. (2000). Information from your doctor: Using oxygen at home. *Patient Care, 34*(10), 74.

Carroll, P. (1998). Closing in on safer suctioning. *RN, 61*(5), 22–26.

Carroll, P. (2002). A guide to mobile chest drains. *RN, 65*(5), 56–60, 65.

Day, T., Franell, S., & Wilson-Barnett, J. (2002). Suctioning: A review of current research recommendations. *Intensive and Critical Care Nursing, 18*(2), 79–89.

Fink, J. B., & Hunt, G. E. (1999). *Clinical practice in respiratory care.* Philadelphia: Lippincott Williams & Wilkins.

Goodfellow, L. T., & Jones, M. (2002). Bronchial hygiene therapy. *American Journal of Nursing, 102*(1), 37–43.

Griggs, A. (1999). Tracheostomy: Suctioning and humidification. *Emergency Nurse, 6*(9), 33–40.

Harman, R. (1999). Management of COPD with oxygen therapy at home. *Community Nurse, 5*(7), 25–26.

Little, C. (2000). Manual ventilation. *Nursing, 30*(3), 50–51.

McConnell, E. A. (2000). Dos & don'ts: Suctioning a tracheostomy tube. *Nursing, 30*(1), 80.

McConnell, E. A. (2002). Dos & don'ts: Providing tracheostomy care. *Nursing, 32*(1), 17.

Perkins, L. A., & Shortall, S. P. (2000). Ventilation without intubation. *RN, 63*(1), 34–38.

Pope, B. B. (2002). Asthma. *Nursing, 32*(5), 44–45.

Schreiber, D. (2001). Trach care at home. *RN, 64*(7), 43–36.

Schultz, T. R. (2000). Airing differences in pediatric nebulizer therapy. *Nursing, 30*(9), 55–57.

Seay, S. J., Gay, S. L., & Strauss, M. (2002). Tracheostomy emergencies. *American Journal of Nursing, 102*(3), 59, 61, 63.

CHAPTER | 49

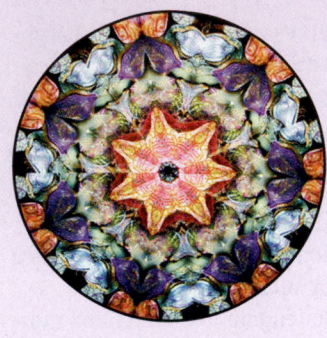

CIRCULATION

LEARNING OUTCOMES

After completing this chapter, you will be able to:

- Outline the structure and function of the cardiovascular system
- Identify factors influencing cardiovascular function.
- Identify major risk factors for the development of coronary heart disease
- Discuss the manifestations of cardiovascular disorders.
- Identify common responses to alterations in cardiovascular status.
- List signs of alterations in cardiovascular function
- Identify and describe nursing measures to promote circulation.
- Describe the critical nature of cardiopulmonary resuscitation.

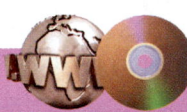

MediaLink

www.prenhall.com/kozier

Additional resources for this chapter can be found on the Student CD-ROM accompanying this textbook, and on the Companion Website at www.prenhall.com/kozier. Click on Chapter 49 to select the activities for this chapter.

CD-ROM
- Audio Glossary
- NCLEX Review
- Animations:
  Anatomy 3D
  A & P Review
  Circulation
  Normal Heart Hemodynamics
  Congenital Heart Defects

Companion Website
- Additional NCLEX Review
- Case Study: Client with Diabetes
- Care Plan Activity: Client Experiencing Pain from Walking
- MediaLink Application: Using Heart Savers Website
- Links to Resources

The circulatory system or cardiovascular system is responsible for transport of oxygen, fluids, electrolytes, and products of metabolism via the blood to and from tissues.

PHYSIOLOGY OF THE CARDIOVASCULAR SYSTEM

The respiratory and cardiovascular systems are closely linked and dependent on one another to deliver oxygen to the tissues of the body. Alterations in function of either system can affect the other and lead to tissue **hypoxia,** or lack of oxygen.

The heart and the blood vessels make up the cardiovascular system. Together with blood, it is the major transport system of the body, bringing oxygen and nutrients to the cells and removing wastes for disposal. The heart serves as the system pump, moving blood through the vessels to the tissues.

The Heart

The heart is a hollow, cone-shaped organ about the size of a fist. It is located in the mediastinum, between the lungs and underlying the sternum. It is enclosed by a double layer of fibroserous membrane known as the **pericardium.** The parietal, or outermost, pericardium serves to protect the heart and anchor it to surrounding structures. The visceral pericardium adheres to the surface of the heart, forming the heart's outermost layer, the **epicardium.** The heart wall contains two additional layers: the **myocardium,** cardiac muscle cells that form the bulk of the heart and contract with each beat, and the **endocardium,** which lines the inside of the heart's chambers and great vessels (Figure 49–1 ■).

Four hollow chambers within the heart, two upper **atria** and two lower **ventricles,** are separated longitudinally by the interventricular **septum,** forming two parallel pumps (Figure 49–2 ■). The atria and ventricles are separated from one another by the **atrioventricular (AV) valves,** the tricuspid valve on the right and the bicuspid or mitral valve on the left. The valves are named for the number of cusps (or leaflets) present on the valve. The ventricles, in turn, are separated from the great vessels (the pulmonary arteries and aorta) by the **semilunar valves** (named for their crescent moon shape): the pulmonic valve on the right and the aortic valve on the left. The valves serve to direct the flow of blood, allowing it to move from the atria to the ventricles, and the ventricles to the great vessels, but preventing backflow.

Deoxygenated blood from the veins enters the right side of the heart through the superior and inferior venae cavae (singular is vena cava). From there, it flows into the right ventricle, which pumps it through the pulmonary artery into the lungs for gas exchange at the alveolar/capillary membrane. Freshly oxygenated blood returns to the left atrium via the pulmonary veins. From here,

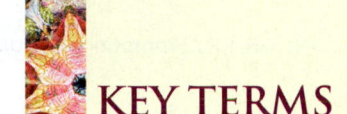
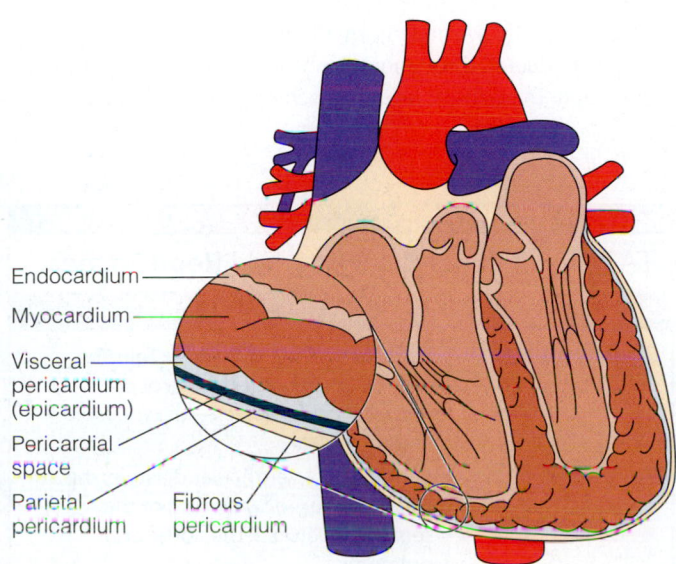

Endocardium
Myocardium
Visceral pericardium (epicardium)
Pericardial space
Parietal pericardium
Fibrous pericardium

Figure 49–1 ■ The layers of the heart: the epicardium, the myocardium, and the endocardium.

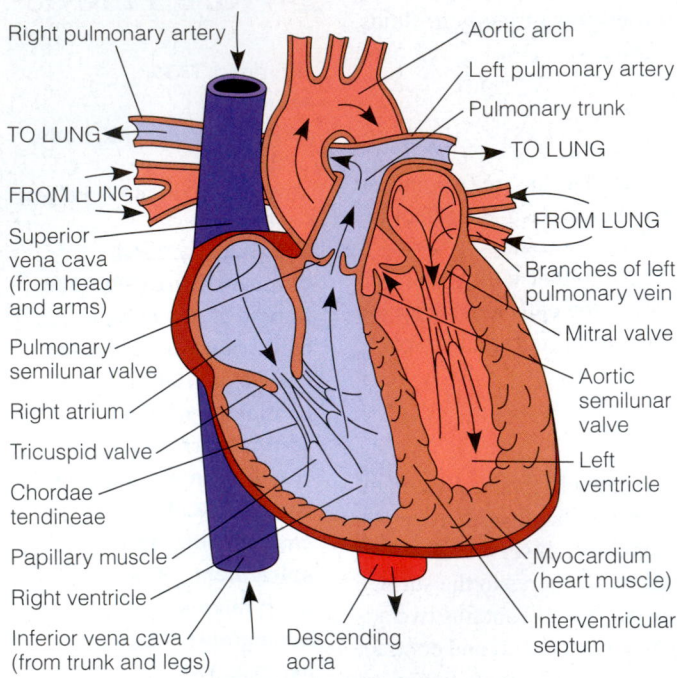

Right pulmonary artery

Aortic arch

Left pulmonary artery

Pulmonary trunk

TO LUNG

TO LUNG

FROM LUNG

FROM LUNG

Superior vena cava (from head and arms)

Branches of left pulmonary vein

Mitral valve

Pulmonary semilunar valve

Aortic semilunar valve

Right atrium

Tricuspid valve

Left ventricle

Chordae tendineae

Papillary muscle

Myocardium (heart muscle)

Right ventricle

Inferior vena cava (from trunk and legs)

Descending aorta

Interventricular septum

Figure 49–2 ■ Structures of the heart. The diagram shows the vena cava, right atrium, tricuspid valve, right ventricle, pulmonic valve, pulmonary arteries, pulmonary veins, left atrium, mitral valve, left ventricle, aortic valve, and the aorta.

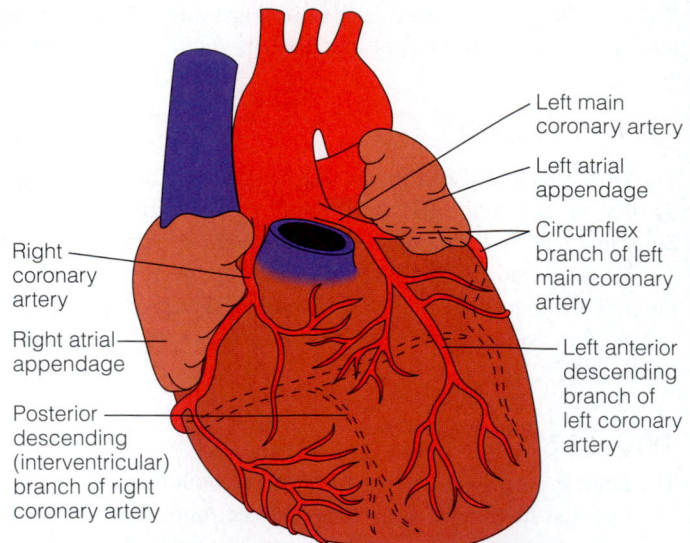

Left main coronary artery

Left atrial appendage

Circumflex branch of left main coronary artery

Right coronary artery

Right atrial appendage

Left anterior descending branch of left coronary artery

Posterior descending (interventricular) branch of right coronary artery

Figure 49–3 ■ The coronary arteries supply the heart muscle with oxygenated blood.

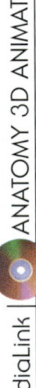

the blood enters the left ventricle to be pumped out to the systemic circulation through the aorta.

Coronary Circulation

The heart muscle moves blood to the lungs and peripheral tissues but receives no oxygen or nourishment from the blood within its chambers. Instead, it is supplied by a network of vessels known as the coronary circulation or more commonly the **coronary arteries.** The coronary arteries originate at the base of the aorta, branching out to encircle and penetrate the myocardium. The coronary arteries fill during ventricular relaxation, bringing oxygen-rich blood to the myocardium (Figure 49–3 ■). If these arteries become clogged with atherosclerotic plaque or are obstructed by a blood clot, the myocardium is deprived of oxygen, and the client may develop chest pain (angina) or experience a myocardial infarction (heart attack). The cardiac veins drain the deoxygenated blood from the myocardium into the coronary sinus, which empties into the right atrium.

Cardiac Cycle

With each heartbeat, the myocardium goes through a cycle of contraction (*systole*) and relaxation (*diastole*). **Systole** is when the heart ejects (propels) the blood into the pulmonary and systemic circulations. **Diastole** is when the ventricles fill with blood. The diastolic phase of the cardiac cycle is twice as long as the systolic phase. This is important because diastole (or ventricular filling) is largely a passive process. The longer diastolic phase allows this filling to occur. At the end of the diastolic phase the atria contract, adding an additional volume to

the ventricles. This volume is sometimes called *atrial kick.* The relationship between the phases of the cardiac cycle and the normal heart sounds is described in Table 49–1.

Cardiac Conduction System

Cardiac muscle contraction is a mechanical event that occurs in response to electrical stimulation. Cardiac muscle is unique in that, unlike skeletal muscle, it can generate an electrical impulse and contraction independently of the nervous system. This unique property of the heart is called **automaticity.** A network of specialized cells and pathways known as the cardiac conduction system normally controls the electrical activity and contraction of the heart.

The primary pacemaker of the heart is the **sinoatrial (SA or sinus) node,** located where the superior vena cava enters the right atrium. The SA node normally initiates electrical impulses that are conducted throughout the heart and result in ventricular contraction. In adults, it usually discharges impulses at a regular

TABLE 49–1 Cardiac Cycle and Heart Sounds

Sound	Phase of Cardiac Cycle
S_1—first sound	Beginning of ventricular systole; the sound is caused by closure of the atrioventricular valves—the tricuspid and the mitral
S_2—second sound	Beginning of ventricular diastole; the sound is caused by closure of the semilunar valves—the aortic and pulmonic

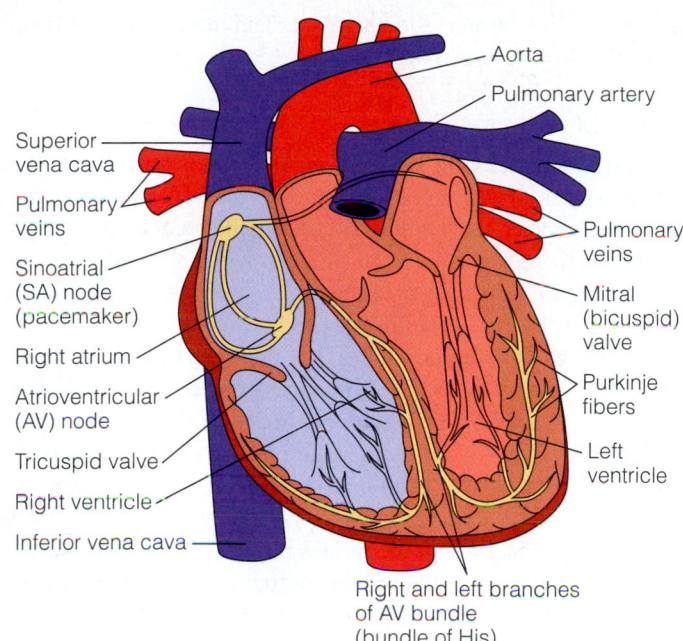

Aorta

Pulmonary artery

Superior vena cava

Pulmonary veins

Sinoatrial (SA) node (pacemaker)

Right atrium

Atrioventricular (AV) node

Tricuspid valve

Right ventricle

Inferior vena cava

Pulmonary veins

Mitral (bicuspid) valve

Purkinje fibers

Left ventricle

Right and left branches of AV bundle (bundle of His)

Figure 49–4 ■ The electrical system of the heart. The impulse is initiated by the SA node, then travels to the AV node, the bundle of His, and finally to the Purkinje fibers.

rate of 60 to 100 times per minute, the "normal" heart rate. The impulse then spreads throughout the atria via the interatrial pathways. These conduction pathways converge and narrow through the **atrioventricular (AV) node,** slightly delaying transmission of the impulse to the ventricles. This delay allows the atria to contract slightly before ventricular contraction occurs. From the AV node, the impulse then progresses down through the intraventricular septum to the ventricular conduction pathways: the **bundle of His,** the right and left bundle branches, and the **Purkinje fibers.** These fibers terminate in ventricular muscle, stimulating contraction (Figure 49–4 ■).

Cardiac Output

As the ventricles contract during systole, blood flows out of the ventricles into the great vessels and systemic and pulmonic circulation. The heart muscle then relaxes (the diastolic phase), allowing the ventricles to refill and cardiac muscle to be perfused. This contraction and relaxation of the heart is known as the *cardiac cycle* or the *heartbeat.* The cycle is repeated 60 to 100 times a minute in the adult, stimulated by impulses generated by the SA node.

With each contraction, a certain amount of blood, known as the stroke volume, is ejected from the ventricles into the circulation. In adults, the average is about 70 mL per beat. **Cardiac output (CO)** is the amount of blood pumped by the ventricles in 1 minute. Cardiac output is calculated by multiplying the **stroke volume (SV),** the amount of blood ejected with each contraction times the heart rate (HR). Thus, SV × HR = CO. The cardiac output is an important indicator of how well the heart is functioning as a pump. If the cardiac output is poor, tis-

sue perfusion suffers and oxygen and nutrients do not reach the cells as needed.

Cardiac output is affected by several factors:

HEART RATE. An increased heart rate increases cardiac output, even if the stroke volume doesn't change. Conversely, cardiac output decreases when the heart rate falls if the stroke volume remains constant. There are physiologic limits to this. For example, very rapid heart rates, more than 150 beats per minute, may not allow adequate time for the ventricles to fill, causing cardiac output to fall. The heart rate is influenced by many factors including the autonomic nervous system, blood pressure, hormones such as thyroid hormone, and some medications.

PRELOAD. **Preload** is the degree to which muscle fibers in the ventricle are stretched at the end of the relaxation period (diastole). Preload largely depends on the amount of blood returning to the heart from the venous circulation: Increased volume causes increased stretch, leading to more forceful contraction of cardiac muscle fibers. This physiologic action is referred to as the Frank-Starling Law of the Heart. The length of the ventricular muscle fibers (stretch) at the end of diastole directly affects the strength (force) of contraction. For example, exercise increases venous return and the amount of blood in the ventricle before contraction; therefore, the heart contracts more forcefully and stroke volume and cardiac output increase during exercise.

CONTRACTILITY. **Contractility** is the inherent ability of cardiac muscle fibers to shorten or contract. Stroke volume decreases if contractility is poor, reducing cardiac output. Contractility also is affected by the autonomic nervous system and certain drugs. Drugs that affect contractility are called inotropic drugs. Positive inotropic drugs increase contractility and negative inotropic drugs decrease the contractile strength.

AFTERLOAD. **Afterload** is the resistance against which the heart must pump to eject the blood into the circulation. Blood flows from an area of higher pressure to an area of lower pressure. To move blood into the circulatory system, the ventricles must generate sufficient pressure to overcome vascular resistance or the pressure within the arteries, known as afterload. The right ventricle pumps blood into the low-pressure, low-resistance pulmonary vascular system; therefore, the pressures generated by the right ventricle are fairly low. The left ventricle, by contrast, pumps blood into the higher pressure systemic arterial system, generating much higher pressures and requiring more work. Systemic vasoconstriction increases the arterial blood pressure and afterload, increasing the cardiac workload; vasodilation, on the other hand, reduces arterial pressure and the workload of the heart. Table 49–2 summarizes the above information.

The Blood Vessels

With each cardiac contraction, blood is ejected into a closed system of blood vessels that transport blood to the tissues and

TABLE 49–2 Factors Related to Cardiac Function

Indicator	Definition
Cardiac output (CO)	Amount of blood ejected from the heart each minute; CO = SV × HR
Stroke volume (SV)	Amount of blood ejected from the heart with each beat
Heart rate (HR)	Number of beats each minute
Contractility	Inotropic state of the myocardium, strength of contraction
Preload	Left ventricular end diastolic volume, stretch of the myocardium
Afterload	Resistance against which the heart must pump

return it to the heart. The heart supports two circulatory systems: the low-pressure pulmonary system and the higher pressure systemic circulatory system.

Deoxygenated blood from the right ventricle enters the pulmonary vascular system through the pulmonary arteries. The pulmonary arteries subdivide into lobar arteries. These lobar arteries follow the main bronchi into the lungs, then branch out to form arterioles and the dense capillary networks that encompass the alveoli. Oxygen diffuses into the blood from the alveoli, and carbon dioxide diffuses into the alveoli from the blood. This diffusion occurs across the alveolar/capillary membrane. The blood then returns to the left side of the heart via venules and the pulmonary veins. Note that the pulmonary vascular system is the only part of the circulatory system in which arteries (which transport blood away from the heart) carry deoxygenated blood and veins (which transport blood toward the heart) contain oxygenated blood.

The muscular left ventricle of the heart pumps oxygenated blood into the aorta. The blood then moves into major arteries that branch from the aorta and into successively smaller arteries, arterioles, and finally into the thin-walled capillary beds of organs and tissues. It is in the capillary beds that oxygen and nutrients are exchanged for metabolic waste products. The deoxygenated blood then returns to the heart through a series of venules and veins that become progressively larger until they empty into the superior and inferior venae cavae.

With the exception of capillaries, blood vessel walls have three distinct layers, or tunics. The innermost layer, the tunica intima, is smooth endothelium that facilitates blood flow. The tunica media is made up of elastic fibers and smooth muscle cells innervated by the autonomic nervous system. This allows vessels to constrict or dilate, depending on the needs of the body. The tunica media of arteries is thicker and more muscular in arteries than in veins, a feature that helps maintain blood pressure and continuous circulation to the tissues. The outermost layer of blood vessels is the tunica adventitia, a layer of connective tissue that supports, protects, and anchors the vessel to surrounding tissues. Capillaries contain only one thin layer of tunica intima, allowing gases and molecules to diffuse between the blood and the tissues.

Arterial Circulation

The arterial circulation moves blood pumped by the heart to the tissues, maintaining a constant flow to the capillary beds despite the intermittent pumping action of the heart.

Blood flow, the volume of blood flowing through a given vessel, organ, or the entire circulation over a specific period, is determined by pressure differences and resistance. Blood always moves from an area of higher pressure to area of lower pressure. The greater the difference between pressures, the greater the blood flow. The **blood pressure (BP)** is the force exerted on arterial walls by the blood flowing within the vessel (see Chapter 27 for a further explanation of blood pressure). The *mean arterial pressure (MAP)* is the pressure that maintains blood flow to the tissues throughout the cardiac cycle. It is a product of the cardiac output times the **peripheral vascular resistance (PVR)**, or CO × PVR = MAP.

Resistance is opposition to flow; peripheral vascular resistance impedes or opposes blood flow to the tissues. PVR is determined by

- The viscosity, or thickness, of the blood
- Blood vessel length
- Blood vessel diameter.

Venous Return

In contrast to the high-pressure arterial system, venous pressure is too low to adequately return blood from peripheral tissues to the heart without assistance. The fall in intrathoracic pressure that occurs with breathing draws blood upward toward the heart, an adaptation known as the respiratory pump. Skeletal muscle activity contributes to the muscular pump, as muscle contractions "milk" blood toward the heart. Venous valves are vital in making these pumps work; once blood passes a valve, it cannot flow backward away from the heart. Figure 49–5 ■ depicts the relationship between arteries and veins and the entire circulatory system.

Blood

Blood serves as the transport medium within the cardiovascular system, bringing oxygen and nutrients from the environment (via the lungs and gastrointestinal system) to the cells. Blood is a complex mixture of living formed elements (the blood cells) suspended in fluid (the plasma). Its primary functions are

- Transporting oxygen, nutrients, and hormones to the cells, and metabolic wastes from the tissues for elimination
- Regulating body temperature, pH, and fluid volume
- Preventing infection and blood loss.

As previously noted, most oxygen is transported bound to hemoglobin. **Hemoglobin** is a major component of red blood cells (erythrocytes), the predominant cell present in blood. Hemoglobin binds easily with oxygen, releasing it in the body

MediaLink CIRCULATION ANIMATION

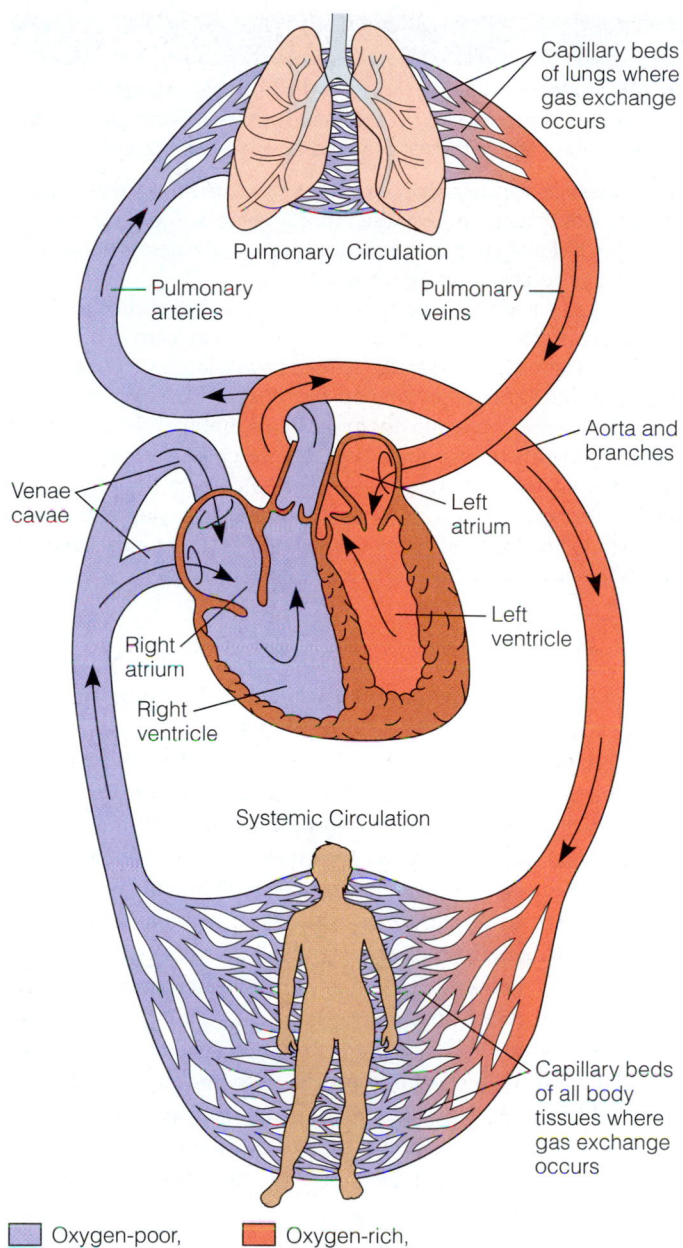

Pulmonary Circulation

Pulmonary arteries

Pulmonary veins

Capillary beds of lungs where gas exchange occurs

Aorta and branches

Venae cavae

Left atrium

Right atrium

Left ventricle

Right ventricle

Systemic Circulation

Capillary beds of all body tissues where gas exchange occurs

☐ Oxygen-poor, CO₂-rich blood   ☐ Oxygen-rich, CO₂-poor blood

Figure 49–5 ■ The heart and blood vessels. The left side of the heart pumps oxygenated blood into the arteries. Deoxygenated blood returns via the venous system into the right side of the heart.

tissues. When all four heme groups of the hemoglobin molecule are bound to oxygen, it is said to be *fully saturated*. Oxygen binding is affected by several factors, including the PO_2, temperature, pH, and PCO_2. Up to a certain point (about 70 mm Hg), the higher the PO_2, the greater the affinity of hemoglobin for oxygen and the more saturated the hemoglobin molecules. The relationship to temperature, pH, and PCO_2 is the opposite: at higher temperatures, greater hydrogen ion concentrations (lower pH), and higher PCO_2 levels, the affinity for oxygen decreases, and hemoglobin releases its oxygen molecules. Because of hemoglobin's importance in oxygen trans-

portation, anemia (too few red blood cells or RBCs that contain too little or abnormal hemoglobin) interferes with oxygen delivery to the tissues, leading to fatigue and activity intolerance.

LIFE SPAN CONSIDERATIONS

At birth, profound changes occur in the cardiovascular systems. As the lungs expand, pressures in the pulmonary vascular system fall, changing pressure relationships within the heart. The foramen ovale between the atria closes as pressures on the right side of the heart fall and pressures on the left side increase. Arterial PO_2 rises and arterial PCO_2 falls, prompting closure of the ductus arteriosus between the pulmonary artery and aorta.

Pulse rates are highest and most variable in newborns. The resting heart rate for a neonate ranges from 80 to 200 beats per minute, decreasing to 80 to 150 in infancy and early childhood, and reaching the adult rate of 55 to 100 by about age 10 years. Irregular heart rates are common in infants and young children, often increasing and decreasing with each breath. This pattern of irregularity is known as sinus arrhythmia, a normal variation of the heart rate.

As the conversion from fetal circulation takes place and pressures in the left side of the heart rise, the arterial blood pressure increases. Immediately after birth (1 to 3 days of age) the blood pressure averages about 65/40. By 1 month the arterial pressure is about 90/55. It rises gradually to the adult "norm" of 120/80 by approximately 16 years of age. With aging, blood pressure may again rise as arteriosclerosis affects the blood vessels, narrowing their lumen and decreasing their compliance (ability to distend).

Congenital heart defects may affect infants and children; however, acquired heart diseases are rare in childhood. Rheumatic fever is an inflammatory disorder that may occur following streptococcal infection (e.g., strep throat). For most people, the heart continues to function effectively well into older adulthood unless the blood supply to the heart muscle is impaired by blood vessel disease. Atherosclerosis, the buildup of fatty plaque within the arteries, is the major contributor to cardiovascular disease, the leading cause of death in North America.

Children rarely are affected by diseases of the blood vessels. During middle adulthood, however, the incidence of hypertension, or an elevated blood pressure, increases significantly. Hypertension, known as the silent killer because of its lack of symptoms, is a major risk factor for sudden cardiac death in middle adulthood.

FACTORS AFFECTING CARDIOVASCULAR FUNCTION

Many factors affect cardiovascular function. Some of these factors are called risk factors, because, if present, they increase the risk of cardiovascular disease. Risk factors have been identified for coronary artery disease, hypertension, and peripheral vascular disease, and the majority are the same.

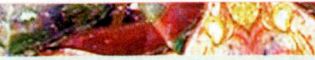

Lifespan Considerations

Elders

Normal changes of aging may contribute to problems of circulation in elders, even when there is no actual pathology:

- Blood vessels become less elastic and have an increase in calcification. This results in a restricted blood flow and a decrease of oxygen and nutrients to tissues (heart, peripheral, and cerebral).
- Impaired valve function in the heart is often the result of increased stiffness and calcification and results in a decrease in cardiac output.
- A decrease of muscle tone in the heart results in a decrease in cardiac output.
- There is a decrease in baroreceptor response to blood pressure changes, making the heart and blood vessels less responsive to exercise and stress. This often results in dizziness, falls, orthostatic hypotension, and mental changes.

- A decrease in conduction ability in the heart also makes the heart less responsive to changes and stresses. This can also result in dizziness, falls, orthostatic hypotension, and mental changes.

All of these factors become important if the person is challenged by stressors, such as exercise, stress, fever, surgery, or other changes. If challenged, the circulatory system of elders is not as effective or as quick to return to normal.

Persons living with normal changes of aging and/or pathologic conditions of the circulatory system need to learn to balance diet, medications, and exercise. Nurses have a large part in working with these clients to develop appropriate interventions and provide teaching to help them maintain optimal functioning. Teaching clients to recognize any changes or worsening of their condition is very important. They need to contact the physician and make any needed changes. Changing lifestyles and fine-tuning medications can be critical, and nurses can be a part of this in every phase of the nursing process.

Risk Factors

Major risk factors for cardiovascular disease in general are classified as *nonmodifiable* (cannot be altered) and *modifiable* (can be reduced) (Table 49–3).

Nonmodifiable Risk Factors

The first nonmodifiable risk factor is *heredity*. There is a genetic link for the development of coronary artery disease. That is, if a client has a parent with heart disease, he or she is at higher risk. The second is *age*. Coronary heart disease is mainly a disease of people over 60. It does occur in younger people as well, but generally risk increases with age. The third nonmodifiable risk factor is *gender*. Through middle adulthood (until menopause), estrogen has a protective effect in women, slowing the progress of atherosclerosis and reducing the risk of cardiovascular disease. This effect is lost at menopause, but hormone replacement therapy (HRT) *may* be beneficial in reducing this risk later in life. Possible benefits from HRT must be weighed against possible risks. This is a complex analysis and requires through discussion between the women and her health care provider. Among people in their 40s and 50s, men have a higher incidence of hypertension than women.

The modifiable risk factors include elevated serum lipid levels, hypertension, cigarette smoking, diabetes, obesity, and sedentary lifestyle.

Elevated Serum Lipid Levels

A strong link exists between elevated serum lipid levels and the development of coronary heart disease. Lipoproteins circulate in the blood and are made up of cholesterol, triglycerides, and phospholipids. A high dietary intake of saturated fats is the most critical factor for the development of elevated serum lipids. The average American diet often contains more than 40% of its calories in fats. The American Heart Association recommends that less than 30% of total calories come from fats.

Hypertension

Hypertension (or increased blood pressure) increases the risk of coronary heart disease in several ways. First, it increases the workload of the heart, increasing oxygen demand and coronary blood flow. The increased workload also causes hypertrophy. Over time this can contribute to heart failure. Secondly, hypertension causes endothelial damage to the blood vessels, which stimulates the development of atherosclerosis.

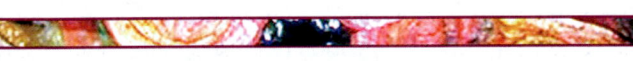

TABLE 49–3 Risk Factors for Coronary Heart Disease

Nonmodifiable Risk Factors
- Heredity
- Age
- Gender (women's risk increases postmenopause)

Modifiable Risk Factors
- Elevated serum lipid level
- Hypertension
- Cigarette smoking
- Diabetes
- Obesity
- Sedentary lifestyle

Other Risk Factors
- Heat and cold
- Previous health status
- Stress and coping
- Dietary factors
- Alcohol intake
- Elevated homocysteine level

Cigarette Smoking

The cardiovascular system also is affected by cigarette smoking. Nicotine increases the heart rate, blood pressure, and peripheral vascular resistance, increasing the heart's workload. Smoking causes vasoconstriction, and in areas where vessels already are narrowed by atherosclerosis, tissue oxygenation can be impaired.

Diabetes

Diabetes mellitus increases the risk of coronary heart disease, myocardial infarction and peripheral vascular disease as well. High blood sugars are linked with accelerated development of atherosclerosis as well as high levels of serum lipids and triglycerides. Closely monitoring blood sugar levels in diabetics and checking blood sugar levels in all clients for the development of increased levels is an important nursing function. Control of blood sugar levels can greatly reduce risk and slow development of atherosclerosis.

Obesity

Obese people have an increased risk for the development of heart disease. Obesity is often accompanied by elevated serum lipid levels, which increase risk. Additionally, obesity places an increased workload on the heart, which increases oxygen demand.

Sedentary Lifestyle

Physical exercise or activity increases the heart rate and hence the supply of oxygen in the body. With regular vigorous exercise, the heart muscle becomes more powerful and efficient. Aerobic exercise slows the atherosclerotic process, reducing the risk of cardiovascular disease. Sedentary people, by contrast, have a higher risk of cardiovascular disease.

Other Factors Influencing Cardiovascular Function

Other factors that may influence cardiovascular function include environmental factors such as heat and cold, previous health status, stress and coping, dietary factors, alcohol intake, and an elevated homocysteine level.

Heat and Cold

In response to heat, the peripheral blood vessels dilate; consequently, blood flows to the skin, increasing the amount of heat lost from the body surface. With vasodilation the lumens of blood vessels enlarge, thus decreasing the resistance to the blood flow. In response the heart increases output to maintain blood pressure. The increased cardiac output requires additional oxygen, which is acquired though increased rate and depth of breathing.

In response to cold environmental temperatures, the peripheral blood vessels constrict. This mechanism helps to conserve heat that is normally lost through the skin.

Health Status

In the healthy person, the cardiovascular system (working together with the respiratory system) is able to provide sufficient oxygen to meet the body needs. Diseases of the cardiovascular system will often affect the delivery of oxygen to the cells of the body, and when any system or tissue does not get the required oxygen for metabolic processes, cellular function will be altered. The body has "compensatory mechanisms" that are activated when oxygen decreases. These mechanisms include increased heart rate, increased strength of cardiac contraction, vasoconstriction, and the release of certain hormones such as aldosterone. The health status of a client may affect how the body tolerates the compensation and the decreased oxygen availability. A client with no significant health history and with good nutritional status will be more likely to tolerate short periods of decreased oxygen and the body's compensation than a client with multiple disorders and poor nutritional status.

Most cardiovascular conditions affect how the blood gets to the tissues. One cardiovascular condition that affects the oxygen-carrying capacity of the blood is anemia, described in the "Blood Alterations" section later in this chapter.

Stress and Coping

Stress causes a neurohormonal response. The stress response involves a number of interrelated responses and effects. One of the major effects of stress is the release of adrenal medullary hormones: epinephrine and norepinephrine. Epinephrine has several effects including causing the heart to contract more forcefully, increasing heart rate, and stimulating peripheral vasoconstriction. Norepinephrine causes widespread vasoconstriction, which increases the blood pressure.

Diet

Diet can also affect cardiovascular function. A healthy diet with adequate calories, protein, and other nutrients is important to maintain good immune function and increase resistance to disease. Along with certain vitamins and minerals, dietary protein is important to prevent anemia. High salt intake can affect blood pressure and contribute to the development of hypertension. High intake of sodium may contribute to hypertension in two ways. First, it may increase the release of a hormone called natriuretic hormone which indirectly contributes to hypertension. Additionally, sodium stimulates vasopressor mechanisms, which cause vasoconstriction. There is also evidence that other factors such as low potassium, calcium, and magnesium intake may contribute to vasoconstriction and the development of hypertension.

Alcohol

Recent studies suggest that moderate alcohol use (1 to 2 oz of alcohol per day) may actually reduce the risk of heart disease; however, excessive alcohol intake affects oxygenation several ways. Alcohol is a respiratory depressant, slowing respirations. Alcohol abusers often are malnourished, increasing their risk of anemia and infections. Excess alcohol intake also increases the risk of hypertension.

Elevated Homocysteine Level

Homocysteine is an amino acid that has been shown to be increased in many people with atherosclerosis. Clients with elevated homocysteine levels may have an increased risk of myocardial infarction and cerebrovascular accidents (stroke). Clients can reduce their homocysteine level by taking folate and vitamin B$_{12}$ (Reeder, Hoffman, Magdic, & Rodgers, 2000).

ALTERATIONS IN CARDIOVASCULAR FUNCTION

Cardiovascular function can be altered by conditions that affect

1. The function of the heart as a pump
2. Blood flow to organs and peripheral tissues
3. The composition of the blood and its ability to transport oxygen and carbon dioxide.

Three major alterations in cardiovascular function are decreased cardiac output, impaired tissue perfusion, and disorders that affect the composition or amount of blood available for transport of gases.

Decreased Cardiac Output

Although the heart normally is able to increase its rate and force of contraction to increase cardiac output during exercise, fever, or other times of need, some conditions interfere with these mechanisms.

The vessels that supply blood to the heart muscle may become occluded by atherosclerosis or a blood clot, shutting off the blood supply to a portion of the myocardium. When this happens, the tissue becomes necrotic and dies, a condition known as a **myocardial infarction (MI)** or *heart attack*. If a large portion of the heart muscle is affected, particularly in the left ventricle, cardiac output falls because the affected muscle no longer contracts. Signs and symptoms of myocardial infarction are variable and may include

- Chest pain; substernal and/or radiating to the left arm, jaw
- Nausea
- Shortness of breath
- Diaphoresis.

Heart failure may develop if the heart isn't able to keep up with the body's need for oxygen and nutrients to the tissues. Heart failure usually occurs because of myocardial infarction, but it may also result from chronic overwork of the heart, such as in clients with uncontrolled hypertension or extensive arteriosclerosis. In left-sided heart failure, the vessels of the pulmonary system become congested or engorged with blood. This may cause fluid to escape into the alveoli and interfere with gas exchange, a condition known as *pulmonary edema*. Signs of heart failure may include

- Pulmonary congestion; adventitious lung sounds
- Shortness of breath
- Increased heart rate
- Increased respiratory rate
- Peripheral vasoconstriction; cold, pale extremities
- Distended neck veins.

TABLE 49–4 Examples of Conditions that May Precipitate Heart Failure

Conditions that Increase Preload
  Hypervolemia
  Valvular disorders such as mitral regurgitation
  Congenital defects such as patent ductus arteriosus
Conditions that Increase Afterload
  Hypertension
Conditions that Affect Myocardial Function
  Myocardial infarction
  Cardiomyopathy
  Coronary artery disease

Other diseases such as myocarditis and cardiomyopathy also can affect the heart muscle, impairing its ability to contract and pump. Table 49–4 gives examples of conditions which may precipitate heart failure.

Very irregular or excessively rapid or slow heart rates can decrease the cardiac output. With irregular or very rapid heart rates, the ventricles may not fill adequately between beats, so the stroke volume (amount pumped with each beat) falls. If the heart rate is too slow, the heart may not be able to increase its stroke volume enough to maintain the cardiac output. Abnormalities of the heart rate and rhythm are known as dysrhythmias and can be identified on the electrocardiogram (ECG).

Alterations in the structure of the heart can affect cardiac output. Congenital heart defects result in abnormal blood flow and may even allow venous and arterial blood to mix. The oxygen supply to the tissues is affected in this case. Acquired heart diseases such as bacterial endocarditis and rheumatic fever may damage the heart valves, affecting the flow of blood within the heart and to the great vessels. For example, if the mitral (bicuspid) valve becomes scarred and stenotic (constricted), it may not open fully, impairing filling of the left ventricle. Or, if the mitral valve doesn't fully close (mitral insufficiency), blood may escape back or regurgitate into the left atrium instead of entering the aorta each time the ventricle contracts.

Impaired Tissue Perfusion

Atherosclerosis is by far the most common cause of impaired blood flow to organs and tissues. As vessels narrow and become obstructed, distal tissues receive less blood, oxygen, and nutrients. **Ischemia** is a lack of blood supply due to obstructed circulation. Any artery in the body may be affected by atherosclerosis, although the effects are often related to coronary arteries, vessels supplying blood to the brain, and arteries in peripheral tissues. Obstruction of the coronary arteries causes myocardial ischemia, often resulting in angina pectoris. If the cerebral vessels are affected, the result may be a *transient ischemic attack (TIA)* or a stroke. Peripheral vascular disease leads to ischemia of distal tissues such as the legs and feet. Gangrene and amputation may result. Signs of impaired peripheral circulation may include

- Decreased peripheral pulses
- Pale skin color
- Cool extremities
- Decreased hair distribution.

The risk factors for peripheral atherosclerosis are similar to those for coronary artery disease and include cigarette smoking, high fat intake, obesity, and a sedentary lifestyle. Hypertension and diabetes also increase the risk for atherosclerosis, particularly if the blood pressure or blood glucose levels are not maintained at near-normal levels.

Although much less common, other disorders such as vessel inflammation, arterial spasm, and blood clots also can occlude blood vessels, leading to ischemia. Tissue edema can impair flow through vessels and can increase the distance oxygen and nutrients must diffuse across to reach cells.

On the venous side, incompetent valves may allow blood to pool in veins, causing edema and decreasing venous return to the heart. Veins also can become inflamed, reducing blood flow and increasing the risk of thrombus (clot) formation. Thrombi may then break loose, becoming emboli. These emboli tend to travel as far as the pulmonary circulation where they become trapped in small vessels (pulmonary emboli), occluding blood supply to the capillary side of the alveolar-capillary-membrane. Although alveolar ventilation to the affected area often remains adequate, no gas exchange occurs there because of impaired blood flow. Signs of acute pulmonary embolism can be nonspecific and variable but may include:

- Sudden onset of shortness of breath
- Pleuritic chest pain.

Blood Alterations

Because most oxygen is transported to the tissues in combination with hemoglobin, the problems of inadequate RBCs, low hemoglobin levels, or abnormal hemoglobin structure can affect tissue oxygenation. Anemia has several different causes: RBCs are lost along with other components because of acute or chronic bleeding; if the diet is deficient in iron or folic acid, hemoglobin and RBCs are not formed adequately; and some disorders cause RBCs to break down excessively. People with sickle-cell disease produce an abnormal form of hemoglobin and may experience tissue ischemia during exacerbations of the disease. Signs of anemia may include

- Chronic fatigue
- Pallor
- Shortness of breath
- Hypotension.

Blood volume also affects tissue oxygenation. If the blood volume is inadequate as in hemorrhage or severe dehydration, the blood pressure and cardiac output fall, and tissues may become ischemic. Conversely, clients with hypervolemia (excess blood volume), which can result from fluid retention or kidney

failure, may develop heart failure and peripheral edema, leading to tissue ischemia.

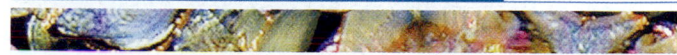

NURSING MANAGEMENT

ASSESSING

Nursing assessment of the cardiovascular system status includes a history, physical examination, cardiac monitoring, and review of relevant diagnostic data.

Nursing History

A comprehensive nursing history should include data regarding

- Current and past cardiovascular problems
- Family history of cardiovascular problems such as high blood pressure, increased cholesterol level, and stroke
- Other medical history including diabetes and respiratory disorders
- Exercise program
- History of cigarette smoking
- Diet, including fat and salt intake, alcohol intake, caffeine intake including soft drinks, and chocolate
- Presence of any symptoms such as pain, shortness of breath, fatigue, palpitations, cough, and fainting
- Medications for heart, blood pressure, circulation, and cholesterol
- Lifestyle, including social support, stressors, and methods of coping.

Physical Assessment

To examine the cardiovascular system, the nurse first evaluates the blood pressure for both arms (the results should be within 10 mm Hg of each other) and palpates peripheral pulses for their strength and equality. The apical pulse is auscultated for rate, rhythm, and the quality of heart sounds. Carotid arteries are auscultated for bruits (a sound of turbulence), which may indicate atherosclerosis and narrowing (see Chapter 27). Also important as an indicator of cardiac function is lung sounds. By auscultating the lungs for adventitious sounds, the nurse assesses for increased pulmonary vessel pressure secondary to decreased cardiac output.

Much information about the cardiovascular system is obtained by assessing the skin for color, temperature, hair distribution, lesions, and edema. Clients with extensive peripheral vascular disease may have cool feet with weak pulses and shiny, nearly hairless shins. Pitting edema of the feet and ankles may be noted in clients with heart failure. See Chapter 28 for specific techniques for assessing the respiratory and cardiovascular systems.

Diagnostic Studies

Many diagnostic studies are available that can help to identify the presence of cardiovascular disease. Diagnostic studies may also be used as screening tools to identify increased risk and then modifications made to reduce the risk of development of cardiovascular dysfunction. An example of this is the

Assessment Interview

CIRCULATION

Current or Past Cardiovascular Problems

- Do you have high blood pressure?
- Do you have any history of heart disease such as angina, heart attack, or heart failure? Have you ever had a cardiac catheterization, angiogram, or angioplasty? Have you ever been diagnosed with rheumatic fever, endocarditis, pericarditis, or other diseases of the heart? If so, when? Have you had cardiac surgery or stent placement?
- Have you ever been told that you have peripheral vascular disease? Do you ever develop pain in the calves of your legs when walking? How far can you walk before it occurs? What do you do to relieve it? Have you had surgery on your blood vessels?
- Do your feet and ankles ever swell or feel very cold, numb, or tingling? Do you experience pain in your feet? Is the pain changed by position?
- Do you become extremely fatigued with activity? Have you ever been told that you are anemic?

Medication History

- Have you taken or do you take any over-the-counter or prescription medications for your heart or blood pressure or to increase blood flow?
- Do you take any anticoagulants or other medications to "thin" your blood?

Lifestyle

- Do you smoke?
- Do you exercise? What kind of exercise and how often?
- How much alcohol do you drink?

---

serum lipid level. If a client has an elevated serum lipid level, he or she should be educated about the effects of diet and the importance of reducing lipids to reduce the risk of coronary heart disease.

Cardiac Monitoring. Cardiac monitoring allows continuous observation of the client's cardiac rhythm. Cardiac monitoring is a recording of the heart's electrical activity. It is used in many instances: for clients who have known or suspected cardiovascular disease, during and after surgery, to monitor responses to drug therapy, and to monitor clients at risk for serious complications such as shock. Electrodes placed on the client's chest are attached to a monitor cable and bedside monitor. The monitor is equipped with alarms used to warn of potential problems such as very fast, very slow, or irregular heart rates. The alarm limits are set for 20 beats higher and lower than the client's baseline rate, often at 100 to 110 and 50 to 55, respectively, for adults. For ambulatory clients (in the hospital or at home), the electrodes connect to a transmitter unit (also called telemetry). This unit electronically sends the signal to a central monitor for display or may store the information to be retrieved later in the physician's office. Another name for this type of ambulatory

---

monitoring is the Holter monitor. Electrodes are attached and the client wears the monitor for 24 hours. A continuous ECG is recorded and later analyzed for irregularities.

Electrocardiography most commonly uses 12 "leads" or 12 different views of the heart. In contrast, cardiac monitoring only uses 1 or 2 leads at any given time. See Chapter 32 ⬧ for more information about ECGs.

> ► **CLINICAL ALERT** *It is important to remember that ECG monitoring is a recording of the electrical activity of the heart; it does not reflect mechanical contraction and cardiac output. ALWAYS remember to check the client to assess for cardiac function. Just looking at the ECG does not give an assessment of the client's status.* ■

Blood Tests. Specimens of venous blood are taken for several tests that may reflect some aspect of cardiovascular functioning.

Because *hemoglobin* is the molecule that oxygen attaches to, it gives an indication of the oxygen-carrying capacity of the blood. A decreased hemoglobin increases the risk of oxygen deficit in the tissues when cardiovascular disease is present.

Measurement of serum electrolytes is important for clients with cardiovascular problems because electrolyte abnormalities such as hyperkalemia (higher than normal potassium) and hypokalemia (lower than normal potassium) can have a critical effect on the heart. Serum levels of magnesium, calcium, sodium, and phosphorus are also important to assess.

Measurement of enzyme levels in the blood are an important part of the diagnostic evaluation of patients with chest pain. Certain enzymes such as **creatine kinase (CK)** and **troponin** are released into the blood during an MI. These enzymes are released into the blood as the cell membrane is damaged. Elevated levels of these enzymes can help differentiate between an MI (when the cells actually die) and chest pain from a different cause such as angina or pleuritic pain.

Hemodynamic Studies. *Hemodynamics* is the study of the forces or pressures involved in blood circulation. Hemodynamic studies or monitoring procedures may be performed to evaluate fluid status and cardiovascular function. Parameters evaluated in hemodynamic studies include heart rate, arterial blood pressure, central venous pressure, pressures in the pulmonary vascular system, and cardiac output. Some of these parameters—for example, heart rate, arterial blood pressure, and venous pressure—are measured directly using an arterial, central venous, or pulmonary artery catheter; others such as the stroke volume and cardiac output are calculated. Hemodynamic studies are performed in a diagnostic cardiac laboratory and require informed consent. Clients in intensive and cardiac care units may undergo continuous hemodynamic monitoring to evaluate cardiovascular status and the effect of interventions. Nurses in these units are responsible for maintaining accurate readings and the integrity of the system.

DIAGNOSING

NANDA includes the following diagnostic labels for clients with circulation problems:

- *Ineffective Tissue Perfusion* (Cardiopulmonary): Decrease in oxygen resulting in the failure to nourish the tissues at the capillary level
- *Decreased Cardiac Output*: Inadequate blood pumped by the heart to meet metabolic (demands) of the body
- *Activity Intolerance*: Insufficient physiological or psychological energy to endure or complete required or desired daily activities.

   Examples of application of these using NANDA, NIC, and NOC designations are shown in Identifying Nursing Diagnoses, Outcomes, and Interventions.

PLANNING

When planning care the nurse identifies nursing interventions that will assist the client to achieve these broad goals:

- Maintain or improve tissue perfusion.
- Maintain or restore an adequate cardiac output.

Obviously, goals will vary according to the diagnosis and defining characteristics for each individual. Appropriate preventive and corrective nursing interventions that relate to these must be identified. Specific nursing activities can be selected to meet the client's individual needs. Examples of NIC interventions related to decreased cardiac output and tissue perfusion include

- Circulatory Care: Arterial Insufficiency
- Cardiac Care
- Hemodynamic Regulation.

To promote the transport of oxygen and carbon dioxide, the nurse can optimize cardiac output by reducing stress, planning appropriate activities, and positioning the client for improved vascular blood flow (see Identifying Nursing Diagnoses, Outcomes, and Interventions).

IDENTIFYING NURSING DIAGNOSES, OUTCOMES, AND INTERVENTIONS
CLIENTS WITH DECREASED CARDIAC OUTPUT

DATA CLUSTER	NURSING DIAGNOSIS/ DEFINITION	SAMPLE DESIRED OUTCOMES [NOC#]/DEFINITION	INDICATORS	SELECTED INTERVENTIONS [NIC#]/DEFINITION	SAMPLE NIC ACTIVITIES
Ed Wallace, a 67-year old retired contractor has a history of an acute myocardial infarction 1 year ago. During the last 2 weeks he has experienced a weight gain of 4 kg (9 lb). He states that he can't walk a flight of stairs without shortness of breath, and he sleeps on three pillows. His ankles are swollen, and his heart pounds at times. Physical exam reveals jugular vein distention above 3 cm; pulse (86); pitting edema in feet, ankles, and lower legs; and crackles in both lung fields.	*Decreased Cardiac Output/Inadequate blood pumped by the heart to meet metabolic demands of the body*	Cardiac Pump Effectiveness. [0400]/*Extent to which blood is ejected from the left ventricle per minute to support systemic perfusion pressure*	Mildly compromised • BP in expected range • Heart rate in expected range • Neck vein distention not present • Peripheral edema not present • Adventitious breath sounds not present • Activity tolerance in expected range	Cardiac Care, [4040]/*Limitation of complications resulting from an imbalance between myocardial oxygen supply and demand for a patient with symptoms of impaired cardiac function.*	• Perform a comprehensive appraisal of peripheral circulation • Monitor respiratory status for symptoms of heart failure • Monitor fluid balance (e.g., intake/output, daily weights) • Arrange exercise and rest periods to avoid fatigue • Monitor the patient's activity tolerance

IMPLEMENTING
Promoting Circulation

Most people in good health give little thought to their cardiovascular function. Changing position frequently, ambulating, and exercising usually maintain adequate cardiovascular functioning. See Teaching: Home Care and Teaching: Wellness Care for other ways to promote a healthy heart.

Immobility is also detrimental to cardiovascular function. Without exercise of the calf and leg muscles, blood pools in the veins of the lower extremities. This stagnant blood flow may allow clots to develop (venous thrombosis). With time, these clots can break loose and become emboli, eventually lodging in the small vessels of the pulmonary vascular system. Blood flow and gas exchange in the lungs is then impaired.

There are many nursing interventions that can help clients maintain cardiac and vascular function. They may be classified as vascular and cardiac.

Vascular

- Position with the legs elevated to promote venous return to the heart. This is particularly important for clients with venous dysfunction. Care should be taken to avoid this position in clients with cardiac dysfunction because it will increase preload and may stress the dysfunctional heart.
- Avoid pillows under the knees or more than 15 degrees of knee flexion to improve blood flow to the lower extremities and reduce venous stagnation.
- Encourage leg exercises (such as flexion and extension of the feet, active contraction and relaxation of calf muscles) for a client on bed rest and promote ambulation as soon as possible.
- Encourage or provide frequent position changes.

Cardiac

- Position the client in a high Fowler's position to decrease preload and reduce pulmonary congestion.

   Monitor intake and output. Fluid restriction is usually not required for patients with mild to moderate cardiac dysfunction. With severe heart failure, a fluid restriction may be ordered.

Medications

Many classes of medications are administered to clients with cardiovascular disorders. Drugs such as nitrates, calcium channel blockers, and angiotensin-converting enzyme (ACE) inhibitors reduce the workload of the heart and prevent vasoconstriction. Various drugs are used to treat cardiac dysrhythmias. Positive inotropic drugs such as digitalis are used to increase the contractile strength of the heart. Beta adrenergic blocking agents such as propranol or metoprolol may be given to block the sympathetic nervous system action on the heart and decrease oxygen consumption. Direct vasodilators may be used for clients with peripheral vascular disease and sometimes hypertension. Often clients are on numerous medications and it is an important role of the nurse to help the patient understand the purposes, effects, and side effects of the different medications.

Administering medications is an important nursing function. The nurse is responsible for assessing for the effects of medications and also for potential complications. Examples include:

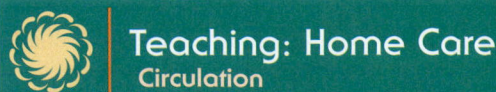

Teaching: Home Care
Circulation

Maintaining Cardiac Output and Tissue Perfusion

- Teach the symptoms of heart failure to the client and family and emphasize when to contact the care provider.
- Teach the client about the importance of maintaining regular physical activity to promote circulation and vascular health. Emphasize the need to increase activity levels gradually with the goal of exercising (walking, swimming, weight training, or aerobic exercise as recommended by the care provider) for at least 20 minutes four to five times per week.
- Instruct the client to avoid exposure to cold, wearing warm clothing as needed.
- Teach cardiopulmonary resuscitation or refer for instruction.

Dietary Alterations

- Instruct the client and family about prescribed dietary restrictions such as a low-sodium diet. Refer to a dietitian as needed for further instruction.
- Discuss dietary measures to reduce the risk of atherosclerosis, including reducing total and saturated fats in the diet, reducing weight if obese, and increasing the intake of dietary fiber.

Medications

- Instruct the client and family about prescribed medications, including effects, side effects, and administration instructions.

- When diuretics are administered, the nurse assesses intake and output and potassium level (because many diuretics can lower potassium level).
- When positive inotropic medications are administered, the nurse should assess blood pressure, heart rate, peripheral pulses, and lung sounds as indicators of cardiac output.

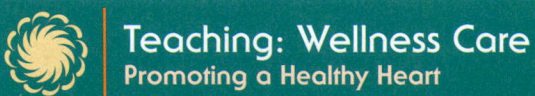

Teaching: Wellness Care
Promoting a Healthy Heart

- Exercise regularly, participating in at least 20 minutes (40 minutes is preferred) of vigorous exercise four to five times a week.
- Do not smoke.
- Maintain your ideal weight.
- Eat a diet low in total fat, saturated fats, and cholesterol.
- Drink alcohol in moderation, if at all, consuming no more than one cocktail or one to one and a half glasses of wine or beer daily.
- Reduce stress and manage anger.
- Effectively manage diabetes and hypertension, maintaining blood glucose and blood pressure levels within normal limits.
- If female, discuss with your health care provider the advantages and risks of hormone replacement therapy after menopause (or after a total hysterectomy).
- Consult your health care provider about the advisability of low-dose aspirin therapy to further reduce the risk of cardiovascular disease.

- When antihypertensive medications are administered, it is critical for the nurse to monitor blood pressure. Additionally, many antihypertensive medications can cause postural hypotension.

Preventing Venous Stasis

When clients have limited mobility or are confined to bed, venous return to the heart is impaired and the risk of venous stasis increases. Immobility is a problem not only for ill or debilitated clients but also for some travelers who sit with legs dependent for long periods in a motor vehicle or an airplane. Venous stasis can lead to thrombus formation and edema of the extremities.

Preventing venous stasis is an important nursing intervention to reduce the risk of complications following surgery, trauma, or major medical problems. Positioning and leg exercises are discussed in Chapter 48 ⚭ and antiemboli stockings in Chapter 35. ⚭ Sequential compression devices are additional measures to help prevent venous stasis.

Sequential Compression Devices. Clients who are undergoing surgery or who are immobilized because of illness or injury may benefit from a sequential compression device (SCD) to promote venous return from the legs. SCDs inflate and deflate plastic sleeves wrapped around the legs to promote venous flow. The plastic sleeves are attached by tubing to an air pump that alternately inflates and deflates portions of the sleeve to a specified pressure. The ankle area inflates first, followed by the calf region, and then the thigh area. This sequential inflation and deflation assists the leg muscles in moving blood toward the heart (Figure 49–6 ■).

Antiemboli stockings are worn under the SCD to provide added support and protect the skin from irritation by the plas-

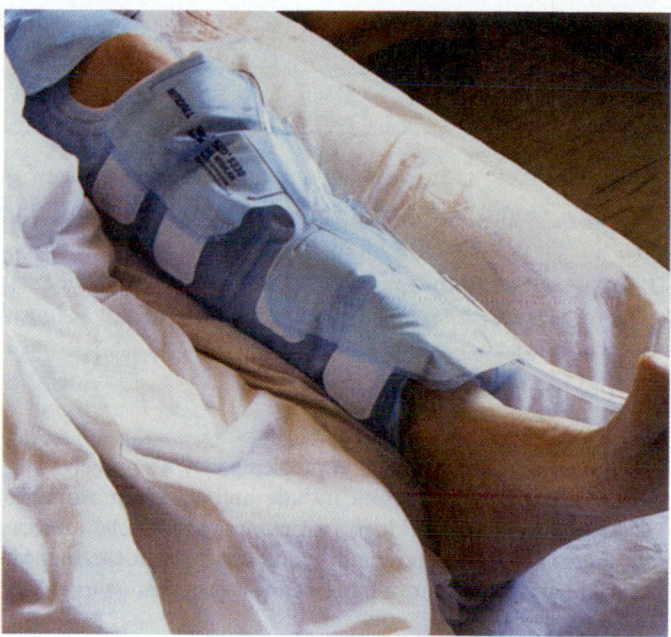

Figure 49–6 ■ The sequential venous compression device enhances venous return. They are available in knee-high or above-the-knee length.

tic. The SCD is removed for ambulation and is usually discontinued when the client resumes activities. SCDs are useful in preventing thrombi and edema from venous stasis, but they are not used for clients who have arterial insufficiency, cellulitis, infection of the extremity, or preexisting venous thrombosis.

Procedure 49–1 outlines how to apply a sequential compression device.

Procedure 49–1 Sequential Compression Devices

Purposes

- To promote venous return from the legs
- To decrease risk of deep vein thrombosis and/or pulmonary embolism

ASSESSMENT

Assess for baseline data:
- Cardiovascular status, including heart rate and rhythm, peripheral pulses, and capillary refill

- Color and temperature of extremities
- Movement and sensation of feet and lower extremities and Homans' sign

PLANNING

Check the physician's order for type of SCD sleeve. *Both knee- and thigh-length sleeves are available.*

Delegation

UAP often remove and reapply the SCD when performing hygiene care. The nurse should check that the UAP knows the correct application process for the SCD. Remind the UAP that the client should

not have the SCD removed for long periods of time because the purpose of the SCD is to promote circulation.

Equipment

- Measuring tape
- Antiemboli stockings
- SCD, including disposable sleeves, air pump, and tubing

continued on page 1346

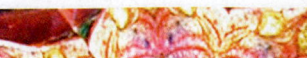

Procedure 49–1 Sequential Compression Devices *continued*

IMPLEMENTATION

Performance

1. Explain to the client what you are going to do, why it is necessary, and the procedure for applying the sequential compression device. *The client's cooperation and comfort will be increased by understanding the rationale for applying the SCD.*
2. Observe appropriate infection control procedures.
3. Provide for client privacy and drape the client appropriately.
4. Prepare the client.
   - Place the client in a dorsal recumbent or semi-Fowler's position.
   - Measure the client's legs as recommended by the manufacturer if a thigh-length sleeve is required. *Knee-length sleeves come in just one size; the thigh circumference determines the size needed for a thigh-length sleeve.*
   - Apply antiemboli stockings (see Procedure 35–2 on page 909). Make sure there are no wrinkles or folds in the stockings. *Antiemboli stockings provide added support and reduce skin irritation from the compression sleeve.*
5. Apply the sequential compression sleeves.
   - Place a sleeve under each leg with the opening at the knee.
   - Wrap the sleeve securely around the leg, securing the Velcro tabs (Figure 49–7 ■). Allow two fingers

to fit between the leg and the sleeve. *This amount of space ensures that the sleeve does not impair circulation when inflated.*

6. Connect the sleeves to the control unit and adjust the pressure as needed.
   - Connect the tubing to the sleeves and control unit, ensuring that arrows on the plug and the connector are in alignment and that the tubing is not kinked or twisted. *Improper alignment or obstruction of the tubing by kinks or twists will interfere with operation of the SCD.*
   - Turn on the control unit and adjust the alarms and pressures as needed. The sleeve cooling control and alarm should be on; ankle pres-

sure is usually set at 35 to 55 mm Hg. *It is important to have the sleeve cooling control on for comfort and to reduce the risk of skin irritation from moisture under the sleeve. Alarms warn of possible control unit malfunctions.*

7. Document the procedure.
   - Record baseline assessment data and application of the SCD. Note control unit settings.
   - Assess and document skin integrity and neurovascular status at least every 8 hours while the SCD is in place. Remove the unit and notify the physician if the client complains of numbness and tingling or leg pain. These may be symptoms of nerve compression.

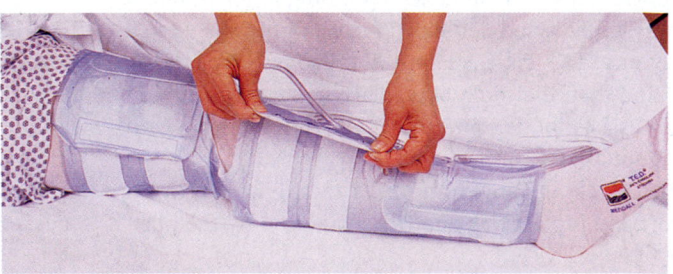

Figure 49–7 ■ Applying a sequential compression device to the leg.

EVALUATION

- Perform appropriate follow-up assessments, such as cardiovascular status including pedal pulses, skin color and temperature, skin integrity, and neurovascular status, including movement and sensation.
- Compare to the baseline data, if available.
- Report significant deviations from normal to the physician.

Lifespan Considerations

Sequential Compression Devices

Children
- The SCD is rarely used on children.

Elders
- The SCD sleeves may become loose as clients move around in bed. Check that the sleeves are secure and properly positioned.

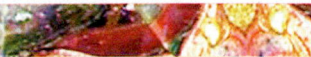

Home Care Considerations

Sequential Compression Devices

■ A sequential compression device may be used in the home. Inform the client or caregiver how to apply the device correctly and how to operate the system, including how to respond to the alarm.

Sequential compression therapy often complements other preventive measures. The client's risk level for DVT or pulmonary embolism often determines the preventive measures used. For example, clients at low risk may require only antiemobli stockings. Clients at moderate risk may have both antiemboli stockings and sequential therapy as part of their treatment. The physician may order antiemboli stockings, sequential therapy, and anticoagulation therapy for the high-risk client.

Cardiopulmonary Resuscitation

Cardiopulmonary resuscitation (CPR) is a combination of oral resuscitation (mouth-to-mouth breathing), which supplies oxygen to the lungs, and external cardiac massage (chest compression), which is intended to reestablish cardiac function and blood circulation. CPR is also referred to as *basic life support (BLS)*.

A cardiac arrest is the cessation of cardiac function; the heart stops beating. Often a cardiac arrest is unexpected and sudden. When it occurs, the heart no longer pumps blood to any of the organs of the body. Breathing then stops, and the person becomes unconscious and limp. Within 20 to 40 seconds of a cardiac arrest the victim is clinically dead. After 4 to 6 minutes the lack of oxygen supply to the brain causes permanent and extensive damage.

The three cardinal signs of a cardiac arrest are apnea, absence of a carotid or femoral pulse, and dilated pupils. The person's skin appears pale or grayish and feels cool. Cyanosis is evident when respiratory function fails before heart failure.

A respiratory arrest (pulmonary arrest) is the cessation of breathing. It often occurs because of a blocked airway, but it can occur following a cardiac arrest and for other reasons. A respiratory arrest may occur abruptly or be preceded by short, shallow breathing that becomes increasingly labored.

It is vital that all nurses be trained to perform CPR so resuscitation measures can be initiated immediately when a cardiac or respiratory arrest occurs. Nurses also can be instrumental in increasing community awareness of the need for CPR training and ensuring its availability.

Each health care facility has policies and procedures for announcing cardiac/respiratory arrest and initiating interventions. In many institutions this emergency is called a **Code Blue,** and the announcement is referred to as "calling a code." Each health care institution has a procedure for calling a code. There may be a special Code Blue button at the head of each bed, sometimes it is a special extension on the phone, or it may be a special phone used to announce the emergency. It is critical that each member of the patient care team know the procedure for announcing a

---

Research Note

Treatment of the Client with Acute Myocardial Infarction: Reducing Time Delays

There is a critical relationship for the patient with myocardial infarction between the time to treatment and the amount of myocardial muscle damage. The purpose of a study by Meils, Kaleta, and Mueller (2002) was to reduce the time to reperfusion of the myocardium with thrombolytic therapy or intervention. There were three target areas: (a) time from the emergency department door to ECG, (b) time to initiation of thrombolytic therapy, and (c) time to the intervention in the catheterization laboratory. Data were collected using the National Registry of Myocardial Infarction data tool as well as an internal data tool developed by the research team. Following data analysis, several key factors were identified that could reduce delays. These included synchronizing the wall clocks and the ECG machines, ongoing staff education regarding presenting symptoms, bedside ECG machines always available, and increasing the availability of a cardiologist.

The researchers were able to significantly decrease the time from the door to the ECG. They were unable to make a significant change in the times to initiation of thrombolytic therapy. Finally, they were able to improve the time to intervention in the catheterization laboratory.

Implications: Reducing time delays is an important issue for hospitals to address. It is clear that the time is critical to outcomes for patients with acute myocardial infarction. This research demonstrated that a multidisciplinary team working together can have an effect that ultimately benefits the client.

Note: From "Treatment of the Client with Acute Myocardial Infarction: Reducing Time Delays," by C. M. Meils, K. A. Kaleta, and C. L. Mueller, 2002, *Journal of Nursing Care Quality, 17*(1), pp. 83–89.

code. Calling the code summons the code team to the location of the emergency. The code team is made up of specially trained staff who can handle the emergency. Persons are needed to perform rescue breathing, deliver chest compressions, administer medications, and make a record of the code activities. One person must be designated as the code leader—the person who directs the activities of the other team members.

Some clients have designated, via an advanced directive, that, should they arrest, they not be resuscitated. It is every person's right to make an advanced directive of their wishes. If it is the client's wish, the physician should designate "no Code Blue," "No CPR," or "Do Not Resuscitate (DNR)" on the medical record.

EVALUATING

Using the overall goals identified in the planning stage, the nurse collects data to evaluate the effectiveness of interventions. Examples of desired outcomes for the identified goals are found in the Identifying Nursing Diagnoses, Outcomes, and Interventions box earlier in this chapter.

If desired outcomes are not achieved, the nurse, client, and support person if appropriate need to explore the reasons before modifying the care plan. For example, if the outcome cardiac pump effectiveness is not achieved, questions to be considered might include the following:

- Have other outcome measures for the goal of maintaining adequate cardiac output been met?
- Are prescribed medications being taken/administered as ordered?
- Are there additional factors which are placing stress on the heart?
- Is there a balance between factors that affect cardiac output, such as preload and afterload?
- Are there signs of fluid overload such as weight gain?

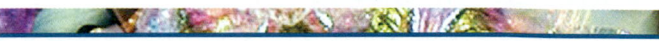

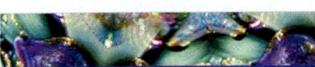

Focus on Critical Thinking

Mrs. Gloria Papadopolis reports that she is having increasing difficulty because she experiences severe pain in her calf muscles after walking for more than a city block. The pain subsides if she rests for a few minutes, but returns with activity. Her feet are cool and pale; pedal and posterior tibial pulses are not palpable, femoral pulses difficulty to palpate. She lives in a downtown apartment and uses public transportation to travel across town to visit her husband's grave weekly.

1. What are the circulatory causes of her leg pain? Which risk factors would you expect to find in her history to support this conclusion?

2. Name two nursing diagnoses appropriate for Mrs. Papadopolis. Which would have the highest priority and why?

3. The physician suggests that Mrs. Papadopolis cease her visits to the cemetery since she has to walk a long way there to reach the grave site. Would you agree with this plan? Why or why not? What considerations or viewpoints influence your choice?

4. Mrs. Papadopolis says that she wears support stockings because her friend told her they help the circulation in her legs. How would you respond to this information?

See Critical Thinking Possibilities in Appendix A.

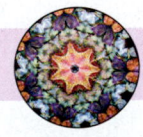 | Chapter Review

EXPLORE MediaLink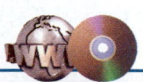

NCLEX review questions, case studies, care plan activities, MediaLink applications, and other interactive resources for this chapter can be found on the Companion Website at www.prenhall.com/kozier. Click on Chapter 49 to select the activities for this chapter.

For animations, more NCLEX review questions, and an audio glossary, access the Student CD-ROM accompanying this textbook.

Chapter Highlights

- The cardiovascular system transports gases in the blood to and from the tissues and facilitates the diffusion of gases between the capillaries and body tissues.
- The heart and the blood vessels make up the cardiovascular system that, together with blood, is the major system for transporting oxygen and nutrients to the tissues, and waste products away from the tissues for elimination.
- The right side of the heart receives deoxygenated blood from the body and pumps it to the lungs via the pulmonary arteries; the left side receives oxygenated blood from the lungs and pumps it out to the body via the aorta.

- Coronary arteries supply oxygen and nutrients to the heart muscle.
- The cardiac cycle is made up of systole and diastole periods.
- The cardiac conduction system controls the electrical activity of the heart and the cardiac cycle: systole, contraction of the heart muscle and ejection of blood, and diastole, the relaxation period during which the heart fills with blood.
- Cardiac output depends on the stroke volume, or amount of blood ejected during systole, and the heart rate.
- The systemic blood vessels carry blood to the tissues through a system of arteries, arterioles, and capillaries and return it to the heart through the venules, veins, and the venae cavae.
- The blood pressure rises gradually from birth to reach the adult range in adolescence.
- Atherosclerosis causes fatty plaque to develop within arteries.
- Decreased cardiac output, impaired tissue perfusion, and disorders affecting the blood are the major cardiovascular problems that may affect oxygenation.

- Cardiac output may fall with a myocardial infarction (MI), heart failure, dysrhythmias, and structural alterations of the heart (e.g., valve deformities).
- The most common cause of impaired blood flow to tissues is atherosclerosis; this can lead to tissue ischemia and pain.
- Cardiac monitoring is used for continuous observation of the heart rate and rhythm.
- Nursing interventions to promote circulation include using antiembolic stockings and sequential compression devices to prevent venous stasis and edema, and also administering cardiopulmonary resuscitation.
- Cardiopulmonary resuscitation (CPR) is used during cardiopulmonary arrest. Each nurse needs to be aware of the hospital's policies and procedures regarding emergencies.

Review Questions

49–1. The home health nurse has developed a teaching guide for a client that focuses on the importance of regular physical activity with gradually increasing activity levels. This teaching guide specifically promotes
   a. cardiac output and tissue perfusion.
   b. renal perfusion and formation of urine.
   c. oxygen-carrying capacity of white blood cells.
   d. effective breathing and airway clearance.

49–2. A goal that the client will "demonstrate adequate tissue perfusion" has been established. Which of the following would most likely be included in evaluation of this goal?
   a. symmetrical chest expansion
   b. uses pursed-lip breathing
   c. has brisk capillary refill
   d. has activity intolerance

49–3. Which of the following clients is most likely to experience poor cardiac output?
   a. A client who has recently completed exercising.
   b. A client who has a stroke volume of 70 mL per beat and a heart rate of 70 beats/minute.

   c. A client with a sustained heart rate of 150 beats/minute.
   d. A client who receives a positive inotropic medication.

49–4. What are the cardinal signs of cardiac arrest?
   a. cool, pale skin; unconsciousness; absence of radial pulse.
   b. cyanosis, slow pulse, dilated pupils.
   c. absent pulses, flushed skin, pinpoint pupils.
   d. apnea, absence of carotid or femoral pulses, dilated pupils.

49–5. The purpose of sequential compression devices is
   a. to promote arterial circulation.
   b. to promote venous return from the legs.
   c. to decrease afterload.
   d. to decrease postoperative pain.

Readings and References

Suggested Readings
Nagle, B., & Nee, C. (2002). Recognizing and responding to acute myocardial infarction. *Nursing, 32*(10), 50–54.
   This article gives an overview of how to recognize when a client is having a myocardial infarction and how to respond. It begins with signs and symptoms and addresses classic symptoms and variations. It includes a good review of serum markers and a fairly in-depth discussion of ECG changes. Every nurse can learn from the discussion of "how to inter-

vene," which is a step-by-step guide for what to do and what the physician will likely order.

Related Research
Segers, P., Belgrado, J. P., Leduc, A., Leduc, O., & Verdonck, P. (2002). Excessive pressure in multichambered cuffs used for sequential compression therapy. *Physical Therapy, 82,* 1000–1008.
Zuzelo, P. R. (2002). Gender and acute myocardial infarction symptoms. *Medsurg Nursing, 11,* 126–137.

References
Johnson, M., Maas, M., & Moorhead, S. (Eds.). *Nursing outcomes classification (NOC)* (2nd ed.). St. Louis, MO: Mosby.
McCloskey, J. C., & Bulechek, G. M. (Eds.). (2000). *Nursing interventions classification (NIC)* (3rd ed.), St. Louis, MO: Mosby.
Meils, C. M., Kaleta, K. A., & Mueller, C. L. (2002). Treatment of the patient with acute myocardial infarction: Reducing time delays. *Journal of Nursing Care Quality, 17*(1), 83–89.

NANDA International. (2003). NANDA *nursing diagnoses: Definitions and classification 2003-2004.* Philadelphia: Author.

Reeder, S. J., Hoffman, R. L., Magdic, K. S., & Rodgers, J. M. (2000). Homocysteine: The latest risk factor for heart disease. *Dimensions of Critical Care Nursing, 19*(1), 22–28.

Selected Bibliography

Anonymous. (2002). ACE inhibitors for heart failure: No race issue here. *Nursing, 32*(11), CC8.

Anonymous. (2002). Excess weight linked to the development of heart failure. *Geriatrics, 57*(10), 16–17.

Anonymous. (2002). Quick blood test identifies heart failure. *Nursing, 32*(6), 34.

Anonymous. (2002). "Resetting" the heart helps heart failure patients. *Nursing, 32*(10), CC8.

Anonymous. (2002). Teaching your patient about cardiovascular tests. *Nursing, 32*(1), 62–64.

Asselin, M. E., & Cullen, H. A. (2001), What you need to know about the new BLS guidelines. *Nursing, 31*(3), 48–50.

Bauer, J. (2002). Implantable defibrillators cut risk of death for MI patients. *RN, 65*(5), 20.

Bosen, D. M. (2002). What you need to know about the new heart failure guidelines. *Nursing, 32*(6), CC8–CC9.

Chorzempa, A. (2002). Post myocardial infarction treatment in the older adult. *Dimensions of Critical Care Nursing, 21*(1), 20–26.

Davis, S. L. (2002). How the heart failure picture has changed. *Nursing, 32*(11), 36–46.

Haddad, A. (2002). Ethics in action: Family presence during codes. *RN, 65*(11), 31–34.

Hohm, S. (2002). Code blue. *Nursing, 32*(4), 64.

Hussar, D. A. (2002). New drugs 2002, part III. *Nursing, 32*(7), 55–64.

Lanza, M. (2002). Right ventricular myocardial infarction: When the power fails. *Dimensions of Critical Care Nursing, 21,* 122–126.

McCance, K. L., & Huether, S. E. (2002). *Pathophysiology: The biologic basis for disease in adults and children* (4th ed.). St. Louis, MO: Mosby.

McConnell, E. A. (2001). Applying cardiac monitor electrodes. *Nursing, 31*(18), 17.

McVeigh, J. P., & Musto, J. (1999). Acute myocardial infarction. *Australian Nursing Journal, 7*(2), CU1–CU4.

Miranda, M. B. (2002). An evidence-based approach to improving care of patients with heart failure across the continuum. *Journal of Nursing Care Quality, 17*(1), 1–15.

Parker, K. P. (2002). Sleep and heart failure. *The Journal of Cardiovascular Nursing, 17*(1), 30–42.

Pope, B. B. (2002). Heart failure. *Nursing, 32*(8), 50–51.

Rodgers, J. M. (2002). Managing heart failure. *Nursing Management, 33*(10), 48A–57A.

Sarter, B. (2002). Coenzyme Q10 and cardiovascular disease: A review. *The Journal of Cardiovascular Nursing, 16*(4), 9–20.

Stryer, D. B. (2002). The development and role of predictive instruments in acute coronary events: Improving diagnosis and management. *The Journal of Cardiovascular Nursing, 16*(3), 1–8.

Vernarec, E. (2002). Clot-buster approved for clearing central caths. *RN, 65*(1), 93.

Walton, J. (2002). Discovering meaning and purpose during recovery from an acute myocardial infarction. *Dimensions of Critical Care Nursing, 21*(1), 36–44.

Williams, J. M. (2002). Family presence during resuscitation: To see or not to see? *Nursing Clinics of North America, 37,* 211–221.

CHAPTER 50

FLUID, ELECTROLYTE, AND ACID–BASE BALANCE

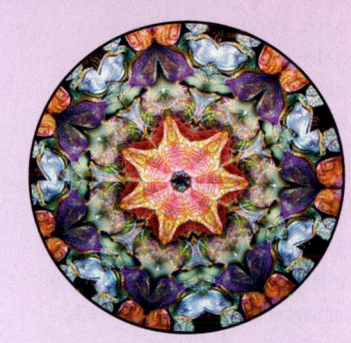

LEARNING OUTCOMES

After completing this chapter, you will be able to:

- Discuss the function, distribution, movement, and regulation of fluids and electrolytes in the body.

- Describe the regulation of acid–base balance in the body, including the roles of buffers, the lungs, and the kidneys.

- Identify factors affecting normal body fluid, electrolyte, and acid–base balance.

- Discuss the risk factors for and the causes and effects of fluid, electrolyte, and acid–base imbalances.

- Collect assessment data related to the client's fluid, electrolyte, and acid–base balances.

- Identify examples of nursing diagnoses, outcomes, and interventions for clients with altered fluid, electrolyte, or acid–base balance.

- Teach clients measures to maintain fluid and electrolyte balance.

- Implement measures to correct imbalances of fluids and electrolytes or acids and bases such as enteral or parenteral replacements and blood transfusions.

- Evaluate the effect of nursing and collaborative interventions on the client's fluid, electrolyte, or acid–base balance.

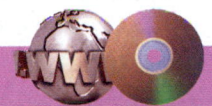

MediaLink

www.prenhall.com/kozier

Additional resources for this chapter can be found on the Student CD-ROM accompanying this textbook, and on the Companion Website at www.prenhall.com/kozier. Click on Chapter 50 to select the activities for this chapter.

CD-ROM
- Audio Glossary
- NCLEX Review
- Animations:
  Membrane Transport
  Filtration Pressure
  Fluid Balance
  Acid-Base Balance
  Inserting A Central Venous Line

Companion Website
- Additional NCLEX Review
- Case Study: Client with Suspected Electrolyte Imbalance
- Care Plan Activity: Client with Heart Failure
- MediaLink Application: Determining Body Fluid Problems
- Links to Resources

In good health, a delicate balance of fluids, electrolytes, and acids and bases is maintained in the body. This balance, or physiologic **homeostasis,** depends on multiple physiologic processes that regulate fluid intake and output and the movement of water and the substances dissolved in it between the body compartments.

Almost every illness has the potential to threaten this balance. Even in daily living, excessive temperatures or vigorous activity can disturb the balance if adequate water and salt intake is not maintained. Therapeutic measures, such as the use of diuretics or nasogastric suction, can also disturb the body's homeostasis unless water and electrolytes are replaced.

BODY FLUIDS AND ELECTROLYTES

The proportion of the human body composed of fluid is surprisingly large. About 46% to 60% of the average adult's weight is water, the primary body fluid. In good health this volume remains relatively constant and the person's weight varies by less than 0.2 kg (0.5 lb) in 24 hours, regardless of the amount of fluid ingested.

Water is vital to health and normal cellular function, serving as

- A medium for metabolic reactions within cells
- A transporter for nutrients, waste products, and other substances
- A lubricant
- An insulator and shock absorber
- One means of regulating and maintaining body temperature.

Age, sex, and body fat affect total body water. Infants have the highest proportion of water, accounting for 70% to 80% of their body weight, but the proportion of body water decreases with aging. In people older than 60 years of age, it decreases to approximately 50%. Fat tissue is essentially free of water, whereas lean tissue contains a significant amount of water. Water makes up a greater percentage of a lean person's body weight than an obese person's. Women, who have proportionately more body fat than men, have a lower percentage of body water.

Distribution of Body Fluids

The body's fluid is divided into two major compartments, intracellular and extracellular. **Intracellular fluid (ICF)** is found within the cells of the body. It constitutes approximately two-thirds of the total body fluid in adults. **Extracellular fluid (ECF)** is found outside the cells and accounts for about one-third of total body fluid. It is subdivided into compartments. The two main compartments of ECF are intravascular and interstitial. **Intravascular fluid,** or **plasma,** is found within the vascular system. **Interstitial fluid** surrounds the cells. The other compartments of ECF are the lymph and transcellular fluids. Examples of **transcellular fluid** include cerebrospinal, pericardial, pancreatic, pleural, intraocular, biliary, peritoneal, and synovial fluids (Figure 50–1 ■).

Intracellular fluid is vital to normal cell functioning. It contains solutes such as oxygen, electrolytes, and glucose, and it provides a medium in which metabolic processes of the cell take place.

Although extracellular fluid is in the smaller of the two compartments, it is the transport system that carries nutrients to and waste products from the cells. For example, plasma carries oxygen from the lungs and glucose from the gastrointestinal tract to the capillaries of the vascular system. From there, the oxygen and glucose move across the capillary membranes into the interstitial spaces and then across the cellular membranes into the cells. The opposite route is taken for waste products, such as carbon dioxide going from the cells to the lungs and metabolic acid wastes going eventually to the kidneys. Interstitial fluid, which composes three-quarters of the ECF, transports wastes from the cells by way of the lymph system as well as directly into the blood plasma through capillaries.

Composition of Body Fluids

Extracellular and intracellular fluids contain oxygen from the lungs, dissolved nutrients from the gastrointestinal tract, excretory products of metabolism such as carbon dioxide, and charged particles called **ions.**

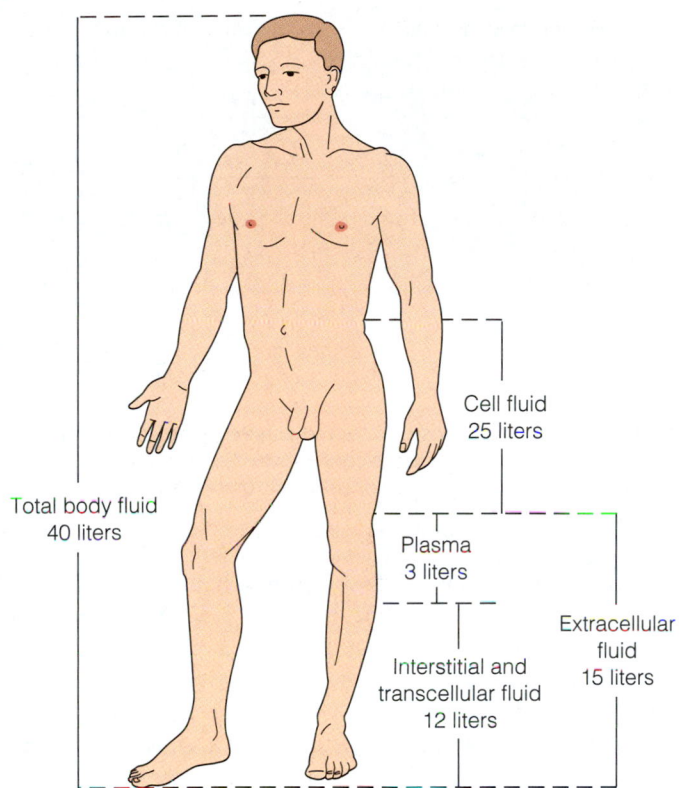

Cell fluid
25 liters

Total body fluid
40 liters

Plasma
3 liters

Extracellular
fluid
15 liters

Interstitial and
transcellular fluid
12 liters

Figure 50–1 ■ Total body fluid represents 40 L in an adult male weighing 70 kg (154 lb).

Many salts dissociate in water, that is, break up into electrically charged ions. The salt sodium chloride breaks up into one ion of sodium (Na^+) and one ion of chloride (Cl^-). These charged particles are called **electrolytes** because they are capable of conducting electricity. Ions that carry a positive charge are called **cations,** and ions carrying a negative charge are called **anions.** Examples of cations are sodium (Na^+), potassium (K^+), calcium (Ca^{2+}), and magnesium (Mg^{2+}). Examples of anions include chloride (Cl^-), bicarbonate HCO_3^- phosphate HPO_4^{2-} and sulfate SO_4^{2-}.

Electrolytes generally are measured in milliequivalents per liter of water (mEq/L) or milligrams per 100 milliliters (mg/100 mL). The term **milliequivalent** refers to the chemical combining power of the ion, or the capacity of cations to combine with anions to form molecules. This combining activity is measured in relation to the combining activity of the hydrogen ion (H^+). Thus, 1 mEq of any anion equals 1 mEq of any cation. For example, sodium and chloride ions are equivalent, since they combine equally: 1 mEq of Na^+ equals 1 mEq of Cl^-. However, these cations and anions are not equal in weight: 1 mg of Na^+ does not equal 1 mg of Cl^-; rather, 3 mg of Na^+ equals 2 mg of Cl^- (Figure 50–2 ■).

Clinically, the milliequivalent system is most often used. However, nurses need to be aware that different systems of measurement may be found when interpreting laboratory results. For example, calcium levels frequently are reported in milligrams per deciliter (1 dL = 100 mL) instead of milliequivalents per liter. It also is important to remember that laboratory tests are usually performed using blood plasma, an extracellular fluid. These results may reflect what is happening in the ECF, but it generally is not possible to directly measure electrolyte concentrations within the cell.

The composition of fluids varies from one body compartment to another. In extracellular fluid, the principal electrolytes are sodium, chloride, and bicarbonate. Other electrolytes such as potassium, calcium, and magnesium are also present but in much smaller quantities. Plasma and interstitial fluid, the two primary components of ECF, contain essentially the same electrolytes and solutes, with the exception of protein. Plasma is a protein-rich fluid, containing large amounts of albumin, but interstitial fluid contains little or no protein.

The composition of intracellular fluid differs significantly from that of ECF. Potassium and magnesium are the primary cations present in ICF, with phosphate and sulfate the major anions. As in ECF, other electrolytes are present within the cell, but in much smaller concentrations.

A Combining Power

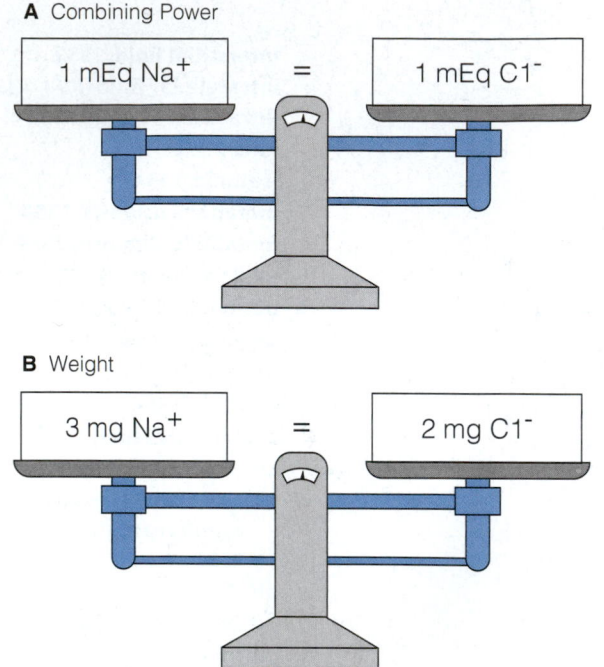

Figure 50–2 ■ Relating sodium (Na$^+$) and chloride (Cl$^-$): *A*, by combining power; *B*, by weight.

Maintaining a balance of fluid volumes and electrolyte compositions in the fluid compartments of the body is essential to health. Normal and unusual fluid and electrolyte losses must be replaced if homeostasis is to be maintained.

Other body fluids such as gastric and intestinal secretions also contain electrolytes. This is of particular concern when these fluids are lost from the body (for example, in severe vomiting or diarrhea or when gastric suction removes the gastric secretions). Fluid and electrolyte imbalances can result from excessive losses through these routes.

Movement of Body Fluids and Electrolytes

The body fluid compartments are separated from one another by cell membranes and the capillary membrane. These membranes are described as **selectively permeable** because substances move across them with varying degrees of ease. Small particles such as ions, oxygen, and carbon dioxide easily move across these membranes, but larger molecules like glucose and proteins have more difficulty moving between fluid compartments.

The methods by which electrolytes and other solutes move are osmosis, diffusion, filtration, and active transport.

Osmosis

Osmosis is the movement of water across cell membranes, from the less concentrated solution to the more concentrated solution (Figure 50–3 ■). In other words, water moves toward the higher concentration of solute in an attempt to equalize the concentrations.

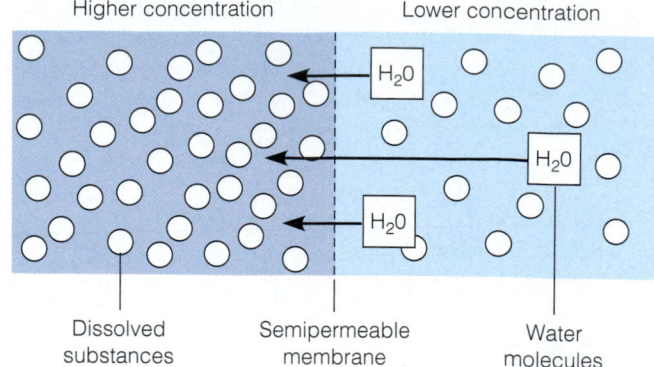

Figure 50–3 ■ Osmosis: Water molecules move from the less concentrated area to the more concentrated area in an attempt to equalize the concentration of solutions on two sides of a membrane.

Solutes are substances dissolved in a liquid. For example, when sugar is added to coffee, the sugar is the solute. Solutes may be **crystalloids** (salts that dissolve readily into true solutions) or **colloids** (substances such as large protein molecules that do not readily dissolve into true solutions). A **solvent** is the component of a solution that can dissolve a solute. In the previous example, coffee is the solvent for the sugar.

In the body, water is the solvent; the solutes include electrolytes, oxygen and carbon dioxide, glucose, urea, amino acids, and proteins. Osmosis occurs when the concentration of solutes on one side of a selectively permeable membrane, such as the capillary membrane, is higher than on the other side. For example, a marathon runner loses a significant amount of water through perspiration, increasing the concentration of solutes in the plasma because of water loss. This higher solute concentration draws water from the interstitial space and cells into the vascular compartment to equalize the concentration of solutes in all fluid compartments. Osmosis is an important mechanism for maintaining homeostasis and fluid balance.

The concentration of solutes in body fluids is usually expressed as the **osmolality**. Osmolality is determined by the total solute concentration within a fluid compartment and is measured as parts of solute per kilogram of water (Figure 50–4 ■).

Osmolality is reported as milliosmols per kilogram (mOsm/kg). Sodium is by far the greatest determinant of *serum osmolality*, with glucose and urea also contributing. Potassium, glucose, and urea are the primary contributors to the osmolality of intracellular fluid. The term *tonicity* may be used to refer to the osmolality of a solution. An **isotonic** solution has the same osmolality as body fluids. Normal saline, 0.9% sodium chloride, is an isotonic solution. **Hypertonic** solutions have a higher osmolality than body fluids; 3% sodium chloride is a hypertonic solution. **Hypotonic** solutions such as one-half normal saline (0.45% sodium chloride), by contrast, have a lower osmolality than body fluids.

Osmotic pressure is the power of a solution to draw water across a semipermeable membrane. When two solutions of different solute concentrations are separated by a semipermeable membrane, the solution of higher solute concentration exerts a

Milliosmols   Milliequivalents

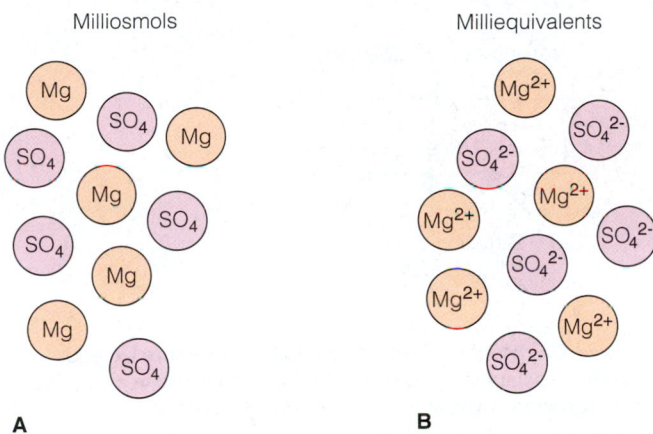

A   B

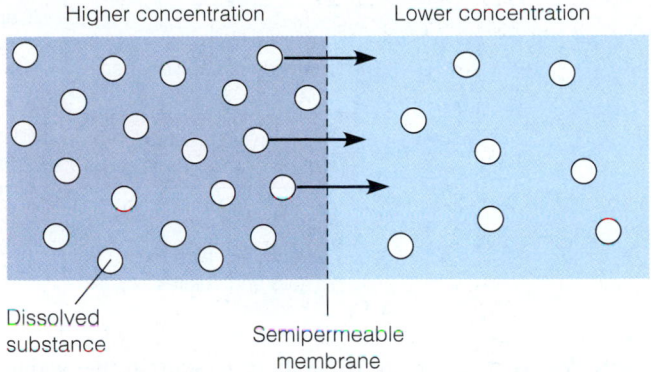

Higher concentration   Lower concentration

Dissolved substance   Semipermeable membrane

Figure 50–5 ■ Diffusion: The movement of molecules through a semipermeable membrane from an area of higher concentration to an area of lower concentration.

Figure 50–4 ■ Comparison of milliosmols and milliequivalents. A, Milliosmols measure osmotic activity as a total of the number of particles present—in this case 10. B, Milliequivalents measure the chemical activity as a total of the number of available electrovalent bonds (− −, + +)—in this case, 20.

higher osmotic pressure, drawing water across the membrane to equalize the concentrations of the solutions. For example, infusing a hypertonic intravenous solution such as 3% sodium chloride will draw fluid out of red blood cells (RBCs), causing them to shrink. On the other hand, a hypotonic solution administered intravenously will cause the RBCs to swell as water is drawn into the cells by their higher osmotic pressure. In the body, plasma proteins exert an osmotic draw called **colloid osmotic pressure** or **oncotic pressure,** pulling water from the interstitial space into the vascular compartment. This is an important mechanism in maintaining vascular volume.

Diffusion

Diffusion is the continual intermingling of molecules in liquids, gases, or solids brought about by the random movement of the molecules. For example, two gases become mixed by the constant motion of their molecules. The process of diffusion occurs even when two substances are separated by a thin membrane. In the body, diffusion of water, electrolytes, and other substances occurs through the "split pores" of capillary membranes.

The rate of diffusion of substances varies according to (a) the size of the molecules, (b) the concentration of the solution, and (c) the temperature of the solution. Larger molecules move less quickly than smaller ones because they require more energy to move about. With diffusion, the molecules move from a solution of higher concentration to a solution of lower concentration (Figure 50–5 ■). Increases in temperature increase the rate of motion of molecules and therefore the rate of diffusion.

Filtration

Filtration is a process whereby fluid and solutes move together across a membrane from one compartment to another. The movement is from an area of higher pressure to one of lower pressure. An example of filtration is the movement of

fluid and nutrients from the capillaries of the arterioles to the interstitial fluid around the cells. The pressure in the compartment that results in the movement of the fluid and substances dissolved in fluid out of the compartment is called **filtration pressure. Hydrostatic pressure** is the pressure exerted by a fluid within a closed system on the walls of a container in which it is contained. The hydrostatic pressure of blood is the force exerted by blood against the vascular walls (e.g., the artery walls). The principle involved in hydrostatic pressure is that fluids move from the area of greater pressure to the area of lesser pressure. Using the example of the blood vessels, the plasma proteins in the blood exert a colloid osmotic or oncotic pressure (see the earlier section "Osmosis") that opposes the hydrostatic pressure and holds the fluid in the vascular compartment to maintain the vascular volume. When the hydrostatic pressure is greater than the osmotic pressure, the fluid filters out of the blood vessels. The filtration pressure in this example is the difference between the hydrostatic pressure and the osmotic pressure (Figure 50–6 ■).

Active Transport

Substances can move across cell membranes from a less concentrated solution to a more concentrated one by **active transport** (Figure 50–7 ■). This process differs from diffusion and osmosis in that metabolic energy is expended. In active transport, a substance combines with a carrier on the outside surface of the cell membrane, and they move to the inside surface of the cell membrane. Once inside, they separate, and the substance is released to the inside of the cell. A specific carrier is required for each substance, enzymes are required for active transport, and energy is expended.

This process is of particular importance in maintaining the differences in sodium and potassium ion concentrations of ECF and ICF. Under normal conditions, sodium concentrations are higher in the extracellular fluid, and potassium concentrations are higher inside the cells. To maintain these proportions, the active transport mechanism (the sodium-potassium pump) is activated, moving sodium from the cells and potassium into the cells.

MediaLink | MEMBRANE TRANSPORT ANIMATION

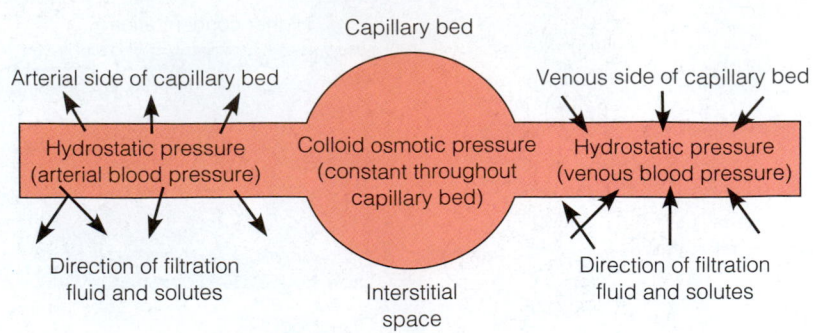

Figure 50–6 ■ Schematic of filtration pressure changes within a capillary bed. On the arterial side, arterial blood pressure exceeds colloid osmotic pressure, so that water and dissolved substances move out of the capillary into the interstitial space. On the venous side, venous blood pressure is less than colloid osmotic pressure, so that water and dissolved substances move into the capillary.

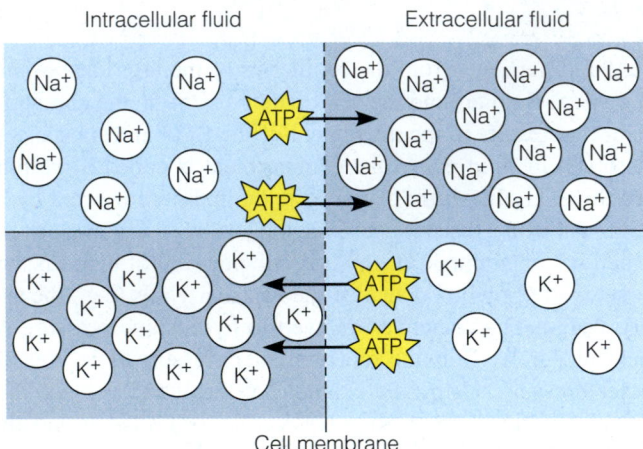

Figure 50–7 ■ An example of active transport. Energy (ATP) is used to move sodium molecules and potassium molecules across a semipermeable membrane against sodium's and potassium's concentration gradients (i.e., from areas of lesser concentration to areas of greater concentration).

Regulating Body Fluids

In a healthy person, the volumes and chemical composition of the fluid compartments stay within narrow safe limits. Normally fluid intake and fluid loss are balanced. Illness can upset this balance so that the body has too little or too much fluid.

Fluid Intake

During periods of moderate activity at moderate temperature, the average adult drinks about 1,500 mL per day but needs 2,500 mL per day, an additional 1,000 mL. This added volume is acquired from foods and from the oxidation of these foods during metabolic processes. Interestingly, the water content of food is relatively large, contributing about 750 mL per day. The water content of fresh vegetables is approximately 90%, of fresh fruits about 85%, and of lean meats around 60%.

Water as a by-product of food metabolism accounts for most of the remaining fluid volume required. This quantity is approximately 200 mL per day for the average adult.

The thirst mechanism is the primary regulator of fluid intake. The thirst center is located in the hypothalamus of the brain. A number of stimuli trigger this center, including the osmotic pressure of body fluids, vascular volume, and angiotensin (a hormone released in response to decreased blood flow to the kidneys). For example, a long-distance runner loses significant amounts of water through perspiration and rapid breathing during a race, increasing the concentration of solutes and the osmotic pressure of body fluids. This increased osmotic pressure stimulates the thirst center, causing the runner to experience the sensation of thirst and the desire to drink to replace lost fluids.

Thirst is normally relieved immediately after drinking a small amount of fluid, even before it is absorbed from the gastrointestinal tract. However, this relief is only temporary, and the thirst returns in about 15 minutes. The thirst is again temporarily relieved after the ingested fluid distends the upper gastrointestinal tract. These mechanisms protect the individual from drinking too much, because it takes from 30 minutes to 1 hour for the fluid to be absorbed and distributed throughout the body. Table 50–1 lists average daily fluid requirements.

Fluid Output

Fluid losses from the body counterbalance the adult's 2500-mL average daily intake of fluid, as shown in Table 50–2. There are four routes of fluid output:

TABLE 50–1 Average Daily Fluid Requirements by Age and Weight		
Age	**Approximate Body Weight (kg)**	**mL/24 hr**
3 days	3.0	250 to 300
1 year	9.5	1,150 to 1,300
2 years	11.8	1,350 to 1,500
6 years	20.0	1,800 to 2,000
10 years	28.7	2,000 to 2,500
14 years	45.0	2,200 to 2,700
18 years (adult)	54.0	2,200 to 2,700

Note: From: Nelson Textbook of Pediatrics (p. 107), by R. E. Behrman, 1992, Philadelphia: Saunders. Adapted with permission.

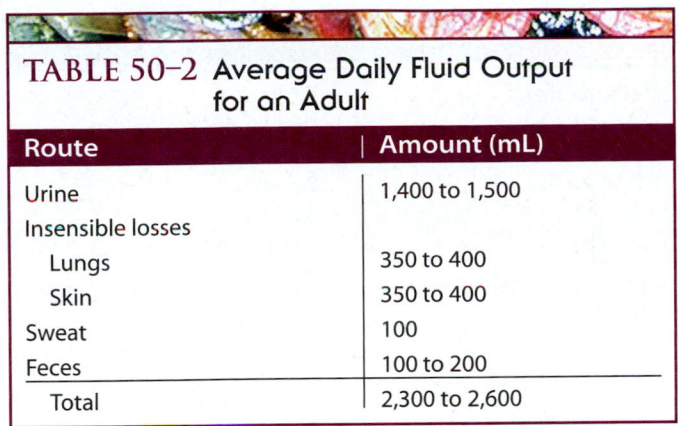

TABLE 50–2 Average Daily Fluid Output for an Adult	
Route	**Amount (mL)**
Urine	1,400 to 1,500
Insensible losses	
Lungs	350 to 400
Skin	350 to 400
Sweat	100
Feces	100 to 200
Total	2,300 to 2,600

1. Urine
2. Insensible loss through the skin as perspiration and through the lungs as water vapor in the expired air
3. Noticeable loss through the skin
4. Loss through the intestines in feces.

URINE. Urine formed by the kidneys and excreted from the urinary bladder is the major avenue of fluid output. Normal urine output for an adult is 1,400 to 1,500 mL per 24 hours, or at least 0.5 mL per kilogram per hour. In healthy people, urine output may vary noticeably from day to day. Urine volume automatically increases as fluid intake increases. If fluid loss through perspiration is large, however, urine volume decreases to maintain fluid balance in the body.

INSENSIBLE LOSSES. **Insensible fluid loss** occurs through the skin and lungs. It is called insensible because it is usually not noticeable and cannot be measured. Insensible fluid loss through the skin occurs in two ways. Water is lost through diffusion and through perspiration (which is noticeable but not measurable). Water losses through diffusion are not noticeable but normally account for 300 to 400 mL per day. This loss can be significantly increased if the protective layer of the skin is lost as with burns or large abrasions. Perspiration varies depending on factors such as environmental temperature and metabolic activity. Fever and exercise increase metabolic activity and heat production, thereby increasing fluid losses through the skin.

Another type of insensible loss is the water in exhaled air. In an adult, this is normally 300 to 400 mL per day. When respiratory rate accelerates, for example, due to exercise or an elevated body temperature, this loss can increase.

FECES. The chyme that passes from the small intestine into the large intestine contains water and electrolytes. The volume of chyme entering the large intestine in an adult is normally about 1,500 mL per day. Of this amount, all but about 100 mL is reabsorbed in the proximal half of the large intestine.

Certain fluid losses are required to maintain normal body function. These are known as **obligatory losses.** Approximately 500 mL of fluid must be excreted through the kidneys of an adult each day to eliminate metabolic waste products from the body. Water lost through respirations, through the skin, and in feces

also are obligatory losses, necessary for temperature regulation and elimination of waste products. The total of all these losses is approximately 1,300 mL per day.

Maintaining Homeostasis

The volume and composition of body fluids is regulated through several homeostatic mechanisms. A number of body systems contribute to this regulation, including the kidneys, the endocrine system, the cardiovascular system, the lungs, and the gastrointestinal system. Hormones such as antidiuretic hormone (ADH; also known as arginine vasopressin or AVP), the renin-angiotensin-aldosterone system, and atrial natriuretic factor are involved, as are mechanisms to monitor and maintain vascular volume.

KIDNEYS. The kidneys are the primary regulator of body fluids and electrolyte balance. They regulate the volume and osmolality of extracellular fluids by regulating water and electrolyte excretion. The kidneys adjust the reabsorption of water from plasma filtrate and ultimately the amount excreted as urine. Although 135 to 180 L of plasma per day is normally filtered in an adult, only about 1.5 L of urine is excreted. Electrolyte balance is maintained by selective retention and excretion by the kidneys. The kidneys also play a significant role in acid–base regulation, excreting hydrogen ion (H^+) and retaining bicarbonate.

ANTIDIURETIC HORMONE. Antidiuretic hormone, which regulates water excretion from the kidney, is synthesized in the anterior portion of the hypothalamus and acts on the collecting ducts of the nephrons. When serum osmolality rises, ADH is produced, causing the collecting ducts to become more permeable to water. This increased permeability allows more water to be reabsorbed into the blood. As more water is reabsorbed, urine output falls and serum osmolality decreases because the water dilutes body fluids. Conversely, if serum osmolality decreases, ADH is suppressed, the collecting ducts become less permeable to water, and urine output increases. Excess water is excreted, and serum osmolality returns to normal. Other factors also affect the production and release of ADH, including blood volume, temperature, pain, stress, and some drugs such as opiates, barbiturates, and nicotine.

RENIN-ANGIOTENSIN-ALDOSTERONE SYSTEM. Specialized receptors in the juxtaglomerular cells of the kidney nephrons respond to changes in renal perfusion. This initiates the **renin-angiotensin-aldosterone system.** If blood flow or pressure to the kidney decreases, renin is released. Renin causes the conversion of angiotensinogen to angiotensin I, which is then converted to angiotensin II by angiotensin-converting enzyme. Angiotensin II acts directly on the nephrons to promote sodium and water retention. In addition, it stimulates the release of aldosterone from the adrenal cortex. Aldosterone also promotes sodium retention in the distal nephron. The net effect of the renin-angiotensin-aldosterone system is to restore blood volume (and renal perfusion) through sodium and water retention.

ATRIAL NATRIURETIC FACTOR. Atrial natriuretic factor (ANF) is released from cells in the atrium of the heart in response to excess blood volume and stretching of the atrial walls. Acting on the nephrons, ANF promotes sodium wasting and acts as a potent diuretic, thus reducing vascular volume. ANF also inhibits thirst, reducing fluid intake.

Regulating Electrolytes

Electrolytes, charged ions capable of conducting electricity, are present in all body fluids and fluid compartments. Just as maintaining the fluid balance is vital to normal body function, so is maintaining electrolyte balance. Although the concentration of specific electrolytes differs between fluid compartments, a balance of cations (positively charged ions) and anions (negatively charged ions) always exists. Electrolytes are important for

- Maintaining fluid balance
- Contributing to acid–base regulation
- Facilitating enzyme reactions
- Transmitting neuromuscular reactions.

Most electrolytes enter the body through dietary intake and are excreted in the urine. Some electrolytes, such as sodium and chloride, are not stored by the body and must be consumed daily to maintain normal levels. Potassium and calcium, on the other hand, are stored in the cells and bone, respectively. When serum levels drop, ions can shift out of the storage "pool" into the blood to maintain adequate serum levels for normal functioning. The regulatory mechanisms and functions of the major electrolytes are summarized in Table 50–3.

Sodium (Na⁺)

Sodium is the most abundant cation in extracellular fluid and a major contributor to serum osmolality. Sodium functions largely in controlling and regulating water balance. When sodium is reabsorbed from the kidney tubules, chloride and water are reabsorbed with it, thus maintaining ECF volume. Sodium is found in many foods, such as bacon, ham, processed cheese, and table salt.

Potassium (K⁺)

Potassium is the major cation in intracellular fluids, with only a small amount found in plasma and interstitial fluid. Just as sodium helps maintain ECF water balance, potassium is important in maintaining ICF water balance. Potassium is a vital electrolyte for skeletal, cardiac, and smooth muscle activity. It is involved in maintaining acid–base balance as well, and it contributes to intracellular enzyme reactions. Potassium is found in many fruits and vegetables, meat, fish, and other foods (see Box 50–1).

Calcium (Ca²⁺)

The vast majority of calcium in the body is in the skeletal system, with a relatively small amount in extracellular fluid. Although this calcium outside the bones and teeth amounts to only about 1% of the total calcium in the body, it is vital in regulating muscle contraction and relaxation, neuromuscular

BOX 50–1 ■ Potassium-Rich Foods

Vegetables	**Fruits**
Avocado	Dried fruits (e.g., raisins
Raw carrot	and dates)
Baked potato	Banana
Raw tomato	Apricot
Spinach	Cantaloupe
	Orange
Meats and Fish	
Beef	**Beverages**
Cod	Milk
Pork	Orange juice
Veal	Apricot nectar

function, and cardiac function. ECF calcium is regulated by a complex interaction of parathyroid hormone, calcitonin, and calcitriol, a metabolite of vitamin D. When calcium levels in the ECF fall, parathyroid hormone and calcitriol cause calcium to be released from bones into ECF and increase the absorption of calcium in the intestines, thus raising serum calcium levels. Conversely, calcitonin stimulates the deposition of calcium in bone, reducing the concentration of calcium ions in the blood.

With aging, the intestines absorb calcium less effectively and more calcium is excreted via the kidneys. Calcium shifts out of the bone to replace these ECF losses, increasing the risk of osteoporosis and fractures of the wrists, vertebrae, and hips. Lack of weight-bearing exercise (which helps keep calcium in the bones) and a vitamin D deficiency because of inadequate exposure to sunlight contribute to this risk.

Milk and milk products are the richest sources of calcium, with other foods such as dark green leafy vegetables and canned salmon containing smaller amounts. Many clients benefit from calcium supplements.

Magnesium (Mg²⁺)

Magnesium is primarily found in the skeleton and in intracellular fluid. It is important for intracellular metabolism, being particularly involved in the production and use of ATP. Magnesium also is necessary for protein and DNA synthesis within the cells. Only about 1% of the body's magnesium is in ECF; here it is involved in regulating neuromuscular and cardiac function. Maintaining and ensuring adequate magnesium levels is an important part of care of patients with cardiac disorders. Cereal grains, nuts, dried fruit, legumes, and green leafy vegetables are good sources of magnesium in the diet, as are dairy products, meat, and fish.

Chloride (Cl⁻)

Chloride is the major anion of ECF. Chloride functions with sodium to regulate serum osmolality and blood volume. The concentration of chloride in ECF is regulated secondarily to sodium; when sodium is reabsorbed in the kidney, chloride usually follows. Chloride is a major component of gastric juice as hydrochloric acid (HCl) and is involved in regulating acid-base bal-

TABLE 50-3 Regulation and Functions of Electrolytes

Electrolyte	Regulation	Function
Sodium (Na$^+$)	• Renal reabsorption or excretion • Aldosterone increases Na$^+$ reabsorption in collecting duct of nephrons	• Regulating ECF volume and distribution • Maintaining blood volume • Transmitting nerve impulses and contracting muscles
Potassium (K$^+$)	• Renal excretion and conservation • Aldosterone increases K$^+$ excretion • Movement into and out of cells • Insulin helps move K$^+$ into cells; tissue damage and acidosis shift K$^+$ out of cells into ECF	• Maintaining ICF osmolality • Transmitting nerve and other electrical impulses • Regulating cardiac impulse transmission and muscle contraction • Skeletal and smooth muscle function • Regulating acid-base balance
Calcium (Ca^{2+})	• Redistribution between bones and ECF • Parathyroid hormone and calcitriol increase serum Ca^{2+} levels; calcitonin decreases serum levels	• Forming bones and teeth • Transmitting nerve impulses • Regulating muscle contractions • Maintaining cardiac pacemaker (automaticity) • Blood clotting • Activating enzymes such as pancreatic lipase and phospholipase
Magnesium (Mg^{2+})	• Conservation and excretion by kidneys • Intestinal absorption increased by vitamin D and parathyroid hormone	• Intracellular metabolism • Operating sodium-potassium pump • Relaxing muscle contractions • Transmitting nerve impulses • Regulating cardiac function
Chloride (Cl$^-$)	• Excreted and reabsorbed along with sodium in the kidneys • Aldosterone increases chloride reabsorption with sodium	• HCl production • Regulating ECF balance and vascular volume • Regulating acid–base balance • Buffer in oxygen–carbon dioxide exchange in RBCs
Phosphate (PO$_4^-$)	• Excretion and reabsorption by the kidneys • Parathyroid hormone decreases serum levels by increasing renal excretion • Reciprocal relationship with calcium: increasing serum calcium levels decrease phosphate levels; decreasing serum calcium increases phosphate	• Forming bones and teeth • Metabolizing carbohydrate, protein, and fat • Cellular metabolism; producing ATP and DNA • Muscle, nerve, and RBC function • Regulating acid–base balance • Regulating calcium levels
Bicarbonate (HCO$_3^-$)	• Excretion and reabsorption by the kidneys • Regeneration by kidneys	• Major body buffer involved in acid–base regulation

ance. It also acts as a buffer in the exchange of oxygen and carbon dioxide in RBCs. Chloride is found in the same foods as sodium.

Phosphate PO$_4^-$

Phosphate is the major anion of intracellular fluids. It also is found in ECF, bone, skeletal muscle, and nerve tissue. Children have much higher phosphate levels than adults, with that of a newborn nearly twice that of an adult. Higher levels of growth hormone and a faster rate of skeletal growth probably account for this difference. Phosphate is involved in many chemical ac-

tions of the cell; it is essential for functioning of muscles, nerves, and red blood cells. It is also involved in the metabolism of protein, fat, and carbohydrate. Phosphate is absorbed from the intestine and is found in many foods such as meat, fish, poultry, milk products, and legumes.

Bicarbonate HCO$_3^-$

Bicarbonate is present in both intracellular and extracellular fluids. Its primary function is regulating acid–base balance as an essential component of the carbonic acid–bicarbonate buffering system. Extracellular bicarbonate levels are regulated by the kidneys: Bicarbonate is excreted when too much is present; if more is needed, the kidneys both regenerate and reabsorb bicarbonate ions. Unlike other electrolytes that must be consumed in the diet, adequate amounts of bicarbonate are produced through metabolic processes to meet the body's needs.

ACID–BASE BALANCE

An important part of regulating the chemical balance or homeostasis of body fluids is regulating their acidity or alkalinity. An **acid** is a substance that releases hydrogen ions (H^+) in solution. Strong acids such as hydrochloric acid release all or nearly all their hydrogen ions; weak acids like carbonic acid release some hydrogen ions. **Bases** or *alkalis* have a low hydrogen ion concentration and can accept hydrogen ions in solution. The relative acidity or alkalinity of a solution is measured as **pH.** The pH reflects the hydrogen ion concentration of the solution: The higher the hydrogen ion concentration (and the more acidic the solution), the lower the pH. Water has a pH of 7 and is neutral; that is, it is neither acidic in nature nor is it alkaline. Solutions with a pH lower than 7 are acidic; those with a pH higher than 7 are alkaline. The pH scale is logarithmic: A solution with a pH of 5 is 10 times more acidic than one with a pH of 6.

Regulation of Acid–Base Balance

Body fluids are maintained within a narrow range that is slightly alkaline. The normal pH of arterial blood is between 7.35 and 7.45 (Figure 50–8 ■). Acids are continually produced during metabolism. Several body systems, including buffers, the respiratory system, and the renal system, are actively involved in maintaining the narrow pH range necessary for optimal function. Buffers help maintain acid–base balance by neutralizing excess acids or bases. The lungs and the kidneys help maintain a normal pH by either excreting or retaining acids and bases.

Buffers

Buffers prevent excessive changes in pH by removing or releasing hydrogen ions. If excess hydrogen ion is present in body fluids, buffers bind with the hydrogen ion, minimizing the change in pH. When body fluids become too alkaline, buffers can release hydrogen ion, again minimizing the change in pH. The action of a buffer is immediate, but limited in its capacity to maintain or restore normal acid–base balance.

The major buffer system in extracellular fluids is the bicarbonate HCO_3^- and carbonic acid (H_2CO_3) system. When a strong acid such as hydrochloric acid (HCl) is added, it combines with bicarbonate and the pH drops only slightly. A strong base such as sodium hydroxide combines with carbonic acid, the weak acid of the buffer pair, and the pH remains within the narrow range of normal. The amounts of bicarbonate and carbonic acid in the body vary; however, as long as a ratio of 20 parts of bicarbonate to 1 part of carbonic acid is maintained, the pH remains within its normal range of 7.35 to 7.45 (Figure 50–9 ■). Adding a strong acid to ECF can change this ratio as bicarbonate is depleted in neutralizing the acid. When this happens, the pH drops, a condition called **acidosis.** The ratio can also be upset by adding a strong base to ECF, depleting carbonic acid as it combines with the base. In this case the pH rises and the client has **alkalosis.**

In addition to the bicarbonate–carbonic acid buffer system, plasma proteins, hemoglobin, and phosphates also function as buffers in body fluids.

Respiratory Regulation

The lungs help regulate acid–base balance by eliminating or retaining carbon dioxide (CO_2), a potential acid. Combined with water, carbon dioxide forms carbonic acid ($CO_2 + H_2O \rightarrow H_2CO_3$). This chemical reaction is reversible; carbonic acid breaks down into carbon dioxide and water. Working together with the bicarbonate–carbonic acid buffer system, the lungs regulate acid–base balance and pH by altering the rate and depth of respirations. The response of the respiratory system to changes in pH is rapid, occurring within minutes.

Carbon dioxide is a powerful stimulator of the respiratory center. When blood levels of carbonic acid and carbon dioxide rise, the respiratory center is stimulated and the rate and depth of respirations increase. Carbon dioxide is exhaled, and carbonic acid levels fall. By contrast, when bicarbonate levels are excessive, the rate and depth of respirations are reduced. This causes carbon dioxide to be retained, carbonic acid levels to rise, and the excess bicarbonate to be neutralized.

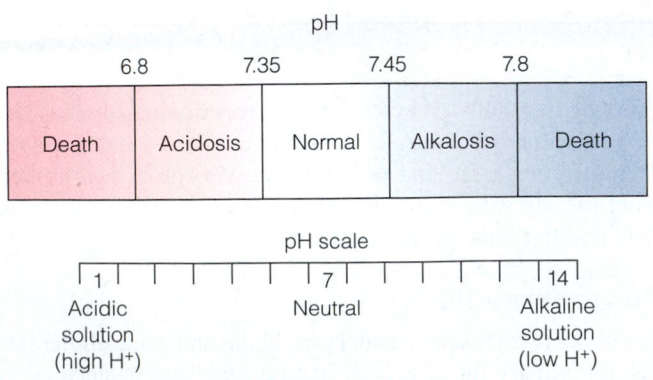

Figure 50–8 ■ Body fluids are normally slightly alkaline, between a pH of 7.35 and 7.45.

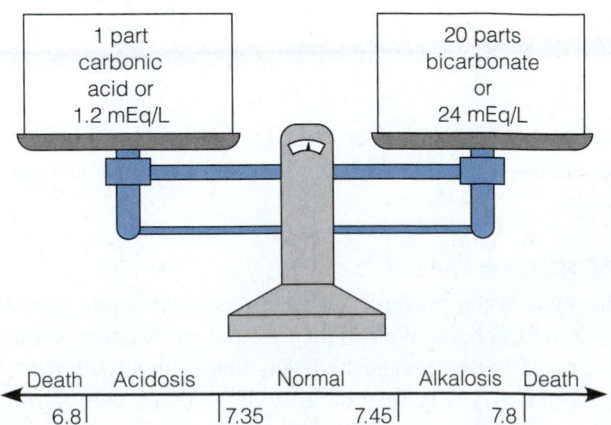

Figure 50–9 ■ Carbonic acid–bicarbonate ratio and pH.

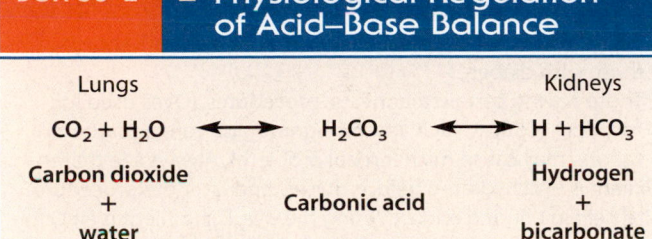

BOX 50–2   ■ Physiological Regulation
of Acid–Base Balance

Lungs   Kidneys

$$CO_2 + H_2O \longleftrightarrow H_2CO_3 \longleftrightarrow H + HCO_3$$

Carbon dioxide   **Hydrogen**
+   **+**
water   **Carbonic acid**   **bicarbonate**

The lungs and kidneys are the two major systems that are working on a continuous basis to help regulate the acid–base balance in the body. In the biochemical reactions above, the processes are all reversible and go back and forth as the body needs change. The lungs can work very quickly and do their part by either retaining or getting rid of carbon dioxide by changing the rate and depth of respirations. The kidneys work much more slowly; they may take hours to days to regulate the balance by either excreting or conserving hydrogen and bicarbonate ions. Under normal conditions, the two systems work together to maintain homeostasis.

Carbon dioxide levels in the blood are measured as the PCO_2, or partial pressure of the dissolved gas in the blood. PCO_2 refers to the pressure of carbon dioxide in venous blood. $PaCO_2$ refers to the pressure of carbon dioxide in arterial blood. The normal $PaCO_2$ is 35 to 45 mm Hg.

Renal Regulation

Although buffers and the respiratory system can compensate for changes in pH, the kidneys are the ultimate long-term regulator of acid–base balance. They are slower to respond to changes, requiring hours to days to correct imbalances, but their response is more permanent and selective than that of the other systems.

The kidneys maintain acid–base balance by selectively excreting or conserving bicarbonate and hydrogen ions. When excess hydrogen ion is present and the pH falls (acidosis), the kidneys reabsorb and regenerate bicarbonate and excrete hydrogen ion. In the case of alkalosis and a high pH, excess bicarbonate is excreted and hydrogen ion is retained. The normal serum bicarbonate level is 22 to 26 mEq/L.

The relationship of the respiratory and renal regulation of acid–base balance is further explained in Box 50–2.

FACTORS AFFECTING BODY FLUID, ELECTROLYTES, AND ACID–BASE BALANCE

The ability of the body to adjust fluids, electrolytes, and acid–base balance is influenced by age, gender and body size, environmental temperature, and lifestyle.

Age

Infants and growing children have much greater fluid turnover than adults because their higher metabolic rate increases fluid loss. Infants lose more fluid through the kidneys because immature kidneys are less able to conserve water than adult kidneys. In addition, infants respirations are more rapid and the body surface area is proportionally greater than that of adults, increasing insensible fluid losses. The more rapid turnover of fluid plus the losses produced by disease can create critical fluid imbalances in children much more rapidly than in adults.

In elderly people, the normal aging process may affect fluid balance. The thirst response often is blunted. Antidiuretic hormone levels remain normal or may even be elevated, but the nephrons become less able to conserve water in response to ADH. Increased levels of atrial natriuretic factor seen in older adults may also contribute to this impaired ability to conserve water. These normal changes of aging increase the risk of dehydration. When combined with the increased likelihood of heart diseases, impaired renal function, and multiple drug regimens, the older adult's risk for fluid and electrolyte imbalance is significant. Additionally, it is important to consider that the older adult has thinner, more fragile skin and veins, which can make an intravenous insertion more difficult.

Gender and Body Size

Total body water also is affected by gender and body size. Because fat cells contain little or no water and lean tissue has a high water content, people with a higher percentage of body fat have less body fluid. Women have proportionally more body fat and less body water than men. Water accounts for approximately 60% of an adult man's weight, but only 52% for an adult woman. In an obese individual this may be even less, with water responsible for only 30% to 40% of the person's weight.

Environmental Temperature

People with an illness and those participating in strenuous activity are at risk for fluid and electrolyte imbalances when the environmental temperature is high. Fluid losses through sweating are increased in hot environments as the body attempts to dissipate heat. These losses are even greater in people who have not been acclimatized to the environment.

Both salt and water are lost through sweating. When only water is replaced, salt depletion is a risk. The person who is salt depleted may experience fatigue, weakness, headache, and gastrointestinal symptoms such as anorexia and nausea. The risk of adverse effects is even greater if lost water is not replaced. Body temperature rises, and the person is at risk for heat exhaustion or heatstroke. Heatstroke may occur in older adults or ill people during prolonged periods of heat; it can also affect athletes and laborers when their heat production exceeds the body's ability to dissipate heat.

Consuming adequate amounts of cool liquids, particularly during strenuous activity, reduces the risk of adverse effects from heat. Balanced electrolyte solutions and carbohydrate-electrolyte solutions such as sports drinks are recommended because they replace both water and electrolytes lost through sweat.

Lifestyle

Other factors such as diet, exercise, and stress affect fluid, electrolyte, and acid–base balance.

Lifespan Considerations

Elders

Certain changes related to aging place the elder at risk for serious problems with fluid and electrolyte imbalance, if homeostatic mechanisms are compromised. Some of the changes are

- A decrease in thirst sensation
- A decrease in ability of the kidneys to concentrate urine
- A decrease in intracellular fluid and in total body water
- A decrease in response to body hormones that help regulate fluid and electrolytes.

Other factors that may influence fluid and electrolyte balance in elders are

- Increased use of diuretics for hypertension and heart disease
- Decrease in fluid and food intake, especially in elders with dementia or who are dependent on others to feed them and offer them fluids
- Preparations for certain diagnostic tests that have the client NPO for long periods of time or cause diarrhea from laxative preps

- Clients with impaired renal function, such as elders and/or those with diabetes
- Those having certain diagnostic procedures. (Dyes used for some procedures, such as arteriograms and cardiac catheterizations, may cause further renal problems. Always see that the client is well hydrated before, during, and after the procedure to help in diluting and excreting the dye. If the client is NPO for the procedure, the nurse should check with the physician to see if IV fluids are needed.)
- Any condition that may tax the normal compensatory mechanisms, such as a fever, influenza, surgery, or heat exposure.

All of these conditions increase elders' risk for fluid and electrolyte imbalance. The change can happen quickly and become serious in a short time. Astute observations and quick actions by the nurse can help prevent serious consequences. A change in mental status may be the first symptom of impairment and must be further evaluated to determine the cause.

The intake of fluids and electrolytes is affected by the diet. People with anorexia nervosa or bulimia are at risk for severe fluid and electrolyte imbalances because of inadequate intake or purging regimens (e.g., induced vomiting, use of diuretics and laxatives). Seriously malnourished people have decreased serum albumin levels, and may develop edema because the osmotic draw of fluid into the vascular compartment is reduced. When calorie intake is not adequate to meet the body's needs, fat stores are broken down and fatty acids are released, increasing the risk of acidosis.

Regular weight-bearing physical exercise such as walking, running, or bicycling has a beneficial effect on calcium balance. The rate of bone loss that occurs in postmenopausal women and older men is slowed with regular exercise, reducing the risk of osteoporosis.

Stress can increase cellular metabolism, blood glucose concentration, and catecholamine levels. In addition, stress can increase production of ADH, which in turn decreases urine production. The overall response of the body to stress is to increase the blood volume.

Other lifestyle factors can also affect fluid, electrolyte, and acid–base balance. Heavy alcohol consumption affects electrolyte balance, increasing the risk of low calcium, magnesium, and phosphate levels. The risk of acidosis associated with breakdown of fat tissue also is greater in the person who drinks large amounts of alcohol.

DISTURBANCES IN FLUID VOLUME, ELECTROLYTE, AND ACID–BASE BALANCES

A number of factors such as illness, trauma, surgery, and medications can affect the body's ability to maintain fluid, electrolyte, and acid–base balance. Clients who are confused or unable to communicate their needs are at risk for inadequate fluid

intake. Vomiting, diarrhea, or nasogastric suction can cause significant fluid losses. Tissue trauma, such as burns, causes fluid and electrolytes to be lost from damaged cells. Decreased blood flow to the kidneys due to impaired cardiac function stimulates the renin-angiotensin-aldosterone system, causing sodium and water retention. Medications such as diuretics or corticosteroids can result in abnormal losses of electrolytes and fluid loss or retention. Diseases such as diabetes mellitus or chronic obstructive lung disease may affect acid–base balance.

Fluid Imbalances

Fluid imbalances are of two basic types: isotonic and osmolar. *Isotonic imbalances* occur when water and electrolytes are lost or gained in equal proportions, so that the osmolality of body fluids remains constant. *Osmolar imbalances* involve the loss or gain of only water, so that the osmolality of the serum is altered. Thus four categories of fluid imbalances may occur: (a) an isotonic loss of water and electrolytes, (b) an isotonic gain of water and electrolytes, (c) a hyperosmolar loss of only water, and (d) a hypo-osmolar gain of only water. These are referred to, respectively, as fluid volume deficit, fluid volume excess, dehydration, and overhydration (hypo-osmolar imbalance).

Fluid Volume Deficit

Isotonic **fluid volume deficit (FVD)** occurs when the body loses both water and electrolytes from the ECF in similar proportions. In FVD, fluid is initially lost from the intravascular compartment, so it often is called **hypovolemia.**

FVD generally occurs as a result of (a) abnormal losses through the skin, gastrointestinal tract, or kidney; (b) decreased intake of fluid; (c) bleeding; or (d) movement of fluid into a third space. See the section on third space syndrome that follows.

For the risk factors and clinical signs related to fluid volume deficit, see Table 50–4.

TABLE 50–4 Isotonic Fluid Volume Deficit

Risk Factors	Clinical Manifestations	Nursing Interventions
Loss of water and electrolytes from • Vomiting • Diarrhea • Excessive sweating • Polyuria • Fever • Nasogastric suction • Abnormal drainage or wound losses Insufficient intake due to • Anorexia • Nausea • Inability to access fluids • Impaired swallowing • Confusion, depression	Complaints of weakness and thirst Weight loss • 2% loss = mild FVD • 5% loss = moderate • 8% loss = severe Fluid intake less than output Decreased tissue turgor Dry mucous membranes, sunken eyeballs, decreased tearing Subnormal temperature Weak, rapid pulse Decreased blood pressure Postural (orthostatic) hypotension (significant drop in BP when moving from lying to sitting or standing position) Flat neck veins; decreased capillary refill Decreased central venous pressure Decreased urine volume (<30 mL/h) Increased specific gravity of urine (<1.030) Increased hematocrit Increased blood urea nitrogen (BUN)	Assess for clinical manifestations of FVD. Monitor weight and vital signs, including temperature. Assess tissue turgor. Assess breath sounds. Monitor fluid intake and output. Monitor laboratory findings. Administer oral and intravenous fluids as indicated. Provide frequent mouth care. Implement measures to prevent skin breakdown. Provide for safety, e.g., provide assistance for a client rising from bed.

THIRD SPACE SYNDROME. In **third space syndrome,** fluid shifts from the vascular space into an area where it is not readily accessible as extracellular fluid. This fluid remains in the body but is essentially unavailable for use, causing an isotonic fluid volume deficit. Fluid may be sequestered in the bowel, in the interstitial space as edema, in inflamed tissue, or in potential spaces such as the peritoneal or pleural cavities.

The client with third space syndrome has an isotonic fluid deficit but may not manifest apparent fluid loss or weight loss. Careful nursing assessment is vital to effectively identify and intervene for clients experiencing third-spacing. Because the fluid shifts back into the vascular compartment after time, assessment for manifestations of fluid volume excess or hypervolemia is also vital.

Fluid Volume Excess

Fluid volume excess (FVE) occurs when the body retains both water and sodium in similar proportions to normal ECF. This is commonly referred to as **hypervolemia** (increased blood volume). Because both water and sodium are retained, the serum sodium concentration remains essentially normal. FVE is always secondary to an increase in the total body sodium content. Specific causes of FVE include (a) excessive intake of sodium chloride; (b) administering sodium-containing infusions too rapidly, particularly to clients with impaired regulatory mechanisms; and (c) disease processes that alter regulatory mechanisms, such as heart failure, renal failure, cirrhosis of the liver, and Cushing's syndrome.

The risk factors and clinical manifestations for FVE are summarized in Table 50–5.

EDEMA. In fluid volume excess, both intravascular and interstitial spaces have an increased water and sodium content. Excess interstitial fluid is known as **edema.** Edema typically is most apparent in areas where the tissue pressure is low, such as around the eyes, and in dependent tissues (known as dependent edema), where hydrostatic capillary pressure is high.

Edema can be caused by several different mechanisms. The three main mechanisms are increased capillary hydrostatic pressure, decreased plasma oncotic pressure, and increased capillary permeability. It may be due to FVE that increases capillary hydrostatic pressures, pushing fluid into the interstitial tissues. This type of edema is often seen in dependent tissues such as the feet, ankles, and sacrum because of the effects of gravity. Low levels of plasma proteins from malnutrition or liver or kidney diseases can reduce the plasma oncotic pressure so that fluid is not drawn into the capillaries from interstitial tissues, causing edema. With tissue trauma and some disorders such as allergic reactions, capillaries become more permeable, allowing fluid to escape into interstitial tissues. Obstructed lymph flow impairs the movement of fluid from interstitial tissues back into the vascular compartment, resulting in edema.

Pitting edema is edema that leaves a small depression or pit after finger pressure is applied to the swollen area. The pit is caused by movement of fluid to adjacent tissue, away from the point of pressure (Figure 50–10 ■). Within 10 to 30 seconds the pit normally disappears.

TABLE 50–5 Fluid Volume Excess

Risk Factors	Clinical Manifestations	Nursing Interventions
Excess intake of sodium-containing intravenous fluids Excess ingestion of sodium in diet or medications (e.g., sodium bicarbonate antacids such as Alka-Seltzer or hypertonic enema solutions such as Fleet's) Impaired fluid balance regulation related to • Heart failure • Renal failure • Cirrhosis of the liver	Weight gain • 2% gain = mild FVE • 5% gain = moderate • 8% gain = severe Fluid intake greater than output Moist mucous membranes Full, bounding pulse; tachycardia Increased blood pressure and central venous pressure Distended neck and peripheral veins; slow vein emptying Moist crackles (rales) in lungs; dyspnea, shortness of breath Mental confusion	Assess for clinical manifestations of FVE. Monitor weight and vital signs. Assess for edema. Assess breath sounds. Monitor fluid intake and output. Monitor laboratory findings. Place in Fowler's position. Administer diuretics as ordered. Restrict fluid intake as indicated. Restrict dietary sodium as ordered. Implement measures to prevent skin breakdown.

Dehydration

Dehydration, or hyperosmolar imbalance, occurs when water is lost from the body without significant loss of electrolytes. Because water is lost while electrolytes, particularly sodium, are retained, the serum osmolality and serum sodium levels increase. Water is drawn into the vascular compartment from the interstitial space and cells, resulting in cellular dehydration. Older adults are at particular risk for dehydration because of decreased thirst sensation. This type of water deficit also can affect clients who are hyperventilating or have prolonged fever or in diabetic ketoacidosis and those receiving enteral feedings with insufficient water intake.

Overhydration

Overhydration, also known as hypo-osmolar imbalance or *water intoxication,* occurs when water is gained in excess of electrolytes, resulting in low serum osmolality and low serum sodium levels. Water is drawn into the cells, causing them to swell. In the brain this can lead to cerebral edema and impaired neurologic function. Water intoxication often occurs when both fluid and electrolytes are lost, for example, through excessive sweating, but only water is replaced. It can also result from the syndrome of inappropriate antidiuretic hormone (SIADH), a disorder that can occur with some malignant tumors, AIDS, head injury, or administration of certain drugs such as barbiturates or anesthetics.

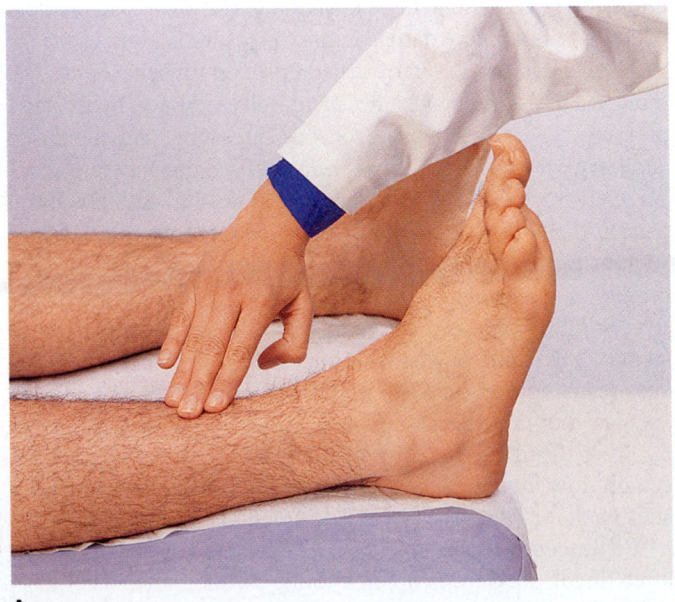

A

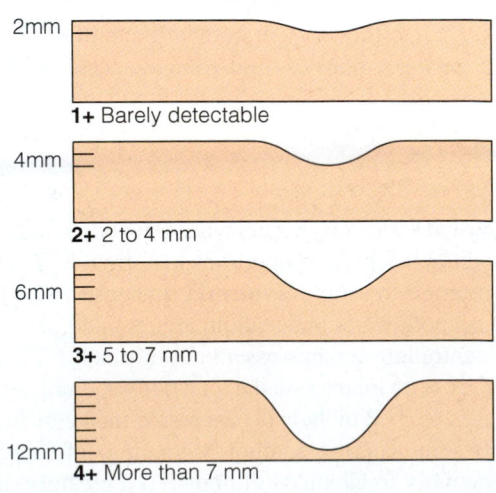

2mm — **1+** Barely detectable

4mm — **2+** 2 to 4 mm

6mm — **3+** 5 to 7 mm

12mm — **4+** More than 7 mm

B

Figure 50–10 ■ Evaluation of edema. *A,* Palpate for edema over the tibia as shown here and behind the medial malleolus, and over the dorsum of each foot. *B,* Four-point scale for grading edema.

Electrolyte Imbalances

The most common and most significant electrolyte imbalances involve sodium, potassium, calcium, magnesium, chloride, and phosphate.

Sodium

Sodium (Na^+), the most abundant cation in the extracellular fluid, not only moves into and out of the body but also moves in careful balance among the three fluid compartments. It is found in most body secretions, for example, saliva, gastric and intestinal secretions, bile, and pancreatic fluid. Therefore, continuous excretion of any of these fluids, such as via intestinal suction, can result in a sodium deficit. Because of its role in regulating water balance, sodium imbalances usually are accompanied by water imbalance.

Hyponatremia is a sodium deficit, or serum sodium level of less than 135 mEq/L. Because of sodium's role in determining the osmolality of ECF, hyponatremia typically results in a low serum osmolality. Water is drawn out of the vascular compartment into interstitial tissues and the cells (Figure 50–11 ■, A), causing the clinical manifestations associated with this disorder.

Hypernatremia is excess sodium in ECF, or a serum sodium of greater than 145 mEq/L. Because the osmotic pressure of extracellular fluid is increased, fluid moves out of the cells into the ECF (Figure 50–11 ■, B). As a result, the cells become dehydrated.

Table 50–6 lists risk factors and clinical signs for hyponatremia and hypernatremia.

Potassium

Although the amount of potassium (K^+) in extracellular fluid is small, it is vital to normal neuromuscular and cardiac function. Potassium is usually excreted by the kidneys. However, the kidneys do not regulate potassium excretion as effectively as they do sodium excretion. Therefore, an acute potassium deficiency can develop rapidly. Of the body's secretions, the gastrointestinal secretions are high in potassium.

Hypokalemia is a potassium deficit or a serum potassium level of less than 3.5 mEq/L. Gastrointestinal losses of potassium through vomiting and gastric suction are common causes of hypokalemia, as are the use of potassium-wasting diuretics, such as thiazide diuretics or loop diuretics (e.g., furosemide).

Hyperkalemia is a potassium excess or a serum potassium level greater than 5.0 mEq/L. Hyperkalemia is less common than hypokalemia and rarely occurs in clients with normal renal function. It is, however, more dangerous than hypokalemia, and can lead to cardiac arrest. Table 50–6 lists risk factors and clinical signs for hypokalemia and hyperkalemia.

> **► CLINICAL ALERT** *Potassium may be given intravenously for severe hypokalemia. It must ALWAYS be diluted appropriately and NEVER given IV push. Potassium that is to be given IV should be mixed in the pharmacy and double checked prior to administration by two nurses. The usual concentration of IV potassium is 20 to 40 mEq/L.* ■

Calcium

Regulating levels of calcium (Ca^{2+}) in the body is more complex than the other major electrolytes so calcium balance can be affected by many factors. Imbalances of this electrolyte are relatively common.

Hypocalcemia is a calcium deficit, or a total serum calcium level of less than 8.5 mg/dL and an ionized calcium level of less than 4.0 mg/dL. Severe depletion of calcium can cause tetany with muscle spasms and paresthesias and can lead to convulsions. Clients at greatest risk for hypocalcemia are those whose parathyroid glands have been removed. This is frequently associated with total thyroidectomy or bilateral neck surgery for cancer. Low serum magnesium levels (hypomagnesemia) and chronic alcoholism also increase the risk of hypocalcemia.

Hypercalcemia, or serum calcium levels greater than 10.5 mg/dL, most often occurs when calcium is mobilized from the bony skeleton. This may be due to malignancy or prolonged immobilization.

The risk factors and clinical manifestations related to calcium imbalances are found in Table 50–6.

Magnesium

Magnesium (Mg^{2+}) imbalances are relatively common in hospitalized clients, although they may be unrecognized. **Hypomagnesemia** occurs more frequently than hypermagnesemia. Chronic alcoholism is the most common cause of hypomagnesemia. Magnesium deficiency also may aggravate the manifestations of alcohol withdrawal, such as delirium tremens (DTs). **Hypermagnesemia** is present when the serum magnesium level rises. It is due to increased intake or decreased excretion. It is often iatrogenic, that is, a result of overzealous magnesium therapy.

Table 50–6 lists risk factors and manifestations for clients with altered magesium balance.

Chloride

Because of the relationship between sodium ions and chloride ions (Cl^-), imbalances of chloride commonly occur in conjunction with sodium imbalances. **Hypochloremia** is a decreased

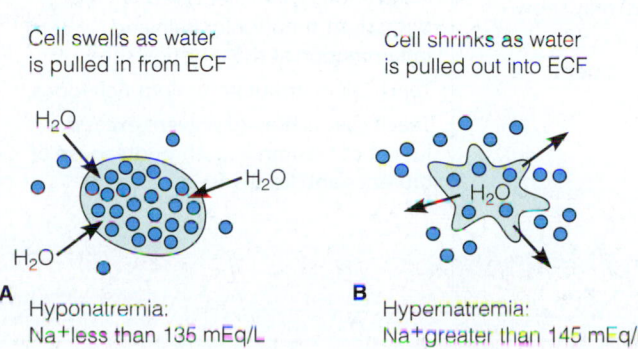

Cell swells as water is pulled in from ECF

Cell shrinks as water is pulled out into ECF

H_2O H_2O H_2O H_2O

A Hyponatremia: Na⁺less than 135 mEq/L

B Hypernatremia: Na⁺greater than 145 mEq/L

Figure 50–11 ■ The extracellular sodium level affects cell size. *A,* In hyponatremia, cells swell; *B,* in hypernatremia, cells shrink in size.

TABLE 50-6 Electrolyte Imbalances

Risk Factors	Clinical Manifestations	Nursing Interventions
Hyponatremia *Loss of sodium* • Gastrointestinal fluid loss • Sweating • Use of diuretics *Gain of water* • Hypotonic tube feedings • Drinking water • Excess IV D5W (dextrose in water) administration *Syndrome of inappropriate ADH (SIADH)* • Head injury • AIDS • Malignant tumors	Lethargy, confusion, apprehension Muscle twitching Abdominal cramps Anorexia, nausea, vomiting Headache Seizures, coma *Laboratory findings:* Serum sodium below 135 mEq/L Serum osmolality below 280 mOsm/kg	Assess clinical manifestations. Monitor fluid intake and output. Monitor laboratory data (e.g., serum sodium). Assess client closely if administering hypertonic saline solutions. Encourage food and fluid high in sodium if permitted (e.g., table salt, bacon, ham, processed cheese). Limit water intake as indicated.
Hypernatremia *Loss of fluids* • Insensible water loss (hyperventilation or fever) • Diarrhea *Water deprivation* Excess salt intake • Parenteral administration of saline solutions • Hypertonic tube feedings without adequate water • Excessive use of table salt (1 tsp contains 2,300 mg of sodium) Conditions such as • Diabetes insipidus • Heat stroke	Thirst Dry, sticky mucous membranes Tongue red, dry, swollen Weakness Postural hypotension, dyspnea Severe hypernatremia: • Fatigue, restlessness • Decreasing level of consciousness • Disorientation • Convulsions *Laboratory findings:* Serum sodium above 145 mEq/L Serum osmolality above 300 mOsm/kg	Monitor fluid intake and output. Monitor behavior changes (e.g., restlessness, disorientation). Monitor laboratory findings (e.g., serum sodium). Encourage fluids as ordered. Monitor diet as ordered (e.g., restrict intake of salt and foods high in sodium).
Hypokalemia *Loss of potassium* • Vomiting and gastric suction • Diarrhea • Heavy perspiration Use of potassium-wasting drugs (e.g., diuretics) Poor intake of potassium (as with debilitated clients, alcoholics, anorexia nervosa) Hyperaldosteronism	Muscle weakness, leg cramps Fatigue, lethargy Anorexia, nausea, vomiting Decreased bowel sounds, decreased bowel motility Cardiac dysrhythmias Depressed deep-tendon reflexes *Laboratory findings:* Serum potassium below 3.5 mEq/L Arterial blood gases (ABGs) may show alkalosis T wave flattening and ST segment depression on ECG	Monitor heart rate and rhythm. Monitor clients receiving digitalis (e.g., digoxin) closely, because hypokalemia increases risk of digitalis toxicity. Administer oral potassium as ordered with food or fluid to prevent gastric irritation. Administer IV potassium solutions at a rate no faster than 10–20 mEq/h; never administer undiluted potassium intravenously. For clients receiving IV potassium, monitor for pain and inflammation at the injection site. Teach client about potassium-rich foods. Teach clients how to prevent excessive loss of potassium (e.g., through abuse of diuretics and laxatives).

TABLE 50–6 Electrolyte Imbalances (continued)

Risk Factors	Clinical Manifestations	Nursing Interventions
Hyperkalemia		
Decreased potassium excretion • Renal failure • Hypoaldosteronism • Potassium-conserving diuretics	Gastrointestinal hyperactivity, diarrhea Irritability, apathy, confusion Cardiac dysrhythmias or arrest Muscle weakness, areflexia (absence of reflexes)	Closely monitor cardiac status and ECG. Administer diuretics and other medications such as glucose and insulin as ordered. Hold potassium supplements and K^+ conserving diuretics.
High potassium intake • Excessive use of K^+ containing salt substitutes • Excessive or rapid IV infusion of potassium Potassium shift out of the tissue cells into the plasma (e.g., infections, burns, acidosis)	Paresthesias and numbness in extremities *Laboratory findings:* Serum potassium above 5.0 mEq/L Peaked T wave, widened QRS on ECG	Monitor serum K^+ levels carefully; a rapid drop may occur as potassium shifts into the cells. Teach clients to avoid foods high in potassium and salt substitutes.
Hypocalcemia		
Surgical removal of the parathyroid glands Conditions such as • Hypoparathyroidism • Acute pancreatitis • Hyperphosphatemia • Thyroid carcinoma *Inadequate vitamin D intake* • Malabsorption • Hypomagnesemia • Alkalosis • Sepsis • Alcohol abuse	Numbness, tingling of the extremities and around the mouth Muscle tremors, cramps; if severe can progress to tetany and convulsions Cardiac dysrhythmias; decreased cardiac output Positive Trousseau's and Chvostek's signs (see Table 50–8) Confusion, anxiety, possible psychoses *Laboratory findings:* Serum calcium less than 8.5 mg/dL or 4.5 mEq/L (total)	Closely monitor respiratory and cardiovascular status. Take precautions to protect a confused client. Administer oral or parenteral calcium supplements as ordered. When administering intravenously, closely monitor cardiac status and ECG during infusion. Teach clients at high risk for osteoporosis about • Dietary sources rich in calcium • Recommendation for 1,000–1,500 mg of calcium per day • Calcium supplements • Regular exercise • Estrogen replacement therapy for postmenopausal women.
Hypercalcemia		
Prolonged immobilization Conditions such as • Hyperparathyroidism • Malignancy of the bone • Paget's disease	Lethargy, weakness Depressed deep-tendon reflexes Anorexia, nausea, vomiting Constipation Polyuria, hypercalciuria Flank pain secondary to urinary calculi Dysrhythmias, possible heart block *Laboratory findings:* Serum calcium greater than 10.5 mg/dL or 5.5 mEq/L (total)	Increase client movement and exercise. Encourage oral fluids as permitted to maintain a dilute urine. Teach clients to limit intake of food and fluid high in calcium. Encourage ingestion of fiber to prevent constipation. Protect a confused client; monitor for pathologic fractures in clients with long-term hypercalcemia. Encourage intake of acid-ash fluids (e.g., prune or cranberry juice) to counteract deposits of calcium salts in the urine.
Hypomagnesemia		
Excessive loss from the gastrointestinal tract (e.g., from nasogastric suction, diarrhea, fistula drainage) Long-term use of certain drugs (e.g., diuretics, aminoglycoside antibiotics)	Neuromuscular irritability with tremors Increased reflexes, tremors, convulsions Positive Chvostek's and Trousseau's signs (see Table 50–8)	Assess clients receiving digitalis for digitalis toxicity. Hypomagnesemia increases the risk toxicity.

continued on page 1368

TABLE 50-6 Electrolyte Imbalances (continued)

Risk Factors	Clinical Manifestations	Nursing Interventions
Conditions such as • Chronic alcoholism • Pancreatitis • Burns	Tachycardia, elevated blood pressure, dysrhythmias Disorientation and confusion Vertigo *Laboratory findings:* Serum magnesium below 1.5 mEq/L	Take protective measures when there is a possibility of seizures. • Assess the client's ability to swallow water prior to initiating oral feeding. • Initiate safety measures to prevent injury during seizure activity. • Carefully administer magnesium salts as ordered. Encourage clients to eat magnesium-rich foods if permitted (e.g., whole grains, meat, seafood, and green leafy vegetables). Refer clients to alcohol treatment programs as indicated.
Hypermagnesemia Abnormal retention of magnesium, as in • Renal failure • Adrenal insufficiency Treatment with magnesium salts	Peripheral vasodilation, flushing Nausea, vomiting Muscle weakness, paralysis Hypotension, bradycardia Depressed deep-tendon reflexes Lethargy, drowsiness Respiratory depression, coma Respiratory and cardiac arrest if hypermagnesemia is severe *Laboratory findings:* Serum magnesium above 2.5 mEq/L Electrocardiogram showing prolonged QT interval; an AV block may occur	Monitor vital signs and level of consciousness when clients are at risk. If patellar reflexes are absent, notify the physician. Advise clients who have renal disease to contact their care provider before taking over-the-counter drugs.

serum chloride level and is usually related to excess losses of chloride ion through the GI tract, kidneys, or sweating. Hypochloremic clients are at risk for alkalosis and may experience muscle twitching, tremors, or tetany.

Conditions that cause sodium retention also can lead to a high serum chloride level or **hyperchloremia.** Excess replacement of sodium chloride or potassium chloride are additional risk factors for high serum chloride levels. The manifestations of hyperchloremia include acidosis, weakness, and lethargy, with a risk of dysrhythmias and coma.

Phosphate

The phosphate anion PO_4^- is found both in intracellular and extracellular fluid. Most of the phosphorus (P^+) in the body exists as PO_4^-. Phosphate is critical for cellular metabolism because it is a major component of adenosine triphosphate (ATP).

Phosphate imbalances frequently are related to therapeutic interventions for other disorders. Glucose and insulin administration and total parenteral nutrition can cause phosphate to shift into the cells from extracellular fluid compartments, leading to **hypophosphatemia,** a low serum phosphate. Alcohol

withdrawal, acid–base imbalances, and the use of antacids that bind with phosphate in the GI tract are other possible causes of low serum phosphate levels. Manifestations of hypophosphatemia include paresthesias, muscle weakness and pain, mental changes, and possible seizures.

Hyperphosphatemia occurs when phosphate shifts out of the cells into extracellular fluids (e.g., due to tissue trauma or chemotherapy for malignant tumors), in renal failure, or when excess phosphate is administered or ingested. Infants who are fed cow's milk are at risk for hyperphosphatemia, as are people using phosphate-containing enemas or laxatives. Clients who have high serum phosphate levels may experience numbness and tingling around the mouth and in the fingertips, muscle spasms, and tetany.

Acid–Base Imbalances

Acid–base imbalances generally are classified as *respiratory* or *metabolic* by the general or underlying cause of the disorder. Carbonic acid levels are normally regulated by the lungs through the retention or excretion of carbon dioxide, and problems of regulation lead to respiratory acidosis or alkalosis.

Bicarbonate and hydrogen ion levels are regulated by the kidneys, and problems of regulation lead to metabolic acidosis or alkalosis. Healthy regulatory systems will attempt to correct acid–base imbalances, a process called **compensation.**

Respiratory Acidosis

Hypoventilation and carbon dioxide retention cause carbonic acid levels to increase and the pH to fall below 7.35, a condition known as **respiratory acidosis.** Serious lung diseases such as asthma and COPD are common causes of respiratory acidosis. Central nervous system depression due to anesthesia or a narcotic overdose can sufficiently slow the respiratory rate so that carbon dioxide is retained. When respiratory acidosis occurs, the kidneys retain bicarbonate to restore the normal carbonic acid to bicarbonate ratio. Recall, however, that the kidneys are relatively slow to respond to changes in acid–base balance, so this compensatory response may require hours to days to restore the normal pH.

Respiratory Alkalosis

When a person hyperventilates, more carbon dioxide than normal is exhaled, carbonic acid levels fall, and the pH rises to greater than 7.45. This condition is termed **respiratory alkalosis.** Psychogenic or anxiety-related hyperventilation is a common cause of respiratory alkalosis. Other causes include fever and respiratory infections. In respiratory alkalosis, the kidneys will excrete bicarbonate to return the pH to within the normal range. Often, however, the cause of the hyperventilation is eliminated and the pH returns to normal before renal compensation occurs.

Metabolic Acidosis

When bicarbonate levels are low in relation to the amount of carbonic acid in the body, the pH falls and **metabolic acidosis** develops. This may develop because of renal failure and the inability of the kidneys to excrete hydrogen ion and produce bicarbonate. It also may occur when too much acid is produced in the body, for example, in diabetic ketoacidosis or starvation when fat tissue is broken down for energy. Metabolic acidosis stimulates the respiratory center, and the rate and depth of respirations increase. Carbon dioxide is eliminated and carbonic acid levels fall, minimizing the change in pH. This respiratory compensation occurs within minutes of the pH imbalance.

Metabolic Alkalosis

In **metabolic alkalosis,** the amount of bicarbonate in the body exceeds the normal 20-to-1 ratio. Ingestion of bicarbonate of soda as an antacid is one cause of metabolic alkalosis. Another cause is prolonged vomiting with loss of hydrochloric acid from the stomach. The respiratory center is depressed in metabolic alkalosis, and respirations slow and become more shallow. Carbon dioxide is retained and carbonic acid levels increase, helping balance the excess bicarbonate.

The risk factors and manifestations for acid–base imbalances are listed in Table 50–7.

NURSING MANAGEMENT

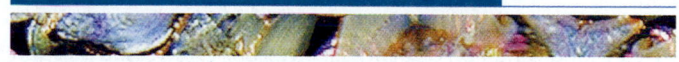

ASSESSING

Assessing clients for fluid, electrolyte, and acid–base balance and imbalances is an important nursing care function. Components of the assessment include (a) the nursing history, (b) physical assessment of the client, (c) clinical measurements, and (d) review of laboratory test results.

Nursing History

The nursing history is particularly important for identifying clients who are at risk for fluid, electrolyte, and acid–base imbalances. The current and past medical history reveal conditions such as chronic lung disease or diabetes mellitus that can disrupt normal balances. Medications prescribed to treat acute or chronic conditions (e.g., diuretic therapy for hypertension) also may place the client at risk for altered homeostasis. Functional, developmental, and socioeconomic factors must also be considered in assessing the client's risk. Older people and very young children, clients who must depend on others to meet their needs for food and fluid intake, and people who cannot afford or do not have the means to cook food for a balanced diet (e.g., homeless people) are at greater risk for fluid and electrolyte imbalances. Common risk factors are listed in Box 50–3.

When obtaining the nursing history, the nurse needs to not only recognize risk factors but also elicit data about the client's food and fluid intake, fluid output, and the presence of signs or symptoms suggestive of altered fluid and electrolyte balance. The Assessment Interview on page 1371 provides examples of questions to elicit information regarding fluid, electrolyte, and acid–base balance.

Physical Assessment

Physical assessment to evaluate a client's fluid, electrolyte, and acid–base status focuses on the skin, the oral cavity and mucous membranes, the eyes, the cardiovascular and respiratory systems, and neurologic and muscular status. Data from this physical assessment are used to expand and verify information obtained in the nursing history. The focused physical assessment is summarized in Table 50–8 on page 1372; refer to Tables 50–5 through 50–8 for possible abnormal findings related to specific imbalances.

Clinical Measurements

Three simple clinical measurements that the nurse can initiate without a physician's order are daily weights, vital signs, and fluid intake and output.

Daily Weights. Daily weight measurements provide a relatively accurate assessment of a client's fluid status. Significant changes in weight over a short time (e.g., days to a week or two) are indicative of acute fluid changes. Each kilogram (2.2 lb) of weight gained or lost is equivalent to 1 L of fluid gained or lost. Such fluid gains or losses indicate changes in total body fluid volume rather than in any specific compartment, such as

TABLE 50–7 Acid-Base Imbalances

Risk Factors	Clinical Manifestations	Nursing Interventions
Respiratory Acidosis Acute lung conditions that impair alveolar gas exchange (e.g., pneumonia, acute pulmonary edema, aspiration of foreign body, near-drowning) Chronic lung disease (e.g., asthma, cystic fibrosis, or emphysema) Overdose of narcotics or sedatives that depress respiratory rate and depth Brain injury that affects the respiratory center	Increased pulse and respiratory rates Headache, dizziness Confusion, decreased level of consciousness (LOC) Convulsions Warm, flushed skin **Chronic:** Weakness Headache *Laboratory findings:* Arterial blood pH less than 7.35 $PaCO_2$ above 45 mm Hg HCO_3^- normal or slightly elevated in acute; above 26 mEq/L in chronic	Frequently assess respiratory status and lung sounds. Monitor airway and ventilation; insert artificial airway and prepare for mechanical ventilation as necessary. Administer pulmonary therapy measures such as inhalation therapy, percussion and postural drainage, bronchodilators, and antibiotics as ordered. Monitor fluid intake and output, vital signs, and arterial blood gases. Administer narcotic antagonists as indicated. Maintain adequate hydration (2–3 L of fluid per day).
Respiratory Alkalosis Hyperventilation due to • Extreme anxiety • Elevated body temperature • Overventilation with a mechanical ventilator • Hypoxia • Salicylate overdose	Complaints of shortness of breath, chest tightness Light-headedness with circumoral paresthesias and numbness and tingling of the extremities Difficulty concentrating Tremulousness, blurred vision *Laboratory findings (in uncompensated respiratory alkalosis):* Arterial blood pH above 7.45 $PaCO_2$ less than 35 mm Hg	Monitor vital signs and ABGs. Assist client to breathe more slowly. Help client breathe in a paper bag or apply a rebreather mask (to inhale CO_2).
Metabolic Acidosis Conditions that increase nonvolatile acids in the blood (e.g., renal impairment, diabetes mellitus, starvation) Conditions that decrease bicarbonate (e.g., prolonged diarrhea) Excessive infusion of chloride-containing IV fluids (e.g., NaCl)	Kussmaul's respirations (deep, rapid respirations) Lethargy, confusion Headache Weakness Nausea and vomiting *Laboratory findings:* Arterial blood pH below 7.35 Serum bicarbonate less than 22 mEq/L $PaCO_2$ less than 38 mm Hg with respiratory compensation	Monitor ABG values, intake and output, and LOC. Administer IV sodium bicarbonate carefully if ordered. Treat underlying problem as ordered.
Metabolic Alkalosis Excessive acid losses due to • Vomiting • Gastric suction Excessive use of potassium-losing diuretics Excessive adrenal corticoid hormones due to • Cushing's syndrome • Hyperaldosteronism Excessive bicarbonate intake from • Antacids • Parenteral $NaHCO_3$	Decreased respiratory rate and depth Dizziness Circumoral paresthesias, numbness and tingling of the extremities Hypertonic muscles, tetany *Laboratory findings:* Arterial blood pH above 7.45 Serum bicarbonate greater than 26 mEq/L $PaCO_2$ higher than 45 mm Hg with respiratory compensation	Monitor intake and output closely. Monitor vital signs, especially respirations, and LOC. Administer ordered IV fluids carefully. Treat underlying problem.

BOX 50–3 ■ **Common Risk Factors for Fluid, Electrolyte, and Acid–Base Imbalances**

Chronic Diseases and Conditions
- Chronic lung disease (COPD, asthma, cystic fibrosis)
- Heart failure
- Kidney disease
- Diabetes mellitus
- Cushing's syndrome or Addison's disease
- Cancer
- Malnutrition, anorexia nervosa, bulimia
- Ileostomy

Acute Conditions
- Acute gastroenteritis
- Bowel obstruction
- Head injury or decreased level of consciousness
- Trauma such as burns or crushing injuries
- Surgery
- Fever, draining wounds, fistulas

Medications
- Diuretics
- Corticosteroids
- Nonsteroidal anti-inflammatory drugs

Treatments
- Chemotherapy
- IV therapy and total parenteral nutrition
- Nasogastric suction
- Enteral feedings
- Mechanical ventilation

Other Factors
- Age: Very old or very young
- Inability to access food and fluids independently

---

the intravascular compartment. Rapid losses or gains of 5% to 8% of total body weight indicate moderate to severe fluid volume deficits or excesses.

To obtain accurate weight measurements, the nurse should balance the scale before each use and weigh the client (a) at the same time each day (e.g., before breakfast and after the first void), (b) wearing the same or similar clothing, and (c) on the same scale. The type of scale (i.e., standing, bed, chair) should be documented.

Regular assessment of weight is particularly important for clients in the community and extended care facilities who are at risk for fluid imbalance. For these clients, measuring intake and output may be impractical because of lifestyle or problems with incontinence. Regular weight measurement, either daily,

---

Assessment Interview

FLUID, ELECTROLYTE, AND ACID–BASE BALANCE

Current and Past Medical History
- Are you currently seeing a health care provider for treatment of any chronic diseases such as kidney disease, heart disease, high blood pressure, diabetes insipidus, or thyroid or parathyroid disorders?
- Have you recently experienced any acute conditions such as gastroenteritis, severe trauma, head injury, or surgery? If so, describe them.

Medications and Treatments
- Are you currently taking any medications on a regular basis such as diuretics, steroids, potassium supplements, calcium supplements, hormones, salt substitutes, or antacids?
- Have you recently undergone any treatments such as dialysis, parenteral nutrition, or tube feedings or been on a ventilator? If so, when and why?

Food and Fluid Intake
- How much and what type of fluids do you drink each day?
- Describe your diet for a typical day. (Pay particular attention to the client's intake of foods high in sodium content, of protein and of whole grains, fruits, and vegetables.)
- Have there been any recent changes in your food or fluid intake, for example, as a result of following a weight-loss program?
- Are you on any type of restricted diet?

- Has your food or fluid intake recently been affected by changes in appetite, nausea, or other factors such as pain or difficulty breathing?

Fluid Output
- Have you noticed any recent changes in the frequency or amount of urine output?
- Have you recently experienced any problems with vomiting, diarrhea, or constipation? If so, when and for how long?
- Have you noticed any other unusual fluid losses such as excessive sweating?

Fluid, Electrolyte, and Acid–Base Imbalances
- Have you gained or lost weight in recent weeks?
- Have you recently experienced any symptoms such as excessive thirst, dry skin or mucous membranes, dark or concentrated urine, or low urine output?
- Do you have problems with swelling of your hands, feet, or ankles? Do you ever have difficulty breathing, especially when lying down or at night? How many pillows do you use to sleep?
- Have you recently experienced any of the following symptoms: difficulty concentrating or confusion; dizziness or feeling faint; muscle weakness, twitching, cramping, or spasm; excessive fatigue; abnormal sensations such as numbness, tingling, burning, or prickling; abdominal cramping or distention; heart palpitations?

TABLE 50-8 Focused Physical Assessment for Fluid, Electrolyte, or Acid–Base Imbalances

System	Assessment Focus	Technique	Possible Abnormal Findings
Skin	Color, temperature, moisture	Inspection, palpation	Flushed, warm, very dry Moist or diaphoretic Cool and pale
	Turgor	Gently pinch up a fold of skin over sternum or inner aspect of thigh for adults, on the abdomen or medial thigh for children	Poor turgor: Skin remains tented for several seconds instead of immediately returning to normal position
	Edema	Inspect for visible swelling around eyes, in fingers, and in lower extremities	Skin around eyes is puffy, lids appear swollen; rings are tight; shoes leave impressions on feet
		Compress the skin over the dorsum of the foot, around the ankles, over the tibia, in the sacral area	Depression remains (pitting): see scale for describing edema in Figure 50–10
Mucous membranes	Color, moisture	Inspection	Mucous membranes dry, dull in appearance; tongue dry and cracked
Eyes	Firmness	Gently palpate eyeball with lid closed	Eyeball feels soft to palpation
Fontanels (infant)	Firmness, level	Inspect and gently palpate anterior fontanel	Fontanel bulging, firm Fontanel sunken, soft
Cardiovascular system	Heart rate	Auscultation, cardiac monitor	Tachycardia, bradycardia; irregular; dysrhythmias
	Peripheral pulses	Palpation	Weak and thready; bounding
	Blood pressure	Auscultation of Korotkoff's sounds	Hypotension
		BP assessment lying and standing	Postural hypotension
	Capillary refill	Palpation	Slowed capillary refill
	Venous filling	Inspection of jugular veins and hand veins	Jugular venous distention; flat jugular veins, poor venous refill
Respiratory system	Respiratory rate and pattern	Inspection	Increased or decreased rate and depth of respirations
	Lung sounds	Auscultation	Crackles or moist rales
Neurologic	Level of consciousness (LOC)	Observation, stimulation	Decreased LOC, lethargy, stupor, or coma
	Orientation, cognition	Questioning	Disoriented, confused; difficulty concentrating
	Motor function	Strength testing	Weakness, decreased motor strength
	Reflexes	Deep-tendon reflex (DTR) testing	Hyperactive or depressed DTRs
	Abnormal reflexes	*Chvostek's sign:* Tap over facial nerve about 2 cm anterior to tragus of ear	Facial muscle twitching including eyelids and lips on side of stimulus
		Trousseau's sign: Inflate a blood pressure cuff on the upper arm to 20 mm Hg greater than the systolic pressure, leave in place for 2 to 5 minutes	Carpal spasm: contraction of hand and fingers on affected side

every other day, or weekly, provides valuable information about the client's fluid volume status.

Vital Signs. Changes in the vital signs may indicate, or in some cases precede, fluid, electrolyte, and acid–base imbalances. For example, elevated body temperature may be a result of dehydration or a cause of increased body fluid losses.

Tachycardia is an early sign of hypovolemia. Pulse volume will decrease in FVD and increase in FVE. Irregular pulse rates may occur with electrolyte imbalances. Changes in respiratory rate and depth may cause respiratory acid–base imbalances or act as a compensatory mechanism in metabolic acidosis or alkalosis.

Blood pressure, a sensitive measure to detect blood volume changes, may fall significantly with FVD and hypovolemia or increase with FVE. Postural, or orthostatic, hypotension may also occur with FVD and hypovolemia.

To assess for orthostatic hypotension, measure the client's blood pressure and pulse in a supine position. Allow the client to remain in that position for 3 to 5 minutes, leaving the blood pressure cuff on the arm. Stand the client up and immediately reassess the blood pressure and pulse. A drop of 10 to 15 mm Hg in the systolic blood pressure with a corresponding drop in diastolic pressure and an increased pulse rate (by 10 or more beats per minute) is indicative of orthostatic or postural hypotension.

Fluid Intake and Output. The measurement and recording of all fluid intake and output (I & O) during a 24-hour period provides important data about the client's fluid and electrolyte balance. Generally, intake and output are measured for hospitalized at-risk clients.

The unit used to measure intake and output is the milliliter (mL) or cubic centimeter (cc); these are equivalent metric units of measurement. In household measures, 30 mL is roughly equivalent to 1 fluid ounce, 500 mL is about 1 pint, and 1,000 mL is about 1 quart. To measure fluid intake, nurses convert household measures such as a glass, cup, or soup bowl to metric units. Most agencies provide conversion tables, since the sizes of dishes vary from agency to agency. Such a table is often provided on or with the bedside I & O record. Examples of equivalents are given in Box 50–4.

Most agencies have a form for recording I & O, usually a bedside record on which the nurse lists all items measured and the quantities per shift (Figure 50–12 ■). Some agencies have another form for recording the specifics of intravenous fluids, such as the type of solution, additives, time started, amounts absorbed, and amounts remaining per shift.

It is important to inform clients, family members, and all caregivers that accurate measurements of the client's fluid intake and output are required, explaining why and emphasizing the need to use a bedpan, urinal, commode, or in-toilet collection device (unless a urinary drainage system is in place). Instruct the client not to put toilet tissue into the container with urine. Clients who wish to be involved in recording fluid intake measurements need to be taught how to compute the values and what foods are considered fluids.

To measure fluid intake, the nurse records on the I & O form each fluid item taken (if the client has not already done so),

specifying the time and type of fluid. All of the following fluids need to be recorded:

- Oral fluids. Water, milk, juice, soft drinks, coffee, tea, cream, soup, and any other beverages. Include water taken with medications. To assess the amount of water taken from a water pitcher, measure what remains and subtract this amount from the volume of the full pitcher. Then refill the pitcher.
- Ice chips. Record the fluid as approximately one-half the volume of the ice chips. For example, if the ice chips fill a cup holding 200 mL and the client consumed all of the ice chips, the volume consumed would be recorded as 100 mL.
- Foods that are or tend to become liquid at room temperature. These include ice cream, sherbert, custard, and gelatin. Do not measure foods that are pureed, because purees are simply solid foods prepared in a different form.
- Tube feedings. Remember to include the 30- to 60-mL water flush at the end of intermittent feedings or during continuous feedings.

			PATIENT LABEL
	Intake and Output Record		
INTAKE	0600-1800	1800-0600	TOTAL
Oral			
Tube feeding			
IV (primary)			
IV Meds			
TPN			
Blood			
TOTAL			24-Hour Total
OUTPUT	0600-1800	1800-0600	TOTAL
Urine			
Emesis			
G.I. Suction			
Stool			
TOTAL			24-Hour Total

Figure 50–12 ■ A sample 24-hour fluid intake and output record.

BOX 50–4   ■ Commonly Used Fluid Containers and Their Volumes

Water glass	200 mL	Creamer	
Juice glass	120 mL	Large	90 mL
Cup	180 mL	Small	30 mL
Soup bowl		Water pitcher	1,000 mL
Adult	180 mL	Jello, custard dish	100 mL
Child	100 mL	Ice cream dish	120 mL
Teapot	240 mL	Paper cup	
		Large	200 mL
		Small	120 mL

- Parenteral fluids. The exact amount of intravenous fluid administered is to be recorded, since some fluid containers may be overfilled. Blood transfusions are included.
- Intravenous medications. Intravenous medications that are prepared with solutions such as normal saline (NS) and are administered as an intermittent or continuous infusion must also be included (e.g., ceftazidime 1 g in 50 mL of sterile water). Most intravenous medications are mixed in 50 to 100 mL of solution.
- Catheter or tube irrigants. Fluid used to irrigate urinary catheters, nasogastric tubes, and intestinal tubes must be measured and recorded if not immediately withdrawn.

To measure fluid output, measure the following fluids (remember to observe appropriate infection control precautions):

- Urinary output. Following each voiding, pour the urine into a measuring container, observe the amount, and record it and the time of voiding on the I & O form. For clients with retention catheters, empty the drainage bag into a measuring container at the end of the shift (or at prescribed times if output is to be measured more often). Note and record the amount of urine output. In intensive care areas, urine output often is measured hourly. If the client is incontinent of urine, estimate and record these outputs. For example, for an incontinent client the nurse might record "Incontinent × 3" or "Drawsheet soaked in 12-in. diameter." A more accurate estimate of the urine output of infants and incontinent clients may be obtained by first weighing diapers or incontinent pads that are dry, and then subtracting this weight from the weight of the soiled items. Each gram of weight left after subtracting is equal to 1 mL of urine. If urine is frequently soiled with feces, the number of voidings may be recorded rather than the volume of urine.
- Vomitus and liquid feces. The amount and type of fluid and the time need to be specified.
- Tube drainage, such as gastric or intestinal drainage.
- Wound drainage and draining fistulas. Wound drainage may be recorded by documenting the type and number of dressings or linen saturated with drainage or by measuring the exact amount of drainage collected in a vacuum drainage (e.g., Hemovac) or gravity drainage system.

Fluid intake and output measurements are totaled at the end of the shift (every 8 to 12 hours), and the totals are recorded in the client's permanent record. In intensive care areas, the nurse may record intake and output hourly. Usually the staff on night shift totals the amounts of I & O recorded for each shift and records the 24-hour total.

To determine whether the fluid output is proportional to fluid intake or whether there are any changes in the client's fluid status, the nurse (a) compares the total 24-hour fluid output measurement with the total fluid intake measurement and (b) compares both to previous measurements. Urinary output is normally equivalent to the amount of fluids ingested; the usual range is 1,500 to 2,000 mL in 24 hours, or 40 to 80 mL in 1 hour (0.5 mL/kg/hour). Clients whose output substantially exceeds intake are at risk for fluid volume deficit. By contrast, clients whose intake substantially exceeds output are at risk for fluid volume excess. In assessing the client's fluid balance it is im-

portant to consider additional factors that may affect intake and output. The client who is extremely diaphoretic or who has rapid, deep respirations has fluid losses that cannot be measured but must be considered in evaluating fluid status.

When there is a significant discrepancy between intake and output or when fluid intake or output is inadequate (for example, a urine output of less than 500 mL in 24 hours or less than 0.5 mL per kilogram per hour in an adult), this information should be reported to the charge nurse, physician, or other care provider.

Laboratory Tests

Many laboratory studies are conducted to determine the client's fluid, electrolyte, and acid–base status. Some of the more common tests are discussed here.

Serum Electrolytes. Serum electrolyte levels are often routinely ordered for any client admitted to hospital as a screening test for electrolyte and acid–base imbalances. Serum electrolytes also are routinely assessed for clients at risk in the community, for example, clients who are being treated with a diuretic for hypertension or heart failure. The most commonly ordered serum tests are for sodium, potassium, chloride, magnesium, and bicarbonate ions. Normal values of commonly measured electrolytes are shown in Box 50–5.

Complete Blood Count (CBC). The complete blood count, another basic screening test, includes information about the hematocrit (Hct). The **hematocrit** measures the volume (percentage) of whole blood that is composed of RBCs. Because the hematocrit is a measure of the volume of cells in relation to plasma, it is affected by changes in plasma volume. Thus the hematocrit increases with severe dehydration and decreases with severe overhydration. Normal hematocrit values are 40% to 54% (men) and 37% to 47% (women).

Osmolality. *Serum osmolality* is a measure of the solute concentration of the blood. The particles included are sodium ions, glucose, and urea (blood urea nitrogen, or BUN). Serum osmolality can be estimated by doubling the serum sodium, because sodium and its associated chloride ions are the major determinants of serum osmolality. Serum osmolality values are used primarily to evaluate fluid balance. Normal values are 280 to 300 mOsm/kg. An increase in serum osmolality indicates a fluid volume deficit; a decrease reflects a fluid volume excess.

Urine osmolality is a measure of the solute concentration of urine. The particles included are nitrogenous wastes, such as creatinine, urea, and uric acid. Normal values are 500 to 800 mOsm/kg. An increased urine osmolality indicates a fluid volume deficit; a decreased urine osmolality reflects a fluid volume excess.

Urine pH. Measurement of urine pH may be obtained by laboratory analysis or by using a dipstick on a freshly voided specimen. Because the kidneys play a critical role in regulating acid–base balance, assessment of urine pH can be useful in determining whether the kidneys are responding appropriately to acid–base imbalances. Normally the pH of the urine is relatively acidic, averaging about 6.0, but a range of 4.6 to 8.0 is

BOX 50–5 ■ Normal Electrolyte Values for Adults*	
Venous blood	
Sodium	135–145 mEq/L
Potassium	3.5–5.0 mEq/L
Chloride	95–105 mEq/L
Calcium (total)	4.5–5.5 mEq/L or 8.5–10.5 mg/dL
(ionized)	56% of total calcium (2.5 mEq/L or 4.0–5.0 mg/dL)
Magnesium	1.5–2.5 mEq/L or 1.6–2.5 mg/dL
Phosphate (phosphorus)	1.8–2.6 mEq/L
Serum osmolality	280–300 mOsm/kg water

*Normal laboratory values vary from agency to agency.

BOX 50–6 ■ Normal Values of Arterial Blood Gases*	
pH	7.35–7.45
PaO_2	80–100 mm Hg
$PaCO_2$	35–45 mm Hg
HCO_3^-	22–26 mEq/L
Base excess	−2 to +2 mEq/L
O_2 saturation	95–98%

*Some normal values will vary according to the kind of test carried out in the laboratory. Nurses are advised to use the normal values issued by the agency when interpreting laboratory results.

considered normal. In metabolic acidosis, urine pH should decrease as the kidneys excrete hydrogen ions; in metabolic alkalosis, the pH should increase.

Urine Specific Gravity. **Specific gravity** is an indicator of urine concentration that can be performed quickly and easily by nursing personnel. Normal specific gravity ranges from 1.005 to 1.030 (usually 1.010 to 1.025). When the concentration of solutes in the urine is high, the specific gravity rises; in very dilute urine with few solutes, it is abnormally low.

Arterial Blood Gases. **Arterial blood gases (ABGs)** are performed to evaluate the client's acid–base balance and oxygenation. Arterial blood is used because it provides a truer reflection of gas exchange in the pulmonary system than venous blood. Blood gases may be drawn by laboratory technicians, respiratory therapy personnel, or nurses with specialized skills. Because a high-pressure artery is used to obtain blood, it is important to apply pressure to the puncture site for 5 minutes after the procedure to reduce the risk of bleeding or bruising.

Six measurements are commonly used to interpret arterial blood gas tests:

- pH, a measure of the relative acidity or alkalinity of the blood
- PaO_2, the pressure exerted by oxygen dissolved in the plasma of arterial blood; an indirect measure of blood oxygen content
- $PaCO_2$, the partial pressure of carbon dioxide in arterial plasma; the respiratory component of acid–base determination
- Bicarbonate HCO_3^- a measure of the metabolic component of acid–base balance
- Base excess (BE), a calculated value of bicarbonate levels, also reflective of the metabolic component of acid–base balance
- Oxygen saturation (SaO_2), the percentage of hemoglobin saturated (combined) with oxygen

Normal ABG values are listed in Box 50–6. Changes seen in common acid–base imbalances are summarized in Table 50–9. Note that although the PaO_2 and SaO_2 are important for assessing respiratory status, they generally do not provide useful

information for assessing acid–base balance and so are not included in this table.

When evaluating ABG results to determine acid–base balance, it is important to use a systematic approach such as the one outlined in Box 50–7. Nurses need to assess each measurement individually, then look at the interrelationships to determine what type of acid–base imbalance may be present.

DIAGNOSING

NANDA includes the following diagnostic labels that relate to fluid and acid–base imbalances:

- *Deficient Fluid Volume:* Decreased intravascular, interstitial, and/or intracellular fluid. This refers to dehydration, water loss alone without change in sodium.
- *Excess Fluid Volume:* Increased isotonic fluid retention
- *Risk for Imbalanced Fluid Volume:* At risk for a decrease, increase, or rapid shift from one to the other of intravascular, interstitial, and/or intracellular fluid. This refers to body fluid loss, gain, or both.
- *Risk for Deficient Fluid Volume:* At risk for experiencing vascular, cellular, or intracellular dehydration.
- *Impaired Gas Exchange:* Excess or deficit in oxygenation and/or carbon dioxide elimination at the alveolar-capillary membrane.

Clinical applications of selected diagnoses are shown in Identifying Nursing Diagnoses, Outcomes, and Interventions and in the Nursing Care Plan and the Concept Map at the end of this chapter.

Fluid, electrolyte, and acid–base imbalances affect many other body areas and as a consequence may be the etiology of other nursing diagnoses, such as

- *Impaired Oral Mucous Membrane* related to fluid volume deficit
- *Impaired Skin Integrity* related to dehydration and/or edema
- *Decreased Cardiac Output* related to hypovolemia and/or cardiac dysrhythmias secondary to electrolyte imbalance (K^+ or Mg^{2+})
- *Ineffective Tissue Perfusion* related to decreased cardiac output secondary to fluid volume deficit or edema

TABLE 50–9 Arterial Blood Gas Values in Common Acid–Base Disorders

Disorder		ABG Values
Respiratory acidosis	pH	< 7.35
	$PaCO_2$	> 45 mm Hg (excess CO_2 and carbonic acid)
	HCO_3^-	Normal; >26 mEq/L with renal compensation
Respiratory alkalosis	pH	> 7.45
	$PaCO_2$	< 35 mm Hg (inadequate CO_2 and carbonic acid)
	HCO_3^-	Normal; < 22 mEq/L with renal compensation
Metabolic acidosis	pH	< 7.35
	$PaCO_2$	Normal; < 35 mm Hg with respiratory compensation
	HCO_3^-	< 22 mEq/L (inadequate bicarbonate)
	BE	< − 22 mEq/L
Metabolic alkalosis	pH	< 7.45
	$PaCO_2$	Normal; > 45 mm Hg with respiratory compensation
	HCO_3^-	> 26 mEq/L (excess bicarbonate)
	BE	> +12 mEq/L

- *Activity Intolerance* related to hypervolemia
- *Risk for Injury* related to calcium shift out of bones into extracellular fluids
- *Acute Confusion* related to electrolyte imbalance.

PLANNING

When planning care the nurse identifies nursing interventions that will assist the client to achieve these broad goals:

- Maintain or restore normal fluid balance.
- Maintain or restore normal balance of electrolytes in the intracellular and extracellular compartments.

- Maintain or restore pulmonary ventilation and oxygenation.
- Prevent associated risks (tissue breakdown, decreased cardiac output, confusion, other neurologic signs).

Obviously, goals will vary according to the diagnosis and defining characteristics for each individual. Appropriate preventive and corrective nursing interventions that relate to these must be identified. Specific nursing activities can be selected to meet the client's individual needs. Examples of application of these using NANDA, NIC, and NOC designations are shown in Identifying Nursing Diagnoses, Outcomes, and Interventions and in the Nursing Care Plan and the Concept Map at the end of

BOX 50–7 ■ Interpreting ABGs

1. Look at the pH:
   a. If the pH is less than 7.35, the problem is acidosis.
   b. If the pH is greater than 7.45, the problem is alkalosis.
2. Look at the $PaCO_2$:
   a. If the $PaCO_2$ is less than 35 mm Hg, more carbon dioxide is being exhaled than normal.
   b. If the $PaCO_2$ is greater than 45 mm Hg, less carbon dioxide is being exhaled than normal.
3. Assess the pH and $PaCO_2$ relationship for a possible respiratory problem:
   a. If the pH is less than 7.35 (acidosis), and the $PaCO_2$ is greater than 45 mm Hg, retained carbon dioxide is causing respiratory acidosis.
   b. If the pH is greater than 7.45 (alkalosis), and the $PaCO_2$ is less than 35 mm Hg, lack of carbon dioxide is causing respiratory alkalosis.
4. Look at the bicarbonate:
   a. If the HCO_3^- is less than 22 mEq/L, bicarbonate levels are lower than normal.
   b. If the HCO_3^- is greater than 26 mEq/L, bicarbonate levels are higher than normal.
5. Assess pH, HCO_3^-, and base excess (BE) values for a possible metabolic problem:

   a. If the pH is less than 7.35 (acidosis), the HCO_3^- is less than 22 mEq/L, and the BE is below −2 mEq/L, low bicarbonate levels are causing metabolic acidosis.
   b. If the pH is greater than 7.45 (alkalosis), the HCO_3^- is greater than 26 mEq/L, and the BE is above +2 mEq/L, high bicarbonate levels are causing metabolic alkalosis.
6. Look for evidence of compensation:
   a. In respiratory acidosis (pH < 7.35, $PaCO_2$ > 45 mm Hg), if the HCO_3^- is greater than 26 mEq/L, the kidneys are retaining bicarbonate to minimize the acidosis: renal compensation.
   b. In respiratory alkalosis (pH > 7.45, $PaCO_2$ < 35 mm Hg), if the HCO_3^- is less than 22 mEq/L, the kidneys are excreting bicarbonate to minimize the alkalosis: again, renal compensation.
   c. In metabolic acidosis (pH < 7.35, HCO_3^- < 22 mEq/L), if the $PaCO_2$ is less than 35 mm Hg, carbon dioxide is being "blown off" to minimize the acidosis: respiratory compensation.
   d. In metabolic alkalosis (pH > 7.45, HCO_3^- > 26 mEq/L), if the $PaCO_2$ is greater than 45 mm Hg, carbon dioxide is being retained to compensate for excess base: again, respiratory compensation.

IDENTIFYING NURSING DIAGNOSES, OUTCOMES, AND INTERVENTIONS

CLIENTS WITH FLUID VOLUME EXCESS

DATA CLUSTER	NURSING DIAGNOSIS/ DEFINITION	SAMPLE DESIRED OUTCOMES [NOC#]/DEFINITION	INDICATORS	SELECTED INTERVENTIONS [NIC#]/DEFINITION	SAMPLE NIC ACTIVITIES
Tom Bricker, a 67-year-old pensioner who has a history of heart disease, has experienced a weight gain of 4 to 5 kg (9 to 11 lb) during the past month. He states his rings are too tight to remove, his ankles are swollen, his heart pounds at times, he gets breathless with exertion, and he feels bloated. Physical findings reveal jugular vein distention above 3 cm, delayed emptying of hand veins, bounding pulse (86), pitting edema in feet, ankles, and lower legs, and moist lung sounds (rales/crackles).	*Excess Fluid Volume/Increased isotonic fluid retention*	Fluid Balance. [0601]/*Balance of water in the intracellular and extracellular compartments of the body*	Not compromised • 24-hour intake and output balanced • Adventitious breath sounds not present • Body weight stable • Neck vein distention not present	Fluid Management [4120]/*Promotion of fluid balance and prevention of complications resulting from abnormal or undesired fluid levels*	• Assess location and extent of edema on scale from 1+ to 4+ • Assess for indications of fluid overload/retention (e.g., crackles, elevated BP, edema, neck vein distention) as appropriate • Maintain accurate intake and output record • Weigh daily and monitor trends • Consult physician if signs and symptoms of fluid volume excess persist or worsen

this chapter. Examples of NIC interventions related to fluid, electrolyte, and acid–base balance include

- Acid–base management
- Electrolyte management
- Fluid monitoring
- Hypovolemia management
- Intravenous (IV) therapy.

Specific nursing activities associated with each of these interventions can be selected to meet the individual needs of the client.

Nursing activities to meet goals and outcomes related to fluid, electrolyte, and acid–base imbalances are discussed in the next section. These include (a) monitoring fluid intake and output, cardiovascular and respiratory status, and results of laboratory tests; (b) assessing the client's weight; location and extent of edema, if present; skin turgor and skin status; specific gravity of urine; and level of consciousness and mental status; (c) fluid intake modifications; (d) dietary changes; (e) parenteral fluid, electrolyte, and blood replacement; and (f) other appropriate measures such as administering prescribed medications and oxygen, providing skin care and oral hygiene, positioning the client appropriately, and scheduling rest periods.

Planning for Home Care

To provide for continuity of care, the client's needs for assistance with care in the home need to be considered. Home care planning includes assessment of the client's and family's resources and abilities for care, and the need for referrals and home health services. The accompanying Home Care Assessment describes the specific assessment data required to establish a home care plan. Based on the data gathered in assessment of the home situation, the nurse tailors the teaching plan for the client and family (see Teaching: Wellness Care and Teaching: Home Care on page 1379).

IMPLEMENTING
Promoting Wellness

Most people rarely think about their fluid, electrolyte, or acid–base balance. They know it is important to drink adequate fluids and consume a balanced diet, but they may not understand the potential effects when this is not done. Nurses can promote clients' health by providing wellness teaching that will help them maintain fluid and electrolyte balance.

Enteral Fluid and Electrolyte Replacement

Fluids and electrolytes can be provided orally in the home and hospital if the client's health permits, that is, if the client is not

IDENTIFYING NURSING DIAGNOSES, OUTCOMES, AND INTERVENTIONS
CLIENTS WITH IMPAIRED GAS EXCHANGE

DATA CLUSTER	NURSING DIAGNOSIS/ DEFINITION	SAMPLE DESIRED OUTCOMES [NOC#]/DEFINITION	INDICATORS	SELECTED INTERVENTIONS [NIC#]/DEFINITION	SAMPLE NIC ACTIVITIES
Fred Boysniak was admitted to emergency after being found with an empty bottle of morphine tablets by his bed. He appears very lethargic and stuporous; pulse is 120, respiration 12 and very shallow. Blood gases reveal pH of 7.28, $PaCO_2$ 49 mm Hg, and HCO_3^- 25 mEq/L.	Impaired Gas Exchange/Excess or deficit in oxygenation and/or carbon dioxide elimination at the alveolar-capillary membrane	Respiratory Status: Ventilation [0403]/ Movement of air in and out of the lungs	Not compromised • Depth of inspiration • Auscultated breath sounds	Acid–Base Management: Respiratory Acidosis [1913]/ Promotion of acid–base balance and prevention of complications resulting from serum pco_2 levels higher than desired	• Monitor respiratory pattern • Monitor ABG levels for decreased pH levels • Monitor neurological status (e.g., level of consciousness) • Provide oxygen therapy if necessary • Provide mechanical ventilatory support if necessary

vomiting, has not experienced an excessive fluid loss, and has an intact gastrointestinal tract and gag and swallow reflexes. Clients who are unable to ingest solid foods may be able to ingest fluids.

Fluid Intake Modifications. Increased fluids (ordered as "push fluids") are often prescribed for clients with actual or potential fluid volume deficits arising, for example, from mild diarrhea or mild to moderate fevers. Guidelines for helping clients increase fluid intake are shown in Practice Guidelines on page 1380.

Restricted fluids may be necessary for clients who have fluid retention (fluid volume excess) as a result of renal failure, congestive heart failure, SIADH, or other disease processes.

Home Care Assessment
FLUID, ELECTROLYTE, AND ACID–BASE BALANCE

Client
- Risk factors for imbalances: The client's age, medications required such as diuretic therapy or corticosteroids, and presence of chronic diseases such as diabetes mellitus, heart disease, lung disease, or dementia (see Box 50–3 on p. 1371)
- Self-care abilities for maintaining food and fluid intake: Mobility; ability to chew and swallow, to access fluids and respond to thirst; to purchase food and prepare a balanced diet
- Current level of knowledge (as appropriate) about: Prescribed diet, any fluid restrictions, activity restrictions, actions and side effects of prescribed medications, regular weight monitoring, gastric tube care and enteral feedings, central line or PICC catheter care, and parenteral fluids and nutrition

Family
- Caregiver availability, skills, and responses: Availability and willingness to assume responsibility for care, knowledge and ability to provide assistance with preparing food and maintaining adequate intake of food and fluids, knowledge of risk factors and early warning signs of problems
- Family role changes and coping: Effect on financial status, parenting and spousal roles, social roles
- Alternate potential primary or respite caregivers: For example, other family members, volunteers, church members, paid caregivers or housekeeping services; available community respite care (e.g., adult day care, senior centers)

Community
- Current knowledge of and experience with community resources: Home health agencies, organizations that offer financial assistance or assistance with food preparation, Meals on Wheels or meal services (e.g., at senior centers, homeless shelters), pharmacies, home intravenous services, respiratory care services

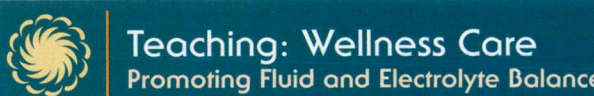

Teaching: Wellness Care
Promoting Fluid and Electrolyte Balance

- Consume six to eight glasses of water daily.
- Avoid excess amounts of foods or fluids high in salt, sugar, and caffeine.
- Eat a well-balanced diet. Include adequate amounts of milk or milk products to maintain bone calcium levels.
- Limit alcohol intake because it has a diuretic effect.
- Increase fluid intake before, during, and after strenuous exercise, particularly when the environmental temperature is high, and replace lost electrolytes from excessive perspiration as needed with commercial electrolyte solutions.

- Maintain normal body weight.
- Learn about and monitor side effects of medications that affect fluid and electrolyte balance (e.g., diuretics) and ways to handle side effects.
- Recognize possible risk factors for fluid and electrolyte imbalance such as prolonged or repeated vomiting, frequent watery stools, or inability to consume fluids because of illness.
- Seek prompt professional health care for notable signs of fluid imbalance such as sudden weight gain or loss, decreased urine volume, swollen ankles, shortness of breath, dizziness, or confusion.

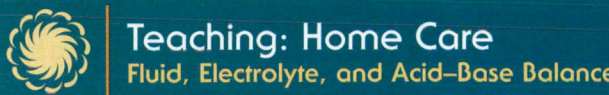

Teaching: Home Care
Fluid, Electrolyte, and Acid–Base Balance

Monitoring Fluid Intake and Output

- Teach the client and family as appropriate how to monitor fluid intake and output, including using a commode or collection device ("hat") in the toilet, emptying and measuring urinary catheter drainage, counting or weighing diapers.
- Instruct the client and family to monitor weight on a regular basis at the same time of day, using the same scale and with the client wearing the same amount of clothing.
- Inform the client and family when to contact a health care professional, such as in the cases of a significant change in urine output; any change of 5 pounds or more in a 1- to 2-week period; prolonged episodes of vomiting, diarrhea, or inability to eat or drink; dry, sticky mucous membranes; extreme thirst; swollen fingers, feet, ankles, or legs; difficulty breathing, shortness of breath, rapid heartbeat; and changes in behavior or mental status.

Maintaining Food and Fluid Intake

- Instruct the client and family about any diet or fluid restrictions, such as a low-sodium diet. Contact a dietitian to provide appropriate teaching.
- Teach family members the importance of offering fluids regularly to clients who are unable to meet their own needs because of age, impaired mobility or cognition, or other conditions such as impaired swallowing due to a stroke.
- If the client is on enteral or intravenous fluids and feeding at home, teach caregivers about proper administration and care. Contact a home health or home intravenous service to provide services and teaching.

Safety

- Instruct the client to change positions slowly if appropriate, especially when moving from a supine to a sitting or standing position.
- Inform the client and family about the importance of good mouth and skin care. Teach the client to change positions frequently and to elevate the feet on a stool when sitting for a long period.
- Teach the client and family how to care for intravenous access sites or gastric tubes. Include what to do if tubes become dislodged.

Medications

- Emphasize the importance of taking medications as prescribed.
- Instruct clients taking diuretics to take the medication in the morning. If a second daily dose is prescribed, they should take it in the late afternoon to avoid disrupting sleep to urinate.
- Inform clients about any expected side effects of prescribed medications and how to handle them (e.g., if a potassium-depleting diuretic is prescribed, increase intake of potassium-rich foods; if taking a potassium-sparing diuretic, avoid excess potassium intake such as using a salt substitute).
- Teach clients when to contact their primary care provider, for example, if they are unable to take a prescribed medication or have signs of an allergic or toxic reaction to a medication.

Measures Specific to Client's Problem

- Provide instructions specific to the client's fluid, electrolyte, or acid–base imbalance, such as
  a. Fluid volume deficit
  b. Risk for fluid volume deficit
  c. Fluid volume excess

Referrals

- Make appropriate referrals to home health or community social services for assistance with resources such as meals, meal preparation and food, intravenous infusions and access, enteral feedings, and homemaker or home health aide services to help with ADLs.

Community Agencies and Other Sources of Help

- Provide information about companies or agencies that can provide durable medical equipment such as commodes, lift chairs, or hospital beds for purchase, for rental, or free of charge.
- Provide a list of sources for supplies such as catheters and drainage bags, measuring devices, tube feeding formulas, and electrolyte replacement drinks.
- Suggest additional sources of information and help such as the American Dietetic Association, the American Heart Association, and the American Lung Association.

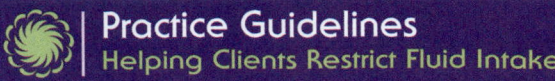

Practice Guidelines
Facilitating Fluid Intake

- Explain to the client the reason for the required intake and the specific amount needed. This provides a rationale for the requirement and promotes compliance.
- Establish a 24-hour plan for ingesting the fluids. For the hospitalized or long-term care client, half of the total volume is given during the day shift, and the other half is divided between the evening and night shifts, with most of that ingested during the evening shift. For example, if 2,500 mL is to be ingested in 24 hours, the plan may specify 7–3 (1,500 mL); 3–11 (700 mL); and 11–7 (300 mL). Try to avoid the ingestion of large amounts of fluid immediately before bedtime to prevent the need to urinate during sleeping hours.
- Set short-term outcomes that the client can realistically meet. Examples include ingesting a glass of fluid every hour while awake or a pitcher of water by 12 noon.
- Identify fluids the client likes and make available a variety of those items, including fruit juices, soft drinks, and milk (if allowed). Remember that beverages such as coffee and tea have a diuretic effect, so their consumption should be limited.
- Help clients to select foods that tend to become liquid at room temperature (e.g., gelatin, ice cream, sherbet, custard), if these are allowed.
- For clients who are confined to bed, supply appropriate cups, glasses, and straws to facilitate appropriate fluid intake and keep the fluids within easy reach.
- Make sure fluids are served at the appropriate temperature: hot fluids hot and cold fluids very cold.
- Encourage clients when possible to participate in maintaining the fluid intake record. This assists them to evaluate the achievement of desired outcomes.
- Be alert to any cultural implications of food and fluids. Some cultures may restrict certain foods and fluids and view others as having healing properties.

Practice Guidelines
Helping Clients Restrict Fluid Intake

- Explain the reason for the restricted intake and how much and what types of fluids are permitted orally. Many clients need to be informed that ice chips, gelatin, and ice cream, for example, are considered fluid.
- Help the client decide the amount of fluid to be taken with each meal, between meals, before bedtime, and with medications. For the hospitalized or long-term care client, half the total volume is scheduled during the day shift, when the client is most active, receives two meals, and most oral medications. A large part of the remainder is scheduled for the evening shift to permit fluids with meals and evening visitors.
- Identify fluids or fluidlike substances the client likes and make sure that these are provided, unless contraindicated. A client who is allowed only 200 mL of fluid for breakfast, for example, should receive the type of fluid the client favors.
- Set short-term goals that make the fluid restriction more tolerable. For example, schedule a specified amount of fluid at one or two hourly intervals between meals. Some clients may prefer fluids only between meals if the food provided at mealtime helps relieve thirst.
- Place allowed fluids in small containers such as a 4-ounce juice glass to allow the perception of a full container.
- Periodically offer the client ice chips as an alternative to water, because ice chips when melted are approximately half of the frozen volume.
- Provide frequent mouth care and rinses to reduce the thirst sensation.
- Instruct the client to avoid ingesting or chewing salty or sweet foods (hard candy or gum), because these foods tend to produce thirst. Sugarless gum may be an alternative for some clients.
- Encourage the client when possible to participate in maintaining the fluid intake record.

Fluid restrictions vary from "nothing by mouth" to a precise amount ordered by a physician. The restriction of fluids can be difficult for some clients, particularly if they are experiencing thirst. Guidelines for helping clients restrict fluid intake are shown in Practice Guidelines.

Dietary Changes. Specific fluid and electrolyte imbalances may require simple dietary changes. For example, clients receiving potassium-depleting diuretics need to be informed about foods with a high potassium content (e.g., bananas, oranges, and leafy greens). Some clients with fluid retention need to avoid foods high in sodium. Most healthy clients can benefit from foods rich in calcium.

Oral Electrolyte Supplements. Some clients can benefit from oral supplements of electrolytes, particularly when a medication is prescribed that affects electrolyte balance, when dietary intake is inadequate for a specific electrolyte, or when fluid and electrolyte losses are excessive as a result of, for example, excessive perspiration.

Corticosteroids and many diuretics can cause too much potassium to be eliminated through the kidneys. For clients taking these medications, potassium supplements may be prescribed. Instruct clients taking oral potassium supplements to take the medication with juice to mask the unpleasant taste and reduce the possibility of gastric distress. Emphasize the importance of taking the medication as prescribed and seeing their primary care provider on a regular basis. Because hyperkalemia can have serious cardiac effects, clients should never increase the amount of potassium being taken without an order to do so. In addition, inform clients that most salt substitutes contain potassium, so it is important to consult with the primary care provider before using salt substitutes.

People who ingest insufficient milk and milk products benefit from calcium supplements. The recommended daily allowance for calcium is 1,000 to 1,500 mg. It is generally recommended that postmenopausal women take 1,500 mg of calcium per day to reduce the risk of osteoporosis. Long-term use of corticosteroid drugs can also cause calcium loss from the bone, and calcium supplements may help reduce this loss.

Research Note
Is Water Intake Adequate Among Nursing Home Residents?

Concerned about the water intake of the elderly, Gaspar (1999) designed a study to explore the adequacy of water intake among nursing home residents and identify the variables associated with water intake.

Data were collected through observation during two 24-hour periods. Additionally data including weight, height, and urine output were obtained through chart review. The researchers used several tools to increase the accuracy and specificity of the data. These included a tool to elicit subjective reports of thirst, fear of incontinence, health and nausea, a situational modifier sheet that included factors such as level of assistance and swallowing ability,

and a pressure sores scale to help determine the general function of the individual. There were a total of 99 subjects, mean age was 85 years. Only 8 of the 99 participants met or exceeded their required water intake standard.

Implications: Ensuring that clients have adequate water intake is an important nursing responsibility. Because this study showed that nursing home residents do not ingest enough water, it can be implied that many elderly clients do not. The author offers several suggestions to improve water intake. These include identifying clients at risk for inadequate water ingestion and increasing water ingestion opportunities.

Note: From "Water Intake of Nursing Home Residents," by P. M. Gaspar, 1999, *Journal of Gerontological Nursing, 25*(4), pp. 22–29.

Clients who take supplemental calcium need to maintain a fluid intake of at least 2,500 mL per day (unless contraindicated) to reduce the risk of kidney stones, which are commonly composed of calcium salts.

Although routine supplements for other electrolytes generally are not recommended, clients who have poor dietary habits, who are malnourished, or who have difficulty accessing or eating fresh fruits and vegetables may benefit from electrolyte supplements. A daily multiple vitamin with minerals may achieve the desired goal. People who engage in strenuous activity in a warm environment need to be encouraged to replace water and electrolytes lost through excessive perspiration by consuming a sports drink such as Gatorade or another commercial fluid and electrolyte solution.

Liquid nutritional supplements are often given to clients who are malnourished or have poor eating habits. They are used with frequency in older adults to bolster nutritional status and caloric intake. It is very important to be a "label reader" of the product and to be aware of the contents of the supplement. Some of them are very high in protein and high in potassium, which may be contraindicated in an individual with impaired renal function.

Parenteral Fluid and Electrolyte Replacement

Intravenous (IV) fluid therapy is essential when clients are unable to take food and fluids orally. It is an efficient and effective method of supplying fluids directly into the intravascular fluid compartment and replacing electrolyte losses. Intravenous fluid therapy is usually ordered by the physician. The nurse is responsible for administering and maintaining the therapy and for teaching the client and significant others how to continue the therapy at home if necessary.

Intravenous Solutions. Intravenous solutions can be classified as isotonic, hypotonic, or hypertonic. Most IV solutions are *isotonic*, having the same concentration of solutes as blood plasma. Isotonic solutions are often used to restore vascular

volume. *Hypertonic* solutions have a greater concentration of solutes than plasma; *hypotonic* solutions have a lesser concentration of solutes. Table 50–10 provides examples of IV solutions and nursing implications.

IV solutions can also be categorized according to their purpose. Nutrient solutions contain some form of carbohydrate (e.g., dextrose, glucose, or levulose) and water. Water is supplied for fluid requirements and carbohydrate for calories and energy. For example, 1 L of 5% dextrose provides 170 calories. *Nutrient solutions* are useful in preventing dehydration and ketosis but do not provide sufficient calories to promote wound healing, weight gain, or normal growth in children. Common nutrient solutions are 5% dextrose in water (D5W) and 5% dextrose in 0.45% sodium chloride (dextrose in half-strength saline).

Electrolyte solutions contain varying amounts of cations and anions. Commonly used solutions are normal saline (0.9% sodium chloride solution), Ringer's solution (which contains sodium, chloride, potassium, and calcium), and lactated Ringer's solution (which contains sodium, chloride, potassium, calcium, and lactate). Lactate is metabolized in the liver to form bicarbonate HCO_3^- Saline and balanced electrolyte solutions commonly are used to restore vascular volume, particularly after trauma or surgery. They also may be used to replace fluid and electrolytes for clients with continuing losses, for example, because of gastric suction or wound drainage.

Lactated Ringer's solution is an *alkalinizing solution* that may be given to treat metabolic acidosis. *Acidifying solutions,* in contrast, are administered to counteract metabolic alkalosis. Examples of acidifying solutions are 5% dextrose in 0.45% sodium chloride and 0.9% sodium chloride solution.

Volume expanders are used to increase the blood volume following severe loss of blood (e.g., from hemorrhage) or loss of plasma (e.g., from severe burns, which draw large amounts of plasma from the bloodstream to the burn site). Examples of expanders are dextran, plasma, and albumin.

TABLE 50–10 Selected Intravenous Solutions

Type/Examples	Comments/Nursing Implications
Isotonic Solutions 0.9% NaCl (normal saline) Lactated Ringer's (a balanced electrolyte solution) 5% dextrose in water (D5W)	Isotonic solutions such as NS and lactated Ringer's initially remain in the vascular compartment, expanding vascular volume. Assess clients carefully for signs of hypervolemia such as bounding pulse and shortness of breath. D5W is isotonic on initial administration but provides free water when dextrose is metabolized, expanding intracellular and extracellular fluid volumes. D5W is avoided in clients at risk for increased intracranial pressure (IICP) because it can increase cerebral edema.
Hypotonic Solutions 0.45% NaCl (half normal saline) 0.33% NaCl (one-third normal saline)	Hypotonic solutions are used to provide free water and treat cellular dehydration. These solutions promote waste elimination by the kidneys. Do not administer to clients at risk for IICP or third-space fluid shift.
Hypertonic Solutions 5% dextrose in normal saline (D5NS) 5% dextrose in 0.45% NaCl (D5 1/2NS) 5% dextrose in lactated Ringer's (D5LR)	Hypertonic solutions draw fluid out of the intracellular and interstitial compartments into the vascular compartment, expanding vascular volume. Do not administer to clients with kidney or heart disease or clients who are dehydrated. Watch for signs of hypervolemia.

Venipuncture Sites. The site chosen for venipuncture varies with the client's age, the length of time the infusion is to run, the type of solution used, and the condition of veins. For adults, veins in the hand and arm are commonly used; for infants, veins in the scalp and dorsal foot veins are often used. Larger veins are preferred for infusions that need to be given rapidly and for solutions that could be irritating (e.g., certain medications).

The metacarpal, basilic, and cephalic veins are commonly used for intermittent or continuous infusions (Figure 50–13 ■, *B*). The ulna and radius act as natural splints at these sites, and the client has greater freedom of arm movements for activities such as eating. Although the basilic and median cubital veins in the antecubital space are convenient sites for venipuncture, they are usually used for blood draws, bolus injections of medication, and insertion sites for a peripherally inserted central catheter line (see Figure 50–13 ■, *A*). See Practice Guidelines for vein selection.

When long-term IV therapy or parenteral nutrition is anticipated or the client is receiving IV medications that are damaging to vessels (e.g., chemotherapy), a central venous catheter may be inserted. **Central venous catheters** usually are inserted into the subclavian or jugular vein, with the distal tip of the catheter resting in the superior vena cava just above the right atrium (Figure 50–14 ■). They may be inserted at the client's bedside or, for longer term access, surgically inserted. Subclavian central venous catheters permit freedom of movement for ambulation; however, there is a risk of pneumothorax on catheter insertion. Assess the client closely for manifestations such as shortness of breath, chest pain, cough, hypotension, tachycardia, and anxiety after the insertion procedure.

With a **peripherally inserted central venous catheter (PICC),** the catheter is inserted in the basilic or cephalic vein just above or below the antecubital space of the right arm. The tip of the catheter rests in the superior vena cava. The risk of pneumothorax is eliminated with PICC. These catheters frequently are used for long-term intravenous access when the client will be managing IV therapy at home.

Implantable venous access devices or ports (Figures 50–15 ■ and 50–16 ■) are used for clients with chronic illness who require long-term IV therapy (e.g., intermittent medications such as chemotherapy, total parenteral nutrition, and frequent blood samples). The device is designed to provide repeated access to the central venous system, avoiding the trauma and complications of multiple venipunctures. Using local anesthesia, implantable ports

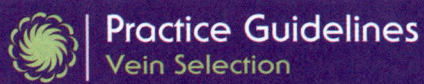

Practice Guidelines
Vein Selection

■ Use distal veins of the arm first.
■ Use the client's nondominant arm whenever possible.
■ Select a vein that is
  a. Easily palpated and feels soft and full
  b. Naturally splinted by bone
  c. Large enough to allow adequate circulation around the catheter.
■ Avoid using veins that are
  a. In areas of flexion (e.g., the antecubital fossa)
  b. Highly visible, because they tend to roll away from the needle
  c. Damaged by previous use, phlebitis, infiltration, or sclerosis
  d. Continually distended with blood, or knotted or tortuous
  e. In a surgically compromised or injured extremity (e.g., following a mastectomy), because of possible impaired circulation and discomfort for the client.

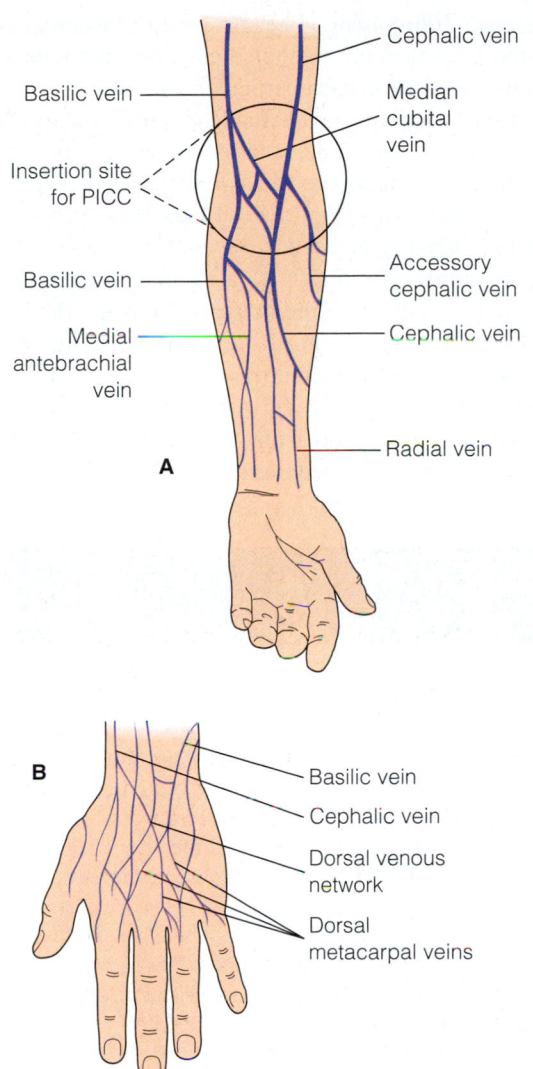

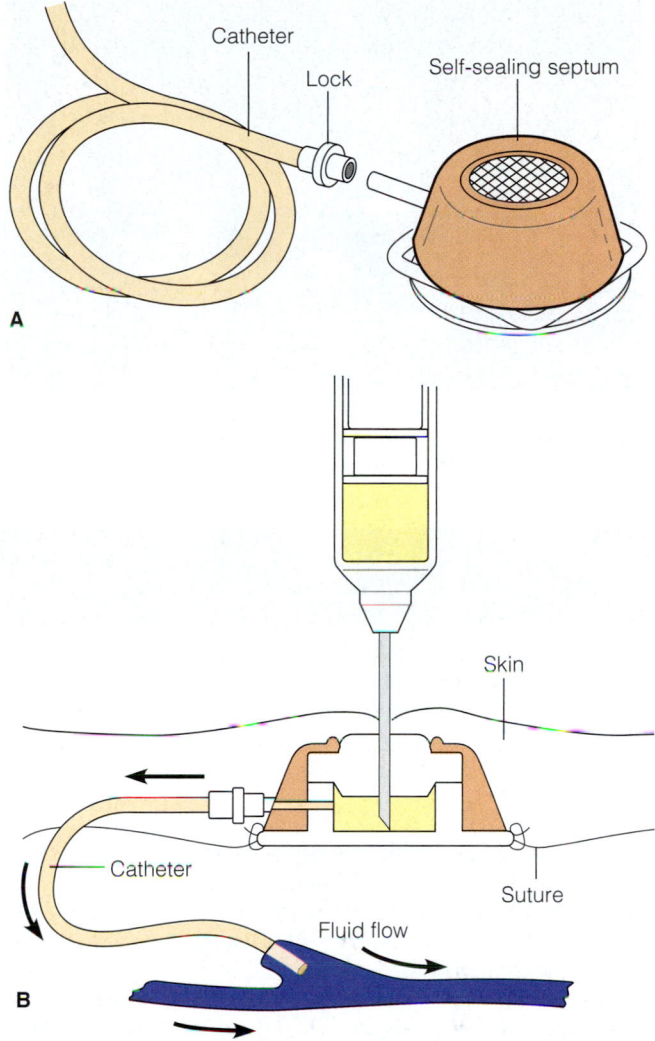

Figure 50–15 ■ An implantable venous access device: *A,* components; *B,* the device in place.

Figure 50–13 ■ Commonly used venipuncture sites of the *A,* arm; *B,* hand. *A* also shows the site used for a peripherally inserted central catheter (PICC).

are surgically placed into a small subcutaneous pocket, usually on the upper chest. The distal end of the catheter is placed in the subclavian or jugular vein. There are different kinds of implantable venous access devices and they may be tunneled or nontunneled.

Special precautions need to be taken with all central lines and venous access ports to ensure asepsis and catheter patency. Nursing care of clients with these devices is outlined in Practice Guidelines.

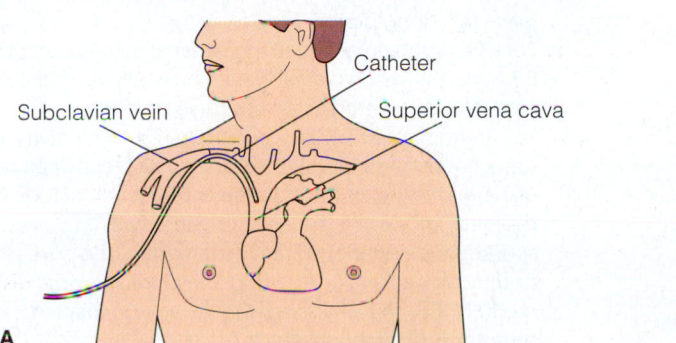

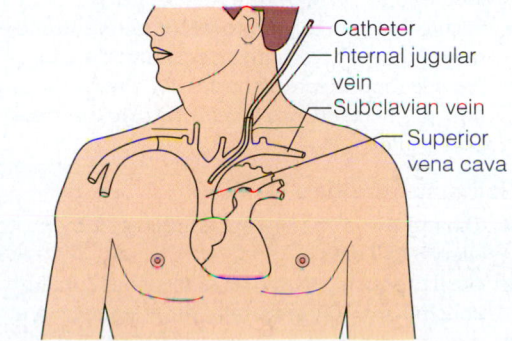

Figure 50–14 ■ Central venous lines with *A,* subclavian vein insertion, and *B,* left jugular insertion.

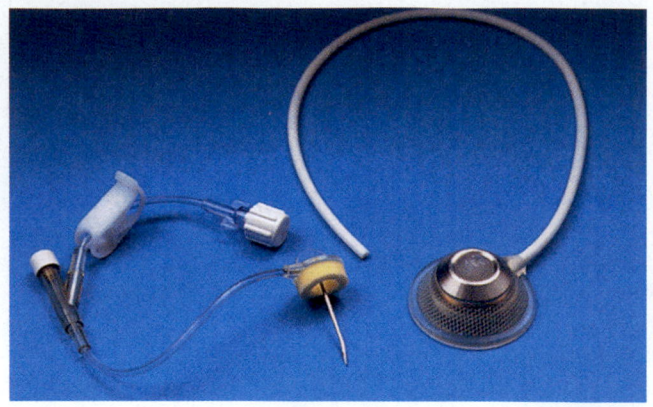

Figure 50–16 ■ An implantable venous access device (right) and a Huber needle with extension tubing.

Intravenous Equipment. Because equipment varies according to the manufacturer, the nurse must become familiar with the equipment used in each particular agency.

Solution containers are available in various sizes (50, 100, 250, 500, or 1,000 mL); the smaller containers are often used to administer medications. Most solutions are currently dispensed in plastic bags (Figure 50–17 ■). However, glass containers may need to be used if the administered medications are incompatible with plastic. Glass containers require an air vent so that air can enter the bottle and replace the fluid that enters the client's vein. Some have a tube inside the bottle that serves as a vent; other containers without air vents require a vent on the administration set. Air vents usually have filters to prevent contamination from the air that enters the container. Air vents are not required for plastic solution contain-

Practice Guidelines
Caring for Clients with a Venous Access Device

■ On insertion, document the date; the site; the brand, gauge, and catheter length; the location of the catheter tip (verified by x-ray); the length of the external segment; and client teaching. Do not utilize the access device until correct placement has been verified by x-ray.

Site Care

■ Use strict aseptic technique when caring for central lines and long-term venous access devices.
■ The frequency of dressing changes may vary from every 3 to 7 days, depending on the site. Dressings also should be changed when loose or soiled.
■ Assess the site for any redness, swelling, tenderness, or drainage. Compare the length of the external portion of the catheter with its documented length to assess for possible displacement. Obtain a chest x-ray to determine the catheter tip's position if in doubt. Report and document any position changes or signs of infection.
■ Follow agency protocol for cleaning solutions and types of dressings. Isopropyl alcohol or a combination of alcohol and acetone followed by povidone-iodine are commonly used to clean the port site.
■ Before accessing the port, clean an area 2 inches in diameter around the site with an alcohol-acetone solution on a sterile cotton swab. Start at the center of the port site, moving outward with a firm, circular motion. Follow with povidone-iodine solution. Allow the site to air dry.
■ Secure the catheter, and cover the entry site and external portion of the catheter with an occlusive dressing.
■ Provide routine care of the incision site for the implant device until it is healed. Once it heals, no care is necessary when the port is idle.

Catheter Care and Flushing

■ Change the catheter cap as indicated by protocol, usually every 3 to 7 days.
■ Flush the port with normal saline, a heparin flush solution (10 units/mL or 100 units/mL), or as agency protocol recom-

mends for the specific type of port being used. After infusing medications or solutions, again flush the port with saline before using heparinized saline.
■ Using a 10-mL syringe, flush the catheter with a solution of 10 units of heparin after each use. The frequency of flushes between uses may vary from every 12 hours to once a week or less, depending on the type of catheter.
■ Remember to flush all lumens for multiple-lumen catheters.
■ Use a specially designed needle to access an implanted port. A needle with a 90-degree angle is generally used for infusions because it is easier to stabilize and more comfortable for the client. Stabilizing the port between the thumb and index finger of the nondominant hand, insert the needle through the center of the port until the resistance of the platform is felt.
■ To remove the needle after a treatment, again stabilize the port and use even pressure to withdraw the needle. Maintain positive pressure by withdrawing the needle as the last milliliter of flush solution is being instilled.
■ Flush idle implanted ports with heparinized saline in accordance with agency protocol or at least every 8 weeks.

Teaching

Provide clients with the following instructions:

■ Do not allow anyone to take a blood pressure on the arm in which a PICC line is inserted.
■ Wear a medic-alert tag or bracelet if the device is to be in place for a long period.
■ For a PICC, you do not need to restrict activities, except do not immerse the arm in water. Showering is allowed if the site and catheter are covered by an occlusive dressing.
■ For an implanted venous port there are no activity restrictions, but remember that the port or catheter tip can become dislodged. Signs of a dislodged catheter tip include pain in the neck or ear on the affected side, swishing or gurgling sounds, or palpitations. Free movement of the port, swelling, or difficulty accessing the port may indicate port dislodgement. Notify the physician should any of these occur or if symptoms of infection develop.

Note: From "Getting a Line on Central Vascular Access Devices," by S. Masoorli and T. Angeles, 2002, *Nursing, 32*(4), pp. 36–43. Adapted with permission.

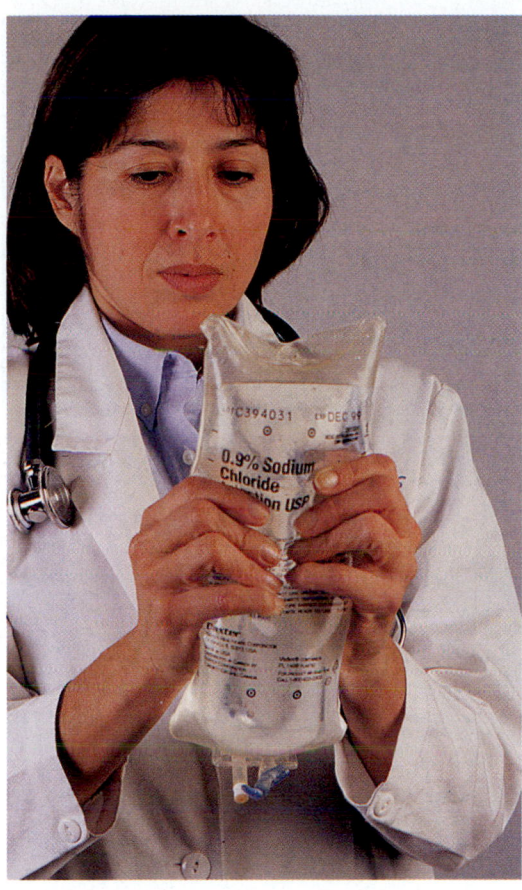

Figure 50–17 ■ A plastic intravenous fluid container.

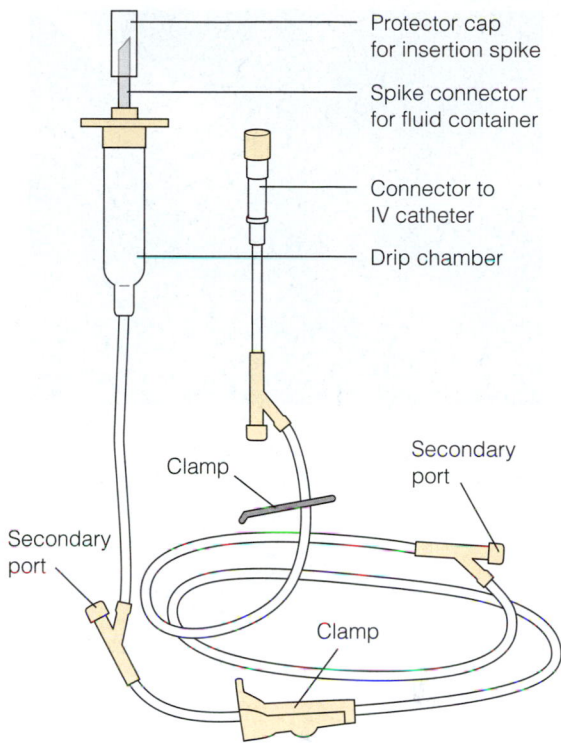

Protector cap
for insertion spike

Spike connector
for fluid container

Connector to
IV catheter

Drip chamber

Secondary
port

Clamp

Secondary
port

Clamp

Figure 50–18 ■ A standard IV administration set.

ers, because plastic bags collapse under atmospheric pressure when the solution enters the vein.

Avoid selecting a container whose volume is greater than the volume ordered. For example, if 750 mL D5NS (750 mL of 5% dextrose in normal saline) has been ordered, the nurse should obtain one 500-mL container and one 250-mL container, which total 750 mL. Do not obtain a 1,000-mL container with the intention of stopping the solution after 750 mL has been administered. Too often, the incorrect amount can be instilled unless an electronic device is used to regulate the volume. If a 1,000-mL solution container must be used, remove 250 mL before starting the infusion.

It is essential that the solution be sterile and in good condition, that is, clear. Cloudiness, evidence that the container has been opened previously, or leaks indicate possible contamination. Always check the expiration date on the label. Return any questionable or contaminated solutions to the pharmacy or IV therapy department.

Infusion sets usually include an insertion spike, a drip chamber, a roller valve or screw clamp, tubing with secondary ports, and a protective cap over the needle adapter (Figure 50–18 ■). The insertion spike is kept sterile and inserted into the solution container when the equipment is set up and ready to start. The drip chamber permits a predictable amount of fluid to be delivered. A commonly used drip chamber is the 10 to 20 drops which delivers macrodrip, per milliliter of solution. This information is found on the package. There are also 60 drops sets, which de-

liver microdrip per milliliter of solution. The roller valve or screw clamp, which compresses the lumen of the tubing, controls the rate of the flow. The protective cap over the needle adapter maintains the sterility of the end of the tubing so that it can be attached to a sterile needle inserted in the client's vein.

Most infusion sets include one or more injection ports for administering IV medications or secondary infusions. Needleless systems are increasingly used because they reduce the risk of needlestick injury and contamination of the intravenous line. With a needleless system, a blunt cannula is inserted into a special injection port or adapter on the IV tubing to administer medications or secondary infusions (Figure 50–19 ■). Many infusion sets include an in-line filter to trap air, particulate matter, and microbes. A special infusion set may be required if the IV flow rate will be regulated by an infusion pump.

Catheters and needles are commonly used for intravenous infusions. Over-the-needle catheters, also known as angiocaths, are commonly used for adult clients. The plastic catheter fits over a needle used to pierce the skin and vein wall (Figure 50–20 ■). Once inserted into the vein, the needle is withdrawn and discarded, leaving the catheter in place. IV catheters allow the client more mobility and rarely infiltrate, that is, become dislodged from the vein and allow fluid to flow into interstitial spaces.

Butterfly, or wing-tipped, needles with plastic flaps attached to the shaft are sometimes used (Figure 50–21 ■). The flaps are held tightly together to hold the needle securely during insertion; after insertion, they are flattened against the skin and secured with tape.

IV poles are used to hang the solution container. Some poles are attached to hospital beds; others stand on the floor or hang from the ceiling. In the home, plant hangers or robe hooks

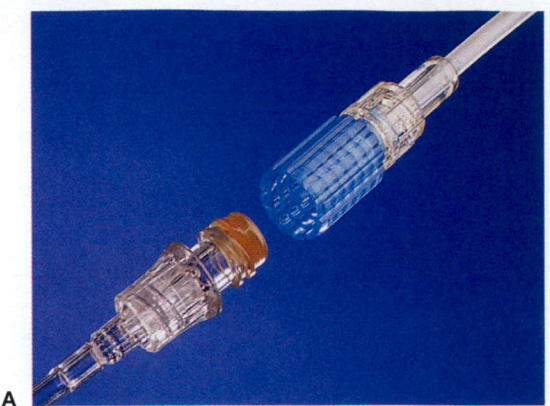

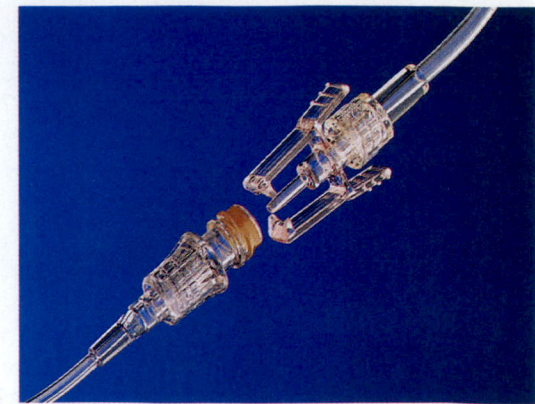

A   B

Figure 50–19 ■ Cannulae used to connect the tubing of additive sets to primary infusions: *A,* threaded-lock cannula; *B,* lever-lock cannula. (Photographs reprinted courtesy of (BD) Becton, Dickinson and Company and courtesy of Baxter Healthcare Corporation. All rights reserved.)

INSERTING A CENTRAL VENOUS LINE ANIMATION

MediaLink

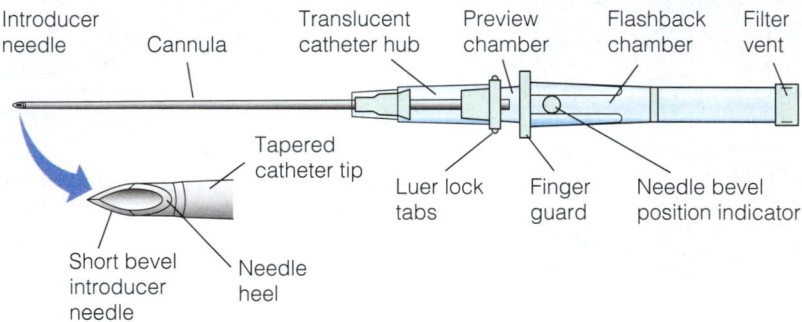

Introducer needle   Cannula   Translucent catheter hub   Preview chamber   Flashback chamber   Filter vent

Tapered catheter tip

Short bevel introducer needle   Needle heel   Luer lock tabs   Finger guard   Needle bevel position indicator

Figure 50–20 ■ Schematic of an over-the-needle catheter.

(even kitchen cabinet knobs or an S-hook over the top of a door) may be used to hang solution containers. The height of most poles is adjustable. The higher the solution container, the greater the force of the solution as it enters the client and the faster the rate of flow.

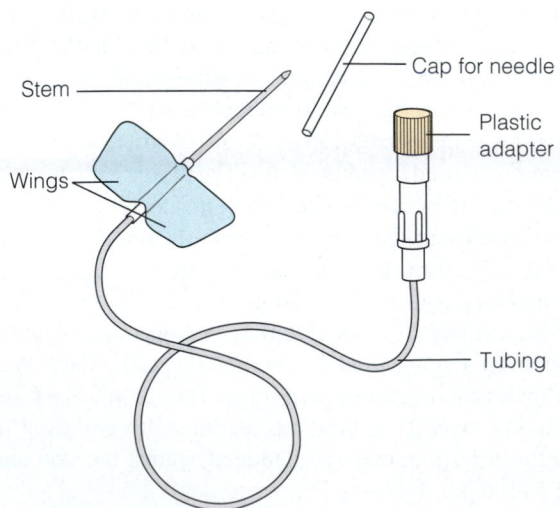

Stem

Wings

Cap for needle

Plastic adapter

Tubing

Figure 50–21 ■ Schematic of a butterfly needle with adapter.

Starting an Intravenous Infusion. Although the physician is responsible for ordering IV therapy for clients, nurses initiate, monitor, and maintain the prescribed IV infusion. This is true not only in hospitals and long-term care facilities but increasingly in community-based settings such as clinics and clients' homes.

Before starting an infusion, the nurse determines the following:

- The type and amount of solution to be infused
- The exact amount (dose) of any medications to be added to a compatible solution
- The rate of flow or the time over which the infusion is to be completed.

If solutions are prepared by the pharmacy or another department, the nurse must verify that the solution supplied exactly matches that which the physician ordered.

Understanding the purpose for the infusion is as important as assessing the client. For example, the nurse may question an order for 5% dextrose in water at 150 mL/h if the client has peripheral edema and other signs of fluid overload.

To perform venipuncture and start an intravenous infusion, see Procedure 50–1.

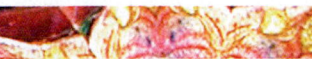

Procedure 50–1 Starting an Intravenous Infusion

Before preparing the infusion, the nurse first verifies the physician's order indicating the type of solution, the amount to be administered, the rate of flow of the infusion, and any client allergies (e.g., to tape or povidone-iodine).

Purposes
- To supply fluid when clients are unable to take in an adequate volume of fluids by mouth

- To provide salts needed to maintain electrolyte balance
- To provide glucose (dextrose), the main fuel for metabolism
- To provide water-soluble vitamins and medications
- To establish a lifeline for rapidly needed medications

ASSESSMENT

- Vital signs (pulse, respiratory rate, and blood pressure) for baseline data;
- skin turgor;
- allergy to tape or iodine;

- bleeding tendencies;
- disease or injury to extremities
- status of veins to determine appropriate venipuncture site.

PLANNING

Prior to initiating the IV infusion, consider how long the patient is likely to have the IV, what kinds of fluids will be infused, and what medications the patient will be receiving or is likely to receive. These factors may affect the choice of vein.

Delegation
This procedure is done by a registered nurse. Due to the use of sterile technique, intravenous infusion therapy is not delegated to unlicensed assistive personnel (UAP). UAP may care for clients receiving IV therapy, and the nurse must ensure that the UAP knows how to perform routine tasks such as bathing and positioning without disturbing the IV. The UAP should also know what complications or adverse signs, such as leakage, should be reported to the nurse. In some states a licensed vocational nurse with special IV therapy training may start intravenous infusions.

Equipment
- Infusion set
- Container of sterile parenteral solution

- IV pole
- Adhesive or nonallergenic tape
- Clean gloves
- Tourniquet
- Antiseptic swabs
- Antiseptic ointment, such as povidone-iodine (optional)
- Intravenous catheter; see Variation at the end of this procedure for a butterfly (winged-tip) needle
- Sterile gauze dressing or transparent occlusive dressing
- Arm splint, if required
- Towel or pad
- Electronic infusion device or pump (The nurse decides what device is needed as appropriate to the client's condition.)

IMPLEMENTATION

Preparation

1. Prepare the client.
   - Explain the procedure to the client. A venipuncture can cause discomfort for a few seconds, but there should be no discomfort while the solution is flowing. Use a doll to demonstrate for children, and explain the procedure to the parents. Clients often want to know how long the process will last. The physician's order may specify the length of time of the infusion, for example, 3,000 mL over 24 hours.
   - Unless initiating IV therapy is urgent, provide any scheduled care before establishing the infusion to minimize movement of the affected limb during the procedure. Moving the limb after the infusion has been established could dislodge the needle.
   - Make sure that the client's clothing or gown can be removed over the IV apparatus if necessary. Some agencies provide special gowns that open over the shoulder and down the sleeve for easy removal.

Performance
- Wash your hands.
1. Open and prepare the infusion set.
   - Remove tubing from the container and straighten it out.
   - Slide the tubing clamp along the tubing until it is just below the drip chamber to facilitate its access.
   - Close the clamp.
   - Leave the ends of the tubing covered with the plastic caps until the infusion is started. *This will maintain the sterility of the ends of the tubing.*
2. Spike the solution container.
   - Remove the protective cover from the entry site of the bag.
   - Remove the cap from the spike and insert the spike into the insertion site of the bag or bottle (Figure 50–22 ■). Follow manufacturer's instructions.

continued on page 1388

Procedure 50–1 Starting an Intravenous Infusion *continued*

IMPLEMENTATION *continued*

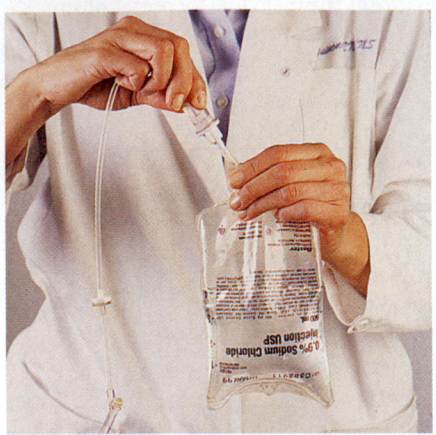

Figure 50–22 ■ Inserting the spike.

3. Apply a medication label to the solution container if a medication is added.
   • In many agencies, medications and labels are applied in the pharmacy; if they are not, apply the label upside down on the container. *The label is applied upside down so it can be read easily when the container is hanging up.*
4. Apply a timing label on the solution container.
   • The timing label may be applied at the time the infusion is started. Follow agency practice. See later discussion of regulating infusion flow rates and Figure 50–30.
5. Hang the solution container on the pole.
   • Adjust the pole so that the container is suspended about 1 m (3 ft) above the client's head. *This height is needed to enable gravity to overcome venous pressure and facilitate flow of the solution into the vein.*
6. Partially fill the drip chamber with solution.
   • Squeeze the chamber gently until it is half full of solution (Figure 50–23 ■).
7. Prime the tubing.
   • Remove the protective cap and hold the tubing over a container. Maintain the sterility of the end of the tubing and the cap.
   • Release the clamp and let the fluid run through the tubing until all bubbles are removed. Tap the tubing if necessary with your fingers to help the bubbles move. *The tubing*

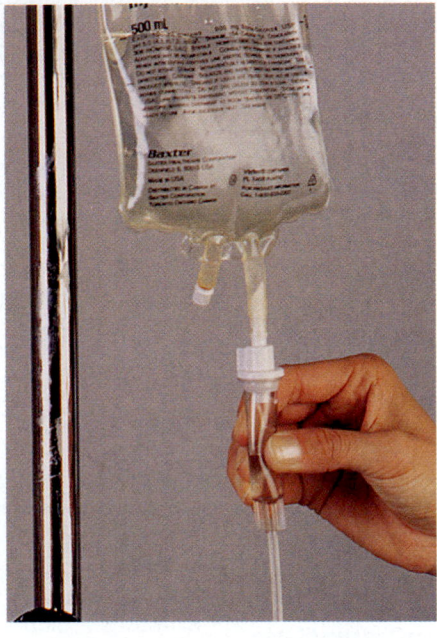

Figure 50–23 ■ Squeezing the drip chamber.

is primed to prevent the introduction of air into the client. Air bubbles smaller than 0.5 mL usually do not cause problems in peripheral lines.
   • Reclamp the tubing and replace the tubing cap, maintaining sterile technique.
   • For caps with air vents, do not remove the cap when priming this tubing. The flow of solution through the tubing will cease when the cap is moist with one drop of solution.
   • If an infusion control pump, electronic device, or controller is being used, follow the manufacturer's directions for inserting the tubing and setting the infusion rate.
8. If indicated, wash your hands again just prior to client contact.
9. Select the venipuncture site.
   • Unless contraindicated, use the client's nondominant arm. Identify possible venipuncture sites by looking for veins that are relatively straight, not sclerotic or tortuous. Consider the catheter length; look for a site sufficiently distal to the wrist or elbow that the tip of the catheter will not be at a point of flexion. *Sclerotic veins may make initiating and maintaining the IV diffi-*

cult. Joint flexion increases the risk of irritation of vein walls by the catheter.
   • Check agency protocol about shaving if the site is very hairy.
   • Place a towel or bed protector under the extremity *to protect linens (or furniture if in the home).*
10. Dilate the vein.
   • Place the extremity in a dependent position (lower than the client's heart). *Gravity slows venous return and distends the veins. Distending the veins makes it easier to insert the needle properly.*
   • Apply a tourniquet firmly 15 to 20 cm (6 to 8 in.) above the venipuncture site (Figure 50–24 ■). Explain that the tourniquet will feel tight. *The tourniquet must be tight enough to obstruct venous flow but not so tight that it occludes arterial flow. Obstructing arterial flow inhibits venous filling.* If a radial pulse can be palpated, the arterial flow is not obstructed.

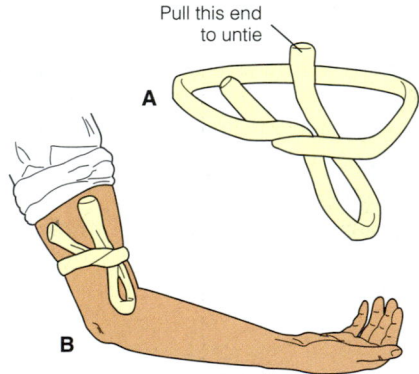

Figure 50–24 ■ Applying a tourniquet.

   • If the vein is not sufficiently dilated:
   a. Massage or stroke the vein distal to the site and in the direction of venous flow toward the heart. *This action helps fill the vein.*
   b. Encourage the client to clench and unclench the fist. *Contracting the muscles compresses the distal veins, forcing blood along the veins and distending them.*
   c. Lightly tap the vein with your fingertips. *Tapping may distend the vein.*

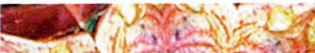 **Procedure 50–1 Starting an Intravenous Infusion** *continued*

IMPLEMENTATION *continued*

- If the preceding steps fail to distend the vein so that it is palpable, remove the tourniquet and apply heat to the entire extremity for 10 to 15 minutes. *Heat dilates superficial blood vessels, causing them to fill.* Then repeat step 11.
11. Put on clean gloves and clean the venipuncture site. *Gloves protect the nurse from contamination by the client's blood.*
    - Clean the skin at the site of entry with a topical antiseptic swab, 2% chlorhexidine, or alcohol. Some institutions use an anti-infective solution such as povidone-iodine (check agency protocol). Check for allergies to iodine or shellfish before cleansing skin with Betadine or iodine products.
    - Use a circular motion, moving from the center outward for several inches. *This motion carries microorganisms away from the site of entry.*
    - Permit the solution to dry on the skin. Povidone-iodine should be in contact with the skin for 1 minute to be effective.
12. Insert the catheter and initiate the infusion.
    - If desired and permitted by policy, inject 0.05 mL of 1% lidocaine intradermally over the site where you plan to insert the IV needle. Allow 5 to 10 seconds for the anesthetic to take effect.
    - Use the nondominant hand to pull the skin taut below the entry site. *This stabilizes the vein and makes the skin taut for needle entry. It can also make initial tissue penetration less painful.*
    - Holding the over-the-needle catheter at a 15- to 30-degree angle with bevel up, insert the catheter through the skin and into the vein in one thrust. Sudden lack of resistance is felt as the needle enters the vein.
    - Once blood appears in the lumen of the needle or you feel the lack of resistance, reduce the angle of the catheter until it is almost parallel with the skin, and advance the needle and catheter approximately 0.5

to 1 cm (about 1/4 in.) further. Holding the needle portion steady, advance the catheter until the hub is at the venipuncture site. The exact technique depends on the type of device used. *The catheter is advanced to ensure that it, and not just the metal needle, is in the vein.* The exact technique depends on the type of catheter used.
    - Release the tourniquet.
    - Remove the protective cap from the distal end of the tubing and hold it ready to attach to the catheter, maintaining the sterility of the end.
    - Carefully remove the needle, engage the needle safety device, and attach the end of the infusion tubing to the catheter hub.
    - Initiate the infusion.
13. Tape the catheter.
    - Tape the catheter by the "U" method or according to manufacturer's instructions. Using three strips of adhesive tape, each about 7.5 cm (3 in.) long:
      a. Place one strip, sticky side up, under the catheter's hub.
      b. Fold each end over so that the sticky sides are against the skin (Figure 50–25 ■).
      c. Place second strip, sticky side down, over catheter hub.
      d. Place third strip, sticky side down, over tubing hub.

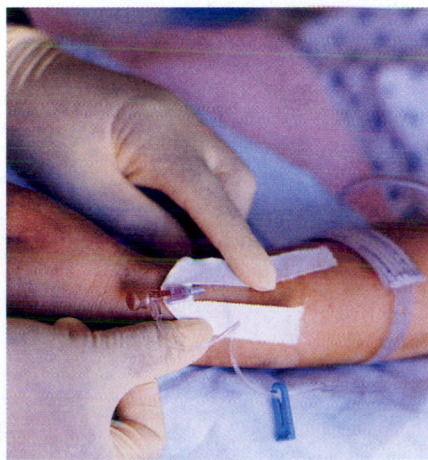

Figure 50–25 ■ Taping an intravenous catheter by the "U" method.

14. Dress and label the venipuncture site and tubing according to agency policy.
    - In some agencies, the nurse puts a small amount of antiseptic ointment, such as povidone-iodine, over the venipuncture site, then a gauze square. In other agencies, a sterile transparent occlusive dressing is applied. This permits assessment of the site without disturbing the dressing. This type of dressing can be left on for 72 hours, then changed.
    - Remove soiled gloves and discard appropriately.
    - Loop the tubing and secure it with tape. *Looping and securing the tubing prevent the weight of the tubing or any movement from pulling on the needle or catheter.*
    - Label the dressing with the date and time of insertion, type and gauge of needle or catheter used, and your initials (Figure 50–26 ■).

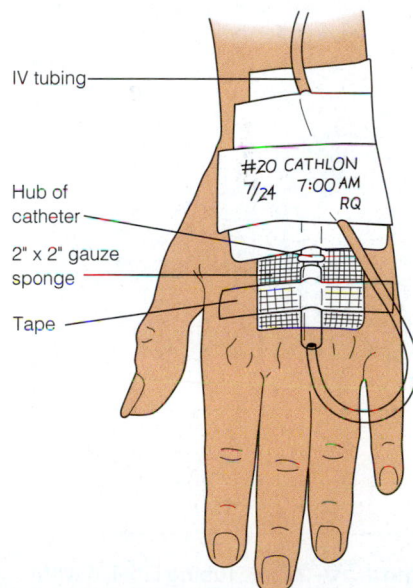

IV tubing

Hub of catheter

2" x 2" gauze sponge

Tape

#20 CATHLON
7/24   7:00 AM
RQ

Figure 50–26 ■ Labeled tape for a venipuncture dressing.

15. Ensure appropriate infusion flow.
    - Apply a padded arm board to splint the joint, as needed.
    - Adjust the infusion rate of flow according to the order.

continued on page 1390

IMPLEMENTATION *continued*

16. Label the IV tubing.
   • Label the tubing with the date and time of attachment and your initials (Figure 50–27 ■). This labeling may also be done when the infusion is started. *The tubing is labeled to ensure that it is changed at regular intervals (i.e., every 24 to 96 hours according to agency policy).*

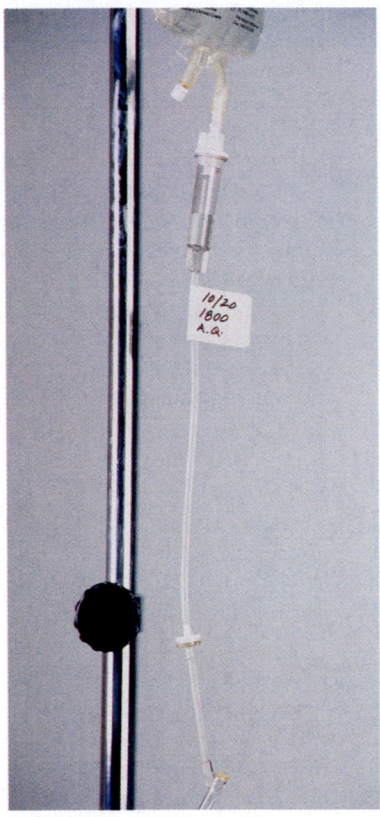

I.V. SET– _72_ HRS.–ONLY
START DATE_ _9/11_ ___ HR. _0800_
DISCARD DATE_ _9/14_ ___ HR. _0800_
R.N. INITIAL_ _LA_ _____

Figure 50–27 ■ Tubing labeled with date, time of attachment, and nurse's initials. Also shown is a preprinted label.

17. Document relevant data, including assessments.
   • Record the start of the infusion on the client's chart. Some agencies provide a special form for this purpose. Include the date and time of the venipuncture; amount and type of solution used, including any additives (e.g., kind and amount of medications); container number; flow rate; type and gauge of the needle or catheter; venipuncture site; and the client's general response.

VARIATION: INSERTING A BUTTERFLY (WINGED-TIP) NEEDLE

■ Hold the needle, pointed in the direction of the blood flow, at a 30-degree angle, with the bevel up, and pierce the skin beside the vein about 1 cm (1/2 in.) below the site planned for piercing the vein.
■ Once the needle is through the skin, lower the needle so that it is almost parallel with the skin. *Lowering the needle reduces the chances of puncturing both sides of the vein.* Follow the course of the vein, and pierce one side of the vein. Sudden lack of resistance can be felt as blood enters the needle.
■ When blood flows back into the needle tubing, insert the needle to its hub.
■ Release the tourniquet, attach the infusion, and initiate flow as quickly as possible. *Attaching the tubing quickly prevents blood from clotting and obstructing the needle.*

■ Secure the butterfly needle by taping it securely by the crisscross (chevron) method (Figure 50–28 ■). Place a small gauze square under the needle, if required. *The gauze keeps the needle in position in the vein.*

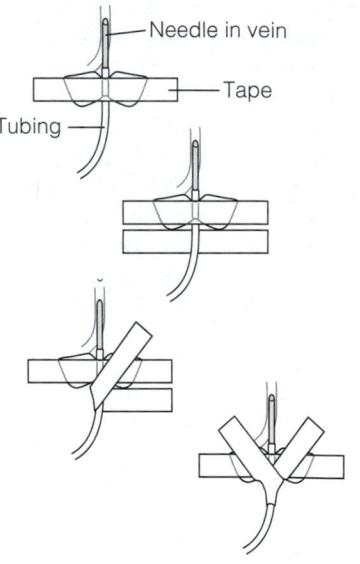

Needle in vein
Tape
Tubing

Figure 50–28 ■ Taping the butterfly needle by the chevron method.

EVALUATION

■ Skin status at IV site (warm temperature and absence of pain, redness, and swelling);
■ Status of dressing;
■ IV flow rate consistent with that ordered;

■ Ability to perform self-care activities; understanding of any mobility limitations;
■ Vital signs compared to baseline level.

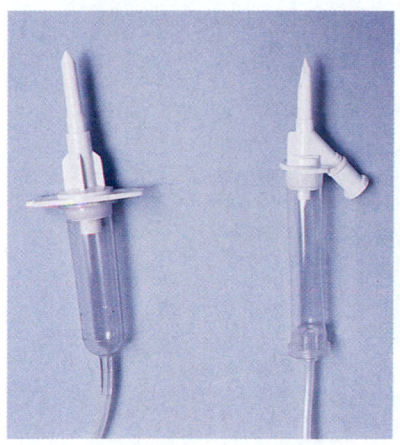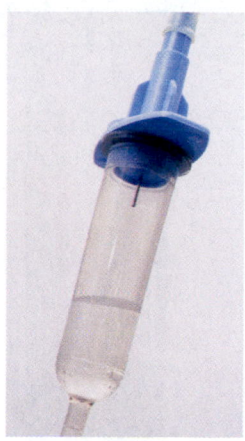

Figure 50–29 ■ Infusion set spikes and drip chambers: nonvented macrodrip, vented macrodrip, nonvented microdrip.

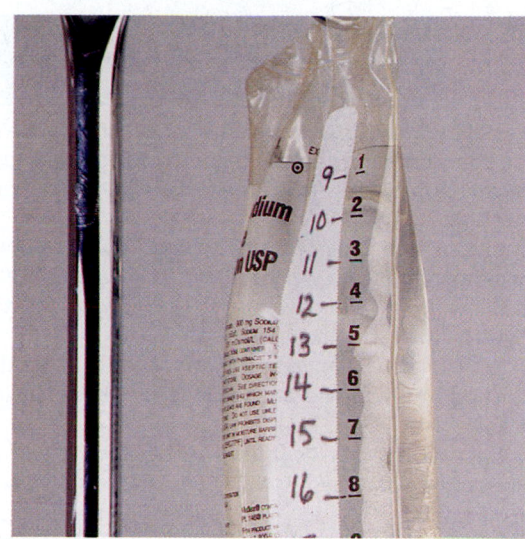

Figure 50–30 ■ Timing label on an intravenous container. The first time marked (0900 hours) would be correct for a bag hung at 0800 hours with a rate of 100 mL per hour.

Regulating and Monitoring Intravenous Infusions. Orders for IV infusions may take several forms: "3,000 mL over 24 hours"; "1,000 mL every 8 hours × 3 bags"; "125 mL/h until oral intake is adequate." The nurse initiating the IV calculates the correct flow rate, regulates the infusion, and monitors the client's responses. Unless an infusion control device is used, the nurse manually regulates the drops per minute of flow using the roller clamp to ensure that the prescribed amount of solution will be infused in the correct time span. If the flow is incorrect, problems such as hypervolemia, hypovolemia, or inadequate medication administration can result.

The number of drops delivered per milliliter of solution varies with different brands and types of infusion sets. This rate, called the **drip factor** (sometimes called the *drop factor*), generally is printed on the package of the infusion set. Macrodrops commonly have drop factors of 10, 12, 15, or 20 drops/mL; the drop factor for microdrip is always 60 drops/mL (Figure 50–29 ■).

To calculate flow rates, the nurse must know the volume of fluid to be infused and the specific time for the infusion. Two commonly used methods of indicating flow rates are designating the number of milliliters to be administered in 1 hour (mL/h) and the number of drops to be given in 1 minute (gtt/min). Because 1 milliliter of fluid displaces 1 cubic centimeter of space, the volume to be infused in the first method may also be designated as cubic centimeters per hour (cc/h).

Milliliters per Hour. Hourly rates of infusion can be calculated by dividing the total infusion volume by the total infusion time in hours. For example, if 3,000 mL is infused in 24 hours, the number of milliliters per hour is

$$\frac{3,000 \text{ mL (total infusion volume)}}{24 \text{ h (total infusion time)}} = 125 \text{ mL/h}$$

Nurses need to check infusions at least every hour to ensure that the indicated milliliters per hour have infused and that IV patency is maintained. A strip of adhesive marking the exact time and/or amount to be infused may be taped to the solution container. Some agencies make premarked labels available (Figure 50–30 ■).

DROPS PER MINUTE. The nurse initiating and monitoring an infusion must regulate the drops per minute to ensure that the prescribed amount of solution will infuse. Drops per minute are calculated by the following formula:

$$\text{Drops per minute} = \frac{\text{Total infusion volume} \times \text{drop factor}}{\text{Total time of infusion in } \textit{minutes}}$$

If the requirements are 1,000 mL in 8 hours and the drip factor is 20 drops/mL, the drops per minute should be

$$\frac{1,000 \text{ mL} \times 20}{8 \times 60 \text{ min (480 min)}} = 41 \text{ drops/min}$$

Approximating this rate as 40 drops/min, the nurse regulates the drops per minute by tightening or releasing the IV tubing clamp and counting the drops for 15 seconds, then multiplying that number by 4 (e.g., 10 drops/15 sec).

A number of factors influence flow rate (see Box 50–8).

Devices to Control Infusions. A number of devices are used to control the rate of an infusion. *Electronic infusion devices* (EIDs) regulate the infusion rate at preset limits. They also have an alarm that is triggered when the solution in the IV bag is low, when there is air in the tubing, or when the tubing is not high enough. The *Dial-A-Flo* in-line device (Figure 50–31 ■) is a regulator that controls the amount of fluid to be administered. Hospitals may stock the Dial-A-Flo for use in situations where a pump is not required, but prevention of fluid overload is important. It is preset at the volume to be infused and can be attached at the time the infusion is set up or when the tubing is changed. Another variation is a *volume-control set,* or *Volutrol,* which is used if the volume of fluid administered is to be carefully controlled. The set, which holds a maximum of 100 mL

BOX 50–8 ■ Factors Influencing Flow Rates

- The position of the forearm. Sometimes a change in the position of the client's arm decreases flow. Slight pronation, supination, extension, or elevation of the forearm on a pillow can increase flow.
- The position and patency of the tubing. Tubing can be obstructed by the client's weight, a kink, or a clamp closed too tightly. The flow rate also diminishes when part of the tubing dangles below the puncture site.
- The height of the infusion bottle. Elevating the height of the infusion bottle a few inches can speed the flow by creating more pressure.
- Possible infiltration or fluid leakage. Swelling, a feeling of coldness, and tenderness at the venipuncture site may indicate infiltration.
- Relationship of the size of the angiocath to the vein. A catheter that is too large may impede the infusion flow.

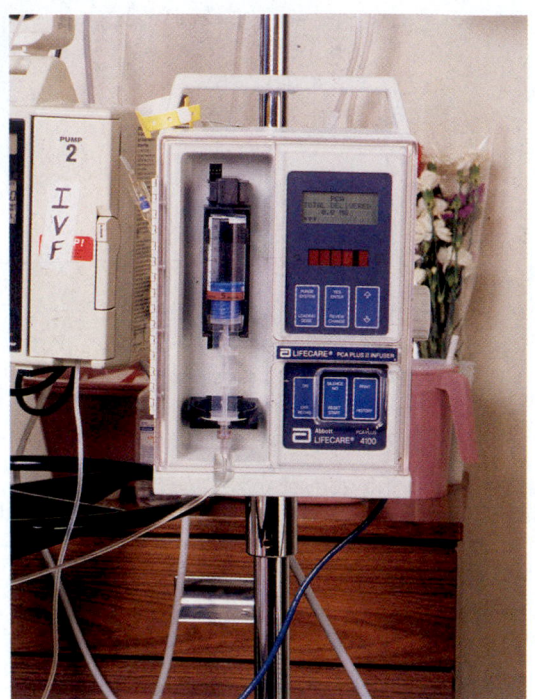

Figure 50–32 ■ An intravenous infusion pump.

of solution, is attached below the solution container, and the drip chamber is placed below the set. Volume-control sets are frequently used in pediatric settings, where the volume administered is critical.

> ► **CLINICAL ALERT**   *A flow rate control device should be used when administering IV fluid to elderly or pediatric clients. Both of these age groups are especially at risk for complications of fluid overload, which can occur with rapid infusion of IV fluids.* ■

An infusion pump (Figures 50–32 ■ and 50–33 ■) delivers fluids intravenously by exerting positive pressure on the tubing or on the fluid. In situations where the fluid flow is unrestricted, the pump pressure is comparable to that of gravity flow.

However, if restrictions develop (increased venous resistance), the pump can maintain the fluid flow by increasing the pressure applied to the fluid.

A controller, by contrast, operates solely by gravitational force. The delivery pressure depends on the height of the container in relation to the venipuncture site. The container must be at least 76 cm (30 in.) above the venipuncture site for a controller to work. A controller does not have the ability to add pressure to the line and to overcome resistances to fluid flow.

Procedure 50–2 outlines the steps involved in monitoring an intravenous infusion.

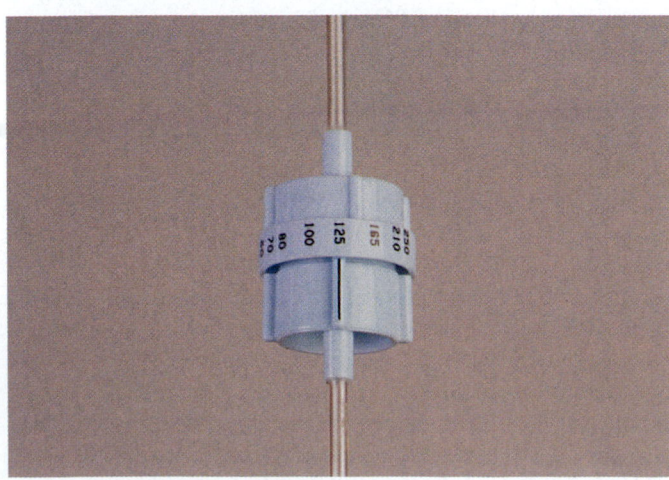

Figure 50–31 ■ The Dial-A-Flo in-line device.

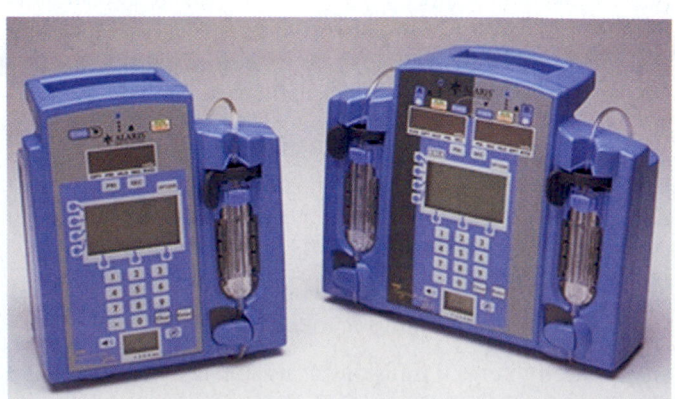

Figure 50–33 ■ Programmable infusion pumps. (Courtesy of ALARIS Medical Systems, Inc., San Diego, California.)

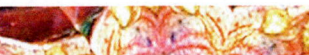 **Procedure 50–2 Monitoring an Intravenous Infusion**

Purposes

- To maintain the prescribed flow rate
- To prevent complications associated with IV therapy

ASSESSMENT

- Appearance of infusion site; patency of system;
- type of fluid being infused and rate of flow;
- Response of the client.

PLANNING

Review the type of equipment used outside the client's room. Read all appropriate materials and confirm the type of tubing, controller, or pump being used.

Delegation

This procedure should be done by the nurse because it is an important part of assessment and complications may occur.

IMPLEMENTATION

Preparation

1. Gather the pertinent data.
   - From the physician's order, determine the type and sequence of solutions to be infused.
   - Determine the rate of flow and infusion schedule.

Performance

1. Ensure that the correct solution is being infused.
   - If the solution in incorrect, slow the rate of flow to a minimum to maintain the patency of the catheter. *Stopping the infusion may allow a thrombus to form in the IV catheter. If this occurs, the catheter must be removed and another venipuncture performed before the infusion can be resumed.*
   - Change the solution to the correct one. Document and report the error according to agency protocol.
2. Observe the rate of flow every hour.
   - Compare the rate of flow regularly, for example, every hour, against the infusion schedule. *Infusions that are off schedule can be harmful to a client.*
   - If the rate is too fast, slow it so that the infusion will be completed at the planned time. *Solution administered too quickly may cause a significant increase in circulating blood volume (which is about 6 L in an adult). Hypervolemia may result in pulmonary edema and cardiac failure.* Assess the client for manifestations of hypervolemia and its complications, including dyspnea; rapid, labored breathing; cough; crackles (rales) in the lung bases; tachycardia; and bounding pulses.

   - If the rate is too slow, check agency practice. Some agencies permit nursing personnel to adjust a rate of flow by a specified amount. Adjustments above this rate require a physician's order. *Solution that is administered too slowly can supply insufficient fluid, electrolytes, or medication for a client's needs.*
   - If the rate of flow is 150 mL/h or more, check the rate of flow more frequently, for example, every 15 to 30 minutes.
3. Inspect the patency of the IV tubing and needle.
   - Observe the position of the solution container. If it is less than 1 m (3 ft) above the IV site, readjust it to the correct height of the pole. *If the container is too low, the solution may not flow into the vein because there is insufficient gravitational pressure to overcome the pressure of the blood within the vein.*
   - Observe the drip chamber. If it is less than half full, squeeze the chamber to allow the correct amount of fluid to flow in.
   - Open the drip regulator and observe for a rapid flow of fluid from the solution container into the drip chamber. Then partially close the drip regulator to reestablish the prescribed rate of flow. *Rapid flow of fluid into the drip chamber indicates patency of the IV line. Closing the drip regulator to the prescribed rate of flow prevents fluid overload.*
   - Inspect the tubing for pinches or kinks or obstructions to flow. Arrange the tubing so that it is

   lightly coiled and under no pressure. Sometimes the tubing becomes caught under the client's body and the weight blocks the flow.
   - Observe the position of the tubing. If it is dangling below the venipuncture, coil it carefully on the surface of the bed. *The solution may not flow upward into the vein against the force of gravity.*
   - Lower the solution container below the level of the infusion site and observe for a return flow of blood from the vein. *A return flow of blood indicates that the needle is patent and in the vein. Blood returns in this instance because venous pressure is greater than the fluid pressure in the IV tubing. Absence of blood return may indicate that the needle is no longer in the vein or that the tip of the catheter is partially obstructed by a thrombus, the vein wall, or a valve in the vein.*
   - Determine whether the bevel of the catheter is blocked against the wall of the vein. If it is blocked, pull back gently, turn it slightly, or carefully raise or lower the angle of insertion slightly, using a sterile gauze pad underneath to protect the skin and change the position of the catheter bevel.
   - If there is leakage, locate the source. If the leak is at the catheter connection, tighten the tubing into the catheter. If the leak cannot be stopped, slow the infusion as much as possible without stopping it, and replace the tubing with a new sterile set. Estimate the amount of solution lost, if it was substantial.

continued on page 1394

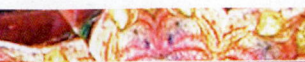

Procedure 50–2 Monitoring an Intravenous Infusion *continued*

IMPLEMENTATION *continued*

4. Inspect the insertion site for fluid infiltration.
   - When an IV needle becomes dislodged from the vein, fluid flows into interstitial tissues, causing swelling. This is known as *infiltration* and is manifested by localized swelling, coolness, pallor, and discomfort at the IV site.
   - If an infiltration is present, stop the infusion and remove the catheter. Restart the infusion at another site.
   - Apply a warm compress to the site of the infiltration. *Warmth promotes comfort and vasodilation, facilitating absorption of the fluid from interstitial tissues.*
5. If infiltration is not evident but the infusion is not flowing, determine whether the needle is dislodged from the vein.
   - Gently pinch the IV tubing adjacent to the needle site. This will cause blood to flow (flash back) into the tubing if the needle is in the vein.

- Use a sterile syringe of saline to withdraw fluid from the port near the venipuncture site. If blood does not return, discontinue the intravenous solution.
6. Inspect the insertion site for phlebitis (inflammation of a vein).
   - Inspect and palpate the site at least every 8 hours. Phlebitis can occur as a result of injury to a vein, for example, because of mechanical trauma or chemical irritation. Chemical injury to a vein can occur from intravenous electrolytes (especially potassium and magnesium) and medications. The clinical signs are redness, warmth, and swelling at the intravenous site and burning pain along the course of a vein.
   - If phlebitis is detected, discontinue the infusion, and apply warm compresses to the venipuncture site. Do not use this injured vein for further infusions.
7. Inspect the intravenous site for bleeding.

- Oozing or bleeding into the surrounding tissues can occur while the infusion is freely flowing but is more likely to occur after the needle has been removed from the vein.
- Observation of the venipuncture site is extremely important for clients who bleed readily, such as those receiving anticoagulants.
8. Teach the client ways to maintain the infusion system, for example:
   - Avoid sudden twisting or turning movements of the arm with the needle or catheter.
   - Avoid stretching or placing tension on the tubing.
   - Try to keep the tubing from dangling below the level of the needle.
   - Notify a nurse if
     a. The flow rate suddenly changes or the solution stops dripping.
     b. The solution container is nearly empty.
     c. There is blood in the IV tubing.
     d. Discomfort or swelling is experienced at the IV site.
9. Document all relevant information.

EVALUATION

- Amount of fluid infused according to the schedule;
- Intactness of IV system;
- Appearance of IV site (e.g., dry, tissue infiltration, discomfort);
- Urinary output compared to urinary intake;
- Tissue turgor; specific gravity of urine;
- Vital signs and lung sounds compared to baseline data.

Changing Intravenous Containers, Tubing, and Dressings. Intravenous solution containers are changed when only a small amount of fluid remains in the neck of the container and fluid still remains in the drip chamber. However, all IV bags should be changed every 24 hours, regardless of how much solution remains, to minimize the risk of contamination. IV tubing is changed every 48 to 96 hours, depending on agency protocol, as is the site dressing. Procedure 50–3 provides guidelines for changing an IV solution container, tubing, and the IV site dressing.

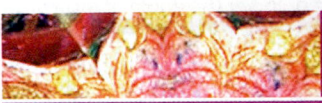

Procedure 50–3 Changing an Intravenous Container, Tubing, and Dressing

Purposes

- To maintain the flow of required fluids
- To maintain sterility of the IV system and decrease the incidence of phlebitis and infection
- To maintain patency of the IV tubing
- To prevent infection at the IV site and the introduction of microorganisms into the bloodstream

ASSESSMENT

- Presence of fluid infiltration, bleeding, or phlebitis at IV site;
- Allergy to tape or iodine;
- Infusion rate and amount absorbed;
- Blockages in IV system;
- Appearance of the dressing for integrity, moisture, and need for change;
- The date and the time of the previous dressing change.

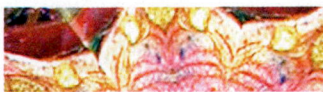

Procedure 50–3 Changing an Intravenous Container, Tubing, and Dressing *continued*

PLANNING

Review physician's orders for changes in fluid administration.

Delegation

This procedure includes assessment of the IV site and should be completed by a registered nurse. In some states, licensed vocational nurses with IV certification may complete the procedure.

Equipment

- Container with the correct kind and amount of sterile solution
- Administration set, including sterile tubing and drip chamber
- Timing label
- Sterile gauze square for positioning the needle

FOR THE DRESSING

- Clean gloves
- Sterile 2-in. × 2-in. or 4-in. × 4-in. gauze or transparent dressing
- Adhesive remover
- Povidone-iodine swabs
- Alcohol swabs
- *Optional:* Antiseptic ointment (e.g., povidone-iodine or other recommended by the agency)
- Tape
- Towel

IMPLEMENTATION

Preparation

1. Obtain the correct solution container.
   - Read the label of the new container.
   - Verify that you have the correct solution, correct client, correct additives (if any), and correct dose (number of bags or total volume ordered).

Performance

1. Wash your hands.
2. Set up the intravenous equipment with the new container and label all. See Procedure 50–1, steps 1 to 8.
   - Apply a timing label to the container.
   - Prime the tubing.
   - Label the tubing as shown in Figure 50–27.
3. Prepare the IV needle or catheter tape and the dressing equipment near the client.
   - Prepare strips of tape as needed for the type of needle or catheter. For the butterfly needle, two or three strips of 1.25-cm (1/2-in.) tape are needed. For a catheter, three strips of 1.25-cm (1/2-in.) tape are needed. These will be used later to secure the needle or catheter without covering the insertion site.
   - Hang the pieces of tape from the edge of a table. *This places the tape in readiness for use without disrupting the adhesive.*
   - Open all equipment: swabs, dressing and adhesive bandage, and ointment. *This facilitates access to supplies after gloves are donned.*
   - Place a towel under the extremity. *This prevents soiling of bed linens.*
   - Apply clean gloves.

4. Remove the soiled dressing and all tape, except the tape holding the catheter or IV needle in place.
   - Remove tape and gauze from the old dressing one layer at a time. *This prevents dislodgement of the catheter or needle in case tubing becomes entangled between layers of dressing.*
   - Remove adhesive dressings in the direction of the client's hair growth when possible. *This minimizes discomfort when adhesive is removed from the skin.*
   - Discard the used dressing materials in the appropriate container.
5. Assess the IV site.
   - Inspect the IV site for the presence of infiltration or inflammation. *Inflammation or infiltration necessitates removal of the IV needle or catheter to avoid further trauma to the tissues.*
   - Go to step 6, or discontinue and relocate the IV site if indicated. See Procedures 50–1 and 50–4.
6. Disconnect the used tubing.
   - Place a sterile swab under the hub of the catheter. *This absorbs any leakage that might occur when the tubing is disconnected.*
   - Clamp the tubing.
   - Holding the hub of the catheter with the nondominant hand, loosen the tubing with the dominant hand, using a twisting, pulling motion. *Holding the catheter firmly but gently maintains its position in the vein.*
   - Remove the used IV tubing.
   - Place the end of the tubing in the basin or other receptacle.

7. Connect the new tubing, and reestablish the infusion.
   - Continue to hold the catheter and grasp the new tubing with the dominant hand.
   - Remove the protective tubing cap and, maintaining sterility, insert the tubing end securely into the needle hub. Twist it to secure it.
   - Open the clamp to start the solution flowing.
8. Remove the tape securing the needle or catheter.
   - When removing this tape and while cleaning the site, stabilize the needle or catheter hub with one hand. *This prevents inadvertent dislodgement of the needle or catheter.*
9. Clean the IV site.
   - Start with adhesive remover to remove adhesive residue. *Removal of adhesive residue facilitates adherence of the new dressing.*
   - Then, using chlorhexidine swabs or alcohol and povidone-iodine swabs, clean the site, beginning at the catheter or needle and cleaning outward in a 2-in. diameter. *Cleaning in this manner prevents contamination of the IV site from bacteria on the peripheral skin areas. Antiseptics reduce the number of microorganisms present at the site, thus reducing the risk of infection.*
   - Follow agency protocol about cleaning procedures.
10. Retape the needle or catheter.
    - For a butterfly needle, apply strips of tape to the wings of the butterfly using the crisscross (chevron) method (Figure 50–28).

continued on page 1396

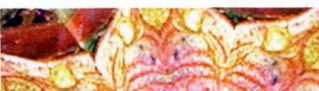

Procedure 50–3 Changing an Intravenous Container, Tubing, and Dressing *continued*

IMPLEMENTATION *continued*

- For a catheter; apply the tape using the U method (Figure 50–25).
11. Apply antiseptic ointment or solution if indicated and apply the dressing.
    - Place povidone-iodine ointment or solution at the entry site in accordance with agency protocol. *This reduces skin bacteria and risk of infection. Solution is preferred to ointment when transparent dressings are used because the former facilitates the dressing's adherence; however, solution can traumatize the skin.*

- Apply a sterile gauze or transparent dressing over the site.
- Remove gloves.
12. Label the dressing and secure IV tubing.
    - Place the date and time of the dressing change and your initials either on the label provided or directly over the top of the dressing.
    - Secure IV tubing with additional tape as required.
13. Regulate the rate of flow of the solution according to the order on the chart.

14. Document all relevant information.
    - Record the change of the solution container, tubing, and/or dressing in the appropriate place on the client's chart. Also record the fluid intake according to agency practice. Record the number of the container if the containers are numbered at the agency. Also record your assessments.

EVALUATION

- Status of IV site;
- Patency of IV system;

- Accuracy of flow.

When an IV infusion is no longer necessary to maintain the client's fluid intake or to provide a route for medication administration, the infusion is either discontinued and the catheter removed or the catheter is left in place and converted to a saline or heparin lock. Guidelines for discontinuing an IV infusion or converting the catheter to a lock are outlined in Procedures 50–4 and 50–5, respectively.

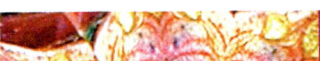

Procedure 50–4 Discontinuing an Intravenous Infusion

Purpose

- To discontinue an intravenous infusion when the therapy is complete or when the IV site needs to be changed

ASSESSMENT

- Appearance of the venipuncture site;
- Any bleeding from the infusion site;

- Amount of fluid infused;
- Appearance of IV catheter.

PLANNING

Review physician's orders.

Delegation
This procedure should be done by a registered nurse. In some states, licensed vocational nurses may initiate and discontinue IV therapy.

Equipment
- Clean gloves
- Dry or antiseptic-soaked swabs, according to agency practice
- Small sterile dressing and tape

IMPLEMENTATION

Performance

1. Prepare the equipment.
   - Clamp the infusion tubing. *Clamping the tubing prevents the fluid from flowing out of the needle onto the client or bed.*

- Loosen the tape at the venipuncture site while holding the needle firmly and applying countertraction to the skin. *Movement of the needle can injure the vein and cause discom-*

fort to the client. Countertraction prevents pulling the skin and causing discomfort.
- Don clean gloves and hold a sterile gauze above the venipuncture site.

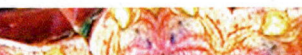

Procedure 50–4 Discontinuing an Intravenous Infusion *continued*

IMPLEMENTATION *continued*

2. Withdraw the needle or catheter from the vein.
   - Withdraw the needle or catheter by pulling it out along the line of the vein. *Pulling it out in line with the vein avoids injury to the vein.*
   - Immediately apply firm pressure to the site, using sterile gauze, for 2 to 3 minutes. *Pressure helps stop the bleeding and prevents hematoma formation.*
   - Hold the client's arm or leg above the body if any bleeding persists. *Raising the limb decreases blood flow to the area.*

3. Examine the catheter removed from the client.
   - Check the catheter to make sure it is intact. *If a piece of tubing remains in the client's vein it could move centrally (toward the heart or lungs) and cause serious problems.*
   - Report a broken catheter to the nurse in charge or physician immediately.
   - If a broken piece can be palpated, apply a tourniquet above the insertion site. *Application of a tourniquet decreases the possibility of the piece moving until a physician is notified.*

4. Cover the venipuncture site.
   - Apply the sterile dressing. *The dressing continues the pressure and covers the open area in the skin, preventing infection.*
   - Discard the IV solution container properly, if infusions are being discontinued, and discard the used supplies appropriately.
5. Document all relevant information.
   - Record the amount of fluid infused on the intake and output record and on the chart, according to agency practice. Include the container number, type of solution used, time of discontinuing the infusion, and the client's response.

EVALUATION

- Appearance of the venipuncture site;
- The pulse;

- Respirations, skin color, edema, sputum, cough, and urine output;
- And how the person feels physically and psychologically.

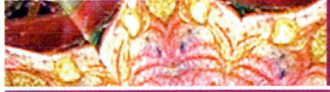

Procedure 50–5 Changing an Intravenous Catheter to an Intermittent Infusion Lock

Purpose

- To permit IV administration of medications or fluids on an intermittent basis

ASSESSMENT

- Patency of the IV catheter,

- Appearance of the site (evidence of inflammation or infiltration).

PLANNING

Review physician's order.
- A specific order may be written to convert an intravenous access to a heparin or saline lock. The order also may be implied, for example, IV fluids are to be discontinued but the client has orders for an IV antibiotic every 6 hours or is receiving analgesics intravenously.

Delegation

Due to the need for sterile technique and technical complexity, this procedure is not delegated to UAP. UAP may care for clients with such devices, and the nurse must ensure that the UAP knows what complications or adverse signs should be reported to the nurse.

Equipment
- Intermittent infusion cap or device
- Clean gloves
- Sterile 2-in. × 2-in. or 4-in. × 4-in. gauze
- Sterile saline for injection (without preservative) or heparin flush solution (10 units/mL or 100 units/mL) in a prefilled syringe, a 3-mL syringe with a needleless infusion device
- Isopropyl alcohol wipe
- Tape
- Clean emesis basin

continued on page 1398

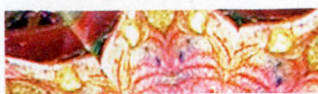

Procedure 50–5 Changing an Intravenous Catheter to an Intermittent Infusion Lock *continued*

IMPLEMENTATION

Preparation

1. Prepare the client.
   - Explain the procedure to the client and the reason for leaving the IV catheter in place. Changing an IV to a heparin or saline lock should cause no discomfort other than that associated with removing tape from the IV tubing.

Performance

1. Prepare the equipment.
   - Wash your hands.
   - Assess the IV site (if visible) and determine the patency of the catheter (see Procedure 50–2). If the catheter is not fully patent or there is evidence of phlebitis or infiltration, discontinue the catheter and establish a new IV site.
   - Expose the IV catheter hub and loosen any tape that is holding the IV tubing in place or that will interfere with insertion of the intermittent infusion plug into the catheter.
   - Clamp the IV tubing to stop the flow of IV fluid.

   - Open the gauze pad and place it under the IV catheter hub.
   - Open the alcohol wipe and intermittent infusion plug, leaving the plug in its sterile package.

2. Remove the IV tubing and insert the intermittent infusion plug into the IV catheter.
   - Put on gloves.
   - Stabilize the IV catheter with your nondominant hand and use the little finger to place slight pressure on the vein above the end of the catheter. Twist the IV tubing adapter to loosen it from the IV catheter and remove it, placing the end of the tubing in a clean emesis basin.
   - Pick up the intermittent infusion plug from its package and remove the protective sleeve from the male adapter, maintaining its sterility. Insert the plug into the IV catheter, twisting it to seat it firmly or engage the Luer lock.

3. Instill saline or heparin solution per agency policy. *Saline or heparin are used to maintain patency of the IV*

catheter when fluids are not infusing through the catheter.

4. Tape the intermittent infusion plug in place using a chevron or U method. *Tape provides added security to prevent the infusion plug from coming out of the intravenous catheter. It also promotes comfort, preventing the plug from catching on clothing or bedding.*

5. Teach the client how to maintain the lock.
   - Avoid manipulating the catheter or infusion plug and protect it from catching on clothing or bedding. A gauze bandage such as Kerlix or Kling may be wrapped over the plug when it is not in use to protect it.
   - Cover the site with an occlusive dressing when showering; avoid immersing the site.
   - Flush the catheter with saline or heparin solution as directed.
   - Notify the nurse or primary care provider if the plug or catheter comes out, if the site becomes red, inflamed, or painful, or if any drainage or bleeding occurs at the site.

6. Document all relevant information.

EVALUATION

- Patency of the catheter;
- Appearance of the site;
- Ease of flushing.

Blood Transfusions

Intravenous fluids can be effective in restoring intravascular (blood) volume; however, they do not affect the oxygen-carrying capacity of the blood. When red and white blood cells, platelets, or blood proteins are lost because of hemorrhage or disease, it may be necessary to replace these components to restore the blood's ability to transport oxygen and carbon dioxide, to clot, to fight infection, and to keep extracellular fluid within the intravascular compartment. A blood transfusion is the introduction of whole blood or blood components into the venous circulation.

Blood Groups.

Human blood is commonly classified into four main groups (A, B, AB, and O). The surface of an individual's red blood cells contains a number of proteins known as **antigens** that are unique for each person. Many blood antigens have been identified, but the antigens A, B, and Rh are the most important in determining blood group or type. Because antigens promote *agglutination* or clumping of blood cells, they

are also known as **agglutinogens.** The A antigen or agglutinogen is present on the RBCs of people with blood group A, the B antigen is present in people with blood group B, and both A and B antigens are found on the RBC surface in people with group AB blood. Neither antigen is present in people with group O blood.

Preformed **antibodies** to RBC antigens are present in the plasma; these antibodies are often called **agglutinins.** People with blood group A have B antibodies (agglutinins); A antibodies are present in people with blood group B; and people with blood group O have antibodies to both A and B antigens. People with group AB blood do not have antibodies to either A or B antigens (Table 50–11). When blood is transfused, the blood group of the donor and recipient must match to avoid an antigen-antibody reaction and destruction (hemolysis) of RBCs.

Rhesus (Rh) Factor.

The Rh factor antigen is present on the RBCs of approximately 85% of the people in the United States. Blood that contains the Rh factor is known as Rh-positive

TABLE 50–11 The Blood Groups with Their Constituent Agglutinogens and Agglutinins

Blood Types	RBC Antigens (Agglutinogens)	Plasma Antibodies (Agglutinins)
A	A	B
B	B	A
AB	A and B	—
O	—	A and B

(Rh$^+$); when it is not present the blood is said to be Rh-negative (Rh$^-$). In contrast to the ABO blood groups, Rh$^-$ blood does not naturally contain Rh antibodies. However, on exposure to blood containing Rh factor (e.g., an Rh$^-$ mother carrying a fetus with Rh$^+$ blood, or transfusion of Rh$^+$ blood into a client who is Rh$^-$), Rh antibodies develop. Subsequent exposures to Rh$^+$ blood place the client at risk for an antigen–antibody reaction and hemolysis of RBCs.

Blood Typing and Crossmatching. To avoid transfusing incompatible red blood cells, both blood donor and recipient are typed and their blood crossmatched. *Blood typing* is done to determine the ABO blood group and Rh factor status. This test is also performed on pregnant women and neonates to assess for possible intrauterine exposure of either to an incompatible blood type (particularly Rh factor incompatibilities).

Because blood typing only determines the presence of the major ABO and Rh antigens, *crossmatching* also is necessary prior to transfusion to identify possible interactions of minor antigens with their corresponding antibodies. RBCs from the donor blood are mixed with serum from the recipient; a reagent (Coombs' serum) is added, and the mixture is examined for vis-

ible agglutination. If no antibodies to the donated RBCs are present in the recipient's serum, agglutination does not occur and the risk of transfusion reaction is small.

Selection of Blood Donors. Screening of blood donors is rigorous. Criteria have been established to protect the donor from possible ill effects of donation and to protect the recipient from exposure to diseases transmitted through the blood. Blood donors are unpaid volunteers. Potential donors are eliminated by a history of hepatitis, HIV infection (or risk factors for HIV infection), heart disease, most cancers, severe asthma, bleeding disorders, or convulsions. Donation may be deferred for people with malaria or who have been exposed to malaria or hepatitis or in situations of pregnancy, surgery, anemia, high or low blood pressure, and certain drugs.

Blood and Blood Products for Transfusion. Most clients do not require transfusion of whole blood. Most often transfusion of a particular blood component is more appropriate. Table 50–12 lists some of the common blood products that may be transfused.

Transfusion Reactions. Transfusion of ABO- or Rh-incompatible blood can result in a **hemolytic transfusion reaction** with destruction of the transfused RBCs and subsequent risk of kidney damage or failure. Other forms of transfusion reaction also may occur, including febrile, allergic, circulatory overload, and sepsis. Because the risk of an adverse reaction is high when blood is transfused, clients must be frequently and carefully assessed before and during transfusion. Many reactions become evident within 30 minutes of initiating the transfusion; clients are closely monitored during this period. Stop the transfusion immediately if signs of a reaction develop. Possible transfusion reactions, their clinical signs, and nursing implications are listed in Table 50–13.

TABLE 50–12 Blood Products for Transfusion

Product	Use
Whole blood	Not commonly used except for extreme cases of acute hemorrhage. Replaces blood volume and all blood products: RBCs, plasma, plasma proteins, fresh platelets, and other clotting factors.
Red blood cells	Used to increase the oxygen-carrying capacity of blood in anemias, surgery, disorders with slow bleeding. One unit raises hematocrit by approximately 4%.
Autologous red blood cells	Used for blood replacement following planned elective surgery. Client donates blood for autologous transfusion 4–5 weeks prior to surgery.
Platelets	Replaces platelets in clients with bleeding disorders or platelet deficiency. Fresh platelets most effective.
Fresh frozen plasma	Expands blood volume and provides clotting factors. Does not need to be typed and crossmatched (contains no RBCs).
Albumin and plasma protein fraction	Blood volume expander; provides plasma proteins.
Clotting factors and cryoprecipitate	Used for clients with clotting factor deficiencies. Each provides different factors involved in the clotting pathway; cryoprecipitate also contains fibrinogen.

TABLE 50-13 Transfusion Reactions

Reaction: Cause	Clinical Signs	Nursing Intervention*
Hemolytic reaction: incompatibility between client's blood and donor's blood	Chills, fever, headache, backache, dyspnea, cyanosis, chest pain, tachycardia, hypotension	1. Discontinue the transfusion immediately. **NOTE:** When the transfusion is discontinued, the blood tubing must be removed as well. Use new tubing for the normal saline infusion. 2. Keep the vein open with normal saline, or according to agency protocol. 3. Send the remaining blood, a sample of the client's blood, and a urine sample to the laboratory. 4. Notify the physician immediately. 5. Monitor vital signs. 6. Monitor fluid intake and output.
Febrile reaction: sensitivity of the client's blood to white blood cells, platelets, or plasma proteins	Fever; chills; warm, flushed skin; headache; anxiety, muscle pain	1. Discontinue the transfusion immediately. 2. Give antipyretics as ordered. 3. Notify the physician. 4. Keep the vein open with a normal saline infusion
Allergic reaction (mild): sensitivity to infused plasma proteins	Flushing, itching, urticaria, bronchial wheezing	1. Stop or slow the transfusion, depending on agency protocol. 2. Notify the physician. 3. Administer medication (antihistamines) as ordered.
Allergic reaction (severe): antibody–antigen reaction	Dyspnea, chest pain, circulatory collapse, cardiac arrest	1. Stop the transfusion. 2. Keep the vein open with normal saline. 3. Notify the physician immediately. 4. Monitor vital signs. Administer cardiopulmonary resuscitation if needed. 5. Administer medications and/or oxygen as ordered.
Circulatory overload: blood administered faster than the circulation can accommodate	Cough, dyspnea, crackles (rales), distended neck veins, tachycardia, hypertension	1. Place the client upright, with feet dependent. 2. Administer diuretics and oxygen as ordered. 3. Notify the physician. 4. Stop or slow the transfusion.
Sepsis: contaminated blood administered	High fever, chills vomiting, diarrhea, hypotension	1. Stop the transfusion. 2. Send the remaining blood to laboratory. 3. Notify the physician. 4. Obtain a blood specimen from the client for culture. 5. Administer IV fluids, antibiotics. 6. Keep the vein open with a normal saline infusion.

*Nurses should follow agency's protocol regarding interventions. These may vary among agencies.

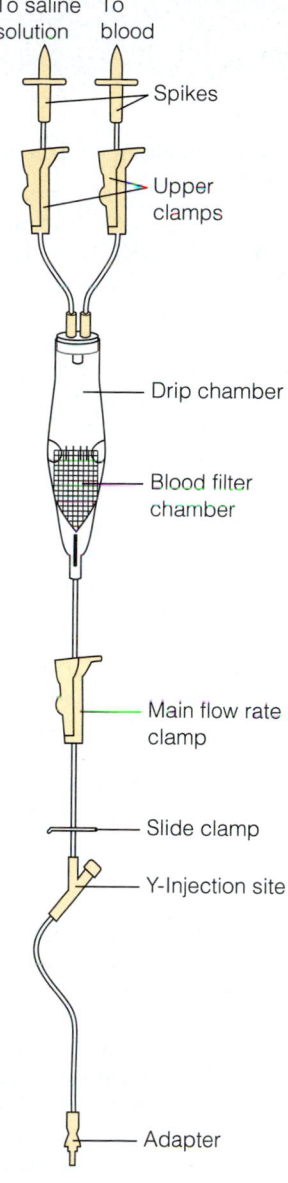

To saline solution   To blood

- Spikes
- Upper clamps
- Drip chamber
- Blood filter chamber
- Main flow rate clamp
- Slide clamp
- Y-Injection site
- Adapter

Figure 50–34 ■ Schematic of a Y-set for blood administration.

Administering Blood. Special precautions are necessary when administering blood.

When a transfusion is ordered, obtain the blood from the blood bank just before starting the transfusion. Do not store the blood in the refrigerator on the nursing unit; lack of temperature control may damage the blood. Follow agency policies for verifying that the unit is correct for the client. Blood is administered through a #18- or #19-gauge intravenous needle or catheter; using a smaller needle may slow the infusion and damage blood cells (although a smaller gauge needle may be necessary for small children or clients with small, fragile veins). A Y-type blood transfusion set with an in-line or add-on filter is used when administering blood (Figure 50–34 ■). One arm of the administration set connects to the blood; normal saline (0.9% NaCl) is attached to the other arm of the Y-type set. Saline is used to prime the set and flush the needle before administering blood. It also provides a means to keep the vein open should a transfusion reaction occur. No other IV solutions should be administered with blood; they may cause the blood cells to clump or cause clotting. A transfusion should be completed within 4 hours of initiation. The risk of sepsis increases if blood hangs for a longer period. Blood tubing is changed after every 4 to 6 units per agency policy; new intravenous tubing is used following a transfusion.

To initiate, maintain, and terminate a blood transfusion, see Procedure 50–6.

> **CLINICAL ALERT** *Normal saline should always be used when giving a blood transfusion. If the client has an infusion of dextrose, stop that infusion and flush the line with saline prior to initiating the transfusion. Solutions other than saline can cause damage to the blood components.* ■

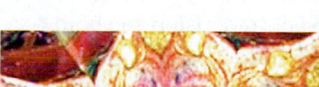

Procedure 50–6 Initiating, Maintaining, and Terminating a Blood Transfusion Using a Y-Set

Purposes

- To restore blood volume after severe hemorrhage
- To restore the capacity of the blood to carry oxygen
- To provide plasma factors, such as antihemophilic factor (AHF) or factor VIII, or platelet concentrates, *which prevent or treat bleeding*

ASSESSMENT

- Clinical signs of reaction (e.g., sudden chills, fever, nausea, itching, rash, low back pain, dyspnea);
- Manifestations of hypervolemia;
- Status of infusion site;
- Any unusual symptoms.

continued on page 1402

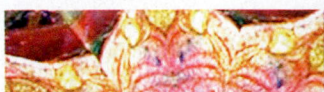

Procedure 50–6 Initiating, Maintaining, and Terminating a Blood Transfusion Using a Y-Set *continued*

PLANNING

- Verify physician order for transfusion
- Verify client consent and obtain baseline data before the transfusion.
- Verify that a signed consent form was obtained.
- Assess vital signs for baseline data, including blood pressure, pulse, respiratory rate and depth, and temperature.
- Determine any known allergies or previous adverse reactions to blood.
- Note specific signs related to the client's pathology and the reason for the transfusion. For example, for an anemic client, note the hemoglobin and hematocrit levels

Delegation

Due to the need for sterile technique and technical complexity, blood transfusion is not delegated to UAP. The nurse must ensure that the UAP knows what complications or adverse signs can occur and should be reported to the nurse.

Equipment

- Unit of whole blood, or packed RBCs
- Blood administration set
- 250 mL normal saline for infusion
- IV pole
- Venipuncture set containing a #18- or #19-gauge needle or catheter (if one is not already in place) or, if blood is to be administered quickly, a #15-gauge needle or a larger catheter (e.g., #14)
- Povidone-iodine solution or scrub pad
- Alcohol swabs
- Tape
- Clean gloves

IMPLEMENTATION

Preparation

1. Prepare the client.
   - Explain the procedure and its purpose to the client. Instruct the client to report promptly any sudden chills, nausea, itching, rash, dyspnea, back pain, or other unusual symptoms.
   - If the client has an intravenous solution infusing, check whether the needle and solution are appropriate to administer blood. The needle should be #18 or #19 gauge, and the solution must be normal saline. Dextrose (which causes lysis of RBCs), Ringer's solution, medications and other additives, and hyperalimentation solutions are incompatible. Refer to step 5 below if the infusing solution is not compatible.
   - If the client does not have an IV solution infusing, check agency policies. In some agencies an infusion must be running before the blood is obtained from the blood bank. In this case, you will need to perform a venipuncture on a suitable vein (see Procedure 50–1) and start an IV infusion of normal saline.

Performance

1. Obtain the correct blood component for the client.
   - Check the physician's order with the requisition.
   - Check the requisition form and the blood bag label with a laboratory technician or according to agency policy. Specifically, check the client's name, identification number, blood type (A, B, AB, or O) and Rh group, the blood donor number, and the expiration date of the blood. Observe the blood for abnormal color, RBC clumping, gas bubbles, and extraneous material. Return outdated or abnormal blood to the blood bank.
   - With another nurse (the agency may require an RN), compare the laboratory blood record with
     a. The client's name and identification number
     b. The number on the blood bag label
     c. The ABO group and Rh type on the blood bag label.
   - If any of the information does not match exactly, notify the charge nurse and the blood bank. Do not administer blood until discrepancies are corrected or clarified.
   - Sign the appropriate form with the other nurse according to agency policy.
   - Make sure that the blood is left at room temperature for no more than 30 minutes before starting the transfusion. *RBCs deteriorate and lose their effectiveness after 2 hours at room temperature. Lysis of RBCs releases potassium into the bloodstream, causing hyperkalemia.* Agencies may designate different times at which the blood must be returned to the blood bank if it has not been started. *As blood components warm, the risk of bacterial growth also increases.* If the start of the transfusion is unexpectedly delayed, return the blood to the blood bank. Do not store blood in the unit refrigerator. *The temperature of unit refrigerators is not precisely regulated and the blood may be damaged.*

2. Verify the client's identity.
   - Ask the client's full name.
   - Check the client's arm band for name and ID number. Do not administer blood to a client without an arm band.

3. Set up the infusion equipment.
   - Ensure that the blood filter inside the drip chamber is suitable for whole blood or the blood components to be transfused. Attach the blood tubing to the blood filter, if necessary. *Blood filters have a surface area large enough to allow the blood components through easily but are designed to trap clots.*
   - Put on gloves.
   - Close all clamps on the Y-set: the main flow rate clamp and both Y-line clamps.
   - Using a twisting motion, insert the piercing pin (spike) into a container of 0.9% saline solution.
   - Hang the container on the IV pole about 1 m (36 in.) above the planned venipuncture site.

4. Prime the tubing.
   - Open the upper clamp on the normal saline tubing and squeeze the drip chamber until it covers the filter and one-third of the drip chamber above the filter.

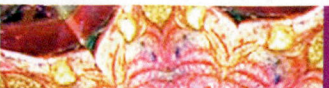

IMPLEMENTATION *continued*

- Tap the filter chamber to expel any residual air in the filter.
- Remove the adapter cover at the tip of the blood administration set.
- Open the main flow rate clamp, and prime the tubing with saline.
- Close both clamps.

5. Start the saline solution.
- If an IV solution incompatible with blood is infusing, stop the infusion and discard the solution and tubing according to agency policy.
- Attach the blood tubing primed with normal saline to the intravenous catheter.
- Open the saline and main flow rate clamps and adjust the flow rate. Use only the main flow rate clamp to adjust the rate.
- Allow a small amount of solution to infuse to make sure there are no problems with the flow or with the venipuncture site. *Infusing normal saline before initiating the transfusion also clears the IV catheter of incompatible solutions or medications.*

6. Prepare the blood bag.
- Invert the blood bag gently several times to mix the cells with the plasma. *Rough handling can damage the cells.*
- Expose the port on the blood bag by pulling back the tabs (Figure 50–35 ■).

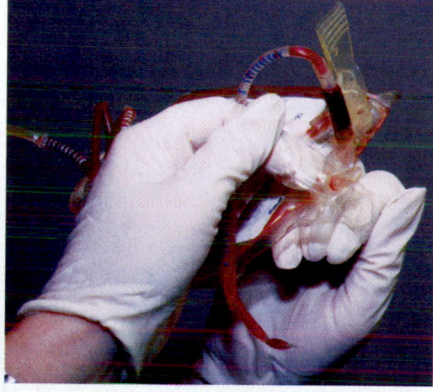

Figure 50–35 ■ Exposing the port on the blood bag by pulling back the tabs.

- Insert the remaining Y-set spike into the blood bag.
- Suspend the blood bag.

- Close the upper clamp below the IV saline solution on the Y-set.
- Open the clamp on the blood arm of the Y-set and prime the tubing.

7. Establish the blood transfusion.
- The blood will run into the saline-filled drip chamber. If necessary, squeeze the drip chamber to reestablish the liquid level with drip chamber one-third full. (Tap the filter to expel any residual air within the filter.)
- Readjust the flow rate with the main clamp.

8. Observe the client closely for the first 5 to 10 minutes.
- Run the blood slowly for the first 15 minutes at 20 drops per minute.
- Note adverse reactions, such as chilling, nausea, vomiting, skin rash, or tachycardia. *The earlier a transfusion reaction occurs, the more severe it tends to be. Identifying such reactions promptly helps to minimize the consequences.*
- Remind the client to call a nurse immediately if any unusual symptoms are felt during the transfusion.
- If any of these reactions occur, report these to the nurse in charge and take appropriate nursing action (see Table 50–13).

9. Document relevant data.
- Record starting the blood, including vital signs, type of blood, blood unit number, sequence number (e.g., no. 1 of three ordered units), site of the venipuncture, size of the needle, and drip rate.

10. Monitor the client.
- Fifteen minutes after initiating the transfusion, check the vital signs of the client. If there are no signs of a reaction, establish the required flow rate. Most adults can tolerate receiving one unit of blood in 1 1/2 to 2 hours. Do not transfuse a unit of blood for longer than 4 hours.
- Assess the client including vital signs every 30 minutes or more often, depending on the health status, until 1 hour post-transfusion. If the client has a reaction and the

blood is discontinued, send the blood bag to the laboratory for investigation of the blood.

11. Terminate the transfusion.
- Don clean gloves.
- If no infusion is to follow, clamp the blood tubing and remove the needle. If another transfusion is to follow, clamp the blood tubing and open the saline infusion arm. Blood administration sets are changed within 24 hours or after 4 to 6 units of blood per agency protocol.
- If the primary IV is to be continued, flush the maintenance line with saline solution. Disconnect the blood tubing system and reestablish the intravenous infusion using new tubing. Adjust the drip to the desired rate. Often a normal saline or other solution is kept running in case of delayed reaction to the blood.
- Discard the administration set according to agency practice. Needles should be placed in a labeled, puncture-resistant container designed for such disposal. Blood bags and administration sets should be bagged and labeled before being sent for decontamination and processing. See agency policy.
- Remove gloves.
- Again monitor vital signs.

12. Follow agency protocol for appropriate disposition of the blood bag.
- On the requisition attached to the blood unit, fill in the time the transfusion was completed and the amount transfused.
- Attach one copy of the requisition to the client's record and another to the empty blood bag.
- Return the blood bag and requisition to the blood bank.

13. Document relevant data.
- Record completion of the transfusion, the amount of blood absorbed, the blood unit number, and the vital signs. If the primary intravenous infusion was continued, record connecting it. Also record the transfusion on the IV flow sheet and I & O record.

EVALUATION

■ Changes in vital signs or health status;

■ Presence of chills, nausea, vomiting, or skin rash.

EVALUATING

Using the overall goals identified in the planning stage of maintaining or restoring fluid balance, maintaining or restoring pulmonary ventilation and oxygenation, maintaining or restoring normal balance of electrolytes, and preventing associated risks of fluid, electrolyte, and acid–base imbalances, the nurse collects data to evaluate the effectiveness of interventions. Examples of desired outcomes for the identified goals are found in Identifying Nursing Diagnoses, Outcomes, and Interventions on pages 1377 and 1378.

If desired outcomes are not achieved, the nurse, client, and support person if appropriate need to explore the reasons before modifying the care plan. For example, if the outcome "Urine output is greater than 1,300 mL per day and within 500 mL of intake" is not achieved, questions to be considered might include

- Have other outcome measures for the goal of achieving fluid balance been met?
- Does the client understand and comply with planned fluid intake?
- Is all urinary output being measured?
- Are unusual or excessive amounts of fluid being lost by another route (e.g., gastric suction, excessive perspiration, fever, rapid respiratory rate, wound drainage)?
- Are prescribed medications being taken or administered as ordered?

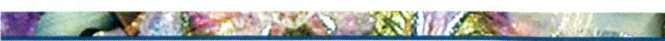

NURSING CARE PLAN FOR DEFICIENT FLUID VOLUME

ASSESSMENT DATA		NURSING DIAGNOSIS	DESIRED OUTCOMES [NOC #]/INDICATORS*
Nursing Assessment Merlyn Chapman, a 27-year-old sales clerk, reports weakness, malaise, and flu-like symptoms for 3–4 days. Although thirsty, she is unable to tolerate fluids because of nausea and vomiting, and she has liquid stools 2–4 times per day.	**Physical Examination** Height: 160 cm (5'3") Weight: 66.2 kg (146 lb) Mild fever: 38.6C (101.5F) Pulse: 86 BPM Respirations: 24/minute Scant urine output BP: 102/84 mm Hg Dry oral mucosa, furrowed tongue, cracked lips **Diagnostic Data** Urine specific gravity: 1.035 Serum sodium 155 mEq/L Serum potassium 3.2 mEq/L Chest x-ray negative	*Deficient Fluid Volume* related to nausea, vomiting, and diarrhea as evidenced by decreased urine output, increased urine concentration, weakness, fever, decreased skin/tongue turgor, dry mucous membranes, increased pulse rate and decreased blood pressure	Electrolyte & Acid/Base Balance [0600] as evidenced by not compromised serum electrolytes within normal limits. Fluid Balance [0601] as evidenced by - Maintains urine output >1,300 mL/day - Maintains normal blood pressure, pulse, and body temperature - Maintains elastic skin turgor, moist tongue, and mucous membranes - Explains measures that can be taken to treat or prevent fluid volume loss - Describes symptoms that indicate the need to consult with health care provider

NURSING INTERVENTIONS [NIC#]/SELECTED ACTIVITIES*	RATIONALE
Electrolyte Management: Hypokalemia [2007] - Obtain specimens for analysis of altered potassium levels (e.g., serum and urine potassium) as indicated.	*Urine and serum analysis provides information about extracellular levels of potassium. There is no practical way to measure intracellular K^+.*
- Administer prescribed supplemental potassium (PO, NG, or IV) per policy.	*Low potassium levels are dangerous and Mrs. Chapman may require supplements.*

NURSING CARE PLAN FOR DEFICIENT FLUID VOLUME *continued*

NURSING INTERVENTIONS [NIC#]/SELECTED ACTIVITIES*	RATIONALE
• Monitor for neurologic and neuromuscular manifestations of hypokalemia (e.g., muscle weakness, lethargy, altered level of consciousness).	Potassium is a vital electrolyte for skeletal and smooth muscle activity.
• Monitor for cardiac manifestations of hypokalemia (e.g., hypotension, tachycardia, weak pulse, rhythm irregularities).	Many cardiac rhythm disorders can result from hypokalemia. It is critical to monitor cardiac function with hypokalemia.
Electrolyte Management: Hypernatremia [2004]	
• Obtain specimens for analysis of altered sodium levels (e.g., serum and urine sodium, urine osmolality, and urine specific gravity) as indicated.	Urine analysis provides information about retention or loss of sodium and the ability of the kidneys to concentrate or dilute urine in response to fluid changes.
• Provide frequent oral hygiene.	Oral mucous membranes become dry and sticky due to loss of fluid in the interstitial spaces.
• Monitor for neurologic and neuromuscular manifestations of hypernatremia (e.g., lethargy, irritability, seizures, and hyper-reflexia).	Hypernatremia, as a result of low fluid volume, creates a hypertonic vascular space, which causes water to move out of the cells, including brain cells. This accounts for neurologic symptoms.
• Monitor for cardiac manifestations of hypernatremia (e.g., tachycardia, orthostatic hypotension, and flat neck veins.)	The heart responds to a loss of fluid by increasing the heart rate to compensate with an increase in cardiac output. Low fluid volume leads to a fall in blood pressure and flat neck veins.
Fluid Management [4120]	
• Weigh daily and monitor trends.	Weight helps to assess fluid balance.
• Maintain accurate I & O record.	Accurate records are critical in assessing the patient's fluid balance.
• Monitor vital signs as appropriate.	Vital sign changes such as increased heart rate, decreased blood pressure, and increased temperature indicate hypovolemia.
• Give fluids as appropriate.	As her nausea decreases encourage her oral intake of fluids as tolerated, again to replace lost volume.
• Administer IV therapy as prescribed.	Mrs. Chapman has signs of severe fluid volume deficit. She will probably require intravenous replacement of fluid. This is especially true because her oral intake is limited because of nausea and vomiting.

EVALUATION

Outcomes met. Mrs. Chapman remained hospitalized for 48 hours. She required fluid replacement of a total of 5 L. Her blood pressure increased to 122/74, pulse rate decreased to a resting level of 74, and respirations decreased to 12/minute. Her urine output increased as the fluid was replaced and was adequate at > 0.5 mL/kg/hour by the time of discharge. She was taking oral fluids and was able to discuss symptoms of deficient fluid volume that would necessitate her calling her health care provider.

*Outcomes, interventions, and activities selected are only a sample of those suggested by NOC and NIC and should be further individualized for each client.

Applying Critical Thinking

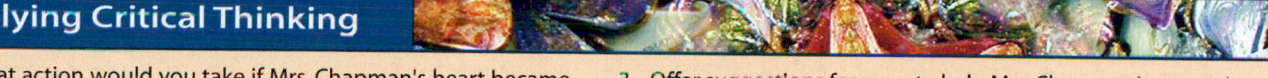

1. What action would you take if Mrs. Chapman's heart became irregular?
2. Mrs. Chapman is responding inappropriately to your questions; she seems to be confused. What do you think is happening?
3. Offer suggestions for ways to help Mrs. Chapman increase her oral intake.
4. Mrs. Chapman asks why you weigh her every morning. How do you respond?

See Critical Thinking Possibilities in Appendix A.

CONCEPT MAP Deficient Fluid Volume

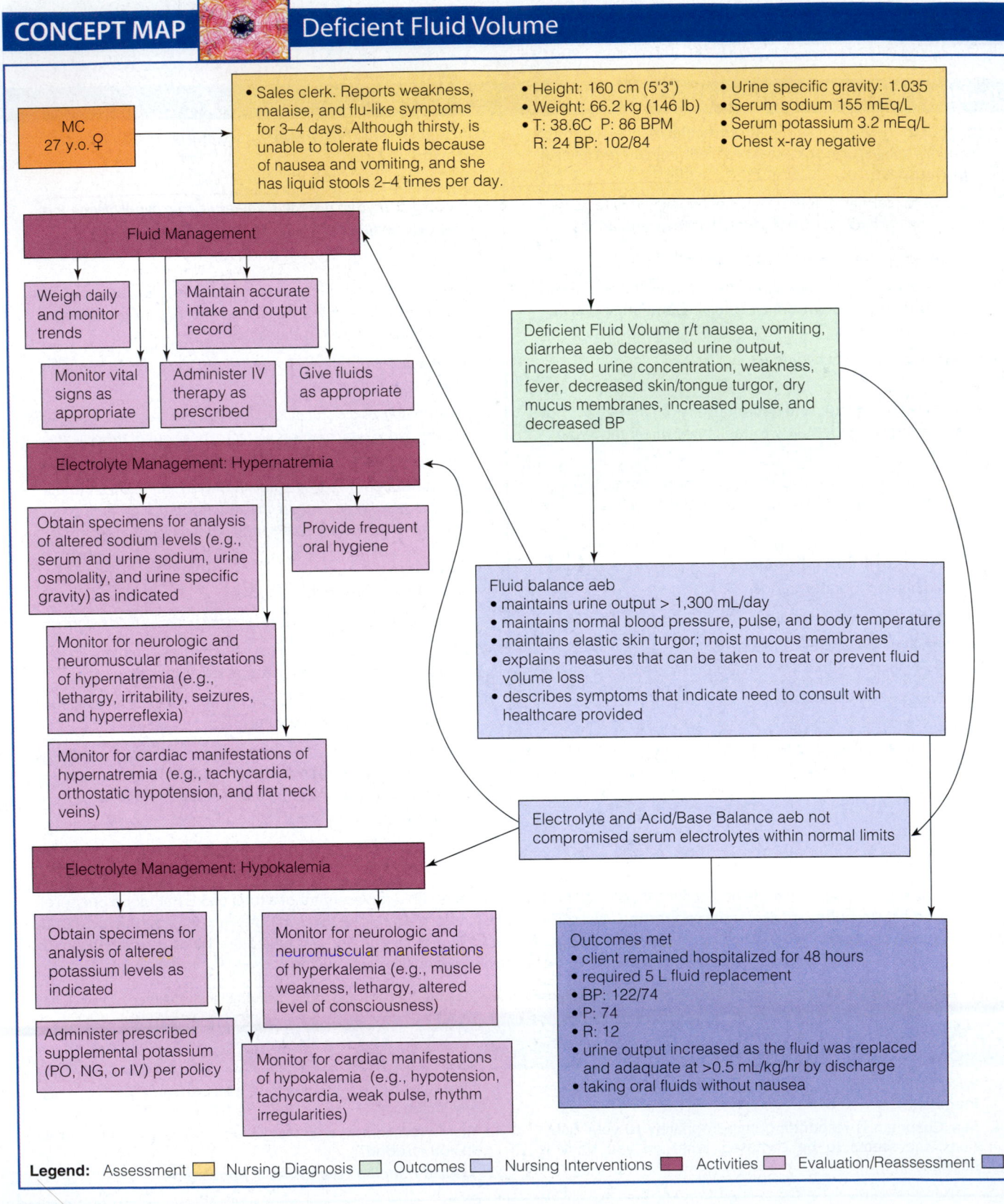

MC
27 y.o. ♀

- Sales clerk. Reports weakness, malaise, and flu-like symptoms for 3–4 days. Although thirsty, is unable to tolerate fluids because of nausea and vomiting, and she has liquid stools 2–4 times per day.

- Height: 160 cm (5'3")
- Weight: 66.2 kg (146 lb)
- T: 38.6C P: 86 BPM
  R: 24 BP: 102/84

- Urine specific gravity: 1.035
- Serum sodium 155 mEq/L
- Serum potassium 3.2 mEq/L
- Chest x-ray negative

Fluid Management

Weigh daily and monitor trends

Maintain accurate intake and output record

Monitor vital signs as appropriate

Administer IV therapy as prescribed

Give fluids as appropriate

Electrolyte Management: Hypernatremia

Obtain specimens for analysis of altered sodium levels (e.g., serum and urine sodium, urine osmolality, and urine specific gravity) as indicated

Provide frequent oral hygiene

Monitor for neurologic and neuromuscular manifestations of hypernatremia (e.g., lethargy, irritability, seizures, and hyperreflexia)

Monitor for cardiac manifestations of hypernatremia (e.g., tachycardia, orthostatic hypotension, and flat neck veins)

Deficient Fluid Volume r/t nausea, vomiting, diarrhea aeb decreased urine output, increased urine concentration, weakness, fever, decreased skin/tongue turgor, dry mucus membranes, increased pulse, and decreased BP

Fluid balance aeb
- maintains urine output > 1,300 mL/day
- maintains normal blood pressure, pulse, and body temperature
- maintains elastic skin turgor; moist mucous membranes
- explains measures that can be taken to treat or prevent fluid volume loss
- describes symptoms that indicate need to consult with healthcare provided

Electrolyte and Acid/Base Balance aeb not compromised serum electrolytes within normal limits

Electrolyte Management: Hypokalemia

Obtain specimens for analysis of altered potassium levels as indicated

Monitor for neurologic and neuromuscular manifestations of hyperkalemia (e.g., muscle weakness, lethargy, altered level of consciousness)

Administer prescribed supplemental potassium (PO, NG, or IV) per policy

Monitor for cardiac manifestations of hypokalemia (e.g., hypotension, tachycardia, weak pulse, rhythm irregularities)

Outcomes met
- client remained hospitalized for 48 hours
- required 5 L fluid replacement
- BP: 122/74
- P: 74
- R: 12
- urine output increased as the fluid was replaced and adaquate at >0.5 mL/kg/hr by discharge
- taking oral fluids without nausea

Legend: Assessment ▢ Nursing Diagnosis ▢ Outcomes ▢ Nursing Interventions ▢ Activities ▢ Evaluation/Reassessment ▢

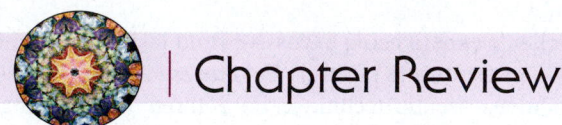

Chapter Review

EXPLORE MediaLink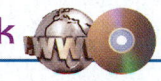

NCLEX review questions, case studies, care plan activities, MediaLink applications, and other interactive resources for this chapter can be found on the Companion Website at www.prenhall.com/kozier. Click on Chapter 50 to select the activities for this chapter.

For animations, more NCLEX review questions, and an audio glossary, access the Student CD-ROM accompanying this textbook.

Chapter Highlights

- A balance of fluids, electrolytes, acids, and bases in the body is necessary for health and life.
- The body fluid is divided into two major compartments: the intracellular fluid (ICF) inside the cells and extracellular fluid (ECF) outside the cells.
- Extracellular fluid is subdivided into two compartments: intravascular (plasma) and interstitial. It constitutes about one-fourth to one-third of total body fluid.
- ECF is in constant motion throughout the body. It is the transport system that carries nutrients to and waste products from the cells.
- The percentage of total body fluids varies according to the individual's age, body fat, and sex. The younger the person, the higher the proportion of water in the body. The less body fat present, the greater the proportion of body fluid. Postadolescent females have a smaller percentage of fluid in relation to total body weight than do men.
- There are two types of body electrolytes (ions): positively charged ions (cations) and negatively charged ions (anions).
- The principal ions of ECF are sodium and chloride; the principal ions of ICF are potassium and phosphate.
- Fluids and electrolytes move among the body compartments by osmosis, diffusion, filtration, and active transport.
- The major fluid pressures exerted as part of the movement of fluid and electrolytes from one compartment to another are osmotic pressure and hydrostatic pressure.
- The three sources of body fluid are fluids taken orally, food ingested, and the oxidation of food. Fluid intake is regulated by the thirst mechanism.
- Fluid output occurs chiefly through excretion of urine, although body fluid is also lost through sweat, feces, and insensible vapor loss.
- In healthy adults, measurable fluid intake and output should balance (about 1,500 mL per day). The output of urine normally approximates the oral intake of fluids. Water from food and oxidation is balanced by fluid loss through the skin, respiratory process, and feces.
- A number of body systems and organs are involved in regulating the volume and composition of body fluids: the kidneys, the endocrine system, the cardiovascular system, the lungs, and the gastrointestinal system. The kidneys are the primary regulator of fluid and electrolyte balance.

- Substances such as the antidiuretic hormone, the renin-angiotensin-aldosterone system, and the atrial nutriuretic factor are also involved in maintaining fluid balance.
- Fluid imbalances include
  a. Fluid volume deficit (FVD), also referred to as hypovolemia
  b. Fluid volume excess (FVE), also referred to as hypervolemia
  c. Dehydration, a deficit in water only
  d. Overhydration, an excess of water only.
- The most common electrolyte imbalances are deficits or excesses in sodium, potassium, and calcium.
- The acid–base balance (pH range) of body fluids is maintained within a precise range of 7.35 to 7.45.
- Acid–base balance is regulated by buffers that neutralize excess acids or bases; the lungs, which eliminate or retain carbon dioxide, a potential acid; and the kidneys, which excrete or conserve bicarbonate and hydrogen ions.
- Acid–base imbalance occurs when the normal 20-to-1 ratio of bicarbonate to carbonic acid is upset. Imbalances may be either respiratory or metabolic in origin; either can result in acidosis or alkalosis.
- Factors that influence an individual's fluid, electrolyte, and acid–base balance include age, gender and body size, environmental temperature, and lifestyle. Illness, trauma, surgery, and certain medications can place individuals at risk for fluid, electrolyte, and acid–base imbalances.
- Fluid, electrolyte, and acid–base imbalance is most accurately determined through laboratory examination of blood plasma.
- Assessment relative to fluid, electrolyte, and acid–base balances includes (a) a nursing history; (b) physical examination of the skin, oral cavity, eyes, jugular vein, veins of the hand, and the neurologic system; (c) measurement of body weight, vital signs, and fluid intake and output; and (d) various diagnostic studies of blood and urine.
- A nursing history includes data about the client's fluid and food intake; fluid output; signs of fluid, electrolyte, and acid–base imbalances; and medications, therapies, or disease processes that may disrupt these balances.
- NANDA-approved nursing diagnoses that relate specifically to fluid, electrolyte, and acid–base imbalances include *Deficient Fluid Volume, Excess Fluid Volume, Risk for*

Imbalanced Fluid Volume, Risk for Deficient Fluid Volume, and *Impaired Gas Exchange.* Other diagnoses that may be relevant are *Impaired Oral Mucous Membrane, Impaired Skin Integrity, Decreased Cardiac Output, Impaired Tissue Perfusion, Activity Intolerance, Risk for Injury,* and *Acute Confusion.*

- In many instances, fluids and electrolytes can be provided orally to clients who are experiencing or at risk of developing fluid deficits. The nurse needs to establish with the client a 24-hour plan for ingesting the necessary fluids and to respect the client's fluid preferences.
- For clients with fluid retention, fluids may need to be restricted; a schedule and short-term goals that make the fluid restriction more tolerable need to be developed.

- For clients experiencing excessive fluid losses, the administration of fluids and electrolytes intravenously is necessary. Meticulous aseptic technique is required when caring for clients with intravenous infusions.
- Preventing complications such as infiltration, phlebitis, hypervolemia (circulatory overload), and infection are an important aspect of intravenous therapy.
- The administration of blood transfusions involves accurately matching and identifying the blood for the individual, correctly identifying the recipient, and monitoring the client throughout the procedure for transfusion reactions.

Review Questions

50–1. What are two principal electrolytes found in intracellular fluid?
  a. sodium and bicarbonate
  b. chloride and calcium
  c. potassium and phosphate
  d. albumin and magnesium

50–2. Which electrolyte helps regulate cardiac impulse transmission and muscle contraction?
  a. sodium
  b. calcium
  c. chloride
  d. potassium

50–3. A client shows signs of isotonic fluid deficit, but his weight is stable and he does not have an obvious source of fluid loss. The most likely problem is
  a. Fluid Volume Deficit.
  b. Fluid Volume Excess.
  c. dehydration.
  d. third space syndrome.

50–4. A client's weight has increased by 4.5 pounds during the past 3 days. Approximately how many liter(s) of fluid does this mean the client has gained?
  a. 2
  b. 1
  c. 0.5
  d. 3

50–5. A client with congestive heart failure (weight 80 kg) has had a fluid intake of 500 mL and has voided 10 mL over a 4-hour period. What action should the nurse take?
  a. Insert an indwelling urinary catheter.
  b. Continue monitoring intake and output.
  c. Notify the physician or charge nurse.
  d. Increase the client's intake.

Readings and References

Suggested Readings

Cooper, A., & Moore, M. (1999). IV fluid therapy. *Australian Nursing Journal, 7*(5), 1–5.
  This article presents the physiologic basis for IV fluid choices. The author discusses the principles of fluid and electrolyte balance including water distribution in the body, fluid movement, and hormonal influence in fluid balance. Additionally, it addresses patient assessment as an important factor in understanding fluid administration. An excellent review article.

Fitzpatrick, L. (2002). When to administer modified blood products. *Nursing, 32*(5), 36–42.
  This article begins with a question: Do you understand why your patient is receiving this type of blood? Blood transfusion therapy can be complicated and confusing. Additionally, it poses significant risks to clients. This review article will help the nurse understand which blood components are a threat to patients and when it is appropriate to administer modified blood products. Specifically it covers irradiation, blood washing, leukocyte reduction, and CMV-negative blood components.

Masoorli, S., & Angeles, T. (2002). Getting a line on central vascular access devices. *Nursing 2002, 32*(4), 36–43.
  This article reviews common types of central lines. It addresses location of different catheters, insertion techniques, and uses for each type of catheter. The author focuses on nursing care and presents critical clinical information including dressings, flushing, obtaining blood specimens, and troubleshooting.

Related Research

Creamer, E., McCarthy, G., Tighe, I., & Smyth, E. (2002). A survey of nurses' assessment of peripheral intravenous catheters. *British Journal of Nursing, 11,* 999–1007.

References

Behrman, R. E. (1992). *Nelson textbook of pediatrics.* Philadelphia: Saunders.

Gaspar, P. M. (1999). Water intake of nursing home residents. *Journal of Gerontological Nursing, 25*(4), 23–29.

Johnson, M., & Maas, M., & Moorhead, S. (Eds.). (2000). *Nursing outcomes classification (NOC).* St. Louis, MO: Mosby.

Masoorli, S., & Angeles, T. (2002). Getting a line on central vascular access devices. *Nursing, 32*(4), 36–43.

McCloskey, J. C., & Bulechek, G. M. (Eds.). (2000). *Nursing interventions classification (NIC)* (3rd ed). St. Louis, MO: Mosby.

NANDA International. (2003). *NANDA nursing diagnoses: Definitions and classification 2003-2004.* Philadelphia: Author.

Selected Bibliography

Anonymous. (1999). Understanding imbalances caused by GI fluid loss. *Nursing, 29*(8), 72.

Aschenbrenner, D. S. (2000). A matter of practice: Skin preps and protocols. *American Journal of Nursing, 100*(4), 78.

Beyerle, K. (2001). Focus on autotransfusion: Recycling blood lost from a chest wound eliminates incompatibility risk and saves precious time. *Nursing, 31*(12), 49–51.

Burke, S. (2001). Boning up on osteoporosis. *Nursing, 31*(10), 38.

Carlson, K. R. (1999). Correct utilization and management of peripherally inserted central catheters and midline catheters in the alternate care setting. *Journal of Intravenous Nursing, 22*(6 Suppl.): S46–S50.

Centers for Disease Control and Prevention. (2002). Guidelines for the prevention of intravascular catheter-related infections. *Mortality and Morbidity Weekly Report, 51*(10), 1–29.

Cook, N. (1999). Central venous catheters: Preventing infection and occlusion. *British Journal of Nursing, 8,* 980, 982, 984, 986–988.

Cooper, A., & Moore, M. (1999). IV fluid therapy. *Australian Nursing Journal, 7*(5), 1–5.

Copstead, L. C., & Banasik, J. L. (2000). *Pathophysiology: Biological and behavioural perspectives* (2nd ed.). Philadelphia: Saunders.

Dougherty, L. (2000). Central venous access devices. *Nursing Standard, 14*(43), 45–50, 53–54.

Drewett, S. R. (2000) Complications of central venous catheters: Nursing care. *British Journal of Nursing, 9,* 466, 468, 470–478.

Hadaway, L. C. (2002). IV Rounds: Choosing the right vascular access device, Part I. *Nursing, 32*(9), 75.

Hadaway, L. C. (2002) IV Rounds: Choosing the right vascular access device, Part II. *Nursing, 32*(10), 74.

Hadaway, L. C. (2002). What you can do to prevent catheter related infections. *Nursing, 32*(9), 46–48.

Josephson, D. L. (1999). *Intravenous infusion therapy for nurses: Principles and practice.* Albany, NY: Delmar.

Klein, T. (2001). PICCs and midlines—fine tuning your care. *RN, 64*(8), 26–29.

Kobriger, A. M. (1999). Dehydration: Stopping a sentinel event. *Nursing Homes, 48*(10), 60–65.

Lee, C. A. B., Barrett, C. A., & Ignatavicius, D. D. (1996). *Fluids and electrolytes: A practical approach* (4th ed.). Philadelphia: F. A. Davis.

Leigh, G. (2001). Securing an IV insertion site. *Nursing, 31*(4), 46–47.

McConnell, E. A. (1999). Vascular access devices: Lines to live by. *Nursing Management, 30*(12), 49–52.

McConnell, E. A. (2000). Clinical do's and don'ts: Changing a central venous catheter dressing. *Nursing, 30*(4), 24.

McConnell, E. A. (2000). Clinical do's and don'ts: Infusing packed RBC's. *Nursing, 30*(2), 17.

McConnell, E. A. (2000). Infusion perfusion: IV pumps for every need. *Nursing Management, 31*(4), 53–55.

Mentes, J. C. (2000). Hydration management protocol. *Journal of Gerontological Nursing, 26*(10), 6–15.

Metheny, N. M. (2000). *Fluid and electrolyte balance: Nursing considerations* (4th ed.). Philadelphia: Lippincott.

Milliam, D. A., & Hadaway, L. C. (2000). On the road to successful IV starts. *Nursing, 30*(4), 34–48.

Pagana, K. D., & Pagana, J. P. (2002). *Mosby's manual of diagnostic and laboratory tests* (2nd ed.). St. Louis, MO: Mosby-Year Book.

Parker, L. (1999). IV devices and related infections: Causes and complications. *British Journal of Nursing, 8,* 1491, 1493, 1495, 1497–1498.

Przybylek, C. (2002), Two ways to avoid a "sticky" IV situation. *Nursing, 32*(11), 47–49.

Todd, J. (1999). Peripherally inserted central catheters and their use in IV therapy. *British Journal of Nursing, 8,* 140, 142, 144, 146–148.

Workman, B. (1999). Peripheral intravenous therapy management. *Nursing Standard, 14*(4), 53–60, 62.

Appendix A

CRITICAL THINKING POSSIBILITIES for Critical Thinking Exercises

CHAPTER 2: Nursing Education and Research

1. It will be important to gather the following information to allow you to give the person the best response:

   - What is their knowledge of nursing? Is it accurate or based on a stereotype or the media's image of nursing? Do they know the differences between the types of nursing education?
   - Do they have any experience with the health care system? If yes, how has that experience influenced them?
   - Do they have prior educational experience or degrees? For example, if they have a baccalaureate degree, they may be interested in a generic master's program.
   - What are their professional goals and what kind of time frame are they considering?
   - What is their personal situation? For example, some students have a professional goal of becoming a nurse practitioner; however, they wish to enter the nursing field as soon as possible. They elect to first complete a practical nursing program to allow them to work in nursing while completing course work for an RN program and finally advancing to a graduate program.
   - What is the availability and accessibility to nursing programs in their area? People in rural areas may not have as many choices as individuals who live in an urban area.

   Obtaining answers to these questions will provide you needed information that will enable you to provide direction for the individual.

CHAPTER 3: Nursing Theories and Conceptual Frameworks

1. Some of the many concepts that can be identified are illness, disease, wellness, and nutrition.
2. The physician seems to view Tony as someone who has some choices in his own care. He also appears to be making a statement related to quality of life (wellness) that reflects a belief that the client would not be getting better and intravenous nutrition was, therefore, not indicated. The nurse appears to have expanded the definition of client to include family and friends and has a different prognosis in mind.
3. Florence Nightingale would focus Tony's care on the need for a clean environment, good water, and light as necessary for his health.
4. None of the nursing models supports the physician's plan of care. All of them recognize an interdependence of systems and relationships that would make controlling diarrhea a top priority. None of the nursing models is any more powerful than the others as a foundation for the nurse's plan of care.

CHAPTER 4: Legal Aspects of Nursing

1. The nurse needs to verify that the client received information from the physician and that she understands the information. Can the client explain in her own words what the doctor told her? Does she have any questions?
2. The three exceptions of people who cannot provide consent are minors, persons who are unconscious or injured in such a way that they are unable to give consent, and mentally ill persons judged to be incompetent. If this client is an alert, competent adult, she can provide consent.
3. The nurse will need to read the form to the client.
4. Unless the husband is the appointed guardian or has power of attorney for health care decisions, the client should sign the form. The client will need assistance as to where to sign the form. The client could even mark an "X." Remember, the nurse witnesses that the client gave her consent voluntarily and that the signature is authentic.
5. The nurse needs to include the following:

   - The consent form was read to the client before she signed it.
   - A reference to the client's understanding of the procedure (e.g., "able to state reasons for surgery, pro's and con's of surgery. Stated she had no questions. Aware that she can change her mind").
   - If the husband helped the client sign (e.g., guided her hand), this information should be documented.
   - Record any teaching as a result of nursing-related questions by the client (e.g., "discussed and demonstrated techniques for coughing and deep breathing after surgery").

CHAPTER 5: Values, Ethics, and Advocacy

1. Personal values are often based on family, cultural, religious, or other beliefs and attitudes. The nurse must not assume any particular values based on these characteristics, however. They must be validated with the individual. What appear to be the client's values must be confirmed with him through open and supportive discussion.
2. The client's values and decisions are influenced by a variety of factors such as family support, previous experience with health care situations, the meaning of illness (and of the foot) to the person, and his personal goals. The surgeon has information about the client's overall health status, possibly previous experiences with this client, and personal values and beliefs about the impact of an amputation.

Conduct a thorough health history on the client if not already completed, and review the content related to the factors influencing the client's values and decision. Review the medical history and physical examination for additional data. Gather missing information from the client or surgeon as indicated.

3. The nurse's responsibility is to ensure that the client has all the accurate information required for him to make an informed decision. This may include information beyond his physiologic condition such as facts about his health insurance coverage for acute and rehabilitative care. The nurse's personal beliefs about what the client should do or what the surgeon should recommend must not influence the nurse in carrying out this responsibility.

4. It is sometimes difficult to find the middle ground between advocating for the client and interfering in the client–physician relationship. Also, the client's informed decision may be counter to standard or recommended medical practice.

5. The Code of Ethics for Nurses or a patient bill of rights can help the nurse recall the standards that apply in guiding nurse decision making during possible ethical dilemmas. The nurse's actions should be based on ethical theory and standards, not on personal opinion.

CHAPTER 6: Health Care Delivery Systems

1. It does not seem as though the client has used many health-promotion or prevention services. He would have used secondary prevention services extensively in seeing the physician for his blood pressure and joint problems and having surgery. His time at the skilled nursing facility, with the home health nurse, and the physical therapist visits were tertiary preventive care.

2. He has visited the physician's office, which is useful for monitoring existing problems and screening for new ones; the hospital has the expert staff for performing his surgery and the nursing personnel for caring for him during the perioperative period. They have laboratories, therapeutic (e.g., physical therapy), and nutrition services to meet his needs. Examples of other agencies would include the skilled nursing facility and home health care.

3. This client has health care needs in a variety of areas. His age and health problems suggest that he will continue to need health care for the foreseeable future. The case manager can become very familiar with the client and family situation so that the appropriate levels of care can be provided when he needs them and within his insurance coverage. He would have Medicare but may also have supplemental coverage. Should he become unable to continue living in the current house, the case manager may assist with determining the type of living facility most appropriate. If the client needs to be readmitted to the hospital, the case manager serves as an excellent facilitator in the communication needed among the physician, hospital, rehabilitative setting, and home health care personnel.

4. Examples include these: Pharmacist—elders often take many different medications. During an acute illness there is a particular need to ensure that newly ordered medications that may be required for the current condition do not interfere with medications used for chronic conditions. Spiritual support—although we do not know Mr. Mendel's religious preference, he may be experiencing some spiritual concerns, for example, about dying. If he and his wife have a relationship with a church or other similar institution, it would be important to include this aspect in his care. Many other professionals may be included on the team.

CHAPTER 7: Community-Based Nursing and Care Continuity

There can be no traditional answers to these questions. What follow below are aspects to consider.

1. Overall, decreasing the time clients spend in dependent situations such as being patients in acute care hospitals is consistent with the agenda's aims at health care reform. However, the nurse must also consider the culture of the client and the environment. Active decision making by the client is a Western view that may not be shared by clients from Eastern, African American, or Latino backgrounds. In European health care systems, clients often spend as much as five times longer in a hospital than do American patients. The client may not be accustomed to community-based care and have very different views of the health care professionals who provide community-based care. Also, the scenario does not address outcomes. A primary concern would be to measure the incidence of complications, need for rehospitalization, and client satisfaction with the short stays.

2. Individuals will have unique responses to this question. Answers should reflect consideration of the views and skills of nurses, clients, and systems.

3. In an integrated health care system, the client would move easily from the diagnostic phase through treatment and rehabilitation—possibly using a case manager to assess the client and family and follow her though the entire episode. A community coalition would focus more on the risk factors leading to the health problem and initiatives to educate the population on wellness, prevention, and early detection.

4. Communication with the client, family, and other health care providers would be key to determining that a particular client is appropriate for this "fast-track" approach to the surgery. If the parties disagree, shared decision making should be used in establishing the details of how the care will actually be provided. Mutual respect and trust are key—that the health care providers are skilled and knowledgeable about the procedure and that the client and family can carry out their respective roles once the decisions have been made and communicated. Collaboration with third-party payers can be more complex. Investigate their chain of command and try to find nurses with whom to discuss the case.

CHAPTER 8: Health Promotion

1. Key points to remember include, but are not limited to, the following:

   - Active listening is very important because it strengthens the rapport between the client and nurse. Careful listening can help check your understanding of what the client is saying or meaning with the responses.
   - It is important to emphasize that the client has personal choice and control. The client should decide what behavior, if any, to focus on.
   - Readiness to change, including importance and confidence, needs to be continually assessed.
   - It is not unusual for individuals to recycle through the stages of change.

2. Questions to consider include these:

   - "Take me through a typical day in your life and tell me where your [behavior] fits in."
   - "You have mentioned smoking, exercise, food, and losing weight. Would you like to talk about one of these topics or is there something else you would prefer to talk about?" [This gives the client the opportunity to choose the topic most important to them at the time.]
   - "Which of these behaviors do you feel most ready to think about changing?"
   - "Sometimes it can be helpful to examine the pros and cons of [behavior]—would this be helpful?"
   - "What concerns you the most about [behavior]?"
   - "Would you like to know more about [behavior]?"
   - "How do you see the connection between [behavior] and [behavior]?"

3. Mr. W. is in the contemplation stage, because he wonders about changing and is willing to discuss it. Contemplators want to change; however, at the same time, they have a resistance to change. Consciousness-raising is important during this stage. Find out if the client wants more information. Assist the client to increase his awareness of the behavior—why does he want to change, the pros and cons of changing, and so on.

CHAPTER 9: Home Care

1. Many aspects of the nurse's role will be the same. The techniques such as intravenous medication administration will have the same steps but they may need to be modified to apply in situations where not all usual supplies or equipment are available (e.g., using a door hook for an IV pole). More so than in the acute care setting, the nurse needs to consider the client's family as a client in addition to the patient.

2. The client has all the same rights of any patient but, in addition, has the right to direct that care be administered in a way that is acceptable within his or her environment, to decline to accept the nurse's recommendations, and to decline the nurse's assistance and care.

3. Safety issues: Any aspects of his home or daily activities that could worsen his diabetes (e.g., inadequate heating/cooling) or potentially cause injury (unsafe railings). Infection control issues: lack of access to needed hygiene facilities, inability to participate in dressing changes and wound care due to poor vision, reduced dexterity, or other factors. Lack of adequate care giver support.

4. In addition to the intangible savings of emotional comfort provided by being in one's own home, the client is able to maintain many of his personal contacts and activities—including such important tasks as paying bills and caring for pets.

CHAPTER 10: Nursing Informatics

1. Consider the uses of the computer in the following areas: searching the Internet and literature for research or case studies that might relate; sending queries to experts identified through university medical centers of excellence; e-mailing colleagues from relevant professional nursing organizations;

2. Ask the client to share exactly the nature of the concern. Discuss with the client whether any unique identifiers will be associated with the photos or query, for example, name, Social Security number. Suggest that your colleagues will be asked to delete the photo files as soon as the consultation is complete. Would the client find fax or hardcopies more acceptable?

3. Use one of the documents available to critique the website yourself. Share with the client the criteria for determining the usefulness of the information found on websites and discuss how they apply to the specific site. Also provide the client with other reliable sources of health information such as printed pamphlets or referenced articles.

4. Consider issues such as the ability to do your studying and assignments at a time (and place) of your choosing rather than in a classroom on specific days and times; whether you prefer to work alone or in "real place" groups (online programs also use groups that may do synchronous or asynchronous work); how self-directed you are; the availability of local quality education programs; privacy regarding your academic records and financial aid information; and so on.

CHAPTER 11: Health, Wellness, and Illness

1. Jerry has a positive outlook and views himself as "well" while Joe has a negative outlook and views himself as "ill." Identify and compare data indicating the psychologic dimension (self-concept, mind-body interactions, emotional response to health) for both clients. Speculate about how their differences in perception may affect their continuing recovery process.

2. Jerry is most likely an "internal" because he has taken charge of his own health by changing his diet, initiating an

exercise program, and attempting to lower his stress. Joe is more likely an "external" because he has been unable to take control of his health. Joe may believe that his health is largely controlled by outside forces and is beyond his control.

3. The data suggest that Jerry has more positive external variables (e.g. a supportive wife).

4. Joe's perception of his illness, and thus his ability to respond in a positive manner, may be affected by a family history of heart disease and his perception that he is at high risk and there is nothing he can do to change his pattern of health.

   - Joe's perceived barriers to action (cost, time, lack of social support).
   - Perhaps the benefit of assuming the sick role outweighs the benefit of recovery.

5. Verifying that Jerry values the planned outcome achieved from smoking cessation; verifying Jerry's knowledge about the effects of smoking and providing needed information or correcting misconceptions; demonstrating genuine concern for Jerry and positively reinforcing positive changes that Jerry does make; allowing Jerry to make his own decisions, thereby demonstrating trust and respect. Many other interventions are possible.

CHAPTER 12: Individual, Family, and Community Health

1. Many illnesses can be affected by the client's emotional state. If her arthritis is the type called rheumatoid, it can flare when the client is under stress. Also, some medications used to treat arthritis can cause mood changes and other distressing adverse effects. Any aspect of the illness that interferes with daily functioning of a family member will affect the coping of all members.

2. The family is affected because Linda's role functioning is impaired. Others might need to take on additional tasks Linda would normally perform. In addition, Linda's emotional response to her illness can interfere with her ability to provide psychological support to her children and spouse and thus cause them severe distress.

3. Facing illness as a family often draws the members, including those normally at some physical or emotional distance, closer together. A disadvantage of facing an illness with the family is the additional stress, cost, and responsibilities members may have to take on. The ill member may feel great guilt about the extra work that falls to others. Members may become fatigued and be unable or unwilling to support the ill person.

4. Each family member exists as a part of the whole. They interact with each other and with their human and nonhuman environment. The family has become a more closed system (and with thicker boundaries) than usual due to the parents desire to avoid assistance or interference from previous spouses. Linda's biological systems may be malfunctioning,

leading to altered function of her other systems and those of the family. For example, feedback in the form of pain will serve as input to her in deciding how much and what types of physical activity she can perform.

5. Linda's health problem is an individual one rather than the type that reflects the health of the community (as a contagious disease would). She and her family require individualized attention and care—that which the home health nurse is particularly suited to provide.

CHAPTER 13: Culture and Heritage

1. Rachel's culture (values, beliefs, norms, and life practices that guide thinking, decisions, and actions) is mixed and can be referred to as bicultural because she has integrated practices and values from both her mother and father who were of different backgrounds.

   - Rachel's ethnicity (consciousness of belonging to a group that is differentiated from others by symbolic markers) is most strongly associated with her Jewish background as evidenced by her return to the Jewish religion as an adult and by her obvious connection with this group.
   - Rachel's race (shared biologic characteristics, genetic markers, or features) is unknown since we do not know the race of her parents. Jewish persons who come from similar national origins (e.g., Eastern Europe or the Middle East) may share racial traits.

2. Cultural values often determine the roles of family members, their interactions, who has authority to make decisions on the client's behalf, and family involvement in the client's care. Without clear guidelines on the cultural practices Rachel adheres to, it may be difficult to provide culturally sensitive care.

3. Rachel's beliefs and values will strongly affect her approach to death and the way her family reacts toward her before and during the death process.

   - Rachel's culture may dictate her choice of dying with family members present, rites, or rituals to be performed, and the degree of knowledge she wishes about the dying process.
   - Rachel's religion is likely to strongly influence the care of her body after death and burial procedures.

4. A cultural assessment is particularly important at this time in Rachel's life so that her death can be congruent with her beliefs and traditions. It is also important to determine her primary support systems, to preserve her preferences, and to offer support to Rachel and her family in culturally acceptable ways.

5. All aspects of client care are influenced by the nurses' and the clients' cultures. When the beliefs are different, misunderstandings can occur, the relationship can suffer, and client outcomes may be adversely affected. Self-awareness can enable nurses to successfully cope with client practices they themselves might not believe in or value.

CHAPTER 14: Complementary and Alternative Healing Modalities

1. Tim's name suggests that he may be of Asian descent (and cancer of the stomach is more common in Asian populations than in some other ethnic groups). Tim's parents do not speak English and this suggests that they are not from a North American culture. Many Asian people use CAM as a regular part of their health activities. Tim's gastric cancer appears to be quite serious. Often, cancer patients whose disease is not responding to conventional therapy seek CAM to treat the disease or to cope with symptoms.

2. Certainly, touch, biofeedback, prayer, music, meditation, and similar CAM therapies might help Tim's ability to cope with his pain and even increase his nutritional intake. There may also be herbs, homeopathic, and TCM products that are safe to use with his Western therapy although the nurse must investigate these carefully. Where would you look for this information?

3. The nurse may ignore finding the bags of "tea," but there is a risk that the substance could be contraindicated with other medications Tim currently takes. The nurse can ask Tim or his wife what is in the bags and determine the safety of their use.

4. If the nurse is strongly in favor of or opposed to CAM, this may color interactions with the client and family. The nurse should review these biases and ensure that he or she can still provide professional care considering personal perspectives. The nurse should be open minded to hearing the client's beliefs and supporting the client's right to act in accordance with his beliefs.

CHAPTER 15: Critical Thinking and the Nursing Process

1. Examples include these: What evidence supports the assumption? What are other possible explanations for his condition? What might another nurse who sees this situation differently think? What evidence would suggest a different assumption?

2. This attitude says that critical thinking will lead to appropriate conclusions. It requires that you trust yourself, examine the influence of emotions on your thinking, and use logic to reach conclusions. Suggest how you can show that you have considered these things.

3. If your conclusion is correct and acted on, you have helped keep the client's problems at a minimum through early intervention. He can receive proper treatment and the nurse can develop a plan of care to assist the client and family with the impact of the condition. If you are incorrect in your assumption and do not consider what was the correct conclusion, time may be wasted and the real condition could worsen. Increased cost, emotional frustration, and other negative outcomes may result.

4. How does the client feel about his recent retirement? What is the impact of his retirement while his wife continues to work. Do the coming holidays play a role in his illness?

CHAPTER 16: Assessing

1. Extremely important areas include at least allergies, comorbidities (other health problems or diseases), and previous experience with surgery.

2. Because the musculoskeletal system is the reason she is in the hospital, it would be given priority. Due to her age and the immobility that will follow surgery, other priority systems would be cardiopulmanary and integumentary.

3. Many answers may be correct. The question should be open-ended and prompt for the desired information (for example, it would not be helpful to ask her where she lives). One example would be "It may not be possible for you to be alone when you go home from the hospital. Tell me about who might be available to assist you?"

4. Consider family, friends, clergy, and her old charts.

CHAPTER 17: Diagnosing

1. Examples would include insomnia; fidgeting; dry mouth; increased pulse, blood pressure, and respirations; and poor attention span.

2. Examples include the uncertainty of his prognosis, lack of knowledge about his condition and its treatment, and fear of pain.

3. *Ineffective Individual Coping, Sorrow, Spiritual Distress, Hopelessness, Impaired Adjustment, Ineffective Airway Clearance* or *Breathing Pattern, Anticipatory Grieving.*

4. Although this may be a true statement, lung cancer is a medical diagnosis—not a nursing diagnosis, which is a response to health status or a health problem. In addition, the stressor (related to) should be something the nurse can treat independently.

CHAPTER 18: Planning

1. The nurse assumes that the standardized care plan is comprehensive enough for this client with the individualization that is applied to it.

2. The last outcome for *Anxiety*, "Freely expressing concerns and possible solutions about work and parenting roles," and the associated orders are examples because the roles described occur between the client and her family in the home rather than in the hospital setting.

3. Several possibilities exist. The nurse needs to set aside time to discuss the plan with the client, alone or with other family and health care team members. The plan can be presented verbally or in writing. It can be initiated by the nurse who seeks validation from the client, or the problem list, nursing diagnoses, goals, outcomes, and interventions can be decided on by the client and nurse together after the nurse presents assessment data.

4. If agency guidelines delineate the frequency of nursing interventions and the care plan does not require these more often than specified, no time frame is required. Also, if the intervention is performed during every interaction (e.g., the

nurse remains calm and appears confident), no frequency need be written.

5. Nursing diagnoses related to airway are often highest priority since they represent life-threatening conditions. In reassessing priorities, the nurse considers new problems as well as progress toward meeting existing goals. If the airway problem is in the process of improving, other diagnoses may become higher priority.

CHAPTER 19: Implementing and Evaluating

1. For *Ineffective Airway Clearance,* the overall outcome is not met. Although the client is able to cough productively, the care plan requires modification and continuation in order to achieve all of the goals. For *Anxiety,* the overall outcome is mostly met. Ongoing assessment and data collection are indicated.

2. Some possibilities are that the interventions have not been adequately implemented (and still are needed) or more time is needed for their effects to be apparent.

3. It might be good to keep the diagnosis so it can be followed in case it reoccurs. On the other hand, the outcomes remaining may be accomplished through plans for other nursing diagnoses (such as respiratory rate) or are ongoing (teaching).

4. Data collected are recorded in the chart on graphic records and nurses notes (see Chapter 20). 🔗

CHAPTER 20: Documenting and Reporting

1. No date. Do not know if the hospital policy requires military time. Used assumption and bias with use of the term "complainer". Not complete (e.g., what did the nurse listen to. . . would that information be helpful in the care of the client? Were the BP's taken in two different positions or two different times). No information as to why the client refused lunch. Another assumption that client fell out of bed. . . did the nurse see it or walk in and find the client lying on the floor. No evidence of using the nursing process as a framework for documentation.

2. Use the nursing process as a framework. Document assessment findings that relate to the defining characteristics of pain. Chart those interventions that were done to help relieve the pain. Document the client's response to those interventions. If any teaching was done, be sure to document what the teaching was and the client's response.

3. 6/6/03 #1 Pain
   S: "sharp, stabbing pain in lower back that radiates to left leg"
   States pain is 8 out of 10
   "I didn't sleep last night"
   "I feel better" (after interventions)
   O: BP 210/90, P, 72, R, 18
   Last medicated 5 hours previously
   Medicated with ordered analgesic

Heating pad applied to lower back
Positioned on side with pillows behind back
A: Continues to need narcotic medication to progress toward goal of pain relief
P: Add to plan of care to offer analgesic around the clock q4hr versus PRN

4. 6/6/03 Pain
   D: "sharp, stabbing pain in lower back that radiates to left leg"
   States pain is 8 out of 10
   "I didn't sleep last night"
   BP 210/90, P. 72, R. 18
   Last medicated 5 hours previously
   Continues to need narcotic medication to progress toward goal of pain relief
   A: Medicated with ordered analgesic
   Heating pad applied to lower back
   Positioned on side with pillows behind back
   Add to plan of care to offer analgesic around the clock q4hr versus PRN
   R: "I feel better" (after interventions)

CHAPTER 21: Concepts of Growth and Development

1. Brandon is in the early childhood stage, 18 months to 3 years.

   • His central task is autonomy vs. shame and doubt.
   • The goals of this stage are to
   • Learn self-control without loss of self-esteem.
     • Can gain the ability to cooperate with others.
     • Express one's self.
   • A nursing intervention: Encourage Mr. Scott to find ways to give Brandon limited choices.

2. According to Piaget, Brandon is in the preconceptual phase.

   • He uses an egocentric approach to accommodate the demands of the environment.
   • At this age, everything is significant and relates to "me." Children explore the environment and rapidly develop language as they associate words with objects.
   • A nursing intervention: Allow safe exploration of this "new" environment (the clinic) and use this time as a learning experience to learn the names of the equipment and objects in the room.

3. Advise Mr. Scott to:

   • Give the child limited and safe choices.
   • Allow for supervised exploration of the child's world.
   • Try short time-outs (e.g., sitting in a chair or room for 1 to 2 minutes as a consequence of bad behavior) or distraction to limit acting out.
   • Provide a wide variety of experiences and stimuli.
   A nursing intervention: Review the principles of growth and development with Mr. Scott and develop a behavior plan that is suitable to this child and his family.

CHAPTER 22: Promoting Health from Conception through Adolescence

1. Bridget is showing establishment of identity and the need for independence. Her peer groups assume a great importance and provide a sense of belonging, pride, social learning, and sexual roles. Have Bridget explore her own feelings of identity and independence. Maybe have her list her goals and her plan for attaining those goals. Also, ask if she feels safe in her home environment and in her relationship with her boyfriend.

2. Bridget is in the formal operations stage and can think beyond the present and beyond the world of reality. This type of thinking requires logic, organization, and consistency. Reasoning is deductive and futuristic. Help Bridget visualize herself in 10 years. What is she doing? Where is she living? Is she with someone or alone? How did she get there?

3. First, find out if she is pregnant and then encourage her to tell her boyfriend and family. If she is pregnant, give her options for prenatal care. If she is not pregnant, give her and her boyfriend options for birth control methods. Encourage Bridget to have regular dental and physical assessments. Provide information on the importance of a healthy diet and factors that may lead to nutritional problems.

CHAPTER 23: Promoting Health in Adults and Older Adults

1. Osteoporosis means "porous bone," or bone that has gotten thinner and greatly increases the risk of fractures, particularly in older women. Pictures or actual x-rays can be shown to the client to facilitate learning the basics of osteoporosis. The seriousness of the condition should be stressed, but at the same time, it should be stressed that following preventive measures and participating in treatment regimes, if this is indicated, will help to maintain bone health.

2. Risk factors should include physical factors such as early menopause, small thin frame, use of steroids, history of rheumatoid arthritis, family history of disease, history of fractures.

3. Some risk factors are considered to be modifiable, including smoking, diet low in calcium, lack of exposure to sun (sunlight helps to increase Vitamin D), increased intake of caffeine and alcohol, lack of exercise.

4. Most of the medications used to treat osteoporosis help to reduce bone resorption, which means that bone mass is at least maintained. Some of these medications have serious gastrointestinal side effects and some increase the risk of formation of blood clots. It is essential for the client to know the possible side effects and call the physician if any unusual symptoms are experienced. If the medication is an experimental medication, bone density scans may be done at regular intervals to determine effectiveness of the treatment.

5. Measures to discuss for a decrease risk of fractures include these: assessment of home environment to see what safety measures need to be instituted, making sure that hallways and stairwells are well lit, wearing well-fitting shoes with nonskid soles, removing loose rugs in the house, and keeping the floor free of cords (electrical and telephone) to prevent tripping over them. Measures to maintain bone mass include increasing calcium in the diet and taking a calcium supplement, increasing the amount of weight-bearing exercise, and taking medications to prevent further bone loss.

CHAPTER 24: Caring, Comforting, and Communicating

1. Mrs. Manasovitz's nonverbal behavior may include changes in posture, facial expression, lack of verbal expression, and so on. Mrs. Manasovitz's nonverbal communication most likely represent fear, disappointment, loss, anxiety, devastation, and so on.

2. The nurse conveyed the following caring actions: sitting with Mrs. Manasovitz, listening to her, and giving her undivided attention. The nurse also conveyed comforting actions: using a soothing voice, reassuring, touching, offering presence, and offering a cup of coffee. The nurse's actions did communicate caring and comforting as evidenced by Mrs. Manasovitz's willingness to share her feelings.

3. It is important to provide essential information and establish a trusting relationship during emotional stressful times. Other advantages of effective communication are helping families with stress reduction, helping them understand treatment options, helping them with decision making.

4. The nurse conveyed attentive listening by sitting with Mrs. Manasovitz, paying attention to both her verbal and nonverbal language, remaining silent, and focusing solely on Mrs. Manasovitz. Other examples may include not interrupting the client, noting the congruency between verbal and nonverbal language, encouraging the client to talk, thinking before responding, and so on.

CHAPTER 25: Teaching

1. Mrs. Yorty seems preoccupied, so this may not be the ideal time to proceed with teaching. She needs time to adjust to the news that has been given to her and to come to terms with how her heart condition is going to affect her life. When she is ready to learn, she will give you her full attention, ask questions, talk to others, and show interest.

2. A needs assessment provides information about numerous factors that affect learning, not just cognitive ability. Don't assume that well-educated persons have all the information they need to make decisions about their health, or that persons who are not as well educated do not have the capacity to understand.

   • A needs assessment would provide such information as Mrs. Yorty's baseline knowledge of cardiac disease, any health beliefs or cultural factors that may impact her acceptance or rejection of needed changes, the method of learning she prefers to use, and the support systems available to her.

3. Using your learning needs assessment, consider how Mrs. Yorty perfers to learn.

   - Consider leaving material for Mrs. Yorty to read or videos for her to view.
   - Schedule short learning sessions rather than overwhelming long sessions, use teaching aids, repeat information often, allow active learning. Allow Mrs. Yorty to set the pace.

4. If Mrs. Yorty is able to accurately select foods in accordance with her prescribed diet, is able to accurately plan an exercise program, and can offer suggestions for stress reduction, your teaching has most likely been effective.

   - Don't confuse the client's lack of compliance with ineffective teaching. Clients may choose not to follow a prescribed regimen even though they have thorough knowledge of the regimen.

5. Teaching strategies may differ depending on the availability of equipment; however, the principles of teaching would be similar.

   - A learning needs assessment would still be useful, the person's learning readiness and motivation remain important, and learning objectives would continue to serve as evaluation criteria.
   - The client and family would be more in control of the teaching setting, including scheduling, time limits, and place.

CHAPTER 26: Delegating, Managing, and Leading

1. Mr. Caruso has characteristics of democratic or participative leadership. He is complimentary of his staff's ability to set goals and make decisions. He encourages your input and ideas. Mrs. Turner has characteristics of the autocratic leader. She explains her expectations and speaks of implementing her programs.

2. Not sure which characteristics of your admired manager/leader you might want for yourself? If you didn't already, consider how they influence people; their interest in exploring new ideas; their ability to relate to others; how much freedom they allow or control they exert over others; their use of authoritarian, democratic, or laissez-faire style; their energy level; and their creativity.

3. Strategies for dealing with change may include acknowledging that some resistance to change is normal, examining the reasons for the change, focusing on the positive impact of the change, forming a support group, and examining the steps of the change process. Review Boxes 26–5 and 26–6 for more ideas.

4. In both primary care and team nursing, registered nurses may delegate tasks to other nurses or to UAPs. However, in primary nursing, the nurse generally provides as much direct care as possible while present, accepts supervisory responsibility for the client's 24-hour care, and, by definition, delegates care to the other shifts. In team nursing, a designated set or pair of providers is assigned to care for a group of clients. These members will share care for the clients according to agreed-on assignments that include delegation of appropriate tasks by the nurse.

CHAPTER 27: Vital Signs

1. You need to determine the source of the client's concern. Is this just a bad time for her? Inquire if she has ever had her blood pressure taken previously. If so, what was the experience like for her? What does she imagine will happen if you take her blood pressure?

   - Discuss factors that influence clients' views of having vital signs measured—especially factors such as setting: long-term care, hospitals, clinics, physician offices.

2. Each nurse develops his or her own style for addressing problems such as this with clients. You need to develop yours or it will sound insincere. As a general rule, however, explain the situation without assigning fault. For example, you might say "I wasn't able to hear your blood pressure that time," rather than "I'm really new at this and not very good yet."

   - If you are confident that your equipment is functioning properly, you may wish to retake the pressure using palpation rather than auscultation since you will be able to establish the presence of the peripheral pulse before you begin.
   - If you are very new at taking blood pressures, you may wish to ask another nurse to take the blood pressure for you this time. If a teaching stethoscope is available, use it so both of you can listen at the same time.
   - Role-play this situation with fellow students or friends. Try several different responses until you feel comfortable and the "patient" expresses trust in your approach.

3. When you take a client's blood pressure for the first time, you need to relate it to previous or expected values. Determine the client's most recent BP—although this reading is elevated, it might actually be lower than previous readings. Also assess for any stressors or medications that might currently be influencing the reading.

4. The oxygen saturation value is inconsistent with her other vital signs. Begin by determining if the pulse oximeter equipment is functioning properly and you have applied it to an appropriate location correctly.

CHAPTER 28: Health Assessment

1. A focused neurologic system assessment must be conducted, including determining her mental status, motor and sensory function, and pupillary reactions. The client may

have had a stroke or have injured her head when/if she fell. The musculoskeletal system is also a priority since she may have injured herself or broken a hip either before or after falling. In an older adult who has apparently been injured, the integumentary system is a priority because of the high risk for skin damage, bruising, and skin breakdown. Assessment of other systems may also be justifiable.

2. Be sure that you are asking open-ended questions that cannot be answered with yes or no. Open-ended questions often begin with the words "how" or "what" or "tell me about." Use good nonverbal communication skills such as being at her level when you speak and making eye contact.

3. Although you should still use the head-to-toe approach, it may be best to do all of the anterior assessment first and then turn her to perform posterior assessments. You can assess her upper extremities and much of her lower extremities without turning her at all. Do not omit the posterior assessment, however, just to reduce her discomfort. It is extremely important to determine if abnormal findings are there such as lung consolidation or skin breakdown.

4. Begin with family members. Although she lives alone, there may be children, grandchildren, or other relatives who are in contact with her regularly. Also ask about the source of her regular health care. Another community source may be neighbors or organizations with which she is affiliated (e.g., church, social groups). If she has a primary care physician, ensure that he or she has been notified of the client's admission and determine if she was seen recently or if the office can provide pertinent medical history data.

CHAPTER 29: Asepsis

1. Examples include age (reduced immune defenses), dehydration and nutritional deficit (decreased ability to synthesize antibodies), and the chronic respiratory problem.

2. A full history and physical assessment are indicated.

   - In particular, explore her immunization status, chronic illnesses, exposure to others who may have had an infection, medications that could increase susceptibility to infection, stress level, and history of previous infections of any kind.
   - Assess her skin and mucous membranes and check vital signs that could indicate infection.
   - Determine spiritual, cultural, and educational characteristics that may influence her beliefs and understandings, care preferences, and practices.

3. Use of Standard Precautions (SP) alone will not prevent transmission of her respiratory infection (if contagious) to others since SP are designed to prevent the transmission of bloodborne pathogens. As such, SP do not apply to sputum, nasal secretions, or urine unless contaminated with blood.

4. Depending on the type of organism infecting Mrs. Cortez's respiratory tract, she may need to be placed on specific isolation precautions. Identification of the organism will determine the type of mask and other precautions needed.

- Interventions that protect all clients from the spread of disease include consistent and thorough hand washing, encouraging clients to cover their mouths with tissues when coughing or sneezing, disposal of soiled tissues in an appropriate bedside receptacle, making sure that reusable equipment is cleaned or sterilized appropriately, and handling soiled linens to prevent cross-contamination.

5. The assistant should be complimented on knowing the need to wash her hands after contact with the client. However, her technique could be improved through the use of paper towels on the faucet handles and increasing the time spent washing to at least 10 seconds.

CHAPTER 30: Safety

1. Restraints should only be used as a last resort. Some of the reasons include, but are not limited to, the following: Research has not proven that restraining clients prevents falls or injury; they lessen the client's movement and independence, which infringes on their rights; restraints can increase agitation of the client; the restraints can cause injury (pressure ulcers, skin tears, or death); restraints can interfere with the client's treatment; restraints can potentially cause health problems such as poor circulation; and restraints can be embarrassing to both client and family members.

2. Several factors that could affect Mr. Moore's safety include, but are not limited to, the following.

   - He is greater than age 65; he has a history of falls; recent surgery for a hip fracture may impair his mobility; he may be weaker now than before his surgery; his medications may affect his safety (e.g., antihypertensives, diuretics, analgesics).
   - Mr. Moore may resume normal activities before he is strong enough.
   - Mr. Moore may not be able to meet his nutritional needs because he will need to prepare all but one meal per day. He is at greater risk for injury while preparing his own food.
   - Mr. Moore may not understand the precautions necessary to protect his own safety.

3. You need to perform a home hazard appraisal. Suggestions for safety enhancement include the following:

   - Because the majority of adult injuries stem from falls, caution Mr. Moore about using area rugs and to be aware of where his pets are when he is up moving about.
   - Use grip handles in the bathtub and toilet.
   - All rooms should be well lighted. Use night-lights.
   - Carpets should be in good condition and hardwood floors should not be waxed.
   - The house should have smoke alarms; telephones should be easily accessible in case of emergency.

4. He has been physically and socially active and independent; he has a strong family support system (his son will visit

daily); he has access to community resources; his rooms are on one level and his house is small; he has pets to decrease his loneliness; he has no other chronic illnesses that would interfere with his healing process.

CHAPTER 31: Hygiene

1. After reviewing the defining characteristics and related factors, there is little data to support that the client actually has an impaired ability to perform her own bathing and hygiene. She has been providing for her own needs, has been ambulating, and has no physical impairments.

   - The following factors influence an individual's hygienic practices: culture, religion, environment, developmental level, health and energy, and personal preference.

2. Assess the client for discomfort/pain, fatigue, embarrassment, cultural beliefs, or personal preferences that may affect her decision to omit her personal care.

   - Suggested questions for the client: "Are you uncomfortable?" "Are you more tired today than yesterday?" "Do you want to wait until you go home?"

3. In general, bathing and personal care are essential for maintenance of skin integrity and mucous membranes, decreasing potential for infections, enhancing comfort, fostering a feeling of well-being, enhancing relaxation, minimizing odor, increasing circulation, and so on.

   - Benefits of personal care to the client include, but are not limited to, decreasing her risk of surgical wound infection and enhancing her comfort and ability to relax; cleaning her teeth decreases the risk for infection and enables her to enjoy her food.

4. Offer the client several explanations regarding the benefits of proceeding with her bath and personal care, emphasizing the need to prevent infections.

   - Offer to assist her and seek her input on where she wants to bathe (e.g., at the bedside or in the bathroom); gather her toiletries and provide for privacy.
   - Make sure she has warm water and clean linens.
   - Provide intervention, if appropriate, depending on her reason for not wanting to perform personal care (e.g., pain medication).

5. You can gather information and perform assessments during the bathing process.

   - You can convey to clients that you have the time and the interest to make them feel better.

CHAPTER 32: Diagnostic Testing

1. Consider the possible causes. Is the finger vasoconstricted because of decreased blood volume? Would warming it with a warm cloth and having the client hold her hand in a de-

pendent position help? Check the equipment (e.g., lancet injector) to see that it is operating correctly. Was it poor technique? Frequently, a novice nurse does not use enough force to press the injector firmly against the skin and/or have the injector in a perpendicular position relative to the skin. Both are needed to obtain a deep, clean puncture. After you have ascertained the cause, you will need to do another finger stick to obtain a large enough drop of blood to obtain an accurate reading.

2. The lab results suggest an infection is present and dehydration. Having a previous Hct for comparison would be helpful. Nursing interventions would relate to both infection and dehydration: VS TPR, check for orthostatic hypotension, obtain urine for C&S, interventions to promote hydration.

3. Consider that Ms. Angyal has had no fluids for 3 days. There is no information about the antibiotic (e.g., route and classification) which can also be factors. Some antibiotics can be nephrotoxic. It is important to obtain a specimen for C&S before starting antibiotics, otherwise the results may not be accurate. Therefore, priorities would be to first start the IV fluids, because this will begin rehydrating her and may also help with obtaining the urine specimen. Second, obtain the urine specimen. You will need to assess how much assistance she may need with providing the clean-catch urine specimen because of expected weakness as a result of not eating or drinking for 3 days. Assistance may include placing her on a bedpan with the nurse doing the cleansing of the area and collecting the sample. Finally, the third priority would be administration of the antibiotic. All of these priorities would take place quickly because they are all important as is the order of the priorities.

4. The reduction in Hct reflects that she was dehydrated and the first Hct was elevated due to hemoconcentration. After being rehydrated, this Hct is more accurate. The WBC indicates that the infectious process is subsiding.

5. Assess her knowledge about an MRI and explain, if necessary, the purpose, procedure, benefits, and risks. Sedation is provided if the client is claustrophobic or unable to lie still during the procedure. Assure her that two-way communication is provided so that the client can provide feedback and be monitored. Inform her that there is a loud knocking noise during the procedure and earplugs are available if she desires. Document her concerns and the teaching you provided. If she continues to be anxious, inform the physician.

CHAPTER 33: Medications

1. Differences between an allergic reaction and a drug side effect can include:

   - Side effects are not related to an allergic reaction and do not produce the same symptoms as are produced by allergies. Allergic reactions have a distinct pattern of reaction (e.g., skin rash, pruritus, angioedema, rhinitis, tearing, nausea, vomiting, wheezing, dyspnea, or diarrhea).

- A severe reaction is called *anaphylaxis* and can produce respiratory collapse if emergency treatment is not immediately instituted.
- Drug hypersensitivity or drug allergy is often listed as a systemic side effect in drug handbooks.

2. Mr. Ketron may have allergies to either of the drugs; he may be on another prescribed drug, tobacco, alcohol, or nonprescription drug that interferes with or potentiates one of the prescribed drugs; he may have a medical condition that limits the kinds of drugs he can take safely, he could be allergic to penicillin, and so on.

3. Make the following assessments:

- Inspect and palpate the IV insertion site for signs of infection, infiltration, or a dislocated catheter.
- Inspect the surrounding skin for redness, pallor, or swelling.
- Palpate the surrounding tissues for coldness and the presence of edema, which could indicate leakage of the IV fluid into the tissues.
- Take vital signs for baseline data, especially respiratory rate.
- Determine if the client has allergies to the medication.
- Check the compatibility of the medication and IV fluid.
- Determine specific drug action, side effects, normal dosage, recommended administration time, and peak action time of the morphine.
- Check patency of the IV line by assessing flow rate.

4. All the same precautions should be taken with intravenous medications as with other medications; correct client, correct dose, correct route, and so on. Additional precautions include, but are not limited to, confirming that the antibiotic is compatible with the intravenous fluid infusing, verifying sterility of the system and integrity of the medication bag, verifying that there is no air in the system, cleaning the port prior to placing a needle, and reviewing Mr. Ketron's medication history for possible allergies.

5. Some drugs are better absorbed when given on an empty stomach, whereas others cause gastrointestinal irritation and should be given with meals or after meals.

CHAPTER 34: Skin Integrity and Wound Care

1. Mr. Johns' age, his decreased activity and mobility, his decreased sensation on the right, his incontinence, and his nutritional status (thin for his height) suggest he is vulnerable. In fact, he has evidence of a stage I pressure ulcer over his hips and coccyx.

2. You should assess the degree of his loss of sensation, his ability to recognize if he is incontinent, the frequency of his incontinence, how often he ambulates and his capacity for ambulation, his serum protein as an indicator of his nutritional status, and his ability to attend to his own needs.

3. You should undertake measures that include, but are not limited to, providing nutritious meals and snacks; assisting

him if necessary; changing his position every 2 hours; avoiding shearing or friction when moving and positioning him; keeping his skin clean and dry; using pressure-relieving support devices; encouraging activity. Discuss the benefit of each of these measures. Consider their cost and the amount of caregiver time required. Prioritize the measures and include rationales.

4. Although the skin is not yet broken, he meets the description of having a stage I ulcer and will progress to further stages (and probably more areas of breakdown) if interventions are not initiated.

CHAPTER 35: Perioperative Nursing

1. Factors that may increase Mr. Teng's risk include, but are not limited to, he is 77 years old, placing him at greater risk than younger adults; his respiratory status is compromised and he runs a greater risk for developing postoperative atelectasis or lung infection; and he may be taking medications that will slow healing, such as corticosteroids.

2. A major disadvantage of general anesthesia is that it depresses the respiratory and circulatory systems, so the surgeon and anesthesiologist probably chose not to further complicate Mr. Teng's respiratory status. A client's preference for a particular anesthesia is also considered when selecting the type of anesthesia to use.

3. Mr. Teng's preoperative preparation most likely included, but was not limited to, preoperative teaching regarding preparation for surgery; what to expect following surgery; deep-breathing, coughing, and leg exercises; how to splint his abdomen when moving or coughing; fluid and nutritional support; a bath or shower; antiemboli stockings, and medications to enhance rest the night prior to the scheduled surgery.

4. Even though Mr. Teng had spinal anesthesia and is awake, the same general assessments will be made to detect actual or potential problems. He will not go through the stages of anesthesia arousal or experience altered gag reflexes. He will be assessed for return of feeling to his lower extremities to evaluate remaining spinal anesthesia effect. His postoperative monitoring will not differ from that of other clients.

5. Specific precautions may include, but are not limited to, promoting adequate hydration to replace fluids lost during surgery or fluid limitations prior to surgery, early movement and ambulation to foster maximum lung expansion and prevent lung infection, deep-breathing exercises to remove mucus and prevent stasis of lung secretions, pain control so that he can ambulate and cough more effectively, and leg exercises to prevent thrombophlebitis.

CHAPTER 36: Sensory Perception

1. Mrs. Dodd is at greatly increased risk for sensory overload due to her environment (critical care unit). She is being bombarded by the noise of her monitors and ventilator, which may be distorted and meaningless due to the sedation

she is receiving. Her pain and inability to communicate also contribute to her sensory overload because they contribute to her feelings of being overwhelmed and out of control.

2. Signs of sensory overload may include, but are not limited to, restlessness, agitation, confusion, disorientation, hallucinations, or inability to sleep or rest. Signs of sensory deprivation may include apathy, emotional detachment, and depression. Many times the signs of sensory deprivation and overload are the same; consequently, the nurse must assess the client for factors that may be contributing to one problem over the other.

3. Interventions include, but are not limited to, reducing and dimming lights; decreasing noise to the degree possible (close doors or curtains); providing comfort measures; explaining all procedures; orienting the client to person, place, and time; speaking in a soft, unhurried manner; and limiting visitors.

4. Clients cared for at home may experience either sensory deprivation or overload depending on the environment. If it is a busy, active environment with several family members, they may experience overload. If clients live alone, have few supportive family members, or are seldom contacted, they are more likely to experience social isolation and become withdrawn or uncommunicative, or lose interest in their usual activities. Interventions for home care or ICU clients are similar and adapted to the specific needs of the client, regardless of setting.

CHAPTER 37: Self-Concept

1. Because of his age, Craig's basic self-concept should be fairly well set and is not likely to be negatively affected. Body image and self-esteem, however, may be altered by his amputation. Body image is at risk because the amputation will change the way he views his body. Personal identity is at risk because he sees himself as an athlete.

2. Craig's mood, inability to look at the stump, unwillingness to discuss rehabilitation. If they continue or new negative responses develop, a negative change in his self-esteem may be occurring. Since his father is also having difficulty with the loss, a strong source of support is unavailable to Craig.

3. There are many possibilities including his nurses' attitudes; rehabilitation team and primary caregiver abilities; family and friends' support; and his internal ability to be adaptable, revise his goals, and use his resources. Craig's mother's presence is likely to be supportive unless she offers assistance while encouraging dependency.

4. Adapting to change may be more difficult for elders. Elders fear dependence more than younger clients, therefore, a large loss such as this puts them at greater risk for altered self-esteem. In addition, elders do not heal and progress as quickly as younger clients—the additional time required may seem to them a negative factor. Much care, however, will be similar: encouragement and support, participation in their own care, identifying personal strengths, and so on.

5. Clients with chronic mental illnesses, cancer, socially stigmatized diseases (AIDS, TB, obesity, sexually transmitted diseases), and other sources of disfigurement.

CHAPTER 38: Sexuality

1. Many people are uncomfortable discussing such a private matter with strangers (such as their nurses) unless they are made to feel that sexuality is normal and okay. They need to be given permission to openly discuss their concerns without fear of being belittled or made fun. Discuss the benefits of "permission giving." How would you feel about discussing your sexuality with a stranger?

2. Factors include nurses' knowledge and comfort with their own sexuality, recognition and acceptance of sexuality as normal and important human function, understanding of how health impacts sexuality, and nurses' ability to communicate in general.

3. There is a direct relationship between health and ability to function sexually in that the healthier you are the more likely you are to have the desire and ability to function sexually.

   - Both physical and mental status affects the ability to function sexually
   - Diseases such as heart disease, hypertension, diabetes, renal failure, spinal cord injury, or pain can lessen both sexual desire and ability. Mental disorders such as depression can lessen desire.

4. You will need to perform a complete sexual health assessment to provide baseline data.

   - Two primary problems need to be addressed: his fear of resuming sexual activity and the effects of his antihypertensive medication.
   - Specific interventions may include providing information, correcting misconceptions, reassurance that resuming sexual activity is safe, suggesting alternative positions for sex that require less energy than other positions if sexual activity causes him fatigue.
   - Consult with Mr. Curry's primary care provider regarding antihypertensive medications that are less likely to produce sexual dysfunction.

CHAPTER 39: Spirituality

1. Being religious means being part of an organized system of worship such as a church or synagogue. Terry may mean that he no longer attends the Methodist church or participates in organized religion.

   Spirituality refers to belief in or a relationship with some higher power, creative force, divine being, or infinite source of energy, such as God or Allah. Clients can be deeply spiritual without belonging to an organized system of worship. Terry admits that he is not very religious; however, there are no data to suggest that he is not spiritual. In fact, Terry's statement that he is being punished is evidence that he believes in a higher power who is punishing him for not going to church.

2. He states "I can't see any reason for going on," "I know I'm not going to get well," "I guess I'm being punished." Terry's spiritual distress is related to both his physiologic situation as well as his concern over not being religious.

3. Spiritual beliefs and religious beliefs can assume greater importance during times of illness. Many persons will return to their religious roots during times of illness in hopes that they will be cured through divine intervention.

4. A spiritual assessment will help both you and Terry by providing information relative to his spirituality, his religion, and his degree of spiritual distress, so that appropriate interventions can be planned and implemented.

Possible benefits may include, but are not limited to, helping Terry draw on inner resources more effectively to deal with his present physical and emotional situation, helping him find meaning in living and hope for the future even though he is presently very ill, and providing appropriate spiritual resources such as a minister or priest.

CHAPTER 40: Stress and Coping

1. It is difficult to know whether Ruby's coping would differ if only a portion of the breast were going to be removed or whether this is merely the focus of her difficulty in coping with the diagnosis and need for surgery. It might depend on how large her breasts are and if the lump represented a significant portion of the breast. Persons may have very different emotional reactions to situations in which they can or cannot hide their condition or if the impact is directly linked to their role (such as the fact that she is a dress designer).

2. Ruby's situation fits with a stimulus-based model since the stressors of diagnosis, surgery, and implications of having cancer serve as stress stimuli causing physical and emotional outcomes (such as her ineffective mothering). However, her situation would also fit the response model since the surgery and any further cancer treatment required plus her alcohol use would create stress reactions in the mind and body.

3. The nurse will validate that she cannot know exactly what Ruby is experiencing (assuming the nurse has not actually had a mastectomy), but has worked with many clients undergoing extremely distressful and possibly life-threatening conditions. One of the interventions will include making a connection with other women who have/had breast cancer, but that is a response to the content of her message. The nurse first needs to respond to the emotional part of the message—Ruby's anger, frustration, and lack of control.

4. The suddenness of this diagnosis and Ruby's extreme reaction of alcohol abuse and neglecting her children certainly may qualify the situation as a crisis. Her inability to discuss her feelings or plans supports the presence of a crisis situation. Under these circumstances, caregivers may need to be more assertive in providing her care and mak-

ing decisions. She may benefit from referral for psychological therapy/counseling.

5. Many answers may be correct. She does not appear to be using denial. She might use projection in attempting to find a cause of her cancer, which could be maladaptive since, most commonly, the cause of breast cancer is unknown.

CHAPTER 41: Loss, Grieving, and Death

1. The eldest son most nearly approximates the "awareness of loss" phase. He is experiencing the loss but is able to resume normal activities. The middle son has characteristics of the "conservation/withdrawal" phase. He has a need to be alone, and is experiencing both physical and psychologic symptoms of bereavement. The younger son is experiencing "shock." He is having difficulty believing that his mother is dead and is experiencing several physical symptoms.

2. Factors include amount of conflict or closeness each brother felt to the mother, amount of time/caring each was able to provide, significance/meaning of the mother to each, spiritual beliefs and practices, amount of guilt each felt related to meeting mother's needs during her later years or illness.

3. Cues might include wanting to talk about death, reminiscing or reviewing one's life, emotional withdrawal or becoming quite and pensive, allowing others to take over physical care, voicing a sense of urgency about seeing loved ones, and so on.

4. The primary factor is the client's desire for pain relief rather than the family's wishes or concern for hastening death. If the client has diminished ability to communicate desires, other sources of data about current level of pain and previously expressed desires must be considered. An advance directive can assist in this area.

5. If you have had mostly positive experiences, or ones similar to those the client is experiencing, these can be shared with others. Consider characteristics of the losses (e.g., if they were expected or unexpected, your age and that of the deceased) and effectiveness of sources of support during grieving.

CHAPTER 42: Activity and Exercise

1. His dyspnea on mild exertion is a worrisome sign and his activity intolerance will worsen if he remains immobile. His edema indicates inadequate venous return, especially with his amount of time spent sitting, and will lead to other problems.

2. Check environment for possible safety hazards, get a walker light enough to handle easily and be sure it has been adjusted for proper height, keep the tips in good shape, do exercises to keep strength in the hands and arms.

3. Being overweight certainly contributes to his difficulties and should be addressed. More assessment is needed regarding how long he has been overweight and his eating patterns.

4. There is a relationship between physical and emotional health; that the client "wants" to be healthier.
5. With chronic illness, because the condition has existed for a longer time, the outcomes may require more time to achieve than with acute illnesses. Outcomes should be in smaller increments. Lower levels of expectations are often appropriate since full return to earlier levels of health is unlikely.

CHAPTER 43: Rest and Sleep

1. A sleep diary would help him identify factors that may be interfering with his ability to establish and maintain good sleep habits. Many times, people are unaware of the relationship between what they do at bedtime and ability to sleep. A sleep diary would also help Mr. Harrison better estimate the actual amount of sleep he is or is not getting.
2. Other data that may be helpful include, but are not limited to, activities and bedtime habits, degree of noise in the environment, what foods or drinks he consumes just prior to bedtime, if he uses over-the-counter medications to help him sleep, if he has a regular pattern of arising, and whether or not he is a smoker.
3. Suggest that he read a book or other quiet activity (not watching TV or exercising) before going to sleep, maintain regular sleep and waking hours, explore nonpharmacologic sleep remedies, and so on.
4. Mr. Harrison's history is suggestive of insomnia, a primary sleep disorder. If pain from his arm was keeping him from sleeping, or if he was found to have post-stress disorder, he would be experiencing a secondary sleep disorder.
5. Common causes of difficulty in sleeping are physical distress, noisy environment, severe fatigue, changing work shifts, emotional distress, alcohol and other stimulants, weight loss, and smoking.

CHAPTER 44: Pain Management

1. There is subjective data (rating her pain as 5) and objective data (vital signs, position, holding abdomen, lying in rigid position) to support that Mrs. Lundahl is experiencing pain; however, no conclusions can be drawn about the intensity, location, quality, or pattern of Mrs. Lundahl's pain.
2. It would be incorrect to assume that Mrs. Lundahl needs no interventions for her pain. People rate their pain differently based on their past pain experiences, their pain tolerance, their ethnic/cultural values, and so on. Mrs. Lundahl should be asked if she needs pain intervention.
3. Mrs. Lundahl is most likely experiencing acute pain from her surgery. Depending on the amount of manipulation of bowel, blood vessels, and so on, within her abdomen, she may also be experiencing visceral pain.
4. Numerous interventions may be helpful, such as changing her body position, a back massage, use of a cutaneous stimulator, distraction (e.g., soft music), and so on.
5. The most reliable method of determining that Mrs. Lundahl's pain has been relieved is for her to tell you that her pain has been relieved. Objective data may include decreased pulse, blood pressure, and respirations when compared to preintervention values; Mrs. Lundahl resting quietly or sleeping; pink color, absence of nausea or perspiration; relaxed facial expression, and so on.

CHAPTER 45: Nutrition

1. Being a woman means that her distribution of fat is generally higher than a man's. At age 59, she is beginning to enter the age range when the body configuration changes somewhat, fewer calories are needed to maintain weight, but nutrients are still very important. Being alone contributes to poor eating habits since meals are often a social event. We do not know her ethnicity but this can influence her view of nutrition and weight.
2. What were her eating patterns before her husband died? What foods do she like and dislike most? What kinds of snacks is she eating? Does she have the financial means to buy food? Does her living situation allow her to make and store food?
3. Suggestions may be many such as keeping busy with her hands while watching TV (e.g. folding laundry), choosing healthy snacks like carrot and celery sticks, and not buying snacks at the store.
4. Although there are many ways to determine her ideal weight from tables, charts, and calculators, her best weight is influenced by many other factors that are difficult to include in these (specific activity level, BMR, body configuration). Since she states she formerly was "petite," she may wish to return to this state—as much as is possible as she ages. It is important that the nurse not tell her a specific weight that she should achieve. Goal setting must be collaborative.

CHAPTER 46: Fecal Elimination

1. Ask her about the number and amount of stool she has in order to determine if she is actually having diarrhea or has an impaction. Assess her usual diet, daily fluid intake, amount of fiber in the diet, daily activities, medications, or other factors that could be contributing to constipation and possible impaction.
2. A digital examination may be performed to verify or rule out the presence of a fecal impaction. Other interventions may include administering an oil retention enema followed by a cleansing enema, suppositories, or stool softeners. If all else fails, manual removal of the fecal impaction may be necessary.
3. Consider interventions to promote regular defecation such as increasing intake of fluids, maintaining a regular schedule for defecation, paying attention to the urge to defecate, and so on. To add more fiber to the diet, teach the client about foods that are high in fiber; go through her kitchen with her pointing out what foods qualify. Suggest she interface with others in her complex to plan good menus, eat together, and so on. Also consider referral to physical therapy or other resources to increase activity appropriate for elders such as water exercises.

4. The chronic use of laxatives will actually make her more prone to constipation and impaction because she loses muscle tone. Increased fiber, fruits, and vegetables and other ways of naturally dealing with constipation are safer and more appropriate.

CHAPTER 47: Urinary Elimination

1. Urinary frequency could be a sign of infection due to causes other than prostate hypertrophy. No other data are given about his other health problems including medications that might be contributing factors. A thorough assessment is indicated.
2. The nurse needs to ensure that the client completely understands what is proposed and the intended outcomes. There is always a balance between the expected positive result and the risk of the intervention. Is this surgery considered culturally appropriate? Although you may not know a great deal about the actual surgery, you realize that not every procedure is completely successful. How would the client react if he continued to have some incontinence following the operation?
3. Often, there is a medical standard of care that is followed unless there are contraindications. If the physician determines that the hypertrophy is severe, and knows that this is not a reversible condition, surgery may be the only logical option. Investigate what other treatments may be used in this situation and propose why they may be seen as less desirable than surgery.
4. The nurse should fully explore the client's understanding of his condition and what measures can be taken to diminish its impact on his ADLs and quality of life. If the client truly understands and makes this informed choice, it is the nurse's responsibility to support the client.

CHAPTER 48: Oxygenation

1. The physical assessment reveals fever, use of accessory muscles, adventitious lung sounds, and yellow sputum all of which suggest more than an average cold. The nurse certainly would have suspected a more significant underlying condition.
2. Ms. Singh has quite a stressful lifestyle with work and school plus her physical stressors of a poor diet and smoking for more than 20 years. The nurse should perform discharge teaching that includes examination of which of these modifiable risk factors may be addressed in both short- and long-term plans.
3. Alteration in mental status may be a very useful sign that the client is hypoxic. Also, increased respiratory and cardiac rates and substantial shortness of breath would be negative signs. If not already in place, continuous oxygen saturation monitoring should be initiated, frequent assessments, and notification of the physician are required. The nurse should have nasotracheal suction equipment available. The client may require transfer to a higher acuity nursing station.

4. Standard precautions must always be in place. The nurse is careful to glove whenever coming into direct contact with the client's secretions. The nurse will also wear a mask if the client is unable to control her secretions and may cough or spit in the nurse's face.
5. A face mask may be uncomfortable or cause the client to feel confined or claustrophobic. If she is not wearing it, it cannot help her. Discuss the face mask with her and determine why she is taking it off. If the mask cannot be modified to address these reasons, consider arranging for her to have oxygen by nasal cannula instead (with an appropriate change in the flow rate).

CHAPTER 49: Circulation

1. This client has decreased arterial circulation to her feet. When the tissues become ischemic, lactic acid builds up and causes the discomfort. The pain she describes is consistent with the medical condition *intermittent claudication*. Risk factors for peripheral vascular disease include cigarette smoking, high fat intake, obesity, sedentary lifestyle, hypertension, and diabetes.
2. *Ineffective Tissue Perfusion (Peripheral)* and *Activity Intolerance* are two likely diagnoses. Of these two, *Activity Intolerance* may be of highest priority for the nurse since there is a greater likelihood of developing a nursing care plan that can substantially affect her desired level of function and quality of life. Desired outcomes and interventions for the *Ineffective Tissue Perfusion* will focus on implementing the medical treatment plan and protection from injury. However, remember that for a care plan to be effective, the client must be an active participant in the process. Thus, the diagnoses of highest priority can only be suggested without her input.
3. The physiological impact of the plan must be weighed against the psychological impact—always a difficult thing to do. The nurse must explore the client's response to the recommendation. If it is unacceptable to her, consider if any compromises such as less frequent visits or use of a wheelchair are more agreeable.
4. Support stockings help increase venous return. This client has impaired arterial circulation. If the stockings are tight, they could actually interfere with the flow of arterial blood to her extremities. She requires client teaching explaining the differences at a level she can comprehend.

CHAPTER 50: Fluid, Electrolyte, and Acid-Base Balance

1. Cardiac dysrhythmias can be a result of hypokalemia. If cardiac irregularities occur, it is an emergency and requires notifying the physician and the charge nurse immediately. Emergency orders may be instituted. As you are assessing her cardiac irregularity, notice whether there is a pattern to the irregularity and the rate. It is also important to assess blood pressure as an indicator of cardiac function and the effects of the dysrhythmia.

2. Fluid volume deficit creates a hypertonic vascular space, which causes water to move out of the cells, including brain cells. This is what causes neurologic symptoms—intracellular dehydration.

3. Suggestions may be many such as finding a fluid that she likes or helps her nausea, making sure fluids are served at the appropriate temperature, using a straw, and starting with small amounts. Administering an antiemetic medication as ordered may also help improve her oral intake.

4. Although there are many indicators of fluid balance, daily weights are an important way to provide more data about fluid. You can explain that a loss of 1 kg (2.2 lb) indicates a fluid loss of approximately 1 liter. It is an easy, quick way to get more information about fluid balance.

Appendix B

Measurement Scales Used in NOC

Scale Number

1	Extremely compromised	Substantially compromised	Moderately compromised	Mildly compromised	Not compromised
2	Extreme deviation from expected range	Substantial deviation from expected range	Moderate deviation from expected range	Mild deviation from expected range	No deviation from expected range
3	Dependent, does not participate	Requires assistive person and device	Requires assistive person	Independent with assistive device	Completely independent
4	No motion	Limited motion	Moderate motion	Substantial motion	Full motion
5	Not at all	To a slight extent	To a moderate extent	To a great extent	To a very great extent
6	Not adequate	Slightly adequate	Moderately adequate	Substantially adequate	Totally adequate
7	Over 9	7–9	4–6	1–3	None
8	Extensive	Substantial	Moderate	Limited	None
9	None	Limited	Moderate	Substantial	Extensive
10	None	Slight	Moderate	Substantial	Complete
11	Never positive	Rarely positive	Sometimes positive	Often positive	Consistently positive
12	Very weak	Weak	Moderate	Strong	Very strong
13	Never demonstrated	Rarely demonstrated	Sometimes demonstrated	Often demonstrated	Consistently demonstrated
14	Severe	Substantial	Moderate	Slight	None
15	No evidence	Limited evidence	Moderate evidence	Substantial evidence	Extensive evidence
16	Extreme delay from expected range	Substantial delay from expected range	Moderate delay from expected range	Slight delay from expected range	No delay from expected range
17	Poor	Fair	Average	Good	Excellent

Note: From *Nursing Outcomes Classification (NOC),* 2nd ed., by M. Johnson, M. Maas, and S. Moorhead, Eds., St. Louis, MO: Mosby, 2000, pp. 48–60. Used with permission.

Appendix C

Answers to Review Questions

Chapter 1 1. D 2. C 3. B 4. B 5. D 6. A   **Chapter 2**
1. C 2. B 3. A 4. C 5. D   **Chapter 3** 1. C 2. B 3. D 4. A
5. B   **Chapter 4** 1. C 2. D 3. B 4. A 5. D   **Chapter 5**
1. A 2. B 3. A 4. C 5. D   **Chapter 6** 1. C 2. B 3. A 4. B
5. D   **Chapter 7** 1. C 2. A 3. B 4. B 5. D   **Chapter 8**
1. C 2. B 3. D 4. A 5. D   **Chapter 9** 1. C 2. A 3. B 4. A
5. D   **Chapter 10** 1. A 2. C 3. D 4. C 5. A   **Chapter 11**
1. C 2. B 3. A 4. A 5. A   **Chapter 12** 1. C 2. D 3. A
4. B 5. D   **Chapter 13** 1. C 2. B 3. C 4. D 5. C
Chapter 14 1. B 2. D 3. C 4. A 5. B   **Chapter 15** 1. B
2. A 3. D 4. A 5. D   **Chapter 16** 1. A 2. C 3. B 4. C
5. D   **Chapter 17** 1. B 2. C 3. A 4. D 5. A   **Chapter 18**
1. D 2. A 3. B 4. C 5. C   **Chapter 19** 1. B 2. D 3. A
4. B 5. B   **Chapter 20** 1. C 2. A 3. B 4. D 5. D
Chapter 21 1. C 2. D 3. B 4. B 5. A   **Chapter 22** 1. B
2. A 3. C 4. A 5. A   **Chapter 23** 1. C 2. B 3. C 4. B
5. C   **Chapter 24** 1. C 2. B 3. A 4. A 5. B   **Chapter 25**
1. B 2. C 3. B 4. A 5. C   **Chapter 26** 1. A 2. A 3. B
4. C 5. D   **Chapter 27** 1. B 2. C 3. D 4. B 5. A
Chapter 28 1. B 2. D 3. A 4. A 5. B   **Chapter 29** 1. B
2. A 3. C 4. A 5. D   **Chapter 30** 1. B 2. A 3. C 4. C
5. D   **Chapter 31** 1. C 2. C 3. B 4. A 5. D   **Chapter 32**
1. B 2. C 3. B 4. D 5. C   **Chapter 33** 1. C 2. D 3a. D
3b. A 4. D 5a. B 5b. C 5c. A 5d. D   **Chapter 34** 1. B
2. A 3. C 4. A 5. C   **Chapter 35** 1. C 2. B 3. D 4. B
5. C   **Chapter 36** 1. D 2. C 3. B 4. B 5. D   **Chapter 37**
1. A 2. C 3. B 4. A 5. D   **Chapter 38** 1. D 2. A 3. C
4. B 5. D   **Chapter 39** 1. D 2. C 3. C 4. C 5. B
Chapter 40 1. C 2. D 3. A 4. C 5. B   **Chapter 41** 1. D
2. B 3. A 4. C 5. C   **Chapter 42** 1. B 2. A 3. A 4. D
5. C   **Chapter 43** 1. C 2. A 3. B 4. C 5. D   **Chapter 44**
1. C 2. B 3. C 4. A 5. D   **Chapter 45** 1. B 2. C 3. A
4. C 5. A   **Chapter 46** 1. A 2. B 3. D 4. C 5. B
Chapter 47 1. D 2. C 3. B 4. A 5. C   **Chapter 48** 1. D
2. C 3. A 4. C 5. B   **Chapter 49** 1. A 2. C 3. D 4. C
5. D   **Chapter 50** 1. C 2. D 3. D 4. A 5. C

Evaluating Your Response

Chapter 1   Answers to Review Questions

1. The term *patient* implies passive acceptance of decisions
   made by health care professionals. Consumer is an individual, group of people or community that uses a service
   or commodity.

2. Answer **a** is an example of illness prevention. Answers
   b and **d** are examples of restoring health.

3. A clinical nurse specialist is an expert in a specialized
   field and often works in a hospital setting. The nurse
   midwife provides primary care (e.g., prenatal care, Pap
   smears), but also manages delivery of normal
   pregnancies. The nurse-entrepreneur manages a health-
   related business.

4. The advanced beginner demonstrates marginally acceptable performance. The proficient practitioner has 3 to 5
   years of experience and has developed a holistic
   understanding of the client. The expert practitioner
   demonstrates highly skilled intuitive and analytic ability
   in new situations.

5. The National Student Nurses' Association developed the
   Code of Academic and Clinical Conduct for nursing students in 2001. ANA developed *Standards of Clinical
   Nursing Practice* and a code for nurses. NLN focuses on
   nursing education. The American Association of Colleges
   of Nursing (AACN) identifies values essential to the professional nurse.

6. All will impact nursing but not necessarily the supply
   and demand issue. Aging of the nurse workforce, aging
   of nursing faculty, and the aging population contribute to
   more elders needing specialized care (increasing the demand). Fewer nursing faculty to educate students and
   fewer nurses practicing because of retirement contribute
   to the decreasing supply.

Chapter 2   Answers to Review Questions

1. Continuing education refers to formalized experiences
   designed to enlarge the knowledge or skills of practitioners. The other answers are examples of in-service education, which is designed to upgrade the knowledge or
   skills of *employees* and is less formal in presentation.

2. Naturalistic inquiry is the philosophical basis for qualitative research. Positivism and logical positivism is the
   philosophical basis for quantitative research, which uses
   a specific plan to collect numerical data. Testing tip: two
   answers using a similar word usually means neither is
   correct.

3. Quantitative research collects numerical data. Sleep deprivation can be defined by X number of hours without
   sleep and wound healing can be measured by size of
   wound. The other answers investigate subjective experiences of clients.

4. This study investigates the subjective experience of stress
   and would be collected through narrative data. The other
   answers are examples of quantitative research.

5. The right of self-determination means that subjects should feel free from constraints, coercion, or any undue influence to participate in a study. There is not enough information given to indicate if any of the other rights have been violated.

Chapter 3   Answers to Review Questions

1. A supposition or system of ideas proposed to explain a given phenomenon is a theory.

2. A group of related ideas or statements is a conceptual framework.

3. A set of shared understandings and assumptions about reality and the world is a pardigm.

4. Disciplines that do not have performance as their primary focus are not practice disciplines. One can study physics but not apply that knowledge in actuality.

5. The concepts in the nursing metaparadigm are person/client, environment, health, and nursing.

Chapter 4   Answers to Review Questions

1. This is the best answer because the nurse is assessing the client's level of knowledge as a result of the discussion with the physician. Based on this assessment, the nurse may initiate other actions (e.g., call the doctor if the client has many questions). In answer **a,** the nurse is not assessing if the client received enough information to give consent. Answer **b** is one way to assess the client's level of knowledge regarding the procedure. However, it is not the *best* approach because it is a closed-ended question, asking for only a "yes" or "no" response. Answer **c** provides more information from the client in his/her own words. The statement in answer **d** is true, however, the nurse should first verify if the client received enough information to give consent. After the assessment, this statement may be appropriate but the assessment needs to be done first.

2. Battery is the willful touching of a person without permission. An unintentional tort in answer **a** is malpractice. The example is an intentional tort because the nurse executed the act on purpose. Assault (answer **b**) is the attempt or threat to touch another person unjustifiably. The nurse in this case, actually touched the client without permission. Answer **c,** invasion of privacy, injures the feelings of the person.

3. Anytime a nurse questions an order, the nurse should call the person who wrote the order for clarification. Answer **a** is incorrect because knowing the dose is outside the normal range and not questioning the order could lead to client harm and liability for the nurse. Answer **c** is not the best answer because the nurse needs to obtain clarification from the person who wrote the order, and answer **d** is not the best answer because the nurse should *first* call the physician. The physician may have made a mistake or may provide the rationale for why the unusual dosage needs to be given.

4. All elements, including harm, must be present for malpractice to be proven. Notifying the physician does not exempt the nurse from liability. A medication error occurred by the nurse prior to calling the physician. A breach of duty does exist and foreseeability is present, however, no harm occurred to the client.

5. An invasive procedure is outside the scope of practice of a UAP. The UAP, even though a nursing student, must follow the agency job description while working as a UAP. The job description is the standard of care in this situation.

Chapter 5   Answers to Review Questions

1. A nurse's actions in an ethical dilemma must be defensible according to moral and ethical standards. The nurse may have strong personal beliefs but distancing oneself from the situation does not serve the client. A team is not always required to reach decisions and the nurse is not obligated to automatically follow the client's wishes when they may have negative consequences for self or others.

2. A nurse is ethically bound to act on knowledge of another provider's unsafe or incompetent actions. Many medical practices are controversial but not necessarily unethical. Although some may view nurses' strikes as unethical, supporting others who are striking is a personal decision. Although a client statement in confidence to a nurse may have ethical overtones, it does not automatically constitute an ethical dilemma.

3. Autonomy is the client's (or surrogate's) right to make his or her own decisions. Remember, the nurse is obliged to respect a client's informed decision. These parents may modify their decision as time goes on and the child's condition, or their feelings, change. This situation is not clearly one of nonmaleficence (do no harm) or beneficence (do good) since there are many aspects of both. If the child appeared to be suffering or an effective treatment was being denied, these principles might apply. Justice (fairness) generally applies when the rights of one client are being balanced against those of another client.

4. In values clarification, clients are assisted to think about the factors that influence their beliefs and decisions. Any statement from the nurse that passes judgment on the rightness or wrongness of the client's thoughts or actions will impede this reflection.

5. A major role of the client advocate is to mediate between conflicting parties. Although a competent client may have the right to decide for herself and the physician may agree, understanding and cooperation among family members is a crucial goal. Legal action should be a last resort.

Chapter 6   Answers to Review Questions

1. Actions that help to prevent an illness or detect it in its early stages are primary prevention. Treatment of a disease is secondary prevention, while rehabilitation efforts are considered tertiary prevention.

2. City, county, state, or federal government funds pay for health department and agency activities aimed at the global health of the community. Hospitals may provide a variety of wellness and clinic programs in addition to inpatient services. Surgery may be performed in outpatient surgery centers and physicians' offices in addition to within hospitals. Skilled nursing, extended care, and long-term care facilities provide care to persons of all ages who require rehabilitation or subacute care. This is not necessarily related to insurance coverage for hospital stays.

3. Primary care providers are generally limited to physicians and nurses, and not all of those practitioners qualify. For example, in some cases a gynecologist may qualify as a primary care physician and in other cases not. Hospitals and clinics, as agencies, are not primary care providers. Pharmacists and case managers are not responsible for providing direct client care.

4. When people have inadequate insurance for health costs, they tend to avoid early and preventive care. This results in eventual use of much more costly resources. Methods to provide minimum levels of insurance coverage have been successful in other countries. The number of older adults is increasing but this is a nonmodifiable factor. There is currently a significant shortage of nurses and maldistribution of physicians. Competition among manufacturers is more likely to cause costs to fall than to rise.

5. A health maintenance organization involves a set monthly membership fee and predictable visit or deductible costs. Medicare does not cover many preventive and outpatient services. Individual fee-for-service insurance is perhaps the most costly, with potentially large differences between the coverage paid and the provider's charges. PPOs are less costly that fee-for-service but more expensive than HMOs.

Chapter 7   Answers to Review Questions

1. Nursing's Agenda for Healthcare Reform (ANA, 1991) called for case management of those with ongoing health care needs. It also proposed that primary care be community based and that essential services be paid for by a combination of public and private funding sources and be phased in gradually.

2. The Pew Commission identified the need for modern health care providers to be proficient in the use of technology. No mention is made of financial competencies beyond the attention to cost-effective care. The commission also identified the need for contemporary (not traditional) clinical strategies and for collaborative decision making with clients.

3. In community-based health care, clients are cared for according to their geographical locations that facilitate access such as where they live or work, rather than at a major medical center or similar provider setting. Emphasis is more on client wellness and prevention than on illness and may be paid for through any of the usual forms of insurance or payment (including managed care, private pay, or welfare).

4. In collaboration, each member of the team, including the client, participates in sharing ideas and reaching consensus on the best plan of care. The team is generally led by the health care professional most skilled in the client's specific need areas. Once the plan is established, it may be implemented by any member of the team or a designate at an appropriate time and place.

5. Effective discharge planning would have included an assessment of home care needs prior to the client leaving the hospital. Following a thorough assessment, the client would be taught self-care strategies and a basic plan of care for the coming days. If the client will need care at home, those referrals would be made by the discharge planner and communicated to the client. Answer **d** indicates the client knows and accepts these referrals.

Chapter 8   Answers to Review Questions

1. Answer **a** reflects the precontemplation stage. Answer **b** reflects the planning stage, and **d,** the maintenance stage.

2. Perceived self-efficacy is the confidence the person has for achieving the desired outcome. Answer **a** is a person's perceptions about available time, inconvenience, expense, and difficulty performing the activity; **c** is the person's perceptions concerning the behaviors, beliefs, or attitudes of others; and **d** refers to the person's perception of the environment and how it assists or detracts from the healthy behavior.

3. See Box 8–7. The death of a spouse is a score of 100 on the Life-Change Index by Holmes and Rahe (1967). Answer **a** is a score of 50, **b** is a score of 47, and **c** is a score of 26.

4. Answer **b** is a strategy for the contemplation stage, **c** is a strategy for the preparation stage, and answer **d** is a strategy for the maintenance stage.

5. Change is a complex process and a nurse should not give up or assume that the client doesn't want to change. People often resist a tough approach because it can make them feel cornered. This approach may work for some people but not for everyone. The goal of teaching is to try to help the client become the expert as well.

Chapter 9   Answers to Review Questions

1. Although hospitals have recently become more hospitable to families, a major strength of home care is the involvement and proximity of loved ones. Curative and lifesaving approaches may be used at home or in the hospital. A strength of home care nurses is their ability to manage complex symptoms. This includes expertise in pain management but the same legal strategies are available in either hospice or hospitals.

2. Assuming the client is medically stable, feeding and bathing are tasks within the aide's abilities. Teaching the

client about or adjusting medications and performing assessments are duties restricted to the registered nurse.

3. The nurse needs to encourage the client to express feelings or thoughts that lead to the refusal so that misunderstandings can be clarified and other possible solutions explored. Answers **a** and **c** do nothing to help get at the reasons for the client's behavior. Answer **d** is almost a threat and has a paternalistic implication. Clients are entitled to make informed decisions to perform or not perform recommended activities.

4. If the caregiver's own health is becoming threatened, it may be a sign of overload. It would be appropriate for the caregiver to ask for assistance from others or to ask for clarification of ways he or she can assist the client. Sadness related to a poor prognosis would be a normal and expected response as long as it does not evolve into depression.

5. A physician's authorization of the plan of care is needed before home health care by a nurse can be initiated. Insurance coverage is not required although the agency may need proof of the client's ability to pay if insurance is not available or adequate. Many clients benefit from home health care even if there is no in-home caregiver present or needed. The health problem for which home care is needed may be chronic or acute and may necessitate preventive, curative, or palliative therapy.

Chapter 10 Answers to Review Questions

1. Most CD-ROMs cannot be changed by the user. Some CDs are "rewriteable" but not commonly. RAM is random-access memory that is gone when the computer is turned off. A floppy diskette is more fragile than a CD and even files on a locked disk are easily erased since it can be unlocked by any person. A network is a communication method and not data storage.

2. Control over who has access to computerized data is the greatest concern. Computer systems become less expensive over time. With some built-in programs, computerized data can be much more accurate than paper and pencil. Due to ease of making copies and backups, electronic data can last forever.

3. Since learners may do their online work at different times and do most of their work offline, it is harder for them to feel and act like a class group. Through audio and video file sharing, learners can see and hear the faculty and each other. Some learners move more quickly through online courses than in face-to-face classes, others take longer.

4. Although all steps of the research process can be accomplished without computers, electronic data analysis helps ensure accuracy and speeds the analysis immensely.

5. Many websites are sponsored by legitimate organizations such as the National Cancer Institute. They often report results of extensive research. However, each site is different and the practitioner is compelled to evaluate the site and the treatment to determine if it is safe and appropriate for the client.

Chapter 11 Answers to Review Questions

1. Frustration is an example of an emotion. The client who chooses healthy foods represents the physical component, taking parenting classes enhances the intellectual component, and the bowling league is both the physical and social components.

2. The mother has taken on the sick role by expecting to be excused from her usual role responsibilities. The sick role states that persons are not answerable for their illness, contrary to the obese client's perspective. In the sick role, the client tries to get better as opposed to the man who misses his physical therapy appointments. The elder is not following the sick role expectation to rely on competent help.

3. While Mrs. Parajh probably has beliefs about the seriousness of her illness, which are influencing her actions, the health belief model is most useful to determine who is likely to participate in health-promoting activities. She is already taking action. The clinical model focuses on signs and symptoms of illness, which are not mentioned. The role performance model relates to the client's ability to act in her roles or work. The agent–host–environment model focuses on predicting illness.

4. Education has not been shown to be a factor in predicting adherence. There is good evidence that a trusting relationship with her provider, evidence supporting the effectiveness of the medication, and a less complex dosing regime are important predictors.

5. Although not always practical, direct observation is the best method to measure adherence (for example, watching heroin addicts actually take their methadone dose). Adherence to treatment regimens does not always ensure the client will be without complications or that lab values will respond to proper medication administration. Client report or recall is not always accurate, even if the client believes he or she is telling the truth.

Chapter 12 Answers to Review Questions

1. Holism implies consideration of all aspects of the client's life, not just their physiologic problems. Although arranging for home care, facilitating spirituality, and offering coping resources may be appropriate, the nurse begins a holistic approach to care by examining, with the client, in what ways the illness influences the various segments of her life.

2. Because the child's behavior results in a change in the father's behavior, it is considered feedback. It is also a type of negative feedback in that, the more the child cries, the

less the father leaves. In some ways, the child's behavior is also input because it is used by the father in making a decision (throughput).

3. The health history of the client's current living partners is critical information since many illness are communicable or environmental. Giving this advice, the nurse also validates that family is whoever the client says they are. History of illness data of blood relatives is also extremely valuable and should always be included.

4. When a person feels strongly enough, a lower level need (rest) can be postponed until a higher level need (success, safety) is met. It is very likely that no one else can meet that need for him and the lower need must still be met eventually.

5. The community health nurse will focus on activities that influence the larger group of individuals affected. These include prevention and monitoring of infectious disease plus actions that will promote health for multiple affected persons (e.g., food and shelter). The home health nurse more commonly works with single persons or families at one time—addressing their particular needs that may be similar to or different from those of others.

Chapter 13   Answers to Review Questions

1. There is an ongoing, natural shift in the population; one need only compare the 1990 and 2000 census data to see evidence that demographic change continues. The birthrate is actually decreasing, immigration has increased, and limited access to health care is a complex issue that is not the major factor here.

2. Culturally sensitive implies that the nurse possesses some basic knowledge of and constructive attitudes toward the diverse cultural groups found in the setting in which they are practicing. Answer **a** is incorrect because to be prepared in transcultural nursing implies that one has completed an advanced degree in this discipline, has passed a certification examination, and so forth. Answers **c** and **d** apply to nursing care in general and are irrelevant to this question.

3. The nurse should indicate that he or she is open to diverse views and practices. Answer **a** assumes the client follows this particular cultural practice, which may not be the case. It may be good to learn more about the culture (answer **b**), but that is not the best starting place to care for the client. Answer **d** reflects an incorrect approach to culturally appropriate care.

4. *Culturally competent* implies that within the delivered care the nurse understands and attends to the total context of the client's situation including awareness of immigration, stress factors, and cultural differences.

5. Culture is not physical. It is not limited to group membership. In addition, it is not only learned behavior.

Chapter 14   Answers to Review Questions

1. While CAM is a broad term encompassing treatments from several cultures, many treatments are related to each other and parts of larger healing systems such as TCM. CAM does include chiropractic, traditional Chinese medicine, touch therapies, naturopathy, and homeopathy, but is not limited to these. There are instances where Western medical treatments are certainly more effective than many CAM therapies, but this is not always the case. In some diseases it makes sense to start with CAM and then move to Western medicine if CAM fails rather than starting with Western medicine and, if it fails, moving to CAM.

2. This is one of the main problems when people using CAM do not feel comfortable talking about it to physicians. It is true that nurses are in a position to provide increased support for patient decisions about CAM and that some CAM treatments may prove more beneficial than the Western treatment. However, the main reason to ask these questions during the history is to protect against the harm that can occur with herbal and pharmaceutical combinations that are contraindicated.

3. Clients do not gain *conscious control* over processes like cardiac blood flow, blood pressure, or the heart rate. Rather, physiologic feedback helps patients learn to relax, and this has secondary effects on bodily processes.

4. The breath is not controlled in meditation, but rather observed. Achieving peace, promoting healing and relaxation, releasing fears, anxieties, and doubts are all possible beneficial outcomes of meditation, but the purpose is to quiet and focus the mind. Any other approach to meditation is referred to as "instrumental" (perform an activity to produce an effect). With meditation, the practice and the purpose are the same.

5. Yin, yang, thoughts, emotions, and social relationships are also important in TCM, but the primary focus is on the flow of qi.

Chapter 15   Answers to Review Questions

1. The nurse has concluded something that is beyond the available information (and in this case may not be accurate). The order and the diarrhea are facts. It would be judgment and opinion if the nurse stated that the laxative would make the diarrhea worse and should not be given. (*Note:* Critical thinking will cause this nurse to examine the assumptions made and gather more data before acting.)

2. The nurse recognizes that many assumptions could interfere with the client eating—such as that the food presented is culturally appropriate. These assumptions must be clarified. Answers **b** and **c** reach conclusions not supported by the facts. In answer **d**, the nurse has made a judgment or has an opinion that may not be accurate.

3. The critical-thinking approach should include persever-ance until a reasonable solution or answer is determined. Giving in, over questioning self or poor trust in one's own beliefs, or bypassing normal routes of authority vio-late the desirable attitudes of integrity, intellectual courage, and confidence in reason.

4. The scientific method uses a research study-based approach to problem solving. Trail and error and intuition would not involve the same type of data gathering and experimentation. The nursing process generally uses ap-plication of known interventions, previously determined by the scientific (research) process.

5. It is important to project what problems might interfere with the plan and have responses to those problems in mind. The purpose for the decision should have been clear enough at the outset as to not require reexamination at this point. Clients and families should be consulted early—in the purpose-setting and criteria-setting steps. Considering various means for reaching the outcomes is the same as examining alternatives.

Chapter 16   Answers to Review Questions

1. Because nursing diagnosis involves establishing the im-plications of the data, it may also be called analysis.

2. During assessment, data are collected, organized, validated, and documented. Hypotheses are generated during diagnosing, outcomes are set during planning, and care is documented during implementing.

3. Primary data come from the client, whereas secondary data come from any other source (chart, family). Subjective data are covert (reported or an opinion), whereas objective data can be measured or validated (weight, edema). If the spouse states the client has eaten only toast and tea, this would be secondary objective (measured) data.

4. Eliciting feelings requires an open-ended question that cannot be answered with a single word (**b**) or factual in-formation (**a**). Although exploring family reactions (**d**) may eventually give the desired data, it is not the best way to determine the client's own feelings.

5. Other members of the health care team may use very dif-ferent conceptual organizing frameworks than do nurses. The framework is somewhat constraining (not creative) in order to serve as a reference to the nurse in considering all important aspects of assessment. Cost-ef-fective care is more likely to occur with systematic appli-cation of the nursing process but use of a framework for assessment alone may not accomplish this goal.

Chapter 17   Answers to Review Questions

1. In diagnosing, data from assessment are analyzed and problems, risks, and strengths are identified before diag-nostic statements can be established. Interventions are more commonly part of the planning and implementing phases of the nursing process.

2. Pallor, hypertension, and tachycardia could be defining characteristics—ways the nurse can validate the presence of the diagnostic condition. Of those listed, only malnu-trition could be a risk or causative factor.

3. The nurse must ensure that the diagnostic statement does not say the same thing as the related factor (falls and col-lapse) and that the related factor is not a defining charac-teristic of the diagnostic statement (emesis is a sign of nausea). The statement must be specific and guide the plan of care (fatigue may be a result of sleep deprivation and does not direct intervention).

4. The **S** in PES stands for signs and symptoms of the prob-lem. The statement will be longer than a one- or two-part statement. Any properly worded statement will be accu-rate but with this type, the author's thought process is made overt. A risk diagnosis cannot have three parts be-cause there are no signs or symptoms.

5. A collaborative (multidisciplinary) problem is indicated when both medical and nursing interventions are needed to prevent or treat the problem. If nursing care alone can treat the problem, a nursing diagnosis is indicated. If medical care alone can treat the problem, a medical diag-nosis is indicated.

Chapter 18   Answers to Review Questions

1. The client requires admission planning since he has just arrived on the orthopedic unit for the first time. He also requires the ongoing type of planning necessary to deter-mine the care appropriate for this shift. Discharge planning is continuous and must be started as soon as the client is admitted in order for appropriate post-hospital care to be adequately orchestrated.

2. Standardized care plans, standards of care, and protocols are written for groups of clients with similar medical or nursing diagnoses. They generally do not address questions such as hospital routines and nonmedical client needs. Policy and procedure documents provide data about how certain situations are handled. *Note:* Even hospital policies are not absolute. Each situation must be analyzed and responded to individually.

3. Although more detailed assessment data would be needed to absolutely confirm the priority, postoperative nausea to the level of inhibiting oral intake has the great-est likelihood of leading to complications and requires nursing intervention now. The client's pain level is not extreme considering the recency of the surgery and pain intervention can be assumed to be effective. Although the constipation is probably bordering abnormal, nursing in-tervention would most likely begin with oral treatment, which is not possible due to the nausea. More invasive interventions such as an enema or suppository would not be commonly administered the first day postoperative. Wound infection can occur but there are no data to indi-cate that this requires a change in the current plan.

4. The goal or outcomes should reflect the positive condition of the problem: that *Impaired Skin Integrity* does not occur. Turning in bed, applying lotion, and using a special mattress are all interventions that may result in achieving the goal.

5. Although there may be standard policies or routines for measuring intake and output, the nursing order should specify if this is to be done "routinely" or at specific intervals (e.g., q4h). The nurse is also aware, however, that critical thinking indicates that the intake and output should be monitored more frequently than ordered if assessment reveals abnormal findings.

Chapter 19   Answers to Review Questions

1. Just prior to carrying out any nursing order or intervention, the nurse reassesses the client to determine that the activity is still indicated and safe. The next action would be to determine if assistance is required, then implement the activity, and last document the activities.

2. It is never acceptable practice for the nurse to document a nursing activity before it is carried out. This would be very unsafe because many things can cause an activity to be postponed or canceled and prior charting would be inaccurate, misleading, and potentially dangerous. In a few situations, it may be permissible to chart frequent or routine activities some time following the activities such as at the end of a shift or after a particular interval (e.g., every 4 hours) rather than immediately following the activity.

3. The desired outcomes and indicator statements reflect the parameters by which success will be measured. The goal can be met even if the nursing activities were not carried out or were ineffective. Although the desired outcome, by definition, indicates a change in the client's condition (behavior, knowledge, or attitude), only specific changes (desired outcomes) reflect the success of the care plan.

4. There is no reason to delete or alter the nursing diagnosis or its priority since the risk factors that prompted it are still present.

5. Because this assessment focuses on *how* care is provided, it is a process evaluation. A structure evaluation would focus on the setting (e.g., how well equipment functions), and outcome evaluations focus on changes in client status (e.g., whether reported satisfaction levels vary with type of person who answers the call light). An audit would be a chart or document review.

Chapter 20   Answers to Review Questions

1. All of the other answers endanger the client's confidentiality.

2. Critical pathways work best for clients with one diagnosis. Answer **b** is a possibility, however, there may be many individualized needs. Because that information is not available, the *best* answer is **a**. Answers **c** and **d** have too many diagnoses to work well with a critical pathway.

3. ii = two; gtts = drops; OD = right eye although it could mean overdose but that abbreviation would not make sense in this order; ac = before meals and qd = every day.

4. It is the most complete answer. You may see error written above a mistake even though many authors suggest not writing it. It is important to also put your name or initials next to the words *mistaken entry*.

5. **D** is the "best" answer although it could be more complete by adding the response of the physician. Answer **a** is too vague because it is not clear if the nurse found the client or was present when the client fell. Also, there is no need to write the word *client* because it is the client's chart. Answer **b** is judgmental revealing a negative attitude toward the person. It would be better to describe specific signs and symptoms such as staggering, slurred speech, and smell of alcohol on breath. Answer **c** is too general and can be more specific by charting "2 cm × 3 cm bruise on mid-inner thigh."

Chapter 21   Answers to Review Questions

1. The sequence of each stage of development is predictable, although the time of onset, the length of the stage, and the effects of each stage vary with the person. For answer **a,** the word *exactly* is incorrect. Answer **b** is incorrect because the order or sequence is predictable. In answer **d,** each child is unique, however, the pattern of developmental sequences is predictable.

2. The study of growth (physical) and development (function and skills) needs to have both components to be complete. Answer **a** addresses only the growth aspects. Answer **b** addresses only developmental aspects and answer **c** addresses only the environmental factors that might influence growth and development.

3. This stage includes the preadolescent period. The peer group increasingly influences behavior. Physical, cognitive, and social development increases and communication skills improve. With this age group, one needs to allow time and energy for the school-age child to pursue hobbies and school activities and to recognize and support the child's achievement. Answer **a** is a judgmental statement as this is not unusual and not indicative of problems in the home. For answer **c,** it is good to be supportive of the school-age child, however, making her stay home with her family might cause anger and resentment. Answer **d** is also a judgmental statement. Even though this is normal development, calling the father "silly" is not therapeutic communication.

4. Erikson's late childhood stage focuses on initiative versus guilt. During this stage, the children are beginning to have the ability to evaluate one's own behavior and are learning the degree to which assertiveness and purpose

influence the environment. Answer **a** is incorrect because Fowler's focus is spiritual development. Both answers **c** and **d** are adult theorists.

5. Piaget identifies this phase as the intuitive thought phase with the following significant behaviors occurring: Egocentric thinking diminishes, thinks of one idea at a time, includes others in the environment, words express thoughts. Erikson identifies this developmental stage as industry versus inferiority and the children learning the degree to which assertiveness and purpose influences the environment. They have the beginning ability to evaluate their own behavior. Fowler identifies this stage as intuitive-projective, a combination of images and beliefs given by trusted others, mixed with the child's own experience and imagination. Given all of these theorists, the nurse knows that this child has a normal imagination and needs to explore this new piece of equipment and to understand in language appropriate to his age. For answer **b,** imagination is normal for this age group and telling him that his thoughts are "silly" and to be a "big boy" are counter productive. Answer **c** is incorrect because his language skills are developing and he needs to understand the world around him. Answer **d** is incorrect because feeding into his fears will only increase his anxiety level and decrease his trust in you as a nurse.

Chapter 22   Answers to Review Questions

1. Many newborn babies have a misshapen head because of the molding made possible by fontanelles in the bone structure of the skull and overriding of the sutures. This asymmetry is usually corrected within the first 7–10 days. Answer **a**—Side-lying does take pressure off the fetus, but sitting does not contribute to the head molding seen in infants. Answer **c**—Much erroneous information is given to parents, however, immediate correction is not always indicated. Answer **d**—Not all babies have misshapen heads, and not all are corrected in one week.

2. Although toddlers like to explore the environment, they always need to have a significant person nearby. Parents need to know that young children experience acute separation anxiety and that abandonment is their greatest fear. Answer **b**—This is normal toddler development. Answer **c**—There are no signs of manipulation. Answer **d**— Regression or reverting to an earlier developmental stage is not indicated in this action.

3. Some activities may need to be limited or modified to allow for proper healing to take place. Answer **a**—Some activities do need to be limited and/or modified. Answer **b**—Limiting a preschooler to only sitting activities is unrealistic. Answer **d**—Riding a bike and jumping rope may be too aggressive, especially at first.

4. During the phase of concrete operations, children change from egocentric interactions to cooperative interactions. They also develop an increased understanding of concepts that are associated with specific objects. They

learn to add and subtract and understand cause-and-effect relationships. Answer **b**—This action is indicative of the preconceptual phase — an egocentric approach that uses magical thinking. Answer **c**—This action is indicative of the formal operations phase—reasoning is deductive and futuristic. Answer **d**—This is indicative of physical growth.

5. Often the first noticeable sign of puberty in females is the appearance of the breast bud, although the appearance of hair along the labia may precede this. Answer **b**—In boys, the growth spurt, sudden and dramatic physical changes, usually begins between ages 12 to 16. The growth spurt in girls is between ages 10 and 14. Answer **c**—The eccrine glands are found over most of the body and produce sweat. The apocrine glands develop in the axillae, anal and genital areas, external auditory canals, and around the umbilicus and the areola of the breasts. Answer **d**—The leading causes of death in adolescents are motor vehicle crashes, suicide, homicide, and unintentional accidents.

Chapter 23   Answers to Review Questions

1. The incidence of lung cancer has been increasing in women, which is thought to be due to the increase in the number of women who smoke. The cancers listed in the other answers are serious health concerns, but statistically, the increase in lung cancer in women is much greater and can be reduced with an increase in public awareness and encouragement of smoking cessation.

2. Grieving is a normal behavior after the death of a loved one and the behaviors listed in the other answers would indicate signs of normal grieving. When the behavior becomes extreme, and signs of self-neglect are obvious, ineffective coping may be a problem. Then it would be the responsibility of the nurse to be attentive to the problem and engage appropriate resources for her, if needed.

3. Many older adults have degenerative changes in the inner ear that result in decreased hearing. The changes are usually irreversible and the hearing loss associated with these age-related changes is called *presbycusis*. Persons with this problem often lose the ability to hear high-pitched tones, but can hear low-pitched tones if the speaker adjusts his or her voice. The changes usually occur in the inner ear, rather than the middle ear. Hearing aids are not appropriate for all persons with hearing problems—they should be carefully evaluated by a specialist to determine their usefulness.

4. Reminiscence about past life events, doing a "life review" of past experiences, especially, if they were positive, is considered to be a normal psychosocial activity of elderly adults. It helps them focus on past accomplishments and contributions to society, thus increasing their self-concept. If behavioral or significant memory problems had been noted, then a geriatric psychiactric consult would be appropriate, but not in this

situation. Other activities and conversations should certainly be encouraged, but not to the point of demeaning the importance of his life stories.

5. When a patient with dementia becomes agitated, the main interventions are to decrease the stimuli, but not to leave them alone. Distracting them, staying with them, and the use of a calm, gentle manner will usually decrease the agitation. Touching must be done in a gentle way, not to surprise or alarm them.

Chapter 24   Answers to Review Questions

1. Nonverbal, gentle touch is an important tool here. A loud voice can offend, written directions may not be helpful, and lack of facial expression may increase fear.

2. Study of distance in relationships.

3. Only answer **a** is a listening behavior; the others are barriers to listening.

4. Respect is correct because the nurse is validating the client's feeling. It is not genuineness because the nurse is giving information versus being genuine. Concreteness is giving a specific example. The nurse is not confronting but supporting through respect for the client's feelings.

5. Powerlessness is correct; the other answers are tangential to the situation described.

Chapter 25   Answers to Review Questions

1. Answers **a** and **c** are psychomotor and **d** is under the cognitive domain.

2. Answers **a** and **b** are passive learning strategies. Learning is faster and retention better when the learner is actively involved. Answer **d** promotes affective learning about adapting to a chronic health condition and is important. However, the question asks about learning diet information.

3. There will be no separation anxiety because the parents are present. The story book may allow for the child to learn information about the hospital and ask questions. The client in answer **a** will be preoccupied by his illness. The **c** client is most likely still in pain. It would be better to wait until the pain is resolved. It would also be important to check if the client is too sleepy because pain medication can have that effect also. Client **d** may be too tired after his physical therapy treatment. This would need to be assessed.

4. Answer **b** is a literacy test, a factor in learning; however, a is the best answer. Answers **c** and **d** involve others and it is best to ask the client.

5. Answer **a** is an old diagnosis, which has been changed. The data would need to address that the client is seeking health information and why to be answer **b.** The diagnosis of *Noncompliance* is associated with the intent to comply, but situational factors make it difficult. The data in the questions don't support answer **d.**

Chapter 26   Answers to Review Questions

1. The staff in this situation require direction. A democratic style could waste time in discussion and group participation in decision making. A laissez-faire leader would not provide the control and responsibility needed. A bureaucratic leader, with emphasis on rules and institutional policies, might not provide the situational decisions that will be required.

2. Transformational leaders are creative and use collaboration and group empowerment. Subgroups or task forces would be found in shared governance structures. Transactional leaders use rewards as incentives. Situational leaders vary their approach depending on the context.

3. In answer **a,** the manager has authority but not accountability; in answer **c,** only responsibility; and in answer **d,** both authority and accountability. Only in answer **b** does the manager have accountability (evaluates staff) but not authority (can't hire or fire).

4. A UAP should be able to perform the transfer safely with a new wheelchair or elderly client since these are variations that are considered typical (unless there were additional aspects of the new chair or the specific client not identified in the question). There is also no reason to believe that an absence from work would impair the UAP's skills. However, a fresh postoperative patient is, by definition, in somewhat unstable condition and the nurse must assess and supervise this initial transfer.

5. Although explaining the reasons for the desired change is useful, overemphasis on the rationale may not be useful since resistance is often more emotional than rational. A manager who has determined the need for a change would have their power undermined if either answer **b**— the autocratic mandate—or answer **c**—the caving-in— were allowed to occur. Hopefully, the opponents and proponents can discuss their opinions and reach a compromise. The manager should be open to modification of the proposal if justified.

Chapter 27   Answers to Review Questions

1. This temperature is pretty low, even for the morning. It would be best to see what the client's "usual" temperature has been. Maybe he or she usually has a low temperature. Depending on that finding, you might want to retake it with another thermometer to see if yours is functioning correctly. If everything checks out, chart it and check that the client has no signs of hypothermia.

2. If the cardiac rhythm is irregular, the apical pulse is the most accurate and informative. For clients in shock, use the carotid or femoral pulse. The radial pulse is adequate for determining change in orthostatic heart rate and for routine postoperative vital sign checks for clients with regular pulses.

3. Postponing the assessment may seem a controversial answer to some nurses and is definitely a judgment requiring critical thinking. Unless the client is leaving for the test immediately and respiration rate is a critical aspect of the pretest assessment, it is probably not necessary to invade privacy and require the client to end the phone call nor to waste the nurse's time waiting at the bedside for the call to be completed. Because respirations should be counted with the client "at rest," counting during a pause in the conversation doesn't really qualify. Agency policy would dictate if the deferral should be charted or just the accurate measurement once it has been obtained.

4. If the cuff is inflated to about 30 mmHg over previous systolic pressure, that would be 168. To ensure that the diastolic has been determined, the cuff should be released slowly until the mid-60s mmHg (and then completely) for someone with a previous reading of 74. Thus, a range of 90 mmHg at a rate of 2 to 3 mm per second will require 30 to 45 seconds.

5. Vital signs measurement may be delegated to UAP if the client is in stable condition, the findings are expected to be predictable, and the technique requires no modification. Only the preoperative client meets these requirements. In addition, UAP are not delegated to take apical pulse measurements for the client with an irregular pulse.

Chapter 28   Answers to Review Questions

1. Tympany would be heard over the stomach (air filled), hyperressonance is never a normal finding, and dullness would be heard below (not above) the 10th intercostal space.

2. For palpation of the abdomen, heart, and breast, the client should be supine.

3. In order for absence of bowel sounds to be considered abnormal, they must be silent for 3 to 5 minutes. Continuous bowel sounds are heard over the ileocecal valve following meals. Bowel sounds are more commonly irregular than they are regular.

4. If a pedal pulse, which is more distal than the popliteal, is present, then adequate arterial circulation to the leg is present even though the popliteal artery has not been located. Presence of a femoral pulse would not provide confirmation that arterial flow exists below that point. Taking a thigh BP requires locating the popliteal pulse. Since the purpose of finding the popliteal pulse is to provide information about arterial circulation to the leg, checking the distal pulse before requesting assistance from another nurse is appropriate.

5. Visual acuity often lessens with age. Facial hair is likely to become coarser. The sense of smell becomes less acute. The respiratory rate and rhythm should be regular at rest. However, both may change quickly with activity and be slow to return to the resting level.

Chapter 29   Answers to Review Questions

1. Blocking the movement of the organism from the reservoir will succeed in preventing the infection of any other persons. Since the carrier person is the reservoir and the condition is chronic, it is not possible to eliminate the reservoir. Blocking the entry into a host or decreasing the susceptibility of the host will be effective for only that one single individual and, thus, is not as effective as blocking exit from the reservoir.

2. Regular and routine hand washing is the most effective way to prevent movement of potentially infective materials. Personal protective equipment is indicated for situations requiring standard precautions, and isolation precautions are used for clients with known communicable diseases. Routine use of antibiotics is not effective and can be harmful due to the incidence of superinfection and development of resistant organisms.

3. Standard precautions include all aspects of contact precautions with the exception of placing the client in a private room. A mask is indicated when working over a sterile wound rather than an infected one. Disposable food trays are not necessary, nor would sterile technique (surgical asepsis) be indicated for all contact with the client.

4. Unless overly contaminated by material that has splashed in the nurse's face and cannot be effectively rinsed off, goggles may be worn repeatedly. A gown should be used only once and then discarded or washed. Surgical masks and gloves are never washed or reused.

5. It should not be necessary to unroll this small edge of the cuff. The most important consideration is the sterility of the fingers and hand that will be used to perform the sterile procedure. The rolled under portion is now contaminated and should not be unrolled by the nurse or colleague since it would then be contiguous with the sterile portion of the glove.

Chapter 30   Answers to Review Questions

1. The client's safety (protecting and evacuating the client if possible) is always the priority. Answer **a** would mean leaving the client and would not promote safety. Answers **c** and **d** are also important, but would be done after rescuing the client.

2. Answer **b** is the leading cause for school-age children. Answer **c** is the leading cause for older adults, and answer **d** relates to adolescents.

3. Answer **a**, leaving the bathroom light on, would help but the client could still fall as she may be in a hurry because of the diuretic. Thus, answer **c** helps the client with the client's reason for getting up and promotes safety. The nurse cannot withhold a client's medication without consultation with the physician. Providing a bedside commode is an independent nursing action. Answer **d** often promotes falls, rather than preventing them.

4. Remember that toddlers are active and like to explore and as a result are at risk for poisoning (e.g., lead poisoning, toxic substances under the sink or in a drawer). The risk for suffocation could happen but is more likely with a newborn or infant, which is the reason parents are taught not to prop the bottle, to cut food in small pieces, and to use toys with no small detachable pieces. Answer **b** is the general diagnosis that is the umbrella for the seven subdiagnoses. Answer **d** is more applicable to the older adult who is on total bedrest.

5. Answer **a** can increase agitation and confusion and removes the client's independence. Answer **b** would help but may not be a realistic answer. Answer **c** is also not a realistic answer for a nurse. Answer **d** is an intervention that can allow the client to feel independent and also alert the nurse and nursing staff when the client needs assistance. It is the most realistic answer that promotes client safety.

Chapter 31   Answers to Review Questions

1. The client fits the descriptors for semidependent functional level (see Table 31–2).

2. The client will be positioned in a side-lying position with the head of the bed lowered because the client is at risk for aspiration. The absence of gag reflex lets the nurse know that the client has no natural defense (cough) and is at a higher risk for aspiration. All other answers are assessments more appropriate prior to bathing the client.

3. A lotion will help moisten the skin. Perfumed lotions contain alcohol, which is drying to the skin. Soaking the feet for a long time or frequently also causes dry skin. Applying foot powder is appropriate to prevent or control unpleasant foot odor. Elastic stockings may decrease circulation.

4. Check that the battery is in the hearing aid. Turn off the hearing aid and make sure the volume is turned all the way down because a too loud volume is distressing. An in-the-ear hearing aid is cleaned with a damp cloth.

5. Both the placement of the linens for a surgical bed and placing the bed in high position facilitate the client's transfer from a stretcher into the bed. The linens for a closed bed are drawn up to the top of the bed and under the pillows.

Chapter 32   Answers to Review Questions

1. All of the other answers are within normal range. Answer **b** is very low and can lead to death.

2. Answer **a** is incorrect because you want to discard the first voiding. A clean receptacle is used to collect the urine; and the specific test will determine if the urine specimen needs to be refrigerated.

3. Answer **b** is an x-ray of the kidneys, ureters, and bladder. An IVP and retrograde pyelography use injections of contrast media. A cystoscopy uses a lighted instrument (cystoscope) inserted through the urethra.

4. All of the other answers provide anatomic information.

5. Answer **a** is for a liver biopsy, **b** is for a thoracentesis, and **d** is for a lumbar puncture.

Chapter 33   Answers to Review Questions

1. Answer **a** is every hour. Answer **b** is twice a day, and answer **d** is every day. If you are ever unsure of an abbreviation it is safer to ask than to guess.

2. **D** is the best response for the safety of the client. Listen to the client. Find out any other information the client may have about that certain medication, for example, does he know the dosage of the medication taken at home. Do not administer the medication. Inform the client that you will check the chart first. You do not want to leave medications at the bedside. Review the chart to make sure there is no discrepancy between the physician's order and the MAR. Review the physician's progress notes because the medication may have been increased or reduced as part of the treatment plan. Check with the pharmacist because sometimes a pill may be a different color or shape based on the pharmaceutical company. Inform the client of your findings. The client will appreciate that you took the time to make sure that he received the correct medication. While it takes time to check out the client's statement, you will be glad that you avoided a potential medication error.

3a. Remember that the half—life is the time interval required for the body's elimination processes to reduce the concentration of the drug in the body by one-half. If the half-life for digoxin is 36 hours, it would take 1.5 days or 36 hours to have a 50% concentration in the body. The question asked for 24 hours, which is before the half-life time and would be more than 50%.

3b. This is a matter of doing the math:
36 hours = 50%
72 hours = 25%
108 hours = 12.5%
144 hours = 6.25%
180 hours = 3.125%
180 hours ÷ 24 hours = 7.5 days

4. You should question answer **d** because no dosage is given. All of the other answers include the medication, dosage, route, and frequency.

5a. Five milliliters is too great an amount to inject into one site. The nurse needs to divide the amount into two 2.5-mL injections. A 3-mL syringe could be used. The length of the needle will depend on the muscle development of the client. The nurse needs to assess the client. The presumption, based on the information provided, is that this client's muscle mass is within normal limits. The needle length would need to be 1½ inches because the medication is ordered to be given "deep IM." This also suggests that the medication should be given in the preferred site for IM injections—the ventrogluteal site—because it provides the greatest thickness of gluteal muscle. The gauge of the needle for an IM injection into the ventrogluteal muscle can range between #20 and #23 gauge. The nurse needs to assess the viscosity of the medication. Smaller gauges (e.g., #23) produce less tissue trauma; however, viscous solutions may require a larger gauge (e.g., #20–#21).

5b. The type of syringe for subcutaneous injections depends on the medication to be given. This situation does not indicate that the medication is insulin and, thus, another syringe is needed. Generally a 2-mL syringe is used for most subcutaneous injections. Needle size and length are based on the client's body mass, the intended angle of insertion, and the site of the injection. Generally, a #25-gauge, ⅝-inch needle is used for adults of normal weight and the needle is inserted at a 45-degree angle. Because 2 inches of tissue can be grasped or pinched at the site of the injection, the nurse should administer the medication at a 90-degree angle to ensure the medication reaches subcutaneous tissue.

5c. A tuberculin test is given by intradermal injection. A tuberculin syringe is used because the dosage will most likely be 0.1 mL. A short, fine needle is needed to avoid entering the subcutaneous tissue. The needle should have a short bevel and usually be between #25 and #27 gauge. The needle should be between ¼- to ⅝-inch long.

5d. If the nurse goes by the amount of the medication (0.5 mL) only, the deltoid muscle would be the site. However, knowing and assessing the client is critical. The muscles of an elderly, emaciated client will most likely be diminished or atrophied. The nurse should consider the ventrogluteal site because that site will have the most muscle mass.

Chapter 34 Answers to Review Questions

1. An adult who scores 18 or below is considered at risk and a turning schedule is appropriate. Scores of 13–14 indicate moderate risk, 10–12 high risk, and 9 or less very high risk.

2. Wound culture specimens should be obtained from a clean area of the wound. Collected drainage contains old and mixed organisms. The nurse does not generally debride the wound to obtain a specimen. Once systemic antibiotics have been begun, the interval following a dose will not significantly affect the concentration of wound organisms.

3. Hydrocolloid dressings protect shallow ulcers and maintain an appropriate healing environment. Alginates are used for wounds with significant drainage; dry gauze will only stick to new granulation tissue. A dressing is needed to protect the wound and enhance healing.

4. The heating pad needs to be removed. After 30 minutes of either heat or cold application, the blood vessels in the area will begin to exhibit the rebound effect—the opposite of what is desired.

5. Immobile and dependent persons should be repositioned at least every 2 hours. Red areas that do not return to normal skin color should be reported. It would be correct to use a sheepskin to help relieve pressure. Warm water and moisturizing damp skin are correct techniques.

Chapter 35 Answers to Review Questions

1. Answer **a** evaluates fluid and electrolyte status. Answer **b** evaluates renal status, and **d** evaluates nutritional status.

2. *Anticipatory grieving* is the state in which an individual experiences reactions in response to an expected significant loss. The definition for answer **a** is "confusion in mental picture of one's self" and is often characterized by negative responses such as shame, embarrassment, guilt, revulsion. Answer **c**, *Fear*, is usually characterized by feelings of dread, fright, apprehension, alarm. *Ineffective Coping,* answer **d**, is usually characterized by verbalization of inability to cope or ask for help or inappropriate use of defense mechanisms or inability to meet role expectations.

3. Answer **a** is incorrect because of the new ASA guidelines for preoperative fasting. Answer **b** is incorrect because clients are taught how to cough and also how to splint their incision to prevent complications. Answer **c** is incorrect because anticoagulants are one of the medications that is stopped a few days before surgery to avoid excessive bleeding postoperatively.

4. The symptoms describe decreased cardiac output and not any of the other listed complications.

5. Answers **a** and **b** are not the right answers because a client usually has PCA (patient controlled analgesia) of some form during the initial postoperative period. Pain usually decreases after the second or third postoperative day, which is why **d** is not the best answer.

Chapter 36 Answers to Review Questions

1. A sudden, unexpected admission for surgery may involve many experiences (e.g., lab work, x-rays, signing of forms) while the client is in pain or some form of discomfort. The time for orientation will thus be lessened. After surgery, the client may be in pain and possibly in a critical care setting. Answers **a** and **b** reflect a greater risk for sensory deprivation, and **c** is a normal activity for a teenager.

2. The transfer to a different setting can change the amount or patterning of incoming stimuli accompanied by a diminished, exaggerated, distorted, or impaired response to such stimuli. Answer **a** is incorrect because there are no data to reflect that the client has a long-standing or progressive deterioration of intellect and

personality. Answer **d** is incorrect because *Altered Thought Processes* is applied when a person's cognitive abilities (e.g., dementia) interfere with the ability to accurately interpret stimuli.

3. Because of the paraplegia (paralysis of lower body), the client is unable to feel discomfort. The client will be taught to lift self using chair arms every 10 minutes if possible. Answer **a** is an actual problem versus a potential problem. In answer **c**, the client wears glasses that help correct the poor vision. Answer **d** is more of a *Risk for Injury* diagnosis.

4. This client could use an assistive device that flashes a light when the doorbell is rung. Answer **a** relates to safety of the environment rather than sensory alteration. Answers **c** and **d** reflect how the client adapts to the sensory alteration.

5. Answer **d** is the only response that helps orient the client and treats the client with respect.

Chapter 37 Answers to Review Questions

1. Sally has an inappropriate view of her physical self. Personal identity is a sense of uniqueness; self-expectation are those things one believes the self should be able to do; and core self-concept are the most vital central beliefs about one's identity.

2. This is role conflict—several different roles are competing for the person's time, energy, and abilities. Role ambiguity results when there are unclear expectations of the role. Role strain exists when there are feelings of inadequacy in performing a role. Role enhancement is a nursing intervention.

3. Restored self-esteem is vague and not measurable. Teaching is an intervention, not an outcome. Decreased preoccupation with altered self relates to body image rather than self-esteem.

4. This response encourages the client to say more and focuses on the positive. Answer **b** is condescending and closes the discussion. Both answers **c** and **d** ignore the emotional component of the client's statement and do not address the person's feelings of valuelessness.

5. A person who asserts independence (rather than follow the crowd) is demonstrating successful resolution of this task. Inability to express desires is symptomatic of unresolved toddlerhood autonomy versus shame and doubt, while difficulty being a team player suggests unresolved early school-age industry versus inferiority.

Chapter 38 Answers to Review Questions

1. There is still a great deal of shame and discomfort regarding sexuality. Most people assume that providers have a great deal of information and many patients have questions and concerns. While talking with someone of the same gender may make it easier for some women, it is not a requirement for assessment and intervention.

2. Being clear and calling the client on his behavior sets limits while attempting to understand what the client is trying to communicate. Scolding the client is nontherapeutic as are threatening the client rather than trying to understand or ignoring what the client is trying to communicate.

3. Women still do most of the household and child-rearing activities, compared to men. Men are not "allowed" to wear women's clothing and are not encouraged to be nurturing. Women are expected to express their feelings in an energetic manner

4. Antidepressants may decrease sex drive. If the depression lifts, there may be an improvement but the focus is on the partner rather than the patient. Retrograde ejaculation and skin hypersensitivity are not side effects of antidepressant medications.

5. This acknowledges what the client is saying and is exploring to get further information. Answer **a** provides false reassurance. Although the client may need to speak with the physician, she brought the topic up to you and you need to respond. Answer **d** represents feeding into her negative self-concept and inappropriate self-disclosure.

Chapter 39 Answers to Review Questions

1. Answers **a** and **b** are about assessment and diagnosis, not planning. As to **c**, simply keeping the client busy does not necessarily contribute to feeling fulfilled or purposeful.

2. The best initial response is to assess. Answer **a** may be interpreted as distancing by the client. Answer **b** inserts the nurse's experience, which is generally inappropriate. Answer **d** is not appropriate for someone in spiritual distress.

3. Answer **c** is correct, based on the information discussed in the chapter. Answer **a** would be inadequate; answer **b** is only partial presencing; and answer **d** is transcendent presencing.

4. This client portrays no distress or risk for distress, but rather the potential for enhanced spiritual health as a result of the transformative illness experience. Answer **d** is not a valid diagnosis.

5. For answer **a**, a client may not agree, but may still benefit from an open discussion with the nurse. For answer **c**, few, if any, nurses could deliver this outcome—and besides, it's not what the client requested. Answer **d** indicates the nurse may have skirted the issue and not entered into a therapeutic discussion of the client's question; making a referral doesn't necessarily solve all spiritual distress such as this.

Chapter 40 Answers to Review Questions

1. Effective coping may include verbalizing feelings (one-on-one or in groups) or distraction. However, taking on

additional work would only serve as an additional stressor. In addition, a nurse who has not begun resolution of these feelings in unlikely to be able to meet clients' emotional needs.

2. Wearing glasses is another example of beginning a new strategy to assist with what will be a lifelong health need. Interviewing for a job is a very short-lived situational stressor. Coping strategies effective while a teenager may not be relevant at age 50. Experiencing the stress of a divorce is a social/role stressor quite unlike that of a health problem.

3. In the transaction model, stress is a very personal experience and varies widely among individuals. Answer **b** represents the stimulus model and **c** the response model of stress. External resources and support are a factor in determining stress levels but omit the key aspects of internal/personal influences.

4. With stress, respirations increase, pupils dilate, peripheral blood vessels constrict, and the heart rate increases.

5. It is too soon for *Caregiver Role Strain* to appear, especially since the child is not at home. *Denial* and *Fear* are common reactions to this type of threat. The father demonstrates *Compromised Family Coping* by his difficulty in being supportive.

Chapter 41   Answers to Review Questions

1. Dysfunctional grief is unresolved or inhibited and pathologic. Abbreviated is normal grief that is briefly experienced. Anticipatory grief is experienced before the loss/death but is appropriate. In disenfranchised grief, the emotions are felt privately, just not expressed in public.

2. When possible, modifications of policy that demonstrate respect for individual differences should be explored. The physician is in no position to modify the implementation of the policy. Moving the patient and assigning an aide are inappropriate solo decisions and use of staff.

3. **(a)** This statement acknowledges the family's grief simply. Avoid statements that may be interpreted as overly impersonal **(b)**, false support **(c)**, or harsh **(d)**. Other responses may also be correct.

4. A DNR order only controls CPR and similar life-saving treatments. All other care continues as previously ordered. Competent clients can still decide about their own care (including the DNR order). Nothing about the DNR order is related to when the client may die. Because clients' medical conditions and their views of their lives can change, a new DNR order is required for each admission to a health care agency. Once admitted, that order stands until changed or until it expires according to agency policy.

5. Until children are about 5 years old, they believe that death is reversible. Between ages 5 and 9, the child knows death is irreversible but believes it can be avoided. Between 9 and 12 years of age, the child recognizes that he, too, will someday die. At 12 to 15 years old, the child builds on previous beliefs and may fear death, but often pretends not to care about it.

Chapter 42   Answers to Review Questions

1. Broadening the stance increases stability. Leaning backward takes the line of gravity off the base of support. Tensing the abdominal muscles and bending the knees are useful when lifting heavy objects.

2. Isotonic exercises increase muscle tone. Isometric and aerobic exercises increase endurance, isokinetic exercises increase muscle size, and depleting oxygen occurs with anaerobic exercises (and is not desirable).

3. Vital signs that do not return to baseline 5 minutes after exercising indicate intolerance of exercise at that time. This is a real problem, not "at risk for." There is no evidence that the client requires assistance (impaired mobility) or is immobile (disuse syndrome).

4. The client sits on the edge of the chair and then moves back into the seat. The client should never grasp the nurse's neck because this can throw the nurse off balance and cause neck injury. The nurse rocks from front to rear foot, not the reverse. The chair should be placed parallel to the bed.

5. All of the other statements are correct. Although the crutches (or cane) are always used along with the weaker leg, the weaker leg only goes first going down stairs.

Chapter 43   Answers to Review Questions

1. REM sleep is paradoxical and too much leads to restless and poor sleep overall. Relaxation is common to Stage I of non-REM sleep, persons in Stage II are easily awakened, and Stage III may include lowered blood pressure.

2. Sleep apnea may lead to cardiac problems. Nasal obstruction, chest pain, and insomnia are not found with sleep apnea.

3. The goal is for the client to feel rested. Elders often require only 6 hours per night. It may not be realistic for the client to have a plan to alleviate all of his financial difficulties. The client should also maintain normal sleep patterns, not initiate new activities before bed or go to bed earlier or later than usual.

4. Using proper technique, lotion should be poured into the nurse's hand first rather than onto the client's skin and the palm of the hand is used to provide firm, continuous pressure for about 3 to 5 minutes.

5. Barbiturate hypnotics taken for a lengthy time cannot be stopped abruptly but should be tapered by thirds. There is no evidence that a client cannot be tapered off the sleeping pills or that discontinuing on a weekend is efficacious.

Chapter 44   Answers to Review Questions

1. During the transduction phase, tissue injury triggers the release of biochemical mediators such as prostaglandin. Ibuprofen works by blocking the production of prostaglandin. The adjuvant medication in answer **a** would affect the modulation phase because they inhibit the reuptake of norepinephrine and serotonin, which increases the modulation phase that helps inhibit painful ascending stimuli. In answer **b**, opioids block the release of neurotransmitters, particularly substance P, which stops the pain at the spinal level that occurs during the transmission phase. In **d**, distraction is best used during the perception phase when the client becomes conscious of the pain. Distraction (e.g., music, guided imagery, TV) can help direct the client's attention away from the pain.

2. Answers **a** and **c** are also appropriate but you need to assess the client's pain intensity for effective pain management. Answer **a** is important and many now consider pain intensity as the fifth vital sign. Answer **b**, however, is the best answer because is specifically addresses pain intensity and in a postoperative client it is important to assess pain intensity frequently to manage the acute pain experience. Answer **c**: Yes, this is important, but you need to know the client's pain intensity first for effective pain management. Answer **d**: This information is important but not for a client in acute pain. The priority would be to assess the pain intensity. Clients in acute pain may not want to answer pain history questions. You can ask when they are more comfortable.

3. A rating of 6 or more demands immediate attention. None of the other answers addresses this urgency.

4. This indicates an increasing level of sedation, which can be an early sign of impending respiratory depression. Answer **b** is normal. Answer **c** can indicate increasing sedation; however, answer **a** describes a higher level of sedation and an intervention such as notifying the physician. Answer **d** indicates pain management that may be tolerable for the client.

5. The client's perception/intensity rating of his pain is the most important even though other signs may suggest he is not having pain. His pain rating warrants a higher dose of the prn morphine. With answer **a,** you would be undermedicating the client based on the most important data when assessing a client's pain, his perception or rating of the pain. Answer **b**: Research shows that few clients become addicted, plus there is no information to indicate signs of addiction. This answer, based on the data, would be undermedicating the client. Answer **c** does not address the intensity as well as **d.**

Chapter 45   Answers to Review Questions

1. A BMI of 31 to 40 indicates moderate to severe obesity. A BMI of less than 20 indicates underweight. The client is not at risk for imbalance since it already exists. There is no evidence to support a diagnosis of *Deficient Knowledge.*

2. The food pyramid indicates that the client should have 2–3 servings of dairy, 2–4 servings of fruit, 3–5 servings of vegetables, and 6–11 servings of grains daily.

3. Scrambled eggs are not permitted until the client advances to a soft diet. Pudding, juices, and hard candy are permitted on a full liquid diet.

4. Gastric secretions are acidic as evidenced by a pH of less than 6. If the tube were in the client's airway, speaking would be impaired. Gagging during insertion is common and does not indicate that the tube is in the stomach. Ability to easily instill fluid into the tube does not relate to its placement.

5. For proper flow, the feeding bag hangs 1 foot above the tube insertion. Feedings may be administered if there is less than 100 mL of residual volume. The client should be placed in Fowler's position during feeding and the feeding should be warmed to room temperature before administration to decrease cramping and diarrhea.

Chapter 46   Answers to Review Questions

1. Habitually ignoring the urge to defecate can lead to constipation through loss of the natural urge and the accumulation of feces. Diarrhea will not result—if anything, there is increased opportunity for water reabsorption because the stool remains in the colon, leading to firmer stool. Ignoring the urge shows a strong voluntary sphincter, not a weak one that could result in incontinence. Hemorrhoids would occur only if severe drying out of the stool occurs and, thus, repeated need to strain to pass stool.

2. Saline laxatives can be very irritating and are not the preferred treatment for occasional constipation in older adults. In addition, a normal stool pattern for an older adult may not be daily elimination.

3. To cleanse the distal bowel, rectum, and anus a prepackaged small volume enema is frequently used. An oil retention enema is used to soften hard stool, a return flow enema helps expel flatus, and a high, large-volume enema is used to try to evacuate the transverse and upper colon.

4. An established stoma should be dark pink like the color of the buccal mucosa and is slightly raised above the abdomen. The skin under the appliance may remain pink/red for a while after the adhesive is pulled off. Feces from an ascending ostomy are very liquid, less so from a transverse ostomy, and more solid from a descending or sigmoid stoma.

5. Once the cause of diarrhea has been identified and corrected, the client should return to his or her previous elimination pattern. This is not an example of an allergy to the antibiotic but a common consequence of

overgrowth of bowel organisms not killed by the drug. Antidiarrheal medication is usually not indicated and would not be taken routinely around the clock. Increasing intake of soluble fiber such as oatmeal or potatoes may help absorb excess liquid but insoluble fiber will not.

Chapter 47   Answers to Review Questions

1. The capacity of the bladder may decrease with age but the muscle is less strong and can cause urine to be retained. Elders do not ignore the urge to void and may have difficulty in getting to the toilet in time. The kidney becomes less able to concentrate urine with age.

2. Antihistamines can cause urinary retention rather than incontinence. The perineum may become irritated by the presence of urine. Normal fluid intake is at least 1,500 mL/day and clients often decrease their intake to try and minimize urine leakage. Urinary tract infections can contribute to incontinence.

3. The penis and condom should be checked one-half hour after application to ensure that it is not too tight. A 1-in. space should be left between the penis and the end of the condom. The condom is changed every 24 hours and the tubing is taped to the leg or attached to a leg bag. An indwelling catheter is taped to the lower abdomen or upper thigh.

4. The catheter in the vagina is contaminated and cannot be reused. If left in place, it may help avoid mistaking the vaginal opening for the urinary meatus. A single failure to catheterize the meatus does not indicate that another nurse is needed although sometimes a second nurse can assist in visualizing the meatus.

5. Soaking in a bathtub can increase the risk of exposure to bacteria. The other statements indicate correct knowledge of caring for an indwelling catheter.

Chapter 48   Answers to Review Questions

1. A bluish tinge to mucous membranes is called cyanosis. Hypoxia is more commonly represented by pale skin color. Hypoxemia requires blood oxygen saturation to be confirmed, and dyspnea is difficult breathing.

2. Huff coughing helps keep the airways open and secretions mobilized. Deep breathing and coughing should be performed at the same time. Extended forceful coughing fatigues the client. Diaphragmatic and purse-lip breathing are techniques used for clients with obstructive airway disease.

3. Clients with chronic lung disease may have only low levels of supplemental oxygen, generally not over 2 liters per minute.

4. Suction catheters may only be lubricated with water or water-soluble lubricant (Vaseline is an oil base). No suction should ever be applied while the catheter is being inserted because this can traumatize tissues. The client

should be hyperoxygenated for only a few minutes before and after suctioning and this is generally limited to clients who are intubated or have a tracheostomy.

5. Proper use of an SMI requires the client to take slow, steady inhalations, every hour or two, 5 to 10 breaths each time. Only the mouthpiece can be successfully rinsed or wiped. The device should not be submerged in water.

Chapter 49   Answers to Review Questions

1. Regular physical activity will help promote healthy cardiac functioning and will also promote tissue perfusion. Improving tissue perfusion may also improve renal perfusion but it is not the primary goal. Answer **c** is incorrect because it is the red blood cells that carry oxygen.

2. Capillary refill is an assessment of capillary blood flow and thus tissue perfusion. Symmetrical chest expansion is an assessment of respiratory function, and pursed-lip breathing is a technique used to assist clients with obstructive lung diseases.

3. Very rapid heart rates do not allow adequate time for the ventricles to fill causing cardiac output to fall. Answer **a** is normal. Exercise increases venous return and the amount of blood in the ventricle before contraction and therefore the heart contracts more forcefully and stroke volume and cardiac output increase during exercise. Answer **b** is a normal cardiac output of 4900 mL/min. The formula is $SV \times HR = CO$ is about 5 L/min. In answer **d**, positive inotropic drugs (e.g., Digoxin), increase contractility of the cardiac muscle and thus increase stroke volume which increase cardiac output.

4. The three cardinal signs of cardiac arrest are absence of heart beat, cessation of breathing (apnea), and the absence of circulation reflected in dilated pupils.

5. The sequential compression devices help to promote venous return from the legs. They inflate and deflate plastic sleeves wrapped around the legs to promote venous flow. This sequential inflation and deflation counteract blood stasis in the lower extremities.

Chapter 50   Answers to Review Questions

1. Potassium and phosphate are both major intracellular ions. Another major intracellular ion is magnesium. Calcium is largely found in the skeletal system, sodium and chloride are major extracellular ions, and bicarbonate is present in both intracellular and extracellular fluids. Albumin is a major determinant of colloid osmotic pressure and is found in the intravascular space (ECF).

2. Potassium is an important part of regulation of cardiac impulse transmission and muscle contraction. Although not one of the answers, magnesium is also involved in cardiac function. Sodium is involved in transmission of nerve impulses and has a large effect on the regulation of ECF volume and distribution. Chloride also functions to

regulate ECF balance, but also acts as a buffer in the regulation of acid–base balance. Calcium is a major ion involved in the formation of bones and teeth, regulating muscle contraction, and maintaining the automaticity of the cardiac pacemaker.

3. The client is demonstrating signs of fluid deficit such as weak, rapid pulse, decreased blood pressure, orthostatic hypotension, flat neck veins, and decreased urine volume. But because his weight is stable, this indicates that the fluid is still in his body (because weight is a good indicator of fluid status). Thus, third space syndrome is the appropriate answer. If the client had a fluid volume deficit or dehydration, the weight would be decreased. Weight would be increased with fluid volume excess.

4. Each kilogram (2.2 lb) of weight gained is equivalent to 1 L of fluid gained. Recall that this fluid gain indicates change in total body fluid, not any specific compartment.

The client's weight increased by 4.5 pounds. The increase of 4.5 pounds converts to approximately 2 kilograms, which calculates to indicate a 2-L fluid gain.

5. The client has voided 100 mL over a 4-hour period, which converts to 25 mL per hour. This is below the guideline of 30 mL per hour or 0.5 mL per kilogram per hour. Based on the client's weight, a urine output of 40 mL per hour would indicate adequate renal perfusion and function. At this time the nurse should notify either the physician or the charge nurse that the urine output is low. The nurse would also continue to monitor intake and output, but it is most important that the nurse recognize the urine output as low and make a notification. Insertion of an indwelling urinary catheter may be ordered by the physician, but is not an independent nursing action. Finally, increasing the client's intake could be dangerous if he or she is retaining fluid and has heart failure.

Appendix D

2003–2004 NANDA-Approved Nursing Diagnoses

Activity Intolerance
Activity Intolerance, Risk for
Adaptive Capacity: Intracranial, Decreased
Adjustment, Impaired
Airway Clearance, Ineffective
Anxiety
Anxiety, Death
Aspiration, Risk for
Attachment, Parent/Infant/Child, Risk for Impaired
Body Image, Disturbed
Body Temperature: Imbalanced, Risk for
Bowel Incontinence
Breastfeeding, Effective
Breastfeeding, Ineffective
Breastfeeding, Interrupted
Breathing Pattern, Ineffective
Cardiac Output, Decreased
Caregiver Role Strain
Caregiver Role Strain, Risk for
Communication, Readiness for Enhanced
Communication: Verbal, Impaired
Confusion, Acute
Confusion, Chronic
Constipation
Constipation, Perceived
Constipation, Risk for
Coping: Community, Ineffective
Coping: Community, Readiness for Enhanced
Coping, Defensive
Coping: Family, Compromised
Coping: Family, Disabled
Coping: Family, Readiness for Enhanced
Coping (Individual), Readiness for Enhanced
Coping, Ineffective
Decisional Conflict (Specify)
Denial, Ineffective
Dentition, Impaired
Development: Delayed, Risk for
Diarrhea
Disuse Syndrome, Risk for
Diversional Activity, Deficient
Dysreflexia, Autonomic
Dysreflexia, Autonomic, Risk for
Energy Field, Disturbed
Environmental Interpretation Syndrome, Impaired
Failure to Thrive, Adult
Falls, Risk for
Family Processes, Dysfunctional: Alcoholism
Family Processes, Interrupted
Family Processes, Readiness for Enhanced
Fatigue
Fear
Fluid Balance, Readiness for Enhanced
Fluid Volume, Deficient
Fluid Volume, Deficient, Risk for
Fluid Volume, Excess
Fluid Volume, Imbalanced, Risk for
Gas Exchange, Impaired
Grieving, Anticipatory
Grieving, Dysfunctional
Growth, Disproportionate, Risk for
Growth and Development, Delayed

Health Maintenance, Ineffective
Health-Seeking Behaviors (Specify)
Home Maintenance, Impaired
Hopelessness
Hyperthermia
Hypothermia
Identity: Personal, Disturbed
Infant Behavior, Disorganized
Infant Behavior: Disorganized, Risk for
Infant Behavior: Organized, Readiness for
    Enhanced
Infant Feeding Pattern, Ineffective
Infection, Risk for
Injury, Risk for
Knowledge, Deficient (Specify)
Knowledge (Specify), Readiness for Enhanced
Latex Allergy Response
Latex Allergy Response, Risk for
Loneliness, Risk for
Memory, Impaired
Mobility: Bed, Impaired
Mobility: Physical, Impaired
Mobility: Wheelchair, Impaired
Nausea
Neurovascular Dysfunction: Peripheral, Risk for
Noncompliance (Specify)
Nutrition, Imbalanced: Less than Body
    Requirements
Nutrition, Imbalanced: More than Body
    Requirements
Nutrition, Imbalanced: More than Body
    Requirements, Risk for
Nutrition, Readiness for Enhanced
Oral Mucous Membrane, Impaired
Pain, Acute
Pain, Chronic
Parenting, Impaired
Parenting, Readiness for Enhanced
Parenting, Risk for Impaired
Perioperative Positioning Injury, Risk for
Poisoning, Risk for
Posttrauma Syndrome
Posttrauma Syndrome, Risk for
Powerlessness
Powerlessness, Risk for
Protection, Ineffective
Rape-Trauma Syndrome
Rape-Trauma Syndrome: Compound Reaction
Rape-Trauma Syndrome: Silent Reaction
Relocation Stress Syndrome
Relocation Stress Syndrome, Risk for
Role Conflict, Parental
Role Performance, Ineffective
Self-Care Deficit: Bathing/Hygiene
Self-Care Deficit: Dressing/Grooming
Self-Care Deficit: Feeding
Self-Care Deficit: Toileting
Self-Concept, Readiness for Enhanced
Self-Esteem, Chronic Low
Self-Esteem, Situational Low
Self-Esteem, Risk for Situational Low
Self-Mutilation

Self-Mutilation, Risk for
Sensory Perception, Disturbed (Specify: Visual,
    Auditory, Kinesthetic, Gustatory, Tactile,
    Olfactory)
Sexual Dysfunction
Sexuality Patterns, Ineffective
Skin Integrity, Impaired
Skin Integrity, Risk for Impaired
Sleep Deprivation
Sleep Pattern Disturbed
Sleep, Readiness for Enhanced
Social Interaction, Impaired
Social Isolation
Sorrow, Chronic
Spiritual Distress
Spiritual Distress, Risk for
Spiritual Well-Being, Readiness for Enhanced
Spontaneous Ventilation, Impaired
Sudden Infant Death Syndrome, Risk for
Suffocation, Risk for
Suicide, Risk for
Surgical Recovery, Delayed
Swallowing, Impaired
Therapeutic Regimen Management: Community,
    Ineffective
Therapeutic Regimen Management, Effective
Therapeutic Regimen Management: Family,
    Ineffective
Therapeutic Regimen Management, Ineffective
Therapeutic Regimen Management, Readiness for
    Enhanced
Thermoregulation, Ineffective
Thought Processes, Disturbed
Tissue Integrity, Impaired
Tissue Perfusion, Ineffective (Specify: Renal,
    Cerebral, Cardiopulmonary, Gastrointestinal,
    Peripheral)
Transfer Ability, Impaired
Trauma, Risk for
Unilateral Neglect
Urinary Elimination, Impaired
Urinary Elimination, Readiness for Enhanced
Urinary Incontinence, Functional
Urinary Incontinence, Reflex
Urinary Incontinence, Stress
Urinary Incontinence, Total
Urinary Incontinence, Urge
Urinary Incontinence, Risk for Urge
Urinary Retention
Ventilatory Weaning Response, Dysfunctional
Violence: Other-Directed, Risk for
Violence: Self-Directed, Risk for
Walking, Impaired
Wandering

Source. NANDA Nursing Diagnoses: Definitions and Classification, 2003–2004. Philadelphia: North American Nursing Diagnosis Association. Used with permission.

Glossary

24-hour food recall   client recall of all the food and beverages consumed during a typical 24-hour period

Abdominal paracentesis   removal of fluids from the peritoneal cavity

Absorption   the process by which a drug passes into the bloodstream

Accommodation   a process of change whereby cognitive processes mature sufficiently to allow a person to solve problems that were previously unsolvable

Accountability   the ability and willingness to assume responsibility for one's actions and to accept the consequences of one's behavior

Acculturation   the blending of attitudes and beliefs; process by which members of a foreign culture learn the values and behaviors of a culture to which they have immigrated

Acid   a substance that releases hydrogen ions (H+) in solution

Acidosis   a condition that occurs with increases in blood carbonic acid or with decreases in blood bicarbonate; blood pH below 7.35

Acquired immunity   *see* Passive immunity

Action stage   occurs when a person actively implements behavioral and cognitive strategies to interrupt previous behavior patterns and adopt new ones; this stage requires a great commitment of time and energy

Active euthanasia   actions that directly bring about the client's death with or without consent

Active immunity   a resistance of the body to infection in which the host produces its own antibodies in response to natural or artificial antigens

Active ROM exercises   isotonic exercises in which the client moves each joint in the body through its complete range, maximally stretching all muscle groups within each plane over the joint

Active transport   movement of substances across cell membranes against the concentration gradient

Activities   the specific nursing actions needed to carry out the interventions (or nursing orders)

Activity theory   the best way to age is to stay active physically and mentally

Activity tolerance   the type and amount of exercise or daily activities an individual is able to perform

Activity-exercise pattern   refers to a person's pattern of exercise, activity, leisure, and recreation

Actual loss   can be identified by others and can arise either in response to or in anticipation of a situation

Acupressure   a form of healing in which the therapist exerts finger pressure on specific sites

Acute illness   typically characterized by severe symptoms of relatively short duration

Acute infection   those that generally appear suddenly or last a short time

Acute pain   pain that lasts only through the expected recovery period (less than six months), whether it has a sudden or slow onset and regardless of the intensity

Adaptation   the process of modifying to meet new, changing, or different conditions

Adaptive mechanism   learned behaviors that assist an individual to adjust to the environment

Adherence   the extent to which an individual's behavior (for example, taking medications, following diets, or making lifestyle changes) coincides with medical or health advice; commitment or attachment to a regimen

Adjuvant analgesic   medication that may enhance the effects of other analgesics or have its own analgesic properties

Adolescence   the period during which a person becomes physically and psychologically mature and acquires a personal identity

Adolescent growth spurt   the period during puberty when sudden and dramatic physical changes occur

Advance health care directive   a variety of legal and lay documents that allow persons to specify aspects of care they wish to receive should they become unable to make or communicate their preferences

Adventitious breath sounds   abnormal or acquired breath sounds

Adverse effects   more severe side effects that may justify the discontinuation of a drug

Advocate   individual who pleads the cause of another or argues or pleads for a cause or proposal

Aerobic   living only in the presence of oxygen

Aerobic exercise   any activity during which the body takes in more or an equal amount of oxygen than it expends

Afebrile   absence of a fever

Affective domain   known as the "feeling" domain and is divided into categories that specify the degree of a person's depth of emotional response to tasks; includes feelings, emotions, interests, attitudes, and appreciations

Afterload   the resistance against which the heart must pump to eject blood into the circulation

Agglutinins   specific antibodies formed in the blood

Agglutinogens   a substance that acts as an antigen and stimulates the production of agglutinins

Agnostic   a person who doubts the existence of God or a supreme being or believes the existence of God has not been proved

Agonist   a drug that interacts with a receptor to produce a response

Agonist analgesic   full agonists which are pure opioid drugs that bind tightly to mu receptor sites, producing maximum pain inhibition, an agonist effect

Agonist-antagonist analgesic   mixed agonist-antagonist drugs that can act like opioids and relieve pain (agonist effect) when given to a client who has not taken any pure opioids

Airborne precautions   methods used to reduce exposure to infectious agents transmitted by airborne droplet nuclei smaller than 5 microns

Airborne transmission   infectious agent transmitted by droplets or dust

Alarm reaction   the initial reaction of the body to stress, which alerts the body's defenses

Algor mortis   the gradual decrease of the body's temperature after death

Alkalosis   a condition that occurs with increases in blood bicarbonate or decreases in blood carbonic acid; blood pH above 7.45

Alopecia   the loss of scalp hair (baldness) or body hair

Alternative medicine   an unrelated group of nonorthodox practices, often with explanatory systems that do not follow conventional biomedical explanations

Amblyopia   reduced visual acuity in one eye

Ambulation   the act of walking

Ambulatory surgery center (ASC)   facilities where surgeries that do not require hospital admission are performed

Ampule   a small glass container for individual doses of liquid medications

Anabolism   a process in which simple substances are converted by the body's cells into more complex substances (e.g., building tissue, positive nitrogen balance)

Anaerobic   living only in the absence of oxygen

Anaerobic exercise   involves activity in which the muscles cannot draw out enough oxygen from the bloodstream; used in endurance training

Anaphylactic reaction   a severe allergic reaction that usually occurs immediately after the administration of a drug

Andragogy   the art and science of helping adults learn

Anemia   a condition in which the blood is deficient in red blood cells or hemoglobin

Anger   an emotional state consisting of a subjective feeling of animosity or strong displeasure

Angiography a diagnostic procedure enabling x-ray visual examination of the vascular system after injection of a radiopaque dye

Angle of Louis the junction between the body of the sternum and the manubrium; the starting point for locating the ribs anteriorly

Anions ions that carry a negative charge; includes chlorine (Cl^-), bicarbonate (HCO_3^-), phosphate (HPO_4^{2-}), and sulfate (SO_4^-)

Ankylosed permanently immobile joints

Anorexia lack of appetite

Anorexia nervosa a disease characterized by a prolonged inability or refusal to eat, rapid weight loss, and emaciation in persons who continue to believe they are fat

Anoscopy visual examination of the anal canal using an anoscope (a lighted instrument)

Answer (legal) a written response made by the defendant

Antibodies immunoglobulins, part of the body's plasma proteins, defend primarily against the extracellular phases of bacterial and viral infections

Anticipatory grief grief experienced in advance of the event

Anticipatory loss the experience of loss before the loss actually occurs

Antigen a substance capable of inducing the formation of antibodies

Antihelix the anterior curve of the auricle's upper aspect

Antiseptics agents that inhibit the growth of some microorganisms

Anuria the failure of the kidneys to produce urine, resulting in a total lack of urination or output of less than 100 mL per day in an adult

Anxiety a state of mental uneasiness, apprehension, or dread producing an increased level of arousal caused by an impending or anticipated threat to self or significant relationships

Apgar scoring system a scoring system to assess newborn babies

Aphasia any defects in or loss of the power to express oneself by speech, writing, or signs, or to comprehend spoken or written language due to disease or injury of the cerebral cortex

Apical pulse a central pulse located at the apex of the heart

Apical-radial pulse measurement of the apical beat and the radial pulse at the same time

Apnea a complete absence of respirations

Apocrine glands sweat glands located largely in the axillae and anogenital areas; they begin to function at puberty under the influence of androgens

Approximated closed tissue surfaces

Arrhythmia a pulse with an abnormal rhythm

Arterial blood gases specimen of arterial blood that assesses oxygenation, ventilation, and acid–base status

Arterial blood pressure the measure of the pressure exerted by the blood as it pulsates through the arteries

Arteriosclerosis a condition in which the elastic and muscular tissues of the arteries are replaced with fibrous tissue

Ascites the accumulation of fluid in the abdominal cavity

Asepsis freedom from infection or infectious material

Asphyxiation lack of oxygen due to interrupted breathing

Aspiration the withdrawal of fluid that has abnormally collected (e.g., pleural cavity, abdominal cavity) or to obtain a specimen (e.g., cerebral spinal fluid)

Assault an attempt or threat to touch another person unjustifiably

Assessing the process of collecting, organizing, validating, and recording data (information) about a client's health status

Assignment a downward or lateral transfer of both the responsibility and accountability of an activity from one individual to another

Assimilation *see* Acculturation

Assisted suicide a form of active euthanasia in which clients are given the means to kill themselves

Astigmatism an uneven curvature of the cornea that prevents horizontal and vertical rays from focusing on the retina

Atelectasis a condition that occurs when ventilation is decreased and pooled secretions accumulate in a dependent area of a bronchiole and block it

Atheist one who denies the existence of God

Atria two upper hollow chambers of the heart

Atrioventricular (AV) node conduction pathways that slightly delay transmission of the impulse from the atria to the ventricles of the heart

Atrioventricular (AV) valves between the atria and ventricles of the heart, the tricuspid valve on the right and the bicuspid or mitral valve on the left

Atrophy wasting away; decrease in size of organ or tissue (e.g., muscle)

Attentive listening listening actively, using all senses, as opposed to listening passively with just the ear

Attitudes mental stance that is composed of many different beliefs; usually involving a positive or negative judgment toward a person, object, or idea

Auditory related to or experienced through hearing

Auricle flap of the ear

Auscultation the process of listening to sounds produced within the body

Auscultatory gap the temporary disappearance of sounds normally heard over the brachial artery when the sphygmomanometer cuff pressure is high and the sounds reappear at a lower level

Authoritarian leader the individual who makes decisions for the group

Authority the power given by an organization to direct the work of others; the right to act

Autoantigen an antigen that originates in a person's own body

Autocratic leader *see* Authoritarian leader

Automaticity an electrical impulse and contraction independent of the nervous system and generated by the cardiac muscle

Autonomy the state of being independent and self-directed, without outside control, to make one's own decisions

Autopsy an examination of the body after death to determine the cause of death and to learn more about a disease process

Awareness the ability to perceive environmental stimuli and body reactions and to respond appropriately through thought and action

Bacteremia bacteria in the blood

Bacteria the most common infection-causing microorganisms

Bactericidal bacteria-killing action

Bacteriocins substances produced by some normal flora (e.g., enterobacteria) that can be lethal to related strains of bacteria

Bandage a strip of cloth used to wrap some part of the body

Basal metabolic rate (BMR) the rate of energy utilization in the body required to maintain essential activities such as breathing

Base of support the area on which an object rests

Bases (alkalis) have low hydrogen ion concentration and can accept hydrogen ions in solution

Battery (legal) the willful or negligent touching of a person (or the person's clothes or even something the person is carrying), which may or may not cause harm

Bed rest strict confinement to bed (complete bed rest), or the client may be allowed to use a bedside commode or have bathroom privileges

Bedpan a receptacle for urine and feces for clients who are restricted to bed

Behaviorist theory includes the careful identification of what is to be taught and the immediate identification of and reward for correct responses

Beliefs interpretations or conclusions that one accepts as true

Beneficence the moral obligation to do good or to implement actions that benefit clients and their support persons

Bereavement a subjective response of a person who has experienced the loss of a significant other through death

Bevel the slanted part at the tip of a needle

Bicultural used to describe a person who crosses two cultures, lifestyles, and sets of values

Bier block *see* Intravenous block

Binder a type of bandage applied to large body areas (abdomen or chest) or for a specific body part (arm sling); used to provide support

Bioethics ethical rules or principles that govern right conduct concerning life

Biofeedback a stress management technique that brings under conscious control bodily processes normally thought to be beyond voluntary command

Biomedical health belief *see* Scientific health belief

Biopsy the removal and examination of tissue from the living body

Biorhythms inner rhythms that appear to control a variety of biologic processes

Biotransformation process by which a drug is converted to a less active form; also called *detoxification*

Biot's respirations shallow breaths interrupted by apnea

Bladder training client postpones voiding, resists or inhibits the sensation of urgency, and voids according to a timetable rather than according to the urge to void

Blanch test a test during which the client's fingertip is temporarily pinched to assess capillary refill and peripheral circulation

Blood chemistry a number of tests performed on blood serum (the liquid portion of the blood)

Blood pressure (BP) the force exerted on arterial walls by blood flowing within the vessel

Blood urea nitrogen (BUN) a measure of blood level of urea, the end product of protein metabolism

Bloodborne pathogens those microorganisms carried in blood and body fluids that are capable of infecting other persons with serious and difficult-to-treat viral infections, namely, hepatitis B virus, hepatitis C virus, and HIV

Body image how a person perceives the size, appearance, and functioning of his or her body and its parts

Body mass index (BMI) indicates whether weight is appropriate for height

Body substance isolation (BSI) generic infection control precautions for all clients except those with diseases transmitted through the air

Body temperature the balance between the heat produced by the body and the heat lost from the body

Bodymind a state of integration that includes body, mind, and spirit

Bottle mouth syndrome describes the decay of an infant's teeth caused by constant contact with sweet liquid from a bottle

Boundary the real or imaginary lines that differentiate one system from another system or a system from its environment

Bowel incontinence loss of voluntary ability to control fecal and gaseous discharges through the anal sphincter

Bradycardia abnormally slow pulse rate, less than 60 beats per minute

Bradypnea abnormally slow respiratory rate, usually less than 10 respirations per minute

Brand name the name given to a drug by the drug's manufacturer

Breach of duty a standard of care that is expected in the specific situation but that the nurse did not observe; this is the failure to act as a reasonable, prudent nurse under the circumstances

Bronchoscopy visual examination of the bronchi using a bronchoscope

Bruit a blowing or swishing sound created by turbulence of blood flow

Buccal pertaining to the cheek

Buffers prevent excessive changes in pH by removing or releasing hydrogen ions

Bulimia an uncontrollable compulsion to eat large amounts of food and then expel it by self-induced vomiting or by taking laxatives

Bundle of His the right and left bundle branches of the ventricular conduction pathways

Burden of proof the duty of proving an assertion

Bureaucratic leader does not trust self or others to make decisions and instead relies on the organization's rules, policies, and procedures to direct the group's work efforts

Burn results from excessive exposure to thermal, chemical, electric, or radioactive agents

Burnout a complex syndrome of behaviors that can be likened to the exhaustion stage of the general adaptation syndrome; an overwhelming feeling that can lead to physical and emotional depletion, a negative attitude and self-concept, and feelings of helplessness and hopelessness

Calculi renal stones

Callus a thickened portion of the skin

Caloric value the amount of energy that nutrients or foods supply to the body

Calorie (c, cal, kcal) a unit of heat energy equivalent to the amount of heat required to raise the temperature of 1 kg of water 1C

Cannula a tube with a lumen (channel) that is inserted into a cavity or duct and is often fitted with a trocar during insertion

Carbon monoxide an odorless, colorless, tasteless gas that is very toxic

Cardiac arrest the cessation of heart function

Cardiac output (CO) the amount of blood ejected by the heart with each ventricular contraction

Cardinal signs *see* Vital signs

Caregiver a role that has traditionally included those activities that assist the client physically and psychologically

Caregiver burden responses to long-term stress, such as chronic fatigue, sleeping difficulties, and high blood pressure, in family members who undertake the care of a person in the home for a long period

Caregiver role strain physical, emotional, social, and financial burdens that can seriously jeopardize the caregiver's own health and well-being

Caries tooth cavities

Caring intentional action that conveys physical and emotional security and genuine connectedness with another person or group of people.

Carminative an agent that promotes the passage of flatus from the colon

Carrier a person or animal that harbors a specific infectious agent and serves as a potential source of infection, yet does not manifest any clinical signs of disease

Case management a method for delivering nursing care in which the nurse is responsible for a caseload of clients across the health care continuum

Case manager a nurse who works with the multidisciplinary health care team to measure the effectiveness of the case management plan and monitor outcomes

Catabolism a process in which complex substances are broken down into simpler substances (e.g., breakdown of tissue)

Cataracts opacity of the lens or capsule of the eye

Cathartics drugs that induce defecation

Cations ions that carry a positive charge; includes sodium (Na^+), potassium (K^+), calcium (Ca^{2+}), and magnesium (Mg^{2+})

Causation a fact that must be proven that the harm occurred as a direct result of the nurse's failure to follow the standard of care and the nurse could have (or should have) known that failure to follow the standard of care could result in such harm

Cell-mediated defenses *see* Cellular immunity

Cellular immunity also known as cell-mediated defenses, occur through the T-cell system

Center of gravity the point at which the mass (weight) of the body is centered

Central processing unit (CPU) the processor/microprocessor that performs the computer program instructions, located in the box that contains the computer hardware

Central venous catheter catheter that is usually inserted into the subclavian or jugular vein, with the distal tip of the catheter resting in the superior vena cava just above the right atrium

Cephalocaudal proceeding in the direction from head to toe

Cerebral death the higher brain center or cerebral cortex is irreversibly destroyed

Cerumen the wax-like substance secreted by glands in the external ear canal

Change agents persons (or groups) who initiate change or who assist others in making modifications in themselves or in the system

Change-of-shift report a report given to nurses on the next shift

Charismatic leader characterized by an emotional relationship between the leader and the group members; personality of the leader evokes strong feelings of commitment to both the leader and the leader's cause and beliefs

Chart a formal, legal document that provides evidence of a client's care

Charting the process of making an entry on a client record

Charting by exception (CBE) a documentation system in which only significant findings or exceptions to norms are recorded

Chemical name the name by which a chemist knows a drug; describes the constituents of the drug precisely

Chemical restraints medications used to control socially disruptive behavior

Chemical thermogenesis the stimulation of heat production in the body through increased cellular metabolism caused by increases in thyroxine output

Chemotaxis the action by which leukocytes are attracted to injured cells

Cheyne-Stokes respirations rhythmic waxing and waning of respirations from very deep breathing to very shallow breathing with periods of temporary apnea, often associated with cardiac failure, increased intracranial pressure, or brain damage

Chiropractic from the Greek meaning "done by hand"; involves adjustments of the spine and joints and is grounded in the assumption that maintaining the alignment of the spine and joints facilitates the flow of energy throughout the body, including the nervous, circulatory, respiratory, gastrointestinal; and limbic systems

Cholesterol a lipid that does not contain fatty acid but possesses many of the chemical and physical properties of other lipids

Chronic illness illness that lasts for an extended period of time, usually greater than 6 months

Chronic infection infection that occurs slowly, over a very long period, and may last months or years

Chronic pain prolonged pain, usually recurring or persisting over 6 months or longer, and interferes with functioning

Chyme digested products that leave the stomach through the small intestine and then pass through the ileocecal valve

Cicatrix scar

Circadian synchronization the person is awake when the physiologic and psychologic rhythms are most active and is asleep when the physiologic and psychologic rhythms are most inactive

Circulating immunity see Humoral immunity

Circulating nurse assists scrub nurses and surgeons during surgery

Civil action deals with the relationship between individuals in society

Civil law the body of law that deals with relationships among private individuals; also known as *private law*

Clara Barton a schoolteacher who volunteered as a nurse during the Civil War. Most notably, she organized the American Red Cross, which linked with the International Red Cross when the U.S. Congress ratified the Geneva Convention in 1882

Clean free of potentially infectious agents

Clean voided urine specimens for routine urinalysis

Clean-catch specimen (CC) urine specimens for urine culture

Cleaning bath a type of bath given chiefly for hygiene purposes

Client a person who engages the advice or services of another person who is qualified to provide this service

Client advocate an individual who pleads the cause of clients' rights

Client record see Chart

Climacteric the point in development when reproduction capacity in the female terminates (menopause) and the sexual activity of the male decreases (andropause)

Clinical aromatherapy the controlled use of essential oils for specific measurable outcomes

Closed awareness a type of awareness in which the client is unaware of impending death

Closed questions restrictive question requiring only a short answer

Closed system system that does not exchange energy, matter, or information with its environment

Closed wound drainage system consists of a drain connected to either an electric suction or a portable drainage suction, such as a Hemovac or Jackson-Pratt

Clubbing elevation of the proximal aspect of the nail and softening of the nail bed

Cochlea a seashell-shaped structure found in the inner ear; essential for sound transmission and hearing

Code blue emergency announcing cardiac/respiratory arrest and initiating interventions

Code of ethics a formal statement of a group's ideals and values; a set of ethical principles shared by members of a group, reflecting their moral judgments and serving as a standard for professional actions

Coercive power power based on a fear of retribution or withholding of rewards

Cognitive development refers to the manner in which people learn to think, reason, and use language

Cognitive domain the "thinking" domain, includes six intellectual abilities and thinking processes beginning with knowing, comprehending, and applying to analysis, synthesis, and evaluation

Cognitive skills intellectual skills that include problem solving, decision making, critical thinking, and creativity

Cognitive theory recognition of developmental levels of learners, and acknowledgments of the learner's motivation and environment

Coinsurance an insurance plan in which the client pays a percentage of the payment and some other group (e.g., employer, government) pays the remaining percentage

Collaboration a collegial working relationship with another health care provider in the provision of client care

Collaborative care plans see Critical pathways

Collaborative interventions actions the nurse carries out in collaboration with other health team members, such as physical therapists, social workers, dietitians, and physicians

Collagen a protein found in connective tissue; a whitish protein substance that adds tensile strength to a wound

Colloid osmotic pressure a pulling force exerted by colloids that help maintain the water content of blood

Colloids substances such as large protein molecules that do not readily dissolve into true solutions

Colonization the presence of organisms in body secretions or excretions in which strains of bacteria become resident flora but do not cause illness

Colonoscopy visual examination of the interior of the colon with a colonoscope

Colostomy an opening into the colon (large bowel)

Comfort a renewal, an amplification of power or sense of control, an invigorating influence, a positive mind-set, and a readiness for action

Comforting a group of nursing interventions based on clients' cues of distress, with the goal of achieving client comfort

Commode a portable, chairlike structure used as a toilet

Common law the body of principles that evolves from court decisions

Communicable disease a disease that can spread from one person to another

Communication a two-way process involving the sending and receiving of messages

Communicator nurses identify client problems and then communicate these verbally or in writing to other members of the health team

Community a collection of people who share some attribute of their lives

Community health nursing the synthesis of nursing and public health practice as applied to promoting and preserving the health of populations

Community nursing centers (CNCs) provide primary care to specific populations and are staffed by nurse practitioners and community health nurses

Community-based health care (CBHC) a system that provides health-related services within the context of people's daily lives; that is, in places where people spend their time in the community

Community-based nursing (CBN) nursing care directed toward a specific population or group within the community; primary, secondary, or tertiary care may be provided to individuals or groups.

Compact disc (CD) a thin optical disk that can be read by the laser in a computer's CD-ROM drive

Compensation defense mechanism in which a person substitutes an activity for one that they would prefer doing or cannot do

Compensatory counterbalancing

Complaint (legal) a document filed by a plaintiff

Complementary and alternative medicine (CAM) those practices that do not form part of the dominant system for managing health and disease

Complementary therapies therapeutic practices that are not currently considered an integral part of conventional allopathic medical practice

Complete blood count (CBC) specimens of venous blood; includes hemoglobin and hematocrit measurements, erythrocyte (RBC) count, leukocyte (WBC) count, red blood cell indices, and a differential white cell count

Complete proteins a protein that contains all of the essential amino acids as well as many nonessential ones

Compliance the extent to which an individual's behavior coincides with medical or health advice

Compress a moist gauze dressing applied frequently to an open wound, sometimes medicated

Compromised host any person at increased risk for an infection

Computed tomography (CT) a painless, noninvasive x-ray procedure that has the unique capability of distinguishing minor differences in the density of tissues

Computer-based patient records (CPRs) electronic client data retrievable by caregivers, administrators, accreditors, and other persons who require the data

Concept map a visual tool in which ideas or data are enclosed in circles or boxes of some shape and relationships between these are indicated by connecting lines or arrows

Concepts abstract ideas or mental images of phenomena or reality

Conceptual framework a group of related concepts

Conceptual model a graphic illustration of the relationships among concepts

Conduction the transfer of heat from one molecule to another in direct contact

Conduction hearing loss the result of interrupted transmission of sound waves through the outer and middle ear structures

Confidentiality any information a subject relates will not be made public or available to others without the subject's consent

Congruent communication the verbal and nonverbal aspects of the message match

Conjunctivitis inflammation of the bulbar and palpebral conjunctiva

Conscious sedation a minimal depression of level of consciousness during which the client retains the ability to consciously maintain a patent airway and respond appropriately to verbal and physical stimuli

Consequence-based (teleological) theories the ethics of judging whether an action is moral

Constant fever a state in which the body temperature fluctuates minimally but always remains above normal

Constipation passage of small, dry, hard stool or passage of no stool for an abnormally long time

Consultative leader see Democratic leader

Consumer an individual, a group of people, or a community that uses a service or commodity

Contact precautions methods used to reduce exposure to infectious agents easily transmitted by direct client contact or by contact with items in the client's environment

Contemplation stage stage in which a person acknowledges having a problem, seriously considers changing a specific behavior, actively gathers information, and verbalizes plans to change the behavior in the near future

Continuing education (CE) formalized experiences designed to enlarge the knowledge or skills of practitioners

Continuity of care the coordination of health care services by health care providers for clients moving from one health care setting to another and between and among health care professionals

Continuity theory people maintain their values, habits, and behavior in old age

Contract a written or verbal agreement between two or more people to do or not do some lawful act

Contract law the enforcement of agreements among private individuals or the payment of compensation for failure to fulfill the agreement

Contractility the inherent ability of cardiac muscle fibers to shorten or contract

Contractual obligations duty of care established by the presence of an expressed or implied contract

Contractual relationships vary among practice settings; may be as an independent or employer-employee relationship

Contracture permanent shortening of a muscle and subsequent shortening of tendons and ligaments

Convection the dispersion of heat by air currents

Coordinating the process of ensuring that plans are carried out and evaluating outcomes

Coping mechanism an innate or acquired way of responding to a changing environment or specific problem or situation

Coping strategy see Coping mechanism

Cordotomy surgical severing that obliterates pain and temperature sensation below the level of the spinothalamic portion of the anterolateral tract severed; usually done for pain in the legs and trunk

Core self-concept the beliefs and images that are most vital to the person's identity

Core temperature the temperature of the deep tissues of the body (e.g., thorax, abdominal cavity); relatively constant at 37C (98.6F)

Corn a conical, circular, painful, raised area on the toe or foot

Coronary arteries a network of vessels known as the coronary circulation

Coroner a public official, not necessarily a physician, appointed or elected to inquire into the causes of death

Costal (thoracic) breathing use of the external intercostal muscles and other accessory muscles, such as the sternocleidomastoid muscles

Counseling the process of helping a client to recognize and cope with stressful psychologic or social problems, to develop improved interpersonal relationships, and to promote personal growth

Countershock phase second part of the alarm reaction in which the changes the body experienced during the shock phase are reversed

Covert data (systems, subjective data) information (data) apparent only to the person affected that can be described or verified only by that person

Creatine kinase (CK) enzyme that is released into the blood during a myocardial infarction (MI)

Creatinine a nitrogenous waste that is excreted in the urine

Creatinine clearance a test uses 24-hour urine and serum creatinine levels to determine the glomerular filtration rate, a sensitive indicator of renal function

Creativity thinking that results in the development of new ideas and products

Credentialing the process of determining and maintaining competence in practice; includes licensure, registration, certification, and accreditation

Credé's maneuver manual exertion of pressure on the bladder to force urine out

Crepitation (1) a dry, crackling sound like that of crumpled cellophane, produced by air in the subcutaneous tissue or by air moving through fluid in the alveoli of the lungs; (2) a crackling, grating sound produced by bone rubbing against bone

Crime an act committed in violation of public (criminal) law and punishable by a fine and/or imprisonment

Criminal actions deal with disputes between an individual and the society as a whole

Criminal law deals with actions against the safety and welfare of the public

Crisis counseling   therapy focused on solving immediate problems involving individuals, groups, or families in crisis

Crisis intervention   a short-term helping process of assisting clients to work through a crisis to its resolution and restore their precrisis level of functioning

Critical analysis   a set of questions one can apply to a particular situation or idea to determine essential information and ideas and discard superfluous information and ideas

Critical pathways   multidisciplinary guidelines for client care based on specific medical diagnoses designed to achieve predetermined outcomes

Critical theory   describes theories that help elucidate how social structures affect a wide variety of human experiences from art to social practices

Critical thinking   a cognitive process that includes creativity, problem solving, and decision making

Crystalloids   salts that dissolve readily into true solutions

Cues   any piece of information or data that influences decisions

Cultural care deprivation   lack of culturally assistive, supportive, or facilitative acts

Cultural deprivation   *see* Cultural care deprivation

CulturalCare   professional health care that is culturally sensitive, culturally appropriate, and culturally competent and is essential for the new millennium

Culturally appropriate   application of underlying background knowledge that must be possessed to provide a given client with the best possible health care

Culturally competent   within the delivered care the nurse understands and attends to the total context of the client's situation and uses a complex combination of knowledge, attitudes, and skills

Culturally sensitive   care that demonstrates basic knowledge of and constructive attitudes toward the health traditions observed among the diverse cultural groups found in the setting

Culture   a world view and set of traditions used and transmitted from generation to generation by a particular group, includes related attitudes and institutions

Culture shock   a disorder that occurs in response to transition from one cultural setting to another

Cultures   laboratory cultivations of microorganisms in a special growth medium

Cumulative effect   the increasing response to repeated doses of a drug that occurs when the rate of administration exceeds the rate of metabolism or excretion

Cutaneous pain   pain that originates in the skin or subcutaneous tissue

Cyanosis   bluish discoloration of the skin and mucous membranes caused by reduced oxygen in the blood

Cystoscope   a lighted instrument used to visualize the interior of the urinary bladder

Cystoscopy   visual examination of the urinary bladder with a cystoscope

Dacryocystitis   inflammation of the lacrimal sac

Damages   if malpractice caused the injury, the nurse is held liable for damages that may be compensated

Dandruff   a dry or greasy, scaly material shed from the scalp

Data   information

Data warehousing   the accumulation of large amounts of data that are stored over time

Database   all information about a client, includes nursing health history and physical assessment, physician's history, physical examination, and laboratory and diagnostic test results

Debridement   removal of infected and necrotic tissue

Decision   (legal) outcome made by a judge

Decision making   the process of establishing criteria by which alternative courses of action are developed and selected

Decode   to relate the message perceived to the receiver's storehouse of knowledge and experience and to sort out the meaning of the message

Decubitus ulcers   *see* Pressure ulcers

Deductive reasoning   making specific observations from a generalization

Deep somatic pain   pain that arises from ligaments, tendons, bones, blood vessels, and nerves

Defamation   (legal) a communication that is false, or made with careless disregard for the truth, and results in injury to the reputation of another

Defecation   expulsion of feces from the rectum and anus

Defendant   (legal) person against whom a plaintiff files a complaint against

Defense mechanism   any reaction that serves to protect against something physically or psychologically harmful

Defining characteristics   client signs and symptoms that must be present to validate a nursing diagnosis

Dehiscence   the partial or total rupturing of a sutured wound; usually involves an abdominal wound in which the layers below the skin also separate

Dehydration   insufficient fluid in the body

Delegation   the transfer of responsibility for the performance of an activity from one person to another while retaining accountability for the outcome

Demand feeding   child is fed when hungry

Dementia   a global impairment of cognitive function that usually is progressive and may be permanent; interferes with normal social and occupational activities

Democratic leader   encourages group discussion and decision making

Demography   the study of population, including statistics about distribution by age and place of residence, mortality, and morbidity

Dental caries   tooth decay

Denver Developmental Screening Test (DDST)   a screening test used to assess children from birth to 6 years of age

Dependent functions   with regard to medical diagnoses, physician-prescribed therapies and treatments nurses are obligated to carry out

Dependent interventions   those activities carried out on the order of a physician, under a physician's supervision, or according to specified routines

Dependent variable   the behavior, characteristic, or outcome that the researcher wishes to explain or predict

Depression   feelings of sadness and dejection, often accompanied by physiologic change such as decreased functional activity

Descriptive statistics   procedures that summarize large volumes of data; used to describe and synthesize data, showing patterns and trends

Desire phase   part of the response cycle, which starts in the brain, with conscious sexual desires

Desired effect   *see* Therapeutic effect

Detoxification   *see* Biotransformation

Detrusor muscle   the smooth muscle layers of the bladder

Development   an individual's increasing capacity and skill in functioning, related to growth

Developmental task   skill or behavior pattern learned during stages of development

Diagnosis   a statement or conclusion concerning the nature of some phenomenon

Diagnosis-related groups (DRGs)   a Medicare payments system to hospitals and physicians that establishes fees according to diagnosis

Diagnostic labels   title used in writing a nursing diagnosis; taken from the North American Nursing Diagnosis Association (NANDA) standardized taxonomy of terms

Dialysis   a technique by which fluids and molecules pass through a semipermeable membrane according to the rules of osmosis

Diapedesis   the movement of blood corpuscles through a blood vessel wall

Diaphragmatic (abdominal) breathing   contraction and relaxation of the diaphragm, observed by the movement of the abdomen, which occurs as a result of the diaphragm's contraction and downward movement

Diarrhea   defecation of liquid feces and increased frequency of defecation

Diastole   the period during which the ventricles relax

Diastolic pressure   the pressure of the blood against the arterial walls when the ventricles of the heart are at rest

Diet history a comprehensive assessment of a client's food intake that involves an extensive interview by a nutritionist or dietitian

Diffusion the mixing of molecules or ions of two or more substances as a result of random motion

Digital video disc (DVD) stores and plays digital information, such as a movie; similar in size to a CD

Directing a management function that involves communicating the task to be completed and providing guidance and supervision

Directive interview a highly structured interview that uses closed questions to elicit specific information

Dirty denotes the likely presence of microorganisms, some of which may be capable of causing infection

Disaccharides sugars that are composed of double molecules

Discharge planning the process of anticipating and planning for client needs after discharge

Discovery (legal) pretrial activities to gain all of the facts of a situation

Discrimination the differential treatment of individuals or groups

Discussion an informal oral consideration of a subject by two or more health care personnel to identify a problem or establish strategies to resolve a problem

Disease an alteration in body function resulting in a reduction of capacities or shortening of the normal life span

Disengagement theory aging involves mutual withdrawal (disengagement) between the older person and others in the elderly person's environment

Disinfectants agents that destroy pathogens other than spores

Distance learning learning in which people communicate effectively across long distances

Distribution the transportation of a drug from its site of absorption to its site of action

Diuresis the production of large amounts of urine by the kidneys without an increased fluid intake

Diuretics agents that increase urine secretion

Diversity the fact or state of being different

Documenting *see* Charting or Recording

Do-not-resuscitate (DNR) order a physician's order that specifies no effort be made to resuscitate the client with terminal or irreversible illness in the event of a respiratory or cardiac arrest

Dorsal position a back-lying position without a pillow

Dorsal recumbent position a back-lying position with the head and shoulders slightly elevated

Drip factor (drop factor) the number of drops per milliliter of solution delivered for a particular drip chamber

Droplet nuclei residue of evaporated droplets that remains in the air for long periods of time

Droplet precautions methods used to reduce exposure to infectious agents transmitted by particle droplets larger than 5 microns

Drug a chemical compound taken for disease prevention, diagnosis, cure, or relief or to affect the structure or function of the body

Drug abuse excessive intake of a substance either continually or periodically

Drug allergy an immunologic reaction to a drug

Drug dependence inability to keep the intake of a drug or substance under control

Drug habituation a mild form of psychologic dependence on a drug

Drug half-life the time required for the elimination process to reduce the concentration of a drug to one-half what it was at initial administration

Drug interaction the beneficial or harmful interaction of one drug with another drug

Drug polymorphism a client's variation in response to a drug is influenced by age, gender, size, and body composition

Drug tolerance a condition in which successive increases in the dosage of a drug are required to maintain a given therapeutic effect

Drug toxicity the quality of a drug that exerts a deleterious effect on an organism or tissue

Dullness a thudlike sound produced during percussion by dense tissue of body organs such as the liver, spleen, or heart

Durable medical equipment (DME) companies companies that provide health care equipment for the client at home

Duration the length of time that a sound is heard

Duty the nurse must have (or should have had) a relationship with the client that involves providing care and following an acceptable standard of care

Dysfunctional grief the state in which an individual or group experiences prolonged, unresolved grief and engages in detrimental activities

Dysmenorrhea painful menstruation

Dysphagia difficulty or inability to swallow

Dyspnea difficult or labored breathing

Dysrhythmia a pulse with an irregular rhythm

Dysuria painful or difficult voiding

Eccrine glands glands that produce sweat; found over most of the body

Echocardiogram a noninvasive test that uses ultrasound to visualize structures of the heart and evaluate left ventricular function

Ectoderm the outer layer of tissue formed in the second week of life

Edema the presence of excess interstitial fluid in the body

Effectiveness a measure of the quality or quantity of services provided

Efficiency a measure of the resources used in the provision of nursing services

Effleurage a stroking massage technique

Ego includes consciousness and memory, which serve to mediate between primitive instinctual drives (id), internal social prohibitions (superego), and reality

Ego defense mechanisms (Freud) mental mechanisms that develop as the personality attempts to defend itself, establish compromises among conflicting impulses, and allay inner tensions

Ejaculation expulsion of seminal fluid and sperm

Elasticity of the arterial wall expansibility or stretching of the vessels

Elective surgery performed when surgical intervention is the preferred treatment for a condition that is not imminently life threatening or to improve the client's life

Electric shock occurs when a current travels through the body to the ground rather than through electric wiring, or from static electricity that builds up on the body

Electrocardiogram (ECG, EKG) a graph of the electric activity of the heart

Electrocardiography provides a graphic recording of the heart's electrical activity

Electroencephalogram (EEG) a graph of the electrical activity of the brain

Electrolytes chemical substances that develop an electric charge and are able to conduct an electric current when placed in water; ions

Electronic medical records (EMRs) *see* Computer-based patient records (CPRs)

Elimination half-life *see* Drug half-life

Embolus a blood clot (or a substance such as air) that has moved from its place of origin and is causing obstruction to circulation elsewhere (*plural:* emboli)

Embryonic phase the phase during which the fertilized ovum develops into an organism with most of the features of a human

Emergency surgery surgery that is performed immediately to preserve function or the life of the client

Emigration process in which leukocytes move through the blood vessel wall into the affected tissue spaces

Emmetropic normal refraction so that the eyes focus images on the retina

Empathy the ability to discriminate what the other person's world is like and to communicate to the other this understanding in a way that shows that the helper understands the client's feelings and the behavior and experience underlying these feelings

Emphysema   a chronic pulmonary condition in which the alveoli are dilated and distended

Empirical data   information collected from the observable world

Encoding   involves the selection of specific signs or symbols (codes) to transmit the message, such as which language and words to use, how to arrange the words, and what tone of voice and gestures to use

Endocardium   a layer of the heart wall lining the inside of the heart's chambers and great vessels

Endoderm   the inner layer of tissue formed in the second week of life

End-of-life care   care provided in the final weeks before death

Endogenous   developing from within

Enema   a solution introduced into the rectum and sigmoid colon to remove feces and/or flatus

Enteral   through the gastrointestinal system

Entoderm   *see* Endoderm

Enuresis   bedwetting; involuntary passing of urine in children after bladder control is achieved

Environment   all of the conditions, circumstances, and influences surrounding and affecting the development of an organism or person

Enzymes   biologic catalysts that speed up chemical reactions

Epicardium   the visceral pericardium adhering to the surface of the heart, forming the heart's outermost layer

Epidural   commonly used route for parenteral administration into the epidural space (the area inside the spinal column but outside the dura mater)

Epidural anesthesia   the injection of an anesthetic agent into the epidural space

Equianalgesia   equal analgesia; used when referring to the doses of various opioid analgesics that provide approximately the same pain relief

Equilibrium   a state of balance

Erectile dysfunction   the inability to achieve or maintain an erection sufficient for sexual satisfaction for oneself or one's partner

Erythema   a redness associated with a variety of skin rashes

Erythrocytes   red blood cells, or RBCs

Eschar   thick necrotic tissue produced by burning, by a corrosive application, or by death of tissue associated with loss of vascular supply, bacterial invasion, and putrefaction

Essential amino acids   amino acids that cannot be manufactured in the body and must be supplied as part of the protein ingested in the diet

Ethics   the rules or principles that govern right conduct

Ethnic   belonging to a specific group of individuals who share a common social and cultural heritage

Ethnography   research that provides a framework to focus on the culture of a group of people

Etiology   the causal relationship between a problem and its related or risk factors

Eupnea   normal, quiet breathing

Eustachian tube   the part of the middle ear that connects the middle ear to the nasopharynx; stabilizes air pressure between the external atmosphere and the middle ear

Euthanasia   the act of painlessly putting to death persons suffering from incurable or distressing disease

Evaluating   a planned ongoing, purposeful activity in which clients and health care professionals expected outcomes are compared to actual outcomes

Evaluation statement   a statement that consists of two parts: a conclusion and supporting data

Evisceration   extrusion of the internal organs

Exacerbation   the period during a chronic illness when symptoms reappear after remission

Excitement/plateau phase   part of the response cycle, involves vasocongestion and myotonia

Excoriation   loss of the superficial layers of the skin

Excretion   elimination of a waste product produced by the body cells from the body

Exercise   a type of physical activity; a planned, structured, and repetitive bodily movement done to improve or maintain one or more components of physical fitness

Exhalation   (expiration) the movement of gases from the lungs to the atmosphere

Exogenous   developing from without

Exophthalmus   a protrusion of the eyeballs with elevation of the upper eyelids, resulting in a startled or staring expression

Expectorate   to cough and spit up mucus or other materials

Expert power   power attained through respect for one's abilities, knowledge, and/or skills

Expert witness   one who has special training, experience, or skill in a relevant area and is allowed by the court to offer an opinion on some issue within that area of expertise

Expiration   *see* Exhalation

Express consent   an oral or written agreement

Extended family   family that includes the relatives of the nuclear family (e.g., grandparents, aunts, uncles)

External auditory meatus   the entrance to the ear canal

External respiration   the interchange of oxygen and carbon dioxide between the alveoli of the lungs and the pulmonary blood

Extinction   the failure to perceive touch on one side of the body when two symmetric areas of the body are touched simultaneously

Extracellular fluid (ECF)   fluid found outside the body cells

Exudate   material, such as fluid and cells, that has escaped from blood vessels during the inflammatory process and is deposited in tissue or on tissue surfaces

Fabiola   a wealthy Roman matron; viewed by some as the patron saint of early nursing who used her position and wealth to establish hospitals for the sick

Fad   a widespread but short-lived interest, or a practice followed with considerable zeal

Failure to thrive   a unique syndrome in which an infant falls below the fifth percentile for weight and height on a standard growth chart or is falling in percentiles on a growth chart

Faith   an active "mode of being-in-relation" to another or others in which we invest commitment, belief, love, and hope

False imprisonment   the unlawful restraint or detention of another person against his or her wishes

Family   the basic unit of society that consists of those individuals, male or female, youth or adult, legally or not legally related, genetically or not genetically related, who are considered by others to represent their significant persons

Family-centered nursing   nursing that considers the health of the family as a unit in addition to the health of individual family members

Fasciculation   an abnormal contraction or shortening of a bundle of muscle fibers

Fats   lipids that are solid at room temperature

Fat-soluble vitamins   A, D, E, and K vitamins that the body can store

Fatty acids   the basic structural units of most lipids made up of carbon chains and hydrogen

Fear   an emotional response to an actual, present danger

Feasibility   the availability of time as well as the material and human resources needed to investigate a research problem or question

Febrile   pertaining to a fever; feverish

Fecal impaction   a mass or collection of hardened, putty-like feces in the folds of the rectum

Fecal incontinence   *see* Bowel incontinence

Feces   (stool) body wastes and undigested food eliminated from the bowel

Feedback   the response or message that the receiver returns to the sender during communication

Felony a crime of a serious nature, such as murder, punishable by a term in prison

Fetal phase characterized by a period of rapid growth in the size of the fetus; both genetic and environmental factors affect its growth

Fever elevated body temperature

Fever spike a temperature that rises to fever level rapidly following a normal temperature and then returns to normal within a few hours

Fibrin an insoluble protein formed from fibrinogen during the clotting of blood

Fibrinogen a plasma protein that is converted to fibrin when it is released into the tissues and, together with thromboplastin and platelets, forms an interlacing network making a barrier to wall off an area

Fibrous (scar) tissue connective tissue repair of wounds with tissue that can proliferate under conditions of ischemia and altered pH

Fidelity a moral principle that obligates the individual to be faithful to agreements and responsibilities one has undertaken

Fifth vital sign pain assessment

Filtration process whereby fluid and solutes move together across a membrane from one compartment to another

Filtration pressure the pressure in a compartment that results in the movement of fluid and substances dissolved in fluid out of the compartment

First-level manager a manager responsible for managing the work of non-managerial personnel and the day-to-day activities of a specific work group or groups

Fissures deep grooves that occur as a result of dryness and cracking of the skin

Fixation immobilization or the inability of the personality to proceed to the next developmental stage because of anxiety

Flaccid weak or lax

Flatness an extremely dull sound produced, during percussion, by very dense tissue, such as muscle or bone

Flatulence the presence of excessive amounts of gas in the stomach or intestines

Flatus gas or air normally present in the stomach or intestines

Florence Nightingale considered the founder of modern nursing, she was influential in developing nursing education, practice, and administration

Flowsheet a record of the progress of specific or specialized data such as vital signs, fluid balance, or routine medications; often charted in graph form

Fluid volume deficit (hypovolemia) loss of both water and electrolytes in similar proportions from the ECF

Fluid volume excess (FVE) (hypervolemia) retention of both water and sodium in similar proportions to normal ECF

Focus charting a method of charting that uses key words or foci to describe what is happening to the client

Folk medicine beliefs and practices relating to illness prevention and healing that derive from cultural traditions rather than from modern medicine's scientific base

Fontanelles unossified membranous gaps in the bone structure of the skull of a newborn that makes molding of the head possible

Food diary a detailed record of measured amounts (portion sizes) of all food and fluids a client consumes during a specified period, usually 3 to 7 days

Food frequency record a checklist that indicates how often general food groups or specific foods are eaten

Foreseeability a link that must exist between the nurse's act and the injury suffered

Formal leader an appointed leader selected by an organization and given official authority to make decisions and act

Formal nursing care plan a written or computerized guide that organizes information about the client's care

Fowler's position a bed-sitting position with the head of the bed raised to 45 degrees

Frail elderly and elderly individual who has significant physiologic and functional impairment, whatever the age

Friction rubbing; the force that opposes motion

Full disclosure a basic right, which means that deception, either by withholding information about a client's participation in a study or by giving the client false or misleading information about what participating in the study will involve, must not occur

Fungi infection-causing microorganisms that include yeasts and molds

Gait the way a person walks

Gastrocolic reflex increased peristalsis of the colon after food has entered the stomach

Gastrostomy an opening through the abdominal wall into the stomach

Gastrostomy tube a tube that is surgically placed directly into the client's stomach and provides route for administering nutrition and medications

Gauge diameter of a shaft

Gender indicates biologic male or female status

Gender identity a person's sense of being masculine or feminine, as distinct from being male or female

General adaptation syndrome (GAS) (Selye) a general arousal response of the body to a stressor characterized by certain physiologic events and dominated by the sympathetic nervous system

General anesthesia the induced loss of all sensation and consciousness

Generativity concern for establishing and guiding the next generation

Generic name a drug name not protected by trademark and usually describing the chemical structure of the drug

Geragogy the term used to describe the process involved in stimulating and helping elderly persons to learn

Gingival of or relating to the gums

Gingivitis red, swollen gingiva (gums)

Glaucoma a disturbance in the circulation of aqueous fluid; causes an increase in intraocular pressure

Global self refers to the collective beliefs and images one holds about oneself; the most complete description that individuals can give of themselves at any one time

Global self-esteem how much one likes one's perceived self as a whole

Glomerulus a tuft of capillaries in the kidney surrounded by Bowman's capsule

Glossitis inflammation of the tongue

Glycerides the most common form of lipids consisting of a glycerol molecule with up to three fatty acids

Glycogen the chief carbohydrate stored in the body, particularly in the liver and muscles

Glycogenesis the process of glycogen formation

Goals/desired outcomes a part of a care plan that describes, in terms of observable client responses, what the nurse hopes to achieve by implementing the nursing interventions

Goniometer a device used to measure the angle of a joint in degrees

Governance the establishment and maintenance of social, political, and economic arrangements by which practitioners control their practice, self-discipline, working conditions, and professional affairs

Grand theories articulate a broad range of the significant relationships among the concepts of a discipline

Granulation tissue young connective tissue with new capillaries formed in the wound healing process

Grief emotional suffering often caused by bereavement

Gross negligence involves extreme lack of knowledge, skill, or decision making that the person clearly should have known would put others at risk for harm

Grounded theory research to understand social structures and social processes; this method focuses on the generation of categories or hypotheses that explain patterns of behavior of people in the study

Group two or more people with shared purposes and goals

Group dynamics forces that determine the behavior of the group and the relationships among the group members

Growth   physical change and increase in size

Guaiac test   a test performed for occult (hidden) blood to detect gastrointestinal bleeding not visible to the eye

Gustatory   referring to the sense of taste

Habit training   attempts to keep clients dry by having them void at regular intervals; also referred to as *timed voiding* or *scheduled toileting*

Hardware   the physical parts a computer

Harm   the client or plaintiff must demonstrate some type of harm or injury (physical, financial, or emotional) as a result of the breach of duty owed the client; the plaintiff will be asked to document physical injury, medical costs, loss of wages, "pain and suffering," and any other damages

Harriet Tubman   known as "the Moses of Her People" for her work with the Underground Railroad; during the Civil War she nursed the sick and suffering of her own race

Haustra   pouches that form in the large intestine when the longitudinal muscles are shorter than the colon

Haustral churning   (shuffling) movement of the chyme back and forth within the haustra in the large intestine

HEALTH   the balance of the person, both within one's being, physical, mental, and spiritual—and in the outside world—natural, communal, and metaphysical

Health behaviors   the actions a person takes to understand his or her health state, maintain an optimal state of belief, prevent illness and injury, and reach his or her maximum physical and mental potential

Health beliefs   concepts about health that an individual believes are true

Health care proxy   a legal statement that appoints a proxy to make medical decisions for the client in the event the client is unable to do so

Health care system   the totality of services offered by all health disciplines

Health maintenance organization (HMO)   a group health care agency that provides basic and supplemental health maintenance and treatment services to voluntary enrollees

Health promotion   any activity undertaken for the purpose of achieving a higher level of health and well-being

Health protection   behavior motivated by a desire to actively avoid illness, detect it early, or maintain functioning within the constraints of illness

Health risk assessment (HRA)   an assessment and educational tool that indicates a client's risk for disease or injury during the next 10 years by comparing the client's risk with the mortality risk of the corresponding age, sex, and racial group

Health status   the health of a person at a given time

Heart failure   a condition that develops if the heart cannot keep up with the body's need for oxygen and nutrients to the tissues; usually occurs because of myocardial infarction, but it may also result from chronic overwork of the heart

Heart-lung death   the traditional clinical signs of death: cessation of the apical pulse, respirations, and blood pressure

Heat balance   the state a person is in when the amount of heat produced by the body exactly equals the amount of heat lost

Heimlich maneuver   subdiaphragmatic abdominal thrusts used to clear an obstructed airway

Helix   the posterior curve of the auricle's upper aspect

Helping relationships   the nurse–client relationship

Hematocrit   the proportion of red blood cells (erythrocytes) to the total blood volume

Hematoma   a collection of blood in a tissue, organ, or space due to a break in the wall of a blood vessel

Hemoglobin   the red pigment in red blood cells that carries oxygen

Hemoptysis   the presence of blood in the sputum

Hemorrhage   excessive loss of blood from the vascular system

Hemorrhagic exudate   *see* Sanguineous exudate

Hemorrhoids   distended veins in the rectum

Hemostasis   cessation of bleeding

Hemothorax   a collection of blood in the pleural cavity

Heritage consistency   the degree to which one's lifestyle reflects his or her respective tribal culture

Heritage inconsistency   the observance of the beliefs and practices of one's acculturated belief system

Hernia   a protrusion (such as of the intestine through the inguinal wall or canal)

High Fowler's position   a bed-sitting position in which the head of the bed is elevated 90 degrees

Higher brain death   *see* Cerebral death

Hirsutism   abnormal hairiness, particularly in women

Holism   all living organisms are seen as interacting, unified wholes that are more than the sums of their parts

Holistic health belief   holds that the forces of nature must be maintained in balance or harmony

Holistic health   a model of health based on the belief that the whole is more than the sum of its parts

Holistic health care   a system that considers all components of health: health promotion, health maintenance, health education and illness prevention, and restorative–rehabilitative care

Holistic nursing   nursing practice that has as its goal the healing of the whole person

Holy day   a day set aside for special religious observance

Homans' sign   calf pain produced by dorsiflexion of the foot

Home care   providing care in the clients' home

Home care nursing   *see* Home health nursing

Home health clinical specialists   advanced nurse practitioners who can provide direct care, manage client care, and engage in consulting, education, administrative, and research activities for clients in the home

Home health nursing   services and products provided to clients in their homes that are needed to maintain, restore, or promote their physical, psychologic, and social well-being

Homeopathy   an alternative therapy based on the theory that the cure for the disease lies in the disease itself; thus, treatment is with highly diluted amounts of substances that at a higher concentration would produce the same symptoms as the disease

Homeostasis   the tendency of the body to maintain a state of balance or equilibrium while continually changing; a mechanism in which deviations from normal are sensed and counteracted

Hope   a multidimensional concept that includes perceiving realistic expectations and goals, having motivation to achieve goals, anticipating outcomes, establishing trust and interpersonal relationships, relying on internal and external resources, having determination to endure, and being oriented to the future

Hordeolum (sty)   a redness, swelling, and tenderness of the hair follicle and glands that empty at the edge of the eyelids

Hospice   the delivery of care for terminally ill clients either in health care facilities or in the client's home

Hospice nursing   care frequently given to terminally ill clients in their home; often considered a subspecialty of public health nursing

Hospital information system (HIS)   computer software program suite used to manage client, financial, and administrative data

Hub   the part of a needle that fits onto a syringe

Humanism   learning that focuses on the feelings and attitudes of learners, the importance of the individual in identifying learning needs and taking responsibility for them, and the self-motivation of the learners to work toward self-reliance and independence

Humidifiers   devices that add water vapor to inspired air

Humoral immunity   antibody-mediated defense; resides ultimately in the B lymphocytes and is mediated by the antibodies produced by B cells

Hydrostatic pressure   the pressure a liquid exerts on the sides of the container that holds it; also called *filtration force*

Hygiene   the science of health and its maintenance

Hyperalgesia   extreme sensitivity to pain

Hypercalcemia   an excess of calcium in the blood plasma

Hypercapnia   a condition in which carbon dioxide accumulates in the blood

Hypercarbia   *see* Hypercapnia

Hyperchloremia   an excess of chloride in the blood plasma

Hyperemia   increased blood flow to an area

Hyperinflation   giving the client breaths that are 1 to 1.5 times the tidal volume through the ventilator circuit or via a manual resuscitation bag

Hyperkalemia   an excess of potassium in the blood plasma

Hypermagnesemia   an excess of magnesium in the blood plasma

Hypernatremia   an excess of sodium in the blood plasma

Hyperopia   abnormal refraction in which light rays focus behind the retina, farsightedness

Hyperoxygenation   done with a manual resuscitation bag or through a ventilator; increases oxygen flow (usually to 100%) before suctioning and between suction attempts

Hyperphosphatemia   an excess of phosphate in the blood plasma

Hyperpyrexia   *see* Hyperthermia

Hyperresonance   an abnormal booming sound produced during percussion of the lungs

Hypersomnia   excessive sleep

Hypertension   an abnormally high blood pressure; over 140 mm Hg systolic and/or 90 mm Hg diastolic

Hyperthermia   an extremely high body temperature (e.g., 41C [105.8F])

Hypertonic   solutions that have a higher osmolality than body fluids

Hypertrophy   enlargement of a muscle or organ

Hyperventilation   very deep, rapid respirations

Hypoactive sexual desire disorder   involves a persistent or recurring absence of sexual thoughts or disinterest in sexual activity

Hypocalcemia   deficiency of calcium in the blood plasma

Hypochloremia   deficiency of chloride in the blood plasma

Hypodermic   under the skin

Hypodermic syringe   a type of syringe that comes in 2-, 2.5-, and 3-mL sizes; the syringe usually has two scales marked on it: the minim and the milliliter

Hypokalemia   deficiency of potassium in the blood plasma

Hypomagnesemia   deficiency of magnesium in the blood plasma

Hyponatremia   deficiency of sodium in the blood plasma

Hypophosphatemia   deficiency of phosphate in the blood plasma

Hypotension   an abnormally low blood pressure; less than 100 mm Hg systolic in an adult

Hypothalamic integrator   the center in the brain that controls the core temperature; located in the preoptic area of the hypothalamus

Hypothermia   a core body temperature below the lower limit of normal

Hypotonic   solutions that have a lower osmolality than body fluids

Hypoventilation   very shallow respirations

Hypovolemia   an abnormal reduction in blood volume

Hypoxemia   reduced oxygen in the blood

Hypoxia   insufficient oxygen anywhere in the body

Iatrogenic disease   disease caused unintentionally by medical therapy

Iatrogenic infections   infections that are the direct result of diagnostic or therapeutic procedures

Id   the source of instinctive and unconscious psychologic urges

Ideal body weight (IBW)   the optimal weight recommended for optimal health

Ideal self   how we would prefer to be; the individual's perception of how one should behave based on certain personal standards, aspirations, goals, or values

Identification   perceiving one's self as similar to and behaving like another person

Idiosyncratic effect   a different, unexpected or individual effect from the normal one usually expected from a medication; the occurrence of unpredictable and unexplainable symptoms

Ileostomy   an opening into the ileum (small bowel)

Illicit drugs   drugs that are sold illegally; street drugs

Illness   a highly personal state in which the person feels unhealthy or ill, may or may not be related to disease

Illness behavior   the course of action a person takes to define the state of his or her health and pursue a remedy

Imagery   the internal experience of memories, dreams, fantasies, and visions that serve as a bridge connecting body, mind, and spirit

Imagination   an important part of preschoolers' life (the preschooler has an active imagination and fantasizes in play)

Imitation   copying the behaviors and attitudes of another person

Immobility   prescribed or unavoidable restriction of movement in any area of a person's life

Immune defenses   *see* Specific (immune) defenses

Immunity   a specific resistance of the body to infection; it may be natural, or resistance may develop after exposure to a disease agent

Immunoglobulins   *see* Antibodies

Impaired nurse   a nurse whose practice has deteriorated because of chemical abuse

Implementing   the phase of the nursing process in which the nursing care plan is put into action

Implied consent   consent that is assumed in an emergency when consent cannot be obtained from the client or a relative

Implied contract   a contract that has not been explicitly agreed to by the parties but that the law nevertheless considers to exist

Impotence   *see* Erectile dysfunction

Incentive spirometers   devices that measure the flow of air inhaled through the mouthpiece

Incomplete proteins   protein that lacks one or more essential amino acids; usually derived from vegetables

Incus   the anvil bone of the middle ear

Independent variable   the presumed cause or influence on the dependent variable

Independent functions   areas of health care unique to nursing, separate and distinct from medical management

Independent interventions   activities that the nurse is licensed to initiate as a result of the nurse's own knowledge and skills

Independent practice associations (IPAs)   provide care in offices; clients pay a fixed prospective payment and IPA pays the provider; earnings or losses are assumed by the IPA

Indicator   an observable patient state, behavior, or self-reported perception or evaluation;   similar to desired outcomes in traditional language

Individualized care plan   a plan tailored to meet the unique needs of a specific client—needs that are not addressed by the standardized plan

Inductive reasoning   making generalizations from specific data

Infection   the disease process produced by microorganisms

Inferences   interpretations or conclusions made based on cues or observed data

Inflammation   local and nonspecific defensive tissue response to injury or destruction of cells

Influence   an informal strategy used to gain the cooperation of others without exercising formal authority

Informal care plan   a strategy for action that exists in the nurse's mind

Informal leader   an individual selected by the group as its leader because of seniority, age, special abilities, or charisma

Information transduction   the conversion or transformation of information or energy from one form to another

Informed consent   a client's agreement to accept a course of treatment or a procedure after receiving complete information, including the risks of treatment and facts relating to it, from the physician

Ingestion the act of taking in food or medication

Ingrown toenail the growing inward of the nail into the soft tissues around it, most often results from improper nail trimming

Inhalation (inspiration) the act of breathing in; the intake of air or other substances into the lungs

Inhibiting effect the decreased effect of one or both drugs

Injury *see* Harm

Input consists of information, material, or energy that enters a system

Insensible fluid loss fluid loss that is not perceptible to the individual

Insensible heat loss heat loss that occurs from evaporation (vaporization) of moisture from the respiratory tract, mucosa of the mouth, and the skin

Insensible water loss continuous and unnoticed water loss

In-service education education that is designed to upgrade the knowledge or skills of employees

Insomnia inability to obtain a sufficient quality or quantity of sleep

Inspection the visual examination, that is, assessment by using the sense of sight

Inspiration *see* Inhalation

Insulin syringe similar to a hypodermic syringe, but the scale is specially designed for insulin: a 100-unit calibrated scale intended for use with U-100 insulin

Integrated delivery system (IDS) a system that incorporates acute care services, home health care, extended and skilled care facilities, and outpatient services

Integrated health care system one that makes all levels of care available in an integrated form—primary care, secondary care, and tertiary care

Intensity the loudness or softness of a sound, amplitude

Intention tremor involuntary trembling when an individual attempts a voluntary movement

Intercessory prayer prayer offered in favor of another

Intermittent fever a body temperature that alternates at regular intervals between periods of fever and periods of normal or subnormal temperatures

Internal respiration the interchange of oxygen and carbon dioxide between the circulating blood and the cells of the body tissues

Internet a worldwide computer network

Interpersonal skills all verbal and nonverbal activities people use when communicating directly with one another

Interpreter an individual who mediates spoken communication between people speaking different languages without adding, omitting, or distorting meaning or editorializing

Interstate compact an agreement between two or more states

Interstitial fluid fluid that surrounds the cells, includes lymph

Interview a planned communication; a conversation with a purpose

Intracellular fluid (ICF) fluid found within the body cells, also called *cellular fluid*

Intractable pain pain that is resistant to cure or relief

Intradermal under the epidermis (into the dermis)

Intradermal (ID) injection the administration of a drug into the dermal layer of the skin just beneath the epidermis

Intramuscular into the muscle

Intramuscular (IM) injections injections into muscle tissue that are absorbed more quickly than subcutaneous injections because of the greater blood supply to the body muscles

Intraoperative phase begins when the client is transferred to the operating table and ends when the client is admitted to the postanesthesia care unit

Intrapleural pressure pressure in the pleural cavity surrounding the lungs

Intrapulmonary pressure pressure within the lungs

Intraspinal into the spinal cord

Intrathecal *see* Intraspinal

Intravascular fluid plasma

Intravenous within a vein

Intravenous block anesthesia used most often for procedures involving the arm, wrist, and hand

Intravenous pyelography (IVP) x-ray filming of the kidney and ureters after injection of a radiopaque material into the vein

Introjection the assimilation of the attributes of others

Intuition the understanding or learning of things without the conscious use of reasoning

Invasion of privacy a direct wrong of a personal nature, it injures the feelings of the person and does not take into account the effect of revealed information on the standing of the person in the community

Ions atoms or group of atoms that carry a positive or negative electric charge; electrolytes

Iron deficiency anemia a form of anemia caused by inadequate supply of iron for synthesis of hemoglobin

Irrigation (lavage) a flushing or washing-out of a body cavity, organ, or wound with a specified solution that may or may not be medicated

Ischemia deficiency of blood supply caused by obstruction of circulation to the body part

Isokinetic (resistive) exercises muscle contraction or tension against resistance

Isolation practices that prevent the spread of infection and communicable disease

Isometric (static or setting) exercise tensing of a muscle against an immovable outer resistance that does not change muscle length or produce joint motion

Isotonic solutions that have the same osmolality as body fluids

Isotonic (dynamic) exercise exercise in which muscle tension is constant and the muscle shortens to produce muscle contraction and active movement

Jaundice a yellowish color of the sclera, mucous membranes, and/or skin

Jejunostomy an opening through the abdominal wall into the jejunum

Justice fairness

Kardex the trade name for a method that makes use of a series of cards to concisely organize and record client data and instructions for daily nursing care—especially care that changes frequently and must be kept up to date

Keloid a hypertrophic scar containing an abnormal amount of collagen

Kilocalorie (kcal) *see* Calorie

Kilojoule (kJ) a metric measurement referring to the amount of energy required when a force of 1 newton (N) moves 1 kg of weight 1 m of distance

Kinesthetic refers to awareness of the position and movement of body parts

Knights of Saint Lazarus an order of knights that dedicated themselves to the care of people with leprosy, syphilis, and chronic skin conditions

Korotkoff's sounds a series of five sounds produced by blood within the artery with each ventricular contraction

Kosher acceptable or prepared according to Jewish law

Kussmaul's breathing hyperventilation that accompanies metabolic acidosis in which the body attempts to compensate (give off excess body acids) by blowing off carbon dioxide through deep and rapid breathing

Kyphosis excessive convex curvature of the thoracic spine

Laissez-faire (nondirective, permissive) leader recognizes the group's need for autonomy and self-regulation

Lanugo the fine, woolly hair or down on the shoulders, back, sacrum, and earlobes of the unborn child that may remain for a few weeks after birth

Large calorie (Calorie, kilocalorie [kcal]) *see* Calorie

Laryngoscopy visual examination of the larynx with a laryngoscope

Lateral position a side-lying position

Lavage an irrigation or washing of a body organ, such as the stomach

Lavinia L. Dock a nursing leader and suffragist who was active in the protest movement for women's rights that resulted in the U.S. Constitution amendment allowing women to vote in 1920

Law a rule made by humans that regulates social conduct in a formally prescribed and binding manner

Laxatives medications that stimulate bowel activity and assist fecal elimination

Leader a person who influences others to work together to accomplish a specific goal

Leadership style describes traits, behaviors, motivations, and choices used by individuals to effectively influence others

Leading question a question that influences the client to give a particular answer

Learning a change in human disposition or capability that persists over a period of time and cannot be solely accounted for by growth

Learning need a desire or a requirement to know something that is currently unknown to the learner

Legitimate power power related to the authority associated with a specific position or role

Leukocytes white blood cells

Leukocytosis an increase in the number of white blood cells

Liability the quality or state of being legally responsible for one's obligations and action and to make financial restitution for wrongful acts

Libel defamation by means of print, writing, or pictures

Libido urge or desire for sexual activity

License a legal permit granted to individuals to engage in the practice of a profession and to use a particular title

Licensed vocational (practical) nurse (LVN/LPN) a nurse who practices under the supervision of a registered nurse, providing basic direct technical care to clients

Lifestyle the values and behaviors adopted by a person in daily life

Lift an abnormal anterior movement of the chest related to enlargement of the right ventricle

Lillian Wald founder of the Henry Street Settlement and Visiting Nurse Service, which provided nursing and social services and organized educational and cultural activities; considered the founder of public health nursing

Line of gravity an imaginary vertical line running through the center of gravity

Lipids organic substances that are greasy and insoluble in water but soluble in alcohol or ether

Lipoproteins soluble compounds made up of various lipids

Litigation the action of a lawsuit

Living will a document that states medical treatments(s) the client chooses to omit or refuse in the event that the client is unable to make these decisions

Livor mortis discoloration of the skin caused by breakdown of the red blood cells; occurs after blood circulation has ceased; appears in the dependent areas of the body

Lobule earlobe

Local adaptation syndrome (LAS) the reaction of one organ or body part to stress

Local anesthesia an anesthetic agent used for minor surgical procedures that is injected into a specific area

Local area network (LAN) personal computers (PCs) linked directly to or nearby PCs and servers by wires or wireless communication devices

Local infection an infection that is limited to the specific part of the body where the microorganisms remain

Locus of control (LOC) a concept about whether clients believe their health status is under their own or other's control

Logrolling a technique used to turn a client whose body must at all times be kept in straight alignment (like a log)

Long-term memory the repository for information stored for periods longer than 72 hours and usually weeks and years

Lordosis an exaggerated concavity in the lumbar region of the vertebral column

Loss an actual or potential situation in which a valued ability, object, or person is inaccessible or changed so that it is perceived as no longer valuable

Low Fowler's position a bed-sitting position in which the head of the bed is elevated between 15 and 45 degrees, with or without knee flexion

Lumbar puncture a procedure where cerebrospinal fluid (CSF) is withdrawn through a needle that is inserted into the subarachnoid space of the spinal canal between the third and fourth lumbar vertebrae or between the fourth and fifth lumbar vertebrae

Lung compliance expansibility of the lung

Lung recoil the tendency of lungs to collapse away from the chest wall

Lung scan records the emissions from radioisotopes that indicate how well gas and blood are traveling through the lungs; also known as a *V/Q* (ventilation/perfusion) *scan*

Maceration the wasting away or softening of a solid as if by the action of soaking; often used to describe degenerative changes and eventual disintegration

Macrominerals any of the minerals that people require daily in amounts over 100 mg

Macrophages large phagocytes

Magico-religious health belief view a belief system in which people attribute the fate of the world and those in it to the actions of God, the gods, or other supernatural forces for good or evil

Magnetic resonance imaging (MRI) a noninvasive diagnostic scanning technique in which the client is placed in a magnetic field

Maintenance stage stage at which a person integrates newly adopted behavior patterns into his or her lifestyle

Major surgery surgery that involves a high degree of risk for a variety of reasons; it may be complicated or prolonged; large losses of blood may occur; vital organs may be involved; postoperative complications may occur

Malleus hammer bone of the middle ear

Malnutrition a disorder of nutrition; insufficient nourishment of the body cells

Malpractice the negligent acts of persons engaged in professions or occupations in which highly technical or professional skills are employed

Managed care a method of organizing care delivery that emphasizes communication and coordination of care among all health care team members

Management information system (MIS) software designed to facilitate the organization and application of data used to manage an organization or department

Manager one who is appointed to a position in an organization that gives the power to guide and direct the work of others

Mandated reporters a role of the nurse in which he or she identifies and assesses cases of violence against others, and in every case the situation must be reported to the proper authorities

Manometer an instrument used to measure the pressure of fluids or gases

Manslaughter second-degree murder

Manubrium the handle-like superior part of the sternum that joins with the clavicles

Margaret Higgins Sanger considered the founder of Planned Parenthood, was imprisoned for opening the first birth control information clinic in Baltimore in 1916

Margination the aggregating or lining up of substances along a surface or edge (e.g., the lining up of white blood cells against the wall of a blood vessel during the inflammatory process)

Mary Breckinridge a nurse who practiced midwivery in England, Australia, and New Zealand; founded the Frontier Nursing Service in Kentucky in 1925 to provide family-centered primary health care to rural populations

Mass peristalsis involves a wave of powerful muscular contraction that moves over large areas of the colon; usually occurs after eating

Mastoid a bony prominence behind the ear

Maturity the state of maximal function and integration; the state of being fully developed

Mean a measure of central tendency, computed by summing all scores and dividing by the number of subjects; commonly symbolized as X or M

Measures of central tendency measures that describe the center of a distribution of data, denoting where most of the subjects lie; include the mean, median, and mode

Measures of variability   measures that indicate the degree of dispersion or spread of the data; include range, variance, and standard deviation

Meatus   an opening, passage, or channel

Meconium   the first fecal material passed by the newborn, normally up to 24 hours after birth

Median   a measure of central tendency, representing the exact middle score or value in a distribution of scores; the median is the value above and below which 50% of the scores lie

Medicaid   a U.S. federal public assistance program paid out of general taxes and administered through the individual states to provide health care for those who require financial assistance

Medical asepsis   all practices intended to confine a specific microorganism to a specific area, limiting the number, growth, and spread of microorganisms

Medical examiner   a physician who usually has advanced education in pathology or forensic medicine who determines causes of death

Medicare   a national and state health insurance program for U.S. residents older than 65 years of age

Medication   a substance administered for the diagnosis, cure, treatment, a relief of a symptom or for prevention of disease

Meditation   mental exercise that directs the mind to think inwardly by closing the sense organs to external stimulation

Menarche   onset of menstruation

Meniscus   the crescent-shaped upper surface of a column of fluid

Menopause   cessation of menstruation

Menstruation   the monthly discharge of blood through the vagina occurring in nonpregnant women from puberty to menopause

Mentor   a person who serves as an experienced guide, adviser, or advocate and assumes responsibility for promoting the growth and professional advancement of a less experienced individual

Mesoderm   middle layer of the embryonic tissue that forms during the first three weeks of life

Metabolic acidosis   a condition characterized by a deficiency of bicarbonate ions in the body in relation to the amount of carbonic acid in the body, the pH falls to less than 7.35

Metabolic alkalosis   a condition characterized by an excess of bicarbonate ions in the body in relation to the amount of carbonic acid in the body; pH rises to greater than 7.45

Metabolism   the sum of all physical and chemical processes by which a living substance is formed and maintained and by which energy is made available for use by the organism

Metabolites   end products or enzymes

Metaparadigm   originates from the Greek *meta*, meaning "with," and *paradigm*, meaning "pattern;" based on four theoretical concepts of nursing: person, environment, health, and nursing

Metered-dose inhaler (MDI)   a handheld nebulizer, which is a pressurized container of medication that can be used by the client to release the medication through a mouthpiece

Microminerals   a vitamin or mineral

Micturition   *see* Urination

Mid-arm circumference (MAC)   a measure of fat, muscle, and skeleton

Mid-arm muscle circumference (MAMC)   calculated by using reference tables or by using a formula that incorporates the triceps skinfold and the MAC

Middle-level manager   a manager who supervises a number of first-level managers and is responsible for the activities in the departments supervised

Midlevel theories   focus on exploration of concepts such as pain, self-esteem, learning, and hardiness

Midstream urine specimen   *see* Clean-catch specimen

Milliequivalent   one-thousandth of an equivalent, which is the chemical combining power of a substance

Mind modulation   the process by which the brain converts neural messages (thoughts, attitudes, feelings, and emotions) into neurohormonal messenger molecules and communicates them to all body systems that evoke states of health or illness

Minded body   the qualities associated with the mind (including knowledge, emotions and consciousness) are distributed throughout the body

Minerals   a substance found in organic compounds, as inorganic compounds and as free ions

Minim   the basic unit of measure in the apothecary system, equal to 0.0616 mL

Minor surgery   surgery that involves little risk, produces few complications, and is often performed in a "day surgery" facility

Miosis   constricted pupils

Misdemeanor   a legal offense usually punishable by a fine or a short-term jail sentence, or both

Mixed hearing loss   a combination of conduction and sensorineural loss

Mobility   ability to move about freely, easily, and purposefully in the environment

Mode   the score or value that occurs most frequently in a distribution of scores

Modeling   observing the behavior of people who have successfully achieved a goal that one has set for oneself and, through observing, acquiring ideas for behavior and coping strategies

Modern   one's acculturated belief system; the opposite of traditional

Monosaccharides   sugars that are composed of single molecules

Monotheism   belief in the existence of one God

Monounsaturated fatty acids   a fatty acid with one double bond

Moral   relating to right and wrong

Moral behavior   the way a person perceives the requirements necessary for people to live together and how he or she responds to them

Moral development   process of learning to tell the difference between right and wrong and of learning what ought and ought not to be done

Moral rules   specific prescriptions for actions

Morality   a doctrine or system denoting what is right and wrong in conduct, character, or attitude

Mortician   a person trained in the care of the dead; also called an *undertaker*

Motivation   the desire to learn

Mourning   the process through which grief is eventually resolved or altered

Multidisciplinary care plan   a standardized plan that outlines the care required for clients with common, predictable—usually medical—conditions

Music therapy   the behavioral science concerned with the systematic application of music to produce relaxation and desired changes in emotions, behavior, and physiology

Mutual pretense   a type of awareness in which the client, family, and health personnel know that the prognosis is terminal but do not talk about it and make an effort not to raise the subject

Mutual recognition model   a new regulatory model developed by the National Council of State Boards of Nursing (NCSBN), which allows for multistate licensure

Mydriasis   enlarged pupils

Myocardial infarction (MI)   heart attack; cardiac tissue necrosis owing to obstruction of blood flow to the heart

Myocardium   a layer of the heart wall; cardiac muscle cells that form the bulk of the heart and contract with each beat

Myopia   abnormal refraction in which light rays focus in front of the retina (nearsightedness)

Narcolepsy   a condition in which an individual experiences an uncontrollable desire for sleep or attacks of sleep during the day

Narrative charting   a descriptive record of client data and nursing interventions, written in sentences and paragraphs

Nasoenteric tube   a tube inserted through one of the nostrils, down the nasopharynx, and into the alimentary tract

Nasogastric tube   a tube inserted by way of the nasopharynx and placed into the client's stomach for the purpose of feeding the client or to remove gastric secretions

Naturopathy   practice that focuses on nutrition, herbs, homeopathy, acupuncture, hydrotherapy, physical medicine, counseling, and minor surgical interventions

Negative feedback   feedback that inhibits change

Negligence   failure to behave in a reasonable and prudent manner; an unintentional tort

Nerve block   chemical interruption of a nerve pathway effected by injecting a local anesthetic

Network   linkages

Networking   a process by which people develop linkages throughout the profession to communicate, share ideas and information, and offer support and direction to each other

Neurectomy   surgery in which peripheral or cranial nerves are interrupted to alleviate localized pain

Neurogenic bladder   interference with the normal mechanisms of urine elimination in which the client does not perceive bladder fullness and is unable to control the urinary sphincters; the result of impaired neurologic function

Neuropathic pain   the result of a disturbance of the peripheral or central nervous system that results in pain that may or may not be associated with an ongoing tissue-damaging process

Neuropeptides   amino acid messenger molecules produced at various sites throughout the body

Neutral question   a question that does not direct or pressure a client to answer in a certain way

Nitrogen balance   a measure of the degree of protein anabolism and catabolism; net result of intake and loss of nitrogen

Nociception   the physiologic processes related to pain perception

Nociceptor   a pain receptor

Nocturia   voiding two or more times at night

Nocturnal emissions   orgasm and emission of semen during sleep

Nocturnal enuresis   involuntary urination at night

Nocturnal frequency   the need for older adults to arise during the night to urinate

Nondirective interview   an interview using open-ended questions and empathetic responses to build rapport and learn client concerns

Nondirective leader   *see* Laissez-faire (nondirective, permissive) leader

Nonessential amino acids   an amino acid that the body can manufacture

Nonmaleficence   the duty to do no harm

Nonspecific defenses   bodily defenses that protect a person against all microorganisms, regardless of prior exposure

Nonsteroidal anti-inflammatory drugs (NSAIDs)   drugs that relieve pain by acting on the peripheral nerve endings to inhibit the formation of the prostaglandins that tend to sensitize nerves to painful stimuli; have analgesic, antipyretic, and anti-inflammatory effects; include aspirin and ibuprofen

Nonverbal communication   communication other than words, including gestures, posture and facial expressions

Norm   an ideal or fixed standard; an expected standard of behavior of group members

Normocephalic   normal head size

Normocephaly   normal head circumference at birth; usually 35 cm (14 in)

Nosocomial infections   infections associated with the delivery of health care services in a health care facility

NPO   from the Latin *nil per os* meaning "nothing by mouth"

NREM (non-REM) sleep   a deep restful sleep rate; also called *slow wave sleep*

Nuclear family   a family of parents and their offspring

Nurse informaticist   an expert who combines computer, information, and nursing science to develop policies and procedures that promote effective use of computerized records by nurses and other health care professionals

Nursing   the attributes, characteristics, and actions of the nurse providing care on behalf of, or in conjunction with, the client

Nursing diagnosis   the nurse's clinical judgment about individual, family, or community responses to actual and potential health problems/life

processes to provide the basis for selecting nursing interventions to achieve outcomes for which the nurse is accountable

Nursing ethics   ethical issues that occur in nursing practice

Nursing informatics   the science of using computer information systems in the practice of nursing

Nursing intervention   any treatment, based on clinical judgment and knowledge, that a nurse performs to enhance patient/client outcomes

Nursing Interventions Classification (NIC)   a taxonomy of nursing actions each of which includes a label, a definition, and a list of activities

Nursing leadership   purposes include (a) improving the health status of individuals or families, (b) increasing the effectiveness and level of satisfaction among professional colleagues, and (c) improving the attitudes of citizens and legislators toward the nursing profession and their expectations of it

Nursing orders   instructions written on the care plan to direct the specific nursing activities that help the client achieve desired outcomes/goals

Nursing Outcomes Classification (NOC)   a taxonomy for describing client outcomes that respond to nursing interventions

Nursing process   a systematic rational method of planning and providing nursing care

Nutrients   organic or inorganic substances found in food

Nutrition   the sum of all interactions between an organism and the food it consumes

Nutritive value   the nutrient content of a specified amount of food

Obese body   (obesity) weight greater than 20% of the ideal for height and frame

Objective data   information (data) that is detectable by an observer or can be tested against an accepted standard; can be seen, heard, felt, or smelled

Obligatory losses   essential fluid losses required to maintain body functioning

Occult blood   hidden blood

Occupational exposure   skin, eye, mucous membrane, or parenteral contact with blood or other potentially infectious materials that may result from the performance of an employee's duties

Official name   the name under which a drug is listed in one of the official publications (e.g., the *United States Pharmacopeia*)

Oils   lipids that are liquid at room temperature

Oliguria   production of abnormally small amounts of urine by the kidney

Oncotic pressure   *see* colloid osmotic pressure

One-point discrimination   the ability to sense whether one or two areas of the skin are being stimulated by pressure

Online   connected to a computer network

Onset of action   the time after drug administration when the body initially responds to the drug

Open awareness   a type of awareness in which a client and people around know about the impending death

Open system   system in which energy, matter, and information move into and out of the system through the system boundary

Open-ended questions   questions that specify only the broad topic to be discussed and invite clients to discover and explore their thoughts and feelings about the topic

Operational definitions   definitions that specify the instruments or procedures by which concepts will be measured

Ophthalmic   referring to the eye

Opportunistic pathogen   a microorganism causing disease only in a susceptible individual

Oral   referring to the mouth

Organizing   determining responsibilities, communicating expectations, and establishing the chain of command for authority and communication

Orgasmic disorder   a difficulty or inability to achieve orgasm in spite of stimulation and arousal

Orgasmic phase   part of the response cycle, the involuntary climax of sexual tension, accompanied by physiologic and psychologic release

Orthopnea   ability to breathe only when in an upright position (sitting or standing)

Orthopneic position   a sitting position that relieves respiratory difficulty; the client leans over and is supported by an overbed table across the lap

Orthostatic hypotension   decrease in blood pressure related to positional or postural changes from lying to sitting or standing positions

Osmolality   the concentration of solutes in body fluids

Osmosis   passage of a solvent through a semipermeable membrane from an area of lesser solute concentration to one of greater solute concentration

Osmotic pressure   pressure exerted by the number of nondiffusible particles in a solution; the amount of pressure needed to stop the flow of water across a membrane

Ossicles   the three middle ear bones of sound transmission

Osteoporosis   demineralization of the bone

Ostomy   a suffix denoting the formation of an opening or outlet such as an opening on the abdominal wall for the elimination of feces or urine

Otic   referring to the ear

Otoscope   an instrument used to examine the ears

Outcome evaluation   focuses on demonstrable changes in the client's health status as result of nursing care

Output   energy, matter, or information from a system given out by the system as a result of its processes

Overhydration   occurs when water is gained in excess of electrolytes, resulting in low serum osmolality and low serum sodium levels, also known as *hypo-osmolar imbalance* or *water intoxication*

Overnutrition   a caloric intake in excess of daily energy requirements, resulting in storage of energy in the form of adipose tissue

Overt data   *see* Objective data

Overweight   a BMI of 26–30 kg/m^2

Oxyhemoglobin   the compound of oxygen and hemoglobin

Pace   number of steps taken per minute or the distance taken in one step when walking

Packing   filling an open wound or cavity with a material such as gauze

Pain   whatever the experiencing person says it is, existing whenever he or she says it does

Pain reaction   the autonomic nervous system and behavioral responses to pain

Pain sensation   can be considered the same as pain threshold

Pain threshold   the amount of pain stimulation a person requires before feeling pain

Pain tolerance   the maximum amount and duration of pain that an individual is willing to endure

Palliative care   symptom care of clients for whom disease no longer responds to cure-focused treatment

Pallor   the absence of underlying red tones in the skin; may be most readily seen in the buccal mucosa

Palpation   the examination of the body using the sense of touch

Papanicolaou (Pap) test   a method of taking a sample of cervical cells for microscopic examination to detect malignancy

Paradigm   a pattern of shared understandings and assumptions about reality and the world

Parasites   microorganisms that live in or on another from which it obtains nourishment

Parasomnia   a cluster or pattern of waking behavior that appears during sleep, such as somnambulism (sleepwalking), sleeptalking, and enuresis (bed-wetting)

Parenteral   drug administration occurring outside the alimentary tract; injected into the body through some route other than the alimentary canal (e.g., intramuscularly)

Parotitis   inflammation of the parotid salivary gland

Partial pressure   the pressure exerted by each individual gas in a mixture according to its percentage concentration in the mixture

Partially complete proteins   proteins that contain less than the required amount of one or more essential amino acids; cannot alone support continued growth

Participative leader   *see* Democratic leader

Passive euthanasia   allowing a person to die by withholding or withdrawing measures to maintain life

Passive immunity   a resistance of the body to infection in which the host receives natural or artificial antibodies produced by another source

Passive ROM exercises   another person moves each of a client's joints through its complete range of movement, maximally stretching all muscle groups within each plane over each joint

Pathogenicity   the ability to produce disease; a *pathogen* is a microorganism that causes disease

Pathologic fractures   spontaneous fractures to which elderly persons are prone

Patient   a person who is waiting for or undergoing medical treatment and care

Patient Self-Determination Act (PSDA)   legislation requiring that every competent adult be informed in writing on admission to a health care institution about his or her rights to accept or refuse medical care and to use advance directives

Patient-controlled analgesia (PCA)   a pain management technique that allows the client to take an active role in managing pain

Patient-focused care   delivery model that brings all services and care providers to the client

Peak level   indicates the highest concentration of the drug in the blood serum

Peak plasma level   the concentration of a drug in the blood plasma that occurs when the elimination rate equals the rate of absorption

Pedagogy   the discipline concerned with helping children learn

Pediculosis   infestation with head lice

Peer groups   assume great importance and have a number of functions: provides a sense of belonging, pride, social learning, and sexual roles; most peer groups have well-defined, sex-specific modes of acceptable behavior and in adolescence, the peer groups change with age

Penrose drain   a flexible rubber drain

Perceived loss   the loss experienced by a person that cannot be verified by others

Perception   the ability to interpret the environment through the senses

Percutaneous   through the skin

Percussion   a method in which the body surface is struck to elicit sounds that can be heard or vibrations that can be felt

Percutaneous endoscopic gastrostomy (PEG)   feeding catheter inserted into the stomach through the skin and subcutaneous tissues of the abdomen

Percutaneous endoscopic jejunostomy (PEJ)   feeding catheter inserted into the jejunum through the skin and subcutaneous tissues of the abdomen

Perfusion   passage of blood constituents through the vessels of the circulatory system

Pericardium   double layer of fibroserous membrane of the heart; the parietal, or outermost, pericardium serves to protect the heart and anchor it to surrounding structures

Peridural anesthesia   *see* Epidural anesthesia

Periodontal disease   disorder of the supporting structures of the teeth

Perioperative period   refers to the three phases of surgery: preoperative, intraoperative, and postoperative

Peripheral pulse   a pulse located in the periphery of the body (e.g., foot, wrist)

Peripheral vascular resistance (PVR)   impedance or opposition to blood flow to the tissues; determined by viscosity, or thickness, of the blood; blood vessel length; blood vessel diameter

Peripherally inserted central venous catheter (PICC)   catheter inserted in the basilic or cephalic vein just above or below the antecubital space

Peripherals   at the edge or outward boundary

Peristalsis   wavelike movements produced by circular and longitudinal muscle fibers of the intestinal walls; the movement propels the intestinal contents onward

Permissive leader *see* Laissez-faire (nondirective, permissive) leader

Personal computers (PCs) individual microcomputer systems referred to as a desktop, portable, laptop, notebook, or handheld computer

Personal space the distance people prefer in interactions with others

Personal values values internalized from the society or culture in which one lives

Personality the outward expression of the inner self

PES format the three essential components of nursing diagnostic statements including the terms describing the problem, the etiology of the problem, and the defining characteristics or cluster of signs and symptoms

pH a measure of the relative alkalinity or acidity of a solution; a measure of the concentration of hydrogen ions

Phagocytes cells that ingest microorganisms, other cells, and foreign particles

Phagocytosis the process by which cells engulf microorganisms, other cells, or foreign particles

Phantom pain pain that remains after the perceived location has been removed, such as pain perceived in a foot after the leg has been amputated

Pharmacist a person licensed to prepare and dispense drugs and prescriptions

Pharmacodynamics the process by which a drug alters cell physiology

Pharmacokinetics the study of the absorption, distribution, biotransformation, and excretion of drugs

Pharmacology the scientific study of the actions of drugs on living animals and humans

Pharmacopoeia a book containing a list of drug products used in medicine, including their descriptions and formulas

Pharmacy the art of preparing, compounding, and dispensing drugs; also refers to the place where drugs are prepared and dispensed

Phenomenology research that investigates people's life experiences and how they interpret those experiences

Philosophy an early effort to define phenomena that serves as the basis for later theoretical formulations

Phlebotomist a person from a laboratory who performs venipuncture, collecting the blood specimen for the tests ordered by the physician

Physical activity bodily movement produced by skeletal muscles that requires energy expenditure and produces progressive health benefits

Physical restraints any manual method or physical or mechanical device, material, or equipment attached to the client's body that restrict the client's movement

Physiologic dependence biochemical changes occurring in the body as a result of excessive use of a drug

PIE an acronym for a charting model that follows a recording sequence of problems, interventions, and evaluation of the effectiveness of the interventions

Pinna *see* Auricle

Pitch the frequency or number of vibrations heard during auscultation

Pitting edema edema in which firm finger pressure on the skin produces an indentation (pit) that remains for several seconds

Placebo any form of treatment (e.g., medication) that produces an effect in the client because of its intent rather than its chemical or physical properties

Placenta a flat, disc-shaped organ that is highly vascular and normally forms in the upper segment of the endometrium of the uterus; exchanges nutrients and gases between the fetus and the mother

Plaintiff a person claiming infringement of legal rights by one or more persons

Planned change an intended, purposive attempt by an individual, group, organization, or larger social system to influence its own status quo or that of another organism or situation

Planning an ongoing process that involves (a) assessing a situation, (b) establishing goals and objectives based on assessment of a situation or future trends, and (c) developing a plan of action that identifies priorities, delineates who is responsible, determines deadlines, and describes how the intended outcome is to be achieved and evaluated

Plantar wart a wart on the sole of the foot

Plaque an invisible soft film consisting of bacteria, molecules of saliva, and remnants of epithelial cells and leukocytes that adhere to the enamel surface of teeth

Plasma the fluid portion of the blood in which the blood cells are suspended

Plateau a maintained concentration of a drug in the plasma during a series of scheduled doses

Pleximeter in percussion, the middle finger of the nondominant hand placed firmly on the client's skin

Plexor in percussion, the middle finger of the dominant hand or a percussion hammer used to strike the pleximeter

Pneumothorax collection of air in the pleural space

Point of maximal impulse (PMI) the point where the apex of the heart touches the anterior chest wall

Policies rules developed to govern the handling of frequently occurring situations

Polycythemia a condition in which clients with chronic hypoxia may develop higher than normal counts of red blood cells

Polydipsia excessive thirst

Polypnea abnormally fast respirations

Polysaccharides a branched chain of dozens, sometimes hundreds, of glucose molecules; starches

Polysomnography a cluster or pattern of waking behavior that appears during sleep, such as somnambulism (sleepwalking), sleeptalking, and enuresis (bed-wetting)

Polytheism the belief in more than one God

Polyunsaturated fatty acids fatty acid with more than one double bond (or many carbons not bonded to a hydrogen atom)

Polyuria *see* Diuresis

Population includes all possible members of a group who meet the criteria for a study

Positive feedback feedback that stimulates change

Positive reinforcement giving rewards such as praise for a learner's achievements

Positron emission tomography (PET) a noninvasive radiologic study that involves the injection or inhalation of a radioisotope

Possible nursing diagnosis one in which evidence about a health problem is incomplete or unclear

Postmortem examination *see* Autopsy

Postoperative phase begins with the admission of the client to the postanesthesia area and ends when healing is complete

Postural drainage the drainage, by gravity, of secretions from various lung segments

Potentiating effect the increased effect of one or both drugs

Power capacity to influence another person in some way or to produce change

Practice discipline field of study in which the central focus is performance of professional role (nursing, teaching, management, making music)

Prayer human communication with divine and spiritual entities

Preceptor an experienced nurse who assists the novice nurse in improving nursing skill and judgment

Precontemplation stage a person typically denies having a problem and instead views others as having a problem and therefore wants to change the other person's behavior

Precordium an area of the chest overlying the heart

Preemptive analgesia the administration of analgesics prior to an invasive or operative procedure in order to treat pain before it occurs

Preferred provider arrangements (PPAs) similar to PPOs, but PPAs can contract with individual health care providers; the plan can be limited or unlimited

Preferred provider organization (PPO) a group of physicians or a hospital that provides companies with health services at a discounted rate

Prefilled unit-dose system   injectable medications that are disposable and are available as (a) prefilled syringes ready for use or (b) prefilled sterile cartridges and needles that require the attachment of a reusable holder (injection system) before use

Prejudice   a negative belief or preference that is generalized about a group and that leads to "prejudgment"

Preload   the degree to which muscle fibers in the ventricle are stretched at the end of diastole

Preoperative phase   begins when the decision to have surgery is made and ends when the client is transferred to the operating table

Preparation stage   occurs when the person undertakes cognitive and behavioral activities that prepare the person for change

Presbycusis   loss of hearing related to aging

Presbyopia   loss of elasticity of the lens and thus loss of ability to see close objects as a result of the aging process

Prescription   the written direction for the preparation and administration of a drug

Presencing   being present, being there, or just being with a client

Pressure   a compressing downward force on a body area

Pressure ulcers   any lesion caused by unrelieved pressure that results in damage to underlying tissue; formerly called decubitus ulcers, bed sores, pressure sores

Primary care (PC)   the point of entry into the health care system at which initial health care is given

Primary health care (PHC)   essential health care based on practical, scientifically sound and socially acceptable methods and technology made universally accessible to individuals and families in the community through their full participation and at a cost that the community and country can afford to maintain at every stage of their development in the spirit of self-reliance and self-determination

Primary intention healing   tissue surfaces are approximated (closed) and there is minimal or no tissue loss, formation of minimal granulation tissue and scarring

Primary prevention   activities directed toward the protection from or avoidance of potential health risks

Primary sexual characteristics   relate to the organs necessary for reproduction, such as the testes, penis, vagina, and uterus

Primary sleep disorders   the person's sleep problem is the main disorder; include insomnia, hypersomnia, narcolepsy, sleep apnea, and sleep deprivation

Principles-based (deontological) theories   emphasize individual rights, duties, and obligations

Priority setting   the process of establishing a preferential order for nursing strategies

Private (civil) law   the body of law that deals with relationships between private individuals

Prn order   "as needed order"; permits the nurse to give a medication when, in the nurse's judgment, the client requires it

Problem solving   obtaining information that clarifies the nature of the problem and suggests possible solutions

Problem-oriented medical record (POMR)   data about the client are recorded and arranged according to the client's problems, rather than according to the source of the information

Problem-oriented record (POR)   see Problem-oriented medical record (POMR)

Procedures   steps used in carrying out policies or activities

Process evaluation   a component of quality assurance that focuses on how care was given

Process recording   the verbatim (word-for-word) account of a conversation

Proctoscopy   the viewing of the rectum

Proctosigmoidoscopy   the viewing of the rectum and sigmoid colon

Productivity   in health care, frequently measured by the amount of nursing resources used per client or in terms of required versus actual hours of care provided

Profession   an occupation that requires extensive education or a calling that requires special knowledge, skill, and preparation

Professional values   values acquired during socialization into nursing from codes of ethics, nursing experiences, teachers, and peers

Professionalism   a set of attributes, a way of life that implies responsibility and commitment

Professionalization   the process of becoming professional; acquiring characteristics considered to be professional

Progress notes   chart entries made by a variety of methods and by all health professionals involved in a client's care for the purpose of describing a client's problems, treatments, and progress toward desired outcomes

Prompted voiding   supplements habit training by encouraging the client to try to use the toilet (prompting) and reminding the client when to void

Prone position   face-lying position, with or without a small pillow

Proprioceptors   sensory receptors that are sensitive to movement and the position of the body

Protein-calorie malnutrition   problem of clients with long-term deficiencies in caloric intake; characteristics include depressed visceral proteins (e.g., albumin), weight loss, and visible muscle and fat wasting

Protocols   a predetermined and preprinted plan specifying the procedure to be followed in a particular situation

Proxemics   the study of distance between people in their interactions

Psychologic dependence   a state of emotional reliance on a drug to maintain one's well-being; a feeling of need or craving for a drug

Psychologic homeostasis   emotional or psychologic balance or state of mental well-being

Psychomotor domain   the "skill" domain; includes motor skills such as giving an injection

Psychoneuroimmunology   area of study in mind–body research that focuses on the relationships among stress, the immune system, and health outcomes

Puberty   the first stage of adolescence in which sexual organs begin to grow and mature

Public law   refers to the body of law that deals with relationships between individuals and the government and governmental agencies

Pulse   the wave of blood within an artery that is created by contraction of the left ventricle of the heart

Pulse deficit   the difference between the apical pulse and the radial pulse

Pulse oximeter   a noninvasive device that measures the arterial blood oxygen saturation by means of a sensor attached to the finger

Pulse pressure   the difference between the systolic and the diastolic blood pressure

Pulse rhythm   the pattern of the beats and intervals between the beats

Pulse volume   the strength or amplitude of the pulse, the force of blood exerted with each heart beat

Pureed diet   a modification of the soft diet; liquid may be added to the food, which is then blended to a semisolid consistency

Purkinje fibers   fibers of the ventricular conduction pathways that terminate in ventricular muscle, stimulating contraction

Purulent exudates   an exudate consisting of leukocytes, liquefied dead tissue debris, and dead and living bacteria

Pus   a thick liquid associated with inflammation and composed of cells, liquid, microorganisms, and tissue debris

Pyogenic bacteria   bacteria that produce pus

Pyorrhea   purulent periodontal disease

Pyrexia   a body temperature above the normal range, fever

Qi   body's vital energy reflexology

Qualifiers   words that have been added to some NANDA labels to give additional meaning to the diagnostic statement

Quality   a subjective description of a sound (e.g., whistling, gurgling)

Quality improvement   an organizational commitment and approach used to continuously improve all processes in the organization with the goal of meeting and exceeding customer expectations and outcomes; also known as total quality management (TQM) and continuous quality improvement (CQI)

Quality-assurance (QA) program   an ongoing systematic process designed to evaluate and promote excellence in the health care provided to clients

Race   classification of people according to shared biologic characteristics and physical features

Radiating pain   pain perceived at the source and in surrounding or nearby tissues

Radiation   the transfer of heat from the surface of one object to the surface of another without contact between the two objects

Radiopharmaceutical   a pharmaceutical (targeted to a specific organ) labeled with a radioisotope, administered through various routes, to determine hyperfuction or hypofunction of the organ

Random access memory (RAM)   data and instructions stored on chips; RAM storage is temporary and lost when the computer is turned off

Range   a measure of variability, consisting of the difference between the highest and lowest values in a distribution of scores

Range of motion (ROM)   the degree of movement possible for each joint

Rapid ejaculation   when a man is unable to delay ejaculation long enough to satisfy his partner

Rapport   a relationship between two or more people of mutual trust and understanding

Rationale   the scientific reason for selecting a specific action

RBC indices   may be performed as part of the CBC to evaluate the size, weight, and hemoglobin concentration of red blood cells

Retrograde pyelography   a radiographic study used to evaluate the urinary tract

Reactive hyperemia   a bright red flush on the skin occurring after pressure is relieved

Readiness   behaviors or cues that reflect a learner's motivation to learn at a specific time

Read-only memory (ROM)   program and information stored on chips that cannot be altered by the user

Reagent   substance used in a chemical reaction to detect a specific substance

Recent memory   deals with activities of the recent past of minutes to a few hours

Reconstitution   the technique of adding a solvent to a powdered drug to prepare it for injection

Record   a written communication providing formal, legal documentation of a client's progress

Recording   the process of making written entries about a client on the medical record

Referent power   the power associated with the admiration and respect for a leader because of that leader's charisma and success

Referred pain   pain perceived to be in one area but whose source is another area

Reflex   an automatic response of the body to a stimulus

Reflexology   a treatment based on massage of the feet to relieve symptoms in other parts of the body

Reflux   backward flow

Regeneration   renewal, regrowth, the replacement of destroyed tissue cells by cells that are identical or similar in structure and function

Regional anesthesia   the temporary interruption of the transmission of nerve impulses to and from a specific area or region of the body; the client loses sensation in an area of the body but remains conscious

Regression   a defense mechanism in which one adapts behavior that was comforting earlier in life to overcome the discomfort and insecurity of the present situation

Regurgitation   the spitting up or backward flow of undigested food

Reiki   a Japanese word meaning "universal life-force-energy." In this therapy, the practitioner places the hands on the client and energy flows from one to the other

Relapsing fever   the occurrence of short febrile periods of a few days interspersed with periods of 1 or 2 days of normal temperature

Relationship-based (caring) theories   stress courage, generosity, commitment, and the need to nurture and maintain relationships

Reliability   the degree to which an instrument produces consistent results on repeated use

Religion   an organized system of worship

REM sleep   sleep during which the person experiences rapid eye movements

Remission   a period during a chronic illness when there is a lessening of severity or cessation of symptoms

Remittent fever   the occurrence of a wide range of temperature fluctuations (more than 2C (3.6F) over the 24-hour period, all of which are above normal

Renin-angiotensin-aldosterone system   system initiated by specialized receptors in the juxtaglomerular cells of the kidney nephrons that respond to changes in renal perfusion

Report   whether oral or written, it should be concise, including pertinent information but no extraneous detail

Repression   a defense mechanism in which painful thoughts, experiences, and impulses are removed from awareness

Res ipsa loquitur   "the thing that speaks for itself"; a legal doctrine that relates to negligence in which the harm cannot be traced to a specific health care provider or standard but does not normally occur unless there has been a negligent act

Researchability   the problem can be subjected to scientific investigation

Reservoir   a source of microorganisms

Resident flora   microorganisms that normally reside on the skin, mucous membranes, and inside the respiratory and gastrointestinal tracts

Residual urine   the amount of urine remaining in the bladder after a person voids

Resolution phase   the part of the response cycle period of return to the unaroused state, which may last 10 to 15 minutes after orgasm, or longer if there is no orgasm

Resonance   a low-pitched, hollow sound produced over normal lung tissue when the chest is percussed

Respiration   the act of breathing; transport of oxygen from the atmosphere to the body cells and transport of carbon dioxide from the cells to the atmosphere

Respiratory acidosis   (hypercapnia) a state of excess carbon dioxide in the body

Respiratory alkalosis   a state of excessive loss of carbon dioxide from the body

Respiratory character   *see* Respiratory quality

Respiratory membrane   where gas exchange occurs between the air on the alveolar side and the blood on the capillary side; the alveolar and capillary walls form the respiratory membrane

Respiratory quality   refers to those aspects of breathing that are different from normal, effortless breathing, includes the amount of effort exerted to breathe and the sounds produced by breathing

Respiratory rhythm   refers to the regularity of the expirations and the inspirations

Respondeat superior   a legal term meaning "let the master answer"; the employer assumes responsibility for the conduct of the employee and can also be held responsible for malpractice by the employee

Responsibility   the specific accountability or liability associated with the performance of duties of a particular role

Rest   calmness, relaxation without emotional stress, and freedom from anxiety

Resting energy expenditure (REE)   the amount of energy required to maintain basic body functions

Resting tremor   a tremor that is apparent when the client is at rest and diminishes with activity

Restraints   protective devices used to limit physical activity of the client or a part of the client's body

Retarded ejaculation   the inability to ejaculate into the vagina, or a delayed ejaculation of semen

Review of systems   *see* Screening examination

Reward power power based on the incentives a leader can offer

Rhizotomy interruption of the anterior or posterior nerve root between the ganglion and the cord; generally performed on cervical nerve roots to alleviate pain of the head and neck

Right (legal) a privilege or fundamental power to which an individual is entitled unless it is revoked by law or given up voluntarily

Right of self-determination subjects feel free from constraints, coercion, or any undue influence to participate in a study

Rigor mortis the stiffening of the body that occurs after death

Risk factors factors that cause a client to be vulnerable to developing a health problem

Risk management having in place a system to reduce danger to clients and staff

Risk nursing diagnosis clinical judgment that a problem does not exist, but the presence of risk factors indicates that a problem is likely to develop unless nurses intervene

Risk of harm exposure to the possibility of injury going beyond everyday situations

Role the set of expectations about how a person occupying a specific position behaves

Role ambiguity unclear role expectations; people do not know what to do or how to do it and are unable to predict the reactions of others to their behavior

Role conflict a clash between the beliefs or behaviors imposed by two or more roles fulfilled by one person

Role development involves socialization into a particular role

Role mastery performance of role behaviors that meet social expectations

Role performance what a person does in a particular role in relation to the behaviors expected of that role

Role strain a generalized state of frustration or anxiety experienced with the stress of role conflict and ambiguity

S₁ the first heart sound; occurs when the atrioventricular valves (mitral and tricuspid) close

S₂ the second heart sound; occurs when the semilunar valves (aortic and pulmonic) close

Safety monitoring device a position-sensitive switch that triggers an audio alarm when a client attempts to get out of the bed or chair

Sairy Gamp a character in the Charles Dickens book *Martin Chizzlewit* who represented the negative image of nurses in the early 1800s

Saliva the clear liquid secreted by the salivary glands in the mouth, sometimes referred to as *spit*

Sample segment of the population from whom data will actually be collected

Sanguineous exudate an exudate containing large amounts of red blood cells

Saturated fatty acids those in which all carbon atoms are filled to capacity (i.e., saturated) with hydrogen

Scabies a contagious skin infestation caused by an arachnid, the itch mite

Scald a burn from a hot liquid or vapor, such as steam

Scientific health belief based on the belief that life and life processes are controlled by physical and biochemical processes that can be manipulated by humans

Screening examination (review of systems) a brief review of essential functioning of various body parts or systems

Scrub nurses nurses who assist surgeons

Sebaceous glands active under the influence of androgens in both males and females, which secrete sebum and become most active on the face, neck, shoulder, upper back, and chest; are often the cause of an increased incidence of acne

Sebum the oily, lubricating secretion of sebaceous glands in the skin

Secondary intention healing wound in which the tissue surfaces are not approximated and there is extensive tissue loss; formation of excessive granulation tissue and scarring

Secondary prevention activities designed for early diagnosis and treatment of disease or illness

Secondary sexual characteristics physical characteristics that differentiate the male from the female but do not relate directly to reproduction

Secondary sleep disorders sleep disturbance caused by another clinical disorder

Seizure a sudden onset of a convulsion or other paroxysmal motor or sensory activity

Seizure precautions safety measures taken by the nurse to protect clients from injury should they have a seizure

Selectively permeable cell membranes that allow substances to move across them with varying degrees of ease

Self-concept the collection of ideas, feelings, and beliefs one has about oneself

Self-esteem the value one has for oneself; self-confidence

Self-regulation homeostatic mechanisms that come into play automatically in the healthy person

Semicircular canals in the inner ear; contain the organs of equilibrium

Semi-Fowler's position *see* Low Fowler's position

Semilunar valves crescent moon-shaped valves between the cardiac ventricles and the pulmonary artery (pulmonic valve) and the aorta (aortic valve)

Sensorineural hearing loss the result of damage to the inner ear, the auditory nerve, or the hearing center in the brain

Sensoristasis the need for sensory stimulation

Sensory deficit partial or complete impairment of any sensory organ

Sensory deprivation insufficient sensory stimulation for a person to function

Sensory memory momentary perception of stimuli by the senses

Sensory overload an overabundance of sensory stimulation

Sensory perception the organization and translation of stimuli into meaningful information

Sensory reception process of receiving environmental stimuli

Separation anxiety the fear and frustration experienced by young children that comes with parental absences

Sepsis the presence of pathogenic organisms or their toxins in the blood or body tissues

Septicemia occurs when bacteremia results in systemic infection

Septum a dividing structure such as that between the cardiac chambers or between the two sides of the nose

Serous exudates inflammatory material composed of serum (clear portion of blood) derived from the blood and serous membranes of the body such as the peritoneum, pleura, pericardium, and meninges; watery in appearance and has few cells

Serum osmolality a measure of the solute concentration of the blood

Sex the term most commonly used to identify biologic male or female status

Sexual arousal disorder when a woman is unable to attain or maintain adequate vaginal lubrication and/or has decreased clitoral and labial sensations

Sexual health the integration of the somatic, emotional, intellectual, and social aspects of sexuality, in ways that are positively enriching and that enhance personality, communication, and love

Sexual orientation the preference of a person for one sex or the other

Sexual pain disorders include dyspareunia, vaginismus, and genital pain

Sexual self-concept how one values oneself as a sexual being

Sexuality the collective characteristics that mark the differences between the male and female, the constitution and life of the individual as related to sex

Shaft the part of a needle that is attached to the hub

Shaken baby syndrome (SBS) violent shaking of the infant by the arms or shoulders causing a whiplash, which can lead to severe injury in infants

Shared governance a method that aims to distribute decision making among a group of people

Shared leadership a contemporary theory of leadership that recognizes the leadership capabilities of each member in a professional group and assumes that appropriate leadership will emerge in relation to the challenges that confront the group

Shearing force a combination of friction and pressure that, when applied to the skin, results in damage to the blood vessels and tissues

Shock phase first part of the alarm reaction in which the stressor may be perceived consciously or unconsciously by the person

Short-term memory information held in the brain for immediate use or what one has in mind at a given moment

Shroud a large piece of plastic or cotton material used to enclose a body after death

Side effect the secondary effect of a drug that is unintended; usually predictable and may be either harmless or potentially harmful

Significance the potential to contribute to nursing science by enhancing client care, testing or generating a theory, or resolving a day-to-day clinical problem

Signs *see* Overt data

Sims' position side-lying position with lowermost arm behind the body and uppermost leg flexed

Single order common medication order that is a "one-time order"; medication is to be given once at a specified time

Sinoatrial (SA or sinus) node the primary pacemaker of the heart located where the superior vena cava enters the right atrium

Situational leader adapts style according to consideration of the staff members' abilities, knowledge of the nature of the task to be done, and sensitivity to the context or environment in which the task takes place

Sitz bath used to soak a client's pelvic area; also referred to as a *hip bath*

Skinfold measurement an indicator of the amount of body fat, the main form of stored energy

Slander defamation by the spoken word, stating unprivileged (not legally protected) or false words by which a reputation is damaged

Sleep an altered state of consciousness in which the individual's perception of and reaction to the environment are decreased

Sleep apnea periodic cessation of breathing during sleep

Sleep deprivation a syndrome caused by decreases in amount, quality, and consistency of sleep; produces a variety of physiologic and behavioral symptoms, the severity of which depend on the degree of deprivation

Small calorie (c, cal) the amount of heat required to raise the temperature of 1 g of water 1C

SOAP an acronym for a charting method that follows a recording sequence of subjective data, objective data, assessment, and planning

Socialization a process by which a person learns the ways of a group or society in order to become a functioning participant

Socratic questioning a technique one can use to look beneath the surface, recognize and examine assumptions, search for inconsistencies, examine multiple points of view, and differentiate what one knows from what one merely believes

Sojourner Truth an abolitionist, Underground Railroad agent, preacher, and women's rights advocate, she was a nurse for more than 4 years during the Civil War and worked as a nurse and counselor for the Freedman's Relief Association after the war

Solutes substances dissolved in a liquid

Solvent the liquid in which a solute is dissolved

Sordes accumulation of foul matter (food, microorganisms, and epithelial elements) on the teeth and gums

Source-oriented clinical record a record in which each person or department makes notations in a separate section or sections of the client's chart

Spastic describing the sudden, prolonged involuntary muscle contractions of clients with damage to the central nervous system

Specific antagonists drugs that have no special pharmacologic action of their own but that inhibit or prevent the action of an agonist

Specific (immune) defenses immune functions directed against identifiable bacteria, viruses, fungi, or other infectious agents

Specific gravity the weight or degree of concentration of a substance compared with that of an equal volume of another, such as distilled water, taken as a standard

Specific self-esteem how much one approves of a certain part of oneself

Spinal anesthesia anesthesia produced by injecting an anesthetic agent into the subarachnoid space surrounding the spinal cord; also referred to as a *subarachnoid block (SAB)*

Spinal cord stimulation (SCS) involves the insertion of a cable that allows the placement of an electrode directly on the spinal cord and is used with nonmalignant pain that has not been controlled with less invasive therapies

Spiritual distress a disturbance in or a challenge to a person's belief or value system that provides strength, hope, and meaning to life

Spiritual health *see* Spiritual well-being

Spiritual well-being a feeling of inner peace and of being generally alive, purposeful, and fulfilled; the feeling is rooted in spiritual values and/or specific religious beliefs

Spirituality belief in or relationship with some higher power, creative force, driving being, or infinite source of energy

Spreadsheet programs that manipulate primarily numbers

Sputum the mucous secretion from the lungs, bronchi, and trachea

Stage of exhaustion the third stage in the GAS and LAS syndromes that occurs when the adaptation that the body made during the second stage cannot be maintained

Stage of resistance the second stage in the GAS and LAS syndromes when the body's adaptation takes place

Standard a generally accepted rule, model, pattern, or measure

Standard deviation the most frequently used measure of variability, indicating the average to which scores deviate from the mean; commonly symbolized as SD or S

Standardized care plan preprinted guides for giving nursing care of clients with common needs (e.g., a nursing diagnosis)

Standards of care detailed guidelines describing the minimal nursing care that can reasonably be expected to ensure high-quality care in a defined situation (e.g., a medical diagnosis or a diagnostic test)

Standards of clinical nursing practice descriptions of the responsibilities for which nurses are accountable

Standing order a written document about policies, rules, regulations, or orders regarding client care; gives nurses the authority to carry out specific actions under certain circumstances

Stapes stirrups bone of the middle ear

Stat order common medication order which indicates that the medication is to be given immediately and only once

Statistically significant term applied after data have been analyzed to determine whether the results had a probability less than 0.05, which is considered the acceptable level of significance

Status epilepticus continuous seizures

Statutory law a law enacted by any legislative body

Steatorrhea an excessive amount of fat in the stool, which can indicate faulty absorption of fat from the small intestine

Stereognosis the ability to recognize objects by touching and manipulating them

Stereotyping assuming that all members of a culture or ethnic group are alike

Sterile field a specified area that is considered free from microorganisms

Sterile technique practices that keep an area or object free of all microorganisms

Sterilization a process that destroys all microorganisms, including spores and viruses

Sternum the breastbone

Stimulus-based stress model stress is defined as a stimulus, life event, or set of circumstances that arouses physiologic and/or psychologic reactions that may increase the individual's vulnerability to illness

Stoma an artificial opening in the abdominal wall; it may be permanent or temporary

Stool *see* Feces

Strabismus squinting or crossing of the eyes; uncoordinated eye movements

Stress   an event or set of circumstances causing a disrupted response; the disruption caused by a noxious stimulus or stressor

Stress electrocardiography   uses ECGs to assess a client's response to an increased cardiac workload during exercise

Stressor   any factor that produces stress or alters the body's equilibrium

Stridor   a harsh, crowing sound made on inhalation caused by constriction of the upper airway

Strike   an organized work stoppage by a group of employees to express a grievance, enforce a demand for changes in condition of employment, or solve a dispute with management

Stroke volume (SV)   the amount of blood ejected with each cardiac contraction

Structure evaluation   focuses on the setting in which care is given

Subarachnoid block (SAB)   *see* Spinal anesthesia

Subculture   usually composed of people who have a distinct identity and yet are related to a larger cultural group

Subcutaneous   beneath the layers of the skin; hypodermic

Subjective data   data that are apparent only to the person affected; can be described or verified only by that person

Sublingual   under the tongue

Subsystems   system components

Suctioning   the aspiration of secretions by a catheter connected to a suction machine or wall outlet

Sudden infant death syndrome (SIDS)   the sudden and unexpected death of an infant

Sudoriferous glands   glands of the dermis that secrete sweat

Superego   the conscience of personality; the source of feelings of guilt, shame, and inhibition

Supine position   *see* Dorsal position

Supplemental Security Income (SSI)   special payments for people with disabilities, those who are blind, and people who are not eligible for Social Security; these payments are not restricted to health care costs

Suppositories   solid, cone-shaped, medicated substances inserted into the rectum, vagina, or urethra

Suppuration   the formation of pus

Suprapubic catheter   catheter inserted through the abdominal wall above the symphysis pubis into the urinary bladder

Suprasystem   the system above another system

Surface anesthesia   *see* Topical anesthesia

Surface temperature   the temperature of tissue, the subcutaneous tissue, and fat

Surfactant   a surface-active agent (e.g., soap or a synthetic detergent); in pulmonary physiology, a mixture of phospholipids secreted by alveolar cells into the alveoli and respiratory air passages that reduces the surface tension of pulmonary fluids and thus contributes to the elastic properties of pulmonary tissue

Surgical asepsis   *see* Sterile technique

Suture   a thread used to sew body tissues together

Sutures   junction lines of the skull bones

Sweat glands   *see* Sudoriferous glands

Sympathectomy   severance of the pathways of the sympathetic division of the autonomic nervous system; eliminates vasospasm, improves peripheral blood supply, and is effective in treating painful vascular disorders

Symptoms   *see* Covert data

Syndrome diagnosis   a diagnosis that is associated with a cluster of other diagnoses

Synergistic effect   *see* Potentiating effect

System   a set of interacting identifiable parts or components

Systemic infection   occurs when pathogens spread and damage different parts of the body

Systole   the period during which the ventricles contract

Systolic pressure   the pressure of the blood against the arterial walls when the ventricles of the heart contract

Tachycardia   an abnormally rapid pulse rate; greater than 100 beats per minute

Tachypnea   abnormally fast respirations; usually more than 24 respirations per minute

Tactile   related to touch

Tartar   a visible, hard deposit of plaque and dead bacteria that forms at the gum lines

Taxonomy   a classification system or set of categories, such as nursing diagnoses, arranged on the basis of a single principle or consistent set of principles

Teacher   a nurse who helps clients learn about their health and the health care procedures they need to perform to restore or maintain their health

Team nursing   the delivery of individualized nursing care to clients by a team led by a professional nurse

Technical skills   "hands-on" skills such as those required to manipulate equipment, administer injections, and move or reposition patients

Telecommunications   the transmission of information from one site to another, using equipment to transmit information in the forms of signs, signals, words, or pictures by cable, radio, or other systems

Telemedicine   technology used to transmit electronic medical data about clients to persons at distant locations

Teratogen   anything that adversely affects normal cellular development in the embryo or fetus

Termination stage   the ultimate goal where the individual has complete confidence that the problem is no longer a temptation or threat

Territoriality   a concept of the space and things that individuals consider their own

Tertiary prevention   activities designed to restore individuals with disabilities to their optimal level of functioning

Theory   a system of ideas that is proposed to explain a given phenomenon (e.g., theory of gravity)

Therapeutic baths   given for physical effects, such as to soothe irritated skin or to treat an area (e.g., the perineum)

Therapeutic communication   an interactive process between nurse and client that helps the client overcome temporary stress, to get along with other people, to adjust to the unalterable, and to overcome psychologic blocks that stand in the way of self-realization

Therapeutic effect   the primary effect intended of a drug; reason the drug is prescribed

Therapeutic touch (TT)   a process by which energy is transmitted or transferred from one person to another with the intent of potentiating the healing process of one who is ill or injured

Third space syndrome   fluid shifts from the vascular space into an area where it is not readily accessible as extracellular fluid

Thoracentesis   insertion of a needle into the pleural cavity for diagnostic or therapeutic purposes

Thrill   a vibrating sensation over a blood vessel that indicates turbulent blood flow

Thrombophlebitis   inflammation of a vein followed by formation of a blood clot

Thrombus   a solid mass of blood constituents in the circulatory system; a clot (*plural:* thrombi)

Throughput   a transformation that occurs after input is absorbed by the system and is then processed in a way that is useful to the system

Ticks   small gray-brown parasites that bite into tissue and suck blood and transmit several diseases to people, in particular Rocky Mountain spotted fever, Lyme disease, and tularemia.

Tidal volume   the volume of air that is normally inhaled and exhaled

Tinea pedis   athlete's foot (ringworm of the foot), which is caused by a fungus

Tissue perfusion   passage of fluid (e.g., blood) through a specific organ or body part

Topical   applied externally (e.g., to the skin or mucous membranes)

Topical anesthesia   (surface anesthesia) applied directly to the skin and mucous membranes, open skin surfaces, wounds, and burns

Torr   millimeters of mercury

Tort a civil wrong committed against a person or a person's property

Tort law law that defines and enforces duties and rights among private individuals that are not based on contractual agreements

Trademark *see* Brand name

Traditional observance of the beliefs and practices of one's heritage or cultural belief system

Traditional Chinese medicine (TCM) based on the premise that the body's vital energy circulates through pathways or meridians and can be accessed and manipulated through specific anatomical points along the surface of the body

Tragus the cartilaginous protrusion at the entrance to the ear canal

Transactional leader a contemporary theory of leadership in which resources are exchanged as an incentive for loyalty and performance

Transactional stress theory a theory that encompasses a set of cognitive, affective, and adaptive (coping) responses that arise out of person–environment transactions; the person and the environment are inseparable and affect each other

Transcellular fluid compartment of extracellular fluids; includes cerebrospinal, pericardial, pancreatic, pleural, intraocular, biliary, peritoneal, and synovial fluids

Transcendence a person's recognition that there is something other or greater than the self and a seeking and valuing of that greater other, whether it is an ultimate being, force, or value

Transcutaneous electrical nerve stimulation (TENS) a noninvasive, nonanalgesic pain control technique that allows the client to assist in the management of acute and chronic pain

Transdermal patch a particular type of topical or dermatologic medication delivery system

Transformational leader leader who fosters creativity, risk-taking, commitment, and collaboration by empowering the group to share in the organization's vision

Translator a person who converts written material (such as patient education pamphlets) from one language into another

Tremor an involuntary trembling of a limb or body part

Trial the period during which all relevant facts are presented to a jury or judge

Triangular fossa a depression of the antihelix

Triglycerides substances that have three fatty acids; they account for more than 90% of the lipids in food and in the body

Trigone a triangular area at the base of the bladder marked by the ureter openings at the posterior corners and the opening of urethra at the anterior corner

Trimesters the three-month periods during pregnancy marking certain landmarks for developmental changes in mother and the fetus; three trimesters occur during a pregnancy

Tripod (triangle) position the proper standing position with crutches; crutches are placed about 15 cm (6 in.) in front of the feet and out laterally about 15 cm (6 in.), creating a wide base of support

Trocar a sharp pointed instrument that fits inside a cannula and is used to pierce body tissues

Troponin enzyme that is released into the blood during a myocardial infarction (MI)

Trough level represents the lowest concentration of a drug in the blood serum

Tuberculin syringe originally designed to administer tuberculin; a narrow syringe, calibrated in tenths and hundredths of a milliliter (up to 1 mL) on one scale and in sixteenths of a minim (up to 1 minim) on the other scale

Two-point discrimination *see* One-point discrimination

Tympanic membrane the eardrum

Tympany a musical or drumlike sound produced during percussion over an air-filled stomach and abdomen

Ultrasonography the use of ultrasound to produce an image of an organ or tissue

Unconscious mind the mental life of a person of which the person is unaware

Undernutrition an intake of nutrients insufficient to meet daily energy requirements because of inadequate food intake or improper digestion and absorption of food

Undertaker *see* Mortician

Universal precautions (UP) techniques to be used with all clients to decrease the risk of transmitting unidentified pathogens; currently, Standard Precautions incorporate UP and BSI

Unplanned change haphazard change that occurs without control by any person or group

Unprofessional conduct one of the grounds for action against the nurse's license; includes incompetence or gross negligence, conviction of practicing without a license, falsification of client records, and illegally obtaining, using, or possessing controlled substances

Unsaturated fatty acid a fatty acid that could accommodate more hydrogen atoms than it currently does

Upper-level (top-level) managers organizational executives who are primarily responsible for establishing goals and developing strategic plans

Urea a substance found in urine, blood, and lymph; the main nitrogenous substance in blood

Urgency the feeling that one must urinate

Urinary frequency the need to urinate often

Urinary hesitancy a delay and difficulty in initiating voiding; often associated with dysuria

Urinary incontinence a temporary or permanent inability of the external sphincter muscles to control the flow of urine from the bladder

Urinary reflux backward flow of urine

Urinary retention the accumulation of urine in the bladder and inability of the bladder to empty itself

Urinary stasis stagnation of urinary flow

Urination (micturition, voiding) the process of emptying the bladder

Urine osmolality a measure of the solute concentration of urine, a more exact measurement of urine concentration than specific gravity

Utilitarianism a specific, consequence-based, ethical theory that judges as right the action that does the most good and least amount of harm for the greatest number of persons; often used in making decisions about the funding and delivery of health care

Utility *see* Utilitarianism

Validation the determination that the diagnosis accurately reflects the problem of the client, that the methods used for data gathering were appropriate, and that the conclusion or diagnosis is justified by the data

Validity the degree to which an instrument measures what it is intended to measure

Valsalva maneuver forceful exhalation against a closed glottis, which increases intrathoracic pressure and thus interferes with venous blood return to the heart

Value set all of the values (e.g., personal, professional, religious) that a person holds

Value system the organization of a person's values along a continuum of relative importance

Values something of worth; a belief held dearly by a person

Values clarification a process by which individuals define their own value

Vaporization continuous evaporation of moisture from the respiratory tract and from the mucosa of the mouth and from the skin

Variance a variation or deviation from a critical pathway; goals not met or interventions not performed according to the time frame

Vasoconstriction a decrease in the caliber (lumen) of blood vessels

Vasodilation an increase in the caliber (lumen) of blood vessels

Vector-borne transmission a vector is an animal or flying or crawling insect that serves as an intermediate means of transporting the infectious agent

Vehicle-borne transmission a vehicle is any substance that serves as an intermediate means to transport and introduce an infectious agent into a susceptible host through a suitable portal of entry

Venipuncture   puncture of a vein for collection of a blood specimen or for infusion of therapeutic solutions

Ventilation   the movement of air in and out of the lungs; the process of inhalation and exhalation

Ventricles   two lower chambers of the heart

Veracity   a moral principle that holds that one should tell the truth and not lie

Verbal communication   use of verbal language to send and receive messages

Verdict   the outcome made by a jury

Vernix caseosa   a protective covering that develops over the unborn fetus' skin; a white, cheese-like substance that adheres to the skin and can become 1/8-inch thick by birth

Vestibule   contains the organs of equilibrium; found in the inner ear

Vial   a medication container with a sealed rubber cap, for single or multiple doses

Vibration   a series of vigorous quiverings produced by hands that are placed flat against the chest wall to loosen thick secretions

Virulence   ability to produce disease

Viruses   nucleic acid-based infectious agents

Visceral   internal organs

Visceral pain   results from stimulation of pain receptors in the abdominal cavity, cranium, and thorax

Viscous   thick, sticky

Vision   the mental image of a possible and desirable future state

Visiting nursing   delivery of services in the client's home

Visual   related to sight

Visual acuity   the degree of detail the eye can discern in an image

Visual fields   the area an individual can see when looking straight ahead

Vital capacity   the maximum amount of air that can be exhaled after a maximum inhalation

Vital signs   measurements of physiologic functioning, specifically body temperature, pulse, respirations, and blood pressure; may include pain and pulse oximetry

Vitamin   an organic compound that cannot be manufactured by the body and is needed in small quantities to catalyze metabolic processes

Vitiligo   patches of hypopigmented skin, caused by the destruction of melanocytes in the area

Voiding   *see* Urination

Volume control infusion set   small fluid containers (100 to 150 mL in size) attached below the primary infusion container so that the medication is administered through the client's IV line

Volume expanders   used to increase the blood volume following severe loss of blood (e.g., from hemorrhage) or loss of plasma (e.g., from severe burns, which draw large amounts of plasma from the bloodstream to the burn site)

Water-soluble vitamins   vitamins that the body cannot store, so people must get a daily supply in the diet; include C and B-complex vitamins

Well-being   a subjective perception of balance, harmony, and vitality

Wellness   a state of well-being; engaging in attitudes and behaviors that enhance quality of life and maximize personal potential

Wellness diagnosis   (NANDA) describes human responses to levels of wellness in an individual, family, or community that have a readiness for enhancement

White blood cells (WBCs)   *see* Leukocytes

Wide area network (WAN)   computers linked across large distances

World Wide Web (WWW)   refers to the complex links among webpages or websites, accessed through "addresses" called *universal resource locators* (URLs)

Yoga   a type of meditation that is a system of exercises for attaining bodily or mental control and well-being

Photographic and Illustration Credits

All photographs/illustrations not credited on page, under or adjacent to the visual, or not credited below, were photographed/rendered on assignment and are property of Pearson Education/Prentice Hall Health.

Photographer: Elena Dorfman

Figures 11–1, 22–1, 22–2, 22–9, 22–12, 23–1, 23–2, 23–3, 23–5, 24–5, 25–3, 27–6, 27–12, 27–13, 27–22, 27–23, 27–30, 28–98, 29–2, 29–3, 29–4, 29–5, 29–17, 29–18, 31–29, 31–30, 32–5 A & B, 32–12, 33–10, 33–15, 33–21, 33–22, 33–24, 33–25, 33–32, 33–33, 33–34, 33–40, 33–53, 33–54, 33–55, 34–7, 34–20, 34–21, 35–4, 35–5, 35–6, 35–7, 42–58, 42–59, 42–61, 42–66, 42–67, 42–68, 42–69, 42–73 A, 45–7, 45–13, 45–18, 46–9, 46–11, 46–15, 48–10, 48–11, 48–23, 48–26, 50–17, 50–22, 50–23, 50–27, 50–30, 50–31.

Photographer: Jenny Thomas

Figures 27–8, 27–9, 27–14, 27–35, 29–31, 29–32, 29–33, 29–34, 29–35, 30–10, 30–11, 30–13, 30–17, 31–1, 31–2, 31–11, 31–31, 32–6, 33–30, 33–31, 33–43, 33–63, 33–64, 33–65, 33–68, 33–69, 33–72, 33–83, 33–84, 34–12, 35–21, 42–53, 42–54, 42–60, 42–62, 42–70, 44–14, 46–10, 48–9, 48–12, 48–13, 48–27, 48–32, 48–36, 48–37, 49–7, 50–32.

Index